SECOND EDITION

EMT COMPLETE

A Comprehensive Worktext

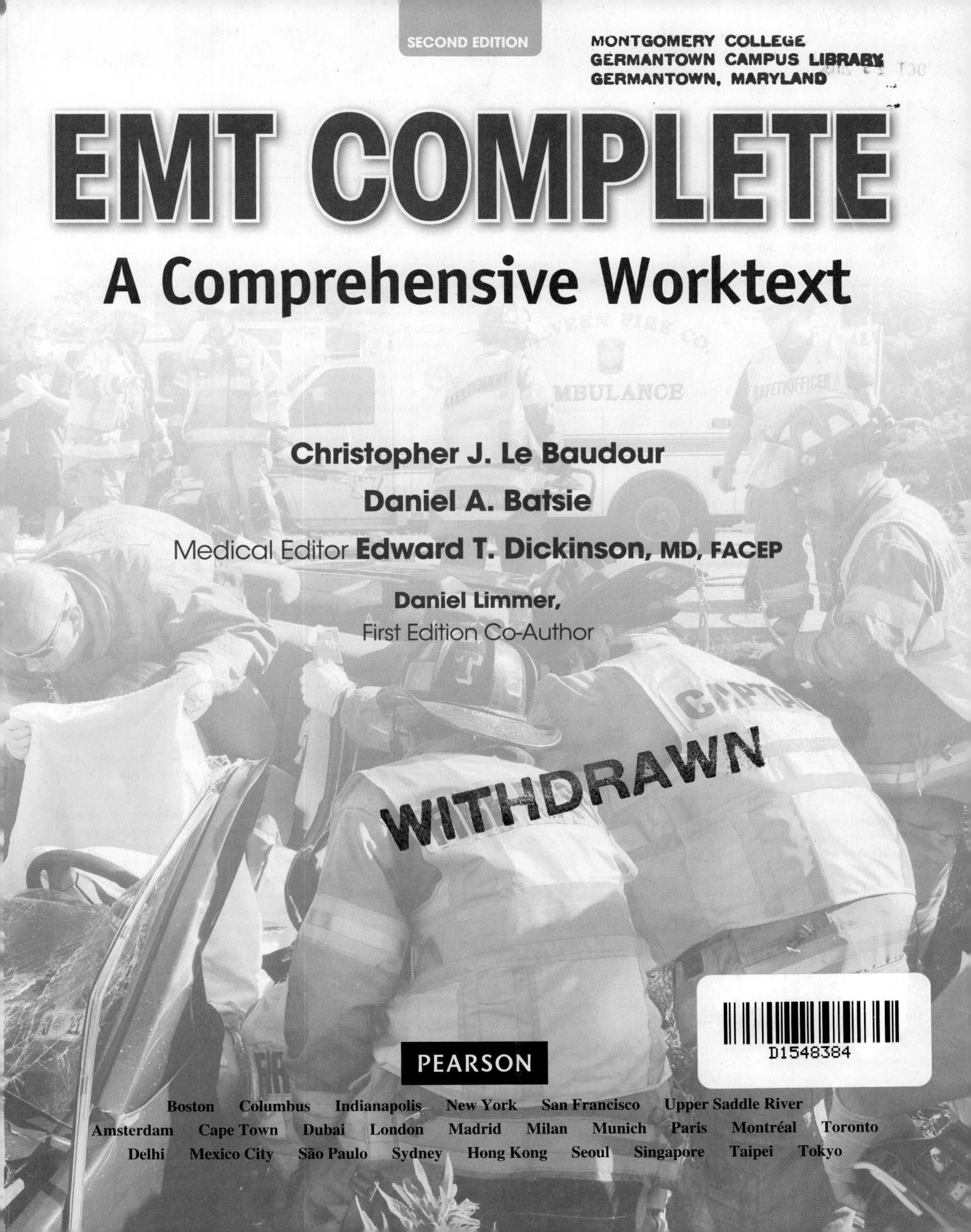

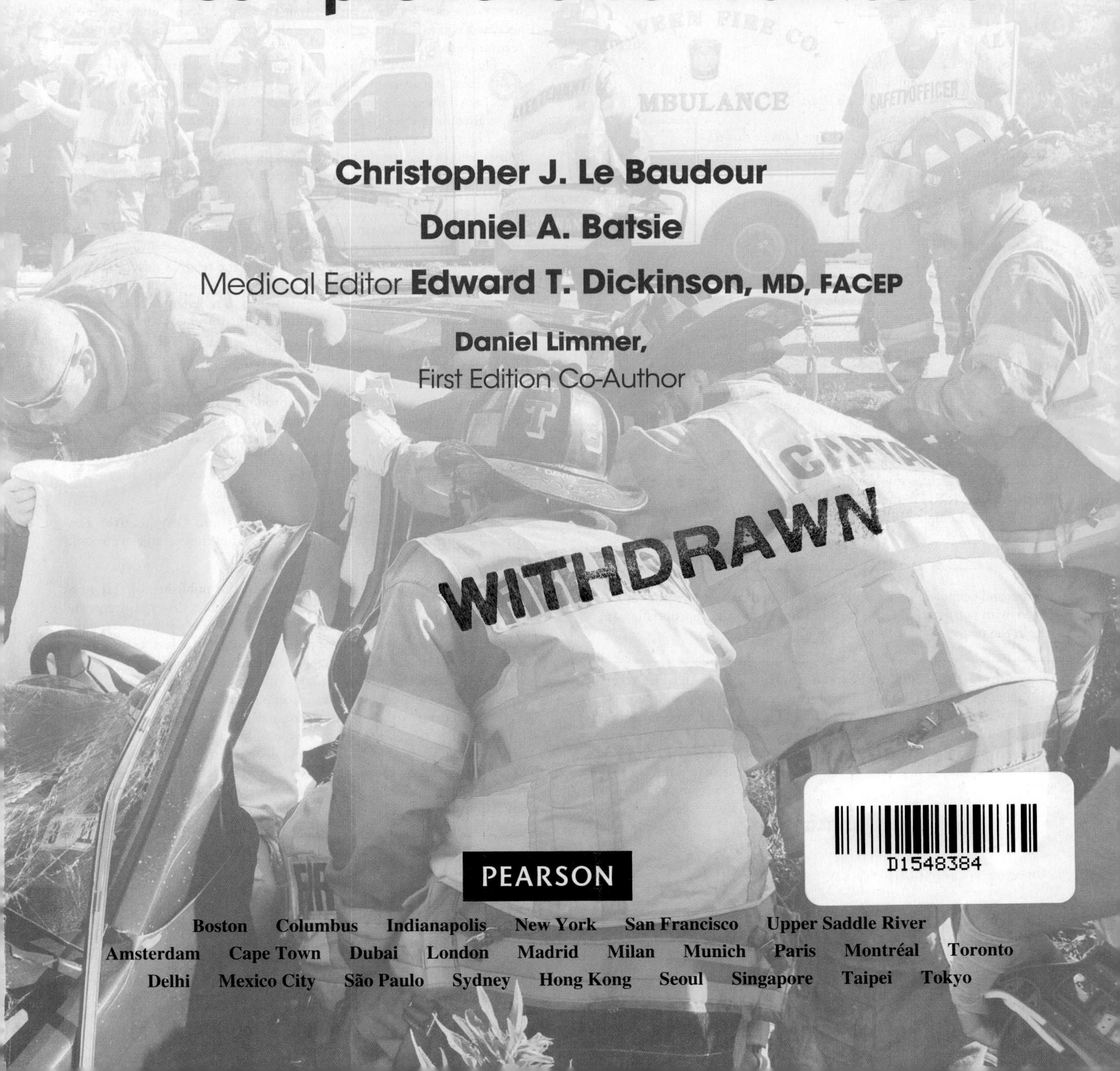

Christopher J. Le Baudour

Daniel A. Batsie

Medical Editor **Edward T. Dickinson, MD, FACEP**

Daniel Limmer,
First Edition Co-Author

PEARSON

Boston Columbus Indianapolis New York San Francisco Upper Saddle River
Amsterdam Cape Town Dubai London Madrid Milan Munich Paris Montréal Toronto
Delhi Mexico City São Paulo Sydney Hong Kong Seoul Singapore Taipei Tokyo

Library of Congress Cataloging-in-Publication Data

Le Baudour, Chris.

EMT complete a comprehensive worktext / Christopher J. Le Baudour, Daniel Batsie, Edward T. Dickinson. — 2nd ed.

p. cm.

Rev. ed. of: EMT complete / Daniel Limmer, Christopher J. Le Baudour; medical editor, Edward T. Dickinson.

Includes index.

ISBN-13: 978-0-13-289777-8

ISBN-10: 0-13-289777-6

1. Emergency medical technicians—Outlines, syllabi, etc. 2. Emergency medicine—Outlines, syllabi, etc. I. Batsie, Dan. II. Dickinson, Edward T. III. Limmer, Daniel. EMT complete. IV. Title.

RC86.92.L56 2013

616.02'5—dc23

2012026113

Publisher: Julie Levin Alexander
Publisher's Assistant: Regina Bruno
Editor-in-Chief: Marlene McHugh Pratt
Acquisitions Editor: Sladjana Repic
Senior Managing Editor for Development: Lois Berlowitz
Editorial Project Manager: Josephine Cepeda
Assistant Editor: Jonathan Cheung
Director of Marketing: David Gesell
Marketing Manager: Brian Hoehl
Marketing Specialist: Michael Sirinides
Managing Editor for Production: Patrick Walsh
Production Liaison: Faye Gemmellaro
Production Editor: Emily Bush, S4Carlisle Publishing Services
Manufacturing Manager: Lisa McDowell
Senior Art Director: Maria Guglielmo
Cover and Interior Design: Wee Design/Wanda Espana
Cover Image: Vincenzo Lombardo, Getty Images USA, Inc.
Managing Photography Editor: Michal Heron
Interior Photographers: Nathan Eldridge, Michael Gallitelli, Michal Heron, Ray Kemp/Triple Zilch Productions, Kevin Link, Richard Logan, Scott Metcalfe
Editorial Media Manager: Amy Peltier
Media Project Managers: Lorena Cerisano, Ellen Martino
Composition: S4Carlisle Publishing Services
Printer/Binder: R.R. Donnelley/Willard
Cover Printer: Lehigh-Phoenix Color/Hagerstown

Credits and acknowledgments borrowed from other sources and reproduced, with permission, in this textbook appear on the appropriate pages within the text.

DISCLAIMERS

Notice on Trademarks Many of the designations by manufacturers and sellers to distinguish their products are claimed as trademarks. Where those designations appear in this book, and the publisher was aware of a trademark claim, the trademark symbol appears next to the trademark at the first mention and the trademark name is printed in initial caps in subsequent mentions.

Notice on Care Procedures It is the intent of the authors and publisher that this textbook be used as part of a formal EMT education program taught by qualified instructors and supervised by a licensed physician. The procedures described in this textbook are based on consultation with EMT and medical authorities. The authors and publisher have taken care to make certain that these procedures reflect currently accepted clinical practice; however, they cannot be considered absolute recommendations.

The material in this textbook contains the most current information available at the time of publication. However, federal, state, and local guidelines concerning clinical practices, including, without limitation, those governing infection control and universal precautions, change rapidly. The reader should note, therefore, that the new regulations may require changes in some procedures. It is the responsibility of the reader to become thoroughly familiar with the policies and procedures set by federal, state, and local agencies as well as the institution or agency where the reader is employed. The authors and the publisher of this textbook and the supplements written to accompany it disclaim any liability, loss, or risk resulting directly or indirectly from the suggested procedures and theory, from any undetected errors, or from the reader's misunderstanding of the text. It is the reader's responsibility to stay informed of any new changes or recommendations made by any federal, state, or local agency as well as by the reader's employing institution or agency.

Notice on Gender Usage The English language has historically given preference to the male gender. Among many words, the pronouns "he" and "his" are commonly used to describe both genders. Society evolves faster than language, and the male pronouns still predominate in our speech. The authors have made great effort to treat the two genders equally, recognizing that a significant percentage of EMTs are female. However, in some instances, male pronouns may be used to describe both males and females solely for the purpose of brevity. This is not intended to offend any readers of the female gender.

Notice on "Emergency Dispatch" Features and "Perspective" Features The names used and situations depicted in these features throughout this text are fictitious.

Notice on Medications The authors and the publisher of this book have taken care to make certain that the equipment, doses of drugs, and schedules of treatment are correct and compatible with the standards generally accepted at the time of publication. Nevertheless, as new information becomes available, changes in treatment and in the use of equipment and drugs become necessary. The reader is advised to carefully consult the instruction and information material included in the page insert of each drug or therapeutic agent, piece of equipment, or device before administration. This advice is especially important when using new or infrequently used drugs. Prehospital care providers are warned that use of any drugs or techniques must be authorized by their medical director, in accord with local laws and regulations. The publisher disclaims any liability, loss, injury, or damage incurred as a consequence, directly or indirectly, of the use and application of any of the contents of this book.

Brady
is an imprint of

PEARSON

www.bradybooks.com

10 9 8 7 6 5 4 3 2 1

ISBN 10: 0-13-289777-6
ISBN 13: 978-0-13-289777-8

Dedications

This edition is dedicated to the men and women of Freedom House Ambulance. Starting from a base in Presbyterian and Mercy Hospitals in 1968, they became the first paramedics in the United States.

— C.J.L.

To the exceptional people who have taken the time to give me guidance, counsel, and confidence on this wild ride I call a career. My success will truly be measured by following your magnanimous examples.

— D.A.B.

To Debbie, Stephen, and Alex for their endless love and extraordinary patience throughout this and many other projects.

— E.T.D.

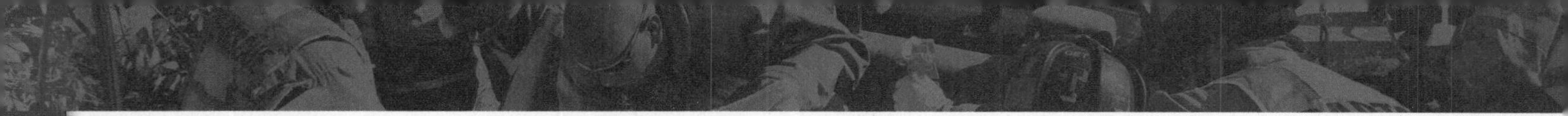

BRIEF CONTENTS

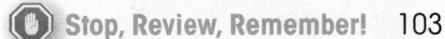

CONTENTS

PHOTO SCANS

PREFACE

There are two things that Brady Publishing understands very well—EMS students and EMS education. *EMT Complete: A Comprehensive Worktext*, Second Edition, is a product of that understanding. What you hold in your hands is the result of over eight years and many thousands of hours of labor and collaboration. In its first edition *EMT Complete: A Basic Worktext* was the first primary EMT textbook to combine the elements of the traditional textbook and a workbook into one easy-to-use student resource. Combined with Brady's online resources, the *EMT Complete: A Comprehensive Worktext*, Second Edition, learning package cannot be beat.

Conceived, written, and reviewed by some of the most dedicated professionals in EMS education today, *EMT Complete: A Comprehensive Worktext*, Second Edition, has been designed to help you develop the critical thinking skills you will need to get the best outcomes possible for your patients. Toward that goal, we have updated and expanded the content to meet the latest national standards and treatment guidelines. New features have been added, too—all to offer you the quality you have come to expect from Brady.

Rest assured that the foundation for the content of this new edition is the most current EMS Education Standards for the EMT and includes pertinent changes in science and practice, including new American Heart Association recommendations affecting EMS. Our goal is simply to assist in the evolutionary process of EMS education by placing a greater focus on you, the student, and the development of critical thinking skills that will result in better patient care.

We have added several new features to this edition of *EMT Complete: A Comprehensive Worktext* and kept the well-established ones you have come to expect from Brady. They are as follows:

What's New in This Edition

NEW! Education Standards and Competencies

This worktext represents the most up-to-date information and content as it relates to the National Department of Transportation EMS education standards. In addition, it incorporates the latest guidelines and recommendations from the American Heart Association for both resuscitation and emergency care.

NEW! Learning Objectives

The foundation of this textbook is built on a completely new set of learning objectives that reflect the EMS Education Standards mentioned above. The new objectives were written with the student in mind and represent the most important content necessary to become a competent EMT who can successfully pass the state or national exam.

Updated! Emergency Dispatch

For this new edition, *Emergency Dispatch* has been updated to reflect current standards and practice. A familiar Brady feature, this chapter-opening scenario helps to get you into the mind-set of an EMT who has just been dispatched to an emergency. It sets the stage for the context of the chapter and allows you to begin the all-important "what-would-I-do" critical-thinking process. Note that each scenario wraps up at the end of the chapter with the *Emergency Dispatch Summary*.

As you will see, the people in the scenarios do not always say or do the "right" thing. Many of the emergencies described have been inspired by actual events involving actual people. So, we allowed the human side to show through now and then, even when it does not model the recommended behavior.

Updated! Perspective

Updated to reflect current standards and practice, the *Perspectives* woven through a chapter are narrated by the many "characters" described in the *Emergency Dispatch*. They take you inside the minds of frightened patients, angry and anxious family members, and concerned neighbors. They also provide a glimpse into the thoughts of EMTs and their partners, fire captains, and other rescue personnel on scene. It is through these insights that you can begin to comprehend how your actions affect those for whom you care and with whom you work.

Updated! Clinical Clues

Within each chapter the *Clinical Clues* offer bits of wisdom that reflect the best possible clinical practice. These pearls come from many years of actual field experience and provide insight beyond the standard curriculum.

NEW! Practical Pathophysiology

A big addition to the *EMT Complete: A Basic Worktext*, Second Edition, is the expanded content related to pathophysiology. Throughout the chapters, *Practical Pathophysiology* offers important information specifically related to a topic at hand, deepening understanding while reinforcing the why behind what the patient may be experiencing.

Updated! Stop, Review, Remember!

Updated to match new content and current standards and practice, *Stop, Review, Remember!* offers opportunities for self-assessment and reinforcement immediately following major sections of text. Each opportunity to *Stop, Review, Remember!* is composed of a minimum of three workbook elements: multiple-choice questions, an activity such as matching or fill in the blank, and critical thinking questions. In most chapters, case studies with questions challenge you to further engage in the learning process.

Updated! Module Review and Practice Examinations

At the end of each of the six learning modules, you will find a *Module Review and Practice Examination.* These are multiple-choice questions modeled after both state- and national-style certification exams to give you valuable practice for your own certification exam. Note that Appendix A offers a "final exam" with even more review and practice questions.

New and Expanded Photography

The medical photography contained in *EMT Complete: A Comprehensive Worktext*, Second Edition, has been refreshed and expanded to expose the reader to more medical and educational images. It includes more than 100 new images that further enhance the educational impact of the text.

New and Expanded Chapters

The content of *EMT Complete: A Comprehensive Worktext*, Second Edition, is summarized in the following paragraphs. Look for the **NEW!** or **Expanded!** flags to see what has been added or changed. As you do, keep in mind that this new edition represents the most current Educational Standards for EMS!

Module 1 Fundamentals

- **Expanded!** *Chapter 1 You and the EMS System*. This chapter still begins with the history of EMS and goes on to cover the scope of practice and standard of care for each level of EMS provider, the role of medical direction in EMS, the 911 system, the EMT's roles and responsibilities, plus quality improvement and its role in the EMS system. **NEW!** In this new edition, also covered are the components of the Technical Assistance Program Assessment Standards, public health and EMS, disaster medical assistance teams and EMS, and the role of research in EMS.
- **Expanded!** *Chapter 2 Workforce Safety and Wellness*. This chapter focuses on the well-being of the EMT and how to manage the many stresses of the job. It also now has expanded coverage of the ways an EMT can be protected from disease and the risks of hazardous materials, rescue, traffic-related injuries, violence, and crime.
- **Expanded!** *Chapter 3 Legal and Ethical Considerations of Providing Care*. This chapter covers the EMT's scope of practice as well as the legal aspects of providing emergency care, such as duty to act, Good Samaritan Laws, consent and refusal, advance directives, negligence, abandonment, assault and battery, patient confidentiality, and special reporting situations. **NEW!** In addition, this chapter now includes content on a patient's capacity (as well as competency) to refuse care, statutes of limitations, contributory negligence, durable power of attorney for health care and physician orders for life-sustaining treatment, the differences between a civil and a criminal lawsuit, the Emergency Medical Treatment and Active Labor Act, and the legal risks of transporting and transferring patient care.
- **NEW!** *Chapter 4 Medical Terminology*. New to this edition, this chapter covers terms for the structures of the body, points of reference, planes and lines, body systems, and location and position, as well as a discussion of effective communication.
- **Expanded!** *Chapter 5 Anatomy and Physiology*. This chapter has been reorganized and expanded to cover the musculoskeletal and integumentary systems; the cardiorespiratory system, including a section on the "Life Support Chain"; the nervous system, which now also addresses the autonomic nervous system; the endocrine system, with additional discussion on the pancreas and adrenal glands; and the gastrointestinal, renal, and reproductive systems.
- **NEW!** *Chapter 6 Pathophysiology*. New to this edition, this chapter covers the topics of the cellular environment and fluid balance, cardiopulmonary system dysfunction and compensation mechanisms, and the pathophysiology of shock and the nervous, endocrine, gastrointestinal, immune, and integumentary systems.
- **NEW!** *Chapter 7 Life Span Development*. New to this edition, this chapter covers the characteristics of human development, including newborns and infants, toddlers, preschoolers, school-age children, adolescents, and early, middle, and late adulthood.

- **Expanded!** *Chapter 8 Lifting, Moving, and Positioning Patients*. This chapter still covers the principles of lifting and moving, emergent and nonemergency moves, patient positioning, and specific lifting and moving devices. **NEW!** Expanded discussion on those topics includes the relationship between health and posture; communication as a key safety component; how to plan a move or lift; how to properly and safely reach, push, and pull; and rapid extrication.
- *Chapter 9 Obtaining Vital Signs and a Medical History*. This chapter covers baseline vital signs, trending, and the assessment of breathing, pulse, blood pressure, skin signs (**NEW!** including how to assess skin turgor), and the eyes. It also offers content on orthostatic vital signs, reassessment of vital signs, capnography, and pulse oximetry. The chapter concludes with a detailed description of how to obtain a patient's medical history.
- **Expanded!** *Chapter 10 Communications*. This chapter covers the role of communications and communication systems, as well as medical communication with the hospital, medical direction, and verbal reports. **NEW!** Expanded discussion on those topics includes the four types of communication, the communication process, strategies for effective communication, therapeutic communication, strategies for interviewing patients including question construction, and communication and transfer of care. You will also find updates on the discussion of technology with information on mobile data terminals, tablets, and cell phones.
- **Expanded!** *Chapter 11 Documenting Your Assessment and Care*. This chapter covers the components of prehospital care reports, confidentiality, HIPAA, corrections and falsification, and special issues such as patient refusal and MCIs. **NEW!** Also covered is what happens when transfer of care is necessary before documentation is complete.

Module 2 Patient Assessment

- *Chapter 12 Performing a Scene Size-up and Primary Assessment*. Two chapters in the previous edition, this one chapter covers scene size-up (including personal protective equipment and scene safety, nature of illness and mechanism of injury, number of patients and additional resources) and the primary assessment (including the general impression and chief complaint, identifying immediate life threats, and patient priority). **NEW!** The Glasgow Coma Scale is described.
- **Expanded!** *Chapter 13 Managing Your Patient's Airway and Ventilation*. This chapter covers the types of respiration, assessing for adequate and inadequate breathing, managing the airway, suctioning, airway adjuncts, ventilation techniques, and supplemental oxygen. **NEW!** Expanded discussion on those topics includes the sounds of airway obstruction, assisted ventilation and dental appliances, risks of positive pressure ventilation, hazards of overventilation, automatic transport ventilators, noninvasive positive pressure ventilation (CPAP and Bi-PAP), and the different types of oxygen delivery masks.
- **NEW!** *Chapter 14 Performing a Secondary Assessment*. Instead of three separate chapters as in the previous edition, this one new chapter covers the rapid and focused secondary assessments for the medical patient and the rapid secondary assessment for the trauma patient, as well as the reassessment process.

Module 3 Medical Emergencies

- **NEW!** *Chapter 15 Your Approach to the Medical Patient*. This new chapter introduces you to specific tips and tricks related to the assessment and management of the medical patient.
- **Expanded!** *Chapter 16 Pharmacology*. This chapter addresses the names of medications and routes by which they are administered, and offers expanded descriptions of specific medications (oxygen, aspirin, epinephrine, nitroglycerin, activated charcoal, oral glucose, and inhaled bronchodilators), the "five rights," documentation, medical direction, and safety and clinical judgment.
- **Expanded!** *Chapter 17 Caring for Patients with Breathing Difficulty*. This chapter offers a review of respiratory anatomy and physiology; assessment of the patient in respiratory distress, including discussion of abnormal breathing patterns and lung auscultation; respiratory diseases and conditions; steps in emergency care of the patient; and respiratory medications and devices. **NEW!** Also covered are the medulla and pons and their role in controlling inspiration and expiration; discussion on respiratory distress vs. respiratory failure; positioning the patient in respiratory distress; beta2 agonists; and descriptions of pneumonia, pulmonary embolism, pulmonary edema, pneumothorax, hyperventilation syndrome, epiglottitis, exposure to poisons, and vital respiratory infections.
- **Expanded!** *Chapter 18 Caring for Patients with Cardiac Emergencies and Resuscitation*. Opening with a review of the circulatory system, this chapter covers the chain of survival, cardiac compromise, assessment of the cardiac patient, emergency care of the patient with cardiac compromise, and defibrillation. **NEW!**

Expanded discussion on those topics includes the relationship between the nervous system and the heart; the heart's electrical and mechanical functions; the concept of "loss of time is loss of muscle"; integrated post-cardiac arrest care; signs and symptoms of cardiogenic shock; resuscitation devices; therapeutic hypothermia; fibrinolytic therapy; and percutaneous transluminal coronary angiography.

- **NEW!** *Chapter 19 Caring for Patients with Seizures and Syncope*. New to this edition, this chapter covers the pathophysiology of seizures, types of seizures, and emergency care and reassessment of the seizure patient. It also covers the types of syncope and emergency care of the syncope patient.
- **Expanded!** *Chapter 20 Caring for Patients with Altered Mental Status, Stroke, and Headache*. This chapter covers assessment and emergency care of both the patient with an altered mental status and the stroke patient. **NEW!** The assessment and emergency care of the headache patient is included.
- **NEW!** *Chapter 21 Toxicology*. New to this edition, this chapter covers assessment and emergency care of the poisoning patient; poison control centers; the portals of entry, plus signs and symptoms and emergency care for each one; and additional aspects of toxicology, including substance abuse, carbon monoxide, nerve agents and organophosphates, and poison antidotes.
- **NEW!** *Chapter 22 Caring for Patients with Acute Abdominal Emergencies*. New to this edition, this chapter covers the anatomy, physiology, and pathophysiology of the abdomen; assessment and emergency care of the acute abdomen patient; differential diagnosis and pattern recognition for gastrointestinal bleeding, abdominal aortic aneurysm, appendicitis, pancreatitis, cholecystitis, gastroenteritis, bowel obstructions, urinary system causes of abdominal pain, and dysfunction of reproductive organs.
- **NEW!** *Chapter 23 Caring for Patients with Acute Diabetic Emergencies*. New to this edition, this chapter covers the body's regulation of glucose, types of diabetes, blood glucose monitoring, acute diabetic emergencies, and assessment and emergency care of the diabetic patient.
- **Expanded!** *Chapter 24 Caring for Patients with Allergy-Related Emergencies*. This chapter covers the immune response as well as the assessment and emergency care of the patient having an allergic reaction. **NEW!** Expanded discussion on those topics includes the concepts of antigens, sensitization, immunoglobulin E (IgE), histamine, and angioedema.
- **NEW!** *Chapter 25 Caring for Patients with Hematologic and Renal Emergencies*. New to this edition, this chapter covers the hematologic system, including blood clotting, coagulopathies, and the assessment and emergency care of patients with clotting disorders and sickle cell disease. The chapter also covers the diseases of the renal system, hemodialysis and peritoneal dialysis, and medical emergencies associated with end-stage renal disease.
- **Expanded!** *Chapter 26 Caring for Patients with Behavioral Emergencies*. This chapter covers the types of behavioral emergencies and assessment and care of the behavioral emergency patient. **NEW!** Expanded discussion on those topics includes scene safety and the behavioral patient, the agitated delirium patient, and documentation.
- **Expanded!** *Chapter 27 Obstetrics and Care of the Newborn*. This chapter covers obstetrical emergencies, normal childbirth, post-delivery care, and complications during pregnancy. **NEW!** Added to this new edition are female reproductive anatomy and physiology and key changes in bodily systems during pregnancy; assessment of a female patient and descriptions of specific gynecological emergencies, including sexual assault; preterm labor, premature rupture of membranes, and uterine rupture; predicting the need for neonatal resuscitation; post-delivery embolism; the precipitous delivery; shoulder dystocia; and the post-term pregnancy.

Module 4 Trauma Emergencies

- **NEW!** *Chapter 28 Your Approach to the Trauma Patient*. This new chapter introduces students to specific tips and tricks unique to the assessment and management of a trauma patient.
- **Expanded!** *Chapter 29 Recognition and Care of the Shock Patient*. This chapter covers personal safety, perfusion, types of shock, internal bleeding, and the assessment and emergency care of the shock patient. **NEW!** Added to this edition are the causes of shock and shock in geriatric patients.
- *Chapter 30 Controlling Bleeding*. This chapter offers a review of the cardiovascular system and covers types of external bleeding and bleeding control. **NEW!** Expanded discussion on those topics includes new standards for bleeding control, the use of hemostatic dressings, and commercial tourniquets.
- *Chapter 31 Caring for Patients with Soft-Tissue Injuries*. This chapter offers a review of skin function and describes the types of injuries to soft tissues; assessment

and emergency care of both closed and open injuries: and the different types and uses of dressings and bandages.

- **Expanded!** *Chapter 32 Caring for Patients with Burn Injuries*. This chapter covers the common sources of burns, burn classifications, assessment and emergency care of the burn patient, establishing patient priority, and special considerations. **NEW!** Added to this new edition is burn pathophysiology and new photographs to better illustrate burn injuries.
- **Expanded!** *Chapter 33 Caring for Patients with Chest, Abdominal, and Genital Trauma*. This chapter covers the anatomy and physiology of the chest and breathing, both open and closed chest injuries and their assessment and emergency care; abdominal anatomy and physiology and closed and open wounds and their assessment and emergency care. **NEW!** Also covered are pulmonary and cardiac contusions, commotio cordis, open pneumothorax, and pericardial tamponade; assessment of closed chest injuries; closed wounds to the abdomen and their assessment and emergency care; and external genitalia trauma.
- **Expanded!** *Chapter 34 Caring for Patients with Musculoskeletal Injuries*. This chapter offers a review of the musculoskeletal system, identifies common MOIs, describes soft-tissue and skeletal injuries, and covers assessment and immobilization. **NEW!** Expanded discussion on those topics includes the use of the long backboard for immobilization and the identification and management of compartment syndrome.
- *Chapter 35 Caring for Patients with Head Injuries*. This chapter describes the anatomy and physiology of the head and brain, identifies head injury classifications, and covers assessment and emergency care. **NEW!** CT scans and medical images have been added to illustrate key concepts.
- **Expanded!** *Chapter 36 Caring for Patients with Spine Injuries*. This chapter describes the anatomy and pathophysiology of the spine and nervous system, covers assessment and emergency care of the patient suspected of spine injury, and outlines special considerations including the needs of pediatric patients and helmet removal. **NEW!** Expanded discussion on those topics includes the role of the spinal cord in regulating vital bodily functions; primary and secondary injuries to the spinal cord; non-transecting spinal-cord injuries; principles of spinal immobilization; immobilization of children found in car seats; and the negative effects of spinal immobilization.
- **Expanded!** *Chapter 37 Caring for Patients with Environmental Emergencies*. This chapter covers localized and generalized hypothermia and its assessment and emergency care, as well as assessment and care in heat emergencies. **NEW!** Expanded discussion on those topics includes descriptions of how the body maintains a normothermic status; active core rewarming; the three major events of a classic drowning, trauma in the setting of drowning, and responding to immersion/submersion emergencies; specific types of heat emergencies; specific types of animal and insect bites and stings and emergency care for each; and assessment and emergency care for lightning and dive injuries.

Module 5 Special Populations

- **Expanded!** *Chapter 38 Caring for Pediatric Patients*. This chapter covers pediatric development and developmental characteristics, the pediatric airway, and assessment of the pediatric patient; common medical problems, airway management, and emergency care; trauma assessment and emergency care; child abuse and neglect; and patients with special needs. **NEW!** Expanded discussion on those topics includes normal pediatric vital signs; specific respiratory and cardiac illnesses and emergencies; gastrointestinal disorders; apparent life-threatening events; and pediatric injury prevention programs.
- **Expanded!** *Chapter 39 Caring for Geriatric Patients*. This chapter covers age-related physical changes, assessment, common medical problems, and elder abuse and neglect. **NEW!** Expanded discussion on those topics includes characteristics of geriatric patients and advocating for the elderly.
- **NEW!** *Chapter 40 Caring for Patients with Special Challenges*. New to this edition, this chapter covers assessment and management of patients with special challenges, causes and types of disability, and up-to-date medical technology that may be encountered on the emergency scene.

Module 6 Ambulance Operations

- **Expanded!** *Chapter 41 Operating and Maintaining Your Ambulance*. This chapter covers the phases of an ambulance call, from preparing for it to terminating it. **NEW!** Expanded discussion on those topics includes readiness check of crew members, safe driving, specific driving hazards, the risk of carbon monoxide exposure, and ambulance security.

- **Expanded!** *Chapter 42 Overview of Incident Command and Incident Management Systems*. This chapter covers NIMS as per the U.S. Department of Homeland Security and all the components of an incident command system.
- **Expanded!** *Chapter 43 Responses to Multiple-Casualty Incidents.* This chapter covers the goals of MCI management, the "Five S's" as initial actions, and the START triage system. **NEW!** Expanded discussion on those topics includes command structure at an MCI, the treatment area at an MCI, staging and transportation, communications, and rescuer health and stress management.
- **Expanded!** *Chapter 44 Responses Involving Hazardous Materials*. This chapter covers hazmat responses to buildings and transportation accidents, general procedures for identifying and approaching the hazmat scene, operations at the site, hazmat training, decontamination, and how certain hazardous materials harm the body. **NEW!** Expanded discussion on those topics includes the special considerations at radiation and WMD incidents.
- *Chapter 45 Vehicle Extrication and Air Medical Response*. This chapter covers rescue incidents and the fundamentals of patient extrication. **NEW!** Added to this edition is coverage of air medical operations.
- **Expanded!** *Chapter 46 Responses Involving Terrorism*. This chapter covers preoperational considerations and the assessment and emergency care of victims of WMDs. **NEW!** Expanded discussion on those topics includes a section on preplanning, incendiary weapons, explosives, and emergency care of victims of radiological weapons.

This Is EMS

Now that we have provided a glimpse of what's inside this new learning package and its new approach to EMS education, sit back, lace up your boots, and hang on as you begin the incredible journey of becoming an EMT. We, as your authors, are honored and excited to be a part of your training. Collectively with Ed Dickinson, MD, the medical editor, we have been fortunate enough to call EMS our career for nearly 80 years. We want to share our experiences with you, the highs and the lows, the successful resuscitations and the loss of life, because this is *our* life. *This is EMS*!

Chris Le Baudour
Dan Batsie
Ed Dickinson

ACKNOWLEDGMENTS

Content Contributors

The authors would like to thank the following contributors for their part in making *EMT Complete: A Comprehensive Worktext*, Second Edition, the best EMT resource on the market:

Donald R. Adams, BS, EMT-P I/C, Emergency Services Education Manager, McLaren Regional Medical Center, Flint, MI

Jamie K. Adams, BA, EMT-P, Deputy/Paramedic, Office of the Genesee County Sheriff

Melissa R. Alexander, Ed.D., NREMT-P, Lake Superior State University, Sault Sainte Marie, MI

Brian D. Bricker, Director of Communications, REACH Air Medical Services

Kristin Burgess McBride PhD, NREMT-P, Lead Instructor, EMT Program, San Francisco Paramedic Association, San Francisco, CA

Laura A. Cathcart, MA, EMT, Adjunct Faculty, Howard Community College; EMS Instructor, Maryland Fire and Rescue Institute; EMT and Firefighter, Laurel Volunteer Fire Department No. 1, Inc., Laurel, MD

Dawn Johnston, NREMT-P, CFRN, BSN, Flight Nurse, West Michigan Air Care, Kalamazoo, MI

John C. La Bare, NREMT, EMT/BLS Instructor, verihealth Inc.

Derek Parker, BS, EMT-P, Program Director, Sacramento State University Prehospital Education Program, Sacramento, CA

Phillip T. Sanderson, NREMT-P, BS, MHA, Manager, EMS Operations, Methodist Le Bonheur Healthcare Systems–Methodist University Hospital, Memphis, TN

Reviewers

We wish to thank the following reviewers for providing invaluable feedback, insight, and suggestions in the preparation of *EMT Complete: A Comprehensive Worktext*, Second Edition:

Jerry Biggart, NREMT-P, Paramedic, Milwaukee Fire Department Training Center, Milwaukee, WI

Marie T. Bliss, NREMT-P, EMSI, Captain, Suffield Volunteer Ambulance Association, Suffield, CT

James A. Brady, BA, NREMT-P, CCEMT-P, Captain, Albemarle County Fire Rescue, Charlottesville, VA

James Brasiel, MD, MHA, MICP, Physician, Consultant, Paramedic Educator, Ready Enterprises, Antioch, CA

HM1 (SCW) Shawn M. Buxton, NREMT-P, EMT-T, U.S. Navy, Manchester, NH

Jackie Carey, NREMT-P, Paramedic, EMT Instructor, CPR Instructor, Newark Volunteer Fire Company, Wor-Wic Community College, Newark, MD and Salisbury, MD

Harold Thomas Carter, BS, MS, Paramedic, Commander, U.S. Navy (retired), Belfast Fire Department, Dixmont, ME

William H. Clark, NREMT-P, AAS, Chief, Escatawpa VFD, Board of Directors for Mississippi EMT Association, Moss Point, MS

Paul H. Coffey, BS, EMT-I, Basic EMT Training Coordinator, MA Dept. of Public Health, Office of EMS, Boston, MA

Judith Crawford, CAEMT-P, Director-Emergency Medical Care Department, Skyline College, San Bruno, CA

Malcolm Dean, Jr., BS, Captain, Stamford EMS, Stamford, CT

John L. Deboard, BSOSH, ASOSH, Instructor-Educator, NREMT, The Breath of Life Training Solutions, Goose Creek, SC

Diane C. Flint, MS, NREMT-P, CCEMT-P, Visiting Associate Clinical Professor, University of Maryland, Baltimore County, Baltimore, MD

Scott A. Gano, BS, NREMT-P, FP-C, CCEMT-P, Faculty Instructor, Columbus State Community College, Columbus, OH

Joseph A. Gilligan, EMT-P, EMSI, Paramedic, Firefighter, EMS Instructor, Mt. Orab Fire Department, Mt. Orab, OH

John Gosford, MS, EMT-P, Assistant Professor, College of Southern Maryland, La Plata, MD

Ian Harmon, NREMT-P, Chief of EMS and Technical Rescue Ops, Lexington, SC

John S. Holloway, Sr., MBA, FF/NREMT-P, Vice-President and CFO, Education Program Director, Benchmark Medical Services, LLC, Seymour, TN

Michael Hunter, NREMT-P, PI, Education Coordinator, Harrison County Hospital EMS, Corydon, IN

Deb Kaye, BS, NREMT, Director, Instructor, EMT, Dakota County Technical College, Sunburg Ambulance, Lakes Area Rural Responders, Rosemount, MN

Lawrence Linder, PhD(c), NREMT-P, Hillsborough Community College, EMS Program, Ruskin, FL

Catherine L. Martin, M.Ed., CHES, Salter College, West Boylston, MA

Jaclyn Nemcik, NREMT, AEMT, EMS-I, Director of Community Outreach, Harwinton Ambulance, Harwinton, CT

Karen Petrilla, RN, EMS Specialist, Riverside County EMS Agency (REMS), Riverside, CA

Paul A. Phillips, DO, NREMT-P, Dante Rescue Squad and Virginia State Police Med Flight II, Dante, VA

Cheryl Pittman, PhD, EMT-B, EMT, First Responder Program Director, East Los Angeles College, Monterey Park, CA

E. Jay Potter, AHS, BA, MM, NREMT-P, Adjunct Instructor, EMT-Basic Adjunct Instructor, Greenville Technical College, Field Training Officer, Laurens County EMS, Corporate & Career Development, Greenville, SC and Laurens, SC

Brian Rechkemmer, AAS, NREMT-P, Program Manager, Kirkwood Community College, Cedar Rapids, IA

Marit Saltrones, Curriculum Development Consultant, Sands Avenue Consulting, Bainbridge Island, WA

Carl W. Seitz, MA, EMT-P, EMS IC, Director, Public Service Institute, Macomb Community College, Clinton Township, MI

Michael A. Smalheer, BS, EMT-P, EMSI, Cleveland Clinic EMS Academy, Euclid, OH

William H. Stack, EMT-B, Instructor, Coordinator, Forsyth Technical Community College, Winston-Salem, NC

Michael Swiman, BS, Lieutenant, Instructor, Wake Forest Fire Department and Durham Technical Community College, Wake Forest, NC and Durham, NC

Jack L. Taylor, BS, EMT-P, I/C, Paralegal, CEO, Taylor Medical Legal Consultant Firm, Kalamazoo, MI

Ken Walters, BS, EMT-P, Hinds Community College, Jackson, MS

Leah Warden, BA, EMT-B, EMT Skills Lab Instructor, Kansas City Kansas Community College, Strum, WI

Brian J. Wilson, BA, NREMT-P, Education Director, Texas Tech University School of Medicine, El Paso, TX

Jason O. Wilson, NREMT-P, Paramedic, Spartanburg County EMS and Rutherford County EMS, Spartanburg, SC and Rutherford, NC

Fred W. Wurster III, AAS, NREMT-P, Director of Training, Good Fellowship Ambulance and EMS Training Institute, West Chester, PA

Photo Credits

All photographs not credited adjacent to the photograph or in a photo credit section were photographed on assignment for Brady/Prentice Hall/Pearson Education.

Organizations

We wish to thank the following organizations for their valuable assistance in creating the photo program:

Canandaigua Emergency Squad, Canandaigua, NY
Winter Park Fire-Rescue, Winter Park, FL, Chief James E. White, Deputy Chief Patrick McCabe
City of Winter Park, FL, Kenneth W. Bradley, Mayor
City Of Orlando Fire Department, Fire Chief John Miller

Technical Advisors

Thanks to the following people for providing technical support during the photo shoots in The City Of Orlando, FL:

Hezedean A. Smith, District Chief, Orlando Fire Department, EMS Division
Felix J. Marquez, Jr., President/CEO Orlando Medical Institute

Thanks to the following people for providing technical support during the photo shoots in Winter Park, FL:

Andrew Isaacs, EMS Captain
Tod Meadors, EMS Captain
Dr. Tod Husty, Medical Director
Richard Rodriguez, EMS Captain
Jeff Spinelli, Engineer-Paramedic

ABOUT THE AUTHORS

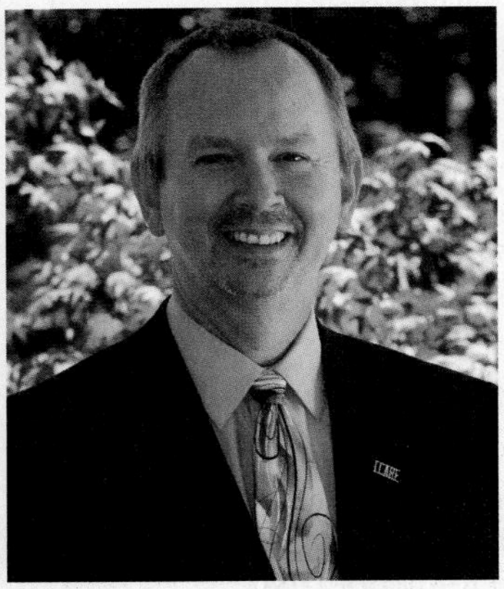

Christopher J. Le Baudour

Christopher Le Baudour has been working in the EMS field since 1978. He has worked as an EMT and an EMT-II in both the field and clinical settings. In 1984 he began his teaching career in the Department of Public Safety—EMS Division at Santa Rosa Junior College in Santa Rosa, CA.

Mr. Le Baudour holds a Master's Degree in Education with an emphasis in online teaching and learning as well as numerous certifications. He has spent the past 28 years mastering the art of experiential learning in EMS and is well known for his innovative classroom techniques and his passion for teaching and learning in both traditional and online classrooms.

Mr. Le Baudour is very involved in EMS education at the national level as a board member of the Distributed Learning Subcommittee of the National Association of EMS Educators. He is a frequent presenter at both state and national conferences and a prolific EMS writer. He currently serves as the Program Director for verihealth Inc. in Petaluma, California.

Mr. Le Baudour is also author, co-author, or contributor to these other Brady texts: *Emergency Medical Responder*, 9th Edition; *Emergency Medical Responder Workbook*, 9th Edition; *Advanced First Aid for Non-EMS Personnel; The Active Learning Manual: EMT*; and *Emergency Care 360—Online EMT Program*.

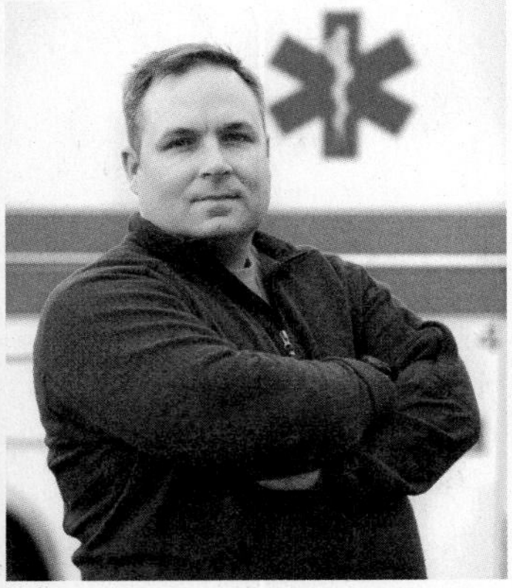

Daniel Batsie

Dan Batsie has been involved in EMS for more than 20 years. He started his career as a paramedic in upstate New York and continued on that path as a paramedic firefighter after moving to Maine in 1999. Mr. Batsie began teaching EMT classes in 1994 and has continued in various capacities as an EMS educator ever since. He is currently the Education Director for Atlantic Partners EMS in Bangor, Maine. In that capacity he oversees licensure education for two regions of Maine EMS. Mr. Batsie also serves as department chair for EMS at Eastern Maine Community College and as an adjunct faculty member for the Kennebec Valley Community College paramedic program.

Mr. Batsie graduated from Hobart College in 1993 and also served in the U.S. Marine Corps. He has participated as a member of the National Association of EMTs Education Committee and has been a contributing author for numerous Brady EMS texts.

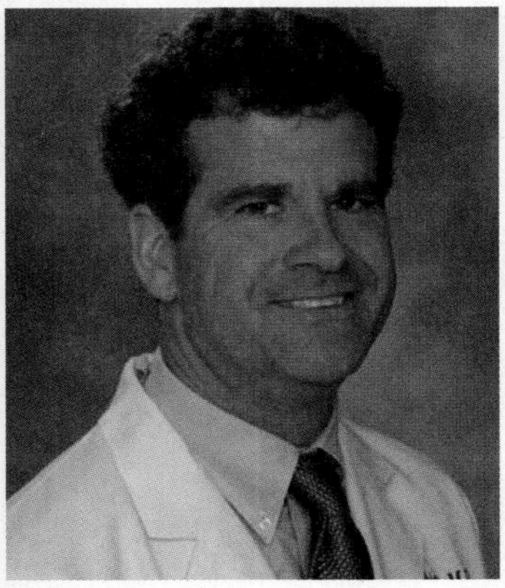

Medical Editor
Edward T. Dickinson

Edward T. Dickinson, MD, NREMT-P, FACEP, is currently Professor and Director of EMS Field Operations in the Department of Emergency Medicine of the Perelman School of Medicine of the University of Pennsylvania School of Medicine in Philadelphia. He is Medical Director of the Malvern, Berwyn, and Radnor Fire Companies, and the Township of Haverford paramedics in Pennsylvania. He is a residency-trained, board-certified emergency medicine physician who is a Fellow of the American College of Emergency Physicians.

Dr. Dickinson began his career in emergency services in 1979 as a firefighter-EMT in upstate New York. He has remained active in fire service and EMS for the past 34 years. He frequently responds with EMS and Fire units and has maintained his certification as a National Registry Paramedic since 1983.

He has served as medical editor for numerous Brady EMT-B and First Responder texts and is the author of *Fire Service Emergency Care* and co-author of *Emergency Care, Fire Service Edition*, and *Emergency Incident Rehabilitation*. He is co-editor of *ALS Case Studies in Emergency Care*.

Welcome to

EMT COMPLETE

A Comprehensive Worktext

SECOND EDITION

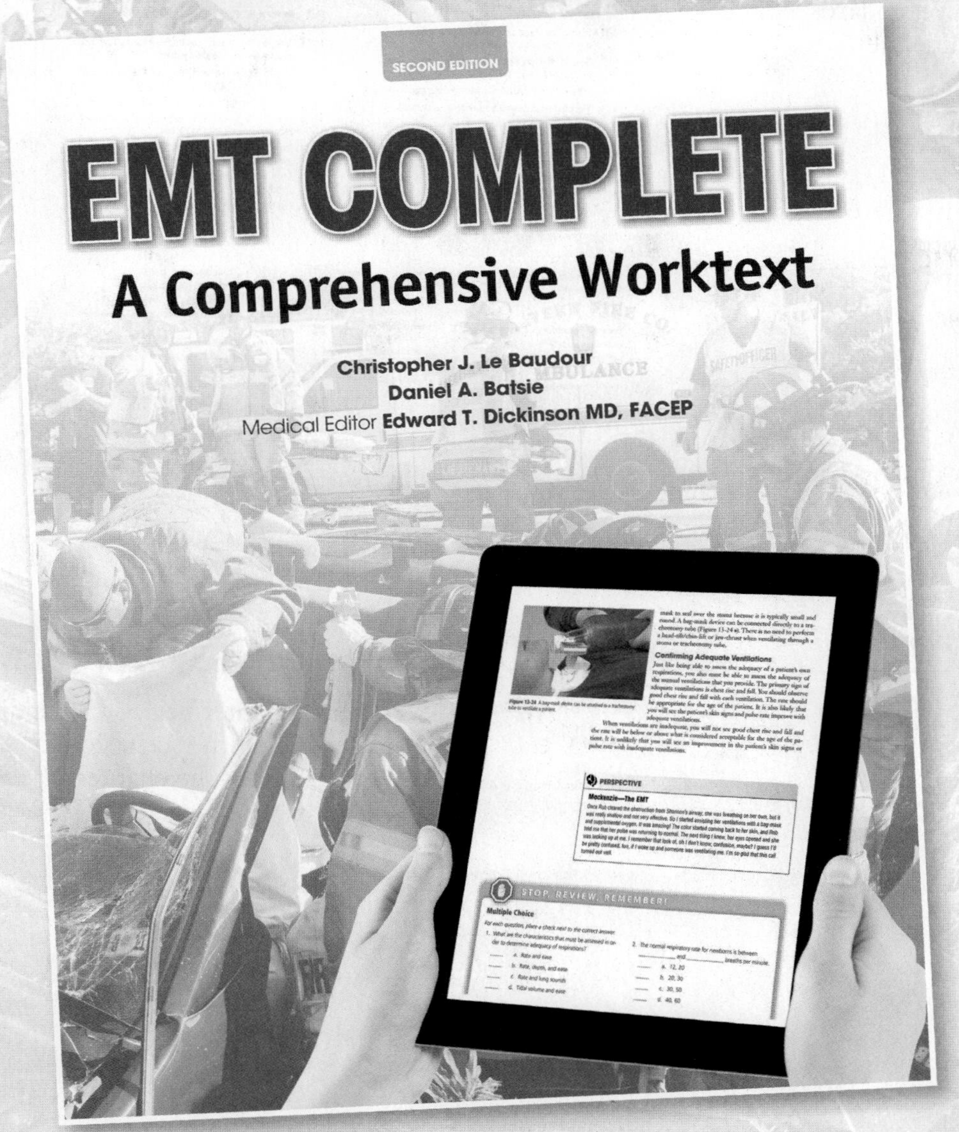

A Guide to Key Features

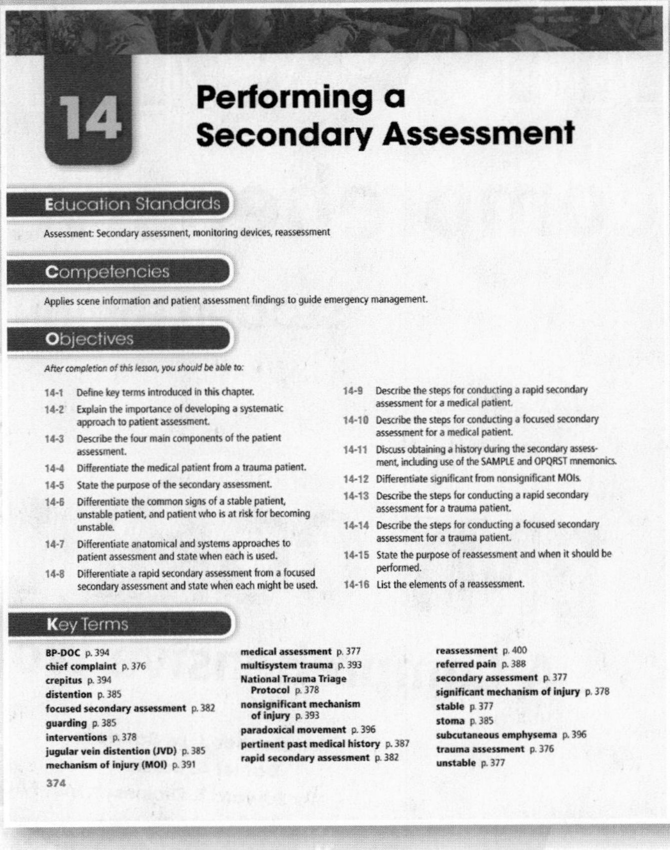

14

Performing a Secondary Assessment

Education Standards

Assessment: Secondary assessment, monitoring devices, reassessment

Competencies

Applies scene information and patient assessment findings to guide emergency management.

Objectives

After completion of this lesson, you should be able to:

14-1 Define key terms introduced in this chapter.
14-2 Explain the importance of developing a systematic approach to patient assessment.
14-3 Describe the four main components of the patient assessment.
14-4 Differentiate the medical patient from a trauma patient.
14-5 State the purpose of the secondary assessment.
14-6 Differentiate the common signs of a stable patient, unstable patient, and patient who is at risk for becoming unstable.
14-7 Differentiate anatomical and systems approaches to patient assessment and state when each is used.
14-8 Differentiate a rapid secondary assessment from a focused secondary assessment and state when each might be used.
14-9 Describe the steps for conducting a rapid secondary assessment for a medical patient.
14-10 Describe the steps for conducting a focused secondary assessment for a medical patient.
14-11 Discuss obtaining a history during the secondary assessment, including use of the SAMPLE and OPQRST mnemonics.
14-12 Differentiate significant from nonsignificant MOIs.
14-13 Describe the steps for conducting a rapid secondary assessment for a trauma patient.
14-14 Describe the steps for conducting a focused secondary assessment for a trauma patient.
14-15 State the purpose of reassessment and when it should be performed.
14-16 List the elements of a reassessment.

Key Terms

BP-DOC p. 394
chief complaint p. 376
crepitus p. 394
distention p. 385
focused secondary assessment p. 382
guarding p. 385
interventions p. 378
jugular vein distention (JVD) p. 385
mechanism of injury (MOI) p. 391
medical assessment p. 377
multisystem trauma p. 393
National Trauma Triage Protocol p. 378
nonsignificant mechanism of injury p. 393
paradoxical movement p. 396
pertinent past medical history p. 387
rapid secondary assessment p. 382
reassessment p. 400
referred pain p. 388
secondary assessment p. 377
significant mechanism of injury p. 378
stable p. 377
stoma p. 385
subcutaneous emphysema p. 396
trauma assessment p. 376
unstable p. 377

374

Chapter Objectives

Objectives form the basis of each chapter and were developed around the Education Standards and Instructional Guidelines.

Key Terms

Page numbers identify where each key term first appears, boldfaced, in the chapter.

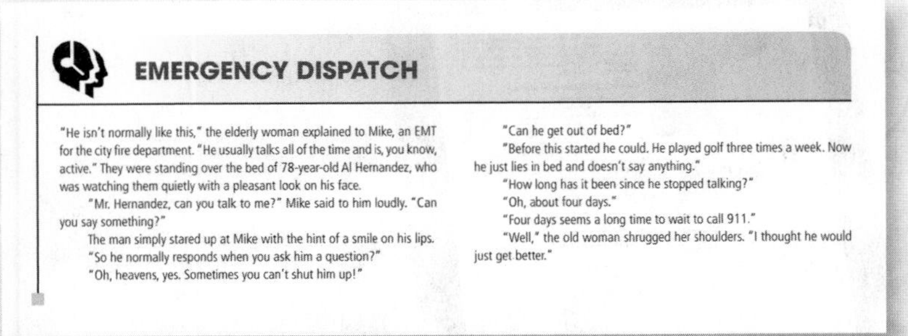

EMERGENCY DISPATCH

"He isn't normally like this," the elderly woman explained to Mike, an EMT for the city fire department. "He usually talks all of the time and is, you know, active." They were standing over the bed of 78-year-old Al Hernandez, who was watching them quietly with a pleasant look on his face.

"Mr. Hernandez, can you talk to me?" Mike said to him loudly. "Can you say something?"

The man simply stared up at Mike with the hint of a smile on his lips.

"So he normally responds when you ask him a question?"

"Oh, heavens, yes. Sometimes you can't shut him up!"

"Can he get out of bed?"

"Before this started he could. He played golf three times a week. Now he just lies in bed and doesn't say anything."

"How long has it been since he stopped talking?"

"Oh, about four days."

"Four days seems a long time to wait to call 911."

"Well," the old woman shrugged her shoulders. "I thought he would just get better."

Emergency Dispatch

Each chapter begins with a dispatch describing the scenario that will be followed throughout the chapter's *Perspectives*.

Perspective

Points of view from people on the scene, whether it be the EMT, the EMT's partner, the patient, other rescuers, bystanders, family members, or the ER doctor. Perspectives show the reader what may be going on in the minds of all participants at a call. This helps the EMT gain a greater understanding of her impact on the scene overall, making for better patient care.

PERSPECTIVE

Mike—The EMT

How are you supposed to do a mental status evaluation, or gather any sort of good history, or even evaluate a chief complaint, when the patient can't communicate at all? And the way that he just smiled at me, I honestly thought that he was just being difficult! At first, that actually made me kind of angry until I realized that there was something really serious going on.

STOP, REVIEW, REMEMBER!

Multiple Choice

For each question, place a check next to the correct answer.

1. It is essential for the EMT to develop a systematic approach to patient assessment because it helps to ensure that the:
   _____ a. patient is transported to the appropriate facility.
   _____ b. patient will receive the appropriate care sooner.
   _____ c. proper personal protective equipment is used at all times.
   _____ d. patient is always assessed from head-to-toe.
2. The four main components of patient assessment in order are:
   _____ a. scene size-up, primary assessment, secondary assessment, and reassessment.
   _____ b. scene size-up, primary assessment, focused assessment, and secondary assessment.
   _____ c. scene size-up, primary assessment, vital signs, and secondary assessment.
   _____ d. scene size-up, primary assessment, secondary assessment, and vital signs.
3. The first time that a patient's mental status is assessed is during the:
   _____ a. scene size-up.
   _____ b. primary assessment.
   _____ c. rapid secondary assessment.
   _____ d. focused secondary assessment.
4. You are caring for a patient who missed the last step on a short flight of stairs and twisted her ankle. This patient would initially be categorized as a ____________ patient.
   _____ a. medical
   _____ b. trauma
   _____ c. stable
   _____ d. unstable
5. You are caring for a patient who is complaining of chest pain similar to the pain he had with a previous heart attack. He is alert and does not complain of shortness of breath. You should categorize this patient as:
   _____ a. critical. _____ c. stable.
   _____ b. noncritical. _____ d. unstable.

Matching

Correctly identify the following signs and symptoms as either consistent with a stable patient or with an unstable patient. Write an "S" for stable or a "U" for unstable.

Sign or Symptom	Category
1. Alert and oriented	
2. No major complaint of chest or abdominal pain	
3. Significant MOI	

(continued on next page)

Stop, Review, Remember!

The "work" part of the Worktext, these exercises are integrated throughout the chapters, enabling readers to assess their learning before going on. Write-in multiple-choice, fill-in-the-blank, matching, and critical-thinking questions provide readers with immediate feedback.

Running Objectives

Objectives are repeated next to the text in which they're first covered.

Patient Assessment

Without question, the patient assessment is the foundational skill that all EMTs must learn and master. It requires hours of memorization and practice of the steps on simulated patients. One of the most important concepts to understand regarding your development of a good assessment is that it must be developed as a systematic routine.

14-2 Explain the importance of developing a systematic approach to patient assessment.

Regardless of the type of patient, developing a systematic approach to patient assessment is essential to ensuring that all of the steps of the assessment will be addressed and in the correct order. Developing a consistent approach and routine also will minimize wasted time and allow you to begin providing the appropriate care sooner.

There are four main components to a patient assessment, they are:

14-3 Describe the four main components of the patient assessment.

- Scene size-up
- Primary assessment
- Secondary assessment
- Reassessment

Running Glossary

Definitions for key terms are provided in the margins, next to the text in which they're first introduced.

rapid secondary assessment the part of the secondary assessment that is performed on unstable patients and on patients who have sustained a significant mechanism of injury.

focused secondary assessment the part of the secondary assessment that is performed on stable medical and trauma patients.

- The **rapid secondary assessment** is used for unstable patients, whether medical or trauma. Though the path is the same for both, the specific signs and symptoms you will be looking for differ slightly.
- The **focused secondary assessment** is used mostly on stable patients, whether medical or trauma. It is designed to focus in on the chief complaint (medical patient) or injury (trauma patient). The focused secondary assessment is much more detailed than the rapid secondary assessment, and includes a thorough medical history.

Practical Pathophysiology

Found in the clinical chapters, this feature relates to specific medical conditions and disease processes, promoting in-depth understanding that helps providers make the best decisions in the field.

PRACTICAL PATHOPHYSIOLOGY

The assessment of the jugular veins is an indirect indicator of the status of the cardiopulmonary system. It is most often an indicator of right-sided heart failure. When assessing a patient for the presence of jugular vein distention, you must have the patient in a semi-sitting position (between 30 and 45 degrees), because it is normal to see such distention in patients who are supine.

Clinical Clue

This feature provides need-to-know information regarding contraindications, criteria, safety, tips, and other clinical background—to help the practitioner make decisions in the field.

CLINICAL CLUE

Scars

Always be on the lookout for scars as you expose and visually inspect the body. Scars may be a sign of prior injury or surgery. For example, many patients with a cardiac history have the classic "zipper" scar down the center of the sternum, indicating a history of open heart surgery. It is always appropriate to ask the history behind a particular scar.

Scans

Procedures performed step by step with explanations and photographs.

SCAN 14-2 Reassessment

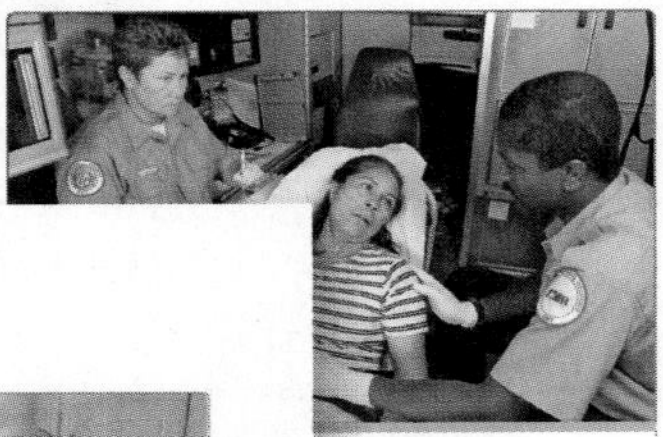

...ssessment.

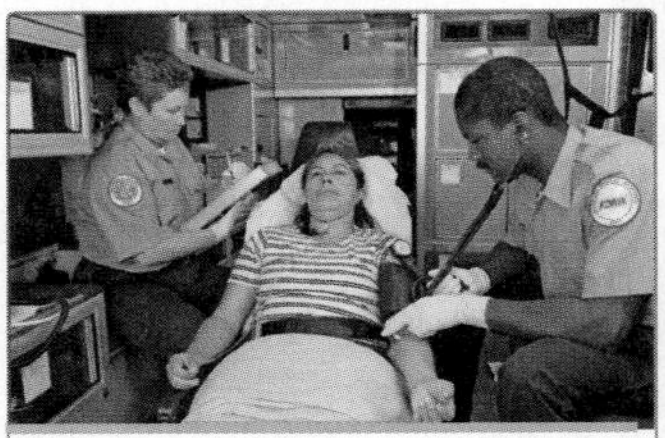

14-2-2 Recheck vital signs and compare with the baseline set.

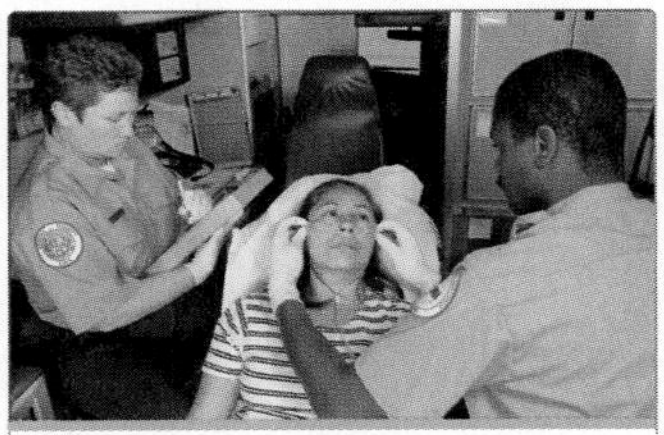

14-2-3 Check the effectiveness of your interventions.

SCAN 14-1 Rapid Secondary Assessment (Medical Patient)

14-1-1 Perform a scene size-up as you approach the scene.

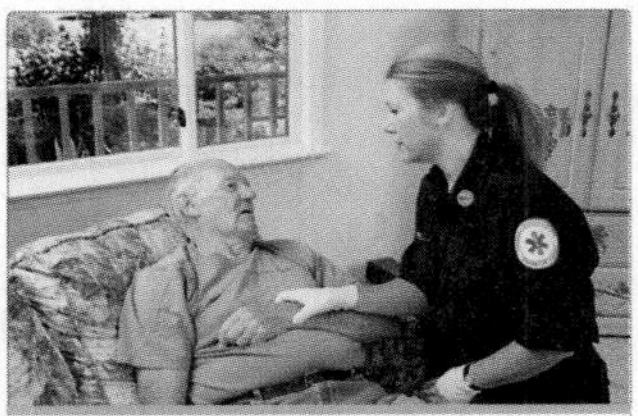

14-1-2 Perform a primary assessment and care for immediate life threats.

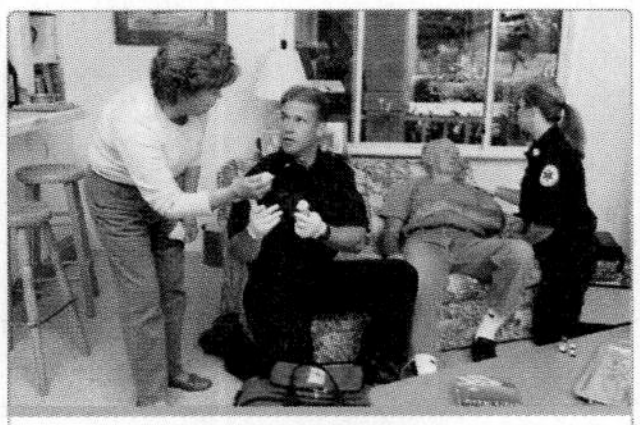

14-1-3 Obtain a chief complaint and make a stable/unstable determination.

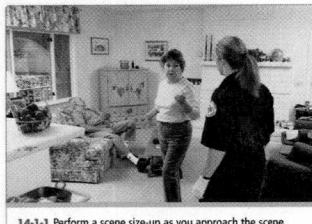

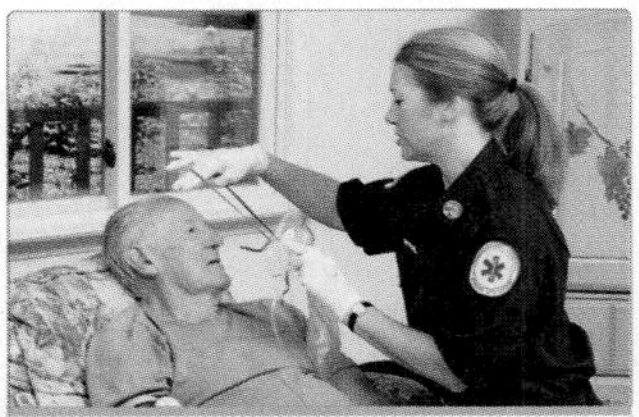

14-1-4 Apply oxygen and prepare for transport.

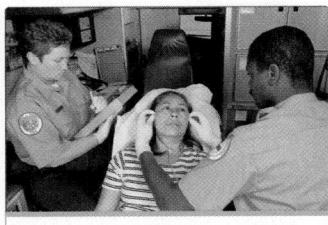

Dispatch Summary

Completion of the call that began at the start of the chapter. This allows the reader to see resolution and follow-up care, as appropriate.

EMERGENCY DISPATCH SUMMARY

Al Hernandez was transported without incident to Saint Anthony Hospital on Broadway and First. Subsequent tests showed that Mr. Hernandez had suffered an ischemic stroke, but with the extended time before help was sought, he was not considered a candidate for fibrinolytic therapy. He has since been placed into the Spring County Advanced Care Facility for follow-up care, but he has so far showed no signs of regaining either his ability to speak or move successfully.

Chapter Review

Each chapter ends with a summary of key points and a review containing multiple-choice, matching, labeling, and critical-thinking questions and case studies.

CHAPTER 14 PERFORMING A SECONDARY ASSESSMENT 405

Chapter Review

To the Point

- It is very important to develop a systematic approach to your patient assessment. It will help ensure a consistently thorough assessment each time and an efficiency that helps ensure the patient will receive prompt care.
- The four main components of the patient assessment are the scene size-up, primary assessment, secondary assessment, and reassessment.
- Patients are categorized first as medical (illness) or trauma (injury) patients.
- The purpose of the secondary assessment is to identify and care for signs and symptoms not previously found or addressed in the primary assessment.
- Patients are further categorized as stable, unstable, or likely to become unstable. Unstable patients must receive more rapid assessment, care, and transport because their condition could worsen rapidly.
- There are two basic approaches used for patient assessment, the anatomical and the systems approach. The anatomical approach is a head-to-toe approach, while the systems approach focuses on the specific body system or systems related to the chief complaint.
- The rapid secondary assessment is used for unstable patients, while the focused assessment is used for stable patients.
- The SAMPLE and the OPQRST memory aids are tools used to obtain a more detailed history based on the patient's chief complaint.
- When caring for trauma patients, you must carefu ate the mechanism of injury and have a high index cion for multisystem trauma.
- Once you have completed the secondary assessn must perform regular reassessments. The reassessn sists of reevaluating the patient's ABCs includin status, rechecking vital signs and looking for trer sessment of the chief complaint, checking the effe of your interventions, and changing patient pr appropriate.

Chapter Questions

Multiple Choice

For each question, place a check next to the correct answer.

1. Which one of the following patients best meets the criteria for a rapid secondary assessment?
   ____ a. 16-year-old who fell 20 feet
   ____ b. 23-year-old who twisted an ankle
   ____ c. 41-year-old with severe chest pain
   ____ d. 77-year-old who fainted during a meal
2. After performing a rapid secondary assessment and taking vital signs for a trauma patient, you should obtain a:
   ____ a. mental status.
   ____ b. detailed assessment.
   ____ c. SAMPLE history.
   ____ d. focused assessment.
3. Which one of the following would *not* be a normal finding of a chest assessment?
   ____ a. Paradoxical movement
   ____ b. Distention
   ____ c. Crepitation
   ____ d. Tenderness
4. All of the following are factors that should be evaluated when assessing the MOI of a fall victim *except*:
   ____ a. height of fall.
   ____ b. speed of fall.
   ____ c. the position in which he landed.
   ____ d. whether or not he lost consciousness.
5. A fall greater than ____ feet is considered a significant MOI for an adult patient.
   ____ a. 5
   ____ b. 10
   ____ c. 15
   ____ d. 20

406 MODULE 2 PATIENT ASSESSMENT

6. Reassessments for the stable patient should be performed about every ____ minutes.
   ____ a. 5
   ____ b. 10
   ____ c. 15
   ____ d. 20
7. Which one of the following best defines the term *multisystem trauma*?
   ____ a. Obvious injuries to multiple bones
   ____ b. Multiple patients
   ____ c. Multiple mechanisms of injury
   ____ d. Trauma to multiple body systems
8. Which one of the following elements of the patient assessment is *not* common to all assessments?
   ____ a. Focused secondary assessment
   ____ b. Vital signs and history
   ____ c. Scene size-up
   ____ d. BSI precautions
9. Which one of the following best represents a significant MOI?
   ____ a. Badly sprained ankle
   ____ b. Vehicle collision at 30 mph
   ____ c. Eight-foot fall from a ladder onto asphalt
   ____ d. Crush injury to a hand
10. The criterion for determining the most appropriate assessment path for a medical patient is:
    ____ a. the chief complaint.
    ____ b. the level of pain.
    ____ c. whether he is stable or unstable.
    ____ d. the mechanism of injury.
11. Which one of the following is the most appropriate assessment tool for evaluating the chief complaint of a medical patient?
    ____ a. SAMPLE
    ____ b. OPQRST
    ____ c. AVPU
    ____ d. DCAP-BTLS
12. Swelling that is found in the ankles of some medical patients with a cardiac history is called:
    ____ a. pedal distention.
    ____ b. ascites.
    ____ c. subtle deformity.
    ____ d. pedal edema.
13. In the unresponsive medical patient, vital signs should be obtained:
    ____ a. following the rapid secondary assessment.
    ____ b. before the rapid secondary assessment.
    ____ c. as often as possible.
    ____ d. every 15 minutes.
14. The vital signs of an unstable patient should be reassessed at least every ____ minutes.
    ____ a. 5
    ____ b. 10
    ____ c. 15
    ____ d. 20
15. You are caring for a 22-year-old patient following what was described as a seizure. The patient is alert but confused. You should:
    ____ a. obtain vital signs and perform a rapid secondary assessment.
    ____ b. administer oxygen and perform a rapid secondary assessment.
    ____ c. administer oxygen and obtain vital signs.
    ____ d. perform a focused secondary assessment and administer oxygen.

Matching

Match the definition on the left with the applicable term on the right.

1. ____ The grating sound or feeling of broken bones rubbing together
2. ____ Displacement of the trachea laterally from the midline
3. ____ Bulging of the neck veins
4. ____ Movement of a part of the chest wall in the opposite direction to the rest of the chest during inhalation and exhalation
5. ____ Air trapped beneath the skin

A. Paradoxical movement
B. Subcutaneous emphysema
C. Tracheal deviation
D. Jugular vein distention
E. Crepitus

The Last Word

Good patient care depends on a thorough assessment. Once you have determined that the scene is safe and you have donned the appropriate personal protection equipment (PPE) for the situation, you must perform a primary assessment on each and every patient.

Trauma and medical patients require slightly different approaches to the secondary assessment. The specific assessment path for the trauma patient is determined by the significance of the mechanism of injury. A rapid secondary assessment is used for the patient who has suffered a significant MOI or has serious injury potentially affecting multiple body systems. In contrast, the focused secondary assessment is used for patients with an injury that is isolated to a noncritical area of the body, such as an extremity.

The specific assessment path for the medical patient is based on how stable the patient appears to be. A rapid secondary assessment is used for the patient who is unstable or unable to provide any meaningful history pertaining to his condition or chief complaint. In contrast, the focused secondary assessment is used for the patient who is responsive and able to provide a meaningful history of his problem.

Reassessment of the ABCs, vital signs, and interventions must be conducted at frequent intervals until the patient is delivered to an appropriate receiving hospital—every 15 minutes for a stable patient and every 5 minutes for an unstable patient.

The Last Word

Found at the conclusion of Chapter Review, this ties together important chapter understandings.

Module Review and Practice Examination

After each of the modules, a test is provided to ensure that learning is cumulative throughout the text.

Module 2: Review and Practice Examination for Chapters 12–14

DIRECTIONS: Assess what you have learned in this module by placing a check mark in the blank beside the best answer for each multiple-choice question. When you are done, check your answers against the Answer Key at the back of the book.

1. Which one of the following is part of the scene size-up?
 ____ a. Determining the number of patients
 ____ b. Checking the patient's airway
 ____ c. Determining the patient's chief complaint
 ____ d. Performing a primary assessment

2. Determining the need for body substance isolation (BSI) precautions is part of the:
 ____ a. dispatch information.
 ____ b. primary assessment.
 ____ c. scene size-up.
 ____ d. general impression.

3. The best way to protect yourself and your crew from hazards at the scene of an emergency is to:
 ____ a. rely on dispatch information.
 ____ b. always respond with a crew of at least three EMS providers.
 ____ c. wear body armor.
 ____ d. observe the scene.

4. You are approaching the porch of a house to which you have been dispatched for an "injured person." Suddenly, the door swings open and you are confronted by a man in his 60s who is armed with a shotgun. You should:
 ____ a. immediately call for law enforcement.
 ____ b. retreat immediately to a safe location.
 ____ c. explain that you were called here to help someone who is injured.
 ____ d. throw your oxygen bag at the man to try to disarm him.

5. The time to call for additional resources at the scene of an emergency is:
 ____ a. after you receive the dispatch information.
 ____ b. as you are performing the scene size-up.
 ____ c. after you have triaged your patients.
 ____ d. during the primary assessment.

6. In addition to looking for signs of danger, the scene size-up can give clues about:
 ____ a. whether the patient is chronically ill.
 ____ b. the patient's past medical history.
 ____ c. how the patient was injured.
 ____ d. the patient's medications.

7. After ensuring personal safety, the first priority in patient care is:
 ____ a. checking the patient's pulse.
 ____ b. getting a medical history from the patient.
 ____ c. assessing the patient's airway.
 ____ d. administering oxygen.

8. Your adult patient has fallen 15 feet off a roof and onto his side. According to the National Trauma Triage Protocol, the patient's fall would be classified as:
 ____ a. nonsignificant mechanism of injury.
 ____ b. nature of illness.
 ____ c. significant mechanism of injury.
 ____ d. chief complaint.

9. Which one of the following is the primary muscle(s) used for breathing under normal conditions?
 ____ a. Intercostal muscles between the ribs
 ____ b. Abdominal muscles
 ____ c. Latissimus dorsi muscle of the back
 ____ d. Diaphragm

10. Your patient is a three-year-old toddler. You should consider her respiratory rate to be normal if it is ____________ per minute.
 ____ a. 38 ____ c. 42
 ____ b. 24 ____ d. 16

11. Your patient is a seven-year-old boy. You should consider his respiratory rate normal if it is ____________ per minute.
 ____ a. 60 ____ c. 28
 ____ b. 48 ____ d. 12

411

Pearson Solutions and Services

MyBradyLab™

www.mybradylab.com

What Is MyBradyLab?

MyBradyLab is a comprehensive online program that gives you the opportunity to test yourself on basic information, concepts, and skills to see how well you know the material. From the test results, the program builds a self-paced, personalized study plan unique to your needs. Remediation in the form of e-text pages, illustrations, animations, exercises, and video clips is provided for those areas in which you may need additional instruction or reinforcement. You can then work through the program until material is learned and mastered. MyBradyLab is available as a standalone program or with an embedded e-text.

MyBradyLab maps objectives created from the National EMS Education Standards for the EMT level to each learning module. With MyBradyLab, you can track your own progress through the entire course. The personalized study plan material supports you as you work to achieve success in the classroom and on certification exams.

How Do Students Benefit?

MyBradyLab helps you:

- Keep up with the new, complex information presented in the text and lectures.
- Save time by focusing study and review on just the content you need.
- Increase understanding of difficult concepts with study material for different learning styles.
- Remediate in areas in which you need additional review.

Key Features of MyBradyLab

Pre-tests and **Post-tests** Using questions aligned to EMT Education Standards, quizzes measure your understanding of topics and expected learning outcomes.

Personalized Study Material Based on the topic pre-test results, you will receive a personalized study plan highlighting areas where you may need improvement. Study tools include:

- Skills and animation videos.
- Links to specific pages in the e-text.
- Images for review.
- Interactive exercises.
- Audio glossary.
- Access to full chapters of the e-text.

How Do Instructors Benefit?

- Save time by providing students a comprehensive, media-rich study program.
- Monitor student activity with viewable student assignments.
- Provide consistent delivery of material across all courses and instructors.
- Track student understanding of course content in the program Gradebook.
- Increase student retention.
- Meet the needs of the wide range of learners in your classroom.

Where Can Instructors Get More Information?

Contact your local Brady representative or visit **www.mybradylab.com** for more information.

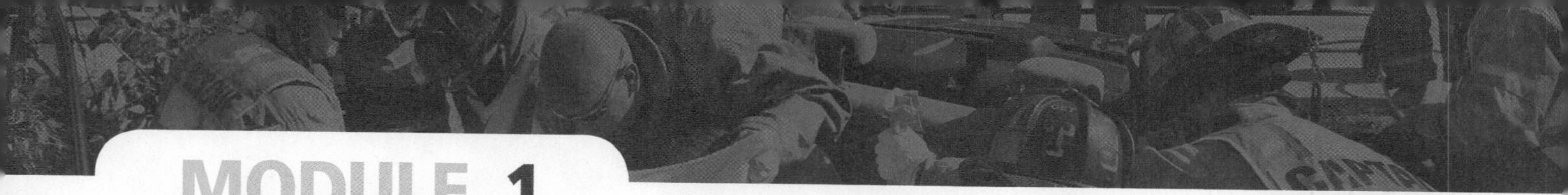

MODULE 1
Fundamentals

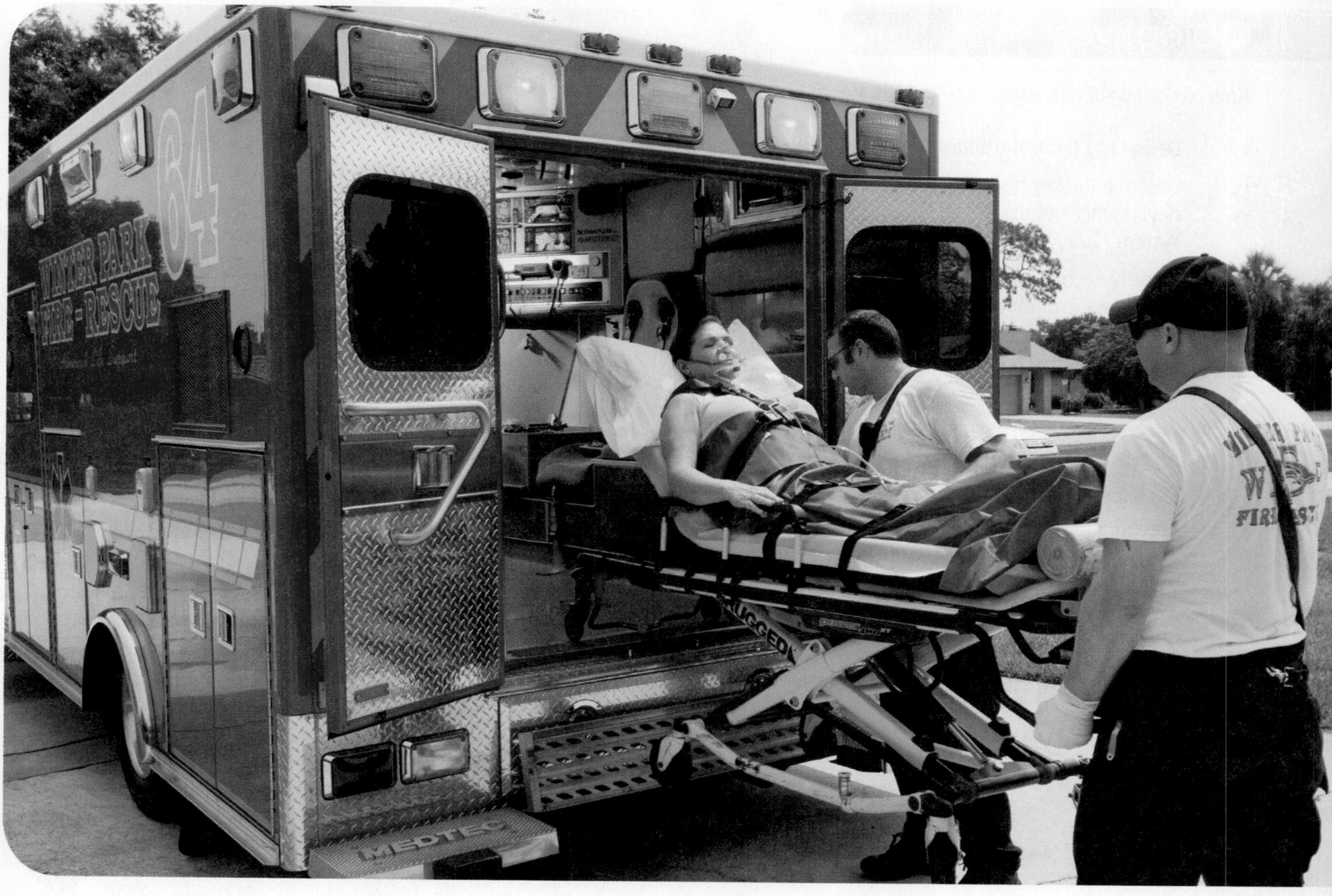

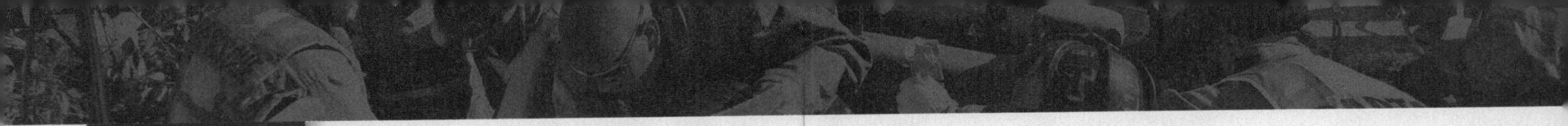

1 You and the EMS System

Education Standards

Preparatory: EMS Systems, Research, Public Health

Competencies

Applies fundamental knowledge of the EMS system, safety/well-being of the EMT, medical/legal issues, and ethical issues to the provision of emergency care.

Maintains an awareness of local public health resources and the role EMS personnel play in public health emergencies.

Uses simple knowledge of the principles of illness and injury prevention in emergency care.

Objectives

After completion of this lesson, you should be able to:

1-1 Define key terms introduced in this chapter.

1-2 Describe the key historical events that have shaped the development of the emergency medical services (EMS) system.

1-3 Identify each of the components of the Technical Assistance Program Assessment Standards.

1-4 Compare and contrast the scopes of practice of the following levels of EMS providers: emergency medical responder (EMR), emergency medical technician (EMT), advanced emergency medical technician (Advanced EMT), and paramedic.

1-5 Describe the role of medical direction/oversight in an EMS system.

1-6 Differentiate between basic 911 and E-911 EMS access systems.

1-7 Give examples of how EMTs can carry out each of the following roles and responsibilities: personal and patient safety, patient assessment and emergency care, transport and transfer of care, record keeping and data collection, and patient advocacy.

1-8 Describe what is expected of EMTs in terms of each of the following professional attributes: appearance, knowledge and skills, physical demands, personal traits, and maintaining certification and licensure.

1-9 Describe the purpose of quality improvement/continuous quality improvement programs in EMS.

1-10 Explain the EMT's roles and responsibilities in quality improvement.

1-11 Describe the relationship between EMS and public health.

1-12 Explain the role of public health systems and their relationship to EMS, disease surveillance, and injury prevention.

1-13 Explain the role that disaster medical assistance teams (DMAT) play and how they integrate with EMS systems.

1-14 Explain the role that research plays in EMS and the ways that an EMT might identify and support research.

Key Terms

advanced EMT p. 9
emergency medical dispatcher (EMD) p. 12
emergency medical responder (EMR) p. 9
emergency medical services (EMS) system p. 6
emergency medical technician (EMT) p. 9
medical direction p. 11
medical director p. 8
off-line medical direction p. 12
on-line medical direction p. 12
paramedic p. 9
protocols p. 11
public safety answering point (PSAP) p. 12
quality improvement (QI) p. 14
standing orders p. 11

Introduction

Congratulations on your decision to enter the world of EMS to become an emergency medical technician (EMT). Becoming an EMT will provide you with knowledge and skills that will carry over into all aspects of your life for many years to come. Not everyone who takes this course intends to work on an ambulance or in an emergency department at a local hospital. Some of you might be taking this course because you will be working as a camp counselor, lifeguard, firefighter, or police officer. What is common to all who learn the skills of an EMT is that they are willing to serve those in need. Albert Schweitzer once said, "One thing I know: The only ones among you who will be really happy are those who will have sought and found how to serve." Serving others in their time of need is an honor, a privilege, and not something everyone desires to do.

Your choice to take this course and become a part of the team of people who are called to assist an ill or injured person brings with it great responsibility. Make no mistake, making decisions about another person's care during a sudden illness or injury can be very stressful and sometimes may even involve life-and-death decisions. However, with that responsibility comes great rewards including the opportunity to save a life.

This chapter will introduce you to the development and growth of the modern-day emergency medical services (EMS) system and the many components that work together to ensure a safer world for all of us.

EMERGENCY DISPATCH

"Dad, why is there a fire truck out front?"

Mark Bennett stopped trying to find his daughter Amy's favorite Dr. Seuss bedtime book and joined her at the window. A large red fire truck was parked across the street, its emergency strobe lights flashing rhythmically, bouncing off the houses up and down the street.

"It's at the Hansons' house." Mark's son, Jared, was now at the window next to them.

"Well, I don't see any signs of a fire," Mark said, peering into the dark evening sky. "I'm sure everything is okay."

Just then, several sirens screamed into range and rapidly grew louder. More emergency lights careened around the neighborhood as an ambulance and a police car joined the fire truck over at the Hansons'.

A Brief History of Modern EMS

1-2 Describe the key historical events that have shaped the development of the emergency medical services (EMS) system.

Where there is life, there is illness and injury. What has not always existed is an organized and efficient means of caring for those illnesses and injuries. Our ability to care for one another has developed slowly over time. It began with simple care provided by those closest to the ill or injured person. Family members provided shelter and necessities such as warmth, food, and water to the person who needed care. This simple care would be given until the injury healed or the illness ran its course. There was little if any care that directly affected the specific illness or injury.

Through trial and error certain individuals became especially skilled at caring for others. Eventually, the ill or injured person would be taken to one of those skilled individuals or the individual would be brought to the patient. Those early caregivers were the forerunners of our modern medical professionals, including EMTs.

Much of the emergency medical experience throughout history has been gained during wars. For example, early Greeks and Romans would transport the injured by chariot from the battlefield to waiting physicians. The first formal ambulance system in the United States was developed during the Civil War when the Union army began training soldiers to provide first aid to the wounded directly on the battlefield. Those "corpsmen" were trained to care for the most immediate life threats, such as bleeding. After initial care, the injured were transported by horse-drawn wagon to waiting physicians.

At the turn of the twentieth century, the few ambulance services that existed were mostly operated by hospitals and staffed by medical interns. Those who drove the vehicles had little or no formal training and generally did not assist with medical care. It was around 1909 when the American Red Cross began offering first-aid classes to the general public. And then in 1928 Julian Stanley Wise founded the nation's first official rescue squad, the Roanoke Life Saving and First Aid Crew (Figure 1-1 ■). Mr. Wise dedicated much of his life to spreading the concept of the volunteer rescue squad around the nation and is credited with starting the first-aid and rescue movement in the United States.

PERSPECTIVE

Pat Hanson—The Patient's Wife

A fire truck, the police, and an ambulance. I just don't get why so many people showed up. I only called 911 because Bill fell and cut his head. They're probably waking up the whole darn neighborhood. And now what'll everyone think? I can just hear it, "Did you see that police car over at Pat's house? I wonder what's *really* going on over there?" This is all so embarrassing!

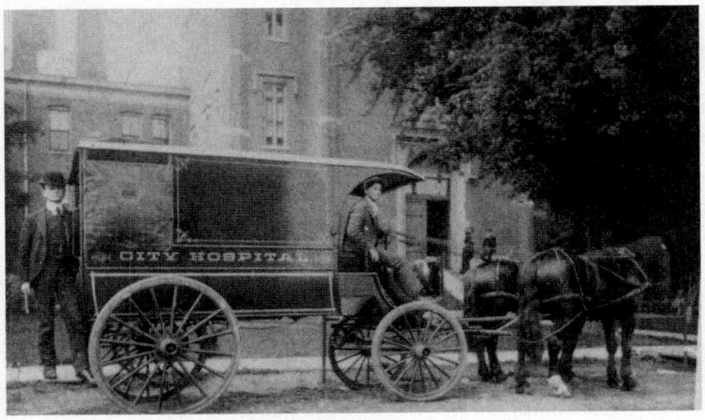

Figure 1-1 An ambulance parked at the entrance of City Hospital, which would later become Wishard Memorial Hospital, circa 1901–1903. The first City Hospital ambulance began carrying sick and injured Indianapolis-area patients in 1887. (Courtesy of Wishard Health Services.)

While the rescue-squad and first-aid movement gained momentum, little emphasis was placed on training the rescuers. Their primary job was to reach the patients as quickly as possible and return them to the hospital for care. In fact, many funeral home vehicles doubled as ambulances during this time.

It was not until the late 1950s and early 1960s that an emphasis on improving prehospital care began. It was during this period that oxygen made its first appearance on ambulances, and cardiopulmonary resuscitation (CPR) was introduced as a life-saving measure.

In 1966 the National Academy of Sciences published a report called *Accidental Death and Disability: The Neglected Disease of Modern Society.* That report detailed many weaknesses in the nation's ability to prevent and manage injuries from accidents. In the prior year, nearly 50,000 people in the United States had died on the nation's roads and highways, more casualties than occurred during the entire eight years of the Vietnam War. The report also offered many recommendations, including standards for ambulance construction and the preparation of nationally accepted textbooks and training programs for fire, police, and ambulance personnel. That same year Congress passed the Highway Safety Act, which led to the formation of the National Highway Traffic Safety Administration (NHTSA). NHTSA has since helped many communities plant the seeds of their own coordinated EMS programs.

In 1972 the television series *Emergency!* made the word *paramedic* a household term. Based on the real-life paramedic program started in 1969 in Los Angeles County, California, the television show created an awareness and demand that is credited in great part with the rapid increase in paramedic programs across the nation.

In 1973 Congress passed the Emergency Medical Services Systems (EMSS) Act, which provided federal funding for the establishment of the emergency medical services (EMS) system all across the nation. The U.S. Department of Transportation developed training and equipment standards for EMS personnel, and state EMS offices began to spring up around the country.

The 1980s and 1990s saw the formation of several national organizations such as the National Association of State EMS Directors and the National Association of EMS Physicians. Those organizations were formed to develop and improve EMS systems throughout the nation. Similarly, the National Association of EMS Educators was formed to enhance the quality and content of EMS education on a national level.

The 1990s also saw the further development of EMS education with the revision of the DOT national standard curricula for all levels of prehospital care. In 1996 the *EMS Agenda for the Future* was released, creating for the first time a vision for EMS that industry leaders, educators, and field personnel could embrace (Figure 1-2 ■).

In 2005 NHTSA published the *National EMS Core Content*, a document that defined the breadth of knowledge that was to be applied to the four levels of EMS training defined by the National Scope of Practice Model.

The Vision of EMS

as written in the *EMS Agenda for the Future*

Emergency medical services (EMS) of the future will be community-based health management that is fully integrated with the overall health care system. It will have the ability to identify and modify illness and injury risks, provide acute illness and injury care and follow-up, and contribute to treatment of chronic conditions and community health monitoring. This new entity will be developed from redistribution of existing health care resources and will be integrated with other health care providers and public health and public safety agencies. It will improve community health and result in more appropriate use of acute health care resources. EMS will remain the public's emergency medical safety net. To learn more about the EMS Agenda for the Future, go to: http://www.nhtsa.dot.gov/people/injury/ems/agenda/emsman.html.

Figure 1-2 The vision of EMS as written in the *EMS Agenda for the Future* (1996).

In 2006 a specialized task force led by the National Association of State EMS Directors and the National Council of State EMS Training Coordinators focused on redefining *The National Scope of Practice Model*. The purpose was to make suggestions for change that would reflect the future of EMS and make recommendations for how EMS systems can best meet the needs of the populations they serve.

In 2009 NHTSA released the National EMS Education Standards, which replaced the National Standard Curricula for all levels of EMS training. The new standards currently define the competencies, clinical behaviors, and judgments that must be met by entry-level EMS personnel. Content and concepts defined in the National EMS Core Content also are integrated within the new standards.

A Systematic Approach to Saving Lives

You may have heard it before and will likely hear it again and again throughout your training as an EMT: Injury is the leading cause of death in the United States for people age 1 to 35. It is also the most common cause of hospitalizations for those under the age of 40.

Each year approximately 40,000 people lose their lives on the nation's roads with approximately 56% of those deaths occurring on rural highways. The cost of those deaths to society is staggering in hard dollars and in the suffering that families who have lost a loved one must endure. The federal agency charged with reducing accidental injury and deaths on the nation's highways is the National Highway Traffic Safety Administration (NHTSA), which was formed out of the Highway Safety Act revision of 1970. Among its many programs are the EMS Technical Assistance Program and the development of the National Standard Curricula for all four levels of EMS providers. (The four levels of EMS providers are discussed later in this chapter.)

Key Components of an EMS System

emergency medical services (EMS) system a highly specialized chain of resources designed to minimize the impact of sudden injury and illness on our society.

1-3 Identify each of the components of the Technical Assistance Program Assessment Standards.

An **emergency medical services (EMS) system** is a highly specialized chain of resources designed to minimize the impact of sudden injury and illness on our society. Scan 1-1 shows how this chain can work.

To make the best use of its limited resources, NHTSA's EMS Technical Assistance Program focuses on helping individual states with the development and evaluation of their emergency medical services. NHTSA also has identified 10 key components of an integrated EMS system and assists states in developing and assessing those components. The 10 components are listed below along with a brief description of each:

- ***Regulation and policy:*** To provide a high-quality, effective system of emergency medical care, each state must have in place legislation that identifies and supports a lead EMS agency. That agency has the authority to plan and implement an effective EMS system and to create appropriate rules and regulations for each recognized component of the EMS system.
- ***Resource management:*** Each state must have in place a centralized method to coordinate all system resources.
- ***Human resources and training:*** The lead state EMS agency must have a mechanism to assess current human resource needs and establish a comprehensive plan for stable and consistent EMS training programs. Programs must be routinely monitored to ensure that instructors meet certain requirements, the curriculum is standardized throughout the state, and valid and reliable testing procedures are utilized.
- ***Transportation:*** Each state must have a comprehensive transportation plan that includes provisions for uniform coverage, including a protocol for air medical dispatch and a mutual aid plan.

SCAN 1-1 The EMS Chain of Resources

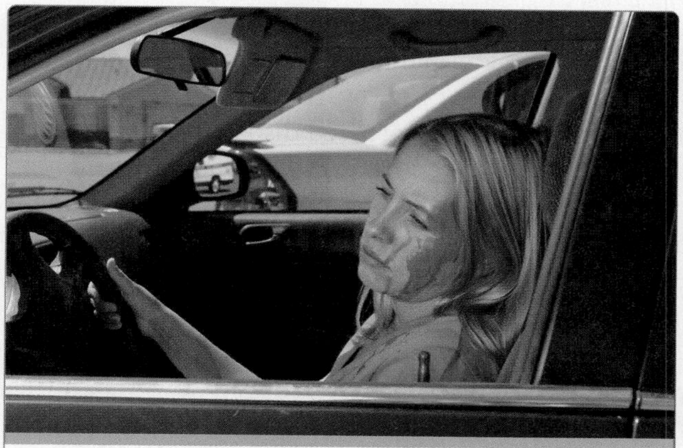

1-1-1 The EMS system is designed to help those in need of immediate medical care.

1-1-2 The EMS system is activated by a call to 911.

1-1-3 A trained dispatcher receives the call and deploys the appropriate resources.

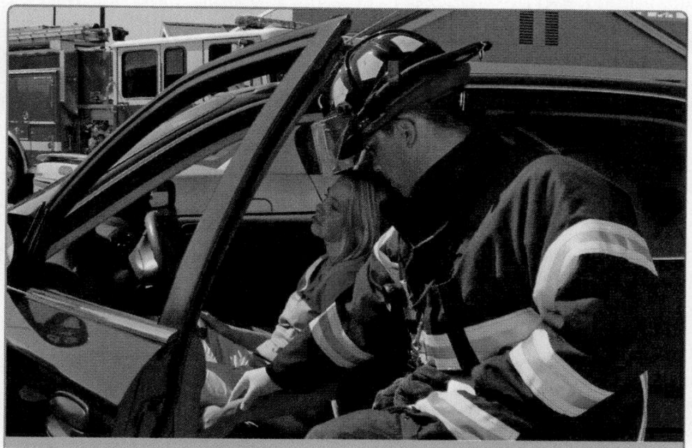

1-1-4 Emergency medical responders often are the first to arrive and begin care.

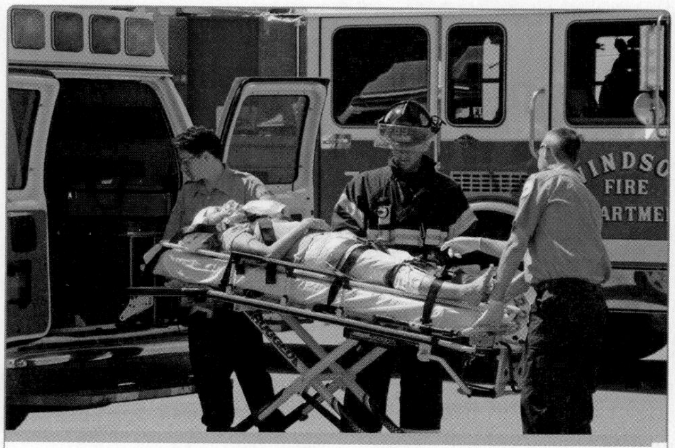

1-1-5 EMTs continue the care and provide transport to the most appropriate facility.

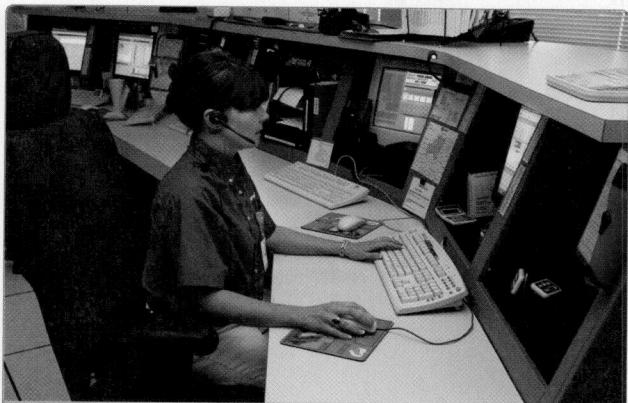

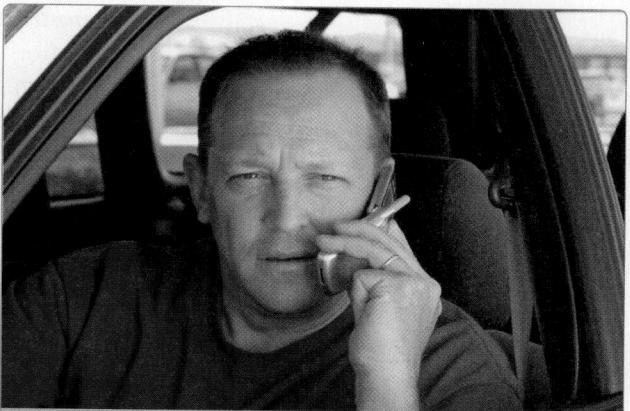

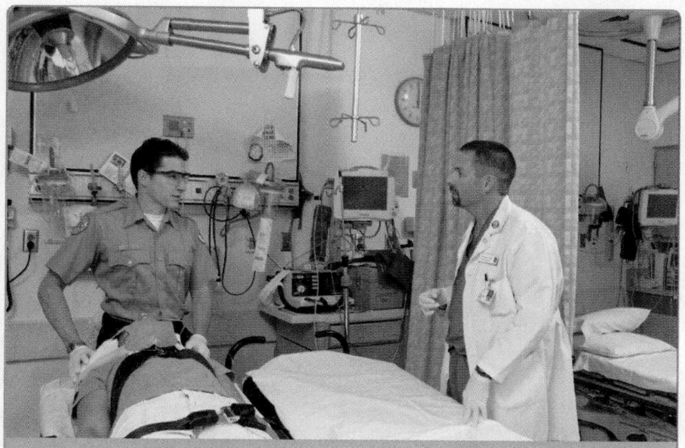

1-1-6 The patient is transferred to more definitive care at an appropriate receiving hospital.

- *Facilities:* It is imperative that the seriously ill patient be delivered in a timely manner to the closest appropriate facility. The lead agency must have a system for categorizing the functional capabilities of all individual health care facilities that receive patients from the prehospital setting.
- *Communications:* The lead agency in each state is responsible for the central coordination of EMS communications. The public must be able to access the EMS system with a single, universal emergency phone number, such as 911, and the communications system must provide for prioritized dispatch.
- *Public information and education:* Each state must develop and implement an EMS public information and education (PI&E) program. The PI&E component of the state EMS plan ensures consistent, structured programs that enhance the public's knowledge of the EMS system, support appropriate EMS system access, demonstrate essential self-help and appropriate bystander care actions, and encourage injury prevention.
- *Medical direction:* Each state must ensure that physicians are involved in all aspects of the patient care system. The role of the EMS **medical director** must be clearly defined, with legislative authority and responsibility for EMS system standards, protocols, and evaluation of patient care. A comprehensive system of medical direction for all prehospital emergency medical care providers must be used to evaluate the provision of medical care as it relates to patient outcome, appropriateness of training programs, and medical direction.

medical director a physician who assumes ultimate responsibility for the patient care aspects of an EMS system.

PERSPECTIVE

Mark—The Neighbor

I wonder if I should call over to the Hanson's house to ask if there is anything that I can do. I mean, with all of those police, firemen, and emergency vehicles, it has to be pretty major. And speaking of the police, why are they there? Don't they only show up if there's a crime?

- *Trauma systems:* To provide a high-quality, effective system of trauma care, each state must have trauma care components that are clearly integrated with the overall EMS system. Legislation should be in place for the development and implementation of the trauma care component of the EMS system. It should include trauma center designation, triage and transfer guidelines for trauma patients, data collection and trauma registry definitions and mechanisms, mandatory autopsies, and quality improvement for trauma patients. (In many systems, it is the EMT who determines which patients go to which hospitals by following local policies and protocols.)
- *Evaluation:* Each state EMS system is responsible for evaluating the effectiveness of services provided to victims of medical or trauma emergencies. A uniform, statewide data-collection system must exist to capture the minimum data necessary to measure compliance with standards. It also must ensure that data are consistently and routinely provided to the lead agency by all EMS providers and that the lead agency performs routine analysis of that data. (Your participation in the evaluation process will help drive the improvement of the EMS system and the care that patients receive.)

In addition to complying with the 10 components just listed, many states also implement and evaluate their own disaster systems in order to be better prepared to respond to large-scale events within their borders.

National Levels of EMS Training

At the present time there are four nationally recognized levels of care as defined by the Department of Transportation (DOT), the parent agency for NHTSA. As part of the redefinition of *The National Scope of Practice Model* mentioned earlier, the four levels of care recently underwent a detailed review and revision. In addition, many states have further divided the levels of training to meet the unique and specific needs of their own systems.

1-4 Compare and contrast the scopes of practice of the following levels of EMS providers: emergency medical responder (EMR), emergency medical technician (EMT), advanced emergency medical technician (Advanced EMT), and paramedic.

The four levels of training are supported by a document known as the *National Standard Curriculum (NSC)*. Each level has its own curriculum, which defines that level's scope of practice. (The concept of *scope of practice* will be discussed more in Chapter 3.) The four levels of training are:

- ***Emergency medical responder:*** This is the most basic level of nationally recognized care and the NSC for this level represents approximately 40 hours of training. The **emergency medical responder (EMR)** is most often the first person on the scene of an emergency. So, he is trained to identify potential hazards, identify and treat immediate life threats, and assist other EMS personnel at the scene. The EMR is trained to function with a minimum of equipment. This level of training was formerly called "First Responder."
- ***Emergency medical technician:*** The NSC for the **emergency medical technician (EMT)** represents approximately 110 hours of training, which is in nearly all areas of the United States the minimum level of training for providing care on an ambulance. The EMT receives training in the assessment and care of many of the most common injuries and illnesses and provides care for patients while at the scene and during transport to an appropriate receiving facility. The level of care provided by EMTs is known as *basic life support (BLS)*.
- ***Advanced EMT:*** The NSC for the **advanced EMT** represents between 300 and 400 hours of instruction and is the first level that is referred to as *advanced life support (ALS)*. In addition to all the BLS skills of an EMT, the advanced EMT can administer certain medications, start intravenous lines, interpret and shock specific heart rhythms, and provide advanced airway management.
- ***Paramedic:*** The NSC for the **paramedic** level of training represents between 1,000 and 1,200 hours and is currently the most advanced level of nationally recognized EMS care. Performing ALS skills in addition to BLS skills, the paramedic can administer a wide variety of medications, initiate intravenous lines, interpret and shock specific heart rhythms, insert advanced airway devices, and perform a variety of other advanced procedures.

emergency medical responder (EMR) a level of EMS training designed for the person who often is first at the scene of an emergency. The emphasis is on activating the EMS system and providing immediate care for life-threatening injuries or illnesses, controlling the scene, and preparing for the arrival of the ambulance.

emergency medical technician (EMT) a level of EMS training with emphasis on assessment and care of the ill or injured patient and in most areas is considered the minimum level of certification for ambulance personnel.

advanced EMT a level of EMS training that is the same as the EMT with additional training in order to provide a minimum level of advanced life support (ALS), such as the initiation of intravenous (IV) lines, advanced airway techniques, and administration of some medications beyond those the EMT is permitted to administer.

paramedic a level of EMS training that requires significantly more training than an EMT, specifically in advanced life support procedures including invasive procedures such as the insertion of endotracheal tubes, initiation of IV lines, administration of a variety of medications, interpretation of electrocardiograms, and cardiac defibrillation.

Most EMS systems are *tiered EMS systems*. That is, it is common to find two or more levels of provider working closely together. A typical tiered system has firefighters trained as emergency medical responders arriving first at the scene, followed closely behind by an ambulance staffed with an EMT and a paramedic. Regardless of your level of training, you must remember that you are an important link in the EMS chain.

PERSPECTIVE

Jared—The Neighbor's Child

It's really scary. Lights are flashing everywhere. Everything is turning red and blue, and it looks like the people are moving in slow motion. I can see our neighbors all up and down the street looking out their windows. I don't ever want the police and firemen to come to my house!

STOP, REVIEW, REMEMBER!

Multiple Choice

For each question, place a check next to the correct answer.

1. Which of the following is one of the 10 essential elements of an EMS system and deals specifically with the creation of appropriate rules and regulations for each recognized component of the EMS system?

_____ a. Communication

_____ b. Regulation and policy

_____ c. Human resources

_____ d. Evaluation

2. Which one of the following essential components of an EMS system deals with categorizing the functional capabilities of all individual health care facilities?

_____ a. Trauma systems

_____ b. Evaluation

_____ c. Facilities

_____ d. Human resources

3. Which one of the following levels of care is considered basic life support (BLS)?

_____ a. Advanced practice paramedic

_____ b. Paramedic

_____ c. Advanced EMT

_____ d. EMT

Fill in the Blank

1. Using a minimal amount of equipment, the ______________________ must identify and care for immediate life threats and assist other EMS personnel.

2. The ______________________ is responsible for developing the standards for each level of training.

3. The ______________________ is a highly specialized chain of resources designed to minimize the impact of sudden injury and illness on our society.

4. The ______________________ receives training at the BLS level on the assessment and care of patients while at the scene and during transport.

5. ______________________ identifies 10 key components of an integrated EMS system and assists states in developing and assessing those components.

Critical Thinking

Develop your awareness and understanding of the EMS system where you live or in which you plan on working by answering the following questions.

1. Identify and list as many components as you can that make up the EMS system where you live or plan to work.

____

____

____

____

2. What is the fundamental difference between the Emergency Medical Responder level of training and the three other levels?

3. To what level are firefighters and law enforcement personnel trained in your system?

EMS and the Health Care System

1-5 Describe the role of medical direction/oversight in an EMS system.

The EMS system is just one small component of a much larger health care system designed to manage and care for patients over a period of time. The EMS system cares for patients and delivers them to the most appropriate facility, which is staffed with skilled professionals who continue the care patients need. The U.S. health care system is constantly becoming more specialized, and many large metropolitan areas now have hospitals with personnel specifically trained and equipped to manage such things as major trauma, burns, pediatric emergencies, and spinal-cord injuries.

Medical Direction

One of the 10 essential components of an EMS system and certainly one that is vital to quality patient care is medical direction. Simply stated, **medical direction** is the oversight of all patient care aspects of an EMS system by the physician designated as the medical director (Figure 1-3 ▪).

As an EMT, you will be acting as an "agent" of the medical director while you are caring for patients in the prehospital setting. You will have completed a training program and must follow written guidelines or **protocols** that have been approved by the medical director. Protocols are written guidelines for patient care. In essence, you are providing care under the authority of the physician medical director, and the extent and nature of this authority can vary from state to state and region to region. In most EMS systems, EMTs rarely interact directly with the medical director but simply provide care based on written protocols or **standing orders.** Standing orders are a type of protocol that allows the EMT to provide specific types of treatment or medications for specific patients. For instance, an EMS system may have a standing order that allows EMTs to administer epinephrine for all patients presenting with a severe allergic reaction. The

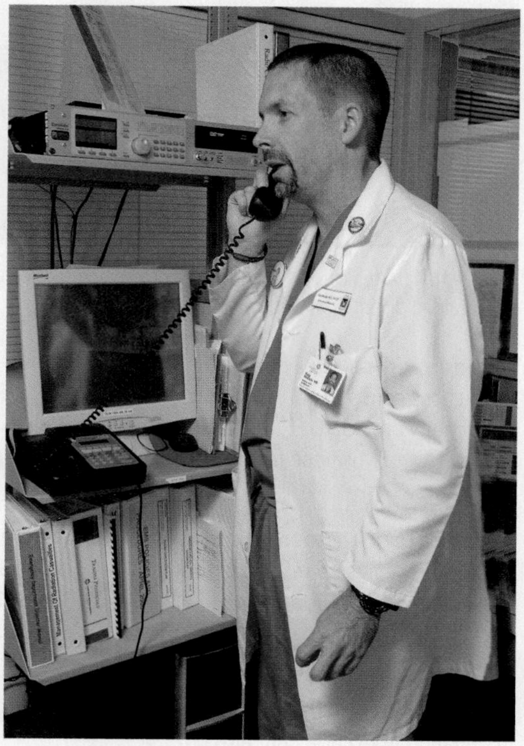

Figure 1-3 Oversight of all aspects of patient care belongs to a designated physician called the *medical director.*

medical direction oversight of the patient-care aspects of an EMS system by a licensed physician referred to as the *medical director*.

protocols written guidelines for patient care approved by the medical director of an EMS system.

standing orders a type of protocol that allows the EMT to provide specific types of treatment or medications for specific patients.

off-line medical direction instructions consisting of the medical director's standing orders, which allow EMTs to give certain medications or perform certain procedures without speaking directly to the medical director or another physician.

written protocols and standing orders guide the EMT and assist in determining how care should be delivered. They are referred to as **off-line medical direction** because there is no real-time direct interaction with the medical director.

When an EMT must interact directly with medical direction regarding patient care, such as by radio or telephone, this is known as **on-line medical direction.** In on-line medical direction, the physician or his designee is providing real-time instructions for care of a patient. Advanced EMTs and paramedics in many EMS systems routinely consult medical direction from the field because they often provide advanced care not covered by the system's protocols and standing orders.

In addition to establishing the minimum standards for patient care within their city, county, region, or state, medical directors are responsible for the continued quality assurance of their EMS systems.

Access to the EMS System

1-6 Differentiate between basic 911 and E-911 EMS access systems.

Accessing emergency services has not always been as easy as dialing 911. In fact it is only within the past 20 years that most 911 systems became operational around the country. In 1999 President Bill Clinton signed into law Senate Bill 800 designating 911 as the official nationwide emergency number (Figure 1-4 ■). To this day, approximately 10% to 15% of the nation is still not covered by 911 services and must access emergency services the old-fashioned way by dialing the appropriate seven-digit number.

Every agency responsible for answering 911 calls is referred to as a **public safety answering point (PSAP).** The PSAPs are typically, but not always, law enforcement dispatch centers and are staffed 24/7 by trained emergency dispatchers. As EMS continues to evolve, the training some dispatchers receive is becoming more and more specialized. A special designation of dispatcher is the **emergency medical dispatcher (EMD)** who is trained to take calls for medical assistance, determine the most appropriate resources, and provide pre-arrival care instructions over the phone until EMS arrives.

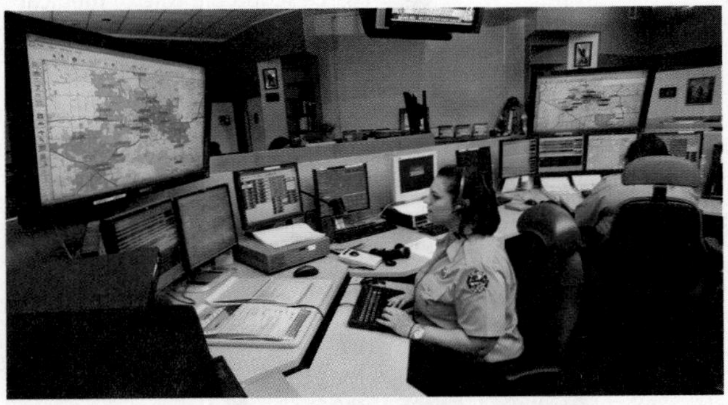

Figure 1-4 A typical 911 emergency communications center staffed with trained dispatchers and call takers.

The technology behind 911 systems continues to improve. Today, there are two main types of 911 systems in place—standard (911) and enhanced (E-911). The standard system is capable of routing all calls to the most appropriate PSAP, where an emergency dispatcher must take the information from the caller. With the enhanced systems, the address and phone number of the caller are automatically displayed on the 911 terminal screen, making it less likely that information will be lost or errors made during the subsequent dispatch.

on-line medical direction instructions consisting of orders from the on-duty physician or designee given directly to an EMT in the field by radio or telephone.

public safety answering point (PSAP) the agency responsible for answering 911 calls.

emergency medical dispatcher (EMD) specially trained dispatchers who not only obtain the appropriate information from callers but also provide medical instructions for emergency care, including instructions for CPR, artificial ventilation, and bleeding control.

PERSPECTIVE

Police Officer

Man, that lady demanded to know why I showed up. She had called for an ambulance and, apparently, only wanted an ambulance. I tried to explain that in a lot of communities, fire crews and law enforcement show up to medical calls. Believe me, these calls can be so odd and unpredictable at times that it's a help to have a lot of people available.

The introduction of the cell phone has created more problems than solutions for many of the busiest 911 systems around the country. In most areas of the country, cell phone calls are funneled through a central dispatch center, which often covers a large geographical area. This makes it difficult for dispatchers to accurately locate the caller and the emergency. In the not too distant future, a new technology will be able to route cell phone calls to the most appropriate PSAP, as with a standard (landline) telephone. Global positioning system (GPS) technology is an important tool used by EMS communication centers and allows 911 dispatchers to pinpoint a caller's exact location.

Roles and Responsibilities of the EMT

As an EMT, you will be required to fulfill many roles. Safety officer, patient care provider, quality assurance officer, patient advocate, and record keeper are just a few of the many hats an EMT is likely to wear. To be as effective as possible, you must have a basic understanding of each role and the responsibilities that go along with it.

1-7 Give examples of how EMTs can carry out each of the following roles and responsibilities: personal and patient safety, patient assessment and emergency care, transport and transfer of care, record keeping and data collection, and patient advocacy.

The EMT as Safety Officer

The importance of safety in EMS cannot be overstated. To be able to do the job safely and effectively, every member of the EMS team must continually have safety in mind. It is not enough to ensure that the scene is safe for you personally. You must constantly be concerned for the safety of everyone else at the scene, including your patients, team members, and bystanders. Emergency scenes are dynamic, and the safety status of an emergency scene can change in an instant.

As an EMS professional, you have no obligation, legal or otherwise, to put yourself at unreasonable risk to assist someone who is ill or injured. Later in this course, you will learn some of the more common risks associated with managing emergency scenes and how best to minimize them.

Simply stated, risk is a hazard or a source of danger. Risk can affect you, the EMT, or it can affect the patients you serve. While not everything you do as an EMT brings with it significant risk, there are specific activities that have significant risk if not properly managed. For instance, lifting and moving patients is a high-risk activity. This poses a risk for both the EMT as well as the patient. If the EMT attempts to lift a patient who is too heavy, he is at great risk for back injury. If the EMT drops the patient during a lift, the patient can be harmed.

Caring for patients brings with it an inherent risk of infection. Many patients have illnesses caused by communicable disease. If you do not take specific precautions to minimize exposure to a patient's blood or body fluids, you could become exposed to a dangerous pathogen. It is your responsibility to recognize the risks and develop habits and practices that minimize negative outcomes for you and your patients.

The EMT as Care Provider

Providing appropriate emergency care promptly and effectively is at the core of an EMT's job. You have a responsibility to provide the best care possible based on a thorough assessment of the patient. You are responsible for safely moving the patient from the scene to the ambulance and then transporting the patient to the most appropriate medical facility. Once at the hospital, you must transfer the care of the patient to the hospital staff by way of a detailed verbal report followed by a written report. You have a responsibility to be clear, concise, and as objective as possible to ensure that the patient continues to receive the best possible care.

The EMT as Record Keeper

Everything you do and see pertaining to the care you provide must be accurately documented. You have a responsibility to document all details of every patient contact in an accurate and timely manner. Those records serve many purposes, including data collection for statistical analysis and quality improvement, and also may serve as evidence in a court of law.

The EMT as Patient Advocate

One of your most important roles as a member of the EMS team is that of patient advocate (Figure 1-5 ■). To truly serve another person means to put their needs before

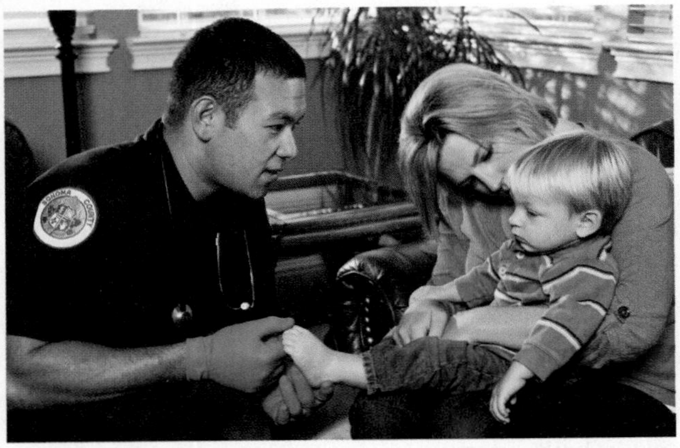

Figure 1-5 Being an advocate for the patient means always showing compassion.

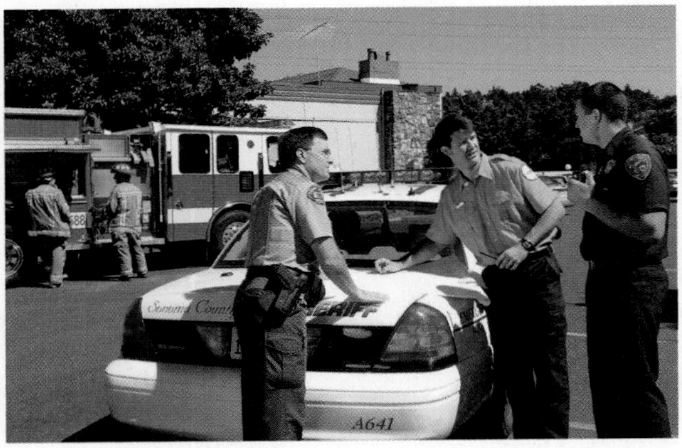

Figure 1-6 As an EMT you will interact with other public service agencies, such as the fire service and law enforcement.

your own, excluding personal safety. This means that you have a responsibility to see that your patients receive the best care possible, even if it interrupts your meals or wakes you during the night. Many patients are not immediately aware of their own needs and therefore must rely on you to make the right decision concerning their well-being. As an EMT you will see patients at their most vulnerable, frightened, and angry moments, when even the most "composed" person may behave irrationally or become incapable of making a rational decision. Often EMTs are called on to assist the patient in making appropriate choices regarding his immediate care and well-being.

The EMT as an EMS Professional

As an EMT, you are a highly visible symbol of the EMS profession and will be interacting with all aspects of your community. It is essential that you present in a professional manner at all times. You have a responsibility to your agency as well as to the profession to appear neat and well groomed at all times and maintain a caring and respectful attitude.

You will be interacting on a regular basis with the other professions related to public safety, law enforcement, and the fire service. It is important to remember that you are just one part of a larger public safety team and that you must consider yourself an ambassador for EMS when interacting with other agencies (Figure 1-6 ▪).

Another responsibility of being an EMS professional means staying abreast of the most current laws and issues affecting your job as an EMT. You have a responsibility to maintain both your knowledge and skills and attend all required training to maintain your certification or license to practice.

1-8 Describe the expectations of EMTs in terms of each of the following professional attributes: appearance, knowledge and skills, physical demands, personal traits, and maintaining certification and licensure.

1-9 Describe the purpose of quality improvement/continuous quality improvement programs in EMS.

1-10 Explain the EMT's roles and responsibilities in quality improvement.

quality improvement (QI) a process of continuous self-review with the purpose of identifying and correcting aspects of the system that require improvement.

The EMT as Quality Improvement Officer

Quality improvement (QI) is a complex system of internal and external reviews of all aspects of an EMS system. It is designed first to identify aspects that need improvement and then to implement the needed improvements, all in an effort to ensure the public receives the highest quality prehospital care.

Each and every member of the EMS team plays an important role in the quality improvement process. You will ensure the continued quality improvement of the system in which you work by fulfilling your responsibility as an EMT, which is to maintain accurate documentation, attend formal reviews of recent calls, participate in the gathering of feedback from patients and other health care professionals, maintain your equipment in top operating condition, attend required continuing education sessions, and keep up on less-frequently used skills.

Knowing Your EMS System

As a member of the EMS team, you have a responsibility to learn and understand the unique qualities of the system in which you work. Your instructor can address specific aspects of your system, but you must not rely entirely on what you learn during your formal training. You must take responsibility for learning the laws, guidelines, and protocols that govern the functions of EMTs in your system. You also must take responsibility for learning all of the available resources within your system, such as specialty rescue teams, hazmat teams, air ambulances, and specialty hospitals.

STOP, REVIEW, REMEMBER!

Multiple Choice

For each question, place a check next to the correct answer.

1. Which one of the following is *not* a typical emergency specialty hospital?
   _____ a. Trauma
   _____ b. Neurosurgery
   _____ c. Pediatric
   _____ d. Geriatric

2. An EMS medical director must be a:
   _____ a. physician.
   _____ b. trauma surgeon.
   _____ c. former paramedic.
   _____ d. registered nurse.

3. The best example of off-line medical direction is orders given via:
   _____ a. radio.
   _____ b. telephone.
   _____ c. fax.
   _____ d. written protocols.

4. The 911 dispatchers who are trained to provide pre-arrival instructions are referred to as _____________ dispatchers.
   _____ a. pre-arrival
   _____ b. emergency medical
   _____ c. advice
   _____ d. advance directive

5. Maintaining accurate documentation, attending formal reviews of recent calls, attending required continuing education sessions, and keeping up on less-frequently used skills fall under which one of the following EMT responsibilities?
   _____ a. Safety
   _____ b. Care provider
   _____ c. Quality improvement
   _____ d. Patient advocate

Matching

Match the definition on the left with the applicable term on the right.

1. _____ The oversight of all patient care aspects of an EMS system by a specifically designated physician
2. _____ Written guidelines or treatment plans for patient care
3. _____ Preauthorized orders that allow the EMT to provide specific types of treatment or medications for specific patients
4. _____ Medical direction involving no real time direct interaction with the medical director
5. _____ Agencies responsible for answering 911 calls
6. _____ Specially trained dispatchers who determine the most appropriate resources and provide pre-arrival care instructions over the phone until EMS arrives

A. Standing orders
B. Medical direction
C. Protocols
D. Emergency medical dispatchers
E. Public safety answering point (PSAP)
F. Off-line medical direction

(continued on next page)

(continued)

Critical Thinking

1. What hospitals in your city, region, or state have specific treatment specialties such as trauma, burns, or pediatrics?

2. Which EMT responsibilities do you feel might be the most difficult for you to learn, and why?

3. EMTs must meet specific requirements to maintain and renew their EMT license or certification. What are those requirements in your state or region?

The Role of the Public Health System

1-11 Describe the relationship between EMS and public health.

1-12 Explain the role of public health systems and their relationship to EMS, disease surveillance, and injury prevention.

Each county, region, and state has people and resources that serve as part of the public health system. The public health system dedicates those resources to promoting optimal health and quality of life for the people it serves. By doing so, it helps ensure quality of life by monitoring the health of the population, providing health care, and educating the populace about disease and injury prevention (Figure 1-7 ■). It also serves to advance population-based health programs and policies.

The following are just some of the areas that a public health agency can help monitor and promote for the health of citizens within its community:

- Health education
- Injury prevention and surveillance
- Disease surveillance
- Vaccinations
- Health screening

As a member of the EMS system you may have the opportunity to participate in one or more of those important initiatives.

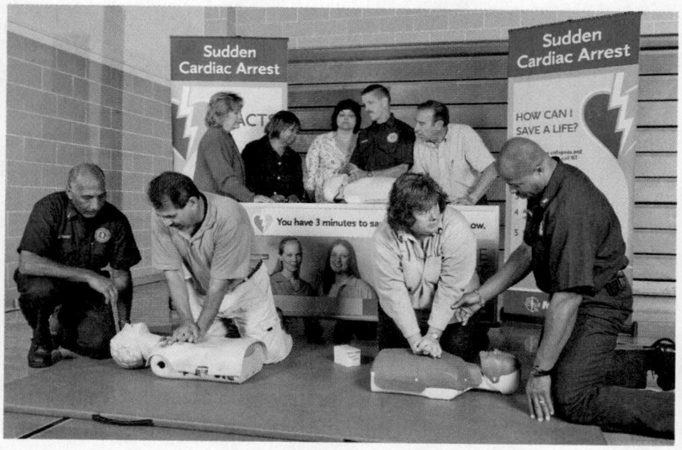

Figure 1-7 One of the roles of an EMS provider is to assist in educating the public.

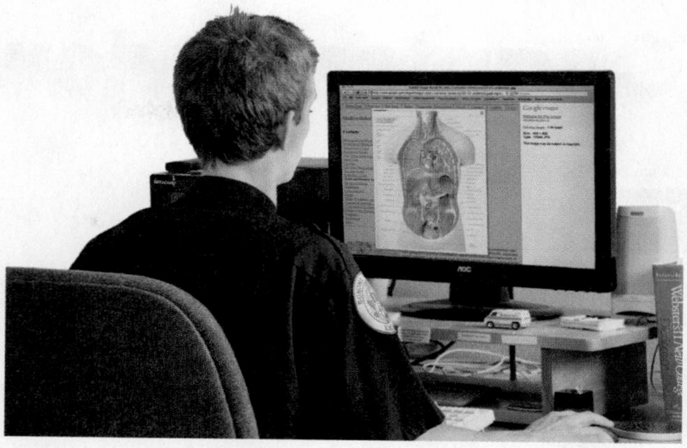

Figure 1-8 Staying current with the latest research is an important aspect of good patient care.

Disaster Assistance

1-13 Explain the role that disaster medical assistance teams (DMAT) play and how they integrate with EMS systems.

Each state has identified specific individuals already working in its EMS systems to participate in specialized teams designed to provide medical care following a disaster. Those teams are called disaster medical assistance teams, or simply DMAT teams for short. State DMAT teams receive significant support, funding, and oversight from the federal government. The individuals who make up the teams are highly experienced EMS personnel who receive specialized training and can be deployed on a moment's notice should a disaster strike anywhere in the United States. Immediately following hurricane Katrina, for example, DMAT teams from across the nation descended on New Orleans. After DMAT teams arrive in an area following a disaster, they are quickly integrated into local EMS resources.

The Role of Research in EMS

1-14 Explain the role that research plays in EMS and the ways that an EMT might identify and support research.

Research is systematic investigation to establish facts. Each year more and more new research is being conducted and old traditions in EMS that were never based in research are being challenged. In late 2010 the American Heart Association released its new guidelines for resuscitation and emergency care. Those new guidelines—and many other changes in emergency care—are now based on the concept of "evidenced-based medicine." That means the new standards and recommendations are based on thorough research and documented evidence. In addition, several organizations around the globe have spent the past five years gathering and verifying data that is defining how EMS will practice emergency care for the next several years. The military also has been conducting research that is influencing how EMS provides care for those who are ill or injured in the civilian world. It is our hope that you will play an active role in searching for, reading, and evaluating research that affects your job as an EMT (Figure 1-8 ■).

EMERGENCY DISPATCH SUMMARY

The EMTs on scene controlled Bill's bleeding and bandaged his head before transporting him to the Glenfield Medical Center in Iverton. After eight stitches and a series of tests, he was released home in good spirits. Over the next several days, the Hansons' neighbors knocked on their door in ones and twos, asking if there was any way to be of help.

Chapter Review

To the Point

- The shape of the modern EMS system has been influenced by many events throughout history with the primary goal of minimizing death and disability for victims of sudden illness and injury.
- EMS systems must address 10 specific areas as defined by the U.S. National Highway Traffic Safety Administration (NHTSA).
- The 911 number is the single point access number for EMS in the United States.
- There are four standardized levels of care identified by the National Scope of Practice model: emergency medical responder (EMR), EMT, advanced EMT, and paramedic.
- Each member of the EMS system must hold safety as the highest priority when performing the duties of an EMS professional. Other responsibilities include proper patient care, patient advocacy, transportation, and record keeping.
- As an EMT you are expected to maintain a professional appearance at all times as well as keep your knowledge and physical condition at your best.
- Members of the EMS system must function under the direction of a licensed physician known as a *medical director*.
- EMS systems are required to monitor effectiveness and develop quality assurance and quality improvement systems.
- You, as an EMT, will play an important role in quality assurance and quality improvement.
- EMS systems work closely with local and state public health systems and initiatives, such as disease surveillance and injury prevention, to help maintain the general health of the community.
- Some EMS providers may serve on disaster medical assistance teams (DMAT) and be deployed to assist in other regions or states when disasters strike.
- Research plays an important role in improving patient care and shaping the care that all EMS personnel provide.

Chapter Questions

Multiple Choice

For each question, place a check next to the correct answer.

1. Which one of the following is *not* typically a component of an EMS system?

_____ a. Ground ambulances
_____ b. Dispatchers
_____ c. Air ambulances
_____ d. Doctors' offices

2. Which one of the following definitions best describes an EMS system?

_____ a. Specialized chain of resources designed to minimize the impact of sudden injury and illness
_____ b. Communication systems that connect dispatchers with field personnel
_____ c. Chain of resources contained within a major hospital
_____ d. Ambulance and emergency department personnel

3. Which of the following levels of EMS personnel are able to start an IV on an ill or injured patient?

_____ a. EMT
_____ b. EMT and paramedic
_____ c. Advanced EMT and paramedic
_____ d. Advanced EMT and EMT

4. Which one of the following is the EMT's primary role at the scene of any emergency?

_____ a. Patient care
_____ b. Safety
_____ c. Transportation
_____ d. Extrication

5. Which one of the following best defines the term *quality improvement* as it pertains to the EMT?
_____ a. Lifelong learning
_____ b. Participation in continuing education
_____ c. Complex system of internal and external reviews
_____ d. Process of asking patients for feedback

6. The 10 standards for EMS systems as defined by NHTSA address all of the following *except*:
_____ a. transportation and resource management.
_____ b. regulation and policy.
_____ c. communications.
_____ d. organ donor programs.

7. One whose training emphasizes care of immediate life threats and assisting other EMS providers is a(n):
_____ a. emergency medical responder (EMR).
_____ b. EMT.
_____ c. advanced EMT.
_____ d. paramedic.

8. Which one of the following is *not* a responsibility of an EMT?
_____ a. Participating in quality improvement programs
_____ b. Designing patient care protocols
_____ c. Ensuring the safety of the crew, bystanders, and patient
_____ d. Consulting with medical direction

9. The EMT acts as an agent of the _______________ when providing care in the prehospital setting.
_____ a. paramedic partner
_____ b. EMS director
_____ c. medical director
_____ d. base station hospital

10. The written guidelines for patient care are called:
_____ a. advanced directives.
_____ b. standing orders.
_____ c. on-line direction.
_____ d. protocols.

Matching

Match the definition on the left with the applicable term on the right.

1. _____ Specially trained personnel who answer calls for help and provide pre-arrival instructions to callers
2. _____ A type of protocol that allows the EMT to provide specific types of treatment or medications for specific patients
3. _____ The complex system of internal and external reviews of all aspects of the EMS system to identify areas of weakness and recommend ways to improve
4. _____ The highest level of EMS training
5. _____ Written guidelines or treatment plans for patient care

A. Paramedic
B. Emergency medical dispatcher
C. Standing orders
D. Protocols
E. Quality improvement

Critical Thinking

1. Describe how staying up on the latest research in resuscitation techniques might affect the way you as an EMT provide care to a victim of sudden cardiac arrest.

____

____

____

____

(continued on next page)

(continued)

2. As an EMT, how might you begin to play a part in the education of the public about what EMS is and how it functions?

3. In what ways does the job of the EMT differ from that of the emergency medical responder (EMR)? How does it differ from that of the advanced EMT and paramedic?

4. List at least four types of specialty hospitals that might be available to receive patients on an emergency basis.

5. Medical direction can exist in a variety of forms. List as many examples of medical direction as you can think of.

6. What is the difference between a traditional dispatcher and one designated as an emergency medical dispatcher (EMD)?

Case Studies

Case Study 1

You are an EMT with a small ambulance company and are working standby at a fair when an obese woman in her 60s approaches you and asks that you help her with some blisters that have formed on her feet. You have her sit down at the first aid station and take a look. You see several good-size blisters on the sides and bottom of both feet. She asks that you please just pop them so that she can go about her way.

1. Because draining blisters is not within the scope of practice for an EMT, how will you respond to this woman's request?

2. If you were not sure how to care appropriately for this woman, who would you consult?

3. Why would it be important to carefully document any care that you might provide to this patient?

Case Study 2

It's 2100 hours. You are in the ambulance on your way back to the station following mutual aid training at a nearby fire department when you happen upon a two-car collision with injuries. The collision has occurred at a blind curve on a well-traveled two-lane highway. You and your partner are the first ones on scene.

1. What will be your primary concern at this scene?

(continued on next page)

(continued)

2. What are the immediate hazards at this scene, and how will you mitigate them?

____

____

____

____

3. Is it ethical to deal with any issue before caring for the injured? Why or why not?

____

____

____

____

The Last Word

EMS systems have been developing and improving for many years and will continue to do so for many more. Find a way that you can make a difference in each of the 10 core areas of your EMS system. Once you have been an EMT for a while, challenge yourself to learn more and understand more about the next levels of providers, the advanced EMTs and paramedics.

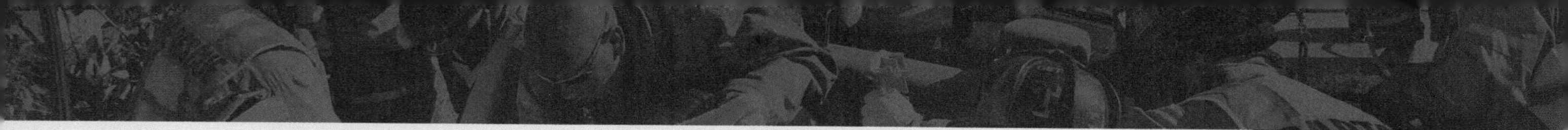

Workforce Safety and Wellness

2

Education Standards

Preparatory: Workforce Safety and Wellness
Medicine: Infectious Diseases

Competencies

Applies fundamental knowledge of the safety/well-being of the EMT to the provision of emergency care.

Objectives

After completion of this lesson, you should be able to:

2-1 Define key terms introduced in this chapter.

2-2 List examples of common stressors the EMT may encounter.

2-3 Describe responses your friends and family may have to your work in EMS.

2-4 Describe common signs and symptoms of stress reactions.

2-5 Compare and contrast the characteristics of acute, delayed, and cumulative stress reactions.

2-6 Describe lifestyle changes you can make to help you deal with stress.

2-7 Discuss the components of a comprehensive system of critical incident stress management.

2-8 Given a description of a patient or family member's behavior, identify the stage of grief it most likely represents.

2-9 Explain the principles for interacting with patients and family members in situations involving death and dying.

2-10 Describe measures you can take to protect yourself from exposure to diseases caused by pathogens.

2-11 Describe the personal protective equipment that may be used by EMS personnel.

2-12 Explain the role of immunizations and tuberculosis testing in maintaining good health.

2-13 Discuss the risks and preventive measures for specific infectious diseases of concern to EMTs, including hepatitis B and C, tuberculosis (TB), human immunodeficiency virus (HIV), and multi-drug-resistant organisms (MDRO).

2-14 Explain the risks and measures that can be taken to protect yourself against the following hazards: hazardous materials, hazardous rescue situations, traffic-related injuries, and violence and crime.

Key Terms

acute stress response p. 26
body substance isolation (BSI) precautions p. 34
critical incident stress debriefing (CISD) p. 30
critical incident stress management (CISM) p. 30
cumulative stress response p. 26
defusing p. 30
delayed stress response p. 26
pathogens p. 34
personal protective equipment (PPE) p. 34
standard precautions p. 34
stress p. 24

Introduction

Responding to an emergency can be both risky and stressful, regardless of your level of training or experience. Many laypeople are reluctant to receive even the most basic training in first aid and CPR because they fear they will not be able to respond appropriately during a medical emergency. They are afraid of making a mistake or making the wrong decision. For EMTs emergencies often are a daily routine. The stress associated with them can be overwhelming. In addition, EMTs face many hazards when responding to emergency scenes, not the least of which is exposure to infectious disease. Without a thorough understanding of the risks and stressors and the mechanisms for minimizing their effects, you can quickly become overwhelmed or injured.

This chapter covers some of the more common stressors as well as many of the hazards encountered in the prehospital setting. It also describes several methods for coping with job stress and ways for staying safe and minimizing exposure to risk while caring for victims of illness and injury.

EMERGENCY DISPATCH

"Unit ninety-nine, headquarters." The dispatcher's voice exploded from the speakers, startling the two EMTs after almost five hours of absolute silence.

"Oh, my gosh, that scared me," Arnell grinned as he picked up the microphone. "Go ahead to ninety-nine."

"Ninety-nine, respond priority one to 2001 Wildwood Lane for an adult male vomiting blood."

"Ten-four, show us en route to 2001 Wildwood." Arnell took a deep breath and slid the ambulance into gear. Several minutes later, Arnell and his partner, Jeff, were met at the front door by a sobbing woman who identified herself as Natasha.

"Come quick," she said, grabbing at Arnell's uniform shirt. "My uncle's back here. He's been sick for a few months, but now he . . . he started throwing up blood. I think he's dying!"

In the back room they found an approximately 50-year-old man named Raymond lying on a hospital bed. The sheets and pillow were soiled red and a small bowl on the nightstand contained fresh blood.

While Arnell began preparing the man for transport, Jeff quickly gathered medical information from Natasha including that her uncle suffers from end-stage liver disease due to hepatitis B (HBV) and has been on the liver transplant list for almost a year. In addition, he has a do not resuscitate (DNR) order.

"Can't you just give me somethin' for the pain?" Raymond said through clenched blood-stained teeth. "Please, you gotta help."

Emotional Aspects of Emergency Care

Emotions are a fact of life. Everyone experiences them many times each and every day. Like most things in life, there are both positive and negative emotions, healthy emotions and not-so-healthy emotions. Think for a moment of a recent time when you were very happy and excited. Perhaps it was a birthday party or the birth of a child. The emotions you felt were likely strong feelings of happiness and joy. Now think back to your most recent bad customer-service experience. Perhaps it was at a restaurant when nothing seemed to go right and the server did not seem to care, or maybe it was when you tried to get something fixed that should have been covered under warranty and the salesperson could do nothing to help you. Both situations are burned into memory by the emotions they aroused.

stress any event or situation that places extraordinary demands on a person's mental or emotional resources.

Stress can be defined as any event or an accumulation of events that places extraordinary demands on a person's mental or emotional resources. It is no secret; the job of the EMS professional is stressful. Being an EMT can be an emotional roller coaster, as you attempt to manage your own feelings as well as those of patients and their loved ones. Over time, the job can take its toll on mental and emotional resources, leaving the EMT unable to cope with the job or with the normal activities of life. Recognizing the aspects of the job that cause stress and learning to manage that stress is an essential skill that every EMS professional must learn early on.

PERSPECTIVE

Natasha—The Niece

No one ever warned us that this kind of thing could happen! We were just watching TV and all of a sudden Uncle Raymond started throwing up blood. Could his liver problem cause this? Is he dying? I don't know and I just want someone to help him.

Common Causes of Stress in EMS

It may seem ironic, but many of the factors that attract people to EMS are the very factors likely to cause job stress. Such things as responding to emergencies, keeping long hours, and working independently all can be stressors. The following is a partial list of some of the situations an EMT responds to that are both stressful and emotional:

2-2 List examples of common stressors the EMT may encounter.

- First encounter with the death of another human being
- Multiple-casualty incidents (multiple patients)
- Emergencies involving infants and children
- Incidents involving major trauma, such as an amputation
- Incidents involving abuse and/or neglect
- Death or injury of a coworker or colleague

It is possible for an EMT to become overwhelmed by stress following a single event, such as a plane crash, vehicle collision with multiple casualties, or a terrorist attack (Figure 2-1 ■). More commonly, stress is cumulative and builds gradually over time. If the buildup of stress is not managed properly along the way, it can result in an emotional breakdown.

Effects on Family and Loved Ones

More than many typical jobs, the job of an EMS professional can cause unexpected stress at home. One reason is this: Responding to emergencies and caring for others in their time of need is very satisfying. Most EMS personnel cannot get enough, especially when new to the job, and tend to spend as much time as possible at the station, even working extra hours. Friends and family do not always understand such

2-3 Describe responses your friends and family may have to your work in EMS.

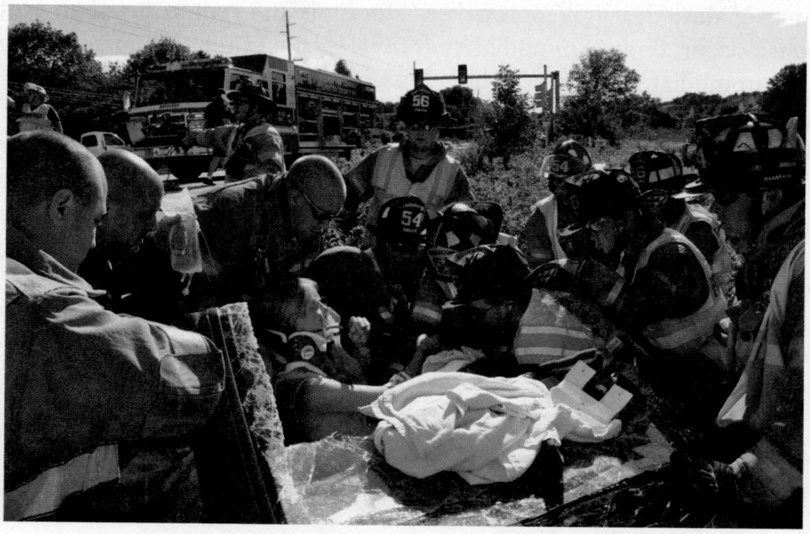

Figure 2-1 A range of stressful reactions can result from working at emergency scenes such as a multiple-vehicle collision. (© Edward T. Dickinson, MD)

passion and may experience anger and frustration when their loved one is always at work or volunteering his or her time.

In addition, shift work causes many EMTs to be away from home for 24 and 48 hours at a time, leaving others to pick up the slack around the house. Being on call also causes tension when family members may be left alone on a moment's notice while the EMT responds to an emergency. While this may seem fun and exciting for friends and family in the beginning, the novelty can soon wear off and cause feelings of anger, resentment, abandonment, and jealousy.

Signs and Symptoms of Stress

2-4 Describe common signs and symptoms of stress reactions.

Although everyone responds to stress a little differently, most people will display at least a few signs that stress is present in their lives. The following is a list of some of the more common warning signs of stress:

- Increased irritability
- Inability to concentrate
- Increased levels of anxiety
- Difficulty sleeping
- Nightmares
- Increased indecisiveness
- Decreased appetite
- Feelings of guilt
- Decreased sex drive
- Wanting to be alone more
- Lack of interest in work
- Increased negative attitude

It is important to remember that not all stress is caused by a person's job. People carry the effects of stress from one aspect of their lives to another. They will bring the effects of stress from school, home, relationships, and other jobs with them to their job as an EMT.

Three Common Reactions to Stress

2-5 Compare and contrast the characteristics of acute, delayed, and cumulative stress reactions.

When we encounter stress, we respond by changing our behavior in predictable ways. In other words, stress causes a normal response to an abnormal event. Response to stress can be divided into three categories—acute, delayed, and cumulative:

- ***Acute stress response.*** Acute stress reactions are most commonly linked to sudden, unexpected catastrophic events such as large earthquakes, plane crashes, or the line-of-duty death of a coworker. The signs and symptoms of an **acute stress response** occur almost immediately following the event and, in some cases, may require immediate intervention.
- ***Delayed stress response.*** The triggers for a delayed stress reaction are similar to those for an acute stress reaction; however, the signs and symptoms may not appear until days, months, or even years later. Because of the delay in the onset of symptoms, victims often are confused about why they are feeling the way they do. This confusion often leads to a delay in treatment and can result in years of drug and alcohol abuse. A **delayed stress response** can be diagnosed as a condition called *posttraumatic stress disorder* and often requires professional treatment.
- ***Cumulative stress response.*** Unlike the other categories of stress response, a **cumulative stress response** is not caused by a single event. Instead it results from the accumulation of recurring low-level stressors over many years. Commonly called *burnout*, cumulative stress is usually the result of stress from more than one aspect of a person's life.

acute stress response stress reactions that are most commonly linked to sudden, unexpected catastrophic events.

delayed stress response stress reactions that may not appear for days, months, or even years following an event.

cumulative stress response a type of stress reaction that results from the accumulation of recurring low-level stressors over many years.

STOP, REVIEW, REMEMBER!

Multiple Choice

For each question, place a check next to the correct answer.

1. Which one of the following is the best definition of stress?

_____ a. Any response for which you are not prepared

_____ b. Any event or situation that places extraordinary demands on a person's mental or emotional resources

_____ c. The uncontrolled increase in vital signs as a result of seeing something traumatic

_____ d. Any event that causes high emotions

2. The stress of being an EMT can extend to family and friends. Those people may exhibit stress in all of the following ways *except*:

_____ a. jealousy.

_____ b. resentment.

_____ c. anger.

_____ d. elation.

3. Which one of the following most accurately depicts the common signs and symptoms of stress in an EMT?

_____ a. Irritability, insomnia, loss of appetite

_____ b. Irritability, sleepiness, hunger

_____ c. Inability to concentrate, hunger, desire to exercise

_____ d. Inability to concentrate, insomnia, desire to be with others

4. The term *burnout* is associated with which type of stress reaction?

_____ a. Acute

_____ b. Delayed

_____ c. Cumulative

_____ d. Severe

5. Which type of stress response is commonly linked to sudden, unexpected catastrophic events?

_____ a. Acute

_____ b. Delayed

_____ c. Cumulative

_____ d. Sudden

Matching

Match the description on the left with the applicable type of response on the right.

1. _____ Any event or situation that places extraordinary demands on a person's mental or emotional resources
2. _____ This is commonly linked to sudden, unexpected catastrophic events
3. _____ Stress reactions that may not appear for days, months, or even years after the stressful event
4. _____ This results from the accumulation of recurring low-level stressors over many years

A. Delayed stress response

B. Stressor

C. Cumulative stress response

D. Acute stress response

(continued on next page)

(continued)

Critical Thinking

1. Describe the most stressful moment in your entire life. What emotions can you remember feeling at the time? How did you deal with the stress at the time?

____

____

____

____

2. List some of the stressors that you face in your life. How do you deal with those stressors when they appear?

____

____

____

____

3. What is your biggest fear about becoming an EMT? What can you do in advance to help overcome or deal with that fear should it become a reality?

____

____

____

____

Learning to Manage the Effects of Stress

2-6 Describe lifestyle changes you can make to help you deal with stress.

The proper management of stress, regardless of the cause, must be a proactive process and not a reactive one. You must make lifestyle changes to minimize the effects of stress before the signs and symptoms appear. As you will see, the changes are not specific to the EMS profession and could be considered universal for a happy, healthy life regardless of your chosen profession.

Improving Diet

A healthy diet is essential to a healthy mind and body (Figure 2-2 ■). As the old saying goes, "You are what you eat," and many of us would not want to admit what we eat sometimes. Change is difficult for most people. However, if change is made in small steps, it is far less painful. Some of the important first steps for improving one's diet are to reduce sugar, caffeine, and alcohol consumption. Just to get started, eliminate one or two sodas, coffee drinks, or alcohol from your daily routine.

Minimizing foods high in saturated fats (most fast food) is another step toward a healthy diet. It may be difficult for the busiest person to eliminate fatty foods

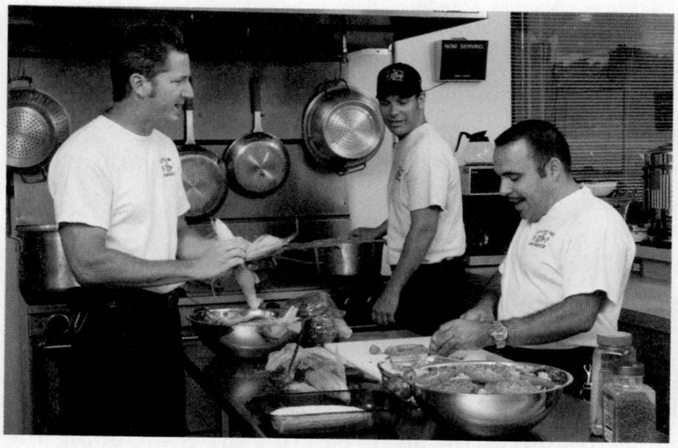

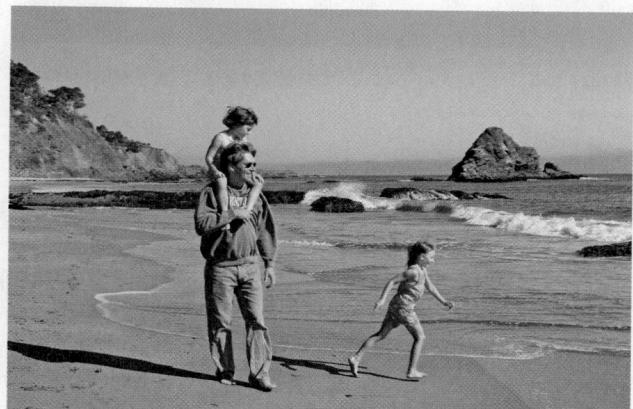

Figure 2-2 A healthy diet helps one cope with the stress of being an EMT.

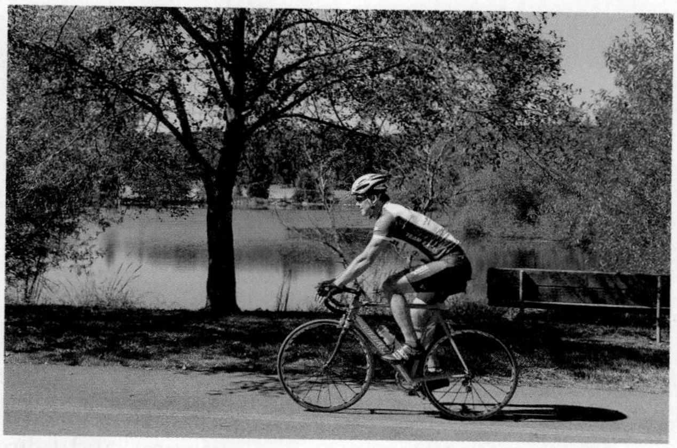

Figure 2-3 A daily exercise program is an important part of a well-balanced life.

altogether, but choosing a salad instead of a burger or not ordering fries with each meal are easy first steps.

Staying well hydrated is another area where many fall short. Keeping a good supply of fresh water handy while on duty and drinking small amounts throughout the shift will help to ensure that you keep plenty of water in your system.

Developing a Daily Exercise Routine

A good diet is only part of a well-balanced life. Exercise is just as important and, to maximize its benefits, must become part of a daily routine. Like most things that take up time in a day, exercise must be scheduled into your daily routine. About 20 to 30 minutes of moderate exercise is all that is needed, but exercise can be more extreme, depending on your level of fitness. Taking time to walk, jog, or bicycle a mile or two a few times a week will do wonders for your ability to work long shifts, miss meals, and still maintain a positive attitude (Figure 2-3 ▪).

Another aspect of an effective exercise routine is allowing personal time for relaxation or meditation. Scheduling personal time to relax and do nothing is as important to a well-balanced life as diet and exercise (Figure 2-4 ▪).

Balance Is the Key

If something in our lives becomes a focal point and we become obsessed, it can create stress and imbalance. Our lives are made up of many aspects that, when balanced, work together to create an enjoyable and joy-filled life. You must bring this new profession into your life and the lives of your friends and family in a balanced manner.

Learning to become an EMT may take you away from some of the other aspects of your life while you are in school, and that is okay. Just do not allow your schooling to become the only priority in your life. Balance school with your job, spiritual life, family, personal time, and exercise. When you are out of school and working as an EMT, do your best to adjust your scale of activities as often as necessary to maintain a healthy balance.

Once you are working in EMS, there are several small things you can do to help maintain that balance. Not working as much overtime, requesting shifts that allow for more time with family, and requesting an assignment in a less busy area are just a few examples. If all of those things fail to provide the balance

Figure 2-4 Allow time for relaxation.

that you are trying to achieve and you find yourself displaying some of the signs and symptoms of stress, it may be time to seek outside assistance. Many employers offer assistance in the form of informal peer counselors as well as more formal professional counseling. It is not a sign of weakness but of wisdom when one seeks outside assistance for coping with stress. Like so many of the things an EMT learns, stress management is just another skill that takes practice in order to do it well.

2-7 Discuss the components of a comprehensive system of critical incident stress management.

critical incident stress management (CISM) a comprehensive, integrated, multicomponent crisis intervention system composed of seven core components: precrisis preparation, support programs, defusing, debriefing, one-on-one intervention, family crisis intervention, and follow-up.

defusing small-group discussion held within hours of a critical incident, designed to address acute symptoms of stress.

critical incident stress debriefing (CISD) a process held 1–10 days after a critical (highly stressful) incident in which teams of professional and peer counselors provide emotional and psychological support to EMS personnel.

Critical Incident Stress Management

According to the International Critical Incident Stress Foundation, **critical incident stress management (CISM)** is a comprehensive, integrated, multicomponent crisis intervention system composed of seven core components: precrisis preparation, support programs, defusing, debriefing, one-on-one intervention, family crisis intervention, and follow-up. It includes resources for all phases of a crisis including the precrisis, crisis, and postcrisis phases. While many EMS systems and large agencies have a CISM system in place, most use only select components.

A **defusing** is a small-group discussion held within hours of a critical incident. It is designed to address acute symptoms of stress.

The term **critical incident stress debriefing (CISD)** is used frequently in EMS to describe any form of crisis intervention. It is important to point out that the terms *CISM* and *CISD* are not interchangeable. CISD is only one component of a multicomponent CISM system designed to help people cope with their feelings before, during, and following a critical incident. If CISD is the only component used, some experts feel that the likelihood of a successful outcome for those involved is minimized.

In a CISD, a skilled facilitator will establish important ground rules, including emphasizing that all discussions remain confidential and should not be shared with others not in attendance. It also is explained that the debriefing is *not* an investigation or an interrogation. Facilitators are there to encourage an open discussion of the event and allow those involved to share their feelings, fears, and reactions in a nonthreatening environment. The ultimate objective for the facilitators is to evaluate the information and responses shared during the CISD and offer suggestions for coping with and eventually overcoming the stress caused by the event. One-on-one counseling also may be helpful in restoring emotional health (Figure 2-5 ■).

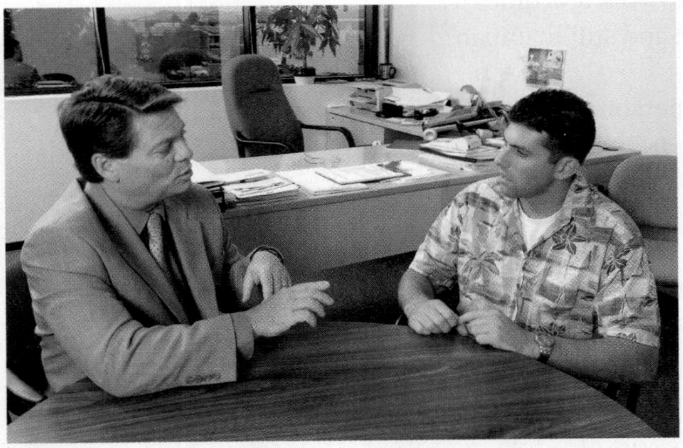

Figure 2-5 One-on-one counseling allows the EMT to discuss feelings in a safe environment.

As an EMT you must become familiar with the CISM system that may be in place in your EMS system and know how to access it. Your instructor can assist you in this process. You also are encouraged to participate in ongoing training and planning as well as to get involved in peer support groups before a crisis occurs. The better prepared you are in advance, the easier it will be to assist others or to overcome the effects of stress yourself.

PERSPECTIVE

Uncle Raymond—The Patient

The pain is killing me! Why can't they give me something for it? I'll tell you what's worse, though: puking blood. Nothing like this has ever happened to me before. Can my liver make me do this? I'm waiting for a new one, you know, but if I'm throwing up blood and feeling pain like this, I doubt if I'll ever live long enough to get one. The pain is so terrible.

Note that recent research is suggesting group debriefings such as those conducted during a traditional CISD may not be as helpful as once thought. Data suggest that personal, symptom-driven support is more successful. A new strategy called the *resiliency model* of stress management is emerging. It is based on prevention and focuses on the development of preexisting personal stress management strategies (strategies that promote resiliency).

Reactions to Death and Dying

You have probably heard it said: "The only sure things in life are death and taxes." As an EMT you are sure to see more than your fair share of the former. You may never get used to it, but you must learn to cope with it, and that takes knowledge and skills developed over time.

2-8 Given a description of a patient or family member's behavior, identify the stage of grief it most likely represents.

Research has revealed that human beings go through predictable emotional stages as they attempt to cope with death, whether it is one's own impending death or the death of a loved one. Dr. Elizabeth Kübler-Ross identified five stages of grief experienced by terminal patients (Table 2-1). Although the five stages of grief provide a helpful framework to understand the cycle of grief, it must be kept in mind that they are not necessarily an orderly step-by-step process. Furthermore, a person may experience more than one stage of grief at the same time, and not everyone goes through all the stages.

There is just no telling when you may encounter death as an EMT. It could be the sudden death of a child struck by a car or the loss of a grandmother after a long and fruitful life. Whatever the circumstances, you must be prepared to offer both the patient and the patient's loved ones a dignified and compassionate response. The following key points will help:

2-9 Explain the principles for interacting with patients and family members in situations involving death and dying.

- ***Assess the situation.*** Identify those most in need of support, given the specific circumstances. In most cases, providing patients with the utmost respect and preserving their dignity will help their loved ones as well. Acknowledge the patient directly and avoid talking about the patient to others in his presence.
- ***Be tolerant.*** You may encounter patients or their loved ones in various stages of coping. Do not take anger that appears to be directed at you personally and, most important, do not become defensive.

TABLE 2-1	KÜBLER-ROSS FIVE STAGES OF GRIEF
1. Denial	This is sometimes called the "not me" stage and is a defense mechanism against the thought of dying.
2. Anger	Patients may become outwardly angry at those around them. An attitude of "why me?" is common during this stage.
3. Bargaining	This is the beginning of acceptance. Patients may attempt to bargain with themselves, God, or others. An attitude of "Okay, but let me first . . ." is common during this stage of coping.
4. Depression	Patients slip into deep mourning depression, often unwilling to communicate with others.
5. Acceptance	Patients appear to have come to accept their fate. In some situations the patient reaches this stage before loved ones, who may need more support at this time.

(Based on the Grief Cycle model first published in On Death & Dying by Elisabeth Kübler-Ross, 1969. Interpretation by Christopher J. Le Baudour.)

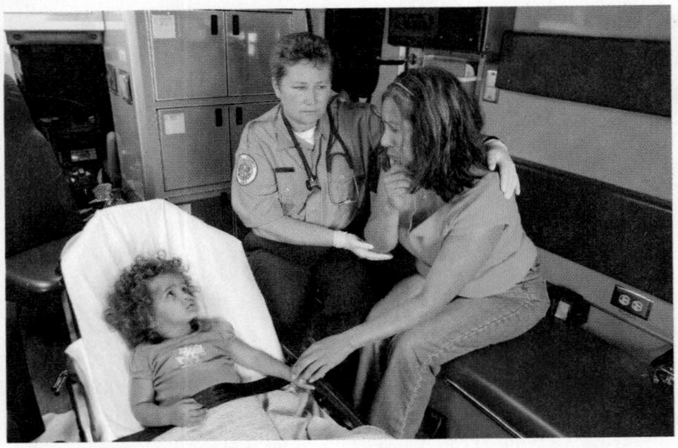

Figure 2-6 Family members should be treated with compassion.

- ***Listen with compassion.*** Listen carefully and empathetically, and be mindful of your body language. Look people in the eyes when speaking to them. You may not be able to fix the situation, but you can offer emotional support. Speak in a confident and compassionate tone (Figure 2-6 ■).
- ***Offer honesty and comfort.*** Let the family know that everything that can be done will be done. If appropriate, a reassuring touch may be helpful in gaining their confidence. Provide as much comfort and support as you can for both patient and his loved ones. Offer to contact additional resources such as hospice support or the clergy if it is appropriate. Most of all, show that you care.

STOP, REVIEW, REMEMBER!

Multiple Choice

For each question, place a check next to the correct answer.

1. Which one of the following is the best definition of CISM?

_____ a. Group of peer counselors who are on call to assist following a critical incident

_____ b. Comprehensive crisis intervention system that includes resources for all phases of a crisis

_____ c. Structured small group discussion that is provided within hours following a critical incident

_____ d. Structured group discussion typically provided 1 to 10 days postcrisis

2. It is recommended that a CISD be conducted between _____________ following a critical incident.

_____ a. 1 and 10 hours

_____ b. 2 and 4 days

_____ c. 1 and 10 days

_____ d. 7 and 14 days

3. According to Kübler-Ross's five stages of grief, which stage is expressed by withdrawal from others, a desire to be alone, and difficulty with communication?

_____ a. Denial

_____ b. Anger

_____ c. Bargaining

_____ d. Depression

4. Which one of the following is *not* a technique the EMT should use when helping loved ones cope with loss?

_____ a. Remain focused on the patient and do not be distracted by loved ones.

_____ b. Remain tolerant of others' feelings and emotions.

_____ c. Listen with compassion.

_____ d. Be honest and do your best to comfort those in need.

5. In which stage of the dying process do patients appear to have come to accept their fate?

_____ a. Denial

_____ b. Anger

_____ c. Acceptance

_____ d. Depression

Matching

Match the description on the left with the applicable term on the right.

1. _____ Comprehensive, integrated, multicomponent crisis intervention system
2. _____ Forum held between 1 and 10 days following a critical incident, facilitated by trained peer counselors and/or mental health professionals
3. _____ Structured small-group discussion that is provided within hours following a critical incident
4. _____ Sometimes called the "not me" stage, it is a defense mechanism against the thought of dying
5. _____ An attitude of, "Okay, but let me first . . ." is common during this stage of coping with dying

A. Defusing
B. CISM
C. CISD
D. Bargaining stage
E. Denial stage

Critical Thinking

1. On a scale of 1 to 10, 10 being totally balanced, how would you rate your life at this point in time? What is the single factor causing the most imbalance?

____

____

____

____

2. What does it mean to be "proactive" versus "reactive" about stress in your life?

____

____

____

____

3. What does the word "resiliency" mean to you and how does it apply to coping with the effects of stress?

____

____

____

____

Personal Safety

2-10 Describe measures you can take to protect yourself from exposure to diseases caused by pathogens.

standard precautions Centers for Disease Control and Prevention (CDC) guidelines and practices based on the awareness that all patients are potentially infectious regardless of diagnosis or presumed infection. Also called *universal precautions*.

body substance isolation (BSI) precautions the practice of using appropriate barriers to infection at the emergency scene, such as gloves, masks, gowns, and protective eyewear.

pathogens organisms that cause disease, such as viruses and bacteria.

2-13 Discuss the risks and preventive measures for specific infectious diseases of concern to EMTs, including hepatitis B and C, tuberculosis (TB), human immunodeficiency virus (HIV), and multi-drug-resistant organisms (MDRO).

As an EMT you will respond to those who are injured and ill in a wide variety of situations and environments. Remaining safe must be your top priority. The exposure or potential exposure to body substances such as blood and vomit is one of the most serious hazards you will face. To assist health care professionals in minimizing exposure to infectious disease, the Centers for Disease Control and Prevention (CDC) have established guidelines and practices known as **standard precautions**. The foundation of standard precautions (also called *universal precautions*) is an awareness that all patients are potentially infectious regardless of diagnosis or presumed infection.

One of the most important aspects of standard precautions is a practice called **body substance isolation (BSI) precautions**. Body fluids can contain organisms known as **pathogens**. Pathogens are organisms such as viruses and bacteria that are capable of causing disease. While it is not realistic to expect that you can perform your duties as an EMT and avoid all contact with body fluids, there are things you can do to greatly minimize your chances of becoming exposed.

The following is a partial list of some of the pathogens likely to be encountered as an EMS professional. As an EMT you will not always know the infectious status of your patients. It is essential that you always observe standard precautions and take the appropriate BSI precautions.

- ***Hepatitis (B and C).*** Bloodborne pathogens such as hepatitis B and C are highly virulent and can spread easily by contact with infected blood. Wear gloves and eye protection, and protect all mucous membranes from exposure.
- ***Tuberculosis (TB).*** TB is a pathogen transmitted by airborne droplets. It can be transmitted easily from an infected patient to a caregiver through coughing. Placing a surgical or HEPA mask on yourself and the patient will provide good protection.
- ***Human immunodeficiency virus (HIV).*** HIV is a virus spread by contact with infected blood and certain other body fluids. Wearing gloves and protecting your eyes and mucous membranes will provide appropriate protection.
- ***Multi-drug-resistant organisms (MDRO).*** Multi-drug resistance is a condition whereby a pathogen has developed resistance to many of the medicines and antibiotics normally used to fight it. Methicillin-resistant *Staphylococcus aureus* (MRSA) is an example of an MDRO. The presence of MDROs is becoming more common and can pose a serious risk to the EMT. Always wear the appropriate protective equipment such as gloves, masks, and eye protection when caring for patients with a known multi-drug-resistant infection.

2-11 Describe the personal protective equipment that may be used by EMS personnel.

personal protective equipment (PPE) equipment that protects the EMS worker from infection and exposure to the dangers of rescue operations.

At the core of proper BSI precautions is appropriate **personal protective equipment (PPE)**. PPE includes anything the EMT might use or wear to minimize risk of illness or injury. The PPE necessary for appropriate BSI precautions are:

- Gloves
- Eye protection
- Masks
- Disposable clothing

Gloves, eye protection, facial protection, and a disposable gown should be donned prior to patient contact when there is reasonable expectation of uncontrolled bleeding or the presence of body fluids such as uncontrolled vomiting.

Gloves

Proper BSI begins with wearing appropriate gloves for all patient contacts (Figure 2-7 ■). Now more than ever, the EMT has a choice in the type and material of gloves worn in the field. The most common gloves are the nonsterile latex type found in most health care settings. As more and more health care professionals are finding they are sensitive to latex, however, they are switching to gloves made of nonlatex materials such as nitrile or vinyl.

Gloves must be donned prior to patient contact when there is an expectation that there will be contact with blood or body fluids (Scan 2-1). Gloves should also be changed between contacts with different patients. Utility gloves, which are thicker and nondisposable, should be worn when decontaminating the ambulance or nondisposable equipment used during the care of the patient.

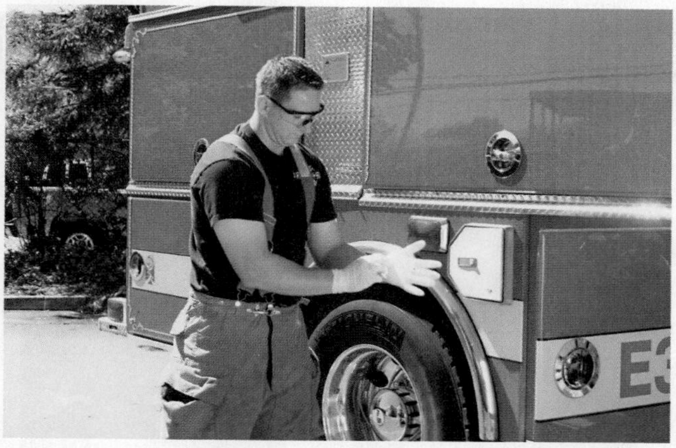

Figure 2-7 Protective gloves are the foundation of good body substance isolation (BSI) precautions.

Microorganisms and bacteria multiply fast in the warm moist environment inside the gloves. It is important to wash hands thoroughly following the removal of protective gloves.

PERSPECTIVE

Jeff—The EMT

This is one of those patients that you gotta be extra careful with. Hep B isn't something to mess with, and he had blood everywhere. Arnell and I both put on our gloves before we even got out of the truck, but my safety glasses are still on the dash where I had thrown them at the start of shift. Have you ever worn those things? They can be uncomfortable and sometimes they fog up, and they'll never make anyone's fashion list. But Arnell's right to make me go back and get them. It's more important to be safe than to get this guy quickly. I'm no good to anyone if I'm messed up.

Eye Protection

The eyes and their surrounding membranes are highly vascular (contain many blood vessels) and are susceptible to exposure to outside elements such as the splatter and spray that accompany many patient contacts. Body fluids that make contact with the eyes and surrounding tissue can be absorbed into the bloodstream and potentially cause an infection. For this reason, the EMT should wear appropriate eye protection for any patient who presents a reasonable risk of infection. Eyewear should be readily available and worn whenever a potential risk is evident (Figure 2-8 ■).

Appropriate eyewear should provide protection against spray and splatter from the front and the sides. If prescription glasses or sunglasses are used as PPE, they should include snap-on side pieces for added protection. In most situations, full goggles are not required but should be available just in case.

Face Protection

The mucous membranes of the nose and mouth are vulnerable, much like the exposed tissues of the eyes. For this reason, it may be necessary in some situations to shield them against the splatter of body fluids. A simple surgical mask worn by the EMT is appropriate for most situations

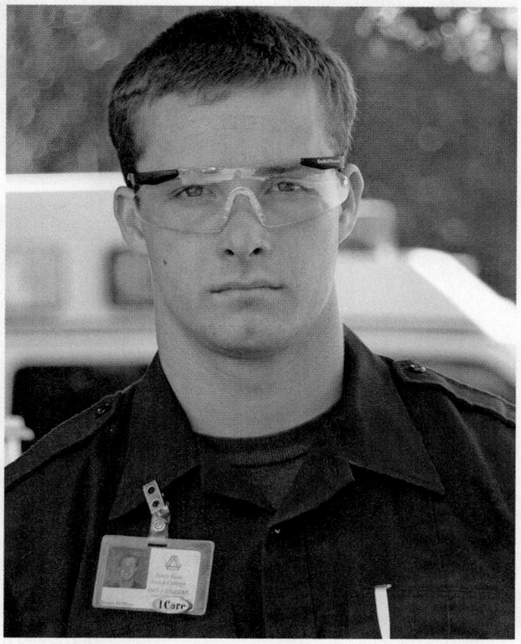

Figure 2-8 Proper eyewear should be comfortable and include protection at the sides of the eyes.

SCAN 2-1 Proper Removal of Gloves

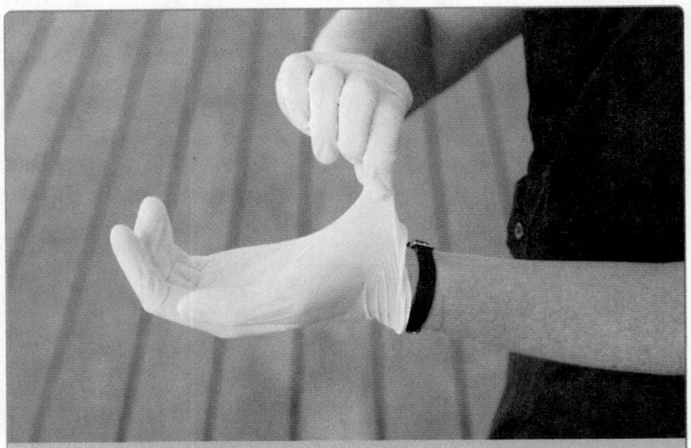

2-1-1 Begin by grasping the outer cuff of the opposite glove.

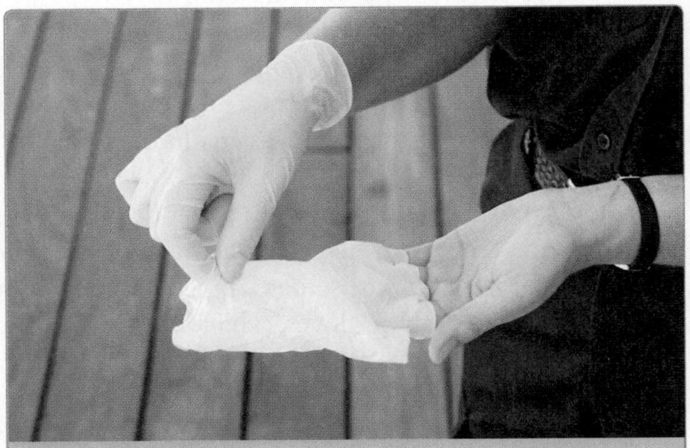

2-1-2 Carefully slip the glove over the hand, pulling it inside out.

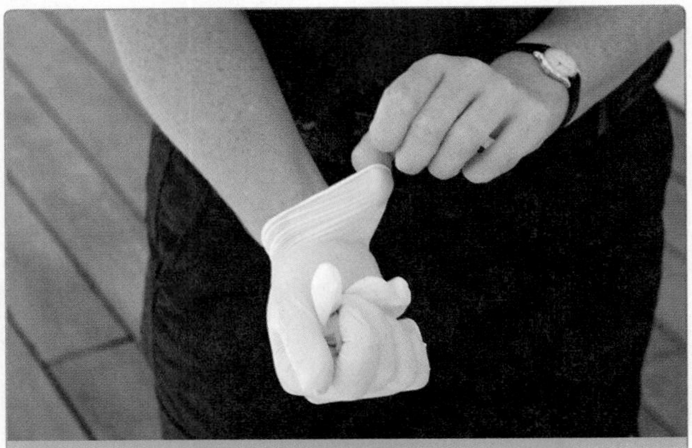

2-1-3 Next, slip a finger of the ungloved hand under the cuff.

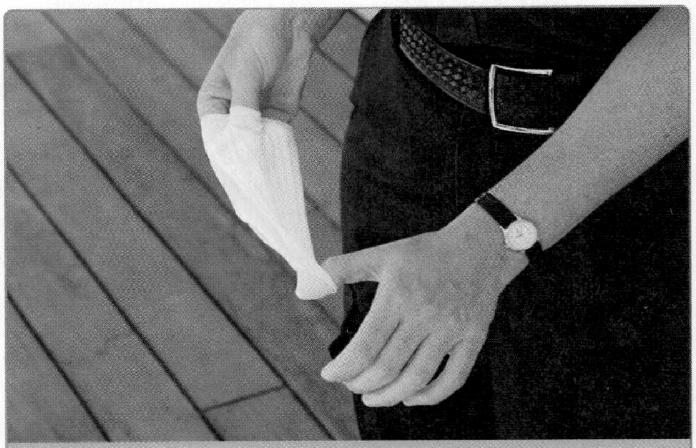

2-1-4 Carefully slip it off, turning it inside out.

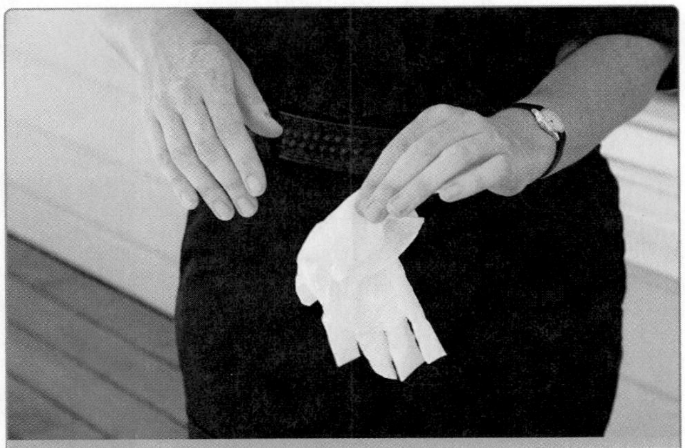

2-1-5 Once removed, both gloves will end up inside out with one inside the other. Dispose of them properly, and then wash your hands.

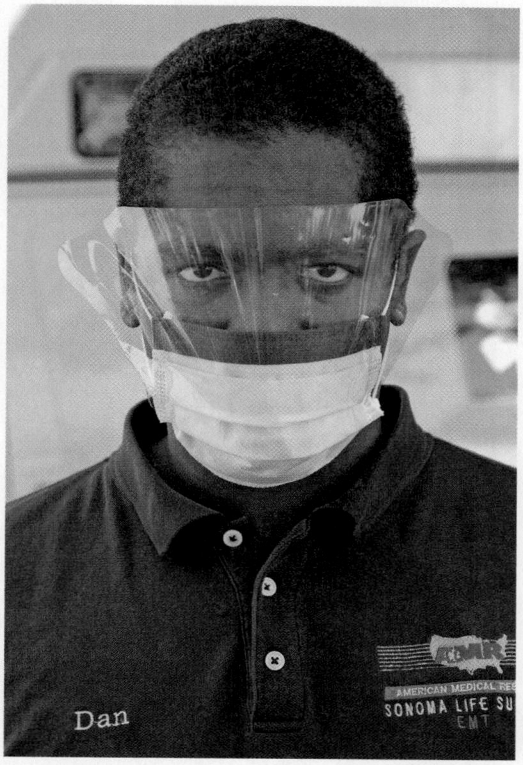

Figure 2-9a The eyes, mouth, and nose should be shielded from the splatter of body fluids. Pictured: Surgical mask with attached eye shield.

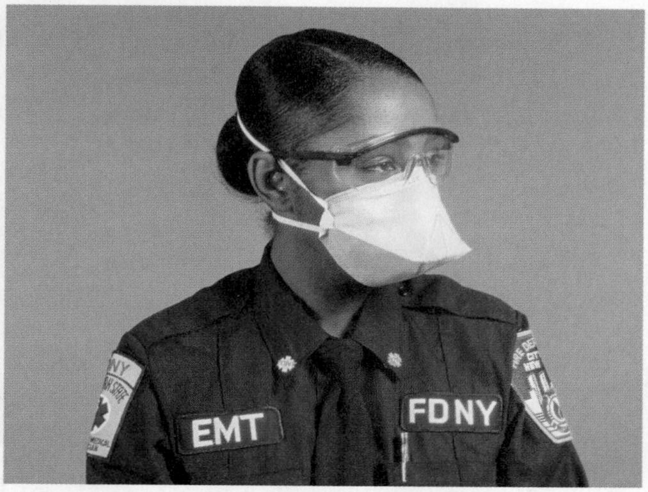

Figure 2-9b An OSHA approved N-95 mask provides a higher level of protection against airborne pathogens.

(Figure 2-9 ■). In situations where it is known or suspected that the patient may have an airborne disease such as tuberculosis, a specialized mask is required. The masks referred to as high-efficiency particulate air (HEPA) respirators and N-95 masks have been approved for this purpose by the National Institute for Occupational Safety and Health (NIOSH).

In cases where you are caring for a patient with a known or suspected airborne infection, it is also helpful to place a similar mask on the patient to further minimize exposure.

Disposable Clothing or Gowns

In rare cases such as major trauma with serious arterial bleeding or field delivery of an infant, the EMT should have access to and consider donning a gown or full disposable clothing (Figure 2-10 ■). This will provide extra protection against body fluids soaking through street clothing to unprotected skin, and will also minimize the chances of a soiled uniform that would require changing.

Hand Washing

In addition to considering the use of PPE, it is necessary to understand the importance of proper hand washing. The CDC states that hand washing is the single most important means of preventing the spread of infection. Whether or not we want to admit it, we carry both good and bad organisms on our hands all the time. Simply wearing gloves is not enough. Once we remove the gloves, we must wash our hands to cleanse them of the organisms that multiplied in the hot damp environment inside the glove.

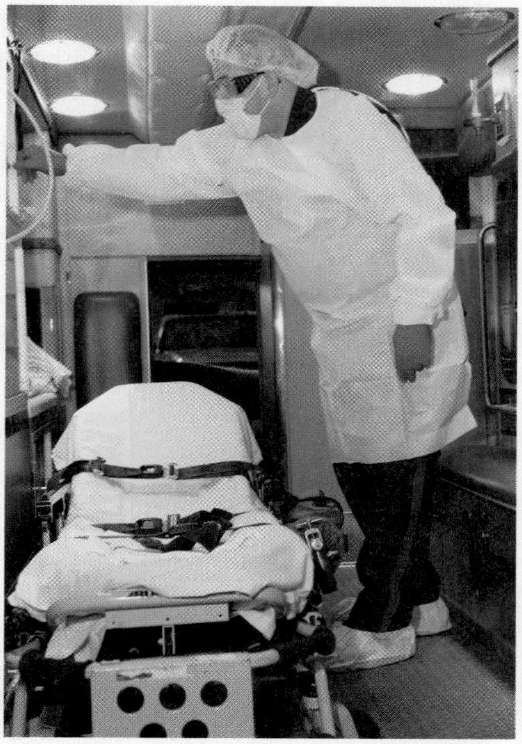

Figure 2-10 A gown should be worn in cases of major trauma or childbirth.

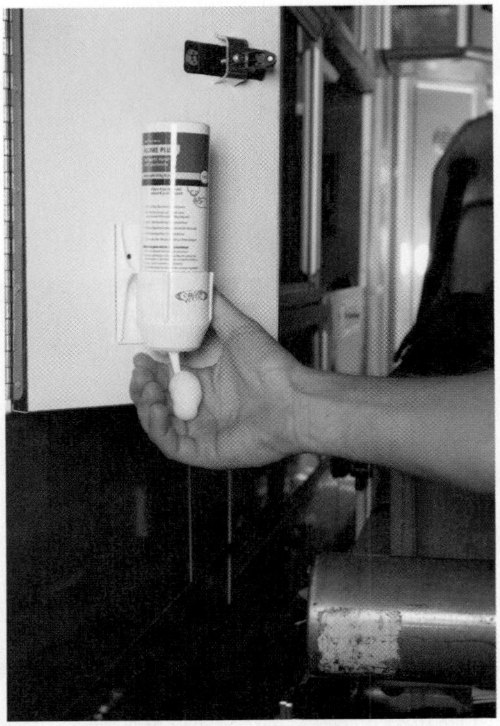

Figure 2-11 Alcohol-based hand sanitizers should be used when running water is not immediately available.

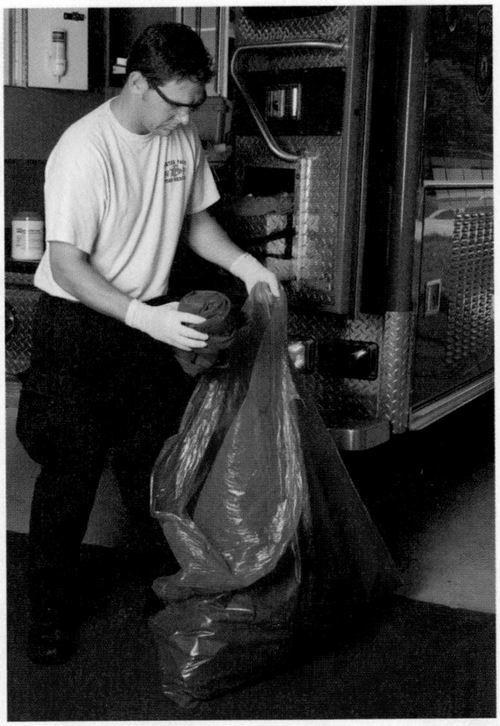

Figure 2-12 OSHA provides clear guidelines on how contaminated materials should be disposed of.

Hands should be washed between patient contacts, after removing gloves, and anytime they are visibly soiled.

In the field, there are essentially two methods the EMT can use to cleanse the hands. The preferred method utilizes soap and warm water and is usually accomplished while at the hospital. Vigorous rubbing with soap and warm water for at least 15 to 30 seconds is adequate. Concentrate on the cuticles, ridges, under the nails, and between the fingers. Remove jewelry prior to washing.

When an adequate supply of water and soap are not available, alcohol-based waterless hand cleaners that are commercially available serve as a good alternative (Figure 2-11 ■). Most alcohol-based cleansers are less effective when they come in contact with visible contaminants. For hand cleaners to be most effective, the hands must first be cleansed of any visible contamination, such as blood or dirt. That may require cleansing your hands twice, once to remove the visible blood, dirt, or other substances and a second time to decontaminate your hands. Place a dime-sized amount of alcohol-based cleanser in the palm of one hand and rub vigorously for several seconds to cover both hands entirely. *Do not* dry your hands but instead allow them to air dry as the alcohol evaporates.

OSHA

The Occupational Safety and Health Administration (OSHA) has one primary focus: to ensure the safety and health of the nation's workforce—and that includes you. OSHA has well-established policies and guidelines that employers must follow to ensure a safe workplace. It is in your best interest to become familiar with those guidelines, follow them, and be sure your employer follows them (Figure 2-12 ■).

Some states have established their own standards and have created even more stringent guidelines pertaining to infection control. Your instructor can provide the specifics of the guidelines established for your state or region. Most if not all states have laws or statutes that require the reporting of a known exposure to an infectious disease. If you think you may have been exposed to a patient's body fluids and you have any reason to suspect the patient could have carried an infectious disease, notify your supervisor immediately and follow your agency's procedure for post-exposure follow-up.

Immunizations

One of the requirements that OSHA has established to minimize the transmission of communicable disease is that employers must offer voluntary, no-cost immunizations. Any employee who has a reasonable risk of being exposed to an infectious disease in the course of normal duties must be offered a free immunization. Of course, EMS professionals fit into this category. The following is a list of recommended immunizations for the EMS professional:

2-12 Explain the role of immunizations and tuberculosis testing in maintaining good health.

- Tetanus
- Hepatitis B
- Measles
- Mumps
- Rubella

More and more of the recommended immunizations are being given as part of a normal childhood immunization series. But even if you were immunized as a child, you may need further immunizations as an adult. Check with a doctor about which ones should be repeated and how often (Figure 2-13 ■).

2-14 Explain the risks and measures that can be taken to protect yourself against the following hazards: hazardous materials, hazardous rescue situations, traffic-related injuries, and violence and crime.

Many EMS agencies accept test results that confirm the immune status of an individual. The tuberculin purified protein derivative (PPD), indicating whether or not the person has been exposed to tuberculosis, is such a test. In cases where the individual is certain that he has had a prior immunization, such as for hepatitis or measles, but cannot produce adequate documentation to support it, he may opt for a blood test that can verify his immune status.

Protection for Specific Emergencies

As mentioned earlier, PPE includes anything the EMT might use or wear to minimize the risk of illness or injury. So far only exposure to body fluids has been discussed. As an EMT you will be responding to many different types of emergencies that will expose you to additional hazards that will need to be identified and likely require specific types of PPE. The following sections discuss types of emergencies that expose the EMT to increased levels of risk, suggestions for identifying the potential hazards, and ways the EMT can minimize exposure to the risks at the scene.

Hazardous Materials Incidents

Confirming that the scene is safe is one of the very first tasks you will perform when arriving on the scene of an emergency. Of course if you know in advance that you are responding to a hazardous material (hazmat) scene, you should remain at a safe distance until trained hazmat personnel have cleared you for entry into the scene. There are times when it is not known in advance that a spill or release has occurred. For this reason have a high index of suspicion when responding to scenes with the potential for hazardous materials. (Chapter 44 covers this topic.)

Observe from a distance for any evidence of a spill or vapor release. Use binoculars, if you have them, to identify any placards that may indicate what

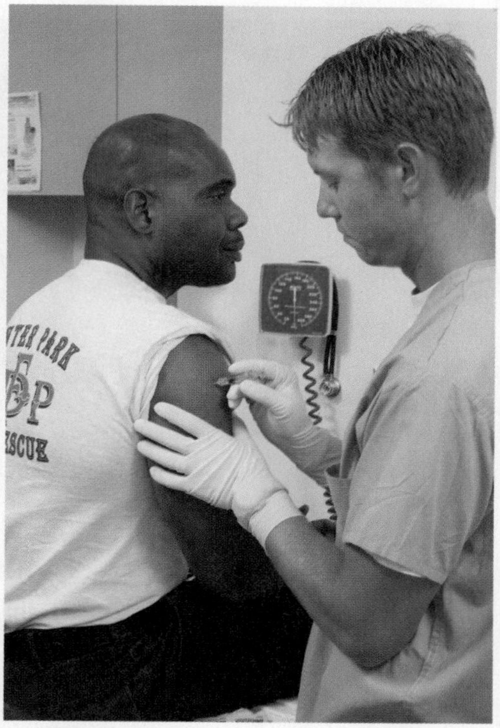

Figure 2-13 Immunizations are an important component of a good risk management plan.

has been spilled. A great resource that should be carried in all emergency vehicles is the *Emergency Response Guidebook*, developed jointly by the U.S. Department of Transportation, Transport Canada, and the Secretariat of Communications and Transportation of Mexico (SCT). It is updated regularly for use by firefighters, police, and other emergency services personnel who may be the first to arrive at the scene of a transportation incident involving a hazardous material. It is primarily a guide to aid first responders in (1) quickly identifying the specific or generic classification of the materials involved in the incident, and (2) protecting themselves and the general public during the initial response phase of the incident. More information, including electronic copies of the guidebook and recent updates, can be found at http://hazmat.dot.gov/pubs/erg/gydebook.htm.

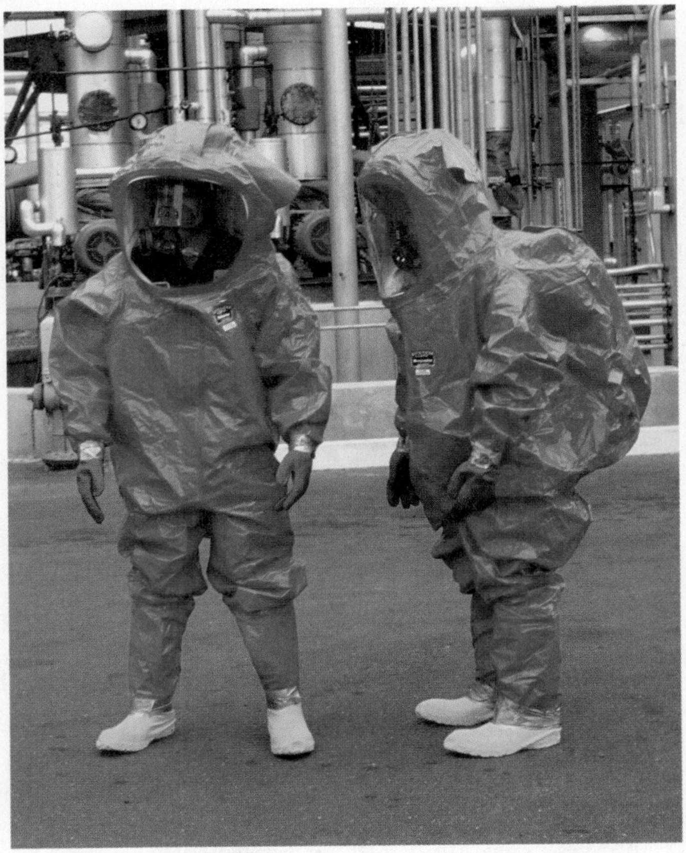

Figure 2-14 Class A protective suits offer the greatest protection at a hazmat scene.

Do not attempt to enter a hazmat scene unless you are specifically trained and equipped. Many hazmat scenes require the donning of specialized suits and self-contained breathing apparatus (SCBA) prior to entry (Figure 2-14 ■). As an EMT your primary role will be one of patient care. In most cases you will have to wait until patients have been removed from the scene and safely decontaminated before you will be allowed to provide emergency care. Rely on those with specialized hazmat training to provide direction and guidance at the scene.

Rescue Operations

Emergency scenes involving rescue operations involve a higher degree of risk than most other types of calls to which an EMT may respond. Rescue operations can involve vehicle extrications, live electrical wires, and fire and explosion hazards as well as hazardous materials. As with hazmat responses, incidents involving rescue operations require specialized training and equipment (Figure 2-15 ■). It is, however, quite common for an EMT to work side by side with the rescuers providing patient care during the rescue process. These situations may require additional PPE not typically found on an ambulance. In addition to protective eyewear, the EMT may want to utilize firefighter style "turnout" clothing as well as puncture-resistant gloves and a helmet.

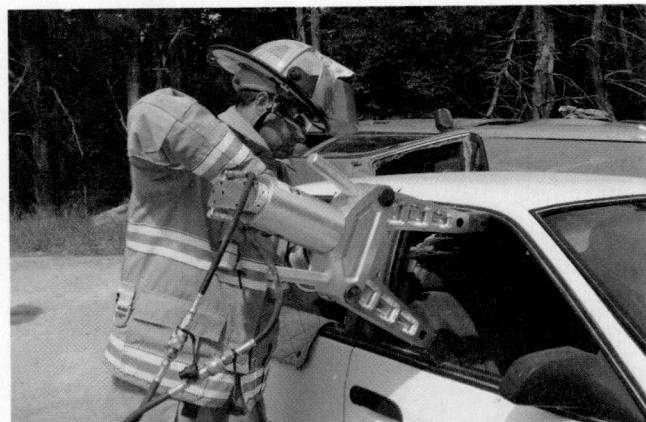

Figure 2-15 The "Jaws of Life" is a tool used for the extrication of patients from wrecked automobiles.

In most cases, once you have arrived on scene and have identified the need for additional resources, you will only do what is safe until a specialized rescue team can bring the patient to safety. (Chapter 45 will cover this information in more detail.)

Violence and Crime Scenes

As an EMT you will be responding to all types of emergencies, including those involving violence. You may respond to the victim of an assault or shooting where the perpetrator is still at large and potentially a risk to you and others at the scene. Bystanders and family members can become violent and begin to lash out at those trying to care for their loved ones. Any time you have any reason to suspect a crime has been committed or that your safety is threatened by another person at the scene, immediately retreat and request law enforcement.

There may be times when you are asked to respond to an incident and "stage" or stand by some distance away until you are cleared by law enforcement to enter. This is usually because they have reason to suspect that additional injuries may occur before the incident is over. Do not enter until you have been specifically requested to do so by law enforcement at the scene. Even after you have been cleared to enter, you should remain very alert for potential hazards.

If you are called to enter a crime scene to care for a patient, be respectful of any potential evidence in or around the scene. Once it is safe for you to enter, the patient is always your top priority. However, be careful to disturb only what is necessary to provide excellent patient care. Do not throw anything away or transport materials with the patient from the scene that may be needed by law enforcement as evidence.

STOP, REVIEW, REMEMBER!

Multiple Choice

For each question, place a check next to the correct answer.

1. Which one of the following is the best description of BSI precautions?

_____ a. Always wearing gloves when in contact with patients

_____ b. Wearing proper PPE only when blood is present

_____ c. Using proper PPE whenever there is a reasonable expectation of exposure to body fluids

_____ d. Using proper PPE only when body fluids such as blood and vomit are present

2. Which one of the following forms of PPE is best for minimizing the exposure to an airborne disease?

_____ a. HEPA mask

_____ b. Gloves

_____ c. Eye glasses

_____ d. Surgical mask

3. Which one of the following represents the greatest risk of exposure for the EMT?

_____ a. Vomit on a gloved hand

_____ b. Splatter of blood in the eyes

_____ c. Blood exposure over intact skin

_____ d. Saliva splatter in the ear

4. The foundation of standard precautions is:

_____ a. that all patients are potentially infectious regardless of diagnosis or presumed infection.

_____ b. that only patients with a known infectious status pose a threat.

_____ c. based on good hand washing.

_____ d. based on getting all immunizations before being exposed.

5. According to the CDC, which one of the following is the single most effective means of preventing the spread of infection?

_____ a. Immunizations

_____ b. Awareness

_____ c. Hand washing

_____ d. Protective gloves

(continued on next page)

(continued)

Critical Thinking

1. Describe the relationship between body substance isolation (BSI) precautions and personal protective equipment (PPE).

2. List the PPE you would want to wear if you were caring for victims following a hazardous materials spill.

3. What are some ways you could help preserve potential evidence while caring for a patient at the scene of a crime?

4. Given the different situations below, choose the appropriate PPE by placing a check in the appropriate column or columns.

Situation	Gloves	Glasses	Mask	Gown
Minor bleed to the left hand				
Suctioning a vomiting patient				
Assisting with a birth				
Cleaning a bloody backboard				
Taking a blood pressure on a medical patient				
Major bleed of the lower leg with spurting blood				
Cleaning the back of the ambulance after a call				

EMERGENCY DISPATCH SUMMARY

Raymond was transported to Sutter Memorial Hospital where he underwent a procedure to repair a broken vessel in his esophagus. He is recovering well, but if his liver continues to weaken and, due to a widespread shortage of organ donors, his chances for survival decline each day.

Chapter Review

To the Point

- Anything that can cause stress for the EMT is known as a *stressor*. EMS exposes the EMT to many stressors on a day-to-day basis.
- Signs and symptoms of stress include irritability, inability to concentrate, insomnia, anxiety, loss of appetite, and a general lack of interest in work.
- Stress can be divided into one of three categories: acute stress, delayed stress, and cumulative stress. Each has its own manifestation that you as an EMT should become familiar with and learn to recognize in yourself and others.
- Maintaining a balanced lifestyle between work and personal time as well as maintaining a balanced diet and regular exercise regimen can help the EMT develop strong resilience and coping mechanisms when stress is high.
- Most EMS systems utilize specific systems and processes to help members cope with stress before, during, and after an event. A common name for this is *critical incident stress management (CISM)*.
- A typical CISM program includes trained personnel who use tools such as talking, debriefings, and defusing to help those affected by stress cope.
- Death is one of the most stressful events a person can face, causing intense grief. There are common responses to this grief that most people experience. They are denial, anger, bargaining, depression, and acceptance.
- It is important for the EMT to recognize the five stages of grief and to learn how to respond appropriately when faced with a patient or family member experiencing grief.
- One of the most common risks associated with caring for patients is exposure to disease-causing organisms called *pathogens*. While there is no way to eliminate exposure, the EMT must understand the modes of transmission and take appropriate precautions to minimize exposure.
- Common types of PPE used by the EMT are gloves, masks, eye protection, and gowns.
- One way the EMT can minimize infection is to obtain all the appropriate immunizations.

Chapter Questions

Multiple Choice

For each question, place a check next to the correct answer.

1. A good strategy for developing resiliency for coping with stress is:
   _____ a. working extra shifts whenever possible.
   _____ b. keeping your thoughts and feelings to yourself.
   _____ c. maintaining a balanced lifestyle.
   _____ d. using alcohol to alleviate distress.

2. The five stages that most dying patients experience are denial, anger, ______________, depression, and acceptance.
   _____ a. resentment
   _____ b. frustration
   _____ c. bargaining
   _____ d. anticipation

3. Irritability with coworkers, inability to concentrate, indecisiveness, and loss of appetite are all warning signs of:
   _____ a. psychosis.
   _____ b. stress.
   _____ c. anxiety.
   _____ d. isolation.

4. You receive a dispatch for a possible assault victim. What other resources will you want to respond as well?
   _____ a. Fire services
   _____ b. Additional ambulance
   _____ c. Field supervisor
   _____ d. Law enforcement

5. One of the best techniques for helping comfort a person who has lost a loved one is to:
   _____ a. just listen.
   _____ b. offer a drink.
   _____ c. suggest a nap.
   _____ d. avoid eye contact.

(continued on next page)

(continued)

6. Hepatitis C is a pathogen likely to be encountered by the EMT by exposure to:

_____ a. saliva.
_____ b. blood.
_____ c. vomit.
_____ d. sweat.

Critical Thinking

1. How do you deal with acute stress? How have you reacted to acute stress in the past and did you react appropriately?

2. What are you doing in your current lifestyle that will help you deal with stress? What areas can you improve?

3. Imagine yourself attending a CISD following a critical incident. Would you be willing or able to talk about your thoughts and feelings in front of your peers? Explain your answer.

Case Studies

Case Study 1

You have arrived at work to find that your regular partner, Tim, has called in sick for the shift and that your new partner for the day is Will. You find out from your supervisor that both Will and Tim were on a double fatality a couple of days earlier that involved two pediatric patients. Your supervisor asks you to be sensitive to the issue and to please alert him if you see any unusual behavior in Will during your shift together. As you and Will begin the shift and complete the ambulance inspection, you notice that Will is definitely not his usual outgoing self.

1. Is it appropriate for you to engage Will in a conversation regarding the call? Why or why not?

2. Describe the typical behavior of someone (such as Will) who has experienced a traumatic event.

3. What can you do as Will's partner to help him deal with the stress he is under?

Case Study 2

You have been working as an EMT for about a year and taking all the overtime shifts that you could get your hands on. At one point you even pulled a 96-hour shift without a break, but most have been 24s and 48s. You are finding it more and more difficult to find the energy to make it to the next call and your partners have been avoiding you while on duty because of your negative attitude. Clearly, stress is taking its toll on you.

1. In what other ways might you find that stress is affecting your life?

2. If you do nothing to change the situation, how will this buildup of stress probably end up affecting you?

3. List at least three things you can do to ease the stress and keep from getting burned out?

The Last Word

The primary goal of this chapter has been to begin preparing you to properly manage the stressors and other hazards that are so much a part of a career as an EMS professional. Balance is the key to managing life's stresses and the stress of EMS is no exception. Establishing a well-balanced diet, an adequate amount of sleep, and a regular exercise routine will do wonders toward preparing you for stress as well as helping you manage its effects.

The top priority for all EMS professionals is personal safety. If the scene is not safe, *do not enter*. Proper BSI precautions are recommended for all patient contacts and include such PPE as gloves, eye protection, and face masks.

Legal and Ethical Considerations of Providing Care

3

Education Standards

Preparatory: EMS Systems, Documentation, Medical/Legal, and Ethics

Competencies

Applies fundamental knowledge of the EMS system, safety/well-being of the EMT, medical/legal issues, and ethical issues to the provision of emergency care.

Objectives

After completion of this lesson, you should be able to:

3-1 Define key terms introduced in this chapter.

3-2 Differentiate between the concepts of *scope of practice* and *standard of care*.

3-3 Explain the EMT's legal obligations with respect to medical direction.

3-4 Describe the ethical responsibilities of EMTs.

3-5 Differentiate between the concepts of *ethics* and *values*.

3-6 Explain the concept of *duty to act*.

3-7 Describe the intent of Good Samaritan laws.

3-8 Explain each of the following types of consent: informed consent, expressed consent, implied consent, and consent to treat minors.

3-9 Define the terms *capacity* and *competency* and how each relates to consent and refusal.

3-10 Discuss the actions you should take when confronted with a patient who refuses care.

3-11 Explain each of the following legal protections for EMTs: sovereign immunity, statutes of limitations, and contributory negligence of the patient.

3-12 Compare and contrast the application of each of the following types of advance directives: do not resuscitate (DNR) order, living will, durable power of attorney, and physician orders for life-sustaining treatment (POLST).

3-13 Differentiate between criminal and civil liability.

3-14 Explain the concept of *negligence*.

3-15 List and explain the elements required for a successful negligence lawsuit.

3-16 Give examples of ways you can avoid a claim of abandonment.

3-17 Describe how the EMT can avoid claims of assault and/or battery and false imprisonment/kidnapping.

3-18 Explain the legal and ethical responsibilities concerning confidentiality and privacy.

3-19 Describe EMTALA provisions as they apply to EMS.

3-20 Describe special considerations for patients who are potential organ donors.

3-21 Describe situations in which the EMT may be mandated to make a report, such as suspected abuse and crimes.

3-22 Discuss special considerations in responding to potential crime scenes.

Key Terms

abandonment p. 51
advance directive p. 58
assault p. 63
battery p. 63
capacity p. 55
competent p. 54
consent p. 54
contributory negligence p. 58
do not resuscitate (DNR) order p. 59
duty to act p. 51
Emergency Medical Treatment and Active Labor Act (EMTALA) p. 63
ethics p. 49
expressed consent p. 54
Good Samaritan laws p. 52
Health Insurance Portability and Accountability Act (HIPAA) p. 64
implied consent p. 55
National EMS Education Standards p. 49
National Highway Traffic Safety Administration (NHTSA) p. 49
National Standard Curriculum (NSC) p. 49
negligence p. 51
scope of practice p. 49
sovereign immunity p. 58
standard of care p. 49
statute of limitations p. 58

Introduction

There is simply no way around it: We live, work, and play in a litigious society. Everywhere we turn we either hear or read about another lawsuit. The reasons go beyond the scope of this textbook, but the fact remains, your choices and actions can greatly influence your chances of being involved in a lawsuit. Suffice it to say that no matter where we live or what our job is, much of our daily lives is influenced in some way by the legal system. This is especially true in EMS. But it is not because the rules are any different for EMS. It is because EMS is a relatively high-profile job, and many pairs of eyes are on EMS personnel as they deliver patient care.

One of your first responsibilities as an EMT is to learn the law as it pertains to providing patient care at the scene of an emergency. That is no different than learning the rules of the road when first learning to drive. Common sense provides much of what you need to know, while training and experience fill in the remaining requisite knowledge.

EMERGENCY DISPATCH

"I think this is it right here," EMT Brandon Gervais said, searching the dilapidated duplex for an address. "I don't see a number, but 212 . . . 214 . . . this has to be 216."

As Brandon and his partner, Jewel, were pulling the cot from the back of the ambulance, a young woman emerged from a doorway and walked quickly up to them. "Oh great, you're here." She glanced at her watch and placed her hand on the cot. "But you won't need this."

"Who are you?" Brandon said, pulling the cot from her hand.

"I'm Janine," the woman said, "Mr. Flowers's caretaker. Look, I just need you guys to help me get him back into bed. He fell onto the floor, I can't lift him, and I'm late for my next appointment."

The house was a mess. Old newspapers, mail, and clothes were strewn everywhere, and the stench of urine was almost caustic. Janine led them back to the only bedroom in the small house. There on the floor next to the bed was Henry Flowers, moaning and clad in nothing but wet undershorts.

"I left about 40 minutes ago to go shopping for him, and when I came back, this is where I found him." She reached down and began pulling on one of his thin arms. "If you'll just help me get him back into bed, we can all go on with our day."

Scope of Practice

The EMT **scope of practice,** sometimes called the *scope of care,* is a detailed description of the specific care and actions EMTs are allowed to perform. It is defined by national standards and state legislation, and enhanced by medical direction through the use of protocols and standing orders.

The scope of practice for the EMT is referenced to documents known as the **National EMS Education Standards** and the **National Standard Curriculum (NSC),** which were developed by the **National Highway Traffic Safety Administration (NHTSA),** a division of the U.S. Department of Transportation (DOT).

3-2 Differentiate between the concepts of scope of practice and standard of care.

scope of practice a detailed description of the specific care and actions EMTs are allowed to perform.

National EMS Education Standards standards developed by NHTSA that define what each level of EMS training must include.

National Standard Curriculum (NSC) the curriculum developed by the U.S. Department of Transportation as the foundation for the scope of practice for all EMS personnel.

National Highway Traffic Safety Administration (NHTSA) a division of the U.S. Department of Transportation (DOT). This agency develops the National Standard Curricula for various levels of EMS providers.

standard of care a modified scope of practice specifically designed to meet the needs of a specific area or region.

Standard of Care

The concept of **standard of care** is somewhat different from the concept of *scope of practice*. One way to explain the difference is that scope of practice is what EMTs are *allowed* to do and standard of care is what they *should* do.

The standard of care is defined as the reasonable care that a prudent person with the same training and experience would be expected to perform. For a specific region it is established by key stakeholders in the EMS system in accordance with local laws and regulations. Those stakeholders are often medical directors, EMS administrators, and experienced field personnel. The local standard of care is most often defined by protocols and standing orders.

Medical Direction

As an EMT providing care within an EMS system, you are acting as an extension of the system's medical director. That means you are required to follow all protocols and provide an appropriate standard of care. As you learned in Chapter 1, all EMS systems are required to have a physician as its medical director. His job is to oversee all aspects of patient care within the EMS system and to ensure continuous quality improvement of the system.

CLINICAL CLUE

Protocols

Each EMS system has a clearly defined set of protocols for each level of care. Understanding those protocols and providing care that is consistent with them will greatly reduce the risk of legal action.

PERSPECTIVE

Brandon—The EMT

Something just doesn't seem right here. Is that caregiver at all concerned about Henry's well-being? Come on! He doesn't seem to be aware of his surroundings or anything, and all she can think of is getting on to her next appointment? I tell you, that's really some standard of care she's providing.

Ethical Responsibilities

3-3 Explain the EMT's legal obligations with respect to medical direction.

As an EMT you will be expected to perform your duties in accordance with both legal and ethical guidelines. While the law may be fairly clear cut, sometimes the ethical side of being an EMT can be somewhat cloudy.

3-4 Describe the ethical responsibilities of EMTs.

Ethics is the study of principles that define behavior as right, good, and proper. Those principles are based on morals and serve as the rules or habits of conduct with regard to standards of right and wrong. Because ethics is based on morals and morals are somewhat subjective, making good ethical choices is not always the same for everyone. In an effort to develop an ethical standard for all EMTs, the National Association of EMTs adopted the EMT Code of Ethics (Figure 3-1 ▪).

ethics the study of principles that define behavior as right, good, and proper.

The EMT Code of Ethics addresses such things as:

- Providing care based on need and without regard for nationality, race, creed, color, or religion

EMT Code of Ethics

Professional status as an EMT is maintained and enriched by the willingness of the individual practitioner to accept and fulfill obligations to society, other medical professionals, and the profession of EMT. As an EMT, I solemnly pledge myself to the following code of professional ethics:

A fundamental responsibility of the EMT is to conserve life, to alleviate suffering, to promote health, to do no harm, and to encourage the quality and equal availability of emergency medical care.

The EMT provides services based on human need, with respect for human dignity, unrestricted by consideration of nationality, race, creed, color, or religion.

The EMT does not use professional knowledge and skills in any enterprise detrimental to the public well being.

The EMT respects and holds in confidence all information of a confidential nature obtained in the course of professional work unless required by law to divulge such information.

The EMT, as a citizen, understands and upholds the law and performs the duties of citizenship; as a professional, the EMT has the never-ending responsibility to work with concerned citizens and other health care professionals in promoting a high standard of emergency medical care to all people.

The EMT shall maintain professional competence and demonstrate concern for the competence of other members of the EMS health care team.

An EMT assumes responsibility in defining and upholding standards of professional practice and education.

The EMT assumes responsibility for individual professional actions and judgment, both in dependent and independent emergency functions, and knows and upholds the laws which affect the practice of the EMT.

An EMT has the responsibility to be aware of and participate in matters of legislation affecting the EMS system.

The EMT, or groups of EMTs, who advertise professional service, do so in conformity with the dignity of the profession.

The EMT has an obligation to protect the public by not delegating to a person less qualified, any service which requires the professional competence of an EMT.

The EMT will work harmoniously with and sustain confidence in EMT associates, the nurses, the physicians, and other members of the EMS health care team.

The EMT refuses to participate in unethical procedures, and assumes the responsibility to expose incompetence or unethical conduct of others to the appropriate authority in a proper and professional manner.

Written by: Charles Gillespie MD

Adopted by: The National Association of EMTs, 1978.

Figure 3-1 The EMT Code of Ethics. (Reprinted with permission of the National Association of Emergency Technicians. http://www.naemt.org)

- Protecting patient confidentiality
- Respecting patient dignity
- Promoting a high standard of care for all
- Assuming responsibility for personal actions and conduct
- Upholding professional standards of practice and education (Figures 3-2 and 3-3 ■)

As an EMT you have an ethical obligation to place the needs of those you are caring for first, so long as it is safe to do so. You must maintain your skills and knowledge of your chosen profession in an effort to continually improve yourself and the system. You also must provide accurate and complete documentation of the care you provide. Making the right choices as an EMT is a serious responsibility, but it is extremely rewarding.

Personal Core Values

3-5 Differentiate between the concepts of ethics and values.

One way to become more aware of your actions as they pertain to ethics is to identify your personal core values. Your values are your beliefs and what you consider important as an individual. Your beliefs are what drive your actions and, in turn, they become the example by which people see and judge you. By identifying and embracing

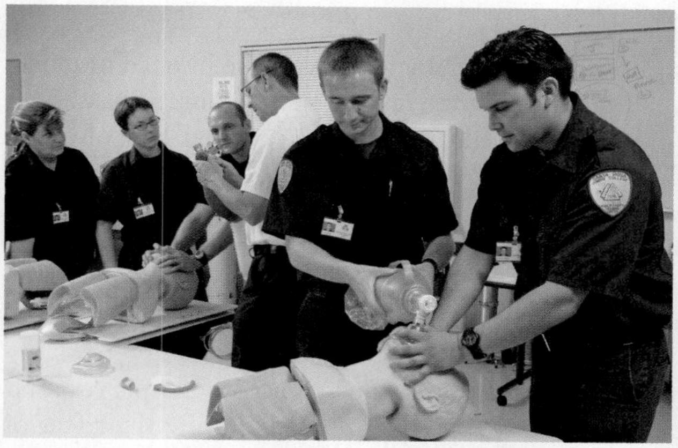

Figure 3-2 Quality training promotes a high standard of care for your patients.

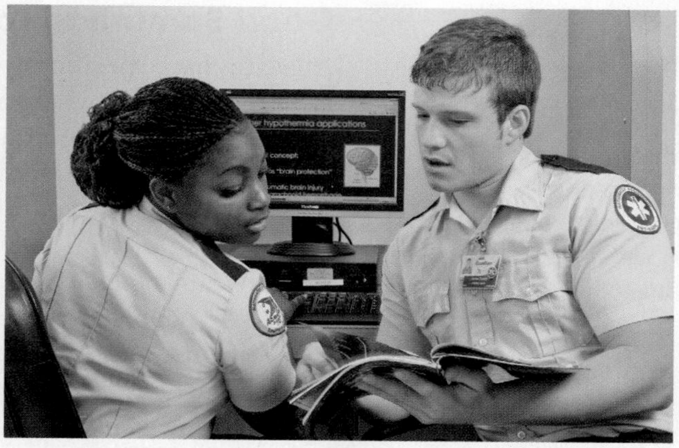

Figure 3-3 As an EMS professional you must do your best to stay informed with the latest research related to patient care.

core values such as integrity, compassion, accountability, respect, and empathy, EMTs will find it easier to make good decisions and do what is right for the patient as well as others in their life. To find out more about exploring your own personal core values, visit *www.icarevalues.org*.

Legal Aspects of Providing Care

3-6 Explain the concept of duty to act.

Once you become an EMT and begin working for an EMS provider, you will have a legal obligation to render care to those in need and to do so to an established standard of care. This obligation is referred to as a **duty to act.** You also must obtain consent from those to whom you offer care and must ensure that those who choose to refuse care understand the consequences of their decision.

duty to act a legal obligation to provide care to a patient.

Duty to Act

An EMT's duty to act can be implied, as in the case of some volunteer rescue and ambulance squads, or it can be contractual, such as when an EMS provider (volunteer or otherwise) has a contract to provide service to an event or a community. The concept of a duty to act becomes less obvious when the trained EMT is not associated with an established EMS agency. For instance, in most states the off-duty EMT has no legal obligation to stop and render care at the scene of an emergency. An EMT who is off duty or one who received his training simply out of personal interest may have no legal obligation to assist those injured in a vehicle collision, even if he witnessed the incident.

The laws pertaining to a duty to act are different in each state, so you must research the laws of your state or region. Your instructor should be able to provide the specifics for your area.

Most states have made it clear that once someone begins to render care to an injured or ill person, a legal duty to act is established. That person must remain at the scene and provide care to the best of his ability and training. Once you have begun to care for the victim of an injury or illness, you *must* remain at the scene and continue to provide care until someone of equal or higher training takes over care. Failure to continue to provide care may be considered **abandonment** and can result in a charge of **negligence.** (More about abandonment and negligence is offered later in this chapter.)

> **CLINICAL CLUE**
>
> **EMS Placards**
>
> It is important to know that the display of signs, placards, or stickers on your vehicle that identify you as a trained medical provider may obligate you to act at the scene of an emergency. Investigate the laws and regulations in your state or region before displaying those symbols on your personal vehicle.

abandonment a legal term referring to leaving a patient after care has been initiated and before the patient has been transferred to someone with equal or greater medical training.

negligence a legal finding of failure to act properly in a situation in which there was a duty to act, needed care as would reasonably be expected of the EMT was not provided, and harm was caused to the patient as a result.

Good Samaritan Laws

3-7 Describe the intent of Good Samaritan laws.

Good Samaritan laws laws, varying in each state, designed to provide limited legal protection for citizens and some health care personnel when they are administering emergency care.

All states have specific laws that encourage passersby to assist those in need of medical attention. Those laws are called **Good Samaritan laws.** They encourage passersby, regardless of training, to stop and provide medical assistance without fear of being held civilly liable for anything they do or do not do while caring for the victim. Good Samaritan laws protect those who "in good faith and not for compensation" render care to those in need and do so as "any prudent man or woman would do" given the same circumstances and training.

Many people state that the reason they would not stop and render care at the scene of an emergency is fear of being sued. The reality is that lawsuits involving passersby who render care are quite rare. Fortunately, the majority of people respond to their ethical and moral obligation to assist someone in need, despite their fear of not knowing exactly what to do.

STOP, REVIEW, REMEMBER!

Multiple Choice

For each question, place a check next to the correct answer.

1. Which one of the following definitions best describes the term *scope of practice?*

_____ a. It is established by state laws and regulations.

_____ b. It is established by local protocols and guidelines.

_____ c. It is the same for EMTs in every state.

_____ d. It is determined by the local physician medical director.

2. The *standard of care* is most often defined by:

_____ a. national leaders in EMS.

_____ b. local protocols and guidelines.

_____ c. national standard curricula.

_____ d. your on-duty supervisor.

3. The obligation you will have as an EMT providing care to the sick and injured is known as a(n):

_____ a. legal obligation.

_____ b. ethical obligation.

_____ c. duty to act.

_____ d. moral responsibility.

4. The National EMS Education Standards were developed by the:

_____ a. National Association of EMS Personnel.

_____ b. National Association of State Program Directors.

_____ c. U.S. Department of Transportation (DOT).

_____ d. National Association of EMS Physicians.

5. Which one of the following best describes the purpose of Good Samaritan laws?

_____ a. They encourage passersby to stop and render care.

_____ b. They discourage untrained passersby from rendering care.

_____ c. They hold passersby exempt from having to stop.

_____ d. They require passersby to stop and render care.

Matching

Match the definition on the left with the applicable term on the right.

1. _____ Detailed description of the specific care and actions EMTs are allowed to perform as defined by state laws and regulations
2. _____ Modified scope of practice specifically designed to meet the needs of a specific area or region
3. _____ Organization responsible for developing the National Education Standards and the scope of practice for EMS
4. _____ Process of overseeing all aspects of patient care within the EMS system and of ensuring continuous quality improvement of the system
5. _____ Study of the principles that define behavior as right, good, and proper
6. _____ Legal obligation to render care to those in need and to do so to an established standard of care
7. _____ Specific laws to encourage passersby to stop and assist those in need of medical attention

A. Good Samaritan laws
B. Medical direction
C. Ethics
D. Duty to act
E. NHTSA
F. Scope of practice
G. Standard of care

Critical Thinking

1. Does the scope of practice differ from the standard of care in the system in which you will be working? How might you find this out?

____

____

____

____

2. Describe the difference between and provide an example of a legal duty and an ethical duty as they pertain to the job of an EMT.

____

____

____

____

3. Describe the purpose and function of Good Samaritan laws.

____

____

____

____

PERSPECTIVE

Henry—The Patient

I just can't seem to get anyone to understand me. My right hip and shoulder are pretty sore, but when I try to tell the ambulance people the words are coming out all wrong. I just want someone to help and to find out what is wrong with me.

Obtaining Consent and Patient Refusal

3-8 Explain each of the following types of consent: informed consent, expressed consent, implied consent, and consent to treat minors.

consent permission from the patient for care or other action by the EMT.

Before you can legally provide care for a patient, you must obtain consent. **Consent,** or permission from the patient to provide care, can take a variety of forms such as verbal, nonverbal, written, and implied. Regardless of the form, it is a legal requirement that the EMT receive consent from the patient before providing care. It is also important to know that a patient may change his mind at any time and refuse care even after having initially given consent. It will be important to understand a patient's reasons for refusal if there is any hope of regaining consent. (There is more about refusal a little later in the chapter.)

Expressed Consent

expressed consent consent given by adults who are of legal age and mentally competent to make a rational decision in regard to their medical well-being.

Consent that is obtained from alert, competent, adult patients who understand the consequences of their choice is referred to as **expressed consent,** also called *informed consent* (Figure 3-4 ▪). Expressed consent can be verbal, nonverbal, or written and can only be obtained from patients who are of legal age and possess the mental capacity to make informed rational decisions about their own care. In most cases, expressed consent is verbal. That is, you introduce yourself and ask the patient if it is okay for you to help. Usually, the patient will respond verbally. However, if he offers no verbal response but does not refuse care, consider that expressed consent has been provided and proceed with the appropriate care.

CLINICAL CLUE

Consent

When you arrive on scene after emergency medical responders (EMRs), such as fire or law enforcement personnel, you should not assume that the patient has given consent. Observe the entire scene carefully and obtain an appropriate briefing from the EMRs before you approach the patient. Is the patient being cooperative or displaying signs of resistance? Observing the interaction between the patient and the EMRs will help determine your best approach. In most cases when a patient is cooperative, you can simply introduce yourself and inform the patient that you will be caring for him. In situations where there may be some resistance on the part of the patient, a slower approach may be best. Introducing yourself and asking permission to treat will usually be a good way to begin.

Competency and Capacity

3-9 Define the terms *competency* and *capacity* and how they each relate to consent and refusal.

competent the ability of an adult to make informed and rational decisions about his own well-being.

An adult who is **competent** is one who is able to make informed and rational decisions about his own well-being. In most states competency is something that is determined by the courts. For example, a person with advanced Alzheimer's dementia may, at the request of his daughter, be deemed by a court as legally no longer competent to make decisions for himself.

Whereas competency is legally determined, **capacity** is medically determined. Capacity becomes an issue when a patient refuses care. A patient who is ill or injured and refusing your care may not be able to make a rational decision because of his medical condition or injury. In order for an adult to refuse care, you must determine if the person has the mental capacity to understand the situation as well as the potential consequences of refusal of care and transport. For this reason you must use great caution when allowing patients to refuse care.

It is also important to understand that an adult who has capacity has the right to refuse care at any time, even after care has been initiated. (Refusal of care will be further discussed later in this chapter.)

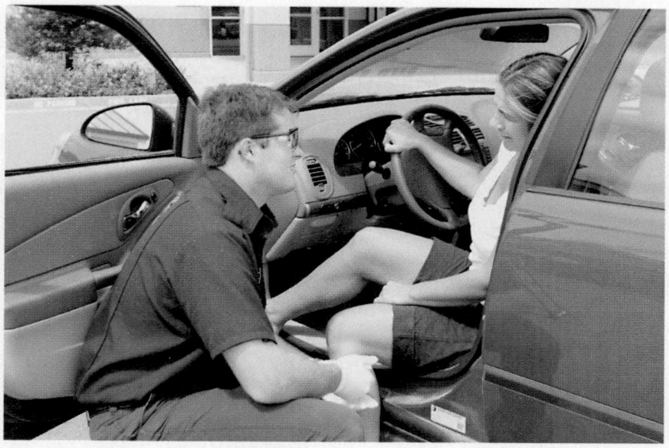

Figure 3-4 Obtaining consent from an adult patient.

Implied Consent

Implied consent is a legal term used to describe an assumed permission to treat. Permission may be assumed when you are caring for the following types of patients:

- Not of legal age (Figure 3-5 ■)
- Unresponsive (Figure 3-6 ■)
- Mentally incompetent

capacity the ability of a patient to fully comprehend the medical situation and the potential consequences of refusal of care or transport.

implied consent the consent it is presumed a patient or patient's parent or guardian would give if he could, such as for an unconscious patient or by a parent who cannot be contacted when care is needed.

PERSPECTIVE

Jewel—The EMT

This poor old guy sure seems confused, and it wouldn't surprise me at all if he really hurt himself falling out of bed like that. We can't just put him back in bed and leave the way that lady wants us to. After all, can't I still take care of a patient even though he can't give consent? I think I can. Right?

In the case of an unresponsive patient, the EMT may provide care because it is assumed that if the patient were aware of his situation, he would consent to be treated. In the case of a minor who is ill or injured, it is assumed that the parents would grant permission to treat if they were present.

Even though the standard legal age in the United States is 18 years, most states allow those between the ages of 14 and 17 to become emancipated, if they meet certain strict requirements, and therefore obtain the full legal rights of an adult. Some of

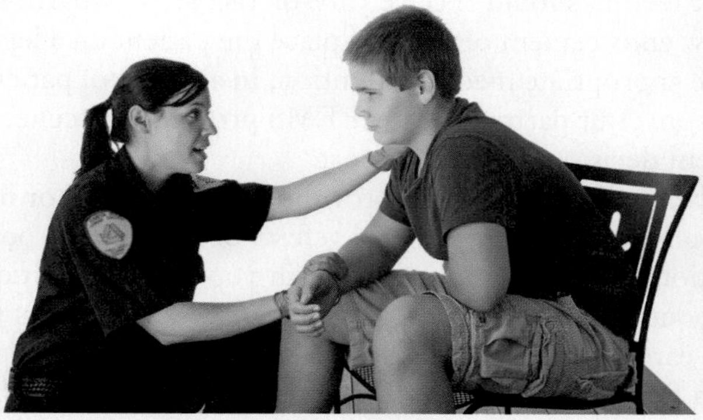

Figure 3-5 Implied consent is used when a pediatric patient requires care and a parent or guardian is not immediately available.

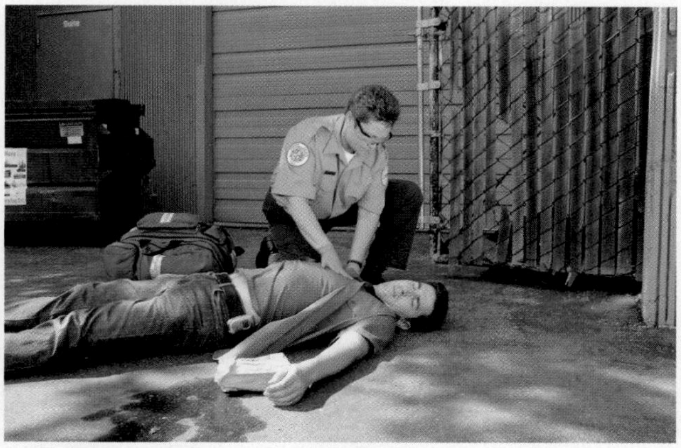

Figure 3-6 Patients who are unresponsive can be cared for based on implied consent.

the more common reasons for the emancipation of a minor are marriage, pregnancy, and enlistment in the armed forces. In most cases, emancipation requires an action by the courts and is rarely encountered.

> **PERSPECTIVE**
>
> **Brandon—The EMT**
>
> You know, I'm not sure if that caregiver can legally refuse care for Mr. Flowers. She may be his legal guardian, but does that give her that right? I really feel that he needs to be seen by a doctor, and it's not like he's the one refusing care.

Patients who do not have capacity because of mental illness or as a result of their illness or injury may be cared for legally based on implied consent. One of the most common reasons for a patient to be deemed not to have the capacity to understand the situation is intoxication from drugs or alcohol. However, although you have the legal right to provide care based on implied consent, the patient may still attempt to refuse your help. In those instances, it is appropriate to call for assistance from law enforcement.

Patients Who Refuse Care

3-10 Discuss the actions you should take when confronted with a patient who refuses care.

As stated earlier, any patient of legal age who is competent and who has capacity may refuse care at any time. Parents and legal guardians may refuse care on behalf of those for whom they are responsible. Competent adults may refuse care even after it has been initiated and they are on the way to the hospital.

As an EMT you have specific responsibilities when dealing with patients who refuse your care. First, you must make every effort to convince the patient that providing consent and allowing you to provide care is in his best interest. You must clearly explain the risks and consequences of the decision to refuse care, and you must feel certain that the patient understands what you are telling him. If all of those conditions are met and a patient still refuses care, it is common practice to ask the patient to sign a release form. The forms are sometimes referred to as *against-medical-advice (AMA) forms* and, in theory, they release the medical team from liability should the patient's condition worsen later (Figure 3-7 ■).

If you are ever in doubt as to whether the patient truly has capacity or if, in your opinion, the patient really needs further medical attention, you should err on the side of caution. Depending on the situation, you may need to contact medical direction, your supervisor, or in extreme cases, law enforcement personnel. In cases where the patient is refusing care but you feel he should receive care or risk serious harm or death, in some jurisdictions a law enforcement officer can place the patient on a legal hold and force him to accept the appropriate medical attention. In all cases of patient refusal, seek a second opinion from your partner or other EMS provider on scene. It is unwise to make an independent decision not to transport.

Proper documentation is always important when providing care for an ill or injured person. It becomes especially important in cases of refusal because of the possibility that the patient's condition may worsen. Be diligent in your documentation of such cases. Include details about your assessment of the patient, your attempts to convince the patient to agree to care, and any witnesses to the patient's refusal. When possible, have the patient sign a form that documents his refusal. In some cases, the patient will even refuse to sign the form. In those instances, have another EMS, fire, or law enforcement official sign the form as a witness to the refusal.

Coastal Valleys EMS Agency

Serving Mendocino, Napa and Sonoma Counties

Applicable for:
✓ Napa County
✓ Sonoma County
✓ Mendocino County

RAS/AMA FORM

Date ____________ ALS # ____________ Dispatch # ____________

Section I Release at Scene (RAS)

I understand that any evaluation and/or emergency treatment I have received by these EMS personnel has been on an emergency basis only and is not intended to be a substitute for complete medical assessment and/or care. I understand it appears that further emergency transportation and/or care does not appear to be needed at this time. I understand that I may have an illness or injury that is unforeseen at this time. I understand that if I change my mind or if my condition changes or becomes worse and I need further treatment/transportation by the Emergency Medical Services System, I can call back and they will respond.

Patient Name (print)____________ Patient Signature____________

Patient / Guardian Signature____________ Relationship____________

Paramedic / EMT signature____________ Witness Signature____________

Comments: ____________

Section II Refusal of Evaluation / Treatment / Transportation Against Medical Advice (AMA)

I, ____________ acknowledge that on ____________
Patient Name (print) Date

____________ / ____________ / ____________
EMT-Paramedic/EMT License/Cert # Service Provider Agency

explained my condition to me and advised me of some of the potential risks and/or complications which could or would arise from refusal of medical care. I have also been advised that other unknown risks and/or complications are possible up to and including the loss of life or limb. Being aware that there are known and unknown potential risks and/or complications, it is still my desire to refuse the advised medical care.

- All Care Refused
- Specific Care Refused: ____________

I do hereby release EMS personnel from all liability resulting from any adverse medical condition(s) caused by my refusal of the recommended medical care.

Patient Signature____________ Paramedic / EMT Signature____________

Patient / Guardian Signature____________ Relationship____________

Witness Name:____________ Witness Signature____________

Comments: ____________

DATE: June 2003 R & T Page 44

Figure 3-7 A patient who refuses care should be asked to sign a release form. (Coastal Valley EMS Agency)

CLINICAL CLUE

Release at Scene

In some EMS systems an additional document called a *Release at Scene (RAS)* is used when both the patient and EMTs feel that ambulance transport is not necessary. This option respects the rights of a competent adult who wishes to seek medical care but does not want to be transported by ambulance. In most cases, specific criteria must be met before a patient can be appropriately released at the scene. It is important to find out if such a form or policy exists in your EMS system. If in doubt, contact medical direction.

PERSPECTIVE

Janine—The Caregiver

I just don't have time for this. I've got 14 patients I have to see each and every day. Henry is fine. Heck, I don't even remember how many times he's fallen down in the past. It's not that big of a deal. These ambulance people must be new or something.

3-11 Explain each of the following legal protections for EMTs: sovereign immunity, statutes of limitations, and contributory negligence of the patient.

statute of limitations the maximum time after an event that legal proceedings based on that event may be initiated.

contributory negligence any behavior on the part of the patient that may have led to the injuries being described in a negligence lawsuit.

sovereign immunity a legal term used to describe the exemption provided to a governmental entity from being sued in its own courts without permission.

Additional Legal Concepts

Statute of limitations is defined as the maximum time after an event that legal proceedings based on that event may be initiated. All 50 states have well-defined laws that govern when and how a lawsuit may be filed. Lawsuits claiming negligence are no exception. When a patient feels that he is the victim of negligence, he has a specified time frame for which to file a lawsuit in order for the courts to recognize and hear the case. The statute of limitations may vary depending on the type of case. A lawsuit that is filed after the statute of limitations has expired may be dismissed by the court.

Some states have laws regarding contributory negligence. **Contributory negligence** is a legal term that refers to any behavior on the part of the patient that may have led to the injuries being described in a negligence lawsuit. If it is discovered that the patient's own behavior contributed to the damages he is claiming, he may not be entitled to compensation.

Sovereign immunity is a legal term used to describe the exemption provided to a governmental entity from being sued in its own courts without permission. Under the concept of sovereign immunity, most EMS services provided by governmental agencies are generally immune from lawsuits from private parties. Private EMS agencies typically do not benefit from the protections offered by sovereign immunity.

3-12 Compare and contrast the application of each of the following types of advance directives: do not resuscitate (DNR) order, living will, durable power of attorney, and physician orders for life-sustaining treatment.

advance directive a legal statement of a patient's wishes regarding his own health care.

Advance Directives

An **advance directive** is a legal statement of a patient's wishes regarding his own health care. It is becoming increasingly common for patients to provide such specific instructions. So, as an EMT it is only a matter of time before you will encounter a patient with one form or another of an advance directive.

Advance directives come in different forms and address a variety of health care issues. In most states, an advance directive must be in writing and in the presence of the patient at all times. Some states will accept an advance directive in the form of medical identification jewelry. Your instructor will provide the details of acceptable advance directives in your state or region.

One form of advance directive is a written document known as a *living will*. In it the patient may provide detailed instructions for his health care in the event he becomes too ill to let his wishes be known. It may describe which treatments and care the patient wants and which he does not want should he be unable to communicate. This document is typically signed by the patient and his physician.

Another type of advance directive is the **do not resuscitate (DNR) order** (Figure 3-8 ■). Its purpose is to advise health care professionals that the patient does not want to be resuscitated in the event of a cardiac or respiratory arrest. There are variations of DNR order that indicate specific care that can or cannot be initiated. For instance, a terminally ill patient may wish to continue to receive pain medication as his condition worsens, but should he go into cardiac arrest he does not want anyone to begin

do not resuscitate (DNR) order a legal document, usually signed by the patient and his physician, which states that the patient has a terminal illness and does not wish to prolong life through resuscitative efforts.

PREHOSPITAL DO NOT RESUSCITATE ORDERS

ATTENDING PHYSICIAN

In completing this prehospital DNR form, please check part A if no intervention by prehospital personnel is indicated. Please check Part A and options from Part B if specific interventions by prehospital personnel are indicated. To give a valid prehospital DNR order, this form must be completed by the patient's attending physician and must be provided to prehospital personnel.

A) ____________ **Do Not Resuscitate (DNR):**
No Cardiopulmonary Resuscitation or Advanced Cardiac Life Support be performed by prehospital personnel

B) ____________ **Modified Support:**
Prehospital personnel administer the following checked options:

____________ Oxygen administration
____________ Full airway support: intubation, airways, bag/valve/mask
____________ Venipuncture: IV crystalloids and/or blood draw
____________ External cardiac pacing
____________ Cardiopulmonary resuscitation
____________ Cardiac defibrillator
____________ Pneumatic anti-shock garment
____________ Ventilator
____________ ACLS meds
____________ Other interventions/medications (physician specify)
____

Prehospital personnel are informed that (print patient name)____________ should receive no resuscitation (DNR) or should receive Modified Support as indicated. This directive is medically appropriate and is further documented by a physician's order and a progress note on the patient's permanent medical record. Informed consent from the capacitated patient or the incapacitated patient's legitimate surrogate is documented on the patient's permanent medical record. The DNR order is in full force and effect as of the date indicated below.

____
Attending Physician's Signature

____
Print Attending Physician's Name

____
Attending Physician's Telephone

____
Date

____
____
____
Print Patient's Name and Location
(Home Address or Health Care Facility)

____
Expiration Date (6 Mos from Signature)

Figure 3-8 An example of an advance directive is the do not resuscitate (DNR) order.

CPR. Another patient may state that he would like to be ventilated should he stop breathing on his own, but if his heart stops he does not want anyone initiating chest compressions.

As an EMT who is called to the scene of a patient with a DNR order, you must insist on seeing a written copy of the order to determine the specifics and nature of the order. Without documented proof of a DNR order, you will be compelled to begin resuscitative efforts. In any case where there is confusion regarding the presence of a DNR order, it is best to begin care until the DNR order can be confirmed or you have transferred care to the hospital.

All states have provisions that allow a family member or other designated individual to make decisions regarding the health care of another person. This is usually in the form of a legal document known as a *durable power of attorney for health care (DPAHC)*. DPAHCs are common when the patient is diagnosed with a terminal illness and is likely to become incapacitated prior to succumbing to the illness.

Another document that is becoming more and more common is known as *physician orders for life-sustaining treatment (POLST)*. Many states have developed or are developing standardized documents that define the specific care that should be provided during the last days and hours of a patient's life. The instructions contained in a POLST are a collaboration between the patient, the patient's family or other loved ones, and caregivers, and are designed to improve the quality of care during the end of life.

STOP, REVIEW, REMEMBER!

Multiple Choice

For each question, place a check next to the correct answer.

1. Which one of the following is the best example of expressed consent?

_____ a. Confused drunken 20-year-old who agrees to allow you to provide care

_____ b. Frightened six-year-old who just sits there and allows you to help

_____ c. Wife who provides consent for her unresponsive husband

_____ d. 40-year-old who asks for assistance

2. Which one of the following statements about a competent adult with capacity is most accurate?

_____ a. He may refuse care at any time.

_____ b. Once care has begun, he may not refuse.

_____ c. Only a law enforcement officer can determine if he is competent.

_____ d. An EMT may restrain him or any patient who is determined to be incompetent.

3. Which type of consent would be used for an 11-year-old unresponsive patient whose parents are not immediately available?

_____ a. Informed

_____ b. Expressed

_____ c. Implied

_____ d. Assumed

4. Before leaving a patient who is refusing care, the EMT must do all of the following *except*:

_____ a. explain that proper care is in her best interest.

_____ b. threaten to call the police if she does not provide consent.

_____ c. explain to her the risks of a decision to refuse care.

_____ d. have her sign a release form.

5. Which one of the following is the most accurate definition of an advance directive?
   _____ a. Legal statement of a patient's wishes regarding health care
   _____ b. Family's verbal wishes regarding the care of a loved one
   _____ c. Patient's verbal refusal of any further care
   _____ d. Patient's wishes regarding funeral arrangements

6. Leaving a patient before formally transferring care to an appropriate health care provider may be considered:
   _____ a. within the EMT scope of practice.
   _____ b. standard practice.
   _____ c. abandonment.
   _____ d. part of the duty to act.

Matching

Match the definition on the left with the applicable term on the right.

1. _____ Permission from the patient to provide care
2. _____ Consent that is obtained from alert, competent adult patients with capacity
3. _____ Legal term used to describe an assumed permission to treat
4. _____ Term used to describe someone who is able to make informed and rational decisions about his own well-being
5. _____ Situation in which an EMT had a legal duty to provide care but left the patient before turning care of the patient over to someone of equal or higher training
6. _____ Legal statement of a patient's wishes regarding his own health care
7. _____ Form advising health care professionals that the patient does not want to be resuscitated in the event of a cardiac or respiratory arrest

A. Implied consent
B. Competent/capacity
C. Advance directive
D. Abandonment
E. DNR
F. Consent
G. Expressed consent

Critical Thinking

1. In what ways might a responsive adult patient provide consent for treatment? Must it always be verbal?

____

____

____

____

2. In what situations might it be difficult to determine if a patient has the capacity to refuse care?

____

____

____

____

(continued on next page)

(continued)

3. How might you handle a situation in which the family states that there is a DNR order but they cannot produce a copy of it?

____

____

____

____

Negligence

3-13 Differentiate between criminal and civil liability.

There are essentially two types of lawsuits that an EMT may be named in as a defendant. A *criminal lawsuit* is one that is brought against a defendant by the government on behalf of the public. If the defendant of a criminal case is found guilty, he may have to pay a fine and/or serve time in jail or prison. The other type of lawsuit is known as a *civil lawsuit*, or *tort*. In a civil lawsuit an individual known as the plaintiff files a suit against a defendant claiming a breach of some civil duty. The defendant may be an individual EMT, an ambulance agency, or anyone else directly involved in the care of the patient. In a tort case the defendant is accused of committing a wrongful act or omission resulting in injury to the plaintiff (patient). In a successful tort case the plaintiff is usually awarded some form of monetary award as compensation for the damages endured. In EMS the most common tort is one that alleges negligence.

3-14 Explain the concept of *negligence*.

Negligence is another of those fundamental terms that every EMT must understand thoroughly. It refers to the omission or neglect of reasonable care, precaution, or action. As an EMT you must provide what is considered to be a reasonable standard of care for your patient and make every attempt to minimize any further harm.

3-15 List and explain the elements required for a successful negligence lawsuit.

For an accusation of negligence to hold up in a court of law, four specific elements must exist. Those elements are:

- ***Duty to act.*** It must be established that the EMT had a legal duty to provide care to the person making the accusation, in this case the patient.
- ***Breach of duty.*** It must be determined that the EMT breached his duty in some form or manner. A breach is a failure to live up to a legal obligation such as the EMT's duty to provide medical care. Providing care outside one's scope of practice also may be considered a breach of duty.
- ***Damages.*** It must be proven that the patient suffered some form of actual physical or emotional damages.
- ***Causation (proximate cause).*** It must be proven that the actions or lack thereof by the EMT actually caused the damages being alleged. In most unsuccessful negligence suits, this is where the argument falls apart.

The EMT is not expected to become a virtual lawyer, but it is important to develop a good understanding of key legal terms and concepts. Together with an equal dose of common sense and experience, that knowledge will go a long way to help keep you from being named or found guilty in a lawsuit.

Abandonment

3-16 Give examples of ways you can avoid a claim of abandonment.

Abandonment is a legal term that the EMT should study and understand thoroughly. It refers to a situation in which an EMT has a legal duty to provide care but leaves or abandons the patient before turning care of the patient over to someone of equal or higher training. For a case involving an accusation of abandonment to hold up, it must first be established that the EMT had a legal duty to care for the patient.

Although on the surface that may seem obvious, most cases of abandonment are much more subtle. For example, imagine that you and your partner are working a busy EMS system and are on your third call. As you wheel your chest-pain patient into the busy emergency department, you catch the attention of one of the nurses who tells you to put your patient in Room 3 and that she will be right there. While transferring the patient to the hospital bed, you receive a dispatch over your radio for a vehicle collision on the other side of town. You quickly finish getting the patient onto the hospital bed, gather up your supplies and, as you are heading out the door, yell to the nurse that you have another call. However, the nurse is so busy that it is 15 minutes before she gets a chance to check on your patient. When she does, she finds him on the bed without respirations or a pulse.

It will not be difficult for an attorney to establish that you and your partner had abandoned this patient, because you left him without formally transferring care to someone of equal or higher training. Simply yelling at the nurse that you were leaving on another call is not what most would consider a formal transfer of care. You must provide a detailed verbal report directly to the person who is taking over care. In many instances you also will leave a copy of your written report, which becomes part of the patient's permanent medical record.

Assault and Battery

3-17 Describe how the EMT can avoid claims of assault and/or battery and false imprisonment/kidnapping.

Although it is quite rare, an EMT who attempts to force care on a patient may be accused of a tort known as *assault* and/or *battery*. **Assault** is the threat to use force on another, and **battery** is the carrying out of that threat. It is important to understand that assault can be alleged even when no physical contact is made. Simply threatening to inflict physical contact against a patient's wishes can be construed as assault.

assault a legal term referring to the threat to use force on another.

battery a legal term referring to the carrying out of a threat to use force on another.

An accusation of battery requires actual unwanted physical contact between the EMT and the patient. This can occur when attempting to care for a combative patient. Unless law enforcement is there to assist, it is not wise to make contact with a patient who is refusing care. Even a simple touch, if unwanted, can constitute battery. In cases where the patient has become a threat to himself, the EMT, or others, it may become necessary to restrain the patient for safety purposes. Those situations are relatively rare and should be documented thoroughly, including statements from any witnesses at the scene.

It is always best to enlist the assistance of law enforcement before attempting to restrain a patient. A patient for whom you provide care against his will or unlawfully restrain may claim false imprisonment and, if you transport against his will, kidnapping.

Patient Transfers

Emergency Medical Treatment and Active Labor Act (EMTALA)

3-19 Describe EMTALA provisions as they apply to EMS.

In 1986 the U.S. government enacted the **Emergency Medical Treatment and Active Labor Act (EMTALA).** This act is often referred to as the *anti-patient-dumping act*. Patient dumping is the refusal of a hospital to provide care for anyone needing medical attention, or the intentional transfer of a patient to another facility without first providing needed medical care. Patient dumping was a common practice in the early 1980s when a hospital would refuse care or transfer a patient to another facility simply because the patient was unable to pay for medical care.

Emergency Medical Treatment and Active Labor Act (EMTALA) passed in 1986, this act requires hospitals to provide care to anyone needing emergency health care treatment regardless of citizenship, legal status, or ability to pay.

Under EMTALA, any patient who presents at a hospital emergency department is entitled to an appropriate medical screening and any needed medical care regardless of the ability to pay for that care. EMTALA prohibits discrimination based solely on a patient's ability to pay.

EMTALA also prohibits the transfer of a patient from one facility to another without specific permission (acceptance) by the receiving facility. In the early 1980s, hospitals would simply call for an ambulance and transfer a patient to another hospital without first confirming that the receiving hospital could accept the patient. Today, any hospital wishing to transfer a patient regardless of the reason must first receive acceptance from the receiving hospital and confirm that they have both a bed for the patient and a physician willing to care for the patient.

As an EMT who is transporting patients from emergency scenes to hospitals and from hospital to hospital, it is important to understand the laws that govern when a hospital may legally refuse a patient.

Transporting and Transferring Patient Care

An area of legal risk for the EMT involves patient transfers. They can take many forms but the most common include the EMT deciding where to transport a patient and transferring patient care to another health care provider. When deciding how and where to transport a patient, you must always keep the patient's best interest in mind, regardless of his condition or ability to pay for medical services. Choosing the most appropriate facility, typically the closest, is almost always the right choice. If in doubt, follow local protocol or contact medical direction for advice.

Not all hospitals have the same capabilities when it comes to patient care, so you may be called on to transfer a patient from one facility to another. This is known as an *interfacility transfer (IFT)*. Before accepting such a transfer, it is essential that you confirm the care the patient is receiving is within your scope of practice. If the patient is intubated and on a ventilator or has multiple medication drips running, he may require a higher level of care such as a paramedic or nurse. Be certain that the patient's needs are clearly within your scope of practice before accepting the transfer.

Another area of legal risk for the EMT is the transfer of care from one health care provider to another. It is normal and expected for an EMT to hand off the care of a patient to the next level of care whether it be outside a hospital or inside. The important thing to remember is that the transfer of care must be formal and clearly articulated. You must transfer care to someone of equal or higher training, and you must provide a formal verbal report to the person accepting care. You may not simply bring your patient into the emergency department, transfer him to an available bed, and alert the nurse that you left the patient in room "C."

When transferring a patient to another health care provider, whether at the scene or at a hospital to a nurse or physician, you must provide a detailed report about the patient's chief complaint, assessment findings, care provided, and any changes in the patient's condition following your interventions.

Patient Confidentiality

3-18 Explain the legal and ethical responsibilities concerning confidentiality and privacy.

Health Insurance Portability and Accountability Act (HIPAA) federal legislation enacted in 1996 that protects the privacy of patient health care information.

More than ever before in the history of EMS the concept of *patient confidentiality* is being stressed and enforced. Legislation called the **Health Insurance Portability and Accountability Act (HIPAA)** has imposed a number of restrictions on how health care providers may use and share patient information.

PERSPECTIVE

Jewel—The EMT

This whole situation stinks. This old man is definitely not receiving the quality of care that he deserves. Heck, his sheets are just plain nasty. He's got bedsores that are obviously infected, and he doesn't look like he's eaten in days. This is just plain neglect. Pure and simple. Somebody should do something about it!

As an EMT you have access to a significant amount of personal information about patients. This can include information such as where they live, their age, their medical history, their employment, and their insurance status. You must keep in mind that any information you gather about a patient is considered confidential and must not be shared with others except in very specific circumstances.

You may legally share information with other health care providers who will be taking over care of the patient, but you may share only information that directly affects patient care and may not share other, nonmedical information. In order to legally share confidential information with other individuals such as law enforcement officers or attorneys, you may need prior written consent from the patient or receive a legal subpoena for release of the information (Figure 3-9 ■).

It is important to learn what your agency's policy is regarding patient confidentiality. Just to be on the safe side, it may be best to refer all such requests to your supervisor.

Special Reporting Situations

3-21 Describe situations in which the EMT may be mandated to make a report, such as suspected abuse and crimes.

Most states have laws that identify specific situations for which EMTs must report what they see or hear. The most common situations involve cases of known or suspected abuse or neglect that involve a child, the elderly, or a spouse. Should you ever care for someone you suspect is a victim of abuse or neglect, you may be required by law to report it. Immediately discuss any such case with your supervisor, who will probably be more knowledgeable about the reporting laws in your state.

Other mandatory reporting laws regard situations that involve a crime such as sexual assault or injuries sustained from a firearm. It is highly likely that you will be mandated by the laws in your state to report those cases to the proper authorities.

Crime Scenes

3-22 Discuss special considerations in responding to potential crime scenes.

At times you may be called to provide care for someone injured or ill at a known or suspected crime scene. In those instances, a law enforcement officer will probably be dispatched to the scene ahead of the ambulance. Should you arrive at the scene of an emergency and suspect that it may involve a crime, you should request law enforcement immediately. Remember that you do not have an obligation to put yourself at undue risk to assist an injured or ill person. The scene must be safe before you can enter (Figure 3-10 ■).

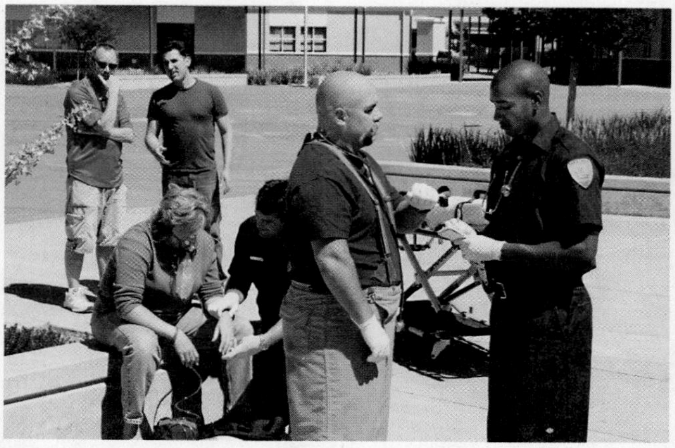

Figure 3-9 To maintain patient confidentiality, discuss your patient only with those who will be continuing patient care.

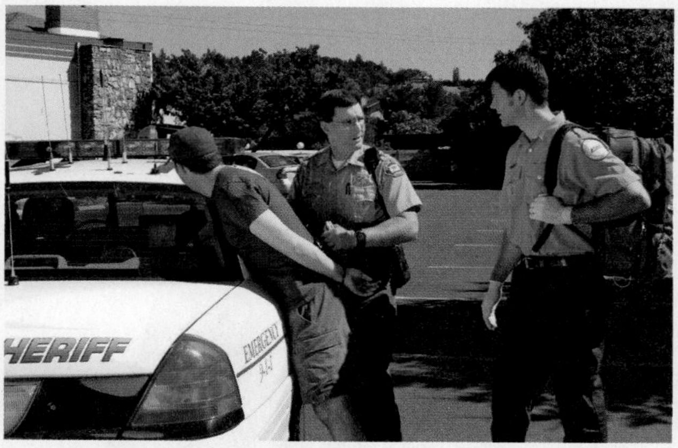

Figure 3-10 A law enforcement officer should be requested at a suspected crime scene.

Once you have been called into the scene by law enforcement, your primary duty is to provide excellent patient care to those who need it without disturbing the scene more than absolutely necessary. You may need to document your findings in more detail than usual, because the call may be involved in a future court case. Pay attention to and document as much detail as you can about the scene as you found it. Document where you entered the scene and where you were at all times within the scene. Observe and document anything that may seem unusual about the scene or the patient. Be careful not to disturb potential evidence at the scene or on the patient. If possible, when removing clothing from your patient, cut around, not through, obvious bullet or stab holes in the patient's clothing.

Potential Organ Donors

3-20 Describe special considerations for patients who are potential organ donors.

More and more people are becoming educated about organ donation and are choosing to be identified as a potential organ donor should they die. The most common form of identification for an organ donor is the card that accompanies the typical driver's license. Sometimes there is a small sticker with the word *Donor* on it that is placed on the front of the driver's license, or there may be a check-off section on the back of the license that indicates the person's wish to be an organ donor.

As an EMT you are likely to encounter patients who have designated themselves as potential donors. Do not let this information change the way in which you care for them. In most instances, the patient is transported to the hospital before death is declared. Continue resuscitative efforts according to your local protocols and advise hospital personnel and/or medical direction of the patient's donor status.

Medical Identification Jewelry

A number of private companies manufacture specialized medical identification jewelry. The most common forms of medical jewelry are the necklace and the bracelet (Figure 3-11 ■). Some people prefer to wear their medical jewelry around the ankle so that it is less obvious to the general public. Medical identification also can take other forms, such as a wallet card or small tag placed on a key ring, watchband, or belt.

The purpose of medical identification jewelry or cards is to alert others to the person's existing medical conditions should the wearer become unresponsive. The most commonly identified are conditions such as diabetes, allergies, epilepsy, and heart conditions.

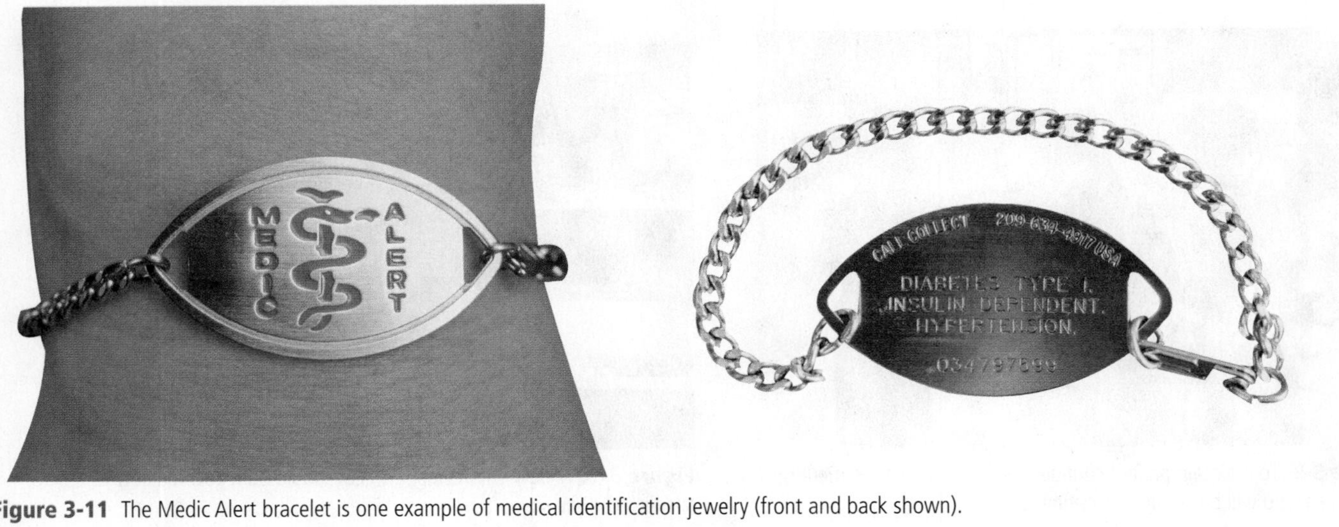

Figure 3-11 The Medic Alert bracelet is one example of medical identification jewelry (front and back shown).

STOP, REVIEW, REMEMBER!

Multiple Choice

For each question, place a check next to the correct answer.

1. Which one of the following definitions best describes the term *assault?*

_____ a. Inflicting physical harm to another person

_____ b. Verbal threat to use force on another person

_____ c. Holding another person against his will

_____ d. Verbal abuse

2. Which one of the following actions could most likely be considered a breach of duty by an EMT?

_____ a. Providing high-flow oxygen to an emphysema patient in acute distress

_____ b. Transporting an unresponsive child without a parent's consent

_____ c. Leaving the scene of one emergency to respond to another emergency before additional help arrives

_____ d. Assisting a chest-pain patient with taking his nitro pills

3. Which one of the following is *not* one of the four elements of a case of suspected negligence?

_____ a. Duty to act

_____ b. Breach of duty

_____ c. Abandonment

_____ d. Causation

4. Which one of the following best describes the EMT's role in regard to patient confidentiality?

_____ a. All information obtained by the EMT may be shared with others so long as it is done in private.

_____ b. Only information documented on the patient care report may be shared with others.

_____ c. The EMT may not share any information about the patient with anyone.

_____ d. The EMT may share information with those who are directly involved with the care of the patient.

5. An EMT who provides care outside the scope of practice could be guilty of:

_____ a. breach of duty.

_____ b. abandonment.

_____ c. causation.

_____ d. scopus exceedus.

Matching

Match the definition on the left with the applicable term on the right.

1. _____ Threat to use force on another
2. _____ Carrying out of a threat to do harm to another
3. _____ Omission or neglect of reasonable care, precaution, or action
4. _____ Legal obligation to provide care
5. _____ Failure to live up to a legal obligation
6. _____ Some form of actual physical or emotional damages
7. _____ Actions or lack thereof that actually caused damage to the patient

A. Causation
B. Negligence
C. Breach of duty
D. Damages
E. Duty
F. Battery
G. Assault

(continued on next page)

(continued)

Critical Thinking

1. Describe the difference between the legal terms *assault* and *battery*.

2. Describe a situation whereby an EMT could be accused of negligence.

3. Describe the steps you would take if you were working as an EMT and suspected that a child or elder is being abused or neglected.

EMERGENCY DISPATCH SUMMARY

Brandon and Jewel argued with Mr. Flowers's caregiver that he needed to be taken to the hospital. She finally relented and then stormed from the house on her way to the "next appointment."

Further evaluation of Henry revealed an elevated blood pressure and marked weakness on his left side. Mr. Flowers was placed on high-flow oxygen and transported to Young America Memorial Hospital where he was treated for a stroke, pneumonia, and gangrenous pressure sores.

Sadly, Mr. Flowers died three weeks later after being moved to a skilled nursing facility.

Chapter Review

To the Point

- The scope of practice is what the EMT is legally allowed to do. The standard of care is the care the EMT is expected to provide as defined by local protocols and regulations.
- As an EMT you work under the direction of a physician known as the *medical director*.
- You must perform your duties to the highest ethical and moral standards based on clearly defined personal and professional values.
- As an EMT you have a legal duty to act and must obtain consent from any patient before providing emergency care.
- Use extreme caution when managing patients who refuse care. Make sure the patient has capacity and fully understands the ramifications of the refusal decision.
- Familiarize yourself with the various forms of advance directives and how you should manage each of them.
- A breach of duty could result in either a criminal or civil action against you. The most common tort is one of negligence.
- A successful negligence suit involves four elements: duty to act, breach of duty, damages, and causation (proximate cause).
- Forcing care on a patient can result in a claim of assault and/or battery. Leaving a patient before transferring care to someone of equal or higher training may result in a claim of abandonment.
- All information related to the care of a patient must be kept confidential and only shared with those who are permitted by law to receive the information.
- You will care for a patient the same as any other patient, regardless if you discover he is an organ donor or not. Follow local protocols and transport to the most appropriate receiving facility.
- It is important to learn the laws in your state regarding your role as a mandated reporter. At a minimum all states have laws requiring EMS personnel to report suspected cases of abuse and neglect.
- Be particularly alert when caring for patients at a crime scene. Do your best not to disturb or destroy potential evidence but remember that patient care comes first.

Chapter Questions

Multiple Choice

For each question, place a check next to the correct answer.

1. A detailed description of the specific care and actions EMTs are allowed to perform based on state laws and regulations is the:
   _____ a. standard of care.
   _____ b. scope of practice.
   _____ c. national standard curriculum.
   _____ d. national scope of care.

2. Physician orders for life-sustaining treatment are designed to ensure:
   _____ a. the quality of care at end of life.
   _____ b. all appropriate life-saving measures are attempted.
   _____ c. that CPR is not performed.
   _____ d. that only oxygen is provided during cardiac arrest.

3. Which one of the following statements about the concept of *consent* is most accurate?
   _____ a. Verbal consent must be obtained from all patients regardless of age.
   _____ b. Parents do not have the right to refuse care for their children.
   _____ c. Consent can come in many forms, including verbal, nonverbal, and written.
   _____ d. It is not necessary to seek consent for treatment of a minor.

(continued on next page)

(continued)

4. An EMT who ceases to provide care to a patient before formally handing off the patient to someone of equal or higher training may be accused of:

_____ a. abandonment.
_____ b. battery.
_____ c. assault.
_____ d. causation.

5. Which of the following are EMTs required to report to the appropriate authorities?

_____ a. Abuse and neglect
_____ b. Abuse and Alzheimer's
_____ c. Negligence and neglect
_____ d. Abandonment and negligence

6. Consent to treat an unresponsive patient is referred to as:

_____ a. parental.
_____ b. expressed.
_____ c. implied.
_____ d. verbal.

7. You are caring for a patient in cardiac arrest and learn from a family member that the patient is an organ donor. You should:

_____ a. transport the patient to the nearest organ transplant center.
_____ b. stop all care and transport to the nearest hospital.
_____ c. continue care and transport to the most appropriate hospital.
_____ d. stop all care and call the coroner.

8. The primary responsibility of an EMT at a crime scene is:

_____ a. preservation of evidence.
_____ b. assisting with the investigation.
_____ c. patient care.
_____ d. collection of evidence.

9. Which organization created the EMS National Education Standards?

_____ a. U.S. Department of Labor
_____ b. World Health Organization
_____ c. Centers for Disease Control and Prevention
_____ d. U.S. Department of Transportation

10. Physically touching another person without that person's consent may be considered:

_____ a. assault.
_____ b. battery.
_____ c. negligence.
_____ d. causation.

Critical Thinking

1. Describe a situation when it might be necessary to use force to restrain a patient you are caring for.

____

____

____

____

2. As a passerby to a motor vehicle collision, are you legally obligated to stop and render care? What is the law in your state?

____

____

____

____

3. How might your care change if you discovered that the patient you were caring for was an organ donor?

Case Studies

Case Study 1

You are on your way home from EMT class one evening on a remote section of a two-lane highway, when you come across an SUV that has rolled over on the side of the road. The wheels on the overturned vehicle are still spinning as you approach the scene. Your heart begins to race as you consider the prospect of stopping and rendering care. You are only three weeks into your EMT class and are very unsure if you will know what to do. As you slowly approach the scene, you see one person lying face down on the opposite side of the road from the vehicle and another person moving about inside the overturned vehicle.

1. What do the laws in your state say about your legal obligation to stop and render aid in situations such as this?

2. What are the legal ramifications if you decide not to stop and just keep going?

3. You have decided to help. Following a brief assessment of the unresponsive victim lying outside the vehicle, you are unable to tell if she is breathing or has a pulse. In a moment of panic you decide to get back in your car and leave the scene. What are the legal ramifications of your actions?

Case Study 2

You have been called to a residence for difficulty breathing. On arrival you find a 56-year-old man with terminal lung cancer. The patient's respirations are shallow and very labored at a rate of 8 per minute. You begin to ventilate the patient using a bag-mask device. After a minute or so, family members advise you that the patient has a DNR order. When you ask to see it, they show you a medical identification bracelet on the patient's wrist indicating a DNR.

1. How would you handle this situation?

____

____

____

____

2. What forms can a DNR take in your state?

____

____

____

____

3. What would you do if the family insists you continue care?

____

____

____

____

The Last Word

Much of what EMTs do is directed or governed by laws, guidelines, protocols, and policies, but they differ from state to state and region to region. Learn and understand those that affect EMT practice in your system. Do not ever forget that first and foremost you are there for the patient. If you make decisions based on what is right for the patient, it will be difficult for others to question your motives. What you see and do at work as an EMT should stay there. Respect patient confidentiality at all times.

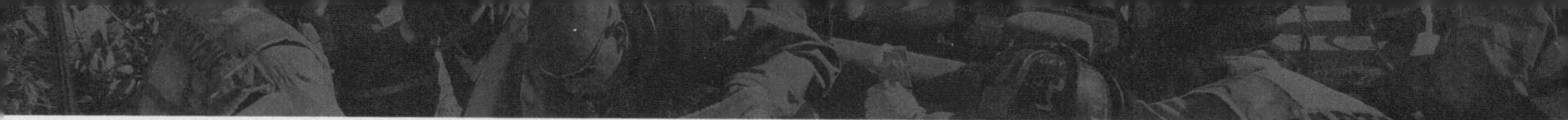

Medical Terminology

4

Education Standards

Anatomy and Physiology: Medical Terminology

Competencies

Applies fundamental knowledge of the anatomy and function of all human systems to the practice of EMS.
Uses foundational anatomical and medical terms and abbreviations in written and oral communication with colleagues and other health professionals.

Objectives

After completion of this lesson, you should be able to:

4-1 Define key terms introduced in this chapter.

4-2 Describe each of the following terms of position: anatomical position, Fowler's position, lateral recumbent position, prone, semi-Fowler's position, shock position, supine, and Trendelenburg position.

4-3 Identify each of the following anatomical terms: abdominal quadrants (right upper quadrant, left upper quadrant, left lower quadrant, right lower quadrant), anterior and posterior, dorsal and ventral, frontal plane, medial and lateral, midaxillary line, midclavicular line, midline, palmar, plantar, proximal and distal, right and left, sagittal plane, superior and inferior, and transverse plane.

4-4 Explain the importance of knowledge of medical terminology in communication among health care team members.

4-5 Apply knowledge of common prefixes, suffixes, and roots to interpret medical terms.

Key Terms

acronym p. 85
anatomical position p. 79
anterior p. 81
bilateral p. 80
cephalic p. 81
combining form p. 74
distal p. 83
dorsal p. 81
Fowler's position p. 83
gastric p. 81
inferior p. 83
lateral p. 80
lateral recumbent position p. 83
left p. 79
medial p. 80
midaxillary line p. 81
midclavicular line p. 81
midline p. 80
palmar p. 81
plane p. 79
plantar p. 81
posterior p. 81
prefix p. 74
prone p. 83
proximal p. 83
right p. 79
root word p. 74
semi-Fowler's position p. 83
shock position p. 83
suffix p. 74
superior p. 83
supine p. 83
Trendelenburg position p. 83
ventral p. 81

Introduction

4-4 Explain the importance of knowledge of medical terminology in communication among health care team members.

As an EMT you will become part of a health care team comprised of different levels of providers. EMTs, nurses, doctors, and other practitioners must work together to provide the highest level of patient care. A key principle of providing excellent care is concise communication. Knowledge of medical terminology forms the basis for a language shared among all health care professionals. Using specific and precise language as an EMT will improve your ability to identify and describe anatomy, and it will assist you in adding precision to your descriptions of patient position and location. Furthermore, a working knowledge of basic medical terminology will make it easier for you to understand more complex terms.

Medical terminology can be challenging. In many ways it is like learning a new language. It is important for you to rise to this challenge because not only is medical terminology useful, it is the language of your new profession.

EMERGENCY DISPATCH

EMTs Heather and her partner, Dan, are just finishing lunch when they hear the dispatcher request their unit. "Control 176, priority two. Respond to 1292 Midland Avenue for a 66-year-old woman with a possible broken ankle."

Heather and Dan secure their seat belts and respond, weaving their way through the crowded midday traffic. When they arrive at the address, they see two to three people crowded around a woman lying next to the front step of a small house. Heather scans the scene as Dan pulls the ambulance up to the curb. Everything seems reasonably safe, so they gather the appropriate equipment and approach the patient.

Heather reaches the patient first and says, "Ma'am, please don't move your head. My name is Heather, and we are going to help you."

Roots of Medical Terminology

root word the main part of a word with all prefixes and suffixes removed.

Many medical terms are created by combining prefixes, suffixes, and common root words. **Root words** are terms that are used to describe or refer to an anatomical system or location. Often root words are developed from a Greek or Latin translation. For example, a common root word used to describe the liver would be *hepat* (or *hepatic*). *Hepat* comes from the Greek word for liver and is frequently used to form other terms referring to the liver or liver function.

It is also common in medicine to see root words used as descriptors. For example, *brady* is derived from the Greek word for *slow* and is frequently used in terms such as *bradycardia* (slow heart rate) to describe things that are slow. *Cyano* is derived from the Greek word for *blue* and is frequently used in terms such as *cyanosis* (blue skin) to describe things that have a bluish tint. Lists of common root words can be found in Tables 4-1 and 4-2.

4-5 Apply knowledge of common prefixes, suffixes, and roots to interpret medical terms.

combining form a root word used to create a compound word.

suffix a word or part of a word added to the end of another word to add description.

prefix a word or part of a word added to the beginning of another word to add description.

Root words are combined with suffixes and prefixes to create larger, more specific terms. When a root word is used with a prefix or suffix and denotes the specific subject of the new compound word, it is often referred to as a **combining form.** In this case, the root word points out what the larger word refers to and then the prefix or suffix adds description. For example, in the term *hepatitis*, *hepa* (a term used to refer to the liver) would be the combining form, and then the suffix *-itis* is added to note inflammation. Therefore, *hepatitis* means inflammation of the liver.

Prefixes and suffixes are commonly added to combining forms (root words) to create a more descriptive term. A **suffix** is added to the end of a word, and a **prefix** is added to the beginning of a word. Consider the term *arteriosclerosis*. *Arterio* is the

TABLE 4-1 ANATOMICAL ROOT WORDS

ANATOMY	ROOT WORD
Artery	arterio-
Back	dorso-/dorsal
Bladder	cyst-
Blood	sanguin-/hemat-
Blood vessel	angio-/vascul-
Bone	osteo-
Brain	encephal-/cerebral
Eye	oculo-/ophthalm-
Gall bladder	cholecyst-
Head	cephal-
Heart	cardio-
Kidney	nephro-
Liver	hepat-/hepatic-
Lungs	pneumo-/pulmon-
Navel (belly button)	umbilic-
Neck	cervic-
Nerve	neuro-
Rib	pleuro-/costal-
Skin	derma-/cut-/cutan-
Skull	cranio-/cranial
Stomach	gastro-/gastric
Throat	pharyng-/laryng-
Uterus	hyster-
Vein	phleb-

TABLE 4-2 DESCRIPTIVE ROOT WORDS

DESCRIPTION	ROOT WORD
Around	peri-/circum-
Bad	mal-
Big	mega-
Black	melano-
Blue	cyano-
Fast	tachy-
Hard	sclero-
Narrow	steno-
Small	micro-
Red	erythro-
Slow	brady-
White	leuk-
Middle	medi-/medial-
Double	diplo-
Many	poly-/multi-

root word that refers to arteries, and *sclerosis* is a suffix that refers to narrowing. So, *arteriosclerosis* means narrowing of the arteries. *Tachycardia* is a combination of the root word *cardia*, which refers to the heart, and the prefix *tachy*, which means fast. Therefore *tachycardia* means fast heart rate. A list of common prefixes and suffixes can be found in Table 4-3.

Because there are many different suffixes and prefixes, it is unlikely that you will remember all of them. As you review the lists provided in this chapter, attempt to identify the key suffixes and prefixes that refer to common phrases and terms. Start with them and work your way toward more complex language. You will find that learning common terms will make it easier to recognize more complex compound words.

You probably already know many suffixes and prefixes (think of *cardio-*, *cerebral-*, and *gastric-*, for example). By learning a few more you will establish a firm foundation to build on. Once you have grasped the basic terms, gradually add the terms you are

TABLE 4-3 COMMON PREFIXES AND SUFFIXES

PREFIX/ SUFFIX	MEANING	PREFIX/ SUFFIX	MEANING	PREFIX/ SUFFIX	MEANING
A-/An-	Absent/without	Endo-	Within/Inside	Naso-	Referring to the nose
Abdomino-	Referring to the abdomen	Enter-	Referring to the intestines	Neo-	New
Ab-	Away	Eryth-	Red/Reddening	Neuro-	Referring to nerves
Ad-	Toward	Ex-	Out/away	Olig-	Little or few
-Algia	Pain	Exo/extra-	Outside	-Osis	Disease or condition
Amnio-	Pertaining to the womb	Gastro-	Pertaining to the stomach	Para-	With/next to
Angio-	Blood vessel	Glosso-	Referring to the tongue	-Paresis	Numbness
Ante-	In front of/before	-Gram/-graph	Recording or tracing	Patho-	Negative condition
Anti-	Against	Gyn-	Woman	Per-	Passing through
Arterio-	Pertaining to an artery	Hemat-	Pertaining to blood	Peri-	Around
Bi-	Double/two	Hemi-	One half	Pharyng-	Pertaining to the throat
Brady-	Slow	Hepat-/Hepatic	Pertaining to the liver	Photo-	Pertaining to light
Bronch-/ Bronchial	Pertaining to the lungs/ bronchial tubes	Hist-	Tissue	-Plegia	Paralysis
Carcin-	Pertaining to cancer	Hydro-	Water	Pleuro-	Referring to the ribs
Cardio-	Referring to the heart	Hyper-	High/above normal	Pneumo-	Referring to the lungs
Cephalo-	Referring to the head	Hypo-	Low/below normal	Poly-	Many
Cerebro-	Pertaining to the brain	Infra-	Below	Post-	After
Cervic-	Referring to the neck	Inter-	In between	Pre/Pro-	Before
Cholecyst-	Pertaining to the gall bladder	Intra-	Within	Pseudo-	False
Circum-	Surrounding	-Ism	Condition or disease	Pyro-	Fever
Co-	With/together	-Itis	Inflammation	Retro-	Behind
-Crine	Referring to secretion	Lacrim-	Tear (as in tear drops)	Sclero-	Hardening
Cutan-	Skin	Laryngeal-/ Laryngo-	Referring to the larynx	Semi-	Partially
Cyst-	Referring to the bladder	Lateral-Latero	To the side	-Stasis	Stoppage
Cyte-	Cell	Leuko-	White	-Staxis	Leak or a drip
Derm-/Dermal	Pertaining to the skin	-Lysis	Destruction	-Stomy	Creation of an opening
Di-	Two/double	Macro-	Big	Sub	Beneath
Digit-	Finger	-Megaly	Enlargement	Super-/Supra-	Above
Dorso-/Dorsal	Referring to the back	Meta-	After	Tachy-	Fast
Dys-	Difficult	Micro-	Small	Therm-	Heat
-Emesis	Vomit	Morph-	Shape	Thoracic-	Referring to the chest
		Myo-	Muscle	Ultra-	Excessive/beyond
				Uni-	One

unfamiliar with. Soon you will have the capability to dissect even the most obscure medical terminology.

The long lists of root words, suffixes, and prefixes may seem daunting. In fact, learning them will take time. The key is to practice, practice, practice and you will quickly improve.

STOP, REVIEW, REMEMBER!

Multiple Choice

For each question, place a check next to the correct answer.

1. The root word *hepat* refers to the:

_____ a. liver.
_____ b. blood.
_____ c. head.
_____ d. kidneys.

2. The root word *pleuro* refers to the:

_____ a. lungs.
_____ b. ribs.
_____ c. diaphragm.
_____ d. throat.

3. The root word that best describes the gall bladder is:

_____ a. hemat-.
_____ b. cyst-.
_____ c. cholecyst-.
_____ d. hepat-.

4. Which one of the following prefixes refers to the neck?

_____ a. cerebral-
_____ b. cephal-
_____ c. coccyc-
_____ d. cervic-

5. Which one of the following prefixes means *against*?

_____ a. anti-
_____ b. bi-
_____ c. di-
_____ d. para-

6. The prefix *dys*- refers to:

_____ a. double.
_____ b. single.
_____ c. small.
_____ d. difficult.

7. Which one of the following suffixes refers to vomiting?

_____ a. -ectopy
_____ b. -asthesia
_____ c. -algia
_____ d. -emesis

Matching

Match the suffix or prefix on the left with the applicable definition on the right.

1. _____ brady-	A. Against
2. _____ tachy-	B. Slow
3. _____ -algia	C. Inflammation
4. _____ anti-	D. Low
5. _____ intra-	E. Fast
6. _____ -itis	F. Within
7. _____ hypo-	G. Pain

(continued on next page)

(continued)

Fill in the Blank

1. A baby that has just been born is known as a ______________________________-nate.
2. A white blood cell is known as a ______________________________-cyte.
3. Inflammation of the gall bladder is known as cholecyst-______________________________.
4. Reddening of the skin is known as ______________________________-ema.
5. An abnormally high body temperature is known as ______________________________-thermia.

Critical Thinking

Use your knowledge of combining forms, suffixes, and prefixes to define the following medical terms.

1. Hydrocephalus

____

____

____

____

2. Aortic stenosis

____

____

____

____

3. Polyuria

____

____

____

____

4. Hematemesis

____

____

____

____

5. Diplopia

____

____

____

____

Medical Terms

Medical terminology is used to provide precise descriptions of anatomy, position, and location. This precision helps EMTs better understand the organization of the body and describe injuries or dysfunction when speaking to other health care providers.

Body Structure

The language of medicine relies on a basic knowledge of anatomy. To describe and document complaints, injuries, and examination findings, you will need to use exact medical terms. Terms you may be accustomed to (such as "around here" or "my stomach hurts") are not appropriate in EMS.

Points of Reference

When describing any part of the body, the first point of reference is the **anatomical position** (Figure 4-1 ▪). The anatomical position is a person standing, facing forward, with arms out to the side and palms forward. All descriptions refer to the body in this position. You will soon see why this is important.

Many terms and descriptions are relative. That means they are meaningless unless you provide a point of reference. Place your right arm down alongside your body. Place your palm forward. There is an inside surface (closest to your body) and an outside surface (farthest away from your body). Now turn your hand so your palm is to the rear. The side that was previously outside is now inside. The inside is now outside. This is why you must always refer to the anatomical position as the standard point of reference, regardless of how you find the patient. It is a standard among health care professionals.

Another important point of reference to remember is that **left** and **right** are always the patient's left and right—*not yours*.

4-2 Describe each of the following terms of position: anatomical position, Fowler's position, lateral recumbent position, prone, semi-Fowler's position, shock position, supine, Trendelenburg position.

anatomical position the standard reference position for the body in the study of anatomy. The body is standing erect, facing the observer, with arms down at the sides and palms of the hands forward.

left refers to the patient's left.

right refers to the patient's right.

Planes and Lines

The body can be divided into planes. A **plane** is a straight line or a flat surface that divides something into sections as if slicing through a solid object. Imagine that the body could be sliced into halves. You could slice the body directly down the middle and have a right half and a left half. Such a slice would be called the *sagittal plane*. You also could slice the body into a front half and a back half. Slicing the body this way would create a *coronal plane* (Figure 4-2 ▪). Finally, you could slice the body into halves at the waist, creating a top and a bottom half to form a *transverse plane*.

Although this might seem like a mere exercise in imagination, planes give you an important frame of reference when considering how to look at anatomy. For example, viewing from front to back would mean looking along the sagittal plane.

plane a flat surface formed when slicing through a solid object.

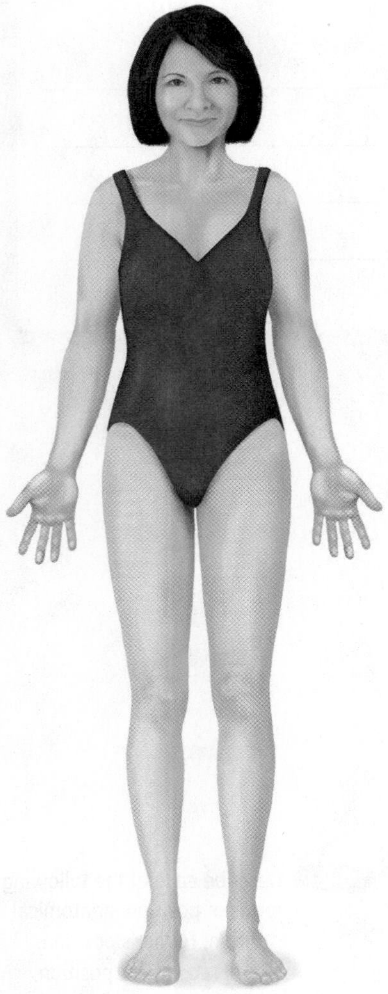

Figure 4-1 The anatomical position.

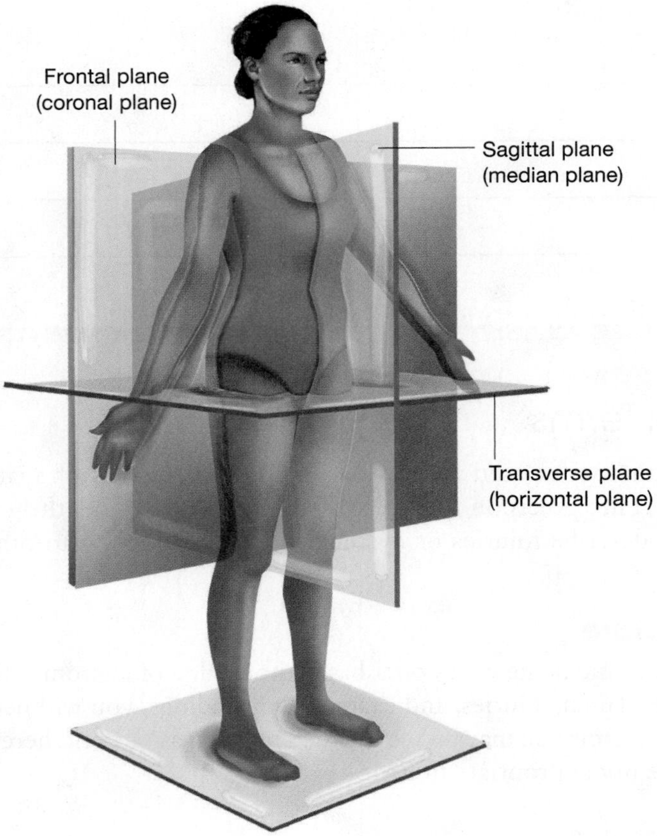

Figure 4-2 Anatomical planes of reference.

Another very important concept is the **midline.** The midline is an imaginary line that is drawn from the top of the head to the bottom of the feet. It is centered on the nose and umbilicus (navel or belly button) and divides the body in half. The midline helps you discuss anatomy and define regions of the body. For example, there are four quadrants of the abdomen. The midline serves as the vertical dividing line (Figure 4-3 ■). The four quadrants are further divided at the umbilicus. Upper quadrants would be above the umbilicus and lower quadrants would be below. The midline would separate left and right.

The midline also is a point of reference for the anatomical terms *medial* and *lateral.* Something that is **medial** is closer to the midline. **Lateral** is farther away from the midline. A laceration might be located on "the medial aspect of the left thigh." A bruise might be on "the lateral aspect of the right upper arm."

The term **bilateral** means both sides. If someone has two broken lower legs, he would have "bilateral lower leg fractures."

midline an imaginary line drawn down the center of the body, dividing it into right and left halves.

medial toward the midline of the body.

lateral to the side, away from the midline of the body.

bilateral on both sides.

midaxillary line an imaginary line drawn vertically from the middle of the armpit to the ankle.

anterior the front of the body or body part. Opposite of *posterior.*

posterior the back of the body or body part. Opposite of *anterior.*

CLINICAL CLUE

Anatomical Position

Understanding the anatomical position is very important for your everyday practice because it will serve as a baseline point of reference for most of your descriptions. EMTs commonly use terms that infer the anatomical position as the point of reference. It is common to hear terms such as "bilateral femur fracture" or "proximal tibia fracture." All those terms require that you understand the starting point.

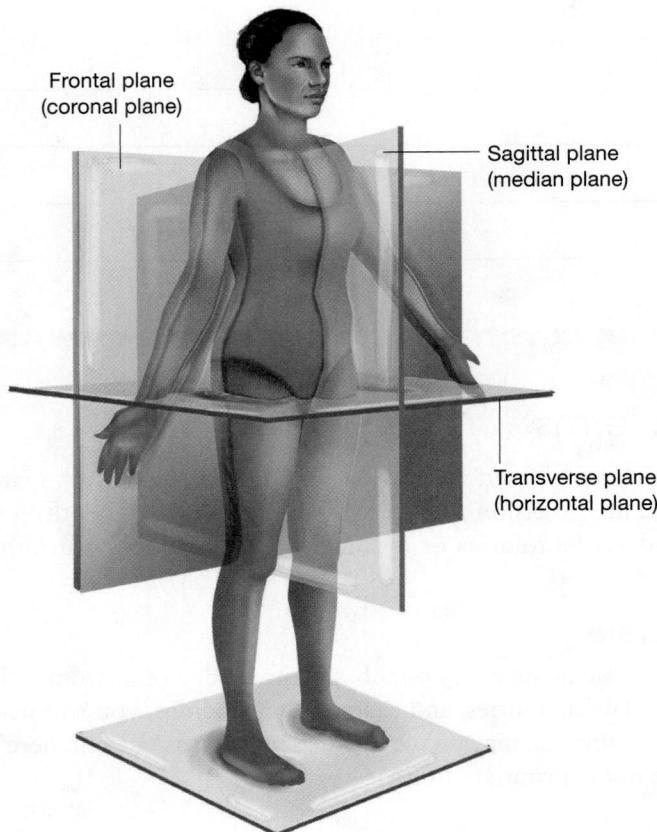

The body also can be divided into a front and back by the **midaxillary line.** This is a vertical line down the side of the body from the armpit to the ankle bone. It divides the body into the **anterior** (front) and **posterior** (rear). If you had a laceration on your shin, it would be on the anterior portion of your leg. If you had a laceration on your lower back, it would be on the posterior of your body. Although uncommon, the anterior is sometimes called **ventral** and the posterior may also be called **dorsal.**

The **midclavicular line** is on the anterior surface of the body and runs vertically through the center of the clavicle (collar bone) down through the nipple. There are two clavicles so there are two midclavicular lines, one on each side of the body. If a patient had a wound in this area, it could be described as "on the midclavicular line at the level of the fifth rib."

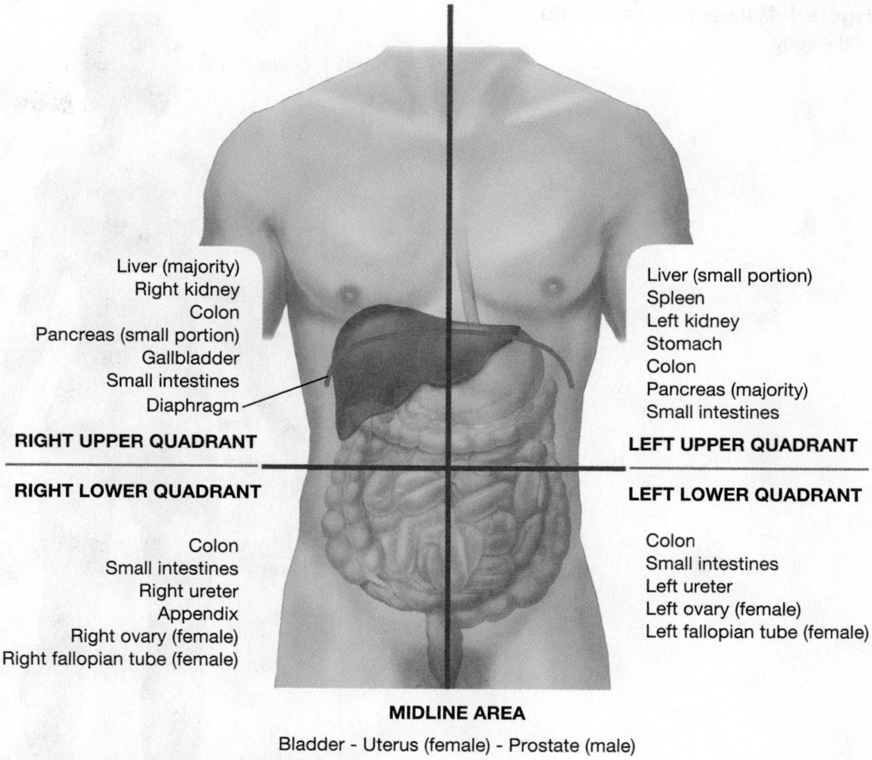

Figure 4-3 The abdominal quadrants.

Body Systems

Organs and organ system terminology are used to specifically describe location or role in the body. For example, you learned in the previous section that the Greek root *hepat* is used to describe liver-related conditions such as hepatitis (inflammation of the liver) or hepatomegaly (enlargement of the liver). As you progress through this text, you will encounter many system-specific terms that will help you understand the anatomy and physiology of the topic at hand. Reviewing all body system terminology is beyond the scope of this chapter, but you should consider the importance of terminology as you move forward.

Specific locations of the body may be referred to by region and by topographic features. Some are common such as "thigh" or "forearm," while others are a bit more technical. The regions and features are shown in Figure 4-4 ▪.

Some anatomical terms can be specific to a certain part of the body. **Plantar** refers to the sole of the foot. **Palmar** refers to the palm of the hand. **Cephalic** refers to the head, and **gastric** refers to the stomach. There are many more terms for organs and body systems, many of which will be brought to your attention when you study each system.

The body also has certain cavities (Figure 4-5 ▪). For example, the heart, lungs, and major blood vessels (the "great vessels," including the aorta and venae cavae) lie within the thoracic cavity. The stomach, intestines, gall bladder, appendix, and other organs lie within the abdominal cavity. The diaphragm separates the thoracic cavity from the abdominal cavity.

Terms of Location and Position

Proper medical terminology aids in the precise description of both patient position and anatomical location.

Terms of Location

Anatomical landmarks and points of reference help us describe specific regions of the body, but there are other terms used to identify location. *Medial* and *lateral* are relative

ventral referring to the front of the body. Synonym for *anterior*.

dorsal refers to the back of the body or the back of the hand or foot. Synonym for *posterior.*

midclavicular line the imaginary line drawn vertically through the center of each clavicle.

4-3 Identify each of the following anatomical terms: abdominal quadrants, anterior and posterior, dorsal and ventral, frontal plane, medial and lateral, midaxillary line, midclavicular line, midline, palmar, plantar, proximal and distal, right and left, sagittal plane, superior and inferior, transverse plane.

plantar refers to the sole of the foot.

palmar refers to the palm of the hand.

cephalic refers to the head.

gastric refers to the stomach.

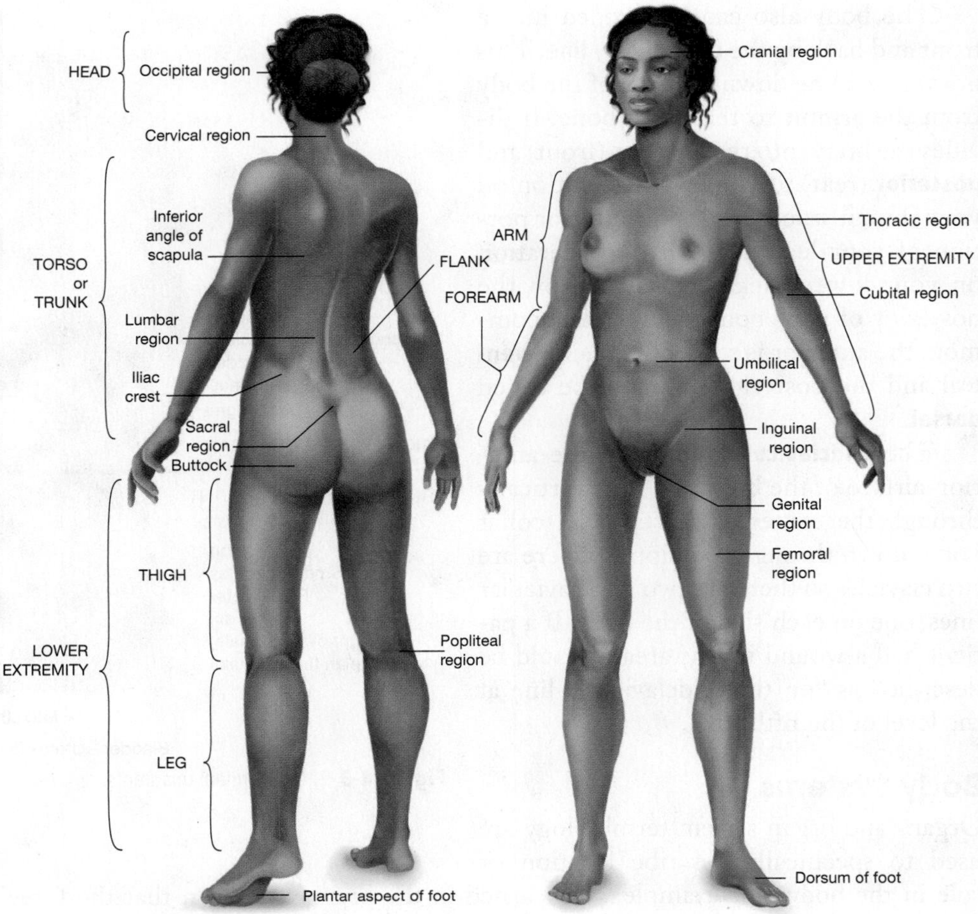

Figure 4-4 The regions and features of the body.

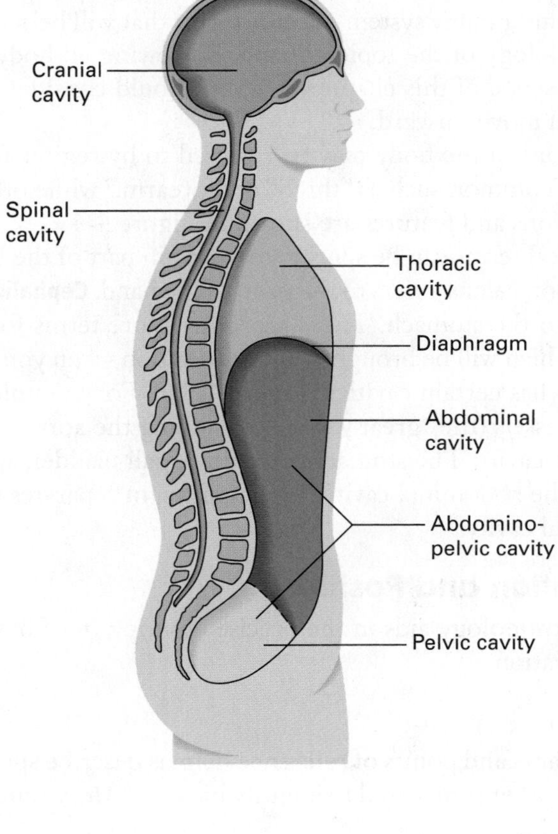

Figure 4-5 The main body cavities.

terms in that they generally require a specific point of reference to best describe a location. *Superior* and *inferior* are similarly relative terms. Simply stated, **superior** is up and **inferior** is down. Remember to identify a point of reference when using these terms. In the example "Your ribs are superior to your belly button," the belly button is the point of reference. In the example, "Your eyes are inferior to your forehead," the forehead is the point of reference.

superior toward the head (e.g., the chest is superior to the abdomen). Opposite of *inferior.*

inferior away from the head; usually compared with another structure that is closer to the head (e.g., the lips are inferior to the nose). Opposite of *superior.*

Two of the most confusing terms (but also two of the most commonly used) are *proximal* and *distal.* **Proximal** means closer to the body (closer to the trunk or heart), and **distal** means farther away. The confusion comes from the fact that a part of the body can be proximal to one part but distal to another. An example is the knee. The knee is distal to the hip (farther away from the torso) but proximal to (closer to the torso than) the ankle. As with the other terms, identifying the point of reference is critical. For example, a patient may have a suspected fracture in the proximal third of the femur or a laceration on the distal forearm. You are now able to picture where those injuries are because of your knowledge of anatomy and terms used to describe it.

proximal closer to the torso. Opposite of *distal.*

distal farther away from the torso. Opposite of *proximal.*

Terms of Position

There are terms that refer to the way the patient is positioned. The position may be the way the patient is found or a position in which you place him for care. There are six major positions (Scan 4-1):

- ***Supine.*** When a patient is **supine,** he is lying on his back (posterior body surface).
- ***Prone.*** When a patient is **prone,** he is lying on his front (anterior body surface).
- ***Lateral recumbent position.*** In the **lateral recumbent position,** the patient is lying on his side. Commonly, you will hear this term further described as a right or left lateral recumbent position. The left or right is determined by which side the patient is lying on. This position is also referred to as the *recovery position.* Unconscious or semi-conscious medical patients who are breathing are often placed in this position to facilitate drainage from the mouth and prevent aspiration of secretions or vomitus into the lungs.
- ***Fowler's position.*** When the patient is in a **Fowler's position,** he is in a sitting position. The **semi-Fowler's position** refers to a semi-sitting position, which typically is defined as a 45 to 60 degree angle, but usually simply means the patient is slightly reclining. Patients with difficulty breathing usually prefer a sitting or semi-sitting position because it often makes breathing easier.
- ***Trendelenburg position.*** When in the **Trendelenburg position,** the patient is lying completely flat with the head lower than the feet. This position is best achieved when a patient is lying on a long backboard or similar device and the foot end is raised slightly.
- ***Shock position.*** A patient in the **shock position** is lying on his back with feet elevated 12 to 18 inches.

supine lying on the back. Opposite of *prone.*

prone lying on the stomach. Opposite of *supine.*

lateral recumbent position lying on the side.

Fowler's position a sitting position.

semi-Fowler's position a semi-sitting position.

Trendelenburg position a position in which the patient's feet and legs are higher than the head. Also called *shock position.*

shock position refers to the patient lying supine with his feet elevated 12 to 18 inches.

Note that the Trendelenburg and shock positions are not recommended for patients who have suffered a traumatic injury. Instead, these positions may be used for patients experiencing signs of shock from a medical origin such as syncope (fainting) and anaphylaxis (a severe allergic reaction).

Effective Communication

Medical terminology can significantly aid communication among health care team members, but there are occasions when it may not be the most effective way to communicate.

SCAN 4-1 Patient Positions

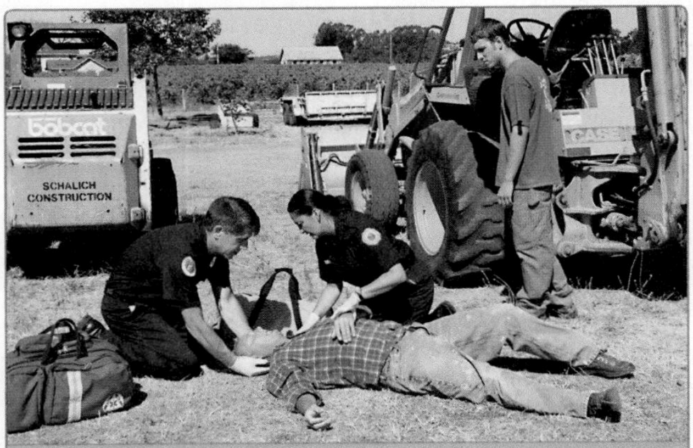

4-1-1 Supine position.

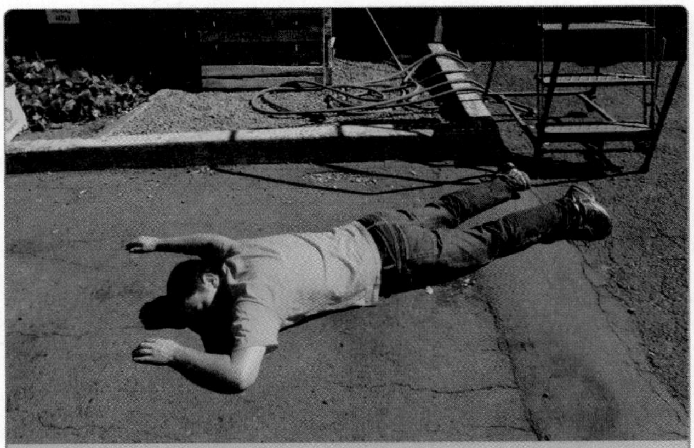

4-1-2 Prone position.

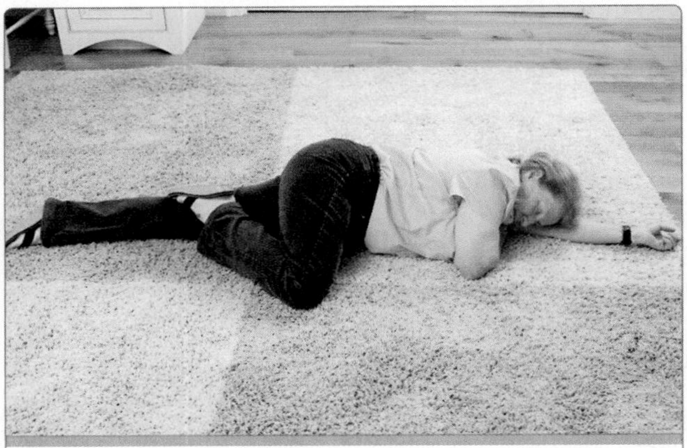

4-1-3 Lateral recumbent (recovery) position.

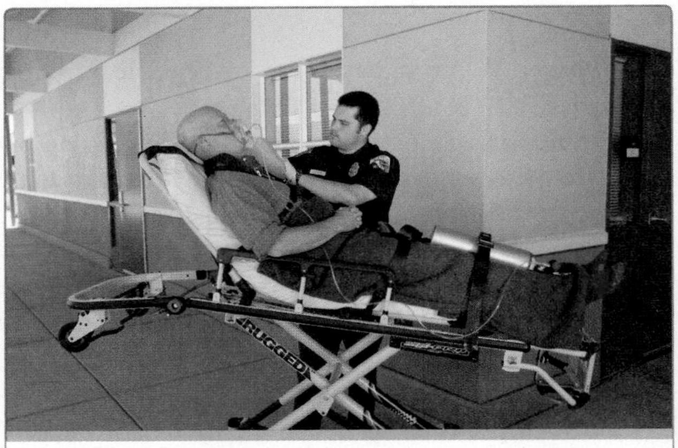

4-1-4 Semi-Fowler's position.

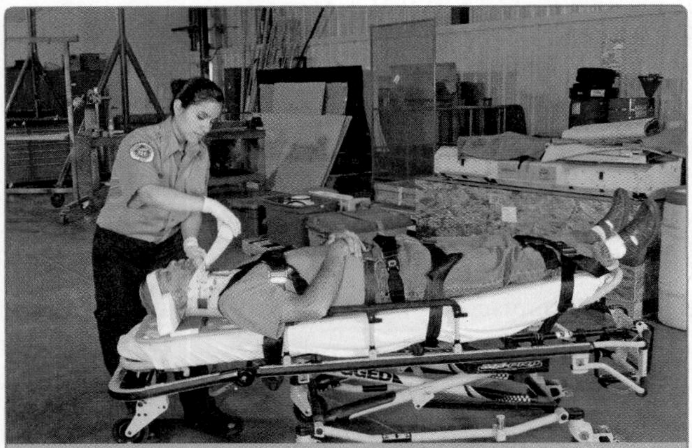

4-1-5 Trendelenburg position.

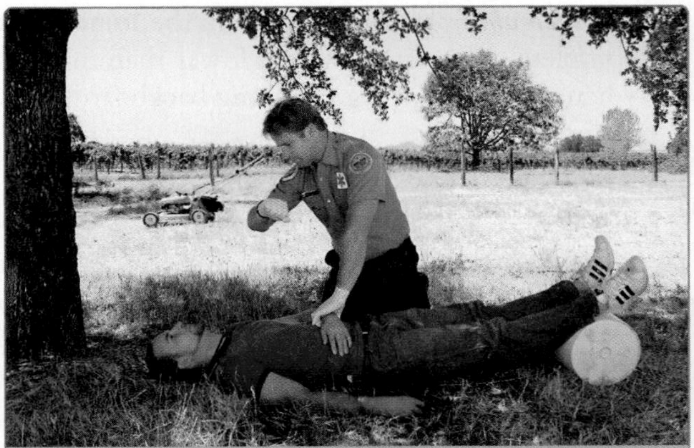

4-1-6 Shock position.

PERSPECTIVE

Violet—The Patient

I heard the EMTs talking on the radio. They were describing my injury using a lot of complex terms I didn't understand. I got scared. When Heather came back to me and explained what was going on in a way I could understand, I felt better. Not understanding what they were talking about made me more frightened.

For instance, when writing a detailed report or describing a specific injury to a physician, medical terminology can be an invaluable tool. However, when assessing a small child or attempting to ease the fears of an anxious parent, medical terminology can be more of a hindrance than a help. As an EMT you must be aware of when and how you use complex medical terms. You must consider your situation and use the most appropriate method to achieve your desired goal. If you ask an untrained bystander if the patient was diaphoretic (perspiring excessively), you may get a very different answer than if you were to ask him if the patient was sweaty. Medical terms can be confusing and sometimes scary for the patient. Terminology can even confuse well-trained providers. If at any time you are unsure of what term to use, remember that you can always fall back on plain language.

Understand that medical terminology is a professional language. In addition to precision, it can bring an air of professionalism. Being able to comprehend terminology shows fellow providers that you speak a common language. Remember that the opposite is true as well. Using slang and improper language can make you appear to be less professional.

CLINICAL CLUE

Medical Terminology

Your use of medical terminology frequently will enhance your ability to precisely describe injuries and patient positions, but sometimes it can be confusing. If you encounter difficulty in communication because of complex terminology, do not hesitate to use simpler language.

Abbreviations and Acronyms

Abbreviations and acronyms are a tricky subject. On the one hand they can speed completion of reports and whittle down long, drawn out terms into fast, usable language. On the other hand, they can be vague or misinterpreted and lead to communication errors.

For years, EMS has relied on abbreviations and catchy acronyms to shorten terminology. An **acronym** is a word created from the first letters of each word in a series of words. Many acronyms are imbedded in the language of EMS. Consider SAMPLE. It is an acronym created from the first letters of signs/symptoms, allergies, medications, past medical history, last oral intake, and event leading to illness/injury, and is used to help the EMT remember important interview questions. Table 4-4 lists common EMS acronyms.

acronym a word created from the first letters of each word in a series of words.

Abbreviations, or the shortening of a longer word, help streamline EMS written reports. Instead of writing *epinephrine*, for example, you might write "epi." Instead of *patients*, you might write "pts." Table 4-5 lists common EMS abbreviations.

TABLE 4-4 COMMON EMS ACRONYMS AND ABBREVIATIONS

ACRONYM	MEANING
CO	Carbon monoxide
C/O	Complains of
CO_2	Carbon dioxide
COPD	Chronic obstructive pulmonary disease
CPAP	Continuous positive airway pressure
CPR	Cardiopulmonary resuscitation
CSF	Cerebrospinal fluid
CVA	Cerebrovascular accident
DNR	Do not resuscitate
DOA	Dead on arrival
DOB	Date of birth
ECG	Electrocardiogram
ED	Emergency department
EMD	Emergency medical dispatcher
EMT	Emergency medical technician
GSW	Gunshot wound
HIV	Human immunodeficiency virus
ICS	Incident command system
LOC	Level of consciousness
MCI	Multiple-casualty incident
NKDA	No known drug allergies
NRB	Nonrebreather mask
O_2	Oxygen
OD	Overdose
PERRL	Pupils equal, round, and reactive to light
PPE	Personal protective equipment
SOB	Shortness of breath

TABLE 4-5 COMMON EMS ABBREVIATIONS AND SYMBOLS

ABBREVIATION	MEANING
$>$	Greater than
$<$	Less than
$\approx$	Approximately
$=$	Equals
$\neq$	Does not equal
$\triangle$	Change
abd.	Abdomen/abdominal
a-fib	Atrial fibrillation
ant.	Anterior
approx.	Approximately
bilat.	Bilateral
CA	Cancer
detox	Detoxification (drug)
Dr.	Doctor
e.g.	For example
exam	Examination
Fx	Fracture
HTN	Hypertension
Hx	History
incl.	Including
info	Information
irreg.	Irregular
neg.	Negative
neur.	Neurological
norm.	Normal
ped.	Pediatric
pos.	Positive
post.	Posterior
Pt.	Patient
reg.	Regular
rehab	Rehabilitation
resp.	Respiration
Sx.	Symptom
syst.	Systolic
temp.	Temperature
unk.	Unknown
w/	With
w/o	Without
y/o	Year old

The problem with acronyms and abbreviations is they can be inconsistent and lead to error. There is little standardization, and too frequently, providers simply make them up on their own. Such abbreviations are of little use if no one else understands them.

Studies have shown that many medical errors occur during *patient transfer* (transferring care from one provider to another). Many mistakes are made due to poor communication. The complete written report (and the verbal report to a lesser degree) is your most important protection against transfer errors. For this reason, many health care providers have chosen to minimize the use of abbreviations and acronyms in the interest of being explicitly clear and avoiding errors. Different EMS systems allow different standards for acronym and abbreviation use. You must learn the common abbreviations and acronyms used in your system.

CLINICAL CLUE

Abbreviations

Beware using abbreviations when transferring care of a patient. Even though abbreviations may be standardized within your organization, they may cause confusion when a patient is handed off to a different organization such as a hospital. Although abbreviations can be helpful in rapidly recording information, it is best to avoid shorthand in patient documentation.

STOP, REVIEW, REMEMBER!

Multiple Choice

For each question, place a check next to the correct answer.

1. Which one of the following terms would be used to describe a location close to the midline?

_____ a. Lateral
_____ b. Medial
_____ c. Distal
_____ d. Dorsal

2. Which one of the following anatomical locations is the border between the upper and lower abdominal quadrants?

_____ a. Midline
_____ b. Diaphragm
_____ c. Umbilicus
_____ d. Midaxillary line

3. The heart, lungs, and great vessels are found in the:

_____ a. abdominal cavity.
_____ b. peritoneal space.
_____ c. retroperitoneal space.
_____ d. thoracic cavity.

4. Your patient is in the anatomical position. When compared to her clavicle, her shoulder would be described as:

_____ a. medial.
_____ b. lateral.
_____ c. proximal.
_____ d. inferior.

5. The midclavicular line passes through the:

_____ a. armpit.
_____ b. umbilicus.
_____ c. nipple.
_____ d. palm.

6. Which one of the following would best describe the direction a patient's palms are facing if she were standing in the anatomical position?

_____ a. Forward
_____ b. Backward
_____ c. Upward
_____ d. Downward

(continued on next page)

(continued)

Labeling

On the following photograph, label the listed anatomical terms, regions, or planes.

Dorsal	Medial	Lateral
Proximal	Distal	Midclavicular
	Midline	

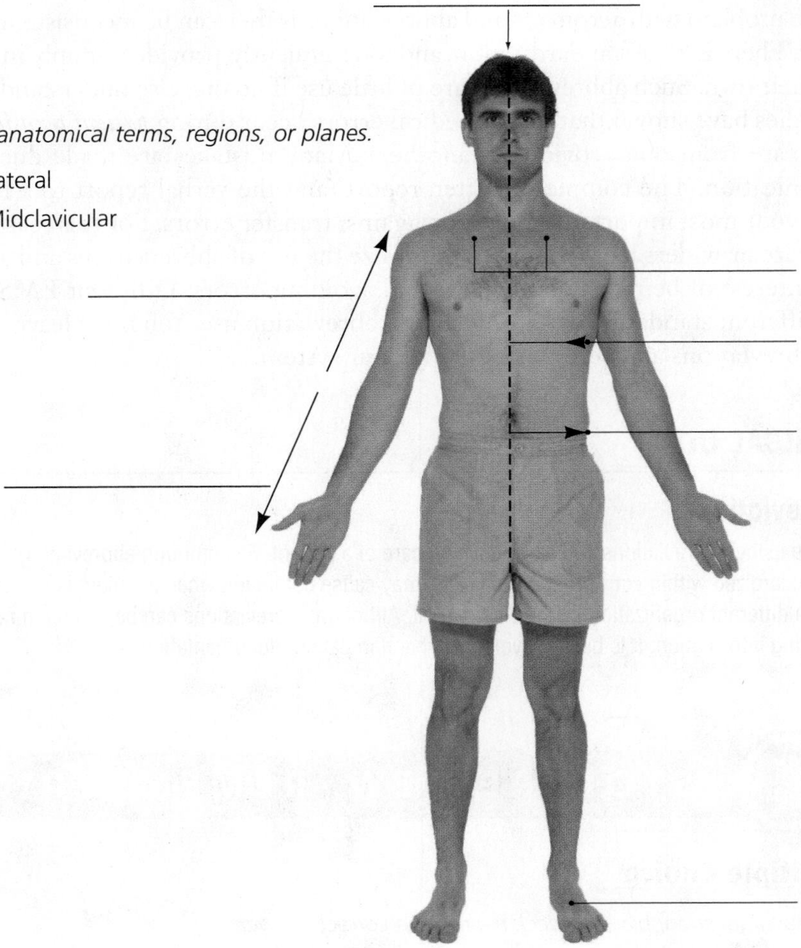

Fill in the Blank

1. The elbow is ______________________ to the wrist and ______________________ to the shoulder.

2. The imaginary line that divides the body into left and right halves is called the ______________________.

3. The ______________________ is the line that is drawn downward from the collar bone.

4. The ______________________ is the line that is drawn through the armpit down through the ankles to divide the body into ______________________ and ______________________.

5. The term ______________________ means "both sides."

Critical Thinking

Each of the following injuries or complaints is stated in common terms. Describe their locations accurately using the anatomical terms and references you learned in this chapter.

1. Your patient has a cut on his left arm near the wrist. It is just about where the face of his watch would cover.

____

____

____

____

2. Your patient has a cut on the back of his leg just below the knee.

____

____

____

____

3. Your patient complains of pain in his lower abdomen on the right side that shoots toward the center of his belly.

____

____

____

____

4. Your patient has a bruise on his forehead above the right eye.

____

____

____

____

5. Your patient stepped on a nail causing a puncture wound on the bottom of his left foot.

____

____

____

____

EMERGENCY DISPATCH SUMMARY

On arrival at the hospital, Heather and Dan carefully transferred their patient to the care of the emergency department staff. Before leaving, Heather gave a verbal report to the attending nurse. In this report she described her assessment of the patient and gave specific details of the injury. Heather also described the treatment she performed in the field. At the conclusion of the call, Heather completed an electronic run report that provided a detailed record of the care provided.

Chapter Review

To the Point

- Understanding medical terminology lends precision to your descriptions and documentation.
- Many medical terms are created by combining prefixes, suffixes, and common root words. Root words form the basis of a term, and prefixes and suffixes add descriptions.
- The anatomical position is a person standing, facing forward, with arms out to the side and palms forward. All descriptions of patients refer to this position.
- Many terms and descriptions are relative. Terms such as *distal* and *proximal* require further description or at least a point of reference.
- Terms of position can be helpful in describing the patient or in identifying specific areas of the body.
- Other anatomical terms refer specifically to the anatomical position. Terms such as *midline*, *lateral*, and *anterior* all refer specifically to that point of reference.
- Know when to use complex terms and when not to. Although they frequently lend precision to descriptions, they also can be confusing and intimidating for those who do not understand them.
- Abbreviations can make documentation easier, but also can lead to confusion and patient error. Use them only when absolutely necessary.

Chapter Questions

Multiple Choice

For each question, place a check next to the correct answer.

1. In medical terminology what is used to relay the basic meaning or reference of a more complex word?
   _____ a. Suffix
   _____ b. Prefix
   _____ c. Root word
   _____ d. Complex form

2. A patient lying on her stomach would be described as lying in what position?
   _____ a. Supine
   _____ b. Prone
   _____ c. Lateral recumbent
   _____ d. Dorsally oriented

3. The ankle is _____________ to the knee.
   _____ a. anterior
   _____ b. posterior
   _____ c. proximal
   _____ d. distal

4. What is added to the beginning of a combining form to add description to its root?
   _____ a. Suffix
   _____ b. Prefix
   _____ c. Preform
   _____ d. Biform

5. Which one of the following prefixes and suffixes would refer to anatomical structures in the throat?
   _____ a. laryngo-
   _____ b. lacrimo-
   _____ c. leuko-
   _____ d. -lytic

6. Your patient has a bruise on the thumb side of his forearm. What side of the arm is that?
   _____ a. Proximal
   _____ b. Lateral
   _____ c. Medial
   _____ d. It depends on how the patient is standing.

7. Which one of the following terms would best describe something that is away from the midline?
   _____ a. Medial
   _____ b. Lateral
   _____ c. Proximal
   _____ d. Planar
8. With reference to the chest, the sternum would be considered:
   _____ a. inferior.
   _____ b. superior.
   _____ c. posterior.
   _____ d. anterior.
9. The abbreviation "Hx" generally stands for:
   _____ a. history.
   _____ b. hysterectomy.
   _____ c. hepatitis.
   _____ d. heat.
10. A reclined sitting position may be described as the _____________ position.
   _____ a. semi-Fowler's
   _____ b. supine
   _____ c. prone
   _____ d. lateral recumbent

Matching

Match the suffix or prefix on the left with the applicable reference on the right.

1. _____	dorso-	A. Bladder
2. _____	cyst-	B. Vein
3. _____	hemat-	C. Bone
4. _____	osteo-	D. Skin
5. _____	cerebral-	E. Back
6. _____	ophthalm-	F. Nerve
7. _____	nephro-	G. Brain
8. _____	neuro-	H. Kidney
9. _____	derma-	I. Skull
10. _____	phleb-	J. Eye
11. _____	cranio-	K. Blood
12. _____	hyster-	L. Around
13. _____	peri-	M. Shape
14. _____	morph-	N. Few
15. _____	olig-	O. Uterus

Critical Thinking

Describe the following patient complaints using correct anatomical and directional terms.

1. A patient has pain just below his ribs on the right side.

____

____

____

____

(continued on next page)

(continued)

2. A patient has a deformity on his left arm near the wrist.

3. A patient has a laceration on his left hand across his knuckles.

Case Study

You are called to a motor-vehicle collision with injuries. You find an injured seven-year-old patient. He was the passenger in a vehicle that was struck directly into the passenger-side door where the patient was sitting. You notice that the door was pushed about a foot into the passenger compartment.

1. The patient complains of pain to the right side of his rib cage over the lower five or six ribs. If you had to relay a report on this injury using anatomical terms, how would you describe it to the on-line medical director?

2. The patient's mother arrives on scene and asks you about her son's injuries. Outline how you would describe those injuries to the mother.

3. Why might it be important to use different language with the mother than you did with the on-line physician?

The Last Word

Medical terminology offers a language of precision. Using such precise terms will improve your accuracy in communication and in the reporting of illness and injury. As with any new language, a full understanding will take time and practice. Adding new vocabulary to your day-to-day practice will improve your ability to use the language of health care. Take care to use it carefully. There is always a time and a place to use simple language instead. Avoid using potentially confusing medical terms when plain language would be more appropriate.

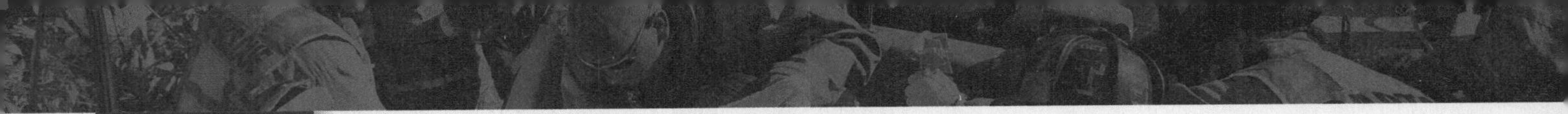

5 Anatomy and Physiology

Education Standards

Anatomy and Physiology: Medical Terminology

Competencies

Applies fundamental knowledge of the anatomy and function of all human systems to the practice of EMS.

Uses foundational anatomical and medical terms and abbreviations in written and oral communication with colleagues and other health professionals.

Objectives

After completion of this lesson, you should be able to:

5-1 Define key terms introduced in this chapter.

5-2 Explain the importance of knowledge of anatomy and physiology to patient assessment and care.

5-3 Define the terms *anatomy* and *physiology*.

5-4 Describe each of the components of the skeleton, including location and function.

5-5 Identify the various types of joints found in the body.

5-6 Describe the function of each of the following musculoskeletal system structures: bone, ligaments, skeletal muscle, and tendons.

5-7 Differentiate between skeletal (voluntary), smooth (involuntary), and cardiac muscle.

5-8 Describe the structure and function of the integumentary system.

5-9 Describe the mechanics and physiology of normal ventilation, respiration, and oxygenation.

5-10 Describe the structures and function of the respiratory system.

5-11 Differentiate between the respiratory system anatomy of adults and children.

5-12 Describe the function of the cardiovascular (circulatory) system.

5-13 Describe the structure and function of the heart.

5-14 Discuss the anatomy and physiology of blood, circulation, perfusion, and metabolism.

5-15 Describe the function of the nervous system.

5-16 Differentiate between the structural components and functions of the central nervous system and peripheral nervous system.

5-17 Differentiate between the functional divisions of the peripheral nervous system: voluntary (somatic) nervous system and involuntary (autonomic) nervous system, including the sympathetic and parasympathetic divisions.

5-18 Describe the structure and function of the endocrine system.

5-19 Describe the general actions of epinephrine and norepinephrine on $beta_1$ and $beta_2$ receptors of the sympathetic nervous system.

5-20 Describe the structure and function of the digestive system.

5-21 Describe the structure and function of the organs of the renal system.

5-22 Describe the structure and function of the organs of the male and female reproductive systems.

Key Terms

aerobic metabolism p. 104
alveoli p. 105
anaerobic metabolism p. 104
anatomy p. 96
aorta p. 109
aortic valve p. 109
arteries p. 110
arterioles p. 110
atria p. 108
automaticity p. 101
autonomic nervous system p. 116
ball-and-socket joints p. 97
bile p. 119
bladder p. 119
blood pressure p. 113
brachial artery p. 110
bronchi p. 105
bronchioles p. 105
capillaries p. 110
carbon dioxide p. 109
cardiac muscle p. 101
cardiovascular system p. 108
carotid artery p. 110
carpals p. 97
cartilage p. 105
central nervous system (CNS) p. 116
cervical vertebrae p. 100
cervix p. 122
clavicles p. 97
coccygeal vertebrae p. 100
conduction system p. 110
conductive tissue p. 110
coronary arteries p. 109
cricoid cartilage p. 105
dermis p. 101
dorsalis pedis artery p. 112
embryo p. 119
epidermis p. 101
epiglottis p. 105
epinephrine p. 116
exhalation p. 107
facial bones p. 97
fallopian tubes p. 119
femoral artery p. 112
femur p. 97
fertilization p. 119
fetus p. 119
fibula p. 97
fused joints p. 97
gall bladder p. 119
gliding joints p. 97
glottic opening p. 105
glucose p. 104
hemoglobin p. 112
hinge joints p. 97
hormones p. 116
humerus p. 97
hypoperfusion p. 113
hypopharynx p. 105
ilium p. 97
implantation p. 119
inhalation p. 106
insulin p. 116
involuntary muscle p. 100
ischium p. 97
islets of Langerhans p. 119
large intestine p. 119
laryngopharynx p. 105
larynx p. 105
ligaments p. 98
lobes p. 105
lumbar vertebrae p. 100
lungs p. 105
mandible p. 97
maxilla p. 97
metacarpals p. 97
metatarsals p. 97
mitral valve p. 109
motor nerves p. 116
nasopharynx p. 105
oropharynx p. 105
ovaries p. 119
ovulation p. 119
pacemaker p. 110
pancreas p. 119
patella p. 97
pelvis p. 97
perfusion p. 104
peripheral nervous system (PNS) p. 116
phalanges p. 97
pharynx p. 105
physiology p. 96
plasma p. 112
platelets p. 112
posterior tibial artery p. 112
pubis p. 97
pulmonary arteries p. 109
pulmonary veins p. 112
pulmonic valve p. 109
pulse p. 108
radial artery p. 112
radius p. 97
red blood cells p. 112
respiration p. 107
retroperitoneal space p. 119
ribs p. 97
sacral spine p. 97
sacral vertebrae p. 100
saturated p. 112
scapulae p. 97
sensory nerves p. 116
skeletal muscle p. 100
small intestine p. 119
smooth muscle p. 100
spinal column p. 100
sternum p. 97
stroke volume p. 113
subcutaneous layer p. 101
systemic vascular resistance (SVR) p. 113
tarsals p. 97
tendons p. 98
thoracic vertebrae p. 100
thyroid cartilage p. 105
tibia p. 97
trachea p. 105
tricuspid valve p. 109
ulna p. 97
ureters p. 119
urethra p. 122
vas deferens p. 122
veins p. 110
vena cava p. 112
ventilation p. 107
ventilation/perfusion match (V/Q match) p. 104
ventricles p. 108
venules p. 110
vertebrae p. 98
voluntary muscle p. 100
white blood cells p. 112

Introduction

5-2 Explain the importance of knowledge of anatomy and physiology to patient assessment and care.

5-3 Define the terms anatomy and physiology.

anatomy the study of the basic structures of the body.

physiology the study of body function.

facial bones bones that combined make up the structures of the face.

maxilla the two fused bones that form the upper jaw.

mandible the lower jaw bone.

clavicles the collarbones.

scapulae the shoulder blades. Singular *scapula*.

humerus the bone of the upper arm, between the shoulder and the elbow.

radius the lateral bone of the forearm.

ulna the medial bone of the forearm.

carpals the wrist bones.

An EMT course in many ways is like assembling a very big puzzle. Each lesson provides you with pieces you can put together to create a larger picture. You will learn how the pieces fit and how the picture should look in the end. You also will learn what happens when pieces are disturbed or missing. **Anatomy,** or the basic structure of the body, constitutes one section of that puzzle, and **physiology,** the study of body function, may be thought of as how those pieces fit together.

Think of any system in the body. Individual cells make up organs, multiple organs make up body systems, and body systems interact with each other to sustain life. Just as the individual pieces of a puzzle must be assembled to see the larger picture, learning the components of any body system will help you understand function.

At all levels of health care, anatomy and physiology provide the basic foundation of knowledge. As you progress through your EMT course and tackle more complex body systems, you will learn more and more anatomy and physiology. Think of it as adding more pieces to the puzzle. These core concepts will help you understand the complex organism that is the human body. Beyond just rote memorization, however, knowledge of anatomy and physiology will help you better assess and treat your patients. Knowing the location of key internal organs will help you decipher external signs and symptoms. Understanding how systems function will help you understand the impact of challenges to those systems and help you predict the results of system failure.

You will constantly use anatomy and physiology as an EMT. Increasing your basic knowledge will only improve your capabilities as a care provider.

This chapter is designed to be an overview of anatomy and physiology, but the discussion does not end at its conclusion. Subsequent chapters will describe the anatomy and physiology of specific systems in greater detail and build on key concepts discussed here. As you review this chapter and work your way through later chapters, keep the basic puzzle pieces in mind. Always think of how they relate to the larger, more comprehensive picture. Knowledge of human anatomy and physiology is an essential component of this course and will continue to be a guiding principle in the decisions you make as an EMT.

EMERGENCY DISPATCH

EMTs Dave Klein and Mike Douglas stood by their ambulance at the weekly community market in the city's downtown area, watching the various vendors, street performers, and wandering families enjoying the warm summer evening when the radio buzzed to life.

"Unit 17, 1-7, respond to Fourth and D Streets for a fall from the parking garage. Showing you dispatched at 1814 hours."

Dave maneuvered the truck away from the curb while Mike whelped the siren several times, parting the crowds so they could make the three-block drive to the scene.

"Oh my God, you've got to hurry," a teen girl was screaming as they pulled up, tears streaming down her face. "I think he's dead!" Dave pulled the gurney stacked with equipment from the back, taking a moment to add the long backboard to the pile, while Mike touched the girl's shoulder and asked where the person fell. She pointed toward a large, concrete planter box about 20 feet away.

"How high up was he?" Dave looked up at the five-story parking structure.

"The top," she sobbed into her shaking hands. "We were just sitting on the edge and he slipped off. Is he dead?"

The two EMTs find the 16-year-old boy lying face down, partially on the raised concrete border of the planter box and partially on the sidewalk. Blood is running in wide sheets across the cement and into the storm drain and there are several glistening bones visible in the tangle of arms and legs.

"He's not breathing," Mike says, crouching down in the pooling blood. "Call for ALS and break out the bag-mask while I try to get an airway."

Musculoskeletal and Integumentary Systems

The skeleton provides the basic framework for the body, and the skin provides the protective covering. In addition to these essential functions, the musculoskeletal and integumentary systems play a variety of other important roles. Protection, movement, and thermal regulation enable many other body functions to be performed. This section reviews important anatomy and physiology of both systems.

Musculoskeletal System

The musculoskeletal system is composed of the bones and skeletal muscles of the body. This system has three major functions:

- To give the body shape
- To protect internal organs
- To provide the ability to move

The Skeleton

Bones provide the structure and shape of the body and can be found literally from head to toe (Figure 5-1 ■). The following is a top-to-bottom description of key areas of the skeleton:

- ***Head.*** The *cranium*, or skull, is a series of bones that are fused together. These bones contain and protect the brain and form the face. **Facial bones,** such as the orbital bones of the eye and the zygomatic bones of the cheeks, give the face structure. The **maxilla** forms the upper jaw and the **mandible** articulates with other bones of the cranium to form the lower jaw (Figure 5-2 ■).
- ***Upper extremities.*** The upper extremities begin with the **clavicles** (collarbones) and **scapulae** (shoulder blades). The **humerus** is the bone of the upper arm, and the **radius** and **ulna** join together to form the forearm. The **carpals** and **metacarpals** make up the bones of the wrist and hand and the **phalanges** are the bones of the fingers.
- ***Torso.*** The **sternum** (breastbone) and the **ribs** form the structure of the chest wall. There are 12 ribs, one attached to each of the 12 thoracic vertebrae of the spinal column and curving anteriorly toward the sternum. Ten of the ribs connect to the sternum. The two not attached to the sternum are called *floating ribs* (Figure 5-3 ■).
- ***Pelvis.*** The **pelvis** is a series of fused bones that include the **ilium, ischium,** and **pubis.** The pelvis is fused with the **sacral spine** posteriorly.
- ***Lower extremities.*** The **femur** (thigh bone) is the largest long bone in the body. It articulates with the pelvis to form the hip joint. The **tibia** and **fibula** are the bones of the lower leg and they articulate with the femur to form the knee joint, which is covered anteriorly by the **patella** (kneecap). The **tarsals** form the ankle, the **metatarsals** are the bones of the foot and, just like the fingers, the phalanges are the bones of the toes.

Bones come together (articulate) with each other to form joints. Some joints are movable and provide motion, while others are only slightly movable or immovable altogether. There are several types of joints (Figure 5-4 ■), including **ball-and-socket joints** (such as the hip and shoulder), **hinge joints** (the knee and elbow, for example), pivot joints (such as the neck and wrist), **gliding joints** (the wrist and ankle, for example), and saddle joints (such as the ankle). In **fused joints** bones come together but do not move (the sutures of the skull bones, for example). Other joints allow some flexibility but move only minimally (such as the vertebrae of the spine).

5-4 Describe each of the components of the skeleton, including location and function.

metacarpals the hand bones.

phalanges bones of the fingers and toes.

sternum the breastbone.

ribs the 12 pairs of bones that help form the thoracic cavity.

pelvis the basin-shaped bony structure that supports the spine and is the point of proximal attachment for the lower extremities.

ilium the superior and widest portion of the pelvis.

ischium the lower, posterior portions of the pelvis.

pubis the medial anterior portion of the pelvis.

sacral spine vertebrae that form the posterior pelvis.

femur the large bone of the thigh.

tibia the medial and larger bone of the lower leg.

fibula the lateral and smaller bone of the lower leg.

patella the kneecap.

tarsals the ankle bones.

metatarsals the foot bones.

5-5 Identify the various types of joints found in the body.

ball-and-socket joints a type of joint in which the ball-shaped head of one bone fits into a rounded receptacle or socket formed by another bone; type of joint with the greatest range of motion.

hinge joints a type of joint that moves in only one direction.

gliding joints a type of joint in which one bone end slides on another.

fused joints a type of joint in which bones meet but do not move.

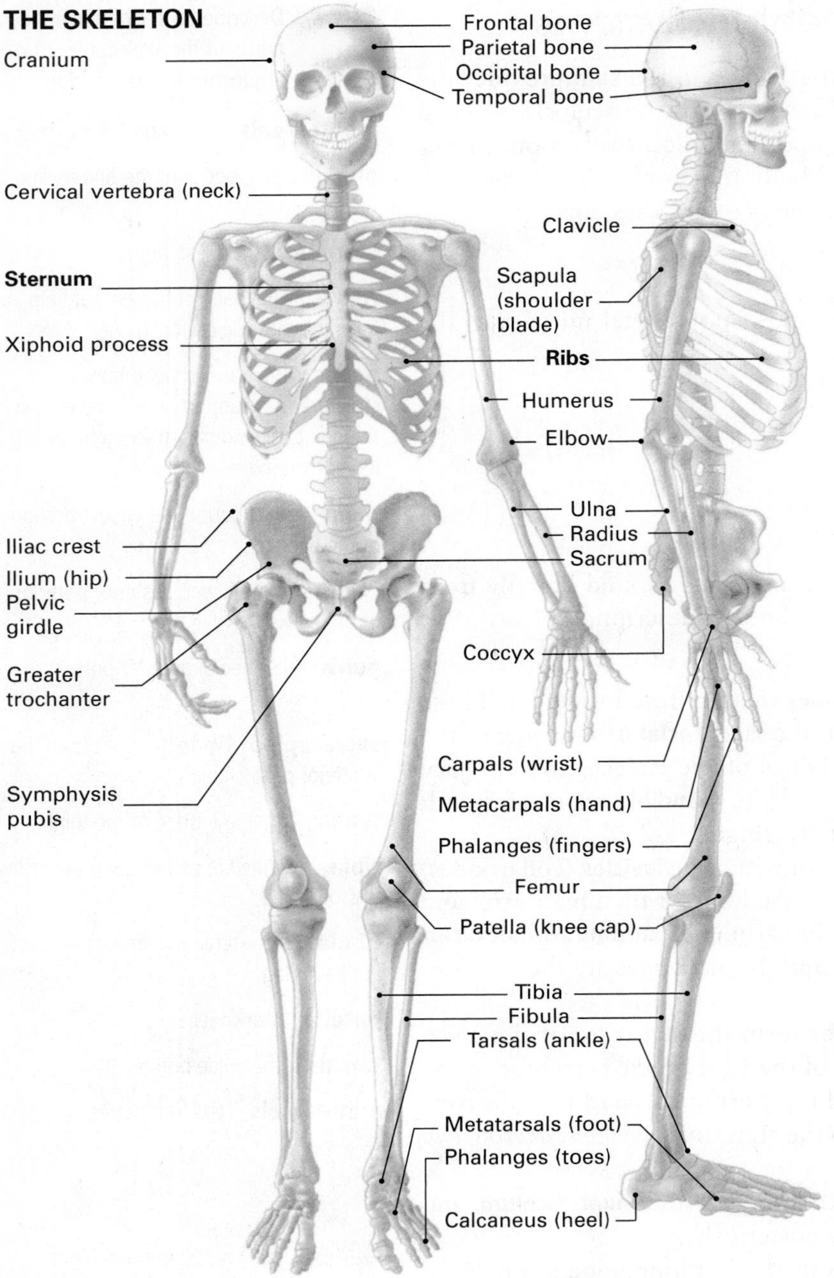

Figure 5-1 The bones of the skeletal system.

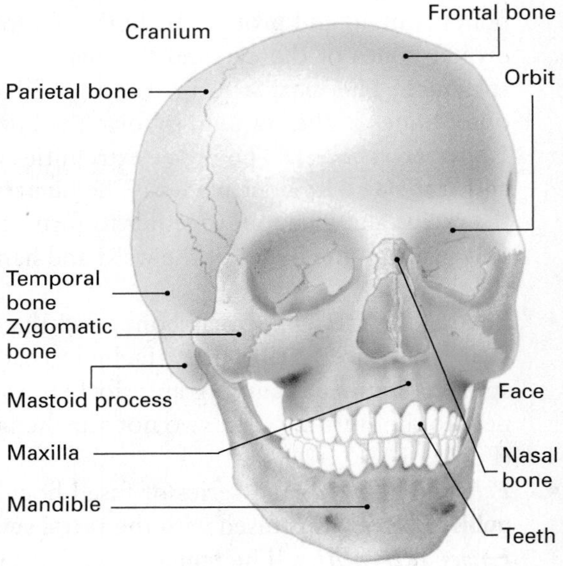

Figure 5-2 The bones of the cranium.

5-6 Describe the function of each of the following musculoskeletal system structures: bone, ligaments, skeletal muscle, tendons.

ligaments tissues that connect bone to bone.

tendons tissues that connect muscle to bone.

Bones and joints have two types of connective tissue: ligaments and tendons (Figure 5-5 ■). They hold the joints together and allow for movement. **Ligaments** connect bones to bones, while **tendons** attach muscle to bone. If you have ever suffered a sprain, you have injured one or more ligaments.

The Spine

The spinal cord is housed within the **spinal column** (sometimes simply called the *spine*). The spinal column is a series of bones called **vertebrae** that are stacked one on top of the other to form the spinal column. The spinal cord runs through a hollow

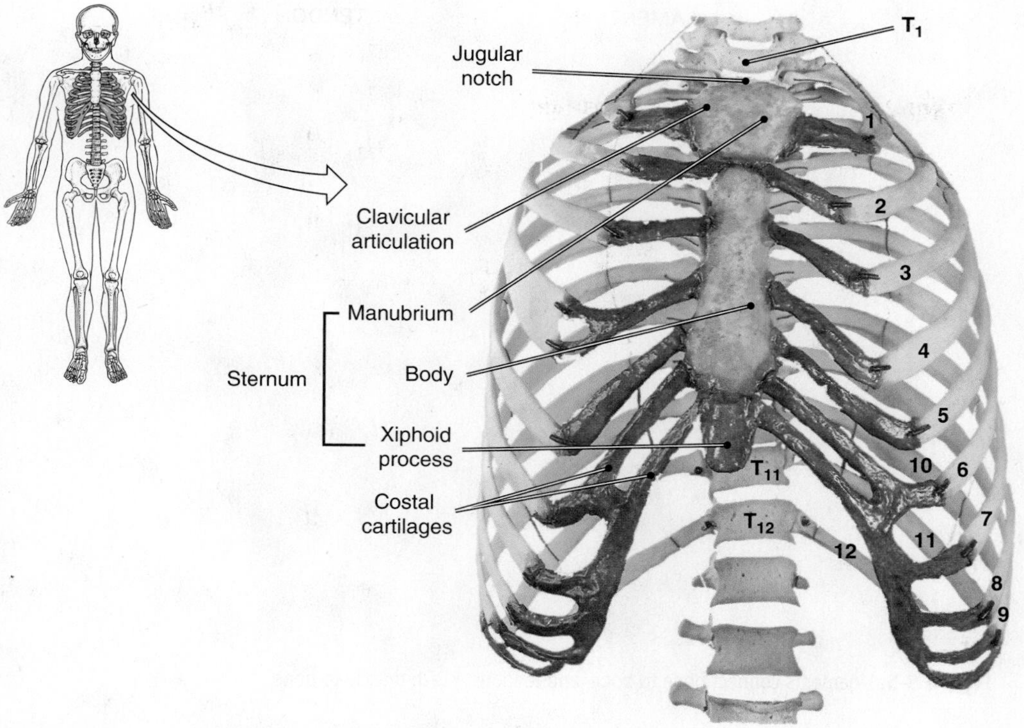

Figure 5-3 The structures of the rib cage.

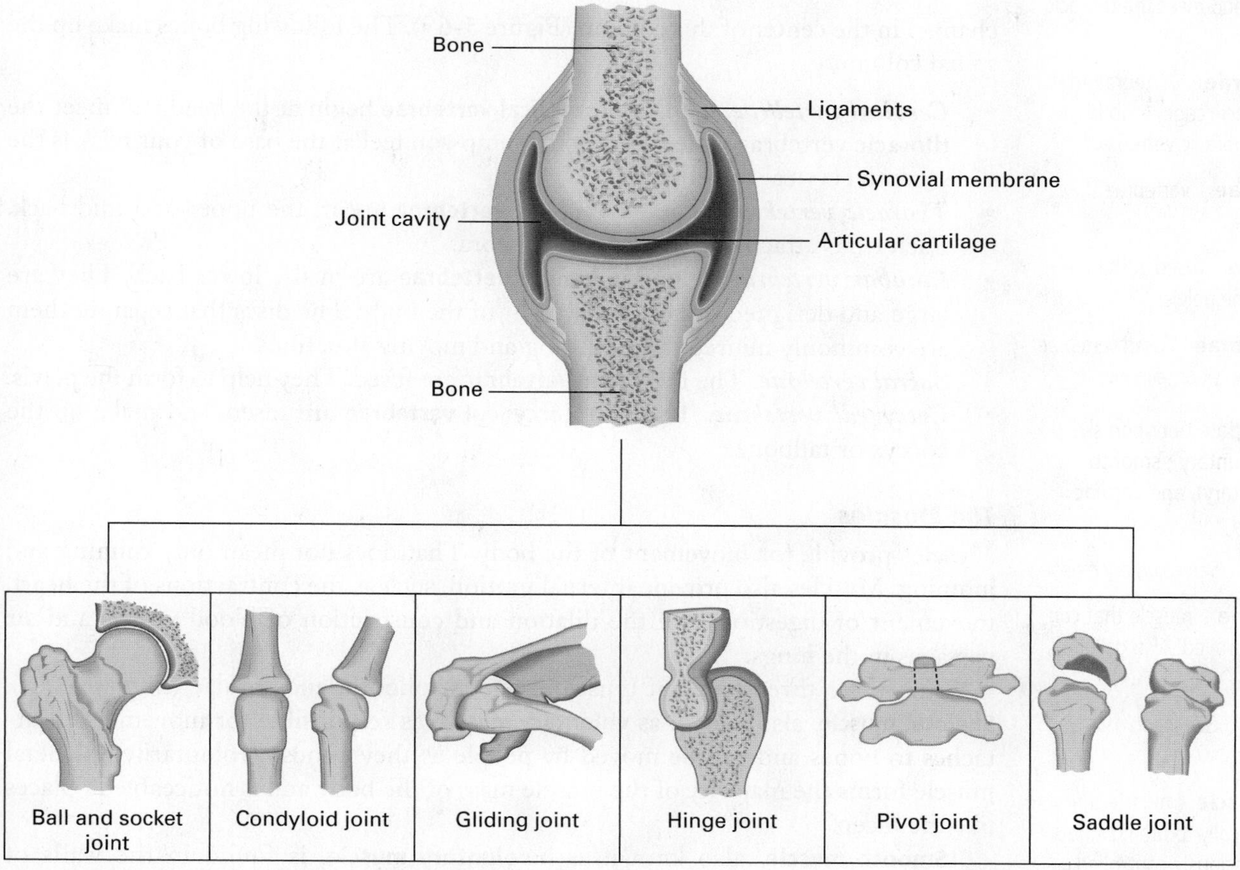

Figure 5-4 The various types of joints within the skeletal system.

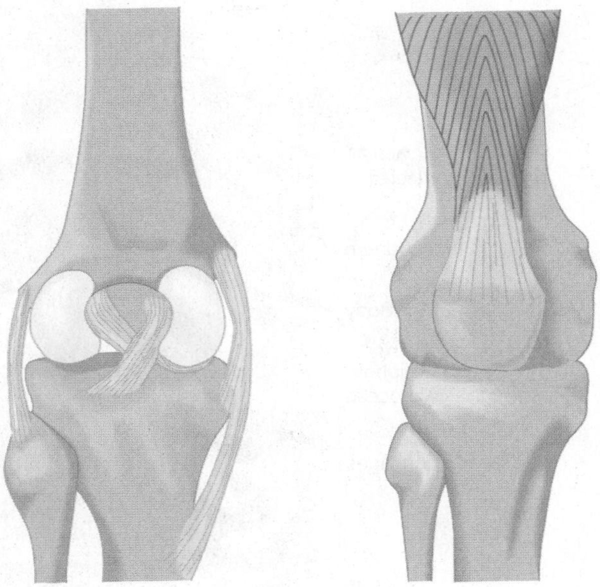

Figure 5-5 Ligaments connect bone to bone, and tendons attach muscle to bone.

PRACTICAL PATHOPHYSIOLOGY

There are 33 separate vertebrae in the spinal column. Because they are interconnected by ligaments, tendons, and muscle tissue, movement of one tends to cause movement of many others. As such, treat spine injuries as if the spinal column was one long bone and immobilize the spine as a whole.

spinal column a series of vertebrae that are stacked one on top of the other to form the column.

vertebrae the 33 bones of the spinal column. Singular *vertebra*.

cervical vertebrae vertebrae that begin at the head and meet the thoracic vertebrae.

thoracic vertebrae vertebrae that help form the thoracic cage. A rib is attached to each thoracic vertebra.

lumbar vertebrae vertebrae that form the lower back.

sacral vertebrae fused vertebrae that help to form the pelvis.

coccygeal vertebrae fused vertebrae that make up the coccyx or tailbone.

5-7 Differentiate between skeletal (voluntary), smooth (involuntary), and cardiac muscle.

skeletal muscle See *voluntary muscle*.

voluntary muscle muscle that can be consciously controlled. Also called *skeletal muscle*.

smooth muscle See *involuntary muscle*.

involuntary muscle muscle that responds automatically to brain signals but cannot be consciously controlled. Also called *smooth muscle*.

channel in the center of this column (Figure 5-6 ■). The following bones make up the spinal column:

- ***Cervical vertebrae.*** The seven **cervical vertebrae** begin at the head and meet the thoracic vertebrae. The slight bony bump you feel at the base of your neck is the seventh cervical vertebra.
- ***Thoracic vertebrae.*** The 12 **thoracic vertebrae** are in the upper and mid back. Each rib is attached to a thoracic vertebra.
- ***Lumbar vertebrae.*** The five **lumbar vertebrae** are in the lower back. They are large and designed to bear the weight of the body. The discs that separate them are commonly injured during lifting and moving situations.
- ***Sacral vertebrae.*** The five **sacral vertebrae** are fused. They help to form the pelvis.
- ***Coccygeal vertebrae.*** The four **coccygeal vertebrae** are fused, and make up the coccyx or tailbone.

The Muscles

Muscles provide for movement of the body. That does not mean only running and jumping. Muscles also provide internal motion, such as the contractions of the heart, movement of digestion, and the dilation and constriction of blood vessels and air passages in the lungs.

There are three types of muscle: skeletal, smooth, and cardiac (Figure 5-7 ■). **Skeletal muscle,** also known as **voluntary muscle,** is responsible for movement. It attaches to bones and can be moved by people as they choose (voluntarily). Skeletal muscle forms the majority of the muscle mass of the body and is noticeable in places like the bicep.

Smooth muscle, also known as **involuntary muscle,** is found in the walls of the intestine and blood vessels, and in the bronchial tubes of the lungs. They

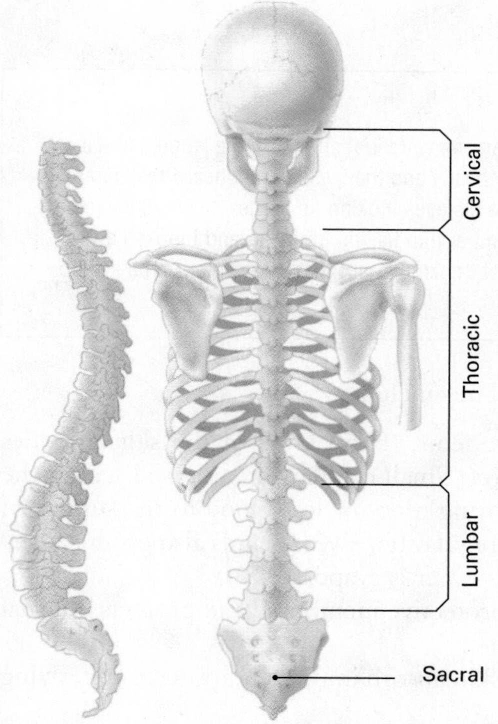

Figure 5-6 The structures of the spinal column.

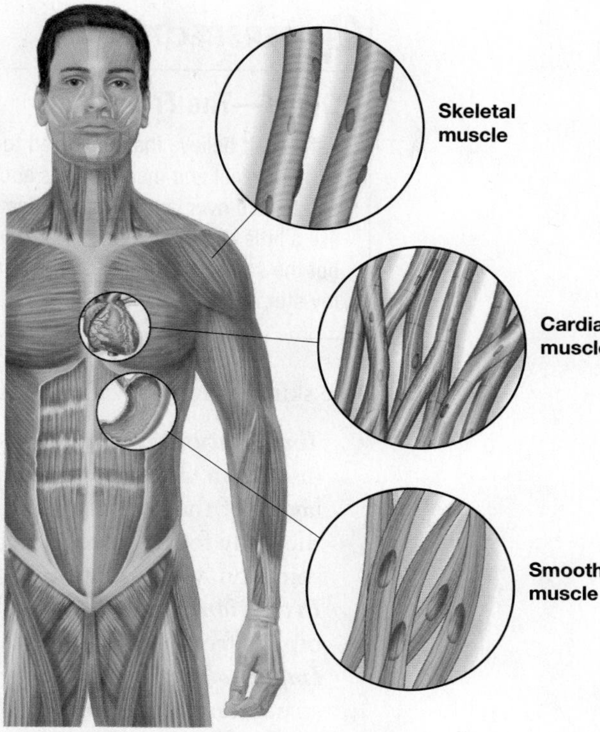

Figure 5-7 The three types of muscle tissue.

constrict (become more narrow) and dilate (become wider) to adjust flow through the structures. For example, when the body senses the need for more oxygen, bronchial tubes dilate to increase the flow of air to the lungs. Smooth muscle also is used to move food through the intestines. The contractions that cause motion are called *peristalsis*.

Cardiac muscle, as the name implies, is found only in the heart. It is involuntary muscle but has the special property of **automaticity.** Automaticity is the ability to stimulate an electrical impulse and contract on its own (without the nervous system). Cardiac muscle is the only muscle in the body that has this ability. The amount of work performed by the heart is truly amazing. The adult heart beats an average of 70 beats per minute, faster in times of stress and slower at rest. That adds up to over 4,000 times per hour and 100,000 times per day.

cardiac muscle specialized involuntary muscle found only in the heart.

automaticity the ability of the heart muscle to generate and conduct electrical impulses on its own.

Integumentary System

5-8 Describe the structure and function of the integumentary system.

The integumentary system is composed of the skin and its protective layers. The skin is the outermost layer of the body, and it covers our bones, muscles, and organs. It protects the body from the outside environment and provides many of our physical characteristics. There are three layers to the skin (Figure 5-8 ■):

- ***Epidermis.*** The **epidermis** is the outermost layer of the skin.
- ***Dermis.*** The **dermis** lies below the epidermis and contains the sweat and sebaceous (oil) glands, hair follicles, nerve endings, and some blood vessels.
- ***Subcutaneous layer.*** The **subcutaneous layer** is the deepest layer and is made up of fatty tissue. It provides shock absorption and insulation for the body.

epidermis the outer layer of the skin.

dermis the inner (second) layer of the skin, found beneath the epidermis. It is rich in blood vessels and nerves.

subcutaneous layer the deepest layer of the skin. It is fatty tissue and provides shock absorption and insulation for the body.

PERSPECTIVE

Diane—The Friend

I still can't believe that happened to Randy. I mean, we were just sitting on the ledge and dangling our feet and making jokes about the people below and then, well, I just heard this scraping and looked over, and he was falling. I can still see his eyes looking up at me. He suddenly looked like a little kid, like he was so scared. I just remember him flailing in the air and I looked away but the sound, just the sound of him landing. Just thinking about that sound makes me sick to my stomach.

The skin performs a variety of functions. They include:

- ***Temperature regulation.*** The subcutaneous (fatty) layer of the skin provides insulation against extreme temperatures. Small capillaries contained within the layers of the skin can change size to bring more or less blood to the surface of the body for purposes of temperature regulation. Sweat glands also produce perspiration, which helps cool the body as water is evaporated.
- ***Protection.*** Skin wraps the body in a protective membrane and protects internal organs from unwanted external invaders.
- ***Impact absorption.*** The layers of the skin absorb impact and protect underlying structures from trauma.

PRACTICAL PATHOPHYSIOLOGY

Always consider the function of the skin when treating patients who have lost skin surface or who have lost the integrity of the skin. Severe traumatic injuries and burns disrupt natural functions of the skin, such as protection from infection and thermoregulation.

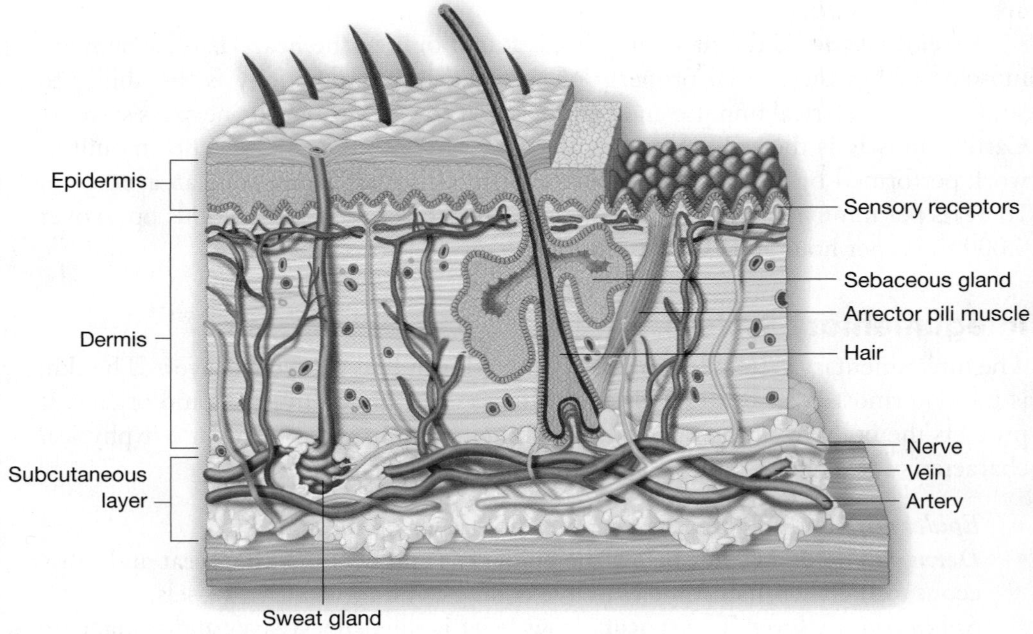

Figure 5-8 The structures of the skin.

STOP, REVIEW, REMEMBER!

Multiple Choice

For each question, place a check next to the correct answer.

1. What is another term for the lower jaw?

_____ a. Maxilla

_____ b. Mandible

_____ c. Orbital bone

_____ d. Zygomatic bone

2. The layer of skin that contains blood vessels, nerve endings, and hair follicles is called the:

_____ a. epidermis.

_____ b. polydermis.

_____ c. subdermis.

_____ d. dermis.

3. The bone of the upper arm is known as the:

_____ a. humerus.

_____ b. fibula.

_____ c. radius.

_____ d. ulna.

4. The bones that form the ankle are known as the:

_____ a. phalanges.

_____ b. metacarpals.

_____ c. tarsals.

_____ d. carpals.

5. The area of the spine that includes the bones in the neck is called the ______________ region.

_____ a. sacral

_____ b. thoracic

_____ c. lumbar

_____ d. cervical

6. The region of the spine designed to bear the weight of the body is the ______________ region.

_____ a. cervical

_____ b. lymphatic

_____ c. thoracic

_____ d. lumbar

7. The kneecap is called the:

_____ a. patella.

_____ b. tibia.

_____ c. femur.

_____ d. periosteum.

Fill in the Blank

1. The bones of the forearm are the ______________________________ and ______________________________.

2. Two ribs are not connected to the sternum. They are called ______________ ribs.

3. The elbow is an example of a ______________________________ joint.

4. The vertebrae that form the tailbone are called the ______________________________.

5. The muscle lining the bronchioles is known as ______________________________ or ______________________________ muscle.

(continued on next page)

(continued)

Critical Thinking

1. List the three functions of the musculoskeletal system.

____

____

____

____

2. List three functions of the integumentary system.

____

____

____

____

The Cardiorespiratory System

The cardiorespiratory system includes both the respiratory and the cardiovascular systems. Although they are separate systems, their functions are so intertwined that often it is useful to think of them as one.

5-9 Describe the mechanics and physiology of normal ventilation, respiration, and oxygenation.

glucose a simple form of sugar that is required by all cells as fuel for metabolic processes.

aerobic metabolism the process of converting glucose to energy by using sufficient supplies of oxygen.

anaerobic metabolism the process of converting glucose to energy by using insufficient supplies of oxygen.

perfusion distribution of blood to all parts of the body to deliver oxygen and remove waste products.

ventilation/perfusion match (V/Q match) the coupling of appropriate amounts of air in the alveoli with a sufficient blood supply so as to promote gas exchange.

The Life Support Chain

The cells of the body require oxygen and **glucose** to complete their normal functions. Glucose is converted by the cells into energy in the form of adenosine triphosphate (ATP). Oxygen is used to effectively fuel this conversion process. The process of converting glucose with the appropriate amount of oxygen is called **aerobic metabolism.** It is very efficient and produces energy (ATP) and minimal waste products such as carbon dioxide and water. In contrast, when oxygen is not in sufficient supply, the process of **anaerobic metabolism** occurs. This process produces less energy (ATP) and more waste products, such as lactic acid. The accumulation of excessive waste products makes the body more acidotic further damaging the body's cells. Acidosis greatly limits the blood's ability to carry oxygen.

Perfusion occurs when oxygen and nutrients are delivered to the cells and waste products are removed. Perfusion is essential to normal cell function. The most important role of the cardiorespiratory system is to maintain perfusion. A number of different elements are required to make perfusion occur. Air must reach the alveoli and match up with a sufficient supply of blood in the pulmonary capillaries. Blood also must reach the alveoli to deliver carbon dioxide and pick up oxygen. That coupling is called a **ventilation/perfusion match (V/Q match).**

In addition to a proper V/Q match, perfusion also requires other important functions. The heart must pump effectively (if the pump fails, blood will not move), and the blood must be capable of carrying oxygen. For example, *anemia* is a condition that in some cases reduces the number of oxygen-carrying red blood cells. Also, there must be enough oxygen in the air that is breathed. Anything that threatens the normal function of the cardiopulmonary system should be considered a threat to perfusion.

The Respiratory System

The respiratory system itself is composed of the lungs and the structures of the airway. It also includes the muscles required to move air. The respiratory system is responsible for bringing oxygen into the body and removing carbon dioxide from the bloodstream. This constant gas exchange is essential to perfusion and is required by all the cells of the body.

The respiratory system (Figure 5-9 ■) begins at the nose and mouth. Air enters and is moved back through the **pharynx.** The pharynx is traditionally divided into three regions. The area behind the mouth is called the **oropharynx,** the area behind the nose is called the **nasopharynx,** and the area in the back of the throat is called the **hypopharynx** or the **laryngopharynx.** Air moves through the pharynx and enters the trachea through the **glottic opening.** The glottic opening rests in the **larynx,** commonly called the *voice box*. The larynx is designed to house and protect the entrance to the trachea and is protected by structures made of **cartilage.** The **thyroid cartilage,** which is commonly referred to as the *Adam's apple*, forms the anterior portion of the larynx, while the **cricoid cartilage,** a complete ring of cartilage at the distal end of the larynx, creates the inferior border. The vocal cords are found just inside the glottic opening and provide protection for the trachea and the ability to make sound.

The glottic opening is protected by a leaf-shaped structure called the **epiglottis.** The epiglottis folds down over the opening of the trachea during swallowing to prevent food and liquids from entering the lungs. When patients are unresponsive, they can lose control of their epiglottis, allowing it to obstruct the glottic opening and block air movement. Additionally, unresponsiveness can result in a failure of the epiglottis to effectively protect the trachea. That failure can allow substances to be breathed (aspirated) into the lungs. For these reasons, you must pay close attention to protecting the airway of unresponsive patients through positioning and suctioning.

The **trachea,** also called the *windpipe*, is the tube through which air passes into the lungs. It has rings of cartilage to maintain its shape and prevent collapse. The trachea splits into two **bronchi,** one traveling to each lung. The bronchi continue to split into smaller and smaller air passages until they reach the smallest level, the **bronchioles.** At the termination of those tiny airways are the **alveoli,** tiny air sacs in which the actual exchange of oxygen and carbon dioxide takes place.

There are millions of alveoli in the lungs, grouped into small grape-like clusters. Each alveolus is covered with microscopic blood vessels called *capillaries*. Through the process of diffusion, oxygen is taken from the air in the alveoli and transferred into the blood. Carbon dioxide is removed from the blood and transferred to alveolar air.

The **lungs** are the primary organs of respiration. There are two. Each lung is divided into **lobes,** or sections. The left lung has two lobes. The right lung has three lobes.

The Act of Breathing

Breathing can be described as a two-step process: inhalation and exhalation. We do it thousands of times a day without thinking about it. One respiratory cycle is one inhalation plus one exhalation. On average an adult breathes 12 to 20 times per minute.

5-10 Describe the structures and function of the respiratory system.

pharynx passageway that extends from nose and mouth to trachea.

oropharynx the area directly posterior to the mouth.

nasopharynx the area directly posterior to the nose.

hypopharynx the back of the throat superior to the opening of the trachea.

laryngopharynx the area in the back of the throat just inferior to the epiglottis. Also called *hypopharynx*.

glottic opening the opening of the trachea in the hypopharynx. Also known as the *glottis*.

larynx the structure that contains the vocal cords and is connected to the superior portion of the trachea.

cartilage tough tissue that covers the joint ends of bones and helps to form certain body parts such as the ear.

thyroid cartilage prominence in the anterior neck. Also called the *Adam's apple*.

cricoid cartilage the ring-shaped structure that circles the trachea at the lower edge of the larynx.

epiglottis a leaf-shaped structure that covers and prevents food and foreign matter from entering the larynx and trachea.

trachea the structure that connects the pharynx to the lungs. Also called the *windpipe*.

bronchi the two large sets of branches that come off the trachea and enter the lungs. There are right and left bronchi. Singular *bronchus*.

bronchioles smallest branches of bronchi.

alveoli the microscopic sacs of the lungs in which gas exchange with the bloodstream takes place.

lungs the primary organs of respiration. There is a left lung and a right lung.

lobes sections of the lung. The left lung has two lobes; the right lung has three lobes.

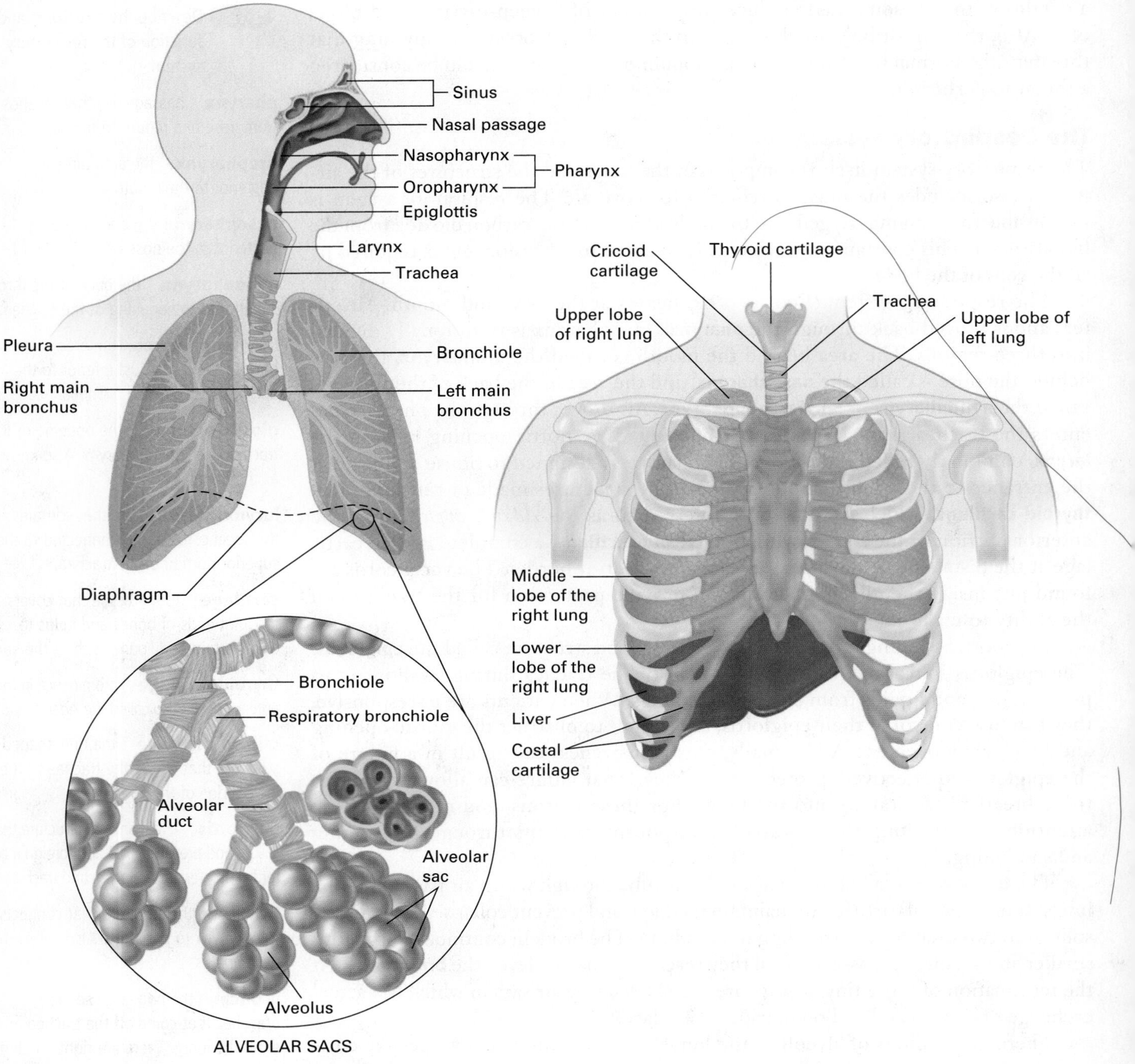

Figure 5-9 The structures of the respiratory system.

inhalation an active process in which the intercostal (rib) muscles and the diaphragm contract, expanding the size of the chest cavity and causing air to flow into the lungs. Also called *inspiration*.

The rate may be a bit slower at rest and a bit faster during exertion and still be considered normal.

Inhalation is an active process. It requires muscle use and energy. During inhalation, the diaphragm muscle contracts and moves downward. The intercostal muscles (muscles between the ribs) contract and move the ribs upward and outward. Those movements increase the size of the chest cavity, creating a negative pressure and causing air to flow into the lungs.

Exhalation is passive and occurs when the diaphragm and intercostal muscles relax. That causes a reduction in size of the chest cavity, creating positive pressure and forcing air out of the lungs.

Through breathing, air is moved into and out of the alveoli. This is referred to as **ventilation.** (As previously mentioned, the alveoli are the site of gas exchange between air and blood.) The pulmonary capillaries bring circulating blood to the outside of the alveoli to be matched up with air. Through the very thin walls of the alveoli, oxygen is transferred from the air to the bloodstream and carbon dioxide is moved from the bloodstream into alveolar air. This movement of gases in the alveoli is called **respiration.**

Oxygenated blood is carried from the lungs to the heart so it can be pumped to the cells of the body. The heart moves that blood to the capillaries that surround each body cell. Oxygen and nutrients then pass to the cells in a process similar to that which occurs in the alveoli. Waste carbon dioxide is picked up and returned to the blood in the capillaries. Capillaries then return it back to the heart where it can be pumped to the lungs for further gas exchange. The process of moving gases (and other nutrients) between the cells and the blood is the foundation of respiration.

Exchanging gas at both the alveolar and at the cellular level is a critical life function. Aerobic metabolism depends on a steady supply of oxygen, and the removal of waste products. This is essential to regulating the body's pH and keeping it at the optimal range of 7.35 to 7.45.

exhalation a passive process in which the intercostal (rib) muscles and the diaphragm relax, causing the chest cavity to decrease in size and air to flow out of the lungs. Also called *expiration.*

ventilation the movement of oxygen and carbon dioxide at the alveolar level.

respiration the movement of oxygen and waste products at the cellular level.

PERSPECTIVE

Dave—The EMT

That kid was bad. And by bad, I mean he was very bad. I have seen people come out of high-speed auto versus pedestrian collisions better off than he. In those cases you just have to remember the ABCs. To be honest, with this kid that's all I could remember initially. You just see this body with tissue and blood and bones that are all supposed to be on the inside, and they're not, you know? I just kept repeating "A-B-C. Airway, breathing, circulation." I knew that the rest would come back to me when I needed it, the immobilization, the splinting, everything. But we had to do first things first.

Breathing in Infants and Children

5-11 Differentiate respiratory system anatomy between adults and children.

Children are generally healthy. If they do suddenly become critically ill, the respiratory system is often the culprit. This means that your attention to an infant or child's respiratory system will be critical, as will your knowledge of the differences between the respiratory structures of children and adults (Figure 5-10 ■). Some of those differences include the following:

- Children's respiratory structures are smaller than those of adults. As a consequence, an obstruction, infection, or swelling can cause a reduction in air flow much more quickly than in an adult.
- The tongues of infants and children take up proportionally more space in the mouth and pharynx than an adult's. This makes it much more likely that a child's airway could become compromised when swelling occurs.
- The trachea is narrower, softer, and more flexible than an adult's. This means the child's trachea will be more easily occluded (blocked) by obstruction or swelling.

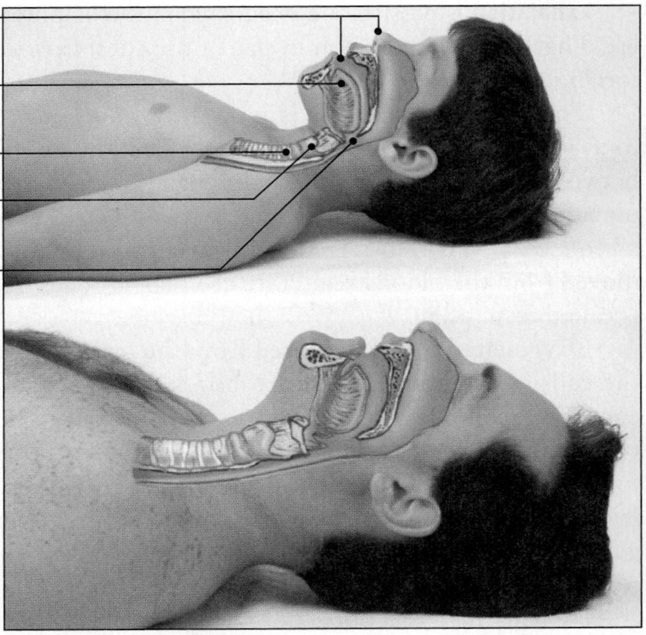
Child has smaller nose and mouth.
In child, more space is taken up by tongue.
Child's trachea is narrower.
Cricoid cartilage is less rigid and less developed.
Airway structures are more easily obstructed.

Figure 5-10 The differences between the adult and pediatric airways.

- The cricoid cartilage is less developed than an adult's, giving less support to the tracheal structure.
- The chest wall is softer, so infants and children tend to rely on the diaphragm to move air in and out. Therefore, abdominal breathing in a child is normal, whereas it would indicate respiratory distress in an adult.
- The respiratory rate in children is much higher than that of an adult. That means they burn oxygen much faster and require a reliable and continual supply to sustain normal function.

5-12 Describe the function of the cardiovascular (circulatory) system.

cardiovascular system the system made up of the heart (*cardio*), the blood vessels (*vascular*), and the blood. Also called the *circulatory system.*

The Cardiovascular System

There are three main components of the **cardiovascular system** (also called the *circulatory system*): the heart, blood vessels, and blood. The purpose of the cardiovascular system is to pump blood to every cell of the body in order to sustain perfusion.

5-13 Describe the structure and function of the heart.

pulse the pumping of the heart as a pressure wave felt over an artery.

atria the two upper chambers of the heart. Singular *atrium.* There is a right atrium (which receives unoxygenated blood from the body) and a left atrium (which receives oxygenated blood from the lungs).

ventricles the two lower chambers of the heart. There is a right ventricle (which sends oxygen-poor blood to the lungs) and a left ventricle (which sends oxygen-rich blood to the body).

The Heart

The heart is a well designed, efficient pump tasked with moving blood to the entire body. It never rests. On average, the heart pumps about 70 times per minute, squeezing blood into circulation each time it pumps. The pressure exerted on the blood vessels as the heart pumps can be felt easily as a **pulse** at the radial artery in the wrist and the carotid artery in the neck.

The heart has four chambers, two on the left side of the heart and two on the right side. The upper chambers are the **atria** (singular *atrium*); the lower chambers are the **ventricles.** They are called the *right atrium, right ventricle, left atrium*, and *left ventricle*. To understand the heart, you must follow blood as it travels through those chambers (Figure 5-11 ▪).

Blood flows toward the heart in vessels called *veins*. The largest of the veins are the venae cavae (singular *vena cava*). The blood from the lower body returns through the inferior vena cava, and blood from the head and neck returns by way of the superior vena cava. These large vessels come together and return blood to

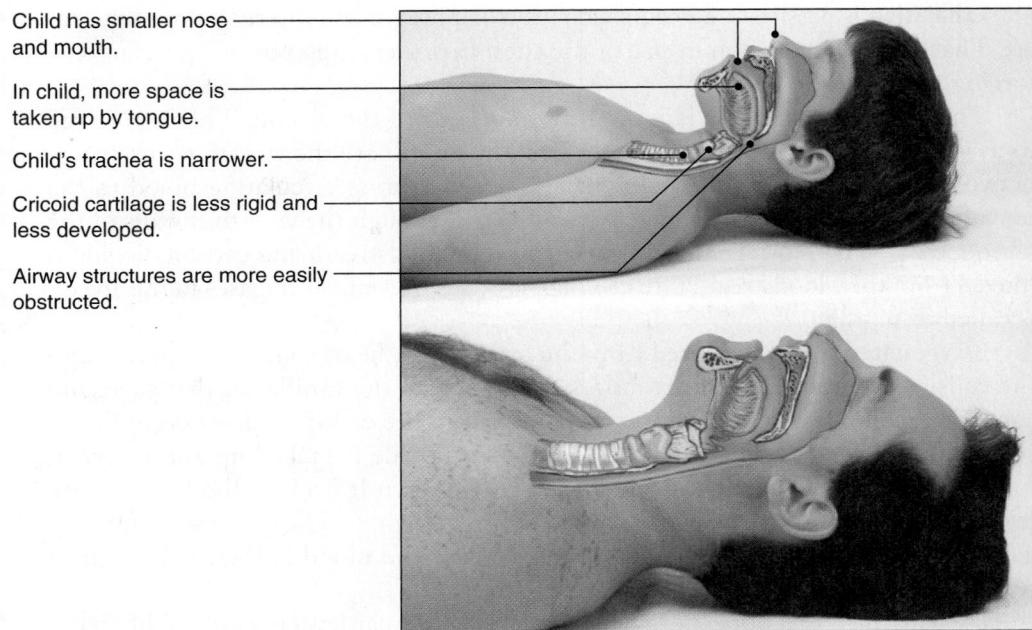

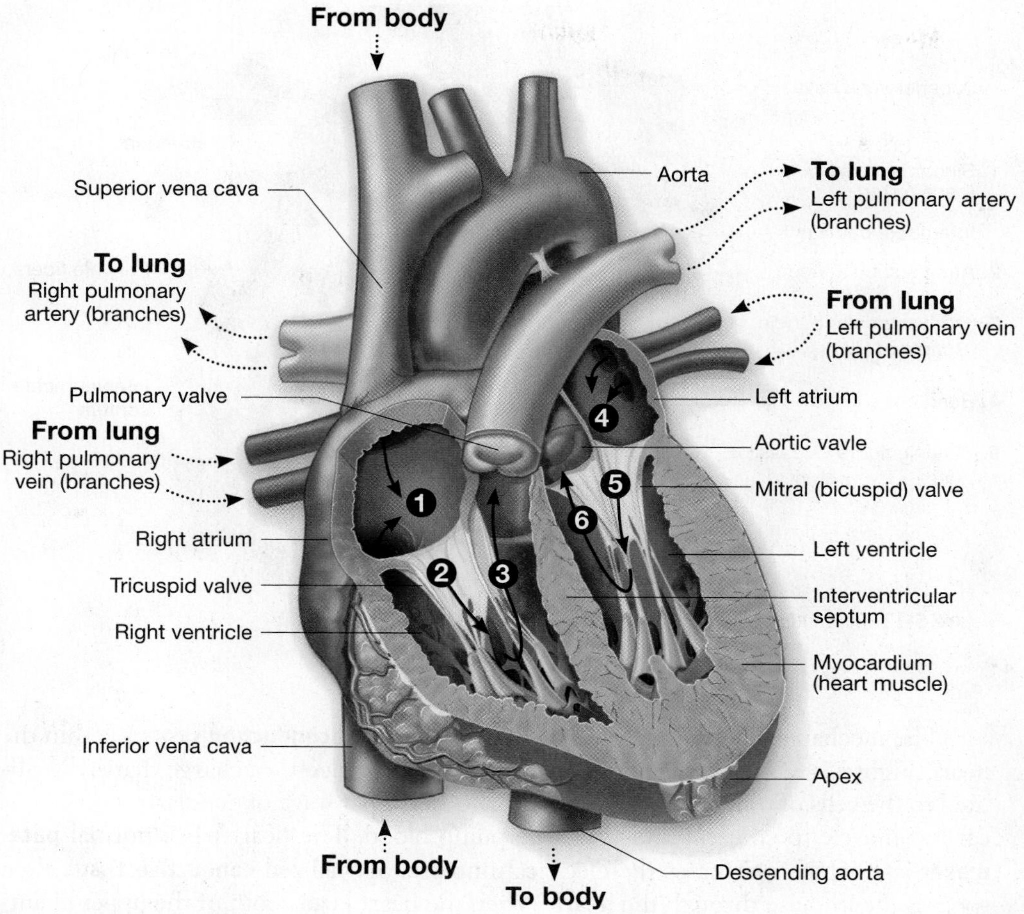

Figure 5-11 The flow of blood and structures of the heart.

the right atrium. Blood is moved from the right atrium through the **tricuspid valve** and into the right ventricle. Blood leaves the right ventricle through the **pulmonic valve** and is pumped to the lungs by way of the **pulmonary arteries.** Since this blood is coming back from the body, it is high in **carbon dioxide** picked up from the cells and low in oxygen. At the lungs, carbon dioxide is off-loaded and exhaled, and oxygen that has been inhaled is moved into the blood. This exchange of oxygen and carbon dioxide is done through the alveoli and the capillaries, as noted in the previous section.

Blood returns from the lungs to the left atrium through the pulmonary veins. This blood is richly oxygenated and ready to be pumped to the body again. The left atrium receives it and pumps it through the **mitral valve** into the left ventricle, the largest and most muscular chamber of the heart. The blood then is passed through the **aortic valve** into the **aorta.** From the aorta blood is moved through a series of branching and gradually smaller arteries, then into the tiny cellular capillaries where oxygen and nutrients are delivered.

The heart is a muscle. Although the heart is filled with blood at all times, it does not receive the blood it needs for its own perfusion from the blood that passes through it. The heart receives its own blood supply through a series of arteries known as the **coronary arteries.** They branch off the aorta as it leaves the left ventricle, and then travel back to the heart to provide essential oxygen and nutrients. When a patient has a heart attack, also known as a *myocardial infarction*, it is caused by the occlusion (blockage) of one or more of the coronary arteries.

tricuspid valve a structure between the right atrium and right ventricle that opens and closes to permit the flow of a fluid in only one direction.

pulmonic valve a structure between the right ventricle and pulmonary arteries that opens and closes to permit the flow of a fluid in only one direction.

pulmonary arteries vessels that carry oxygen-poor blood from the right ventricle to the lungs.

carbon dioxide waste gas found in the blood. This is exchanged with oxygen in the lungs.

mitral valve a structure between the left atrium and left ventricle that opens and closes to permit the flow of a fluid in only one direction.

aortic valve a structure between the left ventricle and aorta that opens and closes to permit the flow of a fluid in only one direction.

aorta the largest artery in the body. It transports blood from the left ventricle to begin systemic circulation.

coronary arteries arteries that branch off the aorta and provide blood supply directly to the heart.

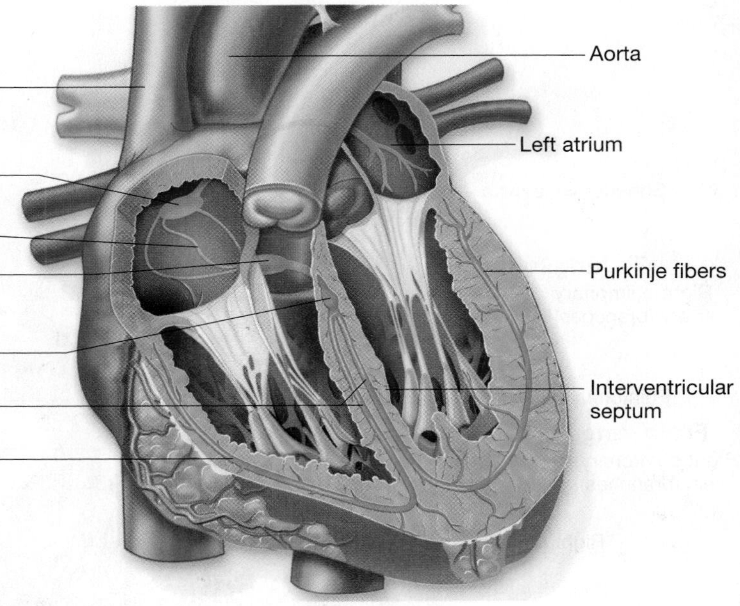

Figure 5-12 The conduction system of the heart.

conduction system specialized tissue that provides the electrical stimulus that makes the heart beat.

pacemaker site within the heart that originates an electrical impulse.

conductive tissue a system of specialized muscle tissues that conduct the electrical impulses that stimulate the heart to beat.

arteries blood vessels that carry blood away from the heart.

veins blood vessels that return blood to the heart.

arterioles the smallest arteries.

capillaries thin-walled, microscopic blood vessels in which oxygen, carbon dioxide, nutrients, and waste are exchanged with the body's cells.

venules the smallest veins.

The mechanical pumping is initiated by a specialized **conduction system** within the heart (Figure 5-12 ▪). Heart cells depolarize to create an electrical charge that is distributed to the cells of the heart in a very specific order. That wave of depolarization causes cardiac muscle to contract and therefore pump blood. The heart has a normal **pacemaker** site, which originates the electrical impulse. Specialized **conductive tissue** then spreads the impulse through the heart. When the heart beats, both of the upper chambers (atria) squeeze at the same time, followed by the two lower chambers (ventricles).

Blood Vessels

Vessels that carry blood away from the heart are **arteries.** Vessels that return blood to the heart are **veins.** As blood leaves the heart, it enters the aorta, the largest vessel in the body. As blood moves away from the heart—toward the toe, for example—it enters smaller and smaller arteries. Eventually, the blood reaches the **arterioles,** the smallest artery branches, which in turn lead to capillaries.

Capillaries are tiny vessels that are found between and connect arterioles and venules. Capillaries have very thin walls that allow the exchange of gases between a cell and the blood. After moving through the capillaries, blood begins its return trip through the venous system back to the heart. Capillaries are followed by **venules,** veins, and eventually, the venae cavae.

Blood in the arteries is under high pressure. This pressure is necessary to move blood to the farthest reaches of the body. Venous blood returning to the heart is under much lower pressure and is kept flowing in one direction by valves that prevent blood from backing up through the system.

There are several arteries and veins that have specific relevance to patient assessment and care (Figure 5-13 ▪). They include the following:

carotid artery the large neck artery that carries blood from the heart to the head. There is one carotid artery on each side of the neck.

brachial artery the major artery of the upper arm.

- ***Carotid artery.*** The **carotid artery** is the major artery of the neck and a primary supplier of blood to the head. It is the artery of choice when checking for a pulse in unresponsive patients.
- ***Brachial artery.*** The **brachial artery** is the artery of the arm that is palpated to obtain a pulse in infants. It is found between the elbow and shoulder. It is also the artery used when obtaining a blood pressure.

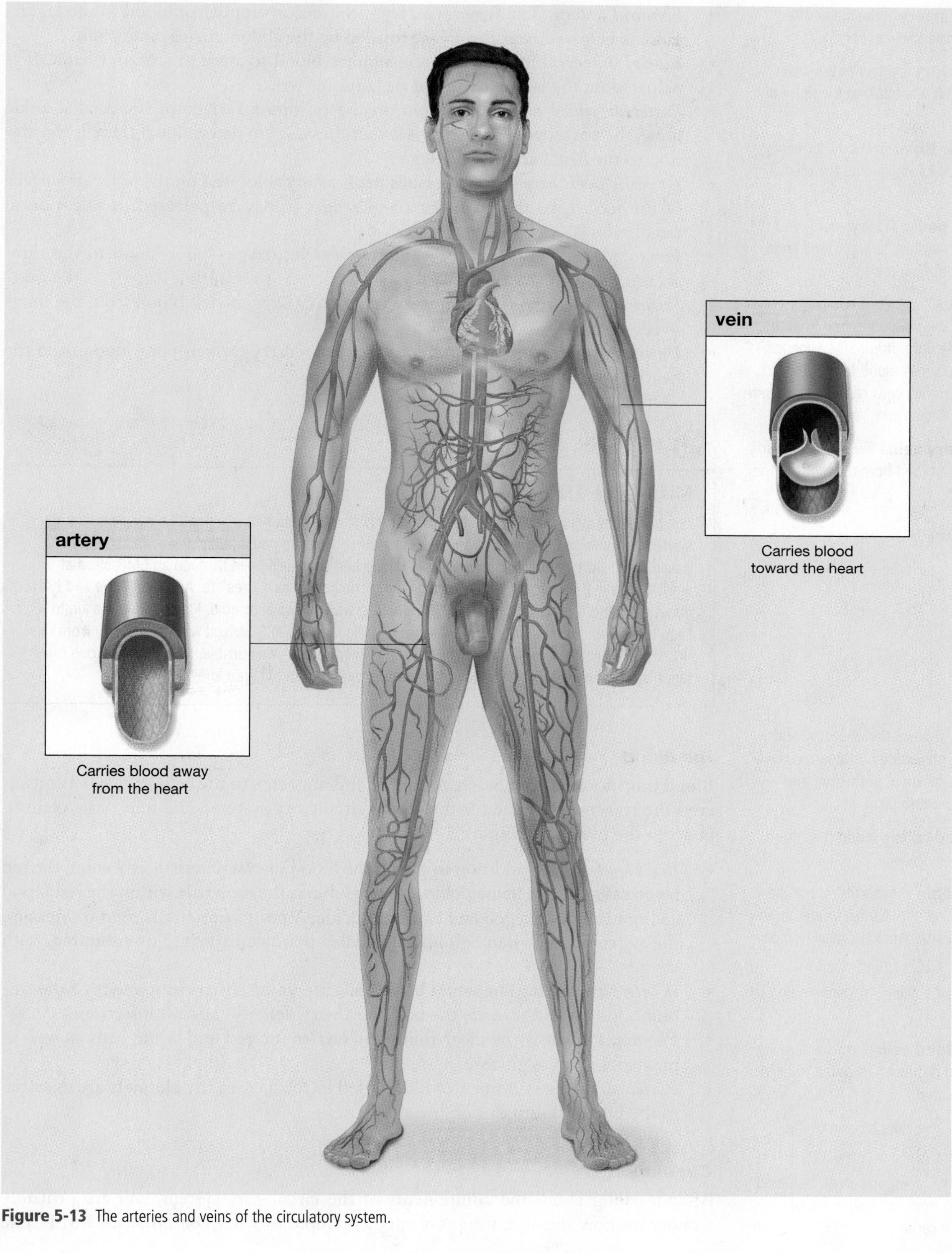

Figure 5-13 The arteries and veins of the circulatory system.

- ***Femoral artery.*** The **femoral artery** is the major supplier of blood to the leg. Its pulse is palpated near the crease formed by the abdomen, leg, and groin.
- ***Radial artery.*** The **radial artery** supplies blood to the forearm and hand. It is palpated on the lateral aspect of the anterior wrist.
- ***Posterior tibial artery.*** Palpated on the posterior surface of the medial ankle bone, the **posterior tibial artery** is sometimes used to determine if there is circulation to the distal areas of the leg.
- ***Dorsalis pedis artery.*** The **dorsalis pedis artery** is located on the anterior surface of the foot. Like the posterior tibial artery, it may be palpated to assess distal circulation.
- ***Vena cava.*** A large vein, the **vena cava** carries oxygen-poor blood to the right atrium of the heart.
- ***Pulmonary veins.*** The **pulmonary veins** carry oxygen-rich blood from the lungs to the heart.
- ***Pulmonary arteries.*** The pulmonary arteries carry oxygen-poor blood from the heart to the lungs.

femoral artery the major artery supplying the lower extremity.

radial artery artery of the lower arm. It is felt when taking the pulse at the wrist.

posterior tibial artery artery supplying the foot, behind the medial ankle.

dorsalis pedis artery artery supplying the foot, lateral to the large tendon of the big toe.

vena cava either of two major veins that carry oxygen-poor blood from the body to the right atrium. The superior vena cava carries blood from the head; the inferior vena cava carries blood from the lower body. Plural *venae cavae.*

pulmonary veins vessels that carry oxygen-rich blood from the lungs to the left atrium.

PERSPECTIVE

Mike—The EMT

The human body is amazing. I got an oral airway in and suctioned a bunch of blood and that guy started breathing so we put him on a nonrebreather. He even had a pulse. It wasn't strong, but it was there. So this guy comes out of the crowd and says he's been through an EMR class at work and asks if he should hold C-spine, which I obviously said "Yes" to. And then Dave and I set about stopping the big bleeds. That one in his leg was definitely arterial. I kept telling the kid to keep breathing, just keep breathing, keep breathing. Just as ALS arrived with the cavalry from the fire department, the guy was actually starting to respond. It was horrible, though, he started crying. I can't even imagine the pain and confusion in that moment, you know?

5-14 Discuss the anatomy and physiology of blood, circulation, perfusion, and metabolism.

The Blood

Blood transports oxygen, waste products, and nutrients to the cells. It may be considered the transport vehicle for the whole circulatory system. The four basic components of the blood are (Figure 5-14 ■):

- ***Red blood cells.*** In addition to giving the blood its characteristic red color, the **red blood cells** contain **hemoglobin.** Hemoglobin is the molecule within the red blood cell that carries oxygen and carbon dioxide. A pulse oximeter is used to measure the percentage of hemoglobin molecules that are carrying, or **saturated,** with oxygen.
- ***White blood cells.*** The **white blood cells** are an essential component of the immune system and provide the body's primary defenses against infection.
- ***Plasma.*** **Plasma** is the clear fluid that carries the red and white cells as well as nutrients, such as glucose.
- ***Platelets.*** The component of blood used to form clots, the **platelets** are essential to the body's ability to stop bleeding.

red blood cells blood cells that contain hemoglobin.

hemoglobin molecule within the red blood cell that carries oxygen to the cells and carbon dioxide away from the cells.

saturated filled, as hemoglobin with oxygen.

white blood cells cells within the blood that produce substances that help fight infection.

plasma the fluid portion of the blood.

platelets components of the blood; membrane-enclosed fragments of specialized cells.

Circulation

After learning about the components of the circulatory system, you are probably wondering how those critical concepts will apply to what you do as an EMT. The answer is: Your evaluation of a patient's circulation will be critical to his survival. Without adequate circulating blood, perfusion stops, cells go without oxygen and nutrients, and waste products accumulate.

Hypoperfusion (also known as *shock*) is inadequate perfusion of the cells. When the body is not perfused properly, shock occurs. The patient will appear pale or blue (cyanotic), the skin will be cool and moist, and the pulse and breathing will increase to compensate for the deficit. The patient may become anxious or restless, and in some cases may have a low blood pressure.

Blood pressure is the pressure exerted by the blood on the walls of an artery. Recall that blood is pumped from the left ventricle under high pressure. When you feel a pulse in the body, the beat you feel corresponds with the compression of the left ventricle sending blood into the aorta.

For each beat of the heart, an average of 70 mL of blood is ejected into the aorta. The amount of blood ejected is called **stroke volume.** The formula for cardiac output is as follows:

heart rate × stroke volume = cardiac output

or

HR × SV = CO

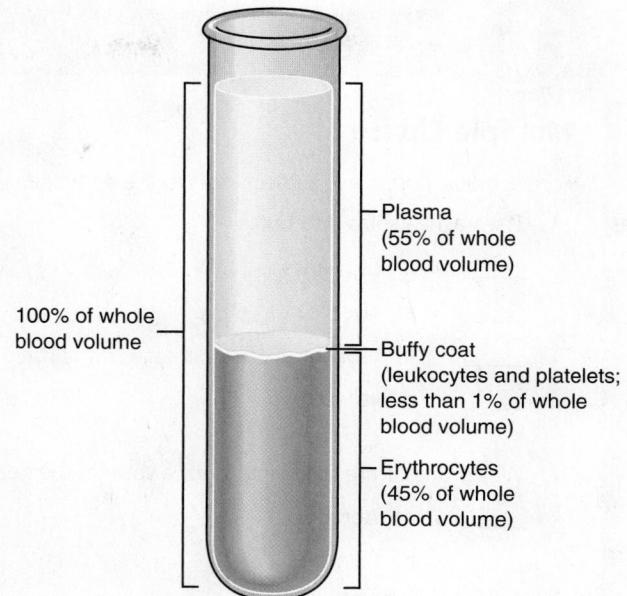

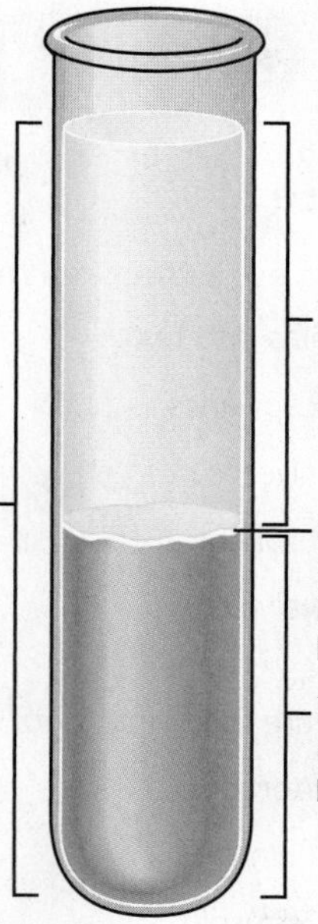

Figure 5-14 Blood is composed of red cells, white cells, plasma, and platelets.

For example, if a normal heart beats 70 times per minute and the average stroke volume is 70 mL per beat, then average cardiac output is 4,900 mL/minute. The body strives to maintain a consistent cardiac output. If the stroke volume falls (as happens with serious blood loss), the body compensates by raising the heart rate. An elevated heart rate is an early sign of hypoperfusion.

Pressure is required to move blood to all parts of the body. The delicate balance of pressure is maintained by the amount of blood in the body, the pumping of the heart, and the size of the blood vessels. Arteries have the ability to increase or decrease their size to compensate for blood loss or to maintain normal pressure within the system. When additional perfusion is needed, arteries can expand and allow more blood to flow. In the event of blood loss, arteries can constrict to help maintain blood pressure. The constriction of blood vessels that supply the skin causes the cool skin often encountered in patients with shock.

Blood pressure is defined as cardiac output times the resistance (also called **systemic vascular resistance [SVR]**) of the blood vessels. That is written as follows:

cardiac output × systemic vascular resistance = blood pressure

or

CO × SVR = BP

If any of the factors in those equations falter, blood pressure falls. If a heart attack causes damage to the left ventricle and cardiac output falls, blood pressure falls. If a patient loses a lot of blood, cardiac output will fall because there will be less blood for the heart to pump. Sometimes the size of the vessels increases. This can be caused by a nervous system disorder or by an allergic reaction. If the blood vessels suddenly expand, the resistance inside the arteries becomes less, and the blood pressure drops.

hypoperfusion inadequate distribution of blood to an organ or organs of the body. Also called *shock*.

blood pressure the pressure exerted by blood against the walls of blood vessels.

stroke volume amount of blood ejected into the aorta with each heartbeat.

systemic vascular resistance (SVR) an indicator of the diameter of the blood vessels.

CLINICAL CLUE

Circulation

Compensation for falling pressure in the circulatory system can be seen externally. Look for rapid heart rates and pale skin due to constricted blood vessels.

STOP, REVIEW, REMEMBER!

Multiple Choice

For each question, place a check next to the correct answer.

1. The trachea splits into two:

_____ a. capillaries.

_____ b. alveoli.

_____ c. bronchi.

_____ d. valves.

2. Which one of the following is *not* a valve in the heart?

_____ a. Aortic

_____ b. Pulmonic

_____ c. Tricuspid

_____ d. Ventral

3. The rings of the trachea consist of:

_____ a. ligaments.

_____ b. bone.

_____ c. cartilage.

_____ d. muscle.

4. What is the formula for determining cardiac output (CO)?

_____ a. $SV \times BP = CO$

_____ b. $SV \times HR = CO$

_____ c. $HR \times BP = CO$

_____ d. $HR \times SVR = CO$

5. How many lobes does the left lung have?

_____ a. One

_____ b. Two

_____ c. Three

_____ d. Four

Fill in the Blank

1. The small, grape-like clusters of air sacs in the lungs are called ________________________________.

2. The area posterior to the nose but superior to the oropharynx is called the ________________________________.

3. ________________________________ carry blood away from the heart.

4. ________________________________ are tiny vessels that connect arterioles and venules.

5. The upper chambers of the heart are called ________________________________ and the lower chambers are called ________________________________.

6. The ________________________________ artery is the artery that produces a pulse in the wrist.

Labeling

On the diagram of the heart below, label each chamber and draw the path of blood as it flows between the chambers to the lung and to the body.

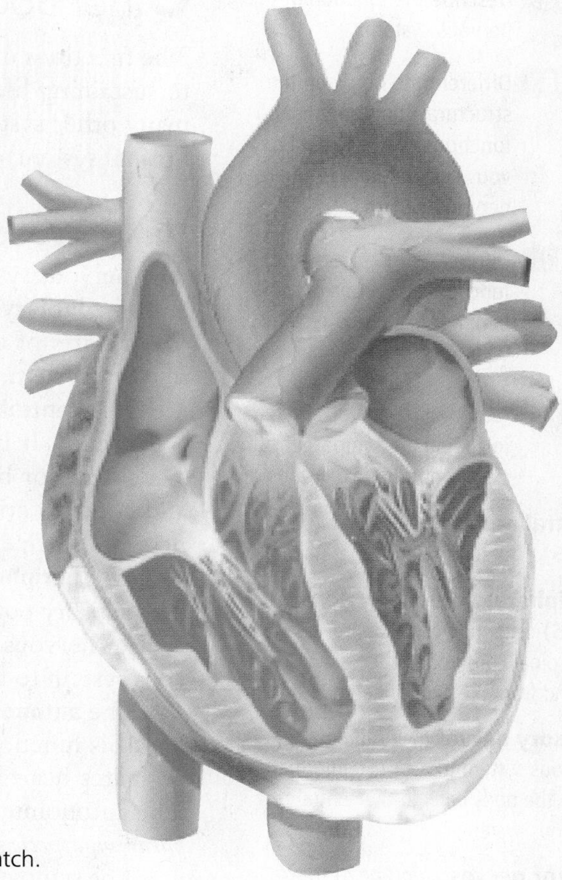

Critical Thinking

1. List the elements that are required for a ventilation/perfusion (V/Q) match.

____

____

____

____

2. Describe the differences between perfusion and hypoperfusion.

____

____

____

____

3. List three ways a child's airway is different from an adult's airway.

____

____

____

____

5-15 Describe the function of the nervous system.

5-16 Differentiate between the structural components and functions of the central nervous system and peripheral nervous system.

5-17 Differentiate between the functional divisions of the peripheral nervous system: voluntary (somatic) nervous system and involuntary (autonomic) nervous system, including the sympathetic and parasympathetic divisions.

central nervous system (CNS) the brain and the spinal cord.

peripheral nervous system (PNS) the nerves that enter and leave the spinal cord and that convey impulses to and from the central nervous system.

sensory nerves portion of the nervous system that carries information from the body back to the central nervous system.

motor nerves portion of the nervous system that carries information from the brain through the spinal cord and to the body.

autonomic nervous system a division of the peripheral nervous system; controls functions that are involuntary.

5-18 Describe the structure and function of the endocrine system.

5-19 Describe the general actions of epinephrine and norepinephrine on $beta_1$ and $beta_2$ receptors of the sympathetic nervous system.

hormones chemicals involved in regulation of body functions.

insulin a hormone produced by the pancreas or taken as a medication by many diabetics that helps the body use glucose as fuel.

epinephrine chemical that stimulates the body in response to stress. Also called *adrenaline.*

Other Body Systems

The functions of the cardiovascular and respiratory systems are incredibly important to sustaining life. However, normal body function also requires the intervention of many other systems. They include the nervous system, endocrine system, gastrointestinal system, renal system, and the reproductive system.

The Nervous System

The nervous system is the messenger system for the body. It controls the voluntary and involuntary actions that make up the functions of everyday life. There are two major parts of our nervous system: the central nervous system and the peripheral nervous system.

The **central nervous system (CNS)** (Figure 5-15 ▪) consists of the brain and the spinal cord. It is called *central* because all the nerves from the body branch off the spinal cord or brain. The brain interprets the sensations brought in from the body and controls critical body functions such as respiratory and pulse rates, consciousness, and temperature.

The **peripheral nervous system (PNS)** contains **sensory nerves** and **motor nerves.** The sensory portion of the nervous system carries information from the body to the central nervous system. The motor nerves carry information from the central nervous system to the body.

The **autonomic nervous system** is a division of the peripheral nervous system and controls functions that are involuntary. For example, the autonomic nervous system regulates heart rate and digestion and does not require conscious thought to do it. The autonomic nervous system can be further broken down into the *sympathetic and parasympathetic nervous systems.*

The sympathetic nervous system is engaged when the body senses trouble. In fact, it is often referred to as the *fight-or-flight response*. Engaging a sympathetic response causes the heart to beat faster, the lungs to breathe deeper, and the blood vessels to constrict to bring more blood to the essential organs of the body.

In contrast, the parasympathetic nervous system often is referred to as a *feed-or-breed response* because it asserts an effect opposite of the sympathetic nervous system. It is engaged in times of relaxation, and stimulation of the parasympathetic system causes decreased heart rate, blood vessel dilation, and increased blood flow to the digestive tract and to the reproductive organs.

The Endocrine System

The endocrine system (Figure 5-16 ▪) is involved in regulation of body functions. This system produces chemicals called **hormones,** which serve as chemical messengers to help control specific system function. Two hormones you may recognize are **insulin,** which helps the body to use glucose as fuel, and **epinephrine,** which helps engage the sympathetic nervous system in response to stress. There are many other hormones, including those that control reproductive functions and metabolism.

One of the key organs of the endocrine system is the pancreas. The pancreas secretes insulin and aids in the process of digestion. Other significant organs of the endocrine system include the adrenal glands, which secrete epinephrine and in turn control the sympathetic nervous system. Epinephrine and norepinephrine are used to signal the sympathetic nervous system to produce the fight-or-flight response. $Beta_1$ receptors in the heart, when stimulated, cause an increase in heart rate and an increase in the force of contractions. $Beta_2$ receptors in the lungs produce a dilation of bronchial tubes, allowing for more air and oxygen to reach the lungs.

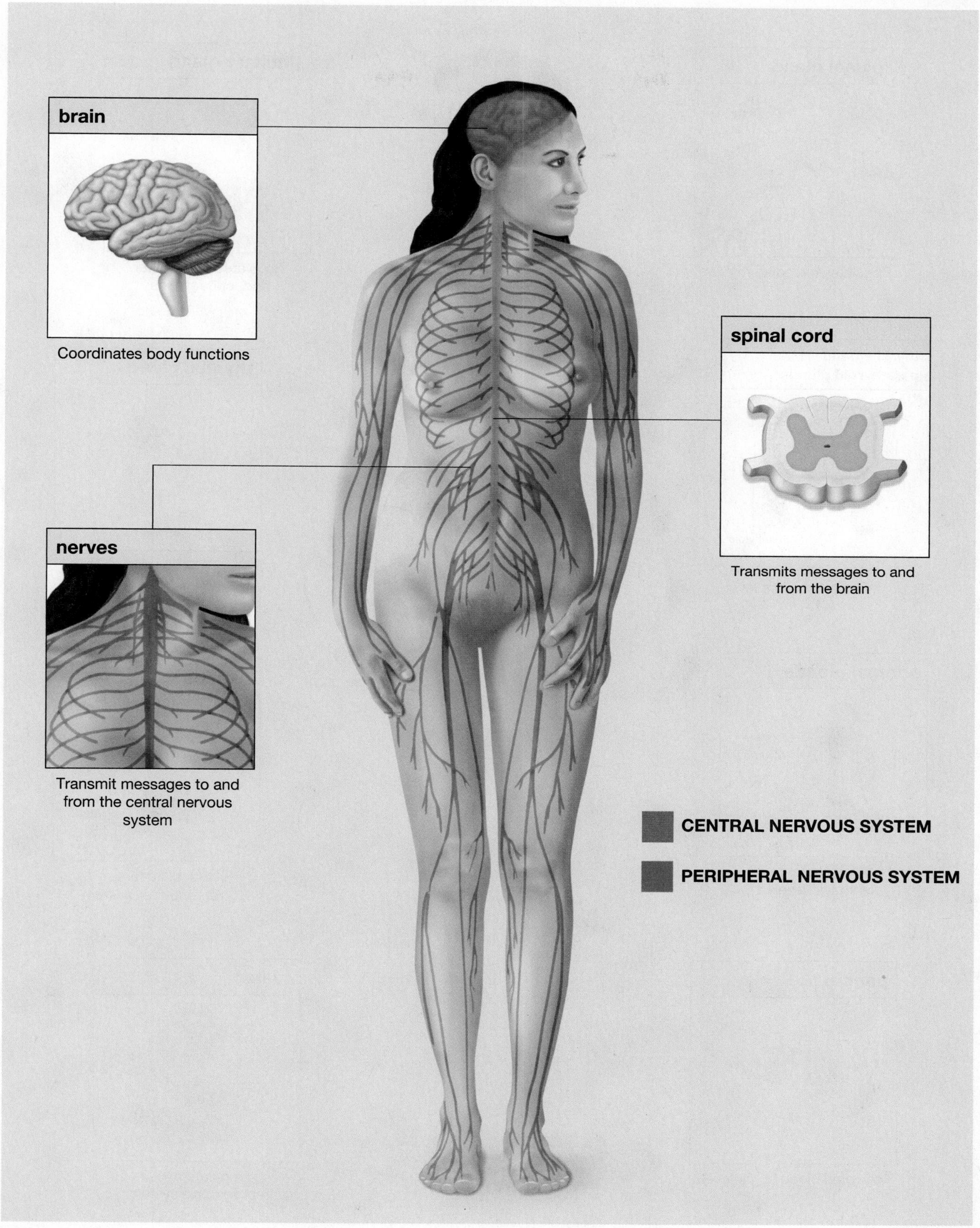

Figure 5-15 The central and peripheral nervous systems.

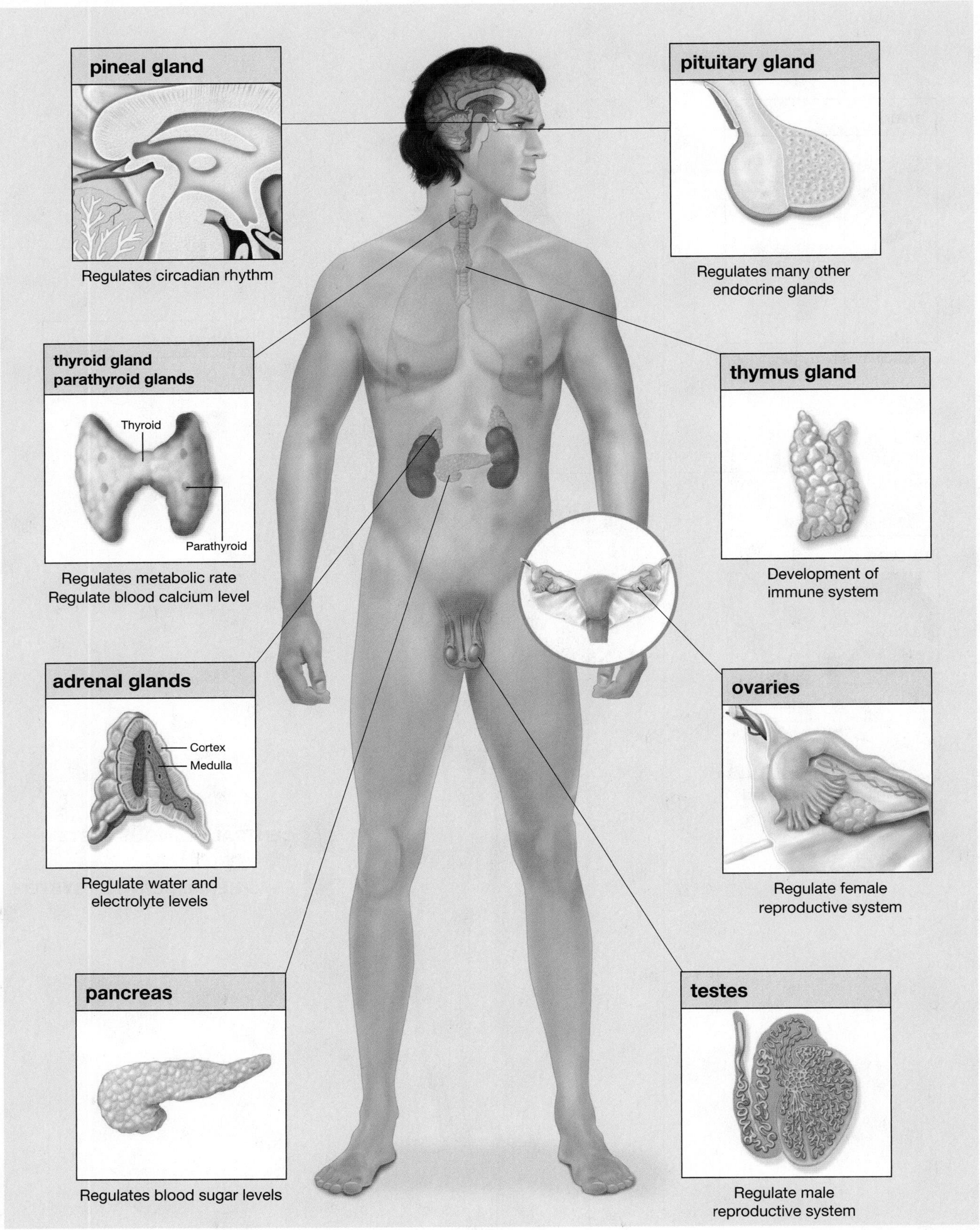

Figure 5-16 The structures of the endocrine system.

The Gastrointestinal System

The gastrointestinal (GI) system controls digestion and the absorption of water and nutrients into the body. The GI system is also partially responsible for the excretion of waste products. Important organs in the GI system include (Figure 5-17 ■):

- ***Esophagus.*** The esophagus is the tube that connects the mouth to the stomach. Food travels through the esophagus as it enters the body.
- ***Stomach.*** The stomach, a tubular organ that expands as it fills, receives food from the esophagus. Gastric juices work to digest the food as it moves to the small intestine.
- ***Small intestine.*** The **small intestine** continues the work of the stomach in digesting solid foods and absorbing nutrients through the intestinal wall. Those nutrients are then transferred into the blood and transported to the cells. The small intestine has three segments: duodenum, jejunum, and ileum.
- ***Large intestine.*** Also known as the *colon*, the **large intestine** absorbs water and moves waste products along for excretion.
- ***Liver.*** The liver secretes **bile** to the small intestine. Bile assists in the digestion of fat. The liver also detoxifies harmful substances (alcohol, for example) and stores a limited amount of glucose.
- ***Gall bladder.*** A small organ located behind the liver, the **gall bladder** stores bile from the liver.
- ***Pancreas.*** The **pancreas** has a digestive function in secreting substances that help digest proteins and carbohydrates. The **islets of Langerhans** are cells in the pancreas that secrete insulin into the blood.

The Renal System

The renal system's primary function is fluid balance, but it also plays an important role in the filtration of waste products and the maintenance of a normal body pH (Figure 5-18 ■). The kidneys are the chief organ of the renal system and play a huge part in regulating the amount of water within the body. When fluid levels are too high, the kidneys decrease the absorption of water and signal for excretion. At times when the fluid levels are too low, the kidneys increase the absorption of water. The kidneys are located in the **retroperitoneal space,** which means they are located behind the abdominal cavity. The abdominal aorta is also located in the retroperitoneal space. This is why patients with an abdominal aortic aneurysm (the ballooning of a weakened section of the wall of an artery) commonly experience back pain.

Other organs of the renal system include the **bladder,** located in the lower abdominal quadrants along the midline and the **ureters,** the tubes that connect the kidneys to the bladder. Each of these structures is used in the elimination of excess fluid in the form of urine.

The Reproductive System

The reproductive systems of men and women are illustrated in Figure 5-19 ■.

Female Reproductive System

The female reproductive system consists of the vagina, uterus, **ovaries,** and **fallopian tubes.** The ovaries produce important hormones and contain ova (eggs). An egg is released every 28 days in a process called **ovulation,** and guided into a fallopian tube by tiny fimbriae (fingerlike projections). Sperm from the male meets the egg during **fertilization,** which usually occurs in the fallopian tube. The fertilized egg then is guided through the fallopian tube to the uterus where **implantation** takes place. The **embryo** will grow into a **fetus** and develop through birth.

PRACTICAL PATHOPHYSIOLOGY

An easy way to differentiate the $beta_1$ and $beta_2$ receptors is to remember that $beta_1$ receptors affect the *one* heart. $Beta_2$ receptors affect the *two* lungs.

5-20 Describe the structure and function of the digestive system.

small intestine organ that digests solid foods and absorbs nutrients through the intestinal wall. The small intestine has three segments: duodenum, jejunum, and ileum.

large intestine organ that is a muscular tube that removes water from waste products received from the small intestine and removes anything not absorbed by the body toward excretion from the body. Also called the *colon*.

bile chemical that assists in the digestion of fat.

gall bladder an organ in the form of a sac on the underside of the liver that stores bile produced by the liver.

pancreas a gland located behind the stomach that produces insulin and produces juices that assist in digestion of food in the duodenum of the small intestine.

islets of Langerhans a group of cells in the pancreas that secrete insulin into the blood.

retroperitoneal space referring to the area behind the abdominal cavity.

bladder organ that stores urine until excretion.

ureters transport urine from the kidneys to the bladder.

ovaries internal gland producing the ovum. Female counterpart to the testicles.

fallopian tubes carries the egg from the ovary to the uterus. Female counterpart to the vas deferens.

ovulation the release of an ovum (egg) from the ovary.

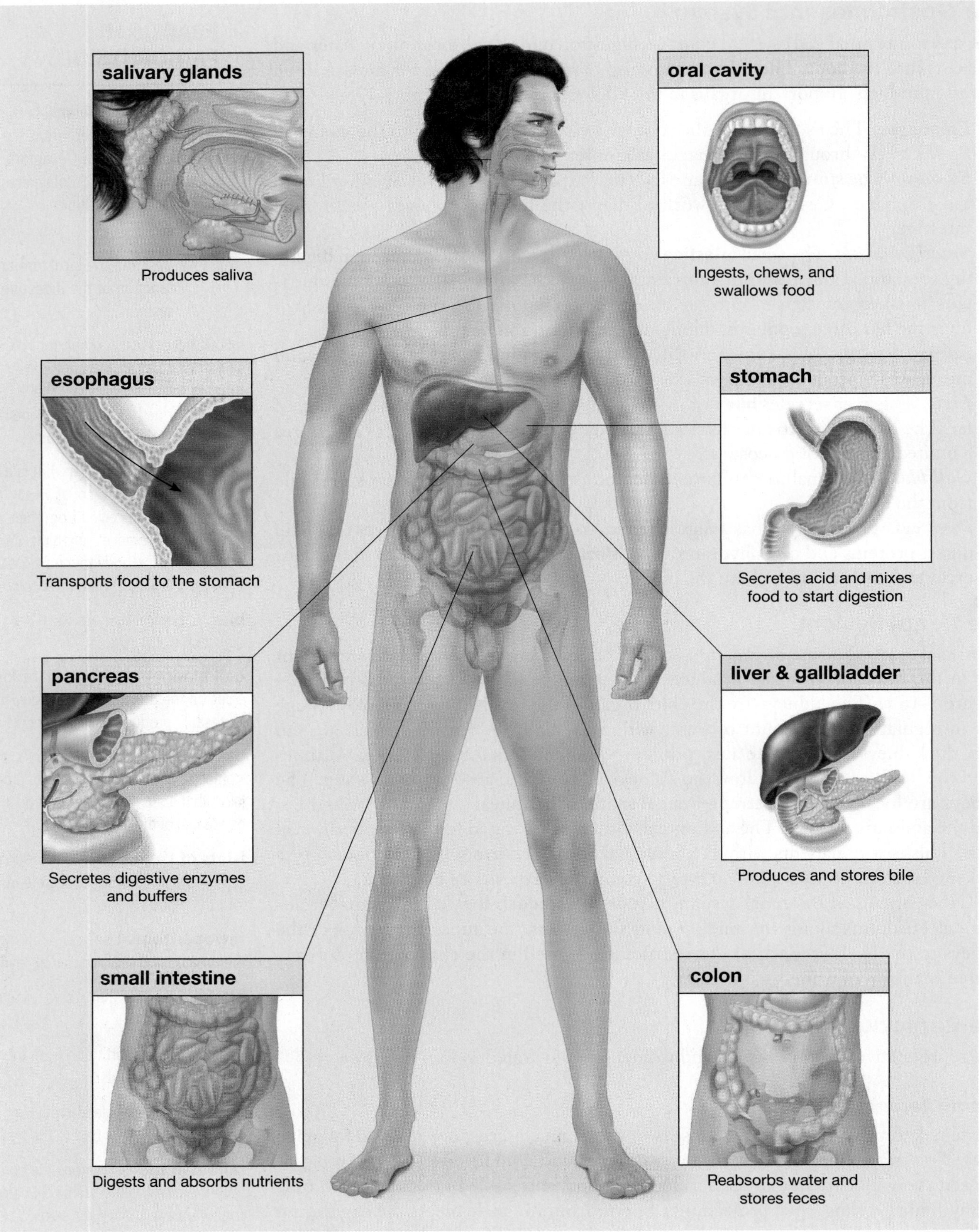

Figure 5-17 The structures of the gastrointestinal (digestive) system.

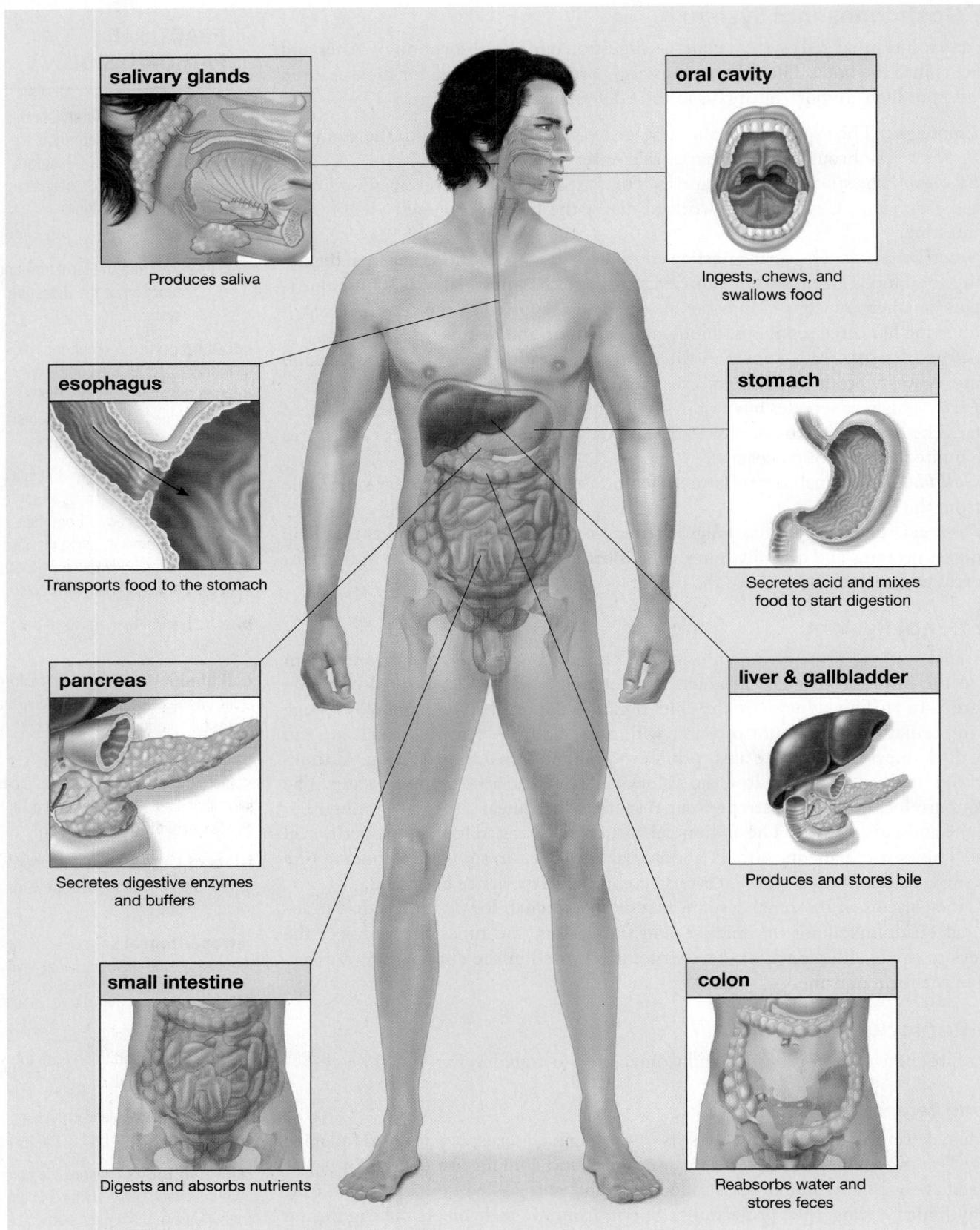

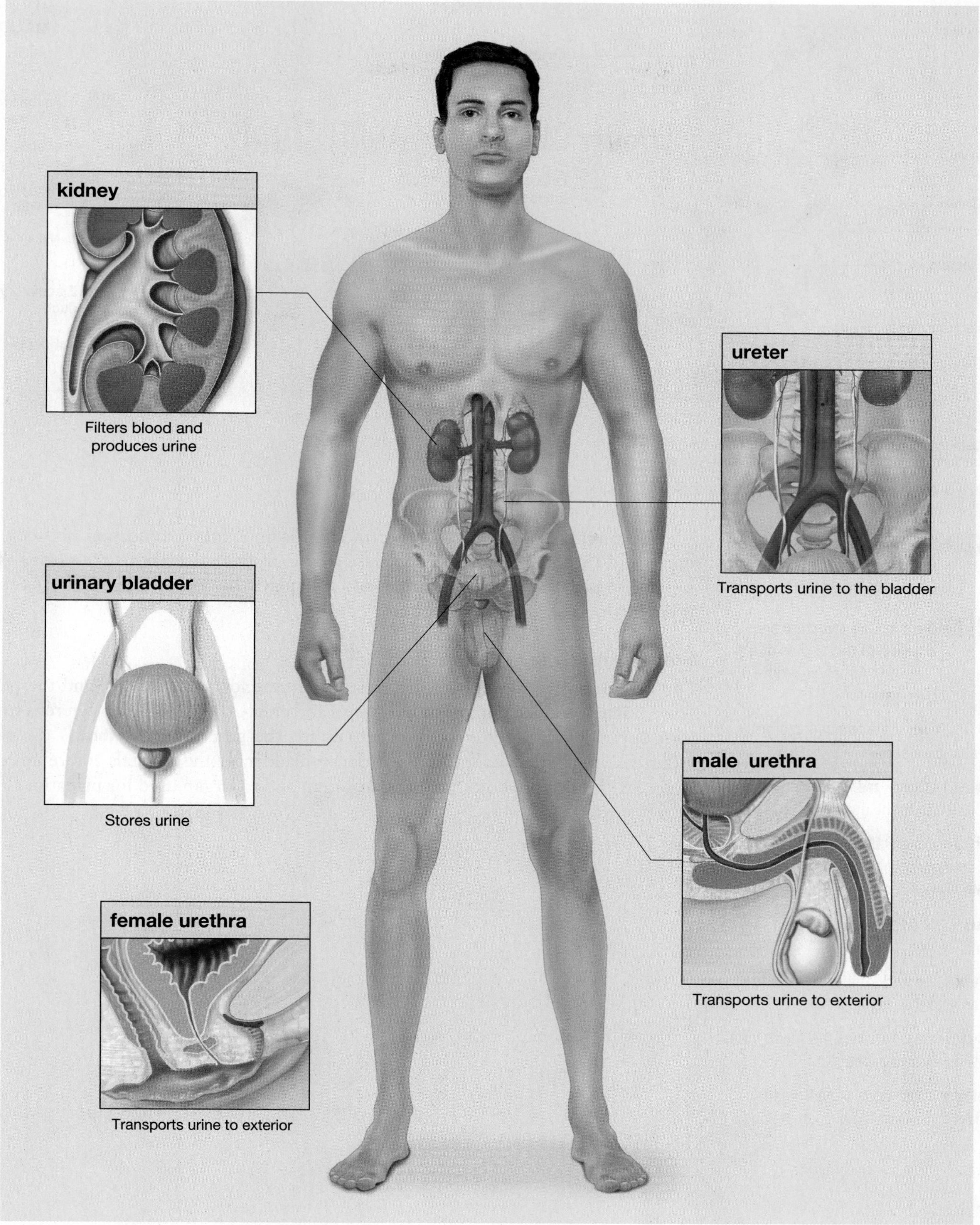

Figure 5-18 The structures of the renal (urinary) system.

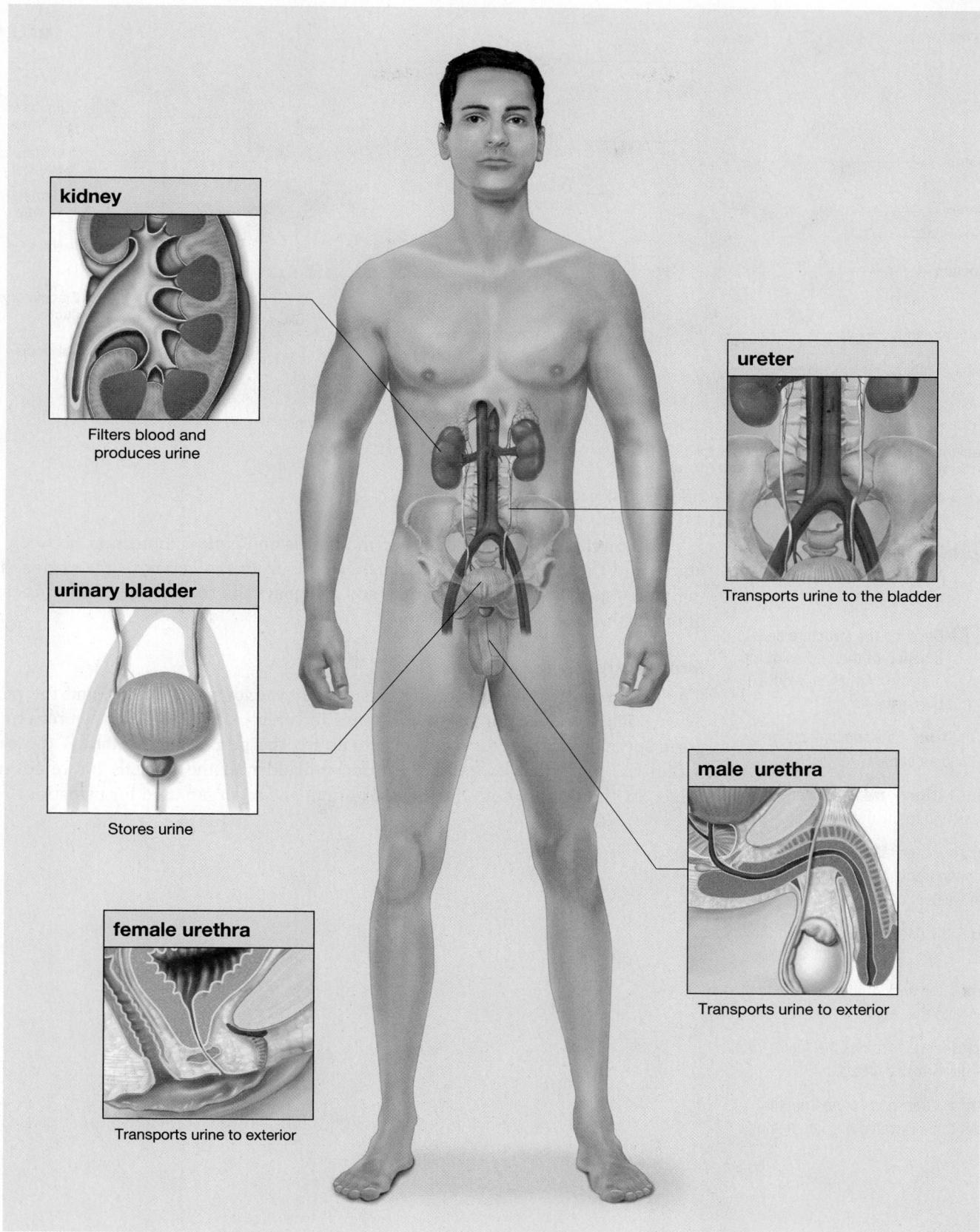

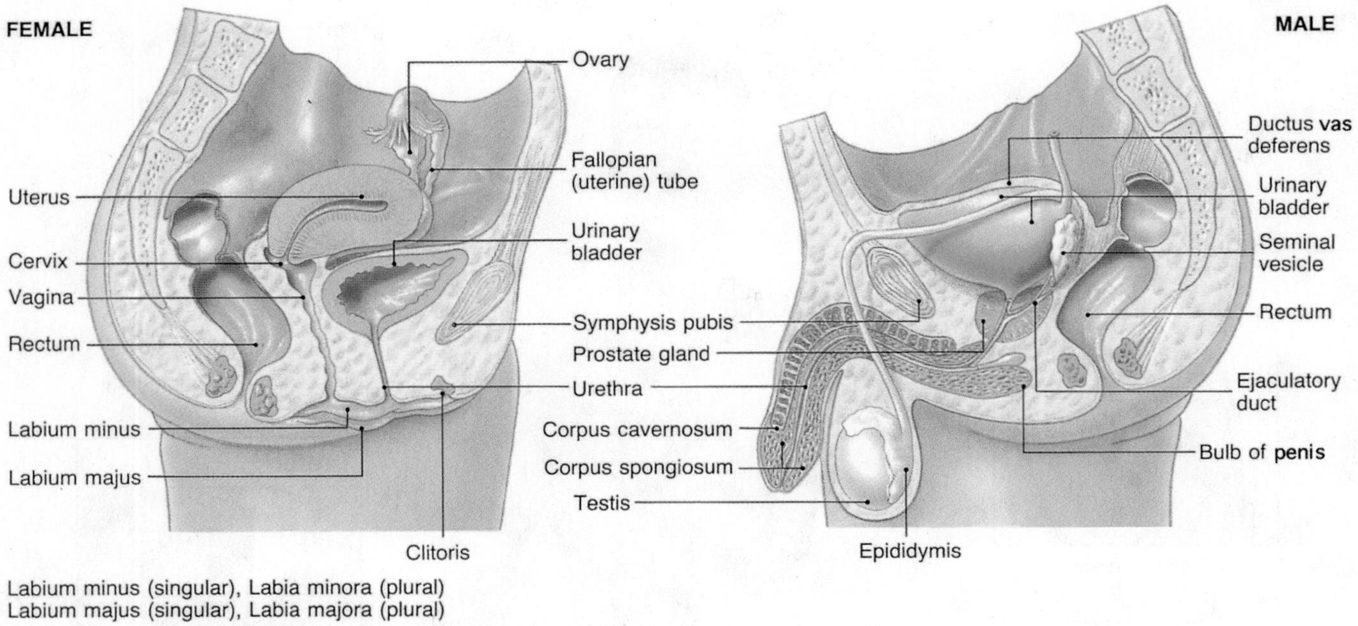

Figure 5-19 The structures of the female and male reproductive systems.

The **cervix** is at the distal end of the uterus and is the connection between the uterus and the vagina. The birth canal extends from the cervix to the vagina. The vagina serves as the female sex organ and also plays the role of the exterior opening of the birth canal.

Male Reproductive System

The male reproductive system consists of the testicles, **vas deferens,** and the penis. The testicles produce important hormones and create sperm. The vas deferens transports sperm to the urethra, and eventually to the penis. The **urethra** is the canal within the penis that connects the urinary bladder to the genitals for removal of urine. So, the penis is both the male sex organ and an organ used for urination.

5-21 Describe the structure and function of the organs of the renal system.

5-22 Describe the structure and function of the organs of the male and female reproductive systems.

fertilization the combining of a sperm and an egg.

implantation the attachment of a fertilized egg to the uterine lining.

embryo prefetal product of conception from implantation to the eighth week of development.

fetus the baby as it develops in the womb.

cervix the neck of the uterus at the entrance to the vagina.

vas deferens carries the sperm from the testicles to the urethra.

urethra transports urine from the bladder to be excreted outside the body.

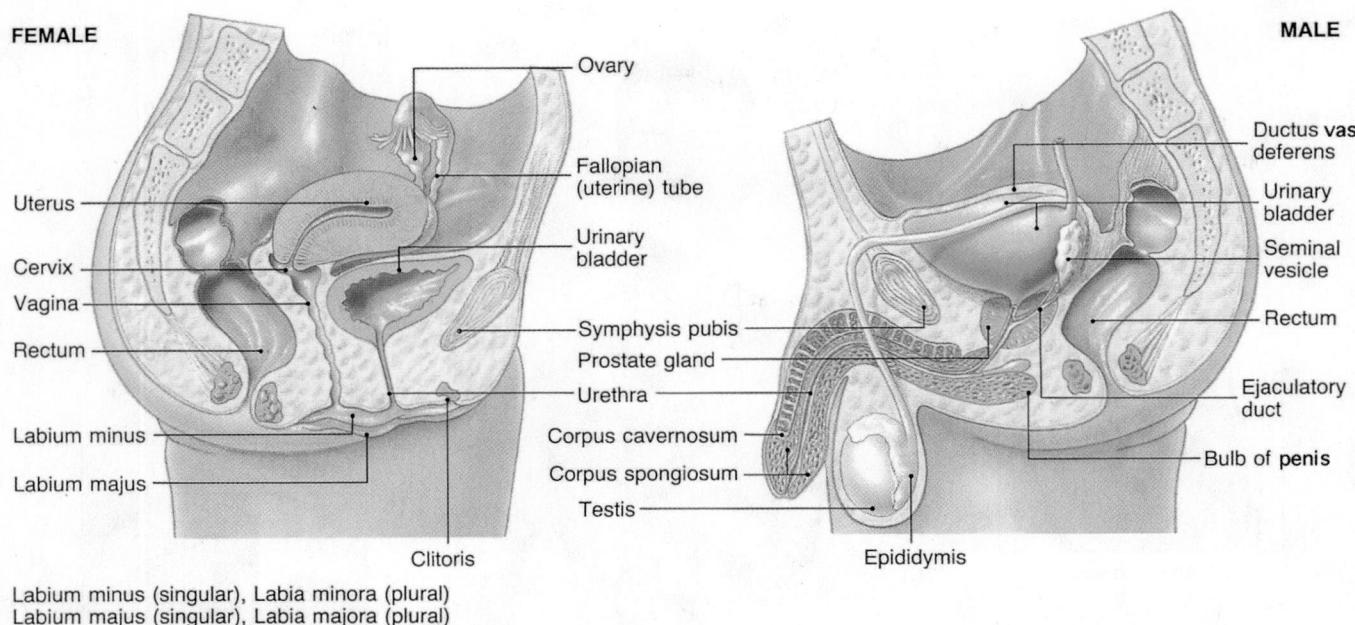

STOP, REVIEW, REMEMBER!

Multiple Choice

For each question, place a check next to the correct answer.

1. Which one of the following carries urine from the kidneys to the bladder?

_____ a. Urethras
_____ b. Capillaries
_____ c. Ureters
_____ d. Uterus

2. Which one of the following organs stores bile to aid digestion?

_____ a. Pancreas
_____ b. Kidney
_____ c. Gall bladder
_____ d. Stomach

3. The organ that secretes insulin and aids in digestion is the:

_____ a. aorta.
_____ b. liver.
_____ c. spleen.
_____ d. pancreas.

4. Which one of the following organs regulates fluid balance for the body?

_____ a. Kidney
_____ b. Ovary
_____ c. Testicle
_____ d. Fallopian tube

5. The endocrine system regulates the body through the use of:

_____ a. hemoglobin.
_____ b. hormones.
_____ c. motor nerves.
_____ d. hematocrit.

6. Which one of the following functions is regulated by the sympathetic nervous system?

_____ a. Blood vessel dilation
_____ b. Decreased heart rate
_____ c. Increased heart rate
_____ d. Increased digestion

7. Which one of the following organs aids in the detoxification of blood?

_____ a. Small intestine
_____ b. Stomach
_____ c. Adrenal gland
_____ d. Liver

Fill in the Blank

1. The ______________________ nervous system controls involuntary function.

2. ______________________ nerves send messages to the brain.

3. ______________________ nerves deliver messages from the brain to the muscles.

4. The hormone ______________________ helps the body use glucose as fuel.

5. The tube that connects the mouth to the stomach is called the ______________________.

6. The central nervous system is composed of the ______________________ and ______________________.

(continued on next page)

(continued)

Critical Thinking

1. Describe the function of the parasympathetic nervous system.

____

____

____

____

2. List three functions of the renal system.

____

____

____

____

EMERGENCY DISPATCH SUMMARY

The entire team on scene was able to quickly and effectively immobilize the patient to the backboard, while the paramedic started two IVs and gave him something for pain. The young man was then loaded into the ALS unit and taken with lights and siren to the regional trauma center, which fortunately was only two miles away. Due to the paramedic calling in a good report from the scene, the trauma team was assembled and waiting when the truck pulled in. Within minutes of being unloaded, the patient was assessed and headed to surgery.

As EMT Dave Klein, who rode along to assist the paramedic, was preparing to leave the hospital emergency department, the charge nurse put her arm around his shoulder and gave him a tight squeeze. "Awesome," she said. "That was a tough one and you guys did a heck of a job. You should be proud." As Dave walked out through the automatic doors to the ambulance bay and into the warm evening, he couldn't help but smile.

Chapter Review

To the Point

- Anatomy and physiology will help you improve patient assessment and care. It provides a baseline and a fundamental blueprint for structure and function in the body.
- Positional and anatomical terms lend precision to assessment and descriptions, and are an essential component of understanding anatomy and physiology.
- The musculoskeletal system provides form, protection, and movement.
- The different joints of the body include ball-and-socket, hinge, pivot, gliding, and saddle.
- The function of the structures of the respiratory system is to move air to the alveoli and exchange oxygen and carbon dioxide.
- Normal ventilation utilizes negative pressure to move air into the lungs.
- The cardiovascular system pairs with the respiratory system to perfuse the body. It circulates blood to remove carbon dioxide and deliver oxygen and nutrients to the cells.
- The nervous system exchanges messages between the outside world and the brain. It also distributes messages from the brain to the body systems. The nervous system has both voluntary and involuntary components.
- The endocrine system is composed of eight major glands. It serves as the chemical messenger system of the body and assists the brain in regulating function of specific body systems.
- The integumentary system protects the body from infection, it regulates body temperature, and it assists the body with elimination of waste. It is composed of the epidermis, dermis, and subcutaneous layer.
- The digestive system absorbs nutrients from food, distributes those nutrients, and eliminates waste.
- The renal system regulates fluid balance and helps eliminate toxins from the body.
- The reproductive system forms the basis for reproduction of our species.

Chapter Questions

Multiple Choice

For each question, place a check next to the correct answer.

1. The molecule in the red blood cell that binds with oxygen is:

_____ a. hormone.
_____ b. hemocult.
_____ c. hemoglobin.
_____ d. hematoglobulin.

2. The bones of the lower leg are called the tibia and the:

_____ a. fibula.
_____ b. radius.
_____ c. ulna.
_____ d. femur.

3. Which one of the following terms refers to the fused vertebrae that form the posterior portion of the pelvis?

_____ a. Sacral
_____ b. Cervical
_____ c. Lumbar
_____ d. Thoracic

4. The area that houses the vocal cords and opens into the trachea is known as the:

_____ a. oropharynx.
_____ b. pharynx.
_____ c. larynx.
_____ d. epiglottis.

(continued on next page)

(continued)

5. The vessels that carry deoxygenated blood from the heart to the lungs are the pulmonary:
   _____ a. arteries. _____ c. capillaries.
   _____ b. veins. _____ d. emboli.
6. Which one of the following terms refers to the valve that separates the left atrium from the left ventricle?
   _____ a. Tricuspid _____ c. Pulmonic
   _____ b. Mitral _____ d. Aortic
7. An increase in epinephrine by the sympathetic nervous system will have which one of the following effects?
   _____ a. Increase in heart rate _____ c. Dilation of blood vessels
   _____ b. Decrease in heart rate _____ d. Drop in blood pressure
8. The hormone that allows glucose to be utilized by the cells is:
   _____ a. cortisol. _____ c. adrenalin.
   _____ b. hemoglobin. _____ d. insulin.
9. Which one of the following organs is considered retroperitoneal?
   _____ a. Spleen _____ c. Kidney
   _____ b. Liver _____ d. Pancreas
10. Smooth muscle is found in all of the following places *except* the:
    _____ a. bicep. _____ c. intestine.
    _____ b. bronchi. _____ d. arterioles.

Matching

Match the bone on the left with the applicable body part on the right.

1. _____	Femur	A. Head
2. _____	Cranium	B. Face
3. _____	Sternum	C. Anterior shoulder
4. _____	Metatarsal	D. Posterior shoulder
5. _____	Maxilla	E. Chest
6. _____	Clavicle	F. Spine
7. _____	Fibula	G. Upper arm
8. _____	Radius	H. Forearm/wrist
9. _____	Tarsals	I. Hand
10. _____	Metacarpal	J. Pelvis
11. _____	Patella	K. Thigh
12. _____	Ischium	L. Knee
13. _____	Humerus	M. Lower leg
14. _____	Scapula	N. Ankle
15. _____	Vertebra	O. Foot

Labeling

In the diagram below, draw the following areas and organs in their proper location: abdominal quadrants, stomach, liver, gall bladder, pancreas, spleen, large intestine, small intestine, and diaphragm.

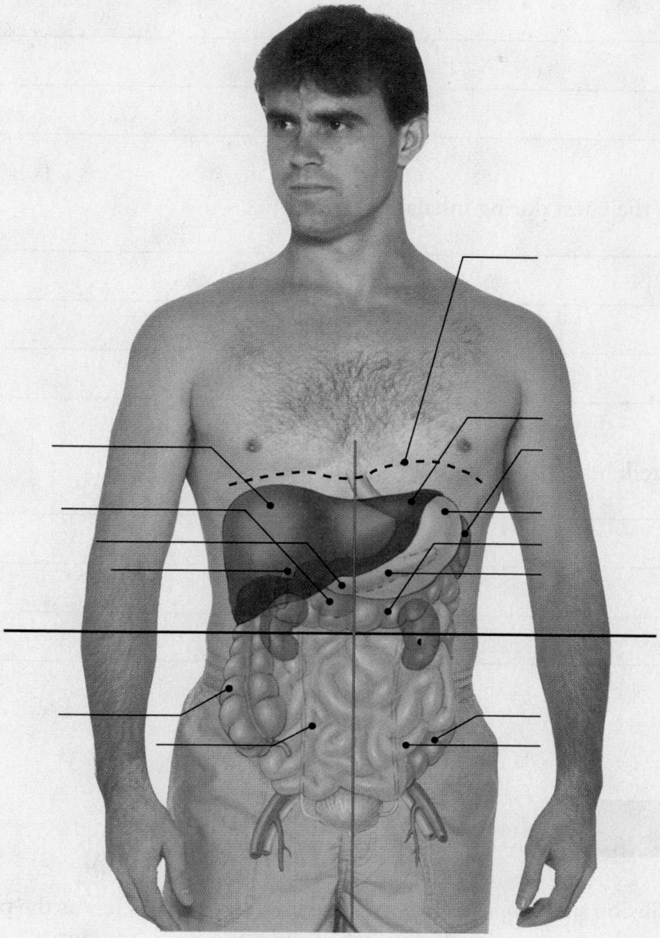

Ordering

Number the following cardiovascular structures in the order in which blood flows when entering the heart from the venae cavae.

_____ Mitral valve

_____ Lung

_____ Left atrium

_____ Left ventricle

_____ Pulmonary artery

_____ Pulmonary vein

_____ Tricuspid valve

_____ Aorta

_____ Right atrium

_____ Right ventricle

_____ Pulmonic valve

_____ Aortic valve

Critical Thinking

1. Describe the relationship between blood pressure and the pulse felt at the radial artery.

2. Describe how air is moved into the chest during inhalation.

3. Describe how perfusion is created. Also list the necessary components that create it.

Case Study

You are called to a motor vehicle collision with injuries. You find one injured patient. He was the passenger in a vehicle that was struck directly into the passenger-side door where he was sitting. You notice that the door was pushed about a foot into the passenger compartment.

1. The patient complains of pain to the right side of his rib cage over the lower five or six ribs. If there were internal injuries, what organs may be affected?

2. The patient also complains of some tenderness to palpation in the right upper abdominal quadrant. What organ or organs could be affected there?

3. What injuries could cause a decrease in perfusion for this patient?

____

____

____

____

The Last Word

Like many of the skills in your EMT training program, learning anatomy and physiology takes time and practice. It is the foundation for the understanding of how the body functions and how you will provide care when it is not functioning properly. You must review this chapter from time to time before this information can become second nature. Then as you observe patient care being performed and discussed, you will see the principles of anatomy and physiology applied in the health care setting. Through diligent study and application, you will be able to use this knowledge to improve the care that you provide.

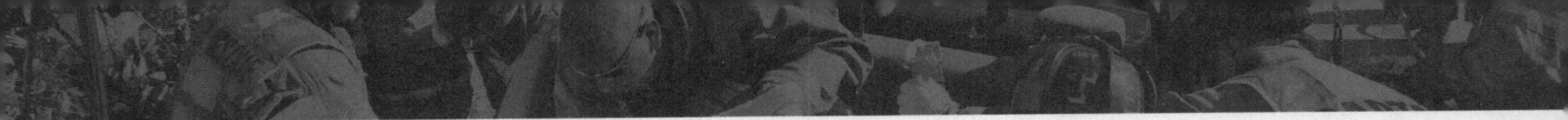

6 Pathophysiology

Education Standards

Pathophysiology

Competencies

Applies fundamental knowledge of the pathophysiology of respiration and perfusion to patient assessment and management.

Objectives

After completion of this lesson, you should be able to:

6-1 Define key terms introduced in this chapter.

6-2 Explain the importance of understanding basic pathophysiology.

6-3 Differentiate between the processes of aerobic and anaerobic cellular metabolism, including explanations of the amount of ATP produced and the removal of by-products of metabolism.

6-4 Describe the consequences of failure of the cellular sodium potassium pump.

6-5 Explain the concept of perfusion, including components necessary to maintain perfusion.

6-6 Describe the composition of ambient air.

6-7 Explain how changes in compliance of the lungs and chest wall and changes in airway resistance affect ventilation.

6-8 Describe the consequences of loss of contact between the parietal and visceral pleura.

6-9 Explain the concept of minute ventilation.

6-10 Differentiate between minute ventilation and alveolar ventilation.

6-11 Describe the roles of chemoreceptors and the nervous system in the control of ventilation.

6-12 Explain the concept of the ventilation/perfusion (VQ) ratio.

6-13 Describe the transport of oxygen and carbon dioxide in the blood.

6-14 Explain the exchange of gases across the alveolar/capillary membrane and the exchange of gases between capillaries and cells.

6-15 Describe the composition of blood, including the function of plasma.

6-16 Explain the effects of changes in hydrostatic pressure and plasma oncotic pressure on the movement of fluid between the cardiovascular system and interstitial spaces.

6-17 Discuss factors that affect cardiac output, including heart rate, stroke volume, preload, and afterload.

6-18 Describe the concept of systemic vascular resistance and its relationship to blood pressure and pulse pressure.

6-19 Summarize the local, neural, and hormonal factors that regulate blood flow through the capillaries.

6-20 Explain the regulation of blood pressure by baroreceptors and chemoreceptors.

6-21 Explain the relationship among ventilation, perfusion, and cellular metabolism.

Key Terms

adenosine triphosphate (ATP) p. 132
aerobic metabolism p. 133
anaerobic metabolism p. 133
baroreceptors p. 142
cardiac output (CO) p. 143
cell membrane p. 132
chemoreceptors p. 140
dead air space p. 138
dehydration p. 134
edema p. 135
electrolytes p. 133
endoplasmic reticulum p. 132
FiO_2 p. 136
hydrostatic pressure p. 140
hypersensitivity p. 150
metabolism p. 133
minute volume p. 137
mitochondria p. 132
nucleus p. 132
patent p. 137
pathophysiology p. 131
perfusion p. 144
plasma oncotic pressure p. 140
sodium potassium pump p. 132
stretch receptors p. 142
stroke volume (SV) p. 143
systemic vascular resistance (SVR) p. 143
tidal volume p. 137
V/Q match p. 145

Introduction

In the complex organism that is the human body, systems constantly interact to sustain life. These highly complicated systems integrate the function of cells, organs, and organ systems in a delicate balancing act to adapt to the changes and challenges of everyday life. Knowing the structure and function (anatomy and physiology) of these systems is important, but a complete understanding also requires that you appreciate what happens when functions fail.

6-2 Explain the importance of understanding basic pathophysiology.

Pathophysiology is the study of how disease processes affect the function of the body. It is the science of change. It looks at major challenges to the body and how the body adapts to them. A basic understanding of anatomy and physiology is the baseline for what *should* be happening in the body, and a working knowledge of pathophysiology helps you recognize how those normal functions change when disrupted. The combination gives you valuable tools for improving your ability to identify key signs and symptoms of patient compromise during patient assessment and for developing an appropriate treatment plan for your patient.

pathophysiology the study of how disease processes affect the function of the body.

Note that a complete review of pathophysiology is a complex topic that exceeds the scope of this text. This chapter is designed to be an overview; it is by no means intended to be comprehensive. Many topics in this chapter have been presented in a simplified

EMERGENCY DISPATCH

EMS dispatcher Sean Sturdevant stretched his back, glanced at his watch, and then sat forward to scan the night's call log. "It's been pretty quiet tonight," he said to his partner Chuck Rowlands. "I thought that it was definitely going to be busier."

Chuck looked around the side of his computer monitor and frowned. "You realize that you just jinxed us, right? And with only an hour to go before shift change!"

Sean's laugh was cut short by a ringing on the emergency line and he shrugged at his partner before answering, "What's your emergency?" Sean had to strain to hear the gasping voice on the other end of the line and initially could only make out the words "can't . . . breathe." He muted his phone and leaned over to Chuck. "I need you to roll an ambulance to this address, code three!"

As Sean returned to the caller, Chuck keyed the radio, "Six-fifty-three, six five three, control, respond code three to 4512 Berry Lane in Jefferson Township for a difficulty breathing. We've got recent history at this address of a 72-year-old male patient with CHF. Showing you dispatched at 0612 hours."

In a back corner of a deserted gas station parking lot across town, EMTs Case Bloomfield and Darin Small secure their seat belts, and as Darin shifts the idling truck into drive, Case acknowledges the dispatch and punches the address into the GPS unit.

manner with the knowledge that there is far more to learn. Anatomy, physiology, and pathophysiology all provide extensive opportunities to continue your quest for knowledge even after your EMT course ends. There are many additional, informative resources on this topic and learning more will only make you a better provider.

The Cellular Environment and Fluid Balance

A cell is the basic building block for the human organism. Each cell exists in an environment that requires a delicate balance of fluids. Understanding basic cell structure and how it interacts with its environment provides a foundation for discussion of how that environment can be disturbed.

The Cell

6-4 Describe the consequences of failure of the cellular sodium potassium pump.

cell membrane outer covering of the cell that protects and selectively allows water and other substances into and out of the cell.

nucleus structure within the cell that contains DNA.

endoplasmic reticulum structure within the cell that synthesizes protein.

mitochondria structure within the cell that produces energy.

adenosine triphosphate (ATP) a byproduct of cellular respiration responsible for the transport of chemical energy for metabolism.

sodium potassium pump element of the cell that is responsible for regulating the concentration of sodium and potassium ions within the cell and uses ATP to power the active transport of those ions.

The most basic unit of the human body is the cell. Many cells have specific functions. When joined together, they create the organs and systems of the body. Individual cells house a series of structures designed to accomplish specific tasks within the cell itself (Figure 6-1 ■).

The **cell membrane** is the outer, protective layer and selectively allows water and other substances into and out of the cell. The cell **nucleus** contains DNA and is the genetic blueprint for reproduction. The **endoplasmic reticulum** plays a key role in synthesizing proteins. The **mitochondria** are responsible for converting glucose and other nutrients into energy in the form of **adenosine triphosphate (ATP),** a critically important process called *cellular metabolism*. It is helpful to think of ATP as the energy for the cell.

The **sodium potassium pump** is a process of the cell that relies on ATP. It uses ATP in a process called *active transport* to regulate the concentration of ions (charged particles) inside the cell itself. Active transport uses energy in the form of ATP to move sodium and potassium ions into and out of the cells against their normal chemical tendencies. This process is critical for the cell because the proper concentrations

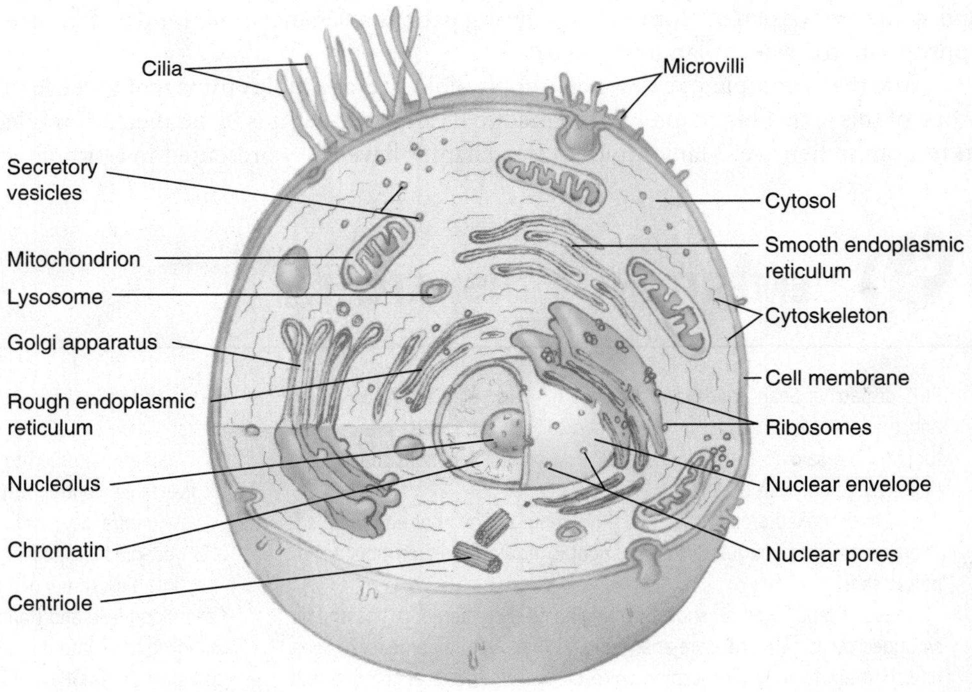

Figure 6-1 The structures of the cell.

of ions allow for an electrical charge to be generated as ions rapidly shift across the cell membrane. This *depolarization* accounts for the creation of mechanical force in the cell. Without ATP, active transport would fail.

All cells have basic needs that must be met in order to accomplish their important functions. Those requirements include:

6-3 Differentiate between the processes of aerobic and anaerobic cellular metabolism, including explanations of the amount of ATP produced and the removal of by-products of metabolism.

- ***Glucose.*** Glucose is a simple sugar converted from food, and it is the basic nutrient of the cell. During normal **metabolism,** the cell converts glucose into ATP to create energy and to power its basic functions. Without glucose, energy is not created and cell functions stop.
- ***Water.*** Cells need a correct balance of water between the inside and outside of the cell membrane. Cells dehydrate and die without enough water. Too much water and cellular function will be interrupted. The cell membrane is a vulnerable element of the cell. Many disease processes alter its *permeability* or its ability to effectively transfer fluids and other substances in and out. An ineffective cell membrane can allow substances into the cell that should not be there (like toxins) and interfere with the regulation of water. Water also influences the concentrations of important chemicals called *electrolytes*. **Electrolytes** are substances that separate into charged particles when dissolved in a solution. The movement of the charged particles creates the electrical function of cells, such as nerve transmission and cardiac depolarization.
- ***Oxygen.*** Oxygen fuels the fire of metabolism. It is a necessary component used by the cell to metabolize glucose into energy. Ordinarily, glucose is converted into ATP with a steady supply of oxygen. This process is called **aerobic metabolism** and it produces an efficient energy yield with minimal by-products (Figure 6-2 ■). One of the by-products of aerobic metabolism is carbon dioxide. **Anaerobic metabolism** occurs when there is not enough oxygen to metabolize glucose. During anaerobic metabolism energy is produced inefficiently and with a great deal more by-products including both carbon dioxide and lactic acid. Anaerobic metabolism is not healthy for the body because the accumulation of waste products makes the body more acidic and creates a toxic environment for the cells.

metabolism the conversion of glucose into energy in the form of adenosine triphosphate (ATP).

electrolytes substances that when dissolved in a solution separate into charged particles.

aerobic metabolism the cellular process by which oxygen is used to metabolize glucose and energy is produced in an efficient manner with minimal waste products.

anaerobic metabolism the cellular process by which glucose is metabolized without oxygen and energy is produced in an inefficient manner with many waste products.

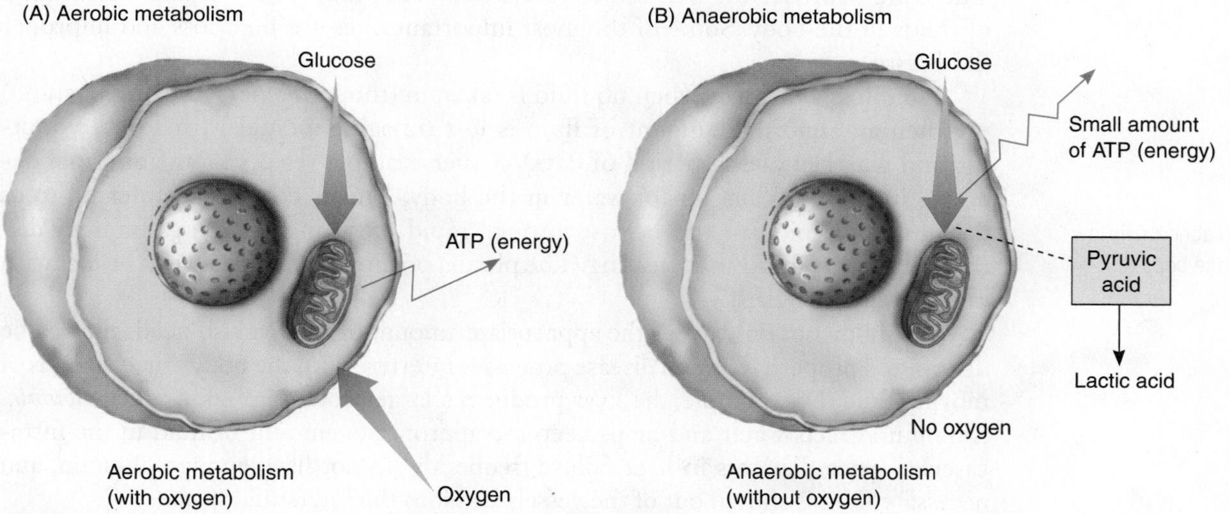

Figure 6-2 (A) Aerobic metabolism: In the presence of oxygen, glucose is broken down and produces a sufficient supply of ATP for the body. (B) Anaerobic metabolism: Without oxygen, glucose produces a very small amount of ATP and the result is pyruvic acid, which converts to lactic acid.

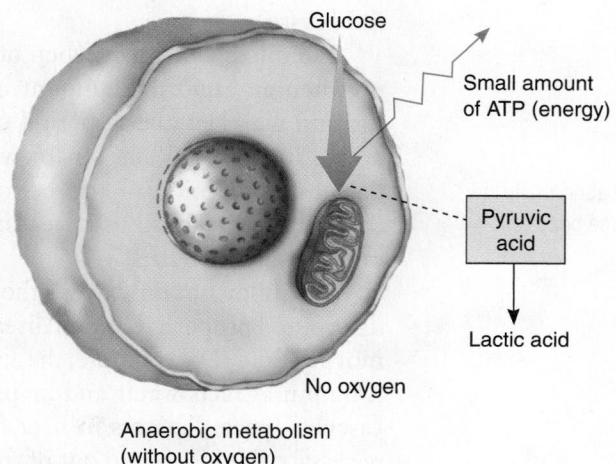

Fluid Balance

Human cells require a constant supply of water. In fact, about 60% of the body is made of water. Fluid is distributed throughout the body, and balancing the distribution is an important part of maintaining normal cellular function. Without an appropriate balance of water, both inside and outside cells, the basic functions of the cells would cease.

Water is divided among three spaces in the body:

- ***Intracellular space (75%).*** This is water that is actually inside the cells.
- ***Intravascular space (7.5%).*** This is water that is in the bloodstream.
- ***Interstitial space (17.5%).*** This water can be found in the space between cells and blood vessels.

6-16 Explain the effects of changes in hydrostatic pressure and plasma oncotic pressure on the movement of fluid between the cardiovascular system and interstitial spaces.

The amount of fluid in each of those spaces is a delicate balancing act that requires constant monitoring and intervention by the body's systems.

Water is introduced into the body by drinking fluids. It is excreted from the body by sweating, breathing, and making urine. These processes allow us to constantly adjust fluid levels based on our levels of activity. Fluid is distributed appropriately through a number of factors:

- The brain and kidneys regulate thirst, the elimination of excess fluid, and the retention of fluid as needed.
- Capillary hydrostatic pressure is the natural tendency for fluid to leave the capillary space by way of the permeable walls of the capillaries.
- Plasma oncotic pressure is the natural opposition to hydrostatic pressure. Large proteins in blood plasma pull fluid into the bloodstream. Because water is attracted to the large molecules and therefore pulled into the vascular space, the hydrostatic pressure of the capillaries is opposed.
- The permeability of both cell membranes and the walls of capillaries help control how much water can be held in and pushed out of cells and blood vessels.

Each of those factors is essential to maintain normal fluid balance. If any one is disrupted, fluid levels and distribution could become problematic.

Disruption of Fluid Balance

There are many factors that can contribute to disrupting the levels and distribution of fluids in the body. Some of the most important ones are fluid loss and improper fluid distribution.

Fluid loss can occur when no fluid is taken in (think of a person dying of thirst) or when an abnormal amount of fluid is lost (imagine a child with severe vomiting and diarrhea over a period of days). Either example results in an abnormal decrease in the total amount of water in the body. This is commonly referred to as **dehydration.** Fluid can also be lost through rapid breathing (as in a respiratory distress patient) and profuse sweating. The plasma portion of blood also can be lost with injuries such as burns.

dehydration an abnormally low amount of water in the body.

The body not only needs the appropriate amount of fluid, it also needs fluid to be distributed properly. Certain disease processes interfere with the body's mechanisms of moving fluid. For example, the liver produces a large protein in blood called *albumin.* Albumin attracts water and helps keep the appropriate amount of fluid in the intravascular space. Patients in liver failure frequently do not have enough albumin, and necessary fluid is shifted out of the vessels and into the interstitial space.

Sepsis is another good example of poor fluid distribution. Massive infection causes changes in capillary membrane permeability. Water migrates out of the bloodstream and cells and into the interstitial space (where it is much less useful). Often this can be seen externally in the form of edema. **Edema** is swelling associated with the abnormal movement of water. Edema can be seen best in *dependent* parts of the body—that is, those parts most subject to gravity such as the hands, feet, and legs. Edema also can occur because of an injury (when your thumb swells up after hitting it with a hammer, for example). In this case, the injury has damaged and altered the permeability of local capillaries resulting in the leakage of blood and a shift in fluid. The larger the injury, the more the fluid shifts.

edema swelling associated with the movement of water into the interstitial space.

Fluids also can be shifted by changing pressures inside the blood vessels. When pressure is high, the tendency will be to move the fluid portion of the blood out. This can be seen in disorders such as acute pulmonary edema.

CLINICAL CLUE

Fluid Balance

A patient's fluid balance can be assessed externally. Dehydration can be seen through dry mucous membranes, sunken eyes, and even through the body's responses, such as tachycardia and low blood pressure. Poor fluid distribution can be recognized through edema accumulation in dependent areas.

STOP, REVIEW, REMEMBER!

Multiple Choice

For each question, place a check next to the correct answer.

1. What is responsible for converting nutrients into energy?
   _____ a. Nucleus
   _____ b. Endoplasmic reticulum
   _____ c. Cytoplasm
   _____ d. Mitochondria

2. The study of how disease processes affect the function of the body is known as:
   _____ a. anatomy.
   _____ b. physiology.
   _____ c. pathophysiology.
   _____ d. kinesiology.

3. During normal metabolism, what does the cell convert into energy in the form of ATP?
   _____ a. Glucose
   _____ b. Water
   _____ c. Oxygen
   _____ d. Lactic acid

4. The process of using sufficient supplies of oxygen to fuel the creation of ATP is called ______________ metabolism.
   _____ a. aerobic
   _____ b. anaerobic
   _____ c. inaerobic
   _____ d. lactic

5. The largest amount of water in the body can be found in the ______________ space.
   _____ a. intracellular
   _____ b. intravascular
   _____ c. interstitial
   _____ d. extracellular

6. A reduction of total body fluid volume below normal levels is known as:
   _____ a. edema.
   _____ b. dehydration.
   _____ c. hypervolemia.
   _____ d. devolumation.

(continued on next page)

(continued)

Fill in the Blank

1. The ______________________ plays a key role in synthesizing proteins inside the cell.

2. ______________________ are substances that separate into charged particles when dissolved in water.

3. ______________________ is swelling associated with the movement of water.

4. The ______________________ space is the area between cells and blood vessels.

5. The ______________________ covers, protects, and selectively allows water and other substances into and out of the cell.

Critical Thinking

1. Describe how aerobic metabolism differs from anaerobic metabolism.

____

____

____

____

2. List three general requirements of normal cell metabolism.

____

____

____

____

3. List three ways the body distributes fluid.

____

____

____

____

The Cardiopulmonary System

6-6 Describe the composition of ambient air.

FiO_2 fraction of inspired oxygen; the concentration of oxygen in the air we breathe.

Aerobic metabolism requires a constant supply of oxygen. The body obtains this oxygen primarily from the air we breathe. Inhaled air contains approximately 21% oxygen. (Nitrogen and a small percentage of other gases make up the other 79%.) The concentration of oxygen in inhaled air is referred to as the *fraction of inspired oxygen*, or **FiO_2**. The respiratory system diffuses oxygen into the bloodstream, and the cardiovascular system transports it out to the body cells. The blood also picks up carbon dioxide from the cells and transports it back to the lungs where it can be eliminated through exhalation.

It is important to remember that both the respiratory and cardiovascular systems must work together. The lungs, heart, blood vessels, and the blood itself must all work in concert to successfully deliver oxygen and nutrients to the cells and remove waste products. Interruption of any part of this balance results in a failure of the cardiopulmonary system.

PERSPECTIVE

Darin—The EMT

I thought I'd been to that address before and when they mentioned "CHF," I knew it. That old man is so nice and I feel so bad for him. He could barely breathe when we arrived and yet he was apologizing for taking us away from "important stuff"! I assured him that at that moment there was nothing more important than helping him. He presented with swollen legs and abdomen and you could hear the fluid in his lungs without a stethoscope. A lot of people with bad CHF sleep sitting up, and I could tell his recliner has had its share of use, but he was in bed when we arrived. Sometimes I think people just need to try to do normal stuff—like sleep in a bed—even if they know it may cause trouble later. I really hope he's going to be okay.

The Respiratory System

The respiratory system includes the structures of the airway, the lungs, and the muscles of respiration. Air enters through the openings of the mouth and nose, travels through the pharynx, and then enters the trachea through the glottic opening. Air travels down the trachea and enters the lungs as it branches into the bronchi. The bronchi divide and subdivide (like branches of a tree) until they reach their endpoints at the alveoli.

Movement of air in and out of the chest requires an open and clear pathway referred to as a **patent** airway. There are a number of potential challenges to maintaining a patent airway due to disease and trauma. They include:

patent open and clear; free from obstruction.

- ***Upper airway obstructions.*** Upper airway obstructions occur above the trachea and prevent air from entering into the lower airway. The most common cause is the tongue. An altered mental status relaxes the muscles of the tongue and other soft tissues, including the tongue and epiglottis, obstructing air flow. Upper airway obstructions are frequently caused by foreign bodies (such as in a choking person) or by swelling caused by infection (such as a child with croup). Trauma or burns also can cause the soft tissues of the larynx to swell. Any of those causes can seriously and significantly impact the flow of air and interrupt the process of moving oxygen in and carbon dioxide out.
- ***Lower airway obstructions.*** The most common lower airway obstruction is bronchoconstriction, or the narrowing of the lower airways. In conditions such as asthma, the small bronchioles spasm and become narrower, causing greater airway resistance and reducing the amount of air that can flow through them to reach the alveoli.

6-7 Explain how changes in compliance of the lungs and chest wall and changes in airway resistance affect ventilation.

6-9 Explain the concept of minute ventilation.

6-10 Differentiate between minute ventilation and alveolar ventilation.

The lungs are the organs of breathing and are filled and emptied by changing pressure within the chest cavity. The diaphragm and chest wall expand and contract to cause those pressure changes and air is pulled in and out of the lungs. The volume of air moved in and out during a single cycle of breathing is called **tidal volume.** To obtain **minute volume,** multiply tidal volume and respiratory rate ($MV = TV \times RR$).

tidal volume the volume of air moved in one cycle of breathing.

minute volume the volume of air moved in one minute by the lungs (tidal volume × respiratory rate).

It is important to remember that minute volume can be affected by changes in either tidal volume or rate (or both). For example:

- A 16-year-old has a normal minute volume of approximately 5,000 mL. (Tidal volume of 500 mL × 10 breaths per minute.) After being struck by a car and sustaining a severe brain injury, his respiratory rate slows to 4 breaths per minute. He is breathing the same tidal volume as he was before, but because his rate is so slow, his minute volume significantly decreases. (Tidal volume of 500 mL × 4 breaths per minute = 2,000 mL minute volume.)
- A 70-year-old woman has a normal minute volume of 6,000 mL. (Tidal volume of 500 mL × 12 breaths per minute = 6,000 mL minute volume.) She has chronic obstructive pulmonary disease (COPD), and because she has been fighting a respiratory infection for the last few days, her tidal volume has decreased to 250 mL. Even though she breathes at the same rate, her minute volume is significantly decreased. (Tidal volume of 250 mL × 12 breaths per minute = 3,000 mL minute volume.)

Not all of the tidal volume gets to the alveoli. In adults, about 150 mL of a normal tidal volume occupies the space between the mouth and alveoli but does not actually reach the alveoli for gas exchange. That space is referred to as **dead air space.** *Alveolar ventilation* occurs only with the air that reaches the alveoli (Figure 6-3 ■).

dead air space air that occupies the space between the mouth and alveoli, but does not actually reach the area of gas exchange.

CLINICAL CLUE

Minute Volume

During your primary assessment, you will assess a patient's breathing rate by counting respirations. Then you will assess tidal volume, which is a bit more subjective. It can be assessed by observing chest rise and fall and listening to lung sounds with a stethoscope.

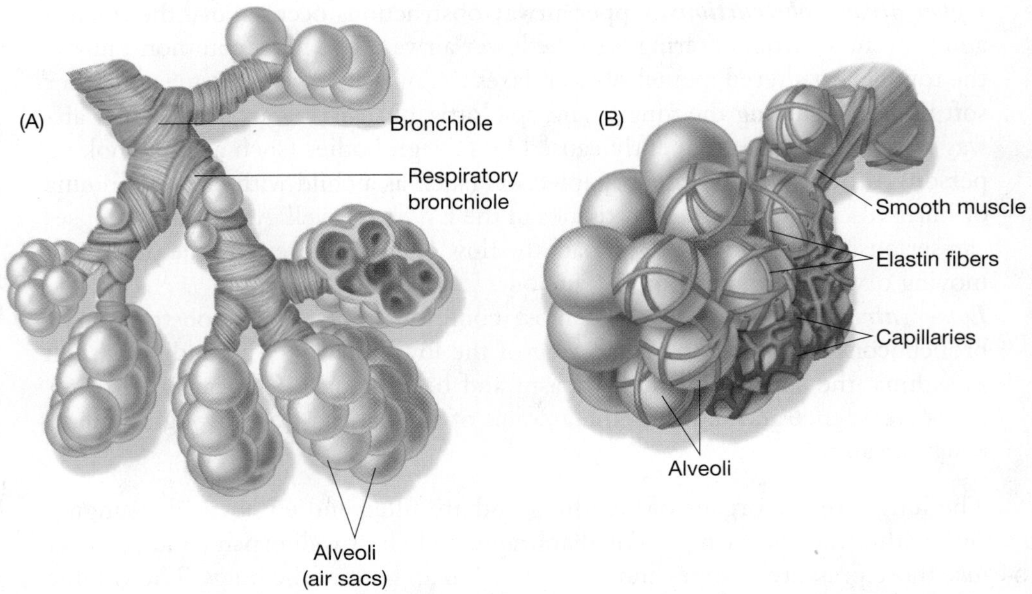

Figure 6-3 (A) Deep within the lungs are tiny structures called *alveoli*. (B) The alveoli are surrounded by capillaries that transfer oxygen and carbon dioxide.

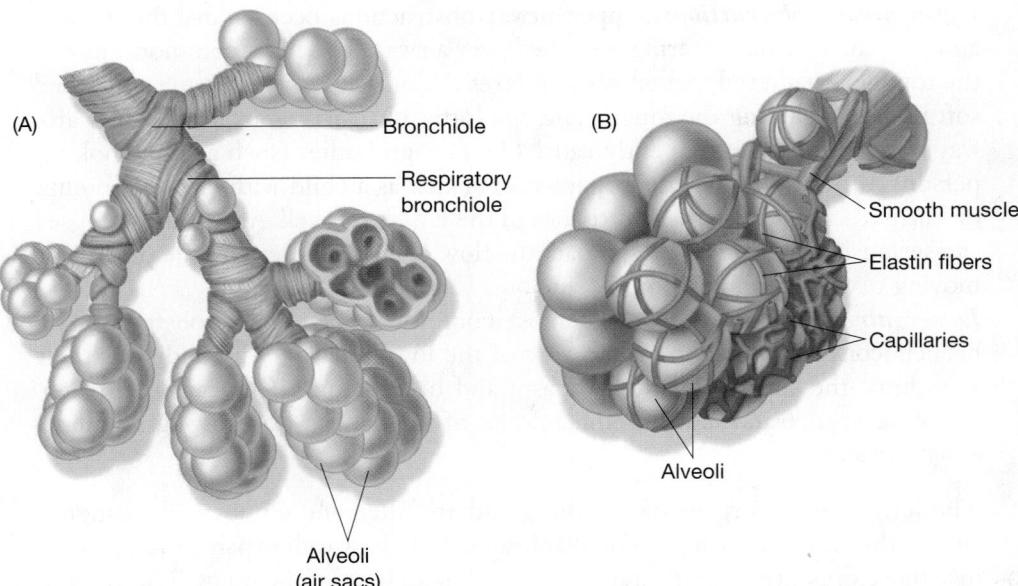

Respiratory System Dysfunction

There are many causes of respiratory system dysfunction. In general normal function is interrupted any time minute volume is negatively impacted. The following examples are common causes of respiratory dysfunction:

6-11 Describe the roles of chemoreceptors and the nervous system in the control of ventilation.

- ***Disruption of respiratory control.*** Breathing is controlled by an area of the brain called the *medulla oblongata*. Disorders that affect this area of the brain can interfere with respiratory function (Figure 6-4 ■). Medical reasons such as stroke, brain tumors, and infection can disrupt the medulla's function and alter the stimulus to breathe. Toxins and drugs also can affect the medulla's ability to regulate breathing by slowing respirations and adversely impacting minute volume. Brain trauma and intracranial pressure can physically harm the medulla and impair its function. Neurological disorders can also impair the brain's ability to send messages to the muscles of respiration. Spinal-cord injuries and neuromuscular diseases such as multiple sclerosis can significantly impair the respiratory system.

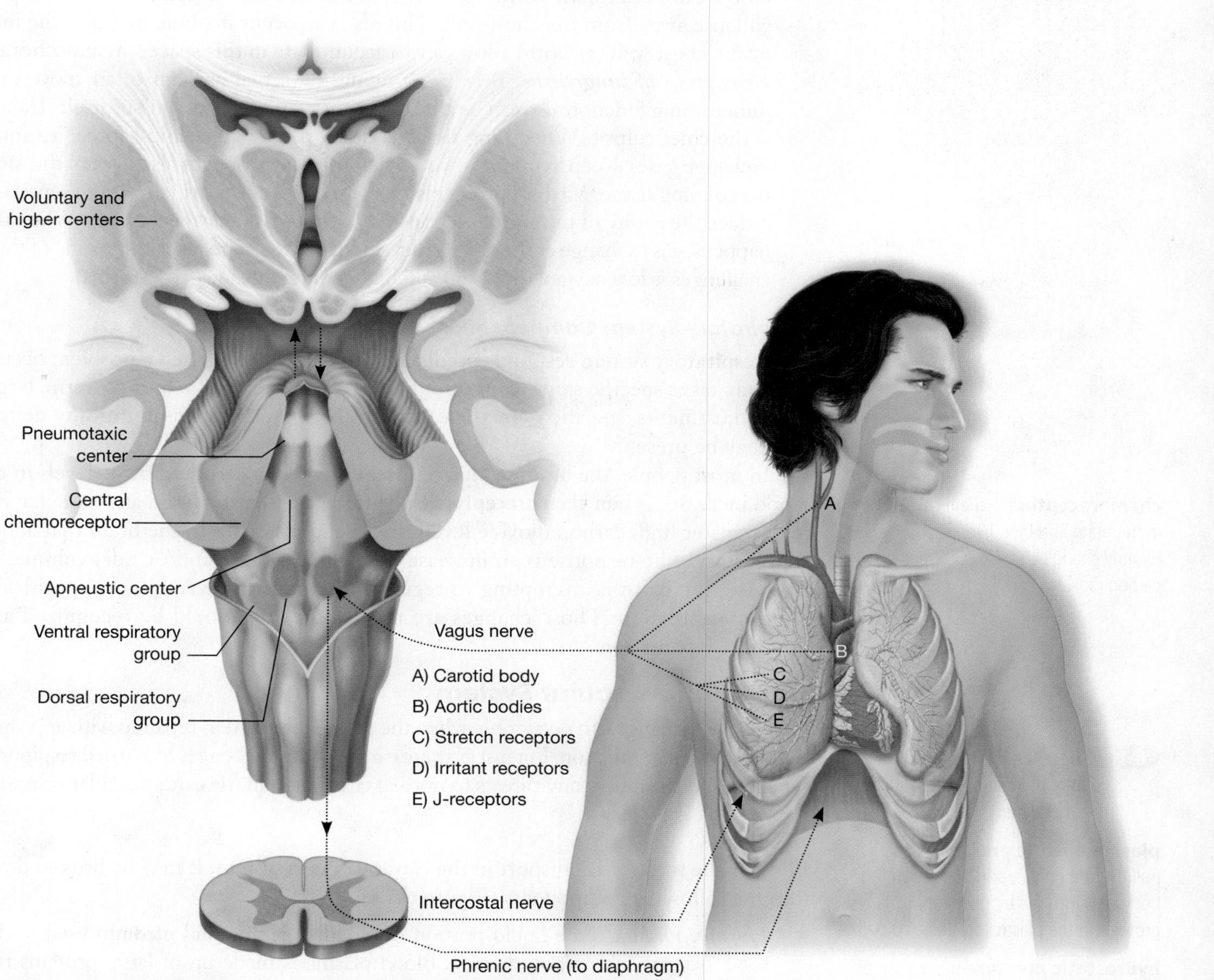

Figure 6-4 Respiration is controlled by the autonomic nervous system. Receptors within the body measure levels of oxygen, carbon dioxide, and hydrogen and send signals to the brain to adjust the rate and depth of respirations as appropriate.

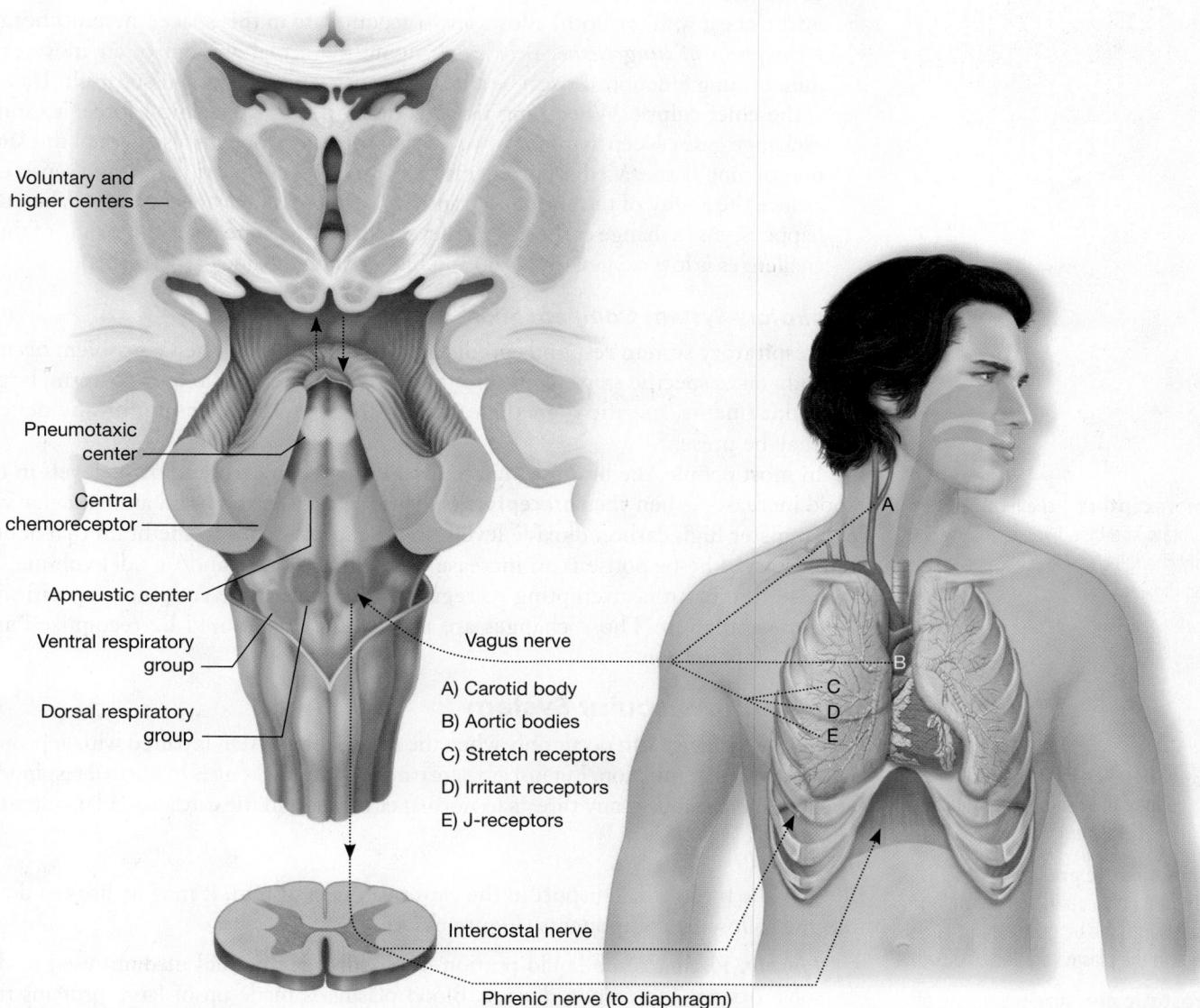

6-8 Describe the consequences of loss of contact between the parietal and visceral pleura.

- ***Disruption of pressure.*** The chest cavity is a closed container. A large muscle called the *diaphragm* forms the lower boundary and combines with the ribs and intercostal muscles to change the container's size. The lungs are adhered to the chest wall by contact between two membranes known as the *parietal pleura* (chest wall) and *visceral pleura* (lung). Even though the two membranes are stuck tightly together, there is a potential space between them called the *pleural space*. A small amount of fluid exists there to lubricate the pleura and help the lungs move and adhere. It is important to remember that the pleural space is a potential space where blood and air can accumulate under the right circumstances.

  When the chest expands, a negative pressure is created inside and air is pulled into the lungs. When the container relaxes and becomes smaller, positive pressure is created inside the chest and air is pushed out. Changing pressures within the chest cavity rely on an intact chest compartment. If a hole is created in the chest wall and air is allowed to escape or be drawn in, the pressure necessary to breathe can be disrupted. Furthermore, if bleeding develops within the chest, blood can accumulate in the pleural space (hemothorax) and force the lung to collapse away from the chest wall. This also can occur if a hole in either the lung or the chest wall (or both) allows air to accumulate in this space (pneumothorax).
- ***Disruption of lung tissue.*** Besides changing the actual amount of air moved per minute, lung function also can be affected by disrupting the lung tissue itself. Trauma is the chief culprit. When lung tissue is destroyed by mechanical force, it cannot exchange gases. Keep in mind, however, that medical problems also disrupt the function of lung tissue. Medical problems such as congestive heart failure and sepsis can reduce the ability of the alveoli to transfer gases across their membranes. When this happens, gas exchange at the alveolar level is disrupted. The net result of any of these challenges is low oxygen (hypoxia) and high carbon dioxide (hypercarbia).

Respiratory System Compensation

The respiratory system responds predictably to challenges. When a problem occurs, the body takes specific steps to attempt to correct it. In addition to long-term, large-scale adjustments, specific immediate changes occur to compensate for any deficits that may be present.

chemoreceptors chemical sensors in the brain and blood vessels that identify changing levels of oxygen and carbon dioxide.

In most people, the brain stimulates breathing when carbon dioxide levels in the blood increase. When **chemoreceptors** (specific sensors in the brain and vascular system) register high carbon dioxide levels, they send messages to the brain that action is necessary. The response is an increase in respiratory rate and/or tidal volume. By doing so, the brain is attempting to regulate minute volume and, more specifically, alveolar ventilation. Those changes are predictable and should be recognized as a sign of compensation.

The Cardiovascular System

6-15 Describe the composition of blood, including the function of plasma.

Proper gas exchange can occur only when the respiratory system is paired with appropriate cardiovascular function. But just as there can be many challenges to normal respiratory function, there can be many threats to normal circulation in the cardiovascular system.

The Blood

plasma oncotic pressure the pull exerted on water in and around the body cells into the bloodstream by large proteins in the plasma portion of blood.

hydrostatic pressure the push of water out of the bloodstream as a result of the pressure within the vessel.

Blood is the means of transport in the cardiovascular system. It may be broken down into the following components (Figure 6-5 ■):

- ***Plasma.*** Plasma is the liquid portion of blood. It is the fluid medium used to dissolve oxygen and carbon dioxide. Blood plasma is made up of large proteins that tend to attract water away from the interstitial space and into the bloodstream. This force is called **plasma oncotic pressure**. It is counterbalanced by **hydrostatic pressure** (increased pressure inside the vessels when the heart beats), which tends to push fluid back out toward the cells. Both types of pressure are important to regulating hydration of the cells. An abnormal change of either one can be devastating (Figure 6-6 ■).

- ***Red blood cells (hemoglobin).*** Red blood cells carry most of the oxygen transported by the blood. Red blood cells must be in sufficient supply and capable of carrying oxygen for the cardiovascular system to be effective.
- ***White blood cells.*** White blood cells are a critical component of the immune system and are used to fight infection.
- ***Platelets.*** Platelets are the components of blood that form clots.

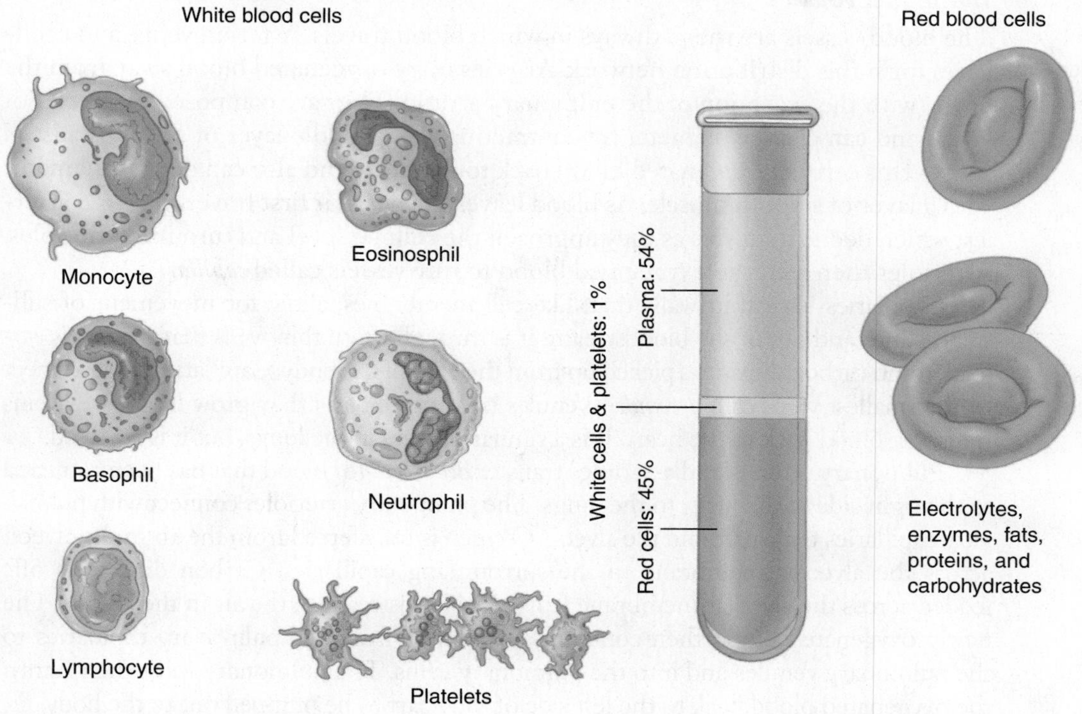

Figure 6-5 The components of blood.

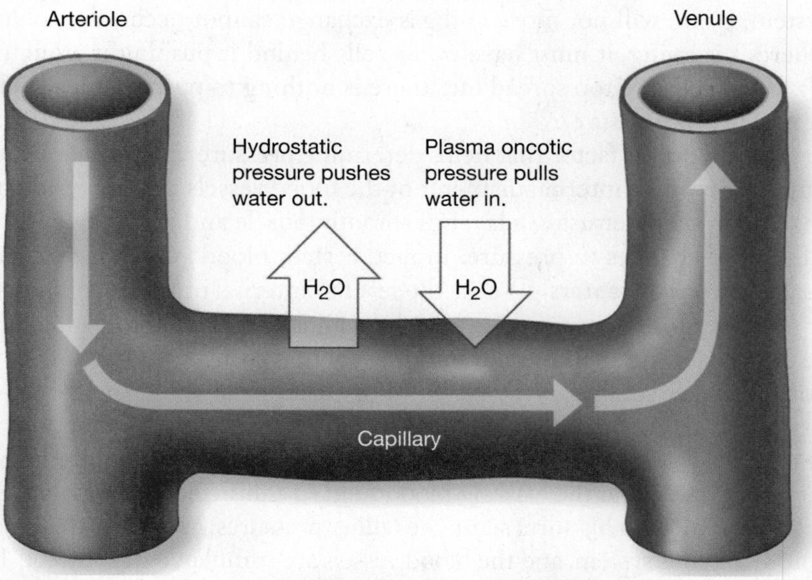

Figure 6-6 Hydrostatic pressure is the force acting to push fluid out of the capillaries. Plasma oncotic pressure pulls water into the capillaries.

The most common dysfunction related to blood is not having enough. Circulation requires a sufficient quantity of blood and when that quantity is not available, circulation fails. Major bleeding is the most likely culprit in this type of problem, but volume also can be lost from the bloodstream by losing water from the plasma as in dehydration.

Other blood dysfunctions include conditions that affect the components of the blood. For example, anemia can decrease the number of red blood cells, and a low body pH (acidosis) can affect their ability to carry oxygen. Other conditions, such as liver failure, can decrease the blood's ability to retain water in plasma.

The Blood Vessels

6-13 Describe the transport of oxygen and carbon dioxide in the blood.

6-14 Explain the exchange of gases across the alveolar/capillary membrane and the exchange of gases between capillaries and cells.

The blood vessels are the pathways in which blood travels. Arteries, veins, and capillaries form this distribution network. Arteries carry oxygenated blood away from the heart (with the exception of the pulmonary artery). They are composed of a series of layers and can change diameter by contracting their middle layer of smooth muscle. Most veins carry deoxygenated blood back to the heart and also can change diameter with a layer of smooth muscle. As blood leaves the heart, it first travels through arteries, which decrease in size as they approach the cellular level and turn into arterioles. Arterioles then feed the oxygenated blood to tiny vessels called *capillaries*.

Capillaries have thin walls that, like cell membranes, allow for movement of substances into and out of the bloodstream. It is through those thin walls that oxygen is offloaded and carbon dioxide is picked up from the cells of the body. Capillaries then connect to the smallest veins called *venules*. Venules become veins as they grow larger and veins transport blood back to the heart. It is a similar process in the lungs, but it is reversed.

Pulmonary arteries and arterioles transfer *deoxygenated* blood that has been returned to the right side of the heart to the lungs. The pulmonary arterioles connect with pulmonary capillaries that surround the alveoli. Oxygen is transferred from the air in the alveoli across the alveolar membrane to the surrounding capillaries. Carbon dioxide is offloaded across the alveolar membrane from the bloodstream to the air in the alveoli. The newly oxygenated blood then continues on its way from the pulmonary capillaries to the pulmonary venules and into the pulmonary veins. The pulmonary veins then return the oxygenated blood back to the left side of the heart to be pumped out to the body.

Blood is moved through the blood vessels by the pressure created by the beating heart. Pressure is an essential element to circulation. Without pressure in the circulatory system, blood will not move and gas exchange cannot occur. For a blood cell to get where it is going, it must have other cells behind it pushing it along (normal pressure). If the cells are too spread out, there is nothing to push that lead cell and it does not move (low pressure).

6-20 Explain the regulation of blood pressure by baroreceptors and chemoreceptors.

stretch receptors specialized sensors in certain blood vessels that sense pressure within the vessel.

One very important factor that helps determine pressure within the cardiovascular system is the relative internal diameter of the blood vessels. Arteries and arterioles can change their diameter using a layer of smooth muscle and will frequently change size to adjust for changes in pressure. In fact, certain blood vessels have specialized sensors called **stretch receptors** to sense the level of internal pressure within itself and transmit messages to the nervous system when adjustments need to be made.

baroreceptors stretch-sensitive sensors in the aorta and carotid arteries that monitor blood pressure.

6-19 Summarize the local, neural, and hormonal factors that regulate blood flow through the capillaries.

Pressure may need to be adjusted for a variety of reasons including loss of volume (blood) or too much volume in the system. For example, imagine an 18-year-old patient who has lacerated his femoral artery. As a result of severe bleeding, the volume of blood in his blood vessels significantly decreases, therefore causing the pressure in the system to decrease and the existing blood to have a difficult time moving. Stretch-sensitive **baroreceptors** in his aorta sense the falling pressures. Messages are transmitted to the central nervous system, and the blood vessels are stimulated to contract. This decreases the container size, and the pressure within the system normalizes (for a while).

The autonomic nervous system plays a major role in controlling vessel diameter. In particular, the sympathetic nervous system in its fight-or-flight response stimulates blood vessels to constrict. In contrast, the parasympathetic nervous system stimulates blood vessels to relax.

A variety of dysfunctions can interfere with the normal operation of blood vessels. The following are common examples:

6-18 Describe the concept of systemic vascular resistance and its relationship to blood pressure and pulse pressure.

- ***Loss of blood vessel tone.*** A major problem related to blood vessels is the inability of a vessel to control its own size (or more specifically its own internal diameter). If blood vessels are unable to constrict when necessary or worse, they are forced into an uncontrolled vasodilation (increase in internal diameter), pressure inside them can drop significantly. Many conditions can cause this loss of vessel tone. Injuries to the brain and spinal cord, uncontrolled infections, and severe allergic reactions all can cause uncontrolled vasodilation.
- ***Permeability problems.*** Certain conditions cause capillaries to become too permeable. In this case, fluid leaks through the capillary walls too easily and the fluid portion of blood leaves the intravascular space too readily. Sepsis and certain diseases are frequently responsible for these problems.
- ***Hypertension.*** The pressure inside the vessel that the heart has to pump against is called **systemic vascular resistance (SVR).** Normally, this pressure is an important element of moving blood. However, in some patients, it is abnormally increased. Chronic smoking, certain drugs, and even genetics can cause abnormal constriction of the peripheral blood vessels and therefore an unhealthy high level of pressure. This increased pressure can be a major risk factor in heart disease and stroke.

systemic vascular resistance (SVR) the pressure in the peripheral blood vessels that the heart must overcome to pump blood.

The Heart

The heart often is described as a simple four-chambered pump. Although its role is fairly simple, the pressure it creates by pumping is critical to the success of the cardiovascular system. The movement of blood and subsequently the transportation of oxygen and carbon dioxide are all dependent on the heart working properly.

The job of the heart is very straightforward: move blood. To do this, it mechanically contracts and ejects blood. The volume of blood ejected in one squeeze is known as **stroke volume (SV).** Stroke volume is dependent on a series of factors. They are:

stroke volume (SV) the volume of blood ejected from the heart in one contraction.

- ***Preload.*** Preload is how much blood is returned to the heart prior to the contraction, or how much it filled.
- ***Contractility.*** Contractility is the force of a contraction, or how hard it squeezed. The more forcefully the muscle squeezes, the greater the stroke volume.
- ***Afterload.*** This is a function of systemic vascular resistance, and describes how much force the heart has to overcome to pump. The greater this force, the lower the stroke volume.

Cardiac output (CO) is the amount of blood ejected from the heart in one minute. Think of it in the same way you think of minute volume. Just as minute volume is a function of both tidal volume and respiratory rate, cardiac output is a function of both stroke volume and heart rate. Just as you could affect minute volume by changing either rate or volume, cardiac output can be changed by altering either heart rate or stroke volume.

6-17 Discuss factors that affect cardiac output, including heart rate, stroke volume, preload, and afterload.

cardiac output (CO) the amount of blood ejected from the heart in one minute (heart rate × stroke volume).

Cardiac output also can be impacted by heart rates that are too fast. Normally, increasing heart rate would increase cardiac output; however, very fast rates (usually >180 in adults) limit the filling time of the heart and can *decrease* stroke volume. Some examples of impaired cardiac output include:

- A 33-year-old woman has tachycardia at a rate of 220. Her tachycardia is not giving her ventricles enough time to fill between contractions. As a result, her stroke volume (and overall cardiac output) has dropped.
- A 67-year-old man has bradycardia (slow heart rate) at a rate of 40. His heart rate has decreased and, because of this, so has his cardiac output.

- A 19-year-old has been stabbed in the abdomen. Because he has severe internal bleeding, not as much blood is returning to his heart and stroke volume is therefore decreased. Cardiac output would drop as a result.
- A 90-year-old man is having his fourth heart attack. In this case the wall of the left ventricle is no longer working. Because his heart has difficulty squeezing out blood, his cardiac output drops.

The autonomic nervous system also plays a large role in adjusting cardiac output. The sympathetic response increases heart rate and the strength of contractions. The parasympathetic response slows the heart down and decreases contractility.

The heart can fail in two different ways—electrically or mechanically. That is, failure can be a result of a muscle (structural) problem or the result of a problem with electrical stimulation of that muscle. Mechanical failure can be caused by a number of factors, including trauma, such as bullet holes and stab wounds; squeezing forces, such as when the heart is squeezed due to bleeding inside its protective pericardial sac; or loss of function of cardiac muscle due to cell death as in a heart attack. Electrical failure can result from problems in the heart's conduction system, which include excessively fast rates (tachycardia), excessively slow rates (bradycardia), and disorganized conduction such as ventricular fibrillation. More information on cardiac dysfunction is discussed in later chapters.

Cardiopulmonary System and Perfusion

6-5 Explain the concept of perfusion, including components necessary to maintain perfusion.

6-12 Explain the concept of the ventilation/perfusion (VQ) ratio.

6-21 Explain the relationship among ventilation, perfusion, and cellular metabolism.

perfusion the constant supply of oxygen and nutrients to the cells by the flow of blood.

Every cell and every organ system requires a constant delivery of oxygen and nutrients and the removal of waste products. This is a function of a continuous supply of blood and is referred to as **perfusion.** Perfusion absolutely relies on the interrelated function of the respiratory and cardiovascular systems.

For oxygen to be delivered and for waste products to be removed, all of the components of the cardiopulmonary system must be functioning together (Figure 6-7 ■). In the respiratory system air movement must bring oxygen all the way to the alveoli and move carbon dioxide back all the way out. There must be a significant quantity of air moving and the alveoli must be capable of exchanging gases. In the cardiovascular system, there must be enough blood, the heart must pump that blood, and there must be enough pressure in the system to move the blood between the body cells and the alveoli. The blood also must be capable of carrying oxygen and carbon dioxide.

PERSPECTIVE

Charlie—The Patient

I used to work oil rigs when I was a young man. I was as strong as an ox, I tell you. Could pull double shifts and still go out with the guys and be the last one standing. Now they tell me my right heart's failing, whatever that means. I thought I only had one to begin with. The thing I find most interesting in all this is how akin to machines our bodies are. I seem to be the victim of fluid dynamics that basically causes the same type of stuff in my plumbing that used to shut down our drilling operations! When fluid backed up on the rig, we'd just blow it off and get back to it, but with my body, it seems it's just a matter of time before I drown in my own lungs and there's not much I can do about it. Sometimes, like this morning, I feel so helpless and tired. And scared. Boy, you'd never catch me admitting that 50 years ago.

An adequate blood pressure is necessary to force blood through the vessels. Blood pressure is derived by multiplying cardiac output (CO) × systemic vascular resistance (SVR). Cardiac output is derived by multiplying heart rate (HR) × stroke volume (SV). Stroke volume is the amount of blood ejected by the left ventricle with

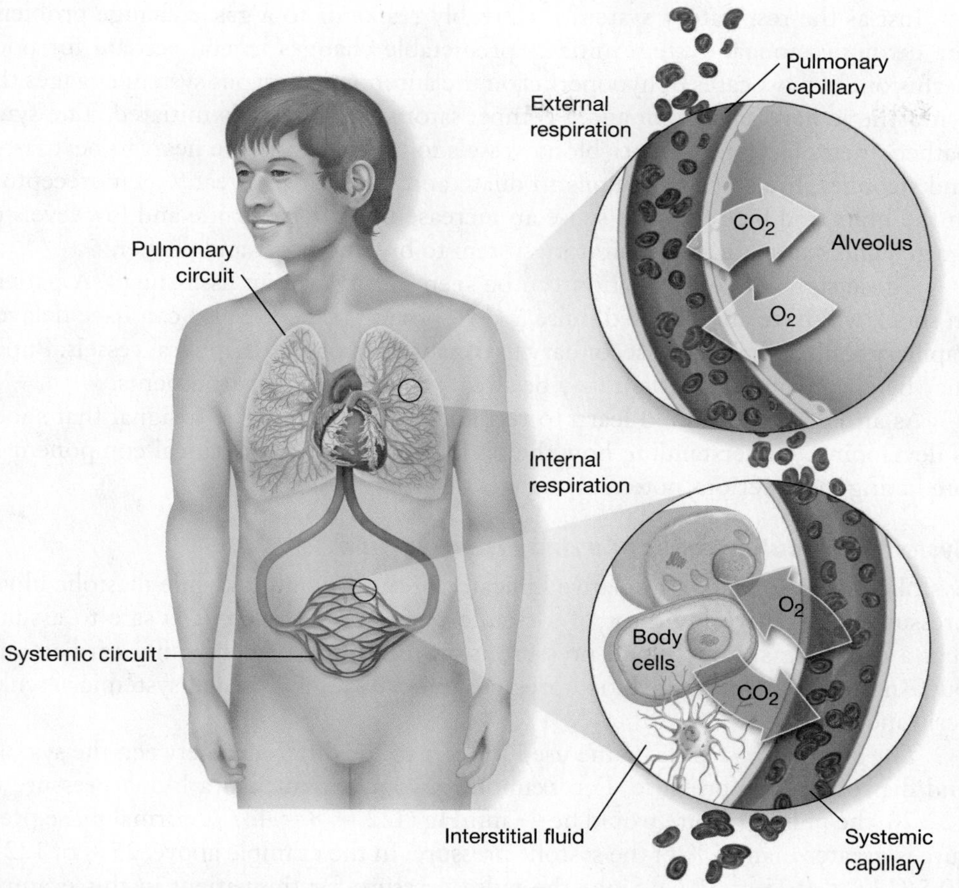

Figure 6-7 Ventilation and perfusion must work together to ensure all cells receive oxygen and nutrients.

each contraction. Systemic vascular resistance is the resistance caused by the vessels as the blood moves through them.

$$CO \times SVR = \text{Blood Pressure}$$

$$HR \times SV = \text{Cardiac Output}$$

When all those functions are in place, a ventilation (V)/perfusion (Q) match occurs. The **V/Q match** is rarely perfect. In fact even in healthy lungs a force as simple as gravity can mean that alveoli in the upper areas of the lungs may not be matched with as much blood as alveoli in the lower areas. As a result, the V/Q match often is expressed as a ratio rather than a true match.

V/Q match ventilation/perfusion match, which implies that the alveoli are supplied with air and that air is matched with sufficient blood in the pulmonary capillaries to exchange oxygen and carbon dioxide.

The V/Q ratio can be disrupted by any challenge that interferes with the cardiopulmonary system. Minute volume problems, cardiac output problems, and structural damage all can disrupt the connection between air and blood.

Hypoperfusion and Shock

Shock occurs when perfusion fails. In other words, shock occurs when the regular delivery of oxygen and nutrients to cells and the removal of their waste products are interrupted. This failure is referred to as *hypoperfusion*. Without a regular supply of oxygen, cells become hypoxic and must rely on anaerobic metabolism. When this type of metabolism occurs, lactic acid and other waste products accumulate and harm the cells. Without the removal of carbon dioxide, the buildup of harmful waste products is accelerated. Unless reversed, the lack of perfusion will kill cells, organs, and eventually the patient.

Just as the respiratory system predictably responds to a gas exchange problem, the cardiopulmonary system initiates predictable changes to compensate for poor perfusion. In most cases of hypoperfusion the autonomic nervous system engages the sympathetic nervous system and a compensatory mechanism is initiated. The sympathetic nervous system causes blood vessels to constrict and the heart to beat faster and stronger. It also causes pupils to dilate and the skin to sweat. Chemoreceptors in the brain and blood vessels sense an increase in carbon dioxide and low levels of oxygen and stimulate the respiratory system to breathe faster and deeper.

Those signs of compensation can be seen during patient assessment. A patient in shock will have an increased pulse and respiratory rate. He also can have delayed capillary refill and pale skin secondary to constriction of the peripheral vessels. Pupils may be dilated and the patient may be sweaty even in cool environments.

As an EMT you should learn to recognize these findings as a signal that shock is developing. Understanding how the body compensates is a critical component in predicting more serious potential changes.

Systemic Vascular Resistance and Pulse Pressure

Systolic blood pressure is a relative indicator of cardiac output, while diastolic blood pressure is a relative indicator of systemic vascular resistance. It is safe to assume that a dropping systolic blood pressure is an indication of decreasing cardiac output. An increase in diastolic blood pressure indicates an increase in systemic vascular resistance.

The *pulse pressure* is the name used to refer to the difference between the systolic and diastolic blood pressure. For example, if your patient had a blood pressure of 122/78, the pulse pressure would be 44 mmHg (122 – 78 = 44). A normal pulse pressure is greater than 25% of the systolic pressure. In the example above, 25% of 122 is 30.5 (122 × 0.25 = 30.5). Since the pulse pressure for the patient in this example is 44 mmHg, it would be considered normal. An abnormal pulse pressure is one that is less than 25% of the systolic pressure.

It is important to monitor pulse pressure in addition to the other vital signs, such as pulse and blood pressure. A narrow pulse pressure may be a significant sign that something is wrong with the patient. For example, in the case of a patient with internal bleeding that goes undetected, the body's normal compensatory response is to constrict the vessels to increase systemic vascular resistance and maintain a good diastolic pressure. On the opposite side, cardiac output is dropping due to the blood loss. A patient such as this may present with a blood pressure of 110/90. While this blood pressure may appear to be normal, when you calculate the pulse pressure (110 × 25% = 27.5 mmHg) you will discover that it is abnormally narrow.

Pediatric Compensation

Children compensate differently than adults do. Children rely more on heart rate and less on increases in contractility to overcome deficits in cardiac output. Because of this, fast heart rates in children should always be considered shock until proven otherwise. Children also rely heavily on vasoconstriction to compensate for volume loss. As a result, they can maintain pressure in their cardiovascular system with relatively less blood than an adult. For this reason, blood pressure is a fairly unreliable indicator of shock in children. Children also have a higher metabolic rate than adults do. That means they burn more oxygen and require more glucose to sustain normal function.

Shock is among the leading killers of pediatric patients. As an EMT, you must learn to adapt your assessment to recognize the specific signs of hypoperfusion and compensation in the younger age groups.

CLINICAL CLUE

Compensation

Recognizing compensation (as manifested by an elevated heart rate) is an important element of trauma patient assessment because it can rapidly identify the patient in shock. Always be on the lookout during your assessment for the telltale signs of hypoperfusion (shock).

STOP, REVIEW, REMEMBER!

Multiple Choice

For each question, place a check next to the correct answer.

1. The concentration of oxygen in inhaled air is referred to as:

_____ a. FiO_2.

_____ b. PaO_2.

_____ c. CO_2.

_____ d. SaO_2.

2. The most common cause of upper airway obstruction is:

_____ a. foreign bodies.

_____ b. infection.

_____ c. the tongue.

_____ d. edema from burns.

3. Minute volume can be found by multiplying _____________ and tidal volume.

_____ a. respiratory rate

_____ b. FiO_2

_____ c. heart rate

_____ d. stroke volume

4. Which one of the following conditions would be an example of a dysfunction of respiratory control?

_____ a. Broken rib that causes decreased movement of the chest wall

_____ b. Stab wound that causes air in the pleural space

_____ c. Pulmonary edema that causes fluid in the aveoli

_____ d. Stroke that causes slowed breathing

5. Specialized sensors in the brain and vascular system that register carbon dioxide and oxygen levels are called:

_____ a. stretch receptors.

_____ b. hypoxic receptors.

_____ c. carboxic receptors.

_____ d. chemoreceptors.

6. The movement of fluid out of the interstitial space and into the bloodstream caused by large proteins in the blood is referred to as what kind of pressure?

_____ a. Hydrostatic

_____ b. Plasma oncotic

_____ c. Perfusion

_____ d. Static osmotic

7. The *smallest* vessel that carries deoxygenated blood from the capillary back to the heart is called a(n):

_____ a. artery.

_____ b. arteriole.

_____ c. venule.

_____ d. vein.

(continued on next page)

(continued)

Fill in the Blank

1. Certain blood vessels have specialized sensors called ______________________ that sense the level of pressure inside the vessels and transmit messages to the nervous system when adjustments need to be made.

2. The pressure inside the vessels caused by the natural dilation and constriction is called ______________________.

3. The term ______________________ refers to the quantity of blood returned to the heart prior to a contraction.

4. ______________________ is another term for the force of a contraction of the heart.

5. Delivery of oxygen and nutrients to a cell and the removal of waste products are referred to as ______________________.

Critical Thinking

1. Describe how the respiratory system compensates for a gas exchange problem. What signs might you see during patient assessment?

____

____

____

____

2. Describe how the cardiopulmonary system compensates for a decreased level of perfusion (shock). What signs might you see during patient assessment?

____

____

____

____

3. Describe how children compensate for shock differently than adults do.

____

____

____

____

Pathophysiology of Other Body Systems

Although the cardiopulmonary system controls many vital body functions, other body systems play an important role in adapting the body to changing conditions. Systems that help the body maintain normal life functions include the nervous system, endocrine system, gastrointestinal system, immune system, and integumentary system.

The Nervous System

The nervous system controls all body functions. Although the brain and spinal cord are well protected, trauma or disease to either of them can disrupt vital processes throughout the body. Examples of the causes of nervous system dysfunction include:

- *Traumatic injuries*, such as blunt force and penetrating trauma to the brain and spinal cord
- *Medical problems*, such as stroke or infection
- *Toxins*, such as alcohol or other poisons that destroy nervous system cells or create an environment in which those cells cannot function properly

Trauma is a leading cause of nervous system dysfunction. Physical destruction of nervous system tissue interrupts message pathways and disrupts function. Furthermore, most nervous system tissue does not regenerate, so injuries often leave permanent damage.

The skull is a closed rigid container that protects the brain. Usually, the brain fills the majority of available space within the cranium. However, when injury occurs, bleeding and swelling can take up space where brain tissue would otherwise be, compressing brain tissue and destroying brain cells. The increase in pressure within the skull [intracranial pressure (ICP)] can have destructive and even fatal effects unless the bleeding and swelling are rapidly controlled.

Mechanical damage (injury) to the spine and other nerve pathways disrupts nervous system communication. When you think of a severed spinal cord, paralysis likely comes to mind, but beyond motor function, the patient may lose sensory and autonomic messaging as well. That means when a nervous pathway is destroyed, movement, sensation, and even automatic functions, such as breathing and blood vessel dilation, may be altered. The swelling of surrounding tissue secondary to trauma is another major threat that can affect the spinal cord.

Medical conditions, both acute and chronic, are also frequently responsible for nervous system dysfunction. Infectious diseases, such as meningitis or encephalitis, can physically harm brain and spinal-cord tissue. Cerebral vascular accidents (strokes) result from blood clots or bleeding in the arteries that perfuse the brain and can deprive nervous system tissue of oxygen and lead to cell death. The net result of damage from any of these causes will depend on the affected area's function.

Certain diseases affect the ability of the nerves to transmit messages. Diseases such as amyotrophic lateral sclerosis (ALS) (also known as Lou Gehrig's disease) and multiple sclerosis (MS) can impair the transmission of messages in the nervous system. When messages cannot be transmitted, functions cannot be carried out.

The Endocrine System

Most body systems are at least in part regulated by the various organs of the endocrine system. Chronic diseases are typically the result of endocrine system disorders, but trauma and other causes also can play a role. Dysfunctions within the endocrine system are primarily related to a specific organ or gland. When that organ is disturbed, its function is interrupted.

The endocrine system is responsible for the production of chemical messengers in the form of hormones. Commonly, endocrine disorders are related to either overproduction or underproduction of a particular hormone. In some disease states, glands produce an excessive amount of hormones. Graves disease, for example, is a condition in which the thyroid gland overproduces its hormones. Patients with this condition can suffer from difficulty regulating temperature and fast heart rates.

More common are endocrine disorders in which glands produce too little of a particular hormone. In diabetes mellitus, for example, the pancreas does not secrete enough of a hormone called *insulin*. Insulin helps move glucose from the bloodstream into the body's cells. Without enough insulin, cells starve for the glucose they need for normal metabolism. At the same time, glucose levels in the bloodstream continue to rise because there is no insulin to carry the glucose out of the blood into the cells.

The Gastrointestinal System

Food and water enter our bodies through the gastrointestinal (GI) system. The esophagus, stomach, intestines, and other organs of this system play an important role in the transfer of nutrients into the bloodstream. The GI system also plays a vital role in the body's fluid balance by absorbing water. Digestive disorders can seriously impact both hydration levels and nutrient transfer.

The most common digestive disorder is vomiting and diarrhea. Vomiting and diarrhea disrupt the GI system's ability to retain solids and fluid long enough to transfer nutrients and absorb water. Although vomiting and diarrhea are not diseases themselves (they are more commonly symptoms of other disorders), their results can be life threatening. Particularly in the pediatric and geriatric populations, nausea and vomiting can lead to severe dehydration and malnutrition.

The Immune System

The immune system is the body's defense against foreign invaders. Its chief role is to fight infection. The immune system responds to specific body invaders by identifying them, marking them, and destroying them. When a foreign body is identified, the body dispatches both white blood cells and antibodies to attack it. Occasionally, the immune system can have an overactive response that actually does harm while fighting the invader.

hypersensitivity an exaggerated response by the immune system to a particular substance.

Hypersensitivity (also known as an *allergic reaction*) can occur in a response to certain foods, drugs, animals, or a variety of other substances. In a hypersensitivity reaction, the immune system releases chemical toxins that cause an exaggerated response. The reaction occurs when the chemicals affect more than just the targeted invader.

Histamine is a chemical released in a hypersensitivity reaction. The release of too much histamine can cause swelling in a variety of tissues including the airway. Other chemicals released by the reaction can cause dilation of the smooth muscles of blood vessels, resulting in a rapid drop in blood pressure. Hypersensitivity reactions range from minor and localized to severe and life threatening. Rapid identification and treatment is often life saving.

The Integumentary System

The integumentary system includes the skin and the body's connective tissues. It plays many vital roles, not the least of which are protection and thermoregulation. Disruption of the integumentary system can lead to infection and an inability to maintain normal body temperature.

Most common integumentary dysfunctions are caused by a loss of the integrity of the skin. Large wounds, burns, and chemical exposures are the most frequent causes. Because of its protective property, a loss of skin integrity can lead to invasion by pathogens (viruses, bacteria, and fungi). Those normally external organisms would then have a route into the body and infection can be the result.

STOP, REVIEW, REMEMBER!

Multiple Choice

For each question, place a check next to the correct answer.

1. The release of ______________ can cause swelling in a variety of tissues including the airway.

_____ a. histamine
_____ b. insulin
_____ c. ATP
_____ d. glucose

2. Which one of the following is a medical cause of nervous system dysfunction?

_____ a. Motor-vehicle crash, resulting in rising intracranial pressure
_____ b. Diving accident, resulting in a partial tear of the spinal cord
_____ c. Stroke, leading to death of brain cells
_____ d. Blow to the head, leading to bleeding in the brain

3. A chemical messenger secreted by an endocrine organ is known as a:

_____ a. glycoprotein.
_____ b. hormone.
_____ c. chemoreceptor.
_____ d. troponin.

4. Which one of the following diseases is a condition in which the thyroid gland overproduces hormones?

_____ a. Addison's
_____ b. Lou Gehrig's
_____ c. Crohn's
_____ d. Graves

5. The hormone secreted by the pancreas that helps cells take glucose from the bloodstream is called:

_____ a. adrenaline.
_____ b. insulin.
_____ c. estrogen.
_____ d. testosterone.

Fill in the Blank

1. The most common digestive disorder is ______________.

2. The immune system dispatches ______________ and ______________ through the bloodstream to attack foreign invaders.

3. In a ______________, the immune system releases chemical toxins that cause more of a reaction than necessary.

4. A ______________ caused by occluded arteries in the brain can deprive nervous system tissue of oxygen and lead to cell death.

5. The ______________ is responsible for production of chemical messengers in the form of hormones.

(continued on next page)

(continued)

Critical Thinking

1. Describe two different causes of dysfunction in the nervous system.

2. Describe two different causes of dysfunction in the endocrine system.

3. Describe how vomiting and diarrhea can negatively impact the digestive system.

EMERGENCY DISPATCH SUMMARY

En route to the hospital, Case noticed the patient was beginning to become lethargic and confused. Through frequent reassessment, Case expected that the patient's severe respiratory distress would soon give way to failure, and he was ready to take over ventilations using a bag-mask device. While he assisted ventilations, Case was careful to frequently reassess the patient's pulse.

At Case's request, a paramedic unit intercepted their ambulance about halfway to the hospital and Case gave the paramedic a detailed report as they transferred care. After an assessment, the paramedic decided to intubate the patient. Case assisted with the procedure and continued to reassess the patient as they continued on to the hospital.

Charlie, the patient, was released back home several days later and is receiving regular in-home visits from a nurse.

Chapter Review

To the Point

- Understanding pathophysiology helps you understand the basic and most important functions of the body and their critical dysfunctions.
- There is a delicate balance of fluid in the body. Levels must be appropriate in the major spaces and balanced constantly to maintain life.
- Aerobic metabolism is the normal way the body converts glucose into ATP. Anaerobic metabolism can be utilized, but is not as efficient and it creates significantly more waste products.
- Perfusion requires the combined function of the respiratory and cardiovascular systems. All functions must be operating correctly in order to deliver oxygenated blood to the cells.
- Oxygen is introduced into the body from the ambient air. This process requires a functioning respiratory system and the ability to move air in and out of the lungs.
- Alveolar ventilation is an essential key to perfusion. Moving air is useless unless it can reach the alveoli.
- Inspired air must be paired with circulating blood for perfusion to occur. Furthermore, appropriate quantities must be matched to ensure adequate delivery of oxygen to the cells.
- The cardiovascular system is the transport mechanism for oxygen, carbon dioxide, and nutrients for the cells. Proper transport requires the presence of appropriate elements of blood, pressure within the system, and a functioning pump.
- Cellular metabolism relies on a constant supply of glucose and oxygen. Therefore, normal metabolism relies on perfusion and the successful operation of the cardiopulmonary system.

Chapter Questions

Multiple Choice

For each question, place a check next to the correct answer.

1. The most basic unit of the human body is the:

_____ a. cell.
_____ b. organ.
_____ c. organ system.
_____ d. quadrant.

2. All cells require a constant supply of glucose, water, and:

_____ a. carbon dioxide.
_____ b. ATC.
_____ c. glycogen.
_____ d. oxygen.

3. Anaerobic metabolism produces carbon dioxide and:

_____ a. lactic acid.
_____ b. carbon monoxide.
_____ c. insulin.
_____ d. hemoglobin.

4. You are caring for a 72-year-old woman with a history of a recent heart attack and heart failure. She appears pale and sluggish, with an increased heart rate and breathing rate. These findings most likely indicate inadequate perfusion caused by a:

_____ a. diabetic problem.
_____ b. nervous system problem.
_____ c. cardiac problem.
_____ d. dehydration problem.

5. While you are in a clinical rotation at the hospital, your nurse preceptor tells you a 71-year-old male patient who has a breathing problem also has a low pH. (He is very acidotic.) The acidosis is most likely caused by:

_____ a. aerobic metabolism.
_____ b. anaerobic metabolism.
_____ c. digestive problems.
_____ d. a nervous system problem.

(continued on next page)

(continued)

6. You are assessing a 68-year-old woman who has liver failure. You note that her legs are very swollen. This is most likely because she:
   _____ a. has been drinking too much fluid.
   _____ b. has a leg injury.
   _____ c. lacks large proteins in her blood.
   _____ d. has too much albumin in her system.

7. A five-year-old has been diagnosed with a respiratory tract infection and sepsis. You notice that her extremities are very swollen. This is most likely caused by:
   _____ a. too much fluid in her system.
   _____ b. not enough large proteins in her blood.
   _____ c. poor ventilation due to the infection.
   _____ d. sepsis, making her capillaries more permeable.

8. A 17-year-old is having an asthma attack. You note that his respiratory rate is 44 (much faster than normal). This rate is most likely caused by:
   _____ a. the body's attempt to regulate minute volume by increasing respiratory rate.
   _____ b. the body's attempt to increase cardiac output by increasing respiratory rate.
   _____ c. the anxiety the patient is experiencing.
   _____ d. pain from the asthma attack.

9. Which one of the following would be a predictable response to hypoperfusion (shock)?
   _____ a. Decreased heart rate
   _____ b. Increased respiratory rate
   _____ c. Vasodilation
   _____ d. Decreased contractility

10. A four-year-old male shock patient has delayed capillary refill time. This is most likely caused by:
   _____ a. vasodilation.
   _____ b. cold ambient temperature.
   _____ c. medicine he has been given.
   _____ d. vasoconstriction.

Matching

Match the system on the left with the applicable dysfunction on the right.

1. _____ Respiratory system
2. _____ Cardiovascular system
3. _____ Nervous system
4. _____ Immune system
5. _____ Endocrine system
6. _____ Gastrointestinal system
7. _____ Integumentary system

A. Underproduction of insulin
B. Multiple sclerosis
C. Massive hemorrhage
D. Severe burn
E. Swelling around the glottic opening
F. Vomiting and diarrhea
G. Hypersensitivity reaction

Critical Thinking

1. Describe how the body regulates and distributes fluid.

____

____

____

____

2. Describe why the respiratory system must work in concert with the cardiovascular system to achieve perfusion at a cellular level.

3. Describe the predictable steps the body takes to respond to shock.

Case Study

A 71-year-old man is suffering from a bout of acute pulmonary edema. Fluid is accumulating in his alveoli and disrupting gas exchange. He has poor oxygenation and poor removal of waste products.

1. Describe how those problems will negatively impact the patient's body systems.

2. What predictable findings would you expect to see when assessing his respiratory system?

The Last Word

When you combine pathophysiology with a fundamental knowledge of anatomy and physiology, you are prepared to take on even the most complex human disorders. Pathophysiology helps point out dysfunction and prepares you for the likely course the patient will take. As an EMT you should always consider pathophysiology when assessing your patient. Consider what is wrong, what systems the problems affect, and what the result of the problem will be on those systems. Furthermore, you should consider what the effect of your treatment will be. Pathophysiology is a complex topic that will require ongoing education to master. Think of it as an ongoing challenge and continue to learn about it throughout your career.

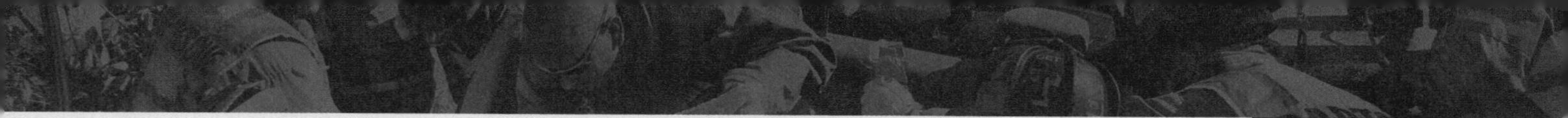

Life Span Development

7

Education Standards

Life Span Development

Competencies

Applies fundamental knowledge of life span development to patient assessment and management.

Objectives

After completion of this lesson, you should be able to:

7-1 Define key terms introduced in this chapter.

7-2 Identify the age ranges associated with each of the following terms: neonate, infant, toddler, preschooler, school age, adolescent, early adulthood, middle adulthood, and late adulthood.

7-3 Describe the physiological changes that occur immediately after birth.

7-4 Describe the key physical, cognitive, and psychosocial characteristics of neonates and infants, toddlers, preschool-age children, school-age children, adolescents, early adulthood, middle adulthood, and late adulthood.

Key Terms

adolescent p. 165
emancipated minor p. 165
geriatrics p. 167
infant p. 159
life expectancy p. 167
neonate p. 159
pediatrics p. 158
preschooler p. 163
puberty p. 165
school-age child p. 165
toddler p. 163

Introduction

7-2 Identify the age ranges associated with each of the following terms: neonate, infant, toddler, preschooler, school age, adolescent, early adulthood, middle adulthood, and late adulthood.

Throughout its life span the human body undergoes significant change as it grows, develops, ages, and matures (Figure 7-1 ■). Those changes occur in three primary areas: biological (the physical body), cognitive (the mind), and psychosocial (how the person interacts with its surroundings). Each phase of development has its unique characteristics that the EMT must become familiar with in order to provide the best care possible.

Life span development spans birth through old age and can be divided into the following phases:

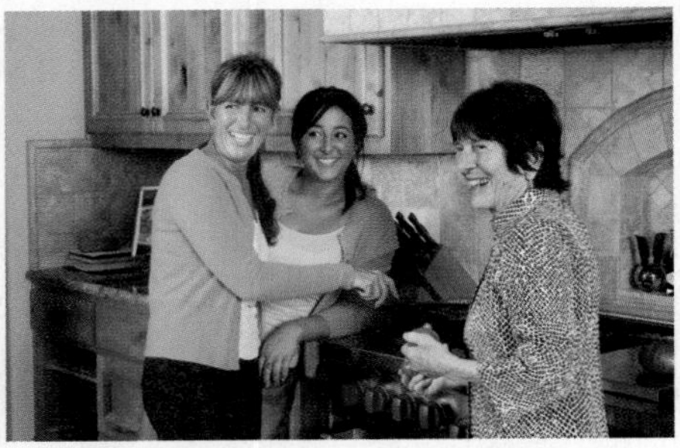

Figure 7-1 A human life often spans several generations.

- Neonate (birth to 28 days)
- Infant (birth up to one year)
- Toddler (1–3 years)
- Preschooler (3–6 years)
- School-age child (6–12 years)
- Adolescent (12–18 years)
- Early adulthood (18–40 years)
- Middle adulthood (40–60 years)
- Late adulthood (60 years to the end of life)

EMERGENCY DISPATCH

EMT Garrett Lincoln stood next to the ambulance and stretched his back, twisting one way and then the other. It had been a slower than usual Sunday afternoon and dispatch had left them posted in an abandoned parking lot for most of the day. He had been watching the MDT screen like a hawk and was comforted that at least the rest of the city units were as stationary as theirs.

"Heads I walk over to the supermarket and get a salad, tails I go to that fast food place," Garrett's partner Jodi McMillan leaned out the window of the truck, holding up a shiny quarter.

"Get a salad, Jodi," Garrett smiled. "I have to work with you the rest of the day."

She glared at him playfully and just as she opened her mouth to deliver a witty response, the MDT alert sounded. "Looks like an MCI at the fairgrounds," Jodi said. "Hop in, I'm driving."

One of the large local companies was hosting an event—a carnival—for employees and their families. Although there were two ambulances standing by at the fairgrounds, one of the rides had malfunctioned, throwing about a dozen people to the ground and quickly overwhelming the two crews on site.

Jodi and Garrett were the first outside team on scene and quickly found EMT Rob Lin, who was currently the incident commander, standing near a small, rickety roller coaster. The train cars were partially derailed and hanging askew at a spot on the track about three feet above the ground and there was a group of 10 patients sitting on the grass in various states of distress.

"Luckily, everyone is green or yellow," Rob said, holding a cell phone to his chest while he directed the arriving EMTs. "We've got all ages for you, a two-year-old up through a great grandfather. Susie will tell you who to help with." He then went back to his telephone conversation, and Garrett and Jodi moved toward the patients.

Childhood Development

pediatrics a term that refers to children up to the age of 18, or more specifically, the branch of medicine dealing with the development and care of children.

Pediatrics is the branch of medicine concerning the development, care, and study of diseases of children from infancy through adolescence. The details of each stage of life span development described in this chapter are meant to serve as guidelines and describe an average patient. No doubt you have met children who do not fit neatly into the developmental category for their age group, or elderly adults who do not suffer from the common ailments of old age. Use your own experiences to supplement the descriptions in this chapter, and remember any particular individual will have his

TABLE 7-1 NORMAL VITAL SIGNS

AGE (YEARS)	PULSE (BEATS PER MINUTE)	RESPIRATION (BREATHS PER MINUTE)	SYSTOLIC BLOOD PRESSURE (mmHg)
At Birth	100–160	40–60	~70
Infant (0–1)	100–160	20–40	70–90
Toddler (1–3)	80–130	20–30	70–100
Preschooler (3–6)	80–120	20–30	80–110
School-age (6–12)	70–110	20–30	80–120
Adolescence (12–18)	55–105	12–20	100–120
Early Adulthood (18–40)	60–100	12–20	~120
Middle Adulthood (40–60)	60–100	12–20	~120
Late Adulthood (>60)	(Depends on individual's physical and health status)		

7-3 Describe the physiological changes that occur immediately after birth.

neonate a child from the moment of birth up until one month of age (28 days). Also called a *newborn*.

infant a child from birth to one year of age.

own somewhat unique developmental timeline. In situations where there are family members or caregivers on scene, they will likely provide the best insight into whether or not the patient is acting normally for himself. This can be especially true for young children. All parents should be able to tell you if their child is behaving abnormally in any way.

In some cases, the age definition of an infant or child will vary depending on the context in which you are providing care. For example, in the context of CPR and AED use, a patient up to the age of one year is referred to as an *infant*, a patient between the age of one year and the onset of puberty is referred to as a *child*, and anyone past puberty is referred to as an *adult*. In other situations, procedures will be dictated by the child's physical size or weight rather than exact age.

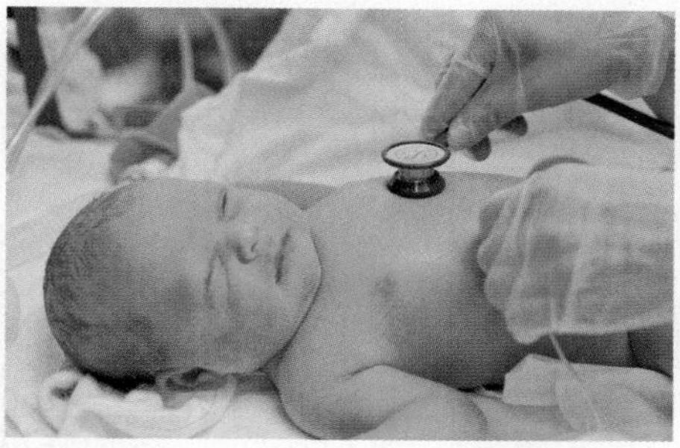

Figure 7-2 Newborn baby (neonate): birth to 28 days.

Pediatric Development Characteristics

Children behave differently at different ages, so it is useful to know something about the stages of development in order to tailor your patient assessment and care. (Particular techniques of pediatric patient assessment will be covered in detail in Chapter 38.)

Table 7-1 displays how typical heart rate, respiratory rate, and blood pressure change from birth through old age. Note that heart rate and respiratory rate tend to decrease with age, while blood pressure increases.

Newborns and Infants

From the moment of birth up until one month of age (birth to 28 days), a child is referred to as a *newborn* or **neonate** (Figure 7-2 ■). An **infant** (Figure 7-3 ■) is a broader category, referring to any child from birth to one year of age.

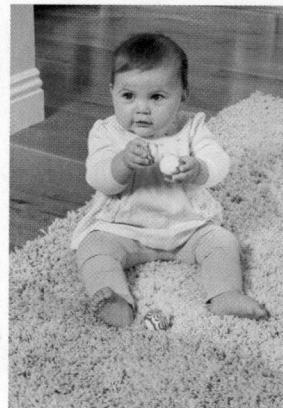

Figure 7-3 Infant: birth to one year.

A neonate typically weighs 3 to 3.5 kg (6.6 to 7.7 lb) at birth but loses 5% to 10% of his body weight in the first two weeks of life as he adjusts to receiving nutrients orally. After the first few weeks, his weight should continuously increase throughout childhood. Infants require breast milk or infant formula to meet their nutritional needs, and many mothers continue to nurse well into the toddler years. Even before their teeth begin to emerge, infants are able to eat soft solid foods, and as their teeth come in, their diet expands considerably. Children typically get their first primary teeth (baby teeth) at around six months. However, they do not receive the full set of 20 primary teeth until the age of two to three years.

CLINICAL CLUE

Kilograms

In medicine documenting patient weight is commonly done in kilograms. As an EMS provider, you should become familiar with how to convert pounds to kilograms (1 kg = 2.2 lb).

The respiratory system of an infant differs from that of an adult in several significant ways. Newborns are primarily nose breathers, and both newborns and infants rely heavily on their diaphragms to breathe. Without fully developed accessory muscles, they can fatigue easily and respiratory distress can quickly progress to respiratory failure. Their airways are proportionally narrower and less rigid, and as a result can more easily become obstructed. (Anatomical differences will be covered in more detail in Chapter 38.)

Babies are born with *fontanels*, or soft spots on their heads. They are open areas in the skull beneath the skin of the scalp where the bones have yet to fuse together. The posterior fontanel closes at around three months, and the anterior fontanel between nine and 18 months. While you should never press directly on a fontanel, gently running your finger along it or carefully observing it can be useful. Bulging or depressed fontanels may be an indication of the patient's fluid status. Bulging fontanels indicate possible increased intracranial pressure. Sunken fontanels indicate possible dehydration.

PRACTICAL PATHOPHYSIOLOGY

Severe dehydration can be a serious condition in any individual, but is especially dangerous in infants because their fluid reserves are so small. In an infant, the most common cause of dehydration is repeated vomiting or severe diarrhea. In addition to sunken fontanels, decreased urine output (dry diaper for longer than six hours), no tears when the child cries, and unexplained irritability or lethargy can all be signs of dehydration.

Many of the bones and muscles in a newborn's musculoskeletal system are soft and not fully developed. As the infant grows, he will begin to develop control and learn to perform increasingly complex actions. The lists that follow describe some of the typical milestones through which many infants progress. Becoming familiar with them will help you determine if an infant is behaving normally. Note that significant deviations from the milestones could suggest new or existing medical conditions or environmental influences such as neglect.

Typically, an infant at two months of age should be able to:

- Track objects with his eyes
- Recognize familiar faces
- Focus on nearby objects
- Smile
- Hear sounds and recognize some familiar sounds
- Move in response to stimuli

At six months, an infant should be able to:

- Sit upright
- Support his upper body with his arms while lying on his stomach
- Try to imitate sounds
- Make some one-syllable sounds (such as "ma" or "da")
- Grasp objects such as toys or your finger
- See and recognize familiar objects at a distance

At 12 months of age, an infant should be able to:

- Walk with help
- Know his name
- Sit up without assistance
- Crawl
- Manipulate objects like spoons and cups
- Feed himself finger foods
- Say and understand the meaning of simple words (such as "no" and "mama")

As an EMT, you will likely discover that an infant cries in response to being taken away from his parent or primary caregiver. Infants who have not yet learned language skills communicate their basic needs through various types of crying. You may even learn to recognize the difference between a basic cry (hungry, wet, tired), an angry cry (being separated from a parent), or a pain cry. It is appropriate for you to ask the infant's caregiver to help identify the type of crying if you are unsure.

By the end of infancy the child should have a relationship with his family. He will recognize favorite objects and people, which can provide him some comfort while you are assessing him. An infant will probably react to the behavior of the parent and respond accordingly. An upset parent usually leads to an upset infant. So, use a calm voice to reassure both infant and parent during patient assessment and care.

STOP, REVIEW, REMEMBER!

Multiple Choice

For each question, place a check next to the correct answer.

1. A typical toddler will have a resting heart rate between:

_____ a. 70 and 110.

_____ b. 80 and 120.

_____ c. 80 and 130.

_____ d. 100 and 160.

2. A neonate is defined as a child:

_____ a. during pregnancy up until birth.

_____ b. from birth through one year old.

_____ c. within his first week of life.

_____ d. up to 28 days old.

(continued on next page)

(continued)

3. Sunken or depressed fontanels in an infant should be regarded as:

_____ a. evidence of a head injury.

_____ b. a sign of possible dehydration.

_____ c. normal in children up to 18 months of age.

_____ d. an indication that the infant is malnourished.

4. A heart rate of 80 beats per minute in an infant should be considered:

_____ a. abnormally low.

_____ b. dangerously fast.

_____ c. normal, depending on the infant's health status.

_____ d. typical for a sleeping infant, but low for an active or crying infant.

5. A child who weighs 50 pounds is approximately how many kilograms?

_____ a. 10

_____ b. 22

_____ c. 26

_____ d. 110

Critical Thinking

1. Describe some of the common behaviors and abilities of a typical six-month-old infant. Include at least two items beyond what is listed in this chapter. You may draw from personal experience, other texts, Internet resources, or stories from an infant caregiver.

____

____

____

____

2. Explain at least two ways in which anatomical differences in the respiratory system of infants could help contribute to serious respiratory conditions.

____

____

____

____

3. Describe the major trends in heart rate, respiratory rate, and blood pressure throughout a person's life span. During which stage(s) do each of the three vital signs go through the fastest changes? By what age have they stabilized at typical adult values?

____

____

____

____

Toddlers

A child is referred to as a **toddler** when he is one to three years of age (Figure 7-4 ■). This is the era of the "terrible twos" and the frustration that can result from the near-instantaneous switch between a smiling and playful child and a screaming, tantrum-beset one. The toddler has begun to develop a sense of independence through walking and talking but is still unable to reason well or communicate complex ideas. The toddler typically does not like to be touched by strangers or separated from parents. Therefore under most circumstances have the alert toddler's caregiver hold him to reduce anxiety during your assessment.

toddler a child between one and three years of age.

As with any pediatric patient, a good part of the assessment can be done visually while you are taking the history from the parent or caregiver. The alert child will be watching and listening to you closely, even when you are not speaking directly to him. Using a calm, reassuring and quiet voice when speaking to adults nearby may even help to calm the toddler. Toddlers may mistakenly understand injury, illness, or separation from family as punishment, so they need reassurance that they are not to blame and that their parents or caregivers are with them or know where they are.

Figure 7-4 Toddler: one to three years.

Throughout early childhood the bones in the skeletal system continue to develop, growing larger, stronger, and more dense. Simultaneously, the muscle mass increases, allowing for more strength and control. It is during this stage that most children are both physiologically and psychologically ready to begin toilet training (though it is not uncommon for children to continue to lose control of their bladder at night for several more years).

Cognitively, children usually master the basics of language by about three years and then continue to refine those skills and develop a more expansive vocabulary throughout childhood. They are able to understand the relationship between cause and effect, though their expectations are not always reasonable. By the age of three years, a child should be able to:

7-4 Describe the key physical, cognitive, and psychosocial characteristics of neonates and infants, toddlers, preschool-age children, school-age children, adolescents, early adulthood, middle adulthood, and late adulthood.

- Walk alone, and begin to run
- Carry toys while walking
- Climb up and down stairs and furniture
- Scribble with crayons
- Recognize body parts
- Sort objects by shape or color
- Form simple sentences, and verbally communicate needs

CLINICAL CLUE

Change Your Approach

When you approach a child, remember to "get low and go slow." You must gain his confidence even if you know that you may have to cause him some pain as you help him. If there are no clear life-threatening conditions, you should first engage the parents. Once the child feels that his parents trust you, he is more likely to trust you as well.

preschooler a child between three and six years of age.

Preschoolers

A child is referred to as a **preschooler** when he is three to six years of age (Figure 7-5 ■). Preschool children have developed concrete thinking skills that allow them to understand and follow instructions and solve basic problems. Like toddlers, preschoolers may mistakenly believe they are being punished for wrongdoing by illness or injury. They are usually very frightened by the thought of potential pain, by the sight of blood, and by the prospect of permanent injury. They need lots of reassurance and

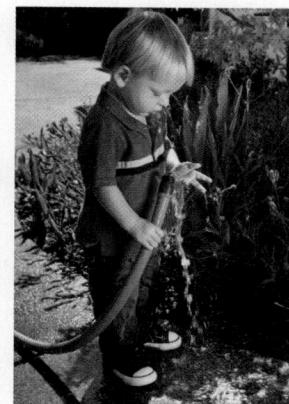

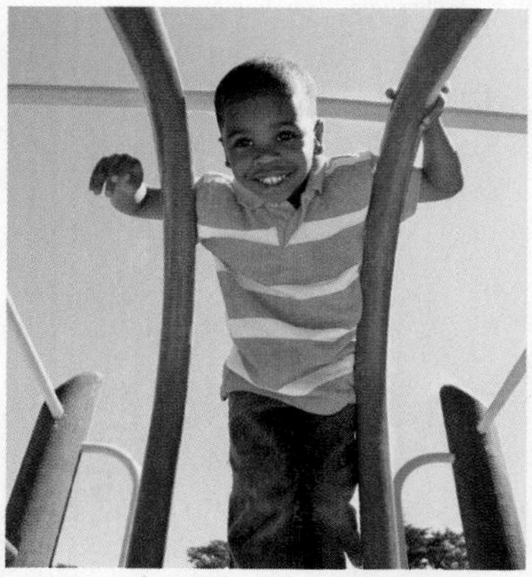

Figure 7-5 Preschooler: three to six years. (Royalty Free/© Masterfile)

respond well to simple explanations that avoid medical or complicated terminology. Though your vocabulary and explanations need to be adjusted to a level they can easily comprehend, you also must make sure not to make them feel minimized or "treated like a baby." It is important to ask them for their version of how they feel and what happened, and to treat them with respect.

Separation from familiarity frequently causes them anxiety, so whenever possible, allow the parent or caregiver to hold or remain near the child as you begin your examination. Taking additional time to build trust and rapport will be an important strategy.

PERSPECTIVE

Terrence—Six-Year-Old Patient

I fell on the worm ride. It was going real fast and then it threw me on the ground and hurt my arm really bad. Look at my cast! I picked the color and the nurse wrote her name there! Granma Jean kept telling me to put my arms inside the car-thing on the worm ride but I kept waving at mom. Did I make everyone fall over? I didn't listen to Granma Jean and she got mad at me a little.

In an effort to foster trust, begin your examination of the alert child with the extremities and then the trunk, followed by the head as he becomes more accustomed to you. Allow the child to touch equipment before you use it on him, and when possible demonstrate on someone else, such as a parent, how it will be used. Never lie to a child (for example, about something you need to do that will cause pain) because you will probably not be able to regain his trust once you have done so.

Children tend to take language literally, so be careful to avoid phrases such as "I'm going to take your blood pressure" when instead you can more precisely explain that you are simply going to "measure your blood pressure."

The preschooler is typically quite modest, so when possible replace items of clothing after taking them off, or allow the child to help you by pulling up his own shirt or exposing the area of injury. Involving preschoolers in simple ways in their care whenever possible can be a great tool because it simultaneously distracts and occupies them, plays into their need for independence, and fosters cooperation in the process.

At this stage, the nervous system develops rapidly and fine motor skills are refined. The brain is the fastest growing part of the body, and by preschool age has reached 90% of its adult size and weight.

By five years of age, a typical preschooler should be able to:

- Balance on one foot for 10 seconds
- Hop, jump, climb, and do somersaults
- Get dressed by himself
- Use forks and spoons appropriately
- Count to 10 (in some cases much higher!)
- Draw simple pictures
- Recall and recount stories

CLINICAL CLUE

First Impressions

Pay close attention to the way the child behaves and responds to your presence. A child responding inappropriately to his environment may be seriously ill.

School-Age Children

School-age children are six to 12 years of age (Figure 7-6 ■). By the time children reach school age, they have a basic understanding of the body and its functions, and they usually understand the need for and try to cooperate with assessment and care. They also develop fundamental problem-solving skills, but often do not yet possess the insight needed to resolve complicated situations on their own. It is during this phase that children develop a deeply personal concept of who they are. They frequently compare themselves with others and many continually seek approval from those around them. It is usually at this age that children also develop self-esteem and morals.

school-age child a child between six and 12 years of age.

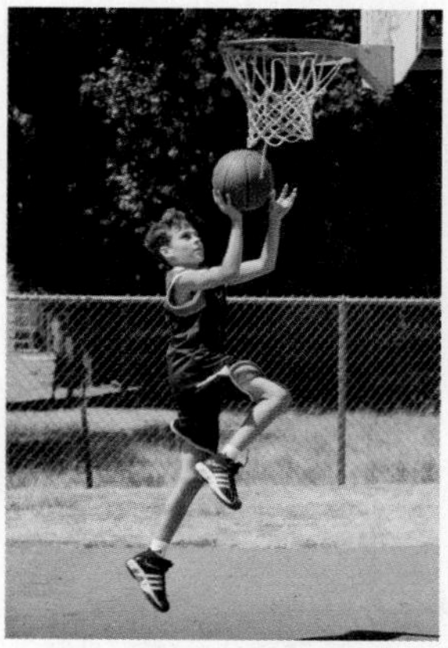

Figure 7-6 School-age child: six to 12 years.

Most school-age children can identify EMS providers as people who can help in an emergency. However, children may have unrealistic expectations of what you can actually do. Even though they are capable of more complex understanding than younger children, it is important to continue to make sure to communicate at a level they can easily understand. They also remain very literal in their interpretation, so pay particular attention to avoiding confusing language and be aware that they are likely listening to every word you say, even if you are not talking to them.

School-age children, just like adults, are aware of and afraid of death and dying as well as pain, deformity, blood, and permanent injury. They benefit from additional reassurance as well as inclusion in discussions involving their care. In many cases, school-age children will turn to a parent or older sibling to help cope with their fears, and it is usually appropriate to allow family members to be involved in care when the child desires.

Physiological development continues to occur at a rapid pace during the grade-school and middle-school years. The strength and agility of the musculoskeletal system continue to improve, primary teeth fall out and are replaced by permanent teeth, and brain function continues to increase in both hemispheres. Additionally, reproductive organs begin to develop and the changes associated with puberty begin toward the end of this stage.

Puberty is the process of physical changes by which a child's body becomes an adult body, capable of reproduction. Technically, puberty refers to changes relating to sexual maturation rather than the psychosocial and cultural aspects of development sometimes grouped with adolescence. Puberty is initiated by hormone signals from the brain to the gonads (the ovaries in females and testes in males). Girls typically begin the process of puberty at age 10–11 and complete it by age 15–17, while boys begin at age 12–13 and complete it by age 16–18. In girls, the onset of puberty is characterized by breast and pubic hair development (average age 10–11) and menstruation (average age 11–12). In boys, changes are hallmarked by testicular enlargement, the growth of facial and underarm hair, and a changing voice.

puberty the process of physical changes by which a child's body matures and becomes capable of reproduction.

adolescent a child between 12 and 18 years of age.

emancipated minor a child under the age of 18 years of age who has become legally independent from his parents or legal guardians.

Adolescents

A child is referred to as an **adolescent** when he is 12 to 18 years of age (Figure 7-7 ■). The adolescent child has a thorough understanding of anatomy and physiology and is able to process and express complex ideas. Despite being afraid of disfigurement and permanent injury, adolescents often believe they are immortal or indestructible. They are frequent risk takers but are often poor judges of consequence, so accidents and injuries are not uncommon.

Adolescents may want to be treated as adults, but you must remember that they are not adults, and in some cases they may even need the same level of support and reassurance as a younger child. Despite this desire to be treated as mature adults, most are not capable of making their own medical decisions nor are they legally entitled to do so. (Notably, an **emancipated minor** is under the age of 18 but may make his own medical decisions.) Therefore, you must obtain a parent or guardian's consent for treatment.

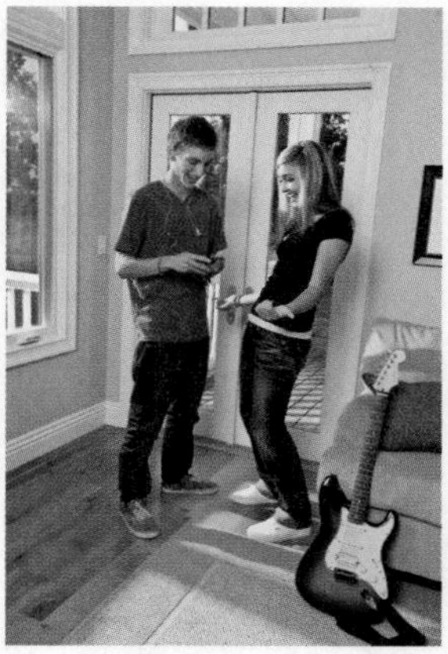

Figure 7-7 Adolescent: 12 to 18 years.

Most adolescents have a strong desire for privacy, and consequently, most will prefer their parents not to be present during the patient interview and examination. If possible, you should try to interview the adolescent in private, or at least consider that you may not be getting a complete or accurate story in the presence of parents. Often, however, the adolescent will be willing to honestly disclose information to EMS or other medical providers once they are alone. Speaking respectfully and non-judgmentally, and helping to protect their privacy and modesty, will be well received by adolescents and usually invites increased cooperation.

PERSPECTIVE

L.J.—15-Year-Old Patient

My dad made me take Tyler on that stupid ride. I was like, "Dad, really? It just goes around in a dumb circle!" and my friends were all laughing at me. That was so embarrassing, not only to have to be on that big neon green cartoon snake thing to begin with, but then to get thrown out onto the ground. When that EMT started asking if I was okay, I was like, "Yeah, I'm fine" and whatever but my favorite shirt was torn, I couldn't find my sunglasses, and I had a humungous grass stain on my butt. My ribs really did hurt on this one side though, I think I'm going to have a monster bruise tomorrow.

In adolescence, self-consciousness, peer pressure, interest in sexuality, and the strong desire for independence all increase dramatically. How they look and feel about themselves can have a profound impact on their sense of identity and self-esteem. Some youths begin to participate in self-destructive behavior such as tobacco, alcohol, or drug abuse. Family conflict is not uncommon. It is at this stage that depression and suicide are more common than in any other age group.

Most teens experience a rapid two- to three-year growth spurt. This development usually begins distally, with enlargement of the hands and feet, and is followed by elongation of the arms and legs, and then ultimately the trunk. Typically, girls are mostly done growing by age 16 and boys by 18. At this time, muscle mass and bone growth are nearly complete, as are the changes begun at puberty. Reproductive maturity is reached.

Adult Development Characteristics

Early Adulthood

A person is classified as being in early adulthood when he is between the ages of 18 and 40 (Figure 7-8 ▪). Early adulthood is often the stage when most complete a formal education, begin careers, and consider starting families. This is the most common stage for childbirth. Lifelong habits and routines are developed, and all body systems are at optimal performance. Adults reach peak physical condition between 19 and 26 years of age, and during this stage are traditionally very active. A leading cause of death at this age is accidents; the majority of young adults are physically quite healthy.

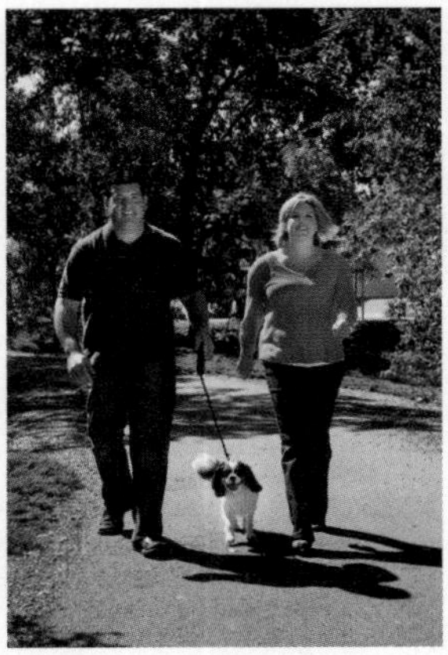

Figure 7-8 Early adult: 18 to 40 years.

Middle Adulthood

A person is classified as being in middle adulthood when he is between the ages of 40 and 60 (Figure 7-9 ▪). It is during middle adulthood that many people develop well-established routines and careers, and the focus of life shifts to the rearing of children. The majority of body systems are still functioning at a high level, though the beginnings of degradation and degeneration commence.

Resulting physiological changes, such as a decrease in the ability to see and hear well, can be difficult to accept. People get shorter, hair begins to turn gray, and permanent wrinkles appear in the skin. Adults of this age become more susceptible to chronic illnesses. Cancer rates rise. Cardiovascular health often first becomes a concern. It is common for cholesterol levels and blood pressure to increase, and cardiac output to decrease. Women in their late 40s and early 50s go through menopause, the permanent end of menstruation and fertility.

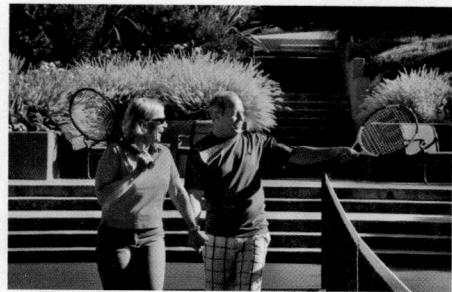

Figure 7-9 Middle adult: 40 to 60 years.

Late Adulthood

A person is classified as being in late adulthood when he is between the ages of 60 and the end of life (Figure 7-10 ■). For many people, late adulthood represents a period in life where they experience pronounced bodily changes. Those changes can be greatly influenced by individual lifestyle but can include a decline in the ability to see, hear, taste, feel, and smell. The awareness of one's own mortality is ever-present, frequently underscored by the death of a spouse or friends.

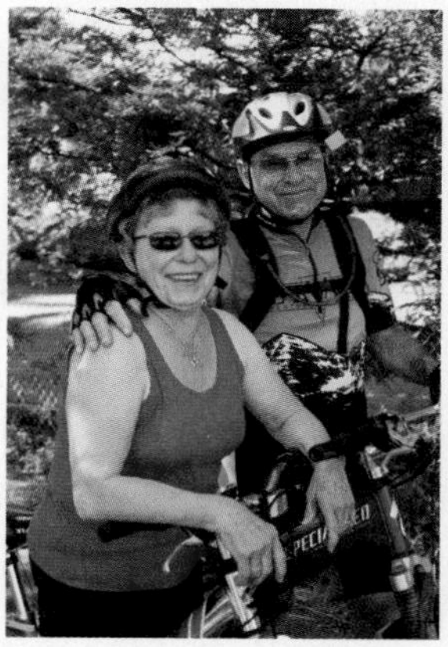

Figure 7-10 Late adult: 60 years to end of life.

Life expectancy is defined as the average number of additional years a person is expected to live. It is a statistical guess, usually based on how old someone is. In the United States today, the average life expectancy at birth is about 78 years. However, there are significant variations once gender, ethnicity, and socioeconomic status are taken into account. **Geriatrics** is the branch of medicine especially devoted to the care of older adults and the study of the diseases commonly affecting them.

life expectancy the average number of additional years a person is expected to live, based on current age.

geriatrics term that refers to older adults, or more specifically, the branch of medicine dealing with care of the elderly.

There are many terms in use that refer to older adults, such as *geriatric*, *senior*, *aged*, and *elderly*. In certain cases those terms carry negative connotations to some people, so use common sense to determine what language is most appropriate to your situation.

The physiological changes during late adulthood follow common patterns. A continuing decline in cardiovascular system function includes thickening and loss of elasticity of the blood vessels, resulting in an increase in peripheral vascular resistance, reduced blood flow to the organs, and degradation of the myocardium. All of these changes work to increase the workload of the heart and decrease the body's ability to compensate for hypoperfusion. Respiratory system changes bring about a decrease in lung function, and endocrine system changes result in a slower and less efficient metabolism.

PERSPECTIVE

Percy—43-Year-Old Patient

That was terrifying! There's this great day going on with food and music and, it's the annual thing that all of us always look forward to, you know? And then we're coming around the bend on this little coaster for the kiddos and BAM, it just lurches sideways and everyone went flying. I'm grateful that there was just grass below and that we were only a few feet up, but with all those kids and grandparents on the ride, it scares me to think how bad it could have been. Those medical folks did a stellar job, though. They jumped right into action and dealt with all of those people amazingly well.

Nervous system changes give rise to some of the ailments most commonly associated with old age. The brain gets smaller and begins to atrophy, resulting in problems with memory, balance, and movement. Mobility and coordination can become difficult, too, leaving patients more prone to falls and more susceptible to injury.

CLINICAL CLUE

What Is Normal?

When a patient with chronic dementia appears to be confused and disoriented, it is important to determine if the behavior is normal for the individual or if it reflects a sudden change in mental status. Determining this by enlisting the help of family members or other bystanders who know the patient can be as simple as asking questions such as "Is Ms. Smith behaving like herself today, or does she seem more confused than usual? Is she usually able to recall her name?"

Typical values for heart rate, respiratory rate, and blood pressure depend heavily on the health status and physical condition of the individual, underlying chronic disease, and in many cases the medications taken to manage those conditions. In particular, both blood pressure and heart rate are affected by many common hypertension medications. Especially in the elderly, you should never discount the possibility of a serious condition simply because the vital signs appear normal.

PRACTICAL PATHOPHYSIOLOGY

Some common high blood pressure medications, such as the so-called "beta blockers," can artificially slow the heart rate. This chemically induced heart rate will persist even in states of shock caused by blood loss or dehydration, when tachycardia would be the body's usual compensatory response. Because the medication is blocking the $beta_1$ receptors of the sympathetic nervous system, the signals that are being sent to increase heart rate are ignored and the usual tachycardic response does not occur.

One characteristic common to late adulthood is a decrease in the ability to perceive pain. This can make it difficult for EMTs to accurately gauge illness and injury during the patient assessment. Furthermore, the fear of being hospitalized or losing one's independence can cause some patients to underreport the seriousness of their condition or even omit symptoms entirely. It also is common for people in this age group to have overlapping illnesses for which they are taking multiple medications, or experiencing simultaneous symptoms. Always be aware of the possibility of underlying ill health, but do not assume that every older patient has physical or mental deficits.

EMERGENCY DISPATCH SUMMARY

A total of five patients were transported from the scene, ranging in age from 6 to 72, all with relatively minor trauma or musculoskeletal complaints. Everyone was released the same afternoon and went on to make full recoveries. The company sponsoring the event held a special awards ceremony for the EMTs who responded and the local EMS agency created a training scenario based on the event to help prepare other responders who could face incidents like this in the future.

Chapter Review

To the Point

- The human body is an amazing machine that begins life as a highly dependent, underdeveloped being that grows in many sophisticated ways biologically, cognitively, and psychosocially. The following is a brief recap of the major developmental stages. Understanding the stages of development will help you better assess and care for your patients.
- Infants range in age from birth to one year. Most of their body systems are underdeveloped, and they are highly dependent on caregivers for every need. Near the end of infancy, the child begins to develop both speech and mobility.
- Toddlers range in age from one to three years. This is the age where children begin to develop a sense of independence. They are often frightened by strangers and respond better when allowed to remain in a caregiver's arms during assessment and care.
- Preschoolers range in age from three to six years. This group can mistake illness or injury as a form of punishment but respond well to reassurance. Pain and the sight of blood are serious fears. Separation from caregivers will often result in increased anxiety.
- School-age children range in age from six to 12 years. This group often is more cooperative with assessment and care but shares many of the same fears as the preschooler. This group responds well to reassurance and often likes to be involved in the assessment and care process.
- The adolescent ranges in age from 12 to 18 years. This is the stage where most of the changes related to puberty take place. They are more self-conscious and are at greater risk for injury due to a perception of being indestructible. Adolescents possess a strong desire for personal privacy with regard to their body.
- Adult stages of development range from 18 to old age with fewer changes during the early and middle stages of development. Late adulthood brings with it a high incidence of illness and injury and a strong fear of a loss of independence. While the majority of older adults live relatively active, healthy lives, they do experience more illnesses than their younger counterparts. The decrease in pain perception and medication use often can lead to a masking of signs and symptoms.

Chapter Questions

Multiple Choice

For each question, place a check next to the correct answer.

1. You are caring for an 85-year-old woman. Based on her age, you would expect her normal resting pulse to be:
   _____ a. determined by her underlying health status and medications.
   _____ b. approximately 70 beats per minute.
   _____ c. slower than 70 beats per minute.
   _____ d. faster than 70 beats per minute.

2. As an adult ages, which one of the following body system changes would you most commonly expect to find?
   _____ a. Increased metabolic rate
   _____ b. Increased lung capacity
   _____ c. Increased bone and muscle elasticity
   _____ d. Increased blood pressure

3. Which stage of life span development is typified by a child's first attempts at communicating his needs in words?
   _____ a. Neonatal
   _____ b. Infant
   _____ c. Toddler
   _____ d. Preschool age

(continued on next page)

(continued)

4. A one-week-old infant presents with a respiratory rate of 40 breaths per minute. You should interpret this rate as:
   _____ a. abnormally slow.
   _____ b. appropriate for this age.
   _____ c. abnormally fast.
   _____ d. indeterminate, without knowing the underlying health status of the infant.

5. During what stage of life span development is menopause most likely to occur?
   _____ a. Adolescence
   _____ b. Early adulthood
   _____ c. Middle adulthood
   _____ d. Late adulthood

Matching

Match the term on the left with the applicable age range on the right.

1. _____ Preschool-age child	A. From birth to one month
2. _____ Infant	B. Up to one year
3. _____ Adolescent	C. Age 1–3
4. _____ Toddler	D. Age 3–6
5. _____ School-age child	E. Age 6–12
6. _____ Neonate	F. Age 12–18

Critical Thinking

1. List several ways you would approach the assessment of an alert three-year-old patient, and several ways you could change this approach to best care for an alert 12-year-old patient.

2. Pick one body system, or a particular component of life span development, and explain how it changes through the course of at least three different stages of a person's lifetime.

3. Imagine that your patient is a 15-year-old girl, accompanied by her parents. She is uncooperative with your physical assessment and initial attempt to question her about her history. Describe your approach to handling the situation.

4. Describe some of the unique challenges EMS providers face when caring for older adults.

Case Studies

Case Study 1

You and your EMT partner have been dispatched to an apartment for an elderly patient who has fallen. When you arrive, the patient's daughter leads you to her 80-year-old father, stating that she has been unable to help him up. You find the patient lying on the tile floor of the bathroom. He is awake but is unable to remember his name or recount the events leading to his fall. As you check his radial pulse, you note that his skin is cool to the touch.

1. List several possible causes for the patient's confused state.

2. How will you go about determining if the patient's confusion is the result of his injury or other sudden illness, or if this is his normal state?

3. The patient's daughter tells you that her father takes several medications to help control his blood pressure. How might those medications affect the patient's vital signs? List as many possibilities as you can think of.

4. Based on the patient's history and what you know of life span development, list at least three reasons this patient may have fallen.

Case Study 2

You respond to the scene of a minivan that collided head-on with a tree. There are four patients in the car: a nine-month-old baby boy, a four-year-old girl, a 30-year-old woman, and an elderly grandmother.

1. For each of the four patients, list the ranges for normal heart rate and respiratory rate.

____

____

____

____

2. For each of the four patients, list the minimum normal value for the systolic blood pressure (that is, below what number would the patient likely be considered hypotensive).

____

____

____

____

The Last Word

There is no telling what the age of your next patient is ever going to be. Understanding the major characteristics that differentiate the various stages of development can be very helpful. Anticipating those differences and adjusting your approach will help ensure the best possible assessment and care. Because it is easy to forget the differences and needs of each age group when you do not encounter them often, review this chapter from time to time to maintain familiarity with them.

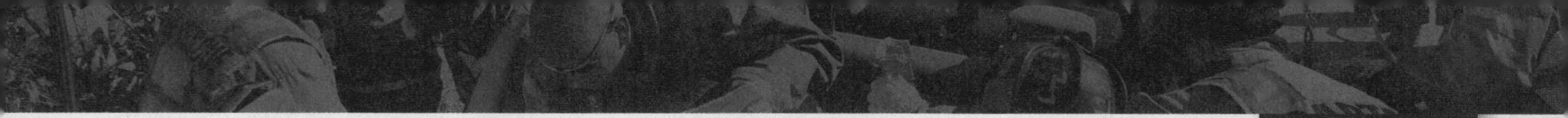

Lifting, Moving, and Positioning Patients

8

Education Standards

Preparatory: EMS Systems, Workforce Safety, and Wellness

Competencies

Applies fundamental knowledge of the EMS system, safety/well-being of the EMT, medical/legal issues, and ethical issues to the provision of emergency care.

Uses knowledge of the principles of illness and injury prevention in emergency care.

Objectives

After completion of this lesson, you should be able to:

8-1 Define key terms introduced in this chapter.

8-2 Explain the importance of always using proper techniques when lifting, carrying, and moving patients and equipment.

8-3 Describe the three principles of body mechanics listed in the text.

8-4 Describe the factors to consider when planning for the safe lifting and moving of patients.

8-5 Explain the roles of proper body posture and physical fitness in preventing injuries resulting from lifting and moving patients.

8-6 Describe considerations in teamwork and communication with partners and patients when lifting and moving patients.

8-7 Discuss the advantages, disadvantages, and steps of each of the following lifting and moving techniques and processes: one-handed equipment carrying, power grip, power lift, pushing and pulling, and reaching.

8-8 Differentiate between emergent and nonemergent moves and when each is indicated.

8-9 Describe the indications and steps for the various emergent and nonemergent moves: armpit-forearm drag, blanket drag, clothes drag, direct carry, direct ground lift, draw-sheet move, extremity lift, and rapid extrication.

8-10 Describe the common positions used for patient transport and when they should be used.

8-11 Describe the proper use, advantages, disadvantages, and limitations of common pieces of equipment used in lifting and moving patients: basket stretcher, flexible stretcher, long backboard, portable (flat) stretcher, scoop stretcher, stair chair, and wheeled stretcher.

Key Terms

basket stretcher p. 191
body mechanics p. 174
emergent moves p. 178
flexible stretcher p. 190
Fowler's position p. 185
lateral recumbent position p. 182
lift-in stretcher p. 189
long backboard p. 190
nonemergent moves p. 180
portable stretcher p. 191
power grip p. 177
power lift p. 176
prone p. 182
rapid extrication p. 178
recovery position p. 182
roll-in stretcher p. 187
scoop stretcher p. 191
semi-Fowler's position p. 182
stair chair p. 189
Stokes basket p. 191
supine p. 182
wheeled stretcher p. 187

Introduction

As an EMT you will be learning many skills that are designed to stabilize or improve the condition of your patient. Those skills are commonly referred to as *interventions*, or things you do to help make your patient feel better. One of the simplest and most common interventions you can provide for your patient is moving him or placing him in a specific or more comfortable position.

Lifting, moving, or positioning ill or injured patients is a tremendous responsibility. If performed properly and at the right time, such interventions can greatly improve safety, reduce pain, and even improve the patient's condition. If performed improperly or at the wrong time, moving a patient can have serious consequences. Just how you choose to move or position a patient will depend on the patient's condition, his location, and even the environment. You do not need to be big and strong to properly move and position patients. Even small EMTs with the proper technique and help from others can lift, move, and position larger patients safely.

Whether your patient has fallen in the bathtub or out in the woods, had a heart attack on a third floor (no elevator), or is found in a car wreck, what you learn in this chapter will help you get the job done safely and efficiently while helping the patient's condition.

EMERGENCY DISPATCH

"Rescue 25, Rescue two-five, respond to 14427 South Orleans. That'll be apartment number 302 for difficulty breathing. Time out 2317 hours."

"Rescue 25 copies," Brent, a new EMT, responds. "Show us en route from Main and Wilmore."

"South Orleans?" Brent's partner, Suki, looks thoughtful for a moment. "Oh wait, I think that's that three-story building where the elevator doesn't work!"

As if on cue, both EMTs sigh and think the same thing: It's been a long, tiring shift. Please don't let this be a big patient.

As Brent navigates the curb in front of the building, he sees that it is the place with the faded out-of-order sign on the elevator door. They take their equipment off the stretcher and climb the three flights of winding stairs to Apartment 302.

They find their patient, 44-year-old Julie Ordeen, on a hospital bed that has been set up in the small, dark front room of her apartment. She is a double amputee—thanks to diabetes—and looks like she weighs well over 350 pounds.

As Brent begins talking to Julie, Suki radios dispatch and requests a lift assist from the local fire crew.

Principles of Safe Lifting and Moving

8-2 Explain the importance of always using proper techniques when lifting, carrying, and moving patients and equipment.

Properly moving, lifting, and positioning patients are important and necessary skills used with every patient that you will encounter. Performing those tasks safely and efficiently is vital for your health and well-being as well as the patient's. EMS personnel are at significant risk for injury on the job, a risk that may be as much as eight times higher than that of municipal and general labor workers. The risk to you is real and of course the risk of adding further injury to an unsuspecting patient who is inadvertently dropped while being carried is just as real. How to minimize those risks is the focus of this chapter.

Body Mechanics

body mechanics the proper use of one's body to facilitate lifting and moving in such a way as to minimize risk of injury.

Body mechanics refers to the proper use of the body for movement and function. Proper body mechanics in EMS involves using specific techniques to help ensure the best mechanical advantage while ensuring safety for the rescuer and the patient.

The following techniques related to proper body mechanics should be used for the moving and lifting of all patients and equipment:

8-3 Describe the three principles of body mechanics listed in the text.

- Keep the object being lifted as close to your body as possible throughout the lift. The further an object is from your body, the more stress and strain it puts on the back.
- Focus on using the larger muscles of the legs and buttocks when lifting. It helps to tighten the muscles of the torso and abdomen when lifting as well.
- Once in the standing position, keep your body as straight as possible with the head over the shoulders, the shoulders over the hips, and the hips over the feet.

Health and Posture

8-4 Describe the factors to consider when planning for the safe lifting and moving of patients.

8-5 Explain the roles of proper body posture and physical fitness in preventing injuries resulting from lifting and moving patients.

The safe lifting and moving of patients and equipment requires both experience and planning. At first it may take several minutes to properly plan the most appropriate move for the situation. However, as you become more experienced you will be able to initiate safe moves quickly and efficiently. One of the most important principles to keep in mind regarding your role when moving and lifting is prevention of injury. You may think that exposure to disease and infection is your biggest risk when performing your duties as an EMT. In reality, the likelihood of becoming injured during a patient move is probably much higher.

The best way to prepare for your role when called on to move or lift a patient is to maintain a high degree of physical fitness. Two of the most important factors in your control that will minimize your exposure to risk are your own physical fitness and posture. A person who is physically fit is more likely to possess the strength required to perform lifts and moves safely. Maintaining good posture during a lift or move also greatly minimizes your risk for injury.

Communication

8-6 Describe considerations in teamwork and communication with partners and patients when lifting and moving patients.

Anytime you have a task that involves more than one rescuer, the need for good communication is essential. When the task involves lifting and moving a patient, the risks from poor communication are significant for both the rescuers and patients. Good coordination and timing of a patient move are achieved through both visual and verbal communication among all rescuers involved in the move.

First and foremost the person coordinating the move must clearly explain exactly what the objective of the move or lift will be. For instance, the objective of a particular move or lift may be to "roll the patient all the way from the prone position to the supine position in two moves." Or the objective might be to "lift the patient from the ground to the stretcher on the count of three." Regardless of the purpose of the move, the person coordinating must ensure that each member of the team knows the specific intent. Next, the coordinator must ensure that each person directly involved in the move or lift knows his specific role in the move. For instance, one rescuer might be in charge of holding the head while another is at the shoulders and another at the hips, and so on.

Once everyone is clear on the purpose of the move and their part in the process, it is time to make the move happen. The coordinator must make eye contact to ensure everyone is paying attention and knows exactly when to initiate the move.

Planning a Move or Lift

One of the most important principles of safe lifting or moving is proper planning. Consider the following factors when planning any move or lift:

- ***Urgency.*** This is often dictated by hazards at the scene or the condition of the patient. You may not have time to wait for the ideal piece of equipment or number of rescuers if the patient is not breathing or is in immediate danger. You must always be prepared to move a patient quickly when necessary.

- ***Size and weight.*** Patients and equipment come in all sizes and shapes. Ensure you have the most appropriate piece of equipment and number of rescuers for the patient.
- ***Number of available rescuers.*** This is in direct correlation to the size and weight of the patient as well as the distance and terrain being encountered. Whenever possible, use an even number of rescuers to help maintain balance during transport.
- ***Distance.*** How far you have to carry a patient must be considered prior to initiating any move. You must make every effort to minimize the distance required to carry your patient.
- ***Terrain.*** A steep hillside, flat asphalt, and a winding staircase are factors that must be considered during the planning of any move. The number of rescuers and the type of equipment will depend on the terrain being covered.

8-7 Discuss the advantages, disadvantages, and steps of each of the following lifting and moving techniques and processes: one-handed equipment carrying, power grip, power lift, pushing and pulling, and reaching.

With experience, many of the decisions you will need to make will come naturally as you size up the scene and assess your patient.

The Power Lift

power lift a lift from a squatting position with weight to be lifted close to the body. Also called the *squat-lift position.*

The **power lift** is one of the most common techniques used by EMTs to lift a patient from the ground or from a low to high position using the stretcher (Figure 8-1 ■). The power lift emphasizes the large muscles of the legs and minimizes the muscles of the back. Use the following guidelines when performing the power lift:

1. Position yourself as close to the device as possible while still maintaining good balance.

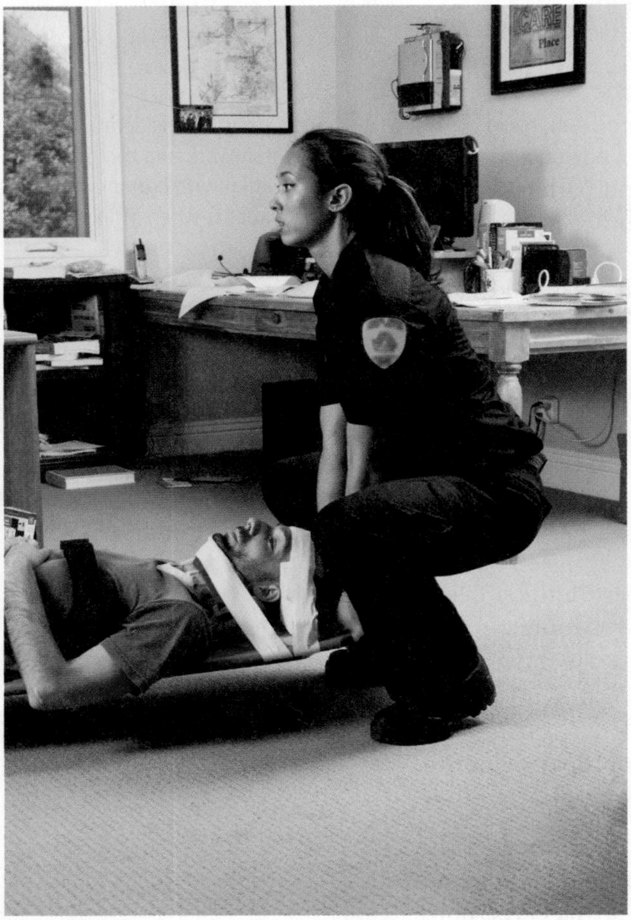

Figure 8-1a To begin the power lift, keep your back straight and eyes on your partner.

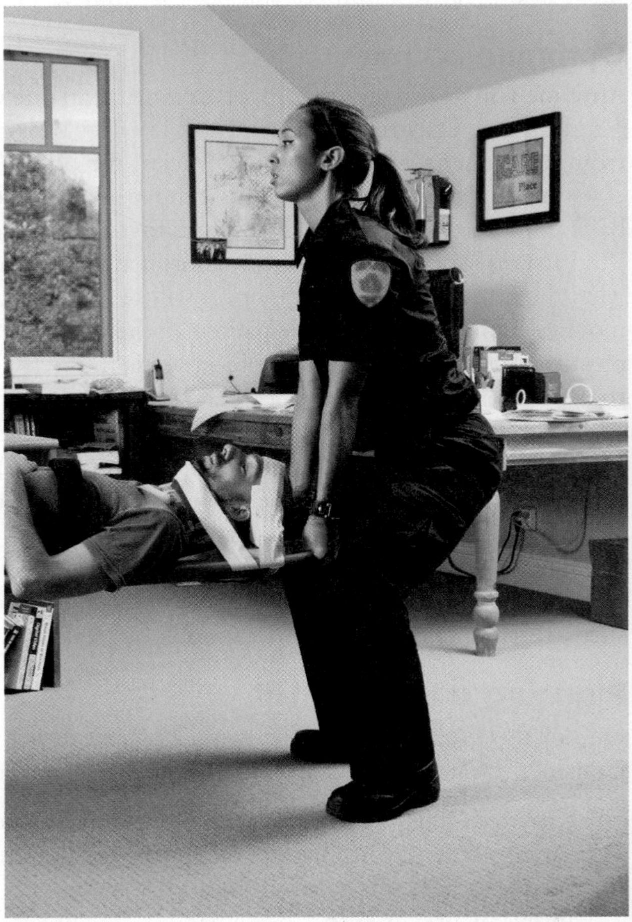

Figure 8-1b Then lift with your legs.

2. Position your feet shoulder width apart or slightly wider.
3. Grip the end of the device with both hands using the **power grip** (Figure 8-2 ■). The power grip involves positioning both hands palm up and gripping as much of the device as possible.
4. Squat down as much as necessary while keeping your back as straight as possible. Your weight should be evenly distributed between both feet.
5. Just prior to the lift, tighten your abdominal muscles.
6. Lift using the large muscles of your legs while keeping your back straight and the weight close to you.

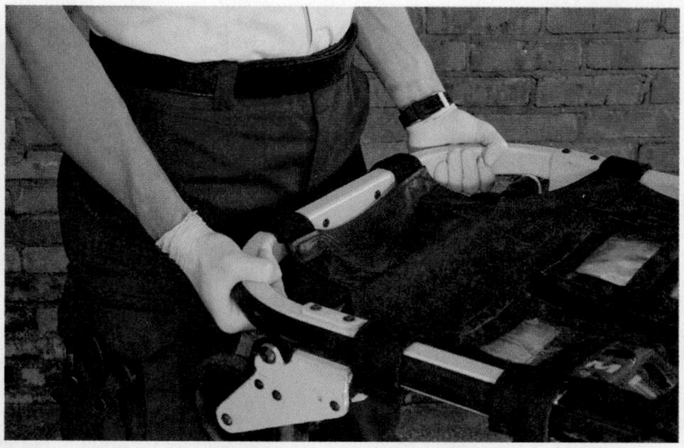

Figure 8-2 The power grip offers the best control during a lift.

At times, you may need to lift and carry a piece of equipment or assist with a stretcher using one hand. To lift with one hand, follow these rules:

1. Stagger your feet with the forward knee up and the rearward knee pointing toward the ground.
2. Bend at the hips, not the waist, and do not lean your torso forward more than 45 degrees.
3. Lift by pushing upward through the arch and heel of the forward foot and the ball of the rearward foot.

power grip gripping with as much hand surface as possible in contact with the object being lifted; all fingers are bent at the same angle, and hands are at least 10 inches apart.

To carry a stretcher or piece of equipment using one hand, keep your back locked. Then, as much as possible, avoid leaning to the opposite side to compensate for the weight imbalance.

Reaching, Pushing, and Pulling

Reaching, pushing, and pulling are common movements that carry a high risk for injury for the EMT. These movements often occur when the EMT is on his knees, standing upright, or sitting in the back of an ambulance. The body is inherently less stable during those maneuvers because they exert forces that are perpendicular to the normal structure of the body.

When reaching, avoid twisting and prolonged, strenuous reaching. Keep your arms low and your back straight and stiff (Figure 8-3 ■). Reaching more than 15 to 20 inches in front of your body places significant strain on your back.

When you are in a position where you have a choice between pushing or pulling a patient who is on a stretcher, keep in mind that pushing poses less risk for injury.

When it is necessary to drag a patient who is on the ground, it is best to pull him, such as in an armpit-forearm drag. Bend your knees and keep the weight being pulled close to your body.

PERSPECTIVE

Julie Ordeen—The Patient

I hate it when things get so bad that I have to call 911. Almost as much as I hate being sick. Have you ever had to be dependent on others for everything? Let me tell you. It's just plain humiliating. You know what I hate most of all though? The looks I get from the ambulance and fire people. I'm not happy that I weigh a little over 400 pounds, but I do. Do I eat too much? Probably. What would you do if you were bedridden, alone in an apartment all of the time, with nothing to do but watch TV? I've also got a thyroid problem. So it's not all my fault. The last time I had to be taken to the hospital, one of the guys from the ambulance made some comment about me eating too many Twinkies. That made me cry for the better part of two days.

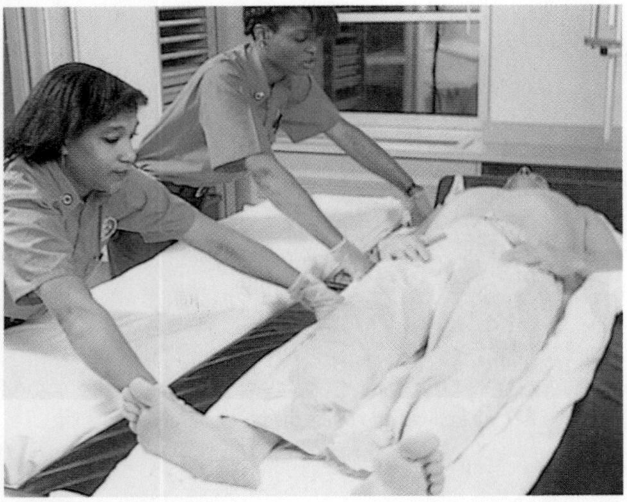

Figure 8-3 When reaching and pulling, keep your arms low and your back straight and stiff.

Patient Moves

Patients require movement for a wide variety of reasons. Some patients may require quick action and immediate movement to correct a life-threatening problem while others require movement that is more routine and controlled. Though there may be many names for the various types of patient moves, all moves fall into one of two broad categories—emergent and nonemergent.

Emergent Moves

Emergent moves are moves that occur in situations that require quick and immediate action, when there is little time to wait for additional rescuers or the appropriate piece of equipment. Common criteria for the use of emergent moves are as follows:

8-8 Differentiate between emergent and nonemergent moves and when each is indicated.

emergent move a category of patient moves performed when there is an immediate risk of death or serious injury to the patient or when access to another patient in need of life-saving care is blocked.

- There is immediate risk of additional injury or death to the patient.
- Access to another patient in need of life-saving care is being blocked.
- It is quickly determined that the risk for further injury outweighs any harm that may come to the patient by moving him quickly.

Examples of situations that may warrant the use of an emergent move include:

- Fire or threat of fire
- Explosives or the presence of other hazardous materials
- Inability to protect the patient from hazards at the scene (such as falling debris at a construction site or oncoming traffic)

Drags and Carries

8-9 Describe the indications and steps for the various emergent and nonemergent moves: armpit-forearm drag, blanket drag, clothes drag, direct carry, direct ground lift, draw-sheet move, extremity lift, and rapid extrication.

Due to the need for rapid movement, emergent moves do not offer the control and coordination offered by nonemergent moves. For example, it might be necessary to drag a patient away from a fire without first stabilizing suspected fractures to extremities. Emergent moves do not have to be reckless, however, and there are ways that the moves can be done quickly, yet with some concern for the spine. A series of emergent moves called *drags* can be employed to move a patient quickly while still being mindful of possible injury.

To drag a patient away from danger, pull from the patient's shoulders while cradling the head. By keeping the body (axis) straight during the drag, you minimize the chance of aggravating existing injuries (Scan 8-1).

Rapid Extrication

rapid extrication the rapid removal of a patient from a vehicle when the patient's condition or the situation does not permit use of a short backboard or vest-type extrication device.

When a patient with a potential spine injury is taken out of a vehicle, the move is normally performed in a very smooth and controlled manner using specialized equipment to protect the spine. In cases where the patient is in serious condition (such as with airway problems or severe shock), taking time to attach a short backboard or vest to the patient would allow his condition to worsen. In this situation, the emergent move called a **rapid extrication** should take place. It is done cautiously but without a short backboard or vest because of the patient's condition. (More about rapid extrication is offered in Chapter 36.)

SCAN 8-1 Emergent Moves

ALWAYS PULL IN THE DIRECTION OF THE LONG AXIS OF THE BODY

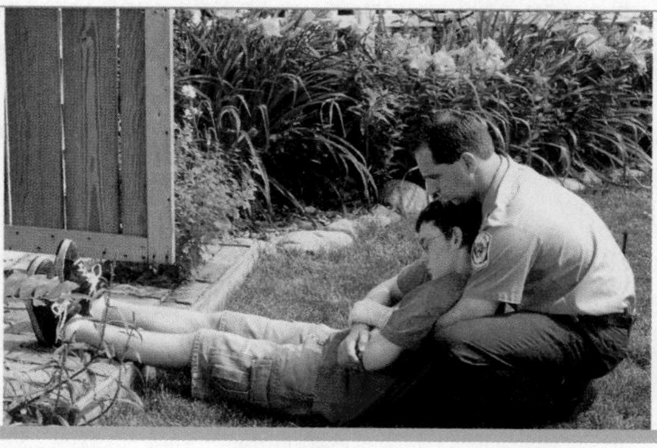

8-1-1 *Armpit-forearm drag*. This drag is ideal for moving an unresponsive patient with a single rescuer.

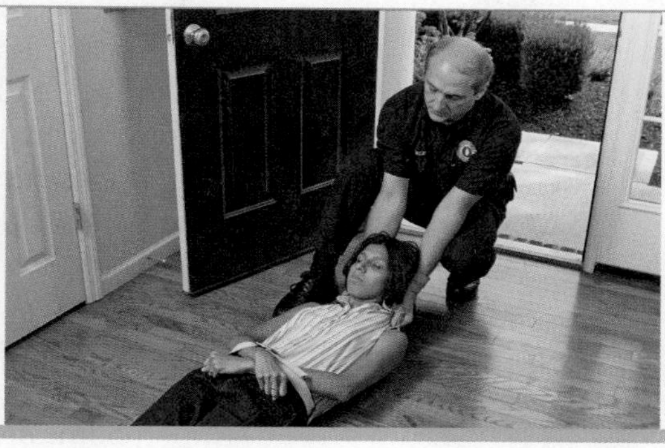

8-1-2 *Clothes drag*. Do not pull a patient sideways. Avoid bending or twisting the patient's trunk.

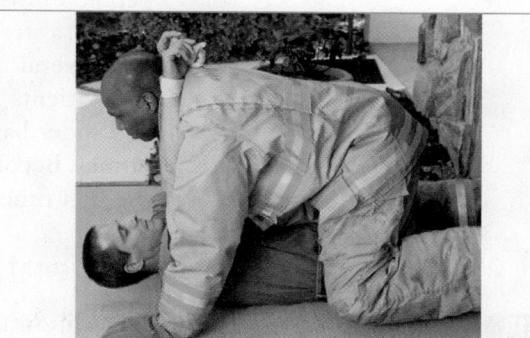

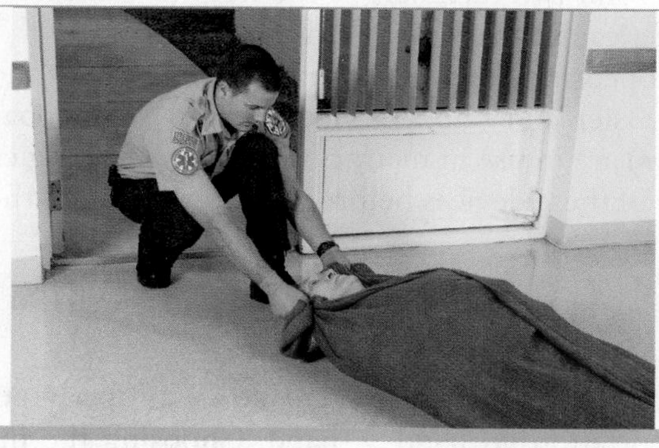

8-1-3 *Blanket drag*. Gather half of the blanket material up against the patient's side. Roll him toward your knees, place the blanket under him, and gently roll him onto the blanket. During the drag, keep the patient's head as low as possible.

8-1-4 *Firefighter's drag*. Place the patient on his back and tie his hands together. Straddle him, crouch, and pass your head through his trussed arms. Raise your body, and crawl on your hands and knees. Keep the patient's head as low as possible.

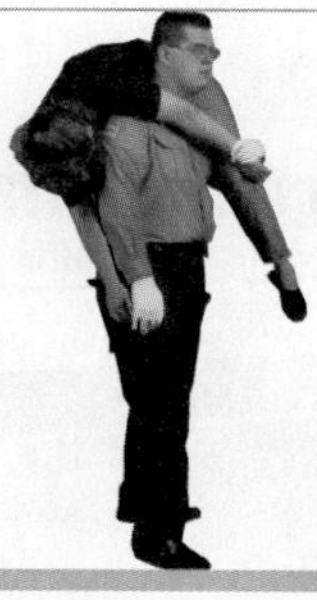

8-1-5 *Firefighter's carry.* Place your feet against her feet and pull patient toward you. Bend at waist and flex knees. Duck and pull her across your shoulder, keeping hold of one of her wrists. Use your free arm to reach between her legs and grasp her thigh. Weight of patient falls onto your shoulders. Stand up. Transfer your grip on thigh to patient's wrist.

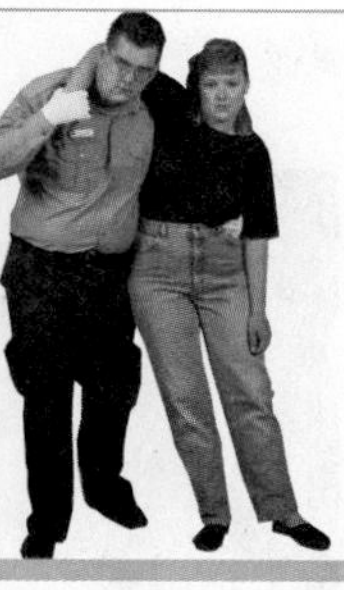

8-1-6 *One-rescuer assist*. Place patient's arm around your neck, grasping her hand in yours. Place your other arm around the patient's waist. Help patient walk to safety. Be prepared to change movement technique if level of danger increases. Be sure to communicate with patient about obstacles, uneven terrain, and so on.

Nonemergent Moves

nonemergent move a category of patient moves performed when there is no need to expedite due to the patient's condition or hazards at the scene.

Nonemergent moves are used when the patient's condition is stable enough to allow for proper planning and coordination of the move. These patients are often alert and responsive and all necessary care has been provided prior to initiating the move.

There are several nonemergent moves the EMT can choose from. The specific move you choose depends on the condition and position of the patient. You will find patients on the floor, in bed, sitting in chairs or standing, even caught between the sink and toilet or in a narrow hallway. The specific move or combination of moves you choose will differ for many of those situations. Keep in mind, however, that patients with spine injuries, even those who are considered nonemergent, must have their spines fully immobilized.

Common nonemergent moves include the *direct ground lift* (Scan 8-2) and the *extremity lift* (Scan 8-3). These moves are commonly used to transfer a patient from the floor or a chair to the stretcher. Do not use the extremity lift if you suspect injury to any of the extremities.

Some moves are used for transferring the patient from a bed to a stretcher (e.g., from the patient's bed at home to the ambulance stretcher or from the ambulance stretcher to a hospital bed). These moves include the *draw-sheet move* (Scan 8-4) and the *direct carry* (Scan 8-5), when there are only two people to make the move. When there are four people to make the move (two EMTs and two members of the hospital staff, for example), a stretcher-to-stretcher transfer can be made using a draw-sheet move.

Several devices have been developed in recent years to make the task of moving patients from stretcher to bed easier and safer. Devices such as slider boards and slider bags (Figures 8-4 and 8-5 ■) are in use in many hospitals and nursing care homes. Become familiar with the use of these devices before you attempt to use them the first time.

Patient Positioning

8-10 Describe the common positions used for patient transport and when they should be used.

In addition to moving your patient, you also will be responsible for properly positioning him. Positioning and transportation go hand-in-hand. Choosing the most appropriate position for your patient is most often determined by the patient's mental status and general condition.

It is important to understand that most conscious patients are quite good at finding a position that is most comfortable for their condition. In other words, unless

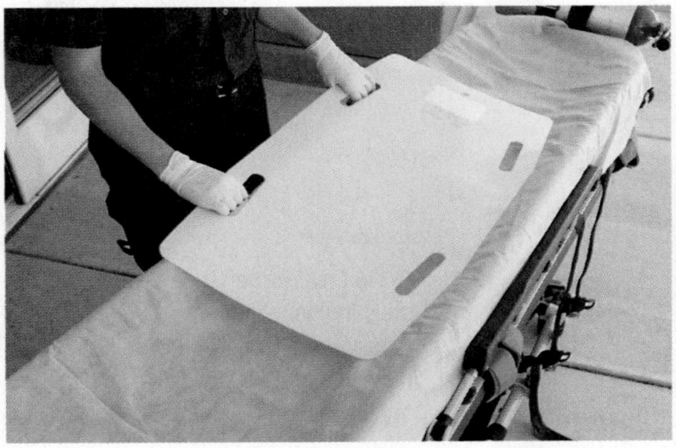

Figure 8-4 A typical slider board is used to help facilitate the transfer of a patient from a bed to stretcher and vice versa.

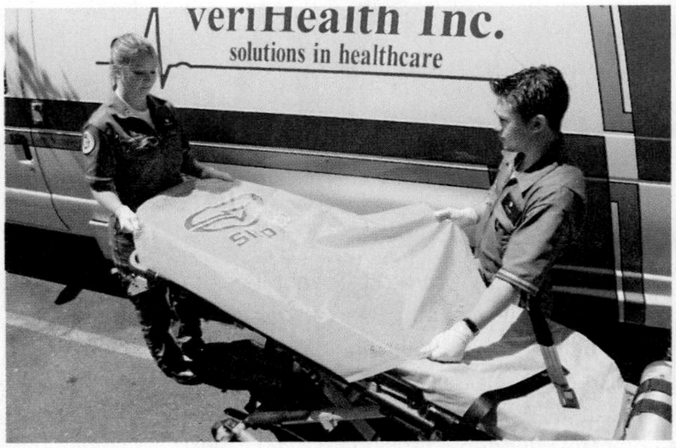

Figure 8-5 A slider bag is another option for facilitating a patient move from bed to stretcher and vice versa.

SCAN 8-2 Direct Ground Lift

NONEMERGENT MOVE TO A STRETCHER OF A PATIENT WITH NO SUSPECTED SPINE INJURY

8-2-1 Position your arms under the patient. Be sure to cradle the head.

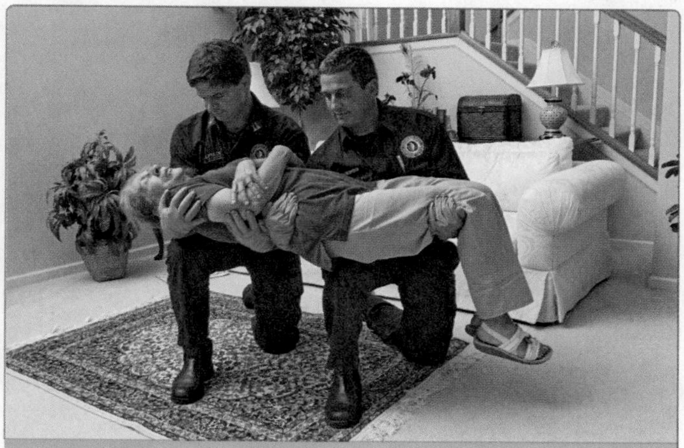

8-2-2 Lift the patient to your knees and roll her toward your chests.

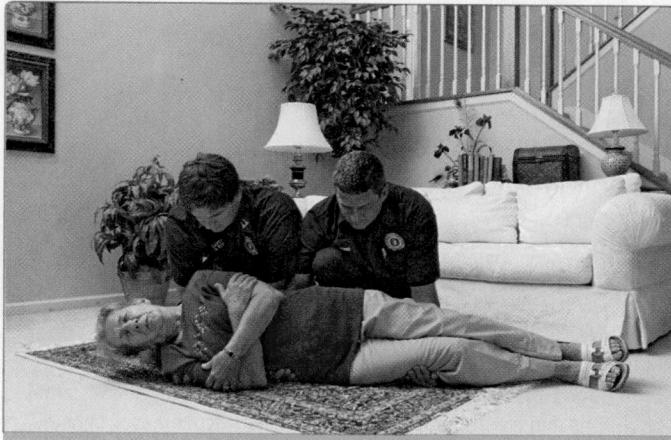

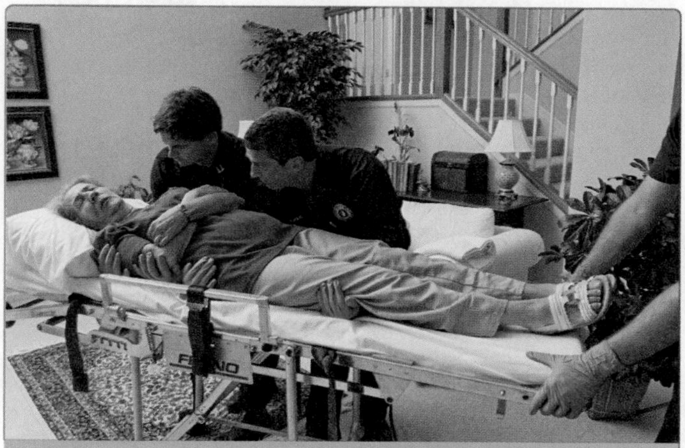

8-2-3 On signal, move the patient to the carrying device.

otherwise needed for patient care, leave them in the position in which you find them. But it is always a good idea to ask the patient if he is comfortable and offer to help him get into a more comfortable position, if needed.

CLINICAL CLUE

Position of Comfort

Most conscious and alert patients will be found in a position of comfort. That is to say they have found a position that is most comfortable for the illness or injury they are experiencing at the moment. It is always a good idea to at least offer to help them into a more comfortable position.

SCAN 8-3 Extremity Lift

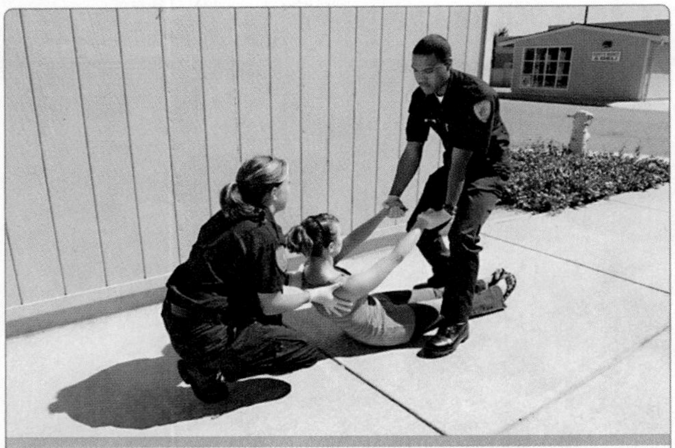

8-3-1 To get the patient into position, one rescuer pushes from behind while the other pulls with the wrists.

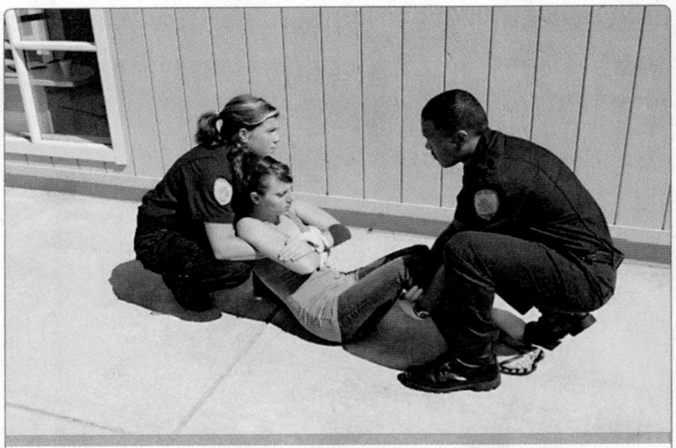

8-3-2 The rescuer at the head places arms under patient's armpits and grasps patient's wrists. Second rescuer grasps behind the knees.

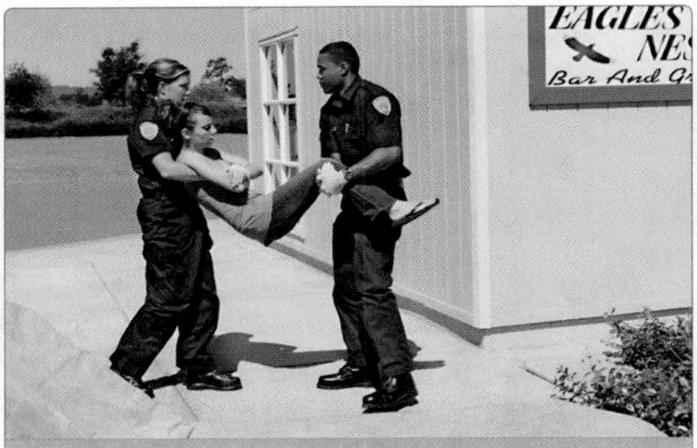

8-3-3 Lifting together you can now move the patient a short distance to a chair or stretcher.

supine a position in which a patient is lying face up. Opposite of *prone*.

recovery position a position in which the patient is lying on one side. Also called a *lateral recumbent position*.

lateral recumbent position lying on one side. Also called the *recovery position*.

prone a position in which the patient is lying face down. Opposite of *supine*.

semi-Fowler's position a semi-sitting position.

The common positions that you may use when caring for a patient include the **supine** position (Figure 8-6 ▪), **recovery position** (or **lateral recumbent position**) (Figure 8-7 ▪), a **prone** position (Figure 8-8 ▪), and a **semi-Fowler's position** (Figure 8-9 ▪). The most appropriate position for your patient will depend on his mental status and general condition. The following are recommendations for specific positions:

- *Unresponsive patients* who do not have a suspected spine injury are placed in the recovery position. Usually the patient is placed on the left side because he will be facing the EMT when placed in most ambulances. This position allows for better management of the airway when the patient is unable to manage his own airway.

SCAN 8-4 Draw-Sheet Move

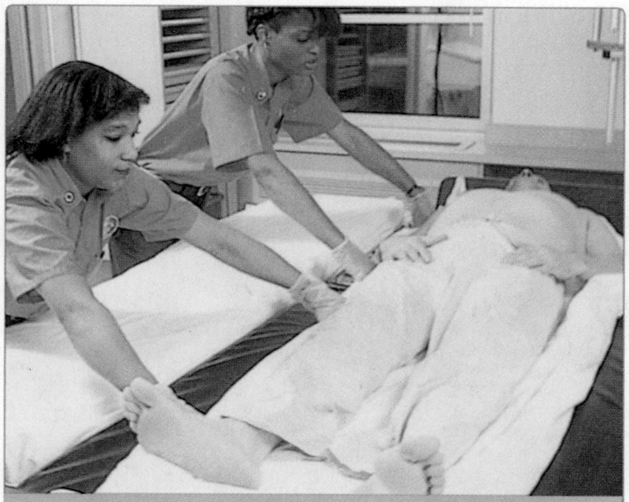

8-4-1 Reach across the stretcher and grasp the sheet firmly.

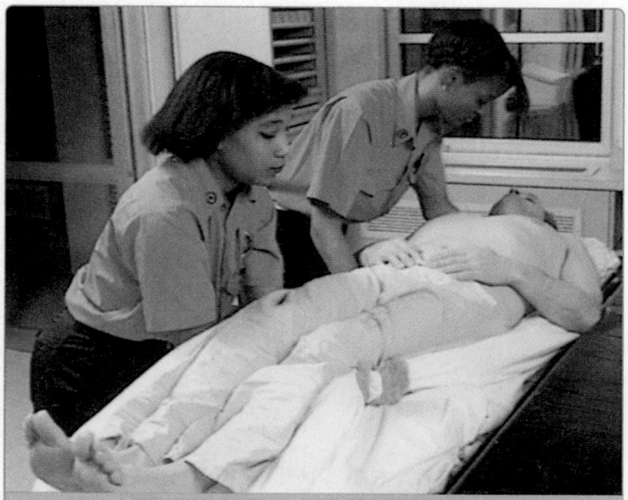

8-4-2 Slide the patient gently onto the carrying device.

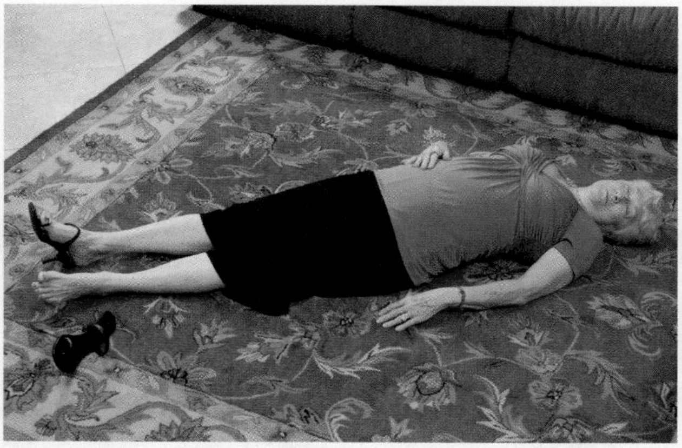

Figure 8-6 The supine position.

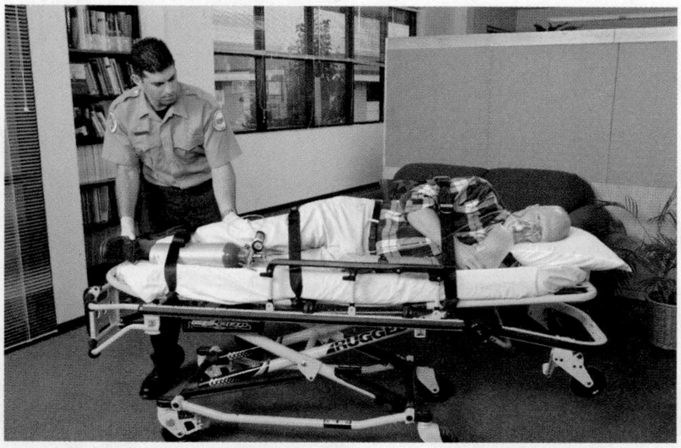

Figure 8-7 The recovery position, which is also called the lateral recumbent position.

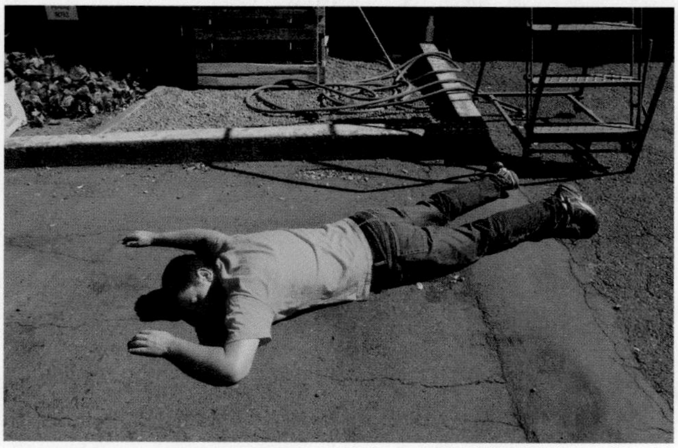

Figure 8-8 The prone position.

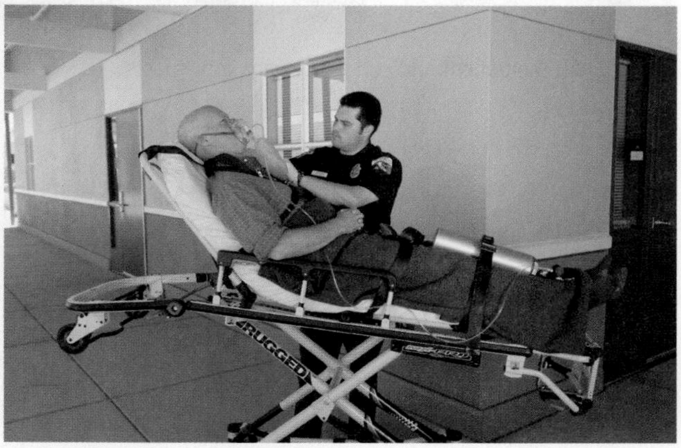

Figure 8-9 The semi-Fowler's position.

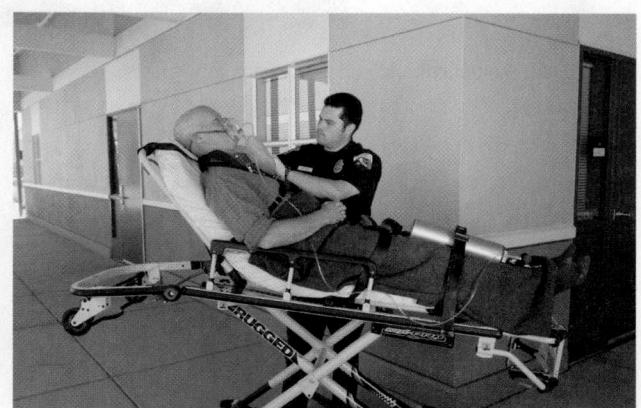

SCAN 8-5 Direct Carry

NONEMERGENT MOVE TO A STRETCHER OF A PATIENT WITH NO SUSPECTED SPINE INJURY

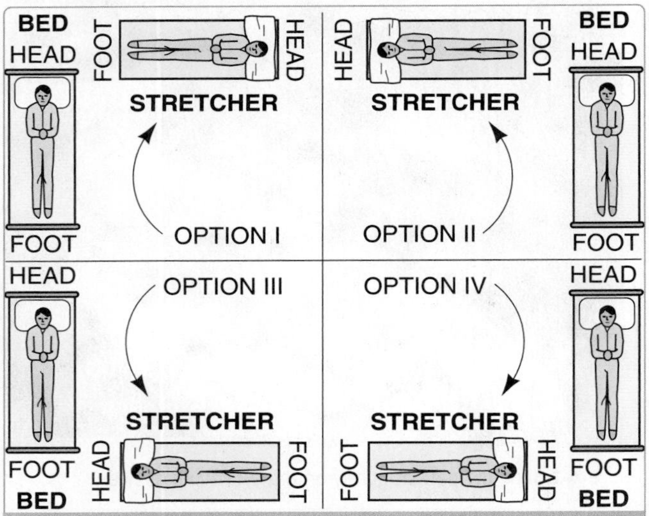

8-5-1 The stretcher is placed at a 90-degree angle to the bed, depending on room configuration. Prepare stretcher by lowering rails, unbuckling straps, and removing other items. Both EMTs stand between the stretcher and the bed, facing patient.

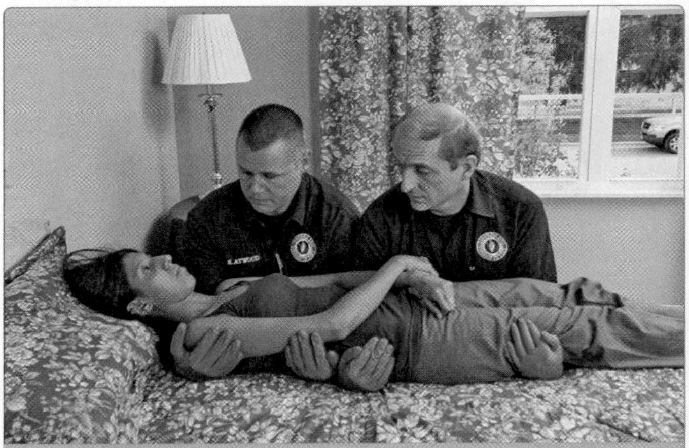

8-5-2 Position your arms under the patient and slide the patient to the edge of the bed.

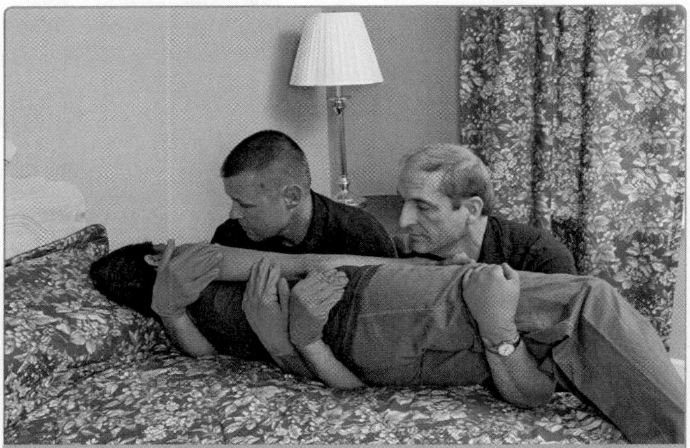

8-5-3 Lift the patient and curl her toward your chests.

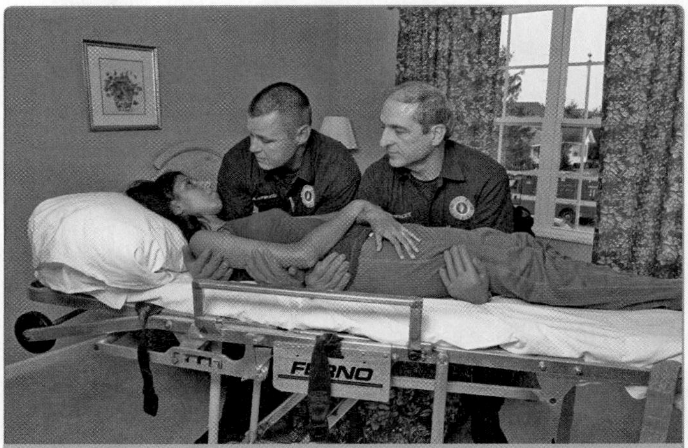

8-5-4 Rotate and place the patient gently on the stretcher.

- *Patients with suspected spine injuries* are immobilized in the supine position on a backboard. The patient found in a sitting position may be immobilized in a vest-type device or short backboard and then moved to a supine position.
- *Patients with chest pain or discomfort or respiratory distress* are allowed to attain a position of comfort. This is usually the **Fowler's position** (sitting upright) or semi-Fowler's, which is a semi-sitting position.
- *Patients who have fainted or who are showing signs of shock but have not suffered an injury* are to be placed in the shock position (supine with legs elevated).
- *Patients who are nauseated or vomiting but alert* may be transported in a position of comfort. Monitor the airway carefully and be prepared to suction, especially if the patient becomes unresponsive.
- *Pregnant patients experiencing low blood pressure* should be transported on their left side to take pressure off the inferior vena cava. Patients with advanced pregnancy (six to nine months) should be transported on their left side during transport. If a spine injury is suspected, immobilize the patient on a long backboard by placing her in a supine position with a towel or blanket under the right side of the board to cause her to shift to the left.

Fowler's position a position in which the patient is sitting fully upright.

CLINICAL CLUE

Fowler's Position

Fowler's position has several variations: a high, standard, semi-, and low sitting position. In the high Fowler's the patient's sitting position is at 80–90 degrees. In the standard Fowler's position, the patient is at 45–60 degrees. In the semi-Fowler's position the patient is at 30–45 degrees. In the low Fowler's position the patient is at 15–30 degrees.

STOP, REVIEW, REMEMBER!

Multiple Choice

For each question, place a check next to the correct answer.

1. For which one of the following situations would the use of a nonemergent move be most appropriate?

_____ a. Moving an alert patient from a vehicle

_____ b. Removing a patient from a car that is on fire

_____ c. Moving a patient away from a wall that is about to collapse

_____ d. Moving a patient with absent breathing down stairs

2. You and your partner are about to lift a patient from the ground to the stretcher. You should:

_____ a. place the patient onto a long backboard.

_____ b. make eye contact prior to the move.

_____ c. perform the move as quickly as possible.

_____ d. first ask the patient to move himself.

(continued on next page)

(continued)

3. To properly move a patient using an emergent drag, you should pull the patient by the:
   _____ a. head.
   _____ b. shoulders.
   _____ c. arms.
   _____ d. waist.

4. You are one of several rescuers using one hand to help lift and carry a patient on a long backboard. You should:
   _____ a. stagger your feet.
   _____ b. bend at the waist.
   _____ c. walk sideways.
   _____ d. lean away from the stretcher.

5. A patient lying on his stomach is said to be in what position?
   _____ a. Supine
   _____ b. Recovery
   _____ c. Prone
   _____ d. Position of comfort

6. You are treating a patient who is unresponsive but breathing adequately. In what position should this patient be placed?
   _____ a. Supine
   _____ b. Prone
   _____ c. Recovery
   _____ d. Comfortable

7. You are transporting a patient who is 33 weeks pregnant and experiencing abdominal pain. You place her on the stretcher in a supine position and in a short time she begins to feel weak and dizzy. You should:
   _____ a. place her in a prone position.
   _____ b. roll her onto her right side.
   _____ c. do nothing; pregnancy normally causes weakness and dizziness.
   _____ d. roll her onto her left side.

8. The EMT should perform an emergent move when the:
   _____ a. patient is alert and stable.
   _____ b. patient is suffering from an immediate threat to life.
   _____ c. patient is too large for just two rescuers.
   _____ d. scene is safe and free of hazards.

9. You and your partner are going to transfer a patient from the ambulance stretcher to the hospital bed. You should:
   _____ a. ask the patient to scoot over.
   _____ b. position the stretcher beside the bed.
   _____ c. wait for at least two more helpers.
   _____ d. perform a direct ground lift.

10. To decrease the risk of injury when lifting and moving patients, you should combine good body mechanics with:
   _____ a. good equipment.
   _____ b. timing.
   _____ c. physical fitness.
   _____ d. good nutrition.

Fill in the Blank

1. A full-term pregnant patient who was involved in a motor vehicle collision is placed on a long backboard. You should place a towel under the ____________________ side of the backboard to cause the patient to roll to the ____________________.

2. A patient found near spilled gasoline at a motor vehicle collision would require a(n) ____________________ move.

3. A patient lying face up is said to be in the ____________________ position.

4. An alert patient with mild respiratory distress can be transported safely in a position of ____________________.

5. An example of an emergent move that is designed to keep the spine in line is called a(n) ____________________ drag.

Critical Thinking

1. Describe one situation in which you would use an emergent move and one situation in which you would use a nonemergent move.

2. List the five factors to consider when planning a patient move.

Specific Devices and Situations

The following text addresses the more common patient transport devices used in the field today as well as common situations when each device can be used.

8-11 Describe the proper use, advantages, disadvantages, and limitations of common pieces of equipment used in lifting and moving patients: basket stretcher, flexible stretcher, long backboard, portable (flat) stretcher, scoop stretcher, stair chair, and wheeled stretcher.

Wheeled Stretcher

Every ambulance is equipped with a device used for patient transport called a **wheeled stretcher** (Figure 8-10 ■). It is exactly as its name suggests: a stretcher with wheels, which is ideally suited for transporting patients over smooth, flat surfaces. Common names for the wheeled stretcher are *cot, gurney, stretcher,* and *pram*. It is probably the most commonly used device for moving patients (Scan 8-6). When there is a choice, it is typically safer to transport a patient using the wheeled stretcher rather than physically carrying the patient from one point to another.

wheeled stretcher the most commonly used device for moving patients. Also called *cot* or *gurney*.

The device is moved by one EMT guiding the foot end of the stretcher while a second EMT pushes the head end (Figure 8-11 ■). The wheeled stretcher has a relatively high center of gravity and should only be moved along its long axis. Sideways or lateral movements should be avoided to minimize the risk of tipping.

There are several manufacturers who produce wheeled stretchers for the EMS market. Each manufacturer produces a wide variety of both manual and automatic-lift stretchers. All stretchers are categorized as either *roll-in* or *lift-in*:

- ***Roll-in stretcher*.** The **roll-in stretcher** is positioned at the back of the ambulance, and the head of the stretcher is secured to a cleat on the floor of the ambulance (Figure 8-12 ■). The undercarriage can then be pulled upward and the gurney

roll-in stretcher a type of wheeled stretcher that can be rolled into the ambulance without lifting; some models can be operated by a single rescuer.

SCAN 8-6 Loading the Wheeled Stretcher into the Ambulance

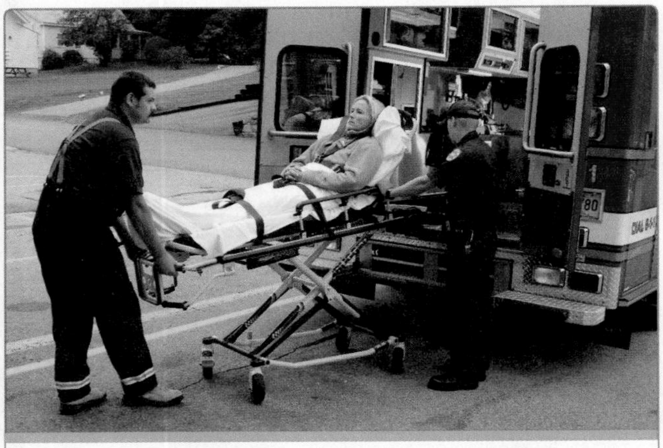

8-6-1 Position the wheels closest to the patient's head at the opening of the ambulance.

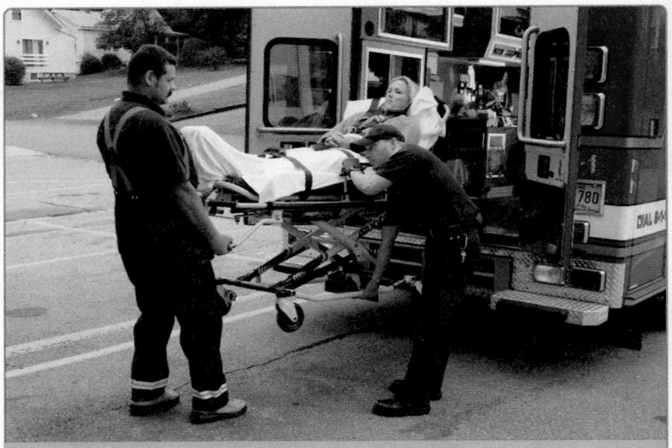

8-6-2 Once the wheels are securely on the ambulance floor, the rescuer at the rear of the stretcher activates the lever to release the wheels. (This may require a slight lift to get the weight off the wheels.) The second rescuer should guide the collapsing carriage, if necessary.

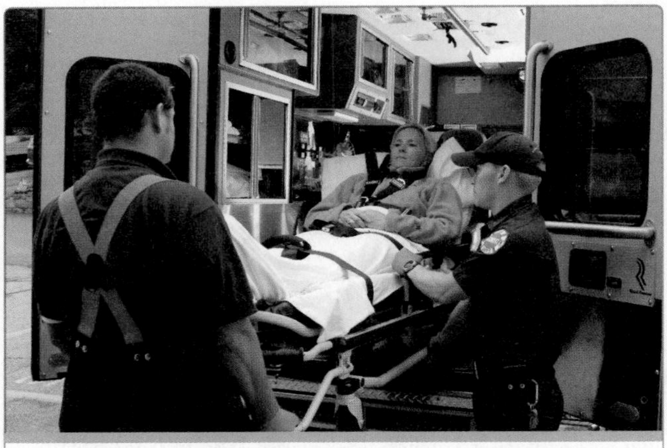

8-6-3 Move the stretcher into the securing device and secure the stretcher in front and rear. Communicate with your partner to achieve balance.

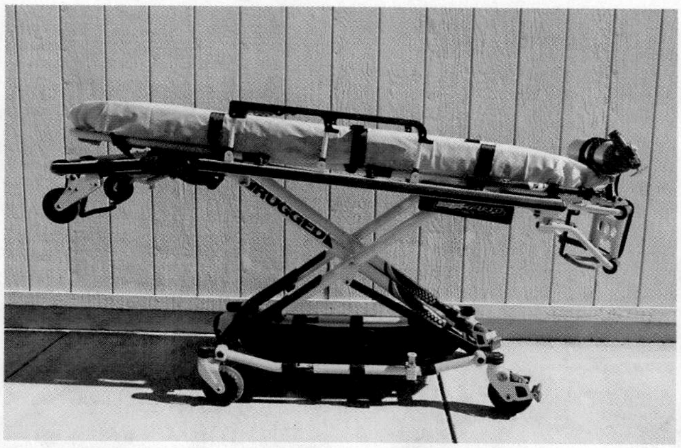

Figure 8-10 Example of a wheeled stretcher.

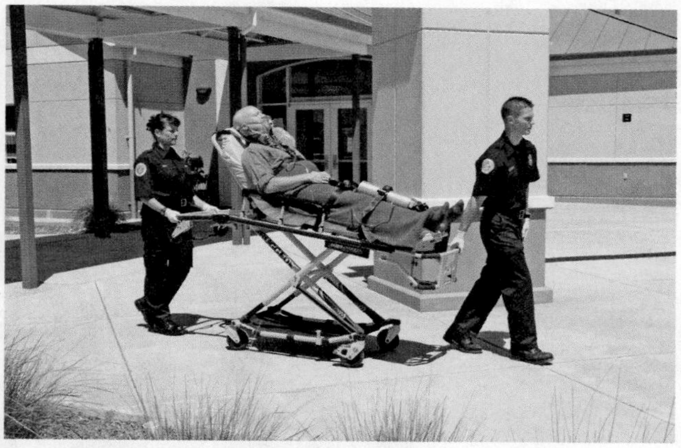

Figure 8-11 One EMT guides the front end of the stretcher while the second EMT pushes from the rear.

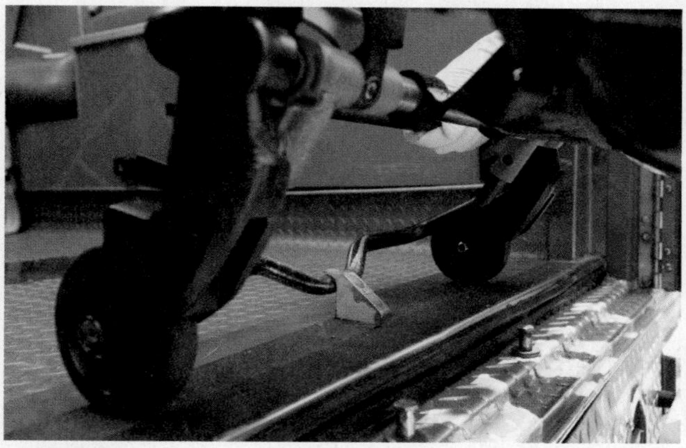

Figure 8-12 A stretcher that attaches to the loading cleat before it is rolled into the ambulance.

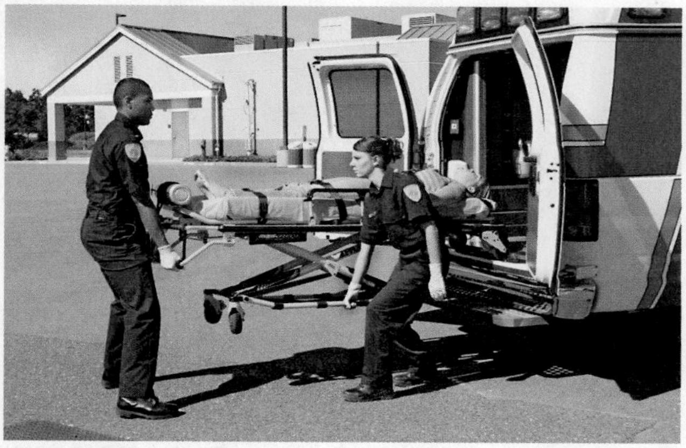

Figure 8-13 One EMT lifts the carriage while the other rolls the stretcher in.

can be rolled into the ambulance. This type of stretcher requires the use of two EMTs but minimizes heavy lifting for the EMTs (Figure 8-13 ■).

- ***Lift-in stretcher.*** The **lift-in stretcher** requires the entire stretcher with the patient on board to be lifted into the ambulance. That requires a significant amount of effort for the EMTs and is much riskier for injury than the roll-in style.

lift-in stretcher a type of wheeled stretcher that must be lifted by at least two rescuers to be placed into the ambulance.

With the increase in the incidence of obese (bariatric) patients, many manufacturers have designed specialty stretchers to accommodate the larger width and weight of these patients. Some ambulances are even equipped with loading ramps and an electric winch, which is used to pull the patient into the ambulance.

Injuries to patients from accidents involving stretchers is a significant cause of lawsuits against EMS providers. You must be alert and diligent when transporting a patient on a stretcher. Be sure that you or your agency maintains the stretcher according to manufacturer's guidelines. Do not exceed the weight limit of your stretcher.

Stair Chair

As the name suggests, the **stair chair** (Figure 8-14 ■) can be used to move patients up and down stairs. Wheeled stretchers are often too bulky and heavy to maneuver stairs and corners. The stair chair is excellent in those situations.

stair chair a chair-style device used to move patients up and down stairs in a sitting position.

A stair chair is only appropriate for patients who are responsive and relatively stable. Patients who are unresponsive, require airway care or ventilation, have spine

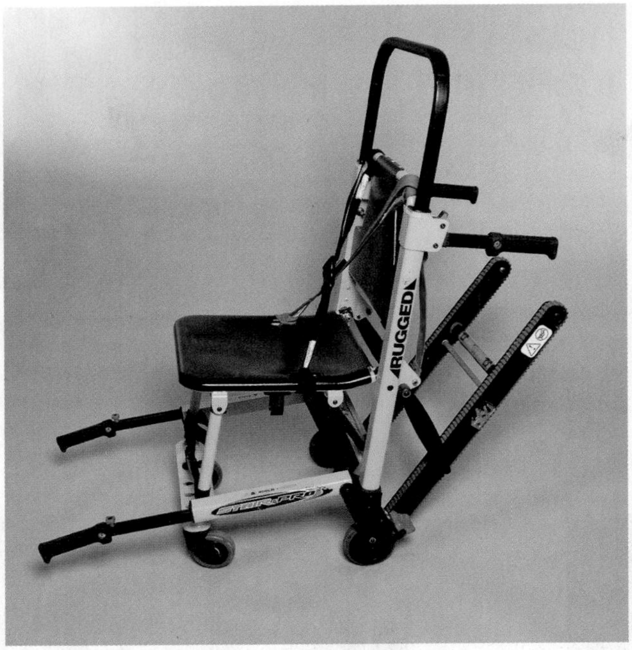

Figure 8-14a Example of a stair chair.

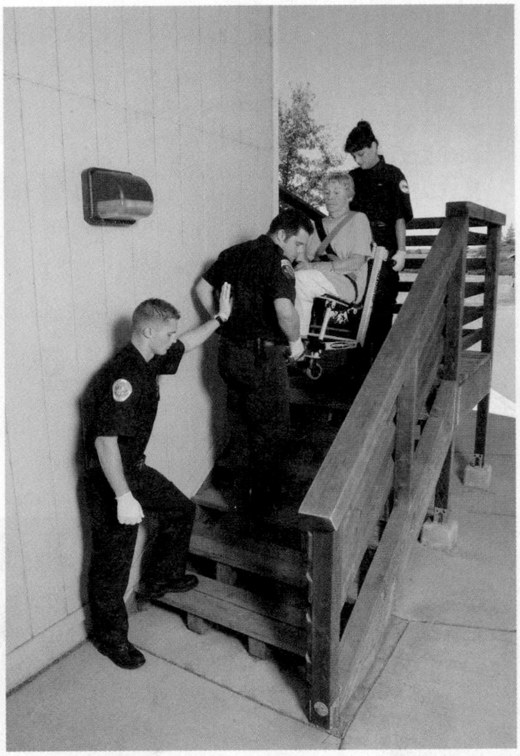

Figure 8-14b The stair chair is used to move the patient up and down stairs.

injuries, or are otherwise unable to be placed in a sitting position are not good candidates for the stair chair. For them, use a flexible stretcher instead. Patients who are responsive and breathing adequately, although with difficulty, are ideal for the stair chair because they are usually most comfortable in a sitting position.

When using the stair chair, be sure to reassure the patient and secure him to the device. The patient may feel awkward or frightened being carried down stairs and may reach out and grab a railing or other object. This can cause the chair to shift, resulting in the patient falling or a back injury to the EMTs carrying the device. Also, because the stair chair is stored in a folded position, it is critical to ensure that the device is fully expanded and locked in position before you seat the patient.

In most cases the patient should be transported feet first. The EMT at the feet will be going down backwards. The EMT nearer the patient's head will face forward. Use the proper methods described earlier in the chapter for lifting. Have someone act as a spotter behind the EMT at the feet to coach him, look for dangers and unstable surfaces, and help ensure good footing with each step.

flexible stretcher a lightweight device used for carrying supine patients down stairs or through tight spaces. Also known as a *Reeves stretcher.*

long backboard a rigid device, usually made of plastic or a composite material, that is used to stabilize a patient with a suspected spine injury. Also called a *long spine board.*

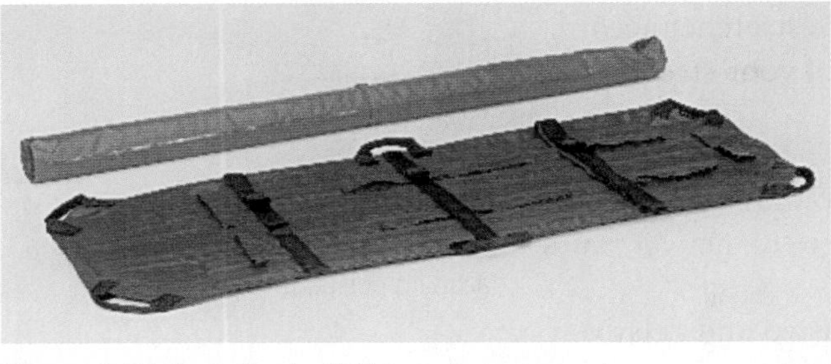

Figure 8-15 Example of a flexible, or Reeves, stretcher.

Flexible Stretcher

The **flexible stretcher,** also called a *Reeves stretcher* (Figure 8-15 ■), is a flat sturdy canvas with handles around the edges. It is ideal for moving patients who must remain supine down stairs or through tight spaces. Some have a rigid aluminum frame for support.

Long Backboard

The **long backboard** or *long spine board* is a rigid device, usually made of a plastic or composite material that is primarily used when the patient has a suspected spine injury

Figure 8-16 Example of a long backboard.

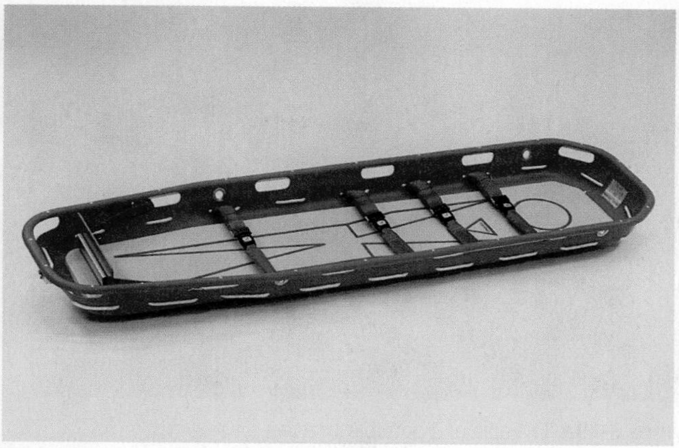

Figure 8-17 Example of the Stokes, or basket, stretcher. (ERNO)

(Figure 8-16 ■). Long backboards also are used to transport patients in cardiac arrest because they provide a firm surface during chest compressions.

The device is called a long backboard because it is designed to support the whole body. That support is designed to restrict motion of the spine and minimize additional spine injury.

Research has shown that rigid backboards, while important in minimizing further spine injury, cause significant discomfort to the patient during transport, at the hospital, and for days after the incident. Chapter 36 describes procedures for applying long and short backboards.

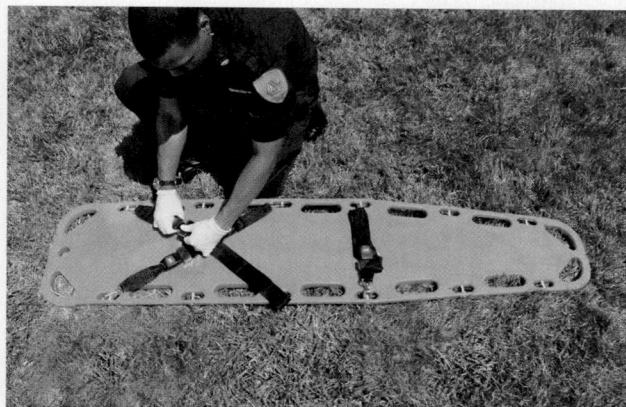

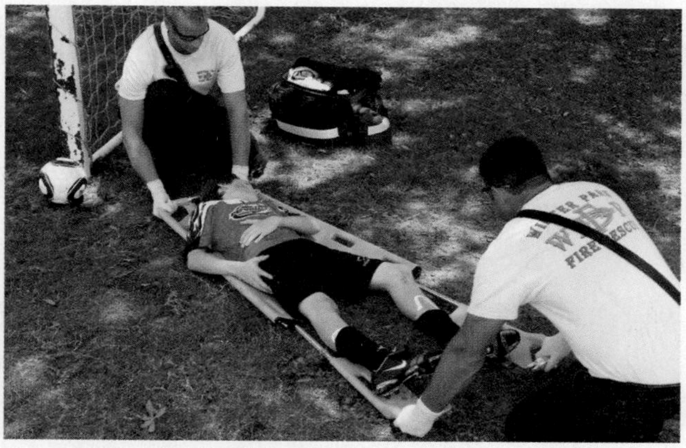

Figure 8-18 Example of the scoop, or orthopedic, stretcher.

Basket Stretcher

Also called a **Stokes basket,** the **basket stretcher** (Figure 8-17 ■) is designed to move patients over rough terrain such as steep grades and cliffs. The basket is made of metal or plastic, which provides protection from hard surfaces on three sides of the patient.

Stokes basket a metal or plastic basket designed to move patients over uneven terrain. Also called a *basket stretcher.*

basket stretcher a metal or plastic basket designed to move patients over uneven terrain. Also called a *Stokes basket.*

Scoop Stretcher

The **scoop stretcher** (Figure 8-18 ■), also called the *orthopedic stretcher,* is so named because it separates in half and comes back together again to literally "scoop" the patient off the ground. This is sometimes used for patients who have suspected hip or pelvic fractures.

scoop stretcher a device that separates in two and can be used to "scoop" the patient off the ground. Also called an *orthopedic stretcher.*

CLINICAL CLUE

Scoop Stretcher

It is important to note that manufacturers of scoop-style stretchers do not recommend them for patients needing spinal immobilization. As you will see by the design of the device, there is no support under the spine of the patient when he is placed on the device. However, it is possible to place a patient who is secured to a scoop stretcher onto a long backboard if you suspect a spine injury.

Portable Stretcher

The **portable stretcher** is sometimes called a *flat stretcher* or simply a *flat*. It is a lightweight aluminum frame covered with canvas or plastic. Portable stretchers are

portable stretcher a lightweight device made of canvas or plastic with two poles extended from each side for easy carrying.

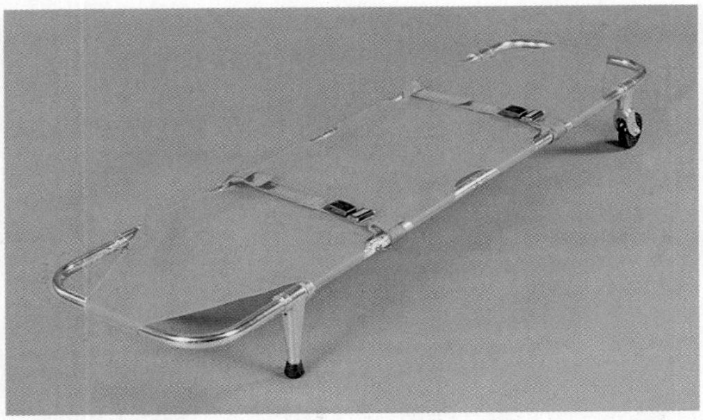

Figure 8-19a Example of a portable stretcher.

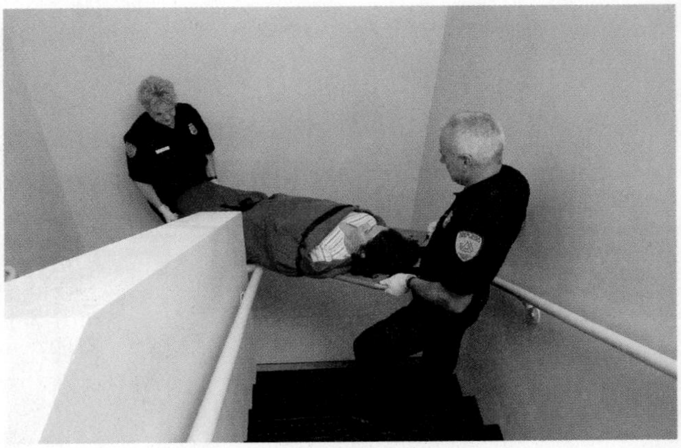

Figure 8-19b A portable stretcher is ideal for transporting a supine patient down narrow stairways.

ideal for transporting supine patients down tight stairwells or through tight spaces. Sometimes it can be split down the middle (breakaway flat) to facilitate removal at the hospital without rolling the patient. Some portable stretchers fold for easy storage (Figure 8-19 ■).

STOP, REVIEW, REMEMBER!

Multiple Choice

For each question, place a check next to the correct answer.

1. Which one of the following statements about lifting is *not* correct?

_____ a. You should communicate with your partner before lifting.

_____ b. An even number of rescuers should be used.

_____ c. You should use your legs, not your back to lift.

_____ d. When practical and safe, patients should be carried rather than wheeled.

2. Which one of the following devices would be most appropriate when transporting an unconscious patient down a flight of stairs?

_____ a. Portable stretcher

_____ b. Long backboard

_____ c. Stair chair

_____ d. Wheeled stretcher

3. You must transport a stable, alert, supine patient across a large parking lot to your waiting ambulance. Which one of the following devices would be the most appropriate for this move?

_____ a. Basket stretcher

_____ b. Stair chair

_____ c. Long backboard

_____ d. Wheeled stretcher

4. You are called to care for a patient who is experiencing difficulty breathing. You find the patient in a second-floor back bedroom of the house. You examine the patient and find him alert. To get this patient downstairs, you would likely use the:

_____ a. basket stretcher.

_____ b. wheeled stretcher.

_____ c. stair chair.

_____ d. flexible stretcher.

5. You and your partner are preparing to transport a patient down two flights of stairs. You should ask the security officer on scene to assist you by:

_____ a. standing at the top of the stairs and watching your steps.

_____ b. standing behind the EMT at the feet and counting off the steps.

_____ c. standing at the bottom of the stairs and watching your steps.

_____ d. keeping everyone off the stairs.

6. When transporting a patient using a wheeled stretcher, the person at the ______________ should only be guiding while the EMT at the ______________ should be pushing/pulling.

_____ a. head, foot

_____ b. foot, head

_____ c. side, head

_____ d. side, foot

Matching

Match the piece of equipment on the left with the applicable situation on the right.

1. _____ Portable stretcher (flat)
2. _____ Basket stretcher (Stokes)
3. _____ Stair chair
4. _____ Wheeled stretcher
5. _____ Scoop (orthopedic) stretcher

A. Moving a patient down a rocky slope
B. Moving a stable supine patient through a narrow hallway
C. Moving a patient on a long backboard a short distance to the ambulance
D. Moving a patient with mild trouble breathing from a second-floor bedroom
E. Moving a patient who has fallen in the bathroom and has a possible hip injury

Critical Thinking

1. Describe the following two lifting techniques.

a. Power grip

____

____

____

____

b. Power lift

____

____

____

____

(continued on next page)

(continued)

2. Describe the role of each person during a stair chair lift down a set of stairs.

____

____

____

____

3. What do you think are the risks of moving a patient too quickly or with the wrong device?

____

____

____

____

PERSPECTIVE

Suki—The EMT

When I walked into the room, my heart just sank. My back started to hurt just thinking about moving that woman down three flights of stairs. It's part of the job though. This wasn't the first—and won't be the last—time for a patient like this. I honestly can't imagine what it's like for the patient though. Brent, my new partner, just stared at her. I don't think he'd ever seen anyone so big. I had to get him started on the assessment while I contacted dispatch for help. It actually turned out okay. We started some oxygen while we waited for fire personnel, and with a heavy-duty stair chair, four carriers, two spotters, and me, we got her to the truck. Ms. Ordeen got safely to the hospital, all of our backs survived, and we returned to the street in no time. I guess planning was the key.

EMERGENCY DISPATCH SUMMARY

Julie was transported to Physician's Hospital on Fifth Street and treated for a urinary tract infection and several diabetes-related issues and released two days later. Due to her condition, and those of several other people in the same apartment building, the management company was ordered to repair the elevator, which it did.

Chapter Review

To the Point

- Body mechanics refers to the proper use of the body for movement and function. It is important to use proper body mechanics when moving and lifting patients and equipment to minimize injury.
- Each and every patient move should be carefully planned to take into consideration the following factors: urgency, size and weight, number of rescuers, distance, and terrain.
- Three important principles to help ensure good body mechanics are to keep the weight to be lifted close to your body, to use the large muscles of the legs to lift, and to keep your body straight when moving.
- All patient moves should be a team effort with communication being clear and concise.
- You should minimize the amount of extended reaching and twisting you do because each leaves you vulnerable to injury.
- An emergent move is one that requires quick action and is used when the patient is in danger or need of immediate care.
- A nonemergent move is more common and used for stable patients.
- There are several positions that can be used for patient transport. First and foremost, use the position that allows for the best patient care. Secondly, use the position that is most comfortable for the patient.

Chapter Questions

Multiple Choice

For each question, place a check next to the correct answer.

1. You are going to carry a 165-pound supine patient 100 yards over rough ground to the ambulance. You should:
   _____ a. use two rescuers with a wheeled stretcher.
   _____ b. use three rescuers and a stair chair.
   _____ c. use four rescuers and a portable stretcher.
   _____ d. use five rescuers and a long backboard.
2. You and two other rescuers are preparing to roll an injured patient onto a long backboard. You should initiate the move on the count of the rescuer:
   _____ a. at the head.
   _____ b. at the waist.
   _____ c. at the feet.
   _____ d. overseeing the entire move.
3. The roll-in style of wheeled stretcher requires a minimum of ______________ rescuer(s) to operate.
   _____ a. one
   _____ b. two
   _____ c. three
   _____ d. four
4. You are required to move an extremely obese patient from a third-floor bedroom to the ambulance. You should first:
   _____ a. ensure that you have enough rescuers.
   _____ b. ask if the patient can walk down the stairs.
   _____ c. check to see if there is an elevator.
   _____ d. call medical direction.

(continued on next page)

(continued)

5. An ideal device for moving a patient with no suspected spine injury down stairs and through tight spaces is a:

_____ a. wheeled stretcher.
_____ b. flexible stretcher.
_____ c. Stokes basket.
_____ d. scoop stretcher.

6. The term *body mechanics* refers to the:

_____ a. mechanical workings of the stretcher.
_____ b. proper use of the patient's weight to facilitate lifting.
_____ c. proper use of the EMT's body while lifting.
_____ d. sum lifting potential (in pounds) of all rescuers on scene.

7. An emergent move is preferred in which one of the following situations?

_____ a. Patient complaining of severe neck pain and partial paralysis from a motor vehicle collision
_____ b. Patient in a motor vehicle collision where the car is on fire and smoke is billowing into the passenger compartment
_____ c. Patient who is found on the ground and appears to have been thrown from a vehicle
_____ d. Patient who pulled to the side of a road while driving because he believed he was having a heart attack

8. A patient with a spine injury from a fall should be placed on a __________ to prevent further injury.

_____ a. stair chair
_____ b. basket stretcher
_____ c. long backboard
_____ d. wheeled stretcher

9. The position of comfort is best described as the position in which the patient:

_____ a. is found following an injury.
_____ b. is placed for transport.
_____ c. feels least comfortable for his illness or injury.
_____ d. feels most comfortable for his illness or injury.

10. In transferring a supine patient with a hip injury from the ground to a stretcher, which one of the following would be the most appropriate?

_____ a. Extremity lift
_____ b. Direct carry
_____ c. Scoop stretcher
_____ d. Draw-sheet move

Matching

Match the patient presentation on the left with the most appropriate position for transport on the right.

1. _____	Patient with spine injuries	A. Recovery position
2. _____	Patient with difficulty breathing	B. Supine with legs elevated
3. _____	Pregnant patient with low blood pressure	C. Supine and rolled to left
4. _____	Patient who fainted	D. Semi-Fowler's
5. _____	Vomiting patients	E. Supine

Labeling

1. Write the position in which each patient is shown in the space below the photo.

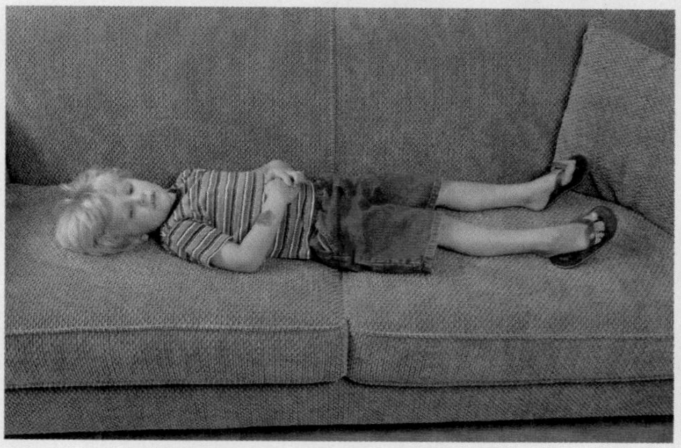

A. ______________________________

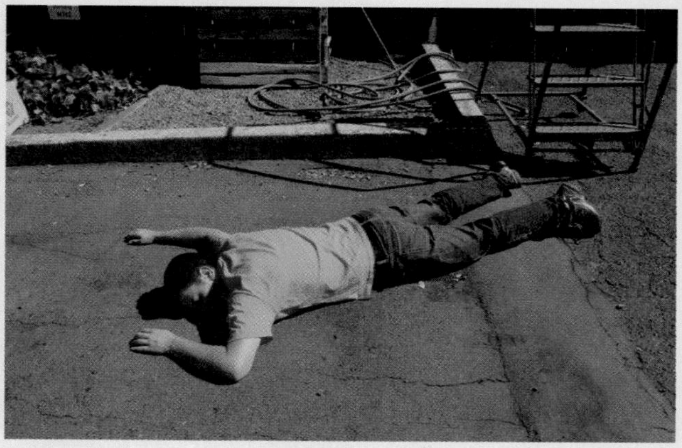

B. ______________________________

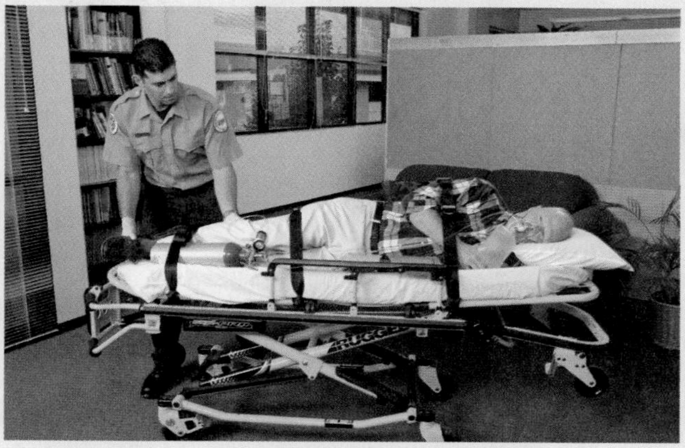

C. ______________________________

2. Write the name of each device in the space below its photo.

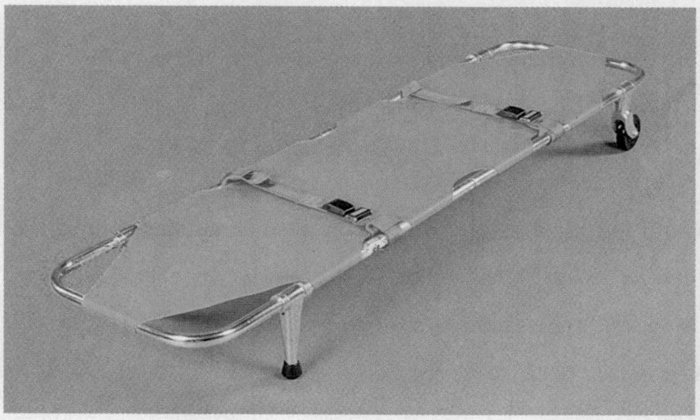

A. ______________________________

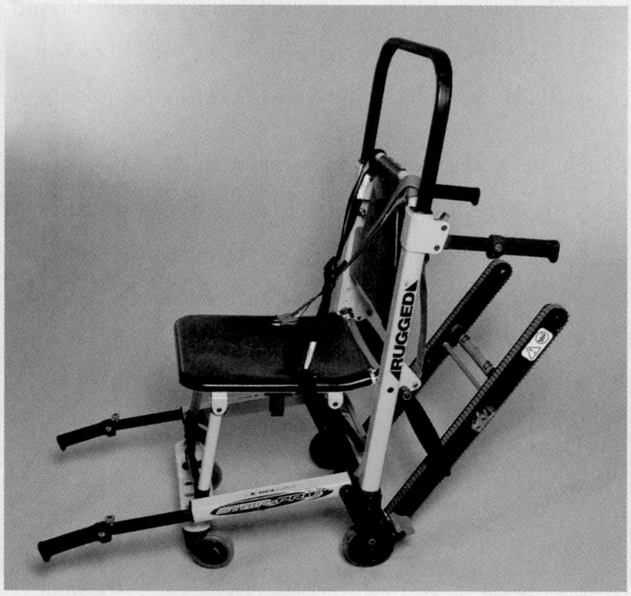

B. ______________________________

(continued on next page)

(continued)

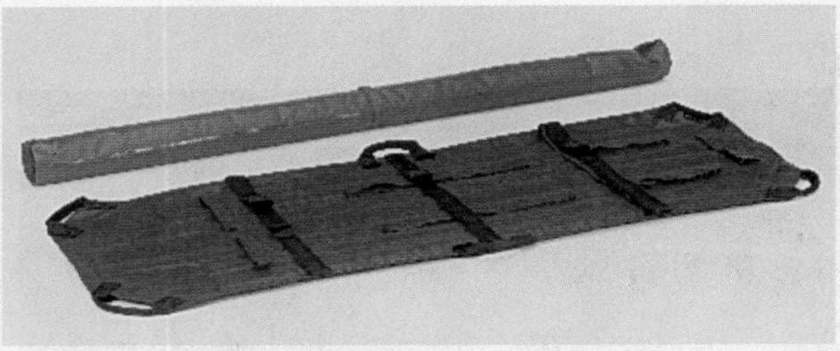

C. ______________________________

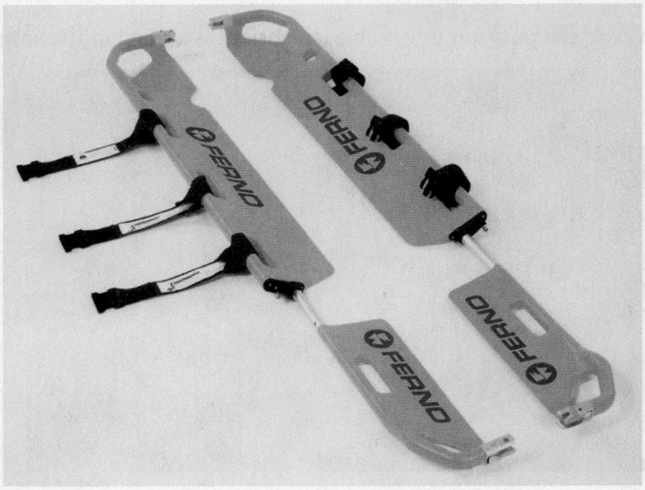

D. ______________________________

Case Studies

Case Study 1

You are called to a motor vehicle collision. You find a badly mangled car with the driver's side wrapped around a tree. You approach the vehicle and find a woman who is alert and able to speak in the front passenger seat. She has pain and deformity to her right arm, but no other complaints. You look past her to the driver's seat and observe an unresponsive man with a head injury and bleeding about the mouth and nose.

1. In reference to the female patient, which one of the following statements is correct?

_____ a. She should be placed in a vest-type extrication device and moved from the vehicle because she appears to be stable.

_____ b. She should be moved from the vehicle via rapid extrication because she is unstable.

_____ c. She should be moved from the vehicle rapidly, but with a vest-type extrication device because she may be unstable.

_____ d. She should be moved from the vehicle via rapid extrication to allow access to the male patient.

2. Which one of the statements in reference to the male patient is correct?

_____ a. He should be placed in a vest-type extrication device and moved from the vehicle because he appears stable.

_____ b. He should be moved from the vehicle via rapid extrication because he is unstable.

_____ c. He should be moved from the vehicle rapidly, but with a vest-type extrication device because he may be unstable.

_____ d. He should be dragged from the vehicle by any means possible because he appears to be unresponsive.

Case Study 2

You are part of a three-person crew performing CPR on a patient in a living room. The patient is placed on a long backboard and CPR must continue as you move him. You have an automated defibrillator, oxygen, and two equipment bags that you have brought into the house.

1. Describe the factors that you must consider when planning this move.

2. Once you exit the house, there is a large grassy lawn that you must pass over. How will you best get the stretcher over the lawn?

3. How would you get your equipment from the house back to the ambulance?

Case Study 3

You have been dispatched to a "sick patient" and find a 532-pound man who feels weak, is unable to stand, and must be transported to the hospital. You are part of a two-person crew.

1. How would you go about getting additional help to move this patient?

2. To what special equipment might you have access to help facilitate a safe move?

The Last Word

A few key points to take away from this chapter include the fact that simple moving and positioning are sometimes very important interventions that can make a big difference for your patient. Even when you think your patient is comfortable, always ask if there is anything more you can do to make him more so. Lifting and moving patients are some of the riskiest tasks you are required to perform as an EMT. Always plan every move carefully and keep yourself physically fit to minimize injuries to both you and the patient.

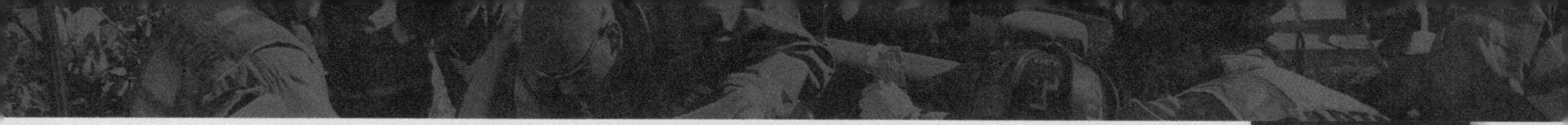

Obtaining Vital Signs and a Medical History

9

Education Standards

Assessment: Secondary assessment, monitoring devices, history taking

Competencies

Applies scene information and patient assessment findings to guide emergency management.

Objectives

After completion of this lesson, you should be able to:

9-1 Define key terms introduced in this chapter.

9-2 Differentiate between a sign and a symptom.

9-3 Explain the importance of taking and recording a patient's vital signs over a period of time to identify trends in the patient's condition.

9-4 Describe the proper technique for assessing breathing.

9-5 Differentiate between normal respiratory rates for adults, children, infants, and newborns.

9-6 Differentiate between normal and abnormal findings when assessing a patient's breathing to include the respiratory rate, depth of respirations, rhythm of respirations, and signs that may indicate respiratory distress or respiratory failure.

9-7 Describe the proper method for auscultating breath sounds to determine their presence, equality, and the likely underlying causes of abnormal breath sounds.

9-8 Describe the proper method for assessing a pulse in both responsive and unresponsive adults as well as pediatric patients.

9-9 Associate pulse abnormalities with possible underlying causes.

9-10 Differentiate between normal and abnormal findings when assessing a patient's pulse to include rate, strength, and rhythm.

9-11 Explain systolic and diastolic blood pressure readings and identify potential causes of abnormal findings or changes.

9-12 Describe the proper method for obtaining blood pressure by both palpation and auscultation.

9-13 Describe normal and abnormal findings in the assessment of skin color, temperature, moisture, capillary refill, and color of mucous membranes, and associate abnormal skin findings with potential underlying causes.

9-14 Describe the proper method for assessing capillary refill time.

9-15 Explain factors that can affect capillary refill findings.

9-16 Describe the proper assessment of the pupils and associate abnormal findings with potential underlying causes.

9-17 Explain the method for assessment of orthostatic vital signs.

9-18 Explain the criteria for determining the frequency with which vital signs should be reassessed.

9-19 Explain what pulse oximetry measures and describe factors and limitations in interpreting pulse oximetry findings.

9-20 Determine a patient's chief complaint.

9-21 Use the mnemonics SAMPLE and OPQRST to ensure a complete prehospital patient history.

Key Terms

auscultation p. 214
baseline vital signs p. 204
brachial pulse p. 211
bradycardia p. 213
capillary refill test p. 222
carotid pulse p. 211
chief complaint p. 230
constricted pupils p. 224
crackles p. 208
cyanotic p. 222
diaphoretic p. 222
diastolic p. 215
dilated pupils p. 224
dorsalis pedis (pedal) pulse p. 211
femoral pulse p. 211
flushed p. 222
general impression p. 230
jaundiced p. 222
OPQRST p. 232
orthostatic vital signs p. 226
pale p. 222
palpation p. 212
PERRL p. 226
popliteal pulse p. 211
posterior tibial pulse p. 211
radial pulse p. 211
SAMPLE p. 231
sign p. 203
stridor p. 208
symptom p. 203
systolic p. 215
tachycardia p. 213
tidal volume p. 207
trending p. 204
wheezing p. 208

Introduction

Taking vital signs and gathering a medical history always fall somewhere in the middle of patient assessment. They are introduced here to give you the opportunity to begin practicing these two very important skills.

During your initial training, you can take vital signs and gather history information on fellow students and perhaps healthy friends and family members. For the most part, you will be obtaining normal vital sign values and histories. It is a whole new experience when you finally get to take vital signs and obtain a medical history on a real patient in the field or clinical setting.

When caring for actual patients, there is a strong likelihood that the values you obtain will not be within normal limits. This can be challenging at first, and you may question the accuracy of your readings. It will be important to take your time and be patient. Ask your partner to check the signs and compare your results. With enough practice on actual patients, you will quickly gain the same confidence you have in the classroom.

What is important to understand is that developing your vital-sign and history-taking skills can take many months and even years before you become confident in all situations.

EMERGENCY DISPATCH

Derrick and Ray, two EMTs assigned to truck #53 on the south side of town, are just finishing the paperwork on a nonemergent transfer from Filmore Assisted Living to Southwest Hospital when their pagers start vibrating. Ray pulls the pager from its clip and reads it.

"They're calling us out for an emergency," he says. Ray replaces the pager on his belt and starts out the door with the stretcher. Once in the truck, Ray keys the radio mic and tells dispatch that they're ready for information on the new call.

"Unit 53, please respond to 2305 South Walker Avenue, 2-3-0-5 South Walker, for a priority-two medical."

Ray pulls the truck out of the Southwest Hospital ambulance parking area, and within minutes they arrive seven blocks away at the South Walker address. The small house is set back off the road with high weeds growing in the front yard, and Derrick and Ray have to fight to get the stretcher, piled with their equipment, to the front door. Derrick knocks on the door and an elderly woman wearing a robe and smoking a cigarette appears.

"My son is back here," she says, leading them to a room in the back of the house. "He's been sick for three days. It's just coming out of both ends, you know? He can't keep anything down."

They find the patient, a thin, pale 55-year-old man named Dick, sitting on the edge of his bed with a garbage can containing vomit on the floor in front of him. Ray gets the stethoscope, blood pressure cuff, and a penlight from the jump bag and approaches the man. "Let's see how you're doing, Dick."

Signs and Symptoms

A lesson on vital signs has to start with a discussion of the difference between signs and symptoms. Just as in your daily life, a **sign** is something that you, the EMT, can see or observe or that has a value that can be recorded. For instance, you can see the stop sign at the intersection near your house or the exit sign near the door in the classroom where you are taking your EMT training. Patients display many signs relating to their current medical condition that you can observe or obtain during assessment. Some of those signs, such as skin color and breathing rate, can be observed without ever touching the patient. Others, such as pulse rate and blood pressure, require you to touch the patient or use a specialized piece of equipment to obtain a reading or value for the sign.

9-2 Differentiate between a sign and a symptom.

sign something that the EMT can see or observe or has a value that can be recorded.

PERSPECTIVE

Ray—The EMT

The first thing that I noticed about this guy was that he was obviously sick. He complained of everything from fatigue and light-headedness to chills and nausea. I could feel that he was running a pretty high fever and, based on the poor turgor of his skin, I could tell that he was very dehydrated.

A **symptom** is very different from a sign. It cannot be seen. The patient alone experiences it and must describe it to you. The most common symptom an EMT encounters is pain. You cannot see pain. You can only see signs of it on a patient's face. The patient must tell you he has pain. Nausea, dizziness, and blurred vision are also symptoms the patient must describe to the EMT. Table 9-1 provides more examples of both signs and symptoms.

symptom something that is experienced and described by the patient as it pertains to his chief complaint.

Vital Signs

Patients can display many signs when they are ill or injured. Some signs are more important than others—so important in fact that if they are absent, it could mean that the patient is clinically dead. The most important of signs are referred to as *vital signs* because they are vital to life. They include:

- Respirations (presence or absence, rate, depth, ease, and lung sounds)
- Pulse (presence or absence, rate, strength, and rhythm)
- Blood pressure

TABLE 9-1 DIFFERENTIATING SIGNS AND SYMPTOMS

EXAMPLES OF SIGNS	EXAMPLES OF SYMPTOMS
Skin color, temperature, and moisture	Fatigue
Pulse rate, strength, and regularity	Nausea
Tenderness	Pain
Blood pressure	Headache
Bruise	Double vision
Deformity	Light-headedness
Swelling	Thirst

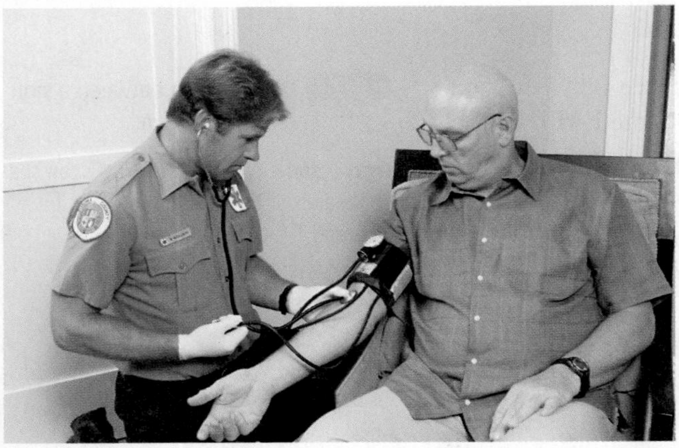
Figure 9-1 Taking vital signs on a seated patient.

- Skin signs (color, temperature, moisture, capillary refill, and turgor)
- Pupils (size and shape, equality, reactivity to light, and sympathetic movement)

While it can be argued that skin and pupil signs are not exactly vital to life, they often are included in the list of vital signs because they are relatively easy to assess and can tell us a great deal about the patient's current condition.

Baseline Vital Signs and Trending

Baseline vital signs is a term commonly used to refer to the very first set of vital signs obtained on the patient during a call. Baseline vital signs are very important because they establish a standard (baseline) to which all subsequent vital signs obtained from the patient will be compared (Figure 9-1 ▪).

baseline vital signs the very first set of vital signs obtained on a patient.

9-3 Explain the importance of taking and recording a patient's vital signs over a period of time to identify trends in the patient's condition.

trending the comparing of multiple sets of vital signs over a period of time in order to reveal a trend in the patient's condition.

Be careful not to jump too quickly to a conclusion after obtaining your baseline vitals. A single set of vital signs gives us nothing more than a quick snapshot of a patient's condition. In fact, it may have very little value unless you can compare it to subsequent sets of vital signs. The taking, documenting, and comparing of multiple sets of vital signs over a period of time is called **trending,** which is the most accurate method of determining a patient's condition or status.

Taking vital signs is only part of this skill. Being able to accurately document your findings to share with other EMS professionals is the other part. Recording the time vitals are taken along with the actual values is essential. Without a time to reference with each set of vitals, it becomes impossible to know which set came first or how much time elapsed between them, which makes them unusable for purposes of trending. Always record the time with each set of vital signs.

CLINICAL CLUE

Trending

A single set of vital signs is an observation, two sets of vital signs is a comparison, and three sets of vital signs reveal a trend. For stable patients, obtain as many sets of vital signs as practical to reveal any trends in the patient's condition. Be sure to document the time each set is taken.

The exact order in which you take and record each of the patient's vital signs is not important. Your instructor will provide a format for recording vital signs that is used in the area or region where you will be working. What is important is that you obtain and record accurate and complete vital signs in a way that will allow for easy comparison.

Figure 9-2 ▪ shows the order and format usually recommended. This format allows for easy comparison of multiple sets of vital signs and presents the first three (the most vital of the vital signs) in the order they are most likely going to be obtained while caring for a patient. However, completeness and consistency is your goal, not format. So, like many of the skills you will be learning throughout your training, deciding on a format and sticking to it will minimize the chances that you will skip or forget something important.

Assessing Breathing

9-4 Describe the proper technique for assessing breathing.

Breathing is typically the first vital sign you will be able to assess as you approach your patient. It can reveal a great deal about a patient in less time and with less effort

TIME	RESPIRATIONS	PULSE	BP	SKIN	PUPILS

Figure 9-2 Suggested form for recording vital signs.

than the other signs. In other words, if your patient is breathing, it is safe to assume he has a pulse and therefore a blood pressure.

9-5 Differentiate between normal respiratory rates for adults, children, infants, and newborns.

In responsive patients, the presence of breathing often can be detected easily from a distance as you first enter the scene and observe the patient. You will be looking for signs of adequate versus inadequate respirations as you approach (Table 9-2).

TABLE 9-2 RESPIRATIONS

NORMAL RESPIRATORY RATES (BREATHS PER MINUTE, AT REST)	
ADULT	12 to 20
	Above 29: Potentially serious
	Below 10: Potentially serious
INFANTS AND CHILDREN	
Adolescent 11–14 years	12 to 20
School age 6–10 years	15 to 30
Preschooler 3–5 years	20 to 30
Toddler 1–3 years	20 to 30
Infant 6–12 months	20 to 30
Infant 0–5 months	25 to 40
Newborn	30 to 50
RESPIRATORY SOUNDS	**POSSIBLE CAUSES/INTERVENTIONS**
Snoring	Airway blocked. Open patient's airway; prompt transport.
Wheezing	Medical problem such as asthma. Assist patient in taking prescribed medications; prompt transport.
Gurgling	Fluids in airway. Suction airway; prompt transport.
Crowing (harsh sound when inhaling)	Medical problem that cannot be treated on the scene. Prompt transport.
Gasping	Gasping breaths by an unresponsive patient are called agonal breaths and should not be considered normal breaths. Assist ventilations as appropriate.

For unresponsive patients, the assessment is not so easy from a distance. You may not be able to perform an adequate assessment until you are right next to the patient. In fact, it may be necessary for you to open the airway and place your ear next to the patient's nose and mouth to listen for breathing as you observe the chest for rise and fall.

CLINICAL CLUE

New CPR Guidelines

Remember that current American Heart Association guidelines recommend that if your primary assessment of an unresponsive patient shows absent or only gasping breaths, you should proceed immediately to a pulse check to assess for cardiac arrest.

As you first begin to practice the skill of assessing respirations in the classroom, it is easiest to have your patient lying flat in a supine position. Then grasp his wrist, as if you were going to take a pulse, and lay it across his abdomen (Figure 9-3 ■). This technique has two benefits. The first is that the patient thinks you are taking his pulse and is less likely to alter his breathing pattern. The second is that you can actually feel the movement of the abdomen as he breathes, and you do not have to stare at his chest, making it obvious that you are counting each breath. Once you have mastered this technique, you can then use the technique for a patient in the sitting position (Figure 9-4 ■).

Characteristics of Respirations

9-6 Differentiate between normal and abnormal findings when assessing a patient's breathing to include the respiratory rate, depth of respirations, rhythm of respirations, and signs that may indicate respiratory distress or respiratory failure.

There are four characteristics of respirations that must be assessed and recorded on each patient. They are as follows: rate, depth, ease, and lung sounds. (You may wish to note that some texts group the characteristics of depth, ease, and sounds under the heading "quality." They are broken out here for ease of understanding.)

Breathing Rate

You must determine an accurate count of how many times the patient is breathing each minute. The normal limits for respiratory rates are as follows:

- ***Adults:*** 10 to 30 (average is 12 to 20) breaths per minute
- ***Children:*** 15 to 30 breaths per minute
- ***Infants:*** 25 to 50 breaths per minute

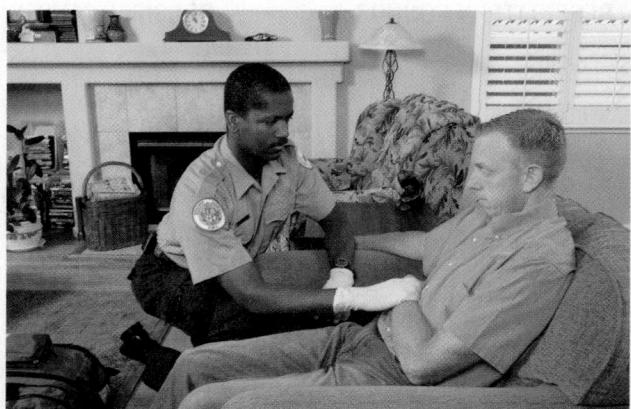

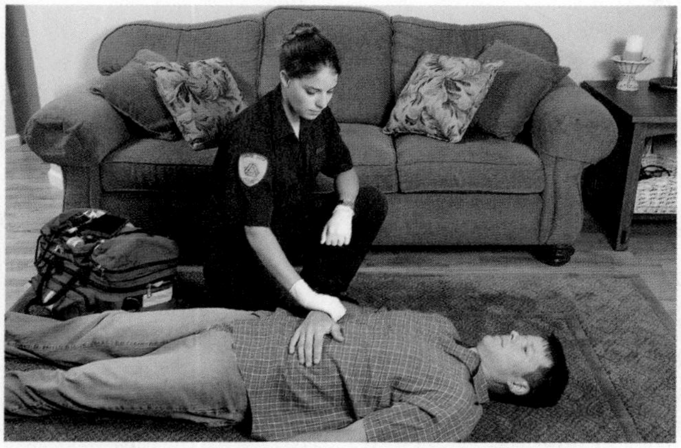

Figure 9-3 Assessing respirations on a supine patient.

Figure 9-4 Assessing respirations on a seated patient.

All breathing rates are recorded as a per-minute value. To obtain the most accurate value possible, the EMT would have to count respirations for an entire minute. However, this wastes valuable time in the field and may delay important interventions.

> **CLINICAL CLUE**
>
> **Calculating Respiratory Rate**
>
> Two common methods for obtaining respiratory rate are as follows:
>
> - Count respirations for 30 seconds × 2 = Minute Rate
> - Count respirations for 15 seconds × 4 = Minute Rate

There are at least two faster methods commonly used for obtaining a breathing rate for patients in the field setting. One method is counting the respirations (one inhalation plus one exhalation = one respiration) for 30 seconds and multiplying that value by 2 to get the minute rate. This often is easier when first learning to assess vital signs. The second method involves counting respirations for 15 seconds and multiplying by 4 to get the minute rate. This method is the one most often used by experienced providers and the one you will likely use once you become more skilled at taking vital signs.

Regardless of which method you use, you should arrive at the same or very similar value. It should be noted that the smaller your sample, the less accurate your value will be. Using samples of less than 15 seconds is not recommended. Also, if your patient has an irregular breathing pattern, you may want to take the time to count the respirations for a full minute to get the most accurate rate.

Every attempt should be made to obtain a respiratory rate without the patient being made aware that you are counting respirations. Once a patient knows you are counting his respirations, he may subconsciously alter his rate. Also, attempting to count respirations while the patient is speaking can result in an inaccurate assessment. You may have to stop asking history questions in order to assess the breathing rate and get an accurate count. Wait for an appropriate time to assess rate.

> **PRACTICAL PATHOPHYSIOLOGY**
>
> There are many factors that contribute to the adequacy of breathing and the oxygenation of the blood during respiration. First and foremost is the amount of air that is being exchanged each minute. This is referred to as "minute volume" and is a factor of both rate (how fast) and tidal volume (how much). When rate and tidal volume are within normal limits, the minute rate is adequate.

Depth of Breathing

Depth of breathing, sometimes referred to as **tidal volume,** is the amount of air moved in and out with each breath. It can be assessed by observing the patient's chest for adequate rise and fall. Assessing for adequate tidal volume (depth) can be difficult for the new EMT, because normal tidal volume is often shallow to begin with. It takes time and practice to learn the difference between normal and shallow respirations.

tidal volume the amount of air moved in and out with each breath.

> **PERSPECTIVE**
>
> **Derrick—The EMT**
>
> I let Ray jump right in and get the vitals on this patient. I always have a really hard time with vitals. I think it's mostly the math that gets me, if you know what I mean. You know, what really bothered me about this call, though, is that the other south side truck, number 48, was available, and yet dispatch sent us. That just didn't make sense, but Derrick explained that we don't always have the big picture. I even made an appointment to sit in our dispatch center next week to get a better understanding of how calls are prioritized.

For some patients, the abdomen moves more than the chest during normal breathing. This is particularly true with infants and small children. For that reason, you must observe both the chest and abdomen when assessing tidal volume.

Depth of respirations can be characterized as one of the following: normal or good tidal volume (GTV), deep, or shallow.

Ease of Breathing

The ease with which a patient is breathing will reveal much about his current respiratory status. A patient who is oxygenating well will breathe easily and show little if any work of breathing. His respirations may be described as unlabored. In contrast, a patient in respiratory distress will likely use accessory muscles and labor much harder to move air. A patient's level of distress can be quantified by the number of words he can speak before having to take another breath. A patient who can only speak two or three words between breaths is in more severe distress compared to a patient who can speak six- to eight-word sentences.

PRACTICAL PATHOPHYSIOLOGY

The increased work of breathing (respiratory distress) is a sure sign that the body is not able to take in an adequate amount of oxygen. The body's way of compensating for an inadequate supply of oxygen is to increase both rate and volume in an attempt to meet the demands of the body.

You must observe for the presence of retractions during inspiration. This is the drawing in of the soft tissues, most commonly in the areas above the clavicles (supraclavicular), between the ribs (intercostal), and below the ribs (subcostal). Retractions are most obvious in thin adults and pediatric patients who are in moderate to severe respiratory distress.

Ease of respirations is described as either unlabored or as labored (mild, moderate, or severe).

Breath Sounds

9-7 Describe the proper method for auscultating breath sounds to determine their presence, equality, and the likely underlying causes of abnormal breath sounds.

wheezing a high-pitched sound that is indicative of lower airway constriction and can be heard during both inspiration and expiration but is more commonly heard during expiration.

stridor a harsh high-pitched sound that generally occurs during inhalation but can also occur during exhalation, indicative of partial upper airway obstruction.

crackles a fine-crackling or bubbling sound heard upon inspiration. The sound is caused as air passes through fluid in the alveoli or by the opening of closed alveoli.

Once you are at the patient's side, you may be able to hear certain sounds associated with his breathing. Be extra alert for noisy respirations, because they are almost always a sign of partial airway obstruction. The following are names and descriptions of some of the abnormal sounds that might be heard when a patient breathes. Some sounds may only be heard when using a stethoscope.

- *Wheezing.* A high-pitched sound, **wheezing** is indicative of lower airway constriction. It can be heard during both inhalation and exhalation but is more commonly heard during exhalation. Mild wheezes may only be heard with a stethoscope. Wheezing is commonly heard when the bronchioles become constricted such as with asthma, bronchitis, or severe allergy.
- *Stridor.* A harsh, high-pitched sound, **stridor** can occur during inhalation or exhalation and is indicative of partial upper airway obstruction. It is most often heard in pediatric patients who have swelling of the larynx.
- *Crackles.* Fine crackling sounds, **crackles** can be heard with a stethoscope during inhalation as air is forced through fluid or mucus in the lower airways. Conditions such as pulmonary edema and pneumonia often cause crackles.

Not all sounds are going to be easily audible. As an EMT you must assess for the presence or absence of sounds deep within the lungs. To adequately assess lung sounds, you must use an appropriate stethoscope. You will use it to listen over several areas of the chest and back for appropriate or abnormal lung sounds (Figure 9-5 ■). Lung sounds are made by air as it moves in and out of the lungs. When assessing lung sounds, you are listening for the presence of air movement in all lung fields; clear sounds free of crackles, stridor, and wheezing; and equal sounds on both sides of the chest.

The following are examples of appropriate ways to document respirations:

16, unlabored with good tidal volume
24, labored and deep

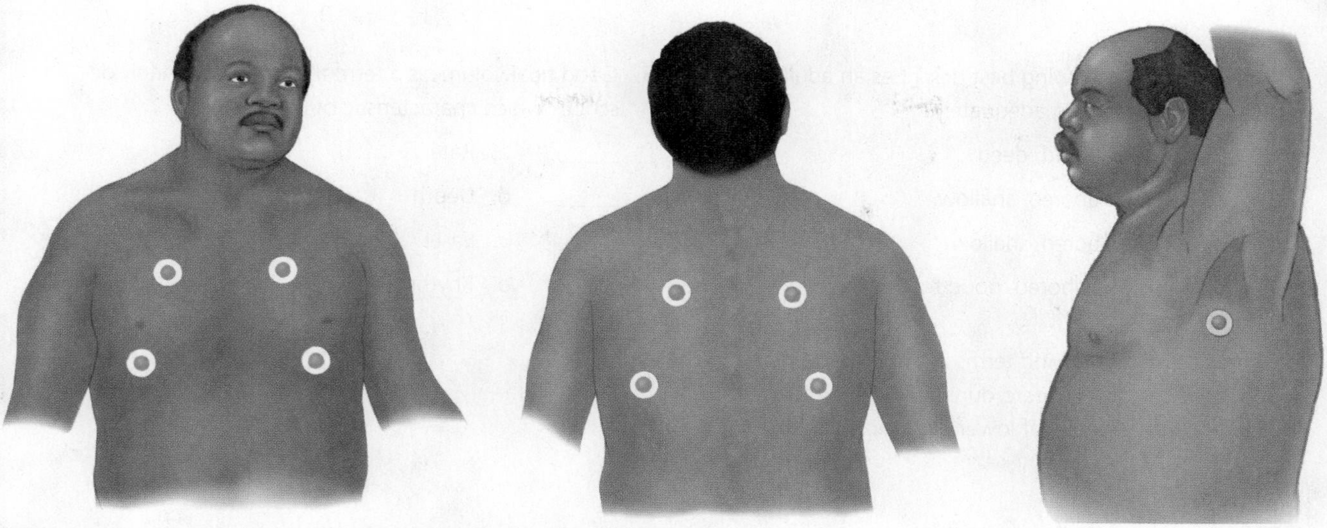

Figure 9-5 Common auscultation points on the chest, back, and midaxillary regions.

8, irregular and shallow

32, labored and shallow

To assess a patient's breathing, follow these steps:

1. Take appropriate BSI precautions.
2. Grasp the wrist of the patient as if you were taking his pulse and place his forearm firmly against the upper abdomen.
3. While looking at your watch, feel the movement of each breath against his forearm as you continue to hold it.
4. Count the number of respirations for 15 or 30 seconds and multiply by the appropriate number to get a minute rate.
5. Note the time and document your findings.

STOP, REVIEW, REMEMBER!

Multiple Choice

For each question, place a check next to the correct answer.

1. Which one of the following best describes the difference between a sign and a symptom?

_____ a. A sign is something the EMT can see or measure, and a symptom is something the patient complains about.

_____ b. A sign is something the patient complains about, and a symptom is something the EMT can see or measure.

_____ c. Assessing signs requires the use of special equipment (blood pressure cuff) while symptoms do not.

_____ d. Signs and symptoms are essentially the same thing.

2. Which one of the following contains the appropriate characteristics of respirations?

_____ a. Rate, depth, and quality

_____ b. Rate, ease, and quality

_____ c. Rate, depth, and ease

_____ d. Rate, depth, and rhythm

(continued on next page)

(continued)

3. Which one of the following best describes an adult patient who is breathing adequately?

_____ a. 18, labored, deep

_____ b. 8, unlabored, shallow

_____ c. 26, labored, shallow

_____ d. 12, unlabored, good tidal volume

4. Which one of the following terms is a high-pitched sound more commonly heard during exhalation than inhalation and is indicative of lower airway constriction?

_____ a. Stridor

_____ b. Wheezing

_____ c. Crowing

_____ d. Grunting

5. Good tidal volume is a term that most accurately describes which characteristic of breathing?

_____ a. Rate

_____ b. Depth

_____ c. Ease

_____ d. Rhythm

Fill in the Blank

1. A ______________________________ is something that you, the EMT, can see or observe.

2. A ______________________________ is something the patient describes or complains of.

3. Skin signs and ______________________________ are not exactly vital to life, but they can tell us a great deal about the patient's current condition.

4. The first set of vital signs taken on any patient is referred to as ______________________________ vital signs.

5. ______________________________ are recorded as a per-minute value.

Critical Thinking

1. Why is recording the time so important when documenting multiple sets of vital signs for the same patient?

____

____

____

____

2. Describe the difference between a sign and a symptom.

____

____

____

____

3. What is meant by the term *baseline vital signs*? Why are baseline vital signs so important?

____

____

____

____

Assessing the Pulse

9-8 Describe the proper method for assessing a pulse in both responsive and unresponsive adults as well as pediatric patients.

A pulse can be thought of as a remote heartbeat. It is the pulsation of the artery as it swells under the pressure of the rushing blood each time the heart pumps. If you could open up the body and see the entire network of arteries, you would see that all arteries pulsate along their entire length. You are able to feel this pulsing only at specific points on the body where the artery lies close to the skin and directly over a firm structure such as a bone. There are *pulse points* throughout the body, some more easily palpated (felt) than others (Figure 9-6 ■). The following is a list of the most common pulse points and their location on the body:

- The **carotid pulse** is located in the anterior neck.
- The **brachial pulse** is felt in two locations: on the inside of the upper arm and over the medial aspect of the anterior elbow.
- The **radial pulse** is located over the lateral aspect of the anterior wrist.
- The **femoral pulse** is located deep in the groin between the hip and the inside of the upper leg.
- The **popliteal pulse** is located over the posterior aspect of the knee.
- The **dorsalis pedis (pedal) pulse** is located over the anterior (dorsal) foot.
- The **posterior tibial pulse** is located over the medial ankle just posterior to the ankle bone.

carotid pulse the pulse point located on either side of the anterior neck lateral to the trachea.

brachial pulse pulse point felt in two locations: on the inside of the upper arm and over the medial aspect of the anterior elbow.

radial pulse pulse point located over the lateral aspect of the anterior wrist.

femoral pulse pulse point located deep in the groin between the hip and the inside of the upper thigh.

popliteal pulse pulse point located over the posterior aspect of the knee.

dorsalis pedis (pedal) pulse pulse point located over the anterior foot.

posterior tibial pulse pulse point located over the medial ankle just posterior to the ankle bone.

The most common pulse point used to assess the pulse of a responsive patient is the radial pulse (Figure 9-7 ■). Palpating the radial pulse is less intrusive than palpating the carotid pulse. The radial pulse is preferred for all responsive patients one year and older.

For unresponsive patients older than one year, the carotid pulse is preferred (Figure 9-8 ■), because the carotid is a *central pulse* (related to the core of the body). It is also one of the last pulses to go away as blood pressure drops and in situations of shock (hypoperfusion). The femoral pulse also is considered a central pulse. In contrast, the brachial, radial, and pedal pulse points are called *peripheral pulses* because they are located in the periphery of the body.

As blood pressure drops, the peripheral pulses become less reliable and can become difficult to palpate. For this reason, the carotid pulse should always be assessed before beginning CPR on any patient over one year old and the brachial pulse for patients younger than one year old (Figure 9-9 ■). Do not assess both carotid pulses at the same time, because this can dangerously reduce the blood flow to the brain.

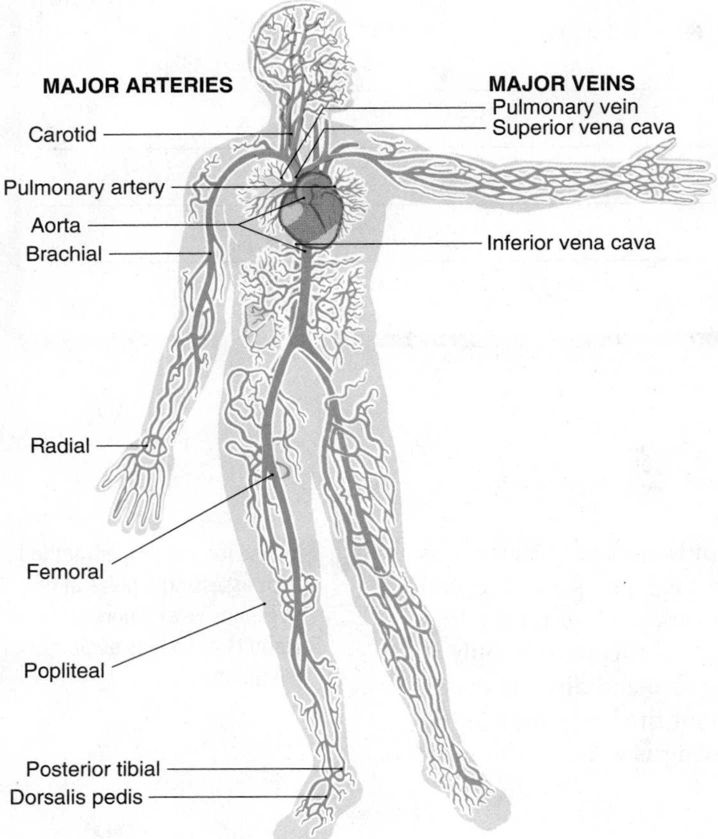

Figure 9-6 Major arteries and pulse points.

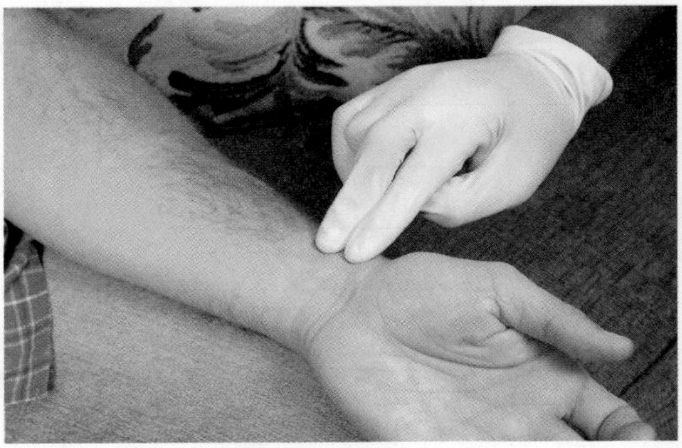

Figure 9-7 Palpating the radial pulse point.

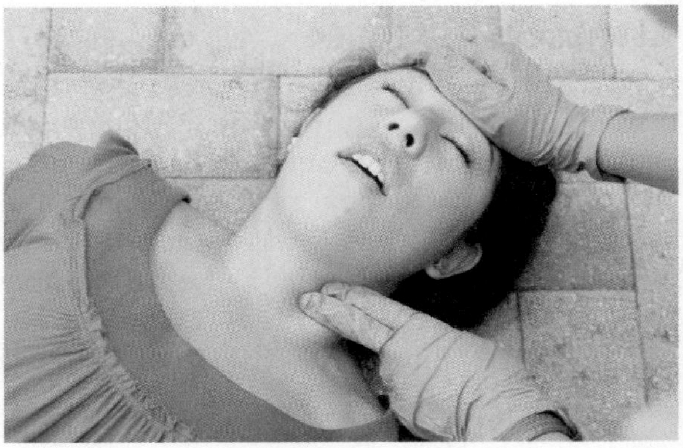

Figure 9-8 Palpating the carotid pulse point on an unresponsive patient.

9-10 Differentiate between normal and abnormal findings when assessing a patient's pulse to include the rate, strength, and rhythm.

palpation the act of examining by feeling with the hands. Also a technique used for obtaining a blood pressure reading.

Becoming proficient at palpating pulses (feeling a pulse with your fingers) requires lots of practice. There are essentially two elements you must master. The first is location. You must place your fingers in the correct place or you will not feel the pulse. The second element is pressure. You must learn to apply the correct amount of pressure for each pulse point or you risk not feeling the pulse. Too much pressure and you can cut off the pulse completely. Too little pressure and you will not feel the pulsations.

When first learning to assess pulses, you must experiment with different techniques of **palpation** (feeling). Some EMTs have better luck using the tips of the fingers, while others prefer the pads of the fingers. Some prefer using two fingers to locate a pulse, while others prefer three fingers. You must try all combinations, and eventually you will find the technique that works best for you.

When assessing a patient's pulse, the EMT should identify the following three characteristics: rate, strength, and rhythm.

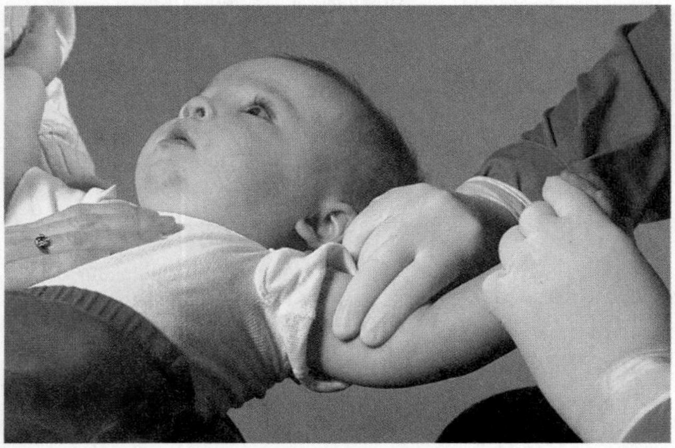

Figure 9-9 Palpating the brachial pulse point in an infant. (© Daniel Limmer)

Pulse Rate

Just as with breathing rate, pulse rate is recorded as the number of pulsations (beats) felt in one minute. The same two methods can be used for determining a minute rate for a pulse as are used for breathing. Count the pulse for either 15 seconds and multiply by 4 or 30 seconds and multiply by 2.

TABLE 9-3 PULSE RATES

NORMAL PULSE RATES (BEATS PER MINUTE, AT REST)	
ADULT	60 to 100
INFANTS AND CHILDREN	
Adolescent 11–14 years	60 to 104
School age 6–10 years	70 to 110
Preschooler 3–5 years	80 to 120
Toddler 1–3 years	80 to 130
Infant 6–12 months	80 to 140
Infant 0–5 months	90 to 140
Newborn	120 to 160
PULSE QUALITY	**SIGNIFICANCE/POSSIBLE CAUSES**
Rapid and regular	Exertion, fright, fever, high blood pressure, first stage of blood loss
Rapid and regular	Shock, later stages of blood loss
Slow	Drugs, some poisons, some heart problems, lack of oxygen in children, and severe head injury
Irregular	Possible abnormal electrical heart activity (arrhythmia)
No pulse	Cardiac arrest (clinical death)

The normal range for pulse rates in adults is between 60 and 100 beats per minute. A pulse rate below 60 is referred to as **bradycardia** and a pulse rate greater than 100 is called **tachycardia** (Table 9-3).

In infants and children, a high pulse rate is not as great a concern as a low pulse. A low pulse rate could indicate imminent cardiac arrest due to lack of adequate oxygen.

9-9 Associate pulse abnormalities with possible underlying causes.

bradycardia a pulse rate below 60 beats per minute.

tachycardia a pulse rate greater than 100 beats per minute.

PRACTICAL PATHOPHYSIOLOGY

Just as we saw with breathing, the body has the ability to adjust pulse rate to meet the immediate needs of the vital organs. Depending on the situation, the heart rate may increase or decrease in order to maintain an appropriate blood pressure. This is all controlled by the part of the brain called the *medulla*, which receives signals from different receptor sites throughout the body.

Strength of Pulse

Pulses can be absent to weak to strong. Many factors contribute to each circumstance. As you learn to assess pulses on your classmates, you will find most to be strong because all of you are likely young and healthy. You may not ever get to feel a weak pulse until you finally work in the field and encounter patients with real medical problems. The key is to practice taking pulses every chance you get with as many different people as possible. Eventually, you will feel pulses that you will describe as weak.

CLINICAL CLUE

Palpation Technique

The strength of a pulse is recorded as either strong or weak. But be careful. Sometimes the reason why you may be feeling the pulse as weak is that you are not directly over the pulse point or you are not using the appropriate amount of pressure.

PRACTICAL PATHOPHYSIOLOGY

The strength of a patient's pulse can be affected by many factors such as environment, level of exertion, and even mood. The strength of a pulse is often directly related to blood pressure. When the blood pressure increases, the strength of the pulse increases, and when the blood pressure drops, the pulse often becomes weaker.

Pulse Rhythm

The rhythm of a pulse is a very important characteristic, because it may reveal a serious heart problem. Normal pulses have a steady, constant, regular rhythm, much like a metronome. Pulses that seem erratic or that skip beats are considered irregular. As an EMT you will record the rhythm of a patient's pulse as either regular or irregular.

To assess the pulse of a patient, follow these steps:

1. Take appropriate BSI precautions.
2. For a responsive patient, grasp the patient's wrist and locate the radial pulse point with the tips of at least two fingers. For an unresponsive patient, locate the carotid artery in the neck.
3. While looking at your watch, count the pulsations of the artery for 15 or 30 seconds. To get the minute rate multiply the number of pulsations by either 4 or 2 as appropriate.
4. Note the time and document your findings.

9-11 Explain systolic and diastolic blood pressure readings and identify potential causes of abnormal findings or changes.

Assessing Blood Pressure

Blood pressure is the pressure inside the arterial system. It is a very dynamic value that changes constantly as we move about our day. Factors such as blood loss, stress, ambient temperature, and exertion all can influence a patient's blood pressure. In general, the better the blood pressure, the better the perfusion.

Blood pressure is most often recorded as two numbers separated by a horizontal line or slash mark, such as 120/80 (Table 9-4). Those two numbers represent two different pressures within the arterial system of the body. Blood pressures are measured in millimeters of mercury (mmHg). *Hg* is the chemical symbol for mercury on the periodic table of elements. The old style of blood pressure gauges (sphygmomanometers) used the heavy metal mercury much as conventional thermometers do today. Because they were not practical for use in the field, newer fluidless (aneroid) gauges had to be developed. Even though the gauges used in the field today do not contain mercury, they are still calibrated in millimeters of mercury.

PRACTICAL PATHOPHYSIOLOGY

Although adequate perfusion with good blood pressure is essential to normal organ function, chronically elevated blood pressure (generally defined in adults as greater than 140/90) can result in increased risk for stroke, heart attacks, and kidney failure.

There are two methods for obtaining a blood pressure in the field. The **auscultation** (hearing) method requires the use of a blood pressure cuff and a stethoscope. The palpation (feeling) method requires only a blood pressure cuff.

auscultation the act of listening for sounds made by internal organs such as the lungs and the heart. Also the technique used to listen for pulse sounds when obtaining a blood pressure.

It is recommended that blood pressure be assessed in all patients over the age of three. Patients under the age of three require an especially small blood pressure cuff,

TABLE 9-4 NORMAL BLOOD PRESSURES IN ADULTS, CHILDREN, AND INFANTS

PATIENT	SYSTOLIC	DIASTOLIC
Adult male	100 + age in years to age 40	60 to 90 mmHg
Adult female	90 + age in years to age 40	60 to 90 mmHg
Adolescent	90 mmHg (lower limit of normal)	2/3 of systolic pressure
Child 1 to 10 years	90 + (2 × age in years) (upper limit of normal)	2/3 of systolic pressure
	70 + (2 × age in years) (lower limit of normal)	
Infant 1 to 12 months	70 mmHg (lower limit of normal)	2/3 of systolic pressure

and because they move around so much, it is difficult to measure their blood pressure in the field. When assessing young pediatric patients, it is advised that you rely on signs and symptoms other than blood pressure, along with your general impression and other exam findings, to determine the indicated care. Those signs and symptoms are often more valuable and take less time to assess.

In a blood pressure reading such as 120/80, which may be spoken as "120 over 80," the top number is called the **systolic** reading. It reflects the pressure inside the artery each time the heart's left ventricle contracts. The bottom number is called the **diastolic** reading and reflects the pressure inside the artery each time the heart rests between beats.

systolic the pressure created when the left ventricle contracts and forces blood out into the arteries.

diastolic the pressure remaining in the arteries when the left ventricle of the heart is relaxed and refilling.

Blood Pressure Equipment

Blood pressure equipment includes the blood pressure cuff and stethoscope (ear pieces, tubing, and head).

BLOOD PRESSURE CUFF

The blood pressure cuff is a simple device consisting of a flat bladder (balloon) with two tubes coming off one side. The bladder is contained within a simple fabric cuff or pouch with a Velcro closure. A bulb-and-valve combination is placed on one tube, and the gauge is placed on the other tube (Figure 9-10 ■).

Cuffs come in many sizes, and it is best to use the correct size when taking a blood pressure. A cuff is the correct size if the bladder inside the cuff can cover approximately 80% of the patient's upper arm. For a child under the age of 13, it should cover 100% of the arm. A cuff that is too narrow will result in high pressure readings.

To properly place the blood pressure cuff on a patient's arm, pick it up with both hands so that you can feel the top corners of the bladder with the thumb and forefinger of each hand. Then, with the labels facing you, place the center of the bladder directly over the brachial artery located on the inside of the upper arm. The cuff should be placed high enough on the arm to allow access to the brachial pulse point on the anterior aspect of the elbow.

STETHOSCOPE

It has been said that the stethoscope is the most important diagnostic tool ever developed. While this may be debatable, what is not debatable is the importance and

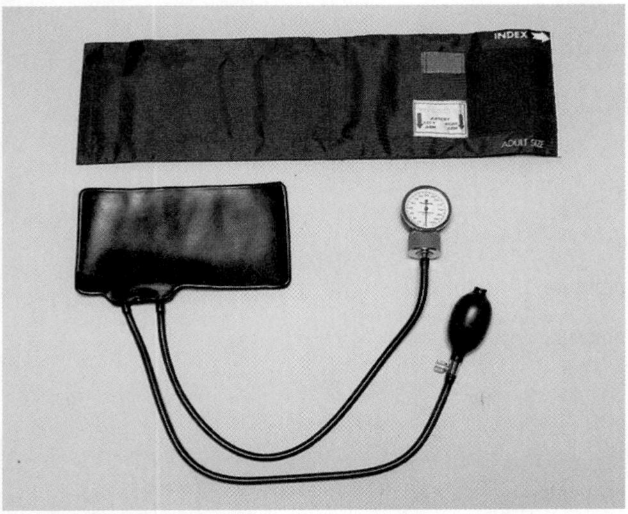

Figure 9-10 Components of a blood pressure cuff.

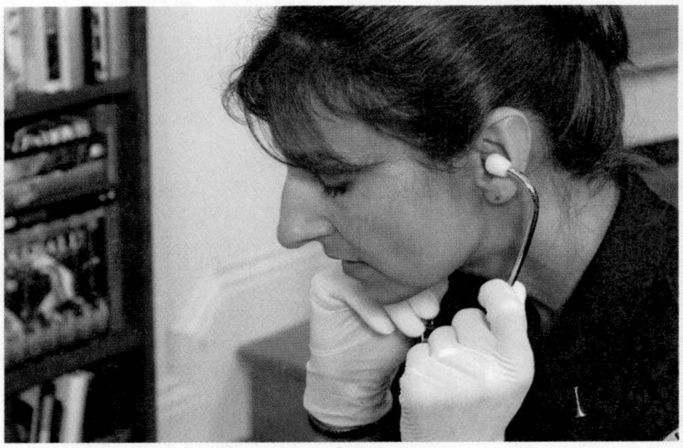

Figure 9-11 Proper positioning of stethoscope ear pieces.

challenge of learning to use it properly. Like any tool, it must be used often if you ever hope to develop mastery (Figure 9-11 ■).

The typical stethoscope has three main parts: ear pieces, tubing, and head. It is important that both ear pieces and the head be adjusted and placed properly to ensure that you will be able to hear the sounds necessary to record a blood pressure.

The ear pieces consist of two metal tubes that are curved at one end with plastic or soft rubber ear tips at the end of each tube. The opposite ends are inserted into the rubber tubing. One of the most important aspects of using a stethoscope properly is the placement of the ear pieces. The ear pieces are adjustable and can easily turn in a circular fashion. Pick up the stethoscope and hold the ear pieces, one in each hand. Then adjust them so that they are both pointing slightly forward or outward away from you. This will help ensure that they seat properly inside your ears. Your ear canals are directed forward toward your nose, and by adjusting the ear pieces, you can ensure that the openings are pointed directly into your ear canal. Ear pieces that are not adjusted properly may be blocked by the ear itself, making it difficult to hear the sounds of the blood pressure. Once the ear pieces are seated comfortably in your ears, tap gently on the diaphragm to ensure that you can hear well. If not, readjust the ear pieces.

Stethoscope tubing comes in two basic styles. The most common is "Y" shaped. Each end of the "Y" attaches to an ear piece and the stem of the "Y" connects to the diaphragm. In the other style, a separate tube comes off each ear piece and they connect at the diaphragm. Regardless of which style your instructor recommends, just ensure that the tubing is straight and has no bends or kinks in it.

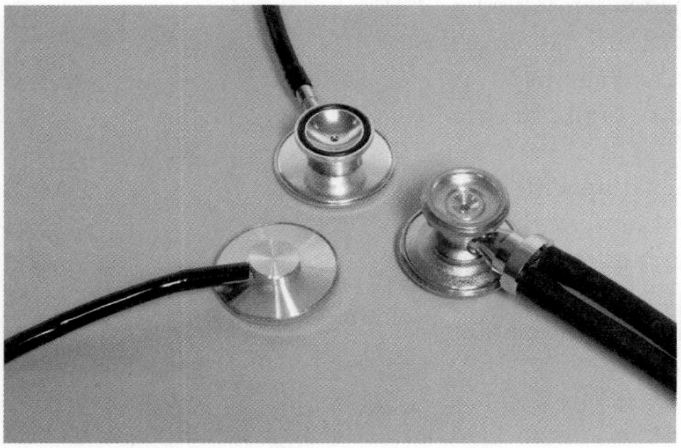

Figure 9-12 Stethoscopes come with various types of heads.

The head also comes in two basic styles, the single head and the double head (Figure 9-12 ■). The single head is the most common and the easiest to use when learning to take blood pressure. It consists of a round, metallic, concave disk that is covered by a plastic diaphragm much like the skin that covers a drum. The diaphragm is held in place over the head by a round threaded ring.

A double head consists of the diaphragm described above on one side and a bell shaped cone on the opposite side. The flat diaphragm is best suited for listening to high-pitched sounds, such as those in the lungs. The bell is used for picking up low-pitched sounds, such as those made by the heart. The diaphragm is the most common side for obtaining a blood pressure; the bell side may also be used for blood pressures, depending on preference.

It is important to realize that the double-headed stethoscope must be adjusted to the side you want to listen with. When one side is turned on, the other side is closed off so no sound can be heard through it. This is accomplished by holding the tubing right at the head and turning the head. You will feel a click when it is positioned properly. Failing to make this adjustment properly is the single most common reason a new EMT has difficulty hearing when using a double-headed stethoscope. In addition, many stethoscopes have a flat side or marking indicating the "active" side. Please make sure you have the proper side turned on so you can hear the appropriate sounds.

Blood Pressure by Auscultation

9-12 Describe the proper method for obtaining blood pressure by both palpation and auscultation.

There are two methods of obtaining a blood pressure: auscultation and palpation. Auscultation is the more accurate of the two methods and requires the use of a stethoscope. Learning to take blood pressure using this method can be very cumbersome and frustrating at first, but with enough practice one becomes quite comfortable using the technique. Taking a blood pressure by auscultation requires a relatively quiet environment in order to hear the necessary sounds. By far the most challenging part of learning to take blood pressure by auscultation is learning to distinguish blood pressure sounds from the multitude of other sounds caused by movement.

Once the blood pressure cuff and stethoscope are in place and the cuff is inflated, you have created a tourniquet and the cuff is restricting all blood flow to the arm. For this reason, do not keep the cuff fully inflated any longer than is absolutely necessary. You must then open the valve near the bulb to release the pressure inside the cuff. At some point as you release the pressure in the cuff, the blood will begin rushing past the cuff with each beat of the heart. This flow of blood past the cuff can be heard through the stethoscope that is placed lower down, over the brachial pulse point. The sound is most often described as a "beat." At the first sound of blood rushing past the cuff or "beat" that you hear, the gauge indicates the systolic blood pressure. You must continue to listen for the sound of the beats and note when the last sound occurs. This is when the pressure on both sides of the cuff equalizes and the gauge reveals the diastolic pressure.

The exact sounds you hear will be slightly different with every patient. Sometimes the sounds are loud and distinct and easily heard. Other times they are distant and faint and difficult to hear. Lots of practice on many different people is the only way to develop mastery at taking blood pressure.

PERSPECTIVE

Ray—The EMT

Listening for Dick's blood pressure was a real challenge on this call. His mother kept talking, Dick kept throwing up or moving his arm to hold onto the garbage can, or I just got the normal junk-noise, like the creaking sound of the cuff as it inflated or deflated. It can get frustrating. I finally ended up just getting his systolic pressure by palpation—and it was very low. You know, when I was new on the streets and was having trouble getting a pressure, I would be tempted to just make it up. That's no lie. But then I realized that we get vitals for a reason. What if I faked it and the seriousness of the patient's condition got overlooked? Now, I always get solid sets of vitals no matter what it takes.

When first learning to take blood pressure in class, have your patient lie down on the floor with his arm out to the side. That will allow you to lay the gauge on the floor next to the cuff or on the patient's abdomen where it can be seen easily. It is a good

SCAN 9-1 Obtaining Blood Pressure by Auscultation

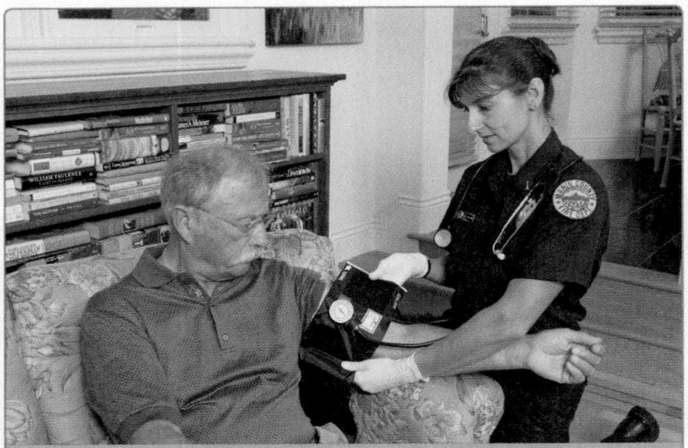

9-1-1 Place the center of the cuff against the inside of the upper arm and secure snugly.

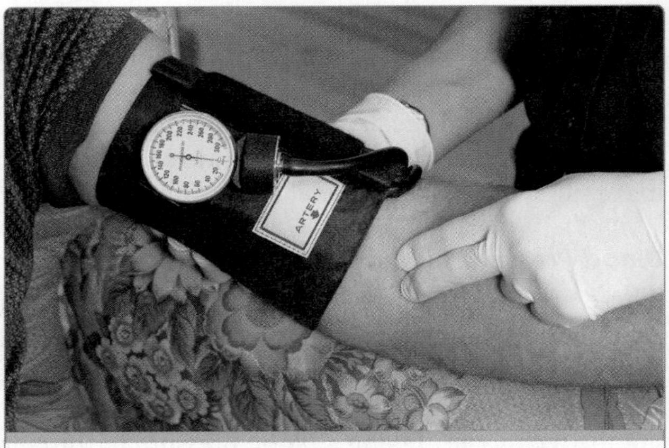

9-1-2 Locate the brachial pulse point on the anterior aspect of the elbow. Place the diaphragm of the stethoscope over the pulse point.

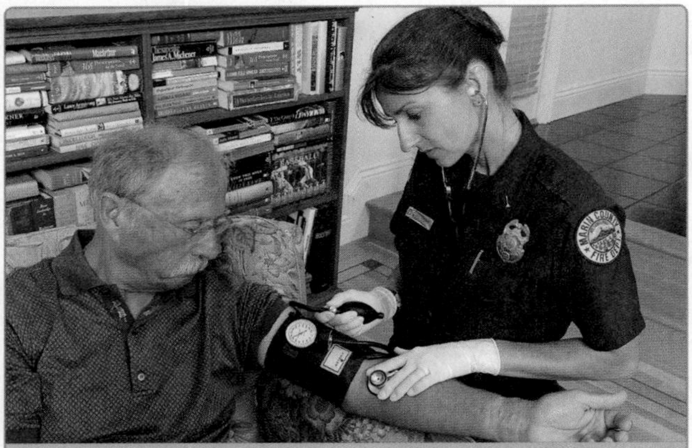

9-1-3 Quickly inflate the cuff then slowly release the air while watching the gauge. Listen for the sounds of the blood pressure.

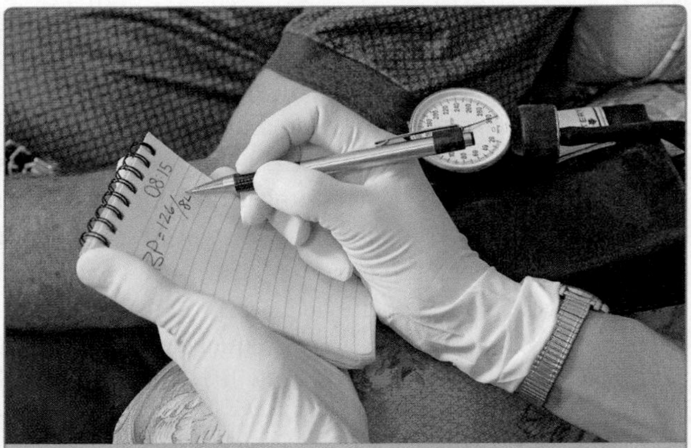

9-1-4 Record your findings along with the time.

idea to switch arms after every two or three attempts, just to give the arms a break. Once you get comfortable taking blood pressure on a person who is lying down, you can then practice on people in other positions, such as sitting and standing.

To assess a patient's blood pressure by auscultation, follow these steps (Scan 9-1):

1. Take appropriate BSI precautions.
2. Place the BP cuff appropriately on the upper arm. Ensure that the gauge remains visible.
3. Ask the patient if he knows what his blood pressure is normally.
4. Place the stethoscope in your ears and the diaphragm over the brachial pulse point on the anterior elbow.
5. Ensure that the valve is closed, and inflate the cuff to approximately 30 mmHg above where the patient indicated his systolic pressure is normally. If in doubt, inflate to 160 mmHg.

SCAN 9-2 Obtaining Blood Pressure by Palpation

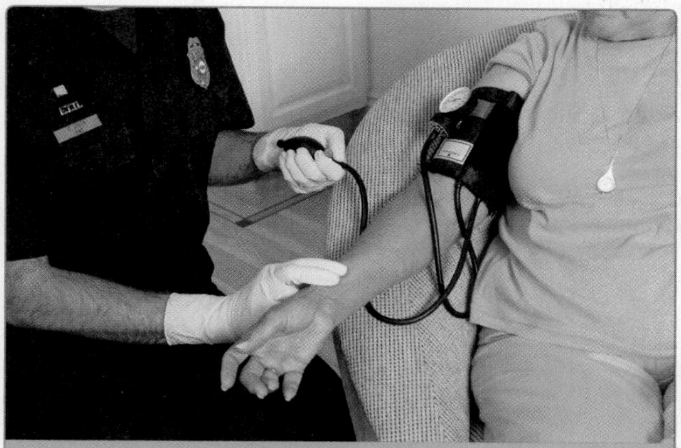

9-2-1 After placing the cuff, locate the radial pulse in the same arm.

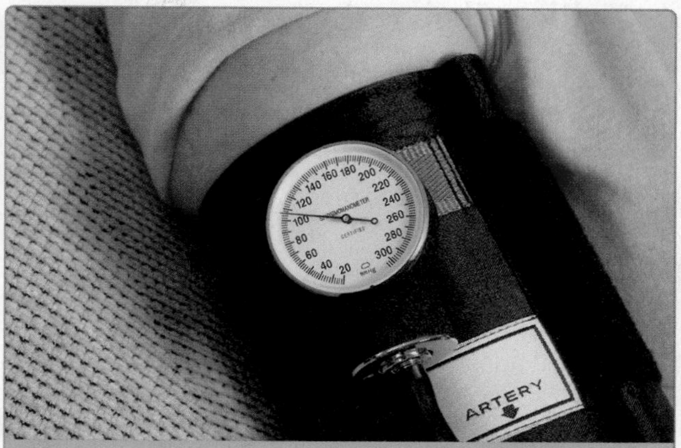

9-2-2 Inflate the cuff until the pulse goes away. Release the pressure and note the pressure when the pulse returns.

6. Open the valve and deflate the cuff slowly, while listening for the pulse sounds.
7. Note where the needle on the gauge is when you hear the first significant sound (systolic) and the last significant sound (diastolic).
8. Note the time and document your findings.

Blood Pressure by Palpation

An alternative to taking a blood pressure by auscultation is taking it by palpation. This is a good alternative when the environment is too noisy or you want to take vitals on multiple patients as quickly as possible. Blood pressures taken by palpation are not as accurate as those taken with a stethoscope but they still can be used to trend a patient if necessary.

Instead of using a stethoscope to hear the blood rushing past the cuff, you will use your fingers placed over the radial pulse to feel the blood as it causes a pulse. Taking a blood pressure by palpation will reveal only the approximate systolic pressure and does not give the diastolic pressure. You will record a blood pressure taken by palpation as the number over the letter P, such as 120/P.

To assess a patient's blood pressure by palpation, follow these steps (Scan 9-2):

1. Take appropriate BSI precautions.
2. Place the BP cuff appropriately on the upper arm. Ensure that the gauge remains visible.
3. Ask the patient if he knows what his blood pressure is normally.
4. Locate the radial pulse in the same arm where you placed the cuff.
5. Ensure that the valve is closed and inflate the cuff to approximately 30 mmHg above where you last felt a radial pulse.
6. Open the valve and deflate the cuff slowly while feeling for the radial pulse to return.
7. Note the location of the needle on the gauge when you feel the first beat return at the radial pulse. This is the approximate systolic blood pressure.
8. Note the time and record your findings.

STOP, REVIEW, REMEMBER!

Multiple Choice

For each question, place a check next to the correct answer.

1. Which one of the following best describes the characteristics you should be looking for when assessing a pulse?

_____ a. Rate, strength, volume

_____ b. Rate, strength, rhythm

_____ c. Rate, regularity, volume

_____ d. Rate, volume, rhythm

2. Which one of the following best describes the most common reason(s) for you to have difficulty in obtaining a pulse on a healthy patient?

_____ a. Wrong finger placement and too many fingers

_____ b. Using the tips instead of the pads of the fingers

_____ c. Using the pads instead of the tips of the fingers

_____ d. Wrong finger placement and pressure

3. Which one of the following is a good question to ask *before* taking a blood pressure on any patient?

_____ a. Is your blood pressure always low?

_____ b. Is your blood pressure always high?

_____ c. What is your blood pressure normally?

_____ d. When is the last time you had your blood pressure taken?

4. When taking a blood pressure by auscultation, you should continue to inflate the cuff until the gauge reads _____________ mmHg higher than the point where the sound of the pulse disappeared.

_____ a. 10

_____ b. 30

_____ c. 50

_____ d. 60

5. Which one of the following statements is most accurate about the value of blood pressure in determining a patient's condition?

_____ a. Multiple readings are necessary to reveal a trend.

_____ b. Blood pressure can reveal very little about a patient's condition.

_____ c. Pulses are more revealing than blood pressures.

_____ d. Trending does not pertain to taking blood pressures.

Matching

Match the term on the left with the applicable definition on the right.

1. _____ Auscultation
2. _____ Brachial pulse
3. _____ Bradycardia
4. _____ Diastolic pressure
5. _____ Palpation
6. _____ Pulse
7. _____ Systolic pressure
8. _____ Tachycardia

A. Pressure wave felt over an artery, caused by contraction of the heart

B. Pressure exerted on the walls of the arteries when the heart is at rest

C. Abnormally rapid heart rate (above 100)

D. Pulse point located at the medial aspect of the upper arm

E. Pressure exerted on the walls of the arteries when the heart is contracting

F. Listening for sounds with a stethoscope

G. Abnormally slow heart rate (below 60)

H. Assessment by touch or feel

Critical Thinking

1. Explain why it is always important to verify the pulse at the carotid artery for patients who are older than one year and do not appear to have a radial pulse.

____

____

____

____

2. What is the value in asking a patient what his blood pressure is normally prior to taking it yourself?

____

____

____

____

3. Explain the meaning of the systolic and diastolic readings of a blood pressure.

____

____

____

____

Assessing Skin Signs

The characteristics of a patient's skin can reveal a lot about his current condition. While skin signs are not always accurate and reliable as a single source of information, they can add to the overall picture of the patient. Skin signs are easy to assess and therefore should be included as part of all baseline vital signs.

9-13 Describe normal and abnormal findings in the assessment of skin color, temperature, moisture, capillary refill, and color of mucous membranes, and associate abnormal skin findings with potential underlying causes.

A patient's skin should be assessed for the color, temperature, moisture, capillary refill, and skin turgor.

Skin Color

Skin color must be assessed in multiple locations to achieve the best overall assessment. In light-skinned patients, it is easy to identify color changes in the skin of the face. In dark-skinned patients, you must rely on the skin in other areas, such as the mucous membranes, conjunctiva, and nail beds for evidence of color change.

Skin color can be assessed in the following areas for evidence of good perfusion: face, nail beds, oral mucosa (inside the lower lip), and conjunctiva (inside the lower eyelid). In pediatric patients, the palms of the hands and soles of the feet also may be assessed. Normal skin color in these locations is pink. Now if you look around and

TABLE 9-5 SKIN TEMPERATURE AND CONDITION	
SKIN TEMPERATURE AND CONDITION	**SIGNIFICANCE/POSSIBLE CAUSES**
Cool, clammy	Sign of shock, anxiety
Cold, moist	Body is losing heat
Cold, dry	Exposure to cold
Hot, dry	High fever, heat exposure
Hot, moist	High fever, heat exposure
"Goose pimples" accompanied by shivering, chattering teeth, blue lips, and pale skin	Chills, communicable disease, exposure to cold, pain, or fear

pale a whitish skin color indicative of poor perfusion.

cyanotic a bluish skin color indicative of poor oxygenation.

flushed a reddish skin color commonly seen when someone is embarrassed or is suffering a heat-related emergency.

jaundiced a yellowish color of the skin and whites of the eyes indicative of poor liver function.

diaphoretic perspiring, sweaty, moist; a characterization of skin condition.

capillary refill test a test used to assess perfusion status in the extremities.

9-14 Describe the proper method for assessing capillary refill time.

pay close attention, you will notice that while everyone's actual skin color is different, it can still be characterized as pink, depending on where you assess.

Abnormal skin colors frequently seen in the field include the following:

- A whitish color is called **pale** skin and is indicative of poor perfusion.
- A bluish skin color indicative of poor oxygenation is described as **cyanotic.**
- An unnatural redness seen primarily in the face is described as **flushed** skin. It is commonly seen when someone is embarrassed or is suffering a heat-related emergency.
- A yellowish color to the skin and whites of the eyes is called **jaundiced** and is indicative of poor liver function.

Skin Temperature

A patient's skin temperature is often relative to his immediate environment. Normal skin temperature is warm (Table 9-5). Skin that is hot, cool, or cold may indicate an underlying medical condition, or it only may be reflecting the environment. So, be aware of this when assessing skin temperature.

Use the back of a nongloved hand placed against the patient's forehead to assess skin temperature (Figure 9-13 ■). Skin temperature is characterized as hot, warm, cool, or cold.

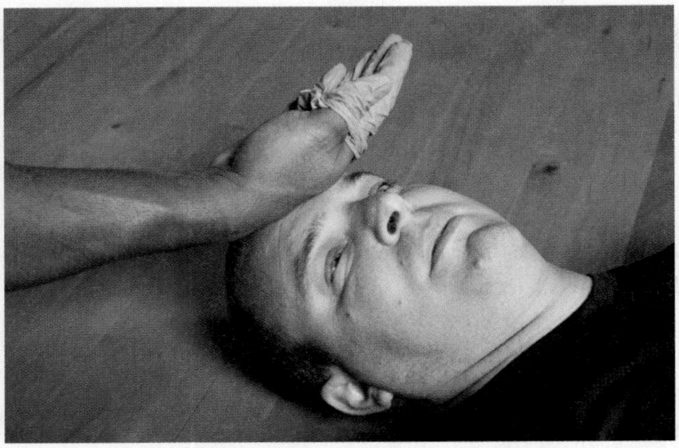

Figure 9-13 Use the back of your ungloved hand to assess skin temperature and moisture.

Skin Moisture

Normal skin is dry to the touch. Skin that is cool and moist or sweaty is called *clammy* or **diaphoretic.** In either case moisture can be caused by physical exertion and may not have anything to do directly with the patient's current medical condition. Skin moisture is most often characterized as dry, diaphoretic, or clammy (cool and moist).

Capillary Refill

The **capillary refill test** is just one tool the EMT can use to assess the perfusion status of a patient. It should be emphasized that the capillary refill test is most reliable in patients younger than six years old and is only one element of an overall assessment that should include pulse rate, blood pressure, and skin signs.

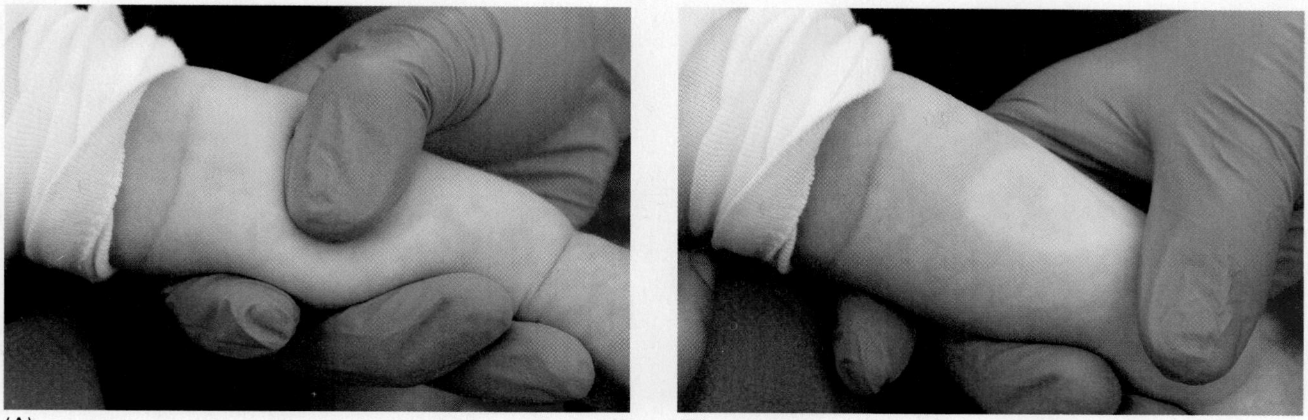

(A) (B)

Figure 9-14 (A) Press firmly against the skin to cause it to blanch. (B) Release the pressure and note the time it takes for the capillaries to refill and the skin to return to normal color.

The capillary refill test is conducted by blanching (pressing until white) a nail bed or the soft tissue of a finger or toe, knee, or upper arm and counting the number of seconds it takes for the capillaries to refill with blood as indicated by the whitened skin turning pink again (Figure 9-14 ■). A capillary refill time of less than two seconds is considered normal. A refill time longer than two seconds is described as delayed and may be an indication of poor perfusion.

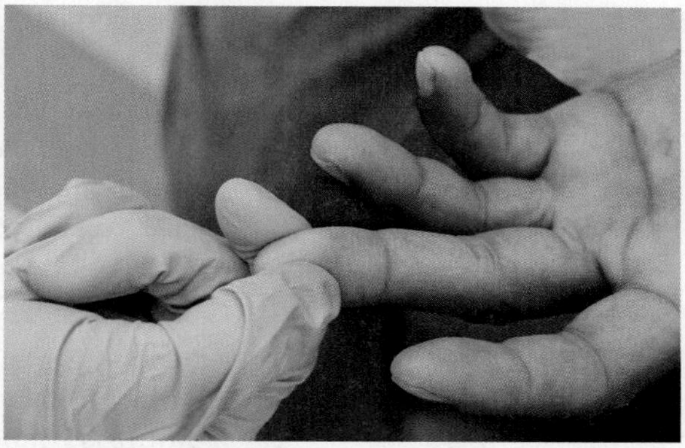

Figure 9-15 Checking capillary refill at the fingertip.

Capillary refill time also can be used to assess the perfusion status of an extremity following an injury. The most common technique for assessing capillary refill time in an adult or child involves pressing a nail bed of the hand or foot and then releasing pressure to observe for refill. This is sometimes difficult, because it requires you to cover the very spot that you are trying to observe for blanching and refill. An alternative method involves squeezing the pad of one finger or toe from both sides (Figure 9-15 ■). This allows the EMT to observe both the blanching and the refill phase of the test for a more accurate assessment.

The capillary refill test requires a well-lit environment in order for you to see the subtle changes in the patient's skin.

9-15 Explain factors that can affect capillary refill findings.

As mentioned earlier, the capillary refill test can be one tool in determining the overall perfusion status of a pediatric patient as well as the perfusion status of a specific extremity in both adults and children. Like any assessment tool, there are several factors that can affect accuracy of the reading. They include underlying medical conditions, prescription medications, and the temperature of the environment.

Skin Turgor

Another assessment that can be performed on the skin is called the *skin turgor test*. This test works best when used on the skin at the back of the hand. It provides some indication of how well or poorly hydrated the patient may be. It is performed by pinching the skin at the back of the patient's hand between your fingers and pulling up slightly (Figure 9-16 ■). If the skin returns to normal position immediately when released, it is a good sign that the patient is likely to be well hydrated. If the skin remains tented, it may indicate a poorly hydrated patient.

> **CLINICAL CLUE**
>
> **Capillary Refill**
>
> Capillary refill alone should not be used to determine the perfusion status of any patient but should be included in your overall assessment of the patient.

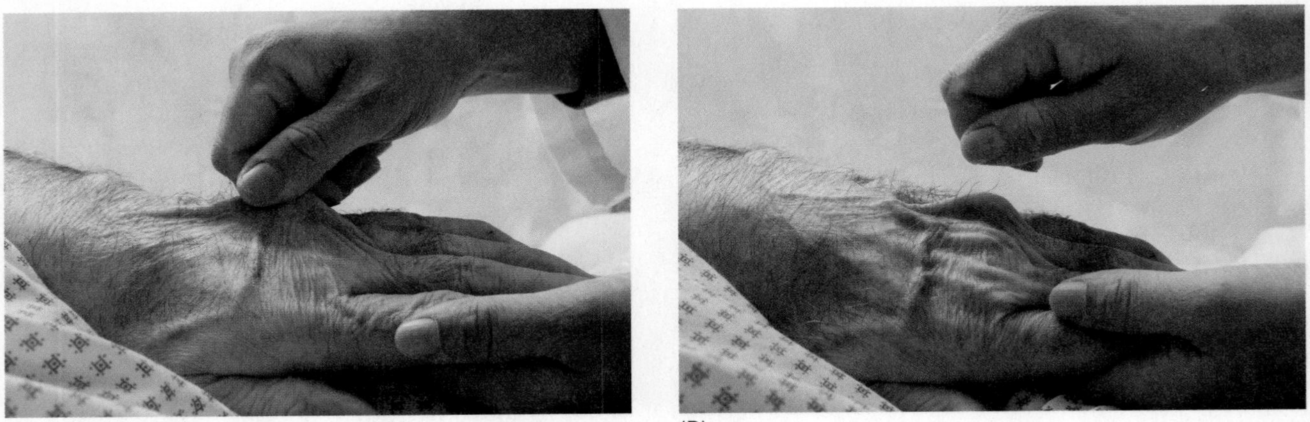

(A) (B)

Figure 9-16 (A) To perform the skin turgor test, gently pinch the skin at the back of the hand and pull up slightly. (B) If the skin remains "tented" it may be a sign of poor hydration.

Assessing the Eyes

9-16 Describe the proper assessment of the pupils and associate abnormal findings with potential underlying causes.

As an EMT you will want to look each and every patient directly in the eyes as you approach him and introduce yourself. This will help you establish an attitude of caring and compassion for the patient that quickly builds rapport and trust. As you examine a patient's eyes, you will be observing for pupil size and shape, equality of pupil size, reactivity to light, and sympathetic movement.

Pupil Size and Shape

As you examine a patient's eyes, look specifically at the pupil, which is the dark circle in the center of the eye. Assess it for approximate size, and note whether or not it is round. To assist in determining approximate pupil size, most EMS-style disposable penlights have a pupil gauge printed on the side. Pupil size can be affected by many things, including medical problems and, of course, ambient light (Figure 9-17 ▪).

Equality of Pupil Size

constricted pupils pupils that are smaller than normal.

dilated pupils pupils that are larger than normal.

The second characteristic of the eyes that must be assessed is the equality of pupil size between both eyes (bilaterally). This is accomplished by observing both pupils and confirming that they are either the same size or not. In some patients you may find that one pupil is larger than the other and this just needs to be noted and documented. Pupils that are small are referred to as **constricted pupils** (Figure 9-18a ▪). When they are large, they are called **dilated pupils** (Figure 9-18b ▪). Pupils that are not of equal size are documented as *unequal* (Figure 9-18c ▪).

Reactivity to Light

Pupils should respond to the sudden introduction of light by constricting and, in contrast, should dilate when light to the pupil is blocked. One of the important signs of good perfusion is pupils that respond briskly to the presence or absence of light. There are at least two methods that can be used to assess pupil reaction, and each depends on the ambient light at the time.

In a well-lit area such as a bright room or the outdoors on a bright sunny day, it may be of no use attempting to shine a light into someone's eyes. The pupils will likely already be constricted due to the large amount of ambient light. In this situation you will have better results covering each of the patient's eyes, one at a time, with

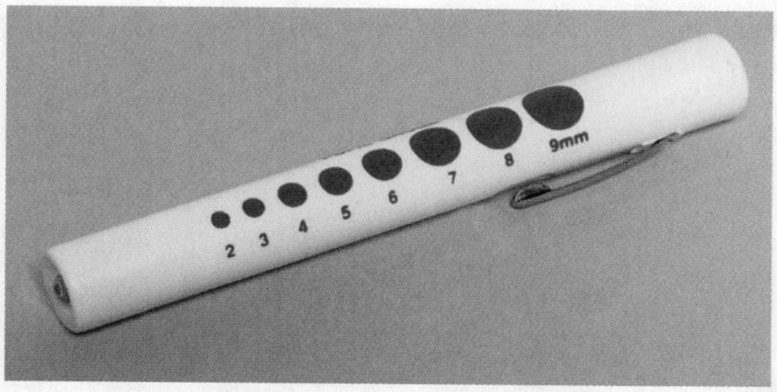

Figure 9-17 A typical disposable penlight with pupil gauge.

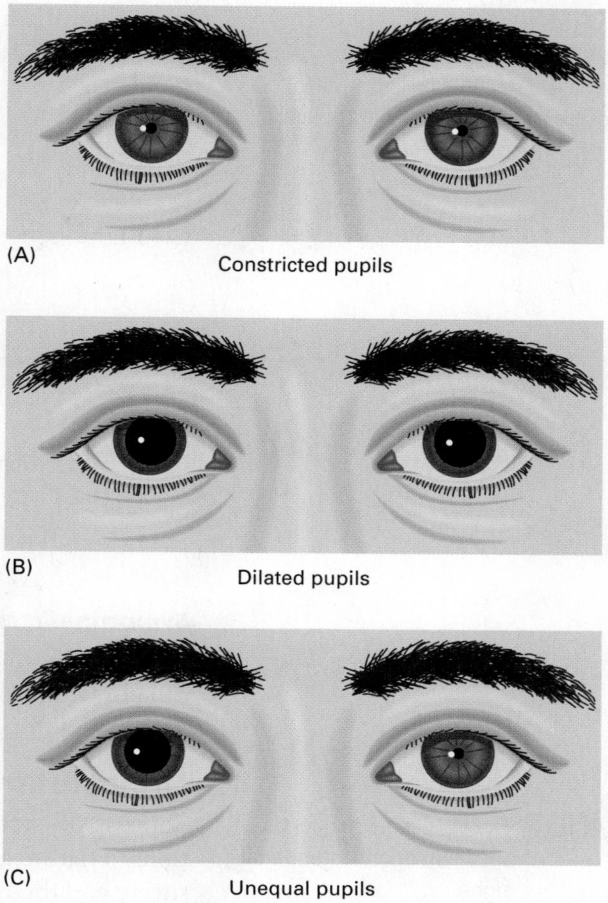

Figure 9-18 (A) Constricted pupils. (B) Dilated pupils. (C) Unequal pupils.

your hand for several seconds, then observing the pupil constrict when you take your hand away. You must learn to be patient when using this method, because it can take some time for the pupil to dilate after you cover the eye. It is a good practice to ask at least two or three questions pertaining to the patient's medical history while you cover each eye. This will allow enough time for the pupil to dilate and not appear as an awkward silence.

In situations where there is not a lot of ambient light, an artificial light source such as a penlight or flashlight will be necessary. Ask the patient to stare straight ahead as you hold the light just outside his field of vision. With the light turned on, quickly move the light from the side directly at his pupil. Watch closely for the pupil to constrict as the light hits it. Then move the light away and watch the pupil dilate slightly and return to its original size.

PERSPECTIVE

Barbara—The Patient's Mother

I didn't understand all the time those two EMTs wasted before getting my son to the hospital. Heart pressures and pulses. They were even looking at his eyes. I'm from the day when if you were sick, then by golly those guys would just load you up and get you to a doctor so he could help you. This poking and prodding in my son's bedroom was an absolute waste of time as far as I'm concerned. It was all just totally unnecessary, absolutely unnecessary.

Both pupils should react to the change in light with the same speed. Pupils that respond slowly to the change in light are documented as *sluggish*. Pupils that do not respond at all are referred to as *fixed*. When a person goes into cardiac arrest, the pupils gradually become fixed and dilated.

PRACTICAL PATHOPHYSIOLOGY

The eyes are very complex structures that demand a constant supply of well-oxygenated blood. When the supply of blood and oxygen is reduced, the ability of the pupils to respond to the presence and absence of light diminishes. Pupils that are not receiving an adequate supply of blood will become increasingly sluggish. Eventually, when perfusion stops, the pupils will become fully dilated and will not respond to light.

An acronym that is widely used in EMS to help EMTs remember the characteristics of pupils is **PERRL**. It stands for:

PERRL a mnemonic used to evaluate a patient's pupils. The letters stand for pupils equal and round reactive to light.

P—Pupils
E—Equal
R—Round
R—Reactive
L—Light

CLINICAL CLUE

PERRL

An earlier version of the PERRL acronym was PERL. The PERRL acronym did not include the "R" for round, which is the shape the pupils should always be. PERRL is now the preferred version.

Sympathetic Movement

Normally, both eyes move together; when one moves so does the other one. This is called *sympathetic movement*. When assessing a patient's eyes or just his pupils, you should look for and confirm that both eyes move together.

Orthostatic Vital Signs

9-17 Explain the method for assessment of orthostatic vital signs.

orthostatic vital signs a test in which vital signs are measured before and after a patient moves from a supine to a sitting or a sitting to a standing position.

Some EMS systems instruct EMTs to obtain **orthostatic vital signs** in certain situations. That means taking blood pressure and pulse readings with a patient lying or sitting and then again when they are sitting or standing. Orthostatic vital signs sometimes reveal that the patient is low on fluid volume. They are typically performed on patients who are not already showing signs of shock but are suspected to be hypovolemic (low fluid volume).

You must first obtain a baseline blood pressure and pulse with the patient lying or sitting. Then have him sit or stand and wait a minute or two for his body to adjust. Retake the blood pressure and pulse. A blood pressure reading that drops more than 20 mmHg, or a pulse that increases more than 20 beats is considered significant and is suggestive of hypovolemia.

Use caution when taking orthostatic vital signs and discontinue if your patient becomes light-headed or dizzy when he sits or stands. Do not attempt to take orthostatic vital signs on trauma patients or on patients with a cardiac history. Do not delay transport for this assessment.

Reassessing Vital Signs

9-18 Explain the criteria for determining the frequency with which vital signs should be reassessed.

Vital signs are dynamic and ever changing, often with little or no outward signs from the patient. Therefore, it is essential that you obtain a thorough and accurate baseline set of vitals as soon as possible and obtain additional sets of vitals as often as appropriate. Each additional set must be immediately compared to the baseline and all previous sets for evidence of a trend.

A patient who you believe is stable may only need additional vital signs taken every 15 minutes or so. A patient who you believe is unstable must have his vitals reassessed every 5 minutes if his condition permits. Do not be concerned about getting additional sets of vitals if the patient requires your immediate care. Patients with a compromised airway or inadequate breathing will need you to perform more important interventions, such as suctioning or assisted ventilations.

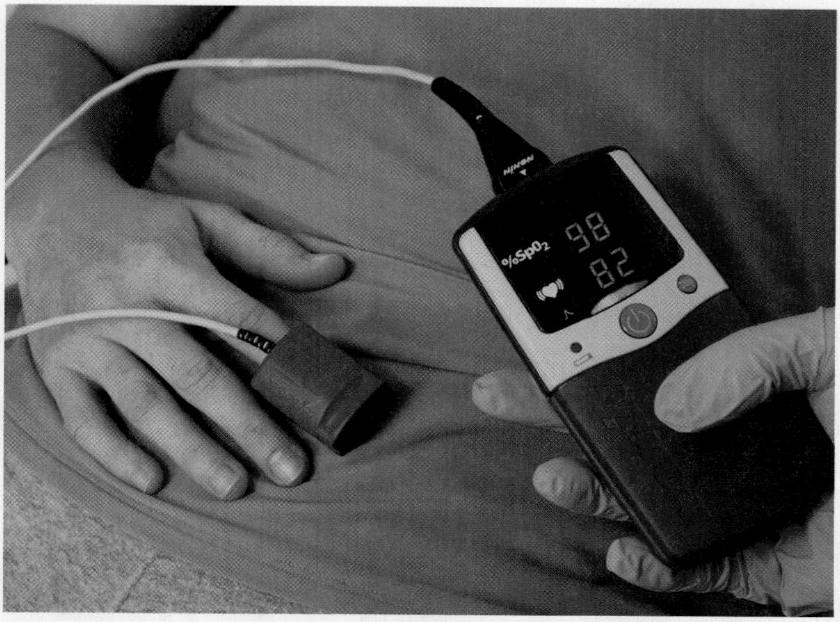

Figure 9-19 A pulse oximeter with probe attached to finger.

These intervals are recommended guidelines and should be modified to suit the patient's needs and to follow local protocols. It also is recommended that you reassess vital signs following all interventions.

Pulse Oximetry

A tool becoming commonplace in many EMS systems is the pulse oximeter. It is a noninvasive device that can monitor the percentage of hemoglobin that is saturated with oxygen. It consists of a probe that attaches to the patient's finger, toe, or earlobe and is linked to a computerized unit (Figure 9-19 ▪). The unit displays the percentage of hemoglobin saturated with oxygen (SpO_2) together with a digital readout of the patient's pulse rate. The device can detect hypoxia (oxygen deficiency) before the patient begins to show outward signs.

9-19 Explain what pulse oximetry measures and describe factors and limitations in interpreting pulse oximetry findings.

Ideally, a patient should be placed on the pulse oximeter prior to receiving supplemental oxygen. Doing so will provide a baseline reading to which later readings with supplemental oxygen can be compared. However, if a patient shows signs of inadequate breathing, do not delay interventions such as supplemental oxygen or manual ventilations for the sake of a baseline pulse oximetry reading. An oxygen saturation (SpO_2) of less than 94% is considered abnormal and may be indicative of early hypoxia.

The pulse oximeter is only one tool in your "assessment toolbox." You must continue to use your assessment skills and vital signs to determine the best care for the patient. Just because the pulse oximeter shows a normal saturation of between 94% and 100% on room air does not mean the patient should not receive supplemental oxygen.

The effectiveness and accuracy of the pulse oximeter depends on a continuous flow of arterial blood to the tissues. For this reason, there are several situations where the pulse oximeter will not be accurate or effective for determining oxygen saturation. The following is a list of these situations:

- Patients who are in shock or have a lower-than-normal body temperature (hypothermia)
- Cases of carbon monoxide poisoning

- Excessive movement
- Nail polish beneath the probe

Pulse oximetry is most useful in revealing a trend in the patient's oxygen saturation. It will tell you when supplemental oxygen is raising the patient's oxygen saturation, and it will reveal when hypoxia is setting in, because the readings will drop.

CLINICAL CLUE

Pulse Oximeter

Do not rely too heavily on the pulse oximeter as the sole indicator of the patient's condition. It is only one piece of the big picture that must include your overall assessment and vital signs.

STOP, REVIEW, REMEMBER!

Multiple Choice

For each question, place a check next to the correct answer.

1. Which one of the following is *not* a typical skin sign?

_____ a. Color
_____ b. Sensitivity
_____ c. Temperature
_____ d. Moisture

2. When assessing skin signs, which one of the following best describes the term *diaphoretic*?

_____ a. Hot and red
_____ b. Cool and moist
_____ c. Hot and moist
_____ d. Cold and dry

3. When assessing a patient's pupils, the two Rs in the mnemonic PERRL refer to:

_____ a. round and reactive to light.
_____ b. responsive and reactive to pain.
_____ c. round and refocusing to light.
_____ d. responsive and reactive to pain.

4. Sympathetic movement of the eyes refers to the ability of the eyes to:

_____ a. open and close together.
_____ b. open and close one at a time.
_____ c. blink.
_____ d. move together.

5. It is recommended to reassess vital signs every 15 minutes for stable patients and every ______________ minutes for unstable patients.

_____ a. 5
_____ b. 10
_____ c. 15
_____ d. 20

Fill in the Blank

1. Skin signs should be assessed for color, ____________________________, moisture, capillary refill, and skin turgor.

2. The ____________________________ is located on the inside of the mouth and can be used to assess tissue perfusion.

3. The conjunctiva is located ____________________.

4. A yellowish color to the skin and whites of the eyes, indicative of poor liver function, is called ____________________.

5. Skin that is moist is often referred to as ____________________.

Matching

Match the definition on the left with the applicable term on the right.

1. _____ Bluish skin color indicative of poor oxygenation
2. _____ Reddish skin color commonly seen when someone is embarrassed or is suffering a heat-related emergency
3. _____ Skin color indicative of poor perfusion
4. _____ Yellowish skin color indicative of poor liver function
5. _____ Skin that is moist (perspiration)

A. Jaundiced
B. Diaphoretic
C. Cyanotic
D. Flushed
E. Pale

Critical Thinking

1. List as many areas on a patient that you can think of for assessing skin color and perfusion status.

2. List a medical condition that can cause each of the following abnormal skin colors: pale, cyanotic, flushed, and jaundiced.

3. Describe the proper method for assessing a patient's skin temperature and moisture and the normal characteristics of each.

Obtaining a Medical History

One of the most important roles that an EMT must learn is that of an investigator. As an investigator, your job is to learn as much about the patient's medical history, both past and present, as possible. This pertains to all patients. However, it is especially important when assessing patients with a medical illness as opposed to an injury.

You will start gathering important history information beginning with the initial dispatch. Dispatches to such common calls as "difficulty breathing," "chest pain," and "unresponsive person" provide at least some insight into the patient's chief complaint. While the dispatch does not always match up with what you find on scene, for the most part it is at least close.

PERSPECTIVE

Ray—The EMT

On the surface, Dick's problem seemed like a pretty common intestinal thing. You know, vomiting, diarrhea, chills, and fever. Stomach flu? Or maybe food poisoning? So I was just going to load him up and head out, but then Derrick was wise to start asking him all of those questions about his medical history. Do you know what? We found out that Dick is diabetic and undergoing chemo for colon cancer. I behaved like a beginner for just assuming this was one of those middle-aged men, living alone with his mom, a hypochondria-type case. This was actually a very, very sick man and I didn't appreciate that. I guess I'm never going to stop learning out here. Let's hope none of us do.

General Impression

general impression an element of the patient assessment that includes assessing approximate age, gender, and level of distress.

Once on scene, your history-taking begins as you approach your patient and begin to form a **general impression** of his condition. The general impression is just one element of your overall patient assessment and includes the following elements: level of responsiveness or level of distress, approximate age, and gender.

As you approach the patient, note his level of responsiveness. Is he sitting up, aware of his surroundings, interacting with those around him? Is he lying supine with eyes closed and unresponsive? A patient who has an altered mental status will require more aggressive airway assessment and management. Next, note his approximate age: Is he elderly, middle-aged, a young adult, or a pediatric patient? Go ahead and estimate his age based on your best guess. You will already know your patient's gender, at least by appearances. The final element of the general impression is the patient's level of distress. Is he in a lot of pain, having difficulty breathing, or simply lying there calm and quiet? Someone with a high level of distress may need immediate attention, so this is an important observation.

Once at the patient's side, introduce yourself and inform him of your level of training and confirm that he has provided permission for you to care for him. This is typically the case if other emergency care providers are already on scene. If you are the first on scene, then you must ask for permission to care for the patient.

9-20 Determine a patient's chief complaint.

chief complaint the patient's perception of the problem in his own words. It is *not* what the EMT perceives to be the problem.

Chief Complaint

After your introduction, determine the patient's **chief complaint** by asking why you were called. The chief complaint is the primary reason the patient feels he needs assistance, usually described in his own words. The chief complaint for an unresponsive patient may be documented as "unresponsive" or simply "none."

SAMPLE History

There are many tools that EMTs can use to help remember all the questions they must ask while obtaining a patient history. The most common of those tools is a memory device—an acronym that spells the word **SAMPLE.** Each letter of the word represents a specific element of a good patient history. They are as follows:

S—Signs and symptoms
A—Allergies
M—Medications
P—Pertinent past medical history
L—Last oral intake
E—Events leading to the injury or illness

9-21 Use the mnemonics SAMPLE and OPQRST to ensure a complete prehospital patient history.

SAMPLE a mnemonic used in obtaining a patient history. The letters stand for signs and symptoms, allergies, medications, past pertinent medical history, last oral intake, and events leading to the injury or illness.

PERSPECTIVE

Dick—The Patient

I don't think I've ever been so sick. That was awful. Just vomiting until every muscle in my body ached. I was so tired, I didn't even want to talk. My mother kept trying to call 911 but I wouldn't let her. I mean, it wasn't until she told me that I was acting just like my father right before he died that I really got concerned. She just lost him two years ago and so how could I argue with her anymore? I may be 55, but she's still my mom. So I let her call for the ambulance and now, I've got to say, I'm glad she did.

Signs and Symptoms

The *S* in SAMPLE stands for signs and symptoms and reminds you to assess or reassess any signs and symptoms relating to the chief complaint. One way that you can begin this process is by asking the patient, "Tell me again where you hurt." When he describes where he has pain (a symptom), you must inspect those areas for any obvious signs of illness or injury. Do not just stop at the most obvious or first place the patient describes as painful. After examining the first painful location, ask if there are any other places that hurt and inspect those as appropriate.

Allergies

All good patient histories include information about known allergies. Known allergies are things the patient is well aware of that have caused an allergic reaction in the past. This is important for several reasons. For instance, the patient may require medication upon arrival at the hospital, but he may be allergic to a specific medication. Discovering known allergies ahead of time should prevent an unnecessary allergic reaction during his treatment and care. It is good practice to ask about all known allergies including allergies to medications, food, and environmental causes such as bites, stings, and plants.

If the patient advises that he does indeed have a known allergy, then it is a good idea to ask him about the last time he had a reaction and what the reaction was like. Was it a minor reaction or was it more severe requiring medical attention? This will provide some insight into how allergic he may be.

Medications

Asking a patient what medications he is currently taking can provide important information about his medical history. As you become more experienced, you will learn the more common prescription medications. They can tell you the type of medical conditions for which the patient is being treated, especially when he is unable to describe his own medical history clearly.

Ask about both prescription and nonprescription medications, including those that do not necessarily pertain to a medical condition, such as birth control pills or patches. Also ask about alternative or holistic medications, dietary supplements, and herbal remedies. Your questioning should include medications from the recent past that the patient may not be currently taking as well as medications he is currently taking. Be sure to confirm he has been taking the prescribed medications as directed.

You are not expected to remember all the names or purposes of the medications the patient is taking. Ask someone to bring them all to you and place them in a paper bag for easy reference and transport to the hospital.

Pertinent Past Medical History

In many situations, the patient's chief complaint relates either directly or indirectly to a past medical complaint or condition. For this reason, a brief assessment of his past medical history is important. Ask about previous or current medical conditions, surgeries, and injuries. It is not for you to decide if the previous history is pertinent or not. Let the physician make that decision. You must include as much detail as possible when transferring or documenting your care.

Last Oral Intake

The question regarding the patient's last oral intake should be asked of all patients but is most important for patients who have suffered a serious injury. Ask the patient when he last had something to eat or drink and an approximate quantity. Should a patient require emergency surgery, it is very important that the surgeons know the time and quantity of food intake, since there is a risk that the stomach contents could be vomited up during surgery.

Events Leading to the Injury or Illness

It may be helpful to know what the patient was doing just prior to the event. For instance, if the chief complaint is chest pain, it will be important to know if the patient was exerting himself prior to the pain or if he was at rest. It also will reveal something important if the patient has no recollection of events prior to your arrival.

OPQRST Assessment

OPQRST a mnemonic for the questions asked to get a description of the present illness. The letters stand for onset, provocation, quality, region and radiate, severity, and time.

Another tool used in EMS to help ensure a thorough assessment and medical history related to a medical patient's chief complaint is the memory aid **OPQRST.** Each of the letters represents a word and each of the words is designed to trigger specific questions that the EMT should ask. The OPQRST memory aid is especially helpful when the chief complaint is related to pain or shortness of breath:

O—Onset. The word *onset* is designed to trigger questions pertaining to what the patient was doing when the pain or symptoms began. For example, "What were you doing when the pain began?" or "What were you doing when you first began to feel short of breath?" are questions you might ask related to onset.

P—Provocation. The word *provocation* is designed to trigger questions pertaining to what might make the pain or symptoms better or worse. For example, "Does anything you do make the pain better or worse?" or "Does it hurt to take a deep breath or when I push here?"

Q—Quality. The word *quality* is designed to trigger questions pertaining to what the pain or symptom actually feels like. For example, "Can you describe how your pain feels?" or "Is it sharp or is it dull?" and "Is it steady or does it come and go?" Be careful not to put words in the patient's mouth. Instead provide him with choices and then be patient and allow him to choose. It is also important to use the patient's own words when documenting the call or handing the patient off to the next level of care. If the patient tells you he feels as though an anvil is sitting on his chest, then use his words rather than paraphrasing and stating that he has pressure on his chest.

R—Region and radiation. The words *region* and *radiation* are designed to trigger questions pertaining to where the pain is originating and to where it may be moving or radiating. For example, "Can you point with one finger to where your pain is the most?" or "Does your pain move or radiate to any other part of your body?" or "Do you feel pain anywhere else besides your chest?"

S—Severity. The word *severity* is designed to trigger questions pertaining to how severe the pain or discomfort is. A standard 1-to-10 scale is typically used and is presented like this: "On a scale of 1 to 10, with 10 being the worst pain you have ever felt, how would you rate your pain right now?" You can take this a step further by asking the patient to describe the severity of his pain when it first began, using the same scale. Once you have been with the patient a while and have provided care, you will want to ask the severity question again to see if his pain is getting better or worse.

T—Time. The word *time* is designed to trigger questions pertaining to how long the patient may have been experiencing his pain or discomfort. A simple question such as "When did you first begin having pain today?" or "How long have you had this pain?" will usually suffice.

It is important to point out that there are many different memory aids that can be used to assist the EMT in performing a more thorough assessment. This chapter has presented only SAMPLE and OPQRST—two of the more common ones currently used in EMS. Your instructor or EMS system may have different or additional memory aids. Find the ones that work best for you.

Medical Identification Jewelry

A valuable resource for medical history is medical identification jewelry (Figure 9-20 ■). Typically a medallion is worn around the patient's neck, wrist, or ankle and provides important medical information about the patient. It should be pointed out that wearing medical identification jewelry is completely optional, and not all patients with a significant history choose to wear it.

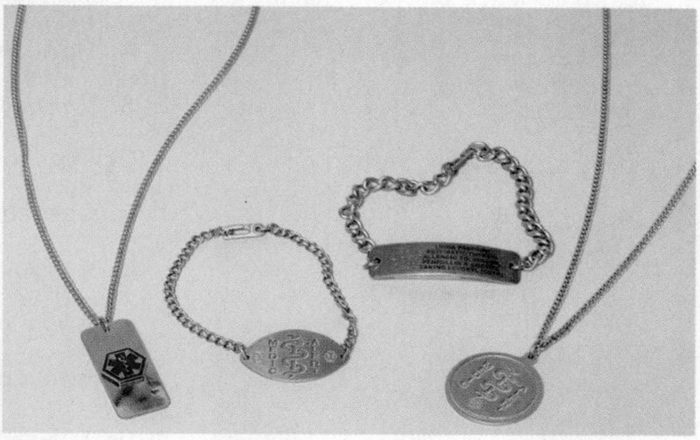

Figure 9-20 Medical identification jewelry comes in many forms.

STOP, REVIEW, REMEMBER!

Multiple Choice

1. An appropriate medical history can begin as early as:

_____ a. with the initial dispatch information.

_____ b. when you arrive on scene.

_____ c. with the SAMPLE history.

_____ d. with the secondary assessment.

2. The general impression of the patient consists of the following elements:

_____ a. approximate age, race, level of responsiveness.

_____ b. approximate age, gender, and level of distress.

_____ c. mechanism of injury, age, and gender.

_____ d. chief complaint, age, and level of distress.

(continued on next page)

(continued)

3. Which one of the following best describes the term *chief complaint*?
   _____ a. What the dispatcher tells you over the radio
   _____ b. What the family member tells you about the patient
   _____ c. What the patient states is his problem
   _____ d. Any past medical history about the patient

4. Which one of the following questions pertains to the "P" in the SAMPLE history?
   _____ a. Do you have any allergies to medications?
   _____ b. When did you last eat?
   _____ c. Do you take any medications?
   _____ d. Do you have any history of chest pain?

5. Which one of the following questions pertains to the "S" in the SAMPLE history?
   _____ a. Do you have pain anywhere?
   _____ b. How severe is your pain?
   _____ c. Where does your pain originate?
   _____ d. What were you doing when the pain began?

Matching

Match the letters of OPQRST on the left with the applicable question(s) on the right. There may be more than one question per letter.

1. _____ O
2. _____ P
3. _____ Q
4. _____ R
5. _____ S
6. _____ T

A. How long have you had this pain/discomfort?
B. Where is your pain/discomfort?
C. Does your pain/discomfort radiate anywhere else?
D. Does anything you do make the pain/discomfort better or worse?
E. Can you describe your pain/discomfort?
F. Is your pain/discomfort sharp or dull?
G. Is your pain/discomfort steady or does it come and go?
H. What were you doing when the pain/discomfort began?
I. How severe is your pain/discomfort now?

Critical Thinking

1. Discuss how you might find out if a patient has a previous medical condition without actually asking the question, "Do you have any previous medical history?"

____

____

____

____

2. List several ways you might ask a patient to describe his pain without leading him to an answer.

EMERGENCY DISPATCH SUMMARY

Based on Dick's vital signs, medical history, and apparent dehydration, Derrick and Ray decided to call for an ALS intercept. When the paramedics arrived, they immediately began two IVs of normal saline and, after evaluating Dick with a 12-lead monitor, began treating him for a cardiac dysrhythmia. The paramedics complimented the two EMTs on calling for ALS care based on their evaluation of Dick's situation. They had done exactly the right thing. Dick spent four days in Southwestern's ICU before being released back to his home and has since completed his chemotherapy.

Chapter Review

To the Point

- A good part of your patient assessment will center around the various signs (what you can see) and symptoms (what the patient tells you).
- It is important to immediately obtain a baseline set of vital signs so that all subsequent readings can be compared in order to establish any trends that indicate the patient is getting better, worse, or remaining the same.
- Normal ranges for vital signs will differ in adults, children, and infants, so it is important to learn the normal ranges for each.
- When assessing breathing, you must evaluate rate, depth, and tidal volume.
- In addition to assessing respirations, you must use your stethoscope to assess for the presence and quality of lung sounds.
- When assessing a pulse you must assess rate, strength, and rhythm. You will locate the carotid pulse for unresponsive adults and children, and the radial pulse for the responsive adults and children. You will locate the brachial pulse point for infants.
- Blood pressure is measured as two numbers, the systolic pressure (when the heart is beating) and the diastolic pressure (when the heart is at rest).
- Blood pressure can be obtained by auscultation (with a stethoscope) or by palpation (feeling the pulse). The palpation method will reveal only an approximate systolic reading.
- When assessing the skin, you must assess for color, temperature, moisture, capillary refill, and skin turgor.
- Capillary refill time should be under two seconds and can be used to evaluate perfusion status in very young children and distal perfusion of an extremity in all patients.
- When assessing pupils, you must evaluate the size and shape, equality of size, reactivity to light, and sympathetic movement.
- Orthostatic vital signs are obtained by measuring the pulse and blood pressure of a patient when he is lying down or sitting and again when he is standing. When the readings change significantly, it can be a sign of hypovolemia.

- Vital signs should be taken more frequently on unstable patients (every 5 minutes) and less often on stable patients (every 15 minutes).
- The pulse oximeter should be used for all patients as a basic vital sign tool. It reveals the oxygen saturation of the peripheral blood supply. A measurement between 94% and 100% is considered normal.
- When obtaining a patient history, you must focus on the patient's chief complaint. This is what the patient states is the primary problem or the reason he called EMS.
- A useful tool that can help ensure a thorough patient history is the SAMPLE memory aid, which stands for signs and symptoms, allergies, medications, past medical history, last oral intake and events leading to the problem.
- Another assessment tool commonly used to further evaluate a complaint of pain is the OPQRST memory aid, which stands for onset, provocation, quality, region and radiation, severity, and time.

Chapter Questions

Multiple Choice

For each question, place a check next to the correct answer.

1. The five most important vital signs are pulse, respirations, blood pressure, pupils, and:
   _____ a. oxygen saturation.
   _____ b. skin signs.
   _____ c. mental status.
   _____ d. capillary refill.
2. The first set of vital signs obtained on any patient is referred to as the ____________ set.
   _____ a. historical
   _____ b. ongoing
   _____ c. baseline
   _____ d. serial
3. ____________ can be assessed by watching and feeling the chest and abdomen move during breathing.
   _____ a. Pulse rate
   _____ b. Blood pressure
   _____ c. Skin signs
   _____ d. Respiratory rate
4. Characteristics of respirations include:
   _____ a. rate, depth, and ease.
   _____ b. rate, rhythm, and strength.
   _____ c. rate, depth, and strength.
   _____ d. rate, ease, and quality.
5. The most appropriate location to obtain a pulse for a responsive adult is the ____________ artery.
   _____ a. brachial
   _____ b. femoral
   _____ c. carotid
   _____ d. radial
6. The pulse located at the top of the foot (dorsal aspect) is called the ____________ pulse.
   _____ a. tibial
   _____ b. pedal
   _____ c. brachial
   _____ d. dorsal
7. The characteristics of a pulse include:
   _____ a. rate, strength, and rhythm.
   _____ b. rate, ease, and rhythm.
   _____ c. rate, depth, and rhythm.
   _____ d. rate, strength, and quality.
8. Skin that is bluish in color is called:
   _____ a. pale.
   _____ b. flushed.
   _____ c. cyanotic.
   _____ d. jaundiced.
9. The term *diaphoretic* refers to:
   _____ a. pupil reaction.
   _____ b. skin temperature.
   _____ c. heart rhythm.
   _____ d. skin moisture.

10. When going from a well-lighted room to a dark room, you would expect the normal pupil to:
_____ a. not react.
_____ b. dilate.
_____ c. constrict.
_____ d. fluctuate.

11. Capillary refill time is most accurate as an assessment tool for perfusion in patients:
_____ a. younger than six years of age.
_____ b. younger than one year of age.
_____ c. older than eight years of age.
_____ d. older than 18 years of age.

12. Which one of the following is most accurate when describing a palpated blood pressure?
_____ a. It includes only the diastolic pressure.
_____ b. It must be taken on a responsive patient.
_____ c. It can be obtained without a stethoscope.
_____ d. It can be obtained without a blood pressure cuff.

13. A respiratory rate that is less than _____________ should be considered inadequate.
_____ a. 4
_____ b. 6
_____ c. 8
_____ d. 10

14. The pressure inside the arteries each time the heart contracts is referred to as the _____________ pressure.
_____ a. diastolic
_____ b. pulse
_____ c. systolic
_____ d. mean

15. A _____________ is something the EMT can see or measure during the patient assessment.
_____ a. symptom
_____ b. history
_____ c. sign
_____ d. chief complaint

Labeling

Correctly label each of the major pulse points.

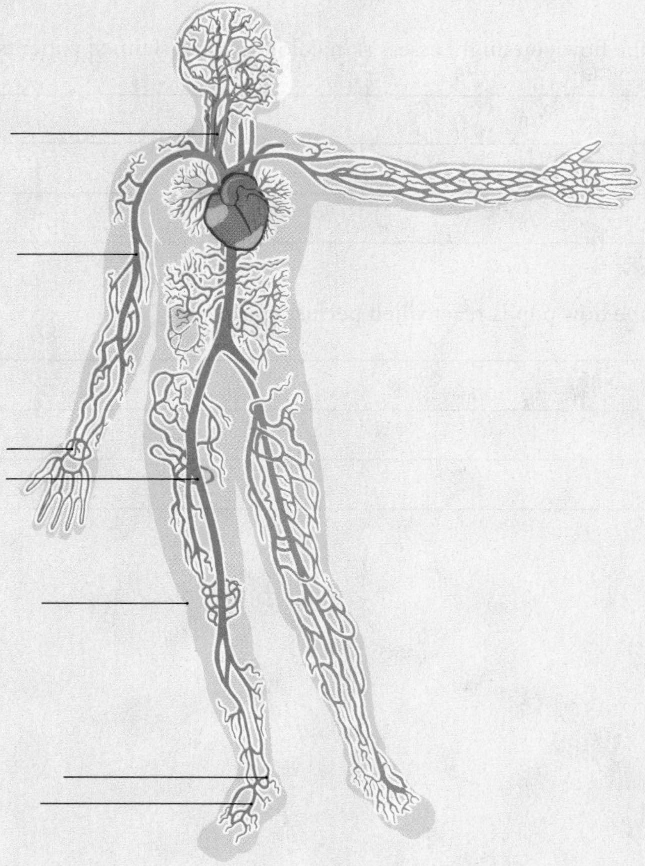

Critical Thinking

1. Describe the importance of recording the time when taking multiple sets of vital signs on an unstable patient.

2. Describe the reasons for not using too small a sample (for example, a 10-second sample versus 15 or 30 seconds) when assessing the pulse rate of a patient.

3. Discuss the differences between an auscultated and palpated blood pressure and when you would use each.

4. Describe how you might assess skin color on dark-skinned patients.

5. Describe how pupils react when perfusion is poor.

Case Studies

Case Study 1

You have been dispatched to the home of an elderly woman for abdominal pain. Your SAMPLE history reveals a long history of bleeding ulcers and recent hip replacement surgery. The patient denies any recent history of bloody stools or vomit. Baseline vitals are as follows: respirations 24 shallow and slightly labored, pulse 96 weak and regular, blood pressure 108/68, skin is pale warm and dry, and pupils are PERRL.

1. What conclusions, if any, can you draw from the patient's baseline vitals?

2. How often will you want to take vital signs on this patient and why?

3. How might you determine what this patient's vital signs are normally?

Case Study 2

You are caring for an approximately 44-year-old male patient who was found on the back porch of his home by his wife. He is alert and oriented on your arrival but is not sure how he ended up on the ground. He has no obvious signs of trauma and is complaining only of moderate pain to his right elbow and shoulder. His wife states that she had seen him approximately 30 minutes earlier at breakfast before he left to go outside to mow the lawn. His wife tells you he may have been stung by a bee, because he passed out the last time he was stung about a year ago. She shows you an Epi-pen (an epinephrine self-injector) that the doctor gave him the last time he was stung. She also tells you that he has high blood pressure and takes a pill once a day for it.

1. Fill in the appropriate information from the scenario above for each letter of the SAMPLE history.

(continued on next page)

(continued)

2. Would this patient be considered stable or unstable and why?

____

____

____

____

The Last Word

Repeated sets of accurate vital signs help the EMT spot trends in a patient's condition. That trend may be stable, for the better, or, in some situations, for the worse. Regardless, vital signs provide valuable information about the patient and should be taken as soon as practical on all patients. Establishing a baseline set of vital signs as early as possible is essential in revealing any trend.

Learning to obtain an excellent medical history is a skill that takes lots of time and experience. Learning to use memory aids such as SAMPLE and OPQRST will help you develop a systematic approach to taking medical histories. Developing a systematic approach will help ensure a complete and thorough history.

Communications

10

Education Standards

Preparatory: EMS System Communication, Therapeutic Communication

Competencies

Applies fundamental knowledge of the EMS system, safety/well-being of the EMT, medical/legal issues, and ethical issues to the provision of emergency care.

Objectives

After completion of this lesson, you should be able to:

10-1 Define key terms introduced in this chapter.

10-2 Discuss the role that effective communication plays in EMS.

10-3 Describe the four types of communication.

10-4 Describe the components of the communication process.

10-5 List several common barriers to communication.

10-6 Discuss several strategies for effective communication.

10-7 Discuss the characteristics of effective interpersonal communication.

10-8 Identify the three objectives of therapeutic communication.

10-9 Discuss strategies for effective interviewing of patients.

10-10 Describe the uses of open-ended and closed-ended questions.

10-11 Discuss the components of an appropriate verbal transfer of care.

10-12 Describe the responsibilities of the Federal Communications Commission.

10-13 Discuss the purposes and characteristics of each of the following EMS system communication components: base station, mobile radios. portable radios, mobile data terminals, and cell phones.

10-14 List key points in an EMS call at which you should communicate with dispatch.

10-15 Discuss the standard ground rules for radio communications.

10-16 Describe the elements of a verbal transfer of care.

Key Terms

base station radios p. 250
communication p. 242
mobile data terminals (MDTs) p. 252
mobile radios p. 250
portable radios p. 250
repeaters p. 250
therapeutic communication p. 247

Introduction

Your ability to communicate clearly and confidently and in a manner that all parties understand will be one of the primary keys to your success as an EMT. This chapter introduces the common elements of effective communication as well as strategies to improve communication with diverse groups. It also introduces you to some of the communication devices commonly used in EMS today.

A wide variety of individuals will interact with you during the course of a typical emergency call or duty shift. Here is a list of just some of the individuals with whom you will likely be expected to communicate on a regular basis:

- Patients
- Your partner
- Other EMS personnel
- Fire personnel
- Law enforcement personnel
- Hospital personnel
- Bystanders
- Family members
- Friends of patients

communication the exchange of common symbols that are written, spoken, or otherwise exchanged, such as through signing and body language.

The task of communicating can be challenging. So, it is extremely important that you understand the characteristics of good **communication** and understand what to do when communication goes bad.

EMERGENCY DISPATCH

"So, what do we have here?" Dr. Orwell had come into the room right after EMTs Jared and Melanie finished transferring their patient to the hospital bed.

"This is Mr. Thompson," Melanie began.

"Tamblyn," the patient winced. "My last name is Tamblyn."

"Okay," Melanie smiled and moved on. "Mr. Tamblyn called because he was having pain on his right."

"Left."

". . . left side . . . and it's gone on for most of the day."

"Most of the week. I told you a week."

"Does he have any allergies?" Dr. Orwell looked over her glasses at Melanie, frowning. Melanie stretched her exam glove between her fingers.

"Uh, yes, I think so," Melanie said, sounding unsure.

"Yes!" the patient roared. "What's wrong with you? I told you that I'm allergic to morphine. Back at my house you asked me, 'Are you allergic to anything?' and I very clearly answered, 'Yes. I'm allergic to morphine' and you wrote it on your glove!"

The doctor looked from one EMT to the other and opened the exam room door. "Thanks for bringing Mr. Tamblyn in. I think I can take it from here."

The Role of Communications

10-2 Discuss the role that effective communication plays in EMS.

Communication is a vital part of being an EMT. Though much of your time in class will be dedicated to acquiring medical knowledge and skills, the role of communication must not be overlooked. Consider the following scenarios:

- You are called to a patient who is hyperventilating. The patient is anxious, breathing rapidly, and getting dizzier and dizzier. You apply oxygen to the patient. You get yourself at a level slightly lower than the patient and use a soft voice to get the patient's attention and then calm her down. You coach her to take slower, deeper breaths. The patient improves.
- You are called to a patient with chest pain. You find a man in his 50s and his wife, who is looking on anxiously. As the man describes his chest pain, you apply some oxygen and reassure him. You note that the man is so worried, he is trembling. You stop briefly

and explain that you are taking care of him and are going to bring him to the hospital. Your calm demeanor provides reassurance throughout treatment and transport. He relaxes somewhat. His pulse comes down a little and his pain diminishes.

- You find a woman who was involved in a motor-vehicle collision with relatively minor front-end damage to her vehicle. She has a minor head injury. She was not wearing a seat belt, and there was no air bag in her vehicle. She is anxious and her pulse is a bit rapid. You recognize this as a sign of possible shock, but also as one of anxiety. You get the patient out of the car with a long backboard and into the ambulance. The entire time you reassure and talk with the patient. She actually jokes with you, so you joke back appropriately. In the ambulance she seems relaxed and calmer. Her pulse has dropped to within normal limits and remains stable.

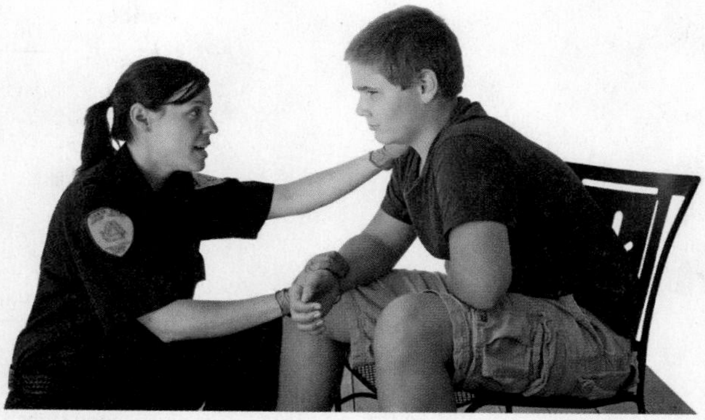

Figure 10-1 The rapport you build with your patient through effective communication skills will greatly improve your ability to provide the appropriate care.

In each of the foregoing cases, communication was a key component of your patient care (Figure 10-1 ■). As in the first case, calming a hyperventilating patient is an established clinical treatment. In the second case, reassurance helped to make a difference in the man with chest pain. Anxiety causes an increased pulse, which causes the heart to work harder and use more oxygen, which causes chest pain. Reassurance is a valuable clinical tool that likely helped to reduce the man's chest pain. In the final case, you were unsure if the woman was simply nervous from the crash or had hidden injuries and shock. Your calming, reassuring manner—plus checking vital signs frequently—led you to answer the question properly: Her nervousness and rapid pulse likely were caused by anxiety.

If you work or volunteer at an ambulance or fire department or have even been a patient, you will find that one of the things patients remember most is the way they were treated. Letters of thanks that come to ambulance squads do not talk primarily of the clinical care. They say things such as, "You took good care of me" or "Thank you for taking such good care of my mother." People remember how they were treated. Something as simple as talking kindly can make a huge difference.

Proper communication and a caring attitude also can reduce legal liability. It is believed that patients are less likely to file a lawsuit if they feel that they were treated well. Good communication also will help you obtain the maximum amount of information from your patient, helping you make better care decisions.

10-3 Describe the four types of communication.

All communication can be placed into one of four broad types. They are:

- *Verbal communication*, which is made up of the words and sounds of language
- *Nonverbal communication*, which is made up of body language, eye contact, and gestures
- *Written communication*, which is made up of the words and letters of language
- *Visual communication*, which is made up of signs, symbols, and designs

Verbal communication can be further broken down into different types, such as interpersonal and therapeutic. As an EMT you also will use specific tools to facilitate communication, such as radios and computer terminals.

The Communication Process

10-4 Describe the components of the communication process.

If someone told you that you were going to communicate, what is the first thing that comes to mind? Likely, it is the word *talking*. While talking is clearly a way by which to communicate, it only represents one half of the total equation. The other half of effective communication involves listening.

There is a lot going on during any communication. There must be a sender, the one who is introducing a new thought or concept or initiating the communication process.

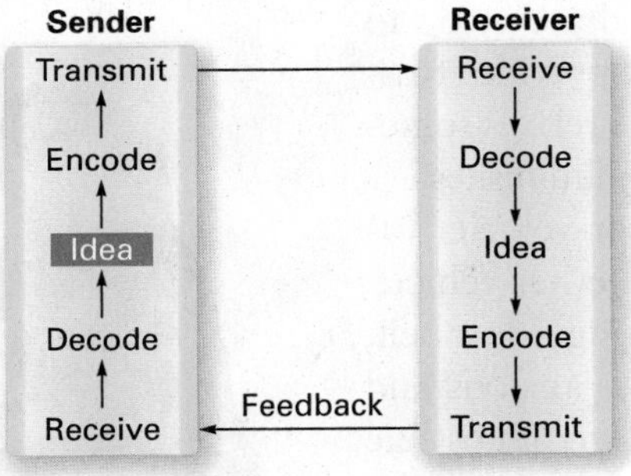

Figure 10-2 The communication process involves many steps.

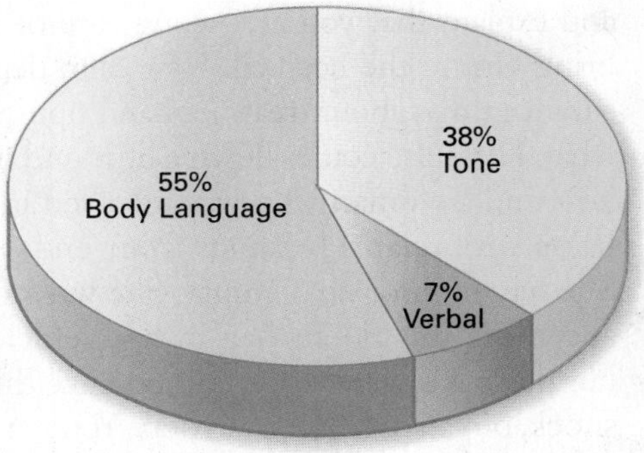

Figure 10-3 The majority of communication is delivered through our body language.

There is the message, which is the thought, concept, or idea being transmitted. There is the receiver, the one for whom the message is intended. The model in Figure 10-2 ▪ illustrates the many steps that a message must go through, regardless of how simple or complex it is. If the message gets blocked or misinterpreted at any one of the steps, the meaning of the message may get misinterpreted or lost. When you are dealing with issues related to safety and patient care, poor communication can be dangerous and even deadly.

Transmitting the Message

Now that you know the mechanics of how messages are processed, it will be helpful to have a basic understanding of how most messages are being transmitted. Take a look at Figure 10-3 ▪ to see how messages are actually getting across to the receiver.

Research suggests that 55% of communication is delivered by way of body language, which includes gestures, expressions, posture, and many other physical manifestations. About 38% of the message is transmitted by way of the voice—its quality, tone, and inflections, which all express important pieces of the message. Only 7% of any given message is transmitted by the specific words used. That can work well when you are physically located next to or in front of the person with whom you are communicating. However, a significant amount of the communication in EMS occurs by way of radio or a computer screen. Knowing this, you can begin to understand how not being able to see a person can create many barriers to effective communication.

Barriers to Communication

10-5 List several common barriers to communication.

There always will be barriers to communication. Dr. Eric Garner is a leading researcher and educator in the area of communication, and he has identified seven barriers to effective communication. They are:

- ***Physical.*** A physical barrier is any barrier either real or perceived that separates the sender and the receiver. Examples of physical barriers include walls, doors, distance, and territories or zones.
- ***Perceptual.*** Everyone brings different experiences to the table. People see things in their own way, or through unique perspectives that can differ in so many ways.
- ***Emotional.*** This can be one of the biggest barriers when dealing with ill and injured patients. It includes fear, mistrust, and suspicion and can be difficult to overcome in the short time EMTs are with patients.
- ***Cultural.*** Each year the United States becomes more culturally diverse. Not understanding some of the basic cultural differences that exist can cause significant barriers that will prevent you from delivering the best care possible.
- ***Language.*** Not being able to communicate with your patient due to language differences can be an overwhelming barrier for many novice EMTs. While no one expects

you to learn several languages, it will be beneficial to learn some common words and phrases related to patient care if you live and work in a culturally diverse environment.

- *Gender.* Simply being a male responding to a female victim of sexual assault or vaginal bleeding can cause barriers the patient is not willing to remove. Gender also can play a role culturally.
- ***Interpersonal.*** A person's attitudes and beliefs or dislike for the sender/receiver can interfere with the message being communicated.

As you can see by the list above, there are many reasons why a message might get blocked or misinterpreted. The first step in becoming a better communicator is simply by gaining an awareness of the many barriers that can interfere with communication.

PERSPECTIVE

Mr. Tamblyn—The Patient

Goodness! How do they let people like that work on an ambulance? She asks questions and then doesn't listen to the answers. I mean, why bother? What if someone was dying? What if she was trying to give someone something that he is allergic to? That's just unbelievable to me.

Your communication will make a difference in the patient's prehospital experience and can even help the patient's clinical condition. One other way to say that is this: Treat every patient the way you would want to be treated. You won't go wrong.

Strategies for Effective Communication

The following are some simple ideas and strategies that will help you become a better communicator:

10-6 Discuss several strategies for effective communication.

- Speak clearly and use words and terminology that the receiver (the patient) will understand. You should not use medical jargon when speaking to a patient, but you should use proper medical terminology when speaking to another medical professional.
- Keep an open mind and resist the urge to be defensive. It is natural to respond defensively when you disagree with a message. However, when this happens, both parties tend to shut down, and any chance of good communication is minimized.
- Become an active listener. Active listening is more than just "paying attention." It means putting your biases aside and making every effort to understand what the other person is saying. Active listening includes using eye contact when appropriate and asking clarifying questions to further define the message.
- Be assertive when appropriate, especially when safety is at stake. Do not passively accept what the other person is saying if you see things differently. Respectfully state your point in a manner that will ensure you are heard.
- Remain aware of the influence that body language plays in effective communication. Pay attention to your own body language, and ensure that it shows you are listening and being attentive to the message.
- Accept the reality of miscommunication. Even the best communicators fail at times. Do not allow yourself to get frustrated, but instead take the miscommunication as a lesson and use it to improve your own communication.
- If you find yourself in a situation where you simply cannot communicate due to a language barrier, use plenty of good eye contact and show the patient everything you will be doing in advance.
- If you find yourself in a situation where the patient is deaf or hard of hearing, try to find someone who can interpret through sign language. If that is not possible, use written communication.

PERSPECTIVE

Jared—The EMT

I just started working with Melanie last week, and what happened today is unfortunately not uncommon. It's like she's so intent on getting through all of the "official" assessment questions that, instead of listening to the answers, she's thinking of the next question. I've tried to talk to her about it—that we ask the questions to get an accurate picture of the patient's overall situation—but she keeps telling me that I'm just new and that she's in paramedic school. At least I can remember my patient's name!

Interpersonal Communication

10-7 Discuss the characteristics of effective interpersonal communication.

One of the most important forms of communication is called *interpersonal communication*. Interpersonal communication most often occurs among three or fewer participants who are in close proximity to one another. This is often the case when two or three EMTs are working a shift together or when the communication occurs between caregivers and a patient. A major characteristic of good interpersonal communication is immediate feedback between the sender and receiver.

Effective interpersonal communication includes:

- ***Listening.*** You cannot communicate without listening. Recall how annoyed you get at a drive-through window when you find that your order is not correct. Now place this annoyance in the context of a life-and-death situation. If you do not listen, you will not appear to care, regardless of how reassuring you sound. In addition, listening will help you obtain vital information in a patient history. It also will help you detect things that are important but not said out loud.
- ***Tone of voice.*** Your demeanor, as noted in the small scenarios at the beginning of this chapter, has a tremendous influence on the patient in both a personal and a clinical sense. It may well be the thing that the patient remembers most about the call.
- ***Clarity of speech.*** Patients will be nervous and confused and may even have an altered mental status. Talk slowly and clearly so the patient can understand. Avoid the unnecessary use of medical abbreviations, jargon, or even big words.
- ***Body language and position.*** Your body language and position tell the patient something. If you are standing above a sitting patient with your arms crossed, you are in a position of authority, appearing disinterested. When it is safe and appropriate to do so, get down to the patient's level, particularly with children. Make eye contact. Looking constantly at the clipboard or elsewhere just establishes poor relations.
- ***Touch.*** There are times when a hand on a shoulder or arm establishes a level of warmth and concern. A handshake shows respect. If a patient refuses transport but promises to call his personal physician, the handshake may "seal the deal."

CLINICAL CLUE

Facial Expressions

Many patients will be distracted by their injury or illness and may not always hear what you are saying. When conveying an important message or asking an important question, be sure to look at the patient in the eyes. Often you will be able to tell from the patient's response and facial expression if he or she understands.

Therapeutic Communication

We have all experienced the effects of a verbal attack and know that words can indeed hurt nearly as much as a broken bone. Likewise, research has shown that what you say to your patient can make a big difference in his ability to manage his illness or injury.

10-8 Identify the three objectives of therapeutic communication.

therapeutic communication the face-to-face communication process that focuses on advancing the physical and emotional well-being of the patient.

Therapeutic communication can be defined as the face-to-face communication process that focuses on advancing the physical and emotional well-being of a patient. How you talk to your patient can make a difference in how he responds to the illness or injury and to you.

There are three objectives of therapeutic communication that you must be aware of to maximize the results for both you and the patient. They are:

- ***Collecting information.*** This is referred to as the patient history. The more information you can gather about the current situation as well as all prior medical history will make it much easier to properly care for the patient.
- ***Assessing behavior.*** Here you are carefully observing the patient's behavior, looking for subtle signs that may offer clues to his condition.
- ***Educating.*** One of your responsibilities as a patient advocate is to inform and educate patients about their condition. The hope is that with proper education patients will make better decisions about their own medical care.

One of the key components of successful therapeutic communication is trust. You will have only a few moments at the beginning of your patient encounter to establish trust. Without trust, the patient may withhold important information about his condition or history, and in the worst case he may refuse care altogether.

Strategies for Successful Interviewing

10-9 Discuss strategies for effective interviewing of patients.

To be sure your patients get the best care possible, you must learn as much about them, their current condition, and any pertinent prior medical history in a very short period of time. To do so, you must develop excellent interviewing skills. The following strategies will help you establish a good rapport with your patients and maximize your effectiveness:

- Immediately introduce yourself and your level of training.
- Obtain the patient's name early, and use it frequently during your interview.
- Position yourself at or below the patient's eye level whenever possible.
- Ask one question at a time, and allow the patient ample time to respond.
- Listen carefully to everything the patient tells you.
- Restate the patient's answers when necessary for clarification.

10-10 Describe the uses of open-ended and closed-ended questions.

Developing your interviewing skills will take some time. Whenever possible, listen in on others who are interviewing the patient and pay attention to their techniques. Notice what works and what does not work and use those lessons to your advantage.

Note that your interviewing strategies may need to be modified, depending on the age of your patient (Figure 10-4 ▪). For instance, obtaining a thorough medical history from a child may be impossible if the child does not know and trust you. In this instance you will need to rely on parents or other caregivers who know the child's history.

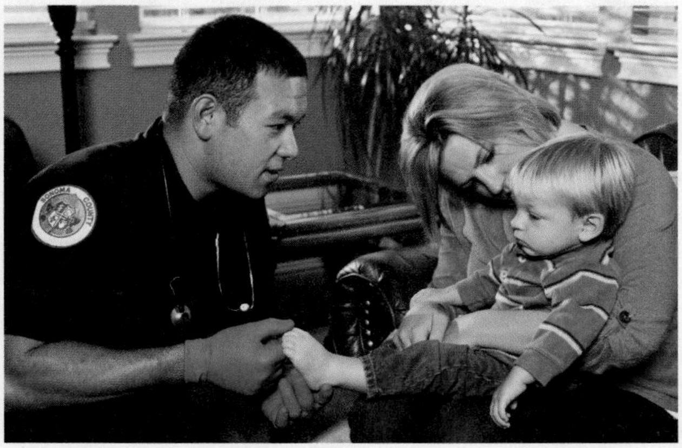

Figure 10-4 You may have to alter your communication approach depending on the age of the patient.

Question Construction

The way you structure your interview questions can have a big impact on the relationship you form with your patients and the accuracy of the information they provide. There is a lot of information that you must gather as an EMT. You need to obtain personal information and sometimes information that your patient may find embarrassing. It is not uncommon for a patient to offer more or different information to different rescuers.

Two types of question construction are helpful: open-ended and closed-ended. Open-ended questions are designed in a way that requires explanation and elaboration from the patient. Examples:

- Tell me about what happened before you had your accident.
- Please explain what the pain in your chest feels like.
- You mentioned you had these pains once before. What happened when you went to the hospital the last time?

Closed-ended questions encourage short or one-word answers. They are appropriate when all you need is follow-up or clarifying information, or if your patient's condition prevents him from going into detail. Examples:

- How old are you?
- When did you eat last?
- Does your knee hurt?
- Tell me again, what time did you take your medication?

As you can see, it is much easier to ask closed-ended rather than open-ended questions in an emergency situation. It is important to stop and think about how you can reformulate your questions in ways that prompt the patient to offer more information.

There is a third type of question, one you should avoid. It is called a *leading question*. It is asked in a way that presents the answer the interviewer is looking for. However, doing so could be the result of making assumptions that may or may not be true. Remember that it is important for the patient to fill in the blanks, not the questioner. An example of a leading question is: "I see you hurt your arm pretty badly. I think it may be broken. What do you think?"

Transfer of Care

10-11 Discuss the components of an appropriate verbal transfer of care.

The verbal transfer of care happens at the scene when care of the patient is transferred from one care provider, the EMT, to the next level of care. Another verbal transfer of care will occur when the ambulance crew turns care of the patient over to the staff at the hospital (Figure 10-5 ■). This is a very important component of what is called *the continuum of care*, and it helps to ensure that medical care is consistent and appropriate as the patient moves from care provider to care provider.

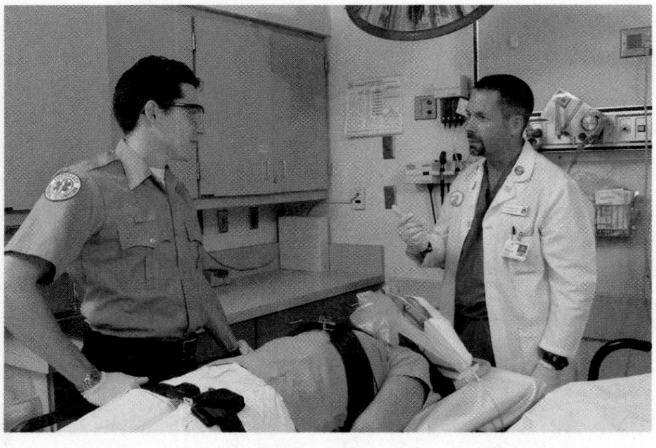

Figure 10-5 Upon arrival at the receiving facility, you must provide a detailed verbal report to those taking over care of the patient.

The verbal transfer of care may be modified based on the patient's condition. If the patient is critical, the transfer of care may be very short and to the point. Do not be offended if the hospital staff does not want to take the time for a complete report when the patient is in need of immediate attention. A good transfer of care should contain all of the following elements, regardless of whether the transfer happens at the scene or at the hospital:

- Patient's name and age
- Chief complaint
- Brief account of the patient's current condition
- Past pertinent medical history

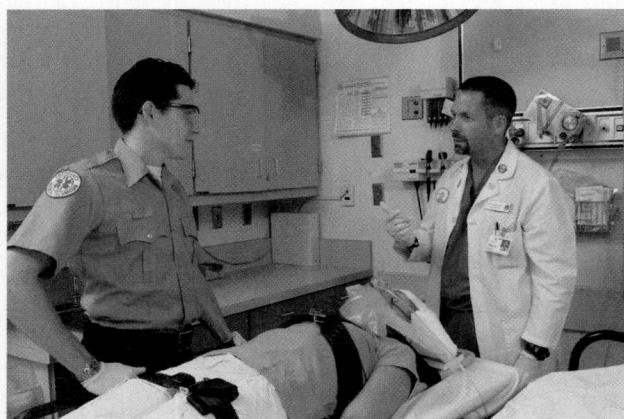

- Vital signs
- Pertinent findings from the physical exam
- Overview of care provided and the patient's response to that care

Keep in mind that you may have to ask for a verbal transfer of care from anyone who may be at the scene before you, such as bystanders, family members, and law enforcement officers. Do not expect them to be able to provide a thorough verbal hand off. You will need to ask specific questions to obtain the information that you need.

STOP, REVIEW, REMEMBER!

Multiple Choice

For each question, place a check next to the correct answer.

1. After suddenly finding it difficult to breathe, your patient starts to panic. How would you use interpersonal communication to help care for her?

_____ a. Hold her hand and speak slowly and softly.

_____ b. Stress the importance of getting to the hospital quickly.

_____ c. Stand above her and tell her to calm down.

_____ d. Lower yourself to her level and fill out paperwork until she can speak easily to you.

2. Your patient may be suffering from a stroke and is quite scared. Which interpersonal communication skill is *most* likely to reassure the patient?

_____ a. Listening

_____ b. Honesty

_____ c. Body language and positioning

_____ d. Touch

3. Which question is going to require your patient to go into the most detail?

_____ a. When did you fall off the ladder?

_____ b. What happened just before you fell off the ladder?

_____ c. Is the ladder rated for someone your weight?

_____ d. Did you get dizzy before you fell off the ladder?

4. Which one of the following is a leading question?

_____ a. What is today's date?

_____ b. Tell me about your medical history.

_____ c. You've had this pain before, right?

_____ d. When did you eat last?

Critical Thinking

1. You are called to a scene and find a deaf adult patient. How will you communicate with the patient? Describe two methods you might try.

____

____

____

____

(continued on next page)

(continued)

2. Your patient is a three-year-old boy who fell and injured his leg. His mother holds him and he is very cooperative as you complete your assessment. However, once in the ambulance, he starts to cry uncontrollably. How will you communicate with the patient? Give two methods you would try.

____

____

____

____

Radio Communication

10-12 Describe the responsibilities of the Federal Communications Commission.

All radio communications in the United States is governed and regulated by the Federal Communications Commission (FCC). The FCC controls and assigns radio frequencies to public service agencies, including EMS, to ensure all agencies can communicate when needed. The FCC also has developed rules regarding proper use of the airwaves and strictly prohibits the use of foul language and profanity.

The FCC does not regulate what the EMT says over the radio about patients, their identity, or the care that is provided. However, it is important to realize that much of your radio traffic can be picked up by most common radio scanners. It is considered inappropriate to use patient names over the radio simply out of respect for patient confidentiality.

10-13 Discuss the purposes and characteristics of each of the following EMS system communication components: base station, mobile radios, portable radios, mobile data terminals, cell phones.

repeaters devices that allow long-distance transmissions by picking up signals from lower-power radio units, such as mobile and portable radios, and retransmitting them at a higher power.

base station radios two-way radios at fixed sites such as a hospital or dispatch center.

mobile radios two-way radios that are used or are affixed in a vehicle.

portable radios handheld two-way radios.

All EMS systems are connected by a very sophisticated system of hardware and software designed to allow all of the resources in the system to communicate with one another. At the heart of those systems are the radios, pagers, and specific frequencies that connect each and every vehicle and person in the system. This system is set in motion when someone initiates an emergency response by calling 911.

A typical radio system is made up of a combination of transmitters, receivers, **repeaters,** and antennae (Figure 10-6 ■). Dispatch centers utilize powerful (80 to 150 watt) **base station radios** that can transmit over a wide area. When terrain is a factor and hills and mountains obstruct radio signals, specialized mountaintop repeaters are used to capture the signal and redirect it to the appropriate receiver.

EMS vehicles are equipped with specialized (20 to 50 watt) **mobile radios** capable of communicating with all aspects of the EMS system (Figure 10-7 ■). EMS personnel in the field often carry both pagers and **portable radios** (1 to 5 watt) that allow them to communicate with the dispatch center and each other (Figure 10-8 ■). Pagers are used to notify response personnel of an emergency call, and portable radios are used to communicate directly with the dispatch center before, during, and after a call.

The use of radios requires a specific protocol when communicating with others within the system. For instance, you cannot simply push the button and speak any time you feel like it. Doing so might interrupt another person using the same frequency. Instead, you should listen first and begin your transmission when there is a break in the "traffic" on your frequency. The term *radio traffic* is the common jargon for the verbal communication that takes place over a radio.

When you use a radio, whether a portable or a mobile one, the following guidelines will help make your radio communications clear:

- Make sure the radio is on and the volume is properly adjusted.
- Listen before transmitting. Do not transmit over someone who is already speaking.

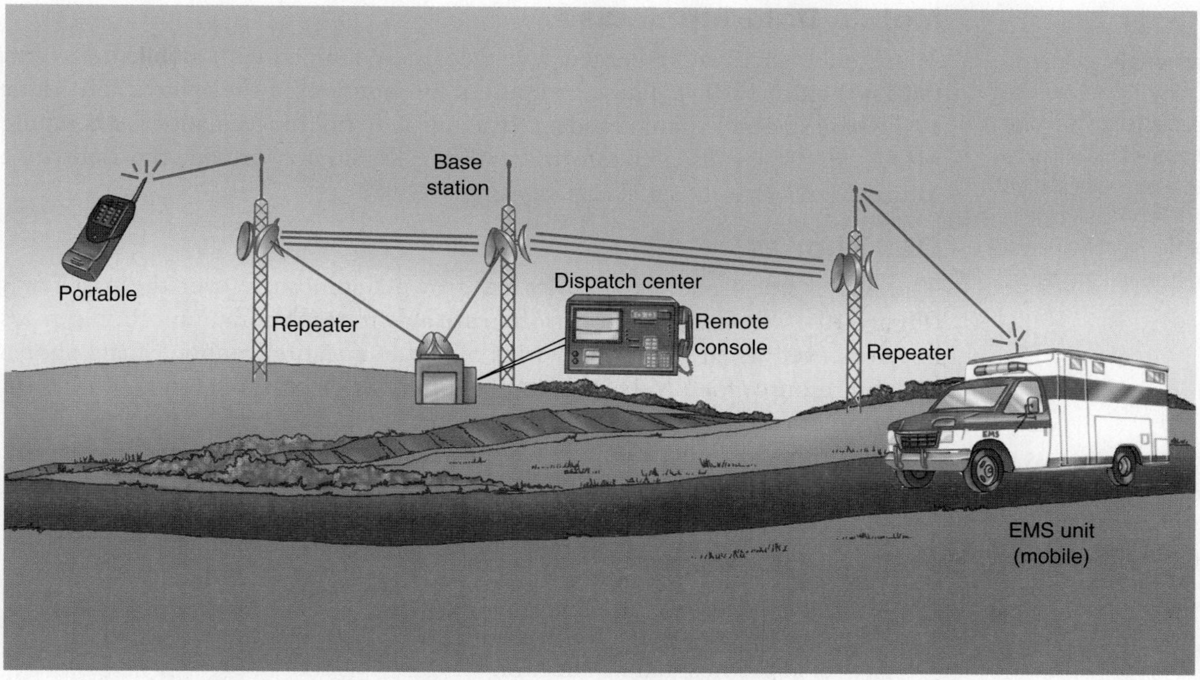

Figure 10-6 A typical EMS communication system is a complex system made up of many components.

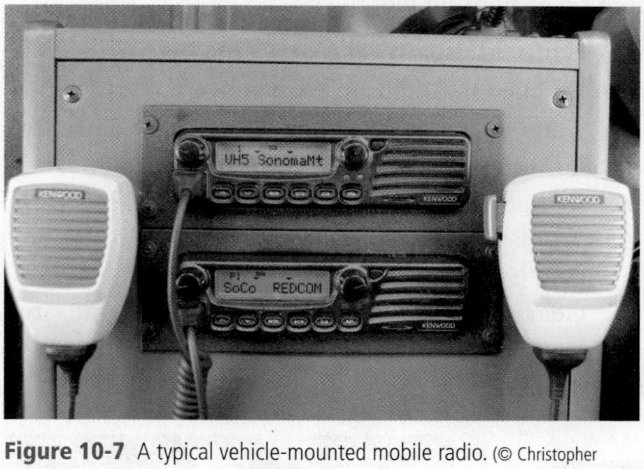

Figure 10-7 A typical vehicle-mounted mobile radio. (© Christopher J. Le Baudour)

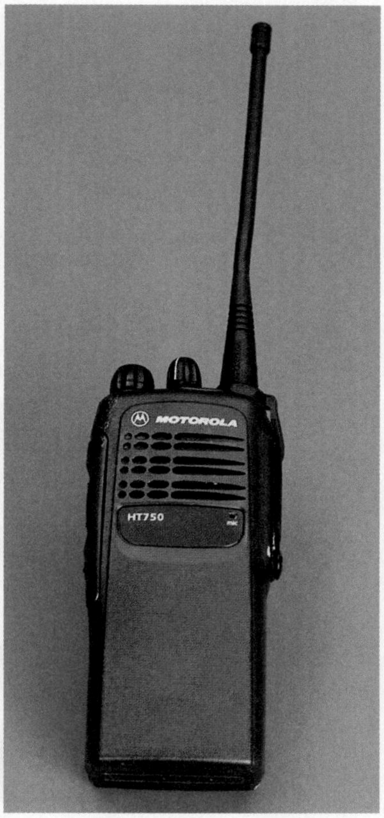

Figure 10-8 A typical hand-held portable radio.

- Press the "push to talk" or "PTT" button for one second before beginning to speak.
- Speak with your mouth about two to three inches from the microphone.
- Address the unit you are calling by its name or radio identifier (for example, its number).
- The unit being called will acknowledge by saying "Go ahead" or another approved code meaning the same thing.
- Speak clearly and slowly.
- Keep transmissions brief.
- Do not use patient names on the air. People with scanners will be able to hear this information. Do not put judgments or negative comments over the air for that same reason.

Mobile Data Terminals

mobile data terminals (MDTs) computers that are mounted in a vehicle and connected to the base station by radio modem. In addition to full functionality as a computer, the MDT will display dispatch information for calls and may provide the ability to enter information for prehospital care reports.

Many ambulances and emergency vehicles are equipped with **mobile data terminals (MDTs)** (Figure 10-9 ■). These computers are mounted in the vehicle and connected to the base station by radio modem. In addition to full functionality as a computer, an MDT will display dispatch information for calls and may provide the ability to enter information for prehospital care reports.

Cell Phones

The use of smart phones in EMS has grown significantly over the past few years (Figure 10-10 ■). Cellular phones often are able to reach communication centers and hospitals even when traditional forms of communication cannot. Smart phones are a useful resource for EMTs because they offer easy access to many resources such as protocols, medical resources, and procedures.

10-14 List key points in an EMS call at which you should communicate with dispatch.

The transmission procedures required of an EMS call vary from agency to agency. Some of the more commonly required transmissions during a call include:

- Dispatch information
- En route notification
- On scene notification
- En route to the hospital notification
- Arrival at the hospital notification
- In service notification
- Back in quarters notification

10-15 Discuss the standard ground rules for radio communications.

Imagine that you are "Rescue One" and you want to ask your dispatch center ("Central Dispatch") to repeat the address where the emergency call is located. The conversation might go something like this:

Rescue One: Central Dispatch, this is Rescue One with a request.

Central Dispatch: Rescue One, Central Dispatch. Go ahead with your request.

Rescue One: Central Dispatch, Rescue One. Can you repeat the address for our call?

Central Dispatch: Rescue One, Central Dispatch. You are responding to 2760 Woolsey Road. That's two seven six zero Woolsey Road. Do you copy?

Rescue One: Central Dispatch, Rescue One. Confirming two seven six zero Woolsey Road.

Central Dispatch: Rescue One, that's affirmative.

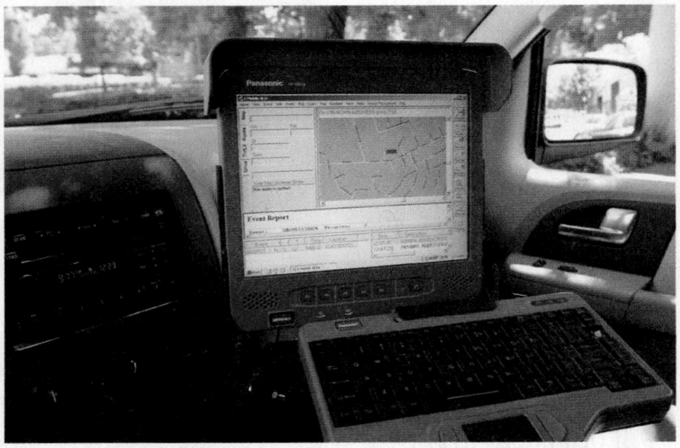

Figure 10-9 A typical vehicle-mounted mobile data terminal.

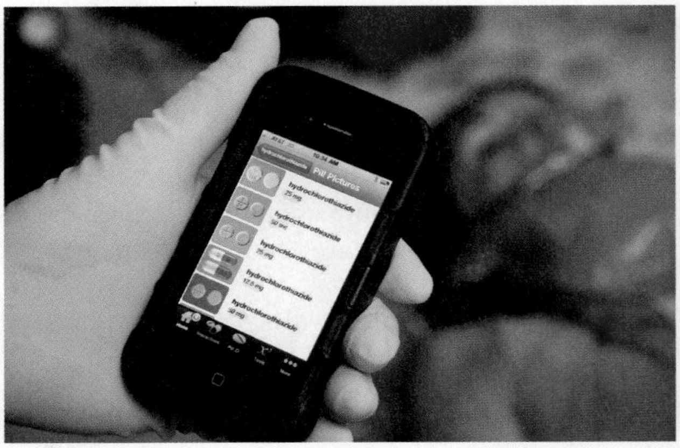

Figure 10-10 Smart phones are becoming useful tools in the prehospital setting.

Do you see the pattern? When you wish to contact another resource in the system, it is standard protocol to state the radio identifier (specified name) of the resource you are calling first (in this case "Central Dispatch"). Follow that with your radio identifier ("Rescue One"). This is especially important when there are several resources using the same frequency, also known as a *channel.*

It is normal to be somewhat shy or intimidated by the prospect of having to talk on the radio in the beginning. Not to worry. It quickly becomes second nature, and you soon will learn to enjoy talking with others on the radio.

One way to become more familiar with radio protocol is to listen to a scanner. A scanner is a specialized radio that only receives radio traffic. Most scanners today can be programmed to receive just about any frequency, so you should be able to program it to the frequencies of the EMS system in your area. If you do not want to purchase a scanner, you can listen on the Internet. A simple Web search should turn up live radio traffic in your area.

STOP, REVIEW, REMEMBER!

Multiple Choice

For each question, place a check next to the correct answer.

1. To ensure the best possible transmission of your message when communicating via portable radio, you should:

_____ a. press the PTT button for one second after you begin speaking.

_____ b. hold the microphone two to three inches from your mouth.

_____ c. transmit your message while seated in the back of the ambulance.

_____ d. begin speaking as soon as you press the PTT button.

2. The radio mounted in the ambulance is called a _____ radio.

_____ a. portable

_____ b. mobile

_____ c. base

_____ d. walkie-talkie

3. Which one of the following statements about repeaters is true?

_____ a. They reduce the signal from radio to radio to reduce interference.

_____ b. They are installed only on base station radios.

_____ c. They boost and retransmit signals a short distance.

_____ d. They boost and retransmit signals a long distance.

4. Which government agency is responsible for allocating EMS radio frequencies?

_____ a. Department of Homeland Security (DHS)

_____ b. Department of Transportation (DOT)

_____ c. Federal Communications Commission (FCC)

_____ d. Federal Emergency Management Agency (FEMA)

5. You have just started your shift. You notify dispatch that your unit is available by saying you are:

_____ a. in quarters.

_____ b. in service.

_____ c. en route.

_____ d. on scene.

(continued on next page)

(continued)

Matching

Match the communication activity described on the left with the type of radio listed on the right.

1. _____ An EMT acknowledges a dispatch from the ambulance. A. Base station
2. _____ An EMT confirms a patient care protocol in the field. B. Mobile radio
3. _____ The dispatcher transmits a call to an ambulance. C. Portable radio
4. _____ An EMT calls for ALS assistance from the patient's living room. D. Smart phone

Critical Thinking

1. Describe the differences among a portable, a mobile, and a base station radio.

____

____

____

____

Medical Communication

Not only will you communicate with your patients, you also will communicate with other medical professionals about each patient you care for and transport. For example, you may call a physician for medical direction, request an advanced life support (ALS) provider, call the hospital on the radio to give a report, and also provide a verbal report to the hospital staff on your arrival. These reports are important because they transfer medical information between health care providers. The reports should be pertinent and concise, while containing all of the appropriate information.

When you contact a busy emergency department by radio or when you drop off a patient, you must provide an accurate, clinically relevant report. That means your report must contain information on the patient's chief complaint and condition, any pertinent medical history, physical exam findings and vital signs, any interventions you have provided, and changes (improvement or worsening) you have seen in the patient's condition.

Communicating with the Hospital

You will contact the hospital for advice or to advise them that you are coming in with a patient so they can prepare. This communication is done from a phone or radio (not in person). It is important that you paint a picture of your patient so the physician can provide any orders or advice accurately.

These reports contain the following information:

- Ambulance identifier and your level of certification—in this case EMT
- Your estimated time of arrival (ETA)
- Patient's age and gender

- Patient's chief complaint
- Brief, pertinent history of the patient's present illness or injury
- Relevant past medical history
- Vital signs including mental status
- Pertinent findings of your examination
- Emergency care you provided
- Patient's response to your care

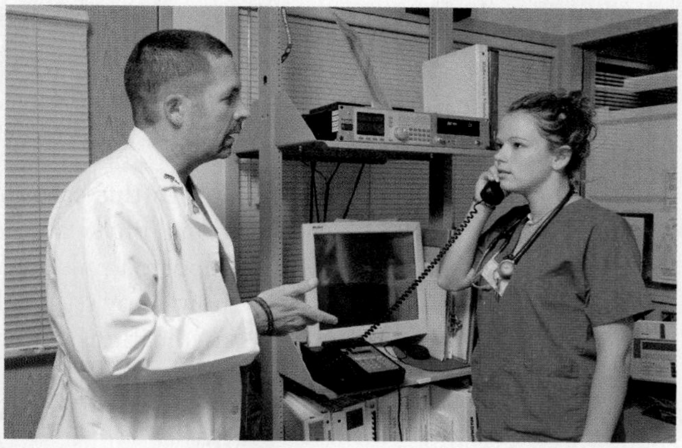

Figure 10-11 A specially trained nurse or physician at the hospital will take your report via radio.

A sample call-in report is as follows (Figure 10-11 ■):

EMT: Mercy Hospital, this is Ambulance 21. How do you copy?

Hospital: This is Mercy 21. Go ahead.

EMT: Mercy, Ambulance 21 is 10 minutes from your location at the EMT level with a 47-year-old male patient who complains of leg pain after a fall from a ladder. The fall was from about four feet. We noted deformity to the left tib/fib. The patient denies other injury. The patient has no past medical history or meds. He is alert and oriented, and never lost consciousness. His pulse is 94 strong and regular, respirations 16, BP 124/86, pupils equal and reactive, skin warm and dry. We have splinted the leg and have good circulation and neuro distal to the injury. We've applied ice. He is in quite a bit of pain but seems stable.

Hospital: Mercy to Ambulance 21. We'll be expecting you. You'll be going to the cast room.

EMT: Ambulance 21, 10-4 and clear.

This is a significant amount of information. Each bit is pertinent and relevant. Read the report above while timing yourself on a watch with a second hand. It should take you 30–40 seconds.

That is what is meant by concise and relevant. There are some things in the patient's medical history that are not important for the radio report. For example, if the patient had hernia surgery seven years ago (and it has been fine since then), that information does not go in the radio report. The fact that he has bunions, occasional indigestion, or broke his arm once as a child also has no significance to his present condition and would only serve to clog an otherwise excellent report with unnecessary facts.

Consider the following report, which describes a more complicated problem:

EMT: Mercy, Ambulance 21. How do you copy?

Hospital: Mercy to Ambulance 21. Loud and clear. Go ahead.

EMT: Mercy, we are en route to your location at the basic level with a 15-minute ETA. We are treating a 64-year-old female patient who complains of difficulty breathing. The difficulty began suddenly and woke her from sleep. She is able to speak five- to six-word sentences before catching her breath. She reports having a heart attack last year and has high blood pressure. She takes furosemide and atenolol. She is alert and oriented, slightly anxious. Pulse is 104 and regular, respirations 24, BP 146/92, skin warm and dry, pupils equal and reactive. We've found that she sleeps on several pillows and has some edema in her ankles. We put her in the Fowler's position and are giving oxygen by nonrebreather mask at 15 liters, which brought her oxygen saturation from 95% to 98% and reduced her anxiety. Over.

Hospital: Okay, Ambulance 21. Sounds good. We'll be awaiting your arrival in 15. Mercy out.

In this case the patient was having difficulty breathing. You also provided additional physical findings, such as the edema and sleeping elevated on pillows, and you reported pulse oximetry readings and your positioning of the patient. The hospital now knows that this is a potentially serious situation based on her cardiac history, medications, and complaint.

Requesting Advice from Medical Direction

There are times you will call a medical direction physician or medical director for advice. There are many reasons this will occur. Some of the most common include when protocols require the contact (for example, to assist a patient with medication administration), patient refusal situations, and any time you feel you would benefit from speaking to a physician.

The format for your report to the physician is similar to the call-in radio report, except you will be asking a question at the end of your report. The question may be specific: "May I assist this patient with the use of her inhaler?" or "Do you think it is appropriate for this patient to refuse transportation?" or "Do you think that this patient should receive nitroglycerin?"

When requesting permission to assist patients with their own medications or to administer medications you carry on the ambulance, there are additional facts a physician will require. You must be very specific. Those facts include answers to the following:

- Do the patient's signs and symptoms match the condition the drug is intended for?
- Has the medication been prescribed specifically to the patient?
- Does the patient have any allergies to medications?
- Has the patient taken any of the medication already? If so, has the patient had any response?
- What are the patient's vital signs? (Vital signs take on increased importance when considering medication orders.)

When you speak to a physician and obtain an order to assist with or administer a medication, you should always repeat the order back to the physician for confirmation. If the physician gives an order that does not make sense to you or suggests a misunderstanding of the information you presented, ask for clarification or explanation before carrying out any order.

The following is an example of a radio report in which the EMT requests an order to administer a medication:

EMT: Mercy Hospital, this is Ambulance 21.

Hospital: This is Mercy. 21, go ahead.

EMT: Ambulance 21 requesting a physician for medical direction request.

Hospital: Stand by, 21.

Hospital: Ambulance 21, this is Dr. Perkins. Go ahead with your report.

EMT: Dr. Perkins, we are en route to your location, 20-minute ETA, with a 32-year-old female patient who complains of shortness of breath after exercising. She reports a history of asthma for which she has an albuterol inhaler. No other health problems or allergies. She is alert, oriented, and anxious. Vitals are pulse 110 strong and regular, respirations 28 and labored. We can hear wheezing without a stethoscope. BP 138/88. Skin is warm but slightly moist. As we said, we have wheezing and also mild accessory muscle use. She is speaking about four-word sentences. Her oxygen sats were 92 when we arrived. Oxygen at 15 L/min via nonrebreather brought that up to 95. Her albuterol inhaler is prescribed to her and is not expired. She used it for "two or three puffs," which caused slight improvement. We'd like to coach her and make sure it is being done properly and administer two more puffs of the albuterol. Over.

Hospital: Okay, 21. Get her to take two more puffs of the albuterol inhaler, timed well and with deep breaths. You said you were 20 minutes out, so give it 5 minutes, and if her vitals remain stable, you can administer two more puffs of the albuterol. Let me know if there are any changes. Monitor her breathing carefully. If I don't hear back, I'll see you in 20 minutes.

EMT: Confirming two puffs of albuterol now. Timed well with deep breaths. Two more in five minutes if vitals remain okay.

Hospital: These orders are confirmed. Please advise of any significant changes in the patient's condition. Mercy out.

EMT: Ambulance 21 out.

There may be times when your medical direction physician may not be at the hospital to which you are taking the patient. In that case, you will need to notify the receiving hospital with a radio report as well.

Verbal Reports at the Hospital

When you arrive at the hospital, the nurse or physician meeting you should already know the information you called in by way of the radio. In that case you will be able to provide a verbal report that summarizes and updates the information given over the radio. If the information has not been relayed to the person you are dealing with, or if partial information was relayed, you will need to provide a full report. Information contained in the verbal report includes:

10-16 Describe the elements of a verbal transfer of care.

- Restatement of the chief complaint
- Significant changes in the patient's condition since the radio report
- History information not previously presented (may include medications)
- Treatments that were administered en route
- Subsequent vital signs taken en route
- Additional pertinent information not presented in the radio report

PERSPECTIVE

Dr. Orwell—The Physician

Most of the ambulance crews are great at communicating with both the patient and us in the emergency department. But sometimes a mistake is made. What if the patient is unresponsive when he is brought in, and I need to make decisions based on the medical information that an EMT gathered at the scene? I could decide on a course of action that kills my patient just because an EMT wasn't actually listening when a family member was talking. And let me tell you, I cannot trust that EMT and will address the mistakes.

An example of a verbal report follows. It pertains to the patient for whom you requested orders from medical direction to administer her prescribed inhaler.

EMT: Hi. This is our patient, Sally Farnsworth. We called in. Did you get the info?

Hospital nurse: Yes, I heard it on the radio.

EMT: Okay. She has a history of asthma and developed shortness of breath after exercising. She says it is similar to previous attacks. She used her albuterol inhaler twice. We did four more puffs en route, spaced five minutes apart as ordered. She has felt considerable relief. Her pulse and respirations have come down a bit. Her sats are up to 98%. Doing better. Do you have any further questions for me?

Hospital nurse: No. Thanks for the report. Very good. Sally, I'm Hal Chapman, the nurse who is going to take care of you today. Let's get you moved over to our stretcher.

Never leave a patient in the emergency department without providing a face-to-face verbal report directly to the staff member who will be assuming care of your patient. Failure to do so could result in potential harm to the patient and would constitute abandonment (as discussed in Chapter 3).

CLINICAL CLUE

Rails Up

When leaving a patient at the hospital, it is always important to make sure the hospital bed is lowered to the lowest position and that the side rails are up. This is for your patient's safety. It is a good idea to document these details in your prehospital care report later.

STOP, REVIEW, REMEMBER!

Multiple Choice

For each question, place a check next to the correct answer.

1. Which one of the following is *not* a part of the hospital radio report?

_____ a. Chief complaint

_____ b. Patient's gender

_____ c. Complete medical history

_____ d. Vital signs

2. Which one of the following items would *not* be appropriate in the radio report to the hospital?

_____ a. Patient's blood pressure

_____ b. You splinted a suspected leg fracture

_____ c. Patient's complete medication list

_____ d. Patient's prior heart attacks

3. Which one of the following statements best describes the content of a radio report?

_____ a. Fair and balanced

_____ b. Concise and relevant

_____ c. Lengthy and complete

_____ d. Short and fast

4. How does a "request for advice" from a physician differ from a basic call-in report?

_____ a. Less medication information is required for physician advice when compared to a call-in.

_____ b. You frequently ask questions at the end of a call-in report.

_____ c. Requests for physician advice may include more than one set of vital signs.

_____ d. Call-in reports are generally longer than requests for advice.

5. Which one of the statements below reflects the differences between the call-in radio report and the in-person hand-off report at the hospital?

_____ a. The hand-off report includes all information from the radio report plus any new information you have obtained.

_____ b. If the person receiving the report at the hospital heard the radio report, no further report is necessary.

_____ c. The verbal report at the hospital is given by the patient. The radio report is given by the EMT.

_____ d. The hand-off report highlights core information, medications, treatments, and changes in the patient's condition.

Critical Thinking

1. List the components of the call-in radio report to the hospital.

____

____

____

____

2. List two differences between the call-in report (radio) and the hand-off report (in person at the hospital).

____

____

____

____

3. How would a physician or nurse at the hospital view you on arrival at the hospital when your radio report was hurried and incomplete?

____

____

____

____

EMERGENCY DISPATCH SUMMARY

Mr. Tamblyn was released later the same day with a diagnosis of a pulled abdominal muscle. He has since recovered fully. Dr. Orwell contacted the Field Supervisor for the ambulance company and made a formal complaint about Melanie's poor communication skills, a third such complaint. Melanie was placed into a remedial training program and is showing marked improvement in her listening and other communication skills.

Chapter Review

To the Point

- Never underestimate the role communication plays in patient care and transfer of care.
- Listening intently to your patient will allow you to build rapport so you will be able to accurately treat and report his condition. A good listener will be able to detect things that may not be said.
- Speaking is done with words and with body language. Convey confidence and speak slowly to the patient to ensure comprehension. If it is safe, go down to the patient's level and make eye contact.
- A reassuring hand on a patient's shoulder or a hand to hold can reassure the patient. Remember, your patient is probably having the worst day of his life. Show you care.
- If you do not speak the same language as your patient, check to see if a member of the family, a neighbor, or a crew member can translate.
- The way you ask questions is important to getting detailed and accurate information from your patient. Note that it is not uncommon for a patient to provide different information to multiple rescuers.
- Therapeutic communication focuses on advancing the physical and emotional well-being of a patient.
- The elements of an appropriate verbal transfer of care include the patient's name and age, chief complaint, brief account of his current condition, past pertinent medical history, vital signs, pertinent findings from the physical exam, overview of the care you provided, and his response to your care.
- Remember that you may have to modify your communication approach, depending on the age of the patient. An elderly patient may be hard of hearing, so you will have to speak louder, and a child may not understand what is going on. Use simple terms and explain everything very carefully ahead of time.
- Radio etiquette is important. Be mindful of others who may be transmitting or need to transmit. Speak clearly, slowly, and briefly.
- When communicating with a hospital to advise them that you are coming in with a patient, it is important that you paint a picture of the patient's condition so the physician can provide any orders accurately and prepare for arrival.
- A physician may be needed for on-line direction and will likely require more patient information than a typical prehospital report. Information such as signs and symptoms, allergies, medications (and when they were taken), and accurate vital signs may be requested.
- Once at the hospital a verbal report should include the patient's chief complaint, changes in the patient's condition since the initial radio report, and any history not provided over the radio.

Chapter Questions

Multiple Choice

For each question, place a check next to the correct answer.

1. You are helping a new EMT with the use of a portable radio. Which piece of advice would *not* be appropriate?

_____ a. Listen before transmitting.
_____ b. Speak with your mouth as close as possible to the microphone for best sound transmission.
_____ c. Do not use the patient's name or other specific identifying information on the air.
_____ d. Push the "PTT" button for one second before you speak.

2. Which one of the following would be the best way to communicate with a patient who is unable to hear?

_____ a. Shouting
_____ b. Speaking quickly to avoid frustration
_____ c. Writing down questions
_____ d. Avoiding speech altogether

3. Which one of the following considerations is *not* included in your request for a physician's order to administer medication?
   _____ a. Do the patient's signs and symptoms match the condition the drug is intended for?
   _____ b. Does the patient have any allergies to medications?
   _____ c. Has the patient taken any of the medication already? If so, has the patient had any response?
   _____ d. Does the patient have any food allergies?

4. Which device boosts the transmission signal from a base station?
   _____ a. Mobile radio
   _____ b. Mobile data terminal (MDT)
   _____ c. Repeater
   _____ d. Remote console

5. What is the best way to communicate with a patient who has a language barrier if no one is available to translate?
   _____ a. Speak louder.
   _____ b. Work quickly and get him to the hospital, where there may be a translator.
   _____ c. Continue to speak to him as if he understood you.
   _____ d. Maintain eye contact, show him the tools you will be using, and motion as to how they work.

Critical Thinking

1. You are called to a 75-year-old patient who is complaining of chest pain. She is extremely anxious and seems fearful of going to the hospital. Describe several things you have learned in this chapter that you will use to calm the patient and help get her to accept transport.

____
____
____
____

2. Why is it important to notify the dispatcher of key events such as arriving on scene, being en route to the hospital, and so on?

____
____
____
____

3. Imagine you are a patient who is being cared for by an EMT. How would you react if the EMT was not listening or making eye contact but stood above you and talked to another person (such as your spouse or your parent) to obtain your medical history and history of the present illness?

____
____
____
____

4. You receive an order from a physician to assist the patient with one sublingual nitroglycerin spray and to have the patient chew four low-dose aspirin. How would you confirm this with the physician? Write down your response.

____
____
____
____

(continued on next page)

(continued)

5. What four additional things (over and above the call-in radio report) will you need to tell the physician when asking for permission to assist a patient with his medication?

____

____

____

____

6. Why is it important to limit the amount of information given in the radio report to the most pertinent information?

____

____

____

____

7. Your grandmother has fallen and is being cared for by EMTs. What would you expect from the EMTs in reference to the way they treat your grandmother?

____

____

____

____

Reconstruct the Radio Report

The following radio reports have been taken apart and placed in individual sentences. Reassemble the reports by numbering the sentences in the most logical order.

Radio Report 1

_____ We have splinted the extremity and applied cold. She has good circulation and sensation distal to the injury.
_____ A 27-year-old female patient.
_____ Her pulse is 86 strong and regular, respirations 16, BP 106/74, pupils equal and reactive, skin warm and dry.
_____ Patient is alert and oriented. She never lost consciousness.
_____ Complains of an ankle injury sustained while hiking. She slipped from a rock and twisted the ankle.
_____ En route to your facility with a 17-minute ETA.
_____ Patient has a history of asthma but has no complaint of difficulty breathing.
_____ She is resting comfortably with minor pain in the ankle.
_____ There is swelling and deformity of the left ankle. Patient did not fall and denies further injury.

Radio Report 2

_____ Vital signs are pulse 104 regular and weak, respirations 26, BP 152/94, skin pale and moist, pupils equal and reactive.
_____ He developed shortness of breath after having an increased cough and sputum production for a week.
_____ We administered oxygen and placed the patient in a position of comfort.
_____ He is alert and oriented.
_____ An 86-year-old male patient.
_____ He is speaking five- to six-word sentences. He has produced some brown sputum. Initial oxygen saturation was 88%.

_____ We are en route to your location with a five-minute ETA.
_____ Complaining of shortness of breath.
_____ His sats came up to 94% with oxygen and he is breathing a little easier.
_____ He has a history of emphysema and MI.

Case Study

You are called to a residence for an unknown medical problem. The dispatcher says she is unable to understand the caller. The police are also dispatched. You arrive on the scene and find the police talking to a male teenager in the doorway. Once you are waved in by the police, you find that the patient does not speak English. The patient, a 50-year-old Hispanic man, was cleaning windows when he fell from the ladder. His wife, who speaks broken English, called for help. You find the son does speak fluent English and will translate.

1. Can you use the son as a translator? Why or why not?

____

____

____

____

2. Would the interpreted information you receive from the son be accurate? How can you ensure accuracy?

____

____

____

____

3. Will you be able to perform an assessment at a normal pace? If not, will it be faster or slower? Why?

____

____

____

____

The Last Word

Communication in EMS is more than talking. The different ways you communicate with patients is important—sometimes therapeutic. It is likely the part of the call the patient will remember most.

Your communication with other health care professionals has a direct relation to the care you give and the care the patient will receive at the hospital. Your communications must be accurate, yet concise.

The radio systems used in your area are vital for communication. Radios, whether they are base stations, mobiles, portables, cell phones, or computers are used for communicating calls and other vital information. Radios must be treated well and maintained so they will be ready when you need them.

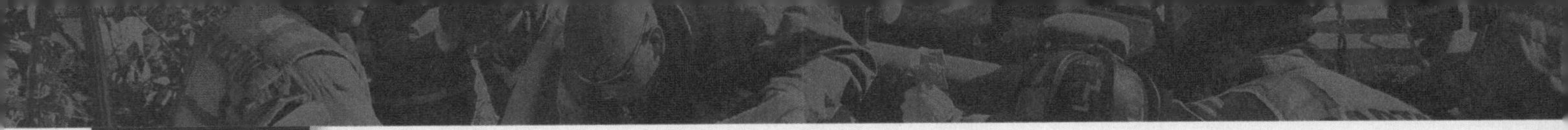

11 Documenting Your Assessment and Care

Education Standards

Preparatory: Documentation

Competencies

Applies fundamental knowledge of the EMS system, safety/well-being of the EMT, medical/legal issues, and ethical issues to the provision of emergency care.

Objectives

After completion of this lesson, you should be able to:

11-1 Define key terms introduced in this chapter.

11-2 Describe each of the following purposes served by the prehospital care report (PCR): continuity of patient care, administrative uses, legal document, education and research, and evaluation and continuous quality improvement (CQI).

11-3 Explain the purposes of the U.S. Department of Transportation (DOT) minimum data set for PCRs.

11-4 List the elements of the DOT minimum data set for PCRs.

11-5 Describe the purpose and contents of each of the following sections of a PCR: administrative data, patient demographics and other patient data, vital signs, narrative, and treatment.

11-6 Give examples of each of the following types of PCR narrative information: chief complaint, pertinent history, subjective information, objective information, and pertinent negatives/positives.

11-7 Describe the elements of the SOAP and CHART methods of documentation.

11-8 Explain each of the following legal concerns with respect to the PCR: confidentiality, allowed distribution of the PCR or information included in it, documenting a patient's refusal of treatment, falsification of the PCR, and correction of errors.

11-9 Discuss how to handle each of the following situations with respect to the PCR:

- Transfer of patient care when returning to service prior to completing the PCR
- Multiple-casualty incidents (MCIs)
- Special reporting situations, such as infectious disease exposure and suspicion of abuse or neglect.

Key Terms

CHART p. 271
error of commission p. 275
error of omission p. 275
falsification p. 275
objective information p. 269
patient data p. 268
prehospital care report (PCR) p. 265
run data p. 268
run report p. 265
SOAP p. 270
subjective information p. 269
timeline narration p. 270

Introduction

Documenting your assessment and care is a vitally important part of your role as an EMT. Your written reports—known as *run reports* or *prehospital care reports (PCRs)*—will follow a patient through the health care system as the only lasting representation of your work. Of course, documentation has many other uses. For example, in the short term it is used by emergency department personnel to reference your assessment findings and what care was given in the field.

Good documentation also plays an important role in minimizing your liability. If someone questions the care you gave, would you want thorough documentation of your quality care, or would a quick and shoddy attempt at writing down a few things be enough? There is no doubt you would want to develop a reputation for thorough, accurate documentation. Good documentation is more than legal protection. Good documentation also should be a matter of pride in what you do.

EMERGENCY DISPATCH

"Mr. Devlin," the attorney said, rolling his pencil on the table and looking at the tiled ceiling for a moment before continuing. "Take us back to that night. Just explain what happened in your own words, and try to be as detailed as possible. Keep in mind that a deposition is just like a trial, and you've sworn to tell the truth."

EMT Joe Devlin looked around the conference table at the others present but dropped his gaze when he encountered the face of the woman who was suing his employer, the North County Ambulance Service.

"Yeah, sure," Joe said. What did he remember about that call? He had been searching his memory ever since the guy showed up with the subpoena at work. He glanced at his copy of the PCR, but the narrative wasn't very helpful, just a couple of hastily written sentences that made this incident sound like every other call that he had ever been on. "Well, we arrived to find the patient, um, that lady's husband in some distress. I guess, um, according to my narrative, we transported him to Midway Hospital."

"Actually, Mr. Devlin," the attorney sat up straight and pointed his pencil at Joe. "You transported Mr. O'Neil to Riverside Community Hospital, not Midway. As a matter of fact, our contention is that had you taken the patient to Midway, he might still be alive today. But please, continue. I might suggest that you don't use that PCR, though. We found that it's full of errors. Just tell us from memory, if you can."

Joe glanced at the patient's address on the PCR: Portland Drive. Why wouldn't he have taken that patient to Midway? Going to Riverside would have added 20 minutes to the transport time. There must have been a reason.

"I'm sorry," Joe shook his head. "I don't remember what happened. It was over a year ago. I just don't know."

"Thanks, Mr. Devlin." The attorney smiled and set his pencil down on a blank legal pad. "We don't have any other questions for you."

Prehospital Care Reports

11-2 Describe each of the following purposes served by the prehospital care report (PCR): continuity of patient care, administrative uses, legal document, education and research, and evaluation and continuous quality improvement (CQI).

run report written documentation of the call and patient encounter. Also called a *prehospital care report*.

prehospital care report (PCR) written documentation of the call and patient encounter. Also called a *patient care report* or a *run report*.

Depending on your agency or region, the report you use to document your care may be called a **run report,** a **prehospital care report (PCR),** or a patient care report (Figure 11-1 ▪). While most reports are still documented on paper, more and more agencies are moving to electronic documentation and reporting (Figure 11-2 ▪).

Whatever your agency calls the report, thorough and complete documentation is necessary. Your report is a direct reflection of your professionalism as an EMT. While you may never see your report again, it will follow the patient through the health care process and be used as a picture of the care you provided from the minute you entered your patient's world until the minute you transferred care.

There are many reasons for accurate and complete documentation. They include:

- ***Continuity of care.*** Your report may be referred to at any time during the hospital care of the patient. After you leave the hospital, the report may be referenced

DATE	TRIP #	UNIT	CALL RECEIVED	DISPATCHED	EN ROUTE	ON SCENE
TRANSPORTING	ARRIVAL	TOTAL MLG	SERVICE PROVIDER VERIHEALTH INC.		(For Billing Use Only)	
BEG MILEAGE	END MILEAGE					

☐ INITIAL TRANSPORT ☐ ADMITTED TO HOSPITAL ☐ DISCHARGED FROM FIRST FACILITY ☐ DISCHARGED

☐ RETURN TRIP ☐ OUTPATIENT (I.E. RADIATION THERAPY, DR. APPOINTMENT) ☐ ADMITTED TO SECOND FACILITY ☐ NON-MEDICAL

SENDING FACILITY/SCENE LOCATION					RECEIVING FACILITY	
PATIENT NAME (LAST, FIRST)	PHONE #	AGE	☐ MO ☐ YR	SEX ☐ M ☐ F	DOB	WEIGHT (kg)
PATIENT ADDRESS (STREET)	(CITY)	(STATE)	(ZIP)		SSN	
ALTERNATE CONTACT (NAME)	(PHONE #)			(RELATION)		

PRIMARY INSURANCE

COMPANY NAME	SUBSCRIBER NAME			POLICY # / GROUP #
ADDRESS (STREET)	(CITY)	(STATE)	(ZIP)	PHONE #

SECONDARY INSURANCE

COMPANY NAME	SUBSCRIBER NAME			POLICY # / GROUP #
ADDRESS (STREET)	(CITY)	(STATE)	(ZIP)	PHONE #

BLS TRANSPORT

MED HX

MEDICAL HX

CURRENT MEDICATIONS — ALLERGIES

MENTAL STATUS	AIRWAY	BREATHING	PULSE	SKIN COLOR	SKIN MOISTURE	SKIN TEMP
☐ ALERT	☐ PATIENT	☐ NORMAL	☐ REGULAR	☐ NORMAL	☐ DRY	☐ NORMAL
☐ ORIENTED X_____	☐ ASPIRATION RISK	☐ DYSPNEA	☐ IRREGULAR	☐ PALE	☐ MOIST	☐ COOL
☐ RESPONDS / VERBAL	☐ SECRETIONS	☐ RETRACTIONS	☐ STRONG	☐ FLUSHED	☐ DIAPHORETIC	☐ HOT
☐ RESPONDS / PAIN	☐ SUCTIONING REQ.	☐ ACC. MUSCLE	☐ WEAK	☐ CYANOTIC		
☐ UNRESPONSIVE				☐ MOTTLED		

IV

LOCATION ☐ N/A ☐ SALINE / HEPARIN LOCK ☐ MONITORED GTT: RATE:________ CC / HR, FLUID TYPE:________

☐ NARCOTIC INFUSION (LOCKED) DRUG:________ RATE:________

ASSESSMENT

CHECK ALL THAT APPLY AND EXPLAIN WHY AND HOW IN THE NARRATIVE

☐ PATIENT BED CONFINED AT TIME OF SERVICE DUE TO:

- ☐ MOTOR CONTROL / MUSCLE TONE PRECLUDES SITTING UP
- ☐ DECUB. ULCERS / WOUNDS REQ. POSITIONING & CAREFUL HANDLING
- ☐ SEVERE CONTRACTURES
- ☐ PAIN INCREASES WITH SITTING / MOVEMENT
- ☐ SPECIAL ORTHOPEDIC DEVICE IN PLACE
- ☐ FRACTURE OR POSSIBILITY OF FRACTURE
- ☐ POST SPINAL INJURY
- ☐ OBESITY (WEIGHT MUST BE NOTED ABOVE)
- ☐ SUPPORTIVE DEVICES REQUIRED (I.E. WEDGE / PILLOWS)
- ☐ REQUIRES MULTIPLE ATTENDANTS
- ☐ PATIENT IN PAIN (SEE DESCRIPTION IN NARRATIVE)
- ☐ REQUIRES OXYGEN DURING TRANSPORT
- ☐ PATIENT SEDATED AT TIME OF SERVICE

RESTRAINTS

- ☐ CHEMICAL (CIRCLE ALL THAT APPLY)
- ☐ PHYSICAL: POSEY VEST WRIST ANKLE BELTS

OBSERVATION / SUPERVISION

- ☐ 5150 – DOCUMENTATION ATTACHED
- ☐ SEVERE DEMENTIA
- ☐ FLIGHT RISK
- ☐ PROTECT MEDICAL MODALITIES

AIRWAY MONITORING

- ☐ REQUIRED SECONDARY TO CONDITION
- ☐ UNABLE TO CONTROL SECRETIONS (ASPIRATION RISK)
- ☐ POOR MUSCLE TONE / CONTROL (QUADRIPLEGIC)

OTHER

- ☐ ISOLATION PRECAUTIONS DUE TO (POSS) INFECTIOUS DISEASE
- ☐ REQUIRED MONITORING BY OTHER LICENSED MEDICAL PROFESSIONAL ACCOMPANYING TRANSPORT
- ☐ TRANSFER TO HIGHER LEVEL OF CARE
- ☐ TRANSFER TO LOCKDOWN FACILITY / WARD

O_2 DELIVERY	CAPILLARY REFILL
LPM ☐ NC ☐ NRB	☐ < 2 SEC ☐ > 2 SEC

VITALS

TIME	BP	PULSE	RR	TIME	BP	PULSE	RR	TIME	BP	PULSE	RR	TIME	BP	PULSE	RR

NARRATIVE

☐ PATIENT SECURED TO GURNEY USING ALL SECURING STRAPS AND GURNEY LOCKED INTO PLACE IN BACK OF AMBULANCE. — CARE TRANSFERRED TO (NAME / TITLE)

MED TEAM

ATTENDANT	EMP #	DRIVER	EMP #
(SIGNATURE)		(SIGNATURE)	
(PRINT)		(PRINT)	

Figure 11-1 A typical paper prehospital care report. Note the various sections and what they contain. (Courtesy of Verihealth Inc., Petaluma, CA)

for the vital signs you obtained early in the call, medications or treatments you administered, or your observations at the scene.

- *Education.* Your written report may be used as an example for others of proper documentation. If you responded to an unusual or challenging call, it may be used as a basis for training other providers who may encounter similar patients or situations.
- *Administrative purposes.* The report will be used for the documentation of billing information. It also may be used to do statistical analysis on issues that affect your agency, such as response times and staffing.
- *Quality improvement.* Prehospital care reports in your agency will be reviewed as part of a continuous quality improvement (CQI), total quality management (TQM), process improvement (PI), or quality assurance (QA) program.
- *Research.* Reports are often used to research important clinical issues in EMS, such as specific treatments for patients with airway problems or shock.
- *Legal purposes.* The report you created is a legal document. It may be called into court as evidence in a legal action where your patient is suing someone for causing his injuries, as evidence in a criminal action where your patient was the victim of a crime, or as documentation when you or another member of the team that treated the patient is accused of improper care of the patient.

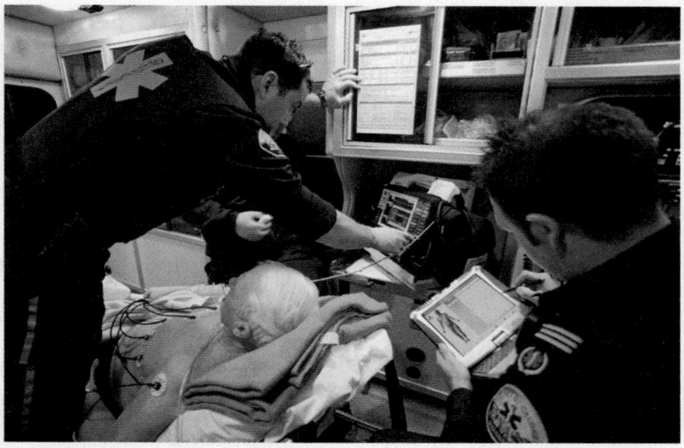

Figure 11-2 An EMT using an electronic tablet to complete his prehospital care report en route to the hospital. (© Kevin Link)

When your report is called to attention in a legal matter, you may be required to provide a pretrial deposition to explain your care and documentation or you may be required to go to court to testify. You may be asked to testify about your observations on the call, what others may have said, details about the care you provided, and that it accurately depicts the events of the call.

Documentation plays a large role in minimizing the exposure to liability for you and your agency. The old saying "If you didn't document it, you didn't do it" is true when it comes to liability. For example, someone may look at your written report and observe that you did not give oxygen to a patient with chest pain. You, of course, recognize that oxygen is a vitally important part of the care for chest pain and are sure you did provide it. However, if it was not documented, the only conclusion a person reading your report could reach is that it was not.

PERSPECTIVE

Joe Devlin—The EMT

Oh man, that couldn't have gone worse. I mean, I'm a good EMT. I really am, and I know for a fact that I just wouldn't have taken a critical patient to a particular hospital if one was closer. Maybe Midway diverted us, or the patient requested Riverside. I don't know. But now I look like the bad guy just because I don't remember and my PCR was a piece of junk.

Good documentation alone will not protect you from liability. One of the most significant ways to minimize liability is to treat people compassionately and provide quality care. Documenting shoddy, incomplete, or inaccurate care will only open the door to lawsuits.

CLINICAL CLUE

Compassionate Care

High quality, compassionate care supported by good documentation can greatly minimize your exposure to liability.

Components of the Prehospital Care Report

11-3 Explain the purposes of the U.S. Department of Transportation (DOT) minimum data set for PCRs.

11-4 List the elements of the DOT minimum data set for PCRs.

11-5 Describe the purpose and contents of each of the following sections of a PCR: administrative data, patient demographics and other patient data, vital signs, narrative, and treatment.

There are two ways prehospital care reports can be completed: on paper and electronically. More and more agencies are moving to an electronic method of documenting patient care because it offers a great deal of standardization and can be easily and quickly shared with others directly involved with the patient's care. Electronic data can also be more easily collected and analyzed to identify trends that may need to be addressed. Regardless of how the reports are completed, the data that goes into each should be consistent and standardized.

Minimum Data Set

In an effort to standardize the data collected about patient care across the nation, the U.S. Department of Transportation (DOT) in conjunction with the National EMS Information System (NEMSIS) has established a minimum data set for prehospital care reports. The goal is to establish a national database of information that can be used to create uniformity in EMS and improve patient outcomes. The elements of the minimum data set are as follows:

- Chief complaint
- Level of responsiveness
- Respiratory rate
- Pulse
- Blood pressure
- Skin color, temperature, and moisture
- Treatment rendered
- Patient demographics
- Call times, as well as response and transport codes

The minimum data set is just that, a minimum. Most prehospital care reports include additional information based on local, regional, and state needs and requirements.

Sections of the Report

Each report has several sections, each of which requires specific, important information. There are sections for run data, patient data, and a narrative.

RUN DATA

run data information about the call itself, such as the name of the unit and crew members responding, the date and time of the call, and the name of the ambulance service.

The **run data** section of the prehospital care report includes information about the call itself, such as the names of the responding unit and crew members, the date and time of the call, the name of the ambulance service, and certification levels of those providing care. Times recorded must be accurate and synchronous (by clocks or watches that show the same time). Be sure to use the time given to you by the dispatcher when noting times on your report, and then make sure the time on your watch does not differ from the dispatch center's official time. Time synchronization is important, especially in determining how long a patient has been in cardiac arrest, documenting trends in the patient's condition, and measurement of system efficiency, such as response times.

PATIENT DATA

patient data all the information about the patient (name, address, date of birth), insurance, and details of the patient's complaint, assessment, care, and vital signs.

The **patient data** section of the prehospital care report includes all the information about the patient, including:

- Name, address, date of birth, sex
- Nature of the call

- Insurance information
- Detailed information on the patient's complaint
- Mechanism of injury, assessment findings
- Care administered before (by bystanders) and after the arrival of the EMT
- Vital signs
- SAMPLE history
- Changes in condition throughout the call

The information in each of the sections of the report can be entered in various ways, depending on the type of report (written or electronic). That information includes:

- ***Fill-in.*** You would write the patient's name, address, date of birth, insurance information, and vital signs in spaces labeled for this use.
- ***Check boxes.*** Some reports have boxes that can be checked for information such as patient history, nature of illness, and care provided.
- ***Drop-down menu.*** This is a common feature of most electronic PCR programs and allows for many choices without taking up too much space on the screen.
- ***Narrative.*** Space is provided for you to write narrative information (your "story" documenting the patient's history, assessment, and care) that does not otherwise fit in check boxes or that requires expansion on the details.

It is easy to get into a routine of simply checking or filling in a box on the prehospital care report with WNL (within normal limits). Do not let that happen. It is important to carefully record your findings because they will guide the ongoing treatment of the patient. Vital signs taken at regular intervals—15 minutes for stable patients and every 5 minutes for unstable patients—show trends in the patient's overall condition. They will allow you to see the effectiveness of your treatment and help guide whomever takes over patient care.

CLINICAL CLUE

WNL

Some medical directors will discourage the use of WNL (within normal limits) when documenting patient care. It often is better to describe what normal is. For instance, rather than describe an abdominal assessment as "WNL," it could be better described as "soft, nontender." Many EMS providers describe WNL as "We never looked" because it can leave the provider open for risk should the PCR ever be called as evidence in a lawsuit.

Narrative Documentation

Narrative portions of the prehospital care report are usually the most challenging to write. When writing the narrative, avoid the use of radio codes and slang. Abbreviations are acceptable, if they are standard and understood by hospital and other EMS personnel. Many agencies have a list of acceptable abbreviations that may be used. Be sure to use proper spelling in your report, even if you must use a medical dictionary. Knowledge of medical terminology and proper spelling of terms will make your reports clearer and more accurate.

The information you write in the narrative should be objective rather than subjective. **Objective information** is that which you have personally observed and can attest to. **Subjective information** is that which is not firsthand or is subject to interpretation. The statement—"The patient has a one-inch laceration on his forehead"—is

objective information information that you have personally observed and can measure or attest to.

subjective information information that is not firsthand or that is subject to interpretation.

objective. Statements that begin with "I think . . ." or "It seems . . ." usually contain subjective information. Examples of subjective statements include "I don't believe this patient is telling the truth" or "His car was probably going 90 miles an hour when it hit the tree." In short, avoid writing conclusions that are not facts.

PERSPECTIVE

Thomas Powell, Esq.—The Plaintiff's Attorney

As soon as I saw that PCR, I knew that we had a slam dunk. Come on. It's been a year since the tragic loss of Mr. O'Neil and that EMT's narrative gave no reason whatsoever for the extended transport. In fact it even named the wrong hospital. This EMT may be good at his job, but I knew he wasn't going to remember anything about this call. His documentation skills, or lack of them, made my job that much easier!

One way to put into your report pertinent items that you may not have witnessed yourself is to put the words of the patient or family member or bystander within quotation marks. For example, you might write: Patient states that he took "40 or 50 sleeping pills." You did not witness him taking the pills. Instead, the information comes from the patient himself, and your report reflects this. Another example might be information from a bystander. You could report: An associate of the patient stated that the patient had "10 or 12 beers" before he fell.

Be sure your narrative includes observations of the scene, such as mechanism of injury, suicide notes, approximate blood loss observed at the scene, living conditions, and care given by bystanders.

One of the most important considerations for your narrative is that it should be written legibly and accurately, and it should contain appropriate information. Some agencies and regions have preferred methods of narrative documentation. They include the **timeline narration** (a sequential method). This method of narration tells the story of the call as it happened in step-by-step, chronological order.

timeline narration method of telling the story of the call as it happened in a step-by-step, chronological narrative. Also called *sequential narration*.

SOAP is another method. The letters stand for subjective, objective, assessment, and plan. It refers to a specific portion of the narrative (Figure 11-3 ■):

11-7 Describe the elements of the SOAP and CHART methods of documentation.

SOAP a method of documentation in which each letter stands for a specific portion of the narrative: subjective, objective, assessment, and plan.

S—*Subjective information.* This includes what the patient says in response to your questions, such as the history of the present illness (including OPQRST). It also includes the patient's medical history and information from family and bystanders.

O—*Objective information.* This is the information you obtain from the physical examination. You may observe a wound or the patient in a posture indicating pain or distress. Vital signs and other physical assessments (such as lung sounds and tenderness to palpation) are also included here.

A—*Assessment.* The assessment section is where you consider the subjective and objective information and make an assessment of the patient's overall condition. Examples might be a patient who developed substernal chest discomfort with nausea and diaphoresis after exertion may have cardiac-related chest pain or a patient who fell and has pain and deformity in the lower leg has a suspected fracture.

P—*Plan.* This is the plan you create for the care of the patient. In the case of the patient with chest discomfort, you would plan to administer oxygen, prevent exertion, and assist him with prescribed nitroglycerin if he has it. In the event of the suspected leg fracture, you would plan on immobilizing the leg, applying ice for pain, and so on.

S: Patient complains of difficulty breathing. She reports that it came on while jogging and was accompanied by a "tightness like I can't breathe." She reports a history of asthma for which she takes an albuterol inhaler. This episode seems to the patient to be exactly like asthma attacks she has had in the past. She reports that she is usually able to breathe easier with an inhaler. She states that she took two puffs from her inhaler without significant relief.

O: Patient appears obviously short of breath and is using accessory muscles to breathe. She is in the tripod position. Wheezes are audible without a stethoscope. Lung sounds and wheezing are present in all fields of the chest by auscultation. Vital signs P: 102 strong and regular, R: 28 and adequate, BP 118/84, skin pink, warm and moist. Pupils equal/react. SaO2 93% before oxygen.

A: Patient has signs and symptoms which are identical to asthma attacks she has had in the past. They also match a clinical picture of asthma.

P: Oxygen administration was begun immediately and medical control was contacted to assist the patient with additional doses of her albuterol inhaler. Dr. Cook from County General approved two puffs, reevaluation and two more puffs. The patient experienced some relief from our first two. After reassessment and stable vital signs (noted above) a second set of puffs was administered with greater relief. SaO2 increased to 98% and the patient was no longer using accessory muscles.

Figure 11-3 Sample documentation using the SOAP format.

Another method is called **CHART,** an acronym that stands for chief complaint, history, assessment, Rx (or treatment), and transport (Figure 11-4 ■).

Remember, it is important to be as thorough as possible when writing your narrative. Information gathered at the scene or en route to the hospital may be lost unless you write it down. The following are examples of specific elements in the narrative that help to paint a picture of the patient:

- ***Chief complaint.*** This is the reason the patient (or someone else) called 911. Typically, you document the chief complaint by using the patient's own words. Example: Pt. states that he feels "a sharp stabbing pain" in his lower abdomen.
- ***Pertinent history.*** This is additional medical information related to the patient's chief complaint. Example: Pt. stated that he had abdominal surgery two days ago.

CHART a method of documentation in which each letter stands for a specific portion of the narrative: chief complaint, history, assessment, Rx (or treatment), and transport.

11-6 Give examples of each of the following types of PCR narrative information: chief complaint, pertinent history, subjective information, objective information, and pertinent negatives/positives.

C: "I'm having an asthma attack."

H: Patient reports difficulty breathing which developed while jogging about 10 minutes ago. It is accompanied by a tightness in her chest when she tried to breathe. Patient has a history of asthma for which she takes an albuterol inhaler. She has taken two puffs with minimal relief. She denies allergies, other medications or additional medical history. She had a light breakfast this AM.

A: Patient exam reveals patient seated on a bench in tripod position using accessory muscles to breathe. Patient is breathing with an adequate tidal volume. She is able to speak 4–5 word sentences. Wheezes are audible without a stethoscope. Lung sounds are equal bilaterally with wheezes in all lobes of the lungs. Initial vital signs P: 102 strong/regular, R: 28 shallow and slightly labored, but adequate, BP 118/84, skin warm and moist. Pupils equal and react. SaO2 93%

R: Oxygen provided via NRB mask at 15 lpm. Dr. Cook at County General contacted via radio who approved 2 puffs of her albuterol inhaler spaced 5 mins apart with reevaluation. The first two puffs were administered with some relief. Vitals stable (noted above) so two additional puffs gave more relief. Patient no longer used accessory muscles, could speak full sentences and SaO2 increased to 98%.

T: Patient transported to County General code 1 with the patient's difficulty breathing improved. Report given to RN in room 4—rails up.

Figure 11-4 Sample documentation using the CHART format.

- ***Subjective information.*** This information is not firsthand and is subject to interpretation. Example: Pt's wife said he ate yesterday but did not eat today.
- ***Objective information.*** This information describes what you have personally observed. Example: As I palpated Pt's upper left quadrant, he grimaced and immediately guarded the area.
- ***Pertinent negatives.*** This documents the absence of a sign or symptom important to the chief complaint. Example: Pt. complains of nausea, but reports no vomiting. The absence of vomiting is the pertinent negative.
- ***Pertinent positives.*** This is the presence of a sign or symptom important to the chief complaint. Example: Pt's chief complaint is chest pain, with shortness of breath. Shortness of breath is the pertinent positive.

STOP, REVIEW, REMEMBER!

Multiple Choice

For each question, place a check next to the correct answer.

1. Prehospital care reports may be used for all of the following *except*:

_____ a. the quality improvement (QI) process.

_____ b. research.

_____ c. as evidence in court.

_____ d. for dissemination to the media.

2. Insurance information is included in which section of the prehospital care report?

_____ a. Run data

_____ b. Patient data

_____ c. Check boxes

_____ d. Assessment data

3. Which one of the following is considered part of the run data?

_____ a. Patient's name

_____ b. Date and time of the call

_____ c. Vital signs

_____ d. Name of the medical direction physician

4. The patient's blood pressure is most commonly recorded in which type of space on the prehospital care report?

_____ a. Fill-in

_____ b. Check boxes

_____ c. Narrative

_____ d. Subjective

5. Which one of the following statements correctly describes subjective and objective information?

_____ a. Objective information is what you hear from others, and subjective information is what you see.

_____ b. Objective information is what you see, and subjective information is information that can be definitively proved by other sources.

_____ c. Objective information is what you reasonably believe to be true, and subjective information is false.

_____ d. Objective information is something you observe, and subjective information is that which is not firsthand or that requires interpretation.

Labeling

Label each of the following statements as either objective (O) or subjective (S).

1. _____ Based on his injuries, the patient must have jumped from the upper floors.
2. _____ The patient has a bone protruding from his midshaft lower leg.
3. _____ The patient has wheezes that are audible without a stethoscope.
4. _____ Due to his high level of intoxication, he obviously had a lot to drink.
5. _____ The patient states she has chest discomfort that radiates to her neck and jaw.
6. _____ The patient has an area of bruising over the fifth to ninth ribs on the left side.

(continued on next page)

(continued)

Fill in the Blank

Fill in the report with the following vital signs.

1117 hours: Respirations 22 and labored, pulse 94 strong and regular, BP 112/74, pupils equal and react to light, skin cool and moist

1122 hours: Respirations 20 and labored, pulse 88 strong and regular, BP 108/70, pupils equal and react to light, skin cool and dry

VITAL SIGNS	TIME	RESP	PULSE	B.P.	LEVEL OF CONSCIOUSNESS	R PUPILS L	SKIN
		Rate: ☐ Regular ☐ Shallow ☐ Labored	Rate: ☐ Regular ☐ Irregular	/	☐ Alert ☐ Voice ☐ Pain ☐ Unresp.	☐ Normal ☐ ☐ Dilated ☐ ☐ Constricted ☐ ☐ Sluggish ☐ ☐ No-Reaction ☐	☐ Unremarkable ☐ Cool ☐ Pale ☐ Warm ☐ Cyanotic ☐ Moist ☐ Flushed ☐ Dry ☐ Jaundiced
		Rate: ☐ Regular ☐ Shallow ☐ Labored	Rate: ☐ Regular ☐ Irregular	/	☐ Alert ☐ Voice ☐ Pain ☐ Unresp.	☐ Normal ☐ ☐ Dilated ☐ ☐ Constricted ☐ ☐ Sluggish ☐ ☐ No-Reaction ☐	☐ Unremarkable ☐ Cool ☐ Pale ☐ Warm ☐ Cyanotic ☐ Moist ☐ Flushed ☐ Dry ☐ Jaundiced
		Rate: ☐ Regular ☐ Shallow ☐ Labored	Rate: ☐ Regular ☐ Irregular	/	☐ Alert ☐ Voice ☐ Pain ☐ Unresp.	☐ Normal ☐ ☐ Dilated ☐ ☐ Constricted ☐ ☐ Sluggish ☐ ☐ No-Reaction ☐	☐ Unremarkable ☐ Cool ☐ Pale ☐ Warm ☐ Cyanotic ☐ Moist ☐ Flushed ☐ Dry ☐ Jaundiced

Critical Thinking

1. Some say, "Documentation is the best way to minimize liability." Defend or disagree with that statement and give your reasons.

____

____

____

____

Confidentiality

11-8 Explain each of the following legal concerns with respect to the PCR: confidentiality, allowed distribution of the PCR or information included in it, documenting a patient's refusal of treatment, falsification of the PCR, and correction of errors.

Your prehospital care reports contain confidential information. Confidentiality is governed by many laws, including the Health Insurance Portability and Accountability Act (HIPAA) that was discussed in Chapter 3. The information in your report may be distributed only to those individuals allowed by law to see the report or to whom the patient has given written authorization to see the report. Generally, the hospital will receive a copy of the report, the EMS agency will keep a copy of it, and often an additional copy goes to a regional or state EMS agency for data collection and research.

Prehospital care reports may be used within an agency or region for quality improvement (QI) review. Patients are often asked to sign a form that allows your agency to share information with insurance companies and billing agencies.

Corrections and Falsification

There will be times when you write something inadvertently or incorrectly on your prehospital care report. Examples might be writing that the pulse was 87 instead of 78, or writing the patient has no medical history, and then finding out she takes medications for diabetes. In those cases you should make a correction. Cross out the incorrect item with a single line, place your initials next to it, and then write the correct information beside or above it (Figure 11-5 ■). It is best to use a single line instead of completely covering the wrong information, because making the entry completely unreadable might look as if you were attempting to hide something.

If an error is discovered after a report has been submitted, make the correction as described above, but note the time and date the correction is made. If the correction is significant to patient care, billing, or research, amended copies should be sent to those affected.

Falsification of a report is very serious. Honesty and integrity are essential traits of an EMT. Never write false information in a prehospital care report. Likewise, never leave out any information from a report, even about something that was done in error.

falsification documentation of false information in a prehospital care report.

There are two types of errors, an **error of omission** and an **error of commission.** Errors of omission are those in which something was not done that should have been. Examples include not giving oxygen when you should have or not asking a patient if he had allergies before giving a medication. Errors of commission are actions that should not have been taken, especially actions that cause harm to a patient. Assisting a patient with a medication that was not his own or using a stretcher in a manner that caused injury to a patient are examples of errors of commission.

error of omission something was not done that should have been.

error of commission action that should not have been taken, especially an action that causes harm to a patient.

PERSPECTIVE

Joe—The EMT

I've been trying to figure out why I wrote the wrong hospital on that PCR. I never do that. The only thing I can think is we must have gotten diverted en route, and I hate the paperwork so much that I always zip through it as soon as I can. I bet I had that sorry excuse for a PCR before we ever got diverted.

If you ever find yourself tempted to document an action that did not take place, don't. It would be considered falsification. One example concerns vital signs. You should take two or more sets of vital signs, even on short transports, because a change over time provides significant clinical information. However, imagine that you took only one set, because you were managing secondary injuries, administering oxygen, or even comforting the patient and lost track of time. Do not write down that you took more than one set. It would be considered falsification. If you were busy performing other important patient care tasks, document those tasks in the narrative.

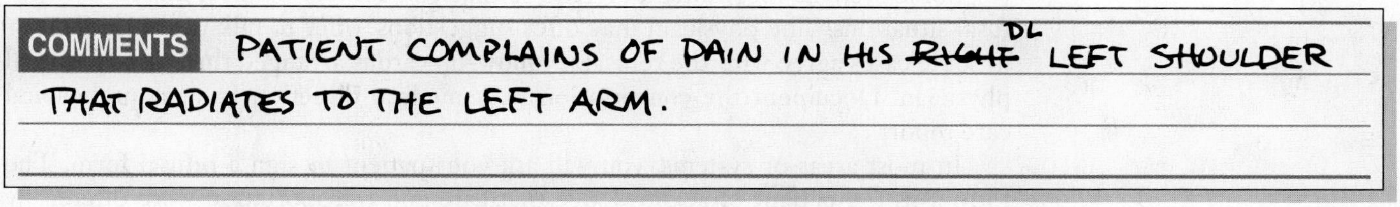
COMMENTS
PATIENT COMPLAINS OF PAIN IN HIS ~~RIGHT~~ DL LEFT SHOULDER
THAT RADIATES TO THE LEFT ARM.

Figure 11-5 Proper method for correcting a documentation error.

Other times you may forget to give oxygen to the patient or the patient will not tolerate the mask or cannula on his face. Never write down that you gave a medication or treatment that was not actually given. Such a falsification could negatively affect patient care decisions later at the hospital.

The run report should not cover up any type of error. If an error occurs, it should be documented. Identify the error and what was done to correct it. The hospital and your supervisor also should be notified of the error.

Give clinically appropriate, patient-centered care at all times. As a human being there always will be the possibility that you will make an error. Work diligently to prevent errors and document them honestly if they do occur.

Special Issues in Documentation

11-9 Discuss how to handle each of the following situations with respect to the PCR: transfer of patient care when returning to service prior to completing the PCR, multiple-casualty incidents (MCIs), and special reporting situations, such as infectious disease exposure and suspicion of abuse or neglect.

There are times when documentation procedures and requirements change or are different than usual. They include instances in which patients refuse care, where there are multiple patients on scene, or when the local jurisdiction requires special reports.

Patient Refusal

In most instances, patients who call for help should go to the hospital. Occasionally, however, you will find patients who do not want to accept your care or transportation. (Chapter 3 offers methods to convince the patient to go to the hospital.) Documentation of your attempts at convincing such a patient is very important, because refusal situations are a significant source of risk and liability for EMTs.

You should take your time when trying to talk your patient into accepting your care and transportation. You may be able to break down barriers or the patient's fears and change his mind. Be prepared to take the time necessary with each patient. Even if your documentation of the patient refusal is meticulous, but the times recorded by the dispatcher show you were only on scene for five minutes, your efforts will appear minimal, regardless of what you document.

In a patient refusal situation, you should document the following information:

- Any assessment and care you performed for the patient
- That the patient has capacity to understand the situation and is of legal age to refuse and has the ability to make an informed decision (he is not intoxicated or otherwise incompetent)
- That the patient was told the risks of refusing care, including worsening of the current problem up to and including death
- That efforts were made to convince the patient to accept care. Those efforts may include (but not be limited to) reassurance, involving family members or friends, offering to call a relative or personal physician, helping arrange care for a pet.
- Any efforts made to protect the patient if he does refuse. Those efforts may include contacting a family member or friend to stay with him, scheduling a visit for that day with a personal physician, or providing phone stickers with EMS access numbers and advising the patient that he can call back at any time.

Some systems recommend or require that you contact medical direction in refusal situations. The physician may offer suggestions, offer to talk to the patient, or in some cases agree with the refusal if follow-up care is arranged through a personal physician. Document the conversation with medical direction in your prehospital care report.

In most areas or systems, you will ask your patient to sign a refusal form. The form asks the patient to acknowledge that care and transportation were offered by EMS and were refused by the patient. It also might mention what you did to persuade the patient to accept your help, including explaining that harm may result with a refusal.

The refusal form is sometimes called a *waiver* or *release*, because it may have legal language releasing the crew and agency from liability if harm comes to the patient (Figure 11-6 ■). Note that the form will not prevent a lawsuit, but it may help to show that the patient was aware of the risks and that you acted appropriately. In addition, some EMS systems have refusal checklists that help EMTs remember and perform all of the necessary steps, both to properly care for the patient and to reduce the potential for liability.

Release At Scene (RAS)
Against Medical Advice (AMA)
Form

Release at Scene (RAS)

I understand that any evaluation and/or emergency treatment I have received by these EMS personnel has been on an emergency basis only and is not intended to be a substitute for complete medical assessment and/or care. I understand it appears that further emergency transportation and/or care does not appear to be needed at this time. I understand that I may have an illness or injury that is unforeseen at this time. I understand that if I change my mind or if my condition changes or becomes worse and I need further treatment/transportation by the Emergency Medical Services System, I can call back and they will respond.

Patient Name (print) ____________ Patient Signature ____________ Date ______

Patient / Guardian Signature ____________ Relationship ____________ Date ______

Paramedic / EMT signature ____________ Witness Signature ____________ Date ______

Comments:

____

____

Section II Refusal of Evaluation / Treatment / Transportation Against Medical Advice (AMA)

I. ______________________________, acknowledge that on ______________
Patient Name (print) Date

______________________ / ____________ / ______________________
EMT–Paramedic/EMT License/Cert # Service Provider Agency

explained my condition to me and advised me of some of the potential risks and/or complications which could or would arise from refusal of medical care. I have also been advised that other unknown risks and/or complications are possible up to and including the loss of life or limb. Being aware that there are known and unknown potential risks and/or complications, it is still my desire to refuse the advised medical care.
All Care Refused__________ Specific Care Refused: ______________________
I do hereby release EMS personnel from all liability resulting from any adverse medical condition(s) caused by my refusal of the recommended medical care.

Patient Signature______________________ Paramedic / EMT Signature______________________

Patient / Guardian Signature______________________ Relationship ______________________

Witness Name:______________________ Witness Signature______________________

Comments:____

____

____

Figure 11-6 An example of an "against medical advice" (AMA) form. (Courtesy of Verihealth Inc., Petaluma, CA)

Multiple-Casualty Incidents

Patients should always receive the best possible care followed by thorough documentation of the care provided. Though in the case of a multiple-casualty incident (MCI), documentation may have to be done later because patient care is a priority, the proper transfer of information from the field to the hospital is still important. Hospital staff would still like to know what the patient's complaint and condition was in the field and if there have been any changes during transport.

PERSPECTIVE

Mrs. O'Neil—The Wife

I actually felt kind of bad for that EMT. I know there are things about Artie's death that even I don't remember now. It seemed that my whole case ended up turning on that hospital issue though, you know? But that could've been Artie's fault. He swore to me that he'd never go to Midway again after the problem with his colonoscopy results there, and I'm the one who told them to take him there. For all I know he asked to go to Riverside once they were driving. Well, I guess the point is my husband of 35 years died and now my life is a wreck. After my attorney said that it may have been the ambulance crew's fault, I had no choice but to sue. Right?

The need for concise but accurate information at MCIs is met by specialized forms such as the triage tag (Figure 11-7 ■). It allows notation of injuries, care, and vital signs in a compact form that stays with the patient. Multiple copies allow one copy to remain at the scene and another to accompany the patient to the hospital.

Specialized Reports

There are special situations for which you will be required to document specific information on your report or to complete a second report. For example, when reporting a crime, such as child or elder abuse, your local social service agencies may have a special form to use. That form will have questions specific to the needs of their agency and investigation of the matter.

Supplemental reports may be needed for calls that were of a very long duration or where there was a significant use of resources. Documentation of those events will be too long to fit in a standard prehospital care report.

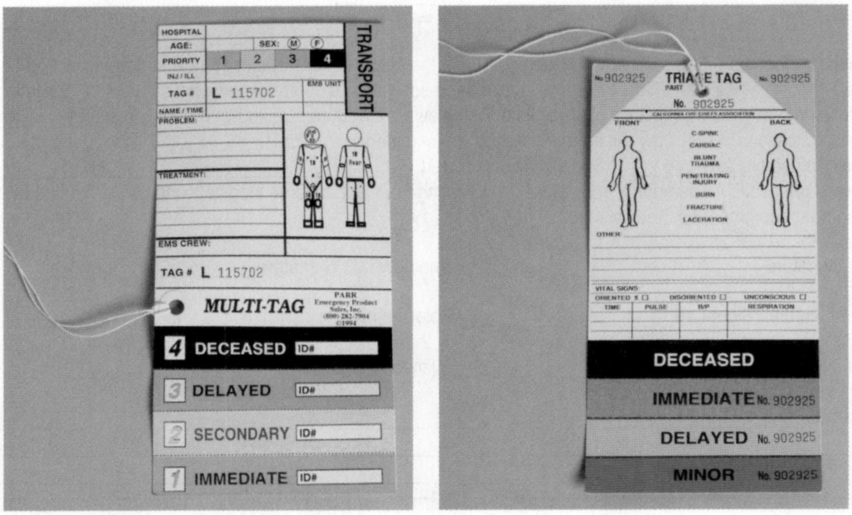

Figure 11-7 Two different examples of common triage tags.

Other times, special documentation is needed because of a motor-vehicle collision involving an EMS vehicle or when there is a conflict between emergency personnel at a scene.

Transferring Care Before Completing the Report

There are times when it may be necessary to leave a patient with emergency department staff without a completed prehospital care report, such as when your district or zone is experiencing an unusually high call volume, other resources have gone out of service, or if your unit provides specialty response. In those situations it is acceptable to notify the facility of your need to leave and provide a nurse or physician with a verbal report. Once you are clear from the urgent call, return to the facility and provide them with the completed written report.

STOP, REVIEW, REMEMBER!

Multiple Choice

For each question, place a check next to the correct answer.

1. The letters *HIPAA* stand for the:

_____ a. Health Insurance Privacy Amendment Act.

_____ b. Health Information Purpose and Accountability.

_____ c. Health Insurance Portability and Accountability Act.

_____ d. Health Industry Perspective and Accountability Access.

2. Prehospital care reports are commonly used for all of the following purposes *except:*

_____ a. maintenance tracking.

_____ b. billing purposes.

_____ c. quality improvement (QI).

_____ d. research.

3. An error in a run report should be corrected by:

_____ a. crossing out all indications of the error.

_____ b. leaving the error as is and noting it at the end of the report.

_____ c. crossing the error out with a single line and writing the correct information near it.

_____ d. covering the error with a thick black marker on all copies and writing the corrected information in at the end of the report.

4. Which one of the following statements about documentation of patient refusal is *not* correct?

_____ a. The patient's age and mental state should be documented.

_____ b. A patient's prior knowledge of the risks of refusing treatment releases an EMT from explaining and documenting them again.

_____ c. For some conditions it is appropriate to tell the patient that serious harm or even death could come from refusing care.

_____ d. You should document any care you did give the patient before he refused transportation.

5. Which one of the following is an example of an error of omission?

_____ a. Giving a patient a medication to which he is allergic

_____ b. Forgetting to document vital signs on the prehospital care report

_____ c. Assisting a patient with a medication from a friend

_____ d. Neglecting to synchronize your watch with dispatch before your shift

(continued on next page)

(continued)

6. Which one of the following is the most appropriate documentation of skin signs?

_____ a. Skin is warm and good.

_____ b. Skin is pink and warm.

_____ c. Skin is pale, cool, and moist.

_____ d. Patient is warm and dry.

7. If your patient refuses to go to the hospital, what should you document?

_____ a. Nothing. No care was provided, so there is nothing to report.

_____ b. Every attempt you made to convince him to go.

_____ c. Only the patient's rational for not wanting to go.

_____ d. Only report care provided and vitals taken, if any.

8. What document must a patient sign if he does not wish to accept your care?

_____ a. Refusal form

_____ b. Narrative acknowledgement

_____ c. HIPAA release

_____ d. Narrative

9. Under what circumstances is it acceptable to document in less detail than you normally would?

_____ a. When your patient is concerned with the level of detail in your report

_____ b. When you have a short distance to transport your patient

_____ c. When you are working a multiple-casualty incident

_____ d. When the computer on which you write your reports stops working

Critical Thinking

1. Your EMS chief read a report you wrote two days ago and in it he found the following statement: "The patient was unconscious and oriented × 3." She was sure you meant "conscious" and brought it to your attention. How should this report be amended two days after it was written?

____

____

____

____

Make It Right

Correct the error in each statement using proper documentation procedure.

1. The patient weighs 90 kg. Yet, you wrote the sentence below. Make the correction.

   The patient weighs approximately 190 kg.

2. The patient is allergic to penicillin. Yet, you wrote the sentence below. Make the correction.

   The patient has no allergies to medications.

3. The patient's blood pressure was lower when the patient stood up. Yet, you wrote the sentence below. Make the correction.

   The blood pressure increased when the patient stood up.

4. The patient's blood pressure was 126/88. Yet, you wrote his vital signs as shown below. Make the correction.

   Pulse 88 strong and regular, respirations 18, blood pressure 88/126, pupils equal and react to light.

5. The patient has equal breath sounds bilaterally. Yet, you wrote the sentences below. Make the correction.

   The respirations are 16 and deep. There are equal sounds bilaterally.

EMERGENCY DISPATCH SUMMARY

Mrs. Arthur O'Neil won a settlement against the North County Ambulance Service for $1.3 million. The case is on appeal. Joe Devlin has since become a paramedic for the same service and is now well known for his clear, concise, and accurate prehospital care reports.

Chapter Review

To the Point

- Documentation is a vital EMS skill that takes time to master. When done right, it paints a complete picture of your patient care and interaction.
- Your prehospital care report is a legal document. It is important that it is accurate and complete, especially if you are called to court.
- Your prehospital care report will have sections for both run data and patient data.
- Data in each section of the prehospital care report can be entered in several different ways: fill-in, check boxes, drop-down menus, and narrative.
- Be careful to write a narrative that is objective, rather than subjective.
- There are different ways to write a narrative. Some agencies have a preference as to which one you use: timeline, SOAP, or CHART.
- The Health Insurance Portability and Accountability Act (HIPAA) outlines how confidential patient information may be used and who may see your report.
- To make a correction on a report, draw a single line through the incorrect information, initial it, and write out the correct information. If the error is discovered after the report is given, make the correction and then add the time and date of the correction or change. Never make the incorrect information illegible.
- A prehospital care report is legal documentation of the care you provided to the patient. Never write false information or omit information that may make you look bad. It is important to create an accurate and complete account of your interaction with your patient.
- Patients have the right to refuse care. It is your job to do everything you can to make your patient aware of the consequences of refusing care and transport, up to and including death.
- In a multiple-casualty incident, complete documentation may not be possible. Triage tags, which allow rescuers to quickly assess and categorize patients, follow the patient to the hospital and provide a snapshot of the patient's injuries, care, and vital signs.

Chapter Questions

Multiple Choice

For each question, place a check next to the correct answer.

1. Which of the following would *not* be legally able to receive a copy of your prehospital care report?
   _____ a. Patient's clergy
   _____ b. State EMS agency
   _____ c. Quality improvement (QI) committee
   _____ d. Ambulance service headquarters

2. You are caring for a patient who has chest pain. You believe she could be experiencing a heart attack. However, the patient is refusing transport. You should:
   _____ a. leave the patient and inform dispatch that she is not being transported.
   _____ b. inform the patient of the consequences of not receiving care.
   _____ c. ask the spouse to transport the patient to the hospital.
   _____ d. insist that the patient see her doctor the next day.

3. You are writing your patient's history on your prehospital care report at the hospital and inadvertently write down a medication not taken by the patient. You should:
   _____ a. leave it as is because you did not give the medication.
   _____ b. cross out the wrong information with a single line.
   _____ c. totally cross out the area where the medication was listed so no one can ever see it.
   _____ d. shred the report you are writing, due to confidentiality issues, and begin again.

4. The patient states he has pain across his upper abdomen. This is a(n) _____________ statement.
   _____ a. sworn
   _____ b. attestable
   _____ c. objective
   _____ d. subjective

5. Giving aspirin to a patient who is allergic to aspirin is an error of:
   _____ a. omission.
   _____ b. operation.
   _____ c. commission.
   _____ d. neglect.

Critical Thinking

1. List three ways you can envision your prehospital care report being used after you complete it.

____

____

____

____

2. You are completing your report at the hospital and realize that you took only one set of vital signs on your patient. He had vomited during the short trip to the hospital and you just did not have time. Your partner says, "Just write down a set that is close to the first. It'll keep the boss off our backs. You know he was stable, and they didn't change anyway." What should you do?

____

____

____

____

3. How is documentation at a multiple-casualty incident (MCI) different from a call with a single patient?

Name That Error

Determine if the errors below are errors of omission (O) or commission (C).

1. _____ You fail to administer oxygen to a patient with chest pain.
2. _____ You fail to identify inadequate breathing in an unresponsive patient.
3. _____ You assist a patient with his prescribed nitroglycerin even though he took Viagra yesterday (a contraindication).
4. _____ You do not immobilize the spine of a person involved in a motor-vehicle collision even though he complains of neck pain.
5. _____ You hit the release mechanism on the stretcher prematurely and it drops from the elevated position to the lowered position in a freefall and injures the patient.

Case Study

Imagine you are a patient who was transported in an ambulance. You are in a coffee shop three days later and hear two EMTs talking about your care. Others in the coffee shop also can hear what is going on.

1. How would you feel about this? What would you do?

2. If you complained about this to the supervisor of the EMTs or a local official, what would happen to the EMTs?

The Last Word

Documentation is a critical skill. It is the only record of the care you provide long after you have dropped the patient off at the hospital. This report, when accurate and complete, will provide a lasting record of quality care. When shoddy, incomplete, or inaccurate, the record kept by your report is not one you would be proud of.

Your documentation is used in court in many different situations. The trial may be one in which you and your report are a witness or a defendant. Accurate and thorough documentation will help you in both situations. The other practice that is vital to your work as an EMT and one that will help in liability prevention is treating each patient carefully and compassionately.

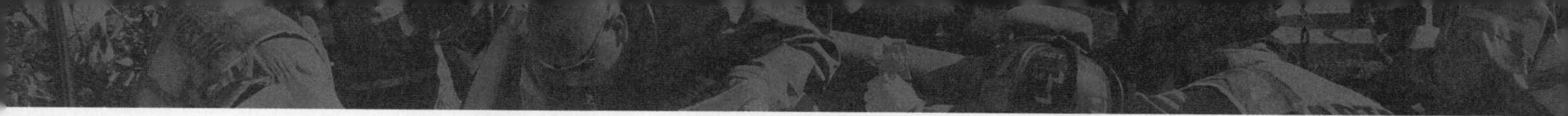

Module 1: Review and Practice Examination for Chapters 1–11

DIRECTIONS: *Assess what you have learned in this module by placing a check mark in the blank beside the best answer for each multiple-choice question. When you are done, check your answers against the Answer Key at the back of the book.*

1. Which one of the following most accurately defines an EMS system?
____ a. Network of injury prevention resources
____ b. Legislation and regulations that govern prehospital care
____ c. All of the EMS provider agencies in a geographical area
____ d. Chain of resources designed to minimize the impact of sudden illness and injury

2. Which one of the following is necessary to help evaluate the effectiveness of an EMS system?
____ a. Review of records by NHTSA
____ b. Statewide uniform data collection system
____ c. Sophisticated computer software
____ d. Court order to release patient information

3. Which of the following is the highest level of nationally recognized EMS training as defined by NHTSA?
____ a. Emergency medical technician
____ b. Emergency medical responder
____ c. Advanced emergency medical technician
____ d. Paramedic

4. Which one of the following is the minimum level of training necessary for providing patient care during ambulance transportation?
____ a. CPR certification
____ b. Emergency medical responder
____ c. Emergency medical technician
____ d. Paramedic

5. Which one of the following is responsible for overseeing all aspects of an EMS system?
____ a. State EMS bureau or agency
____ b. County EMS agency
____ c. Chief trauma surgeon
____ d. EMS officer

6. Which one of the following is an example of on-line medical direction?
____ a. Receiving orders from a physician over the radio
____ b. Receiving direction from a nurse bystander on the scene
____ c. Consulting with a paramedic who is responding to the scene
____ d. Following your system's protocols

7. The EMT's primary concern for safety at the scene of an emergency must be that of:
____ a. patients. ____ c. bystanders.
____ b. yourself. ____ d. fire department.

8. The purpose of a quality improvement program is to:
____ a. identify and discipline individual EMTs for providing inadequate medical care.
____ b. reduce the cost of professional liability insurance.
____ c. ensure that the public receives the best possible prehospital care.
____ d. comply with laws regulating payment for the delivery of medical care.

9. A cumulative stress response is also known as:
____ a. posttraumatic stress disorder.
____ b. burnout.
____ c. an adrenalin rush.
____ d. anguish.

10. Which one of the following changes in your coworker's behavior should make you suspect that he is suffering from an increased amount of stress?
____ a. Increased hunger, excessive sleeping, being overly cooperative
____ b. Increased sleeping, reporting night sweats, decreased appetite
____ c. Irritability, decreased appetite, lack of enthusiasm about work
____ d. Increased social activity, starting a new exercise program, excessive eating

11. The best time to initiate stress management is:
____ a. before a stressful event occurs.
____ b. during the stressful event.
____ c. immediately after the stressful event.
____ d. after the immediate fight-or-flight response has subsided.

12. Which one of the following is a technique that helps family members cope with the sudden loss of a loved one?
____ a. Encouraging denial
____ b. Being tolerant of their anger
____ c. Assuring that everything will be okay
____ d. Deferring all questions to a trained counselor

13. You have been called to the scene of a possible cardiac arrest. On arrival you find an elderly woman with obvious signs of death. When you tell her husband that his wife has died, he asks, "Will she be admitted to the intensive care unit again?" This is an example of which stage of grief?
____ a. Bargaining
____ b. Depression
____ c. Remorse
____ d. Denial

14. The term *standard precautions* applies to:
____ a. traffic hazards.
____ b. crime scenes.
____ c. combative patients.
____ d. exposure to pathogens.

15. You are caring for a patient with a known case of tuberculosis. For the best protection, you should don:
____ a. firefighting turnout gear.
____ b. gloves, mask, and eye protection.
____ c. mask and gown.
____ d. mask only.

16. Your patient has a cut on his forehead and scrapes on his hands and knees. Which one of the following is the best choice of personal protective equipment for caring for this patient?
____ a. HEPA mask, gown, gloves, protective eye wear
____ b. Gloves
____ c. Gloves and protective eye wear
____ d. Protective eye wear and a HEPA mask

17. Which one of the following is the most effective way to prevent the spread of infection?
____ a. Wearing gloves for every patient contact
____ b. Proper hand washing
____ c. Maintaining up-to-date immunizations
____ d. Using all PPE available for every patient

18. The primary agency concerned with the health of the EMS workforce is the:
____ a. National Association of EMTs.
____ b. American Medical Association.
____ c. Occupational Safety and Health Administration.
____ d. Department of Health and Human Services.

19. The primary responsibility of an EMT who responds to an incident involving hazardous materials is:
____ a. identifying the material.
____ b. keeping everyone away.
____ c. evacuating area residents.
____ d. providing patient care.

20. You have been dispatched for an assault at a private residence. Law enforcement has been notified. As you arrive at the scene, you note law enforcement has not yet arrived. You should:
____ a. stage several houses away and await law enforcement.
____ b. stage directly in front of the residence and await law enforcement.
____ c. stage several houses away and approach the residence from the side, rather than from the front.
____ d. approach the house, look in windows, to determine whether it is safe to enter.

21. The specific actions that an EMS provider is legally allowed to perform, based on level of training and state regulations, is best described as:
____ a. standard of care.
____ b. scope of practice.
____ c. duty to respond.
____ d. limit of liability.

22. Which one of the following statements about the practice of EMS is most accurate?
____ a. Protocols are national standards that describe the specific actions EMS providers are allowed to perform.
____ b. Individual states generally allow more skills than those described by the national standard curriculum.
____ c. Standing orders describe the entire standard of care for a given EMS system.
____ d. The standard of care is a modified scope of practice that meets the needs of a given region.

23. Which one of the following is the best example of an ethical responsibility of an EMS provider?
____ a. Remaining within your scope of practice
____ b. Maintaining state licensure or certification
____ c. Serving as the patient's advocate
____ d. Establishing a duty to act

24. An EMT may *not* have a legal obligation to provide emergency care in which one of the following situations?
 ____ a. Off-duty EMT drives up on the scene of a motorcycle collision that has just occurred and no responders have yet arrived at the scene.
 ____ b. Off-duty EMT has stopped to render emergency care but realizes he is now late to work and leaves the patient to avoid being disciplined at work.
 ____ c. On-duty EMT responds to a call and discovers that the patient is not having an emergency but thinks she will be seen more quickly in the emergency department if she arrives by ambulance.
 ____ d. On-duty EMT working for a private ambulance service is assigned to provide care at an outdoor concert.

25. Good Samaritan laws are designed to limit the liability for:
 ____ a. anyone who comes upon an emergency while off duty.
 ____ b. EMTs while working for an ambulance service.
 ____ c. physicians while in the hospital only.
 ____ d. firefighters who may ride in an ambulance.

26. To which one of the following patients does implied consent apply?
 ____ a. Alert and mentally competent
 ____ b. Alert but appears to be intoxicated with alcohol
 ____ c. Unresponsive
 ____ d. Victim of an assault

27. Which one of the following patients has the right to refuse treatment?
 ____ a. 14-year-old whose parents are out of town for the day and cannot be reached by phone
 ____ b. 16-year-old who is married
 ____ c. 12-year-old who is pregnant
 ____ d. 15-year-old who took the GED

28. Mr. Wickett is having chest pain that he describes as "indigestion." He is angry that his wife called EMS and is refusing to allow you to assess or treat him. You should:
 ____ a. leave so as to avoid upsetting him further.
 ____ b. explain that it may be indigestion, but there are also some serious medical problems that feel like indigestion.
 ____ c. tell him that you cannot leave unless he signs a form that he is refusing treatment "Against Medical Advice."
 ____ d. explain that most people who think they are having indigestion may be really having heart attacks and he could go into cardiac arrest at any time and needs to go with you immediately.

29. Your 50-year-old female patient is having severe abdominal cramps. She looks pale and is sweating profusely. She is alert and answers questions appropriately but is embarrassed and is refusing to be transported. You should:
 ____ a. contact law enforcement to put her on a hold.
 ____ b. contact medical direction for advice.
 ____ c. contact your supervisor for assistance.
 ____ d. enlist the assistance of her work supervisor.

30. You are caring for a 22-year-old man who injured his ankle while ice skating. On arrival at the emergency department, the triage nurse asks you to have your patient sit in a wheelchair and to take the patient to the registration desk. Which one of the following is the best action?
 ____ a. Tell the nurse you can only place the patient in a treatment room.
 ____ b. Tell the nurse you cannot leave the patient before he is seen by a physician.
 ____ c. State to the nurse, "I can do that, but I need to give you a report on this patient first."
 ____ d. Transport the patient to a different emergency department.

31. You have arrived at a nursing home where Mr. Jenkins is lying in bed in cardiac arrest. Just as you prepare to perform CPR, the nurse says, "Wait! I think he has a DNR order. Let me go call his doctor." What should you do?
 ____ a. Begin CPR and prepare to transport the patient.
 ____ b. Wait to start CPR and ask the nurse to call Mr. Jenkins's doctor from the room to save time.
 ____ c. Do chest compressions but do not ventilate until you are sure of the patient's DNR status.
 ____ d. Tell the nurse that you cannot honor a DNR under any circumstances.

32. You have just arrived on the scene of a 30-year-old man who reportedly had a seizure. His eyes are closed and he is not responding. The first EMT on the scene appears to believe the patient is "faking" the seizure and unresponsiveness. He says to the patient, "You need to open your eyes and talk to me or we're going to stick a tube down your throat." This could be interpreted as:
 ____ a. battery.
 ____ b. assault and battery.
 ____ c. damages.
 ____ d. assault.

33. Mr. Robertson was shot by his neighbor during an argument. Which one of the following situations is a violation of patient confidentiality?
    ____ a. You describe the location of the wound to law enforcement on the scene.
    ____ b. You discuss this case with your partner to see if there was something you could have done differently to improve patient care.
    ____ c. You discuss the call with your roommate when you get off shift.
    ____ d. You include this information in your documentation, part of which will be used for insurance and billing purposes.

34. A patient with bronchitis is suffering from:
    ____ a. mucus in the lungs.
    ____ b. infection of the trachea.
    ____ c. fluid in the alveoli.
    ____ d. swelling of the bronchioles.

35. The medical term for swelling of the liver is:
    ____ a. nephritis. ____ c. distention.
    ____ b. ascites. ____ d. hepatitis.

36. The term *tachypnea* is used to describe a patient with:
    ____ a. fast heart rate.
    ____ b. slow breathing.
    ____ c. fast breathing.
    ____ d. dilated pupils.

37. Which anatomical reference line begins in the armpit and extends down the side of the torso?
    ____ a. Midclavicular
    ____ b. Midaxillary
    ____ c. Medial aspect
    ____ d. Proximal lateral

38. Cholecystitis is an inflammation of the:
    ____ a. pancreas. ____ c. gall bladder.
    ____ b. liver. ____ d. urinary bladder.

39. The term *vasodilation* refers to:
    ____ a. dilation of the blood vessels.
    ____ b. dilation of the pupils.
    ____ c. inflammation of the blood vessels.
    ____ d. inflammation of the kidneys.

40. The portion of the clavicle (collarbone) that is closest to the sternum (breastbone) is its ____________ end.
    ____ a. distal ____ c. medial
    ____ b. lateral ____ d. plantar

41. The wrist is ____________ to the fingers and ____________ to the elbow.
    ____ a. proximal, distal ____ c. medial, lateral
    ____ b. distal, proximal ____ d. lateral, medial

42. The abdominal cavity is separated from the thoracic cavity by the:
    ____ a. mesentery. ____ c. peritoneum.
    ____ b. ribs. ____ d. diaphragm.

43. Another name for the voice box is the:
    ____ a. pharynx. ____ c. larynx.
    ____ b. epiglottis. ____ d. thyroid cartilage.

44. The structure that transports air from the larynx to the mainstem bronchi is the:
    ____ a. pharynx. ____ c. alveoli.
    ____ b. trachea. ____ d. esophagus.

45. Which one of the following is *true* concerning ways in which a child's respiratory system is different from an adult's?
    ____ a. Children rely more on the diaphragm for breathing.
    ____ b. Child's trachea is short and wide compared to an adult's.
    ____ c. Child's tongue takes up much less space in the mouth.
    ____ d. Cricoid cartilage is very pronounced in a child.

46. The cardiovascular system includes all of the following components *except* the:
    ____ a. heart. ____ c. blood vessels.
    ____ b. blood. ____ d. lungs.

47. The primary function of hemoglobin is to:
    ____ a. help blood clot.
    ____ b. carry oxygen.
    ____ c. carry carbon dioxide.
    ____ d. detoxify waste products.

48. Which one of the following structures transports oxygenated blood?
    ____ a. Pulmonary arteries
    ____ b. Right atrium
    ____ c. Vena cava
    ____ d. Pulmonary veins

49. Which one of the following most directly affects cardiac output?
    ____ a. Tidal volume
    ____ b. Skin signs
    ____ c. Heart rate
    ____ d. Respiratory rate

50. Which one of the following could you use to assess circulation to the foot?
    ____ a. Vena cava
    ____ b. Dorsalis pedis artery
    ____ c. Brachial artery
    ____ d. Femoral vein

51. The skull is made up of the:
____ a. cranium and scalp.
____ b. cranium and face.
____ c. carpals and metacarpals.
____ d. carpals and ilium.

52. A sprain primarily involves an injury to a:
____ a. ligament. ____ c. tendon.
____ b. bone. ____ d. muscle.

53. There are ________ cervical vertebrae in the ________.
____ a. 5, lower back
____ b. 12, posterior chest
____ c. 4, tailbone
____ d. 7, neck

54. In which one of the following structures would smooth muscle be found?
____ a. Bicep ____ c. Heart
____ b. Vessels ____ d. Thigh

55. A muscle that performs without conscious thought is known as a(an) ____________ muscle.
____ a. skeletal ____ c. involuntary
____ b. voluntary ____ d. automatic

56. Which one of the following is part of the central nervous system?
____ a. Vertebrae
____ b. Spinal cord
____ c. Motor nerves
____ d. Sensory nerves

57. Which one of the following is a function of the skin?
____ a. Temperature regulation
____ b. Maintenance of heart rate
____ c. Blood cell production
____ d. Oxygen storage

58. The outermost layer of the skin is the:
____ a. epidermis.
____ b. dermis.
____ c. subcutaneous layer.
____ d. fascia.

59. The organ that secretes insulin is the:
____ a. spleen. ____ c. kidney.
____ b. liver. ____ d. pancreas.

60. Which of the following can be found in the retroperitoneal cavity?
____ a. Gall bladder
____ b. Spleen
____ c. Kidneys
____ d. Abdominal aorta

61. Which one of the following best describes the ventilation/perfusion ratio?
____ a. Amount of air that is moved into and out of the lungs in one minute
____ b. Efficiency with which the body exchanges gases within the alveoli
____ c. Difference between blood pressure and breathing rate
____ d. Ability of the red blood cells to offload oxygen to the cells of the body

62. Which one of the following conditions is most likely to cause acidosis?
____ a. Rapid breathing
____ b. Abnormally slow breathing
____ c. Internal bleeding
____ d. Slow heart rate

63. You are caring for an emphysema patient who is reliant on the hypoxic drive to breathe. You can expect the respiratory rate to increase most when:
____ a. carbon dioxide levels decrease.
____ b. oxygen levels increase.
____ c. oxygen levels decrease.
____ d. both oxygen and carbon dioxide levels increase.

64. Room air produces an FiO_2 of:
____ a. 0.84. ____ c. 1.0.
____ b. 0.99. ____ d. 0.21.

65. A patient with right-sided heart failure will most likely present with:
____ a. crackles in the lungs.
____ b. low diastolic blood pressure.
____ c. pedal edema.
____ d. bradycardia.

66. Which one of the following makes up the by-product(s) of normal cell metabolism?
____ a. Carbon dioxide, water, and heat
____ b. Lactic acid
____ c. ATP in small amounts
____ d. Oxygen and water

67. Middle adulthood is the label applied to which age group?
____ a. 35–55 years
____ b. 30–50 years
____ c. 40–60 years
____ d. 50–55 years

68. A child who has developed thinking skills and can follow directions, but who needs lots of reassurance can be described as being in which age group?
____ a. Toddler ____ c. Adolescent
____ b. Preschooler ____ d. Infant

69. Following birth, a neonate will lose 5% to 10% of body weight. This is caused by:
____ a. the body adjusting to receiving nutrients orally.
____ b. dehydration, as the body adjusts to living in a dry environment.
____ c. the shifting of fat cells to accommodate the rapid growth that starts after week two.
____ d. infection and should be closely monitored.

70. You are caring for an adolescent patient who was discovered by his parents bleeding from self-inflicted wounds to his arms. How might you alter your care to better accommodate your patient?
____ a. Move the patient into the living room so that he can be more accessible to his family.
____ b. Complete your care and questioning in the privacy of the ambulance without family present.
____ c. Invite the parents into the ambulance with the patient to privately talk about the situation and next steps in care.
____ d. Release the patient at the scene because this is most likely a domestic matter.

71. Which one of the following measurements represents a narrowed pulse pressure?
____ a. 108/90 ____ c. 122/88
____ b. 206/136 ____ d. 90/62

72. Perfusion is best described as:
____ a. delivery of oxygen and nutrients to the cells.
____ b. adequate blood pressure for delivery of oxygen to the cells.
____ c. availability of oxygen to the lungs for placement into the blood.
____ d. exchange of oxygen and carbon dioxide between the lungs and blood.

73. Minute volume is best described as the:
____ a. amount of oxygen required by the body each minute.
____ b. number of breaths taken in one minute.
____ c. amount of air moved in and out of the lungs in a minute.
____ d. amount of blood moved by the heart in a minute.

74. Your patient is a conscious and alert 60-year-old man with difficulty breathing. He is nonambulatory and located in a basement apartment in a building without an elevator. Which one of the following would be the best way to get this patient out of his apartment?
____ a. Stair chair
____ b. Basket stretcher
____ c. Long backboard
____ d. Blanket carry

75. Mrs. Johnson fell two days ago in her kitchen. You find Mrs. Johnson lying on her back, complaining of pain in her right leg and hip. Which one of the following devices would most likely cause Mrs. Johnson the least amount of pain in preparing her for transport?
____ a. Scoop stretcher
____ b. Long backboard
____ c. Stokes basket
____ d. Stair chair

76. You are caring for a 29-year-old woman who was the victim of a head-on collision. She is unresponsive and breathing 4 times per minute. The scene is safe. Your patient should be moved using a(n) ____________ move.
____ a. simple ____ c. emergent
____ b. nonemergent ____ d. immediate

77. Your patient has a long history of lung problems and is having difficulty breathing. She is able to maintain her own airway and is breathing on her own. Which one of the following is the best position for transporting this patient?
____ a. Recovery
____ b. Supine
____ c. Supine with legs elevated
____ d. Semi-Fowler's

78. Which one of the following assessment findings is a symptom?
____ a. Hot, dry skin ____ c. Irregular pulse
____ b. Headache ____ d. Bruise

79. Which one of the following assessment findings is a sign?
____ a. Deep respirations
____ b. Nausea
____ c. Chest pain
____ d. Itching on the abdomen

80. The first set of vital signs obtained from a patient is known as the ____________ vital signs.
____ a. trending ____ c. baseline
____ b. size-up ____ d. normal

81. The amount of air that moves in and out of the lungs with each respiration is the ____________ volume.
____ a. tidal ____ c. resting
____ b. minute ____ d. lung

82. With respect to assessing respirations, the term *retraction* refers to:
____ a. abnormal sound heard during inspiration.
____ b. shallow respirations.
____ c. the drawing in of the soft tissues between the ribs.
____ d. prolonged inspiration with short expiration.

83. The presence of wheezing is most indicative of:
____ a. upper airway obstruction.
____ b. partial upper airway obstruction.
____ c. fluid in the airway.
____ d. lower airway obstruction.

84. All of the following are examples of peripheral pulses, *except*:
____ a. femoral. ____ c. pedal.
____ b. popliteal. ____ d. radial.

85. All of the following are characteristics of a pulse, *except*:
____ a. rate. ____ c. duration.
____ b. rhythm. ____ d. strength.

86. The use of a stethoscope to listen to the sounds of the blood pressure is called:
____ a. palpation. ____ c. insufflation.
____ b. auscultation. ____ d. perpetuation.

87. Cyanosis is an indication of:
____ a. poor perfusion.
____ b. liver disease.
____ c. poor oxygenation.
____ d. fever.

88. You are assessing a patient whose skin and whites of the eyes have a yellowish color. This would be documented as:
____ a. pallor. ____ c. jaundice.
____ b. cyanosis. ____ d. turgor.

89. Pupils that do not respond at all to changes in light are described as:
____ a. fixed. ____ c. constricted.
____ b. dilated. ____ d. PERRL.

90. Which one of the following questions should be asked to determine the "P" in OPQRST?
____ a. What were you doing when your pain started?
____ b. Does anything make the pain worse or better?
____ c. Can you describe what your pain feels like?
____ d. Does the pain go anywhere else other than your chest?

91. The process of obtaining and comparing vital signs over time is called:
____ a. trending. ____ c. follow-up.
____ b. profiling. ____ d. verifying.

92. Which one of the following is the primary means of interpersonal communications?
____ a. Gentle touch ____ c. Tone of voice
____ b. Active listening ____ d. Body language

93. The radio that is mounted in a vehicle is a:
____ a. base station. ____ c. mobile radio.
____ b. portable radio. ____ d. repeater.

94. With regards to documentation, which one of the following is the most subjective statement?
____ a. Patient was found sitting at the kitchen table.
____ b. Patient appeared to be in a lot of pain.
____ c. Oxygen was administered at 15 liters per minute with a nonrebreather mask.
____ d. Bystanders were performing CPR when we arrived on scene.

95. HIPAA regulations apply to:
____ a. the radio frequencies assigned to EMS systems.
____ b. decisions about where patients are to be transported.
____ c. the confidentiality and privacy of medical information.
____ d. standard codes that can be used in radio transmissions.

96. While completing your documentation, you inadvertently write that the patient complained of pain to his left leg, when in fact it was his right. Which one of the following is the best way to correct this situation?
____ a. Discard the PCR and start a new one.
____ b. Use correction fluid and write over the mistake.
____ c. Black out the mistake with a marker, make the correction, and initial it.
____ d. Draw a single line through the mistake, make the correction, and initial it.

97. Tidal volume refers to the ____________ of breathing.
____ a. rate ____ c. ease
____ b. rhythm ____ d. depth

98. Hearing crackles when listening to the lungs with a stethoscope is an indication of:
____ a. poor technique of listening to breath sounds.
____ b. lower airway constriction.
____ c. fluid in the alveoli.
____ d. partial upper airway obstruction.

99. In dark-skinned individuals skin color changes can best be detected by observing the:
____ a. inside of the lower eyelid.
____ b. back of the hand.
____ c. nape of the neck.
____ d. medial aspect of the arm.

100. Taking orthostatic vital signs is recommended when:
____ a. a patient's chief complaint is dizziness.
____ b. caring for a trauma patient with possible internal bleeding.
____ c. a patient may have low blood volume but does not have signs of shock.
____ d. caring for a cardiac patient.

MODULE 2

Patient Assessment

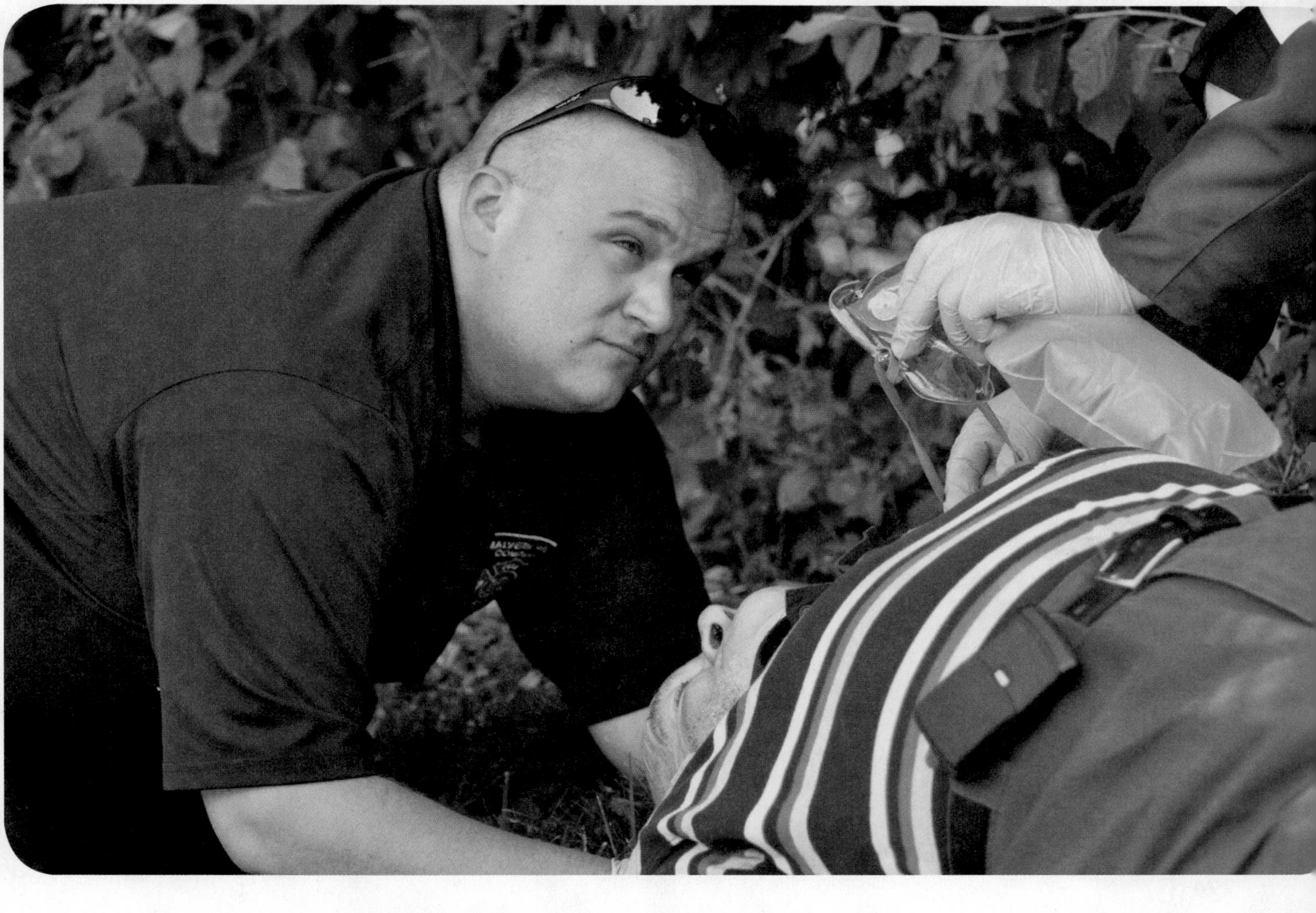

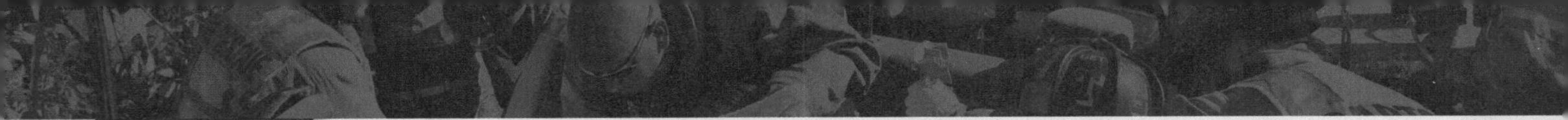

12 Performing a Scene Size-up and Primary Assessment

Education Standards

Assessment: Scene Size-up and Primary Assessment

Competencies

Applies scene information and patient assessment findings to guide emergency management of the patient.

Objectives

After completion of this lesson, you should be able to:

12-1 Define all key terms introduced in this chapter.
12-2 Describe the components of a scene size-up and the importance of each.
12-3 Explain the importance of safety at the scene of an emergency.
12-4 Describe hazards commonly found at emergency scenes (medical and trauma).
12-5 Explain the role that the EMT plays in ensuring the safety of all people at the scene of an emergency.
12-6 Differentiate between mechanism of injury and nature of illness.
12-7 Differentiate between significant and nonsignificant mechanisms of injury.
12-8 Explain the purpose of the primary assessment.
12-9 Describe the components of a primary assessment.
12-10 Explain how encountering a patient in cardiac arrest alters the sequence of the primary assessment.
12-11 Describe how to evaluate each component of the primary assessment.
12-12 Describe how to prioritize and manage problems related to the primary assessment.
12-13 Differentiate patients who are high-priority and low-priority for transport.

Key Terms

AVPU scale p. 308
chief complaint p. 311
confined space p. 302
general impression p. 307
high-angle rescue p. 302
index of suspicion p. 301
low-angle rescue p. 302
mechanism of injury (MOI) p. 300
multiple-casualty incident (MCI) p. 302
nature of illness (NOI) p. 300
patient assessment p. 295
primary assessment p. 295
scene safety p. 298
scene size-up p. 295
secondary assessment p. 295

Introduction

This chapter introduces you to two of the most important duties related to being an EMT: conducting the scene size-up and performing a primary assessment. They are just two of the components that make up a complete **patient assessment.** A complete patient assessment consists of the following elements:

patient assessment overall evaluation of the patient for life-threatening and non-life-threatening conditions.

- Scene size-up
- Primary assessment
- Secondary assessment
- Reassessment

Each of the patient assessment components will be introduced in this Module in logical chunks and in the sequence in which they should be performed. This chapter focuses on scene size-up and the **primary assessment.** The **secondary assessment** and reassessment are introduced in Chapter 14.

A proper scene size-up is an important component of each and every response. It is designed to identify both immediate and potential threats to safety for everyone at the scene of an emergency. It also allows you to identify the need for additional resources and to ensure the most safe and efficient response for the patients involved.

The primary assessment is the component of the patient assessment that is designed to identify all immediate life threats to patients. It is during the primary assessment that you will evaluate the adequacy of the airway, breathing, and circulation and provide immediate interventions as needed to correct any problems.

primary assessment a component of the overall patient assessment. The main objective of the primary assessment is to identify and treat any immediate life threats to the patient.

secondary assessment the component of the patient assessment during which the medical history and physical exam are performed.

EMERGENCY DISPATCH

"Truck 64, this is headquarters."

"Go ahead," C.J., an EMT, said into the mic after pausing a video on his smart phone.

"Truck 64, I need you to respond code three to 377 Grand Avenue for uncontrolled bleeding with a dialysis patient."

"Copy." C.J. dropped the phone into the storage bin between the seats and tapped on the truck's siren to alert his partner to the call. Tammy gathered her cash and receipt from the ATM and climbed into the truck. "There's some sort of bleeding call with a dialysis patient," C.J. told her.

"Oh, great," Tammy said as she pulled her gloves on. "That probably means a laundry list of other medical problems as well."

Upon arrival at the home, they found a shirtless man waving at them from the porch. "I don't know what's wrong with her," the man said frantically, as C.J. and Tammy wheeled the cot and equipment toward the front door. "She's diabetic, on dialysis for renal failure, and having a really, really heavy period."

"Could she be pregnant?" Tammy asked.

"Oh, no! No way. I mean, she's having a period. She can't be pregnant." The man led them to the 32-year-old female patient. She was unresponsive, staring blankly at a wall, and blood was soaking steadily into the couch where she sat.

"How long has she been this way?" Tammy asked, shaking the patient's shoulder.

"About an hour," the man said. "But she always has heavy periods."

"Let's go, C.J." Tammy slid her hands under the woman's arms. "We need to get her on the cot right now!"

Scene Size-up

12-2 Describe the components of a scene size-up and the importance of each.

The **scene size-up** is a process designed to quickly evaluate specific aspects of an emergency scene. While its main purpose is to ensure that the scene is safe for those entering, it includes additional components related to proper management of the emergency. The components of a scene size-up include (Figure 12-1 ■):

scene size-up the component of the patient assessment during which the following factors are assessed: safety, number of patients, need for resources, nature of illness or mechanism of injury, and need for spinal precautions.

- ***Safety.*** Don the appropriate personal protective equipment (BSI precautions) and confirm the scene is free of immediate hazards.

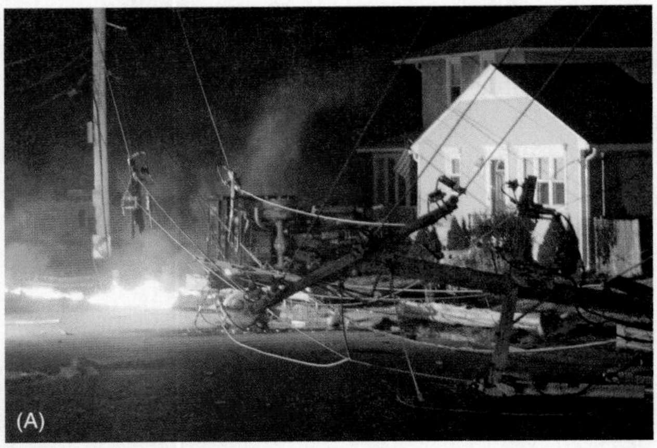

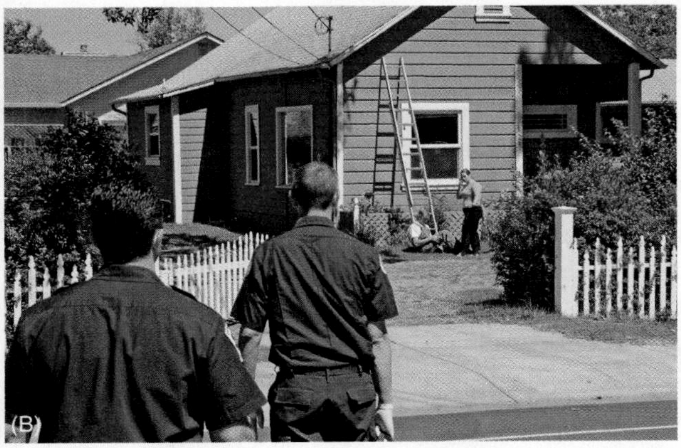

Figure 12-1 (A) Emergency scenes can present with many hazards, both seen and unseen. (© Mark C. Ide) (B) You and your partner must remain alert for hazards as you approach the scene.

- ***Nature of illness (NOI) or mechanism of injury (MOI).*** Determine the nature of the patient's illness or the mechanism that may have caused injury.
- ***Number of patients.*** Determine the number of patients at the scene of the emergency.
- ***Additional resources.*** Determine the need for resources such as law enforcement, additional transport units, advanced life support (ALS) units, specialty response teams, and so on.
- ***Spinal precautions.*** Make an initial determination on whether or not to take spinal precautions based on the mechanism of injury.

Personal Protective Equipment

Proper personal protective equipment (PPE) is designed to minimize the chances of exposure to potentially infectious materials such as blood, vomit, saliva, and so on. Proper PPE is required on every call (Figure 12-2 ■). PPE you must have available at all times include:

- *Gloves* to protect your hands from exposure to body fluids
- *Face protection* to provide protection of the eyes, nose, and mouth (Figure 12-3 ■)
- *Respiratory protection*, such as surgical masks, N95 masks, or HEPA respirators to prevent inhalation of microorganisms (Figure 12-4 ■)
- *Gowns* to protect your clothes from being soiled in circumstances where there are large volumes of blood or other body fluids

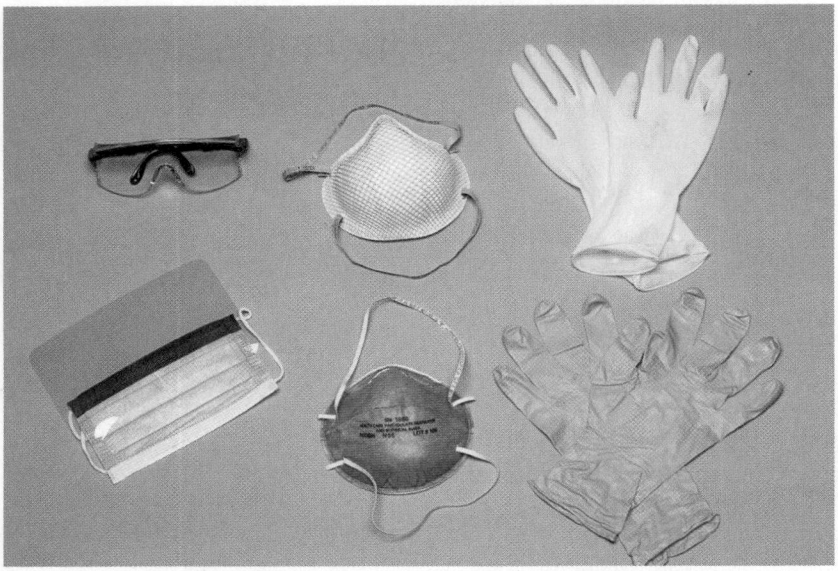

Figure 12-2 Proper personal protective equipment includes face and eye protection, as well as gloves.

Another vitally important part of infection control is hand washing (Figure 12-5 ■). The Centers for Disease Control and Prevention (CDC) suggest that hand washing is the single most effective means of preventing the spread of infection. Proper hand washing should be performed after each and every patient contact. Proper hand washing involves using soap and water with vigorous scrubbing to remove

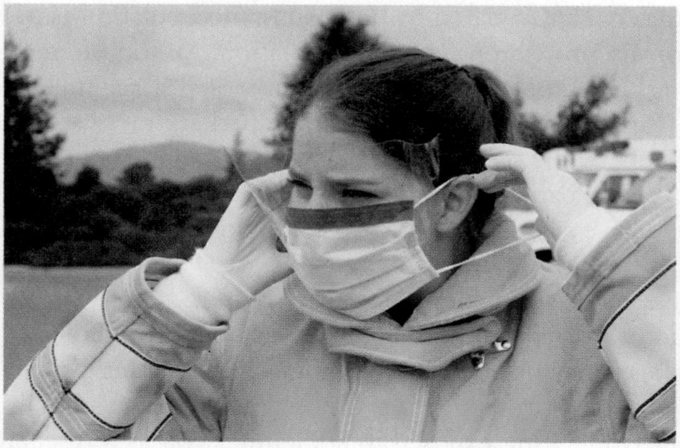

Figure 12-3 A face mask with eye shield is quick and easy to don.

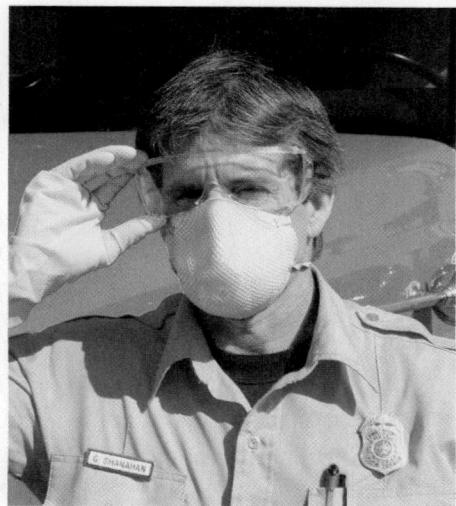

Figure 12-4 In some instances you will want to use an approved N-95 or N-100 mask to minimize exposure to airborne pathogens.

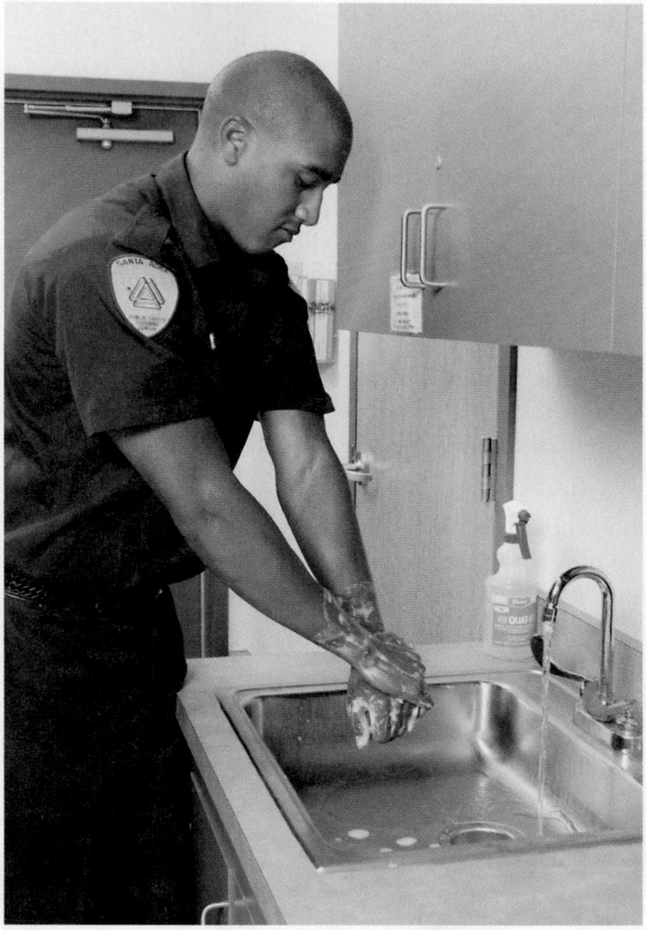

Figure 12-5 Proper hand washing is the single most effective means of preventing the spread of infection.

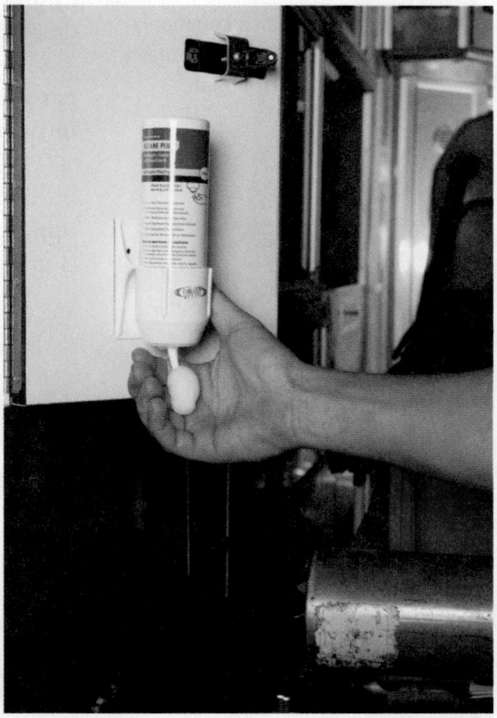

Figure 12-6 An alcohol-based waterless hand cleaner should be used when running water is not immediately available.

visible and nonvisible material and organisms that may be on your hands, wrists, and forearms.

You also should have access to an alcohol-based waterless hand cleaner (Figure 12-6 ■). It allows you to clean your hands in the field when soap and water are not available. The Centers for Disease Control and Prevention (CDC) states that it can be as effective as hand washing for hands that are not visibly soiled.

One of the most important concepts related to body substance isolation (BSI) precautions is choosing the correct protection in a given situation. All too often an EMT dons gloves when leaving the ambulance and never thinks of BSI again. This can be dangerous: Imagine you are responding to a fight in the parking lot of a convenience store. The police have made the scene safe and ask you to look at a patient who has facial trauma. Every time the patient speaks, blood sprays from his mouth. If you are wearing only gloves, you have a high chance of exposure through the mucous membranes of your face—the eyes, nose, and mouth.

Some infectious disease experts do not believe gloves are required on each call. If you respond to a patient who complains of abdominal pain and there are no body fluids or substances present, gloves may not be necessary. However, wearing proper PPE serves two purposes: to protect you from being exposed to a patient's bodily fluid and to protect the patient from being exposed to something you as a rescuer might be carrying. As an EMT, you may come in contact with many patients in a short period of time. You must take standard precautions to ensure that you are not a carrier of pathogens from one patient to another.

12-3 Explain the importance of safety at the scene of an emergency.

scene safety an awareness that you must continually ensure your own and the safety of your crew and your patient. This is done by teamwork, observation, and communication among members of a crew.

12-4 Describe hazards commonly found at emergency scenes (medical and trauma).

Scene Safety

Your ability to determine **scene safety** is perhaps one of the most important nonpatient care skills you will learn as an EMT. If you disregard your own safety and become injured, you will require assistance that diverts available resources and could result in a delay in care for someone else. In short, stay safe for both your sake and your patient's.

The safety of your entire crew is also a concern. You will work together with your partner or crew to remain safe. This is done by teamwork, observation, and communication among members of a crew.

When you approach a scene, do so slowly and carefully. Resist the urge to rush in. Begin your observations long before you arrive on scene. This will give you the opportunity to observe and react to the danger before you get in the middle of it (Figure 12-7 ■). Indications of potential hazards include the following:

- Signs of downed power lines, such as a blackout in an area near a scene. You may also observe asymmetry of telephone poles. Poles are relatively evenly spaced, so if a pole appears to be missing or at an unusual angle, it could indicate that wires are down.
- Large transport vehicles, such as tractor trailer rigs or rail cars, which often carry hazardous materials. Look for hazardous material placards, signs of people injured or down, fire, or threat of explosion.

> **CLINICAL CLUE**
>
> **Scene Safety**
>
> If the scene is not safe, make it safe or call someone who can. Never enter an unsafe scene. As an EMT you are not obligated to assist an ill or injured person if it puts you at unreasonable risk.

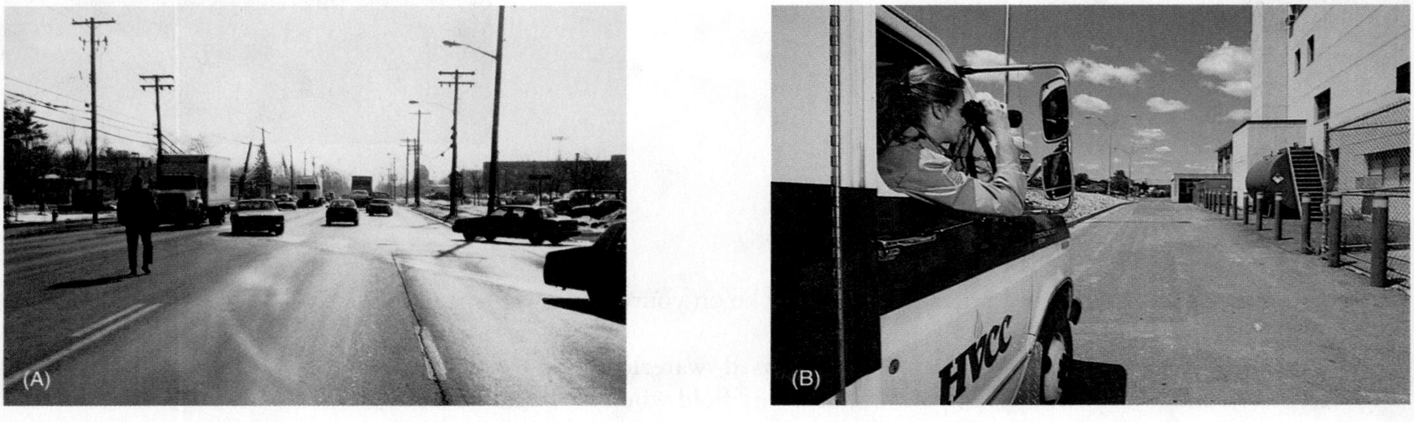

Figure 12-7 (A) Consider both traffic and damaged power poles when entering scenes involving vehicle collisions. (© Dan Limmer)
(B) If possible, use binoculars to assess the scene from a distance.

- Jagged metal at a motor-vehicle collision scene around an area where you will be accessing a patient.
- Agitated persons, hostile crowds, or weapons at a crime scene.
- Signs of potential trouble, such as evidence of alcohol or drugs on the scene or in use, pets, weapons, violent or agitated persons, unruly crowds, injuries that do not match the patient's explanation of how they occurred, and so on.
- Blood or body fluids or situations where you might expect those substances.

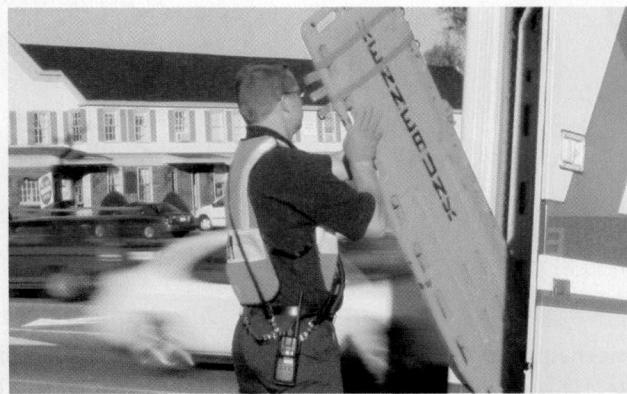

Figure 12-8 Do not approach any patient who is demonstrating violent behavior.

When you encounter what may be an unsafe scene, there are actions you can take to remain safe. In cases involving potential violence:

- Do not enter the scene until law enforcement has made it safe to do so (Figure 12-8 ■).
- Retreat from a scene where there are weapons or violent persons or situations.
- Use your equipment as a distraction to aid your retreat from the scene.
- Take a position of cover or concealment.
- Notify police immediately.

When you are called to the scene of a motor-vehicle collision:

- Wear appropriate personal protective equipment, including turnout gear, gloves, boots, and eye protection (Figure 12-9 ■).
- Be extra alert for traffic and always check both ways before stepping away from your vehicle (Figure 12-10 ■).
- Be alert for leaking fluid, such as gasoline and hazardous materials.
- Be alert for sharp surfaces, such as jagged metal.
- Notify the fire department and hazardous material units as needed.

When you approach the scene of an outdoor emergency:

- Be aware of extremes in weather that may harm you or your patients.
- Do not attempt rescues on or in slopes, heights, confined spaces, or water unless you are trained to do so and have the proper equipment.
- Notify the appropriate rescue teams for those situations.

12-5 Explain the role that the EMT plays in ensuring the safety of all people at the scene of an emergency.

CLINICAL CLUE

Stay Connected

No matter what type of situation you find yourself in, keeping a portable radio with you at all times is essential. It can assist you in rapidly calling for additional resources without having to return to your vehicle to use a mobile radio. Similarly, if a scene turns suddenly violent, your portable radio can be a direct life-saving link to dispatch or law enforcement resources.

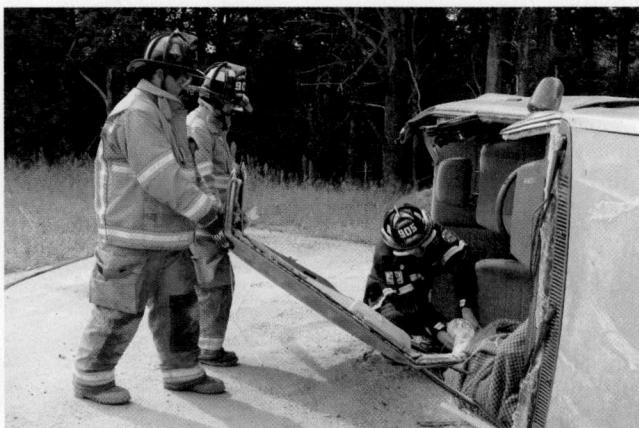

Figure 12-9 Motor-vehicle collision scenes often require specialized personal protective equipment, such as thick gloves and turnout gear.

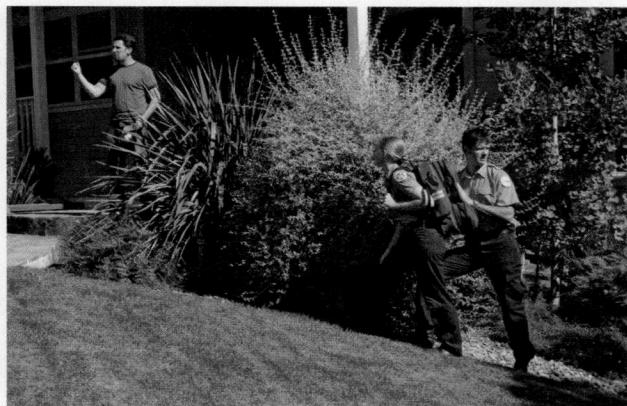

Figure 12-10 Traffic is a major risk for EMTs and rescuers working at the scene of a vehicle collision. (© Dan Limmer)

Nature of Illness or Mechanism of Injury

12-6 Differentiate between mechanism of injury and nature of illness.

After safety has been ensured and it is time to approach the patient, you will shift your focus to assessment and emergency medical care. Experienced EMTs know that they can observe important clues to the patient's condition in the few seconds it takes to move to the patient's side.

Determining the Nature of Illness

nature of illness (NOI) what is medically wrong with a patient.

Determining the exact nature of a patient's illness can be challenging. The **nature of illness (NOI)** is most often directly related to the patient's chief complaint. The chief complaint is best described as the reason why the patient or others at the scene called EMS. While EMTs often enter the scene of a medical emergency with the information obtained from dispatch, such as "chest pain" or "difficulty breathing," you must remain alert for clues that might provide more insight into the patient's condition or medical history (Figure 12-11 ■).

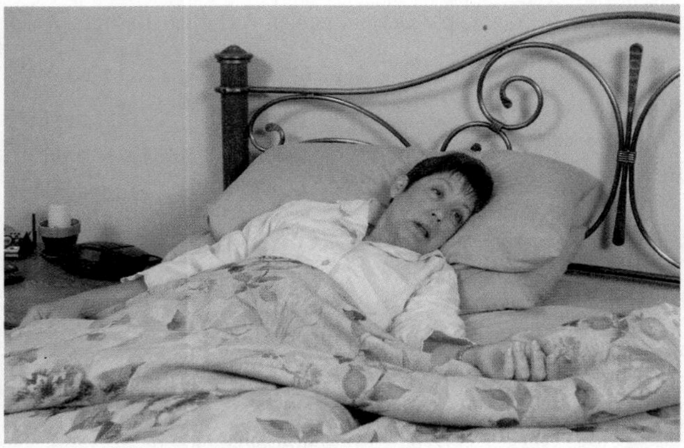

Figure 12-11 An altered mental status is a significant clue to an underlying medical condition.

For example, imagine that you have been dispatched to a call for an "unknown medical problem." You arrive at a residence and are directed into the kitchen. Things appear to be calm and safe. The patient's neighbor tells you he saw the patient working in the yard, when the patient seemed to stumble and clutch his chest. The neighbor called 911 and ran over. He found the patient "dazed" but conscious and got him into the house. You approach the patient and notice that he still has his hand clutched in a fist by his chest. He looks pale and sweaty. As you walk by the kitchen counter, you observe several medications.

You have not even begun to talk to your patient, yet you have identified several clues that could offer insight to the patient's history and affect the care you provide. Those clues include the dispatch information, the neighbor's story, and your own observations. You learned that the patient is probably very ill (he has his hand to his chest and he is pale and sweaty), that he at one point appears to have had some sort of altered mental status (information from the neighbor that the patient was "dazed"), and that he or someone in the residence has a prior medical condition (based on the medications found on the kitchen counter). That information lets you know that the patient's condition is potentially serious. It will affect the way you begin care for the patient, call for additional assistance, and set priorities in the primary assessment.

Other items to consider when determining the nature of illness include:

- Presence of home oxygen devices, which can indicate chronic respiratory conditions
- Presence of hospital beds in a residence, which can indicate a chronic illness
- Condition of the residence in reference to maintenance and cleanliness, which may be a clue to the overall health and abilities of the patient
- Odors including those from feces, spoiled foods, or poor hygiene, which also may be clues to the overall health and abilities of the patient

Mechanism of Injury

mechanism of injury (MOI) a force or forces that may have caused injury.

The **mechanism of injury (MOI)** refers to the forces that may have caused a patient's injuries. Those same forces may still be capable of hurting you. So, upon approaching an injured patient, look for hazards to you, your crew, your patient, and bystanders.

Carefully assessing the patient's mechanism of injury will give you an idea of his potential injuries. Consider the following situations:

- You are called to a motor-vehicle collision. You arrive to find a vehicle on its roof. From the damage, it appears it may have rolled over more than once before it came to rest. You look inside the vehicle and see no one. About 20 feet into a ditch on the side of the road, you see someone lying in an unnatural position.
- You are called to a warehouse for a patient who had his leg crushed between two vehicles. Upon arrival you find an adult male lying on the ground. He is alert and oriented and in significant pain. You observe a deformity to his right leg below the knee. Witnesses confirm that the injury is isolated to his leg and that he did not fall, hit his head, or get knocked out.

The difference between the two mechanisms must be understood. In the first scenario the patient was exposed to significant injury to his entire body as he was tossed around the inside of the overturning car and eventually thrown from the vehicle. That patient has likely suffered injury to the head, chest, abdomen, and pelvis—the areas that contain all the vital organ systems. For that reason you must have a high **index of suspicion** for injury to multiple organ systems.

index of suspicion an awareness or suspicion that there may be injuries based on the evaluation of the mechanism of injury.

In the second scenario the patient suffered a mechanism of injury that was isolated to his lower leg. While this is certainly a serious injury, it does not involve multiple organ systems related to the vital organs. There is a low index of suspicion for a significant life-threatening injury. However, he must receive immediate care to minimize loss of function or loss of limb.

Note that patients who appear to have experienced a significant mechanism of injury are considered to have a serious injury until proven otherwise—even if they appear to be fine. The opposite is *not* true. If the mechanism of injury appears to be nonsignificant, the patient still may have sustained life-threatening injuries.

12-7 Differentiate between significant and nonsignificant mechanisms of injury.

What constitutes a significant mechanism of injury is open to interpretation. Significant mechanisms of injury based on the current recommendations by the Centers for Disease Control in their Field Triage Decision Scheme—The National Trauma Triage Protocol include the following:

- Falls greater than 20 feet for an adult
- Falls greater than 10 feet or more than two or three times the height of the child in pediatrics
- High-risk vehicle crash, which can be identified by the following:
  - Intrusion of more than 12 inches on the occupant side of the crash vehicle or more than 18 inches on any side
  - Death of a passenger within the same compartment of a vehicle
  - Ejection (partial or complete) from a moving vehicle
  - Vehicle telemetry data consistent with high-risk injury. Some newer vehicles have sensors that can capture, record, and transmit vehicle crash data to a service center.
- Vehicle vs. pedestrian or bicyclist thrown, run over, or with significant (more than 20 mph) impact
- Motorcycle crash of more than 20 mph
- Penetrations of the head, chest, abdomen, or pelvis and extremities proximal to the knee or elbow

Number of Patients

A typical emergency response involves a limited amount of resources. In many systems across the country, a call to 911 will initiate a dispatch for an ambulance and a first responder unit. The first responders may be a fire crew composed of three personnel and the ambulance two personnel. This response is based on the assumption that most calls for assistance involve a single patient.

Depending on the specific emergency, it may not be immediately obvious that there are multiple patients. Vehicle collisions can involve patients who have been thrown from the vehicle and may not be immediately obvious, especially at night. A chemical spill or toxic release can affect a wide area and the total number of patients may not be evident for several hours.

The primary reason for wanting to determine the number of patients early on is so that you can ensure all patients receive the appropriate care in a timely manner.

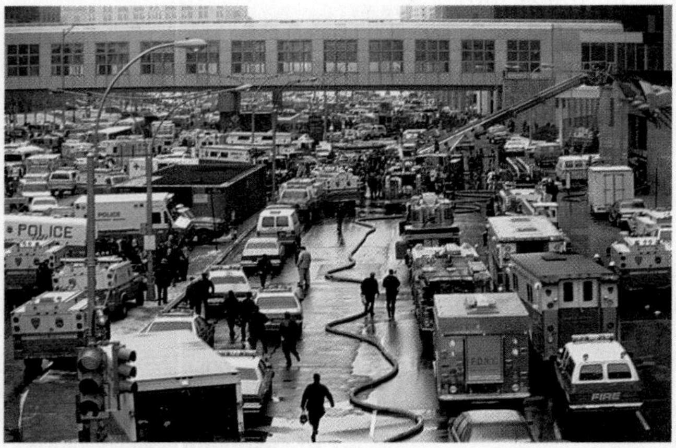

Figure 12-12 Always consider the need for resources as soon as possible. Some incidents require more resources than others. (B.S./Black Star)

Additional Resources

The experiences of countless EMTs have shown one important fact: If you do not call early for the help you need, you are likely to start caring for patients and the call for help may be delayed. The rule here is simple: Call for any help you feel you may need during the scene size-up. If it turns out that you will not need the help, you can always cancel it (Figure 12-12 ■).

Ambulances

If you have multiple patients, you will likely need additional ambulances. Even two patients may require different ambulances if they are being transported to different hospitals. Consider the intoxicated driver who injured others. It may be unwise to transport him with someone he injured.

If there are many patients on scene, you should activate your agency's **multiple-casualty incident (MCI)** plan. Some agencies recommend activation of a plan for as few as three patients. (Chapter 43 discusses multiple-casualty incidents and triage.)

multiple-casualty incident (MCI) any incident involving multiple patients and first-in units/resources being overwhelmed.

Fire Department

There are many types of incidents for which the fire service is called. They include hazardous materials incidents, vehicle extrication, and rescue. Some fire departments have special rescue teams, such as swift-water rescue and high-angle rescue. In many areas the fire department is dispatched for lifting assistance and other situations where additional personnel are necessary.

Law Enforcement

Always consider calling for police when there are immediate threats to scene safety. The police may be of assistance with traffic, patient refusal situations, and situations in which the potential for violence is high. The police also should be called if, in the course of your time on the scene, you discover drugs, weapons, or evidence that a crime has been committed.

Specialized Teams

Experience, training, and the proper equipment are vital when confronted with situations such as hazardous materials, weapons of mass destruction, **confined space** rescue, water rescue, and **high-angle rescue** and **low-angle rescue.** Know what teams are available in your area.

confined space a small, closed-in area with poor access and egress. Rescues involving confined spaces require specialized training and equipment.

high-angle rescue a vertical or above-ground rescue situation requiring specialized training and equipment.

low-angle rescue an off-road rescue situation requiring specialized training and equipment.

Utility Companies

You may need the assistance of the utility company to cut power or safely remove wires from the scene.

STOP, REVIEW, REMEMBER!

Multiple Choice

For each question, place a check next to the correct answer.

1. An appropriate scene size-up:
   _____ a. involves assessing airway, breathing, and circulation.
   _____ b. is completed prior to your arrival on scene.
   _____ c. addresses only issues of safety at the scene.
   _____ d. includes issues of safety and needed resources.

2. Which one of the following would be considered a significant mechanism of injury?
   _____ a. A broken ankle
   _____ b. A fall from 20 feet
   _____ c. Severe chest pain
   _____ d. A dislocated hip from a standing fall

3. A scene where power lines have fallen would require which specialized resource before EMS personnel could safely care for patients?
   _____ a. Fire department
   _____ b. Hazardous materials team
   _____ c. Utility company
   _____ d. Law enforcement

4. You should don personal protective equipment such as gloves and eye protection:
   _____ a. prior to entering the scene.
   _____ b. at the end of the scene size-up.
   _____ c. after determining the nature of illness or mechanism of injury.
   _____ d. just prior to touching the patient.

5. You are caring for patients who were in a vehicle collision when the scene suddenly becomes unsafe. You should:
   _____ a. retreat from the scene and call additional resources.
   _____ b. grab the patients and retreat from the scene.
   _____ c. continue to care for the patients while waiting for additional resources.
   _____ d. direct bystanders to address the hazard while you continue care of the patients.

Short Answer

For each of the following situations, explain how you may be harmed by potential dangers on the scene and what additional resources you may need.

1. A derailed train car carrying hazardous chemicals.

   a. Potential dangers:

   ____

   ____

   ____

   b. Additional resources:

   ____

   ____

   ____

(continued on next page)

(continued)

2. A residence where you hear an intoxicated person yelling.
   a. Potential dangers:

      ____
      ____
      ____

   b. Additional resources:

      ____
      ____
      ____

3. A collision scene where there is an occupied vehicle on its side.
   a. Potential dangers:

      ____
      ____
      ____

   b. Additional resources:

      ____
      ____
      ____

4. A hiker has fallen down a steep slope.
   a. Potential dangers:

      ____
      ____
      ____

   b. Additional resources:

      ____
      ____
      ____

Critical Thinking

1. You have responded to a residence and are caring for a male patient with a laceration to the forearm. It soon becomes apparent that the injury occurred during an altercation with his girlfriend. They begin arguing again while you are at the scene, and the girlfriend threatens the boyfriend. How will you manage this situation?

2. List at least two reasons why you would want to identify the need for additional resources as soon as possible at the scene of an emergency.

PERSPECTIVE

Tammy—The EMT

That poor girl was on her way out. The only thing that she responded to was pain, and then it was only to move her eyes toward me. There was blood everywhere on that couch, even some on the carpet. I know that some women have heavy periods, but this poor girl was bleeding out. All I knew was that we needed to get her to the hospital and fast.

The Primary Assessment

Once you have completed your scene size-up and feel certain that the scene is safe for you and your crew, begin the primary assessment of the patient (Table 12-1). The main objective of the primary assessment is to identify and treat all immediate life threats to the patient. It begins with the formation of a general impression and ends with a decision about the transport priority of the patient.

12-8 Explain the purpose of the primary assessment.

The components of the primary assessment are:

12-9 Describe the components of a primary assessment.

12-11 Describe how to evaluate each component of the primary assessment.

- Forming a general impression
- Evaluating mental status
- Determining the chief complaint
- Ensuring an adequate airway
- Ensuring the adequacy of breathing and administering supplemental oxygen if appropriate
- Ensuring the adequacy of circulation

TABLE 12-1 PRIMARY ASSESSMENT OF ADULTS, CHILDREN, AND INFANTS

	ADULTS	CHILDREN 1–5 YEARS	INFANTS TO 1 YEAR
Mental Status	AVPU: Is patient alert? Responsive to verbal stimulus? Responsive to painful stimulus? Unresponsive? If alert, is patient oriented to person, place, time, and event?	Same as adults	If not alert, shout as a verbal stimulus, flick feet as a painful stimulus. (Crying would be a normal response for an infant.)
Airway	Trauma: jaw-thrust maneuver. Medical: head-tilt/chin-lift maneuver. Both: Consider airway adjunct, suctioning	Same as adults, but see Chapter 13 for special child airway techniques. If performing head-tilt/chin lift, do so without tilting the neck too far.	See Chapters 13 and 38 for special infant airway techniques.
Breathing	If respiratory arrest, perform rescue breathing. If altered mental status and inadequate breathing (slower than 10 per minute), assist ventilations with supplemental oxygen. If alert and respirations are less than 29 per minute, give oxygen by nonrebreather mask.	Same as for adults, but normal rates for children are faster than for adults. (See Chapter 13 for normal child respiration rates.) Parent may have to hold oxygen mask to reduce child's fear of it.	Same as for children, but normal rates for infants are faster than for children and adults. (See Chapter 13 for normal infant respiration rates.)
Circulation	Assess skin, radial pulse, bleeding. If cardiac arrest, perform CPR.	Assess skin, radial pulse, bleeding, capillary refill. See Chapter 9 for normal child pulse rates (faster than for adults). If cardiac arrest, perform CPR.	Assess skin, brachial pulse, bleeding, capillary refill. See Chapter 9 for normal infant pulse rates (faster than for children and adults). If cardiac arrest, perform CPR.

- Identifying and controlling severe bleeding
- Determining priority for transport

There are essentially four conditions that a patient can die from in a matter of minutes that you as an EMT can correct. They are an obstructed airway, absent breathing, absent circulation, and severe bleeding. The core of the primary assessment consists of assessing the patient for each of those potential problems and providing the indicated care as quickly as possible. You should not feel compelled to move beyond the primary assessment and complete an entire patient assessment in each and every situation. In some situations you may be totally occupied with managing a patient's airway on scene and during transport. You will move on from the primary assessment only if all elements identified above are within normal limits and there are no immediate life threats to the patient.

CLINICAL CLUE

The Step-by-Step Approach

It is important to point out that you are learning patient assessment skills in a step-by-step manner, which is meant to help ensure a structured and thorough approach to assessment. This is somewhat different from the approach you will likely see used in the field on actual patients. A two-person EMS team will typically share the duties of the assessment in an effort to complete it more quickly and efficiently.

Forming a General Impression

After ensuring scene safety, your assessment begins as you approach your patient. In many instances you will be able to see him well before reaching his side. As you approach, a first impression of the patient is formed (Figure 12-13 ■). It is called a **general impression** and tells you the type of patient you have and his immediate condition. Forming a general impression involves using a limited amount of information to make a quick "big sick, little sick" decision. This decision can influence the care you provide, as well as the urgency for transport.

The specific elements that form a general impression may vary somewhat from EMT to EMT or system to system. Elements commonly used to help form a general impression of a patient are:

- Level of responsiveness and level of distress
- Approximate age
- Gender

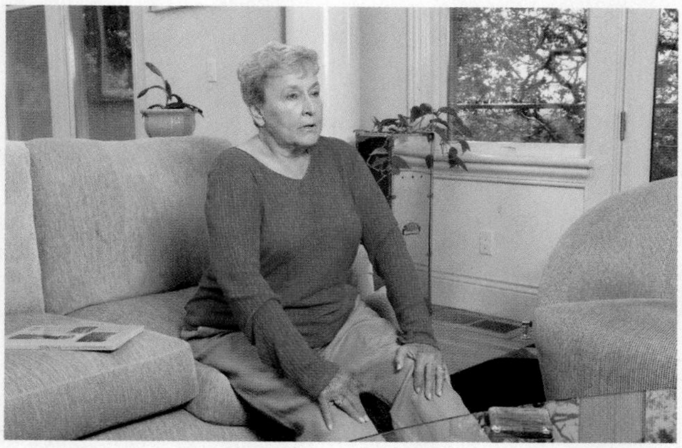

Figure 12-13 Pay close attention to how the patient appears as you approach.

general impression an element of the patient assessment that includes assessing approximate age, gender, and level of distress.

As you approach the patient, note his approximate age: Is he elderly, middle-aged, a young adult, or a pediatric patient? The age of the patient can influence the care you provide. If the patient is responsive, you will be able to ask his age once you get to his side. If the patient is unresponsive or unable to respond verbally, it is appropriate to estimate his age based on your best guess.

You also will notice the patient's level of responsiveness and level of distress. Those two elements will play a large part in making the "big sick, little sick" determination. Is the patient awake or unresponsive? An unresponsive patient is in need of immediate attention. If responsive, does the patient seem to be in a lot of pain, having difficulty breathing, or simply lying there calmly and quietly? Someone who is screaming in pain or clearly struggling to breathe will likely need immediate attention.

When verbalized, a typical general impression might sound something like this: "I observe an approximately 50-year-old male patient who is responsive and in mild distress" or "I observe an approximately 10-year-old female patient who is unresponsive."

CLINICAL CLUE

First Impressions

Although your instructor may ask you to verbalize your general impression as you practice your patient assessment skills in the classroom, it is not typically verbalized during patient care in the field. However, it will likely need to be documented on your prehospital care report.

Assessing Mental Status

Both the scene size-up and the general impression are conducted as you arrive at the scene and approach your patient. Up until that point, you most likely have not made physical contact with your patient. To assess mental status, you are ready to do so and interact with him directly.

It will be helpful to consider the position your patient is in as you approach him. If he is seated, approach him from the front and kneel down to eye level as soon as practical (Figure 12-14 ■). If he is lying down, kneel at his side so that he can see your face. In either case, make eye contact as soon as possible. This approach is less likely to startle the patient and will help establish a good rapport.

If the patient is in a supine position and you suspect a significant mechanism of injury, you may want to gently control his head as you introduce yourself (Figure 12-15 ■). This may prevent him from turning his head in response to your presence and making an existing injury worse. If you are uncertain about the mechanism of injury or if you suspect a spine injury, direct someone to manually hold the patient's head and neck before continuing with the exam.

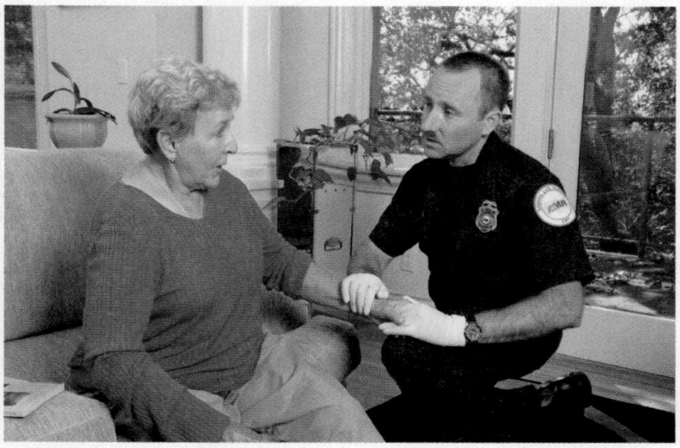

Figure 12-14 If the patient is seated, get down to her eye level as soon as practical.

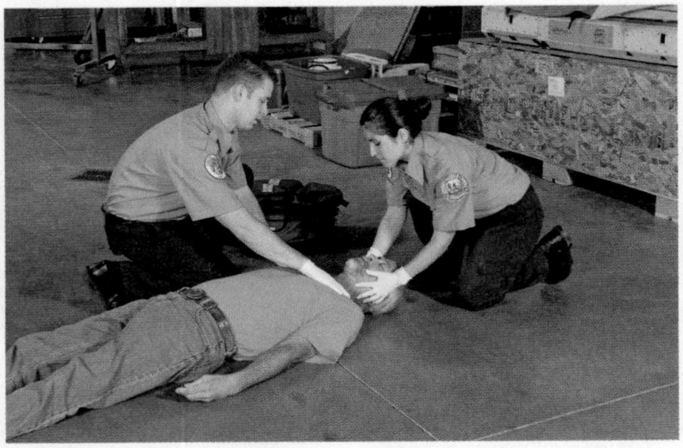

Figure 12-15 Be sure to manage the patient's head and neck if you suspect an injury.

When you make eye contact, introduce yourself and state your level of training. You may start with something like this: "Hello, my name is Chris and I am an EMT. I'm going to be taking care of you." Pay close attention to the patient's response. Does he make eye contact with you? Is he aware of your presence? Does he engage you verbally by speaking to you or crying out in pain? Does it appear that he is going to allow you to care for him? This is your first assessment of his mental status.

The Responsive Patient

For patients who are awake and responsive, determine his level of responsiveness. It is not enough just to know that he is responsive. You also must attempt to determine if he is alert and oriented. This technique is called the *A & O assessment*. The "A" stands for alert and the "O" stands for oriented.

To conduct an A & O assessment, determine the following:

- Person (Does he know who he is?)
- Place (Does he know where he is?)
- Time (Does he know what time it is?)
- Event (Does he know what happened?)

A patient who is oriented to all four is said to be "A & O × 4." A patient who can tell you only his name is "A & O × 1." A patient who can tell you who he is and his location is "A & O × 2." Note that in some EMS systems A & O × 3 (person, place, and time) is considered fully aware and is the normal convention for describing a person's mental status. It is important to learn and use the method unique to your system.

> **CLINICAL CLUE**
>
> **Talk to the Responsive Patient**
>
> One of the best ways of continuously monitoring the airway and breathing status of a responsive patient is to keep him talking. You can attend to other things, such as splinting a suspected fracture or controlling bleeding, while asking him questions. As long as you keep him talking, you know he has an adequate airway and is breathing.

The Unresponsive Patient

AVPU scale a method for classifying a patient's level of responsiveness, or mental status. The letters stand for *alert, verbal, painful,* and *unresponsive*.

Patients are not always fully awake and alert or totally unresponsive. Most patients fall somewhere in between. The **AVPU scale** is another tool used to categorize and document a patient's level of responsiveness. AVPU stands for:

A—*Alert.* The alert patient is one who is responsive and aware of his surroundings and your presence. The A & O scale can be used to further define the level of awareness for responsive patients.

V—*Verbal.* The verbal patient is most likely lying motionless with eyes closed as you approach him. However, when you speak to him or ask him if he can hear you, he responds in some meaningful way. He may respond to the sound of your voice by opening his eyes or trying to speak. When left alone, he may once again appear to be unresponsive. A patient who responds only to verbal stimulus may have a depressed gag reflex and is at risk for airway compromise. Monitor his airway closely.

P—*Painful.* When an apparently unresponsive patient does not respond to the sound of your voice, you may attempt to get a response by inflicting an appropriate painful stimulus. The emphasis here is on "appropriate." Pinching the skin (such as between the finger and thumb or the trapezius muscle) or rubbing the patient's sternum with your knuckles are considered appropriate and not harmful to the patient as long as it is not excessive. An appropriate response to painful stimulus would be movement of the hands toward the point of pain. Sometimes the patient also will moan or groan. A patient who responds only to painful stimulus may have a depressed gag reflex and is at high risk for airway compromise. Monitor his airway closely.

U—*Unresponsive.* The unresponsive patient offers no response to a verbal or a painful stimulus. He may have little to no gag reflex, so airway compromise is a major concern. Any patient found in an unresponsive state with absent or only agonal or gasping breathing should be immediately assessed for the presence of a pulse. If the pulse is absent, then CPR with immediate chest compressions should be initiated.

Continue to assess the patient's mental status throughout your care and transport, and document any change.

PRACTICAL PATHOPHYSIOLOGY

Of all the vital organs in the body, the brain is the most vulnerable to a decrease in adequate perfusion. It needs a constant supply of oxygen and glucose to function at its best. When the supply of oxygen or glucose is disrupted for any reason, the patient may present with an altered mental status.

CLINICAL CLUE

CPR

Any patient found in an unresponsive state with absent or only agonal or gasping breathing should be immediately assessed for the presence of a pulse. If the pulse is absent, then CPR with immediate chest compressions should be initiated.

The Glasgow Coma Scale

The Glasgow Coma Scale (GCS) (Figure 12-16 ■) provides a numerical score that rates a patient's level of responsiveness based on eye opening, speech, and motor function. While it was originally developed as an assessment tool for trauma patients, it is commonly used for medical patients as well.

This assessment tool and its scores, which range from a low of 3 to a high of 15, is valuable in evaluating, trending, and documenting the patient's neurological and mental status. This tool also is used in many EMS systems to assist in the process used to help determine which patients should be transported to a trauma center.

There are three components that ultimately contribute to the final Glasgow Coma Score. They are:

- ***Eye opening.*** Patients are assigned a score based on whether their eyes open spontaneously (4 points), open to voice (3 points), open to painful stimulus (2 points), or not open at all (1 point).
- ***Verbal response.*** Patients are assigned a score based on whether their verbal response is normal and oriented (5 points), confused (4 points), inappropriate words (3 points), incomprehensible (2 points), or none (1 point).
- ***Motor response.*** Patients are assigned a score based on their motor function: patients who follow commands (6 points), localize pain (5 points), withdraw from pain (4 points), display flexion or decorticate posturing (3 points), display extension or decerebrate posturing (2 points), or no response (1 point).

Glasgow Coma Scale	
Eye Opening	
Spontaneous	4
To verbal command	3
To pain	2
No response	1
Verbal Response	
Oriented and converses	5
Disoriented and converses	4
Inappropriate words	3
Incomprehensible sounds	2
No response	1
Motor Response	
Obeys verbal commands	6
Localizes pain	5
Withdraws from pain (flexion)	4
Abnormal flexion in response to pain (decorticate rigidity)	3
Extension in response to pain (decerebrate rigidity)	2
No response	1

Figure 12-16 The Glasgow Coma Scale.

Like other vital signs, it is important to obtain a GCS as soon as possible so that you will be able to trend the patient's condition throughout your care and transport. It is important to remember that any patient with an altered mental status is a high priority for transport. You may not have time to determine an accurate GCS if the patient needs immediate care.

STOP, REVIEW, REMEMBER!

Multiple Choice

For each question, place a check next to the correct answer.

1. You should establish your general impression immediately following the:
   _____ a. determination of the chief complaint.
   _____ b. scene size-up.
   _____ c. primary assessment.
   _____ d. SAMPLE history.

2. A patient who appears to be asleep and only moans when you apply a painful stimulus can be appropriately categorized as:
   _____ a. alert.
   _____ b. verbal.
   _____ c. painful.
   _____ d. unresponsive.

3. A patient who is only able to tell you where he is and who he is can be described as A & O ×:
   _____ a. 1
   _____ b. 2
   _____ c. 3
   _____ d. 4

4. A patient who is apparently asleep but who opens his eyes when spoken to is referred to as ____________ on the AVPU scale.
   _____ a. alert
   _____ b. verbal
   _____ c. painful
   _____ d. unresponsive

5. When caring for an unresponsive patient, it is appropriate for the EMT to have a high index of suspicion for:
   _____ a. absent breathing.
   _____ b. internal bleeding.
   _____ c. airway compromise.
   _____ d. an absent pulse.

Fill in the Blank

1. The primary assessment should be performed immediately following the ____________________.

2. The main objective of the primary assessment is to identify and treat ____________________.

3. The primary assessment begins with the formation of a ____________________.

4. The ____________________ is designed to provide a quick "big sick, little sick" determination.

5. A patient who is A & O × 4 is said to be alert and oriented to person, place, time, and ____________________.

6. A patient who responds to the sound of your voice by opening his eyes or trying to speak is said to be ____________________ on the AVPU scale.

Critical Thinking

1. Describe why the primary assessment is such an important component of the overall patient assessment.

2. How might the fact that a person appears to be unresponsive during the general impression affect what you do for the patient?

3. Describe a patient for whom you may never get to the task of performing a complete patient assessment, one that includes both a primary and the more thorough secondary assessment.

Determining the Chief Complaint

Simply stated, the **chief complaint** is the patient's perception or description of the problem in his own words. It is *not* what you, the EMT, perceive to be the problem. For example, imagine that you have been dispatched to a call for "chest pain." However, when you arrive, your patient states that he is having difficulty breathing. When you ask if he is having any chest pain, he states, "Yes, but I can't seem to catch my breath."

chief complaint the patient's perception of the problem in his own words.

There may be times when the patient has several complaints and does not say that one is worse than the others. With those patients, you must do your best to decide which is the most serious of the complaints and provide care accordingly. One suggested approach to determining the patient's chief complaint is to use the following formula when you initiate contact with the patient: "Hello. My name is Ed and I'm with the rescue squad. What seems to be the problem today?" The first thing out of the patient's mouth will likely be his chief complaint.

CLINICAL CLUE

Safety First

Sometimes there are obvious life threats even before you begin your primary assessment of the patient. Things such as exposure to flames and unstable vehicles must be addressed prior to beginning any formal patient assessment.

PERSPECTIVE

C.J.—The EMT

That lady's airway was fine. I could hear her breathing and grunting as we moved her, but her respiratory rate was a little slow and shallow. When we moved her to our cot, I put a nonrebreather mask on her with 15 liters of oxygen. I figured between her poor breathing and the major blood loss, a bunch of oxygen would be her best bet. Even with the oxygen, I knew we needed to keep an eye on her breathing rate and volume during the transport.

Assessing the Airway

As you introduce yourself to the patient and assess his mental status, you simultaneously will be assessing the status of his airway. This is easier to accomplish for responsive patients, because it can be deduced that if they are talking, they must have a clear airway. If for any reason they do not have a clear airway, such as a patient with snoring or gurgling respirations, you must immediately clear the airway using the appropriate method. Once you are comfortable that your patient has a clear airway, you will be able to assess for adequacy of breathing.

Assessing for an open airway in an unresponsive patient takes a little more work. If you are not certain the airway is open, you must manually open it using the appropriate method. The specific method you use to open the airway will depend on the patient's age and the mechanism of injury. For a patient in whom you do not suspect a spine injury, you will use the head-tilt/chin-lift maneuver. For a patient with an unknown MOI or one in whom you suspect a spine injury, you must perform the jaw-thrust maneuver. (Refer to Chapter 13 for details on how to properly perform both airway maneuvers.)

If for any reason you believe the patient's airway is compromised, you must immediately perform the appropriate procedures to clear it.

Note that it is not enough to know the patient has a clear airway. You also must confirm that he is breathing at an appropriate rate and moving an adequate amount of air (tidal volume) with each breath. The method for initially assessing the adequacy of breathing is the same for all patients. You must assess rate, depth, and ease by observing the chest for rise and fall and looking for signs of difficulty breathing, such as increased rate, a decreased tidal volume, and use of accessory muscles (Figure 12-17 ■). Even if breathing appears adequate, consider the need for supplemental oxygen.

PRACTICAL PATHOPHYSIOLOGY

A person must have an adequate minute volume of air to sustain life. Determining minute volume and thus the adequacy of breathing is a combination of two primary factors: respiratory rate and tidal volume. Too slow of a respiratory rate or too shallow of a tidal volume will result in too low of a minute volume of air.

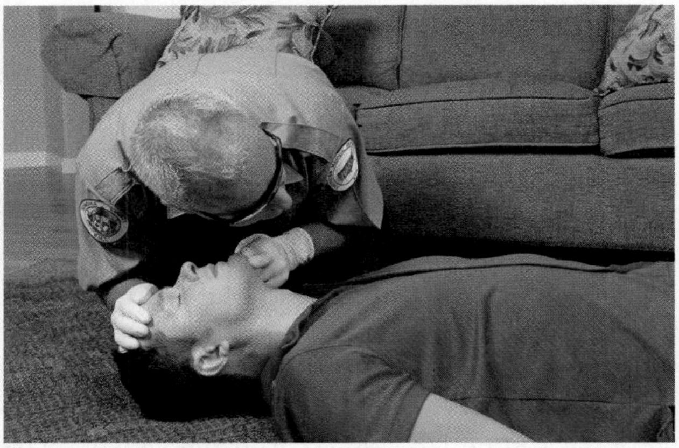

Figure 12-17 Confirm adequacy of breathing by opening the airway and assessing rate and tidal volume.

A respiratory rate that is greater than 29 is considered inadequate, and the patient should receive oxygen by nonrebreather mask at 15 liters per minute. A rate less than 10 is also inadequate and may require assisted ventilations by bag-mask or similar device. Regardless of the device, the use of supplemental oxygen is recommended. For unresponsive patients, consider the need for an appropriate airway adjunct.

PERSPECTIVE

Tammy—The EMT

I'd never seen vaginal bleeding like that, except maybe post delivery. It was just running out. As soon as we got her on the cot, I grabbed a trauma dressing and tried to control the bleeding as best I could, but I knew that the hospital was the only place where this girl was going to have a chance.

Oxygen Therapy

It is during the primary assessment that you will make your first determination of whether the patient would benefit from supplemental oxygen. While it is probably safe to say that all patients will benefit from supplemental oxygen, this does not mean that all patients *must* receive supplemental oxygen. That decision is up to the EMT and may be based on local protocol.

The decision to provide supplemental oxygen is based on many factors, including but not limited to mechanism of injury (MOI) or nature of illness (NOI), level of distress, and signs and symptoms. If you decide initially to not provide oxygen, this does not mean that you cannot change your mind later. Perhaps you will want to initiate oxygen once you have the majority of the history from the patient. The point is that you must constantly reassess the need for appropriate interventions, and oxygen can be initiated at any time.

Assessing Circulation

Once you have determined that the airway is clear and the patient is breathing adequately, assess for adequacy of circulation. To do that, you should first locate the pulse, confirm that it is present, and finally make a quick guess as to rate and rhythm (whether it is regular or irregular).

For responsive patients older than one year of age, use the radial pulse (Figure 12-18 ▪). For responsive patients younger than one year of age, use the brachial pulse in the upper arm (Figure 12-19 ▪).

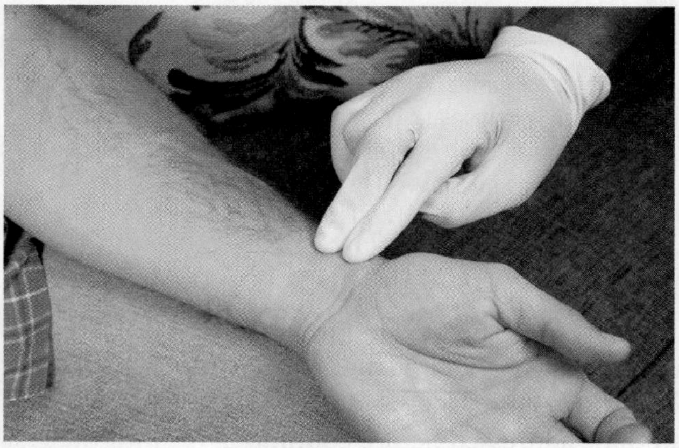

Figure 12-18 Assessing the radial pulse of a responsive patient.

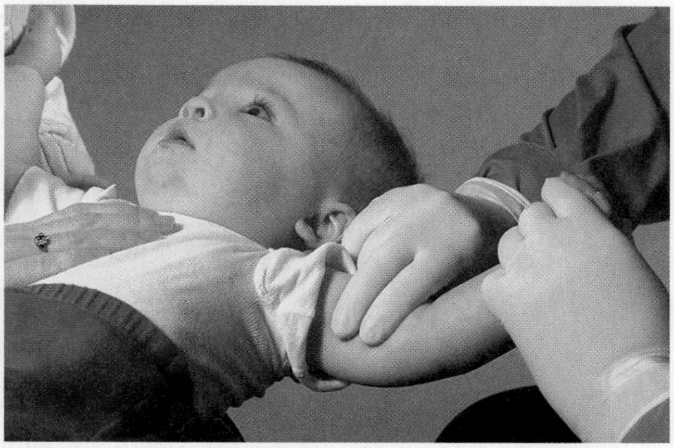

Figure 12-19 Assessing the brachial pulse of an infant. (© Dan Limmer)

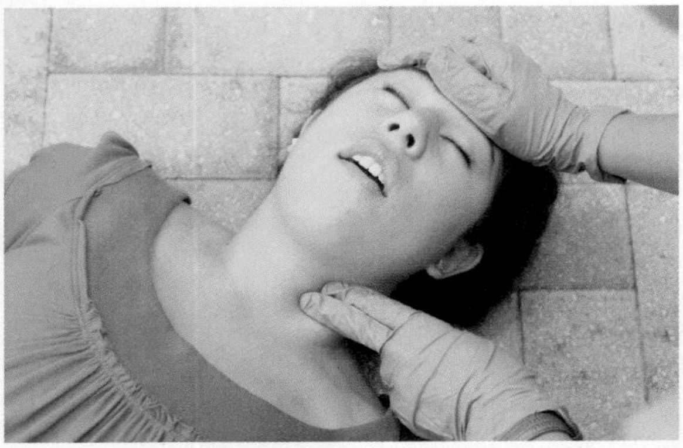

Figure 12-20 Assessing the carotid pulse of an unresponsive patient.

For unresponsive patients older than one year of age, use the carotid pulse (Figure 12-20 ■). For unresponsive patients younger than one year of age, use the brachial pulse.

If a pulse cannot be located, immediately begin CPR beginning with chest compressions. Attach an automated external defibrillator if available (follow local protocol).

CLINICAL CLUE

Capillary Refill for Children

In pediatric patients under the age of six years old, you may use the capillary refill test to help determine the adequacy of perfusion. A capillary refill time of less than two seconds is considered normal. Remember that the capillary refill test is only one component in the overall patient assessment and should not be used as the sole determination of adequate or inadequate perfusion.

12-10 Explain how encountering a patient in cardiac arrest alters the sequence of the primary assessment.

Cardiac Arrest Considerations

In the vast majority of patients you will care for as an EMT, the primary assessment sequence will be airway, breathing, and then circulation—or ABC. However, in patients found to be in cardiac arrest, compressions must begin immediately.

Therefore, in an unresponsive patient who is not breathing or who has only irregular gasping (agonal) breaths, immediately check for a pulse. If a pulse is present (and this will be most of the time), then assess the airway and follow the normal ABC sequence. If no pulse is present, immediately begin a cycle of chest compressions and then open the airway and ventilate the patient.

Identifying and Controlling Severe Bleeding

Quickly assess the patient for evidence of serious external bleeding. Look for obvious blood pooling beneath the patient or blood-stained clothing. Cut away clothing, use a hand sweep beneath the patient, or carefully roll the patient to identify and control obvious bleeding. If you detect serious bleeding, you must take the appropriate measures to control it before moving on with your assessment. (Bleeding control will be addressed in Chapter 30.)

PRACTICAL PATHOPHYSIOLOGY

Adequate perfusion to the vital organs is necessary for life. When the circulatory system is damaged and blood is allowed to spill out, perfusion is immediately compromised. The loss of blood means that there are fewer hemoglobin molecules to carry oxygen to the cells. So, it is essential to identify and control all severe bleeding as soon as possible.

Other Immediate Life Threats

Again, the main purpose of the primary assessment is to identify and care for all immediate life threats. Some of those threats may not be immediately obvious and may not be directly related to the ABCs. Such conditions as open chest wounds, impaled objects, or entrapment may need to be addressed before continuing on with the rest of the primary assessment.

Assessing Skin Signs

Assess the patient's skin color, temperature, and moisture. Begin by looking at and feeling the skin of the patient's face, lips, and conjunctiva (pink tissue around the inside of the eye) (Figure 12-21 ■). Observe for and document any abnormal findings. Normal skin signs are pink, warm, and dry. Abnormal skin signs include skin that is pale, flushed, or a color other than pink. Skin that is sweaty, extremely hot, or cool to the touch also may be a sign of underlying injury or illness.

In addition to the skin signs just mentioned, capillary refill time should be assessed in all pediatric patients. A capillary refill time of less than two seconds is considered normal in most patients. (See Chapter 9 for more information about capillary refill.)

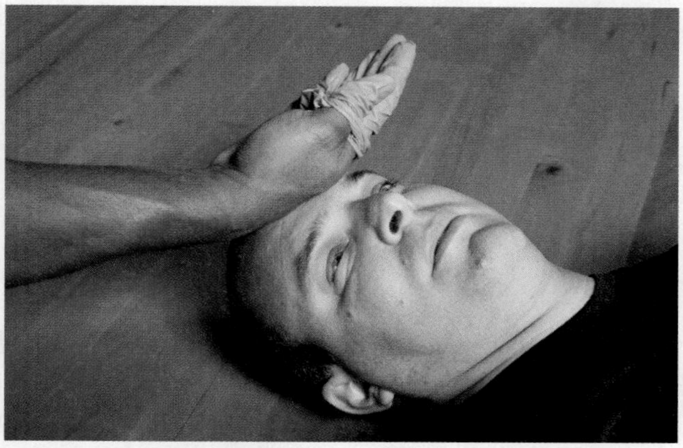

Figure 12-21 Use the back of your ungloved hand to assess skin temperature and moisture.

PERSPECTIVE

The Husband

I've been with her through a lot of medical stuff, you know? Diabetic problems, dialysis, you name it. But I've never seen her so pale and cold. It scared me enough to call 911. She's just never been this bad before.

Determining Patient Priority

12-12 Describe how to prioritize and manage problems related to the primary assessment.

12-13 Differentiate patients who are high-priority and low-priority for transport.

You will use all of the information that you have gathered during your primary assessment to determine the transport priority for your patient. Depending on his condition, a patient can be identified as a high or low priority. The priority will determine such things as how quickly he should receive care and how quickly you will initiate transport to the hospital. The following is a list of factors that might place a patient in a high transport priority category:

- Poor general impression (altered mental status or severe distress)
- Unresponsiveness
- Difficulty breathing
- Signs of shock
- Complicated childbirth
- Chest pain
- Uncontrolled bleeding
- Severe pain anywhere

Patient condition will determine his priority and how quickly he receives care and transport. In some cases, his priority will also determine whether or not an ALS intercept is indicated.

Continuing Assessment

Once you have completed the primary assessment and have identified and cared for all immediate life threats to the patient, you may move on to the next component of the patient assessment process. You may not, however, move on if any of the critical components of the primary assessment still need attention. For instance, if the patient is not breathing adequately, you must assist him accordingly. If there is severe external bleeding, you must perform the appropriate techniques to control the bleeding before doing anything else.

In some situations, you may spend all of your time dealing with issues related to the primary assessment and never complete a full assessment. Do not delay transport simply to complete a full assessment. If the patient is a high priority, consider loading him into the ambulance and continuing care while en route to an appropriate receiving facility.

PERSPECTIVE

Tammy—The EMT

What priority was she? You're kidding, right? Just look at the primary assessment. One, she had a tremendously poor general appearance. Two, she was all but unresponsive. And three, she was losing blood fast and I couldn't stop it. You just don't get to a higher priority than that.

STOP, REVIEW, REMEMBER!

Multiple Choice

For each question, place a check next to the correct answer.

1. You are caring for an unresponsive patient who is ill. She presents with a pulse of 84 and snoring respirations. The appropriate technique for opening this patient's airway is the:

_____ a. jaw-thrust.

_____ b. head-thrust.

_____ c. head-tilt/chin-lift.

_____ d. jaw-tilt.

2. A complete assessment for the adequacy of breathing must include:

_____ a. rate, depth, and ease.

_____ b. rate, strength, and rhythm.

_____ c. rate, depth, and volume.

_____ d. rate, ease, and volume.

3. You have just completed the assessment of your unresponsive patient's breathing status. What should you assess next?

_____ a. The pulse

_____ b. Mental status

_____ c. The airway

_____ d. Bleeding

4. When performing a primary assessment, the control of serious bleeding should occur:

_____ a. before airway and breathing.

_____ b. after assessing circulation.

_____ c. at the end of the primary assessment.

_____ d. immediately upon reaching the patient.

5. The decision to administer supplemental oxygen occurs during which step of the primary assessment?

_____ a. Determination of chief complaint

_____ b. Assessment of mental status

_____ c. Assessment of breathing

_____ d. Determination of priority

Matching

Match the definition on the left with the applicable term on the right.

1. _____ A patient's perception of his problem stated in his own words
2. _____ Identifying life threats is the main objective of this
3. _____ Preferred method for opening the airway of a patient with an unknown MOI
4. _____ Preferred pulse point for assessing circulation in an unresponsive adult
5. _____ Preferred pulse point for assessing circulation in an unresponsive infant

A. Primary assessment
B. Chief complaint
C. Carotid
D. Brachial
E. Jaw-thrust maneuver

Critical Thinking

1. Describe how you would assess the airway of a responsive patient versus an unresponsive patient.

____

____

____

____

2. How would you determine the adequacy of an unresponsive patient's breathing?

____

____

____

____

3. How will you determine if a patient would benefit from supplemental oxygen?

____

____

____

____

EMERGENCY DISPATCH SUMMARY

The patient was placed on a cot in a supine position, covered with a blanket, given oxygen via nonrebreather mask at 15 liters per minute, and rushed to the nearest hospital. The patient was immediately admitted into surgery where her bleeding—determined to have been caused by a miscarriage—was successfully controlled. She was released from the hospital several days later.

Chapter Review

To the Point

- Performing a thorough scene size-up and ensuring your safety as well as the safety of the scene in general is your main concern before patient care.
- Consider the need for additional resources such as hazmat and rescue teams, law enforcement, and utility company personnel early in the call and before entering an unsafe scene.
- Understanding the nature of illness or mechanism of injury will help you focus on the most appropriate care.
- As you approach the patient, form a general impression to begin to make the "big sick, little sick" determination.
- The primary assessment is designed to identify and care for any immediate life threats to the patient. You must ensure there are no problems with the ABCs before moving on to further assess the patient.

Chapter Questions

Multiple Choice

For each question, place a check next to the correct answer.

1. Which one of the following would you identify as a significant mechanism of injury?
   _____ a. Slip and fall to the ground
   _____ b. Fall from the top of a 20-foot ladder
   _____ c. Dislocated knee
   _____ d. A 15 mph vehicle collision

2. You are performing a primary assessment on an alert and oriented patient who was injured. You have just placed him on oxygen. You should next:
   _____ a. form a general impression.
   _____ b. determine the chief complaint.
   _____ c. obtain vital signs.
   _____ d. check circulation.

3. The component of the patient assessment that identifies the patient's age, gender, and level of distress is the:
   _____ a. general impression.
   _____ b. scene size-up.
   _____ c. mechanism of injury.
   _____ d. head-tilt/chin lift.

4. Which one of the following best defines the purpose for forming a general impression?
   _____ a. To determine the level of responsiveness
   _____ b. To determine the patient's chief complaint
   _____ c. To identify any immediate life threats
   _____ d. To formulate a gut sense of the patient's condition

5. A patient who is awake and able to respond appropriately is said to be _____________ on the AVPU scale.
   _____ a. alert
   _____ b. verbal
   _____ c. painful
   _____ d. unresponsive

6. Confirming that a patient is alert and oriented includes establishing that he is aware of person, __________, time, and event.
   _____ a. complaint
   _____ b. place
   _____ c. surroundings
   _____ d. age

Listing

List the components of a scene size-up.

1. ______________________________
2. ______________________________
3. ______________________________
4. ______________________________
5. ______________________________
6. ______________________________

Critical Thinking

1. Four conditions that can cause a person to die in a short period of time are identified in this chapter. List them and briefly note how they would lead to the death of the patient.

____

____

____

____

2. Can you think of any other conditions not included in the above list that can cause the death of a patient in a relatively short period of time?

____

____

____

____

(continued on next page)

(continued)

3. What is the purpose of forming a general impression of each and every patient?

4. Why is it important to use the patient's own words when relaying or documenting the patient's chief complaint?

Case Studies

Case Study 1

You have responded to a single-vehicle rollover. Upon arrival, you are told by bystanders that the car is over the side of the road and against a tree. You safely make your way to the vehicle but are unable to gain access to the patient. You have called for the extrication team and have established verbal contact with the patient.

1. How might you conduct a primary assessment from your position outside the vehicle?

2. What elements of the primary assessment will be most difficult to assess without making patient contact?

Case Study 2

You have been dispatched to a convalescent hospital for an unknown medical problem. Upon arrival, you are escorted back to one of the patient rooms where you find an unresponsive female patient lying on the floor of the bathroom. One of the nursing staff tells you the patient has a history of falling all the time, and they were unable to get her back into bed due to the patient being in too much pain.

1. Describe how you will perform your primary assessment on this patient.

2. The patient remains unresponsive and you are unable to determine if she is breathing adequately. What will you do next?

3. She now appears to be breathing adequately but you are unable to palpate a radial pulse. What will you do next?

The Last Word

If there are only two things you take away from your EMT training, understanding how to assess for and mitigate hazards at the scene and how to properly perform a primary assessment are the most important. Sometimes an EMT can be so focused on helping someone in need that he or she completely neglects or fails to see immediate or potential hazards at the scene of an emergency. You must remain diligent from beginning to end with issues related to scene safety.

When it comes to the primary assessment, you must be just as purposeful and deliberate, and understand that you may need to continue managing issues related to the ABCs or other immediate life threats before even considering moving on to the secondary assessment.

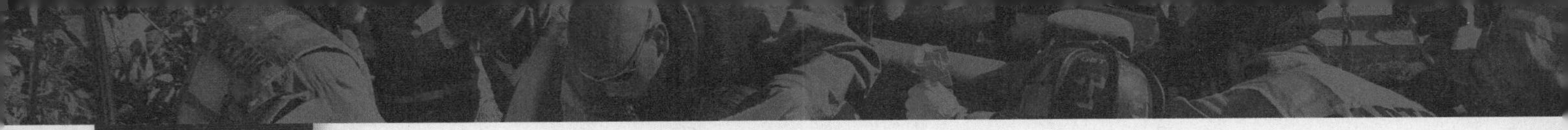

13 Managing Your Patient's Airway and Ventilation

Education Standards

Airway Management, Respiration, and Artificial Ventilation

Competencies

Applies knowledge of general anatomy and physiology to patient assessment and management in order to ensure a patent airway, adequate mechanical ventilation, and respirations for patients of all ages.

Objectives

After completion of this lesson, you should be able to:

13-1 Define key terms introduced in this chapter.

13-2 Distinguish among the terms respiration, ventilation, pulmonary respiration, internal respiration, capillary respiration, and cellular respiration.

13-3 Describe the signs, symptoms, and characteristics of adequate and inadequate breathing, including air flow, breath sounds, flaring of the nostrils, inspection of the chest, minute ventilation, patient's ability to speak, and patient's general appearance.

13-4 Describe the signs and symptoms of inadequate breathing.

13-5 Describe differences between adults and children in the anatomy and physiology of the respiratory system.

13-6 Explain differences between adults and children in the signs of hypoxia.

13-7 Describe the relationship between airway status and mental status.

13-8 Explain the causes of each of the following abnormal upper airway sounds: snoring, crowing, gurgling, and stridor.

13-9 Describe how partial or complete obstruction of the airway leads to hypoxia.

13-10 Describe the proper method of opening the airway for a patient with suspected and no suspected spine injury.

13-11 Describe the proper technique for using both a manual and battery-powered suction device.

13-12 Compare the function of fixed and portable suction devices.

13-13 Compare the use of rigid and soft suction catheters.

13-14 Explain special considerations to be kept in mind when suctioning patients, including signs of hypoxia and patients with copious amounts of vomit that cannot be quickly suctioned.

13-15 Describe the indications, contraindications, limitations, and procedures for the use of oropharyngeal and nasopharyngeal airways.

13-16 Identify patients with indications for supplemental oxygen and positive pressure ventilation.

13-17 Describe the physiological differences between spontaneous and positive pressure ventilation.

13-18 Describe the proper procedures for artificial ventilation using the following methods: mouth-to-mask ventilation and delivery of positive pressure ventilations with a bag-mask device (one-person and two-person), with a demand-valve device, and with an automatic transport ventilator.

13-19 Explain the significance of avoiding gastric inflation when administering positive pressure ventilation.

13-20 Describe indications and methods for administering positive pressure ventilations to a patient who is breathing spontaneously.

13-21 Discuss the indications, contraindications, and methods for administering noninvasive positive pressure ventilation (NIPPV).

13-22 Discuss the hazards of overventilation.

13-23 Discuss special considerations of airway management and ventilation for patients with stomas or tracheostomy tubes, infants and children, and patients with dental appliances.

13-24 Describe the properties of oxygen.

13-25 Differentiate between the various sizes of oxygen cylinders available.

13-26 Describe the hazards associated with oxygen use and safety precautions to be observed when using oxygen or handling oxygen cylinders.

13-27 Describe the purpose and function of pressure regulators.

13-28 Discuss the use of oxygen humidifiers.

13-29 Discuss the administration of oxygen by nonrebreather mask, nasal cannula, simple face mask, partial rebreather mask, Venturi mask, and tracheostomy mask.

Key Terms

bag-mask device p. 350
demand-valve device p. 352
head-tilt/chin-lift maneuver p. 333
jaw-thrust maneuver p. 334
nasal cannula p. 366
nasopharyngeal airway (NPA) p. 339
nonrebreather mask p. 363
oropharyngeal airway (OPA) p. 339
patent airway p. 331
perfusion p. 358
respiration p. 325
respiratory distress p. 327
respiratory failure p. 329
stoma p. 355
tidal volume p. 327

Introduction

This chapter begins discussion on the issues related to patient care and the single most important priority following personal safety—an open and clear airway for the patient. Without a clear airway and adequate air exchange, life quickly comes to an end. People can do without many things for an extended amount of time, such as food, water, and shelter, but the human body cannot tolerate even short intervals without oxygen. In this chapter you will learn how to assess the status of a patient's airway as well as differentiate between adequate and inadequate respiration. You also will be introduced to many of the tools available to the EMT for helping maintain an open and clear airway and ensure adequate oxygen.

EMERGENCY DISPATCH

It is a warm afternoon in late summer and the crew of Unit 281 just started the well-used barbecue at the station when emergency tones chime from the radio: "281, 2-8-1, start emergency for Baker Lake on the east side by the boat ramps for a 23-year-old female who is choking." Mackenzie, an EMT, quickly shuts off the barbecue's propane tank and starts the truck as her partner, Rob, tosses the uncooked chicken back into the refrigerator for the third time today. A quick drive on Baker Parkway brings them to the park entrance by the boat ramp, where a man is waving at them and pointing toward a woman who is lying on the grass at the edge of the lake.

"We were eating lunch and talking and then she just started choking," the man gasps as the ambulance rolls to a stop. "I tried those, um, abdominal thrusts, you know, where you get behind her? It didn't seem to work and then she just passed out."

Rob and Mackenzie approach the woman, stepping over the scattered items of a picnic lunch, and find her cyanotic and unresponsive. Mackenzie turns to the man as she is opening the airway kit. "What's her name and how long has it been since she started choking?"

"It's been about, I don't know, maybe three or four minutes," he says. "And her name is Shannon."

"Okay, Shannon," Rob says as he performs a head-tilt/chin-lift on the woman. "Hang in there."

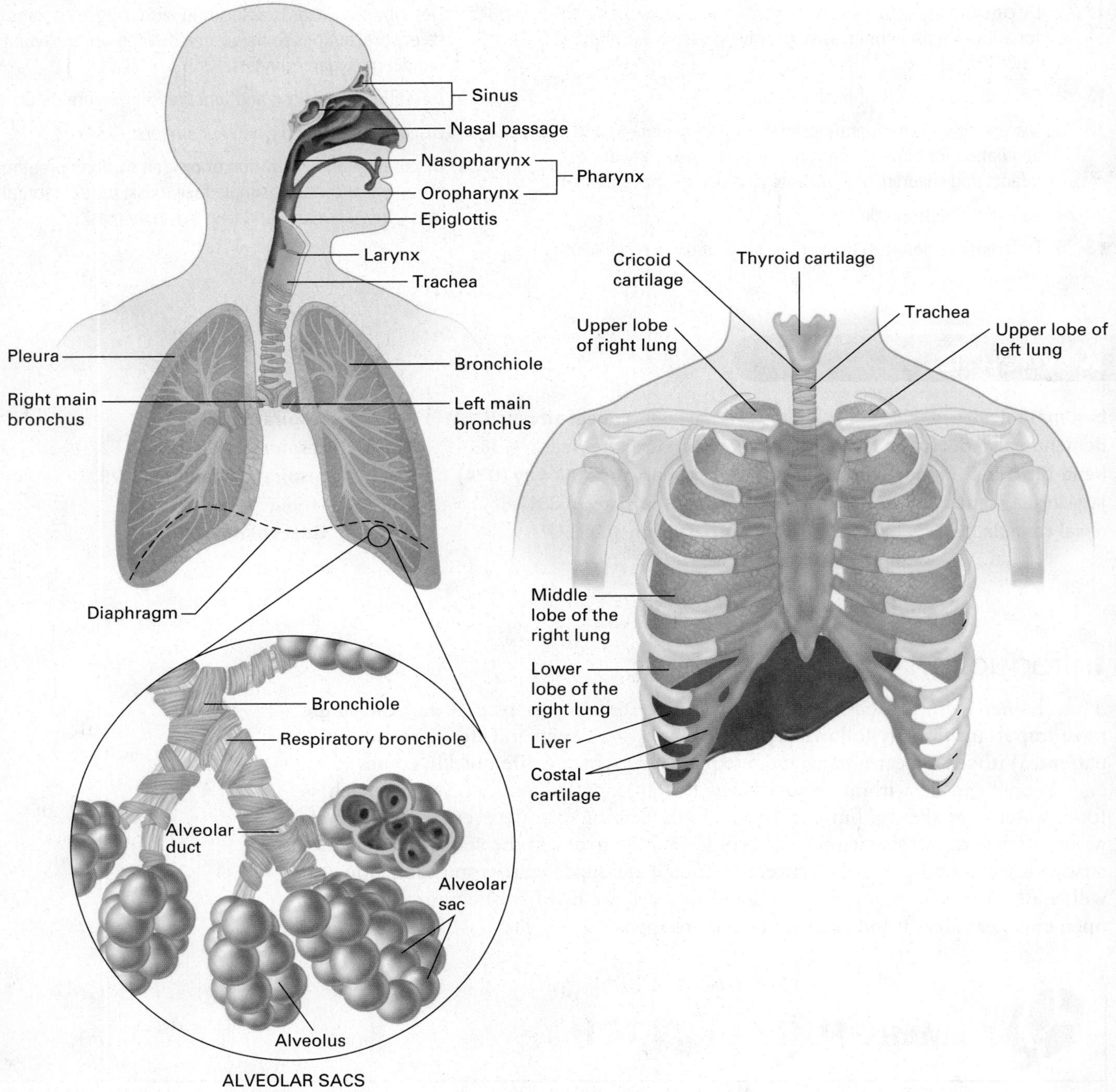

Figure 13-1 Major structures of the respiratory system.

Before going any further with this chapter, it would be helpful for you to review the anatomy and physiology of the respiratory system found in Chapter 5. You must be able to identify the following anatomical structures of the respiratory system (Figures 13-1 and 13-2 ■):

- Nose and mouth
- Pharynx, oropharynx, and nasopharynx
- Epiglottis
- Trachea
- Cricoid cartilage

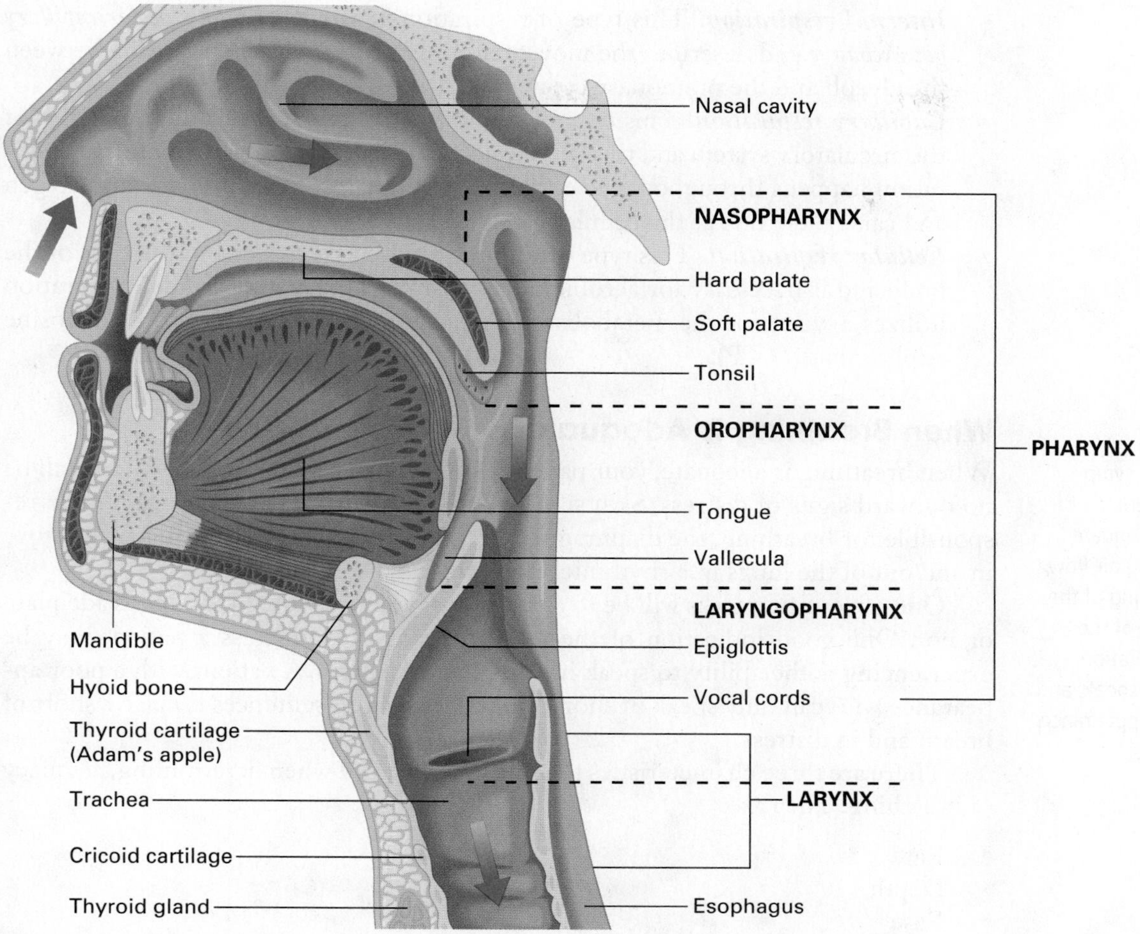

Figure 13-2 Anatomical structures of the upper airway.

- Larynx
- Bronchi and bronchioles
- Lungs
- Diaphragm

Review the physiology of the respiratory system as well, including the process of respiration and how oxygen and carbon dioxide are exchanged at the alveoli and cellular levels. Also review the differences in anatomy between the adult and pediatric patient.

Types of Respiration

It happens nearly 20 thousand times each day and approximately 58 billion times in an average lifetime. It is called *breathing* or **respiration.** When our respiratory system is functioning normally, we hardly notice it and often take it for granted until something goes wrong. Depending on the context, the term *respiration* can mean different things. There are four distinctly different types of respiration. They are:

- ***Pulmonary respiration.*** This is most commonly referred to as *breathing* or sometimes *ventilation*. Pulmonary respiration refers to the mechanical movement of air in and out of the lungs with each breath. The adequacy of pulmonary respiration is commonly quantified by multiplying respiratory rate times tidal volume (the amount of air moved in and out with each breath).

13-2 Distinguish among the terms respiration, ventilation, pulmonary respiration, internal respiration, capillary respiration, and cellular respiration.

respiration inhalation and exhalation. Also called *ventilation*.

- ***Internal respiration.*** This type of respiration is referred to as *alveolar/capillary gas exchange* and describes the movement of oxygen and carbon dioxide between the alveoli and the pulmonary capillaries.
- ***Capillary respiration.*** This type of respiration occurs between the capillaries of the circulatory system and the actual cells needing oxygen for fuel. Internal respiration happens throughout the entire body and involves the exchange of oxygen and carbon dioxide at the cellular level.
- ***Cellular respiration.*** This type of respiration occurs deep within the cells of the body and is necessary for aerobic metabolism to take place. Cellular respiration utilizes oxygen for the metabolism of glucose and the production of adenosine triphosphate (ATP).

When Breathing Is Adequate

13-3 Describe the signs, symptoms, and characteristics of adequate and inadequate breathing, including air flow, breath sounds, flaring of the nostrils, inspection of the chest, minute ventilation, patient's ability to speak, and patient's general appearance.

When breathing is adequate, your patient's appearance will be normal. There will be no outward signs of distress. Skin signs will be normal, and the primary muscle responsible for breathing, the diaphragm, is moving up and down, causing air to move in and out of the lungs in a rhythmic and regular pattern.

One of your first tasks will be to determine if your patient's breathing is adequate or not. One good indication of the level of respiratory distress a patient may be experiencing is the ability to speak in complete sentences. A patient with a poor appearance who can only speak in short two- to four-word sentences is clearly short of breath and in distress.

There are three characteristics that must be assessed when determining adequacy of breathing. They are:

- Rate
- Depth
- Ease

Rate refers to how many times the patient is breathing per minute and is recorded as a numeral. Respiratory rates can be obtained by counting the number of breaths in one minute. (Each inspiration plus expiration equals one respiration.) Average respiratory rates for all developmental age groups are listed in Table 13-1.

Depending on the standard practice in your area, there are at least two common methods for counting respirations. One requires counting the respirations for 30 seconds and multiplying by 2, and the second requires counting for 15 seconds and multiplying by 4. You must understand that the shorter your sample the less

TABLE 13-1 AVERAGE RESPIRATORY RATES

DEVELOPMENTAL AGE	AVERAGE RESPIRATORY RATE
Infant	30 to 60
Toddler	24 to 40
Preschooler	22 to 34
School-age child	18 to 30
Adolescent	12 to 24
Adult	12 to 20

accurate the total rate. For patients with an irregular breathing pattern, it may be best to count for a full minute to get the most accurate rate. Just like a pulse, the breathing rate should be regular and rhythmic. A breathing pattern that is irregular—fast and then slow and then fast again—is typically a sign of serious underlying medical or traumatic problem.

The depth of respirations is referred to as **tidal volume.** When you assess depth, you assess the amount of air the patient is moving in and out with each breath. When an adult patient is breathing adequately, the tidal volume is approximately 400 to 600 mL of air, which can be seen as moderate chest or abdominal rise and fall. Depth is commonly recorded as *deep*, *shallow*, or *normal*, depending on how the patient is breathing. In some areas the term *good tidal volume* is used to describe depth that is normal. A low or inadequate tidal volume may result in an inadequate supply of oxygen and the buildup of dangerous levels of carbon dioxide (CO_2).

tidal volume the depth of respirations.

The ease of breathing refers to the patient's work of breathing. Normal respirations require little to no effort on the part of the patient. Ease can be recorded as *unlabored* or *labored*, depending on the situation.

In addition to rate, depth, and ease, other characteristics that should be assessed with all patients are rhythm and sound. Normal respirations should be steady and regular, much like waves gently crashing on the beach. Irregular respirations are not normal and can be caused by both illness and injury.

Breath sounds should be assessed on all patients as well. Use a stethoscope to listen to both lungs in several places. Normal lung sounds are described as *equal* (same amount of sound) and *clear* (no abnormal sounds) *bilaterally* (on both sides). (More about assessing lung sounds will be discussed in Chapter 17.)

PRACTICAL PATHOPHYSIOLOGY

Minute volume is the total amount of air that is exchanged in and out of the lungs in a single minute. Changes in rate or tidal volume will have a direct effect on minute volume. If a patient's minute volume is not sufficient to meet the demands of the body, hypoxia will be the result.

When Breathing Is Inadequate

13-4 Describe the signs and symptoms of inadequate breathing.

Inadequate breathing is often the result of inadequate gas exchange (oxygen for carbon dioxide) and can result in the development of at least two problems for the patient: an inadequate supply of oxygen and an excessive buildup of carbon dioxide (CO_2). Regardless of the cause, some of the first responses the body makes to inadequate gas exchange are changes in breathing and a change in mental status. Signs of inadequate gas exchange can appear anywhere on a sliding scale from very mild to moderate to severe. In some instances, the buildup of carbon dioxide can occur even with an adequate supply of oxygen.

Signs of inadequate breathing are not always immediately obvious. They can be subtle, such as mild shortness of breath. In those instances, the only way you would know is by asking the patient, "Do you feel short of breath?" Sometimes, if the patient has been short of breath for a while, he may appear to be pale. It is good practice to ask any patient who appears pale if he is having any trouble breathing or if he feels short of breath.

Respiratory Distress

Often the first sign of the patient not receiving an adequate supply of oxygen is an increased respiratory rate. That is the body's way of saying, "If I can't get enough oxygen at the normal rate, I had better increase the rate to try to make up the difference." If the body is unable to compensate simply by increasing the rate, other mechanisms begin to kick in, making the respiratory distress more obvious (Table 13-2). The patient will appear to be working harder to breathe (increased work of breathing) and will be using the muscles of the chest, abdomen, and neck (accessory muscles) to breathe.

Respiratory distress is the body's way of attempting to compensate for an inadequate supply of oxygen (Figure 13-3 ■). In most cases the body does a good job of

respiratory distress the body's attempts to compensate for an inadequate supply of oxygen.

TABLE 13-2 SIGNS OF INADEQUATE GAS EXCHANGE
• Altered mental status (confusion, sleepiness, anxiety) • Increased respiratory rate (tachypnea, an early sign) • Dyspnea (shortness of breath) • Increased work of breathing (labored) • Decreased tidal volume (shallow) • Increased use of accessory muscles (neck, chest, and abdominal) • Nasal flaring (most common in pediatric patients) • Retractions above the clavicles, between the ribs, below the ribs (mostly seen in pediatric patients and very thin adults) • Pale skin that may be moist • Tachycardia (increased heart rate) • Bradycardia (slow heart rate, especially dangerous sign in infants and children) • Slow respirations (a late sign as the patient fatigues)

compensating and, with the assistance of the EMT, some oxygen, and appropriate medications, the patient's respiratory status could return to normal. One of the ways a patient will attempt to compensate when experiencing breathing difficulty is to assume the tripod position (Figure 13-4 ■). This position allows for full expansion of the chest and movement of the diaphragm.

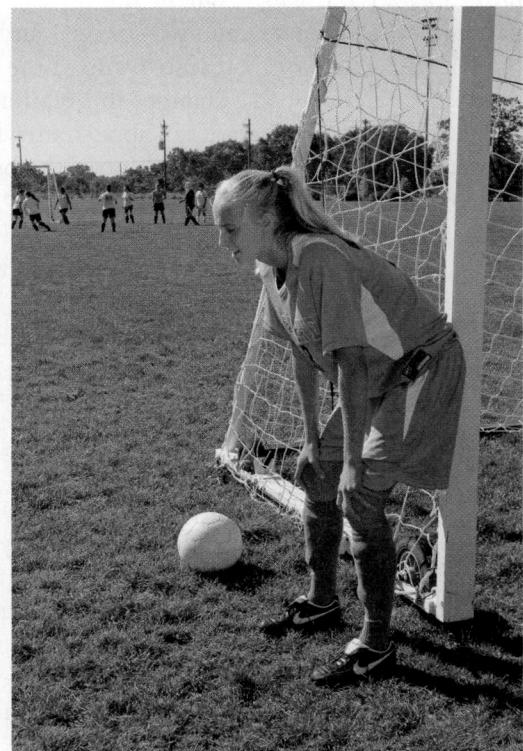

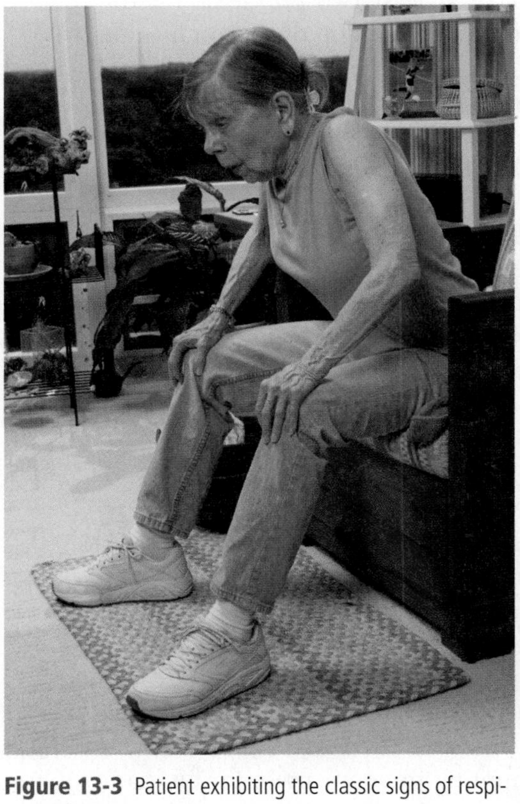

Figure 13-3 Patient exhibiting the classic signs of respiratory distress.

Figure 13-4 A patient using the tripod position to compensate for difficulty breathing.

Respiratory Failure

When the body's normal compensatory mechanisms are not able to provide for adequate gas exchange, the patient is in danger of progressing from respiratory distress to **respiratory failure** (Figure 13-5 ■). Respiratory failure occurs when the body can no longer compensate. Some of the first signs of respiratory failure are a marked decrease in mental status and critical changes in respiratory effort including irregular breathing and a decreased respiratory rate (Table 13-3).

Respiratory failure is an extreme emergency that will result in the patient's death unless the EMT immediately begins providing assisted ventilations (Figure 13-6 ■). (Assisted ventilation will be discussed in more detail later in this chapter.)

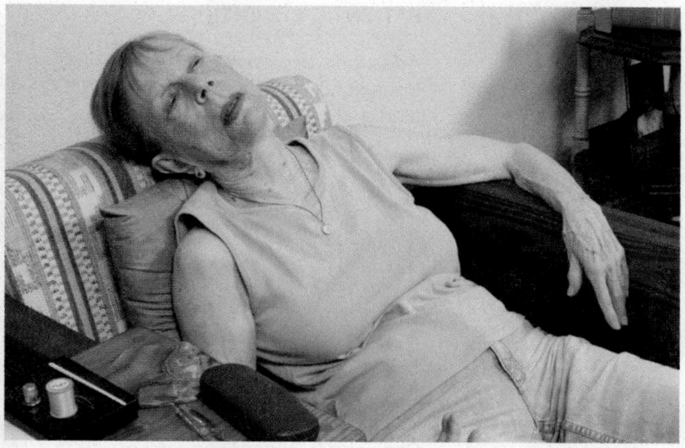

Figure 13-5 A patient in respiratory failure will have an altered mental status and slow gasping breathing.

respiratory failure the reduction of breathing to the point where oxygen intake is not sufficient to support life.

Pediatric Differences

The differences in anatomy between adult and pediatric patients are discussed in Chapter 5. Some of those differences can change the way that you care for the patient. In general, all of the structures of the pediatric respiratory system are smaller and therefore more easily blocked by swelling or foreign material. The tongue takes up proportionately more volume inside the mouth, making it more difficult for the EMT to visualize the back of the throat. The larynx and trachea are much softer and more susceptible to damage. Being soft, the trachea is also susceptible to collapse if the patient's head is tilted too far back during airway management. While this is not damaging to the child, it will cause a partial airway blockage that makes it more difficult to ventilate the patient. Pediatric patients, especially infants, are abdominal breathers, which means that the abdomen moves more than the chest as they breathe (Figure 13-7 ■).

13-5 Describe differences between adults and children in the anatomy and physiology of the respiratory system.

An early sign of hypoxia in infants is an abnormally slow heart rate (bradycardia). Because infants have a heart rate and breathing rate much faster than adults and children, it is easy to be fooled into thinking a heart rate of 80 is normal when caring for an infant. You must become familiar with the normal limits of vital signs for all ages in order to properly care for your patients. Infants and children with significant bradycardia due to respiratory failure will quickly progress to cardiac arrest unless

13-6 Explain differences between adults and children in the signs of hypoxia.

TABLE 13-3 SIGNS OF RESPIRATORY FAILURE

- Decreased mental status
- Decreased respiratory rate (below normal)
- Change in breathing rhythm (irregular)
- Rapid, ineffective breathing (poor minute ventilation)
- Breath sounds that become diminished (less obvious)
- Decreased chest rise and fall (poor tidal volume)
- Skin that may be pale or cyanotic (blue) and cool and clammy
- In infants, possible "seesaw" breathing where the abdomen and chest move in opposite directions
- Slow heart rate (a critical finding in infants and children)
- Agonal respirations (occasional gasping breaths) that may be seen just before death

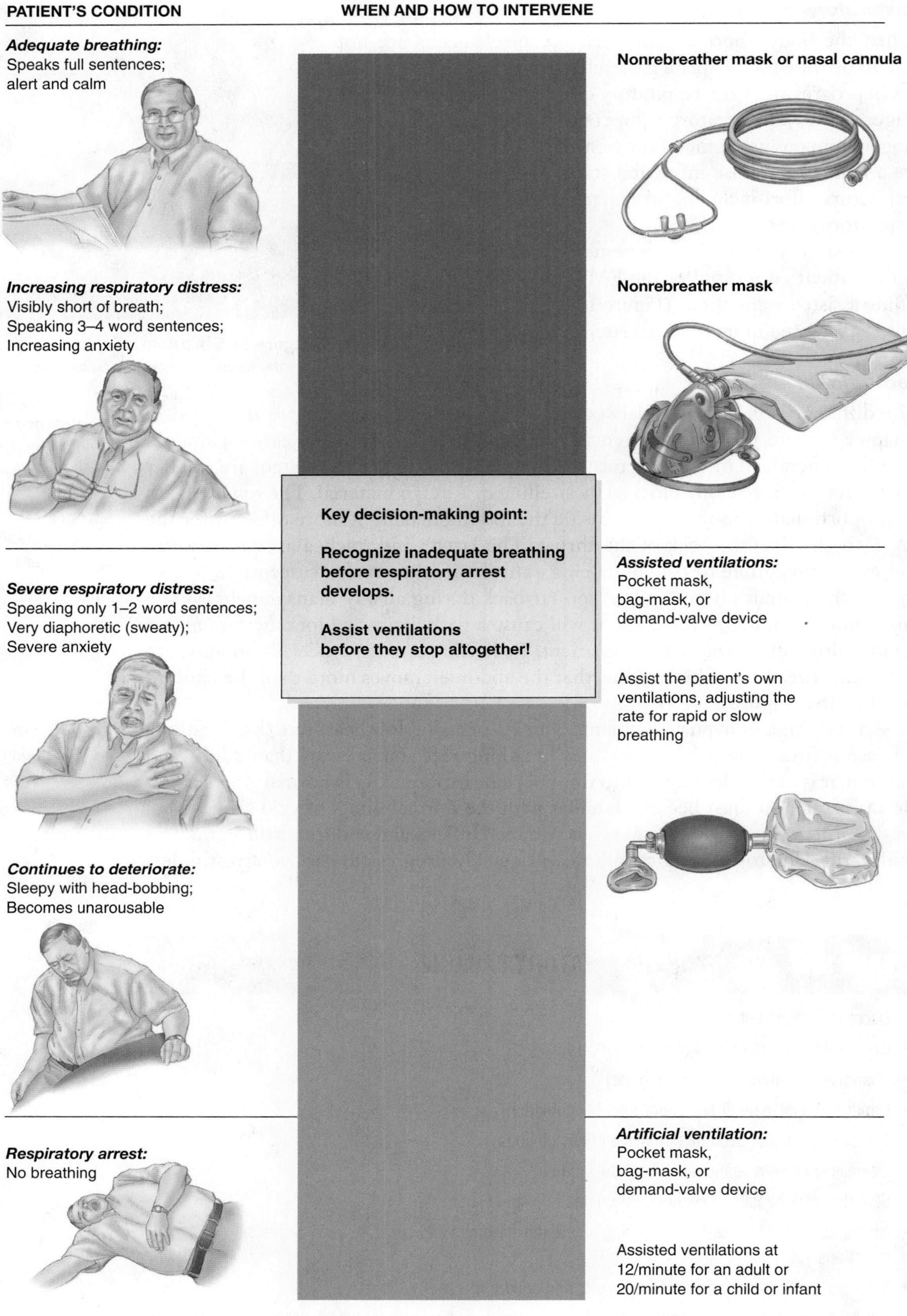
PATIENT'S CONDITION
WHEN AND HOW TO INTERVENE
Adequate breathing:
Speaks full sentences; alert and calm
Nonrebreather mask or nasal cannula
Increasing respiratory distress:
Visibly short of breath;
Speaking 3–4 word sentences;
Increasing anxiety
Nonrebreather mask
Key decision-making point:
Recognize inadequate breathing before respiratory arrest develops.
Assist ventilations before they stop altogether!
Severe respiratory distress:
Speaking only 1–2 word sentences;
Very diaphoretic (sweaty);
Severe anxiety
Assisted ventilations:
Pocket mask, bag-mask, or demand-valve device
Assist the patient's own ventilations, adjusting the rate for rapid or slow breathing
Continues to deteriorate:
Sleepy with head-bobbing;
Becomes unarousable
Respiratory arrest:
No breathing
Artificial ventilation:
Pocket mask, bag-mask, or demand-valve device
Assisted ventilations at 12/minute for an adult or 20/minute for a child or infant

Figure 13-6 Progression and management of a patient with breathing difficulty.

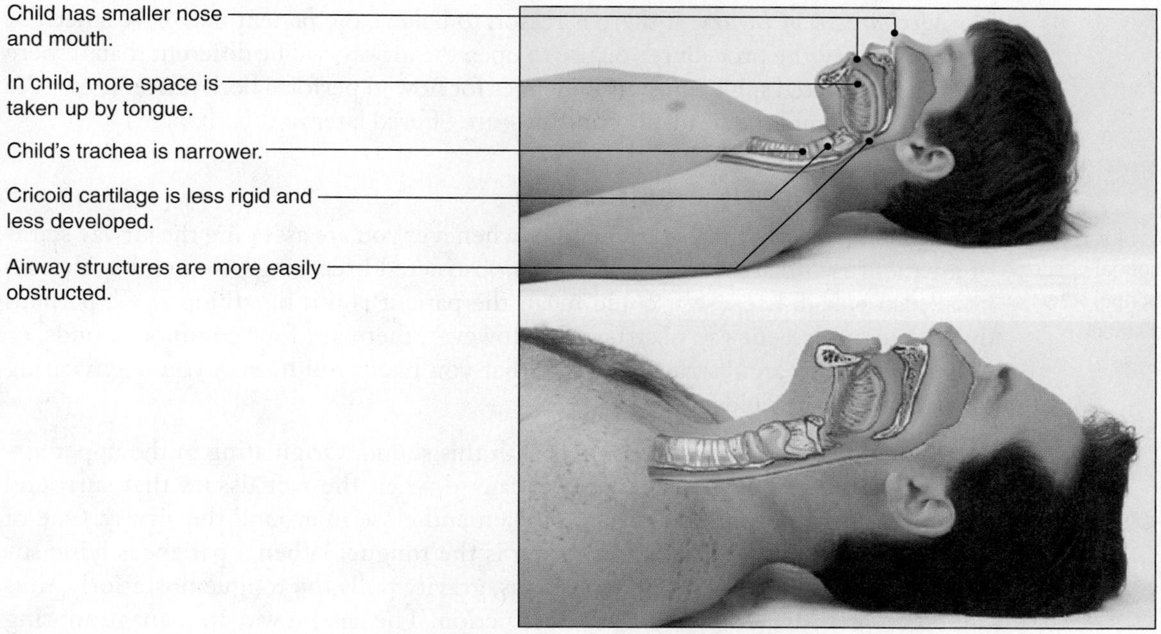
Child has smaller nose and mouth.
In child, more space is taken up by tongue.
Child's trachea is narrower.
Cricoid cartilage is less rigid and less developed.
Airway structures are more easily obstructed.

Figure 13-7 Differences between an adult and pediatric airway.

their hypoxia is immediately reversed by assisting ventilations with an appropriate size bag-mask device connected to high-flow oxygen.

Managing the Airway

Determining whether or not a patient has a **patent airway** (open and clear airway) is an essential skill that all successful EMTs must master. Because the way you manage an airway involves potential motion of the neck, you must determine whether a spine injury is suspected. Your management of that situation is critical and will be among your highest priorities for each patient.

patent airway open and clear, without interference to the passage of air into and out of the body.

Assessing and Opening the Airway

In responsive patients, assessing the airway is achieved quite easily by observing and listening to them speak. If a patient is alert and able to speak, it may be assumed that he has an open and clear airway. What you must assess next is the adequacy of breathing.

13-7 Describe the relationship between airway status and mental status.

In the unresponsive patient, determining whether the airway is patent is much more difficult. Factors that must be considered while managing the airway of an unresponsive patient are presence of a pulse, patient position, and mechanism of injury. Each requires specific procedures to be performed by the EMT, depending on the condition and position of the patient. Those procedures are as follows:

- ***Presence of a pulse.*** In an unresponsive patient who is not breathing or has only gasping breaths, immediately check for a pulse. If a pulse is present (and this will be most of the time), then open the airway. If no pulse is found, immediately begin a cycle of chest compressions and then open the airway and ventilate the patient.
- ***Patient position.*** If the patient is found face down or on his side and appears to be breathing adequately, there may not be an immediate need to move him. If you cannot determine if he is breathing adequately, then you must roll him carefully onto his back to begin managing the airway.

- ***Mechanism of injury.*** If there is reason to believe the patient may have a neck or back injury, the procedure you use to open the airway will be different than if there is no suspected spine injury. (Guidelines for how to perform both procedures—the jaw-thrust and the head-tilt/chin-lift—are offered later in this chapter.)

Sounds of Airway Obstruction

13-8 Explain the causes of each of the following abnormal upper airway sounds: snoring, crowing, gurgling, and stridor.

An excellent rule of thumb to remember whenever you are assessing the airway status of a patient is "noisy breathing is always obstructed breathing." Remember that no noise also is bad, because it could mean the patient is not breathing at all, perhaps due to a complete airway obstruction. However, there are four common sounds, or noises, related to an obstructed airway that you likely will hear as you begin caring for patients in the field. They are:

- ***Snoring.*** You already are familiar with this sound. Originating in the upper airway at the posterior pharynx, it is caused when the soft tissues that surround the pharynx become relaxed or swollen and close in around the airway. One of the most common causes of snoring is the tongue. When a patient is lying supine and either asleep or unconscious, gravity pulls the tongue posteriorly, thus creating a partial upper airway obstruction. The easiest way to manage snoring respirations is to reposition the head or jaw by using either the jaw-thrust or head-tilt/chin-lift maneuver.
- ***Gurgling.*** This sound is very much like the sound one makes when gargling with mouthwash. Gurgling, however, is not intentional. Instead, it represents an immediate threat to life, because it occurs when the airway becomes obstructed by fluid such as blood, vomit, saliva, or other secretions. The presence of gurgling must be managed by suctioning the airway or repositioning the patient to allow for the fluid to drain from the airway.
- ***Stridor.*** This is a high-pitched sound caused by swelling of the tissues or structures of the upper airway. It also can be caused by a foreign body obstruction. Stridor is most often heard during inspiration but also can be heard on expiration in severe cases. It can be a sign of significant airway compromise and should be considered a true emergency. Do not put anything in the patient's mouth because it may cause sudden life-threatening swelling.
- ***Crowing.*** This sound sometimes can resemble a mild barking. It is caused by the spasm of the muscles that surround the larynx and the opening to the trachea. Crowing occurs on inspiration. Both crowing and stridor are sounds that indicate a potential for life-threatening obstruction, so immediate transport is needed.
- ***Wheezing.*** This is a high-pitched sound caused by a narrowing of the bronchioles of the lower airway. Wheezing is most often heard during auscultation of the lungs with a stethoscope but in severe cases can be heard without a stethoscope (called *audible wheezes*).

CLINICAL CLUE

Noisy Breathing

Something to remember that will help you identify and manage airway problems early is that all noisy breathing is obstructed breathing. Sometimes the noise is in the upper airway in the form of snoring, gurgling, or stridor, and sometimes it is in the lower airway in the form of wheezing. Regardless, if it is making noise, there is some form of partial obstruction and the patient will need an intervention of some kind.

Any obstruction of the airway has the potential to affect the patient's ability to breathe adequately. Obstructions also can affect your ability to provide assisted ventilations to a patient who is breathing inadequately. An obstructed airway, even if only obstructed partially, will limit the volume of air the patient needs to maintain adequate oxygenation. If the cause of the obstruction is not identified and cared for quickly, your patient will rapidly develop respiratory failure followed by respiratory arrest.

13-9 Describe how partial or complete obstruction of the airway leads to hypoxia.

No Suspected Spine Injury

In most instances of an unresponsive patient with no suspected spine injury, the **head-tilt/chin-lift maneuver** is the most effective means of opening the airway. The tongue is the most common cause of airway obstruction in the unresponsive patient. Because the tongue is attached to the lower jaw, tilting the head back and moving the jaw upward also lifts the tongue, clearing the back of the throat.

13-10 Describe the proper method of opening the airway for a patient with suspected and no suspected spine injury.

head-tilt/chin-lift maneuver a means of opening the airway by tilting the head back and lifting the chin. It is used when no trauma, or injury, is suspected.

To perform the head-tilt/chin-lift (Figure 13-8 ■), follow these steps:

1. With the patient lying supine on a firm flat surface, kneel beside the patient's head.
2. Place the palm of one hand on the patient's forehead and the index and middle fingers of the other hand on the bony part of the jaw just below the chin.
3. Using equal pressure with both hands, tilt the patient's head back until it is fully extended. Less head tilt is required for the pediatric patient.

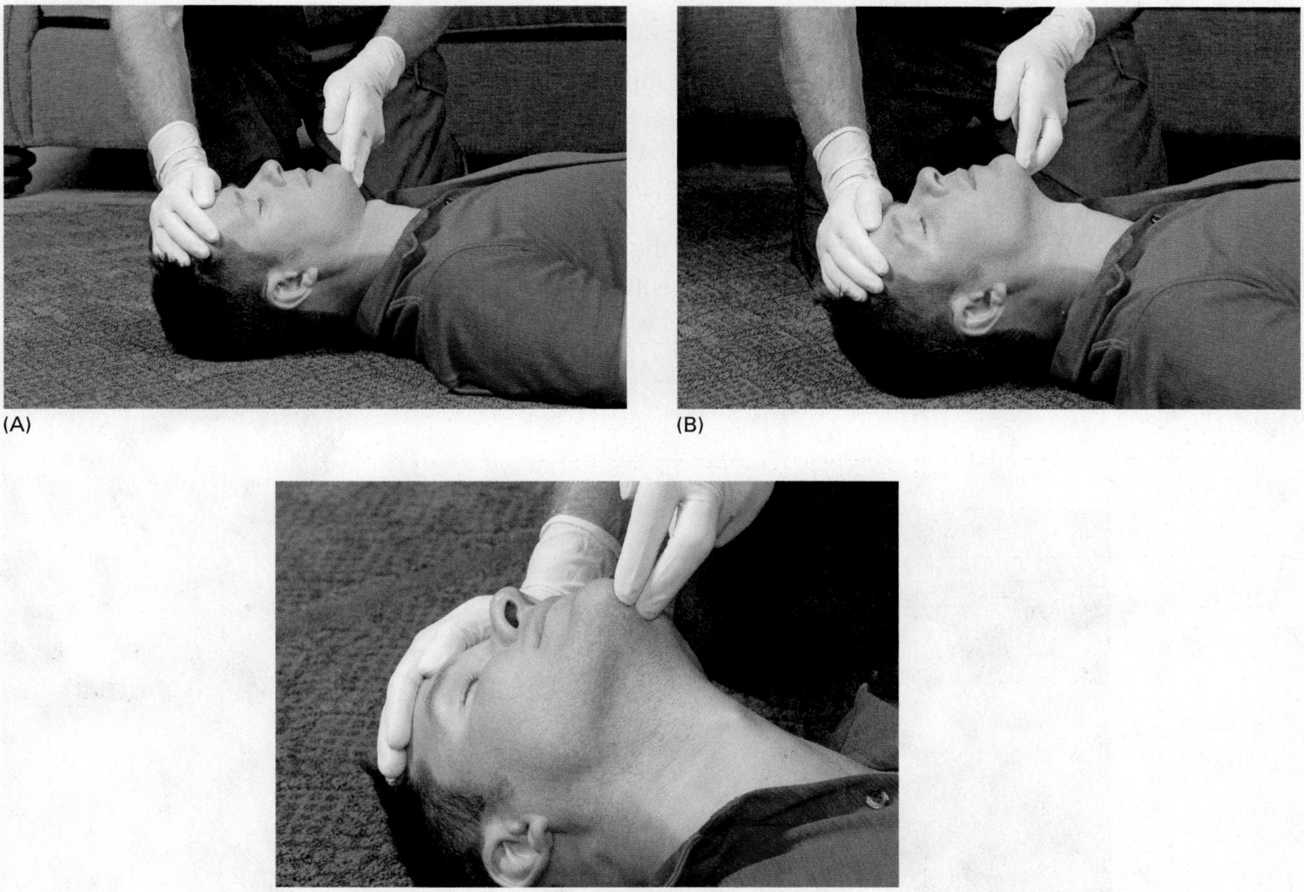

(A) (B) (C)

Figure 13-8 (A) Place the palm of one hand on the patient's forehead and the index and middle fingers of the other hand on the bony part of the jaw. (B) Using equal pressure with both hands, tilt the head back as far as it will comfortably go. (C) Note the fingers on the bony edge of the jaw and NOT on the soft tissue of the neck.

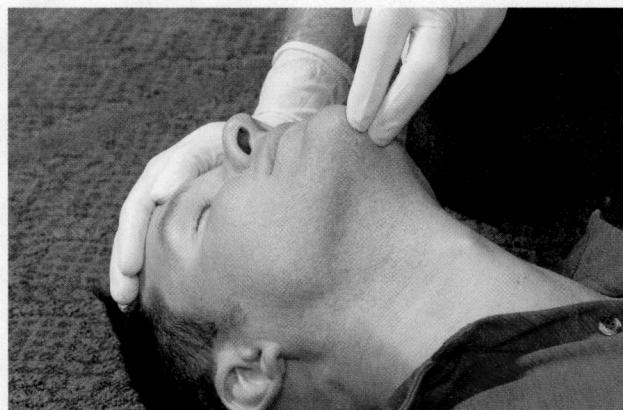

4. Once the head is tilted back, release pressure on the chin to allow the mouth to open slightly.
5. Place your ear next to the patient's nose and mouth to listen for breathing and observe the chest for adequate rise and fall.

Suspected Spine Injury

For any patient with an unknown mechanism of injury, or any patient who you believe may have suffered a spine injury, you must make every attempt to open the airway without compromising the neck or back. To accomplish that goal, you should use the **jaw-thrust maneuver** (Figure 13-9 ■).

jaw-thrust maneuver a means of correcting blockage of the airway by moving the jaw forward without tilting the head or neck. Used when trauma, or injury, is suspected.

PERSPECTIVE

Rob—The EMT

I knew when I heard what happened that this young lady's boyfriend had tried to dislodge the object before she passed out and that she probably wasn't going to have a head or spine injury. It's not like he's just going to drop his girlfriend to the ground when she becomes unresponsive. So, I felt the most effective technique for initially trying to open and look into her airway was the head-tilt/chin-lift. Plus, I knew that we had to get that airway open quickly.

To perform the jaw-thrust maneuver, follow these steps:

1. With the patient lying supine on a firm flat surface, kneel at the top of the patient's head.
2. Place your thumbs on the cheekbones on either side of the patient's face.
3. Using the index and middle fingers of each hand at the angles of the patient's jaw, push the jaw upward.
4. Place your ear next to the patient's nose and mouth to listen for breathing and observe the chest for adequate rise and fall.

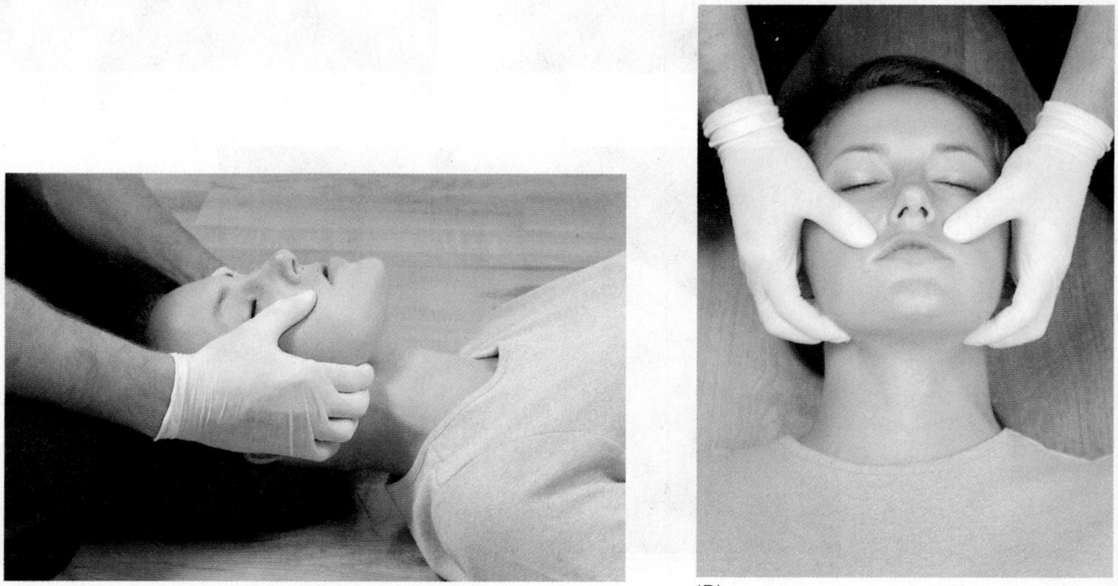

(A) (B)

Figure 13-9 (A) Side view of the proper positioning of the hands for a jaw-thrust maneuver. (B) Top view of the proper positioning of the hands for a jaw-thrust maneuver.

This procedure is best when at least two rescuers are present. If the patient is not breathing adequately, the first rescuer can maintain an open airway, while the second rescuer ventilates the patient. For the single rescuer, a modified jaw-thrust can be performed, so he also can ventilate the patient using the mouth-to-mask technique.

Complications

Several factors can make it difficult to establish a patent airway. Trauma to the face often causes swelling and bleeding that will make it difficult to keep the airway clear. Foreign body airway obstructions (FBAO), such as those caused by food or small objects, are difficult to see and can cause both partial and complete obstructions.

Dental appliances such as crowns, bridges, and dentures can come loose inside the mouth, contributing to the obstruction. Unless they are loose and falling back into the throat, leave them in place. The presence of teeth, real or otherwise, helps with creating a good seal during ventilations. Otherwise remove them with a gloved hand and keep them in a safe place.

PERSPECTIVE

The Boyfriend

That was the scariest thing I've ever been through. One minute we're having this great picnic by the lake, and the next, Shannon is looking at me with this panic in her eyes and she's grabbing at her throat. Do you know what that's like? I mean, here's this person you love more than anything in the world and you're looking into her eyes and all you see is fear, just absolute terror. I can't even imagine what it's like not to be able to breathe. I'm so thankful for that ambulance crew. I don't know what I would've done had they not been there.

STOP, REVIEW, REMEMBER!

Multiple Choice

For each question, place a check next to the correct answer.

1. All of the following are signs of inadequate breathing *except*:
   _____ a. use of accessory muscles.
   _____ b. increased respiratory rate.
   _____ c. use of the tripod position.
   _____ d. good chest rise and fall.

2. Adequate respirations are characterized by:
   _____ a. effortless breathing.
   _____ b. poor chest rise.
   _____ c. nasal flaring.
   _____ d. retractions.

3. You are caring for an unresponsive adult patient. Her respiratory rate is 6, and gurgling can be heard with each breath. You should:
   _____ a. sweep the mouth with your fingers.
   _____ b. roll the patient onto her side.
   _____ c. perform abdominal thrusts.
   _____ d. provide high-flow oxygen.

(continued on next page)

(continued)

4. For which one of the following patients would the jaw-thrust maneuver be most appropriate for opening the airway?
   _____ a. Unresponsive five-year-old in a bicycle collision
   _____ b. Male 56-year-old with chest pain
   _____ c. Unresponsive 27-year-old bee-sting patient
   _____ d. Diabetic patient responsive only to voice

5. What is the most common cause of airway obstruction in the unresponsive patient?
   _____ a. Blood
   _____ b. Foreign body
   _____ c. Tongue
   _____ d. Saliva

Critical Thinking

1. Describe what you would look for to determine if a patient is breathing adequately.

____

____

____

____

2. Discuss the difference between respiratory distress and respiratory failure and how each might be recognized in a patient.

____

____

____

____

3. Describe how you would manage the airway of a trauma patient with a compromised airway.

____

____

____

____

Complete the Table

Identify each sign as one of respiratory distress or one of respiratory failure by placing an "X" in the appropriate column.

Sign	Distress	Failure
Increased respiratory rate		
Decreased respiratory rate		
Altered mental status		
Use of accessory muscles		
Nasal flaring		
Cyanosis		
Agonal respirations		

The Basics of Suctioning

13-11 Describe the proper technique for using both a manual and battery-powered suction device.

It is important to wear the appropriate personal protective equipment (PPE) whenever you are managing a patient's airway because of the strong likelihood that he will vomit or that you are exposed to body fluids. Gloves, a mask, and eye protection are the minimum recommended PPE for airway management.

Suctioning is an important skill that every EMT must learn and practice. The EMT uses suction to assist in maintaining a patent airway that is at risk of becoming blocked by materials such as blood, vomit, and saliva. Noisy respirations are almost always a sign of partial airway obstruction. Gurgling is a strong indication of partial upper airway obstruction caused by fluids. During artificial ventilation, some of the air enters the stomach and may eventually cause the patient to vomit. Use suction to minimize the chances that the vomit could enter the lungs. You must have suction ready at all times when caring for unresponsive patients or when manually ventilating a patient.

Most suction units used in the field are adequate for suctioning fluids and small particles of food but are inadequate at picking up or clearing large objects such as chunks of food or teeth. For those objects, a combination of suctioning and finger sweeps may be necessary.

Suction Devices

13-12 Compare the function of fixed and portable suction devices.

Suction devices are quite simple. They consist of a pump, suction tubing, a catheter, and a reservoir to contain the material being suctioned. Though there are many brands and styles of suction devices in use today, most field suction units fall into three categories: electric, oxygen-powered, and manually operated (Figure 13-10 ■):

- ***Electric.*** An electric suction device may be found permanently mounted in the ambulance for use during transport or it can be a portable battery-powered type used on scene.
- ***Oxygen-powered.*** An oxygen-powered suction device typically is portable and functions as an accessory to an oxygen regulator. It requires an adequate supply of high-pressure oxygen to function.
- ***Manually operated.*** A manually operated suction device is generally the most portable and easy-to-use. Most are operated by squeezing a handle located on the device.

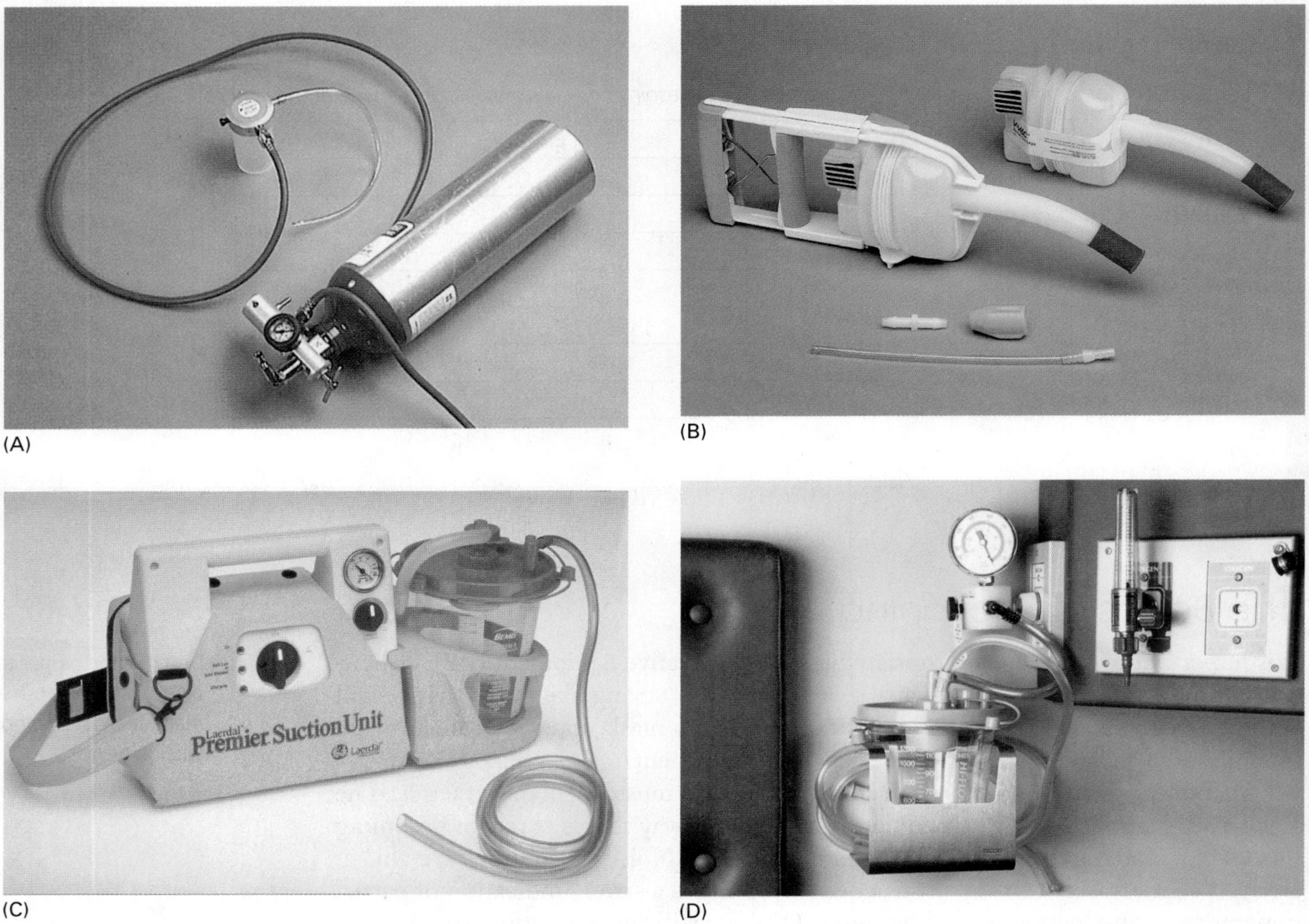

Figure 13-10 (A) Oxygen-powered portable suction unit. (B) Portable manual suction unit (V-VAC® device). (C) Battery-powered portable suction unit. (D) Wall-mounted suction unit in the ambulance.

13-13 Compare the use of rigid and soft suction catheters.

The suction catheter is the part of the suction unit that is placed into the patient's mouth or nose to assist in removing the material from the airway. Catheters come in a wide variety of styles; however, they all fit into one of two basic categories—rigid (hard) or soft (Figure 13-11 ■).

Sometimes called *rigid, hard,* or *tonsil-tip suction catheters*, these catheters are made of nonflexible plastic and can be straight or slightly curved. They are designed primarily for suctioning the mouth (oropharynx) of a semiresponsive or unresponsive patient. In general, catheters used for suctioning the mouth should not be inserted any farther than you can see. Avoid touching the center of the back of the throat, too, because touching can stimulate a gag reflex and cause vomiting.

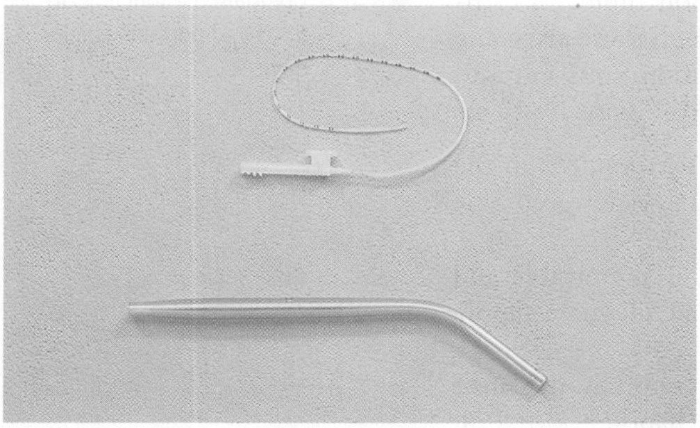

Figure 13-11 Soft (top) and rigid (bottom) suction catheters.

Soft catheters are generally long, narrow tubes made of flexible plastic. They are most useful for suctioning through the nose (nasopharynx) of a semiresponsive or unresponsive patient. A soft catheter used to suction the nose must be measured to ensure it is not placed too far into the airway. Measure it from the tip of the patient's nose to the earlobe prior to insertion. The suction device should be activated only after the catheter is fully inserted into the airway. Soft catheters are also ideal for suctioning the mouths of pediatric patients.

Suctioning Techniques

Like all other equipment on an ambulance, the suction unit should be inspected on a daily basis. Because many units are battery operated, they must regularly be charged or the battery replaced. A properly functioning suction unit is capable of developing approximately 300 mmHg of vacuum power. Use the following guidelines when using suction to help clear a patient's airway.

13-14 Explain special considerations to be kept in mind when suctioning patients, including signs of hypoxia and patients with copious amounts of vomit that cannot be quickly suctioned.

Oral Suctioning

Follow these steps to perform oral suctioning (Scan 13-1):

1. Take appropriate BSI precautions.
2. Attach the appropriate suction catheter to the suction tubing, and then attach the tubing to the device. Turn on the device to confirm you have suction.
3. Place the tip of the catheter into the patient's mouth as far to one side as possible and only as far as you can see.
4. Activate the suction as you move the tip of the catheter around in small circles on one side of the tongue.
5. Remove the tip and insert it in the same manner on the other side of the patient's mouth. Repeat the procedure.
6. For adult patients suction no more than 15 seconds at a time, child patients 10 seconds, and infants 5 seconds.

Nasal Suctioning

Follow these steps to perform nasal suctioning (Scan 13-2):

1. Take appropriate BSI precautions.
2. Attach the appropriate suction catheter to the suction tubing and the tubing to the device. Turn on the device to confirm you have suction.
3. Measure the device from the tip of the patient's nose to the tip of the earlobe.
4. Lubricate the catheter using a water-based lubricant.
5. Carefully insert the catheter into one nostril.
6. Once completely inserted, activate the suction and twist the catheter and slowly remove it.
7. Repeat the procedure for the other nostril.
8. For adult patients suction no more than 15 seconds at a time, child patients 10 seconds, and infants 5 seconds.

Many suction devices have an adjustment that controls the amount of suction being applied. Consider using lower power settings for pediatric patients. When suctioning newborns and infants, it is best to use a bulb-type suction device.

If your patient is producing secretions as fast as you can suction them, suction as best you can for 15 seconds. Then ventilate the patient for two minutes, followed by another 15 seconds of suctioning. Repeat this process as necessary during transport.

Suction catheters, tubing, and most reservoirs are disposable and should be handed off to the hospital personnel taking over care of the patient. Otherwise, they should be disposed of properly.

13-15 Describe the indications, contraindications, limitations, and procedures for the use of oropharyngeal and nasopharyngeal airways.

The Use of Airway Adjuncts

EMTs have two devices (airway adjuncts) they can use to assist in maintaining a patent airway. They are the **oropharyngeal airway (OPA),** sometimes referred to as the *oral airway*, and the **nasopharyngeal airway (NPA),** commonly referred to as the *nasal airway*. It must be clearly understood that both of these devices only *assist* the EMT in maintaining a patent airway. Simply placing either device does

oropharyngeal airway (OPA) a curved device inserted into the patient's mouth and the pharynx to help maintain an open airway.

nasopharyngeal airway (NPA) a soft flexible breathing tube inserted through the patient's nose into the pharynx to help maintain an open airway.

SCAN 13-1 Oral Suctioning Technique

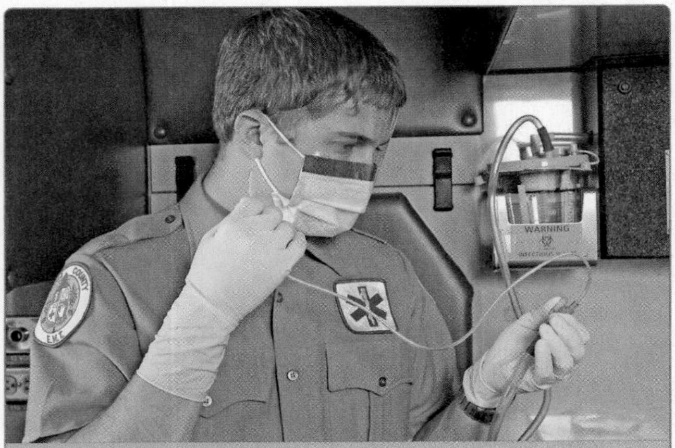

13-1-1 Properly assemble and test the suction unit.

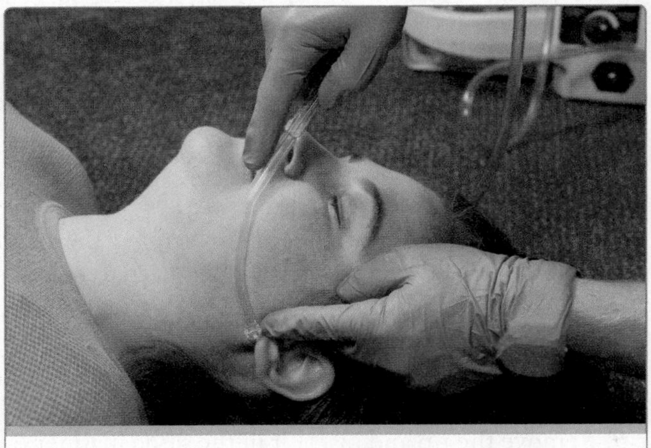

13-1-2 Measure the catheter prior to insertion when appropriate.

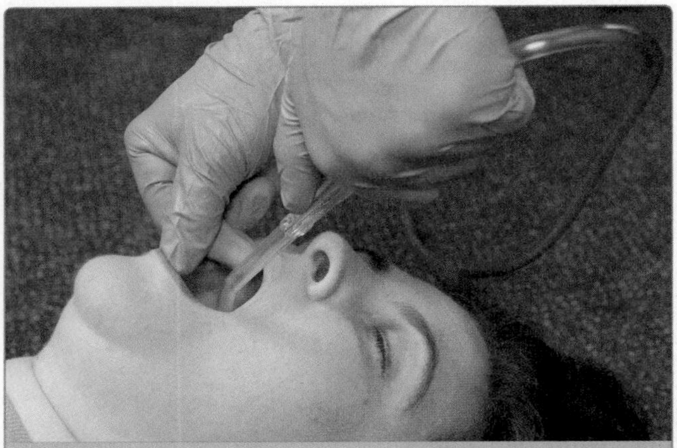

13-1-3 Insert the catheter to one side of the mouth and activate the suction unit.

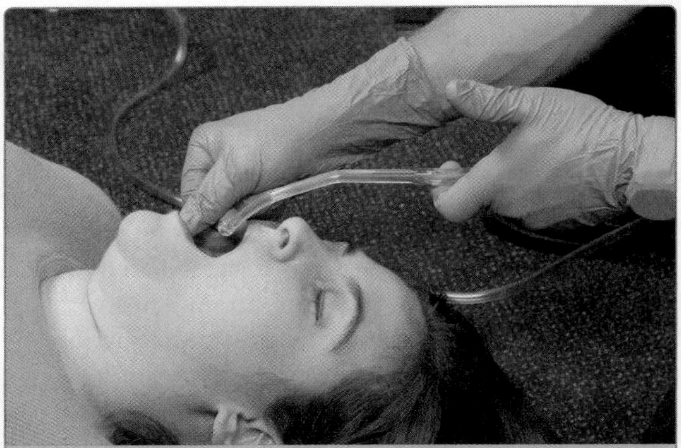

13-1-4 Pull catheter out and repeat on opposite side.

not ensure a patent airway. They should be used in conjunction with good airway management techniques, such as continuous monitoring for adequate chest rise and fall, head-tilt/chin-lift and jaw-thrust maneuvers, and appropriate suctioning when indicated.

Oropharyngeal Airways

Usually, the oropharyngeal airway (OPA) is made of hard plastic and designed to minimize the chances that the patient's airway will become blocked by the tongue (Figure 13-12 ■). Indications for the use of an OPA are unresponsiveness and a missing gag reflex. Sometimes the only way to determine if an unresponsive patient does not have a gag reflex is to attempt the insertion of an OPA. If the patient begins to gag, you must remove it immediately.

SCAN 13-2 Nasal Suctioning Technique

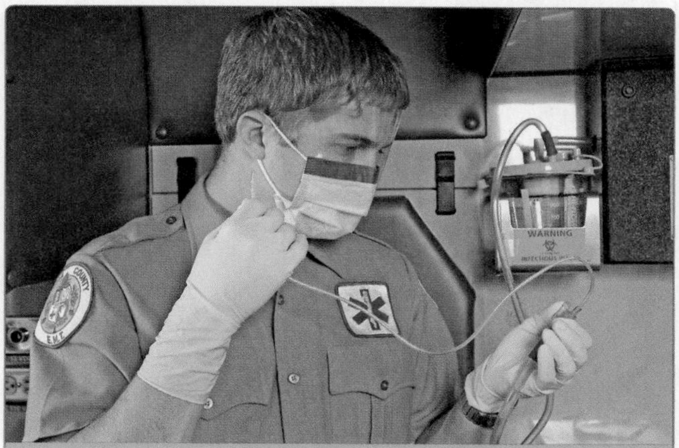

13-2-1 Properly assemble and test the suction unit.

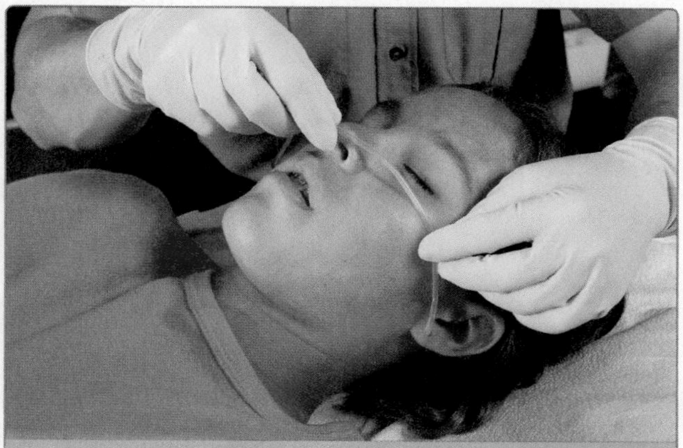

13-2-2 Measure the catheter prior to insertion.

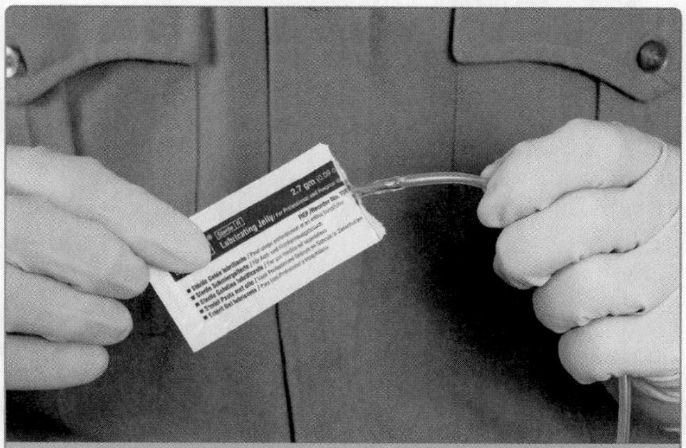

13-2-3 Lubricate the end of the catheter.

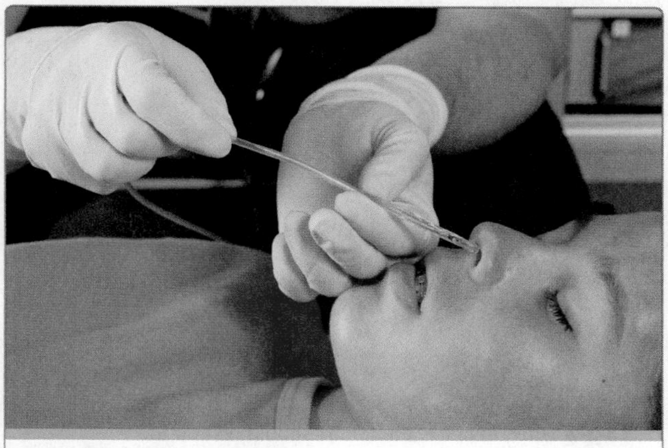

13-2-4 Insert the catheter into the nose.

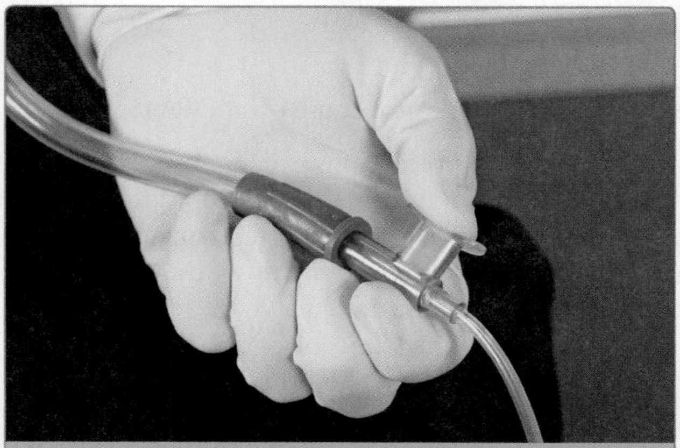

13-2-5 Activate the suction by covering the hole on the catheter (if applicable).

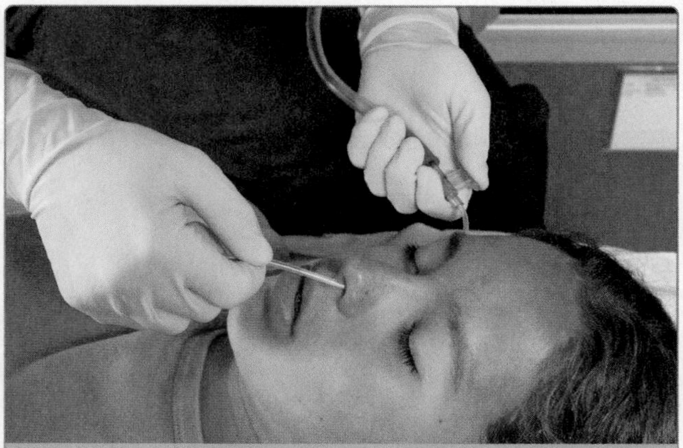

13-2-6 Slowly pull catheter out while twisting and repeat on opposite side.

SCAN 13-3 Insertion of an Oropharyngeal Airway

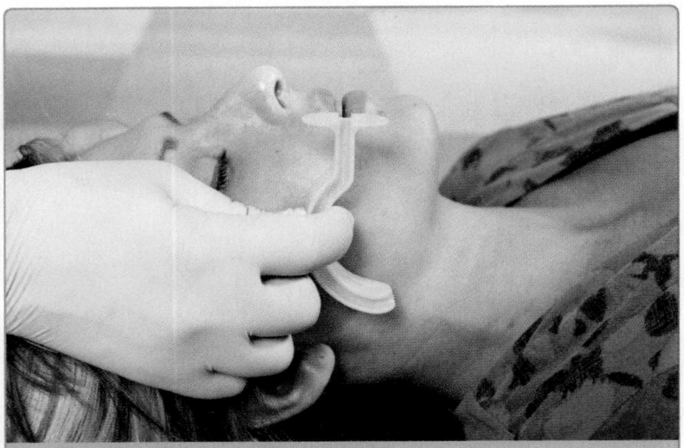

13-3-1 Properly measure the airway prior to insertion.

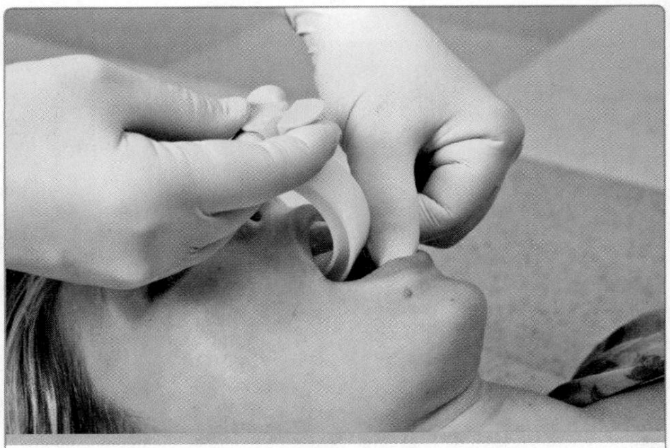

13-3-2 Open the mouth and insert the airway.

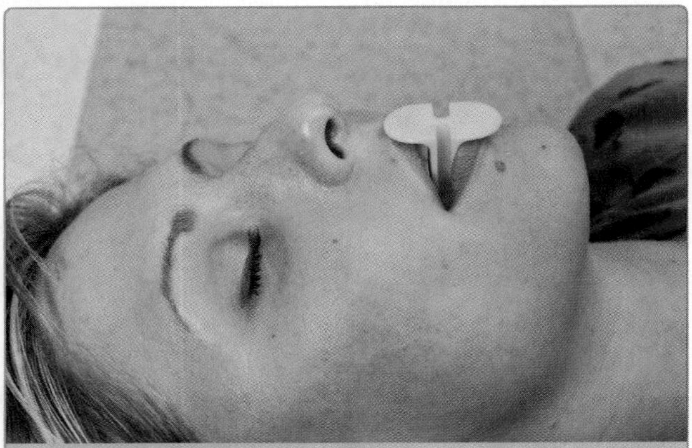

13-3-3 When in place, the flange should rest on the lips and no further than the teeth.

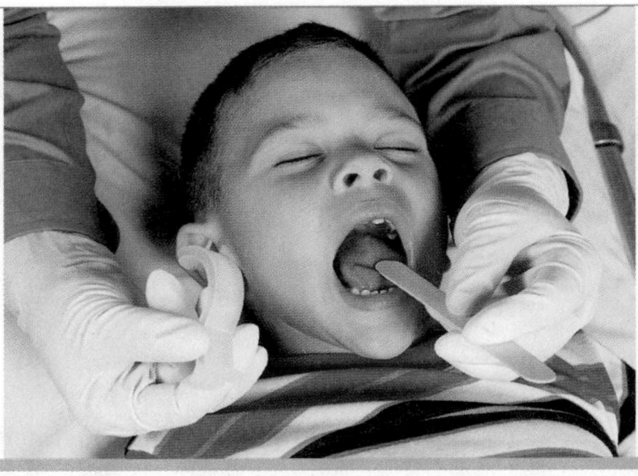

13-3-4 For pediatric patients use a tongue blade to assist with insertion.

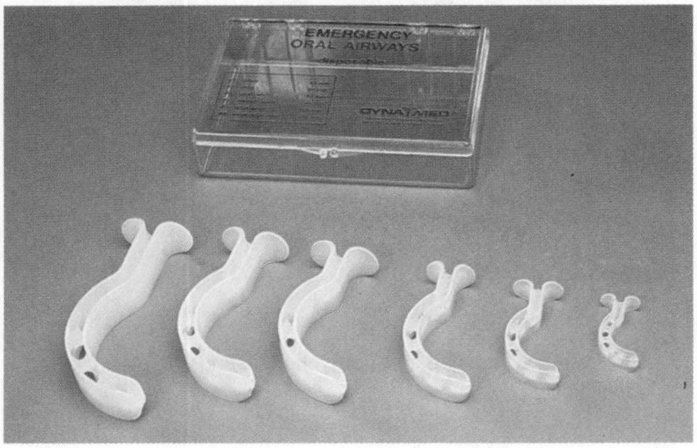

Figure 13-12 Various sizes of oropharyngeal airway (OPA) adjuncts.

Follow these steps for the proper use of an OPA (Scan 13-3):

1. Take appropriate BSI precautions.
2. Manually open the airway, using the appropriate method.
3. Select the appropriate size airway by measuring from the corner of the patient's mouth to the tip of the earlobe.
4. Open the patient's mouth and insert the airway upside down (with the tip facing the roof of the mouth) until it is approximately halfway in. Then rotate it 180 degrees as you insert it the rest of the way.
5. Allow the flange of the airway to come to rest against the outside of the patient's lips. It is acceptable to allow the flange to rest against the patient's teeth; however, if you cannot see the airway, it may have dropped into the mouth and become an obstruction.

CLINICAL CLUE

Alternative OPA Technique

An alternative to the OPA rotation technique is the tongue-blade technique, by which the EMT depresses the tongue with a flat tongue blade and inserts the OPA straight in over the tongue. This is the preferred technique for small children.

CLINICAL CLUE

Important Landmark

There is more than one way to measure the OPA to determine the proper size. Using the corner of the mouth and the tip of the earlobe will always be the easiest, because the angle of the jaw is very difficult to locate on many obese people.

Alternative methods for insertion of an OPA include inserting the airway sideways and rotating it 90 degrees. This is effective as long as you ensure that the OPA is resting behind the tongue and not against it, pushing it further back into the airway. The preferred method for inserting an OPA for an infant or small child is to use a tongue blade to press down on the tongue and then insert the OPA right side up directly over the tongue without rotating it. Proper positioning of an OPA when inserted is illustrated in Figure 13-13 ■.

PERSPECTIVE

Mackenzie—The EMT

I was actually kind of scared on that call. I had never responded to someone who still had the airway obstruction in place when we arrived. I was going through this checklist in my head of things to do for a nonbreathing patient, from which adjuncts to use and how to size them to how fast I should squeeze the bag on the bag-mask device if it came to that. And do you know what I kept forgetting? That this poor girl didn't have a patent airway! Luckily Rob remembered the ABCs and went right for the airway.

Nasopharyngeal Airways

The nasopharyngeal airway (NPA) is a short, round tube made of soft, flexible rubber or vinyl material (Figure 13-14 ■). It has a flange at the top and is beveled at the distal end, and is designed to help maintain an open pathway through the nose and into the nasopharynx. The NPA should not touch the back of the throat, so it is less likely to

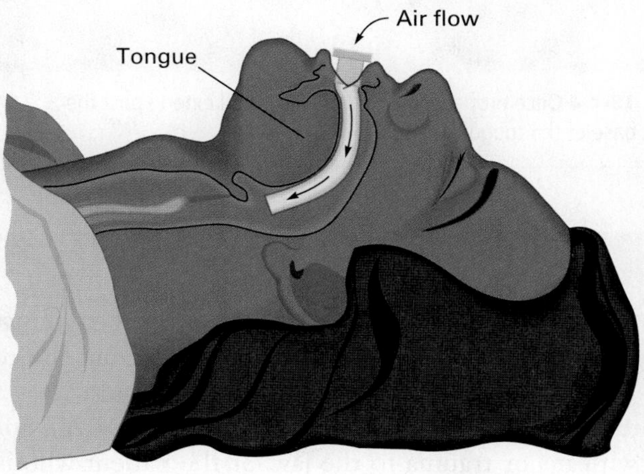

Figure 13-13 When properly placed, the oropharyngeal airway adjunct will hold the base of the tongue from obstructing the patient's airway.

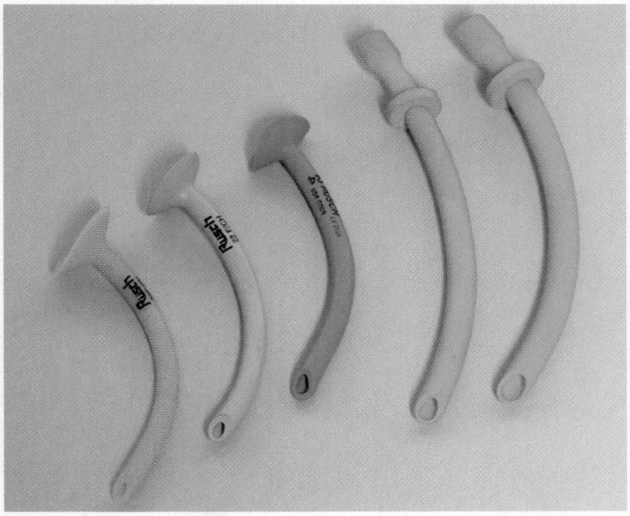

Figure 13-14 Various sizes and types of nasopharyngeal airway (NPA) adjuncts.

SCAN 13-4 Insertion of a Nasopharyngeal Airway

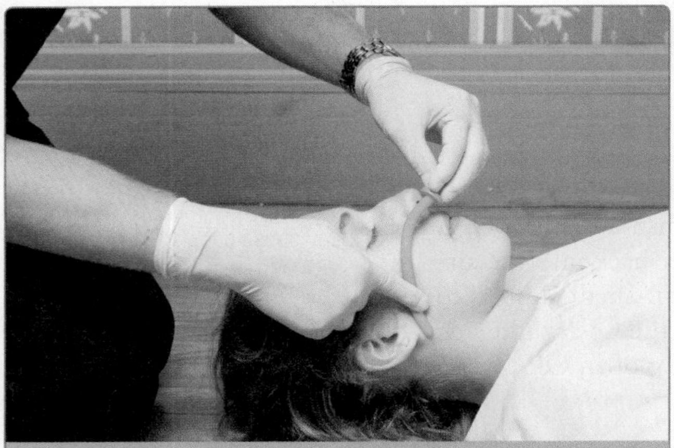

13-4-1 Properly measure the airway prior to insertion.

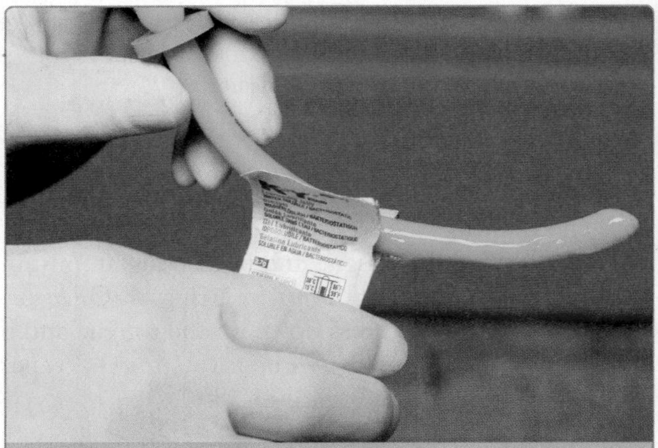

13-4-2 Lubricate the airway prior to insertion.

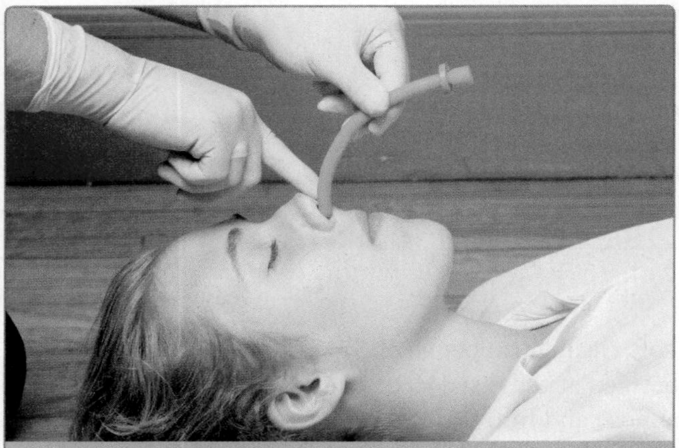

13-4-3 Gently push upward on the tip of the nose to open the nostril and insert the airway until the flange rests against the nostril.

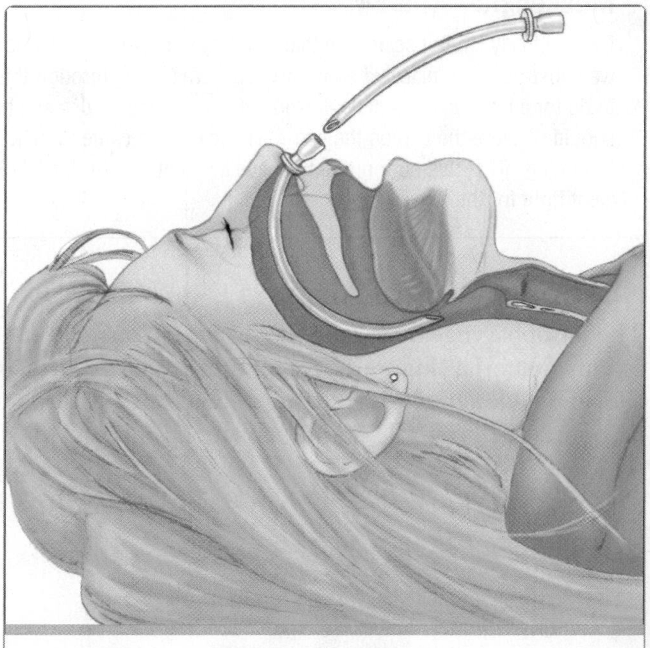

13-4-4 Once properly inserted, the NPA will extend past the base of the tongue.

stimulate the gag reflex than the OPA. However, the NPA does very little, if anything, to keep the tongue from blocking the throat. This is why the NPA is the second choice between the two airway adjuncts for an unresponsive patient with no gag reflex.

NPAs are ideal for the unresponsive or semiresponsive patient who will not tolerate an OPA or the patient with major trauma to the jaw, or the patient who is convulsing, preventing the use of an OPA.

Follow these steps for the proper use of an NPA (Scan 13-4):

1. Take appropriate BSI precautions.
2. Manually open the airway, using the appropriate method.
3. Select the appropriate size airway by first observing the opening of the nostril. Select an airway with a diameter slightly smaller than the opening of the patient's nostril.
4. Next measure from the tip of the nose to the tip of the patient's earlobe. Adjust the flange or cut the airway to the appropriate length.
5. Lubricate the airway using a water-based lubricant.
6. Press gently on the tip of the nose to flare the nostrils, and then insert the NPA posteriorly. Make certain that once inserted, the opening of the bevel is facing inward (toward the septum).
7. Advance the airway until the flange comes to rest against the outside of the nostril.
8. If resistance is felt, try twisting the NPA slightly. If this does not work, then remove it and attempt the same procedure on the opposite side.

It should be noted that all NPAs come from the manufacturer designed for use in the right nostril. This is due to the curvature and the placement of the beveled opening. If the NPA will not easily slide into the right side, then you will have to use a pair of scissors to snip the end and change the direction of the beveled opening. This is simple and does not significantly change the length of the NPA.

CLINICAL CLUE

Facial Trauma

Insertion of an NPA may be contraindicated in patients with significant facial trauma. Fractures to the face and skull could allow the airway to pass into a sinus cavity or in very rare cases, even into the cranium. Follow your local protocols.

STOP, REVIEW, REMEMBER!

Multiple Choice

For each question, place a check next to the correct answer.

1. Which one of the following patients is most in need of immediate suctioning?
   _____ a. Asthma patient with expiratory wheezes
   _____ b. Nonbreathing pediatric patient
   _____ c. Patient with gurgling sounds while breathing
   _____ d. Patient experiencing a severe allergic reaction

2. The most portable and easiest to use of the suction devices is the ______________ device.
   _____ a. manual
   _____ b. battery-operated
   _____ c. oxygen-powered
   _____ d. ambulance-mounted

3. Which of the following are the indications for inserting an oropharyngeal airway adjunct?
   _____ a. Responsive, active gag reflex
   _____ b. Unresponsive, no gag reflex
   _____ c. Responsive, no gag reflex
   _____ d. Unresponsive, active gag reflex

4. Prior to insertion, a nasopharyngeal airway adjunct should be measured from the ______________ to the ______________.
   _____ a. middle of the mouth, earlobe
   _____ b. angle of the jaw, corner of the mouth
   _____ c. tip of the nose, corner of the mouth
   _____ d. tip of the nose, tip of earlobe

(continued on next page)

(continued)

5. The recommended maximum time allowed for suctioning of an adult patient is ______________ seconds.

_____ a. 5

_____ b. 10

_____ c. 15

_____ d. 20

Matching

Match the piece of equipment on the left with the applicable definition on the right.

1. _____ Oxygen-powered suction device
2. _____ Soft suction catheter
3. _____ Bulb-type suction device
4. _____ Oropharyngeal airway adjunct
5. _____ Nasopharyngeal airway adjunct

A. Requires the patient to be unresponsive and have no gag reflex

B. Best suited for suctioning an infant's nose and mouth

C. Contraindicated for patients with face or head trauma

D. Most useful for suctioning through the nose of a semiresponsive or unresponsive patient

E. Typically a portable device that functions as an accessory to an oxygen regulator; requires an adequate supply of high-pressure oxygen to function

Critical Thinking

1. Discuss why it is good practice to have a suction device handy whenever you are performing manual ventilations.

____

____

____

____

2. Discuss why airway adjuncts such as the OPA and NPA cannot be relied on to maintain a patient's airway by themselves.

____

____

____

____

3. What are the contraindications for using an NPA? Why?

____

____

____

____

Positive Pressure Ventilation

Now that you have learned how to assess, establish, and maintain an open and clear airway for your patient, it is time to learn what to do if your patient is not breathing adequately or not breathing at all. Assessing whether an airway is patent is only half of the airway management equation. The other half is assessing the adequacy of the patient's own ventilations and providing the necessary support when needed.

13-16 Identify patients with indications for supplemental oxygen and positive pressure ventilation.

The first thing you will want to assess as you approach a patient is the rise and fall of the chest or abdomen during breathing. Is it obvious that he is breathing or is it difficult to tell? If breathing is obvious, then you may assume tidal volume is adequate and you can move on to assess the adequacy of the rate. If the rate is between 10 and 29 per minute, then the patient is breathing adequately and does not need assisted ventilations, but you may want to consider giving supplemental oxygen.

If tidal volume is low and you cannot easily see the patient's breathing, get more aggressive with your assessment. Kneel beside the patient, establish an open airway using the most appropriate method, and place your ear next to the nose and mouth to listen for breathing while you observe the chest and abdomen for rise and fall. Count the respirations. The chances are that as a patient's respiratory rate gets slower, the respirations will get shallower as well. A respiratory rate that is less than 10 per minute or more than 29 per minute should be a big red flag for a patient in trouble. You need to compare the rate with the tidal volume, and if the tidal volume is shallow, you may need to assist the patient's ventilations using one of the appropriate methods. A respiratory rate below 10 requires immediate intervention with assisted ventilations. Similarly, a respiratory rate greater than 29 per minute with low tidal volume (very shallow breathing) likely will require assisted ventilations.

PERSPECTIVE

Shannon—The Patient

I woke up with a mask on my face, and I was being forced to breathe. It was a totally unnatural feeling, and a pretty frightening one. I can remember taking a bite of my sandwich and laughing, and then suddenly I couldn't get a breath. I've never been so scared in my life! I was looking at my boyfriend and trying so hard to breathe. I really thought I was going to die.

Assisted Ventilations for the Responsive Patient

A patient who is still breathing but not breathing adequately because of rate or tidal volume needs immediate ventilatory assistance. You can accomplish this by assisting or enhancing the patient's own attempts to breathe with manual ventilations. The objective is to breathe into the patient as he takes a breath and to make each of his breaths good full breaths by increasing the tidal volume. The exact techniques will vary somewhat, depending on the device that you use. It is preferred to use supplemental oxygen when providing assisted ventilations.

13-20 Describe indications and methods for administering positive pressure ventilations to a patient who is breathing spontaneously.

Ventilation and Dental Appliances

Many patients have one or more forms of dental appliances such as implants, dentures, or partials. Ventilating a patient with missing or loose appliances can be challenging because it can be difficult to acquire an adequate face seal. Missing teeth or dentures allow the lips to collapse inward toward the mouth, making a good mask seal difficult.

Loose appliances can fall back into the mouth creating an airway obstruction. Make it your standard practice to inspect the mouth prior to initiating ventilations and remove any loose or broken appliances before initiating ventilations.

Risks of Positive Pressure Ventilation

13-17 Describe the physiological differences between spontaneous and positive pressure ventilation.

In the physiology of normal (spontaneous) breathing, air is brought into the lungs through a negative pressure created inside the chest. (See Chapter 5.) So, when a patient needs positive pressure ventilations, you will be forcing air into the lungs without the aid of that negative pressure. In fact, positive pressure ventilations create a positive pressure inside the chest that can potentially reduce the normal volume of circulation of blood that returns to the right side of the heart.

13-19 Explain the significance of avoiding gastric inflation when administering positive pressure ventilation.

Another risk of positive pressure ventilation is gastric distention. The esophagus is a soft tube that naturally closes off during normal inhalation. However, during positive pressure ventilation the patient is at greater risk for air entering the stomach through the esophagus.

Two problems are created when air enters the stomach. First and foremost, air that enters the stomach does not get into the lungs where it is needed. Second, when air accumulates in the stomach, it can cause gastric distention (enlargement of the stomach due to air). That distention can push down against the diaphragm muscle, making ventilations difficult and inadequate. In addition, gastric distention almost always results in the patient vomiting, which puts the patient at great risk for airway obstruction and aspiration.

In order to minimize the amount of air that enters the stomach you must maintain a clear airway and provide each breath slowly over one second. Always have suction ready when providing positive pressure ventilations in case of vomiting.

Hazards of Overventilation

13-22 Discuss the hazards of overventilation.

Too much of anything can be harmful, and ventilations are no exception. There are a few risks that you must be aware of when providing positive pressure ventilations to a nonbreathing patient. The most common error made when ventilating a patient is delivering breaths at too fast a rate. Recent research has shown that too many breaths, too close together do not allow the heart to adequately refill between beats. This is especially true during CPR.

Providing ventilations that are too big will cause an increase in pressure inside the chest, resulting in a reduction in cardiac output. This will have a direct effect on the amount of blood that is leaving the heart and circulating to the vital organs.

Another complication of ventilating patients at too fast a rate is that it can result in constricting the blood vessels in the brain. That can result in decreased blood flow to brain cells that are already being subjected to hypoxia.

It is extremely important to pay close attention when providing positive pressure ventilations. When possible, use a watch or clock to time them. For adults the proper rate is one breath every 5 to 6 seconds. For infants and children the proper rate is one breath every 3 to 5 seconds. Provide a volume with each breath that allows the chest to rise just a little. There is no need to cause full chest rise during ventilations. That is especially true when ventilating with supplemental oxygen.

Ventilation Techniques

Normal breathing occurs as a result of pressure changes within the chest. Any time you provide ventilations for your patient, it requires positive pressure from the outside to force air into the lungs. Positive pressure ventilations can be delivered in a variety of ways, depending on the available equipment and the patient's needs. It is best to follow local protocol when selecting a method of delivering positive pressure ventilations.

Ventilation Devices

There are several devices available to the EMT to assist with ventilating a patient. They are listed below in the order of preference. Though the mouth-to-mouth and mouth-to-stoma techniques are viable options in some situations, they will not be discussed here, but will be covered during your CPR training.

Ventilation devices listed in the order of preference when a single rescuer is present are as follows:

- Mouth-to-mask
- Two-rescuer bag-mask device
- Demand-valve device
- Single-rescuer bag-mask device

When ventilating a patient, regardless of the device being used, deliver approximately 10 to 12 breaths per minute for an adult, and 12 to 20 breaths per minute for pediatric patients. Newborns will require ventilations between 30 and 50 per minute. The delivery of each breath should be slow and delivered over one second. If for any reason you are not able to ventilate using the preferred techniques, consider a possible foreign body airway obstruction and follow the recommended technique for clearing the obstruction.

When providing ventilations during CPR, remember that you will provide two breaths following each cycle of 30 compressions. Also, always remember to take appropriate BSI precautions when managing a patient's airway, including providing ventilations.

13-18 Describe the proper procedures for artificial ventilation using the following methods: mouth-to-mask ventilation and delivery of positive pressure ventilations with a bag-mask device (one-person and two-person), with a demand-valve device, and with an automatic transport ventilator.

Mouth-to-Mask Technique

In most situations the pocket mask is the easiest barrier device to use and the quickest to deploy. Many EMS professionals and firefighters keep a pocket mask or similar barrier device on their person while on duty (Figure 13-15 ■). This is to ensure they will be ready to provide ventilations without delay should they encounter a nonbreathing patient. For maximum protection against exposure to body fluids, a one-way valve should be used in conjunction with the pocket mask or barrier device.

When used by itself, the pocket mask can allow for the delivery of between 10% and 15% oxygen to the patient, because that is how much oxygen remains in each of your exhaled breaths. If possible, use a pocket mask with a supplemental oxygen inlet. It will allow you to deliver much higher concentrations of oxygen when the mask is connected to an oxygen source.

To provide ventilations using a pocket mask, follow these steps (Scan 13-5):

1. Take appropriate BSI precautions.
2. Position yourself at the side or top of the patient's head.
3. Insert an appropriate airway adjunct.
4. Connect the mask to an appropriate oxygen source, if available, at a flow rate of 15 liters per minute (15 L/minute).
5. Place the mask over the patient's face, beginning at the top of the nose and walking the mask down so that it rests just below the lower lip.

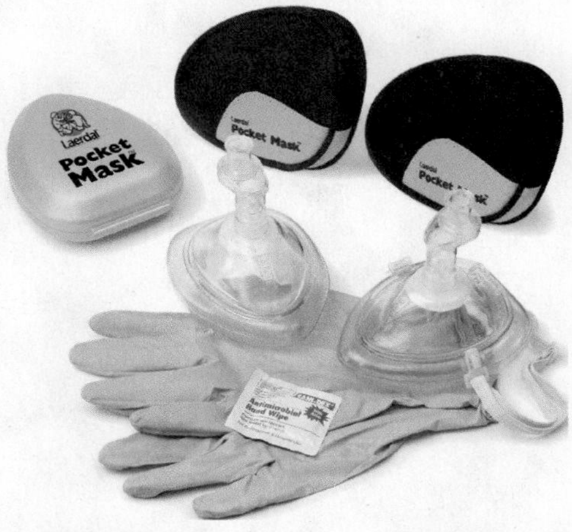

Figure 13-15 Typical pocket mask with one-way valve. (Photo courtesy of Laerdal Medical Corporation)

SCAN 13-5 Ventilations with a Pocket Mask

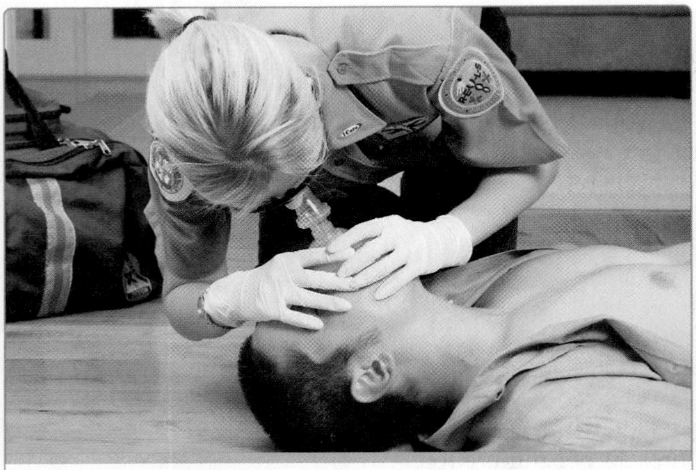

13-5-1 Proper mouth-to-mask technique from the side (lateral) position.

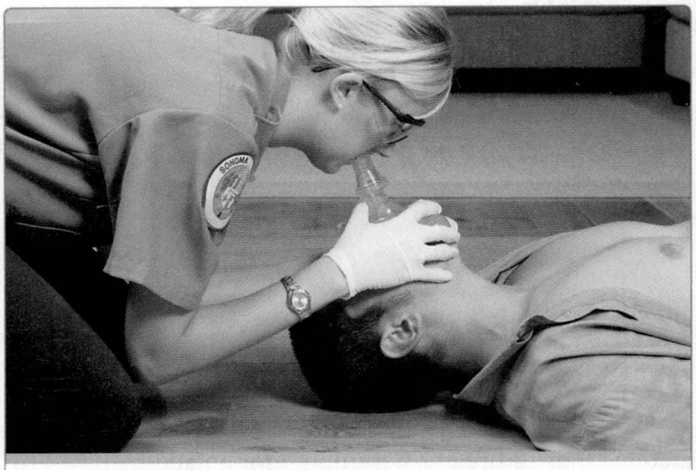

13-5-2 Proper mouth-to-mask technique from the top (cephalic) position.

bag-mask device a handheld device with a face mask and self-refilling bag that can be squeezed to provide artificial ventilations to a patient. It can deliver air from the atmosphere or oxygen from a supplemental oxygen supply.

6. Using both hands, form a tight seal between the mask and the patient's face while maintaining a head-tilt/chin-lift or jaw-thrust.
7. Take a normal breath, and then breathe into the one-way valve at the top of the mask. Watch for chest rise and fall.

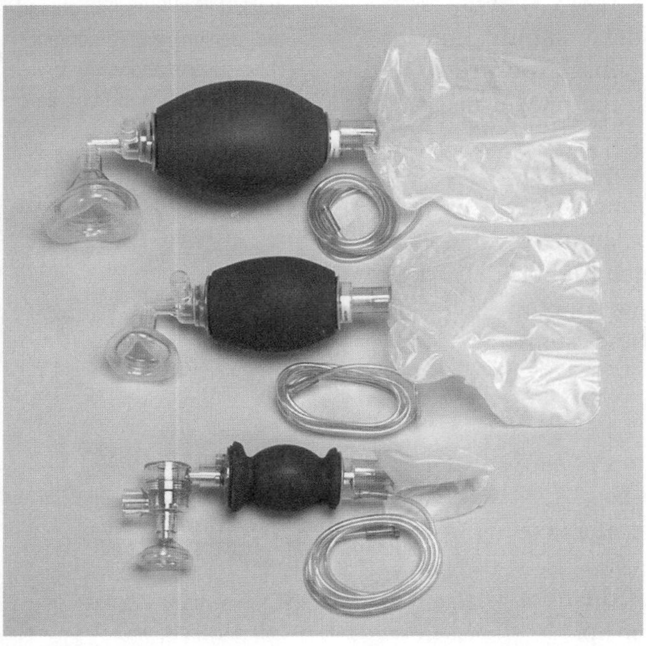

Figure 13-16 Bag-mask devices come in a variety of sizes.

Bag-Mask Device Technique

A **bag-mask device** consists of a self-inflating bag, a one-way valve, and a face mask. Most bag-mask devices have the capacity to be connected to supplemental oxygen and have an oxygen reservoir (Figure 13-16 ■). Regardless of the configuration, all bag-mask devices are most effective when connected to an oxygen source.

When connected to an oxygen source and used by two rescuers, the bag-mask is the preferred device for delivering high concentrations of oxygen up to 100%. Used without oxygen, the bag-mask will deliver room air that is approximately 21% oxygen.

Bag-mask devices come in several sizes, including adult, child, infant, and newborn. The adult-size device has a bag capacity or volume of between 1,000 and 1,600 milliliters. If used improperly, the device has the potential to deliver smaller volumes than a pocket mask. Be sure to watch the chest and abdomen for adequate rise and fall with each breath. A single rescuer attempting to use a bag-mask device will most likely struggle with trying to maintain an adequate seal while squeezing the bag. For this reason it is a preferred device only when there are two rescuers.

SCAN 13-6 Bag-Mask Technique—Single Rescuer

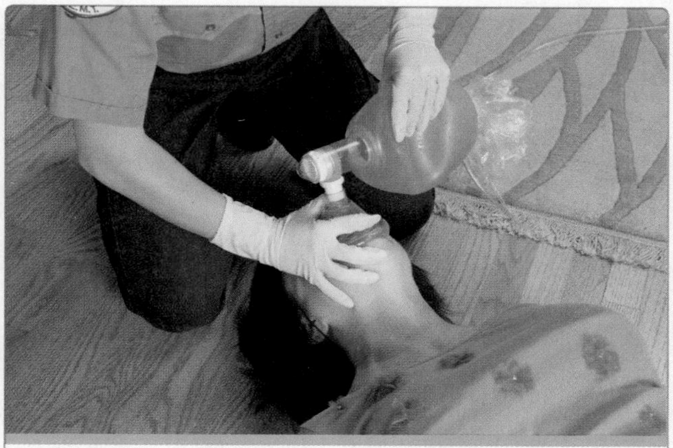
13-6-1 One hand secures the mask firmly to the face while the other had squeezes the bag.

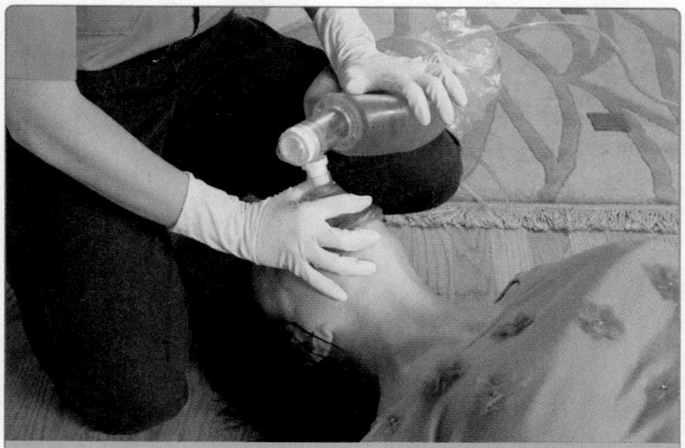
13-6-2 An alternative is to press the bag against the leg to get more volume out.

CLINICAL CLUE

Pop-Off Valve

At one time bag-mask devices were manufactured with "pop-off valves" to prevent overinflation of the patient. It is now known that those valves can release too soon, preventing adequate ventilation. Devices with pop-off valves should be taken out of service and replaced.

To provide ventilations using a bag-mask device with a single rescuer, follow these steps (Scan 13-6):

1. Take appropriate BSI precautions.
2. Insert an appropriate airway adjunct.
3. Connect the device to an appropriate oxygen source, if available, at 15 L/minute.
4. Position yourself at the top of the patient's head and place the mask over the patient's face, beginning at the top of the nose and walking the mask down so that it rests just below the lower lip.
5. Using one hand, form a "C" around the ventilation port with the thumb and index fingers of your hand and place the remaining three fingers on the mandible.
6. Press down firmly on the mask, forming a tight seal between the mask and the patient's face while maintaining a head-tilt/chin-lift or jaw-thrust. Grasp the mandible with the three fingers.
7. With the other hand, squeeze the bag while watching for chest rise and fall.

To provide ventilations using a bag-mask device with two rescuers, follow these steps (Scan 13-7):

1. Take appropriate BSI precautions.
2. Insert an appropriate airway adjunct.

SCAN 13-7 Bag-Mask Technique–Two Rescuers

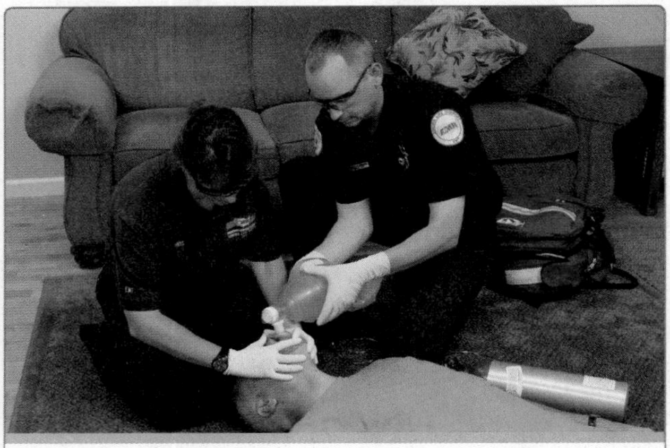

13-7-1 One rescuer uses both hands to ensure a firm mask seal while the other squeezes the bag.

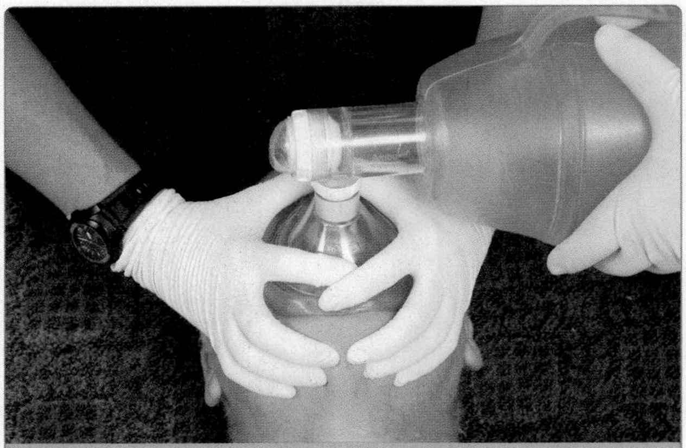

13-7-2 Use the "E," "C," technique to ensure a good mask seal while holding the airway open.

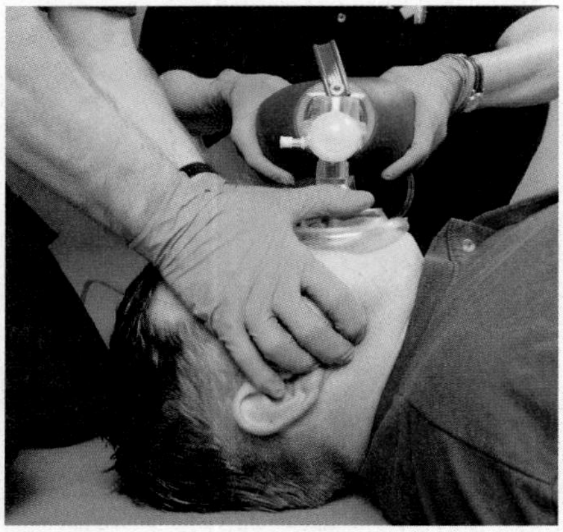

Figure 13-17 For patients with a suspected spine injury, keep the head neutral and use the jaw-thrust maneuver to pull the jaw up against the mask.

3. Rescuer #1 should position himself at the top of the patient's head, and then place the mask over the patient's face, beginning at the top of the nose and walking the mask down so that it rests just below the lower lip.
4. Using both hands, rescuer #1 should form a tight seal between the mask and the patient's face with the thumb and index finger around the ventilation port and the remaining three fingers on the mandible while maintaining a head-tilt/chin-lift or jaw-thrust.
5. Rescuer #2 then connects the device to an appropriate oxygen source, if available, at 15 L/minute.
6. Kneeling at the side of the patient's head, rescuer #2 should connect the device to the mask and squeeze the bag while watching for chest rise and fall.

Be sure to use the jaw-thrust maneuver when ventilating a patient with an unknown mechanism of injury or with a suspected spine injury (Figure 13-17 ▪). This can be accomplished by pulling the lower jaw up toward the mask, rather than tilting the head back (modified jaw-thrust). If the chest does not rise and you are certain there is no airway obstruction, set aside the device and attempt to ventilate using the mouth-to-mask technique.

Demand-Valve Device Technique

demand-valve device a device that uses oxygen under pressure to deliver artificial ventilations to adult patients. It has automatic flow restriction to prevent overdelivery of oxygen to the patient. Also called a *flow-restricted, oxygen-powered ventilation device (FROPVD).*

The **demand-valve device** is an oxygen-powered ventilation device that provides 100% oxygen "on demand" at a peak flow rate of approximately 40 L/minute. The flow of oxygen can be triggered by either the patient or the rescuer. When attached to a mask that is placed tightly over the patient's face, the flow of oxygen can be triggered each time the patient inhales. The device also can be triggered manually by the rescuer by activating a button or lever on the device itself.

Because there is limited control over the pressure delivered by the device, it is recommended that demand valves only be used for adult patients. The demand

SCAN 13-8 Demand-Valve Technique

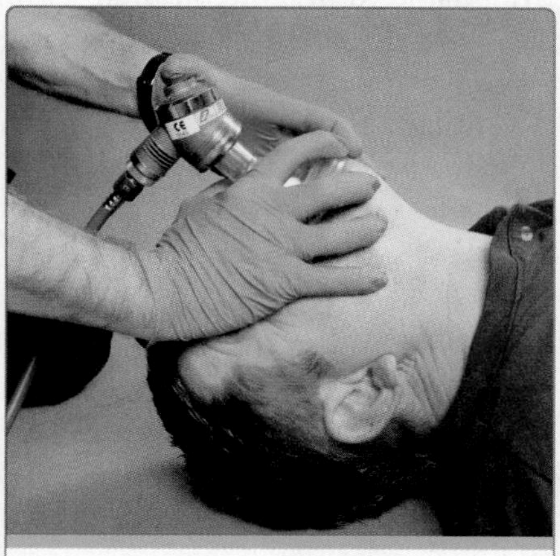

13-8-1 The demand valve is designed to be operated easily by a single rescuer.

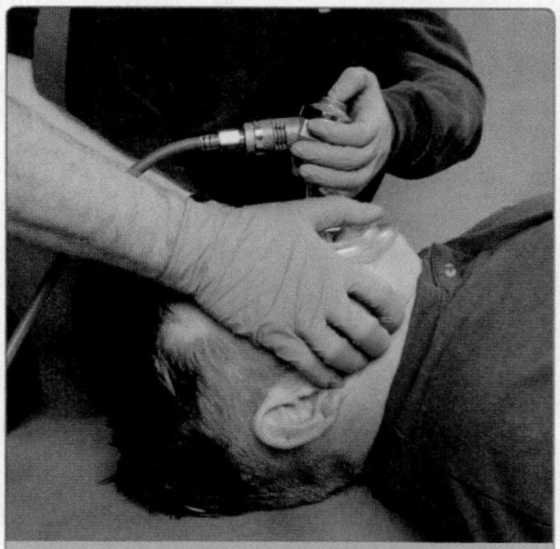

13-8-2 The preferred technique is the two-rescuer technique because it ensures a better mask seal.

valve should not be used on infants and is not recommended for young children. Use with caution and avoid overinflation in patients with chest trauma and chronic lung conditions. Excess or rapid ventilation in any patient will cause gastric distention and subsequent vomiting. All demand valves should be configured with an automatic pressure-relief valve and an audible alarm that sounds whenever the relief valve is activated (Figure 13-18 ▪).

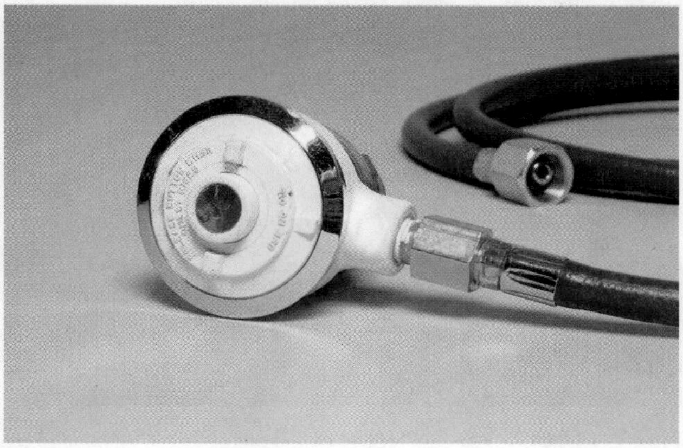

Figure 13-18 Typical demand-valve device.

To provide ventilations using a demand-valve device, follow these steps (Scan 13-8):

1. Take appropriate BSI precautions.
2. Position yourself at the top of the patient's head.
3. Insert an appropriate airway adjunct.
4. Ensure that the valve of the oxygen tank is open and there is plenty of oxygen.
5. Connect a mask to the demand-valve device.
6. Place the mask over the patient's face, beginning at the top of the nose and walking the mask down so that it rests just below the lower lip.
7. Using both hands, form a tight seal between the mask and the patient's face while maintaining a head-tilt/chin-lift or jaw-thrust.
8. Activate the device while watching for chest rise and fall.

Be sure to use the jaw-thrust maneuver when ventilating a patient with an unknown mechanism of injury or with a suspected spine injury. This can be accomplished by pulling the lower jaw up toward the mask, rather than tilting the head back. If the chest does not rise and you are certain there is no airway obstruction, set aside the demand valve and attempt to ventilate using the mouth-to-mask technique.

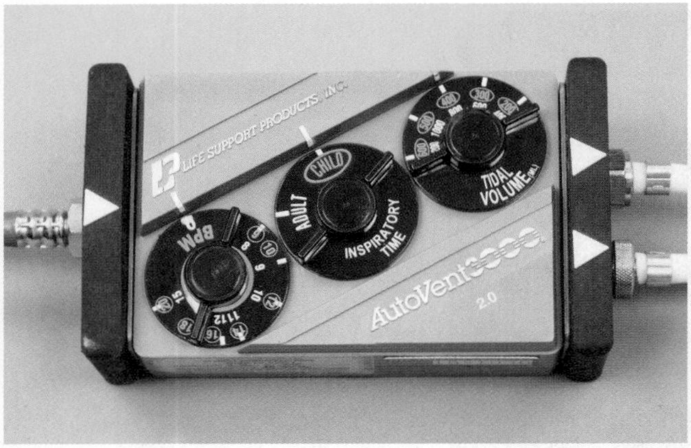

Figure 13-19 Typical transport-type ventilator.

Automatic Transport Ventilators

Automatic ventilators have been commonplace in hospitals for many years. They are used to provide positive pressure ventilations for patients who are unable to breathe on their own. Once properly adjusted, they will deliver ventilations at a prescribed rate, volume, and oxygen concentration indefinitely. A variation of the hospital ventilator that is becoming more common in the prehospital environment is the *automatic transport ventilator (ATV)*. These devices are used when a patient who must remain on a ventilator needs to be transferred from one hospital to another.

The ATV is designed to be connected to an endotracheal tube or a tracheostomy tube. ATVs are powered by oxygen and do not need an external electrical power source to function (Figure 13-19 ▪). The use of ATVs requires specialized training. They should be used only by EMTs who have had that training.

Noninvasive Positive Pressure Ventilation

13-21 Discuss the indications, contraindications, and methods for administering noninvasive positive pressure ventilation (NIPPV).

Another tool that is becoming more common in the prehospital environment is the *continuous positive airway pressure (CPAP) device*. CPAP is a variation of noninvasive positive pressure ventilation (NIPPV) that is used for the responsive patient who is in need of respiratory support. CPAP is used most commonly on patients in severe respiratory distress or failure or patients experiencing heart failure (Figure 13-20 ▪). CPAP is also a common therapy for premature infants with respiratory difficulty and patients with sleep apnea.

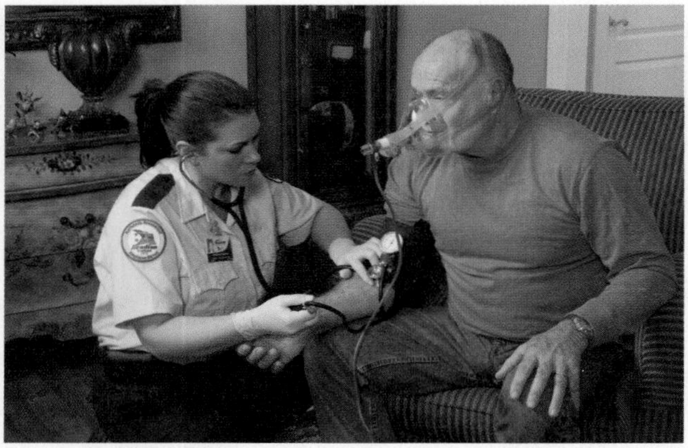

Figure 13-20 Typical CPAP device on a patient.

The CPAP device consists of a small pump attached to a mask that fits tightly over the patient's nose and mouth. The pump provides a continuous flow of pressure through the airways, which helps keep the alveoli inflated and improve internal respiration. The device reduces the amount of effort needed by the patient to breathe and can delay or avert the onset of respiratory failure.

Another form of NIPPV is *bilevel positive pressure ventilation (Bi-PAP)*. Bi-PAP differs from CPAP in that it provides two different airway pressures—one pressure during inhalation and another lower pressure during exhalation. That differs from CPAP, which provides the same constant pressure during inhalation and exhalation. Bi-PAP more naturally parallels normal breathing and can be less fatiguing to the patient over time.

NIPPV devices require specialized training. They are not a part of every EMT's scope of care. You will receive the necessary training if NIPPV is a part of your treatment protocols.

Ventilating Pediatric Patients

13-23 Discuss special considerations of airway management and ventilation for patients with stomas or tracheostomy tubes, infants and children, and patients with dental appliances.

The majority of techniques discussed so far apply to all patients, including infants and children. One exception that should be noted pertains to the head-tilt/chin-lift maneuver. Though it is best to achieve full extension of the neck in adults, children between the ages of one- and eight-years old generally require only moderate hyperextension of the neck to achieve an adequate airway. Infants require only slight extension, sometimes called the *neutral position* or *sniffing position*.

The most important reason for avoiding full extension of the neck in pediatric patients is the possibility that the airway could "kink," causing a partial obstruction.

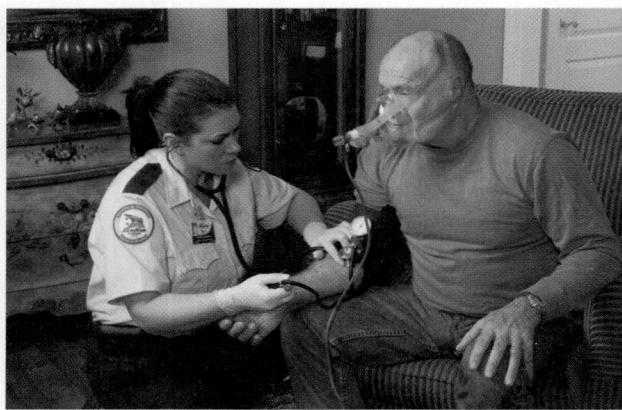

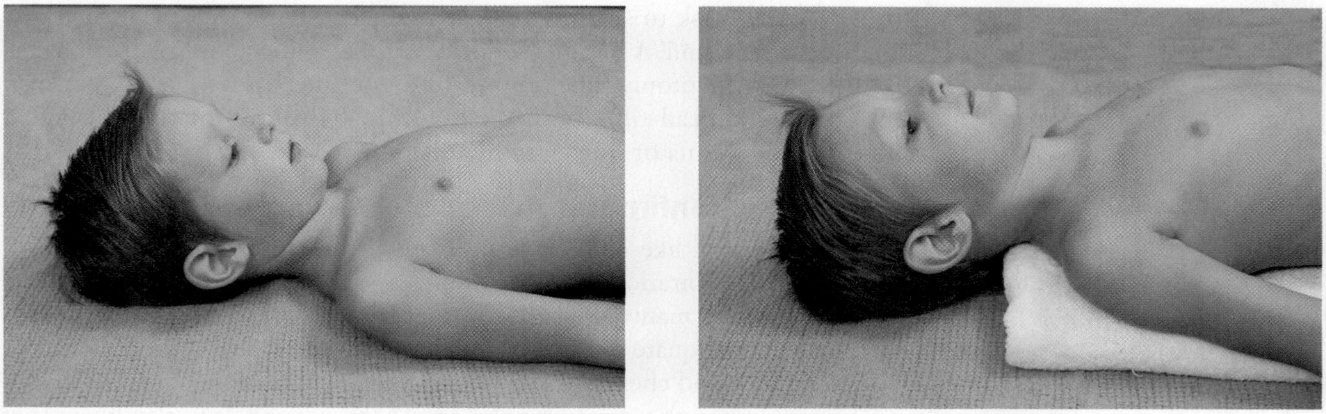

(A) (B)

Figure 13-21 (A) Due to the large occipital region of the pediatric head, the neck naturally flexes causing a high likelihood of airway obstruction. (B) Place folded towels or a similar object beneath the child's shoulders to bring the neck into a more neutral position.

This is possible because the tracheas of children and infants do not have fully developed cartilage rings, which help prevent collapse of the trachea during hyperextension (Figure 13-21 ■).

Pediatric patients also require significantly smaller tidal volumes during ventilation. Care should be taken not to overinflate these patients, because gastric distention occurs more easily in infants and children. Ventilate only until you see adequate chest rise (Figure 13-22 ■).

Ventilating Patients with a Stoma

Some patients may have holes surgically placed in the anterior aspect of the trachea to allow them to breathe. This may have been done secondary to trauma or perhaps the removal of a cancerous tumor. In most instances, there will be an obvious hole, a **stoma,** in the front of the neck inferior to the Adam's apple (Figure 13-23 ■). Sometimes there is a tube inserted into the hole, called a *tracheotomy tube*.

A patient with a tracheotomy or laryngectomy who is having difficulty breathing may have a buildup of secretions at the stoma, causing an obstruction. Use a suction device with a soft catheter to help clear the stoma. If necessary, attempt to ventilate the patient using any one of the techniques mentioned above. It may be necessary to seal the stoma with a gloved hand if air is escaping through the stoma during ventilations. If you have no success with conventional ventilations, seal off the mouth and nose and attempt to ventilate through the stoma. Use an infant

CLINICAL CLUE

Demanding Peds

Due to the small volumes required for pediatric patients when providing assisted ventilations, the use of a demand-valve device is not recommended. When ventilating pediatric patients, use only an appropriate size bag-mask device.

stoma a permanent surgical opening in the anterior aspect of the trachea through which the patient breathes.

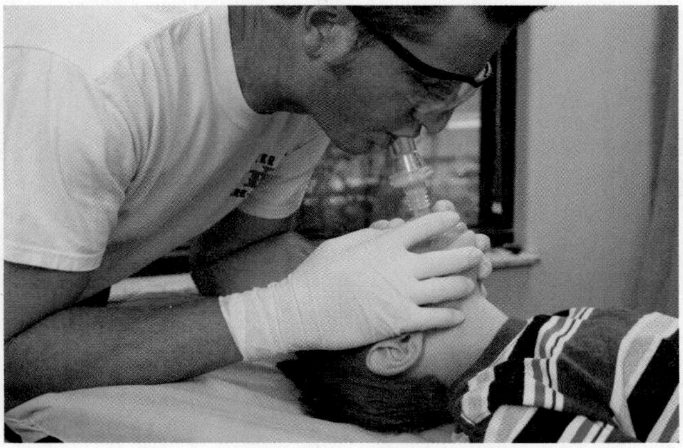

Figure 13-22 Mouth-to-mask technique on a pediatric patient.

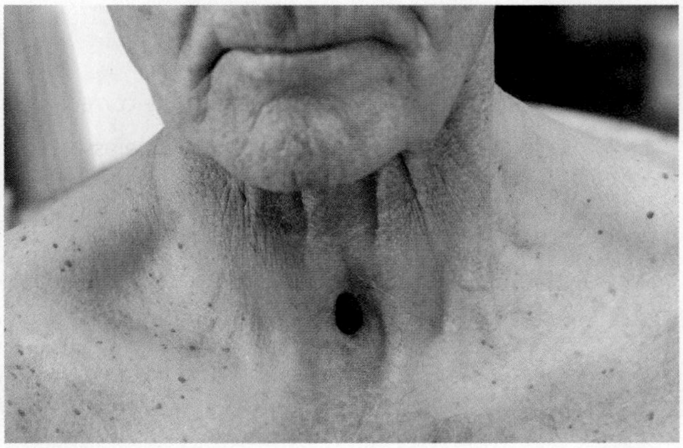

Figure 13-23 Patient with a stoma on the anterior neck.

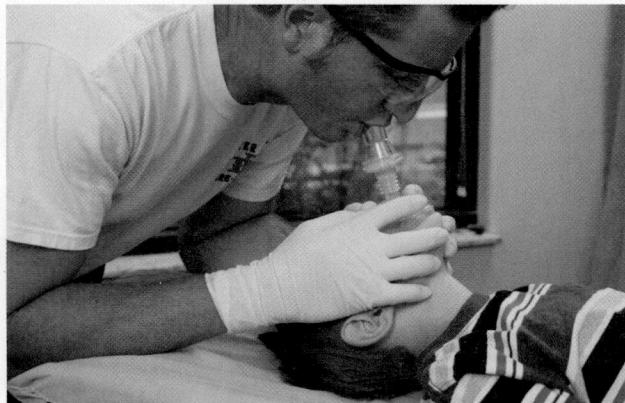

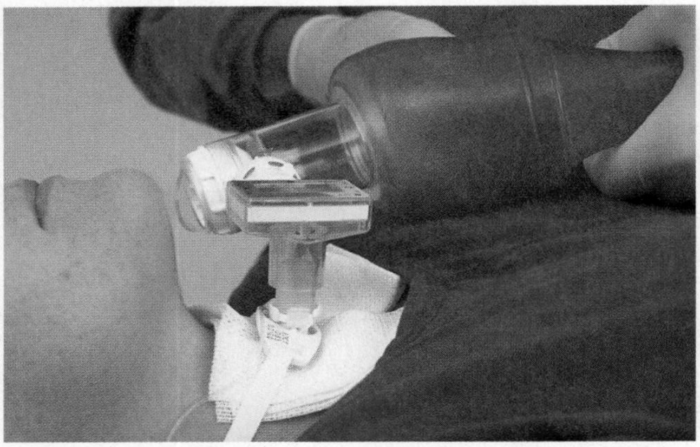

Figure 13-24 A bag-mask device can be attached to a tracheotomy tube to ventilate a patient.

mask to seal over the stoma because it is typically small and round. A bag-mask device can be connected directly to a tracheotomy tube (Figure 13-24 ■). There is no need to perform a head-tilt/chin-lift or jaw-thrust when ventilating through a stoma or tracheotomy tube.

Confirming Adequate Ventilations

Just like being able to assess the adequacy of a patient's own respirations, you also must be able to assess the adequacy of the manual ventilations that you provide. The primary sign of adequate ventilations is chest rise and fall. You should observe good chest rise and fall with each ventilation. The rate should be appropriate for the age of the patient. It is also likely that you will see the patient's skin signs and pulse rate improve with adequate ventilations.

When ventilations are inadequate, you will not see good chest rise and fall and the rate will be below or above what is considered acceptable for the age of the patient. It is unlikely that you will see an improvement in the patient's skin signs or pulse rate with inadequate ventilations.

PERSPECTIVE

Mackenzie—The EMT

Once Rob cleared the obstruction from Shannon's airway, she was breathing on her own, but it was really shallow and not very effective. So I started assisting her ventilations with a bag-mask and supplemental oxygen. It was amazing! The color started coming back to her skin, and Rob told me that her pulse was returning to normal. The next thing I knew, her eyes opened and she was looking up at me. I remember that look of, oh I don't know, confusion, maybe? I guess I'd be pretty confused, too, if I woke up and someone was ventilating me. I'm so glad that this call turned out well.

STOP, REVIEW, REMEMBER!

Multiple Choice

For each question, place a check next to the correct answer.

1. What are the characteristics that must be assessed in order to determine adequacy of respirations?

_____ a. Rate and ease

_____ b. Rate, depth, and ease

_____ c. Rate and lung sounds

_____ d. Tidal volume and ease

2. The normal respiratory rate for newborns is between _____________ and _____________ breaths per minute.

_____ a. 12, 20

_____ b. 20, 30

_____ c. 30, 50

_____ d. 40, 60

3. The primary mechanism for determining if your ventilations are adequate or not is:

_____ a. skin color.
_____ b. lung sounds.
_____ c. mental status.
_____ d. chest rise and fall.

4. Because there is limited control over the pressure delivered by this device, it is recommended that the ____________ be used only for adult patients.

_____ a. demand valve
_____ b. bag-mask device
_____ c. pocket mask
_____ d. pressure regulator

5. When attached to supplemental oxygen, the bag-mask device can deliver oxygen concentrations as high as:

_____ a. 21%.
_____ b. 44%.
_____ c. 60%.
_____ d. 100%.

Critical Thinking

1. Describe how you would manage an unresponsive adult patient whose respirations are 8 times per minute and shallow.

____

____

____

____

2. You are caring for a six-year-old drowning patient who is in respiratory arrest. What will be your device of choice for ventilating this patient? Why?

____

____

____

____

3. List the special factors that must be considered when providing manual ventilations for a pediatric patient.

____

____

____

____

(continued on next page)

(continued)

Complete the Table

Place an "X" in the box indicating the most appropriate ventilation device for the situation.

Situation	Mouth-to-Mask	Two-Rescuer Bag-Mask	Demand Valve	One-Rescuer Bag-Mask
You are alone and off duty with an unresponsive nonbreathing infant.				
You, your partner, and a firefighter are ventilating a patient as you carry him down a flight of stairs on a portable stretcher.				
You and a firefighter are ventilating an adult male patient in the back of an ambulance.				
You are alone in the back of an ambulance and ventilating an eight-year-old near-drowning patient.				
You are ventilating a 20-year-old man who is the third patient from an accidental carbon monoxide poisoning.				

Supplemental Oxygen

13-24 Describe the properties of oxygen.

The U.S. Food and Drug Administration (FDA) has identified medical gases such as oxygen, carbon dioxide, helium, nitrogen, nitrous oxide, medical air, and combinations of them as drugs, and requires them to be dispensed by prescription. In its natural state, oxygen is an odorless, colorless, and tasteless gas. Our atmosphere is made up of approximately 21% oxygen, 78% nitrogen, and 1% other elements. When our bodies are functioning normally, room air provides an oxygen concentration that is more than adequate to support life.

perfusion the supply of oxygen to and removal of wastes from the cells and tissues of the body as a result of the flow of blood through the capillaries.

Good **perfusion** occurs when all cells of the body receive an adequate supply of well-oxygenated blood. When a person experiences a serious illness or injury, his body's ability to utilize oxygen is likely to become compromised. That compromise almost always results in poor perfusion, which can lead to shock and eventually death, if not treated properly.

It is safe to say that all victims of illness or injury can benefit from oxygen. Some will benefit from larger concentrations, while others will respond well to lower concentrations. The point is that oxygen is one of the most important medical interventions the EMT can offer victims of illness and injury.

Oxygen Cylinders

13-25 Differentiate between the various sizes of oxygen cylinders available.

Oxygen is stored under pressure in containers known as *cylinders*, *bottles*, or *tanks*. Cylinders can be made of aluminum, steel, or composite materials. They come in a variety of sizes, with each size designated by a specific letter. Each size also contains a specific amount of oxygen when compressed to approximately 2,015 pounds per square inch (psi). The following list includes the most common cylinder sizes found in EMS along with the approximate volume in liters of oxygen (Figure 13-25 ■):

- D cylinder contains up to 425 liters
- Jumbo D cylinder contains up to 640 liters

- E cylinder contains up to 680 liters
- M cylinder contains up to 3,000 liters
- G cylinder contains up to 5,300 liters
- H cylinder contains up to 6,900 liters

Oxygen cylinders are composed of two main components: the cylinder, which contains the pressurized oxygen, and a valve at the top, which opens and closes the cylinder. The pressure regulator attaches to the cylinder valve when in use.

CLINICAL CLUE

Use of Oxygen

The Food and Drug Administration considers oxygen to be a prescription drug. However, it allows it to be marketed and used as a nonprescription medication under certain criteria:

- That the oxygen unit delivers a minimum of 6 liters per minute for at least 15 minutes
- That the oxygen unit is clearly labeled as emergency oxygen
- That the providers are trained in the safe use and storage of oxygen
- That the oxygen unit is packaged with an appropriate delivery device

Cylinder Safety

13-26 Describe the hazards associated with oxygen use and safety precautions to be observed when using oxygen or handling oxygen cylinders.

Because oxygen is stored under pressure, care must be used when handling and using oxygen cylinders. The valve of the tank is the most vulnerable part. If damaged, it can allow the compressed gas to escape and propel the cylinder at high speed, causing damage to anyone or anything in the way. When not in use, cylinders should be secured so that they cannot fall or roll around (Figure 13-26 ■). When on the

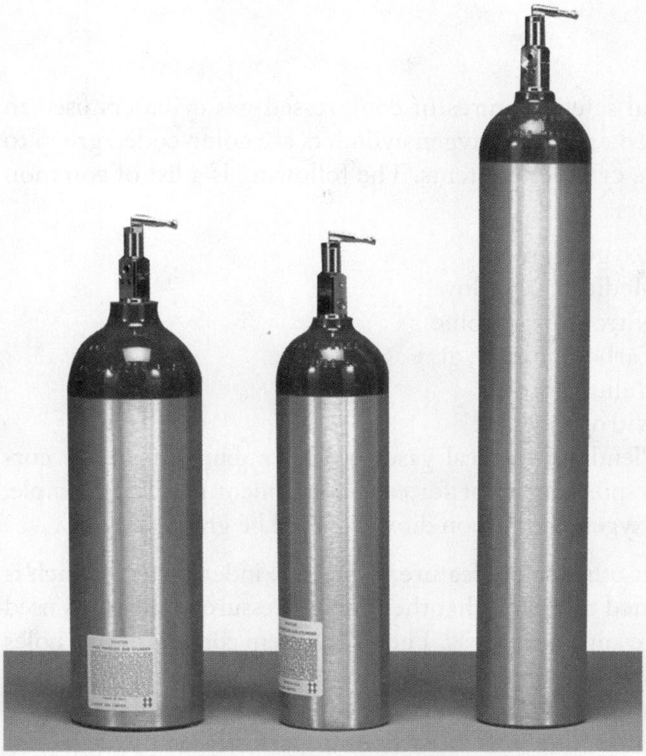

Figure 13-25 Common sizes of portable oxygen cylinders, from left to right, Jumbo D, Standard D, and E.

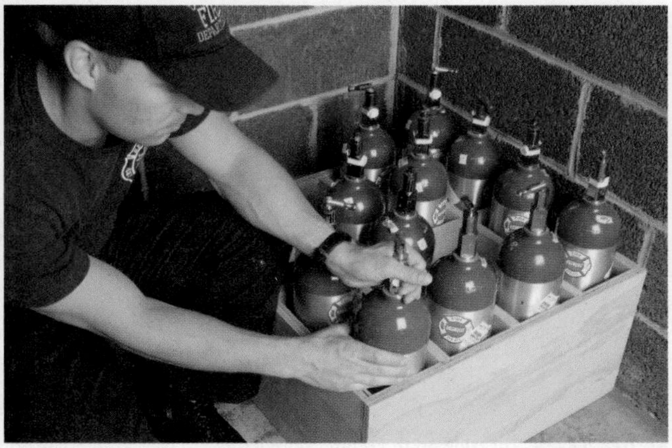

Figure 13-26 Oxygen cylinders must be stored properly when not in use.

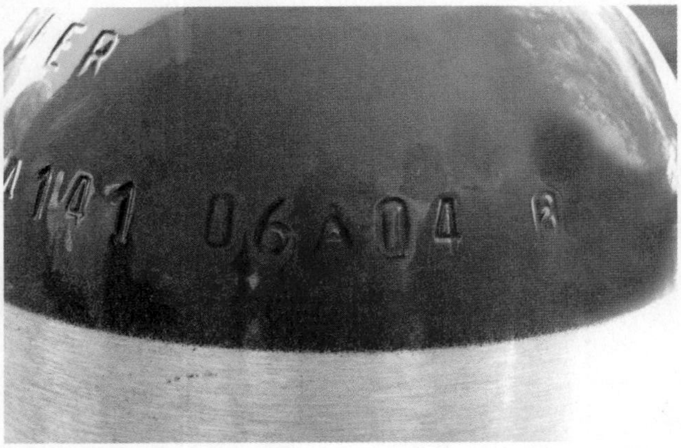

Figure 13-27 Each cylinder is stamped with a date indicating the last time it was hydrotested.

scene of an emergency, portable oxygen cylinders should be kept lying down at all times. Safety features of high-pressure cylinders include hydrostatic testing, color coding, PIN indexing system, and pressure-relief valve.

The DOT requires that all compressed-gas cylinders be inspected and pressure tested at specific intervals. The cylinders used in EMS that contain medical grade oxygen must be tested every five years. This test is commonly referred to as a *hydrostatic test* because, following visual inspection, the tank is filled with water and pressurized to five-thirds the service pressure, or approximately 3,360 psi, to confirm that no leaks exist. The most recent hydrostatic test date must be stamped into the crown of the cylinder and easily readable (Figure 13-27 ▪).

Note that some oxygen cylinders have met more rigorous inspection and testing standards and are allowed to go up to 10 years between test dates. Those cylinders have a five-pointed star immediately following the hydrostatic test date stamped into the crown.

CLINICAL CLUE

Tank Safety

A tank that is in service and still contains oxygen when the hydrostatic test date expires does not have to be taken immediately out of service. It can remain in service until such time that it needs to be refilled. At that time it must be removed from service and testing completed before it can be filled and placed back into service.

There are three additional safety features of compressed-gas cylinders used in EMS. The first is color. All medical grade oxygen cylinders are color-coded green to make easy identification of the cylinder contents. The following is a list of common gases and their associated colors:

- Oxygen, green
- Medical air, yellow
- Nitrous oxide, blue
- Carbon dioxide, gray
- Helium, brown
- Nitrogen, black
- Blends of medical gases use a combination of the corresponding color for each component gas. For example, oxygen and carbon dioxide would be green and gray.

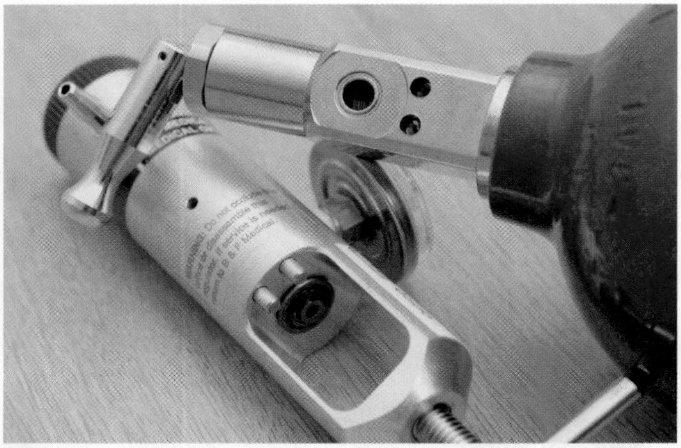

Figure 13-28 The pins on the regulator must match up to the holes on the tank valve for the regulator to fit properly.

Another safety feature is the PIN index system, which is designed to ensure that the proper pressure regulator is used for the appropriate gas. The PIN system consists of two holes strategically placed on the valve of the cylinder. Those holes match up with two pins that extend out from the pressure regulator. The pins must line up perfectly or the regulator will not fit properly onto the cylinder valve (Figure 13-28 ▪).

Still another safety feature is the pressure-relief valve. It is located on the cylinder valve and will allow for escape of the gas should the pressure inside the cylinder exceed a predetermined level. The release of pressure will prevent the cylinder from exploding.

Pressure Regulators

13-27 Describe the purpose and function of pressure regulators.

A full oxygen cylinder is pressurized to approximately 2,015 psi. That pressure will vary somewhat depending on the temperature of the environment. For the oxygen to be used by a patient, the pressure must be reduced to allow for a controlled delivery. An appropriate pressure regulator is used for this purpose. A typical pressure regulator will reduce the pressure to between 40 and 60 psi.

Functions of the Pressure Regulator

Pressure regulators can have several functions in addition to simply regulating the pressure inside the cylinder. Depending on how they are configured they may be able to provide the following functions: pressure gauge, adjustable liter flow outlet, and high-pressure port for use with a demand-valve or oxygen-powered suction device.

PRESSURE GAUGE

It is probably safe to say that all regulators used in EMS have an integrated pressure gauge (Figure 13-29 ■). Once the regulator is placed onto the cylinder valve and the valve turned on, the pressure gauge will display the amount of pressure inside the cylinder. Gauges are calibrated in pounds per square inch (psi), so the dial will reveal the amount of pressure remaining in the cylinder in psi. For practical purposes a cylinder with 2,000 psi is considered full, 1,000 psi is half full, and 500 psi is one-quarter full. In many EMS systems, a tank that has less than 500 psi is either refilled or replaced with a full cylinder.

> **CLINICAL CLUE**
>
> **Faulty Gauge**
>
> Because the gauge utilizes a high-pressure port on the regulator, it is recommended that you not look directly at the gauge while turning on the valve. If the gauge was damaged earlier, there is a slight chance that the gauge could burst when the valve is turned on, causing injury to the user.

ADJUSTABLE LITER FLOW OUTLET

Most, if not all regulators have a means of delivering oxygen at a constant flow rate. Medical oxygen is most commonly measured in liters and the flow rate is in liters per minute. Liter-flow valves vary by manufacturer, but a typical regulator will have a liter-flow valve that is adjustable to the following flow rates: 1, 2, 4, 6, 8, 10, 12, 15, 18, 20, 25 (Figure 13-30 ■). The flow rate that you select will be determined by several factors, including which delivery device you are using and how much oxygen you feel the patient needs. In most cases, the higher the flow rate, the higher the concentration being delivered to the patient.

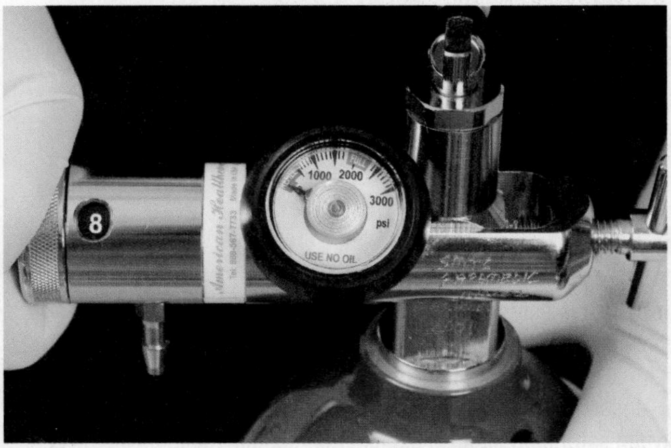

Figure 13-29 Typical oxygen regulator with pressure gauge.

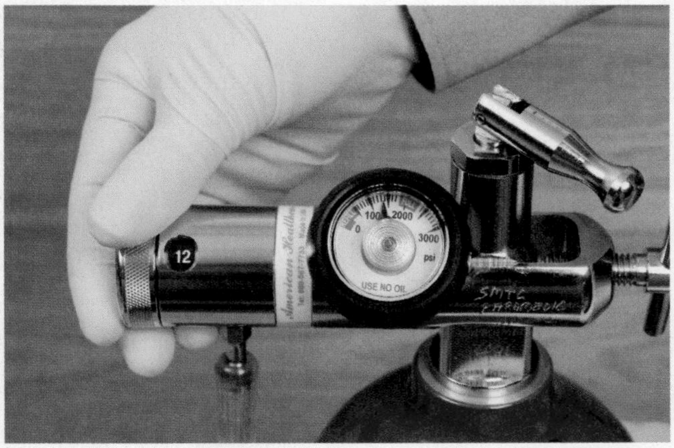

Figure 13-30 A valve on the regulator allows the EMT to adjust the oxygen delivery flow.

REGULATOR ACCESSORIES

Nearly all regulators have additional high-pressure ports that can be used to attach accessories. Two of the most common accessories are the demand-valve and oxygen-powered suction devices. Those devices consume a considerable amount of oxygen and will become less effective as the pressure in the cylinder gets low. Be sure to keep a close eye on the pressure in the cylinder and be prepared to change cylinders if necessary.

Attaching a Regulator to the Cylinder

To properly attach a pressure regulator to an oxygen cylinder, follow these steps (Scan 13-9):

1. Remove the protective seal over the cylinder valve.
2. Inspect the valve for cleanliness.
3. Quickly open and then shut the cylinder valve to expel any particles of dust or debris from the port.
4. Confirm the presence of an "O" ring and slip the yoke of the pressure regulator over the cylinder valve.
5. Line up the pins on the regulator with the holes on the valve and tighten the thumbscrew hand tight.
6. Turn the pressure gauge away from you or others, and open the valve one full turn (counterclockwise).
7. Read the pressure gauge and confirm the pressure in the cylinder.

When you are ready to remove the regulator from the cylinder, turn off the valve (clockwise) and bleed all pressure from the regulator by turning on the liter-flow valve until the flow of oxygen stops. It is up to you whether you store the cylinder with the regulator in place on the valve or off the valve. This is often just personal preference. Some agencies have their own policy concerning how portable oxygen cylinders are stored ready for use. Follow your agency's policy.

Oxygen Delivery Devices

13-29 Discuss the administration of oxygen by nonrebreather mask, nasal cannula, simple face mask, partial rebreather mask, Venturi mask, and tracheostomy mask.

To get the oxygen from the cylinder and to the breathing patient in a usable form, an appropriate delivery device is necessary. The two most common delivery devices used in EMS are the nonrebreather mask and the nasal cannula. The device you choose will depend on several factors, including the amount of oxygen you feel the patient needs and the willingness of the patient to accept or tolerate the device.

Regardless of the liter-flow device being used, it is important to determine that the patient is breathing at an adequate rate and volume. Liter-flow devices provide passive oxygen flow, which means that the patient must be breathing adequately on his own to realize any benefit from the oxygen. The purpose of these devices is to increase the concentration of available oxygen to the patient. Liter-flow devices *do not* provide ventilations for the patient.

PRACTICAL PATHOPHYSIOLOGY

Ensuring good ventilations for your patient is only one part of the equation needed to help ensure your patient is oxygenating and perfusing well. The addition of supplemental oxygen will increase the concentration of inspired oxygen (FiO_2). Increasing the concentration of available oxygen for a patient who is ill or injured will help ensure that the cells receive the oxygen he needs for respiration. To help monitor peripheral oxygen saturation, a pulse oximeter is recommended.

SCAN 13-9 Assembling the Regulator to the Tank

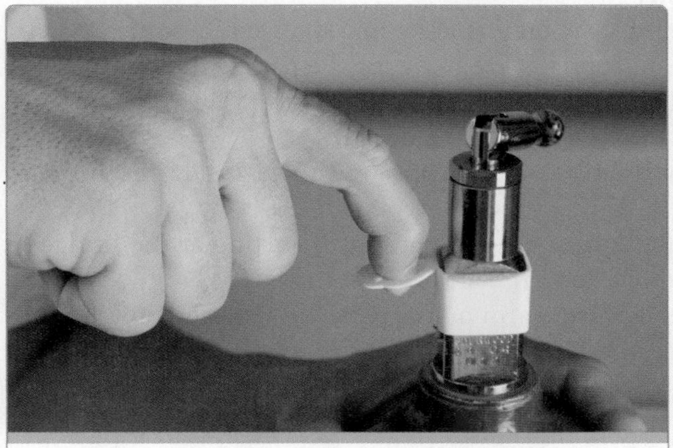

13-9-1 Remove the protective cover on the tank valve.

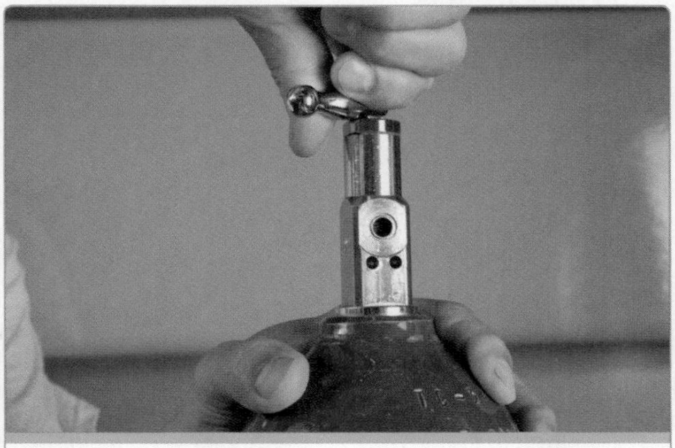

13-9-2 Briefly open the valve to purge any dust that may have accumulated in the valve.

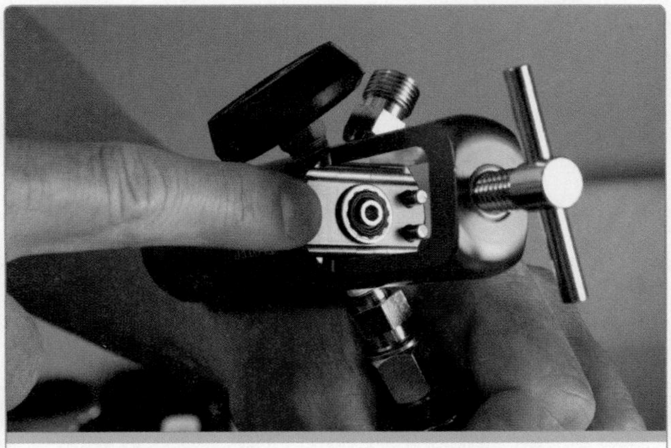

13-9-3 Ensure the presence of an "O" ring on the regulator.

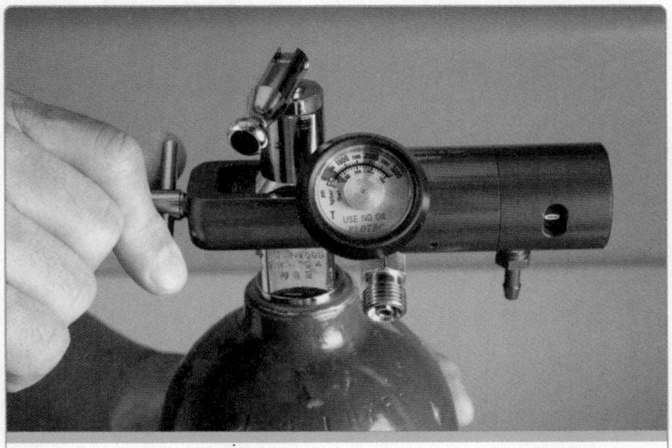

13-9-4 Line up the pins and secure the regulator only hand tight.

Nonrebreather Mask

In most situations in the prehospital setting, the **nonrebreather mask** is the preferred device for delivering a constant flow of oxygen to the breathing patient. It is called a nonrebreather mask because the design allows only minimal rebreathing of the patient's exhaled air. It consists of a clear face mask, a one-way valve, an oxygen reservoir, and the supply tubing (Figure 13-31 ■).

nonrebreather mask a face mask and reservoir bag device that delivers high concentrations of oxygen.

Sometimes referred to as a *high-flow device*, the nonrebreather mask works best at a liter-flow rate of between 10 and 15 L/minute. When properly placed, the nonrebreather mask can increase the concentration of available oxygen to 90%.

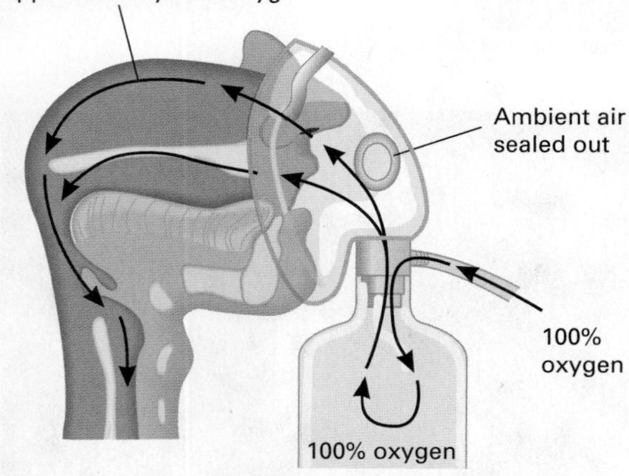

Figure 13-31 Nonrebreather mask and how it functions.

To properly apply a nonrebreather mask to a patient, follow these steps (Scan 13-10):

1. Confirm that the patient is breathing with an adequate rate and tidal volume.
2. Advise the patient that you are going to give him some oxygen.
3. Select the appropriate size mask for the patient.
4. Connect the mask supply tubing to an appropriate oxygen source and adjust the liter flow to the desired rate.
5. Place your thumb over the one-way valve inside the mask to expedite the filling of the reservoir.
6. Place the mask over the patient's face, starting at the bridge of the nose and walking the mask down the face.
7. Place the elastic band around the patient's head and pull the ends through the mask to ensure a snug fit. Squeeze the aluminum nose strap to help seal the mask across the nose.

CLINICAL CLUE

Nonrebreather

Because a nonrebreather mask is not airtight, it will always allow some ambient air in around the seal. For this reason a nonrebreather mask is not capable of providing a breathable oxygen concentration of 100%.

Keep a close eye on the reservoir bag as the patient breathes in and out. The bag should *not* completely deflate when the patient breathes in. The bag also should have enough time to completely refill between breaths. If the reservoir becomes deflated or does not refill completely between breaths, increase the liter-flow rate as appropriate.

PERSPECTIVE

Mackenzie—The EMT

After the patient regained consciousness, I knew that she'd need a good amount of oxygen to help recover from going four or five minutes without any. I chose to put her on a nonrebreather mask with the oxygen set at 15 liters. Because of my nervousness, I forgot to prefill the oxygen reservoir, but Rob was nice enough to remind me.

Additional Oxygen Delivery Devices

There are additional oxygen delivery masks that you may encounter as well, depending on what is common for your system or service. Here is a brief description of each:

- ***Simple mask.*** This is a variation of the nonrebreather mask and does not have an oxygen reservoir attached to it. The design of the simple mask allows for more mixture of ambient air. For this reason the highest concentration that a simple mask can deliver is approximately 60%. The normal flow range for this mask is between 6 and 10 L/minute.

SCAN 13-10 Applying a Nonrebreather Mask

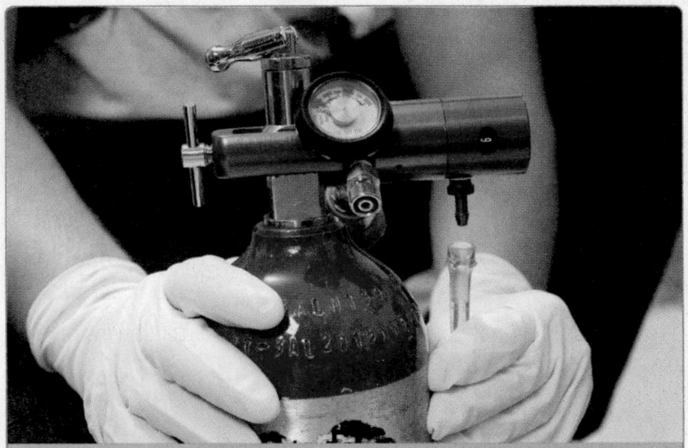

13-10-1 Connect the oxygen tubing from the device to the oxygen regulator.

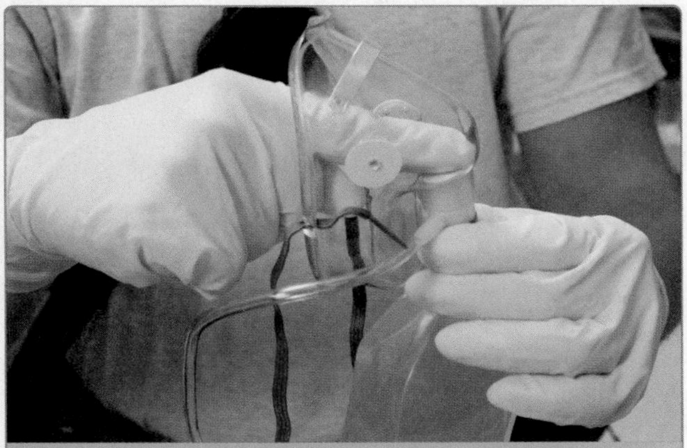

13-10-2 Ensure the reservoir is filled completely before placing on the patient.

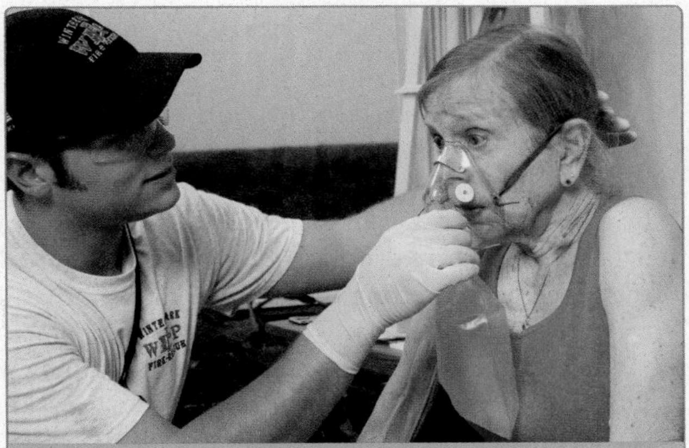

13-10-3 Place the mask on the patient's face and adjust to ensure a good seal all around the mask.

- ***Partial rebreather mask.*** This mask is very similar to the nonrebreather mask, except that it allows the patient to rebreathe more exhaled and ambient air. This mask can facilitate the delivery of oxygen concentrations up to 60% and higher, depending on flow rate. The normal flow range for this device is between 6 and 10 L/minute.
- ***Venturi mask.*** This mask is a high-flow device designed to deliver precise concentrations of oxygen. It contains interchangeable jets that adjust and control the oxygen delivered to the patient (Figure 13-32 ■). It is commonly used for patients with COPD, who must carefully control the amount of oxygen they receive.

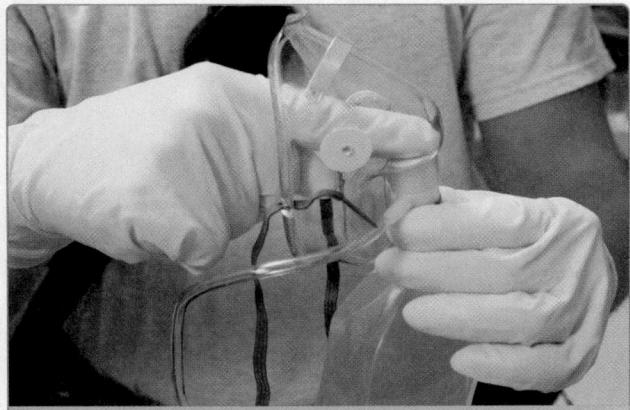

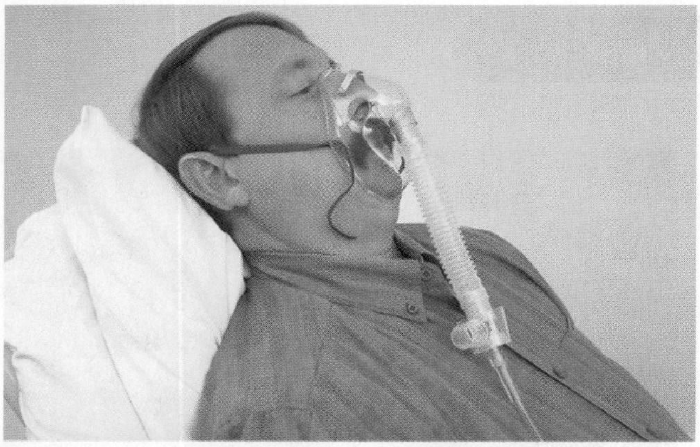

Figure 13-32 Venturi-type mask.

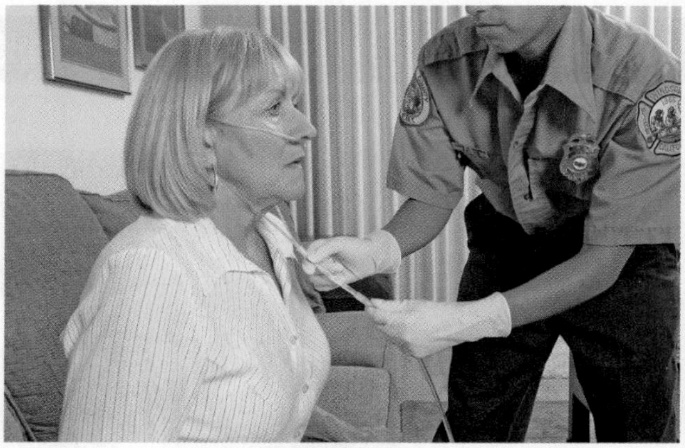

Figure 13-33 A nasal cannula provides lower concentrations of oxygen.

- ***Tracheostomy mask.*** This is a small mask that attaches to a tracheostomy tube and is capable of delivering oxygen concentrations between 25% and 50%. It also can be used to deliver aerosolized medications.

Nasal Cannula

nasal cannula a device that delivers low concentrations of oxygen through two prongs that rest in the patient's nostrils.

A **nasal cannula** is used for patients who are not that critical and may benefit from lower concentrations of oxygen, or who simply do not tolerate the nonrebreather mask (Figure 13-33 ■). Patients sometimes feel that their breathing is being restricted by the nonrebreather mask because it covers their entire face, despite the fact that it is delivering oxygen. Before giving up on the mask, make every attempt to "coach" the patient into getting used to the mask. If that does not work, many patients will tolerate a nasal cannula.

The nasal cannula consists of a loop of tubing with a pair of prongs (short narrow tubes) that are placed into the patient's nostrils. The loop has an adjustable band and is connected to the supply tubing.

Sometimes referred to as a *low-flow device*, the nasal cannula works best at liter-flow rates between 2 and 6 L/minute. When properly placed, the nasal cannula can increase the concentration of available oxygen to approximately 44%.

To properly apply a nasal cannula to a patient, follow these steps (Scan 13-11):

1. Confirm that the patient is breathing with an adequate rate and tidal volume.
2. Advise the patient that you are going to give him some oxygen.
3. Select the appropriate-size cannula for the patient.
4. Connect the cannula supply tubing to an appropriate oxygen source and adjust the liter flow to between 2 and 6 L/minute.
5. Slide the adjusting band downward to allow for full expansion of the cannula loop.
6. Grasp the loop with the thumb and index finger of each hand on either side of the prongs.
7. Advise the patient that the prongs will tickle a little bit but will not hurt. Insert the prongs into the patient's nostrils.
8. Slide your fingers along the loop and wrap each side around the patient's ears.
9. Slide the adjusting band up under the chin to take up any slack in the loop. Advise the patient to breathe through his nose.

SCAN 13-11 Applying a Nasal Cannula

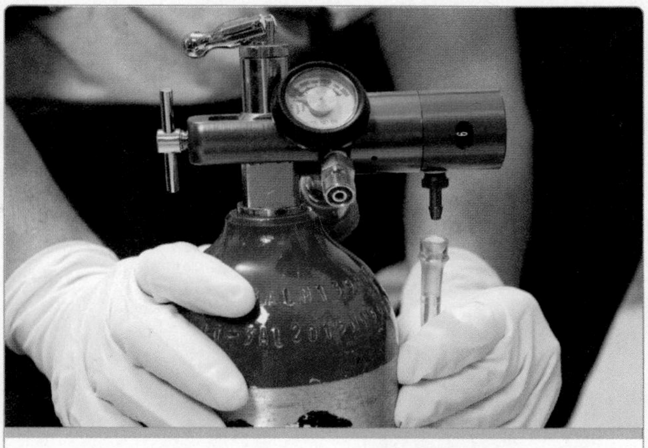

13-11-1 Connect the oxygen tubing from the device to the oxygen regulator.

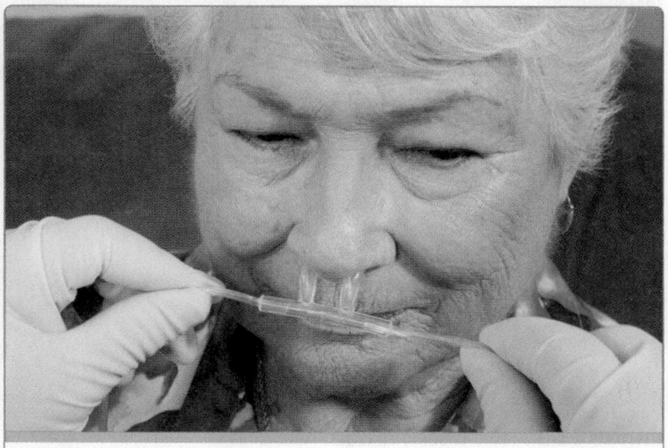

13-11-2 Hold the prongs in both hands as you place them gently in the patient's nostrils.

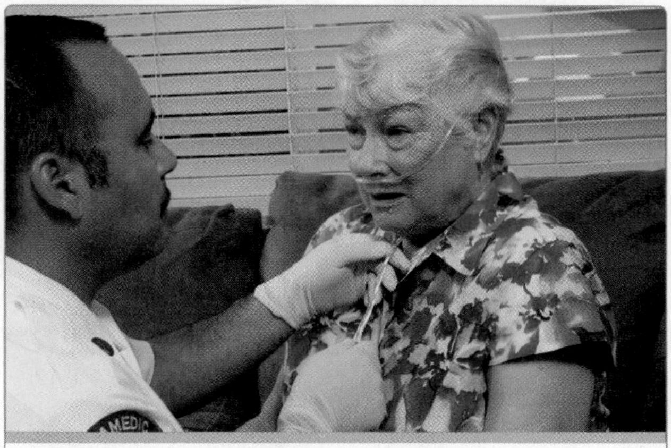

13-11-3 Wrap the tubing around the ears and cinch it up under the chin.

Some EMS professionals prefer the cannula simply because it makes it easier to hear the patient when they are trying to get a medical history. This is not a good reason to choose the cannula. When a patient is in need of supplemental oxygen, the device of choice should be the nonrebreather mask. Only if the patient simply will not tolerate the mask should you attempt a nasal cannula. The device of choice may be specified by your local protocols.

Humidified Oxygen

Compressed oxygen that is stored in cylinders is extremely dry and over time can cause dryness and irritation to the mucous membranes, especially in the nasal

13-28 Discuss the use of oxygen humidifiers.

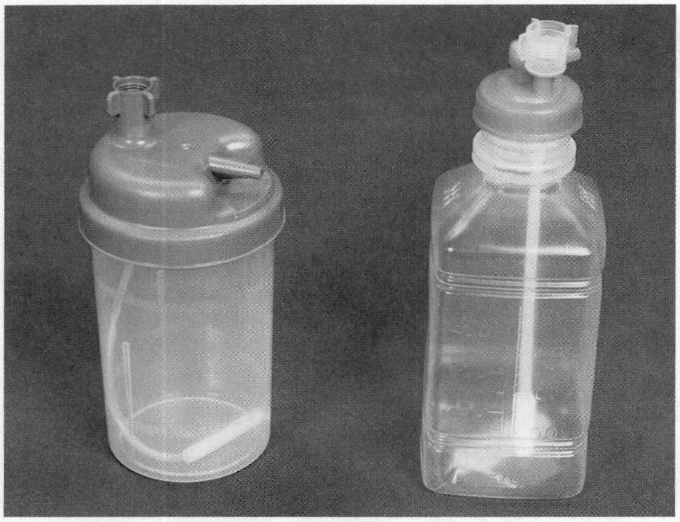

Figure 13-34 Two types of oxygen humidifiers.

passages (Figure 13-34 ■). An oxygen humidifier is a container of sterile water that is connected to the oxygen supply between the patient and the cylinder. As the oxygen passes through the water, it picks up tiny water molecules. This added moisture minimizes the chances of dryness and irritation the patient may experience.

Humidifiers are found in hospitals, rarely on ambulances, and not typically used with portable oxygen cylinders. When humidified oxygen is utilized, a fresh sterile unit must be used each time to prevent the spread of infections from one patient to another.

STOP, REVIEW, REMEMBER!

Multiple Choice

For each question, place a check next to the correct answer.

1. The oxygen concentration that is normally present in the air we breathe is:

_____ a. 19%.

_____ b. 21%.

_____ c. 44%.

_____ d. 78%.

2. In round numbers, an oxygen cylinder is considered full if it contains _____________ psi of pressure.

_____ a. 500

_____ b. 1,500

_____ c. 2,000

_____ d. 3,600

3. Which one of the following is not a safety feature of high-pressure cylinders?

_____ a. Hydrostatic testing

_____ b. Color coding

_____ c. PIN indexing system

_____ d. Round shape

4. The appropriate liter-flow range for a nasal cannula is between _____________ and _____________ L/minute.

_____ a. 2, 6

_____ b. 4, 8

_____ c. 10, 12

_____ d. 12, 15

5. A nonrebreather mask that is set at 15 L/minute will deliver an oxygen concentration of approximately:

_____ a. 30%.

_____ b. 50%.

_____ c. 90%.

_____ d. 100%.

6. An oxygen mask that can deliver precise concentrations of oxygen is the:

_____ a. partial rebreather mask.

_____ b. Venturi mask.

_____ c. simple mask.

_____ d. tracheostomy mask.

7. When providing supplemental oxygen, humidifiers are used to:

_____ a. increase the concentration of oxygen.

_____ b. decrease the concentration of oxygen.

_____ c. moisten the mucous membranes.

_____ d. dry the mucous membranes.

8. Which one of the following oxygen administration devices will provide the patient with the highest concentration of oxygen?

_____ a. Venturi mask at 8 L/minute

_____ b. Nasal cannula at 6 L/minute

_____ c. Simple mask at 10 L/minute

_____ d. Nonrebreather mask at 12 L/minute

9. You are caring for a victim of an automobile collision who is breathing six times per minute and shallow. You should provide:

_____ a. ventilations with a bag-mask device.

_____ b. supplemental oxygen with a nonrebreather mask.

_____ c. supplemental oxygen with a cannula.

_____ d. supplemental oxygen with a humidifier.

10. A cannula set at 6 L/minute will deliver an oxygen concentration of approximately:

_____ a. 21%.

_____ b. 25%.

_____ c. 33%.

_____ d. 44%.

Matching

Match the piece of equipment on the left with the applicable definition on the right.

1. _____	Stoma	A. Low-flow O_2 delivery device that is placed in the nose
2. _____	Oropharyngeal airway adjunct	B. Device used to provide manual ventilations for a nonbreathing patient
3. _____	Nonrebreather mask	C. Curved plastic device used to keep the tongue from blocking the airway
4. _____	Nasal cannula	D. High-flow oxygen delivery device with an inflatable O_2 reservoir
5. _____	Bag-mask device	E. Hole surgically placed in the anterior aspect of the trachea

Critical Thinking

1. What is the difference between medical oxygen and the air that we breathe in the atmosphere?

____

____

____

____

2. Explain how supplemental oxygen can help improve a patient's perfusion status.

____

____

____

____

(continued on next page)

(continued)

3. Explain why a nonrebreather mask is not capable of providing a breathable oxygen concentration of 100%.

EMERGENCY DISPATCH SUMMARY

Once Shannon had regained consciousness and started breathing normally with the nonrebreather mask, Mackenzie urged her to be seen by a doctor in the emergency department. At first Shannon declined, citing embarrassment over the whole incident. She soon changed her mind after Rob explained some of the complications that could arise as the result of having choked to the point of unconsciousness. Rob and Mackenzie then helped Shannon onto their stretcher and into the ambulance where they transported her, still on oxygen and without incident, to Memorial Hospital. Her boyfriend followed them in his own car.

Chapter Review

To the Point

- The word *respiration* has several meanings including the movement of air in and out of the lungs (pulmonary respiration), across the alveolar/capillary bed (external respiration), between the capillaries and the cells (internal respiration), and within the cells (cellular respiration).
- Pulmonary respiration is the easiest to assess and is a factor of rate times volume resulting in minute ventilations.
- Signs of adequate ventilations include appropriate rate, volume, and little to no work of breathing.
- Inadequate ventilations are characterized by altered mental status, increased work of breathing, rapid breathing, decreased tidal volume, and use of accessory muscles.
- The airway structures of a pediatric patient are smaller and more easily obstructed by swelling and foreign objects.
- Inadequate ventilations will lead to hypoxia. Common signs of hypoxia are altered mental status, rapid heart rate (adult), slow heart rate (infants), pale skin, and cyanosis.
- Noisy breathing is always a sign of partial airway obstruction. Noises such as snoring (tongue), crowing (swelling), gurgling (fluid), and stridor (swelling) are signs of partial upper airway obstruction.
- The preferred method for opening the airway of a noninjured patient is the head-tilt/chin-lift maneuver. The jaw-thrust maneuver is recommended for patients with suspected neck or spine injury.
- Patients with an airway obstruction caused by fluid, such as blood or vomit, should be suctioned immediately.
- Patients who are semiresponsive or unresponsive are at high risk for airway compromise. Insertion of a nasopharyngeal or oropharyngeal airway adjunct is appropriate depending on the patient's level of responsiveness.
- Patients who are breathing inadequately or not at all may require positive pressure ventilations using mouth-to-mask, bag-mask, or a demand-valve device technique.

- Ventilations should be provided at the appropriate rate and volume for the size and age of the patient. Overventilation can result in compromise in circulation and perfusion.
- To minimize the chances of gastric distention make sure to maintain an open airway and provide ventilations at an appropriate rate and volume.
- NIPPV is a positive pressure therapy that is used for responsive patients experiencing severe respiratory distress or acute heart failure. CPAP is the most common form of NIPPV used in EMS today.
- Supplemental oxygen is appropriate for most patients who are ill or injured. You must follow local protocol for the appropriate delivery method.

Chapter Questions

Multiple Choice

For each question, place a check next to the correct answer.

1. During the respiratory assessment of the patient, the EMT must ensure that the patient has an open airway and has adequate:

_____ a. capillary refill.
_____ b. skin color.
_____ c. tidal volume.
_____ d. pulses.

2. Which one of the following are structures of the lower airway?

_____ a. Esophagus, bronchi, larynx
_____ b. Trachea, bronchi, alveoli
_____ c. Nasopharynx, larynx, oropharynx
_____ d. Trachea, pharynx, alveoli

3. The natural movement of air in and out of the lungs is called:

_____ a. respiration.
_____ b. exhalation.
_____ c. inhalation.
_____ d. ventilation.

4. Which one of the following best describes the most appropriate way to open the airway of a child with suspected spine injury?

_____ a. Jaw-thrust
_____ b. Head tilt with full extension
_____ c. Sniffing position
_____ d. Head tilt with slight extension

5. The recommended maximum time allowed for suctioning an infant's airway is _____________ seconds.

_____ a. 5
_____ b. 10
_____ c. 15
_____ d. 20

6. Rigid suction catheters are best suited for suctioning the:

_____ a. nose of infants.
_____ b. mouth of an adult patient.
_____ c. nose of an adult patient.
_____ d. mouth of an infant.

7. Ventilating a patient with a bag-mask device is best if performed:

_____ a. by a single rescuer.
_____ b. on responsive patients.
_____ c. by two rescuers.
_____ d. in the prone position.

8. Which one of the following maneuvers is most appropriate for opening the airway of a child with no suspected spine injury?

_____ a. modified chin lift
_____ b. head-tilt/chin-lift
_____ c. jaw-thrust with slight extension
_____ d. cross-finger technique

9. Which one of the following best represents the most appropriate personal protective equipment for suctioning a patient?

_____ a. Gloves and face mask
_____ b. Gloves and gown
_____ c. Gloves and eye protection
_____ d. Gloves, mask, and eye protection

10. An appropriate liter-flow rate for a nonrebreather mask is _____________ L/minute.

_____ a. 6
_____ b. 8
_____ c. 15
_____ d. 30

Critical Thinking

1. How can you determine if the flow rate on a nonrebreather mask is adequate for the patient's condition?

2. A nonrebreather mask and a cannula are sometimes referred to as "passive" delivery devices. Explain what is meant by "passive" and how these devices differ from the demand-valve and the bag-mask device.

3. Explain why a patient on a nonrebreather mask is not receiving a breathable concentration of 100% oxygen.

Case Studies

Case Study 1

You have responded to a scene where a motorcycle has impacted a guardrail at a high rate of speed. The patient is unresponsive and lying face up. His helmet was properly removed by firefighters at the scene, and he has an obvious open fracture of the lower left leg. Your primary assessment finds the man's respirations to be 8 and shallow, and you can hear gurgling as he breathes.

1. What is your first priority for this patient?

2. What will you do to address that priority?

3. What device will you use to ventilate this patient?

Case Study 2

You have responded to a possible overdose at a homeless shelter. Upon arrival you find an approximately 30-year-old female lying on the bathroom floor with some vomit near her mouth. She is breathing approximately 10 times per minute and very shallow.

1. What method will you use to open this woman's airway and why?

2. Will you need to provide assisted ventilations for this patient? If so, what device will you use?

The Last Word

It cannot be overstated how important a patent airway and adequate ventilations are. Once it has been determined that the scene is safe, those two things become your top priority.

The use of airway adjuncts will assist you in maintaining an open airway, but they must be used in conjunction with close monitoring of the airway.

As an EMT you have several options for ventilating a patient with inadequate or absent respirations. Whenever possible, it is strongly suggested that you use supplemental oxygen when ventilating a patient. Supplemental oxygen increases the concentration available to the patient and helps compensate for inadequate perfusion caused by illness and injury.

Constant-flow delivery devices such as the nonrebreather mask and the nasal cannula are passive devices and require the patient to be moving air adequately on his own in order to benefit from them.

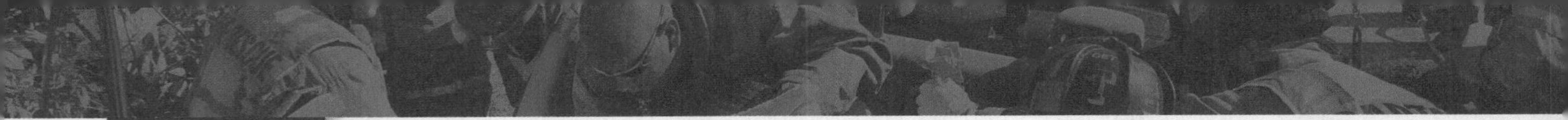

14 Performing a Secondary Assessment

Education Standards

Assessment: Secondary assessment, monitoring devices, reassessment

Competencies

Applies scene information and patient assessment findings to guide emergency management.

Objectives

After completion of this lesson, you should be able to:

14-1 Define key terms introduced in this chapter.

14-2 Explain the importance of developing a systematic approach to patient assessment.

14-3 Describe the four main components of the patient assessment.

14-4 Differentiate the medical patient from a trauma patient.

14-5 State the purpose of the secondary assessment.

14-6 Differentiate the common signs of a stable patient, unstable patient, and patient who is at risk for becoming unstable.

14-7 Differentiate anatomical and systems approaches to patient assessment and state when each is used.

14-8 Differentiate a rapid secondary assessment from a focused secondary assessment and state when each might be used.

14-9 Describe the steps for conducting a rapid secondary assessment for a medical patient.

14-10 Describe the steps for conducting a focused secondary assessment for a medical patient.

14-11 Discuss obtaining a history during the secondary assessment, including use of the SAMPLE and OPQRST mnemonics.

14-12 Differentiate significant from nonsignificant MOIs.

14-13 Describe the steps for conducting a rapid secondary assessment for a trauma patient.

14-14 Describe the steps for conducting a focused secondary assessment for a trauma patient.

14-15 State the purpose of reassessment and when it should be performed.

14-16 List the elements of a reassessment.

Key Terms

BP-DOC p. 394
chief complaint p. 376
crepitus p. 394
distention p. 385
focused secondary assessment p. 382
guarding p. 385
interventions p. 378
jugular vein distention (JVD) p. 385
mechanism of injury (MOI) p. 391
medical assessment p. 377
multisystem trauma p. 393
National Trauma Triage Protocol p. 378
nonsignificant mechanism of injury p. 393
paradoxical movement p. 396
pertinent past medical history p. 387
rapid secondary assessment p. 382
reassessment p. 400
referred pain p. 388
secondary assessment p. 377
significant mechanism of injury p. 378
stable p. 377
stoma p. 385
subcutaneous emphysema p. 396
trauma assessment p. 376
unstable p. 377

Introduction

Good patient care is directly related to a good patient assessment. In other words, if your assessment is thorough and appropriate, it is likely that the care you will be providing will be appropriate as well. If the assessment is poor, it stands to reason that the care provided will be less than optimal. In this chapter, you will be introduced to the concepts related to patient assessment for the medical patient and for the trauma patient.

EMERGENCY DISPATCH

"He isn't normally like this," the elderly woman explained to Mike, an EMT for the city fire department. "He usually talks all of the time and is, you know, active." They were standing over the bed of 78-year-old Al Hernandez, who was watching them quietly with a pleasant look on his face.

"Mr. Hernandez, can you talk to me?" Mike said to him loudly. "Can you say something?"

The man simply stared up at Mike with the hint of a smile on his lips.

"So he normally responds when you ask him a question?"

"Oh, heavens, yes. Sometimes you can't shut him up!"

"Can he get out of bed?"

"Before this started he could. He played golf three times a week. Now he just lies in bed and doesn't say anything."

"How long has it been since he stopped talking?"

"Oh, about four days."

"Four days seems a long time to wait to call 911."

"Well," the old woman shrugged her shoulders. "I thought he would just get better."

Patient Assessment

Without question, the patient assessment is the foundational skill that all EMTs must learn and master. It requires hours of memorization and practice of the steps on simulated patients. One of the most important concepts to understand regarding your development of a good assessment is that it must be developed as a systematic routine.

14-2 Explain the importance of developing a systematic approach to patient assessment.

Regardless of the type of patient, developing a systematic approach to patient assessment is essential to ensuring that all of the steps of the assessment will be addressed and in the correct order. Developing a consistent approach and routine also will minimize wasted time and allow you to begin providing the appropriate care sooner.

There are four main components to a patient assessment, they are:

14-3 Describe the four main components of the patient assessment.

- Scene size-up
- Primary assessment
- Secondary assessment
- Reassessment

The scene size-up and the primary assessment are addressed in Chapter 12. This chapter focuses on the secondary assessment, which is further broken down into the rapid secondary assessment and the focused secondary assessment. A description of the final step in the assessment process—reassessment—follows.

It is important to understand that whether your patient is a trauma patient or a medical patient, you must complete a thorough primary assessment before moving on to a secondary assessment. It is the primary assessment where you will first identify and address most immediate life threats to the patient. In some instances you will be addressing issues revealed in the primary assessment all the way to the hospital and never complete a thorough secondary assessment. Your assessment and care will always be dependent on patient need.

Trauma vs. Medical Patient

14-4 Differentiate the medical patient from a trauma patient.

chief complaint the patient's complaint in his own words.

trauma assessment the part of the secondary assessment that is performed on a patient who has an injury.

While it can be argued that all patients have medical problems, the medical profession, including EMS, divides all patients into one of two fundamental categories. Those categories are based on whether the **chief complaint** is related to an illness (medical problem) or to an injury (trauma). While one can lead to the other, illness and injury are two very different problems.

Patients whose chief complaint is related to an illness such as difficulty breathing, chest pain, or headache are categorized as "medical" patients. Patients whose chief complaint is related to an injury are categorized as "trauma" patients. Simply stated, injury equals trauma and illness equals medical. This differentiation is important, because the specific assessment path you follow will be different for each type of patient.

The flowchart in Figure 14-1 ■ shows all of the components of a patient assessment for both medical and trauma patients. As you will notice, both the **trauma assessment**

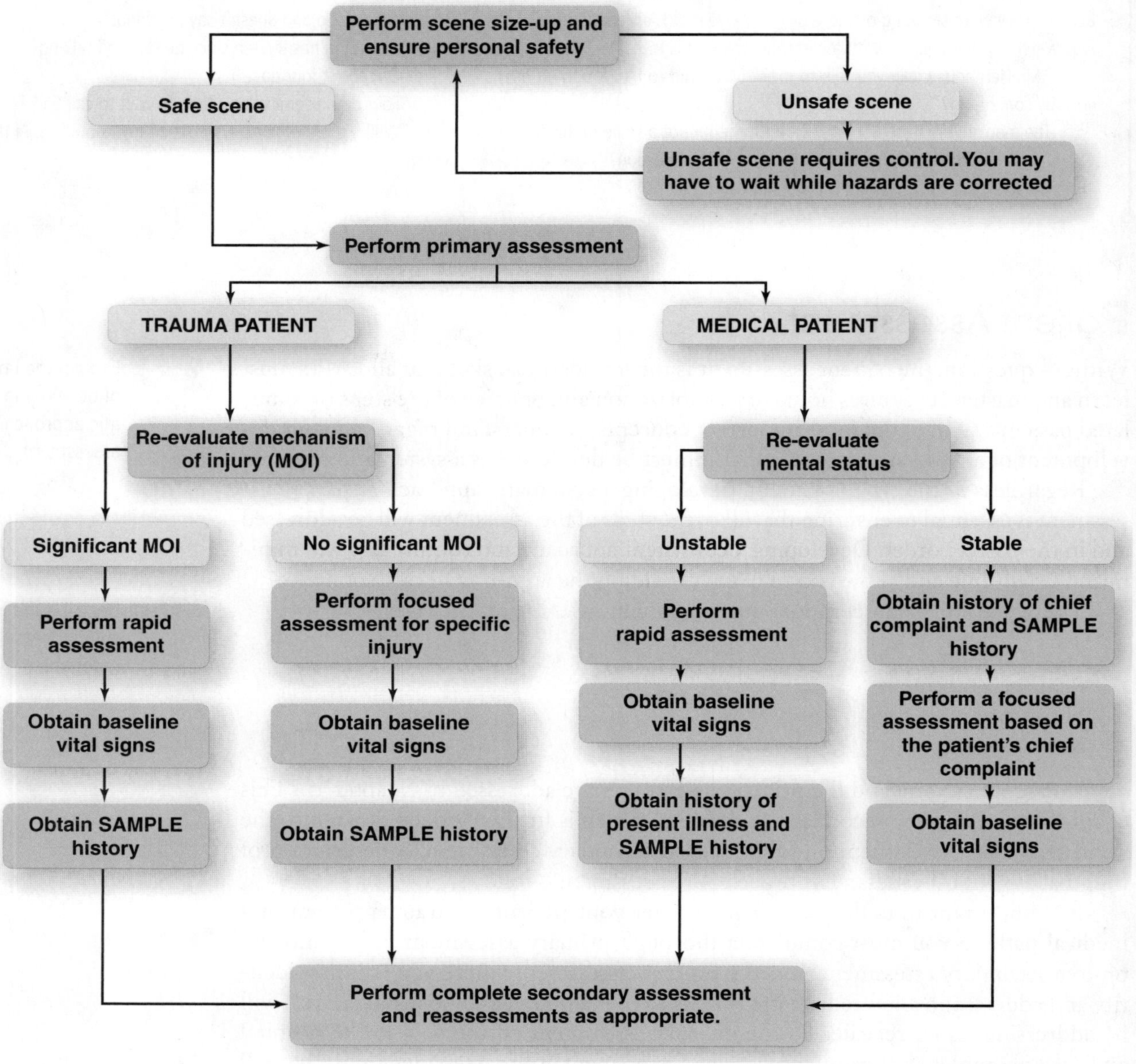

Figure 14-1 The specific path you use for your secondary assessment will differ, depending on the type of patient and other factors.

and the **medical assessment** begin with common elements performed in the same order each time. Those components are as follows:

- BSI precautions
- Scene size-up
- Primary assessment

Other elements, such as vital signs, history, secondary assessment, and reassessment, are common to both but may be performed in a slightly different order depending on the patient type.

It cannot be overstated how important each of the beginning components—BSI precautions, scene size-up, and the primary assessment—is to the well-being of both the EMT and the patient. Only after ensuring that you are protected, the scene is safe, and all aspects of the primary assessment are addressed will you move on to complete the secondary assessment of your patient.

medical assessment the examination of someone with an illness.

The Secondary Assessment

14-5 State the purpose of the secondary assessment.

The purpose of the secondary assessment is to perform a more detailed physical assessment and history of the patient. There are three main considerations when performing a secondary assessment. They are:

- Whether the patient's overall condition is **stable, unstable,** or potentially unstable
- If the patient has a medical complaint
- If the patient has a traumatic injury

stable a term used to describe a patient who is not likely to get worse in the immediate future.

unstable a term used to describe a patient who has a high likelihood of getting worse in the immediate future.

secondary assessment the component of the patient assessment that includes the physical examination and medical history of the patient.

Although patients vary widely in their chief complaints and how they present at the scene, there are two types of **secondary assessment,** or assessment paths: a rapid secondary assessment and a slower, more detailed focused secondary assessment. Those assessment paths apply to both medical and trauma patients. Consider the following examples:

- You are called to a man who was ejected from a vehicle in a high-speed collision. He is unresponsive. Your primary assessment reveals a rapid pulse and cool, moist skin.
- You are called to treat a child who has a laceration on her arm from a rough piece of metal at a playground. The bleeding is not severe and the patient is alert and responsive.
- You are called for a woman who was found by her husband to be "groggy" and with slurred speech.
- You are called for a patient who feels "a little weak" and has had the flu.

The patient ejected from the vehicle is likely to be in shock. The woman who has an altered mental status with slurred speech may have had a stroke (brain attack). Both are high-priority conditions that would require only essential on-scene assessment and care.

The child with the laceration and the general-weakness patient are most likely less severe and a more detailed on-scene assessment at a slower pace is warranted (although you should always be alert for patients in whom severity may be more difficult to recognize).

PERSPECTIVE

Mike—The EMT

How are you supposed to do a mental status evaluation, or gather any sort of good history, or even evaluate a chief complaint, when the patient can't communicate at all? And the way that he just smiled at me, I honestly thought that he was just being difficult! At first, that actually made me kind of angry until I realized that there was something really serious going on.

Stable vs. Unstable Patient

14-6 Differentiate the common signs of a stable patient, unstable patient, and patient who is at risk for becoming unstable.

One of the most significant decisions you will make at the conclusion of your primary assessment is whether the patient is stable or unstable. That determination of the overall status of your patient dictates the pace at which you believe he should be assessed and transported to the hospital.

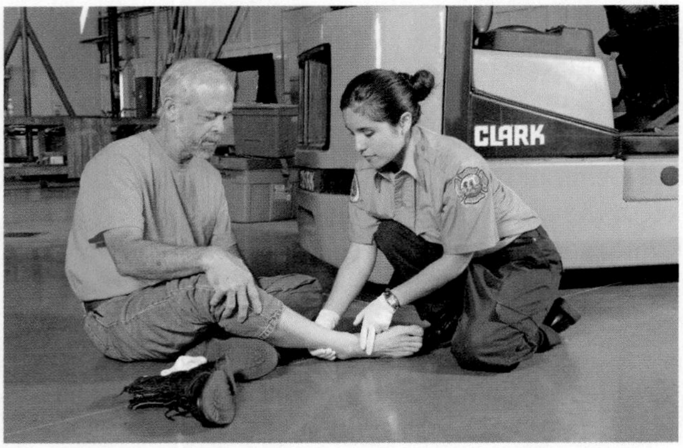

Figure 14-2 A stable patient has no immediate life threats and very little chance of becoming unstable.

A stable patient is one who has no immediate life threats and is in no immediate danger of getting worse or dying (Figure 14-2 ■). If that determination sounds as if it would be quite a challenge for the new EMT to make, you are correct. It is only through experience that one becomes comfortable making this decision. Even when you are confident that someone is "stable," he can become unresponsive or stop breathing without warning.

Signs of a stable patient include:

- Alert and oriented
- No major complaint of chest or abdominal pain
- Absence of recent trauma
- No uncontrolled bleeding or recent blood loss
- Normal breathing characteristics
- Vital signs that are within normal limits

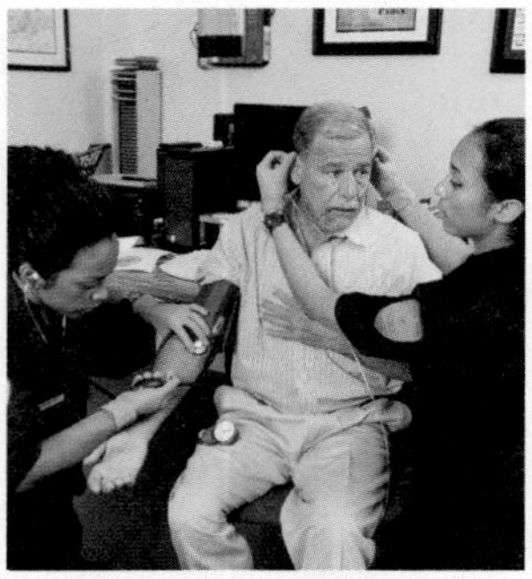

Figure 14-3 An unstable patient is one who is experiencing a significant medical event, such as a possible heart attack or a significant mechanism of injury.

significant mechanism of injury a type of mechanism of injury that has a strong likelihood for multiple organ system injury.

National Trauma Triage Protocol a systematic approach for assessing and categorizing trauma patients developed by the CDC. It is used to determine whether or not the patient should be transported directly to a trauma center.

interventions anything that the EMT does to comfort or provide care for the patient.

A patient who is stable can be cared for more slowly and thoroughly. Since his condition is not likely to get worse immediately, you have time to conduct a more thorough and detailed secondary assessment.

In contrast, an unstable patient is one who may be experiencing a potentially life-threatening problem or one who has suffered a **significant mechanism of injury** (Figure 14-3 ■). Consistent with the **National Trauma Triage Protocol,** signs of an unstable patient are as follows:

- Abnormally altered mental status (GCS <14)
- Significant chest or abdominal pain or discomfort
- Significant mechanism of injury, including physiological and anatomical considerations (Not all patients with a significant MOI will turn out to be unstable, but that ultimate determination is best made at the hospital after advanced evaluation.)
- Uncontrolled bleeding (seen or unseen)
- Moderate to severe breathing difficulty
- Abnormal vital signs

Determining that your patient is unstable will drive the urgency of your assessment and care. An unstable patient will be assessed and transported more rapidly to an appropriate receiving facility. You will *not* have time to complete a thorough physical exam and medical history or to provide valuable **interventions** before transport.

A patient who is often quite difficult to differentiate is the patient who appears stable but has a high likelihood for becoming unstable. These patients can be some of the most challenging because they can be difficult to identify. While it is impossible to always predict which patients are going to get worse, there are some telltale signs to look for. Be alert for the following possible indicators of a patient who may appear stable initially but who is at risk for becoming unstable:

- Unexplained changes in mental status
- Unexplained sudden changes in vital signs
- Patients who develop new (additional) complaints

CLINICAL CLUE

Stable vs. Unstable

The concept of stable vs. unstable can be a difficult one to fully understand as a new EMT. The ability to differentiate between the two will become second nature as you acquire more time and experience caring for actual patients. The bottom line is that you are trying to determine the urgency with which you will want to care for and transport your patient based on his immediate presentation (signs and symptoms).

STOP, REVIEW, REMEMBER!

Multiple Choice

For each question, place a check next to the correct answer.

1. It is essential for the EMT to develop a systematic approach to patient assessment because it helps to ensure that the:

_____ a. patient is transported to the appropriate facility.

_____ b. patient will receive the appropriate care sooner.

_____ c. proper personal protective equipment is used at all times.

_____ d. patient is always assessed from head-to-toe.

2. The four main components of patient assessment in order are:

_____ a. scene size-up, primary assessment, secondary assessment, and reassessment.

_____ b. scene size-up, primary assessment, focused assessment, and secondary assessment.

_____ c. scene size-up, primary assessment, vital signs, and secondary assessment.

_____ d. scene size-up, primary assessment, secondary assessment, and vital signs.

3. The first time that a patient's mental status is assessed is during the:

_____ a. scene size-up.

_____ b. primary assessment.

_____ c. rapid secondary assessment.

_____ d. focused secondary assessment.

4. You are caring for a patient who missed the last step on a short flight of stairs and twisted her ankle. This patient would initially be categorized as a _______________ patient.

_____ a. medical

_____ b. trauma

_____ c. stable

_____ d. unstable

5. You are caring for a patient who is complaining of chest pain similar to the pain he had with a previous heart attack. He is alert and does not complain of shortness of breath. You should categorize this patient as:

_____ a. critical.

_____ b. noncritical.

_____ c. stable.

_____ d. unstable.

Matching

Correctly identify the following signs and symptoms as either consistent with a stable patient or with an unstable patient. Write an "S" for stable or a "U" for unstable.

Sign or Symptom	Category
1. Alert and oriented	
2. No major complaint of chest or abdominal pain	
3. Significant MOI	

(continued on next page)

(continued)

Sign or Symptom	Category
4. Uncontrolled bleeding	
5. Difficulty breathing	
6. Absence of recent trauma	
7. Vital signs that are within normal limits	
8. Abnormal vital signs	
9. Altered mental status	
10. Normal breathing characteristics	

Critical Thinking

1. Describe why it is important to differentiate the condition of your patient as stable vs. unstable early in the assessment process.

2. Describe how you might manage a patient who was originally stable and suddenly became unstable.

PERSPECTIVE

Joanie—The Patient's Wife

Now, that firefighter was a nice enough boy, but he was somewhat annoying. He kept asking about Al's blood pressure history and if he had ever had a stroke or anything like that. He was just all over the map! And what was his little tiff about me waiting a few days to call? It doesn't matter if it was a few days or a few years. My Al was perfectly comfortable and happy! I think he was just having some trouble talking, but that kind of stuff happens when you get as old as we are, right?

Anatomical vs. Body System Approach

14-7 Differentiate anatomical and systems approaches to patient assessment and state when each is used.

There are two basic approaches to performing a patient assessment. The anatomical approach is the most common. It proceeds in a head-to-toe direction, addressing each area or region of the body in a systematic fashion. This approach is a standard part of the secondary assessment of the trauma patient used by EMTs as well as physicians in the emergency department.

The systems approach is used most commonly for the medical patient. It focuses on the specific body systems related to the chief complaint (Tables 14-1 and 14-2). For instance, if the chief complaint is chest pain, the EMT may focus her assessment on the cardiovascular system. Since chest pain also can be caused by injury to bone

TABLE 14-1 EVALUATION OF BODY SYSTEMS BY PATIENT COMPLAINT

PATIENT COMPLAINT	SYSTEMS YOU MAY CHOOSE TO EXAMINE
Difficulty breathing	Respiratory, cardiac
Chest pain or discomfort	Respiratory, cardiac
Altered mental status	Neurological, endocrine, cardiac
Abdominal pain or discomfort	Gastrointestinal, genitourinary
Allergic reaction	Respiratory, circulatory, immune

TABLE 14-2 BODY SYSTEM EXAMINATIONS

TYPE OF COMPLAINT	ADDITIONAL HISTORY	ELEMENTS OF PHYSICAL EXAM
Respiratory	Cough? Fever or chills? Have a prescribed bronchodilator? Pain or discomfort that worsens with deep breaths?	Lung sounds (presence and equality) Wheezing Indications of fluid in the lungs Oxygen saturation
Cardiovascular (cardiac and circulatory)	Chest pain, discomfort, or weakness? Have prescribed nitroglycerin? Taking aspirin? Dyspnea on exertion? Weight gain?	Lung sounds (presence and equality) Pulse Blood pressure Pulse pressure Jugular vein distention Pedal edema Sacral edema Oxygen saturation Orthostatic changes in vital signs
Neurological	Headache? Seizure? Difficulty speaking? Weakness on one side of the body?	Cincinnati Prehospital Stroke Scale (facial asymmetry, slurred or abnormal speech, arm drift) Mental status Pupils Oxygen saturation
Immunological/Allergic	Time of exposure? Time of symptom onset?	Stinger embedded in skin Hives (urticaria) Lung sounds (presence and equality) Edema of the face/neck Oxygen saturation
Abdominal/ Gastrointestinal	Fever? Nausea and vomiting? Diarrhea or constipation? Indications of blood in vomit or stool?	All four quadrants of the abdomen Signs of frank or digested blood in vomit or fecal material
Endocrine	Oral intake? Medication history? Recent illness?	Blood glucose Skin color, temperature, and condition

All exams include a thorough history and evaluation of vital signs and trends in vital signs.

and muscle, the EMT also should include the musculoskeletal system in the assessment to rule out pain related to injury.

With most patients, EMTs tend to begin with an anatomical approach and switch to a systems approach once they narrow down the problem.

The Rapid and Focused Secondary Assessments

14-8 Differentiate a rapid secondary assessment from a focused secondary assessment and state when each might be used.

rapid secondary assessment the part of the secondary assessment that is performed on unstable patients and on patients who have sustained a significant mechanism of injury.

focused secondary assessment the part of the secondary assessment that is performed on stable medical and trauma patients.

The first major decision that needs to be made in the assessment process comes immediately following the primary assessment. At this point you must decide between a rapid secondary assessment and a focused secondary assessment (Figure 14-4 ■). The decision as to which path to follow will be made based on your general impression, evaluation of the patient's primary assessment, chief complaint, history, and mental status.

- The **rapid secondary assessment** is used for unstable patients, whether medical or trauma. Though the path is the same for both, the specific signs and symptoms you will be looking for differ slightly.
- The **focused secondary assessment** is used mostly on stable patients, whether medical or trauma. It is designed to focus in on the chief complaint (medical patient) or injury (trauma patient). The focused secondary assessment is much more detailed than the rapid secondary assessment, and includes a thorough medical history.

Performing a Rapid Secondary Assessment (Medical Patient)

The primary purpose of the rapid secondary assessment is to quickly identify any important signs and symptoms not already addressed by the primary assessment. It involves a rapid head-to-toe physical examination that identifies obvious signs and symptoms related to the patient's condition.

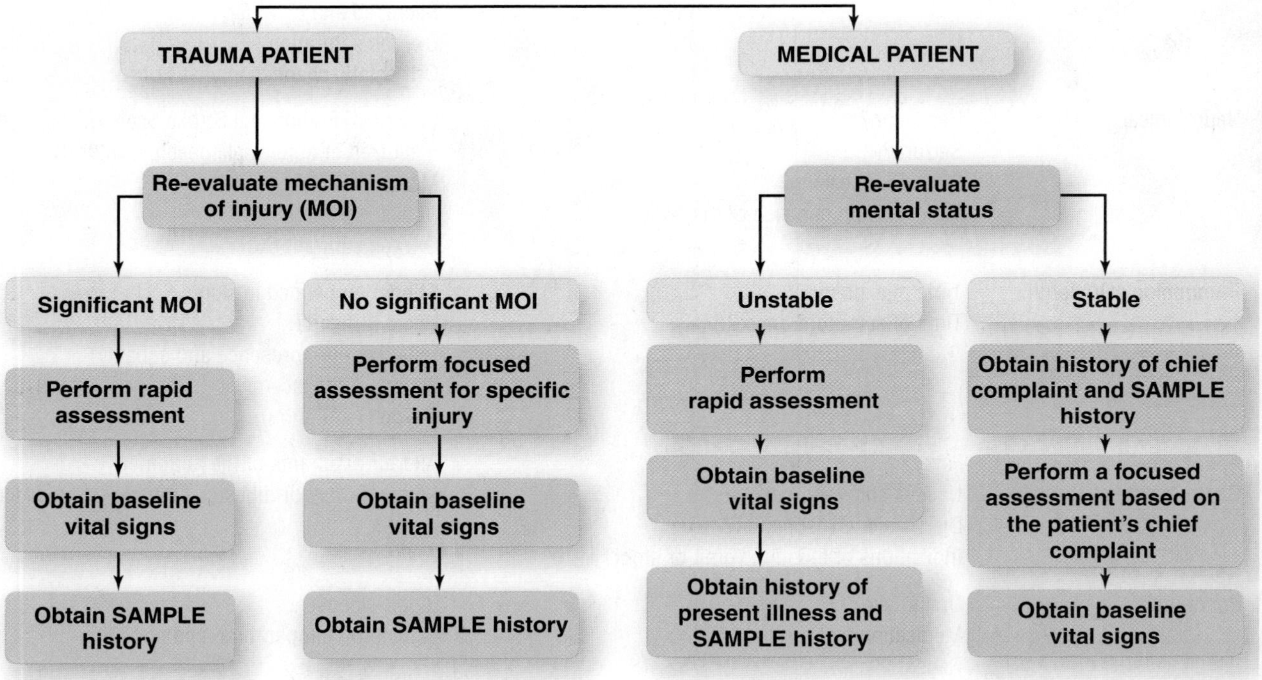

Figure 14-4 Secondary assessment paths differ slightly between medical and trauma patients.

SCAN 14-1 Rapid Secondary Assessment (Medical Patient)

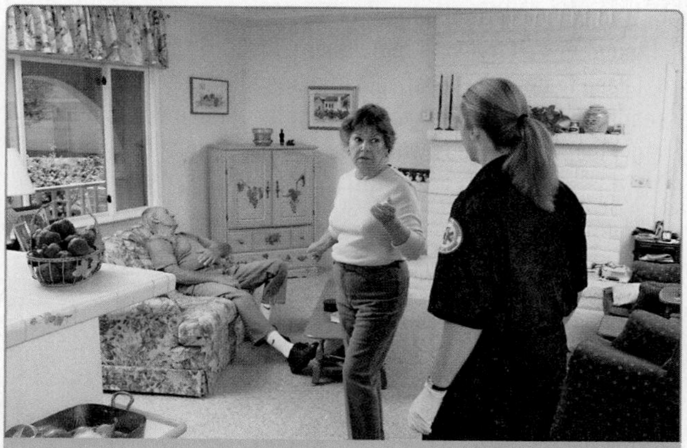

14-1-1 Perform a scene size-up as you approach the scene.

14-1-2 Perform a primary assessment and care for immediate life threats.

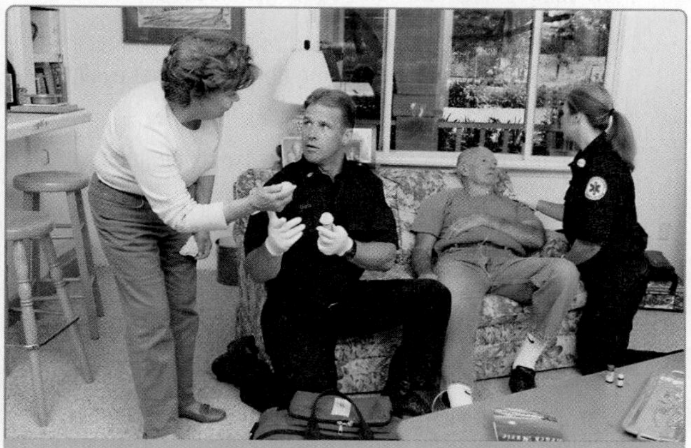

14-1-3 Obtain a chief complaint and make a stable/unstable determination.

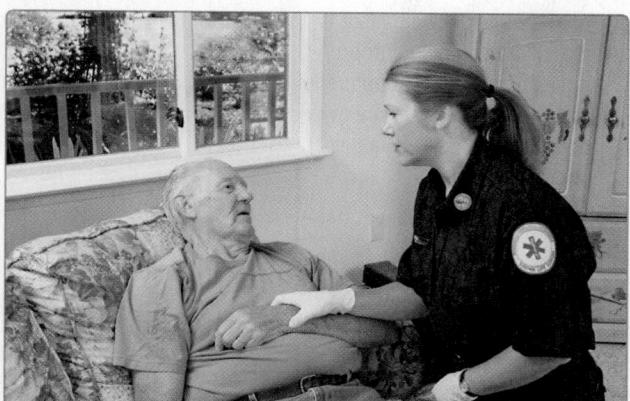

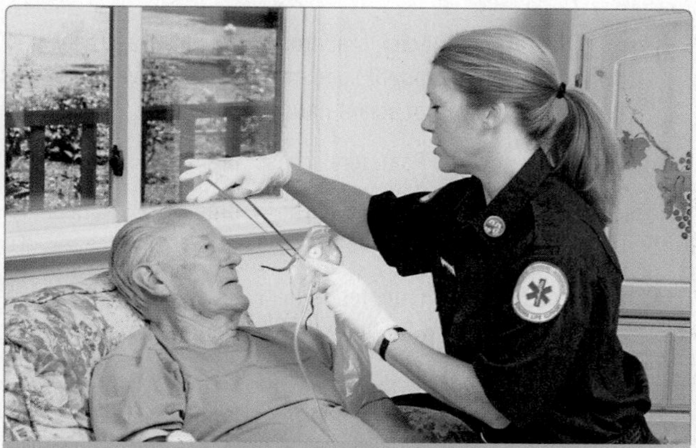

14-1-4 Apply oxygen and prepare for transport.

In the rapid secondary assessment the areas examined are the head, neck, chest, abdomen, pelvis, back, and extremities. If you are caring for what appears to be a medical patient, but you cannot positively rule out an injury to the head, neck, or spine, you must maintain appropriate spinal precautions.

You will be looking for any sign of possible illness (Scan 14-1). When something is discovered, you must decide if it is life threatening or not. For those signs that you suspect could be life threatening, you must stop your exam and provide the indicated care. For non-life-threatening signs, you may proceed with your exam and provide the indicated care when appropriate.

14-9 Describe the steps for conducting a rapid secondary assessment for a medical patient.

To proceed with the rapid secondary assessment (medical patient) in a head-to-toe direction, follow the guidelines listed below. (See also Table 14-3.)

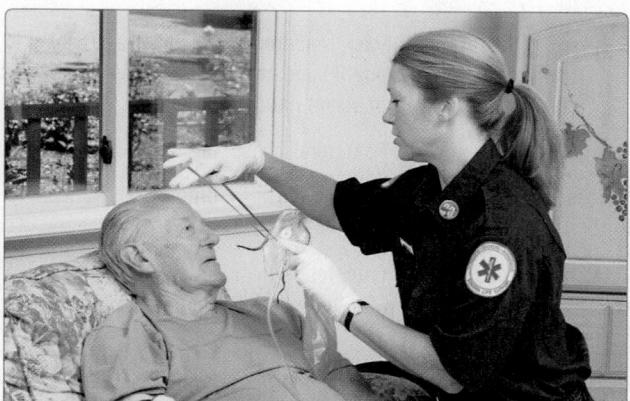

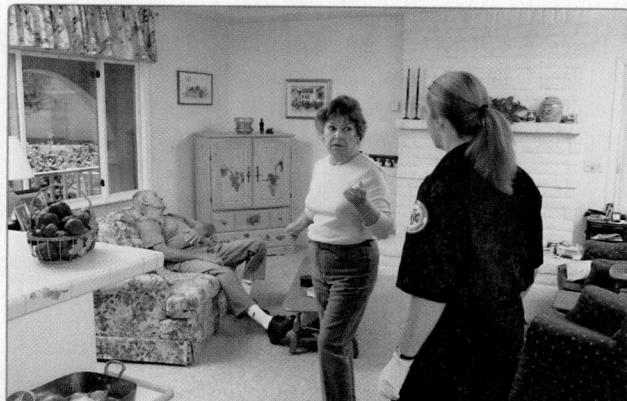

CLINICAL CLUE

Airway

Keep in mind that the airway of an unresponsive patient is at risk of becoming compromised at any time. Continue to monitor the patient's airway and breathing status throughout your exam.

PERSPECTIVE

Mike—The EMT

So here was my conundrum. Al was conscious. His eyes moved, he smiled, he seemed like he was in there, if you know what I mean. I would consider him more or less responsive but he just couldn't communicate with me at all. I found myself trying to remember if my EMT class ever covered a situation like this. It's weird. I keep finding these patients that don't fit neatly into one category or another. It's just another reminder for me to keep focusing on the fundamentals of caring for patients because it's easy to get lost in the weeds when you run into a situation that just doesn't fit.

TABLE 14-3 ELEMENTS OF A SECONDARY ASSESSMENT FOR A MEDICAL PATIENT

AREA/REGION	WHAT	HOW
Head (cranium and scalp)	Pain, tenderness, symmetry, and scars	Run your gloved hands over the scalp and through the hair.
Face	Pain, tenderness, equality of facial muscles	Palpate the face, forehead, and jaw and ask the patient to show you his teeth. Look for equality of facial expression.
Eyes	Pain; tenderness; equality, reactivity, and size of pupils; pink moist conjunctiva; yellow discoloration of sclera (jaundice)	Observe the pupils, using an appropriate light source. Expose the conjunctiva by pulling down the lower eyelid.
Ears	Pain, tenderness, drainage	Observe for drainage of blood or cerebrospinal fluid.
Nose	Pain, tenderness, drainage, nasal flaring	Observe for drainage. Flaring of the nostrils may be a sign of respiratory distress.
Mouth	Pain, tenderness, loose/broken teeth (dentures), foreign material, pink moist mucosa	Observe for damage to the teeth. Remove anything that may cause an obstruction, such as blood or loose dentures. Observe for pink moist mucosa.
Neck	Pain, tenderness, jugular vein distention, accessory muscle use, medical identification jewelry, stoma, scars	Observe for jugular vein distention. Note any retractions above the clavicles.
Chest	Pain, tenderness, chest rise and fall, subcutaneous emphysema, breath sounds, scars, rashes	Palpate the chest with both hands feeling for equal rise and fall, subcutaneous emphysema, listen for equal breath sounds.
Abdomen	Pain, tenderness, distention, rigidity, guarding, scars, and rashes	Palpate each quadrant of the abdomen with both hands. Observe the patient's face for signs of grimacing and note body language for evidence of guarding.
Pelvis	Pain, tenderness, and wetness	Observe for signs of wetness that may be blood or urine.
Legs	Pain; tenderness; distal circulation, sensation and motor function; scars, track marks; medical identification jewelry; edema	Palpate each leg with both hands, assess distal pulses, sensation, and push/pull of both feet simultaneously.
Arms	Pain, tenderness, distal circulation, sensation, and motor function, scars, track marks, medical identification jewelry, edema	Palpate each arm with both hands, assess distal pulses, sensation, and squeeze both hands simultaneously to perform the grip test.
Back	Pain, tenderness, subcutaneous emphysema, scars, and rashes	Palpate as much of the back as you can with both hands, feeling for subcutaneous emphysema. If appropriate, roll the patient and palpate and observe the entire back and buttocks.

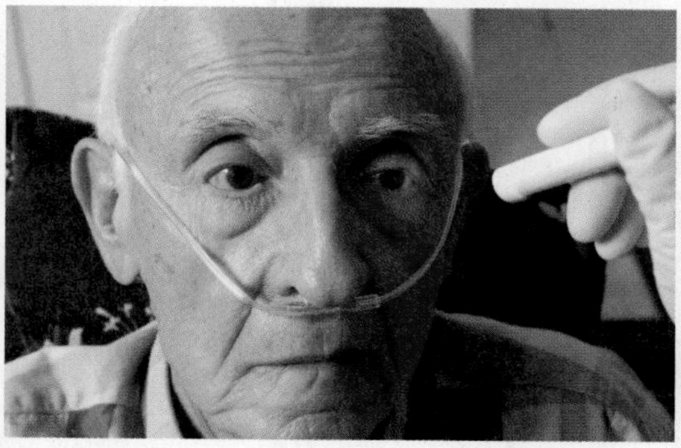

Figure 14-5 Inspect the pupils for equality and reactivity to light.

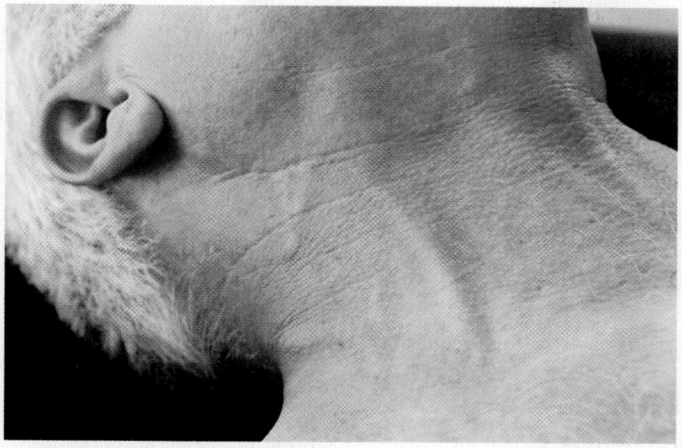

Figure 14-6 Jugular vein distention.

- ***Head.*** Palpate and inspect the head for symmetry and scars. Remember to maintain stabilization of the cervical spine if you suspect any possibility of trauma. While you may not expect to find trauma on a medical patient, always be on the lookout for signs of trauma. Your patient may have fallen several days to weeks prior to you being called. Look for any abnormality of the head such as bumps, bruises, healing wounds, or depressions. Then inspect the mouth and nose for obstruction. Note the color of the oral mucosa. Inspect the ears for drainage. Check the pupils for equality and reactivity to light (Figure 14-5 ▪).
- ***Neck.*** Expose, inspect, and palpate the neck for a **stoma** (breathing hole) and evidence of **jugular vein distention (JVD)** (Figure 14-6 ▪). Distention of the neck veins is an abnormal finding in most patients and may be an indication of heart failure (right-sided or late left-sided). Inspect for medical identification jewelry. Look for scars, which may provide clues regarding prior medical history.

stoma a surgical opening at the anterior neck.

jugular vein distention (JVD) an abnormal bulging of the neck veins commonly caused by a compromise of the circulatory system.

PRACTICAL PATHOPHYSIOLOGY

The assessment of the jugular veins is an indirect indicator of the status of the cardiopulmonary system. It is most often an indicator of right-sided heart failure. When assessing a patient for the presence of jugular vein distention, you must have the patient in a semi-sitting position (between 30 and 45 degrees), because it is normal to see such distention in patients who are supine.

CLINICAL CLUE

Scars

Always be on the lookout for scars as you expose and visually inspect the body. Scars may be a sign of prior injury or surgery. For example, many patients with a cardiac history have the classic "zipper" scar down the center of the sternum, indicating a history of open heart surgery. It is always appropriate to ask the history behind a particular scar.

- ***Chest.*** Expose, inspect, and palpate the chest for equal rise and fall, retractions, rash, and scars. Assessment of the chest also should include bilateral auscultation of breath sounds. You must expose the chest to see retractions, which are most obvious on pediatric patients and thin adults. Retractions are a sign of moderate to severe respiratory distress. Always be on the lookout for any sign of rash because it may be a sign of underlying infection or allergic reaction.
- ***Abdomen.*** Expose, inspect, and palpate the abdomen for **distention,** tenderness, rigidity, **guarding,** scars, rash, or pulsating masses (Figure 14-7 ▪). Grimacing and moaning are also indications that the patient is experiencing pain. A normal abdomen is soft and nontender when palpated. A rigid abdomen may be a sign of pain (guarding) and possible internal bleeding. Distention may be a sign of internal swelling, gas buildup, or tumor growth. Use a systematic approach to palpate all four quadrants of the abdomen. If the patient reports pain in a specific quadrant, palpate that quadrant last. If you feel the presence of a pulsating mass, stop applying pressure, because it may be an indication of an abdominal aortic aneurysm.

distention the state of being stretched beyond normal dimensions.

guarding the act of contracting the abdominal muscles in response to pain.

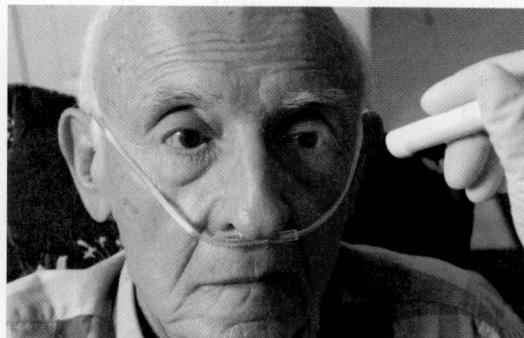

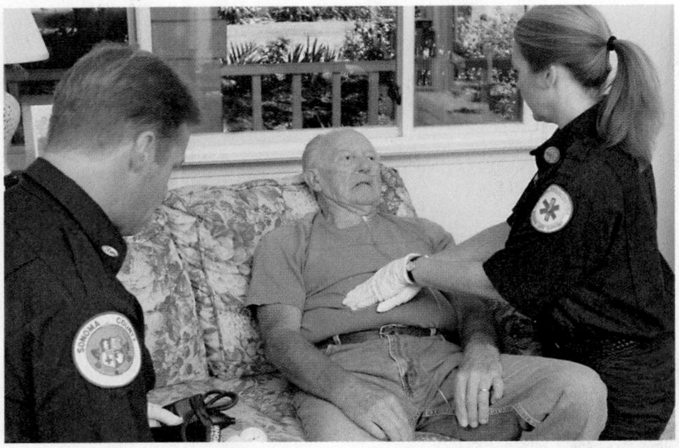

Figure 14-7 Look at the patient's face as you palpate the abdomen with both hands.

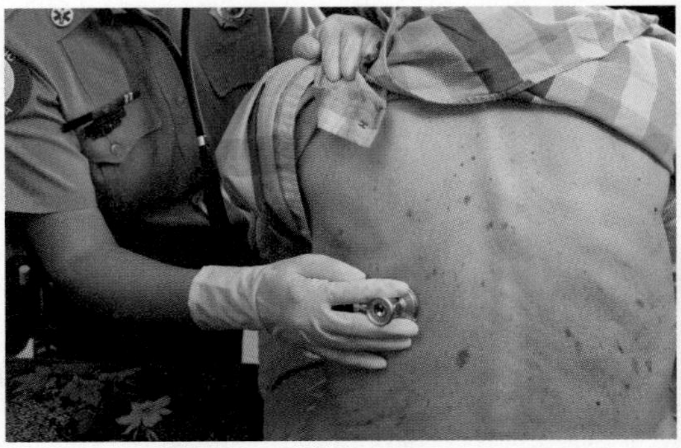

Figure 14-8 Expose and inspect the back for scars and rashes. Auscultate lung sounds.

CLINICAL CLUE

Palpating the Abdomen

When inspecting the abdomen, expose as much of the area as possible while maintaining the patient's modesty. Use both hands, one on top of the other, and press down slowly and firmly in each quadrant. Maintain eye contact with the patient as you palpate. Note any sign of wincing or grimacing, which may indicate the presence of pain.

- ***Pelvis.*** Palpate and inspect the pelvis for evidence of wetness that may be caused by blood or loss of bladder control.
- ***Back.*** Palpate and inspect the back for rash and scars (Figure 14-8 ▪). If necessary, roll the patient to perform a complete assessment of the back. Auscultate lung sounds while you have the back exposed.
- ***Extremities.*** Palpate and inspect each extremity as appropriate. Assess each for circulation, sensation, and motor function (CSM). When evaluating motor function, do so with both hands simultaneously and both feet simultaneously (Figure 14-9 ▪). This will allow you to detect slight differences in strength from one side to the other. Assess for the presence of medical identification jewelry, track marks, scars, and edema of the feet and ankles (pedal edema).

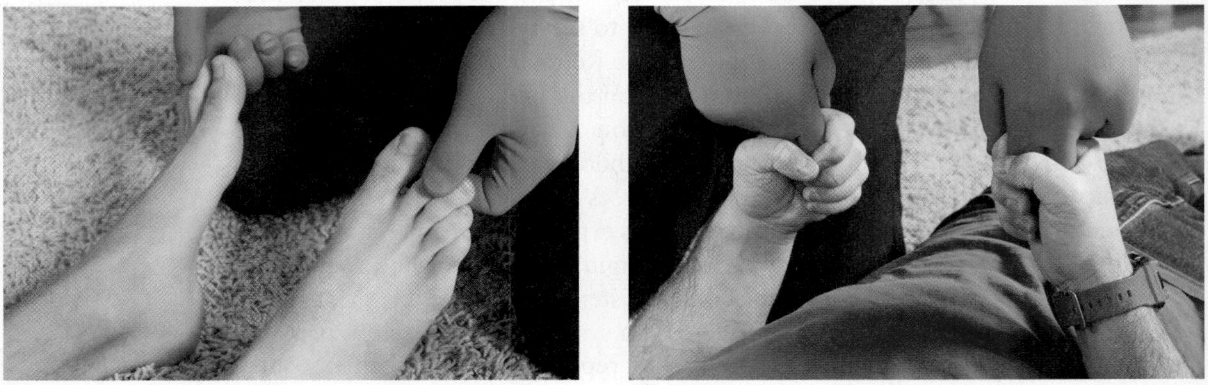

(A) (B)

Figure 14-9 Inspect circulation and sensation in the feet and hands.

If at any point during the rapid secondary assessment you discover what could be a life-threatening injury or condition, you must stop the exam and care for the problem immediately. It is important to remember that all potential life threats must be addressed as they are found.

CLINICAL CLUE

Assessing the Extremities

Not all one-sided weakness is caused by a stroke. Keep in mind that when assessing motor function of the extremities, it is common for pain to be the cause of weakness on one side or the other. When assessing strength of the hands and feet, ask the patient if it is painful to squeeze or push. If so, ask where the pain is and inspect the site of pain if you have not already done so.

Performing a Focused Secondary Assessment (Medical Patient)

When caring for medical patients who are stable, you will perform a focused secondary assessment based on the chief complaint (Figure 14-10 ■). For instance, if your patient has difficulty breathing or chest pain, you would focus your assessment on the signs and symptoms related to the chest pain or difficulty breathing and not waste time completing an exam of the entire body. Keep in mind that it is always good practice to perform a thorough assessment of the entire patient when time allows.

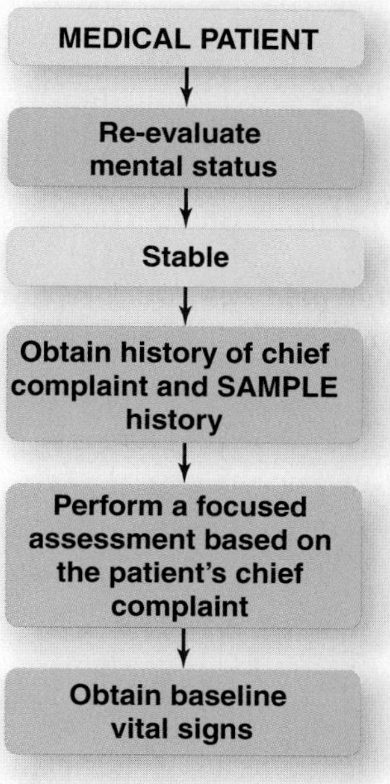

Figure 14-10 The focused secondary assessment path for the medical patient.

14-10 Describe the steps for conducting a focused secondary assessment for a medical patient.

You will use specific components of the secondary assessment that are related to your patient's chief complaint to guide your focused assessment.

During the focused assessment, you will first obtain a detailed history from the patient. The history will include information about the current problem as well as any previous medical issues that may be pertinent.

CLINICAL CLUE

Medical History

In most cases, obtaining a medical history directly from the patient is preferred. In other cases you must rely on family members or caregivers to provide a history. One of the reasons you will want to obtain a history from patients sooner rather than later is because they may become altered or unresponsive, making it impossible to get information from them.

The SAMPLE History

14-11 Discuss obtaining a history during the secondary assessment, including use of the SAMPLE and OPQRST mnemonics.

The core of the focused secondary assessment of the medical patient is a detailed medical history. Note that for the responsive medical patient, the history is obtained first, before the physical exam and vital signs. This is in contrast to the unresponsive medical patient for whom the history is obtained later in the process.

One commonly used tool to assist the EMT in completing a detailed medical history is the acronym SAMPLE. As you may recall from Chapter 9, each letter of the word represents a specific element of a good patient history—signs and symptoms, allergies, medications, **pertinent past medical history,** last oral intake, and events leading to the injury or illness. Each element requires specific questions that should

pertinent past medical history a patient's past illnesses and medical problems that pertain to the current event.

be asked during your history taking. The SAMPLE elements and questions are as follows:

S—Signs and symptoms. Assess or reassess any signs and symptoms relating to the chief complaint. One way to begin is by asking, "Can you tell me where you hurt?" Inspect the areas the patient mentions for any obvious signs of illness or injury. After examining the first painful location, ask if there are any others and inspect those as appropriate. Ask about **referred pain.**

referred pain pain that is perceived at a site other than that of the painful stimulus.

PRACTICAL PATHOPHYSIOLOGY

There are many common nerve pathways within the human body. Sometimes a patient can have an injury to one area and experience pain in a completely different area. This is commonly called "referred pain." For instance, a common example of referred pain is the pain a heart attack patient feels in the neck, jaw, or shoulders even though it is the myocardium that is experiencing the lack of adequate perfusion. Another common example of referred pain is the complaint of pain in the left shoulder, which is often related to an injured or ruptured spleen.

A—Allergies. All good patient histories include information about known allergies. This is important for several reasons. It may be the cause of the patient's chief complaint or he may be allergic to a medication he might be given later at the hospital. Ask about all known allergies, including allergies to medications, food, and the environment (bites, stings, plants). If the patient has a known allergy, ask about the last time he had a reaction and what the reaction was like (a minor reaction or more severe, requiring medical attention).

M—Medications. Ask the patient what medications he is currently taking. They can tell you the type of medical conditions for which the patient is being treated. Ask about both prescription and nonprescription medications, including those that do not necessarily pertain to a medical condition, such as birth control pills or nicotine patches. Also ask about medications from the recent past that he is no longer taking. Confirm he is taking his medications as prescribed. Ask for all the medications the patient is currently taking and place them in a paper bag for easy reference and transport to the hospital.

P—Pertinent past medical history. In many situations, the patient's chief complaint may relate to a past medical complaint or condition. Ask about previous or current medical conditions, surgeries, and injuries. Ask the patient if he has ever had similar symptoms in the past. Inform the physician at the hospital if this information is pertinent. Include as much detail as possible when transferring or documenting your care.

L—Last oral intake. Ask the patient what he last had to eat or drink. Should a patient require emergency surgery, the surgeons need to know the time and quantity of food intake. Stomach contents could be vomited during surgery.

E—Events leading to the injury or illness. What was the patient doing just prior to the event? For instance, if the chief complaint is chest pain, was the patient exerting himself prior to the pain or was he at rest? Or does the patient, perhaps, have no recollection of events prior to your arrival?

The OPQRST Mnemonic

Another mnemonic, or memory aid, that was introduced in Chapter 9 is OPQRST. It can help trigger questions about a patient's pain, discomfort, or difficulty breathing. Examples of questions you might ask for each letter of OPQRST are as follows:

O—Onset. "What were you doing when the pain began?" or "What were you doing when you first began to feel short of breath?"
P—Provocation. "Does anything you do make the pain better or worse?" or "Does it hurt to take a deep breath or when I push here?"
Q—Quality. "Can you describe how your pain feels?" or "Is it sharp or is it dull?" and "Is it steady or does it come and go?" Be careful not to put words in the patient's mouth. Instead provide him with choices and allow him to choose. Use the patient's own words when documenting the call or handing the patient off to the next level of care.
R—Region/radiation. "Can you point to your worst pain?" or "Does your pain move or radiate to another part of your body?" and "Do you feel pain anywhere else?"
S—Severity. A standard 1-to-10 scale is typically used to evaluate the severity of pain or discomfort. You might ask, "On a scale of 1 to 10, with 10 being the worst pain you have ever felt, how would you rate your pain right now?" You also may ask the patient to describe the severity of his pain when it first began, using the same scale. Later, ask the severity question again to see if the pain is getting better or worse.
T—Time. You will want to know how long the patient has been experiencing pain or discomfort. A question such as, "When did you first begin having pain today?" or "How long have you had this pain?" will usually suffice.

Your instructor or EMS system may have different or additional memory aids. Find the ones that work best for you.

CLINICAL CLUE

Pain vs. Tenderness

The terms "pain" and "tenderness" do not mean the same thing. Pain is a symptom and something the patient will describe or complain about when asked. Tenderness is a sign and will often appear during palpation of an area on the body.

STOP, REVIEW, REMEMBER!

Multiple Choice

For each question, place a check next to the correct answer.

1. A patient who is stable should receive which type of assessment?

_____ a. Focused secondary
_____ b. Focused primary
_____ c. Rapid secondary
_____ d. Rapid primary

2. Which one of the following represents the correct assessment path for a trauma patient who has sustained a significant mechanism of injury?

_____ a. Focused secondary assessment, vital signs, SAMPLE history
_____ b. Rapid secondary assessment, vital signs, SAMPLE history
_____ c. Focused secondary assessment, SAMPLE history, vital signs
_____ d. Rapid secondary assessment, SAMPLE history, vital signs

3. The _____________ approach to patient assessment involves a systematic head-to-toe examination of the patient.

_____ a. anatomical
_____ b. secondary
_____ c. systems
_____ d. focused

4. For which one of the following patients would a focused secondary assessment be most appropriate?

_____ a. Patient who was in a high-speed motor-vehicle collision
_____ b. Patient with an altered mental status
_____ c. Patient who is alert and oriented with a mild asthma attack
_____ d. Patient who fell down one flight of stairs

(continued on next page)

(continued)

5. You are caring for an elderly patient who is unresponsive on the floor following a seizure. He has a bleeding wound from the scalp. You should:

_____ a. immediately perform a rapid secondary assessment.

_____ b. stabilize the head and neck as you perform a primary assessment.

_____ c. move the patient to the stretcher while performing a primary assessment.

_____ d. apply oxygen and then perform a primary assessment.

Matching

Match the term on the left with the applicable definition on the right.

1. _____ Stoma
2. _____ Jugular vein distention
3. _____ Tenderness
4. _____ Distention
5. _____ Guarding
6. _____ Referred pain

A. Bulging of the neck veins

B. Pain that is felt in a location other than where the pain originates

C. Opening in the anterior neck that connects to the trachea

D. Condition of being stretched, inflated, or larger than normal

E. Sign that appears when the area being palpated is painful

F. Body defense mechanism, to prevent movement of an injured part

Critical Thinking

1. What are the indications for performing a rapid secondary assessment for a medical patient? Provide a description of a patient who would fit the criteria for this assessment.

____

____

____

____

2. List at least three findings you might observe when assessing the neck of a medical patient.

____

____

____

____

3. List at least three findings you might observe when assessing the abdomen of a medical patient.

____

____

____

____

Performing a Rapid Secondary Assessment (Trauma Patient)

Trauma patients are managed differently than most medical patients in the prehospital setting. Trauma to the body can result in injury to soft tissues, organ systems, and bones and in significant blood loss. For that reason, time is a critical factor in the survival of the trauma patient. As a general rule, it is recommended to limit on-scene time to 10 minutes or less when caring for trauma patients, especially those with serious injuries from a significant mechanism of injury. For many of these patients, the sooner they can get to definitive care the more likely it is that they will survive. The 10-minute rule serves as a guideline only and may not be possible with patients who need significant extrication.

The primary purpose of the rapid secondary assessment for the trauma patient is to quickly identify all areas of injury or suspected injury not already addressed by the primary assessment. It involves a rapid head-to-toe physical examination of the patient, looking for obvious signs of injury. Remember to maintain appropriate spinal precautions with all trauma patients. In most cases, trauma patients will be a high priority for transport. Consider the need for ALS backup or an ALS intercept if appropriate.

14-13 Describe the steps for conducting a rapid secondary assessment for a trauma patient.

Reevaluating the Mechanism of Injury

Evaluation of the **mechanism of injury (MOI)** is critical when caring for the trauma patient. You would make your first assessment of the MOI during the scene size-up and identify to the best of your ability any major MOI, such as a fall, motor-vehicle collision, blunt trauma, or penetrating injury (Figure 14-11 ▪). Now that you have completed the scene size-up and primary assessment, you must take a closer look at the specific factors involved in the MOI and make predictions about potential injury based on those factors.

14-12 Differentiate significant from nonsignificant MOIs.

mechanism of injury (MOI) the event or mechanism that caused the injury.

The following factors that should be assessed during the reevaluation of the MOI are contained in the National Trauma Triage Protocol (Figure 14-12 ▪) and are as follows:

- Falls
    - Adults: more than 20 feet (one story is equal to 10 feet)
    - Children: more than 10 feet or two to three times the height of the child
- High-risk auto crash
    - Intrusion: more than 12 inches at occupant site; more than 18 inches at any site
    - Ejection from vehicle (partial or complete)
    - Death in same passenger compartment
    - Vehicle telemetry data consistent with high risk of injury
- Auto vs. pedestrian/bicyclist thrown, run over, or with significant impact (more than 20 mph)
- Motorcycle crash at more than 20 mph
- All penetrating injuries to the head, neck, torso, and extremities proximal to the elbow or knee
- Flail chest
- Two or more proximal long bone fractures
- Crushed, degloved, or mangled extremity
- Amputation proximal to the wrist or ankle

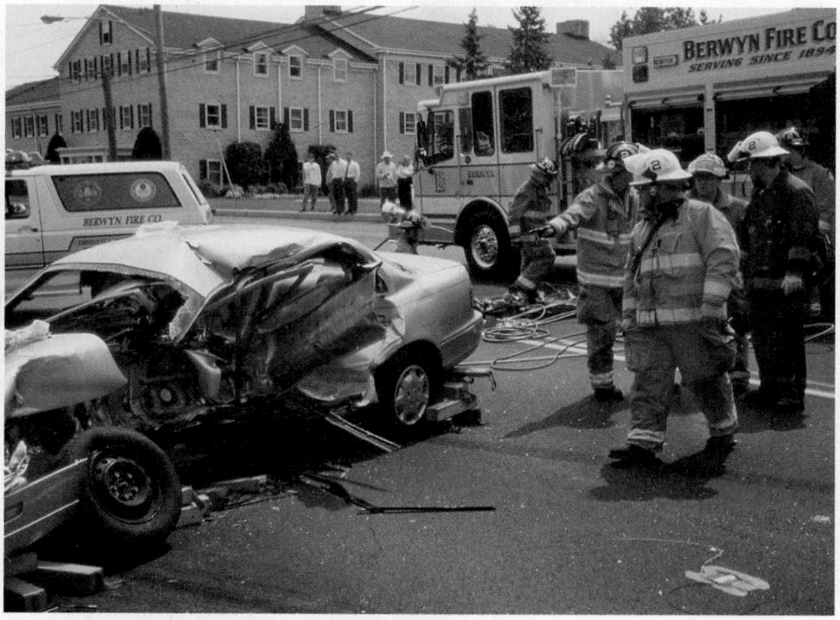

Figure 14-11 Vehicle collisions are a major cause of significant trauma. (© Edward T. Dickinson, MD)

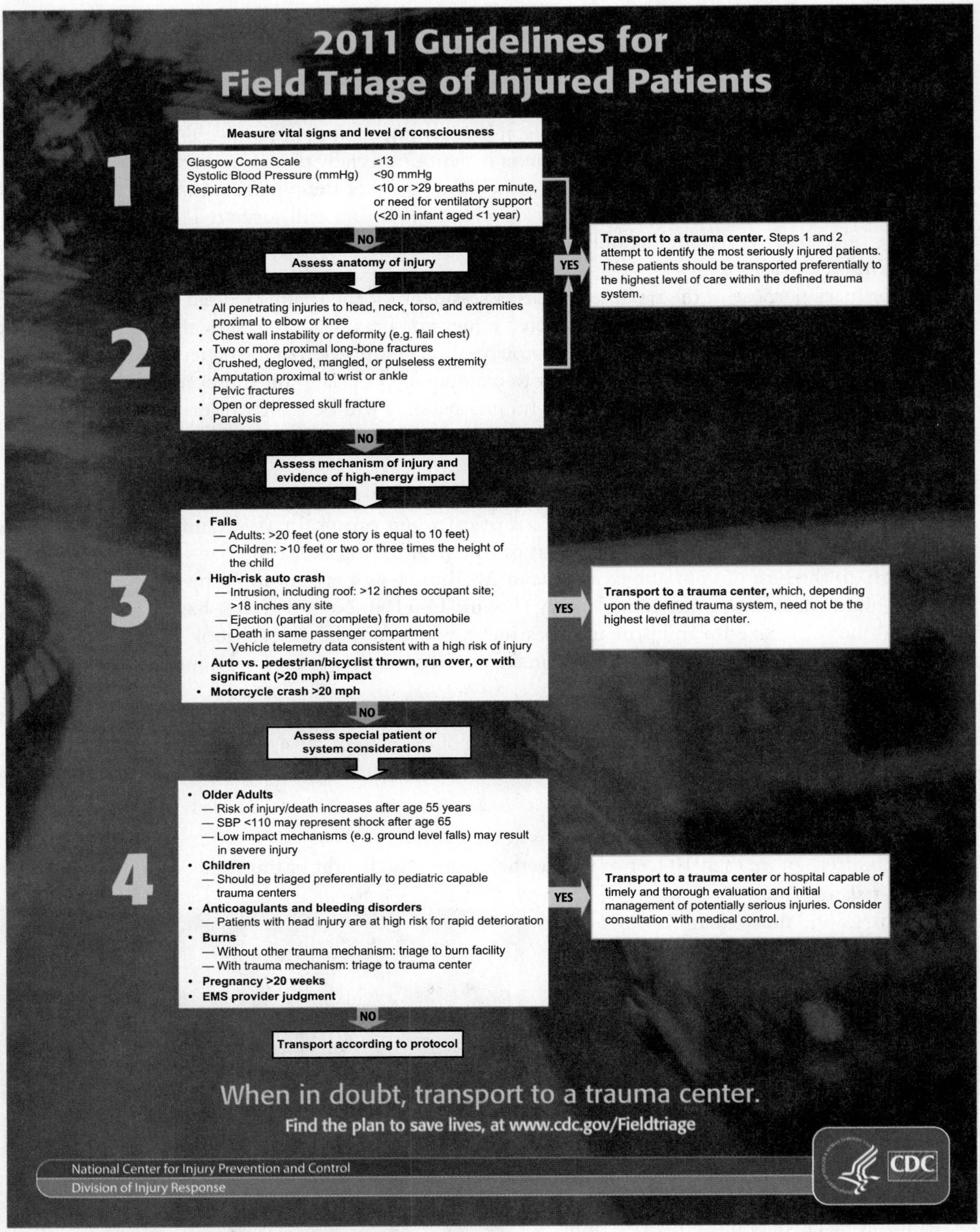

Figure 14-12 National Trauma Triage Protocol. (cdc.gov/Fieldtriage)

- Pelvic fractures
- Open or depressed skull fracture
- Paralysis

Other factors that should be assessed during the reevaluation of the MOI following a fall from height are surface on which the patient landed, position of the patient when he hit the ground (head, feet, or side first, for example), and anything struck on the way down.

CLINICAL CLUE

National Trauma Triage Protocol

The National Trauma Triage Protocol is a document developed by the federal Centers for Disease Control and Prevention (CDC) in consultation with many national organizations involved in trauma care. It is designed to assist prehospital providers in determining the most appropriate type of hospital to transport injured patients to based on vital signs, level of responsiveness, anatomy of injury, and mechanism of injury.

As you will notice when you study the trauma side of the patient assessment flowchart (Figure 14-13 ▪), you will find two parallel assessment paths for the trauma patient. The path that you should follow for a specific trauma patient will depend on the evaluation of one critical piece of information—the mechanism of injury. If the MOI is considered significant, you will follow the path on the left. If the MOI is not significant, you will follow the path on the right.

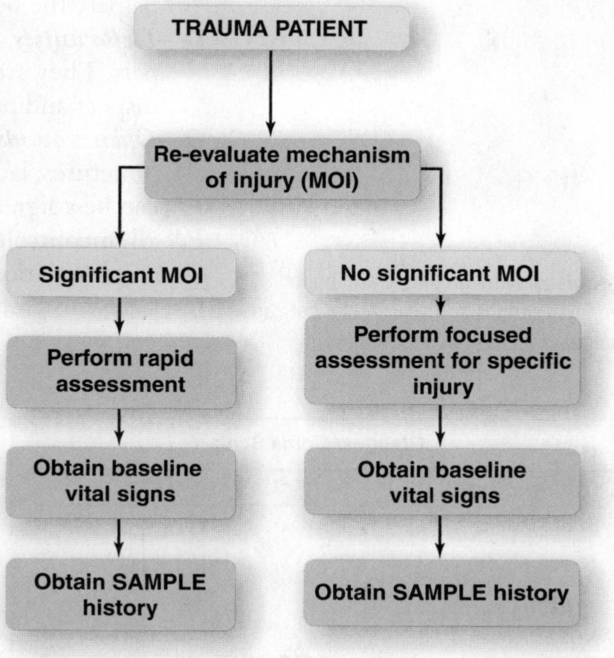

Figure 14-13 The secondary assessment paths for the trauma patient.

Significant Mechanism of Injury

To begin to understand what is meant by a significant MOI, you need to have at least a fundamental understanding of human anatomy. The majority of the body's vital organs are contained within the skull, chest, abdomen, and pelvis. Therefore, when those areas sustain injury, the vital organs that lie within them are at serious risk for damage. The most immediate risk is the loss of blood from tissue and vessel damage. In addition to physical damage to the vital organs, their function can become compromised. When one organ begins to fail, it creates a domino effect and other vital organs begin to fail as well.

A term often associated with victims of significant MOI is **multisystem trauma.** The term *multisystem* refers to the multiple organ systems that are generally affected by significant MOIs.

For a patient who has sustained a mechanism of injury that you suspect could have caused damage to the skull, chest, abdomen, or pelvis, you must consider this a significant MOI and follow the appropriate assessment path. The examples contained above in the National Trauma Triage Protocol are commonly considered significant, but are by no means the only mechanisms that could be considered significant. You must carefully evaluate and reevaluate the MOI and use good common sense when making a determination.

multisystem trauma the damage to multiple organ systems within the body caused by a mechanism of injury.

Nonsignificant Mechanism of Injury

Many patients will have suffered an injury due to a mechanism of injury that is not considered significant. A **nonsignificant mechanism of injury** is one that is isolated to a nonvital area of the body, such as an arm or a leg. While the injury will certainly be significant to the patient, it is not likely to represent a threat to life. Injuries that are isolated to arms and legs are almost always categorized as nonsignificant. One

nonsignificant mechanism of injury an injury with a very low likelihood of involving multiple organ systems.

exception to this rule is injury to both upper arms or both upper legs (thighs) at the same time.

The BP-DOC Mnemonic

BP-DOC an assessment mnemonic, or memory aid, used primarily for the trauma patient. The letters stand for bleeding, pain, deformity, open wounds, and crepitus.

The mnemonic, or memory aid, **BP-DOC** is a tool that can be used by the EMT to assist in remembering the most obvious signs of injury. The letters in BP-DOC stand for the following:

B—Bleeding. Identifying and controlling external bleeding can be difficult at times and must be something you are on the lookout for at all times. It is addressed in the primary assessment and should also be addressed in the secondary assessment. If you find severe uncontrolled bleeding, you must quickly manage it before moving on.

P—Pain. Pain is an obvious indication that something is wrong and possibly injured. Of course, not all patients will be able to tell you they have pain or will respond to pain. First ask the patient if he has pain, and then look for signs of pain as you palpate the body.

D—Deformities. A deformity is a deviation from the normal shape or size of a body part. They are typically caused by broken bones or soft-tissue swelling. You must inspect and palpate all areas of the body, looking for signs of deformity.

O—Open wounds. Inspect the body carefully for any sign of an open wound such as punctures, lacerations, avulsions, eviscerations, burns, and so on. An open wound can be a sign of both external and internal soft-tissue and organ damage. Control all uncontrolled bleeding and cover open wounds to minimize the possibility of contamination.

crepitus the grating, crackling, or popping sounds and sensations that can be heard and felt beneath the skin.

C—Crepitus. **Crepitus** is grating, crackling, or popping sounds and sensations that can be heard and felt beneath the skin. It is commonly associated with broken bone ends rubbing together and the sounds of air trapped beneath the skin. Those sounds and sensations become especially important during the assessment of the unresponsive patient because they can reveal a serious condition, even when the patient is unable to respond to pain.

To find the BP-DOC signs, you will need to expose the patient. That means removing or cutting away clothing in order to see and palpate the area or areas of the body you are assessing. Be sure to tell the patient what you are doing and offer reassurance as necessary. Protect the patient's privacy and take steps to prevent unnecessarily long exposure to cold. Document all appropriate findings.

Glasgow Coma Scale	
Eye Opening	
Spontaneous	4
To verbal command	3
To pain	2
No response	1
Verbal Response	
Oriented and converses	5
Disoriented and converses	4
Inappropriate words	3
Incomprehensible sounds	2
No response	1
Motor Response	
Obeys verbal commands	6
Localizes pain	5
Withdraws from pain (flexion)	4
Abnormal flexion in response to pain (decorticate rigidity)	3
Extension in response to pain (decerebrate rigidity)	2
No response	1

Figure 14-14 Glasgow Coma Scale.

The Glasgow Coma Scale

Once the primary assessment is completed and immediate life threats managed, a common and useful additional tool for determining mental status and patient response is the Glasgow Coma Scale (GCS) (Figure 14-14 ■). It uses three specific assessment findings to arrive at a score that can be used in your documentation and shared with other care providers. The best possible score is 15 and the lowest possible score is 3. A score of 3 indicates the absence of any response to the three GCS assessment areas: eye opening, verbal response, and motor response. The Glasgow Coma Scale score provides a more detailed and thorough assessment than the preliminary AVPU scale. (A more thorough discussion of the Glasgow Coma Scale can be found in Chapter 12.)

The Head-to-Toe Examination

Using appropriate personal protective equipment (PPE), inspect and palpate the following areas of the patient's body, looking for any sign of possible injury. When an injury is discovered, you must decide if it is life threatening or not. For those injuries that you suspect could be life threatening, you must stop your exam and provide the indicated care. For non-life-threatening injuries, you may proceed with your exam and provide the indicated care when appropriate.

The head-to-toe examination should proceed as described in the guidelines below. (Also see Table 14-4.)

TABLE 14-4 ELEMENTS OF A SECONDARY ASSESSMENT FOR A TRAUMA PATIENT

AREA/REGION	WHAT	HOW
Head (cranium and scalp)	BP-DOC	Run your gloved hands over the scalp and through the hair. Note any blood on your gloves.
Face	BP-DOC	Palpate the face, forehead, and jaw.
Eyes	BP-DOC; equality, reactivity, and size of pupils; pink moist conjunctiva (good perfusion)	Observe the pupils using an appropriate light source. Expose the conjunctiva by pulling down the lower eyelid.
Ears	BP-DOC, drainage, bruising behind the ears (Battle's sign)	Observe for drainage of blood or cerebrospinal fluid. Look behind the ears for bruising.
Nose	BP-DOC, drainage, singed nostrils, nasal flaring	Observe for drainage, evidence of smoke inhalation, or burning. Flaring of the nostrils may be a sign of respiratory distress.
Mouth	BP-DOC, loose or broken teeth (dentures), foreign material, pink moist mucosa	Observe for damage to the teeth. Remove anything that may cause an obstruction, such as blood or foreign material. Observe for pink moist mucosa.
Neck	BP-DOC, tracheal deviation, jugular vein distention, accessory muscle use, medical identification jewelry, stoma, scars	Observe for jugular vein distention, run thumb and forefinger along both sides of trachea to confirm proper alignment. Note any retractions above the clavicles.
Chest	BP-DOC, good chest rise and fall, subcutaneous emphysema, paradoxical movement, breath sounds, scars, rashes	Palpate the chest with both hands, feeling for soft spots (paradoxical movement) and crepitation (subcutaneous emphysema). Listen for equal breath sounds.
Abdomen	BP-DOC, distention, rigidity, guarding, scars, and rashes	Palpate each quadrant of the abdomen with both hands. Observe the patient's face for signs of grimacing and note body language for evidence of guarding.
Pelvis	BP-DOC, instability, and wetness	Palpate both sides of the pelvis gently with both hands. Press downward and inward gently. Observe for signs of wetness that may be blood or urine.
Legs	BP-DOC; distal circulation, sensation, and motor function; track marks; medical identification jewelry	Palpate each leg with both hands; assess distal pulses, sensation, and push/pull of both feet simultaneously.
Arms	BP-DOC; distal circulation, sensation, and motor function; track marks; medical identification jewelry	Palpate each arm with both hands, assess distal pulses, sensation, and squeeze both hands simultaneously to perform the grip test.
Back	BP-DOC, paradoxical movement, scars, and rashes	Palpate as much of the back as you can with both hands, feeling for soft spots (paradoxical movement) and crepitation (subcutaneous emphysema). If appropriate, roll the patient, maintaining c-spine precautions, and palpate and observe the entire back and buttocks.

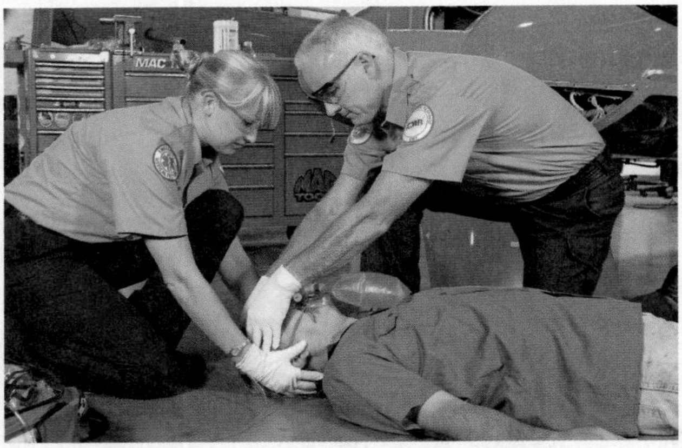

Figure 14-15 Use both hands to palpate and inspect the head.

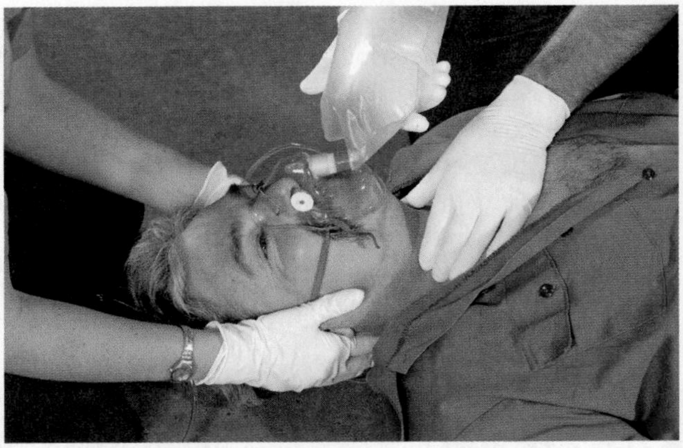

Figure 14-16 Expose and palpate the anterior and posterior neck.

- ***Head.*** Expose, inspect, and palpate the head and face for BP-DOC. Run your fingers through the hair, noting any evidence of blood (Figure 14-15 ▪). You must maintain stabilization of the cervical spine as you palpate and inspect. Inspect the mouth for evidence of obstruction and the ears for drainage. Assess the pupils for equality and reactivity to light.
- ***Neck.*** Expose, inspect, and palpate the anterior and posterior neck for BP-DOC, including tracheal deviation and jugular vein distention (JVD) (Figure 14-16 ▪). Tracheal deviation is the shifting of the trachea to one side of the neck most often caused by a buildup of severe pressure inside the chest due to traumatic chest injury. It can be assessed through palpation of the anterior neck. Jugular vein distention is the abnormal bulging of the neck veins of the anterior neck. It may be a sign of traumatic injury or a problem with the circulatory system.

Immediately following assessment of the neck, apply an appropriate cervical collar in cases of blunt trauma. Tracheal deviation and JVD may be signs of significant chest injury. Assess for wounds on the neck and immediately control any severe bleeding.

PRACTICAL PATHOPHYSIOLOGY

Deviation of the trachea from the midline to one side or the other is a sign of significant injury. It may be caused by direct trauma to the trachea or by injury to a lung. Injury to a lung can cause air to become trapped inside the chest cavity (tension pneumothorax). As the pressure builds, it can cause the structures inside the chest to be pushed to one side, thus causing a shift of the trachea as well. This is a late sign of significant injury and requires rapid intervention by a paramedic or hospital personnel.

paradoxical movement a sign found on the chest wall where a flail segment of the chest moves in a direction opposite from the rest of the chest during inspiration and expiration.

subcutaneous emphysema air that has become trapped beneath the skin; characterized by crepitus.

- ***Chest.*** Expose, inspect, and palpate the chest for BP-DOC, including **paradoxical movement** of the chest wall and **subcutaneous emphysema** (Figure 14-17 ▪). Assessment of the chest also should include bilateral auscultation of breath sounds. (See Chapter 17 for more details on auscultating breath sounds.) Paradoxical movement of the chest wall is commonly discovered as a soft, spongy area of the chest wall. It is often a sign of a flail chest and is quite painful, making breathing difficult. Subcutaneous emphysema is air that has escaped the chest cavity and has become trapped beneath the skin. It is often felt as a crackling (crepitation) beneath the skin when the area is palpated.

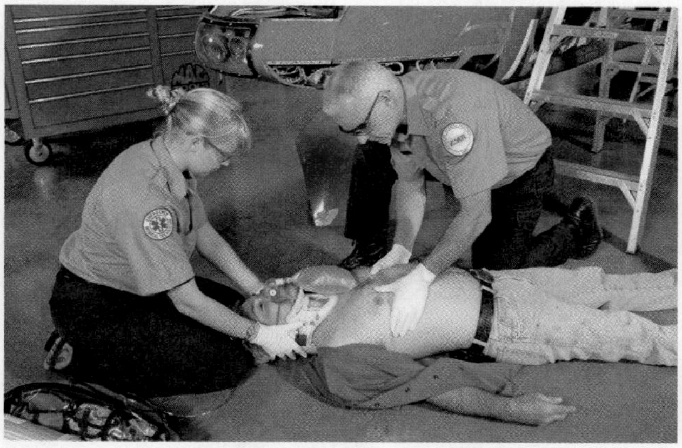

Figure 14-17 Expose the chest and use both hands to palpate the anterior and lateral chest.

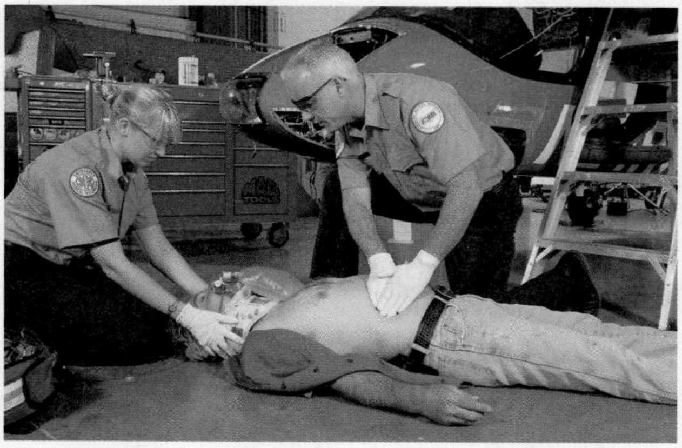

Figure 14-18 Expose the abdomen and use both hands to palpate all four quadrants.

PRACTICAL PATHOPHYSIOLOGY

As you inspect the chest wall, be very deliberate. Palpate for areas that may be soft and spongy which could be a sign of a flail segment. A flail segment occurs when two or more ribs are broken in two or more places causing a "floating" segment of chest wall. When the patient attempts to breathe, the floating segment moves in the opposite direction as the rest of the chest wall, causing the paradoxical movement.

- ***Abdomen.*** Inspect and palpate the abdomen for BP-DOC (Figure 14-18 ▪). Note any rigidity, distention, or guarding, and watch the patient's face for signs of pain (grimacing, for instance) as you palpate. A rigid, abnormally firm abdomen can be caused by both pain and bleeding into the abdomen, both indications of significant injury. Distention or swelling of the abdomen may also be a sign of internal injury. You must ask the responsive patient if his abdomen is the size it normally is. (Many patients have a distended abdomen normally.)

PRACTICAL PATHOPHYSIOLOGY

A normal abdomen is soft and supple on palpation and free of pain. An abdomen that is firm or rigid during palpation may be a sign of underlying injury. A conscious patient with abdominal pain will tighten the abdominal muscles in an attempt to guard against more pain. This is a normal reflex but should be seen as a significant sign of injury. The unresponsive patient who presents with a firm abdomen may have bleeding in the abdomen.

- ***Pelvis.*** Expose, inspect, and palpate the pelvis for BP-DOC, including evidence of wetness that may be caused by blood or loss of bladder control. If there is no major complaint of pain to the pelvis, place one hand on each hip bone and gently compress the pelvis down and inward (Figure 14-19 ▪). Note any pain or instability.
- ***Back.*** Expose, inspect, and palpate the back for BP-DOC including paradoxical movement and crepitation (Figure 14-20 ▪). If you are alone, do your best to palpate as much of the back without rolling the patient or compromising the spine. If necessary, maintain spinal stabilization and roll the patient to perform a complete assessment of the back (Figure 14-21 ▪).

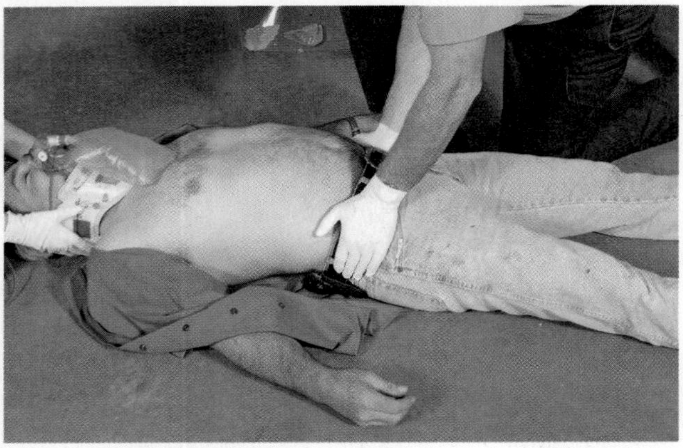

Figure 14-19 Use both hands to palpate the pelvis for injury.

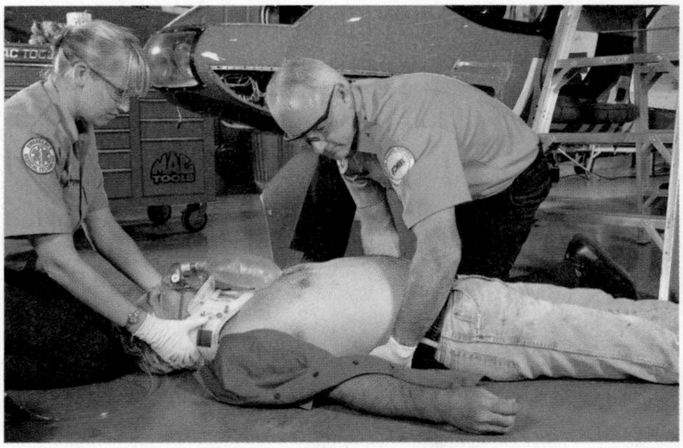

Figure 14-20 Use one hand to slide under the lumbar spine to palpate the lower back.

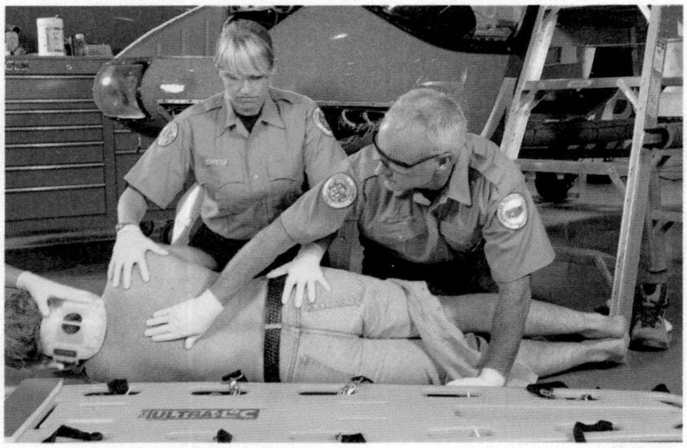

Figure 14-21 Maintain manual stabilization of the head and neck as you roll the patient to inspect and palpate the back.

- ***Extremities.*** Expose, inspect, and palpate each extremity for BP-DOC (Figure 14-22 ■). Assess the hands and feet for circulation, sensation, and motor function (CSM). When evaluating motor function, do so with both extremities simultaneously (Figure 14-23 ■) to allow you to detect slight differences in strength from one side to the other.

If at any point during the rapid secondary assessment for the trauma patient you discover what could be a life-threatening injury not found during the primary assessment, you must stop the exam and provide care for the problem immediately. It is important to remember that all potential life threats must be addressed as they are found. Examples of immediate life threats that need immediate intervention include:

- ***Airway compromise.*** Have suction ready to help clear the airway of blood and other fluids.
- ***Chest wall injuries that result in inadequate breathing.*** Be prepared to provide manual ventilations with a bag-mask device if necessary.
- ***Open wounds with serious uncontrolled bleeding.*** Be prepared to stop and use the appropriate bleeding control steps.

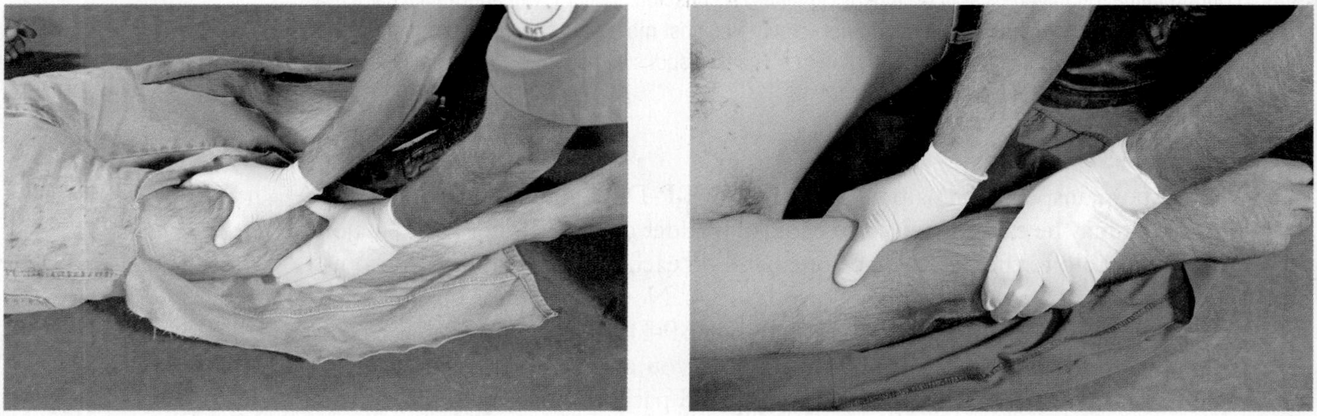

(A) (B)

Figure 14-22 Expose the extremity, and use both hands to palpate it along its entire length.

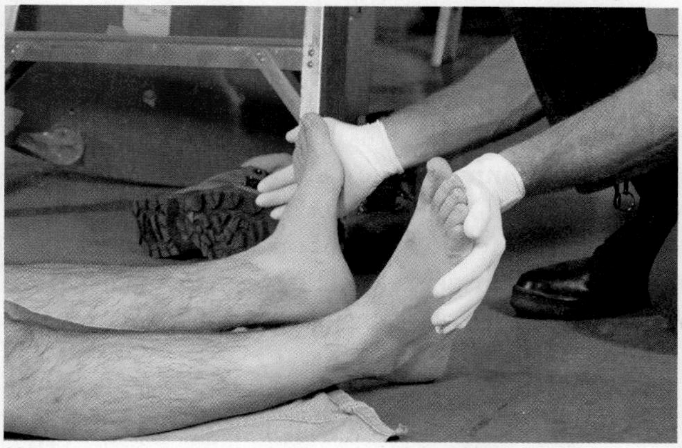

(A)

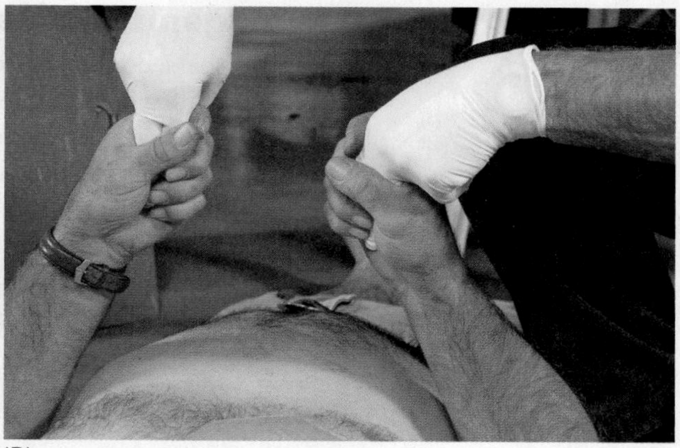

(B)

Figure 14-23 Use both hands to assess circulation, sensation, and motor function in all four extremities.

Performing a Focused Secondary Assessment (Trauma Patient)

When caring for trauma patients who are stable and who have not sustained a significant MOI, perform a focused secondary assessment based on the chief complaint. For instance, if your patient has a lacerated leg or had his foot crushed, you would focus your assessment on the injured extremity and not waste time completing an exam of his entire body.

14-14 Describe the steps for conducting a focused secondary assessment for a trauma patient.

You can use the specific component or components of the secondary assessment that relate to the patient's chief complaint to serve as your focused assessment.

Following the focused secondary assessment, you will obtain a baseline set of vital signs and gather as much of a SAMPLE history as possible. Remember to reassess vital signs every 15 minutes for the stable, noncritical patient.

To see how examination of body systems relates to pathophysiology, see Table 14-5.

TABLE 14-5 RELATING BODY SYSTEM EXAMS TO PATHOPHYSIOLOGY

BODY SYSTEM EXAM FINDING	PATHOPHYSIOLOGY
Dyspnea on exertion (DOE)	The patient has increased difficulty breathing at a level of exertion that previously did not cause a problem. The exertion causes increased oxygen demand, which the body is not able to meet. Heart failure is the common cause of DOE.
Weight gain	Fluid is heavy. When a patient gains two to three pounds/day or more than five pounds/week, it is an indication that congestive heart failure has worsened to a serious level.
Fever	Fever indicates infection. It may be significant. In respiratory distress, it may indicate a condition such as pneumonia. With general weakness or altered mental status, it may indicate sepsis.
Skin color, temperature, and condition	When blood is shunted away from the skin to supply vital organs, the skin becomes cool, pale, and moist. This is most commonly seen as a patient compensates for shock. It also is seen in hypoglycemia (low blood sugar) because the body's response to raise blood sugar uses some of the same hormones as are used to compensate for shock.
Blood glucose readings	Normal blood glucose (BG) is 70 to 120 mg/dL. When BG gets below 60 mg/dL, the patient is hypoglycemic and should receive oral glucose if symptomatic and alert.
Orthostatic changes in vital signs	When a patient moves from a supine position to a standing position (and to some extent from a sitting to a standing position), the patient's cardiovascular system must work harder to pump blood against the change in gravity. If there is low volume or a pump problem, the patient may experience dizziness and an increase in pulse of 20 beats/minute. Note that some elderly patients may experience this routinely.

Management of Secondary Injuries

During the secondary assessment, you will have identified as many signs and symptoms of injury as possible. Once you have completed your exam, you must provide the indicated care for as many of the secondary injuries as appropriate. Small wounds should be covered with dressings and extremity injuries should be immobilized as well as possible. For patients with a significant MOI, extremity injuries are a low priority and can easily be managed by packaging the patient on a long backboard.

For patients with a less significant MOI, suspected fractures can be managed using appropriate splinting techniques. (Splinting will be covered in Chapter 34.)

Reassessment

14-15 State the purpose of reassessment and when it should be performed.

reassessment the component of the patient assessment that is repeated at regular intervals and designed to monitor the status of the ABCs, vital signs, mental status, and effectiveness of interventions.

It can be argued that of all the elements of the patient assessment, the reassessment is second only to the primary assessment in terms of importance and priority. As you will remember from Chapter 12, the purpose of the primary assessment is to identify and care for all immediate life threats to the patient. The **reassessment** is a continuous rechecking of the patient's condition to ensure that everything checked previously is still within normal limits or at least not getting worse.

Just because the patient appeared stable when you first arrived on scene does not mean it will remain the case. A patient's condition can change at any time, and it is critical that you continuously reassess specific elements of the patient assessment, regardless of his injuries or chief complaint.

Elements of the Reassessment Process

14-16 List the elements of a reassessment.

Reassessment is not a repeat of an entire patient assessment. Instead, it is a reassessment of those elements most critical to the well-being of the patient (Scan 14-2). The following are the key components of the reassessment:

- Repeat the primary assessment.
- Recheck vital signs and compare them to the baseline vital signs for trending purposes.
- Repeat assessment of chief complaint or injuries and determine if any new complaints have developed.
- Check the effectiveness of your interventions.
- Confirm the patient's status and transport priority.

Reassessment is a continuous process. You should *not* wait until the end of your secondary assessment to begin performing it. The elements of the more formal reassessment steps should be checked all along the way. For example, when you first arrive at the patient's side, you will assess mental status by asking the patient some simple questions. Based on his response to your questions, you will make an initial evaluation of his mental status, but it does not stop there. As you go on with your assessment, you should be continually asking questions and evaluating his responses. A patient who is talking and responding appropriately is in good shape at that moment. As soon as he begins to get quiet or respond inappropriately, his condition may be changing. By continuously interacting with your patient and asking him questions, you will become immediately aware if his condition changes.

However, once you have completed the majority of your patient assessment, you must look back at the specific elements of reassessment to ensure that the patient's needs are being met. In addition, reassessment will help identify changes in the patient's condition that may require changes in the care you provide.

SCAN 14-2 Reassessment

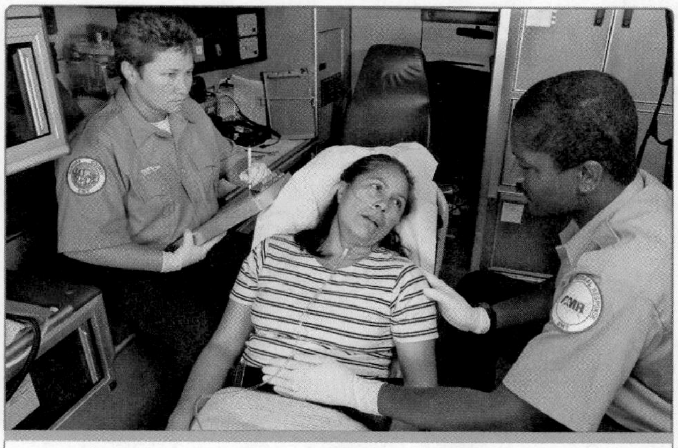

14-2-1 Repeat the primary assessment.

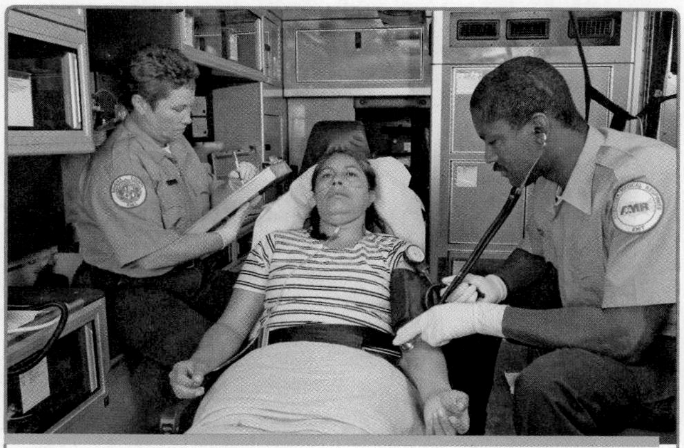

14-2-2 Recheck vital signs and compare with the baseline set.

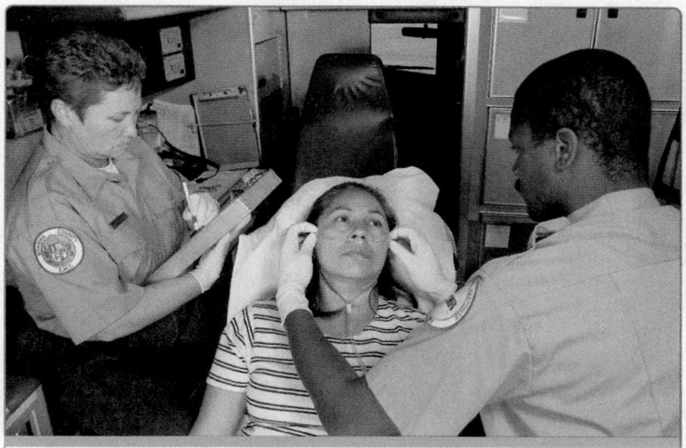

14-2-3 Check the effectiveness of your interventions.

Repeat the Primary Assessment

As you may recall from Chapter 12, the core components of the primary assessment include mental status, airway, breathing, and circulation or pulse and the control of severe bleeding. Your reassessment will include evaluating the patient's mental status, ensuring that the patient is breathing at an acceptable rate and tidal volume, and ensuring that he has an adequate pulse. It may be necessary to perform such interventions as suctioning, insertion of an airway adjunct, administration of oxygen, or perhaps performing CPR, depending on the patient's condition.

You also will need to assess all open wounds for evidence of bleeding, and control any bleeding that has not already been managed.

Recheck Vital Signs

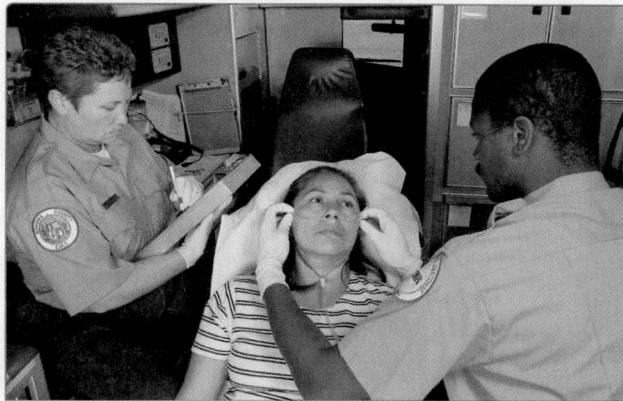

Obtain another set of vital signs. It will be important to compare it to the baseline set and to any additional vital sign measurements obtained earlier. Comparing vital signs helps you identify a trend in the patient's condition and adjust your care as necessary. Remember to document all findings clearly and accurately, including the time at which the signs were obtained.

As you speak with the patient, pay close attention to his skin signs. Often you will see a change in color or moisture that can suggest the patient is getting worse.

Reassess Chief Complaint or Injuries

One thing is certain, a patient's condition is dynamic and may change at any time, including his chief complaint. Pain can get worse or better, bleeding will be controlled or not, and new areas of pain can emerge. As you provide reassurance and care, some of the original symptoms may go away or new and different ones may appear. For instance, on your arrival, a patient may have a chief complaint of chest pain, but after several minutes of oxygen, his pain may be nearly gone and he is now complaining of only shortness of breath. It is important to stay aware of how the patient is feeling and what his complaints are throughout your time with him. An important aspect of your documentation will be to document in detail any changes in the patient's condition (better or worse) or chief complaint while in your care.

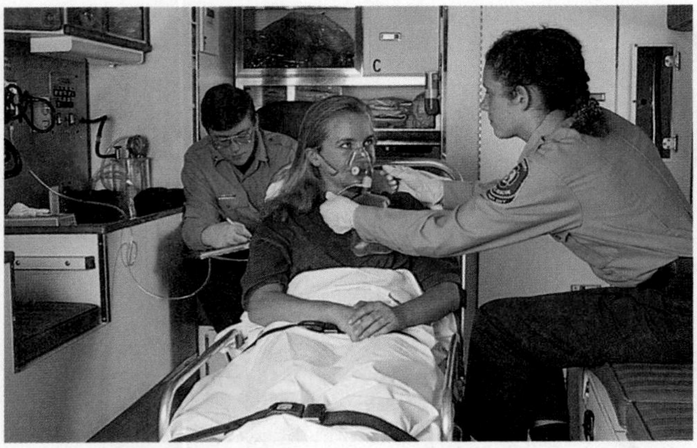

Figure 14-24 Adjust interventions as necessary.

Check Effectiveness of Interventions

It is your goal as an EMT to provide the most appropriate care for the patient based on the patient's condition. For that reason you must constantly evaluate the care you provide (Figure 14-24 ■). For example, you might ask: Is the oxygen set at the right flow rate? Am I using the most appropriate delivery device? Is the bleeding still controlled or has it started to flow again? Is the traction splint still holding traction? These are just some of the things you must constantly be asking yourself relative to the care you are providing. One of the best ways to assess the effectiveness of our interventions is to simply ask the patient how he is feeling.

Confirm Status and Transport Priority

As a patient's condition changes, for better or worse, you must change his priority for care and transport. If you are caring for only one patient, then he should receive your undivided attention, and the only thing you might change is the urgency with which you get him to the hospital. If you are caring for multiple patients, you may have to adjust who gets cared for first and who gets transported first, second, and third, based on each patient's condition.

When to Reassess

Unstable Patients

As previously noted, the vital signs of unstable patients should be reassessed at least every five minutes. However, for unresponsive patients and those patients you feel are unstable or whose condition is likely to deteriorate quickly, reassessment of the status of the patient's airway, breathing, and perfusion is actually a constant ongoing process. That way, if something goes wrong, you will be able to identify it quickly and provide the appropriate care. More frequent vital signs also mean that you are more likely to spot a trend in the patient's condition sooner and therefore anticipate the care he will need before his condition gets too bad.

Stable Patients

Stable patients are those whose condition is not likely to change any time soon. They are typically patients with a non-life-threatening injury or chief complaint but who still need the attention of a higher level of care (Figure 14-25 ▪). Of course vital signs are always important, but more formal reassessment is not typically needed as often for stable patients. It is generally recommended that stable patients be reassessed at least every 15 minutes to observe for and note any significant changes in condition. In addition, they should be reassessed at any time they voice a new or worsening complaint.

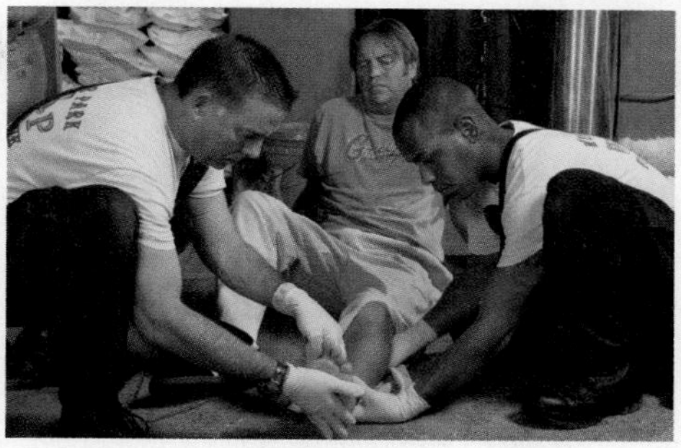

Figure 14-25 A stable patient should be reassessed every 15 minutes.

STOP, REVIEW, REMEMBER!

Multiple Choice

For each question, place a check next to the correct answer.

1. Which one of the following best defines the term *multi-system trauma*?

_____ a. Obvious injuries to more than one bone

_____ b. Suspected injury to more than one body system

_____ c. More than one mechanism of injury

_____ d. More than one patient

2. You are caring for a victim of a motorcycle crash. He is unresponsive and has gurgling respirations. You should:

_____ a. stabilize the head and neck.

_____ b. suction the airway.

_____ c. perform a rapid secondary assessment.

_____ d. apply high-flow oxygen.

3. Which one of the following best represents a significant MOI?

_____ a. Right foot that was run over by a forklift

_____ b. Crush injury to both lower legs

_____ c. 8-foot fall from a ladder onto asphalt

_____ d. 20-foot fall onto concrete

4. Falls greater than _______________ feet should be considered as significant mechanisms of injury for pediatric patients.

_____ a. 2

_____ b. 3

_____ c. 5

_____ d. 10

5. The first time the MOI is assessed is during the:

_____ a. scene size-up.

_____ b. primary assessment.

_____ c. secondary assessment.

_____ d. general impression.

(continued on next page)

(continued)

Critical Thinking

1. Provide two examples each of what would be considered a "medical" patient and a "trauma" patient.

2. If you knew you were responding to a fall victim, what questions would you like to have answered before you arrive on scene?

3. For each of the patients described below, determine whether the MOI is significant or not significant. In the space provided write "S" for significant MOI or "NS" if the MOI is not significant.

_____ a. 57-year-old male patient who was found unresponsive beneath a ladder in his garage.

_____ b. 13-year-old female patient whose arm was run over by a car.

_____ c. 22-year-old female patient who was struck by a car at 25 mph while crossing the street.

_____ d. 32-year-old female patient who was struck by a car at 10 mph while riding a motorcycle.

_____ e. 7-year-old male patient who fell while running and has deformity to his right wrist.

EMERGENCY DISPATCH SUMMARY

Al Hernandez was transported without incident to Saint Anthony Hospital on Broadway and First. Subsequent tests showed that Mr. Hernandez had suffered an ischemic stroke, but with the extended time before help was sought, he was not considered a candidate for fibrinolytic therapy. He has since been placed into the Spring County Advanced Care Facility for follow-up care, but he has so far showed no signs of regaining either his ability to speak or move successfully.

Chapter Review

To the Point

- It is very important to develop a systematic approach to your patient assessment. It will help ensure a consistently thorough assessment each time and an efficiency that helps ensure the patient will receive prompt care.
- The four main components of the patient assessment are the scene size-up, primary assessment, secondary assessment, and reassessment.
- Patients are categorized first as medical (illness) or trauma (injury) patients.
- The purpose of the secondary assessment is to identify and care for signs and symptoms not previously found or addressed in the primary assessment.
- Patients are further categorized as stable, unstable, or likely to become unstable. Unstable patients must receive more rapid assessment, care, and transport because their condition could worsen rapidly.
- There are two basic approaches used for patient assessment, the anatomical and the systems approach. The anatomical approach is a head-to-toe approach, while the systems approach focuses on the specific body system or systems related to the chief complaint.
- The rapid secondary assessment is used for unstable patients, while the focused assessment is used for stable patients.
- The SAMPLE and the OPQRST memory aids are tools used to obtain a more detailed history based on the patient's chief complaint.
- When caring for trauma patients, you must carefully evaluate the mechanism of injury and have a high index of suspicion for multisystem trauma.
- Once you have completed the secondary assessment, you must perform regular reassessments. The reassessment consists of reevaluating the patient's ABCs including mental status, rechecking vital signs and looking for trends, reassessment of the chief complaint, checking the effectiveness of your interventions, and changing patient priority as appropriate.

Chapter Questions

Multiple Choice

For each question, place a check next to the correct answer.

1. Which one of the following patients best meets the criteria for a rapid secondary assessment?
   _____ a. 16-year-old who fell 20 feet
   _____ b. 23-year-old who twisted an ankle
   _____ c. 41-year-old with severe chest pain
   _____ d. 77-year-old who fainted during a meal

2. After performing a rapid secondary assessment and taking vital signs for a trauma patient, you should obtain a:
   _____ a. mental status.
   _____ b. detailed assessment.
   _____ c. SAMPLE history.
   _____ d. focused assessment.

3. Which one of the following would *not* be a normal finding of a chest assessment?
   _____ a. Paradoxical movement
   _____ b. Distention
   _____ c. Crepitation
   _____ d. Tenderness

4. All of the following are factors that should be evaluated when assessing the MOI of a fall victim *except*:
   _____ a. height of fall.
   _____ b. speed of fall.
   _____ c. the position in which he landed.
   _____ d. whether or not he lost consciousness.

5. A fall greater than _____ feet is considered a significant MOI for an adult patient.
   _____ a. 5
   _____ b. 10
   _____ c. 15
   _____ d. 20

(continued on next page)

(continued)

6. Reassessments for the stable patient should be performed about every _____ minutes.
   _____ a. 5
   _____ b. 10
   _____ c. 15
   _____ d. 20
7. Which one of the following best defines the term *multisystem trauma*?
   _____ a. Obvious injuries to multiple bones
   _____ b. Multiple patients
   _____ c. Multiple mechanisms of injury
   _____ d. Trauma to multiple body systems
8. Which one of the following elements of the patient assessment is *not* common to all assessments?
   _____ a. Focused secondary assessment
   _____ b. Vital signs and history
   _____ c. Scene size-up
   _____ d. BSI precautions
9. Which one of the following best represents a significant MOI?
   _____ a. Badly sprained ankle
   _____ b. Vehicle collision at 30 mph
   _____ c. Eight-foot fall from a ladder onto asphalt
   _____ d. Crush injury to a hand
10. The criterion for determining the most appropriate assessment path for a medical patient is:
   _____ a. the chief complaint.
   _____ b. the level of pain.
   _____ c. whether he is stable or unstable.
   _____ d. the mechanism of injury.
11. Which one of the following is the most appropriate assessment tool for evaluating the chief complaint of a medical patient?
   _____ a. SAMPLE
   _____ b. OPQRST
   _____ c. AVPU
   _____ d. DCAP-BTLS
12. Swelling that is found in the ankles of some medical patients with a cardiac history is called:
   _____ a. pedal distention.
   _____ b. ascites.
   _____ c. subtle deformity.
   _____ d. pedal edema.
13. In the unresponsive medical patient, vital signs should be obtained:
   _____ a. following the rapid secondary assessment.
   _____ b. before the rapid secondary assessment.
   _____ c. as often as possible.
   _____ d. every 15 minutes.
14. The vital signs of an unstable patient should be reassessed at least every _____ minutes.
   _____ a. 5
   _____ b. 10
   _____ c. 15
   _____ d. 20
15. You are caring for a 22-year-old patient following what was described as a seizure. The patient is alert but confused. You should:
   _____ a. obtain vital signs and perform a rapid secondary assessment.
   _____ b. administer oxygen and perform a rapid secondary assessment.
   _____ c. administer oxygen and obtain vital signs.
   _____ d. perform a focused secondary assessment and administer oxygen.

Matching

Match the definition on the left with the applicable term on the right.

1. _____ The grating sound or feeling of broken bones rubbing together
2. _____ Displacement of the trachea laterally from the midline
3. _____ Bulging of the neck veins
4. _____ Movement of a part of the chest wall in the opposite direction to the rest of the chest during inhalation and exhalation
5. _____ Air trapped beneath the skin

A. Paradoxical movement
B. Subcutaneous emphysema
C. Tracheal deviation
D. Jugular vein distention
E. Crepitus

Critical Thinking

1. Provide at least three examples each of patients that would be categorized as trauma and medical.

2. Discuss how and why medical patients are cared for differently than trauma patients.

3. What is the purpose of the reassessment?

4. For each of the following patient chief complaints, describe the body system(s) you would focus your assessment on.
   a. "I've been having trouble breathing and my ankles are swollen."

   b. "I've been vomiting for three days."

   c. "My heart is beating funny. Sometimes I think it skips a beat."

(continued on next page)

(continued)

d. "I got stung by a bee and I am starting to feel light-headed."

e. "I have had a very bad headache now for two days."

Case Studies

Case Study 1

You have completed a primary assessment, secondary assessment, vitals, and SAMPLE history on a 66-year-old female patient who has an altered mental status. You are now loaded in the ambulance and en route to the hospital. Your patient becomes unresponsive with gurgling respirations.

1. What might the presence of gurgling say about this patient?

2. How will you alter your assessment to address this new development?

Case Study 2

You have responded to an office building for a man having chest pain. On your arrival, you are escorted to a third-floor office where you find an approximately 50-year-old male patient in moderate distress. The man states that he is experiencing "tightness" in his chest, which started approximately 30 minutes ago and came on while he was walking up the stairs to his office. He also states that he is having difficulty breathing.

1. Which assessment path is most appropriate for this patient and why?

2. List at least two questions for each of the elements of the OPQRST assessment mnemonic.

Case Study 3

You have been dispatched to a vehicle collision on a two-lane highway leading out of the city. En route, you are advised by law enforcement at the scene that there is one fatality and two others with injuries. Once on scene, you are directed over to a two-door sedan with what appears to be an adult female lying across the front seat.

1. What factors can you quickly evaluate that will help you determine the mechanism of injury for this patient?

2. What will be the most appropriate assessment path for this patient?

3. What immediate life threats can you expect?

(continued on next page)

(continued)

Case Study 4

You have been called to a multistory condominium complex for a fall victim. On arrival you are led over to an adult female patient seated on the ground at the base of some stairs. She is alert and in obvious pain. She states that she was carrying some boxes down the stairs and just missed the last step. She has pain and deformity to her right wrist and pain in her right ankle with significant swelling.

1. What questions will you want to ask about the mechanism of injury to rule out an underlying medical condition?

____

____

____

____

2. What assessment path is most appropriate for this patient and why?

____

____

____

____

The Last Word

Good patient care depends on a thorough assessment. Once you have determined that the scene is safe and you have donned the appropriate personal protection equipment (PPE) for the situation, you must perform a primary assessment on each and every patient.

Trauma and medical patients require slightly different approaches to the secondary assessment. The specific assessment path for the trauma patient is determined by the significance of the mechanism of injury. A rapid secondary assessment is used for the patient who has suffered a significant MOI or has serious injury potentially affecting multiple body systems. In contrast, the focused secondary assessment is used for patients with an injury that is isolated to a noncritical area of the body, such as an extremity.

The specific assessment path for the medical patient is based on how stable the patient appears to be. A rapid secondary assessment is used for the patient who is unstable or unable to provide any meaningful history pertaining to his condition or chief complaint. In contrast, the focused secondary assessment is used for the patient who is responsive and able to provide a meaningful history of his problem.

Reassessment of the ABCs, vital signs, and interventions must be conducted at frequent intervals until the patient is delivered to an appropriate receiving hospital—every 15 minutes for a stable patient and every 5 minutes for an unstable patient.

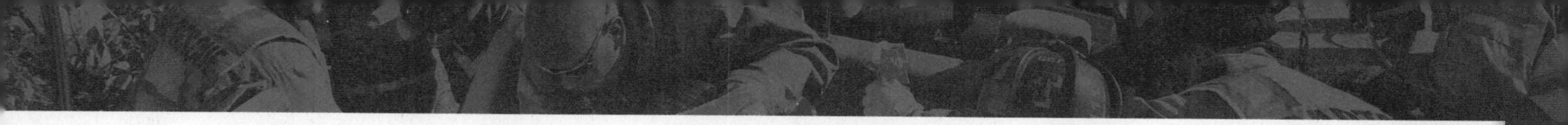

Module 2: Review and Practice Examination for Chapters 12–14

DIRECTIONS: *Assess what you have learned in this module by placing a check mark in the blank beside the best answer for each multiple-choice question. When you are done, check your answers against the Answer Key at the back of the book.*

1. Which one of the following is part of the scene size-up?
____ a. Determining the number of patients
____ b. Checking the patient's airway
____ c. Determining the patient's chief complaint
____ d. Performing a primary assessment

2. Determining the need for body substance isolation (BSI) precautions is part of the:
____ a. dispatch information.
____ b. primary assessment.
____ c. scene size-up.
____ d. general impression.

3. The best way to protect yourself and your crew from hazards at the scene of an emergency is to:
____ a. rely on dispatch information.
____ b. always respond with a crew of at least three EMS providers.
____ c. wear body armor.
____ d. observe the scene.

4. You are approaching the porch of a house to which you have been dispatched for an "injured person." Suddenly, the door swings open and you are confronted by a man in his 60s who is armed with a shotgun. You should:
____ a. immediately call for law enforcement.
____ b. retreat immediately to a safe location.
____ c. explain that you were called here to help someone who is injured.
____ d. throw your oxygen bag at the man to try to disarm him.

5. The time to call for additional resources at the scene of an emergency is:
____ a. after you receive the dispatch information.
____ b. as you are performing the scene size-up.
____ c. after you have triaged your patients.
____ d. during the primary assessment.

6. In addition to looking for signs of danger, the scene size-up can give clues about:
____ a. whether the patient is chronically ill.
____ b. the patient's past medical history.
____ c. how the patient was injured.
____ d. the patient's medications.

7. After ensuring personal safety, the first priority in patient care is:
____ a. checking the patient's pulse.
____ b. getting a medical history from the patient.
____ c. assessing the patient's airway.
____ d. administering oxygen.

8. Your adult patient has fallen 15 feet off a roof and onto his side. According to the National Trauma Triage Protocol, the patient's fall would be classified as:
____ a. nonsignificant mechanism of injury.
____ b. nature of illness.
____ c. significant mechanism of injury.
____ d. chief complaint.

9. Which one of the following is the primary muscle(s) used for breathing under normal conditions?
____ a. Intercostal muscles between the ribs
____ b. Abdominal muscles
____ c. Latissimus dorsi muscle of the back
____ d. Diaphragm

10. Your patient is a three-year-old toddler. You should consider her respiratory rate to be normal if it is ____________ per minute.
____ a. 38 ____ c. 42
____ b. 24 ____ d. 16

11. Your patient is a seven-year-old boy. You should consider his respiratory rate normal if it is ____________ per minute.
____ a. 60 ____ c. 28
____ b. 48 ____ d. 12

12. Often the most obvious sign that someone is *not* receiving enough oxygen is a(n):

____ a. increased tidal volume.
____ b. increased respiratory rate.
____ c. decreased respiratory rate.
____ d. irregular respirations.

13. Which one of the following signs is associated with respiratory failure?

____ a. Flushed skin color
____ b. Increased tidal volume
____ c. Increased respiratory rate
____ d. Decreased respiratory rate

14. If the head of a child is tilted too far back when you open the airway, which one of the following could occur?

____ a. Airway obstruction
____ b. Fracture of the cervical vertebrae
____ c. Damage to the larynx
____ d. Displacement of the tongue into the pharynx

15. A head-tilt/chin-lift maneuver is used to clear the airway from an obstruction caused by:

____ a. a foreign body.
____ b. the tongue.
____ c. swelling due to trauma.
____ d. fluids.

16. The best way to open the airway of a patient with a suspected spine injury is:

____ a. placing him in a prone position.
____ b. using a head-tilt/chin-lift maneuver.
____ c. using a jaw-thrust maneuver.
____ d. placing your gloved hand in the patient's mouth to pull the tongue forward.

17. Which one of the following sets of personal protective equipment (PPE) is recommended when performing airway management procedures?

____ a. Gloves only
____ b. Mask only
____ c. Protective eyewear and gloves
____ d. Gloves, mask, and eye protection

18. Your patient is suspected of taking an overdose of sleeping pills. You note gurgling noises when he attempts to breathe. Which one of the following is most likely responsible for this noise?

____ a. There is fluid in his lungs.
____ b. He has vomited and has fluid in his pharynx.
____ c. His tongue is obstructing his airway.
____ d. His dentures are obstructing his airway.

19. When suctioning an adult, suction should be applied for no more than ____________ seconds.

____ a. 5 ____ c. 15
____ b. 10 ____ d. 20

20. When suctioning an infant, suction should be applied for no more than ____________ seconds.

____ a. 5 ____ c. 15
____ b. 10 ____ d. 20

21. The best device for suctioning the nose or mouth of a pediatric patient is a(n):

____ a. soft suction catheter.
____ b. rigid suction tip.
____ c. bulb syringe.
____ d. large-bore suction tubing.

22. Which one of the following statements regarding airway adjuncts is true?

____ a. Oropharyngeal airway adjuncts must not be used in infants.
____ b. Oropharyngeal airway adjuncts eliminate the need for manually opening the airway, but nasopharyngeal airway adjuncts do not.
____ c. Nasopharyngeal airway adjuncts must never be used in patients with a gag reflex.
____ d. Proper manual positioning of the airway is required with the use of oropharyngeal and nasopharyngeal airway adjuncts.

23. The proper way to measure an oropharyngeal airway is from the:

____ a. tip of the nose to the earlobe.
____ b. nostril to the earlobe.
____ c. corner of the mouth to the tip of the earlobe.
____ d. center of the mouth to the nostril.

24. How do you know when you are having difficulty delivering ventilations to your patient with a bag-mask device?

____ a. You will not see good chest rise and fall.
____ b. The bag squeezes easily.
____ c. Skin signs and pulse rate improve.
____ d. You will see good chest rise.

25. When delivering ventilations to an adult patient, the ideal duration of each ventilation is ____________ second(s).

____ a. 1 ____ c. 1.5 to 2
____ b. 1 to 1.5 ____ d. 2 to 2.5

26. For a single rescuer, the preferred technique for ventilating a nonbreathing patient is:

____ a. bag-mask device.
____ b. mouth to mouth.
____ c. demand-valve device.
____ d. mouth-to-mask.

27. Ventilating a patient with a pocket face mask provides approximately ____________ oxygen with each ventilation.
____ a. over 90% ____ c. 21%
____ b. 45% to 60% ____ d. 10% to 15%

28. Ventilation with a bag-mask device without supplemental oxygen delivers ____________ oxygen with each ventilation.
____ a. over 90% ____ c. 21%
____ b. 45% to 60% ____ d. 10% to 15%

29. Which artificial ventilation technique is *most* appropriate for use in two-rescuer resuscitation?
____ a. Mouth-to-mouth ventilation
____ b. Pocket face mask
____ c. Bag-mask device
____ d. Demand-valve device

30. Which one of the following statements regarding the demand-valve device is true?
____ a. It can be used only on patients who are making a respiratory effort on their own.
____ b. It can be used only by patients who are not breathing on their own.
____ c. It should be used only for adult patients.
____ d. It delivers 40 liters per minute of air flow.

31. Which one of the following is the most immediate danger associated with using too much volume or delivering each breath too quickly when ventilating a pediatric patient?
____ a. Filling the stomach with air
____ b. Creating excessively high oxygen concentrations in the blood
____ c. Airway obstruction
____ d. Damage to the trachea

32. Which one of the following statements regarding airway management in a patient with a stoma is true?
____ a. The EMT must not attempt to suction the stoma; this is a paramedic-level skill.
____ b. The best device for ventilating through the stoma is a bag-mask device using an infant mask.
____ c. When delivering ventilations through the stoma it is necessary to maintain a head-tilt, chin-lift.
____ d. The stoma must be sealed off during ventilations.

33. Which one of the following is used to help identify a gas cylinder containing oxygen?
____ a. Yellow color coding
____ b. Five-pointed star on the crown
____ c. Green/gray color coding
____ d. Letter code from A to H, depending on the concentration of oxygen in the tank

34. Once the hydrostatic test date on an oxygen cylinder has passed, which one of the following statements is true?
____ a. The cylinder may be used until empty but cannot be refilled until the tank is tested.
____ b. The oxygen in the cylinder has expired and the tank now contains mostly carbon dioxide.
____ c. The cylinder must be immediately removed from service for safety testing.
____ d. The cylinder is no longer safe and must be disposed of or recycled.

35. Which one of the following serves to ensure that oxygen is delivered to the patient at a safe pressure?
____ a. PIN index system
____ b. Pressure regulator
____ c. Pressure-relief valve
____ d. O ring

36. The best device for delivering oxygen to a breathing patient who needs a high concentration of oxygen is a(n):
____ a. nasal cannula.
____ b. bag-mask device.
____ c. nonrebreather mask.
____ d. pocket mask.

37. A nonrebreather mask is designed to work best with a minimum liter flow of ____________ liters per minute.
____ a. 6–10 ____ c. 16–24
____ b. 10–15 ____ d. 18–32

38. When setting up the nonrebreather mask, after adjusting the regulator, you should:
____ a. fill the reservoir bag.
____ b. attach the supply tubing.
____ c. adjust the nasal prongs.
____ d. alter the mask shape.

39. A nonrebreather mask, if properly used, can deliver an oxygen concentration of approximately:
____ a. 16%. ____ c. 50%.
____ b. 21%. ____ d. 90%.

40. Your 50-year-old female patient has a long history of lung disease. She is having so much difficulty breathing that she cannot speak. Her respirations are 40 per minute, and she is having trouble keeping her eyes open. Which one of the following is most appropriate for this patient?
____ a. Nasal cannula and administering 15 liters per minute of oxygen
____ b. Nonrebreather mask at 15 liters per minute and administering liters per minute of oxygen
____ c. Assisting her ventilations with a bag-mask device
____ d. Assisting her ventilations with a pocket mask and administering 12 liters per minute of oxygen

41. You have applied a nonrebreather mask to a patient who is complaining of difficulty breathing. The patient complains that the mask is "suffocating" her and that she "can't stand it." You should:
____ a. automatically switch to a nasal cannula with 6 liters per minute flow of oxygen.
____ b. attempt to coach the patient on how to adjust to the nonrebreather mask.
____ c. check to make sure that the reservoir bag is not over inflated.
____ d. remove the mask for 15 seconds every minute to relieve the feeling of suffocation.

42. A nasal cannula can deliver an oxygen concentration of up to approximately:
____ a. 2% to 6%. ____ c. 40% to 45%.
____ b. 10% to 15%. ____ d. 90% to 95%.

43. A nasal cannula is designed to be used with an oxygen flow rate of ____________ liters per minute.
____ a. 2 to 6 ____ c. 6 to 10
____ b. 2 to 10 ____ d. 10 to 15

44. The prongs of a nasal cannula are properly placed when they are:
____ a. resting on the lower lip.
____ b. inside the nostrils.
____ c. resting on the bridge of the nose.
____ d. curving upward.

45. Which one of the following is a drawback to using an oxygen-powered suction device?
____ a. It consumes a great quantity of oxygen.
____ b. It is not as effective as a manual suction device.
____ c. It generates dangerous levels of suction that could injure the patient.
____ d. It requires a special regulator that is expensive and typically difficult to find.

46. Before beginning bag-mask ventilations, you must make sure that the patient:
____ a. is not making any respiratory effort on his or her own.
____ b. has an open airway.
____ c. is completely unresponsive.
____ d. has adequate tidal volume.

47. Your patient is a two-year-old child who is having a severe allergic reaction. He indicates that his throat feels swollen and he is having trouble breathing. Which of the following is a sign of hypoxia that is most common in pediatric patients?
____ a. Tingling in the fingers and toes
____ b. Cyanosis
____ c. Nasal flaring
____ d. Restlessness

48. All of the following are necessary when using a bag-mask device to deliver the highest concentration possible, *except*:
____ a. a good mask seal.
____ b. an oxygen reservoir.
____ c. an oxygen supply.
____ d. pop-off valve.

49. All of the following are required for good central perfusion, *except*:
____ a. blood circulation.
____ b. oxygenation.
____ c. ventilation.
____ d. warm environment.

50. A full oxygen cylinder is pressurized to approximately ____________ pounds per square inch.
____ a. 425 ____ c. 2,000
____ b. 1,000 ____ d. 3,000

51. The most common method for obtaining a respiratory rate is to count the respirations for how many seconds?
____ a. 15 ____ c. 45
____ b. 30 ____ d. 60

52. You are the first EMS provider on the scene of a 30-year-old woman who is breathing inadequately, possibly due to an overdose of prescription medications. Which one of the following should be your primary consideration?
____ a. Airway and breathing status
____ b. Using your radio to find out how far away additional responders are
____ c. Finding out exactly what medication the patient took and how much she took
____ d. Not allowing the patient's family to notice your anxiety

53. Which one of the following is *not* one of the three characteristics that must be assessed when checking a patient's breathing?
____ a. Length of each inspiration
____ b. Respiratory rate
____ c. Depth of respirations
____ d. Ease of respirations

54. Which one of the following is a symptom?
____ a. Hot, dry skin
____ b. Headache
____ c. Irregular pulse
____ d. Bruises

55. Which one of the following is a sign?
____ a. Depth of respiration
____ b. Nausea
____ c. Pain
____ d. Itching

56. The amount of air that moves in and out of the lungs with each respiration is the ______________ volume.

____ a. tidal ____ c. resting
____ b. minute ____ d. lung

57. With respect to assessing respirations, the term *retraction* refers to:

____ a. an abnormal sound heard during inspiration.
____ b. shallow respirations.
____ c. drawing in of the soft tissues between the ribs.
____ d. prolonged inspiration with short expiration.

58. The presence of wheezing is most likely an indication of:

____ a. upper airway obstruction.
____ b. partial upper airway obstruction.
____ c. fluid in the airway.
____ d. lower airway obstruction.

59. When assessing the pulse of a responsive adult, the preferred site of assessment is the ______________ artery, located at the ______________.

____ a. carotid, anterior neck
____ b. femoral, wrist
____ c. radial, wrist
____ d. radial, elbow

60. When assessing the pulse of an unresponsive adult, the preferred site is the ______________ artery, located in/on the ______________.

____ a. brachial, neck ____ c. femoral, groin
____ b. radial, wrist ____ d. carotid, neck

61. The ______________ is the primary reason why the patient summoned EMS, described in his or her own words.

____ a. general impression
____ b. primary assessment
____ c. chief complaint
____ d. pertinent history

62. To determine provocation, which one of the following questions should be asked?

____ a. What were you doing when your pain started?
____ b. Does anything make the pain worse or better?
____ c. Can you describe what your pain feels like?
____ d. Does the pain go anywhere else other than your chest?

63. All of the following elements are used to evaluate a patient's mental status *except*:

____ a. awareness of who she is.
____ b. awareness of what happened to her.
____ c. the ability to calculate a simple math problem.
____ d. awareness of the day and date.

64. The purpose of the primary assessment is to:

____ a. identify and address immediate threats to life.
____ b. get a baseline set of vital signs.
____ c. form a general impression.
____ d. detect any possible hazards at the scene.

65. Which one of the following is considered a significant mechanism of injury?

____ a. Laceration to the lower leg
____ b. Penetration of the torso
____ c. Fall from greater than eight feet
____ d. Being a backseat passenger of an automobile

66. Your patient is a 32-year-old mechanic who dropped an engine block on his right foot. When you arrive, the engine block has been lifted away. He is cursing and yelling at you to "hurry up and give me something for the pain." The most appropriate assessment for this patient is a:

____ a. primary assessment followed by a rapid secondary assessment.
____ b. primary assessment only.
____ c. primary assessment followed by a focused secondary assessment.
____ d. rapid secondary assessment followed by a focused secondary assessment.

67. The rapid secondary assessment for the trauma patient includes:

____ a. vital signs.
____ b. checking the chest for deformities.
____ c. checking the reaction of the pupils.
____ d. formulating a general impression.

68. Your patient is a 50-year-old man who was burned when he poured gasoline into a smoldering pile of leaves to try to "get the fire burning." While your partner and the first-responding EMTs assess the patient, you are trying to get a medical history from his wife. She is impatient with your questions and tells you she does not understand why you need to know all those things. Which one of the following is the best response?

____ a. I'm just trying to do my job.
____ b. Please, ma'am, could you just answer the questions?
____ c. Some medical problems and medications can complicate injuries. The more we know, the better we can help your husband.
____ d. I know this all seems unnecessary. Please, just trust me on this.

69. Which one of the following statements is true regarding the assessment of a stable medical patient?
____ a. A rapid secondary assessment is performed before the history is obtained.
____ b. A thorough, head-to-toe examination is performed.
____ c. A primary assessment is not necessary.
____ d. The history is obtained before performing a focused secondary assessment.

70. When gathering a history of the patient's allergies, you should ask about:
____ a. only allergies to medications.
____ b. allergies to medications and environmental factors, such as bees or wasps.
____ c. allergies to medications and foods.
____ d. allergies to food, medications, and environmental factors, such as bees or wasps.

71. When assessing the severity of pain, you should ask the patient to rate how bad his pain is on a scale from 0 (least severe) to:
____ a. 5. ____ c. 25.
____ b. 10. ____ d. 100.

72. Tidal volume is directly related to the ____________ of breathing.
____ a. rate ____ c. ease
____ b. rhythm ____ d. depth

73. Which one of the following best depicts a patient whose level of responsiveness is described as verbal on the AVPU scale?
____ a. The patient is able to speak, even though the words may or may not make sense.
____ b. The patient is able to speak and the words spoken are appropriate.
____ c. The patient appears to be unresponsive but opens her eyes in response to your voice.
____ d. The patient cries out in response to painful stimulus.

74. Which one of the following is the correct sequence of assessment steps for a trauma patient with *no* significant mechanism of injury?
____ a. Primary assessment, rapid secondary assessment, baseline vital signs, SAMPLE history
____ b. SAMPLE history, primary assessment, baseline vital signs, rapid secondary assessment
____ c. Primary assessment, focused secondary assessment, baseline vital signs, SAMPLE history
____ d. Baseline vital signs, SAMPLE history, focused secondary assessment, primary assessment

75. When palpating a patient's abdomen, you note that the patient tenses up his abdominal muscles. This finding is known as:
____ a. tenderness. ____ c. guarding.
____ b. rigidity. ____ d. distention.

MODULE 3

Medical Emergencies

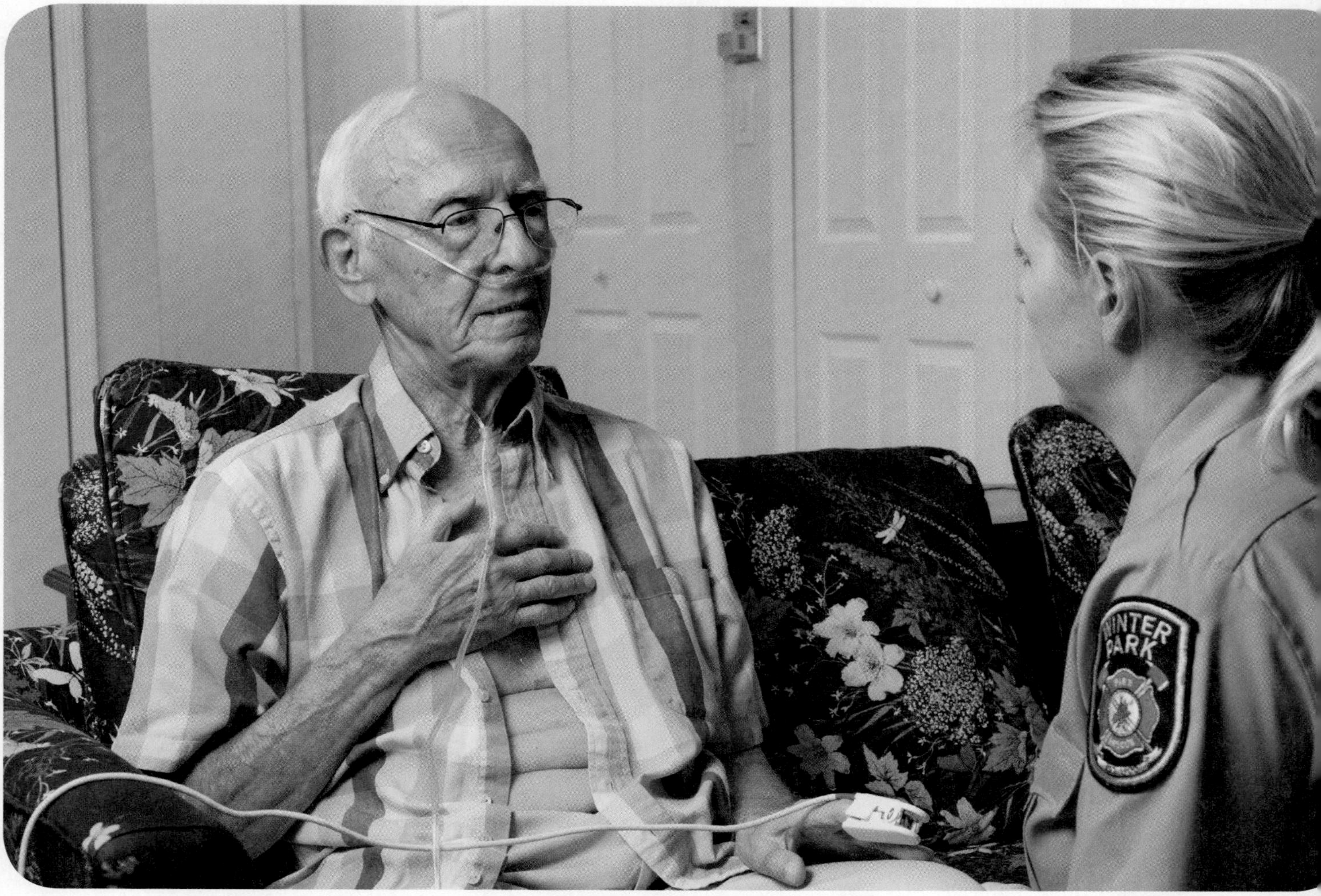

© Edward T. Dickinson, MD

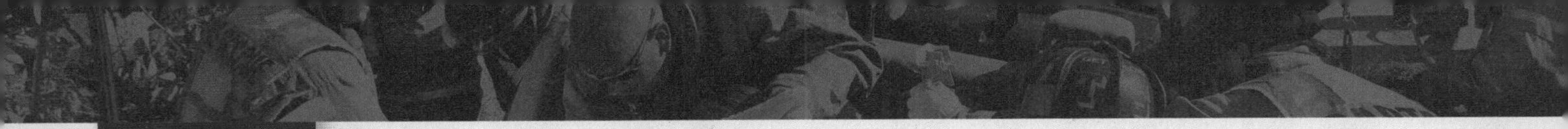

15 Your Approach to the Medical Patient

Education Standards

Assessment: Secondary assessment, monitoring devices, reassessment

Competencies

Applies scene information and patient assessment findings to guide emergency management.

Objectives

After completion of this lesson, you should be able to:

15-1 Define key terms introduced in this chapter.

15-2 Differentiate a medical patient from a trauma patient.

15-3 Discuss the importance of differentiating the medical patient from the trauma patient.

15-4 Discuss the importance of the general impression.

15-5 Describe the elements of the history of the present illness.

15-6 Describe the elements of the past medical history.

15-7 Discuss the role of time on scene with the medical patient.

15-8 Discuss the importance of choosing the appropriate receiving facility when caring for medical patients.

Key Terms

acute medical condition p. 419
chronic medical condition p. 419
history of present illness p. 421
medical patient p. 419
mentation p. 420
past medical history p. 422
time on scene p. 422
trauma patient p. 419

Introduction

In emergency care there are two general categories of patients—those who have an illness (the **medical patient**) and those who have an injury (the **trauma patient**). Your assessment approach to the two general types of patients will differ in both subtle and significant ways.

medical patient a patient whose chief complaint is related to an acute illness or disease process.

trauma patient a patient whose chief complaint is related to a sudden injury.

This chapter describes your approach to the assessment and management of a medical patient who has an acute (sudden) illness. (Chapter 28 reviews your approach to the trauma patient.) As you will see, this chapter differs from other chapters in this textbook in that it is meant to provide only a broad philosophical framework within which you should consider each of the other topics in Module 3, "Medical Emergencies."

Aren't All Patients Medical Patients?

15-2 Differentiate a medical patient from a trauma patient.

As a student in an EMT training program, you are receiving training that will prepare you to manage many of the common medical emergencies for which EMTs get dispatched. The average person tends to refer to all emergencies as "medical emergencies." But as you have likely already discovered, the medical community, including EMS, actually categorizes patients needing medical attention into one of two categories—medical patients or trauma patients.

Medical patients are those patients whose chief complaint is directly related to, or most likely related to, a disease process or illness. Many of the medical patients you treat will have a preexisting underlying medical condition that has been previously diagnosed. They are often already on medications that treat and control their illness. Those preexisting conditions are referred to as **chronic medical conditions.** Examples of chronic medical conditions include diabetes mellitus, high blood pressure (hypertension), and seizure disorders, just to name a few.

chronic medical condition an existing, recurrent medical condition.

Many times medical patients with chronic medical conditions need the services of EMS because their chronic illness suddenly worsens or they have a complication related to it. For example, a seizure patient may have a seizure because he has failed to take his antiseizure medications.

In contrast, certain medical patients you treat will have no known chronic medical condition, yet suddenly develop a medical emergency such as a stroke. Those sudden medical emergencies are often referred to as **acute medical conditions.** There is often a relationship between chronic and acute medical conditions: Many chronic conditions are risk factors for developing new acute medical emergencies. A patient with diabetes and hypertension, for example, is at increased risk of having an acute myocardial infarction (heart attack).

acute medical condition the sudden onset of a new illness or worsening of an existing (chronic) medical condition.

The list of possible signs and symptoms that the medical patient may present with is endless. For this reason, medical patients can be some of the most challenging for the EMT to assess and manage.

Medical Patient or Trauma Patient?

For the great majority of the patients you will encounter, determining which category—medical or trauma—your patient falls into is relatively easy. Things become much more challenging after you confirm you are dealing with a medical patient because there are so many things that can be causing a medical problem. So how will you know how to approach his assessment and management?

Your assessment begins with the information you received from dispatch. Depending on the type of dispatch center, training of the dispatchers, and local dispatch protocols, you might receive dispatches such as the following:

Dispatch example 1: "Unit 531, respond code 3 for difficulty breathing."
Dispatch example 2: "Rescue 33, priority response for an unconscious female."
Dispatch example 3: "Engine 2760, code 3 for an unknown medical."
Dispatch example 4: "Unit 113, respond priority 2 for a man down."

As you can see, you have very little to go on given just the information provided by the dispatch. In most cases, dispatchers are well trained and experienced at staying calm, calming the reporting party, and doing the best they can at getting credible information from frightened and upset family and friends who are faced with an emergency. Not an easy task. The point is that many times you are not given much to go on and, therefore, you must wait until you get on scene and begin your assessment to categorize your patient.

So Why Does It Matter?

15-3 Discuss the importance of differentiating the medical patient from the trauma patient.

Why all the discussion, you ask? Aren't we going to care for all patients the same anyway? Well, yes and no. *Yes*, you will care for all patients in the most appropriate, compassionate, and respectful manner regardless of the underlying problem. *No*, you will not manage medical and trauma patients in the same exact way.

First and foremost when you suspect the emergency is related to a medical condition, your approach will be to center on a complete and thorough patient history. To accomplish that, you must become an expert detective and hone your interviewing skills like a well-sharpened knife. (In contrast, your approach to a trauma patient will center on your physical assessment of the injured body part or area. That approach is discussed in Chapter 28.)

The Medical Patient

The General Impression

15-4 Discuss the importance of the general impression.

You have heard how important first impressions can be. You have also heard that first impressions are usually right. The same holds true in medicine. Medicine is as much intuition as it is science. Back in Chapter 12 you were introduced to the concept of the *general impression* and how it can help determine how you will proceed with the patient. The general impression, also referred to as the *initial impression*, is your gut feeling of how sick your patient is. Some EMS folks call this the "doorway diagnosis" or the "big sick, little sick" decision. While this may be referred to as a "gut" decision or some sort of intuition, it really is more objective than that in most cases.

You are now combining the information from dispatch, your observations at the scene, and your general impression of the patient to further define the type of patient you have. There are several things you will want to look for, or assess, as you enter the scene and make visual contact with your patient. The following three factors play a big part of forming your "big sick, little sick" decision:

mentation the mental activity of a patient.

- *Mentation.* Simply put, **mentation** addresses the question, "Is the patient awake or unresponsive?" If he is awake, how is he responding to the environment? Is he alert and interacting with those around him, or sluggish and confused with little interaction? Position plays a part in this as well. A person who is sitting up will likely be more responsive than someone who is lying supine.

- *Color*. Look at the patient's face if he is light-skinned, or inspect the oral mucosa, nail beds, and palms of the hands of the dark-skinned patient. Check specifically for color. Is it pink as it should be? Or is it pale indicating poor perfusion?
- ***Level of distress.*** Patients are most commonly in distress for two reasons—pain and difficulty breathing. Ask yourself: Does the patient appear to be in immediate distress for either one of those reasons or both?

So, your "gut" is actually responding to a few very important observations or findings that help form your "big sick, little sick" decision.

The Interview

Most new EMTs come to the job without good interviewing skills. During training and thereafter, the only way to develop those skills is through purposeful practice. The good news is your interviewing skills practice does not have to involve actual patients. You can practice obtaining medical histories on just about anyone willing to answer personal questions relating to their own medical history. Family and friends are always willing participants in this process.

Remember to stay focused while you practice your interviewing skills. Your goal will be to develop a comfort with asking strangers very specific and personal questions. You must learn to do so in a clear, concise, efficient, and respectful manner. In addition, an emergency is no time to lose your train of thought or forget what question to ask next. The best way to master this is to practice on anyone and everyone willing to participate.

History of the Present Illness

15-5 Describe the elements of the history of the present illness.

history of present illness the medical history related to the patient's chief complaint.

There are two major categories when it comes to gathering a history for the medical patient—the **history of present illness** and the history of past medical conditions, or past medical history. The place to begin is with the history relating to the present illness or problem by asking questions related to the patient's chief complaint (the reason that you were called in the patient's own words). It is important to remember that you may have to ask the patient directly why you were called, because dispatch may not have gathered that information.

An example of how you might begin this conversation when the chief complaint is not obvious is as follows:

> "Mr. Jones, my name is Chris. I am an EMT and I will be taking care of you today. Can you tell me why you called us today?"

By beginning in this way you allow the patient to tell you in his own words what the issue is. Do this even when a family member or caregiver has already told you that the patient is having chest pain. Many times, experienced EMTs have reported, they were told the problem by someone other than the patient, only to have the patient describe something completely different. So, keep an open mind. Do not depend only on what you are told by dispatch or by others at the scene. Whenever possible, go right to the best source of information—the patient.

You will want to develop a line of questioning that focuses on the signs and symptoms related to the chief complaint. For every question you ask, there are at least two or three related follow-up questions that should be asked. Consider this line of questioning:

EMT: "So tell me, Mrs. Grandie, do you currently take any medications?"
Mrs. Grandie: "Yes, I take insulin and a pill for my high blood pressure."
EMT: "Have you been taking all of your medications as prescribed?"

Mrs. Grandie: "Oh yes, I take them every day."
EMT: "Have you taken them today?"
Mrs. Grandie: "Well no, not today, not yet anyway. I usually take them right after breakfast."

The exchange above is very common and one every EMT has engaged in. You cannot simply ask one question for each element of the SAMPLE history or OPQRST, despite the fact that this is what you will learn to do to successfully pass your patient assessment skills exam. Realize that obtaining a thorough medical history is much more than the questions prompted by the SAMPLE and OPQRST assessment tools.

Past Medical History

15-6 Describe the elements of the past medical history.

past medical history the medical history related to prior illness or events.

After you have gathered the history of the present illness, you will focus your line of questioning on the patient's **past medical history** (also referred to as the *pertinent past medical history*). To gather it, you must venture down a line of questioning that might reveal anything about the patient's past medical conditions that could in any way be related to the current problem. As an EMT, you will not have the knowledge, expertise, or experience to know for certain what information is directly related to the current chief complaint. However, you can remain objective, be thorough, and take good notes.

Your investigation into the patient's past medical history must include questions related to the following:

- Prescribed medications
- Purpose for taking prescribed medications
- Past surgeries
- Recent doctor visits
- Current signs/symptoms similar to those experienced before

Stay and Play, or Load and Go?

15-7 Discuss the role of time on scene with the medical patient.

time on scene the time spent on scene assessing, caring for, and preparing the patient for transport.

Another difference between emergency care of a medical patient and a trauma patient is the amount of time you spend on scene. **Time on scene** is the time you spend assessing, caring for, and preparing a patient for transport. In many instances your assessment of the medical patient will dictate appropriate emergency care, and that care will be initiated best on scene or while preparing for transport.

Interventions such as positioning the medical patient, administering supplemental oxygen, assisting with prescribed medications, or gathering a thorough history are best performed at the scene. Many times those interventions will make an immediate improvement in the medical patient's condition. In addition, you will learn in upcoming chapters that the optimal outcome for two conditions—acute myocardial infarction (AMI) and acute stroke—is directly dependent on how quickly the patient can get to a hospital for very specific care. Therefore, in cases of AMI and acute stroke, scene time must be minimized, resulting in a "load-and-go" situation.

Calling for Advanced Life Support

One of your most important roles as an EMT will be to recognize the need for advanced life support (ALS) care as early in the process as possible. Each and every level of EMS training has its limitations, and each EMT must have a clear understanding of the levels of care beyond his own. Recognizing the need for more advanced care and calling for it will help ensure the patient gets the necessary interventions as soon as possible.

Generally speaking, the medical patient is more likely to benefit from ALS care than the trauma patient. An ALS provider has many assessment tools and medication options that could immediately benefit the medical patient. In contrast, most trauma patients benefit most from immediate care for life threats, support of the ABCs, and rapid transport to an appropriate receiving hospital.

There are at least two options when requesting an ALS response for a medical patient. The first is called a *simultaneous response*, for which a BLS resource (vehicle staffed with EMTs) is dispatched at the same time as an ALS resource. This may occur when the BLS resource is known to be closer and can arrive and begin care while waiting for the ALS resource to arrive.

The second type of request is called an *ALS intercept*. It is recommended when transport is initiated by the BLS ambulance, and somewhere between the scene and the hospital, the two vehicles meet to transfer care. In most instances the patient is transferred to the ALS ambulance and then transported to the hospital.

Determining Your Destination

More and more hospitals are becoming specialized in caring for specific medical emergencies such as strokes, heart attacks, and post-resuscitation care. For that reason it is very important to be familiar with all of the medical facilities in your area or region and their specific specialties. In some instances, it is appropriate to bypass one hospital for the services of a specialty center. Such decisions are often guided by local protocols. Your instructor should be able to tell you about the specialty centers in your area and the protocol for deciding which patients should go where.

15-8 Discuss the importance of choosing the appropriate receiving facility when caring for medical patients.

Chapter Review

The Last Word

In summary, you should understand that in the medical world, especially the world of EMS, patients are categorized as either medical (illness) patients or trauma (injury) patients. Medical patients require sharp investigative and interviewing skills and will often benefit from interventions that you can provide at the scene. Your assessment begins with a deliberate general impression and then a structured and methodical approach to the secondary assessment.

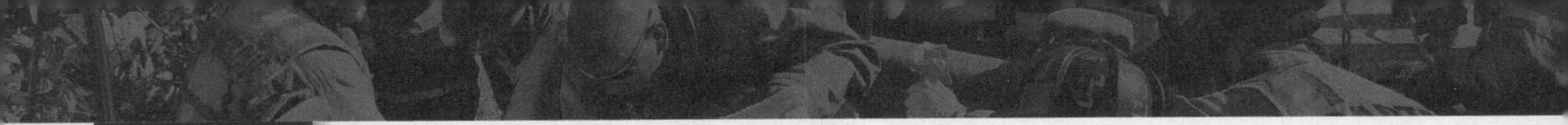

16 Pharmacology

Education Standards

Pharmacology: Principles of pharmacology, medication administration, emergency medications

Competencies

Applies fundamental knowledge of the medications that the EMT may assist/administer to a patient during an emergency.

Objectives

After completion of this lesson, you should be able to:

16-1 Define key terms introduced in this chapter.

16-2 Describe the roles and responsibilities associated with administering and assisting patients with the administration of medications.

16-3 Differentiate between a drug's chemical, generic, and trade names.

16-4 List the medications in the EMT's scope of practice.

16-5 Differentiate the following medication forms: tablet, liquid for injection, gel, suspension, fine powder for inhalation, gas, and liquid for spray and aerosolization.

16-6 Describe the proper administration of drugs by each of the following routes: sublingual, oral, inhalation, and intramuscular (epinephrine auto-injector only).

16-7 Describe the "five rights" related to medication administration.

16-8 Explain the roles of off-line and on-line medical direction with regard to medication administration.

16-9 Document required information regarding medication administration.

16-10 Describe the reassessment of a patient after the administration of a medication.

Key Terms

actions p. 442
activated charcoal p. 434
adsorption p. 434
albuterol p. 426
aspirin p. 431
blood clot p. 427
carbohydrate p. 434
chemical name p. 426
contraindication p. 427
dose p. 441
enteral p. 426
epinephrine p. 431
five rights p. 441
gel p. 426
generic name p. 426
indication p. 427
inhaled bronchodilators p. 437
inhaler p. 426
injection p. 431
intramuscular p. 431
mechanism of action p. 427
nebulized p. 437
nitroglycerin p. 431
oral glucose p. 434
oxygen p. 430
parenteral p. 426
pharmacodynamics p. 427
pharmacology p. 425
route p. 441
side effects p. 442
smooth-muscle relaxant p. 431
sublingual p. 426
suspensions p. 426
tablets p. 426
trade name p. 426
transdermal p. 426
United States Pharmacopoeia (USP) p. 426

Introduction

Prehospital medicine is designed to bring medical therapies into the field. Prehospital providers administer necessary, potentially life-saving treatments to patients before they arrive at the hospital. Medication administration is a vital component of this prehospital strategy.

16-2 Describe the roles and responsibilities associated with administering and assisting patients with the administration of medications.

Increasingly, EMTs are entrusted to administer a growing list of medications outside the hospital. The medications can be of great benefit to the patient and are frequently life-saving, but for all their value, those same medications can be dangerous when given incorrectly. Medication administration is an important trust that is formed with both our patients and with the medical direction physicians who authorize the administration.

The prehospital world is an unpredictable and ever changing environment and at times can present numerous challenges to critical thinking. Despite those challenges EMTs must thoughtfully and carefully process their decisions to administer medications. The results of a medication error can be tragic. Even under the worst circumstances, you must take care to consider the drug's intended effects, side effects, and potential complications before that medication is administered.

Medication administration requires an understanding of pathophysiology, the drug's mechanism of action, and knowledge of how the medication will interact with the normal functions of the patient. The study of drugs—their sources, characteristics, and effects—is called **pharmacology,** and every EMT must understand the pharmacology of the medications they are entrusted to administer.

pharmacology the study of drugs—their sources, characteristics, and effects.

This chapter will introduce you to the principles of pharmacology and the drugs commonly administered by EMTs, including how those medications are named, provided, and administered, how they act, and why one medication can act differently in different patients.

EMERGENCY DISPATCH

EMTs Rebecca and Lorenzo have been dispatched to a house on Butternut Street for a woman with shortness of breath. As they pull up to the scene, they notice a woman standing in the doorway, leaning on the doorframe. Rebecca says, "You go assess her and I'll bring the stretcher around." Because the scene appears to be safe, Rebecca and Lorenzo exit the ambulance and approach the patient.

As Lorenzo arrives beside the patient, he hears her wheezing. She looks at Lorenzo but cannot catch her breath long enough to speak. She is breathing very rapidly and is sweaty.

Rebecca brings the stretcher and Lorenzo assists the patient down onto it. The look on Lorenzo's face tells Rebecca that rapid transport is indicated. At that moment, the patient's daughter arrives and runs over to them. Rebecca introduces herself first and tells the daughter they will be right back, but need to load the patient into the ambulance right away.

Lorenzo climbs into the back of the ambulance with the patient, and Rebecca pauses briefly to talk to the daughter. The patient's daughter tells Rebecca that her mother's name is Susan and that she has asthma. She says that her mother phoned her about 30 minutes ago and said she was having a "bad asthma attack." Rebecca ends the brief medical history by asking the daughter if Susan takes any medications. The daughter hands Rebecca a prescribed inhaler.

Medications

Medications are derived from a variety of sources. Plants, minerals, and synthetic chemicals are commonly refined into compounds that can be beneficial if administered under the right circumstances.

16-3 Differentiate between a drug's chemical, generic, and trade names.

Each medication may have several names—a drug name, a generic name, and a trade name. Each name refers to the same medication, but describes it differently. Any drug can be expressed in a chemical formula also known as the **chemical name,** the scientific expression of the molecules that make up the chemical. For example, oxygen is often referred to using its chemical name O_2. The **generic name** of a drug is the one listed in the **United States Pharmacopoeia (USP),** a comprehensive government listing of all medications. A drug also may have a trade name or brand name. The **trade name** is the name a pharmaceutical company gives to a drug. Consider the following example:

> **Albuterol** is the generic name of a medication commonly administered by EMTs. Its chemical name is α1-[(tert-Butylamino)methyl]-4-hydroxy-m-xylene-α,α′-diol sulfate (2:1) (salt). Manufacturers also have assigned albuterol the trade names Proventil and Ventolin.

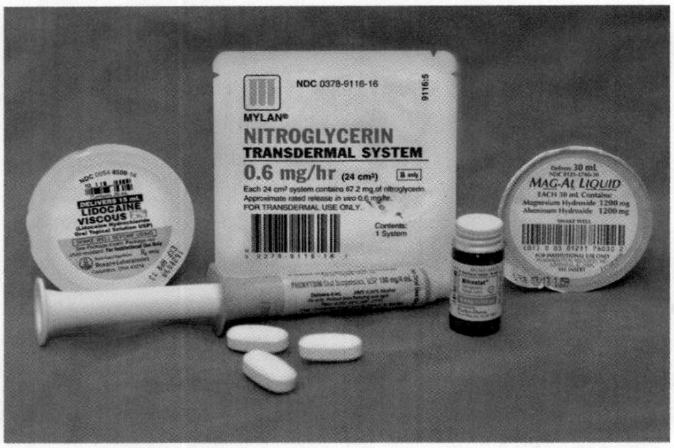

Figure 16-1 Medications come in a variety of forms such as pills, sprays, pastes, patches, and gels. (© Edward T. Dickinson)

16-5 Differentiate the following medication forms: tablet, liquid for injection, gel, suspension, fine powder for inhalation, gas, and liquid for spray and aerosolization.

Medications come in a variety of forms (Figure 16-1 ■). Each form allows a medication to be absorbed at an appropriate rate and achieve its designated effect at the proper time and location. Each form is administered by way of a specific route. Note that injected medications act very quickly. Medications taken orally (by mouth) reach the intended area much more slowly because they require digestion and absorption. Inhaled medications reach the lungs quickly and are absorbed across the alveolar membrane and into the pulmonary capillaries. **Sublingual** medications are administered under the tongue and are absorbed by the mucus membranes in the mouth.

Examples of the forms of medication are as follows:

- ***Pills or tablets.*** Generally, pills or **tablets** are taken orally (by mouth) or sublingually (under the tongue). An example of a pill or tablet is a nitroglycerin pill.
- ***Liquids for use outside the digestive tract.*** This form of medication may be administered by way of the **parenteral** route, which refers to bypassing the GI tract. An example of a parenteral medication is an epinephrine auto-injector.
- ***Liquids to be taken orally.*** This form of medication may be administered by way of the **enteral** route, which refers to using the digestive tract to reach the bloodstream. An example of an enteral medication is cough syrup.
- ***Liquids that are vaporized*** (mixed with air). This form of medication is absorbed in the lungs. It is commonly delivered through a nebulizer device.
- ***Gels.*** This form of medication is usually a viscous (thick and sticky) or jelly-like substance that the patient swallows. An example of a **gel** is oral glucose.
- ***Suspensions.*** A **suspension** is made up of two substances that must be mixed (because they generally separate into their individual parts). An example is activated charcoal. It is made of a powder and water that form a thick slurry, which is administered by mouth.
- ***Fine powder for inhalation.*** This form of medication is mixed with air and inhaled to be absorbed by the lungs. An example is a medication delivered by metered-dose **inhaler**.
- ***Gases.*** This form of medication is inhaled. An example is oxygen.
- ***Patches.*** **Transdermal** medications are placed on patches and applied to the skin through which the medications are absorbed. Examples include nitroglycerin or fentanyl patches.

As an EMT, you will encounter medications in many different ways. There are medications you are authorized to carry and administer, there are medications you may assist patients in taking, and there are medications that patients have been prescribed and take on a daily basis. Although much of your study of pharmacology will

chemical name the name that reflects the chemical structure of the medication.

generic name the medication name found in the United States Pharmacopoeia.

United States Pharmacopoeia (USP) government listing of all medications.

trade name the medication name a pharmaceutical company gives to a drug. Also called *brand name*.

albuterol a medication used to dilate bronchioles in patients who have respiratory disorders.

sublingual beneath the tongue.

tablets small disk-like compressed form of medication.

parenteral administered outside of the GI system.

enteral administered through the GI system.

gel jelly-like form of medication.

suspension solid medication mixed in a fluid; must be shaken before giving.

inhaler a spray device with a mouthpiece that contains an aerosol form of a medication that a patient can spray into his airway.

focus on the medications you are allowed to administer, do not overlook the importance of the prescribed daily medications your patient may be taking. In addition to problems like overdose and drug interactions, prescription medications can assist you in your assessment by providing information on the patient's most likely medical history. For example, a patient who takes insulin is surely a diabetic, and a person who takes nitroglycerin likely has a history of cardiac problems. Even though the patient may not be able to communicate, examining the patient's prescribed medications could provide you with volumes of information about the current condition.

transdermal through or by way of the skin.

16-4 List the medications in the EMT's scope of practice.

Also consider the potential effects of over-the-counter medications. Many patients take a variety of nonprescription medications including vitamins, supplements, and pain relievers. Even though they may be taken without the advice of a physician, they can have potent effects and can interact with other drugs.

PRACTICAL PATHOPHYSIOLOGY

Always consider the underlying impact of a medication before administering it. Recalling anatomy, physiology, and pathophysiology is always important. Consider albuterol, for example. It is an inhaled beta agonist and is given to patients with bronchospasm, a condition that narrows the bronchiole tubes and decreases air flow. Albuterol links with the beta receptor sites in the lungs and, through the sympathetic nervous system, signals the bronchiole tubes to dilate. If this occurs, air flow can be increased. Beware, however, that engaging the sympathetic nervous system also has side effects such as increased heart rate (tachycardia) and increased blood pressure.

By nature, a medication causes specific changes to occur within the body. Most of the time, those changes are designed to cause some therapeutic benefit. For example, albuterol is given to cause the bronchial tubes of the lungs to dilate. This can be beneficial in patients suffering from bronchoconstriction such as in asthma. The **mechanism of action** of a drug is the specific biochemical interaction that produces a pharmacological effect. Different medications can produce different effects from person to person. Often the effects can be altered by factors such as age, weight, or even underlying medical conditions.

mechanism of action the specific biochemical interaction that is caused by a medication to produce a pharmacological effect.

Pharmacodynamics is the study of the effects of medication on the body and is an important consideration for any provider before administering a drug. There is a reason for each medication to be given and that reason is referred to as an **indication.** The same medication may have a variety of different indications. For example, aspirin is often given to relieve the pain of a headache, but also it is given to reduce the chance of a **blood clot** in patients suffering from a heart attack.

pharmacodynamics the study of the biochemical and physiological effects of medications on the body.

indication reason a medication is administered.

blood clot a clumping together of blood cells.

In addition to reasons a particular medication is given (indication), the EMT must consider any reason a medication should *not* be given. This is called a **contraindication.** Most medications have contraindications. For instance, a contraindication for giving nitroglycerin to a patient with chest pain is a systolic blood pressure less than 100. Because one of the effects of nitroglycerin is to lower blood pressure, a patient who already has low blood pressure could experience a further drop in blood pressure that is sudden and dangerous. Another example is the administration of oral glucose to a diabetic patient with an altered mental status. In that case, putting the medication in the mouth of a patient who may not be able to swallow properly or manage his own airway could cause an airway obstruction.

contraindication situation in which a medication should not be administered because it could do more harm than good.

STOP, REVIEW, REMEMBER!

Multiple Choice

For each question, place a check next to the correct answer.

1. A medication's generic name is:
   _____ a. its chemical structure.
   _____ b. its "brand name."
   _____ c. the name listed in the USP.
   _____ d. a name based on the brand name of the medication.

2. A medication found in gel form is:
   _____ a. epinephrine.
   _____ b. oxygen.
   _____ c. nitroglycerin.
   _____ d. glucose.

3. The device that dispenses medication in fine-powder form is the:
   _____ a. nonrebreather oxygen mask.
   _____ b. nebulizer.
   _____ c. metered-dose inhaler.
   _____ d. oxylizer.

4. Albuterol sulfate would be an example of a medication's ______________ name.
   _____ a. generic
   _____ b. brand
   _____ c. trade
   _____ d. pharmacy

5. Sublingual medications are given:
   _____ a. under the tongue.
   _____ b. by injection under the skin.
   _____ c. as an ointment on the skin.
   _____ d. by inhalation or vapor.

Matching

Match the definition on the left with the applicable term on the right.

1. _____ The medication name found in the United States Pharmacopoeia
2. _____ The medication name that reflects the molecular structure of the medication
3. _____ Solid medication mixed in a fluid and must be shaken before administration
4. _____ The medication name a pharmaceutical company gives to a drug, which also could be referred to as a brand name
5. _____ Process of mixing air and medication to produce a vapor

A. Chemical name
B. Generic name
C. Nebulized
D. Trade name
E. Suspension

Critical Thinking

1. What is the difference between a metered-dose inhaler and a nebulizer?

____

2. A member of your family has gone to the cardiologist and received a prescription for nitroglycerin. The prescription was filled at his local pharmacy. Since you are an EMT, he stops by to ask you about his medication. Upon opening the pharmacy bag, you notice the medication container says "Nitrostat." Is there a difference between nitroglycerin and Nitrostat?

____

3. You are in a discussion with another EMT who tells you, "It doesn't matter if you put the nitroglycerin pill under the patient's tongue or if he chews it or swallows it. It all goes to the same place." Do you agree or disagree with this? Why?

____

4. Using this text and a drug reference source for each of the following medication names, list whether it is a trade name, chemical name, or generic name.

   a. Nitrostat _______________

   b. Albuterol sulfate _______________

   c. Activated charcoal _______________

   d. Nitroglycerin _______________

   e. Proventil _______________

   f. Glucose _______________

   g. Actidose _______________

   h. Epinephrine _______________

PERSPECTIVE

Susan—The Patient

I was terrified. I was having the worst asthma attack of my life. My breathing was so bad that I couldn't even speak. I would have used my inhaler, but I left it at my daughter's house. Thank goodness I called her early on. I tried to talk to the EMTs but I just couldn't. All I know is that they showed up in the nick of time. I don't think I would have lasted much longer without them.

Prehospital Medications

16-6 Describe the proper administration of drugs by each of the following routes: sublingual, oral, inhalation, and intramuscular (epinephrine auto-injector only).

The following section provides an introduction to the most common medications you will be allowed to administer as an EMT. Depending on your local system, you may not be allowed to administer all of them and in some systems you may be authorized to administer more. Your instructor and system protocols will tell you what medications are allowed in your area.

Medicine is a constantly evolving science and the appropriate medications of today may be inappropriate tomorrow. Furthermore, as science advances, new medications may be added to the formulary. For example, epinephrine auto-injectors are used to treat severe allergic reactions. EMTs have been allowed to assist patients in using them for many years. But because allergic reactions can be deadly and patients do not always have their auto-injector with them, many ambulances now carry epinephrine auto-injectors as part of their equipment.

A review of common medications is provided in this section, but further detail pertaining to specific drugs will be provided in later chapters. There, drugs will be discussed in the context of specific treatment plans. More information will be provided on how the medication affects the specific system in question. For example, nitroglycerin will be covered in greater detail in the cardiac chapter and inhalers will be covered with more depth in the respiratory emergencies chapter.

Oxygen

oxygen a medication administered to increase the amount of circulating oxygen in the bloodstream.

Oxygen is a naturally occurring gas that is used by our cells in the process of converting glucose into energy. As you read in Chapter 6, hypoxia (not enough oxygen) causes significant problems at a cellular level and is a frequent problem in patients you will encounter. To counteract hypoxia EMTs increase the patient's oxygen levels by administering supplemental oxygen. Supplemental oxygen is the same gas that is found in the air around us, but is in a more concentrated form (Figure 16-2 ■). Typically, supplemental oxygen is carried in a tank and administered through a mask or nasal cannula.

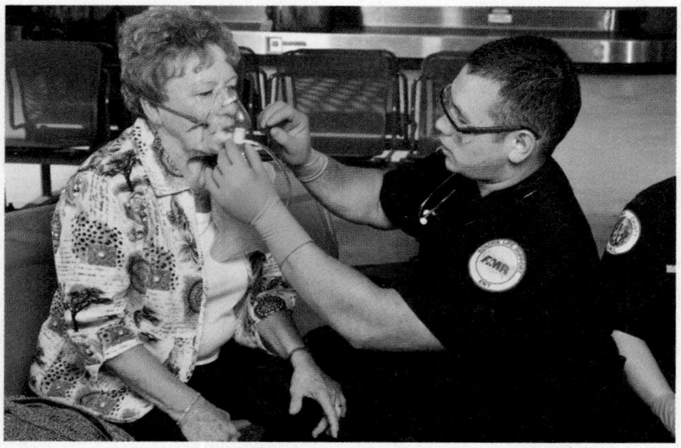

Figure 16-2 Oxygen is the most common drug administered by the EMT.

Although it is naturally occurring, 100% oxygen is a drug and as such it must be handled and administered with care. As with any medication, oxygen has specific indications and important side effects to consider. In fact, some studies demonstrate that there is such a thing as too much oxygen, a condition called *hyperoxia*.

The specifics of oxygen administration are discussed in greater detail in later chapters, but it is important to remember that oxygen should be treated with the same discretion and care you would give to any other medication you administer. Always know the appropriate indications and follow local protocols.

Aspirin

In the prehospital world, **aspirin,** the common household pain reliever, is given to treat acute coronary syndrome. In a heart attack, plaque buildup in the middle layers of a coronary artery gets exposed to passing blood and a clotting response begins. The clotting can obstruct (occlude) blood from getting through the vessel and stop it from perfusing the muscle of the heart. In the case of a heart attack, aspirin can reduce the blood's ability to clot and promote blood flow to help perfuse tissue (Figure 16-3 ■). The American Heart Association recognizes aspirin as one of the best early therapies for myocardial infarction. That means that the medication that has been in America's medicine cabinets for over 100 years now may be the best medicine to administer in the event of a heart attack.

aspirin medication used both during a heart attack and as a method to prevent heart attacks.

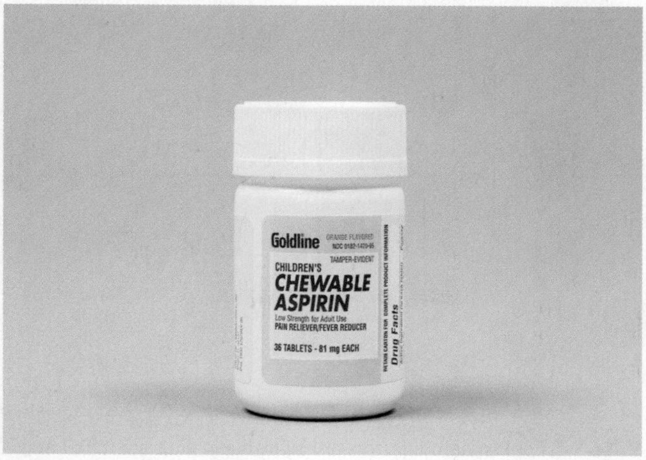

Figure 16-3 Low-dose, chewable aspirin is the type carried on most ambulances.

Although many of us have taken aspirin for headaches through the years, it is not a completely benign drug. Many people have allergies to aspirin and it can exacerbate bleeding problems particularly in the gastrointestinal system. You should always follow local protocols as you administer aspirin and take great care in administering it to patients with previous bleeding disorders. When in doubt, you should contact medical direction to consult on whether administration of aspirin is appropriate in your particular patient.

Epinephrine

Epinephrine is a medication used to treat serious allergic reactions. In an anaphylactic reaction (a life-threatening allergic reaction) epinephrine is administered by **injection** to help constrict blood vessels and dilate bronchial passages. It is a naturally occurring substance that also has a potent effect on the heart. Fast heart rates and increased blood pressures are a frequent side effect of this drug's administration.

epinephrine a medication used to treat serious allergic reactions called anaphylaxis.

injection placement of medication in or under the skin with a needle and syringe.

Epinephrine is commonly administered by **intramuscular** injection by way of an auto-injector (Scan 16-1). In an auto-injector a syringe uses a spring-loaded needle that will release and inject medicine into the muscle when it is pushed against the skin. Epi-Pen® is the trade name of a commonly carried epinephrine auto-injector and Twinject® is the trade name of an auto-injector that contains two doses of epinephrine.

intramuscular within a muscle.

When treating a patient with anaphylaxis, you may be authorized to assist in the administration of a prescribed epinephrine auto-injector. More information on administering medications will be provided later in this chapter and the use of auto-injectors in anaphylaxis will be discussed in detail in future chapters.

Some EMS systems allow EMTs to carry and use an epinephrine auto-injector to treat anaphylaxis. This authority is typically granted by medical direction and is very different than simply assisting a patient in the use of his own auto-injector. Depending on local protocol, such a capability may require additional education and testing.

Nitroglycerin

Nitroglycerin is a **smooth-muscle relaxant** that is used to treat chest pain associated with acute coronary syndrome. It comes in a variety of forms such as tablet, spray, and paste, but tablets and spray are the most common used in EMS. Tablets are placed under the tongue to dissolve, and the spray is sprayed directly under the tongue (Scan 16-2). The smooth-muscle relaxant properties of nitroglycerin are thought to dilate coronary arteries to increase blood flow and also dilate other blood vessels in the body to reduce the workload of the heart, which helps to relieve chest pain.

nitroglycerin a medication used to treat chest pain.

smooth-muscle relaxant a medication that relaxes smooth muscles, for example, as nitroglycerin relaxes the muscle in blood vessels and permits an increased blood flow.

SCAN 16-1 Epinephrine Auto-Injectors

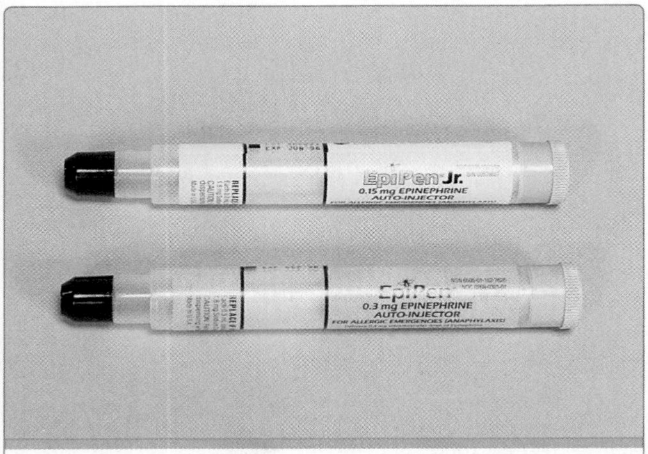

16-1-1 Epi-Pen auto-injectors are available in both adult (0.3 mg) and pediatric (0.15 mg) dosages.

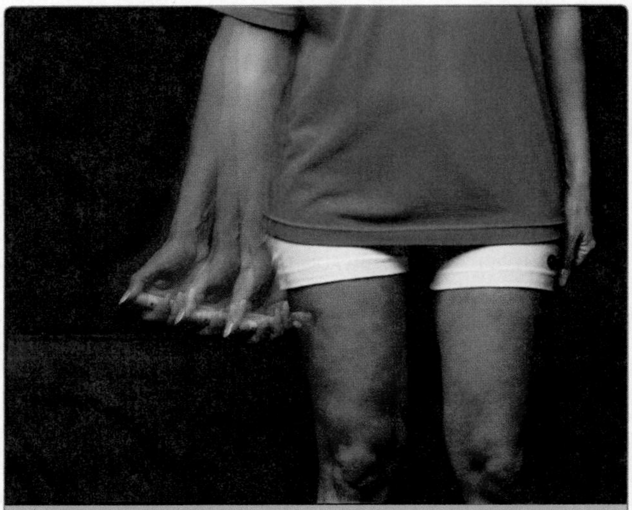

16-1-2 The auto-injector is ideally suited for self injection at the lateral thigh.

MEDICATION NAME

1. **Generic:** epinephrine.
2. **Trade:** Adrenalin®, Epi-Pen®.

INDICATIONS

Must meet the following three criteria:

1. Patient exhibits signs of a severe allergic reaction, including either respiratory distress or shock.
2. Medication is prescribed for this patient by a physician.
3. Medical direction authorizes use for this patient.

CONTRAINDICATIONS

No contraindications when used in a life-threatening situation.

MEDICATION FORM

Liquid form of 1:1,000 concentration. Administered by an automatically injectable needle-and-syringe system.

DOSAGE

Adults: one adult auto-injector (0.3 mg).

Infant and child: one infant/child auto-injector (0.15 mg).

Adult has a yellow label and the pediatric has a white label.

STEPS FOR ASSISTING PATIENT

1. Obtain patient's prescribed auto-injector. Ensure right medication, right dose, right route, right patient, and right time. Note that most auto-injectors have a two-year shelf life. Medication will discolor (yellowish) when expired.
2. Obtain order from medical direction.
3. Remove cap from auto-injector. Then grasp the auto-injector barrel, avoiding placing your thumb over the end of the device.
4. Place tip of auto-injector against patient's lateral thigh, midway between hip and knee. You may inject through clothing if necessary.
5. Push the injector firmly against the thigh until the injector activates.
6. Hold the injector in place until the medication is injected (at least 10 seconds).
7. Document the time and any response to the medication.
8. Dispose of injector in biohazard container.

ACTIONS

1. Dilates the bronchioles.
2. Constricts blood vessels.

SIDE EFFECTS

1. Increased heart rate.
2. Dizziness.
3. Chest pain.
4. Headache.
5. Nausea.
6. Vomiting
7. Excitability, anxiety.
8. Pale skin.

REASSESSMENT STRATEGIES

1. Initiate transport to an appropriate receiving facility as soon as practical.
2. Continue assessment of airway, breathing, and circulatory status. If patient's condition continues to worsen (decreasing mental status, increasing breathing difficulty, decreasing blood pressure):
   a. Obtain medical direction for an additional dose of epinephrine.
   b. Provide care for shock, including administration of oxygen per local protocols.
   c. Prepare to initiate basic life support (CPR, AED).
3. If patient's condition improves, provide supportive care:
   a. Continue oxygen.
   b. Provide care for shock.

SCAN 16-2 Nitroglycerin (Pills and Spray)

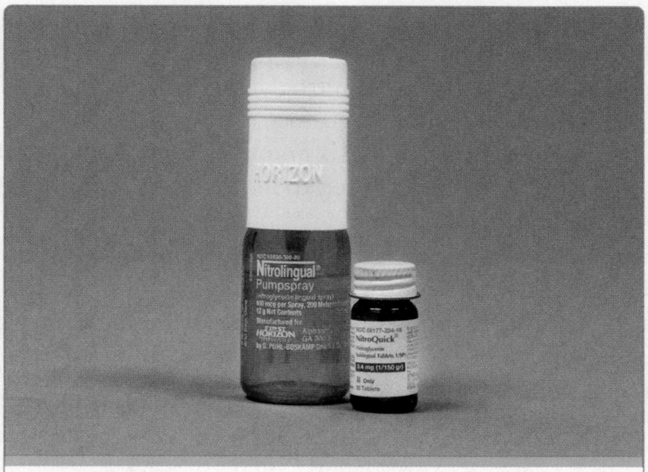

16-2-1 Nitroglycerin is available in both a spray bottle and pill form. Both are administered under the tongue.

MEDICATION NAME

1. **Generic:** nitroglycerin.
2. **Trade:** Nitrostat®, NitroTab®, Nitrolingual®.

INDICATIONS

All of the following conditions must be met:

1. Patient complains of chest pain.
2. Patient has a history of cardiac problems.
3. Patient's physician has prescribed nitroglycerin.
4. Systolic blood pressure is greater than 100 systolic. (Local protocols may vary.)
5. Medical direction authorizes administration of the medication.

CONTRAINDICATIONS

1. Patient has a systolic blood pressure below 100 mmHg. (Local protocols may vary.)
2. Patient has a head injury.
3. Patient has already taken the maximum prescribed dose.

MEDICATION FORM

Tablet or sublingual spray.

DOSAGE

One dose is equal to 0.4 mg. Repeat in three to five minutes. If no relief, if systolic blood pressure remains above 100 (local protocols may vary), and if authorized by medical direction, up to a maximum of three doses. Spray is typically prescribed for one metered spray followed by a second in 15 minutes.

STEPS FOR ASSISTING PATIENT

1. Perform assessment for cardiac patient.
2. Take blood pressure. (Systolic pressure must be above 100; local protocols may vary.)
3. Contact medical direction if no standing orders.
4. Ensure right medication, right dose, right route, right patient, right time.
5. Ensure patient is alert.
6. Question patient on last dose taken and effects. Ensure understanding of route of administration.
7. Ask patient to lift tongue and place tablet or spray dose on or under tongue (while you are wearing gloves) or have patient place tablet or spray under tongue.
8. Have patient keep mouth closed with tablet under tongue (without swallowing) until dissolved and absorbed.
9. Recheck blood pressure within two minutes.
10. Record administration, route, and time.
11. Perform reassessment.

ACTIONS

1. Dilates blood vessels.
2. Decreases workload of heart.

SIDE EFFECTS

1. Hypotension (lowers blood pressure).
2. Headache.
3. Pulse rate changes.
4. Dizziness, light-headedness.

REASSESSMENT STRATEGIES

1. Monitor blood pressure.
2. Ask patient about effect on pain relief.
3. Seek medical direction before re-administering.
4. Record assessments.
5. Provide oxygen as appropriate.

A dangerous side effect associated with nitroglycerin is that it can cause an abnormal drop in blood pressure. Nitroglycerin is generally *not* given to patients whose systolic blood pressures are less than 90 mmHg, or as in some systems, less than 100 mmHg. Erectile dysfunction medications such as Viagra™ or Cialis™ also can cause a dangerous drop in blood pressure when combined with nitroglycerine therapy. Patients, both men and women, should always be questioned about these types of medications prior to nitroglycerin administration and should *not* be given nitroglycerin if they have used them within the last 24 to 72 hours (depending on local protocol).

PRACTICAL PATHOPHYSIOLOGY

Nitroglycerin helps patients in acute coronary syndrome in two ways. First, nitroglycerin dilates coronary arteries to allow more blood to flow to the heart muscle. Second, it dilates the venous side of the circulatory system and therefore decreases blood return to the heart. This decreases the workload of the heart and reduces its oxygen consumption.

Nitroglycerin tablets remain potent for only about six months after the bottle has been opened. They degrade and deactivate when exposed to light, so bottles must be protected accordingly.

Nitroglycerin is a medication that EMTs commonly assist the patient in taking. Frequently, an EMT would identify a previously prescribed bottle of nitroglycerin and after careful consideration and appropriate medical direction authorization, would assist the patient who is having chest pain in taking the medication. In some systems EMTs carry and administer nitroglycerin. Always follow local protocol.

Activated Charcoal

activated charcoal a medication used to treat certain cases of poisoning or overdose.

Activated charcoal is a powder prepared from charred wood. The powder is usually premixed with water to form a suspension that is used to treat certain cases of poisoning or overdose (Scan 16-3). The resulting slurry is administered to some patients who have ingested poisons to prevent the gastrointestinal system from absorbing toxins. Activated charcoal molecules have a very large surface area and many toxins are easily adsorbed by the substance. This **adsorption** prevents the poison from crossing over into the bloodstream.

adsorption the attachment of a substance to the surface of another material.

Activated charcoal is not recommended for all poisonings and should only be administered on the orders of medical direction or a poison control center. Some poisons are not adsorbed well by the charcoal and in some cases the timing of the ingestion may prevent activated charcoal from being effective.

Typically, activated charcoal is administered on the advice of medical direction or the poison control center and should always be used with care. Most commonly, EMTs will mix and administer activated charcoal as a drink given to a conscious patient. Because the aspiration of activated charcoal into the lungs can be a potentially fatal complication, only select patients who are awake and alert and can manage their own airway should be given activated charcoal to drink.

The procedure for administering activated charcoal will be discussed in greater detail in later chapters.

Oral Glucose

Many patients, especially those with poorly managed diabetes, will suffer from low blood sugar (also known as *hypoglycemia*). For a variety of reasons the cells of their body do not have enough glucose to maintain normal cellular metabolism. Many cells, including cells of the brain, are very sensitive to this type of deficiency. As a result, symptoms such as altered mental status are common in patients with low blood sugar.

oral glucose a medication used to treat patients with suspected low blood sugar.

carbohydrate source of fuel for the body.

Oral glucose is a **carbohydrate** used to treat patients with suspected low blood sugar. It is administered to rapidly replace depleted glucose stores and provide cells with the fuel they need to enable normal aerobic metabolism. Oral glucose is a gel that typically comes in a tube (Scan 16-4). It can be ingested or applied to a tongue depressor and placed between the patient's cheek and gum. This allows the glucose to be swallowed and absorbed into the digestive tract and bloodstream. If given under the right circumstances, an amazing improvement in the patient's condition will occur. However, like any other drug, there are considerations that must be accounted for before administration.

SCAN 16-3 Activated Charcoal

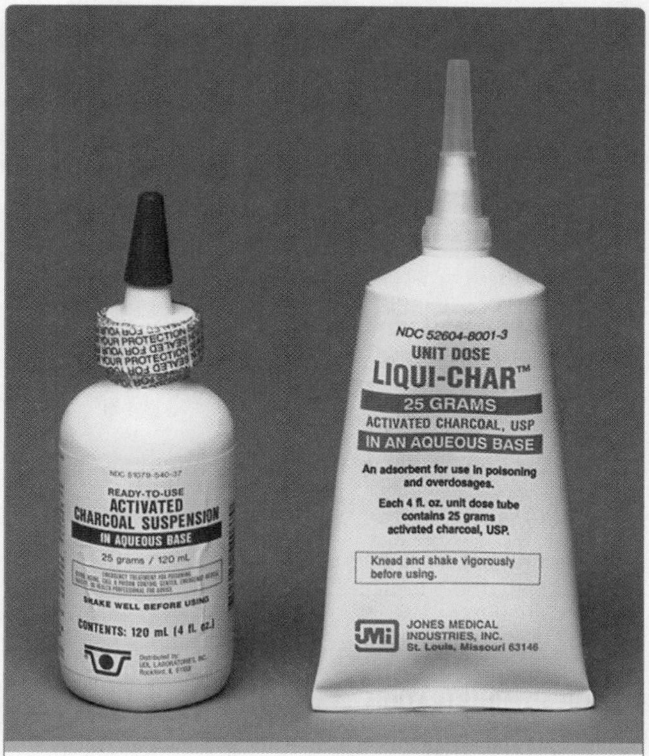

16-3-1 Activated charcoal typically is available in 25 gram dosages.

MEDICATION NAME

1. **Generic:** activated charcoal.
2. **Trade:** SuperChar®, InstaChar®, Actidose®, Liqui-Char™, and others.

INDICATIONS

Poisoning by mouth (ingestion).

CONTRAINDICATIONS

1. Altered mental status.
2. Ingestion of acids or alkalis.
3. Unable to swallow.

MEDICATION FORM

1. Premixed in water, frequently available in plastic bottle.
2. Powder, which should be avoided in field.

DOSAGE

1. **Adults and children:** 1 gram activated charcoal per kg of body weight.
2. **Usual adult dose:** 25 to 50 grams.
3. **Usual pediatric dose:** 12.5 to 25 grams.

STEPS FOR ADMINISTRATION

1. Consult medical direction.
2. Shake container vigorously.
3. Because medication looks like mud, the patient may need to be persuaded to drink it. Providing a covered container and a straw will prevent the patient from seeing the medication and so may improve patient compliance.
4. If patient does not drink the medication right away, the charcoal will settle. Shake or stir it again before administering.
5. Record the name, dose, route, and time of administration of the medication.

ACTIONS

1. Activated charcoal adsorbs (binds) certain poisons in the digestive tract and prevents them from being absorbed into the body.
2. Not all brands of activated charcoal are the same: some adsorb much more than others, so consult medical direction about the brand to use.

SIDE EFFECTS

1. Causes black stools.
2. Some patients, particularly those who have ingested poisons that cause nausea, may vomit. If the patient vomits, repeat the dose once.

REASSESSMENT STRATEGIES

Be prepared for the patient to vomit or further deteriorate. If the patient worsens, provide oxygen as you have been trained to do.

Oral glucose is administered by mouth. This means that the patient must have full control of his airway or risk accidentally aspirating (breathing in) the glucose into his lungs.

Oral glucose is only effective in patients who actually have low blood sugar. Ideally, it should be given only when this problem can be identified. Many EMS

SCAN 16-4 Oral Glucose

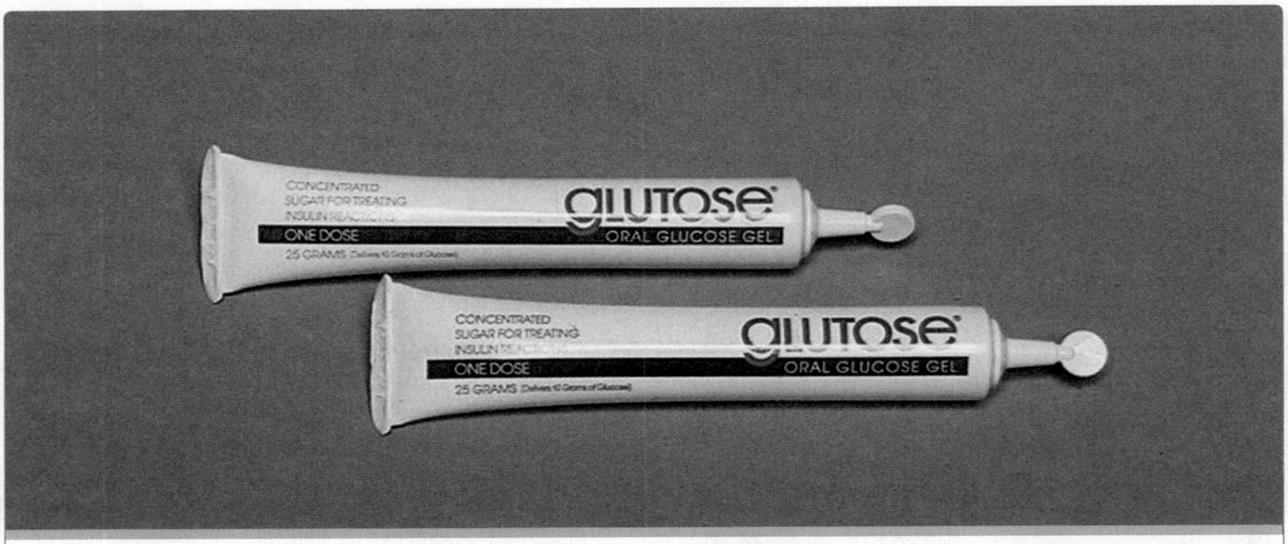

16-4-1 Oral glucose comes in dosages ranging in concentrations from 15 to 45 grams. (Shown are 25 gram tubes.)

MEDICATION NAME

1. **Generic:** glucose, oral.
2. **Trade:** Glutose™, Insta-Glucose®, BD™ Glucose Tablets.

INDICATIONS

1. Patients with altered mental status with a known history of diabetes.
2. Patient has taken insulin but no food recently and may have been very physically active.

CONTRAINDICATIONS

1. Unresponsiveness or unable to swallow or otherwise manage own airway.
2. Known diabetic who has not taken insulin for days.

MEDICATION FORM

Gel, in toothpaste-type tubes; chewable tablets.

DOSAGE

One tube; three 5.0 gram chewable tablets. This dose can be used for both adults and children. Tubes can come in 15, 30, and 45 mg dosages.

STEPS FOR ADMINISTRATION

1. Ensure signs and symptoms of altered mental status with a known history of diabetes.
2. Ensure patient is alert enough to swallow.
3. Administer glucose.
   a. Self-administered into mouth and swallowed.
   b. Place on tongue depressor between cheek and gum.
   OR
   c. Have patient chew one to three tablets.
4. Perform reassessment.

ACTIONS

Increases blood sugar levels.

SIDE EFFECTS

None when given properly.

REASSESSMENT STRATEGIES

Continue to monitor the patient's mental status and signs and symptoms. If patient becomes less responsive, discontinue administration. Continue to provide oxygen as you have been trained to do.

systems allow EMTs to monitor blood sugar. If you have this capability, double check blood sugar before administration. Always follow local protocols.

Inhaled Bronchodilators

Inhaled bronchodilators, as the name implies, open up bronchioles that are constricted due to a respiratory disease such as asthma. In most cases, these medications are prescribed to a patient, and an EMT will assist in their administration. The early administration of bronchodilators can significantly impact the outcomes of patients suffering from bronchoconstriction, so your intervention, even if it is just assisting a patient with his medication, is important.

inhaled bronchodilators medication used to open up bronchioles that are constricted due to a respiratory disease such as asthma.

Typically, bronchodilators are delivered in two ways: through a metered-dose inhaler (Figure 16-4 ▪) or through a small-volume nebulizer. A metered-dose inhaler generally aerosolizes a fine powder that is inhaled by breathing deeply as the inhaler is activated. A nebulizer mixes a liquid medication with air to create a vapor that is inhaled. **Nebulized** medications are generally administered over a longer period of time (Scan 16-5).

nebulized process of mixing air and medication to produce a mist, which is inhaled.

Many bronchodilators can cause an increased heart rate, agitation, and increased blood pressure. Care should be taken when giving these medications to patients who already have a fast heart rate. You will need to keep track of the number and timing of previous doses to avoid administering too much of this type of medication.

The medications used in your EMS system may differ slightly from the medications listed in Table 16-1. Ask your instructor or refer to your local protocols to learn about the medications you may administer.

PERSPECTIVE

Rebecca—The EMT

I could see how sick the patient was. There was a look of fear on her face that was unmistakable. I knew if we didn't act quickly, things would get much worse. The day before we had discussed the value of early bronchodilator administration in asthma, so I was thrilled when the patient's daughter showed up with the inhaler. It gave me an immediate step I could take.

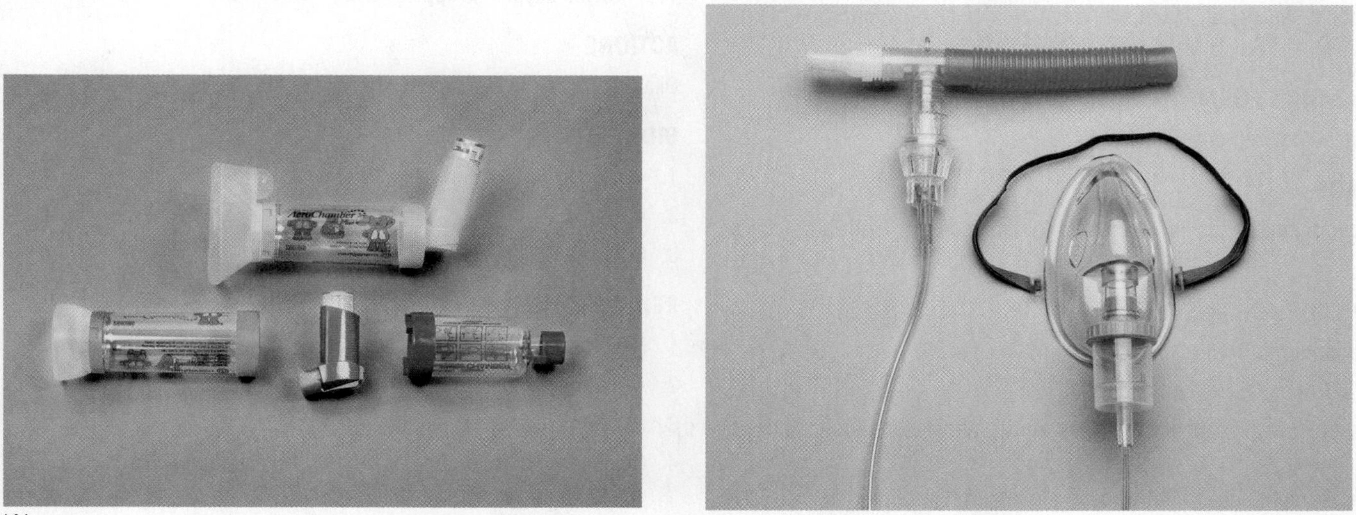

(A) (B)

Figure 16-4 (A) Metered-dose inhalers and the spacers that are sometimes used with them. (B) A small-volume nebulizer typically carried on an ambulance.

SCAN 16-5 Metered-Dose Inhalers

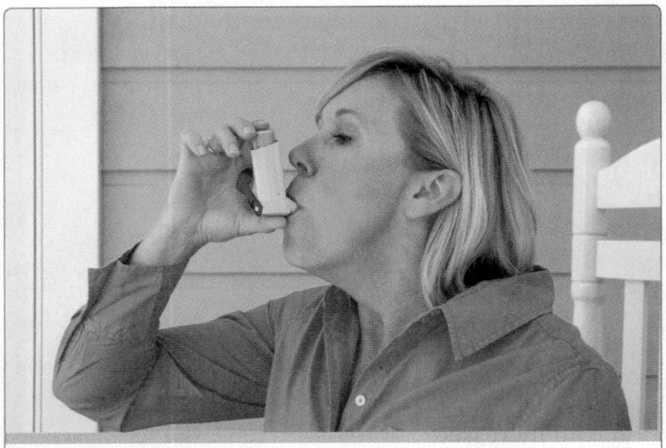

16-5-1 A typical metered-dose inhaler (MDI).

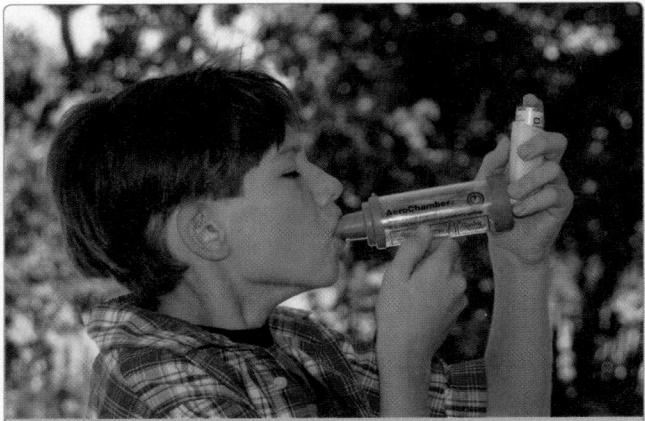

16-5-2 For better results, a spacer is sometimes used with an MDI.

MEDICATION NAME

1. **Generic:** albuterol, ipratropium, metaproterenol.
2. **Trade:** Proventil™, Ventolin™, Atrovent®, Alupent™, Metaprel®.

INDICATIONS

Meets all of the following criteria:

1. Patient exhibits signs and symptoms of respiratory difficulty.
2. Patient has physician-prescribed inhaler.
3. Medical direction gives the EMT specific authorization to use.

CONTRAINDICATIONS

1. Altered mental status (such that the patient is unable to use the device properly).
2. No permission has been given by medical direction.
3. Patient has already taken maximum prescribed dose prior to EMT's arrival.

MEDICATION FORM

Handheld metered-dose inhaler.

DOSAGE

Number of inhalations based on medical direction's order or physician's order.

STEPS FOR ADMINISTRATION

1. Obtain order from medical direction.
2. Confirm patient is alert enough to use inhaler.
3. Ensure it is the patient's own prescription and check expiration date of inhaler.
4. Ensure right dose, right route, right patient, right time.
5. Check if patient has already taken any doses.
6. Shake inhaler vigorously several times.
7. Have patient exhale deeply.
8. Have patient put lips around the opening of the inhaler.
9. Have patient depress the handheld inhaler as he begins to inhale deeply.
10. Instruct patient to hold breath for as long as is comfortable so that medication can be absorbed.
11. Allow patient to breathe a few times and repeat second dose if so ordered by medical direction.
12. If patient has a spacer device for use with the inhaler (device for attachment between inhaler and patient to allow for more effective use of medication), it should be used.
13. Provide oxygen as appropriate.

ACTIONS

Dilates bronchioles, reducing airway resistance.

SIDE EFFECTS

1. Increased pulse rate.
2. Anxiety.
3. Nervousness.

REASSESSMENT STRATEGIES

1. Monitor vital signs.
2. Adjust oxygen as appropriate.
3. Reassess level of respiratory distress.
4. Observe for deterioration of patient. If breathing becomes inadequate, provide artificial ventilations.

TABLE 16-1 PREHOSPITAL MEDICATIONS

MEDICATION	CARRIED ON THE AMBULANCE OR PATIENT'S OWN	FORM	INDICATION (USE)
Epinephrine	Patient's own Carried on the ambulance in many areas	Auto-injector	Severe allergic reactions (anaphylaxis)
Nitroglycerin	Patient's own	Tablet or spray administered under the tongue (sublingually)	Cardiac-related chest pain
Oral glucose	Carried on the ambulance	Gel (oral)	Diabetic patients with suspected low blood sugar
Activated charcoal	Carried on the ambulance	Suspension	Some poisoning and overdose patients
Albuterol (prescribed inhaler)	Patient's own Carried on the ambulance in some areas	Fine powder for inhalation	Asthma, chronic lung conditions
Albuterol (nebulized)	Patient's own Carried on the ambulance in some areas	Nebulized (aerosolized)	Severe asthma and chronic lung conditions
Aspirin	Patient's own Carried on the ambulance	Tablet (chewable)	Chest pain
Oxygen	Carried on the ambulance Patients may be on home oxygen	Gas	Various, including respiratory distress, chest pain, shock, many others

STOP, REVIEW, REMEMBER!

Multiple Choice

For each question, place a check next to the correct answer.

1. Which one of the following medications is supplied as a suspension?

_____ a. Glucose
_____ b. Epinephrine
_____ c. Activated charcoal
_____ d. Aspirin

2. Which one of the following medications is supplied as a tablet?

_____ a. Nitroglycerin
_____ b. Albuterol
_____ c. Activated charcoal
_____ d. Proventil

3. You assist a patient with his inhaler. Almost immediately the patient feels shaky and as if his heart has sped up. Those sensations are called:

_____ a. contraindications.
_____ b. actions.
_____ c. indications.
_____ d. side effects.

4. The medication that is designed to adsorb certain ingested poisons and prevent them from entering the body is:

_____ a. nitroglycerin.
_____ b. activated charcoal.
_____ c. aspirin.
_____ d. albuterol.

(continued on next page)

(continued)

5. Which one of the following would be an absolute contraindication to the administration of oral glucose?

_____ a. Inability to protect the airway
_____ b. Hypotension
_____ c. Altered mental status
_____ d. Tachycardia

Matching

Match the form of medication on the left with the medication on the right that comes in that form.

1. _____ Liquid for injection
2. _____ Gel
3. _____ Tablet
4. _____ Suspension
5. _____ Fine powder for inhalation
6. _____ Sublingual spray
7. _____ Gas
8. _____ Nebulized (vaporized)

A. Oxygen
B. Nitroglycerin
C. Epinephrine
D. Oral glucose
E. Activated charcoal
F. Albuterol
G. Ventolin

Critical Thinking

1. Is nitroglycerin carried on your ambulance? Describe your local protocols regarding administering or assisting in the administration of nitroglycerin.

____

____

____

____

2. Your patient uses an inhaler. What form of medication is in the inhaler? How does the inhaler work?

____

____

____

____

Administering Medications

Administering a medication is a significant responsibility. Although some areas of the country do not require physician interaction for EMTs to assist with medication, there are plenty of areas that do. Furthermore, there are some areas that do not allow EMTs to assist at all. Always follow local protocol related to medication administration.

16-7 Describe the "five rights" related to medication administration.

There are very important rules that apply to the administration of medication. Those rules establish why it is important to administer the medication, how it is best administered, and how much of the medication to give. The rules must be applied whenever a medication is administered to ensure a safe and appropriate use of the drug. Furthermore, medication administration must consider both the positive and negative effects that will occur in the body.

There are many situations in which a medication, no matter how therapeutic it may be, cannot be administered. You must become familiar with the likely effects of a drug so that you can safely weigh the costs and benefits before administration.

Five Rights

The rules described in the previous section are commonly referred to as the **five rights** of medication administration. These concepts will apply each and every time you administer or consider administering a medication. They are a simple way to remember all the elements you must review before administering a medication to the patient. The five rights are as follows:

five rights memory aid for all things you must check when administering a medication to the patient. They include right medication, right dose, right route, right patient, and right time.

- ***Right medication.*** You must first ensure that you have an appropriate indication to administer the medication. An indication is the reason the medication is administered. Is this the right medication for the patient's condition? Is this medication indicated to treat this condition? Is the medication I am about to administer the medication I believe it is? Have I checked and rechecked the label to verify this? Is the medication current (not expired)?
- ***Right dose.*** A **dose** is how much of the medication you will administer. Each medication has a specific dose to safely achieve the desired effect with the minimal number of side effects. Before administering a medication, you should ask, "Am I giving the correct amount of medication?" Incorrect doses can be dangerous to the patient. Do not assist with the administration of medication if you are not certain of the correct dose.

dose the amount of medication that is to be administered.

- ***Right route.*** The **route** refers to how the medication is administered (for example, sublingually, injected, or inhaled) and how the medicine will enter the body. Before administering any medication, you should first ask, "Am I giving the medication through the correct route?" Specific routes regulate the rate at which a medication is absorbed into the body, and incorrect routes can lead to unsafe rates of absorption.

route how the medication is administered.

- ***Right patient.*** Ask yourself, "Does this medication belong to the patient I am about to give it to?" Frequently, you will assist patients in the administration of a previously prescribed medication. Before doing so, you should always be sure the medication has actually been prescribed to the patient. Sometimes patients will use medications that are actually prescribed to friends or family members. This is another opportunity to be sure your indications are correct.
- ***Right time.*** Before administering any medications, you must make sure that you have an appropriate indication to give the drug. Ask yourself, "Is it the right time to give the medication? Will the medication treat the patient's condition?" A contraindication is a reason not to give the medication (such as an allergy).

Before giving any medication, you must be sure you have both an appropriate indication and no contraindications to administration. For example, you should ask, "Are the patient's vital signs appropriate for the medication that will be given? Has the patient taken any other medications that could cause an undesirable side effect?" These are all important considerations and can be thought of as a cost-benefit analysis.

PRACTICAL PATHOPHYSIOLOGY

Consider how underlying conditions may impact the medication you are about to give. For example, if a patient has a very fast heart rate, should you give a medication such as albuterol, which may increase heart rate further? Consider also the patient's ability to metabolize the medication. Poor underlying circulation may make it more difficult for the patient to process the medication you are about to administer.

actions the desired responses in the body a medication may cause. Also called the *desired effect.*

side effects any action of a drug other than the desired action.

You must consider how the medication will affect your patient. All medications have specific actions. **Actions** are the responses in the body that the medication is designed to create. Actions are also called the *desired effect.* In addition to the desired effect, medications can cause side effects. A **side effect** is a negative action other than the desired effect. For example, a side effect of epinephrine administration is an increased heart rate. Sometimes side effects are minor, but there are times when side effects can significantly harm your patient. You should always consider the possibilities before administering a medication.

When considering how a medication will affect your patient, you must consider age and underlying condition. Pediatric patients are frequently smaller and require less medication to achieve the desired effect. Their ability to process the medication may differ significantly from an adult. Older patients may have similar issues. Age can seriously impact how medications affect the body. Special consideration must be given when administering medications to a patient of advanced age. Finally, underlying conditions such as shock, hypothermia, chronic disease, and other medications can change the way drugs interact with body systems. When given unusual circumstances, it is always best to consult on-line medical direction prior to administering medications.

Documentation

16-9 Document required information regarding medication administration.

Documentation is exceptionally important in medication administration. You should document the patient's condition before administration, as well as document the patient's response to the medication after administering it, including a recheck of vital signs. Documentation should also include the specific dose, route, and time that the medication was administered.

Medical Direction

16-8 Explain the roles of off-line and on-line medical direction with regard to medication administration.

When you administer a medication, it will often be after consulting a physician (also sometimes called medical direction) by radio or phone (Figure 16-5 ■). After verbally presenting your patient and his condition to the physician, you may receive an order to administer a medication.

When receiving a medication order, it is important to acknowledge the order, and then repeat it back to the physician for verification. Once it is confirmed, write down the medication, dose, route, and any other specific information. You may be told to administer one sublingual nitroglycerin now and another one in five minutes if the patient's blood pressure remains over 100 mmHg systolic. It is important to remember the order exactly. Writing it down will help ensure that it is done correctly.

After receiving the order and writing it down, you should select the medication from your kit (if it is one that is carried on the ambulance) or obtain it from your patient (if it is one prescribed to the patient). Verify the medication name on the container and the expiration date and all of the five rights. Ensure that the medication is uncontaminated. For example, if it is a liquid, ensure that it is normal (usually clear) and free of particles or impurities. Be sure the patient is not allergic to the medication you wish to administer.

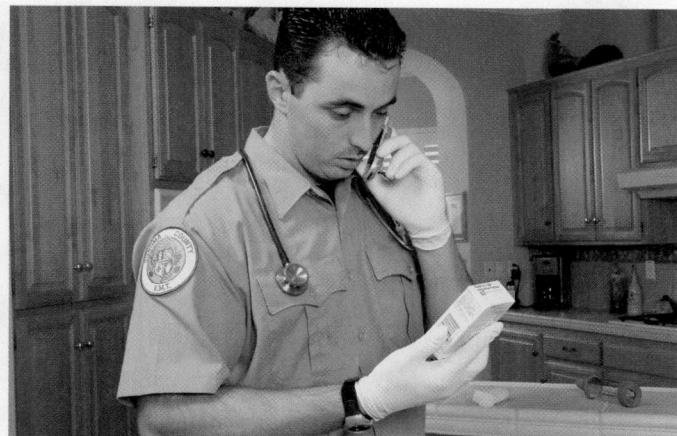

Figure 16-5 Sometimes it is necessary to contact medical direction prior to assisting with the administration of a medication.

After a medication is given, reassess the patient. This will include determining the effect the patient felt from receiving the medication (better, worse, or no change) and reassessing vital signs. This reassessment is often performed as part of a reassessment en route to the hospital.

16-10 Describe the reassessment of a patient after the administration of a medication.

> **CLINICAL CLUE**
>
> **Communicating with Medical Direction**
>
> If an order from a physician does not seem to make sense to you, ask the physician for clarification. Remember that the physician cannot see the patient. His information is based on your radio report. If part of your transmission is distorted or if there is a misunderstanding on either end, an order could be incorrect. It is always better to ask for clarification and express the concerns you have than to administer a medication in error.

Medication Safety and Clinical Judgment

When given incorrectly, medications can cause serious harm to the patient. Therefore, any medication administration is a serious responsibility. Judgment and careful consideration must be used before the patient receives the drug. The world of prehospital medicine is a dynamic place and there are many distractions to your concentration. Regardless of distractions, decisions have to be made. When it comes time to make decisions about medications, you will need to focus.

Medication administration should only be undertaken after a thorough patient assessment and thorough consideration of the five rights. You must understand not only how this medication will impact the patient in general, but also how it will impact your current patient under the current, specific circumstances. Know the medication. If you are unsure about it, or if conditions are unusual, use your references; that is, ask questions, contact medical direction, look up medications, but never guess. Once a medication is administered, it cannot be taken back. Focus, good judgment, and clear thinking all will help ensure proper and safe treatment.

STOP, REVIEW, REMEMBER!

Multiple Choice

For each question, place a check next to the correct answer.

1. With regard to the five rights of medication administration, the "right route" would mean the:

_____ a. route the ambulance takes to the hospital.

_____ b. manner by which the medication is delivered to the patient.

_____ c. urgency of transport for the patient.

_____ d. method by which medications are carried on the ambulance.

2. The reason a medication is administered is known as the:

_____ a. route.

_____ b. mechanism of action.

_____ c. indication.

_____ d. contraindication.

3. A(n) _____________ is a negative action of a medication other than the desired effect.

_____ a. contraindication.

_____ b. action.

_____ c. indication.

_____ d. side effect.

4. You are caring for a patient who has severe anaphylaxis. She has her own auto-injector with her. You should first:

_____ a. confirm the medication has not expired.

_____ b. immediately administer the medication.

_____ c. ask a family member to administer it.

_____ d. request to see the prescription form.

5. Medical direction has asked you to assist with the administration of two puffs of a patient's metered-dose inhaler. The medication has *not* expired. You should:

_____ a. ask a family member to administer the medication.

_____ b. assist the patient with the administration of the medication.

_____ c. immediately spray two puffs into the patient's mouth.

_____ d. ask if the patient is allergic to the medication.

Short Answer

1. With regard to the five rights of medication administration, describe what is meant by right medication.

____

____

____

____

2. With regard to the five rights of medication administration, describe what is meant by right patient.

____

____

____

____

3. With regard to the five rights of medication administration, describe what is meant by right dose.

4. With regard to the five rights of medication administration, please describe what is meant by right route.

5. With regard to the five rights of medication administration, please describe what is meant by right time.

Critical Thinking

1. Explain your local procedure or protocol for obtaining medical direction authorization to administer a medication.

2. You call medical direction because you are treating a patient experiencing a severe allergic reaction and request an order for epinephrine. The doctor approves the order and says, "Okay, go ahead and put the epinephrine in the IV line." What should you do?

(continued on next page)

(continued)

3. Please describe the key elements of documentation following medication administration.

____

____

____

____

EMERGENCY DISPATCH SUMMARY

After placing the patient on high-flow oxygen, Lorenzo contacted medical direction to request authorization to assist the patient with her inhaler. Lorenzo explained the circumstances to the doctor on the radio and provided a complete picture of assessment findings. The doctor concurred with Lorenzo's plan and instructed him to assist with two puffs of the metered-dose inhaler. Lorenzo repeated back the order and wrote it down on his clipboard. He then paused and reviewed the five rights for the administration of this bronchodilator. Yes, he was correct, it was time to give the medication.

The patient was anxious to take the medication and quickly inhaled a puff. Lorenzo then instructed her to take another puff. The oxygen was replaced and Lorenzo recorded the time and dose of the prescribed inhaler. After replacing the oxygen, he reassessed the patient and completed the transport without incident.

Chapter Review

To the Point

- An EMT brings life-saving medications to patients in the prehospital world, but with this capability comes significant responsibility to protect the patient's safety.
- In some cases EMTs assist patients with their prescribed medications, while for others they actually administer medications carried on the ambulance.
- EMTs commonly administer oxygen, aspirin, albuterol, oral glucose, nitroglycerin, epinephrine, and sometimes activated charcoal.
- Medications can come in a variety of forms. Tablets, liquids for injection, liquids to be taken orally, liquids that are vaporized, gels, suspensions, powders for inhalation, patches (transdermal), and gases are all common forms.
- An EMT must be familiar with a drug's generic and trade names and be comfortable with the appropriate resources to obtain further information.
- Medications administered by an EMT utilize the sublingual, oral, inhaled, and intramuscular routes.
- The five rights of medication administration are essential to the safe administration of medications and must be reviewed for each administration, before the drug is given.
- Medical direction is often utilized in the administration of medications. This influence can be seen off-line in the form of protocols and guidelines and on-line as in a direct conversation or authorization prior to the administration of a medication.
- Reassessment of a patient after the administration of a medication is essential.
- Documentation is another essential element of medication administration.

Chapter Questions

Multiple Choice

For each question, place a check next to the correct answer.

1. When receiving an order from medical direction, you should:
   _____ a. write down the order, and then administer the medication.
   _____ b. repeat the order as confirmation, write down the order, and then administer the medication.
   _____ c. write down and repeat the order, confirm it with the patient, and then administer the medication.
   _____ d. confirm the order with a second physician, write down the order, and then administer the medication.

2. A previous anaphylactic reaction to aspirin would be considered a:
   _____ a. contraindication.
   _____ b. desired effect.
   _____ c. mechanism of action.
   _____ d. therapeutic effect.

3. Aspirin, when carried on the ambulance, may be administered by the EMT when ____________ is suspected.
   _____ a. pain
   _____ b. fever
   _____ c. heart attack
   _____ d. infection

4. Assessing a patient's response after administering a medication is often done as part of the:
   _____ a. primary assessment.
   _____ b. scene size-up.
   _____ c. secondary assessment.
   _____ d. reassessment.

5. Which one of the following questions would you ask to determine "right patient" in the five rights?
   _____ a. Is this the correct drug for this patient?
   _____ b. Is this the right amount of the drug for this patient?
   _____ c. Is this patient allergic to this drug?
   _____ d. Is this medication prescribed to the patient?

Matching

Match the term on the left with the definition on the right.

1. _____ Indication	A. What we expect the medication to do within the body
2. _____ Route	B. The reason the medication is administered
3. _____ Dose	C. Situations in which you would not administer a medication
4. _____ Actions	D. Negative effects that may occur
5. _____ Side effects	E. How much of the medication is administered
6. _____ Contraindications	F. How the medication is administered

Critical Thinking

1. What is the difference between a side effect and a contraindication?

____

____

____

____

(continued on next page)

(continued)

2. You have just administered nitroglycerin for chest pain and begin to reassess the patient. For what will you reassess?

3. You are at a high school football game where a student is having breathing difficulty. The patient says he has asthma, but his inhaler is inside the locked school. Another student has an inhaler for asthma. Can you use the other student's inhaler? Why or why not?

4. List the five rights of medication administration and one question you can ask to verify each.

Case Study

You are called to a patient with chest pain. John Gillis is 67 years old. The patient reports that he was mowing the lawn when the pain started. This was about 10 minutes ago. He came in and sat down in the air conditioning. You find him pale, cool, and sweaty. He reports that although his chest pain has subsided, it is still significant. He describes it as "5" on a scale of 0 to 10. Previously it was "8."

His vital signs are pulse 96 strong and regular, respirations 20 and slightly labored, blood pressure 124/86, pupils equal and reactive. Skin as noted above.

The patient has taken one of the nitroglycerin tablets he received after his first and only other bout of chest pain "four or five months ago." Otherwise the patient is healthy. He takes an aspirin a day for prevention of heart attacks and Lipitor for high cholesterol.

Assuming (until you study cardiac emergencies in Chapter 18) that this patient would benefit from nitroglycerin:

1. Compose a radio report to your medical direction physician requesting an order for administration of sublingual nitroglycerin.

2. What side effect(s) might you see from the administration of nitroglycerin?

____

____

____

____

The Last Word

The safety of your patient requires a serious approach to medication administration. As an EMT, you must understand the pharmacology of the medications you are authorized to administer. You must be able to identify the medication and understand the indications, contraindications, actions, and side effects before giving any drug. You also must have a working knowledge of the pharmacodynamics so you can understand how it will affect different types of patients. Most importantly, you must take your time to review and seriously consider the five rights of medication administration before you administer a drug. There is no substitute for good judgment. Remember, a drug cannot be taken back once it has been administered.

There are many medications that EMS providers may administer or assist in administering. They change over time as research reveals additional benefits and risks of a medication. Part of being a professional requires you to stay current with changes and adjust your practice to changing protocols and additional information. Continuing education will be vital.

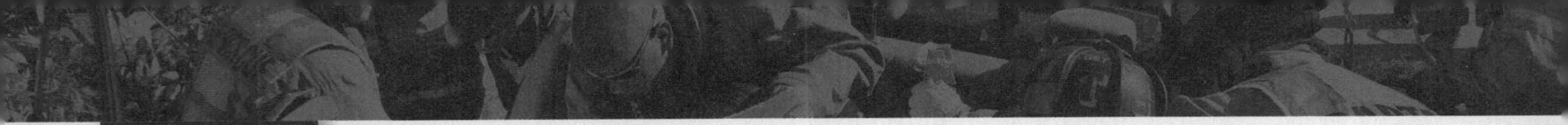

17 Caring for Patients with Breathing Difficulty

Education Standards

Medicine: Respiratory

Competencies

Applies fundamental knowledge to provide basic emergency care and transportation based on assessment findings for an acutely ill patient.

Objectives

After completion of this lesson, you should be able to:

17-1 Define key terms introduced in this chapter.

17-2 Describe the structure and function of the respiratory system.

17-3 Explain the importance of being able to quickly recognize and care for patients with respiratory emergencies.

17-4 Explain the relationship between dyspnea and hypoxia.

17-5 Describe an assessment-based approach for the patient with respiratory distress.

17-6 Describe at least three types of abnormal breathing patterns.

17-7 Describe the term *hypoxic drive* and how it relates to the COPD patient.

17-8 Differentiate respiratory distress, respiratory failure, and respiratory arrest.

17-9 Describe the characteristics of normal and abnormal breath sounds.

17-10 Describe the pathophysiology by which each of the following conditions leads to inadequate oxygenation: epiglottitis, hyperventilation syndrome, obstructive pulmonary diseases (emphysema, chronic bronchitis, and asthma), pneumonia, pneumothorax, poisonous exposures, pulmonary edema, pulmonary embolism, and viral respiratory infections.

17-11 Describe the steps for managing a patient with respiratory distress.

17-12 Describe special considerations in the assessment and management of pediatric patients with respiratory emergencies.

17-13 Describe the indications for administering or assisting a patient with self-administration of bronchodilators by metered-dose inhaler and small-volume nebulizer.

17-14 Differentiate between short-acting beta$_2$ agonists appropriate for prehospital use and respiratory medications that are not intended for emergency use.

17-15 Explain the importance of the reassessment to identify responses to treatment and changes in the patient's conditions.

Key Terms

accessory muscles p. 457
apnea p. 460
aspiration p. 452
asthma p. 463
auscultation p. 462
beta$_2$ agonist p. 474
bronchoconstriction p. 463
central neurogenic hyperventilation p. 460
Cheyne-Stokes respirations p. 460
chronic bronchitis p. 464
crackles p. 463
croup p. 472
dead space p. 452
dyspnea p. 456
emphysema p. 464
epiglottitis p. 467
gurgling p. 458
hypercarbia p. 452
hyperventilation p. 467
hyperventilation syndrome p. 467
hypoxia p. 452
hypoxic drive p. 461
Kussmaul's respirations p. 461
metered-dose inhaler (MDI) p. 474
midaxillary line p. 462
nebulizer p. 471
parietal pleura p. 452
pneumonia p. 464
pneumothorax p. 466
pulmonary edema p. 466
pulmonary embolism p. 465
pulse oximetry p. 460
respiratory arrest p. 462
respiratory failure p. 461
rhonchi p. 463
small-volume nebulizer (SVN) p. 475
snoring p. 458
spontaneous pneumothorax p. 466
stale air p. 464
status asthmaticus p. 464
stridor p. 458
sympathetic nervous system p. 474
tension pneumothorax p. 466
triggers p. 463
tripod position p. 457
visceral pleura p. 452
wheezing p. 458
work of breathing p. 456

Introduction

Patients with respiratory distress will require prompt clinical as well as emotional support. Respiratory distress can be the chief complaint in a variety of serious conditions, such as heart attack, congestive heart failure, and acute asthma or emphysema. The patient experiencing shortness of breath may literally feel he is going to die. The feeling is one of the most frightening sensations there is for both the patient and the loved ones who are with the patient.

This chapter discusses the management of patients experiencing respiratory distress, including some of the conditions that can cause difficulty breathing and the care you will provide to these patients.

EMERGENCY DISPATCH

The light drizzle that had been falling on the ambulance windshield for an hour had just progressed to a steady downpour when the radio broke the silence.

"Unit 2, respond to 1163 Courtside Avenue for an adult male in respiratory distress."

"Unit 2, copy." Brent, a new EMT, switched on the windshield wipers and looked up and down the deserted street before pulling out and activating the emergency lights.

Brent and his partner, Joanne, first saw the patient as they rolled to a stop in front of the address. The man was sitting in the tripod position on the front steps of his home, drenched by the rain and waving his arm feebly.

"You. Gotta. Help. Me." The man struggled with each word as the EMTs approached. The rain poured down on them, soaking everything, including the stretcher.

"Quick, let's get him in the truck," Joanne shouted over the thunder.

Thomas, the patient, was pale and struggling frantically to breathe. His eyes were wide with fear, and with each attempted breath, he pounded on the plastic cabinet doors in the back of the ambulance.

"I'll get a nonrebreather," Brent said, sliding one of the compartment doors aside with a trembling hand.

"Forget that," Joanne said through a tangle of wet hair. "We're going to have to bag him."

Review of Respiratory Anatomy and Physiology

17-2 Describe the structure and function of the respiratory system.

A sound knowledge of respiratory anatomy and physiology will allow you to understand the signs and symptoms presented by your patient. This knowledge will also help you understand some of the basic pathophysiology (disease processes) you will find when you obtain a patient history and find that the patient has had respiratory conditions in the past. (See Chapter 5 for further review of the respiratory system.)

The movement of oxygen into the bloodstream and to the tissues and the removal of waste products generated by normal cell metabolism are essential to life. These are the primary functions of the respiratory system.

The respiratory system is divided into two parts—the upper and lower airway (Figure 17-1 ▪). The anatomical dividing line between the upper and lower airway are the vocal cords. The air we breathe enters the upper respiratory system through the mouth and nose. The area behind the mouth is known as the *oropharynx*. The area behind the nose is the *nasopharynx*. Once air passes through the oropharynx and nasopharynx, it continues past the epiglottis and through the glottic opening. The air then moves into the larynx. The larynx contains the vocal cords and the entrance to the trachea and lower respiratory system. This opening is protected by the epiglottis. When we swallow, the epiglottis folds down over the opening of the trachea to prevent material from entering the lungs. When foreign substances enter the lungs, it is referred to as **aspiration.**

aspiration the drawing of a foreign substance into the lungs during inhalation.

The trachea is the beginning of the lower airway and is made up of C-shaped rings of cartilage. The first and only complete ring of the trachea is called the *cricoid ring*. Farther down, the trachea splits into two branches called *bronchi*. The point where the trachea branches in two is called the *carina*. Each bronchus continues to split into smaller bronchioles, eventually ending at the alveoli. The alveoli are sacs that resemble grape-like clusters. This is where the transfer of oxygen into the bloodstream and the removal of carbon dioxide from the bloodstream take place.

The lungs, also part of the lower airway, are positioned in the chest cavity. The right lung has three lobes and the left lung has two lobes. The inside of the chest wall is covered with a thin membrane called the **parietal pleura.** Each lung is covered by a membrane called the **visceral pleura.** When the lungs are working normally, they sit tightly against the chest wall and both membranes are attached to one another by a slick fluid. Between the two membranes exists a "potential space," which is called the *pleural space*. In the case of a chest injury, air or blood could enter this space and cause a partial or total collapse of a lung. (Chapter 33 will discuss this type of injury in greater detail.)

parietal pleura a membrane that is attached to the chest wall.

visceral pleura a membrane that is attached to the lung surface.

Dead space exists in the airways any place where oxygen is *not* exchanged. Dead space is anywhere other than the alveoli (Figure 17-2 ▪). When air enters the body, it must travel through the mouth and nose, through the oropharynx and nasopharynx, into the larynx, trachea, bronchi, and through bronchioles before the air reaches the alveoli. That means about 150 mL of the air we breathe does not even reach the alveoli where gas exchange can take place.

dead space areas of the lungs outside the alveoli where gas exchange with the blood does not take place.

The average amount of air taken in with an adult's normal breath is approximately 500 mL. Of this, only about 350 mL actually reach the alveoli, and the rest occupies airway dead space. This is normal. A problem develops when the patient begins to breathe too shallowly. If only 200 to 250 mL of air is breathed in, very little air gets to the alveoli for gas exchange. This is one of the many causes of **hypoxia** and the buildup of carbon dioxide, also known as **hypercarbia.**

hypoxia an insufficiency of oxygen in the body's tissues.

hypercarbia excessive carbon dioxide in the blood.

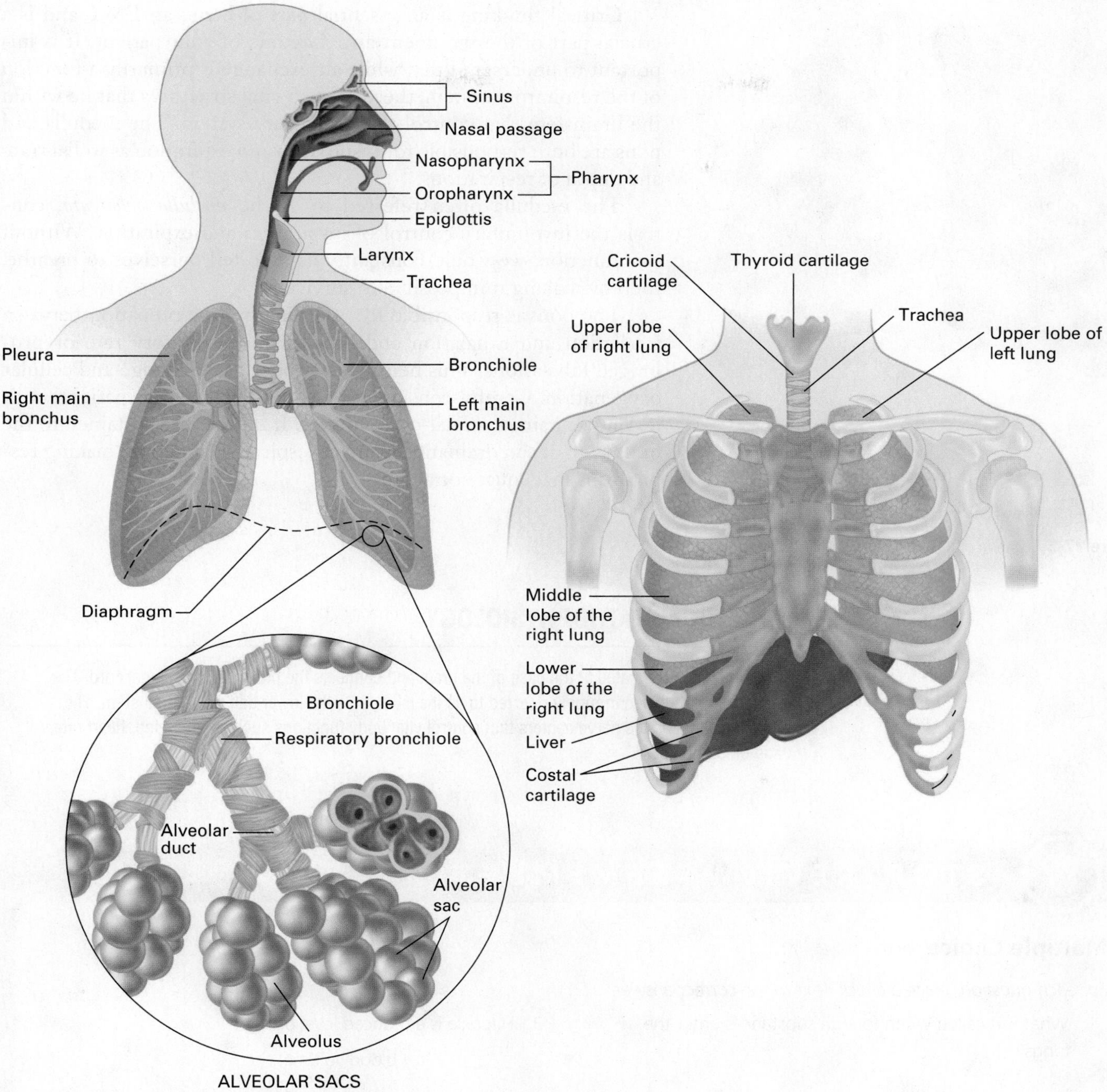

Figure 17-1 The major structures of the respiratory system.

PRACTICAL PATHOPHYSIOLOGY

When there is inadequate ventilation, hypoxia (low blood oxygen) and hypercarbia (high blood carbon dioxide) will eventually result. At high blood levels carbon dioxide (CO_2) has a narcotic-like effect on the brain resulting in lethargy or sleepiness. Always consider hypercarbia from inadequate gas exchange as a possible cause of this type of decreased mental status during your patient assessments.

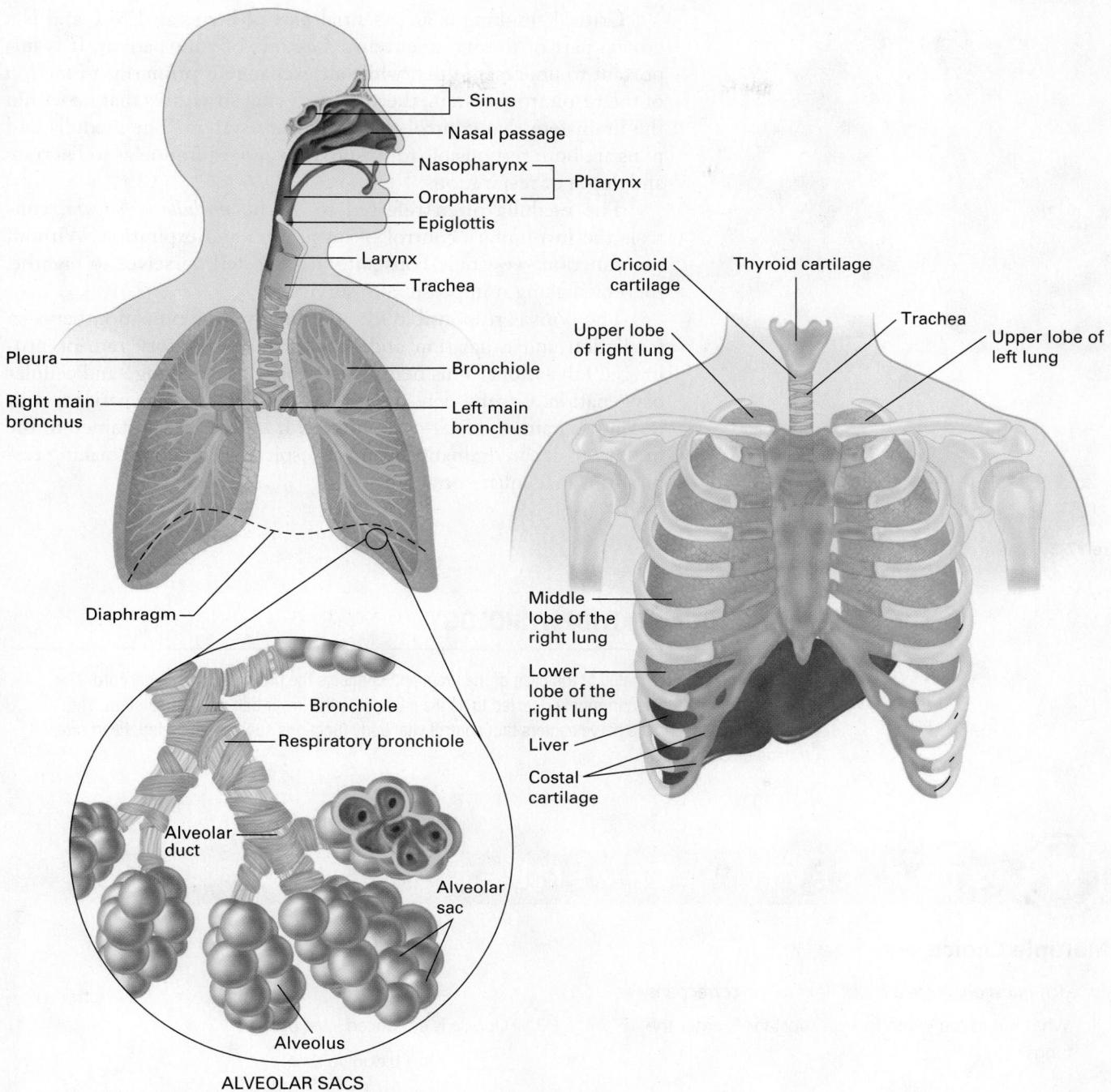

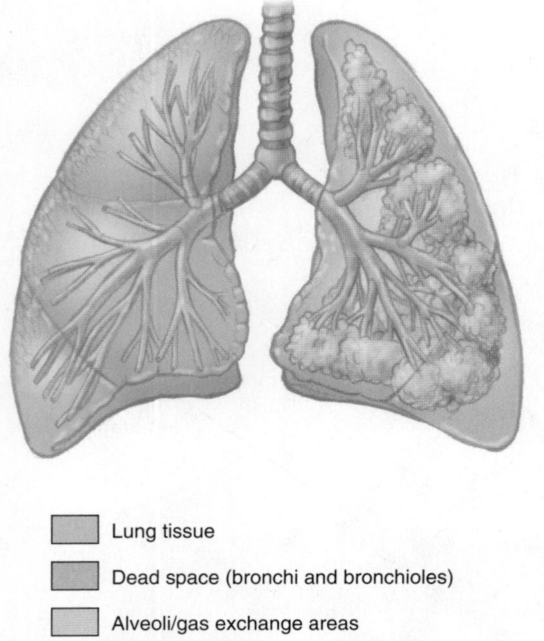

Figure 17-2 Location of dead air space within the respiratory system.

Critical thinking is an essential part of being an EMT and is a crucial part of the treatment and outcome of your patient. It is important to understand that while air exchange is primarily a function of the respiratory system, there are two vital structures that lie within the brainstem that control the respiratory system. The medulla and pons are both responsible for inspiration and expiration as well as rate and depth of respirations.

The medulla often referred to as the *medulla oblongata*, controls the involuntary control of inspiration and expiration. Without this function, we would constantly have to tell ourselves to breathe, thereby making it impossible to survive.

The pons is responsible for coordinating the transition between inhalation and exhalation and defines the respiratory rate or prolonged inhalations. This helps with proper gas exchange and cellular oxygenation. Careful consideration should be given to patients with potential brain or spinal-cord injuries. If injuries are sustained to the brainstem, it can dramatically affect respiratory function, making respirations inadequate or absent.

PRACTICAL PATHOPHYSIOLOGY

The brainstem is located at the base of the brain and connects the brain with the spinal cord. The medulla oblongata, commonly referred to as the *medulla*, is the lower half of the brainstem. The medulla contains the nerve centers that control vital body functions such as breathing, heart rate, and blood pressure.

STOP, REVIEW, REMEMBER!

Multiple Choice

For each question, place a check next to the correct answer.

1. What is it called when foreign substances enter the lungs?

   _____ a. Reflux
   _____ b. Pneumothorax
   _____ c. Inhalation
   _____ d. Aspiration

2. Alveoli are often described as:

   _____ a. multicellular membranes.
   _____ b. grape-like clusters.
   _____ c. pressure-filled vesicles.
   _____ d. venous-pressure driven.

3. Hypoxia is a reduced level of:

   _____ a. blood volume.
   _____ b. carbon dioxide in the blood.
   _____ c. oxygen in the blood.
   _____ d. hemoglobin.

4. What is the only complete ring of the trachea?

   _____ a. Hyoid bone
   _____ b. Cricoid cartilage
   _____ c. Carina
   _____ d. Cricoid ring

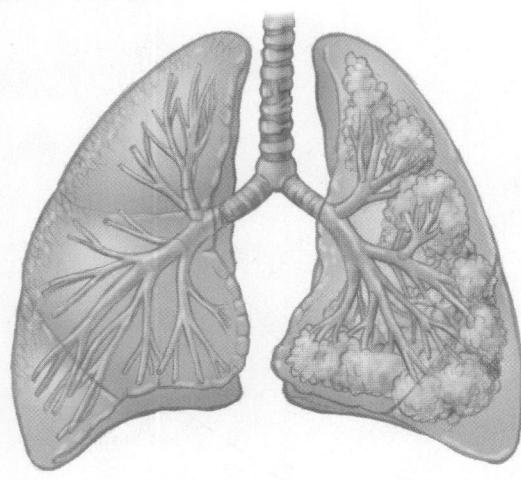

5. The inside of the chest wall is covered with a thin membrane called the:

_____ a. dead space.

_____ b. parietal pleura.

_____ c. visceral pleura.

_____ d. hypercarbia.

6. What is the average amount of air taken in with a normal breath of an adult?

_____ a. 500 mL

_____ b. 350 mL

_____ c. 250 mL

_____ d. 750 mL

Fill in the Blank

1. The area that is posterior to the mouth and above the larynx is called the ____________________.

2. Oxygen is transferred to the blood and waste products are removed in the ____________________.

3. The ____________________ is the tissue that folds over the tracheal opening to prevent solids and liquids from entering the lungs.

4. The lung has two pleura. The ____________________ pleura is attached to the chest wall; the ____________________ pleura is attached to the surface of the lungs.

5. Areas where no transfer of oxygen takes place in the lungs are called ____________________.

6. The ____________________ and ____________________ are where the upper airway begins.

7. The ____________________ is where the lower airway begins.

8. The ____________________ is where the trachea splits into the right and left bronchi.

Critical Thinking

1. Describe the structures that air must pass through from the point it enters the mouth and nose until it gets to the alveoli.

____

____

____

____

2. What is the main purpose of the respiratory system?

____

____

____

____

(continued on next page)

(continued)

3. Describe the function of the medulla and pons relative to respirations.

____

____

____

____

Assessment of the Patient with Respiratory Distress

17-3 Explain the importance of being able to quickly recognize and care for patients with respiratory emergencies.

17-4 Explain the relationship between dyspnea and hypoxia.

dyspnea shortness of breath.

work of breathing effort needed for adequate ventilation.

Patients experiencing difficulty breathing will generally fall into one of three categories: respiratory distress, respiratory failure, or respiratory arrest. Respiratory distress is also called *difficulty breathing*, *shortness of breath*, or **dyspnea.** It is a common complaint seen by EMS providers and extremely frightening for the patient. It almost always indicates some sort of serious underlying condition. It is characterized by difficult or labored breathing and an increase in the **work of breathing** from such things as an asthma attack or an allergic reaction. It also can be a chronic problem caused by disease processes such as bronchitis and emphysema. There are many levels of respiratory distress, ranging from mild to severe.

It is important that you learn to recognize the signs of respiratory distress. A patient in respiratory distress can deteriorate very quickly and may require more advanced care in order to stabilize or reverse the problem. In most cases, a patient in respiratory distress should be considered a high priority for transport. Without quick recognition and treatment by the EMT and intervention from an advanced provider (paramedic), some patients could progress to respiratory failure and ultimately to respiratory arrest. (More about these conditions will be discussed later in this chapter.)

The patient's skin signs, work of breathing, ability to speak, and body position are often key indicators to the severity of a patient's level of distress. Knowing the differences between the different stages of respiratory distress can assist you in making the right choices when treating the patient.

Hypoxia occurs when there is an inadequate supply of oxygen in the blood. It is a result of inadequate gas exchange at the alveolar and cellular levels. The early stage of hypoxia often results in an increased respiratory rate and a mild increase in the work of breathing. If left uncorrected, hypoxia can progress to severe dyspnea. If the underlying cause of the hypoxia is not treated, it can eventually lead to respiratory failure. This is due to the decline or depletion of oxygen at the cellular level. Some patients, depending on their age or medical condition, may shift more rapidly than others from respiratory distress to respiratory failure.

Prolonged hypoxia will eventually lead to respiratory arrest. Respiratory arrest requires immediate intervention with assisted ventilation and supplemental oxygen.

PRACTICAL PATHOPHYSIOLOGY

Respiratory failure occurs when the normal compensatory mechanisms that the body uses to increase air exchange are no longer able to function. As the mechanisms fail, the patient becomes less responsive and breathing generally begins to slow rather than increase. These are significant signs that must be recognized and cared for immediately with assisted ventilations and supplemental oxygen.

PERSPECTIVE

Joanne—The EMT

Sometimes the assessment is quick and simple, you know? Like that guy in the rain. Was he breathing adequately? No. Did he need assistance right away? Definitely! Was I able to determine why he wasn't breathing right? No. Did I need to know the reason before I could help him? Obviously not.

17-5 Describe an assessment-based approach for the patient with respiratory distress.

tripod position a position that may be assumed during respiratory distress to facilitate breathing. The patient usually sits or may stand or crouch, leaning forward with hands placed on the bed, chair, table, or knees.

accessory muscles muscles in the neck, chest, back, and abdomen used to assist ventilations during respiratory distress.

The Assessment-Based Approach

Your assessment of the patient with breathing difficulty will begin as you enter the scene and approach the patient. As you approach, notice if the patient is seated or lying down. Is he alert and interacting with those around him, or is he lying unresponsive? Remember that you will assess breathing adequacy and apply oxygen during the primary assessment.

Scene Size-up

The scene size-up can give you important information about the patient with respiratory distress. As you approach the patient, look for home oxygen devices or medications. Notice if the patient might have been eating prior to the onset of symptoms. Eating could indicate a possible allergic reaction or a partial or complete airway obstruction. Notice what position the patient is in as well. Positions such as the **tripod position** (Figure 17-3 ■) or the appearance of anxiety, restlessness, or altered mental status indicate a patient in serious distress.

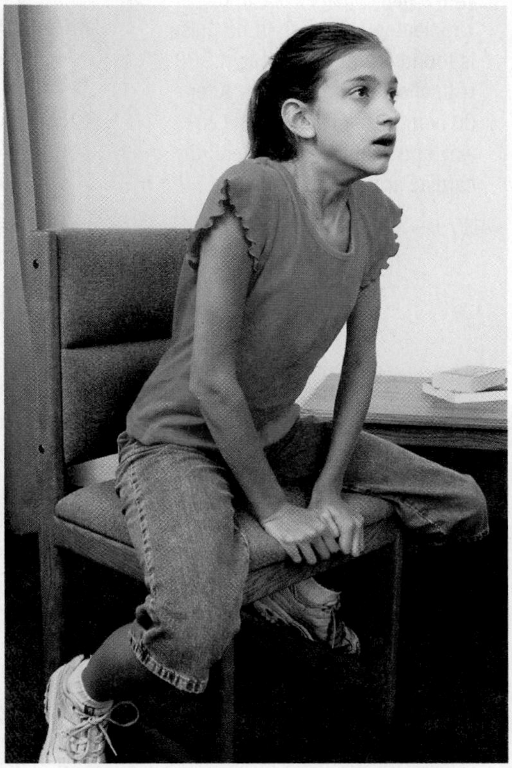

Figure 17-3 A patient in respiratory distress will often assume the tripod position.

Primary Assessment

During the primary assessment note the patient's skin color and mental status. Look for an adequate rate and depth of breathing (Figure 17-4 ■). Note the work of breathing and look for use of **accessory muscles.** You also must listen with a stethoscope to determine if you hear air moving in and out of each lung and if it is equal on both sides (Figure 17-5 ■). Also note any pale skin or cyanosis to the lips and nail beds. A patient who is sweaty (diaphoretic) has likely been struggling to breathe for some time.

If the patient with respiratory distress appears to have a rate and volume within normal limits (approximately 10 to 30 breaths per minute),

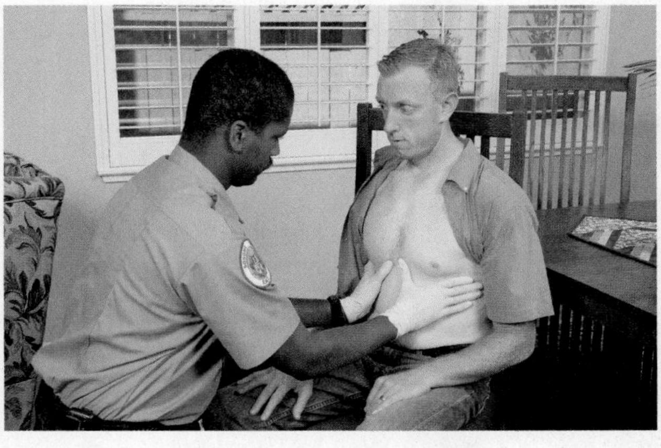

Figure 17-4 Assess both rate and depth of each breath to determine adequacy.

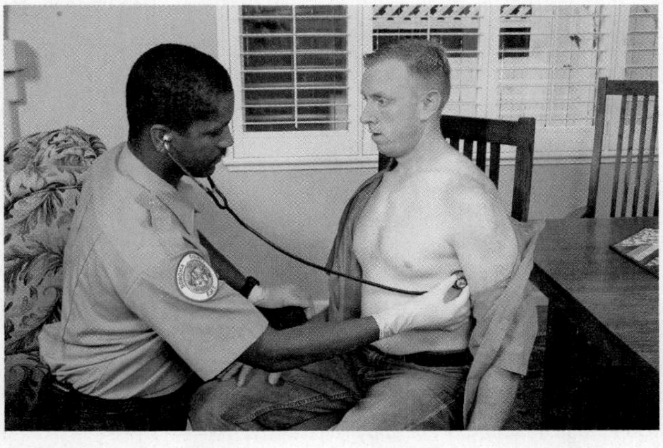

Figure 17-5 Auscultate lung sounds on both sides (bilaterally).

CLINICAL CLUE

ABC and CAB

Remember, in an unresponsive patient who is not breathing or has only irregular gasping (agonal) breaths, immediately check for a pulse. If a pulse is present (and this will be most of the time), then assess the airway and follow the normal ABC sequence by providing ventilations with a bag-mask device and supplemental oxygen. If no pulse is found, immediately begin CPR with chest compressions. After 30 compressions, open the airway and ventilate the patient: the cardiac arrest CAB sequence.

administer oxygen by nonrebreather mask. If the patient is breathing inadequately (has respiration less than 10 or greater than 30), or not at all, provide ventilations with a bag-mask device and supplemental oxygen.

The patient's general appearance provides important clues about the level of respiratory distress. As already noted, poor skin signs such as pale, moist skin may indicate a patient in severe distress. Another indicator of hypoxia or hypercarbia is an altered mental status, which can range from anxiety to combativeness (common with hypoxia) to a sleepy, head-bobbing appearance (common with hypercarbia).

At the conclusion of the primary assessment, make a determination about the priority of your patient for transport. High-priority patients include all patients with moderate to severe respiratory distress. Remember that patients with altered mental status, poor skin color, accessory muscle use, and the inability to speak more than a few words at a time are very sick patients who may require assisted ventilation with a bag-mask device.

History

Obtaining a complete medical history is especially important in the medical patient. Obtain a SAMPLE history. Use the OPQRST mnemonic to obtain information in reference to the patient's shortness of breath and other symptoms. (See Table 17-1.)

The history is important because past conditions could provide clues to current problems. Medications taken by the patient will also be relevant to the patient's condition. You may be able to assist the patient with medications to help his distress. In medical patients, the history is often a greater source of information than the physical examination.

Respiratory problems are often a sign of underlying cardiac problems. Some patients having a heart attack may not have traditional signs and symptoms (such as chest pain or discomfort), but instead have only the symptom of respiratory distress. In some cases the respiratory distress is what the patient notices most, but on being asked, he may indicate that he has pain or discomfort in the chest, neck, jaw, or arm.

CLINICAL CLUE

Severe Respiratory Distress

Clues your patient is in severe distress include:

- Altered mental status including unresponsiveness, sleepiness, head-bobbing, agitation, or anxiety
- Increased work of breathing including the inability to speak in complete sentences
- Poor skin color, diaphoresis
- Use of accessory muscles
- Increased pulse rate (pulse rate will decrease in pediatric patients)
- Shallow respirations with any respiratory rate
- Noisy breathing (usually audible even without a stethoscope) including **wheezing, gurgling, snoring,** and **stridor**

Note that all patients who present with respiratory distress are a high priority. This list describes the patients who are in serious condition and unstable. Patients with any of these signs are serious—all signs do not have to be present.

wheezing high-pitched, musical lung sounds created by air moving through constricted air passages.

gurgling intermittent low-pitched sounds indicative of fluids in the upper airway.

snoring intermittent low-pitched sounds heard during inhalation, and often indicative of partial upper airway obstruction caused by the tongue and associated soft tissue.

stridor a harsh high-pitched sound that usually occurs during inhalation but can also occur during exhalation; a sound indicative of partial upper airway obstruction.

Vital Signs

You will assess vital signs every 5 minutes for the unstable patient and every 15 minutes for the stable patient. Many of your respiratory distress patients will be unstable

TABLE 17-1 MEDICAL HISTORY—RESPIRATORY

SAMPLE HISTORY

S*—Signs and symptoms.* Use the OPQRST mnemonic (below) to obtain this information.

A*—Allergies.* Does the patient have any known allergies? Was the patient eating anything prior to the onset of symptoms? Anaphylaxis (allergic reactions) may cause respiratory distress.

M*—Medications.* Ask the patient if he takes any medications (prescribed or not prescribed). Does he know of any medications he takes specifically for a chronic lung or heart condition? Has he taken all medications as prescribed? Remember that you may be able to assist some patients with a prescribed inhaler.

P*—Pertinent past history.* Does the patient have any prior history of difficulty breathing or other medical problems? Any cardiac problems? Ever experienced anything like this before?

L*—Last oral intake.* When did the patient last eat or drink, and what did he have?

E*—Events.* What was the patient doing when the signs and symptoms first began?

OPQRST

O*—Onset.* What were you doing when the distress began?

P*—Provocation.* Does anything make the distress better or worse?

Q*—Quality.* Do you have any pain? Can you describe what it feels like?

R*—Radiation.* If you do have pain, does it spread to any other part of your body? Do you have pain anywhere else?

S*—Severity.* On a 1–10 scale (where 1 is best and 10 is worst) how would you rate your distress right now? How would you rate it when it first began?

T*—Time.* How long have you had trouble breathing? How long have you been in distress?

OTHER IMPORTANT QUESTIONS/PERTINENT POSITIVES AND NEGATIVES

Do you have chest pain or discomfort?

Do you have pain or discomfort in your neck, jaw, or arms?

Have you ever had a heart problem?

Have you noticed swollen ankles or weight gain recently?

Do you have more difficulty breathing when you lie down?

and require the more frequent vital sign checks. Specific things to look for in vital signs include:

- ***Abnormal pulse rate.*** In response to physiological stress and hypoxia, the heart rate will increase. In adult patients who are near death, and in pediatric patients as an earlier response to hypoxia, the pulse rate may be abnormally slow.
- ***Abnormal respiratory rate or depth.*** The respiratory rate will usually rise in the presence of respiratory distress. But be aware that abnormally high or low rates and low respiratory volumes may require ventilation.
- ***Skin color changes.*** The skin may become pale, cyanotic, cool, and moist.

Remember that it is a trend in vital signs over time that provides the most information.

Physical Examination

Your physical examination of the patient continues what you started in the primary assessment. Patients in respiratory distress should be carefully and frequently

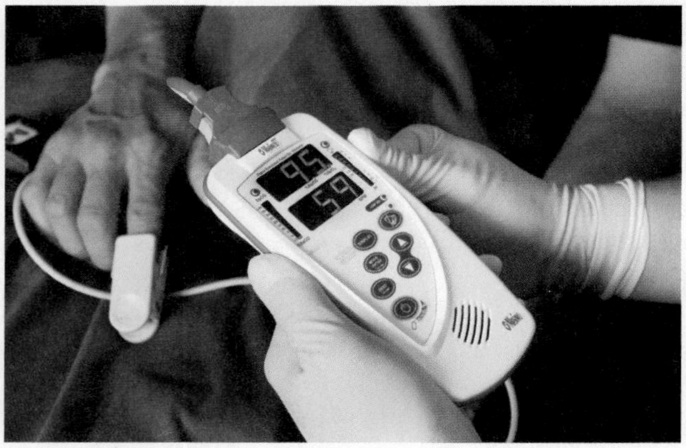

Figure 17-6 A pulse oximeter provides percentage of oxygen saturation as well as heart rate.

monitored to detect inadequate breathing as soon as it begins. Observe the following:

- The patient's overall appearance, which is to be considered in the primary assessment and throughout the call. Look for poor skin signs, altered mental status, increased work of breathing, and tripoding.
- How many words the patient can speak before having to catch his breath. The fewer words spoken, the more serious the distress.
- The patient's use of accessory muscles in the chest and neck.

Listen to the patient's chest with a stethoscope. Listen for lung sounds in both sides of the chest. You should be able to hear air moving in and out on both sides. The sound should be clear and equal on both sides and in all fields. Abnormal lung sounds will be described later in this chapter.

pulse oximetry use of an electronic device, a pulse oximeter, to determine the amount of oxygen carried by the hemoglobin in the blood, known as the oxygen saturation or SpO_2.

Many agencies utilize a **pulse oximeter** as a standard assessment tool (Figure 17-6 ■). It will determine the percent of hemoglobin in the blood that is saturated with oxygen. However, never withhold oxygen from a patient who appears to be in respiratory distress, even when his pulse oximeter readings are normal. The device is useful to show improvement or decline in the patient's condition (for example, improvement in the oxygen saturation after administration of oxygen). Generally, readings below 94% indicate hypoxia. Readings below 90% indicate more severe hypoxia. Note that pulse oximeter readings can be abnormally skewed for patients with a history of respiratory disease, carbon monoxide poisoning, or a long history of smoking.

PRACTICAL PATHOPHYSIOLOGY

A pulse oximeter uses infrared technology to measure the amount of oxygen molecules that are attached (bound) to hemoglobin in the arterial blood. It is measured as a percentage, with the normal range being between 94% and 100%. There are several factors that can affect the accuracy of a pulse oximeter reading. They include temperature of the environment, distal circulation, and the presence of nail polish. You must consider the entire presentation of your patient and not rely just on pulse oximeter readings alone.

17-6 Describe at least three types of abnormal breathing patterns.

apnea absence of any breathing or respiratory effort.

Cheyne-Stokes respirations deep respirations alternating with very shallow respirations, sometimes with a period of apnea in the cycles; seen in patients who have brain injury or end-stage brain tumors.

central neurogenic hyperventilation very rapid, deep respirations usually caused by head injuries or strokes that involve the brainstem.

Abnormal Breathing Patterns

Most patients in respiratory distress will exhibit a normal breathing pattern. Even though breathing is labored, the breaths will remain regular and consistent. There are several specific and identifiable abnormal breathing patterns that indicate serious underlying conditions. The patterns, and the conditions that cause them, are as follows:

- ***Cheyne-Stokes respirations.*** These are deep respirations alternating with very shallow respirations. There also may be periods of **apnea** in the cycles. **Cheyne-Stokes respirations** are seen in patients who have severe brain injury or end-stage brain tumors (Figure 17-7 ■).
- ***Central neurogenic hyperventilation.*** This is seen in severe head injuries or strokes that involve the brainstem. As the name **central neurogenic hyperventilation** suggests, the respirations are very rapid and deep (Figure 17-8 ■).

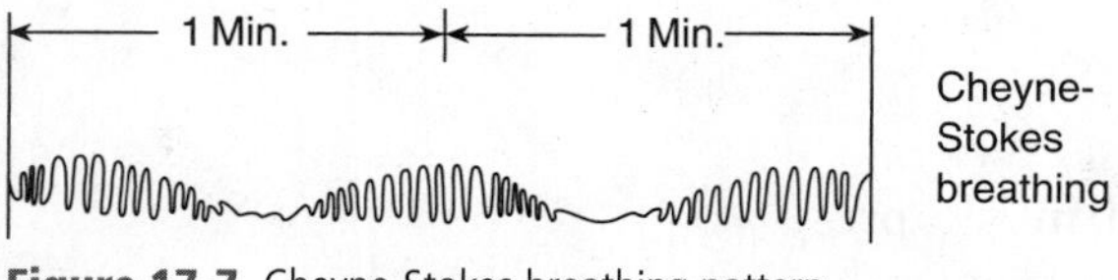

Figure 17-7 Cheyne-Stokes breathing pattern.

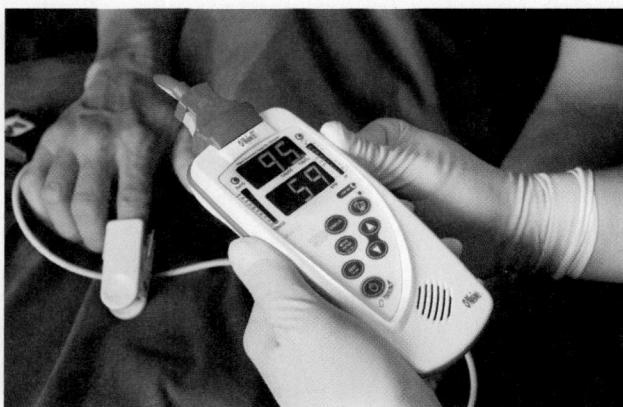

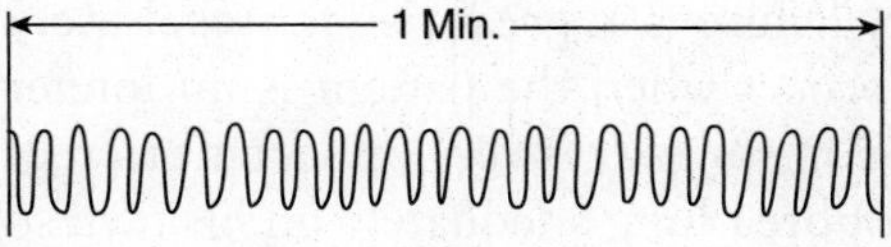

Figure 17-8 Breathing pattern with central neurological hyperventilation.

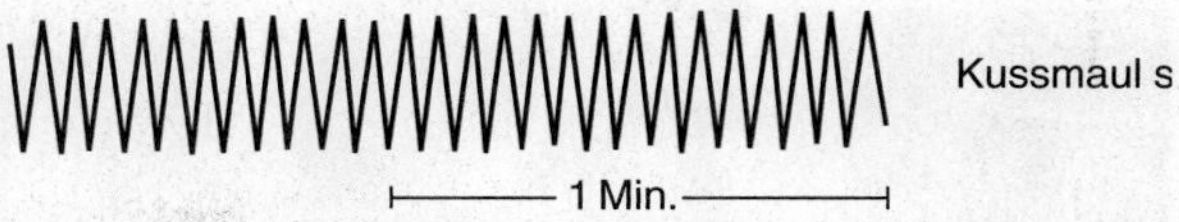

Figure 17-9 Kussmaul's breathing pattern.

- ***Kussmaul's respirations.*** This is another presentation of rapid, deep ventilations, but **Kussmaul's respirations** are usually caused by very acidic blood as in some diabetic conditions and aspirin overdose (Figure 17-9 ▪).

Kussmaul's respirations rapid, deep ventilations usually caused by very acidic blood such as in some diabetic conditions and aspirin overdose.

Hypoxic Drive

17-7 Describe the term *hypoxic drive* and how it relates to the COPD patient.

Normally, the drive to breathe is controlled by carbon dioxide levels in the blood. The body is stimulated to breathe when there is an excess of carbon dioxide. It stops or slows breathing when carbon dioxide levels fall. In some patients with COPD who have chronically elevated levels of carbon dioxide, a **hypoxic drive** develops in which the body is stimulated to breathe by below-normal oxygen levels rather than by elevated carbon dioxide levels. In theory, patients with hypoxic drive may stop breathing with higher than normal oxygen levels in the blood. The concern is that when supplemental oxygen is administered to these patients, it may cause them to stop breathing.

hypoxic drive when the stimulus to breathe is the amount of oxygen in the blood, rather than the normal drive to breathe, which is related to the amount of carbon dioxide in the blood.

Respiratory arrest secondary to hypoxic drive is rare in the field setting. The rule in EMS is to never withhold oxygen from a patient who needs it. This includes patients in respiratory distress with a COPD history. When patients with those conditions have difficulty breathing, they need oxygen. They also can have heart attacks and trauma, both of which are not related to a respiratory problem but require oxygen. In short, never withhold oxygen from a patient who needs it.

PRACTICAL PATHOPHYSIOLOGY

Abnormal breathing patterns are important indicators and warning signs for the patient's condition. The EMT should perform a constant evaluation of the patient's breathing for both rate and depth to monitor regular or irregular patterns. Irregular patterns could be indicative of neurological problems, head or brain injury, subdural or epidural hematomas, a stroke, diabetic emergency, or overdose. Abnormal breathing patterns are very serious and should never be taken lightly. If interventions are not performed, the patient will continue to get worse.

Respiratory Distress vs. Respiratory Failure

17-8 Differentiate respiratory distress, respiratory failure, and respiratory arrest.

The signs of respiratory distress such as increased breathing rate and depth, increased work of breathing, and increased heart rate are ways the body attempts to compensate for a lack of adequate oxygen (hypoxia) or an increase in carbon dioxide (hypercarbia). The signs are the normal ways the body tries to compensate when levels of oxygen and carbon dioxide are out of balance.

In some cases, if the root cause of the respiratory distress is not corrected, it can lead to dangerously low levels of oxygen and high levels of carbon dioxide. When this occurs, the cells convert to anaerobic metabolism and become less efficient. As energy levels diminish, entire organ systems can begin to fail. When this happens, the body is unable to adequately compensate and the patient will experience a drop in respiratory rate, volume, and effort. This is known as **respiratory failure.** The patient also will exhibit a decrease in mental status, becoming very fatigued, lethargic, and confused (Figure 17-10 ▪). When a patient is in respiratory failure, he requires immediate intervention with supplemental oxygen and assisted ventilations.

respiratory failure the condition that occurs when the body is no longer able to adequately compensate for inadequate oxygenation.

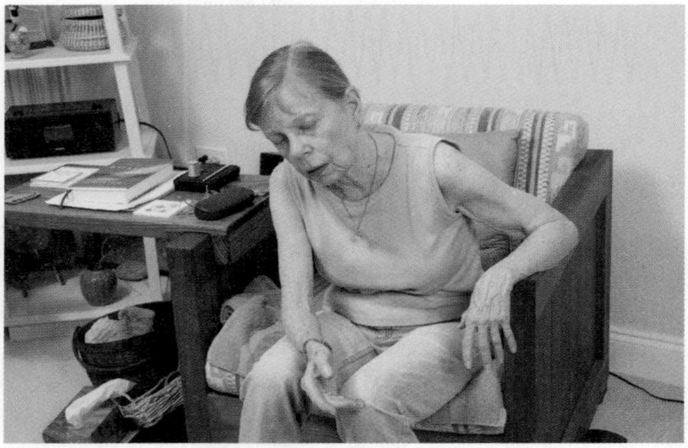

Figure 17-10 A patient in respiratory failure.

A patient in respiratory failure is at great risk for **respiratory arrest.** Respiratory arrest occurs when the patient is no longer breathing spontaneously on his own. It is very important to recognize when a patient is not breathing adequately on his own so that you can intervene with assisted ventilations and hopefully minimize the chances of respiratory arrest.

Lung Auscultation

Listening to the lungs with a stethoscope is called **auscultation.** It is done for two reasons: to listen for air movement in and out and to listen for abnormal sounds. When listening for air movement, note whether the sound of air moving in and out is present as well as equal on both sides. This can be done by listening at the **midaxillary line** over each side of the chest.

17-9 Describe the characteristics of normal and abnormal breath sounds.

respiratory arrest when normal breathing effort stops.

auscultation assessment technique of listening, usually with a stethoscope.

midaxillary line an imaginary line drawn vertically from the middle of the armpit to the ankle.

Listening for abnormal sounds is more difficult. There are many sounds that can be heard in different areas of the chest. In addition, locating and identifying a specific sound is challenging, especially in a moving ambulance.

Auscultating lung sounds must be done in several areas of the lungs. Figure 17-11 ■ shows those areas. You should listen over each area in the front and back. The bases

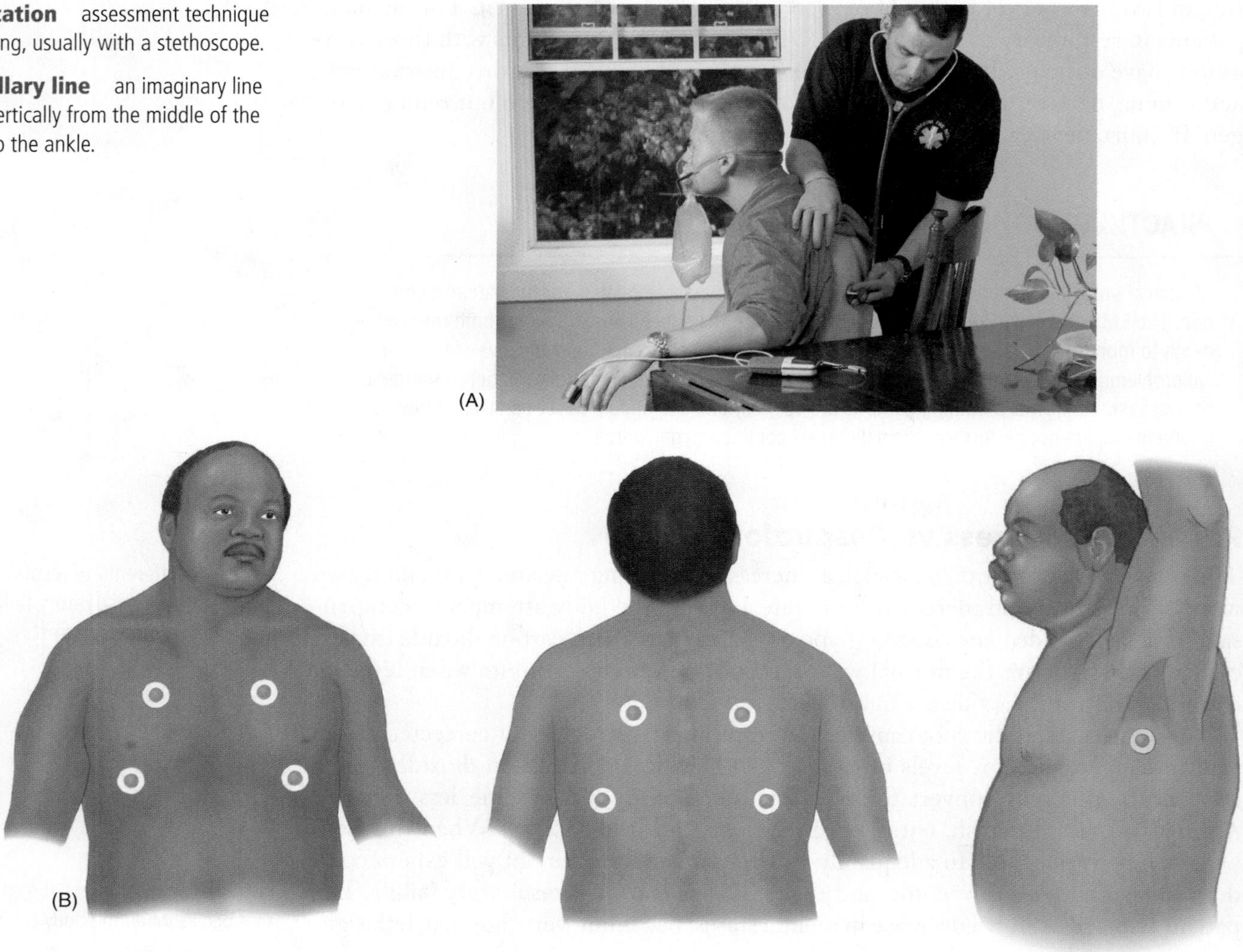

Figure 17-11 (A) Place the stethoscope directly on the skin when auscultating lung sounds. (B) Minimum recommended sites for auscultating lung sounds for a patient in respiratory distress.

of the lungs are auscultated best from the back. The specific abnormal lung sounds you may hear include the following:

- *Wheezing.* Created by air moving through constricted air passages, wheezing produces a high-pitched musical sound. It is heard in asthma, emphysema, and chronic bronchitis. It also can be heard in some cases of pulmonary edema. Wheezing occurs most often during exhalation but also can be heard during inhalation in extreme cases.
- *Crackles.* Sometimes called *rales*, **crackles** are the sounds created in pulmonary edema when alveoli, closed because of fluid, snap open. They are usually heard on inspiration as fine crackling sounds (as the name suggests).
- *Rhonchi.* Low-pitched snoring or rattling sounds caused by secretions in the larger airways, **rhonchi** may be heard in chronic lung diseases and possibly pneumonia.
- *Stridor.* A high pitched sound, stridor is heard on inspiration and expiration. It indicates some sort of obstruction or narrowing of the upper airway (trachea or larynx).

crackles lung sounds created in pulmonary edema when alveoli, closed because of fluid, open; usually heard on inspiration as fine crackling sounds.

rhonchi low-pitched snoring or rattling sounds caused by secretions in the larger airways; may be seen in chronic lung diseases and possibly pneumonia.

PRACTICAL PATHOPHYSIOLOGY

Differentiating between respiratory distress and respiratory failure can be challenging. Respiratory distress begins when the patient complains of shortness of breath and is exhibiting signs of inadequate oxygen exchange. A true sign of respiratory failure is when the patient no longer has the ability to compensate or does not have the ability or strength to maintain normal oxygen levels to perfuse the brain.

The EMT should always listen for adequate air exchange by auscultating the different lung fields, so that conditions such as asthma, upper or lower airway obstruction, pulmonary edema, and other respiratory diseases can be identified.

Listening to and evaluating lung sounds can be challenging. Lung sounds should be evaluated in a quiet area (such as the patient's residence or in the ambulance before leaving the scene, without the additional road noise). If you are going to evaluate lung sounds, realize, as with other vital signs, that it is how the sounds change over time that is important, especially when administering a medication. Listen before and after assisting or administering any medication and note changes.

One pitfall when listening to lung sounds is the "quiet chest." You may have a patient who had wheezes early in the call. Later in the call you note there are no more wheezes. This could be for one of two reasons: The patient has improved (as a result of a medication) or the patient's respirations have become so shallow that there is not enough air moving in and out to make the wheezing noise any more. This means that the patient's respirations are inadequate. If you simply thought "great, no more wheezing," you would falsely assume that the patient was better when he was actually developing inadequate breathing.

17-10 Describe the pathophysiology by which each of the following conditions leads to inadequate oxygenation: epiglottitis, hyperventilation syndrome, obstructive pulmonary diseases (emphysema, chronic bronchitis, and asthma), pneumonia, pneumothorax, poisonous exposures, pulmonary edema, pulmonary embolism, and viral respiratory infections.

Respiratory Diseases and Conditions

There are some common respiratory diseases that you will encounter as an EMT. While it is not necessary to diagnose those conditions as you care for your patient, knowing about the diseases will help you communicate with the patient and health care providers about the patient's history and condition.

Asthma is a chronic lung disease that is characterized by periodic episodes of acute shortness of breath (Figure 17-12 ■). That is, it does not affect the patient every day, but just when there are attacks. Attacks are episodes of **bronchoconstriction** caused by **triggers** such as allergies, respiratory infections, exercise, or strong emotions.

asthma a disease that has attacks involving bronchoconstriction and mucus production with significant difficulty breathing.

bronchoconstriction constriction of the bronchioles in the lungs, caused by allergies, respiratory infections, exercise, or emotion.

triggers allergies, respiratory infections, exercise, or emotion that may cause bronchoconstriction.

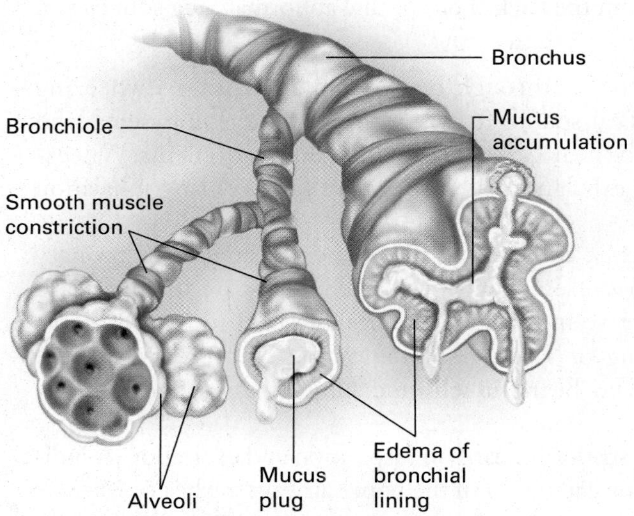

Figure 17-12 Contributing factors for asthma.

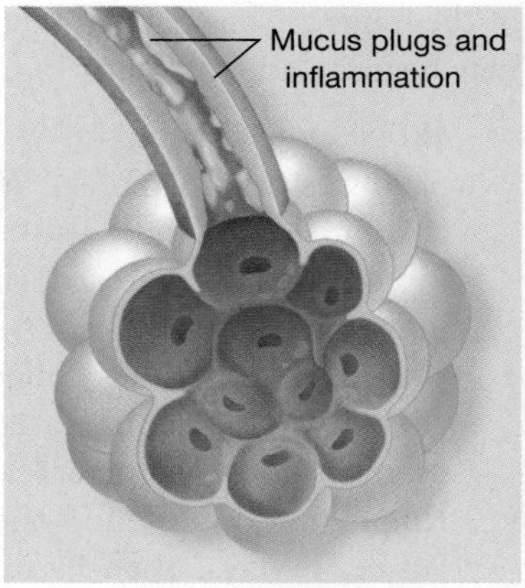

Figure 17-13 Bronchitis is caused by inflammation and swelling of the bronchioles.

status asthmaticus prolonged, life-threatening asthma attack, often not responding to the patient's own medications.

chronic bronchitis condition in which the lining of the bronchiole is inflamed, and excess mucus is formed in the airway, with accumulation becoming severe.

emphysema condition in which the walls of the alveoli break down and lose surface area.

stale air air that has become trapped in the alveoli and contains no oxygen.

pneumonia a respiratory condition caused by inflammation of a lung secondary to infection.

In cases of prolonged constriction, mucus can develop and plug small airways, severely restricting air flow. Asthma attacks can be life threatening. **Status asthmaticus** is a prolonged, life-threatening asthma attack that often does not respond to the patient's own medications.

Chronic bronchitis is a condition in which the lining of the bronchioles become swollen. Excess mucus is formed and remains in the airway (Figure 17-13 ▪). The accumulation of mucus may become severe if the body is unable to clear the mucus from the airway.

Emphysema is a condition in which the walls of the alveoli break down, causing a loss of alveolar surface area (Figure 17-14 ▪). This significantly limits the ability to exchange gases in the alveoli and permits **stale air** to remain in the alveoli, increasing carbon dioxide levels in the lungs and blood. Chronic bronchitis and emphysema are both examples of chronic obstructive pulmonary diseases (COPD).

Pneumonia

Pneumonia is a respiratory disease common to all age groups. However, it is more commonly found in the geriatric population. Pneumonia is characterized by an infection that causes inflammation of the lungs (Figure 17-15 ▪). The infection is a result of bacteria, viruses, or (rarely) fungi. Patients with pneumonia will show signs and symptoms that are similar to the flu, such as fever, cough, chills, chest pain, headache, and fatigue. Patients with pneumonia need prompt medical care and antibiotics to prevent dangerous effects from the illness.

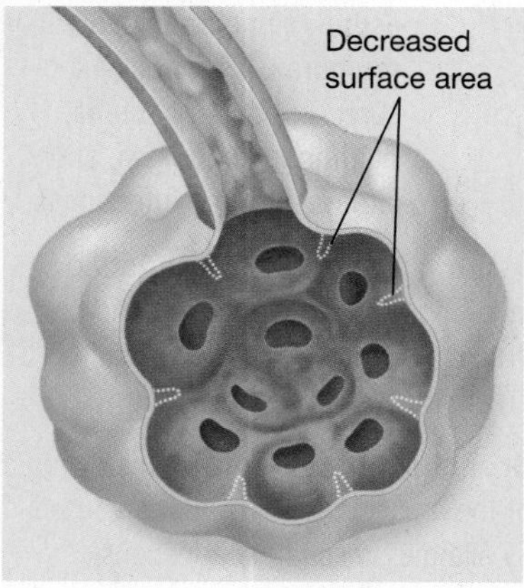

Figure 17-14 With emphysema the alveoli break down and become stiff.

PRACTICAL PATHOPHYSIOLOGY

Pneumonia is an inflammation of the lungs frequently caused by an infection from bacteria, viruses, or fungi. Pneumonia primarily affects the alveoli and causes a buildup of thick pus and fluids in the alveoli, making it difficult for air exchange to occur. Patients with pneumonia will frequently present with a cough, chest pain, fever, and shortness of breath.

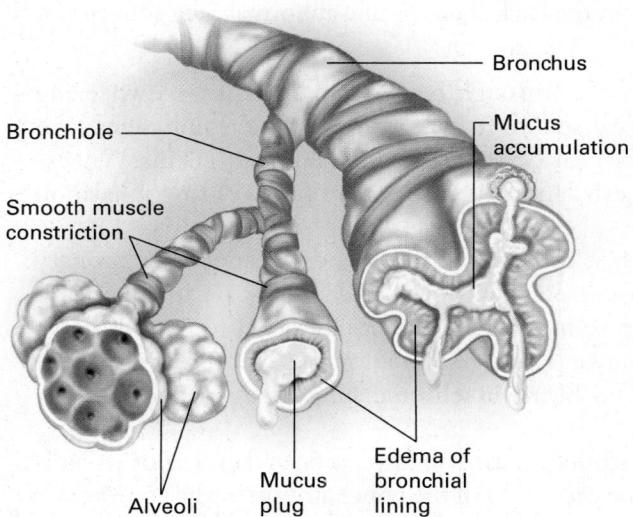

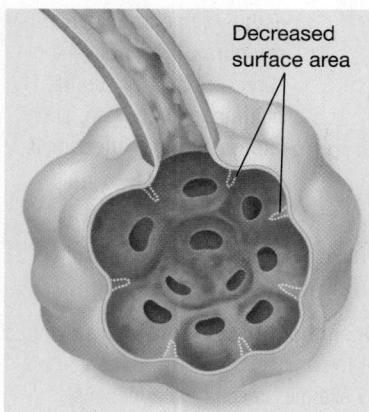

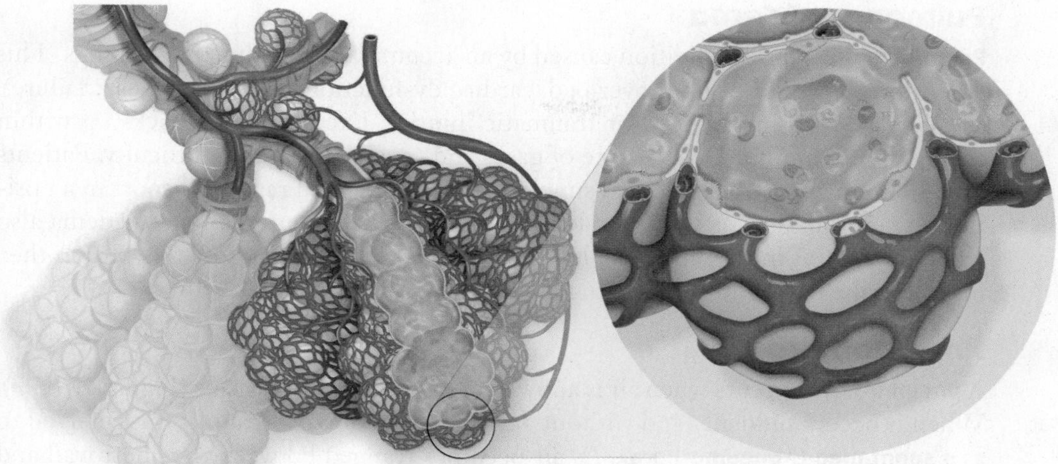

Figure 17-15 Pneumonia causes the alveoli to become inflamed and fill with pus.

Pulmonary Embolism

While many respiratory diseases are directly related to the respiratory system, **pulmonary embolism** actually begins with the circulatory system. Pulmonary embolism is most commonly caused by a *deep vein thrombosis (DVT)*. A DVT is a clot that forms in a vessel somewhere in the body, most commonly in the legs, arms, heart, or pelvis. The clot can become dislodged and travel through the circulatory system. It can sometimes become lodged in one of the tiny vessels of the lungs, causing a complete blockage and subsequent tissue death (Figure 17-16 ■).

pulmonary embolism a blockage of the main artery of the lung.

A pulmonary embolism (PE) is a very serious condition. A patient with a pulmonary embolism will classically exhibit chest pain, shortness of breath, hypoxia (low oxygen saturation), and tachycardia. Patients experiencing breathing difficulty who have had recent surgery, long periods of sitting or travel, trauma, burns, cancer, pregnancy, or obesity should be considered as having a possible pulmonary embolism.

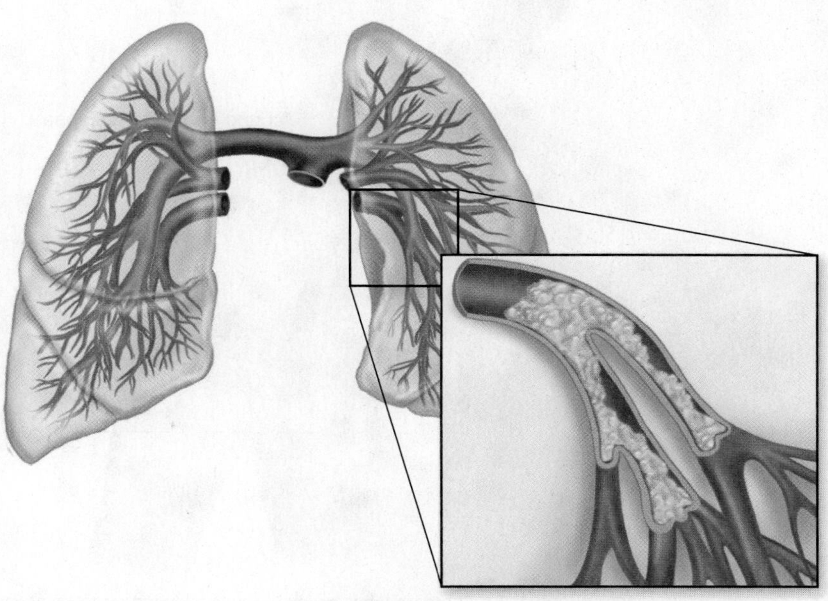

Figure 17-16 Pulmonary embolism is a clot that obstructs one of the pulmonary arteries.

Pulmonary Edema

pulmonary edema a condition of fluid in the lungs.

Pulmonary edema is a condition caused by an accumulation of fluid in the lungs. This condition is a result of fluid overload, cardiac dysfunction (congestive heart failure), sepsis, metabolic imbalances, or traumatic injuries. Excessive fluid backs up within the lungs, disrupting the exchange of gases and causing breathing difficulty. Patients with pulmonary edema will need supplemental oxygen and rapid transport in a position of comfort such as semi-Fowler's. Patients experiencing pulmonary edema also will complain of increased difficulty breathing while lying flat. For this reason they may describe having to sleep sitting up at night.

Pneumothorax

pneumothorax an abnormal collection of air in the pleural space that separates the lung from the chest wall.

spontaneous pneumothorax an abnormal collection of air in the pleural space that occurs with no apparent cause.

tension pneumothorax an abnormal collection of air in the pleural space that results in a build up of pressure significant enough to impair breathing or circulation.

A **pneumothorax** occurs when air is allowed to enter the pleural space (Figure 17-17 ■). When it occurs suddenly and without any direct injury from trauma, it is referred to as a **spontaneous pneumothorax.** As air becomes trapped between the chest wall and the lung, pressure can begin to build up. This increase in pressure, referred to as a **tension pneumothorax,** can put pressure on the lungs, heart, and other structures in the chest. If left untreated, a tension pneumothorax will cause the collapse of both lungs, prevention of normal blood return to the heart, and an eventual shifting of the trachea away from the side of the pressure. Patients with a history of respiratory disease or family history of spontaneous pneumothorax are more likely to experience a pneumothorax.

Because this patient has a decrease in tidal volume and minute volume, he will need assisted ventilations with supplemental oxygen and rapid transport. Always follow your local protocol.

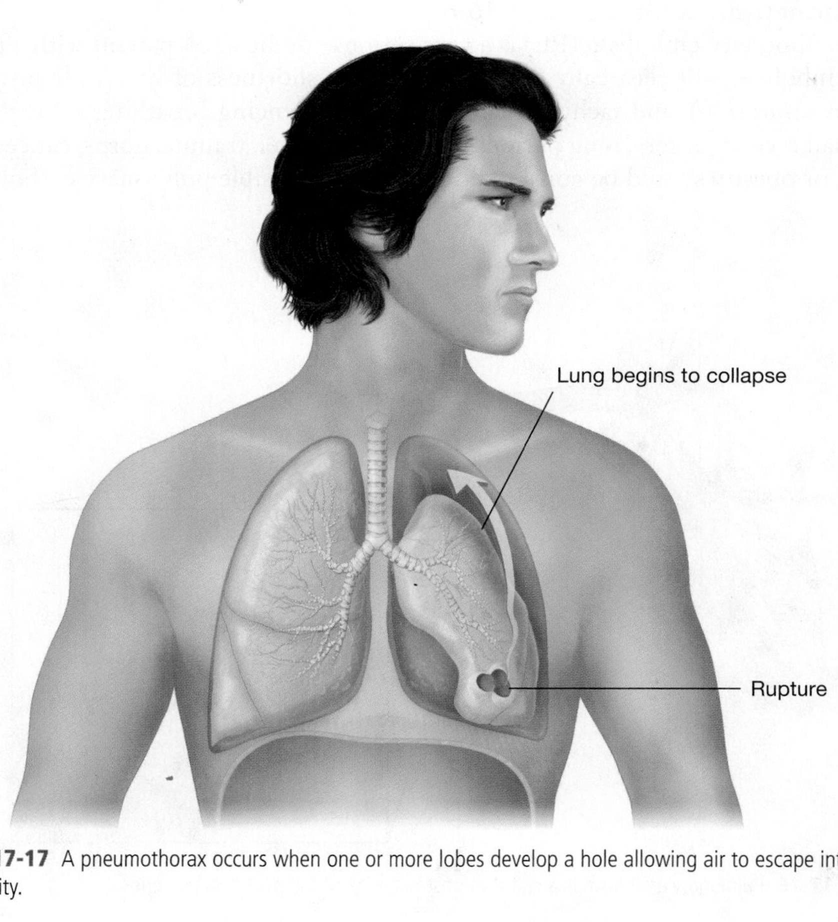

Figure 17-17 A pneumothorax occurs when one or more lobes develop a hole allowing air to escape into the chest cavity.

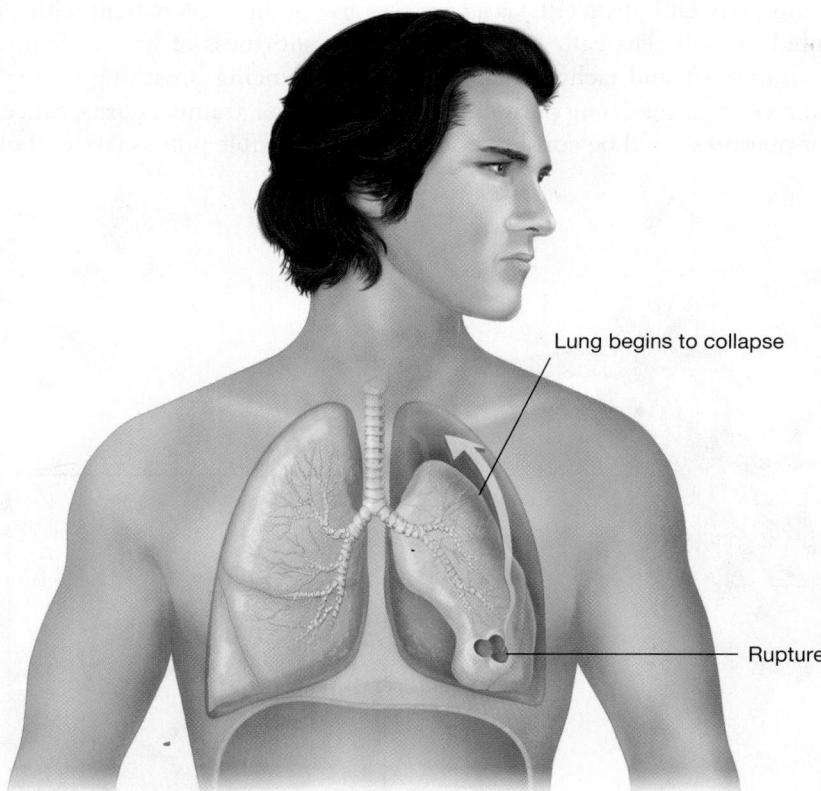

Hyperventilation Syndrome

Hyperventilation syndrome is an abnormal respiratory condition often associated with anxiety that can be psychologically or physiologically based. Patients with hyperventilation syndrome will begin with an erratic breathing pattern called **hyperventilation.** Hyperventilation simply means breathing that is beyond the normal rate and depth. This condition can be brought on by a variety of causes. It is important for the EMT to assist in calming the patient, administering oxygen, and transporting for additional treatment. You should expect your patient to complain of dizziness, tingling in their hands and feet, headache, and fatigue.

hyperventilation syndrome an abnormal respiratory condition characterized by rapid deep respirations; often associated with anxiety that can be psychologically or physiologically based.

hyperventilation breathing that is abnormally rapid and deep.

Remember that patients may be breathing rapidly for many reasons far more serious than hyperventilation syndrome. Never assume you are treating simple hyperventilation syndrome until you have excluded more serious causes of respiratory distress.

PRACTICAL PATHOPHYSIOLOGY

Pulmonary edema, pneumothorax, and hyperventilation syndrome are conditions of very different mechanisms. While hyperventilation syndrome is often a psychologically or physiologically based condition, pulmonary edema is an overload of fluid caused by metabolic imbalance, cardiac dysfunction, sepsis, or traumatic injury. Pneumothorax is the collapse of a lung caused by air trapped in the pleural space. Both pulmonary edema and pneumothorax cause an obstruction within the respiratory system that will result in a decrease in respiratory function. All three conditions are serious emergencies and should be treated rapidly.

Epiglottitis

Epiglottitis is among the least common but most deadly respiratory conditions. Epiglottitis is a rare bacterial infection of the epiglottis, causing excessive edema that can obstruct the airway (Figure 17-18 ■). While epiglottitis was historically more

epiglottitis abnormal swelling of the epiglottis.

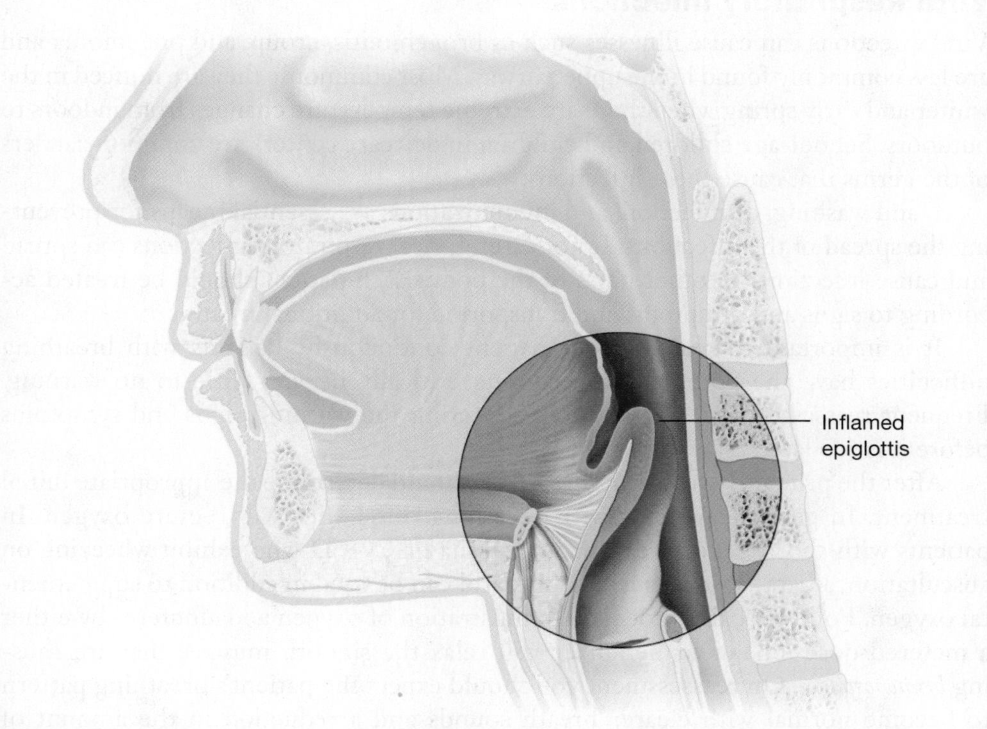

Figure 17-18 Epiglottitis is the swelling of the epiglottis and can result in complete airway obstruction.

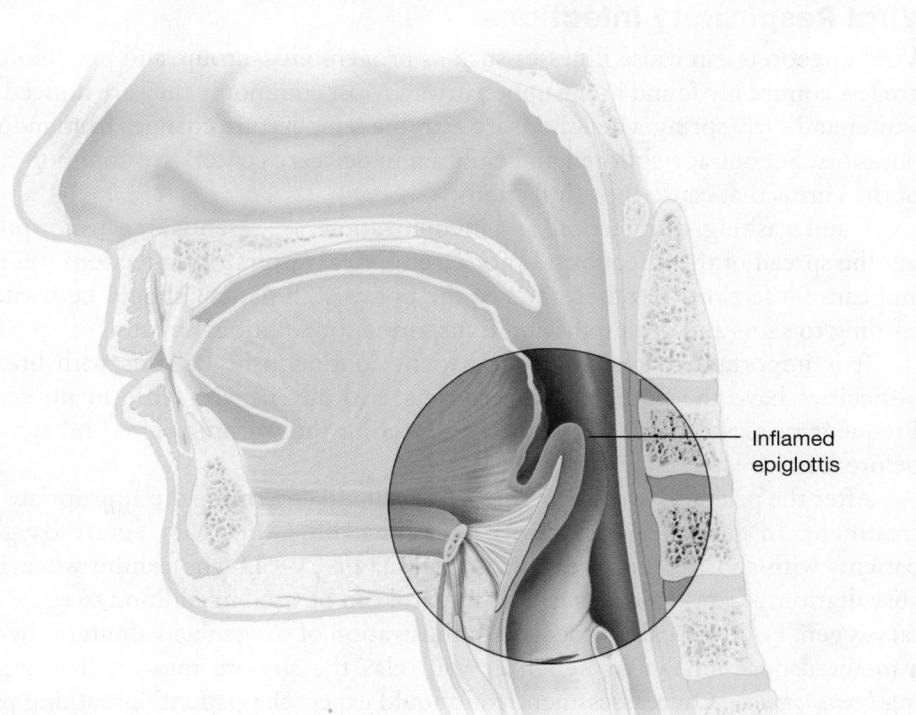

common in children, immunizations have greatly reduced the incidence of pediatric epiglottitis. However, epiglottitis still can occur in adults and children who have not been immunized.

Patients with epiglottitis may complain of hoarseness, excessive drooling, fever, and difficulty swallowing and often exhibit stridor.

Patients with epiglottitis must be handled very carefully. It is extremely important not to agitate patients or force them into an uncomfortable position. Careful consideration should be taken before separating pediatric patients with epiglottitis from their caregivers. This may bring on more stress, causing them to become upset, thus increasing the chances of swelling and further obstructing the airway. When possible, allow the child to remain in the arms of the caregiver and provide blow-by oxygen.

The delivery of oxygen may be challenging. While patients with epiglottitis need oxygen, administering by blow-by may be the best option. Blow-by simply means allowing the patient or caregiver to hold the oxygen mask in front of the patient's face. The EMT should never force the patient to accept oxygen.

Exposure to Poisons

A common symptom of exposure to poisonous or toxic substances is breathing difficulty. Exposures can be from plants, chemicals, medications, or many household items. The effect of the poisonous substances may be different, depending on the substances, amount of exposure, length of time since exposure, and age and current condition of the person exposed. (See Chapter 21.)

In addition, you should take precautions not to become exposed yourself. Each exposure will have its own signs and symptoms. Therefore, it will be important to collect any information possible from the scene and notify poison control for the best treatment.

Viral Respiratory Infections

Viral infections can cause illnesses such as bronchiolitis, croup, and pneumonia and are less commonly found in the upper airway. Most commonly they are noticed in the winter and early spring when there are extreme temperature changes from indoors to outdoors. School-age children and children in day care centers are common carriers of the germs that cause these infections.

Hand washing, disinfection, and immunizations are essential means for preventing the spread of the infections. If not careful, viral respiratory infections can spread and cause infections to other parts of the body. Each patient should be treated according to signs and symptoms and transported for additional treatment.

17-15 Explain the importance of the reassessment to identify responses to treatment and changes in the patient's conditions.

It is important to reassess your patient continuously. Patients with breathing difficulties have the potential of becoming critically ill with little to no warning. Frequent reassessment is the key to discovering the warning signs and symptoms before it is too late.

After the primary assessment, the EMT should determine the appropriate initial treatment. In general, patients with breathing difficulties will require oxygen. In patients with shortness of breath from asthma or COPD who exhibit wheezing on auscultation, a beta$_2$ agonist such as albuterol can be used in addition to supplemental oxygen. Follow local protocols. Administration of oxygen and albuterol by either a metered-dose inhaler or nebulizer will relax the smooth muscles that are causing *bronchospasm*. On reassessment you should expect the patient's breathing pattern to become normal with clearer breath sounds and a reduction in the amount of wheezing.

STOP, REVIEW, REMEMBER!

Multiple Choice

For each question, place a check next to the correct answer.

1. Which one of the following is the *best* indication of severe respiratory distress in adults?

_____ a. Warm, dry skin

_____ b. Speaking two to three words per breath

_____ c. Pulse rate of 110

_____ d. Respiratory rate of 20 per minute

2. You are called to an agitated patient with a respiratory rate of 40 per minute and shallow. You note poor skin color. His wife tells you he began complaining of difficulty breathing about an hour ago and has worsened since. What device would you use to treat this patient's condition?

_____ a. Nasal cannula

_____ b. Simple face mask

_____ c. Nonrebreather mask

_____ d. Bag-mask device

3. Cyanosis is a ______________ color of the skin and/or mucous membranes.

_____ a. black

_____ b. pink

_____ c. pale

_____ d. blue

4. The hypoxic drive is best described as the body:

_____ a. liking carbon dioxide more than oxygen.

_____ b. using increased levels of oxygen as a drive to breathe.

_____ c. using low oxygen levels as the drive to breathe.

_____ d. using low carbon monoxide levels as the drive to breathe.

5. Which one of the following is a chronic obstructive pulmonary disease (COPD)?

_____ a. Emphysema

_____ b. Pneumonia

_____ c. Spontaneous pneumothorax

_____ d. Viral respiratory infection

6. Which one of the following is a condition in which the lining of the bronchiole is inflamed?

_____ a. Emphysema

_____ b. Chronic bronchitis

_____ c. Spontaneous pneumothorax

_____ d. Hyperventilation syndrome

7. The primary cause for a pulmonary embolism is:

_____ a. a collapsed lung.

_____ b. fluid overload.

_____ c. a blood clot.

_____ d. hyperventilation.

8. Minimizing the spread of viral respiratory infections can best be accomplished by:

_____ a. good hand washing techniques.

_____ b. delivering supplemental oxygen.

_____ c. the administration of albuterol.

_____ d. suctioning emesis.

9. Exposure to plants, chemicals, medications, and many household items is often the cause of:

_____ a. respiratory distress.

_____ b. epiglottitis.

_____ c. pneumothorax.

_____ d. viral respiratory infection.

10. Which one of the following is a primary cause of pneumonia?

_____ a. Deep vein thrombosis

_____ b. Bacteria

_____ c. Air trapping in the pleural space

_____ d. Household plants

(continued on next page)

(continued)

Fill in the Blank

1. OPQRST stands for O ____________________,
   P ____________________,
   Q ____________________,
   R ____________________,
   S ____________________,
   T ____________________.

2. A question that would be appropriate for the "O" in OPQRST is: Can you ____________________?

3. A patient who is sitting up and leaning forward with his hands on his knees is said to be in the ____________________ position.

4. When determining whether breathing is adequate or not, it is important to check both ____________________ and ____________________.

5. A patient in moderate respiratory distress with a respiratory rate of 24 should be given oxygen by way of ____________________.

Critical Thinking

1. Why are a patient's medical history and current medications important?

____

____

____

____

2. What generally provides more information for a responsive medical patient—a history or a physical examination? Why?

____

____

____

____

3. Explain the significance of epiglottitis and why it is important not to overstress the patient.

____

____

____

____

PERSPECTIVE

Thomas—The Patient

I honestly thought that I was going to die. It was what I imagine trying to take deep breaths underwater would be like. Just a struggle, you know? At first I can remember being frustrated with the ambulance crew. Then I was just angry. It seemed like it took forever for them to get to my house, and then they started asking me all of those questions. It was no use, though. I just couldn't talk. I know that they were just doing their jobs and all, but while they're going through their checklist steps and hooking up whatever little things that they hook up, I'm losing my life. I had a lot more at stake than they did. All that aside, though, I probably wouldn't be here right now without them. I guess I can't overlook that.

Care of the Patient with Respiratory Distress

17-11 Describe the steps for managing a patient with respiratory distress.

Your care of the respiratory distress patient is vital and begins with your actions in the primary assessment. During the primary assessment, you must ensure a patent airway and evaluate breathing for adequacy. Apply oxygen or administer ventilations as necessary and suction the patient if excess fluids or solids make him unable to maintain his own airway.

The final step in the primary assessment is determining a patient priority. For patients with a high priority for transport, prompt transportation is part of a treatment plan. This should be done concurrently with the secondary assessment and vitals when possible.

To provide emergency care to a patient in respiratory distress, take the following steps:

1. Complete a primary assessment. Suction the patient and provide assisted ventilations if necessary. A patient who is in mild to moderate distress with a normal rate and patent airway should receive oxygen by nonrebreather mask. Follow local protocols.
2. Reassure the patient and provide emotional care and patience as you care for him. Realize that difficulty breathing is very scary to the patient. Patients who are hypoxic may be anxious and argumentative.
3. Determine priority for transport. If the patient is a high priority for transport, begin preparation for transport while completing your assessment.
4. If the patient is breathing adequately, allow him to assume a position of comfort. When on the stretcher, this is often a sitting position or lying with the head elevated. Once a patient's breathing becomes inadequate, you must place him in the best position for assisted ventilations.
5. Perform a secondary assessment. Obtain a SAMPLE history from the patient, family members, or bystanders.
6. Assist the patient with his prescribed inhaler. Some patients may have a home **nebulizer,** with which you may be able to assist. Always follow local protocols.
7. Perform frequent reassessments en route to the hospital.

nebulizer a device used to administer medications in the form of a fine mist.

PERSPECTIVE

Brent—The EMT

That was a scary call for me. I had never seen someone that bad off. Any second I expected him to just die right there in front of me. I know that you can only struggle to breathe for so long before your body just gives up. And if he wasn't at that point, he was right on the line. I was trying to be calm, though, but that kind of backfired. I was moving too slow and I could tell that the patient knew it. And every time that I told him to calm down and try to inhale as I squeezed the bag-mask, he looked up at me, like if he had the energy he'd kick my butt or something! I definitely learned a lot on that call. All in all, though, even though I feel I didn't do everything perfectly, I know that we made a difference for that guy.

Positioning of the Patient

Patient positioning is a key part of patient care for the respiratory distress patient. Attempting to have a patient in this condition lie down may cause considerable anxiety and worsen his condition. Because of this, the choice of how best to position the patient for transport is critical.

There are two basic choices for transporting a patient to the stretcher: sitting up or lying down. The stair chair is the device of choice for patients who are breathing adequately and would be made worse by lying down. Patients who require ventilation are often transported to the stretcher on a portable stretcher or backboard. Remember: *It is inappropriate to have respiratory patients walk to the stretcher.* Any unnecessary exertion could make the condition worse.

Infants and Children

17-12 Describe special considerations in the assessment and management of pediatric patients with respiratory emergencies.

You may be called to help infants and children who experience respiratory distress. There are some significant differences between the adult and child patient. Often the lungs of an adult have undergone years of abuse from smoking or occupational or environmental exposure to substances that harm the lungs. Adults will have more chronic respiratory diseases, such as emphysema and chronic bronchitis. Also, normal breathing rates for infants and children are faster than an adult's rates.

croup viral illness characterized by inspiratory and expiratory stridor and a seal-barklike cough.

You will see certain diseases more often in children. Children experience infectious diseases of the upper airway, such as **croup,** and infections of the lower airway, such as pneumonia. Asthma often begins at an early age. You also must be aware of the potential for foreign body airway obstruction in small children, especially toddlers.

Croup is a respiratory condition of the upper airway caused by a viral infection. The infection causes swelling of the upper airway, which can lead to partial to complete obstruction. It often causes stridor or a barking sound during inhalation or exhalation or both. Croup affects approximately 10% to 15% of children between the ages of six months and six years.

CLINICAL CLUE

Infants and Children

An abnormally low pulse rate in an infant or child with respiratory distress is often a sign of inadequate oxygen (hypoxia) that requires immediate intervention. Increased pulse rate in an infant or child is often a sign of hypovolemia.

Your care for the infant or child patient will be similar to an adult's in that you will provide oxygen, reassurance, assisted ventilations as necessary, and transport. Of course, there will be differences in the way you would comfort an infant or child patient. Many times a younger patient will not tolerate an oxygen mask or understand why it is on his face. Dosages for assisted medications will be less for pediatric patients, or inhalers will dispense a specific pediatric dose. (Chapter 38 covers pediatric respiratory assessment and care in detail.)

Transporting an infant or child can be challenging. When the patient's condition allows, infants and children should be transported in an approved child safety restraint according to age and weight. Many ambulance manufacturers preinstall them

TABLE 17-2 RESPIRATORY MEDICATIONS
EXAMPLES OF MEDICATIONS USED IN EMERGENCIES TO IMPROVE BREATHING
albuterol (Proventil, Ventolin), pirbuterol (Maxair™), ipratropium bromide (Atrovent), albuterol plus ipratropium bromide (Combivent®), terbutaline (Terbulin®), metaproterenol (Alupent)
EXAMPLES OF MEDICATIONS THAT ARE USED FOR LONG-TERM PREVENTION OF BREATHING PROBLEMS (NOT TO BE USED IN ACUTE ATTACKS)
flunisolide (AeroBid®), beclomethasone dipropionate (Vanceril®), fluticasone and salmeterol (Advair®)

in the patient compartment; many EMS services carry them on the units. If possible, transport pediatric patients in their own child safety restraint. When transporting using a portable restraint device such as a child safety seat, the restraint should be secured firmly on the stretcher. It is important to follow the child safety restraint manufacturers' recommendations when transporting infants and children.

Respiratory Medications and Devices

Respiratory medications generally take two forms: medications to help improve breathing immediately by dilating the bronchioles, and medications that help over a longer period of time by preventing attacks (for example, steroids). It is important to be sure that you administer the correct type of medication to a patient who is having difficulty breathing. Medications of each type are listed in Table 17-2. The most common medication used in inhalers and nebulizers is albuterol.

Medications may be administered by inhaler (Figure 17-19 ■) or by small-volume nebulizer (SVN) (Figure 17-20 ■). Both work effectively. Patients with more severe or chronic (long-term) conditions are more likely to have a nebulizer.

17-13 Describe the indications for administering or assisting a patient with self-administration of bronchodilators by metered-dose inhaler and small-volume nebulizer.

Administering or Assisting with Medications

As an EMT, your ability to administer or assist patients with administering respiratory medications is based on local protocols, which vary widely from region to region. Your instructor will explain the protocols and regulations in your area as well as the use of the prescribed inhaler and the small-volume nebulizer (SVN).

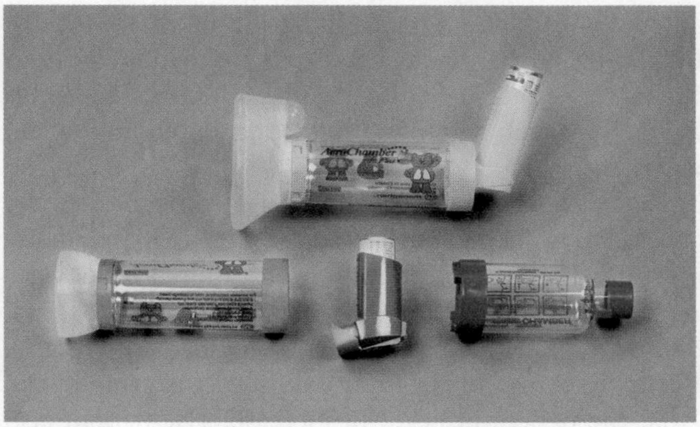

Figure 17-19 Metered-dose inhalers (MDI) and spacers.

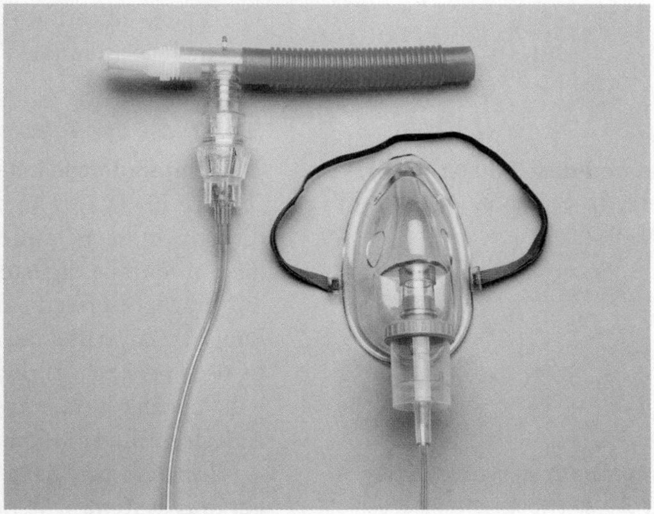

Figure 17-20 Two types of small-volume nebulizers.

17-14 Differentiate between short-acting $beta_2$ agonists appropriate for prehospital use and respiratory medications that are not intended for emergency use.

$beta_2$ agonist a class of medications that cause smooth muscle relaxation resulting in dilation of the bronchioles and vessels.

Prehospital respiratory medications are classified as $beta_2$ agonists. A **$beta_2$ agonist** causes smooth muscle relaxation resulting in the dilation of the bronchial passages. These medications are used in prehospital care as inhaler or nebulizer treatments. Most often they are referred to as short-acting $beta_2$ agonists, whereas maintenance drugs or long-term $beta_2$ agonists are not commonly used in the prehospital setting.

Drugs such as albuterol (Ventolin), levalbuterol (Xopenex®), terbutaline (Terbulin), pirbuterol (Maxair), and metaproterenol (Alupent) are commonly seen in prehospital care because they are fast acting and can be administered by inhalation or by a nebulizer. These medications work fast, giving the patient relief within minutes.

In contrast, respiratory medications that are not intended for emergency use are long-term $beta_2$ agonists or may be commonly referred to as maintenance drugs. Medications such as theophylline (Aerolate®), arformoterol (Brovana®), salmeterol (Serevent™), formoterol (Foradil®), flunisolide (AeroBid), beclomethasone dipropionate (Vanceril), fluticasone and salmeterol (Advair) are used for preventive measures to control the disease process. These medications are not necessarily meant for the prehospital setting because they are given as pills, injections, or by way of inhalation devices. These drugs take longer to act but have a longer duration period to help maintain the disease and comfort of the patient.

Before considering or beginning the administration of any medication, you must consider the "five rights": right medication, right dose, right route, right patient, and right time. (Review them in Chapter 16.)

Administering medications also involves indications and contraindications. Indications for administration of respiratory medications include the following:

- The patient is exhibiting signs of a respiratory emergency (for example, short of breath or wheezing).
- The patient has a medication prescribed to him for this respiratory condition.
- Medical direction (either on-line or by protocol) has approved the use of this medication.

General contraindications include:

- Inability of the patient to use the device (for example, patient is unresponsive or breathing inadequately).
- Device or medication is not prescribed to the patient.
- Medical direction does not approve of the administration.
- The patient has already exceeded the maximum dose.
- The medication is inappropriate for the treatment of acute breathing difficulty, such as an inhaled corticosteroid.

Metered-Dose Inhaler

metered-dose inhaler (MDI) device that patients use to breathe in medication.

The **metered-dose inhaler (MDI)** is a device that patients use to breathe in medication (Figure 17-21 ■). The medication is very effective because it is breathed into the lungs directly and acts immediately, which is much better and faster than a pill that would take time to be digested and absorbed.

The prescribed inhaler contains a fine powder that is inhaled directly into the lungs. Because the medication is a fine powder and not a gas, it is *critical* that the inhaler be used properly. If the inhaler spray is not timed properly with breathing, the powder will deposit on the moist membranes of the mouth and tongue and not enter the lungs. A device called a *spacer* helps eliminate the need for such exact timing (Figure 17-22 ■).

sympathetic nervous system part of the nervous system that activates the fight-or-flight response.

Inhalers can have side effects. Since the medication works on the **sympathetic nervous system,** it is possible that the patient's pulse will increase. The patient also may feel anxious or jittery after taking the medication.

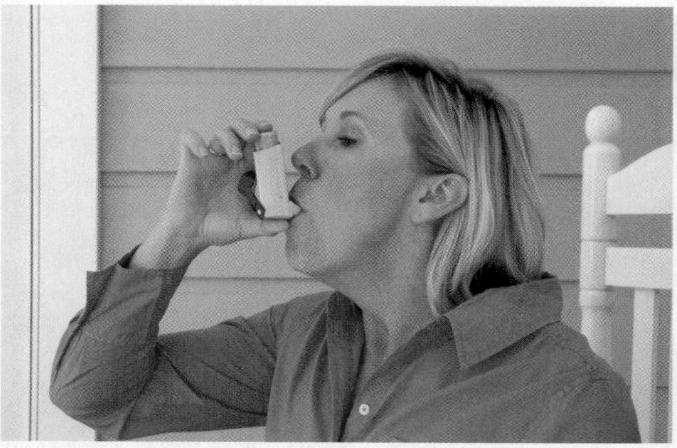

Figure 17-21 An asthma patient using an MDI.

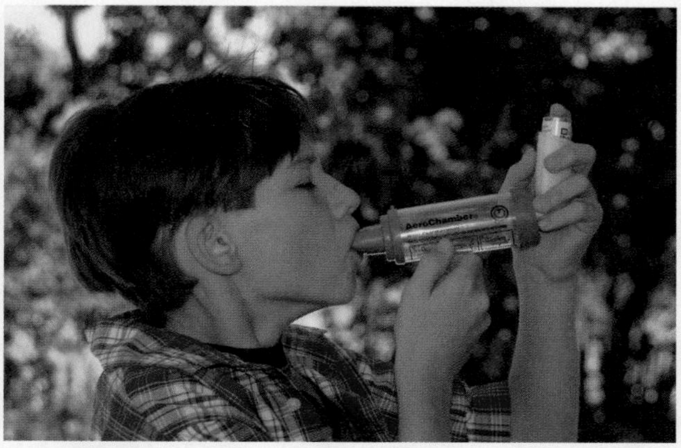

Figure 17-22 A patient using an MDI with a spacer.

To use a prescribed inhaler (Scan 17-1):

1. Obtain an order from medical direction or ensure the patient and medication meet the criteria of your standing orders.
2. Verify the "five rights."
3. Check the inhaler for the expiration date.
4. Verify that the patient has not exceeded the maximum dosage.
5. Ensure that the inhaler is at room temperature or warmer.
6. Shake the inhaler several times.
7. Remove any oxygen mask or device from the patient and have him exhale deeply.
8. Have the patient put his lips around the inhaler and begin to inhale deeply.
9. Have the patient depress the handheld inhaler as he continues to inhale deeply.
10. Instruct the patient to hold his breath for as long as he comfortably can, which allows the medication to be absorbed.
11. Replace the nonrebreather mask or other oxygen device.
12. Wait for several breaths and administer a second dose if approved by medical direction or protocol.

After administering an MDI, or any medication, reassess the patient. Assess the patient's respiratory status. Observe the patient for any changes in work of breathing, accessory muscle use, and ability to speak. Observe for changes in vital signs. Properly document the administration of the medication as well as any changes you observe.

Small-Volume Nebulizer

The **small-volume nebulizer (SVN)** is a method of continuously administering a medication, as opposed to the inhaler that provides a one-time dose. The nebulizer works by having the patient inhale oxygen (or sometimes air) that has been run through a liquid medication. This creates a vapor containing the medication. SVNs are commonly found in the homes of patients with chronic respiratory conditions and those who have frequent attacks of breathing difficulty.

small-volume nebulizer (SVN) a device that continuously administers a vaporized medication, as opposed to the inhaler that provides a one-time dose.

You may be allowed to assist the patient in the setup and use of an SVN. In some regions, EMTs have begun carrying medications such as albuterol on the ambulance to administer to patients by way of an SVN as per protocol or after contacting medical direction.

SCAN 17-1 Using a Metered-Dose Inhaler

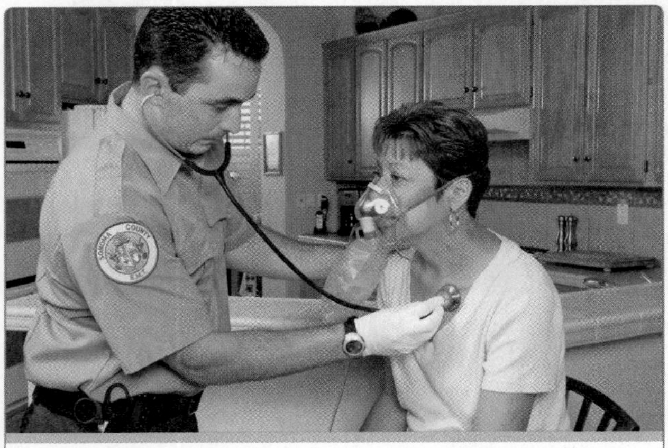

17-1-1 Complete a thorough respiratory assessment and medical history.

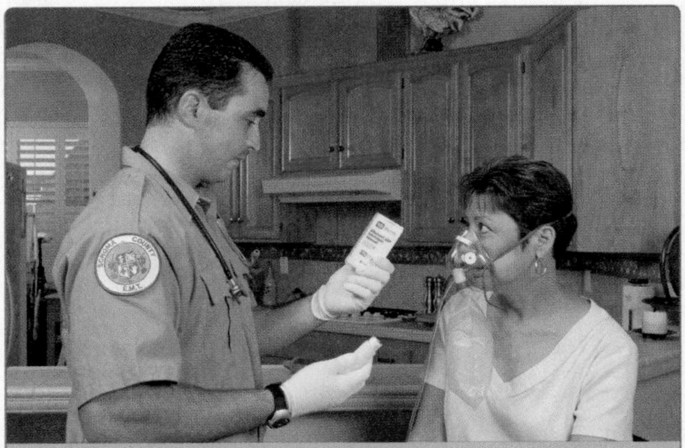

17-1-2 Confirm the medication is the patient's and that it has not expired.

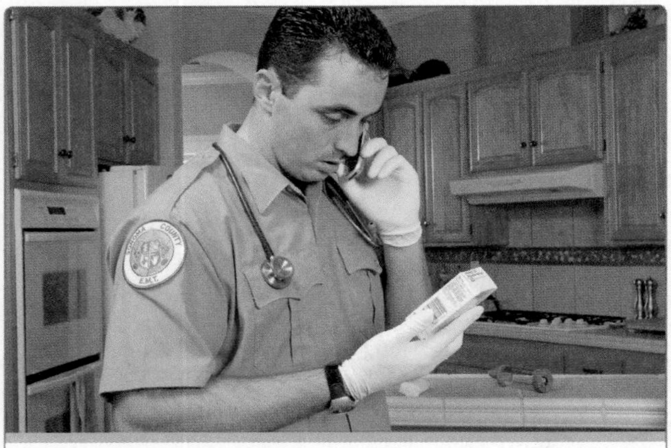

17-1-3 Assist the patient with the administration of the medication based on local protocols.

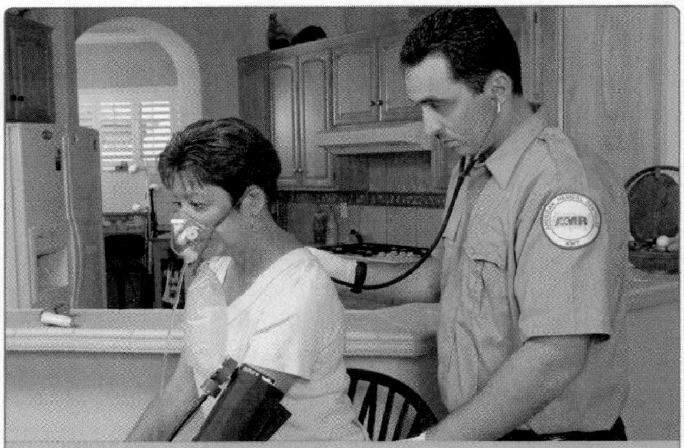

17-1-4 Reassess the breathing status and listen to lung sounds following administration.

The medications given by way of an SVN are often the same medications contained in inhalers, just in a different form. The indications, contraindications, and side effects are similar.

To administer a medication by way of an SVN (Scan 17-2) follow these steps:

1. Obtain an order from medical direction to administer the medication.
2. Ensure the "five rights."
3. Be sure there are no contraindications to administering the medication.
4. Put the liquid medication in the chamber.
5. Attach oxygen tubing to the chamber and set the flow rate at 6 to 8 L/minute.

SCAN 17-2 Using a Small-Volume Nebulizer

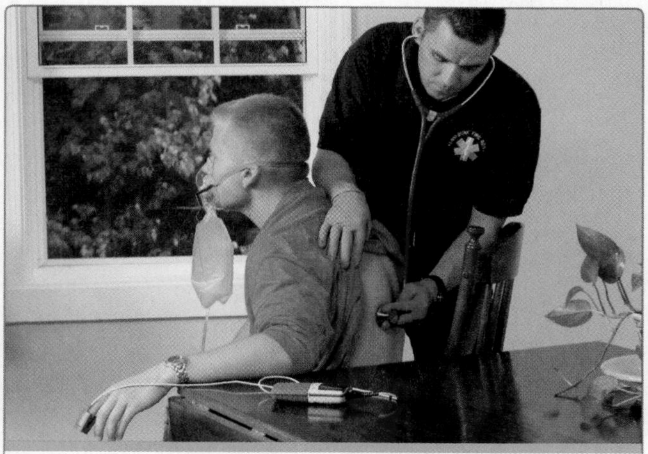

17-2-1 Complete a thorough respiratory assessment and medical history.

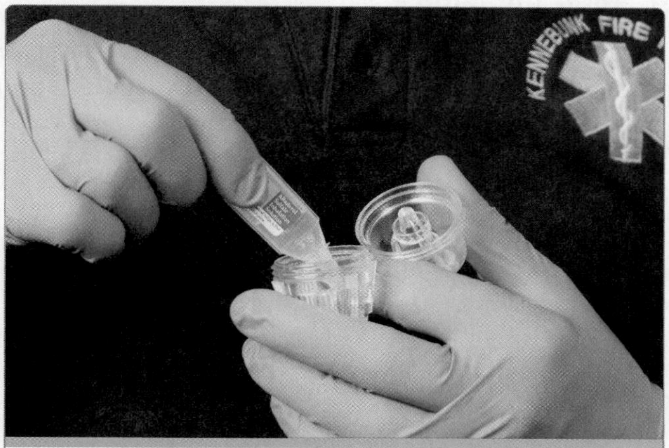

17-2-2 Assemble the device and place the medication into the nebulizer.

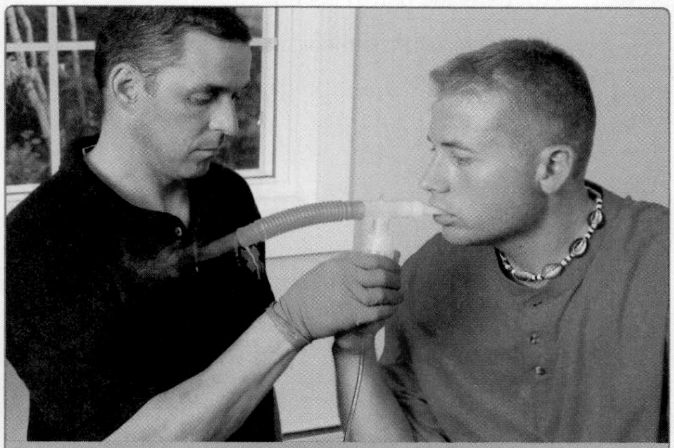

17-2-3 Instruct the patient to breathe through the mouthpiece of the nebulizer.

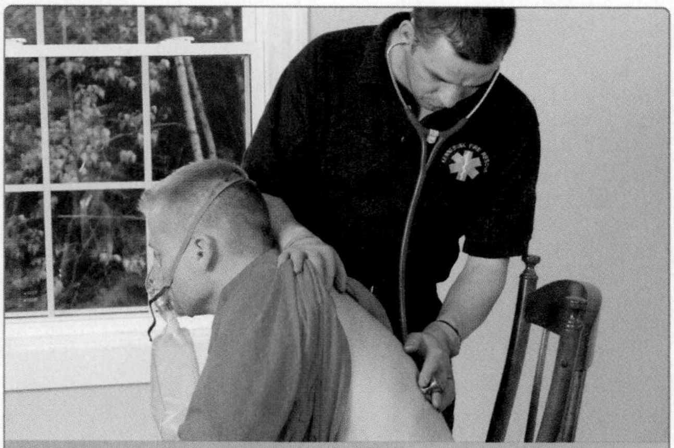

17-2-4 Reassess the breathing status and listen to lung sounds following administration.

6. Observe the medication mist coming from the device.
7. Have the patient seal his lips around the mouthpiece and breathe in deeply.
8. Instruct the patient to hold his breath for a few seconds after breathing if possible.
9. Continue until the medication is gone from the chamber.
10. Reassess the patient's level of distress and vital signs.
11. Document the patient's response to the medication (the sixth "right").

Additional doses may be ordered by medical direction if the patient is still in distress and there have been no adverse effects from the medication.

STOP, REVIEW, REMEMBER!

Multiple Choice

For each question, place a check next to the correct answer.

1. Which one of the following is *not* a common side effect of a prescribed inhaler?

_____ a. Tremors

_____ b. Decreased pulse

_____ c. Jittery feeling

_____ d. Anxiety

2. Why is timing the inhalation important when using an inhaler?

_____ a. To help ensure the medication gets deep into the lungs

_____ b. To ensure the patient inhales a few seconds after the spray

_____ c. The medication has a short half-life once out of the inhaler

_____ d. To ensure the medicine coats the inside of the mouth

3. Which one of the following is *not* a sign of hypoxia?

_____ a. Elevated pulse rate

_____ b. Pink skin color

_____ c. Elevated respiratory rate

_____ d. Anxiety

4. After administering a medication by nebulizer, the patient's pulse will increase and the patient may feel anxious or jittery. This is because the medication is affecting what system?

_____ a. Cardiovascular system

_____ b. Endocrine system

_____ c. Sympathetic nervous system

_____ d. Parasympathetic nervous system

5. You are caring for a patient with breathing difficulty and are about to assist with the administration of an MDI per local protocol. You should first:

_____ a. increase the oxygen flow rate.

_____ b. have the patient lie down.

_____ c. document the medication.

_____ d. verify the expiration date.

Fill in the Blank

1. SVN stands for ______________________________.

2. You may assist a patient with his inhaler with approval from ______________________________.

3. A ______________________________ may be attached to an inhaler to improve the inhalation of medication.

4. Patients with respiratory distress generally prefer being transported in a ______________________________ position.

5. You can assist patients only with medication that is ______________________________ to them.

Critical Thinking

1. List the "five rights" of medication administration.

2. You are caring for a patient with emphysema who is having significant respiratory distress. You begin to administer oxygen, but your partner says, "No, he may have a hypoxic drive." Should you administer oxygen? Why or why not?

EMERGENCY DISPATCH SUMMARY

The patient was loaded into the ambulance and a bag-mask with supplemental oxygen was used to assist his ventilations until an ALS unit could arrive and provide more advanced care. The patient remained in the hospital for several days before being released back home with two inhalers—one to use in an emergency and another (a steroid) to prevent future attacks.

Chapter Review

To the Point

- A sound knowledge of respiratory anatomy and physiology will allow you to understand the signs and symptoms presented by your patient. This knowledge also will help you understand some of the basic pathophysiology.
- The respiratory system is divided into two parts—the upper respiratory system and the lower respiratory system. The vocal cords are the dividing line between the upper and lower airway.
- The average amount of air taken in with a normal breath of an adult is approximately 500 mL. Of this, only about 350 mL actually reach the alveoli.
- The medulla and pons are both responsible for inspiration and expiration, as well as for rate and depth of respirations.
- The patient's skin signs, work of breathing, ability to speak, and body position are often key indicators of the severity of a patient's level of distress. Knowing the differences between

(continued on next page)

(continued)

the different stages of respiratory distress can assist you in making the right choices when treating the patient.

- Dyspnea is characterized by difficult or labored breathing.
- Hypoxia occurs when there is an inadequate supply of oxygen in the blood.
- During the primary assessment, the EMT should note the patient's skin color, mental status, and work of breathing, as well as assess for adequate rate and depth of breathing.
- Cheyne-Stokes respirations are seen in patients who have severe brain injury or end-stage brain tumors.
- Kussmaul's respirations are usually caused by very acidic blood as in some diabetic conditions and aspirin overdose.
- The rule in EMS is to never withhold oxygen from a patient who needs it. This includes patients in respiratory distress with a COPD history.
- Respiratory distress can be determined when the patient complains of shortness of breath and is exhibiting signs of inadequate oxygen exchange. A true sign of respiratory failure is when the patient no longer has the ability to compensate or does not have the ability or strength to maintain normal oxygen levels to perfuse the brain.
- Before considering or beginning the administration of any medication, you must consider the "five rights": right medication, right dose, right route, right patient, and right time.

Chapter Questions

Multiple Choice

For each question, place a check next to the correct answer.

1. The respiratory disease that results in constriction of the bronchioles as a result of allergies, exercise, or emotional stress is called:

_____ a. emphysema.
_____ b. chronic bronchitis.
_____ c. hyperventilation.
_____ d. asthma.

2. Which one of the following is *not* part of the primary assessment of the respiratory patient?

_____ a. Past medical history
_____ b. Administering oxygen
_____ c. Obtaining a pulse rate
_____ d. Determining adequacy of breathing

3. Inhaled medications that open up constricted bronchioles are called:

_____ a. bronchospastics.
_____ b. broncholytic.
_____ c. bronchodilators.
_____ d. bronchocompliant.

4. The grape-like clusters of sacs where gas is exchanged in the lungs are called:

_____ a. alveoli.
_____ b. bronchioles.
_____ c. capillaries.
_____ d. pulmonary venules.

5. You are dispatched to a "sick person." You arrive to find an older man in a chair. His chin is on his chest. He is pale and sweaty. He only groans when you loudly ask him what is wrong. To begin care you should:

_____ a. open his airway in the chair.
_____ b. apply oxygen by nonrebreather mask.
_____ c. move the patient to the floor.
_____ d. determine a history from a family member.

6. Which one of the following is *not* one of the "five rights"?

_____ a. Right medication
_____ b. Right method
_____ c. Right route
_____ d. Right dose

7. A patient is complaining of difficulty breathing. He awoke short of breath. He reports that he has been sleeping on more pillows recently and has noticed weight gain and "puffy" ankles. You suspect his condition is:

_____ a. asthma.
_____ b. chronic bronchitis.
_____ c. congestive heart failure.
_____ d. emphysema.

8. You are called to a 68-year-old man who is complaining of shortness of breath. It began after he ran to the mailbox and back in the rain, and it has not subsided for 15 minutes. He is breathing 24 times per minute. Lung sounds are clear and equal bilaterally. The patient is able to speak about six or seven words before having to catch his breath. He looks a bit anxious. This patient should receive oxygen by:
    _____ a. nasal cannula at 2 L/minute.
    _____ b. nasal cannula at 6 L/minute.
    _____ c. nonrebreather mask at 15 L/minute.
    _____ d. bag-mask device with supplemental oxygen.
9. You are assisting a patient with her prescribed inhaler. You should instruct the patient to do which one of the following before activating the inhaler?
    _____ a. Inhale halfway, and then stop and activate the inhaler.
    _____ b. Exhale fully, and then activate the inhaler.
    _____ c. Activate the inhaler, and then breathe in deeply.
    _____ d. Begin to breathe in deeply, and then activate the inhaler.
10. Which one of the following questions or examinations would be most appropriate in the assessment of a patient with difficulty breathing?
    _____ a. Can you wiggle your fingers and toes?
    _____ b. Checking pupillary reaction
    _____ c. Do you have any chest tightness or discomfort?
    _____ d. Palpating abdominal quadrants

Matching 1

Match the respiratory physical exam finding on the left with the definition on the right.

1. _____	Stridor	A. Sound caused by alveoli snapping open
2. _____	Wheezes	B. High-pitched upper airway sound
3. _____	Rhonchi	C. High-pitched musical sound
4. _____	Crackles	D. Rattling sound

Matching 2

Match the patient presentation on the left with the appropriate oxygen administration device on the right.

1. _____	17-year-old male patient who fell from a moving truck and appears to have multiple fractures	A. Nonrebreather mask at 15 L/minute
2. _____	78-year-old man who complains of chest pain and has a history of emphysema	B. Bag-mask with supplemental oxygen
3. _____	42-year-old male patient who is believed to have overdosed on a pain reliever. He is sleepy and has respirations of 6 per minute and shallow.	C. No oxygen required
4. _____	Extremely anxious 66-year-old female patient with a history of severe congestive heart failure who is breathing 44 times per minute.	
5. _____	82-year-old male patient who was complaining of chest pain and has now stopped breathing	

(continued on next page)

(continued)

6. _____ 32-year-old male with a history of panic attacks who complains of difficulty breathing.
7. _____ 27-year-old man who was hit in the chest with a baseball bat. He is conscious, alert, and breathing deeply at 20 per minute.
8. _____ 13-year-old female patient having an asthma attack. The patient is breathing at 24 per minute. You hear lung sounds bilaterally.
9. _____ 69-year-old woman complaining of fatigue and difficulty breathing. Her respirations are 16 and a bit shallow.
10. _____ 59-year-old man in an automobile collision with a significant MOI. He complains of slight pain to his neck and nothing else. Pulse 104, respirations 20 and deep.

Critical Thinking

1. Why might a patient who is conscious and breathing require ventilation with a bag-mask or pocket mask?

____

____

____

____

2. What are some of the signs of respiratory distress that will be present as you approach your patient?

____

____

____

____

3. Why are pulse and skin color so important as signs of respiratory distress?

____

____

____

____

Case Studies

Case Study 1

Your ambulance is dispatched to a call for a patient experiencing respiratory distress at a local assisted-living facility. You arrive at a safe scene and find the female patient sitting in a wheelchair just inside the door. Her husband is sitting on the couch with his walker nearby.

You introduce yourself to the patient, who seems only slightly short of breath. Her name is Marie. She holds a handful of tissues into which she has been bringing up phlegm. "I haven't been feeling that well," she says. "I've had a cough and some breathing problems." She brings up a sizable wad of phlegm and spits it into the tissues. It is off-white with yellow streaks. "See?" Her skin is pink, warm, and dry. She is talking in full sentences, and her pulse at the wrist feels slightly rapid.

A short distance away, her husband, Frank, is trying to get off the sofa and is reaching for his walker. He is a big man and does not seem very steady on his feet. As you note this, Janice, one of the health aides, comes in with copies of some paperwork for the hospital. She is talking with a patient in the next room. "Okay, Mr. Henry. I'll be right there. Just let me check on Marie."

1. Is Marie breathing adequately? How do you determine this?

2. How much oxygen would you place Marie on and by which device?

3. Do you have any responsibility to help her husband? What help does he need?

4. If the health aide tells you Marie has an inhaler, would you use it? Why or why not?

Case Study 2

You are called to a college running track for a patient with difficulty breathing. You find a 19-year-old woman standing but leaning forward with her hands on her knees. The phys ed teacher tells you that the patient has asthma. The patient is able to speak to you and confirms the history of asthma.

1. Which one of the following would indicate severe respiratory distress in this asthma patient?

_____ a. Pulse of 112 per minute

_____ b. Ability to speak only two or three words without catching her breath

_____ c. Oxygen saturation of 97%

_____ d. Wheezes with adequate air exchange

(continued on next page)

(continued)

2. All of the following are indications for assisting with a prescribed inhaler *except*:

_____ a. patient experiencing respiratory difficulty.

_____ b. patient with inadequate breathing.

_____ c. inhaler prescribed to the patient.

_____ d. medical direction approves of its use.

Case Study 3

You are called to a patient with respiratory distress. You arrive to find a patient sitting in a chair, slumped slightly to the side. You note that the patient is an 80-year-old man who responds only by slight groaning to very loud stimulus. He is limp and his skin is pale, cool, and moist.

1. To assess the airway of the patient above you should:

_____ a. open the airway and evaluate breathing in the chair.

_____ b. open the airway, listen for breathing, and auscultate lung sounds in the chair before moving the patient.

_____ c. move the patient to the floor, open the airway, and evaluate breathing.

_____ d. move the patient to the stretcher and perform the airway and breathing assessments en route to the hospital. This is a critical patient.

2. In this patient you are likely to find:

_____ a. adequate breathing.

_____ b. inadequate breathing.

_____ c. central neurogenic hyperventilation.

_____ d. normal breathing.

3. This patient would receive a reassessment at least every ______________ minutes.

_____ a. 5

_____ b. 10

_____ c. 15

_____ d. 20

The Last Word

Patients experiencing respiratory distress should be considered to be in serious condition, not only because of the medical problems that cause difficulty breathing but also because patients with difficulty breathing sincerely believe that they will die unless they are able to breathe easily again. The feeling of not being able to breathe is terrifying.

In Chapter 13, and again in this chapter, you learned about adequate versus inadequate breathing. This is one of the most important determinations you make as an EMT. You will see patients in various levels of respiratory distress. Remember that anxiety, poor skin color, and an elevated pulse are all signs of significant hypoxia.

Oxygen is the universal treatment for patients with respiratory distress. Provide supplemental oxygen by way of nonrebreather mask for patients with respiratory distress. If you use a pulse oximeter, never withhold oxygen because of a high oxygen saturation reading. You may be allowed to assist a patient with his inhaler or, in some areas, to provide nebulized albuterol as a pharmacological treatment for respiratory distress.

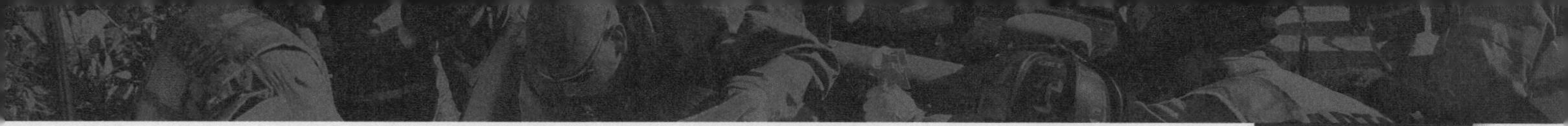

Caring for Patients with Cardiac Emergencies and Resuscitation

18

Education Standards

Medicine: Cardiovascular

Competencies

Applies fundamental knowledge to provide basic emergency care and transportation based on assessment findings for the acutely ill patient.

Objectives

After completion of this lesson, you should be able to:

18-1 Define key terms introduced in this chapter.

18-2 Describe the relationship between chest pain or discomfort, heart disease, and cardiac arrest.

18-3 Describe the structure and function of the circulatory system, including automaticity, cardiac conduction system, coronary arteries, effects of the autonomic nervous system (sympathetic and parasympathetic) on the heart, gross anatomy of the heart, plasma and formed elements of the blood, and systemic and pulmonary circulation.

18-4 Explain the relationship between electrical and mechanical events in the heart.

18-5 Discuss the relationship between hypoxia and damage to the cardiac conduction system.

18-6 Explain each of the links in the Chain of Survival.

18-7 Explain the importance of early recognition of signs and symptoms and the early treatment of patients with cardiac emergencies.

18-8 Explain the pathophysiology and the appropriate assessment and management of the following conditions, which may be classified as cardiac compromise or acute coronary syndrome: angina pectoris, cardiac arrest, cardiogenic shock, congestive heart failure, and myocardial infarction.

18-9 Explain the typical presentation of myocardial ischemia or infarction in women, diabetics, and the elderly.

18-10 Describe the role of advanced cardiac life support (ACLS) in cardiac arrest management.

18-11 Identify situations in which resuscitative attempts should be withheld.

18-12 Explain the assessment-based approach to assessment and emergency medical care for cardiac compromise and acute coronary syndrome.

18-13 Explain the indications, contraindications, forms, dosage, administration, actions, side effects, and reassessment for nitroglycerin and aspirin.

18-14 Discuss the indications and contraindications for fibrinolytic therapy and percutaneous transluminal coronary angiography in patients with acute myocardial infarctions.

18-15 Explain the importance of early defibrillation in cardiac arrest.

18-16 Describe the features, functions, advantages, disadvantages, use, and precautions in the use of automated external defibrillators (AEDs).

18-17 Compare and contrast ventricular fibrillation, ventricular tachycardia, and asystole.

18-18 Describe the various mechanical devices used to enhance the efficiency of resuscitation of the victim of sudden cardiac arrest.

Key Terms

acute p. 497
angina p. 493
arrhythmia p. 512
arteries p. 489
arterioles p. 489
asystole p. 513
atria p. 487
automated external defibrillator (AED) p. 486
automaticity p. 487
capillaries p. 489
cardiac arrest p. 486
chronic p. 497
circulatory system p. 487
conduction pathway p. 487
congestive heart failure (CHF) p. 493
coronary arteries p. 493
dysrhythmia p. 512
fibrinolytics p. 511
fibrinolytic therapy p. 511
jugular vein distention (JVD) p. 497
myocardial infarction (MI) p. 493
percutaneous transluminal coronary angiography (PTCA) p. 511
perfusion p. 490
sinoatrial node p. 487
therapeutic hypothermia p. 500
veins p. 489
ventricles p. 487
ventricular fibrillation (VF or V-fib) p. 512
ventricular tachycardia (VT) p. 513
venules p. 489

Introduction

18-2 Describe the relationship between chest pain or discomfort, heart disease, and cardiac arrest.

cardiac arrest the stopping of the heart, resulting in a loss of effective circulation.

automated external defibrillator (AED) an electrical device that automatically analyzes the heart rhythm and, if appropriate, provides a measured dose of electricity through the heart in an attempt to defibrillate or convert the heart into a normal rhythm.

According to American Heart Association (AHA) statistics, coronary heart disease (CHD) is the single leading cause of death in the United States. CHD is a narrowing or blockage of the coronary arteries that supply blood to the heart. One of every five deaths in the United States is caused by CHD. Coronary heart disease causes both angina (chest pain) and heart attacks. There are approximately 1.2 million new or recurrent cases of cardiac-related chest pain and heart attack each year. The AHA estimates that approximately 13.5 million people (6.9% of the population) in the United States alone suffer from some form or degree of CHD.

Responses to patients whose chief complaint is chest pain is a common occurrence in EMS. For many of those patients, prompt recognition and transport to an appropriate receiving hospital may mean the difference between life and death. For patients suffering **cardiac arrest,** the key to survival may be the prompt application of an **automated external defibrillator (AED).**

EMERGENCY DISPATCH

"Unit 77, Unit 7-7." The dispatcher's voice crackled from D'juan's portable radio, interrupting the relative quiet of the emergency department. "We are at level zero with calls holding. I need you to go en route for an unresponsive patient."

"Copy." D'juan sighed and shrugged his shoulders at the nurse he had been talking to. "What's the address?"

Eight minutes later, D'juan and Tom pulled up to the home in a residential neighborhood. It was one of several housing developments in this city of more than 200,000 people. As they maneuver the stretcher through the front door, they find a fire crew performing CPR on the patient—a 63-year-old woman.

"Her husband says that she was having trouble breathing," a sweating firefighter said, wiping his forehead with the back of a gloved hand. "Then she just screamed and fell down. We got here about two minutes after that and our AED shocked her once. Every time we reanalyzed, no shock was advised. So we've been doing CPR for about 9 or 10 minutes."

Tom quickly looked around the room, assessing the scene. His eyes stopped on the helpless gaze of the patient's husband. "Help her," his eyes begged. "She's all I've got."

"Headquarters, this is 7-7," D'juan said into his portable radio. "Confirming cardiac arrest. We are going to prepare for transport. What is the ETA of the ALS unit?"

Review of Circulatory System

Before continuing with this chapter, it will be helpful to review the basic anatomy and physiology of the **circulatory system** in Chapter 5. Also known as the *cardiovascular system*, the circulatory system comprises three main components: the heart, the blood, and the vessels that carry the blood throughout the body. Certain illnesses as well as injuries can affect one or all of these vital components, thereby reducing the effectiveness of the circulatory system.

18-3 Describe the structure and function of the circulatory system, including automaticity, cardiac conduction system, coronary arteries, effects of the autonomic nervous system (sympathetic and parasympathetic) on the heart, gross anatomy of the heart, plasma and formed elements of the blood, and systemic and pulmonary circulation.

circulatory system the system made up of the heart, the blood vessels, and the blood. Also called the *cardiovascular system* (*cardio* referring to the heart; *vascular* referring to the blood vessels).

PRACTICAL PATHOPHYSIOLOGY

The concept of perfusion is the adequate supply of well-oxygenated blood throughout the entire body, including the vital organs and other tissues. When the circulatory system is functioning properly, a patient is said to be perfusing well. Signs of good perfusion include normal skin signs, normal mental status, and normal vital signs.

When a person is not perfusing well, it is most often due to a malfunction of one or more of the components of the circulatory system. Signs and symptoms of poor perfusion include abnormal skin signs (pale color, cool temperature), altered mental status (sluggishness, confusion, or decreased responsiveness), and abnormal vital signs (increased pulse and respiratory rate, decreased blood pressure).

A properly functioning circulatory system along with an adequate blood pressure is essential for good perfusion.

The Heart

The heart serves as the pump in the system and is responsible for the continuous flow of blood throughout the body (Figure 18-1 ▪). The heart is made up of four interconnected pliable chambers. The top two chambers are the **atria** and the bottom two chambers are the **ventricles.** Deoxygenated blood enters the heart at the right atrium and then flows down into the right ventricle. The right ventricle pumps the blood into the lungs so it can pick up valuable oxygen and rid itself of carbon dioxide. Upon leaving the lungs, the blood reenters the heart at the left atrium, and then flows down into the left ventricle. The left ventricle is the largest and most muscular chamber of the heart because it must then pump blood out to the entire body.

atria the two upper chambers of the heart. There is a right atrium (which receives unoxygenated blood returning from the body) and a left atrium (which receives oxygenated blood returning from the lungs).

ventricles the two lower chambers of the heart. There is a right ventricle (which sends oxygen-poor blood to the lungs) and a left ventricle (which sends oxygen-rich blood to the body).

Conduction System

One of the unique properties of the heart is a characteristic known as **automaticity.** This is the ability of each and every heart muscle cell to independently generate an electrical impulse. When the heart is functioning normally, electrical impulses begin and end along the **conduction pathway** (Figure 18-2 ▪). This pathway begins at the **sinoatrial node** at the top of the heart near the right atrium and flows down the center of the heart, eventually branching across both ventricles. Certain medical conditions can cause damage to this normal electrical pathway. Diseases can cause abnormally fast or abnormally slow or irregular heart rhythms. A heart attack can result in dangerous abnormal electrical heart rhythms and even cardiac arrest.

automaticity the ability of all heart muscle cells to generate an electrical impulse.

conduction pathway the pathway of electrical impulses through the heart, which causes the heart to beat; begins at the sinoatrial node and flows down the center of the heart, eventually branching across both ventricles.

sinoatrial node beginning of the cardiac conduction pathway, located at the top of the heart near the right atrium.

The Vessels

The vessels are the plumbing of the circulatory system. They are often described by their function, location, and whether they carry blood to or from the heart. All vessels

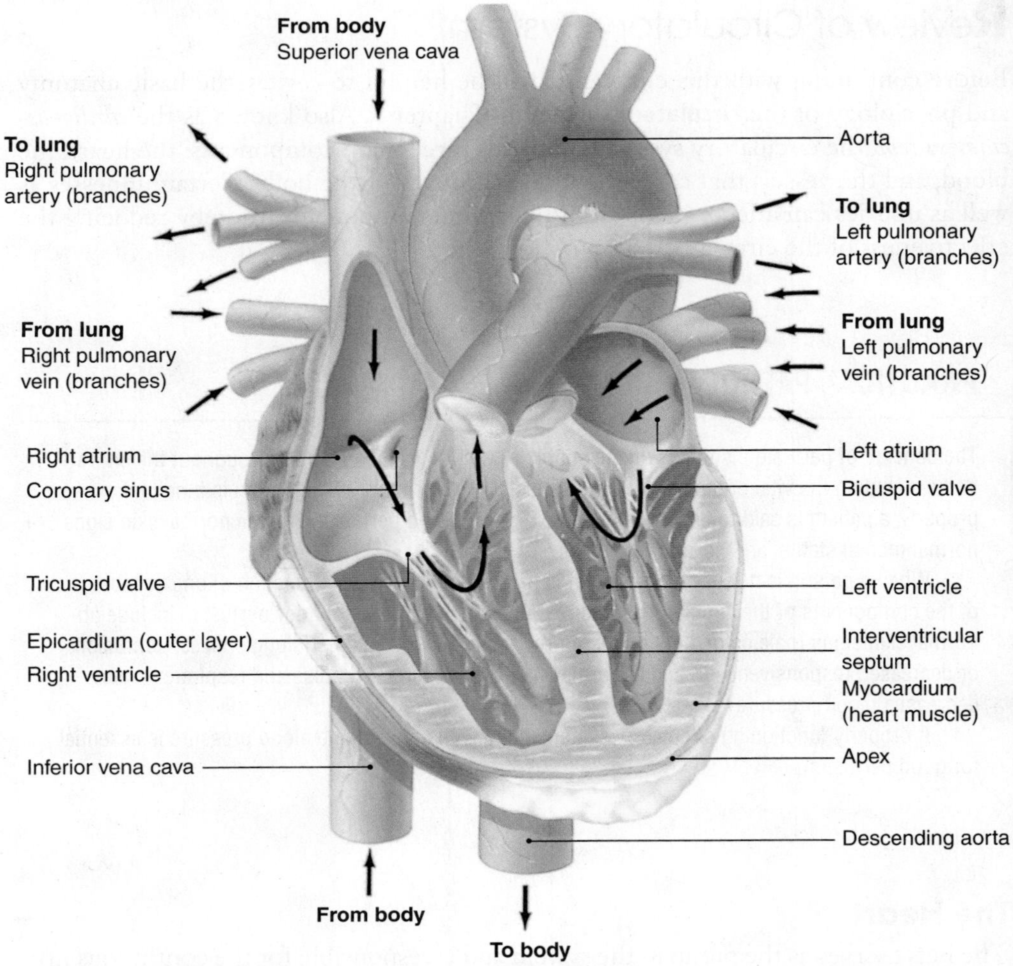

Figure 18-1 Major structures related to the heart and flow of blood.

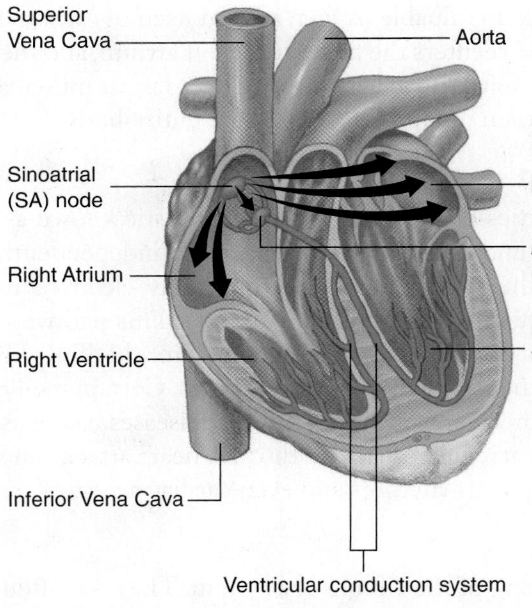

Figure 18-2 The cardiac conduction pathways are highlighted in green.

that carry blood away from the heart are called **arteries,** and vessels that carry blood toward the heart are called **veins.**

Arteries begin as larger vessels and eventually terminate in tiny vessels called **arterioles.** In contrast, veins begin as tiny **venules** that empty into larger vessels before entering the heart. The tiny vessels that join arterioles and venules and where oxygen and nutrients are exchanged for waste products are called **capillaries.** The following is a list of just some of the major vessels of the body, along with their location and function:

- ***Aorta.*** The largest artery in the body, the aorta is attached directly to the left ventricle. It is responsible for carrying oxygenated blood directly from the heart to the major areas of the body.
- ***Venae cavae.*** The venae cavae are the largest veins of the body and deliver deoxygenated blood from the body directly into the heart through the right atrium.
- ***Coronary arteries.*** The coronary arteries are the small arteries that carry oxygenated blood to the heart muscle itself (myocardium). A disruption in flow through these arteries can cause pain (angina) and damage (myocardial infarction) to the heart muscle.
- ***Pulmonary arteries.*** The pulmonary arteries are the only arteries in the body that carry deoxygenated blood. They carry blood from the heart and into the lungs to be oxygenated.
- ***Pulmonary veins.*** The only veins in the body that carry oxygenated blood, the pulmonary veins bring freshly oxygenated blood from the lungs into the left atrium.
- ***Carotid arteries.*** Found in the neck along both sides of the trachea, the carotid arteries carry blood to the head.
- ***Brachial arteries.*** Located on the inside of each arm between the armpit and the elbow, the brachial arteries carry blood to each arm.
- ***Radial arteries.*** Located on the thumb side of the anterior wrist, the radial arteries carry blood to the hands.
- ***Femoral arteries.*** Located in the anterior groin area, the femoral arteries supply blood to the lower extremities.

arteries any blood vessels carrying blood away from the heart.

veins any blood vessel returning blood to the heart.

arterioles the smallest kind of artery.

venules the smallest kind of vein.

capillaries tiny vessels that connect arterioles and venules.

The Nervous System and the Heart

As you may remember from Chapter 5, there are two sets of nerves that assist in the control of all major organs. They are the sympathetic and the parasympathetic nervous systems. The sympathetic nervous system prepares the organs for stress and emergencies and helps stimulate vigorous muscle activity when an emergency occurs. Stimulation of the sympathetic nervous system causes the heart to beat faster and with more force, and causes the dilation of the coronary arteries. All that activity allows the person to respond appropriately in an emergency.

The parasympathetic nervous system controls many of the body's functions when at rest. Stimulation of the parasympathetic nervous system will cause the heart rate to slow and the amount of force with each contraction to be less.

Electrical and Mechanical Functions of the Heart

18-4 Explain the relationship between electrical and mechanical events in the heart.

There is both an electrical and a mechanical function of the heart. When the heart is operating normally, these functions work together perfectly to keep the heart beating so that it can circulate blood. When they work together, the heart's electrical impulses follow a coordinated pathway from the top of the heart to the bottom. This electrical signal stimulates the heart muscle causing coordinated muscle contraction. The muscle contraction causes the heart to move blood forward in the system. The contraction of the right ventricle pushes blood to the lungs and the contraction of the left ventricle pushes blood out to the entire body. It is this mechanical force of blood being pushed out of the left ventricle that causes the pressure wave in the arteries that can be felt as a pulse.

There are conditions that can cause problems with the electrical and the mechanical functions of the heart. An example is a condition known as *atrial fibrillation.* In atrial fibrillation the electrical function of the top two chambers (atria) is affected. The electrical impulses become rapid and chaotic and the atria do not have enough time to adequately fill with blood as well as losing the ability to contract synchronously with the rest of the heart. This condition can decrease cardiac output by as much as 20%.

18-5 Discuss the relationship between hypoxia and damage to the cardiac conduction system.

There are many conditions that can affect the mechanical function of the heart muscle as well. The muscle can become damaged due to trauma or from an event such as a heart attack. In a heart attack, or myocardial infarction, the heart muscle dies due to lack of blood and oxygen. This can severely weaken the muscle, causing a decrease in the heart's ability to pump blood to the body. If the area of the heart that is affected by a heart attack lies over an electrical pathway, this can disrupt or alter the normal electrical function of the heart, causing a dangerous or life-threatening heart rhythm known as a dysrhythmia.

The Function of the Blood

Blood serves many essential functions as it is carried by the circulatory system and flows throughout the body. Its most fundamental duty is to carry oxygen and nutrients to the cells and remove waste products generated by cell metabolism.

Blood is made up of several components, each with a specialized function or functions. The major components of blood are as follows:

- ***Plasma.*** Plasma is the clear, yellowish fluid in which the other components of blood are suspended.
- ***Red blood cells.*** Disc-shaped cells, the red blood cells are responsible for transporting oxygen and carbon dioxide to and from the tissues.
- ***White blood cells.*** The white blood cells help protect the body from infection and disease.
- ***Platelets.*** Irregularly shaped cell fragments, platelets are responsible for promoting rapid blood clotting.

To perform these very important functions and sustain life, blood must be present in a sufficient amount. There is a direct connection between the volume of blood within the circulatory system and blood pressure and **perfusion.** When a patient loses blood from within the circulatory system, blood pressure will eventually fall and perfusion will become inadequate to keep the patient alive.

perfusion the adequate supply of well-oxygenated blood to body tissues, especially the vital organs. (*Hypoperfusion* is inadequate perfusion.)

PRACTICAL PATHOPHYSIOLOGY

The cardiovascular system is made up of three components—the heart (pump), the vessels (container), and the blood (fluid). Each of them must be present and working normally to ensure good circulation to all the vital organs. If any one is damaged or missing, perfusion will suffer.

The Chain of Survival

18-6 Explain each of the links in the Chain of Survival.

You may remember from your CPR training learning about the Chain of Survival. Developed by the American Heart Association and recognized by most, if not all, of the national organizations supporting CPR training, the Chain of Survival consists of five essential components or "links" necessary for the successful care of prehospital cardiac-arrest victims. The five links in the Chain of Survival are:

- Immediate recognition of cardiac arrest and activation of the emergency response system
- Early CPR with an emphasis on chest compressions
- Rapid defibrillation
- Effective advanced life support
- Integrated post-cardiac arrest care

When any one of the five links is weak or missing, the likelihood of a successful patient outcome is greatly diminished. As an EMT in your community, you will likely be involved in some manner with all five links. At the very least, as an EMT working within an EMS system, you will be directly involved in the first three.

Early Recognition and Activation of EMS

18-7 Explain the importance of early recognition of signs and symptoms and the early treatment of patients with cardiac emergencies.

In most emergencies, EMS must rely on willing and informed bystanders to access the EMS system in the most efficient way possible. Thanks to technology, there are more ways to access the EMS system than ever before. You must understand how the system works and when one method is better than another for accessing the system. You must do your part to educate the public on how the system works and encourage them to activate EMS when appropriate.

Due to the vital function of the cardiovascular system, it is especially important to recognize the signs and symptoms when the system is not functioning properly. Cardiac emergencies, such as heart attack and heart failure, are time sensitive. *Loss of time is loss of muscle!*

Cardiac emergencies are most often associated with a lack of oxygen to the heart muscle. As the heart muscle goes without oxygen or when it becomes hypoxic, ischemia and or muscle death (myocardial infarction) may occur. Never forget that the goal of cardiac resuscitation is not simply to return heart function but also to preserve the brain so that the patient can make a full and meaningful recovery without significant disability. Therefore, as an EMT you must place an emphasis on early recognition and transport to an appropriate facility.

The longer a cardiac patient has to wait for recognition and interpretation of signs and symptoms, the longer the delay of transport to the hospital. Advanced life support (ALS) should be initiated based on dispatch information. However, if ALS has not been dispatched, you should request backup immediately.

Early CPR

Early CPR with an emphasis on good compressions is the foundation of successful resuscitation. Beginning CPR immediately and pushing hard and fast is the best way to maintain circulation until more advanced care arrives. As an EMT, you have a duty to keep your skills sharp because you may have to initiate or take over for bystander CPR at the scene of a cardiac arrest. Good CPR, with minimal interruptions has been proven to save more lives than ever before. As a member of the EMS system, you should become an advocate for CPR training and encourage laypersons to become trained.

PERSPECTIVE

Jordan—The Fire Major

Man, it went like clockwork at first. We got there, determined that she was in full arrest, and slapped the AED on. It shocked the first time, but then it said "No shock advised" the rest of the time. She was still in full arrest, so I guess we shocked her into asystole or something. That happens. Most of the time, though, the AED works like a charm. I've even had people go from full arrest to sitting up and talking before the ambulance even gets there.

Rapid Defibrillation

It is important to minimize the time between cardiac arrest and defibrillation. As automated external defibrillators (AEDs) become more common and are used by more and more laypersons, the likelihood that you will have a viable patient when you arrive at the scene of a cardiac arrest is greatly increased.

Effective Advanced Life Support

The fourth link in the chain is early advanced care. In most EMS systems this refers to early access to advanced life support (ALS) by advanced EMTs and paramedics. These individuals possess the advanced skills and equipment necessary to help stabilize a cardiac patient in the field. In most areas of the country, the patient no longer must wait until arrival at the hospital to begin receiving life-saving advanced care. Research has shown that the sooner a patient receives advanced-level care, the better his chances for a positive outcome.

You must know the system you are working in and all the available resources. In some systems, the fastest way to access advanced life support is to simply call dispatch for an ALS backup and have them respond directly to the scene. In more rural systems, it may save valuable time to request an ALS intercept, load the patient, begin transporting toward the hospital, and meet the ALS crew along the way to the hospital. In other systems, it may be that ALS is still not available in the field, and you must initiate rapid transport to the most appropriate facility. Regardless of the type of system you may be working in, ALS care is a vital link in the chain of survival.

Integrated Post-Cardiac Arrest Care

The fifth and final link in the Chain of Survival involves a more formal and organized approach to post-cardiac arrest care and includes neurological support and therapeutic hypothermia. Therapeutic hypothermia is the deliberate and controlled cooling of the body with the intent of slowing the body's demand for oxygen. (This will be discussed more a little later in this chapter.)

Cardiac Compromise

The term *cardiac compromise* (also called *acute coronary syndrome*) is used to describe patients who present with specific signs and symptoms that may indicate some type of emergency relating to their heart. Medical conditions such as **myocardial infarction (MI)** (heart attack), **angina** (chest pain), and **congestive heart failure (CHF)** are some of the most common types of cardiac compromise. The following is a list of some of the more common signs and symptoms of cardiac compromise:

- Chest discomfort, which is typically described as pain or a dull pressure, tightness, or squeezing sensation in the chest. It may also radiate to the arms, shoulders, back, or jaw.
- Sudden onset of sweating (diaphoresis)
- Shortness of breath (dyspnea)
- Nausea, vomiting
- Anxiety, irritability
- Feeling of impending doom
- Abnormal pulse rate (may be slow, rapid, irregular)
- Abnormal blood pressure (may be high or low)
- Upper abdomen (epigastric) pain
- Generalized weakness (especially in older women)

18-8 Explain the pathophysiology and the appropriate assessment and management of the following conditions, which may be classified as cardiac compromise or acute coronary syndrome: angina pectoris, cardiac arrest, cardiogenic shock, congestive heart failure, and myocardial infarction.

myocardial infarction (MI) occlusion or blockage of one or more of the coronary arteries, resulting in damage to the heart muscle. Also called a *heart attack*.

angina literally a pain in the chest; occurs when one or more of the coronary arteries are unable to provide an adequate supply of oxygenated blood to the heart muscle. Also called *angina pectoris*.

congestive heart failure (CHF) an overload of fluid in the body's tissues that results when the heart is unable to pump an adequate volume of blood.

PERSPECTIVE

Ted—The Husband

Joanie has CHF. We've known that for a while. And she's diabetic. But we're very careful about her medications. We really take all of that stuff very seriously. When Joanie was complaining about her breathing, I thought immediately of the CHF, because that happens sometimes. But when she screamed and fell down, I felt, I don't know, like I was a little kid again or something. Just completely helpless.

Cardiac compromise can have many causes and can present with any or all of the above signs and symptoms. The point is, not all patients experience the same signs and symptoms in the same order and therefore will present differently. As an EMT, you must use your assessment skills to quickly perform an appropriate history and physical exam to identify the potential for cardiac involvement. When in doubt, treat for the worst possible scenario and initiate immediate transport and ALS backup if available.

Myocardial Infarction (Heart Attack)

The medical term for heart attack is *myocardial infarction (MI)*. *Myo-* means muscle, *cardial-* means heart, and *infarction* means death of tissue due to a loss of adequate blood supply. It is important to understand that an MI and cardiac arrest are not one and the same. In its simplest definition, a cardiac arrest is the sudden stopping of the heart, resulting in a loss of effective circulation. Patients suffering a cardiac arrest are unresponsive, not breathing, and have no palpable pulses. These patients should receive immediate CPR and the application of an AED. While it is true that many cardiac arrests are the result of an MI, most MIs do not result in a cardiac arrest.

The heart is a living organ that must have an adequate supply of well-oxygenated blood to continue to function properly. The heart receives its blood supply through vessels known as **coronary arteries.** When these arteries become excessively narrow or

coronary arteries small arteries that carry oxygenated blood to the heart muscle itself. A disruption in flow through these arteries can cause pain and damage to the heart muscle.

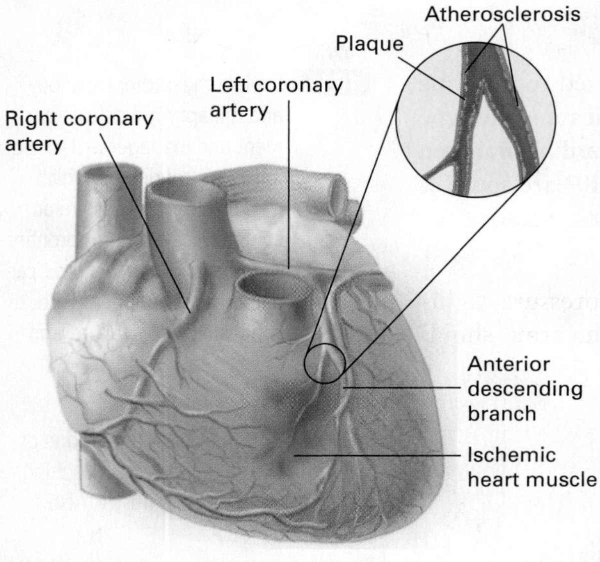

Figure 18-3 The myocardium is fed by the coronary arteries. When a coronary artery becomes blocked, ischemia results.

blocked from disease and can no longer supply the heart with enough oxygenated blood, the tissue of the heart begins to die (Figure 18-3 ▪).

There are many factors that will ultimately determine whether or not an MI will result in a cardiac arrest, but the most common factors are where the damage occurs on the heart and how extensive an area actually dies. Damage that occurs to a large area, over an important electrical pathway, or to the left ventricle is more likely to cause a cardiac arrest than an MI that is very small or occurs to a less critical area of the heart.

Signs and Symptoms of an MI

The signs and symptoms of an MI can occur suddenly—as often portrayed in movies and on television. However, in real life their onset is often more gradual and subtle. It is not unusual for a patient to awaken in the morning with mild chest, back, or arm pain and some shortness of breath. He will often experience nausea, which makes him think it may be the flu. This gradual onset is not consistent with what the patient understands a heart attack is, and therefore he may delay seeking care until symptoms worsen. This delay can be detrimental and may lead to cardiac arrest before he seeks medical care. Chest pain from an MI typically lasts more than a few minutes and is not relieved by rest.

Some studies suggest that nearly half of patients who experience a heart attack do not have chest pain as the primary symptom. Common yet atypical symptoms of an MI include the following:

- Shortness of breath
- Nausea
- Dizziness, weakness, and fainting
- Abdominal pain
- Fatigue

18-9 Explain the typical presentation of myocardial ischemia or infarction in women, diabetics, and the elderly.

Patients most likely to have atypical symptoms of an MI are women, diabetics, and the very elderly (although they certainly can have classic heart attack symptoms as well). During an acute myocardial infarction (AMI), these populations more often experience nausea and vomiting, indigestion, back, neck, or jaw pain, and less often experience the chest pain that is so common in middle-aged men.

As an EMT, you must be very aware of all the possible presentations of cardiac compromise and not just the typical "Hollywood" presentation of the man who suddenly grasps his chest and falls to the ground. You must be very suspicious of the elderly, female, or diabetic patients who may be insisting its just indigestion and will be just fine. You must provide care, presuming the worst possible scenario.

Signs and Symptoms of Cardiogenic Shock

A form of shock that results when the heart becomes damaged and can no longer pump blood efficiently is known as *cardiogenic shock.* It is most often caused by myocardial infarction and results in inadequate perfusion to the vital organs. Signs and symptoms of cardiogenic shock include:

- Anxiety
- Rapid, weak pulse
- Low blood pressure
- Pale, cool skin

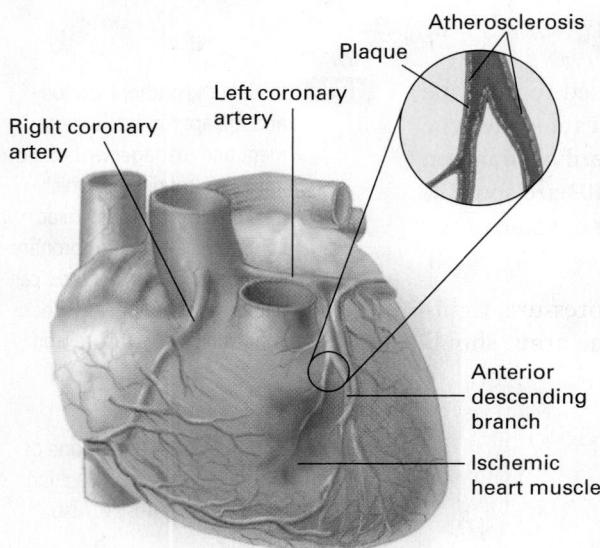

Consider the possibility of cardiogenic shock when the patient presents with signs of shock but without any evidence of trauma or history of internal bleeding.

Angina Pectoris

A slightly less dangerous type of cardiac compromise is *angina pectoris* or, as it is more commonly called, *angina*. Literally translated, it means "pain in the chest." Angina occurs when one or more of the coronary arteries are unable to provide an adequate supply of oxygenated blood to the heart muscle. While this may sound like what happens in an MI, the similarity ends here. With angina there is no actual damage to the heart muscle. The supply of oxygenated blood is never cut off entirely, and the pain is caused by the muscles starving for more blood and oxygen.

Angina often is triggered by exertion. Exertion such as physical activity creates a demand on the heart muscle that the coronary arteries, which have been narrowed by disease or spasm, are unable to meet. The pain increases until the patient must stop the activity and rest. Within a few minutes, the demand on the heart returns to normal and the pain begins to subside and eventually goes away. Some patients are prone to angina attacks and must take medication, such as nitroglycerin, to help increase circulation to the heart. (Nitroglycerin will be discussed in more detail later in this chapter.)

The signs and symptoms of angina are nearly identical to those of an MI. For that reason, it is important to treat all patients experiencing cardiac-related pain as though they were having an MI and seek immediate advanced medical care. Do not try to distinguish between an MI and angina; this must be left up to the doctors and other specialists at the hospital.

STOP, REVIEW, REMEMBER!

Multiple Choice

For each question, place a check next to the correct answer.

1. Which vessels supply blood to the heart muscle?

_____ a. Pulmonary veins

_____ b. Pulmonary arteries

_____ c. Coronary arteries

_____ d. Coronary veins

2. Which chamber of the heart pumps blood to the body?

_____ a. Left atrium

_____ b. Left ventricle

_____ c. Right atrium

_____ d. Right ventricle

3. One out of every _____________ deaths in the United States is attributed to coronary heart disease.

_____ a. 2

_____ b. 5

_____ c. 10

_____ d. 25

4. A sudden cardiac arrest is most likely due to:

_____ a. myocardial infarction.

_____ b. angina.

_____ c. diabetes.

_____ d. trauma.

(continued on next page)

(continued)

5. Compared to a myocardial infarction, chest pain from angina will typically be of ____________ duration.

_____ a. slightly longer
_____ b. similar
_____ c. much longer
_____ d. shorter

Fill in the Blank

1. ______________________ is the flow of well-oxygenated blood throughout the entire body including the vital organs and other tissues.

2. The top two chambers of the heart are called the ______________________ and the bottom two chambers are the ventricles.

3. ______________________ is the ability of all muscle cells in the heart to stimulate an electrical impulse.

4. All vessels that carry blood away from the heart are called ____________________, and vessels that carry blood to the heart are called ____________________.

5. The five links in the Chain of Survival are early recognition, early ______________________, rapid defibrillation, effective ______________________, and integrated post-cardiac arrest care.

6. Conditions such as ____________________ and ____________________ are some of the most common causes of cardiac compromise.

Critical Thinking

1. Describe what you might look for to determine a patient's perfusion status.

____

____

____

____

2. Describe how a myocardial infarction can lead to cardiac compromise.

____

____

____

____

3. Describe the difference between a myocardial infarction and angina.

____

____

____

____

Heart Failure

Heart failure, sometimes referred to as *congestive heart failure (CHF)* is a term used to describe an overload of fluid in the body's tissues that results when the heart is unable to pump adequately. Because the heart is unable to manage the normal amount of fluid volume, fluid begins to back up within the circulatory system. If left untreated, this backup of fluids can result in excessive fluid buildup in the lower extremities and lungs. Patients with CHF usually present with difficulty breathing as a chief complaint, due to the accumulation of fluids in the lungs.

CHF can be both a **chronic** problem and an **acute** one as well. Some of the causes of chronic CHF include diseased heart valves and hypertension. A patient also can experience an acute episode of CHF secondary to an MI because of the heart's inability to pump effectively.

chronic slow-onset or long-term. Opposite of *acute*.

acute sudden-onset. Opposite of *chronic*.

Unlike angina and MI, which typically present with a chief complaint of chest pain or discomfort, the acute CHF patient will typically have difficulty breathing. However, patients with CHF also can develop MIs and angina, and they may present with chest pain or discomfort in addition to shortness of breath. These patients often have a history of cardiac problems and, for that reason, will likely have a long list of prescribed medications.

If the patient is standing or seated, you will usually see obvious swelling of the feet and ankles (pedal edema), because gravity pulls the excess fluids to these areas (Figure 18-4 ■). If the patient is confined to a bed, you may see edema in the sacral area (sacral edema), because this usually is the lowest part of the body and, once again, gravity pulls the excess fluid downward. Depending on the amount of fluid in the lungs, the patient may experience increased shortness of breath while lying down. Be alert for it and be prepared to place the patient in a position of most comfort. Many of these patients will want to sit up. You may see some **jugular vein distention (JVD)** when the patient is in the sitting position as a result of the increased pressure inside the circulatory system (Figure 18-5 ■).

jugular vein distention (JVD) bulging of the neck veins.

Cardiac Arrest

The ultimate cardiac compromise is *cardiac arrest.* The heart has failed completely as a pump and circulation is no longer adequate to support life. While there still may be some electrical activity and movement within the heart, it is not able to circulate blood. The victim of cardiac arrest will be unresponsive, pulseless, and not breathing

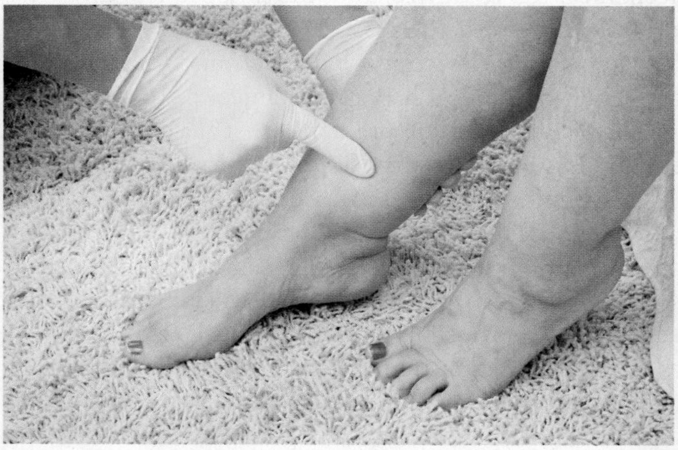

Figure 18-4 One of the signs of possible heart failure is swelling (edema) of the ankles.

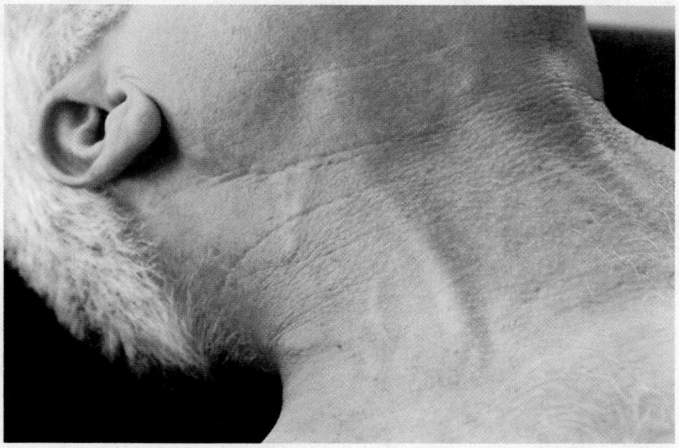

Figure 18-5 Another sign of possible heart failure is jugular vein distention (JVD).

and will require immediate CPR (beginning with chest compressions) and the placement of an AED. AEDs are now being recommended for patients as young as one month old. Be sure to consult your local protocols and the manufacturer's recommendations about the use of AEDs.

18-10 Describe the role of advanced cardiac life support (ACLS) in cardiac arrest management.

In addition to rapid defibrillation, it is important to initiate advanced life support (ALS) care as soon as possible for the victim of cardiac arrest. In addition to providing rapid defibrillation, an ALS provider can deliver a variety of medications that will assist in restoring normal heart function. They also can insert advanced airways to help improve ventilations and the delivery of oxygen to the lungs, heart, and brain. In some areas ALS providers are even initiating therapeutic hypothermia in the field for cardiac-arrest patients who have had return of spontaneous circulation (ROSC).

18-11 Identify situations in which resuscitative attempts should be withheld.

Cardiac arrest is a common occurrence for many EMS systems and the approach to resuscitation is well established. There may be times when resuscitation should not be initiated or perhaps stopped before transport. One such example is when an advance directive is in effect. Some patients with a known terminal illness may request that CPR not be initiated should they go into cardiac arrest. When caring for patients with a terminal illness, it is appropriate to question family and other caregivers to determine if such a directive is in place.

As an EMT, you will initiate resuscitation efforts and transport as soon as possible. However, it is not uncommon for an ALS provider to attempt resuscitation at the scene and if there is no response from the patient after all standard procedures have been followed, to pronounce the patient deceased. The pronouncement of death at the scene following sudden cardiac arrest is driven by carefully designed protocols and is always conducted in direct coordination with medical direction. You must become familiar with the specific protocols used in your area or service.

18-18 Describe the various mechanical devices used to enhance the efficiency of resuscitation of the victim of sudden cardiac arrest.

Resuscitation efforts may be withheld in cases involving signs of obvious death such as when rigor mortis, lividity, or evidence of decay is present. Patients with devastating trauma such as decapitation also are not candidates for resuscitation. Most EMS systems have clearly defined protocols that define when resuscitation may be withheld. Always follow local protocol.

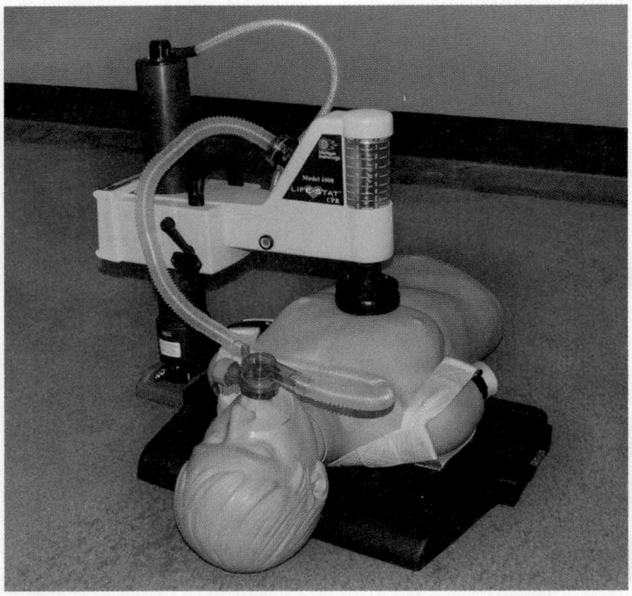

Figure 18-6 The "Thumper®" mechanical CPR device from Michigan Instruments. (© Edward T. Dickinson)

Resuscitation Devices

There are several mechanical devices that are currently being used throughout the country during resuscitation of a sudden cardiac-arrest victim. Two of the more common devices are the mechanical CPR device and the impedance threshold device (ITD).

Mechanical CPR devices have been around for more than 30 years. The first models had a mechanical piston driven by oxygen. The piston could compress the chest at a consistent rate and depth once properly applied (Figure 18-6 ▪). In recent years there have been new entries in this arena with variations of the piston device and the load-distributing vest-type device known as the AutoPulse™ (Figure 18-7 ▪). Devices such as the Lucas™ Device from Jolife can perform both regular CPR or active compression/decompression (suction cup) CPR (Figure 18-8 ▪). Studies have shown that active compression/decompression CPR enhances changes in intrathoracic chest pressures improving CPR and ultimately improving survival rates in cardiac arrest patients. Active compression/decompression CPR has not been approved by the FDA for use in the United States yet.

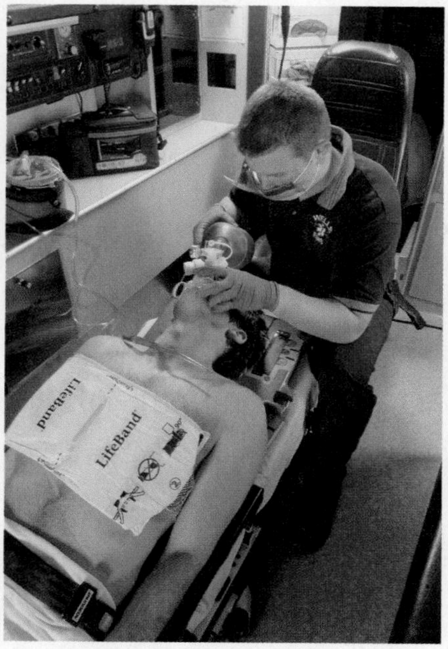

Figure 18-7 The Autopulse Model 100 CPR device by Zoll.

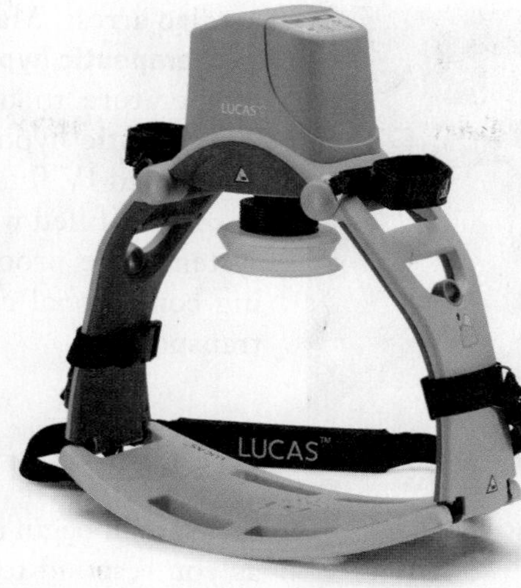

Figure 18-8 The Lucas CPR device. (Image provided by: Physio-Control, Inc. Lucas® 2 Chest Compression System.)

These devices are driven by compressed air, oxygen, or battery power and can be applied quickly to a victim of cardiac arrest. Once applied, these devices can do the job of up to two rescuers and are programmed to provide chest compressions according to the latest AHA resuscitation guidelines. Once properly applied, they can provide compressions at a very consistent rate and depth for an indefinite period of time.

Another device that is gaining acceptance throughout the country and that was highly recommended for use by the American Heart Association in cardiac-arrest patients is the ResQPOD® impedance threshold device (ITD) (Figure 18-9 ■). It is a small device that is placed between a bag-mask device and mask or an advanced airway. The ITD is designed to improve circulation of blood to the heart by increasing the negative pressure inside the chest during CPR, improving the ability of the heart to refill between compressions, thus improving the amount of blood being circulated with each compression. It also helps control the ventilation rate of the rescuer by the use of a flashing LED that directs the rescuer when to deliver a ventilation. Strict control of the rate of ventilation (specifically preventing rescuers from over-ventilating) has shown to improve patient outcome in cardiac arrest.

Several EMS systems around the country are utilizing one or more of these devices in an attempt to improve the return of spontaneous circulation (ROSC) in victims of sudden cardiac arrest.

Therapeutic Hypothermia

Recent research has shown that cooling the post-cardiac-arrest patient improved survival by reducing the likelihood of tissue damage from ischemia following

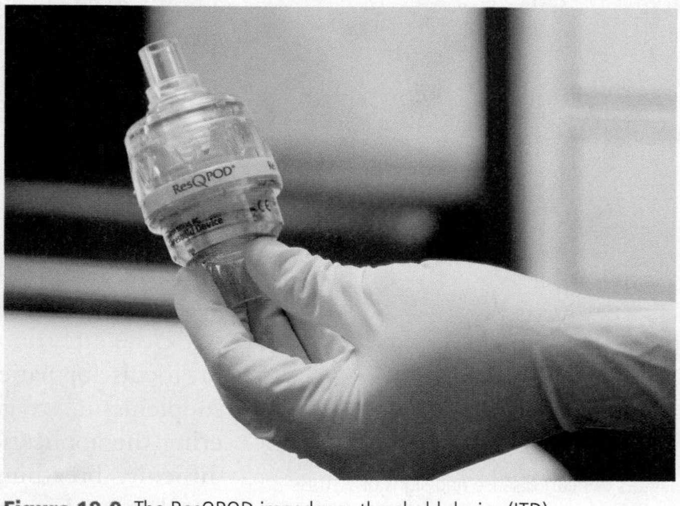

Figure 18-9 The ResQPOD impedence threshold device (ITD).

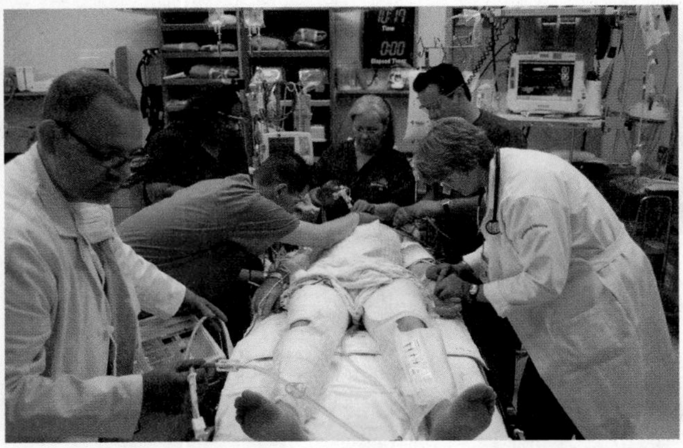

Figure 18-10 A therapeutic hypothermia device. (© Edward T. Dickinson, MD)

cardiac arrest. Many hospitals are employing what is known as **therapeutic hypothermia** to actively cool the patient's core temperature to between 32°C and 34°C or 90°F to 93°F. Therapeutic hypothermia is most often performed by infusing cooled IV fluid and covering the patient's torso with thin envelopes filled with a chilled fluid (Figure 18-10 ■). In some systems, the process of cooling the patient begins by placing commercial cold packs around the patient's core during transport.

therapeutic hypothermia the intentional and controlled cooling of the body in order to slow metabolism and the demand for oxygen.

Assessment of the Cardiac Patient

You should begin thinking about your assessment and care even as you respond to the call. In most cases, it will be a call for chest pain. What personal protective equipment will you want to wear? Who will perform the history and physical exam, you or your partner? What equipment will you want to bring into the scene with you? How will you get a history if the patient is unable to provide one? These are just some of the things you can be thinking about as you safely drive to the scene. Keep in mind that upon your arrival, things may be quite different from information provided in the original dispatch.

18-12 Explain the assessment-based approach to assessment and emergency medical care for cardiac compromise and acute coronary syndrome.

Scene Size-up and the Primary Assessment

Once you have completed an appropriate scene size-up and determined that the scene is safe for you and your partner, you will need to perform a primary assessment. As you enter the scene and approach the patient, pay particular attention to the patient's body language. Is the patient sitting comfortably talking to others or is the patient showing signs of distress—sitting upright, leaning forward with hands on knees (tripod position), perhaps holding a clenched fist to his chest (Figure 18-11 ■) with a troubled or painful facial expression? What is his color like, and does he appear to be diaphoretic or having difficulty breathing? Many of these signs will be obvious as you approach your patient. Trust your gut. If the patient looks bad and you do not like what you see, consider this patient as a high priority for transport. Confirm the patient's chief complaint (nature of illness). Are his signs and symptoms consistent with what he is telling you?

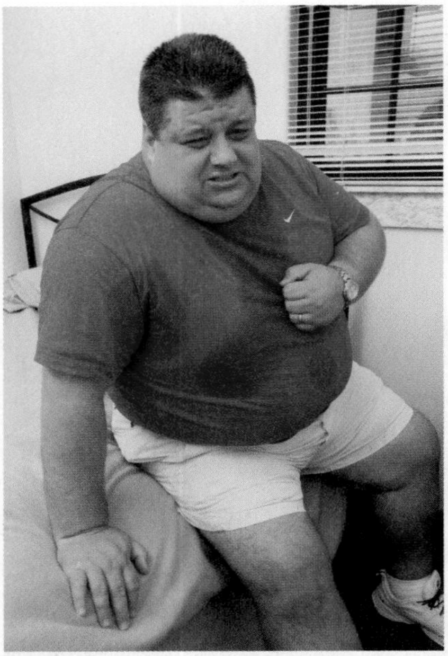

Figure 18-11 A patient with many of the risk factors of heart disease and signs of distress related to chest pain.

Look at the patient's immediate environment. Do you see anything, such as a home oxygen supply or medication bottles on the table or nightstand that may give you clues to his current medical history?

Based on your general impression and your primary assessment, you must make an initial decision regarding transport priority. If ALS is available in your area, you may want to consider calling it to the scene or setting up an intercept en route to the hospital if it has not already been dispatched.

Depending on the level of responsiveness of the patient, airway management may play an important role. If the patient is responsive, it will be easy to determine the status of his airway because he will be talking and relaying information about his history. For patients with a decreased level of responsiveness, you must pay close attention to the status of the airway and adequacy of breathing. Most protocols for patients with cardiac compromise mandate the administration of supplemental oxygen. Do not move past the primary assessment without considering the application of oxygen. Cardiac patients may or may not present with difficulty breathing. However, most suspected cardiac patients should receive supplemental oxygen. It is becoming more common to adjust the flow of oxygen depending on the patient's pulse oximeter reading. Always follow your local protocol when administering oxygen.

PRACTICAL PATHOPHYSIOLOGY

Recent research has shown that too much oxygen may be harmful to heart tissue that is ischemic. One recommendation is to adjust the oxygen delivery using a pulse oximeter. The idea is to adjust the flow of oxygen to achieve a pulse oximetry reading of between 94% and 99%. A patient with acute coronary syndrome who has pulse oximetry readings of between 94% and 99% on room air may not need supplemental oxygen. Always follow local protocol.

SAMPLE History

Based on the chief complaint of chest pain or discomfort, you will want to move directly into your SAMPLE history and focus your questions on the chief complaint. Direct your line of questioning at the chief complaint of chest pain or discomfort. The mnemonic OPQRST is a common tool used to assess chest pain or discomfort. Be sure to look the patient in the eyes as you ask questions and be very sure that he understands your questions (Figure 18-12 ■). Remember that he is likely very frightened and distracted by what is happening with his body. Below is a review of OPQRST and sample questions for each component:

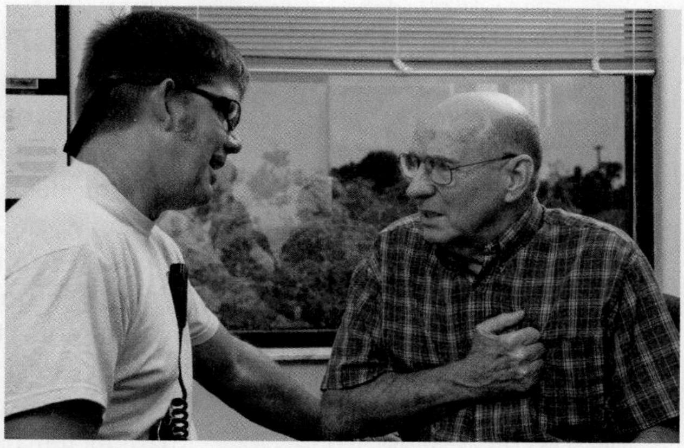

Figure 18-12 Get down at eye level and make eye contact as you obtain a medical history.

- ***Onset: What were you doing when the pain/discomfort began?*** With this question, you are trying to determine if the patient was at rest or may have been involved in some physical activity when the pain began. While it may not change how you treat the patient, this information will be valuable to the physician who will be treating the patient at the hospital.
- ***Provocation: Does anything you do make the pain/discomfort better or worse?*** This question helps to determine if anything the patient does in terms of movement or positioning makes the pain get better or worse. Cardiac-related chest pain is typically a constant pain that will not change with palpation or position. While the patient may feel as though he can breathe easier in one position over another, the pain or discomfort will not usually change. Exertion or strenuous activity may also provoke pain or discomfort.
- ***Quality: Can you describe how your pain/discomfort feels?*** Try to get the patient to describe his pain or discomfort in his own words. Be careful with this one, because it is easy to accidentally lead the patient by your line of questioning. For instance, if the patient is having difficulty finding words to describe what he is experiencing, he may agree with the first suggestion you offer. A better way to explore what he is feeling is to offer contrasting choices and allow him to select the most appropriate word. For example you might ask, "Is your pain or discomfort sharp or dull?" or "Is your pain or discomfort steady, or does it come and go?" You must remember that his mind may be very distracted by what is happening to him, so be patient and allow the patient enough time to process the question and provide an appropriate response. Pay attention and notice any use of the clenched fist to describe his pain. This is a common behavior in patients

experiencing a pressure type of discomfort, which is consistent with cardiac compromise.

- ***Region/radiate: Can you point with one finger where the pain or discomfort is the most? Does your pain or discomfort move or radiate anywhere else?*** The focus of these questions is to determine where the pain or discomfort is located and if it appears to be moving or radiating anywhere else. Watch the patient carefully after you ask this question. Is he able to pinpoint the pain or does he motion with an open hand over his chest or other area suggesting the pain is spread out and perhaps radiating.
- ***Severity: On a scale of 0 to 10, how would you rate your pain/discomfort?*** This question will help you determine just how much pain or discomfort the patient is experiencing from the event. It will be important to ask this question three different times. The first time you ask, try to determine the level of discomfort at that moment. You must then ask, "What level was the pain when it first began?" This will provide insight into whether or not the pain has gotten better, worse, or stayed the same from the time of onset until your arrival. You will want to ask the question again after you have provided some care and comfort or nitroglycerin to the patient—perhaps 5 or 10 minutes after your arrival with the patient having been on oxygen for most of that time. The purpose is to determine if your calming demeanor, and the oxygen or medication are having any effect on the patient's condition.
- ***Time: When did you first begin feeling this pain or discomfort?*** In many cases of cardiac compromise, time plays an important factor. While it will not and should not affect the way you care for your patient, it is a very important part of the history that can affect intervention at the hospital. You will want to ask when the pain or discomfort first began, but you will also want to know if the patient felt bad or had any other symptoms prior to the onset of the pain or discomfort. As mentioned earlier in this chapter, many patients begin feeling nausea, light-headedness, shortness of breath, and fatigue long before the pain or discomfort begins.

> **CLINICAL CLUE**
>
> **Determining Priority**
>
> Not all of the signs and symptoms have to be present in order for you to suspect a cardiac event. Any patient whom you suspect may be experiencing cardiac compromise is a high priority for transport.

Clues your patient is in significant distress, unstable, and a high priority for transport include:

- Altered mental status, including unresponsiveness, sleepiness, head-bobbing, agitation, or anxiety
- Chief complaint of chest, neck, back, or jaw pain or discomfort
- Severe difficulty breathing, including inability to speak or ability to speak only a few words per breath
- Poor skin color, including pale, gray, or cyanotic (blue); cool, moist skin
- Abnormally slow or fast respiratory rates
- Increased pulse rate (greater than 100)
- Decreased pulse rate (less than 60)
- Irregular pulse
- Shallow respirations with any respiratory rate
- Noisy breathing (usually audible even without a stethoscope) including wheezing, gurgling, snoring, stridor

If you have not already done so, consider the use of supplemental oxygen at this time. There are many differing opinions as to whether to use a nasal cannula or a nonrebreather mask for these patients. Which device is not as important as getting the patient on some level of oxygen flow. Follow local protocols.

If the patient is currently taking any medications such as nitroglycerin, you will want to determine if he has taken any of that medication prior to your arrival and what the results were. You also must consider assisting the patient with additional doses if indicated and allowed by local protocol.

Consider the position of the patient if you have not already done so. In most cases, the patient will be in the position of most comfort when you arrive. However, some patients are less able to move on their own, so you must ask if the patient would feel better in a different position. For the majority of patients experiencing chest pain, sitting upright (Fowler's) or slightly reclined (semi-Fowler's) is the position of most comfort. If you find a patient lying down, ask if he would like to try sitting up and assist him into this position if he feels it will help. Do not decide for a patient which position is best.

If he is responsive, always make a suggestion first and allow the patient to decide. Once he decides on a position of comfort, assist him in getting into that position. If your patient is unresponsive or simply unable to remain safely in a seated position, lay him down and place him in the recovery position as appropriate.

Vital Signs

In a typical team of two, one EMT will be getting baseline vital signs while the other completes the SAMPLE/OPQRST history (Figure 18-13 ■). Remember to ask the patient what his blood pressure is normally *before* you take your reading. This will help you know what to expect and be able to determine if it is normal for the patient. Get a complete baseline as soon as possible and take subsequent sets approximately every five minutes. Be sure to document all vitals carefully and compare them for evidence of a trend.

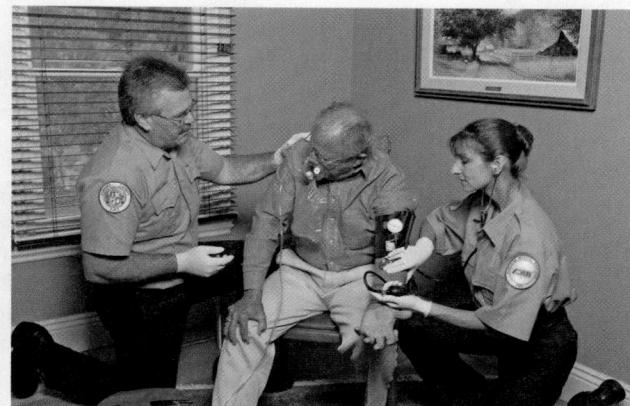

Figure 18-13 Continue with obtaining a medical history while your partner obtains a set of baseline vital signs.

Focused Secondary Assessment

At this point in your patient assessment—after scene size-up and the primary assessment, a SAMPLE history, and vital signs—and assuming your patient is responsive, you will perform a secondary assessment focusing on the patient's chief complaint. In this exam you will be looking and palpating for signs and symptoms of cardiac compromise. Table 18-1 provides specific examples of what to look for when performing your exam as well as what the finding may mean.

Continue to question the patient about his signs and symptoms throughout your examination and during transport. Keep a close eye on whether he appears to be getting better or worse. Consider increasing the oxygen liter flow if his symptoms do not subside at least a little within the first 5 or 10 minutes.

PERSPECTIVE

D'juan—The EMT

The fire-rescue guys were doing a great job with CPR when we arrived. In fact I could feel a great carotid pulse with each compression. As soon as they stopped compressions in order to ventilate, the pulse just stopped. That's always kind of eerie, if you ask me. Just goes to show you that CPR really does circulate blood.

TABLE 18-1 SIGNS AND SYMPTOMS OF CARDIAC COMPROMISE

BODY AREA	ASSESSMENT FINDINGS	POSSIBLE CAUSE
Head	Observe for abnormal skin signs.	Skin that is pale or diaphoretic may be an indication of poor perfusion.
Neck	Observe for jugular vein distention, accessory muscle use, and medical identification necklace.	Jugular vein distention may be a sign that fluid is backing up in the circulatory system. This is often seen in congestive heart failure patients. Use of accessory muscles is frequently an indication of respiratory difficulty. Medical identification jewelry may provide valuable information about the patient's history.
Chest	Observe for adequate chest rise and fall, auscultate breath sounds. Palpate the chest where the patient states it hurts.	Good chest rise and fall is important for all patients. This is an important part of adequate respirations. Listen carefully for lung sounds in all fields. Noisy breath sounds may be an indication of fluid in the lungs, which is often caused by congestive heart failure. Palpate any areas of pain as appropriate to identify if palpation causes more pain or not.
Abdomen	Palpate for pain and pulsating mass.	Be thorough and palpate all four quadrants of the abdomen. Be patient and hold your hands over each area for a few seconds feeling for a pulsating mass. This may be an indication of problems with the abdominal aorta (aneurysm).
Legs and Arms	Assess for distal circulation, sensation, and motor function as well as evidence of pedal edema and medical identification jewelry.	Some of the first areas to show evidence of poor circulation are the extremities. Carefully assess for circulation, sensation, and motor function in all four extremities. Look especially for evidence of swelling in the feet and ankles. This can be an important finding in congestive heart failure patients who spend much of their time sitting or standing. The fluid that backs up from the circulatory system is drawn to the lowest part of the body by gravity. Medical identification jewelry can provide valuable information about the patient's medical history.

STOP, REVIEW, REMEMBER!

Multiple Choice

For each question, place a check next to the correct answer.

1. Asking a patient to describe what his pain or discomfort feels like is associated with which part of the OPQRST assessment mnemonic?

_____ a. Provocation

_____ b. Quality

_____ c. Onset

_____ d. Severity

2. During which phase of your patient assessment should you first consider the need for supplemental oxygen?

_____ a. Scene size-up

_____ b. Primary assessment

_____ c. SAMPLE history

_____ d. Secondary assessment

3. Pedal edema and jugular vein distention are most often seen with which cardiac condition?

_____ a. Myocardial infarction

_____ b. Angina

_____ c. Congestive heart failure

_____ d. Cardiac arrest

4. Which one of the following questions is most appropriate for the "Q" of the OPQRST assessment mnemonic?

_____ a. Can you describe for me what your pain or discomfort feels like?

_____ b. How long have you had this pain?

_____ c. What were you doing when the pain began?

_____ d. Does anything you do make the pain better or worse?

5. The position of comfort is decided by the:

_____ a. EMT. _____ c. medical director.

_____ b. family members. _____ d. patient.

Signs and Symptoms

Complete the chart. List as many signs and symptoms as you can for the following medical conditions and the treatment(s) that would be appropriate for the EMT to provide.

Condition	Signs	Symptoms	Treatment
Congestive heart failure (CHF)			
Myocardial infarction (MI)			
Angina			

Critical Thinking

1. Describe why edema is often found in the ankles and sacral area of patients experiencing CHF.

____

____

____

2. Describe the difference between cardiac arrest and myocardial infarction (heart attack).

____

____

____

____

3. Provide an example of at least one appropriate question to ask a possible cardiac-compromise patient for each letter of the SAMPLE history acronym.

____

____

____

____

Caring for the Patient with Cardiac Compromise

One of the most important aspects of caring for a suspected cardiac patient is a calm professional demeanor and plenty of comfort and reassurance. Remember, it is not important that you determine or diagnose the patient's specific problem, such as MI, angina, or CHF. What is most important is that the EMT recognize and treat the signs and symptoms with which a patient presents. The following steps can be used to provide care for most patients presenting with the signs and symptoms of cardiac compromise (Scan 18-1):

CLINICAL CLUE

Aspirin

Some EMS systems are allowing EMTs to administer chewable low-dose aspirin for patients with suspected cardiac pain. This should be included in your treatment plan if allowed by local protocol.

1. Take appropriate BSI precautions.
2. Perform a primary assessment and consider supplemental oxygen.
3. Obtain a thorough history, using SAMPLE and OPQRST to help you.
4. Obtain a baseline set of vital signs including pulse oximetry.
5. Perform an appropriate secondary assessment.
6. Assist with the administration of the patient's prescribed nitroglycerin or aspirin. (Follow local protocol.)
7. Perform regular reassessments and adjust your care as appropriate.
8. Transport as soon as practical and consider the need for an ALS backup or intercept.

Medical direction plays an important role in every EMS system across the country. This is especially true when you are caring for patients with cardiac emergencies. It has been by the advisement of qualified physician medical directors and through the development of specific treatment guidelines and protocols that EMS has been able to improve the care that these patients receive. As you learn to function as an EMT, make sure you learn the specific protocols that direct the care you will provide.

Assisting with Nitroglycerin

18-13 Explain the indications, contraindications, forms, dosage, administration, actions, side effects, and reassessment for nitroglycerin and aspirin.

During your SAMPLE history, you will have determined if the patient had been prescribed any medications for his condition. One of the most common medications prescribed to patients with a cardiac history is nitroglycerin (Figure 18-14 ▪). A derivative of the explosive, medical nitroglycerin is used to dilate blood vessels in an effort to reduce the workload on the heart and help improve circulation to the heart muscle.

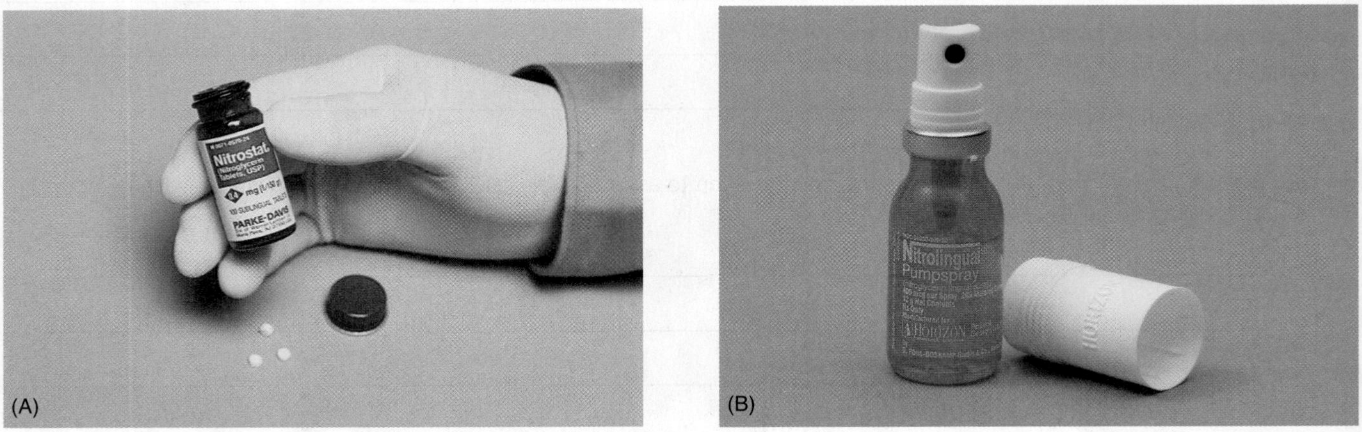

Figure 18-14 Examples of (A) nitroglycerin tablets and (B) nitroglycerin spray.

SCAN 18-1 Caring for a Patient with Suspected Cardiac Compromise

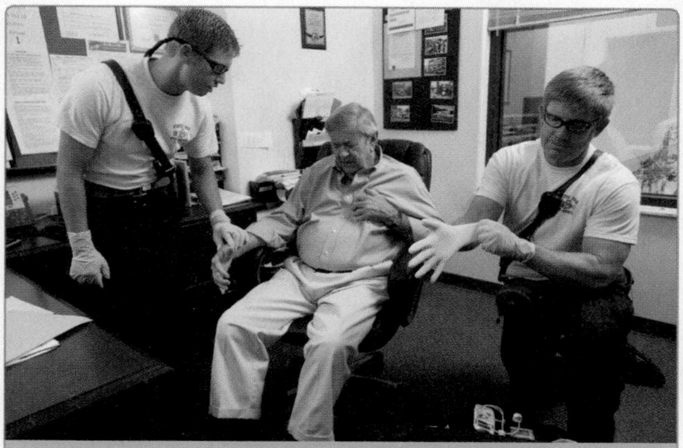

18-1-1 Begin with the primary assessment and the chief complaint.

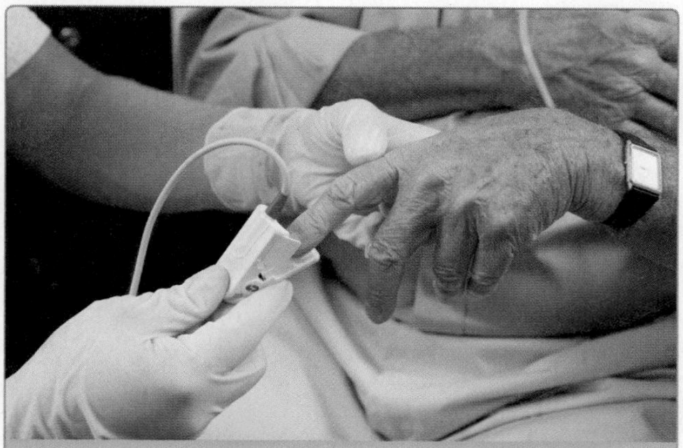

18-1-2 Obtain vital signs, including oxygen saturation, if available.

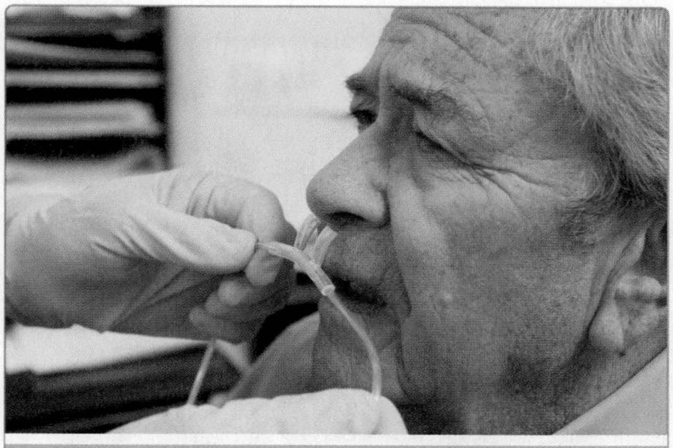

18-1-3 Consider the need for supplemental oxygen.

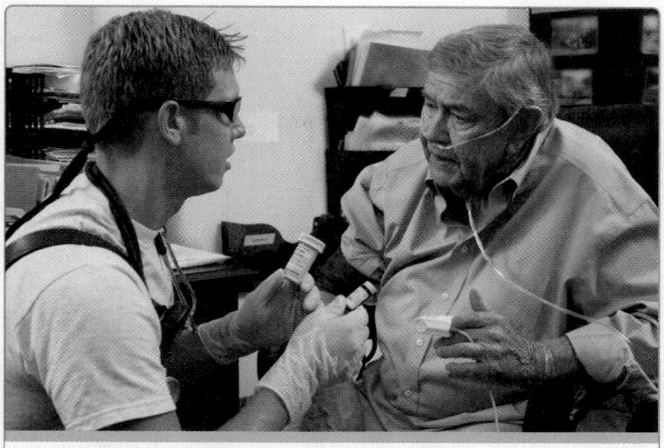

18-1-4 Consider assisting the patient with nitroglycerin, if appropriate.

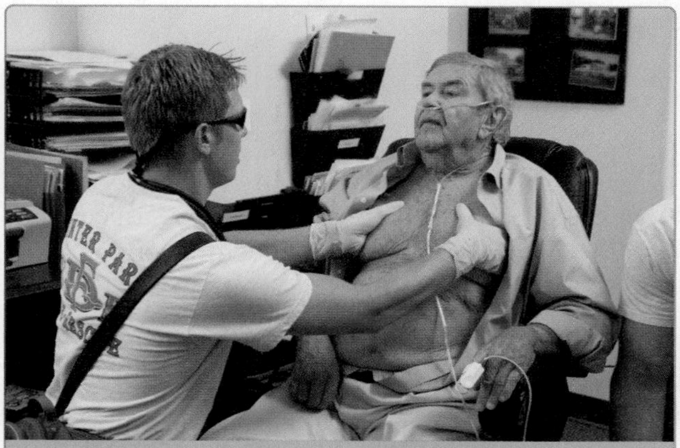

18-1-5 Perform an appropriate secondary assessment.

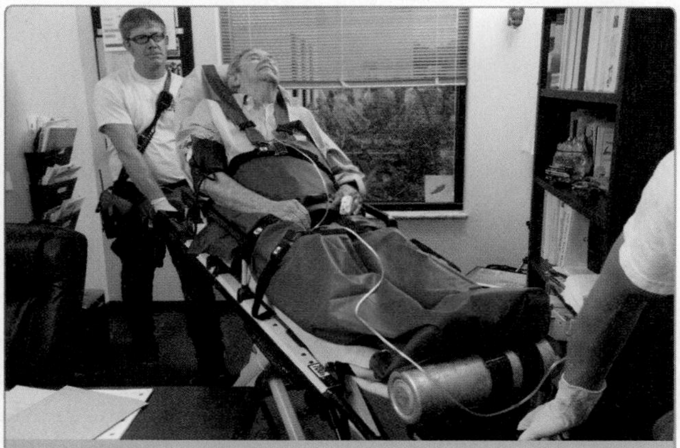

18-1-6 Prepare for transport in the position of comfort.

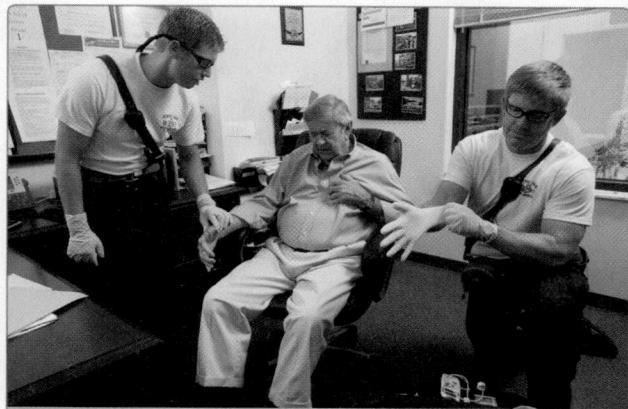

SCAN 18-2 Assisting with the Administration of Nitroglycerin

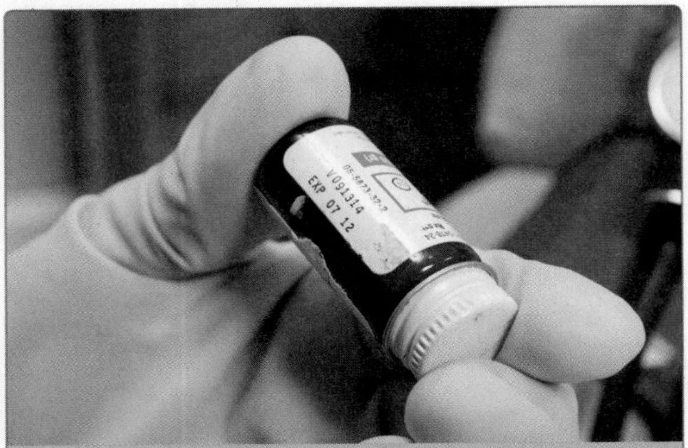

18-2-1 Confirm that the medication is prescribed to the patient and that it has not expired.

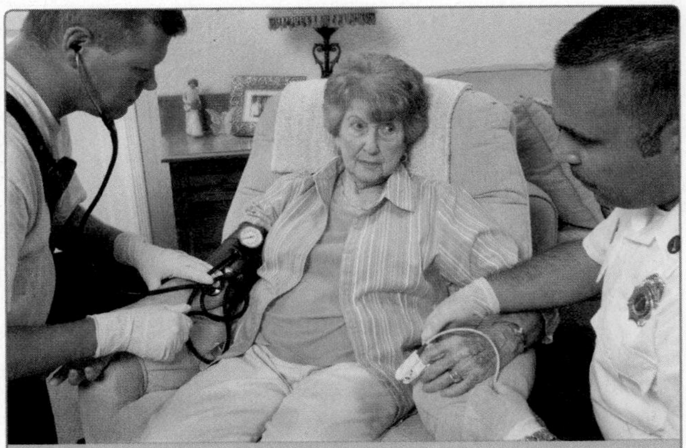

18-2-2 Confirm that the systolic blood pressure is above the minimum required.

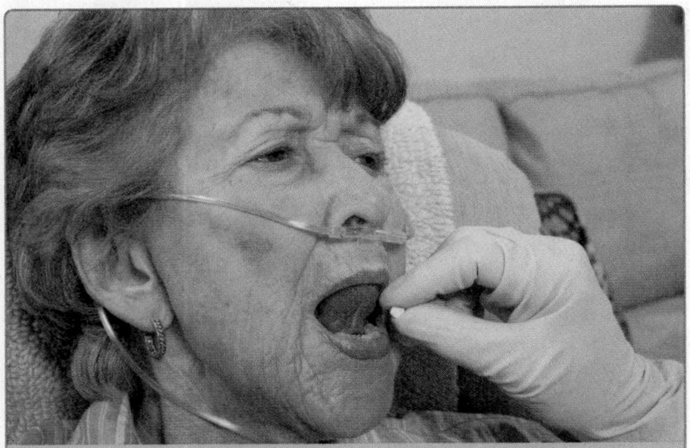

18-2-3 Administer the medication under the tongue.

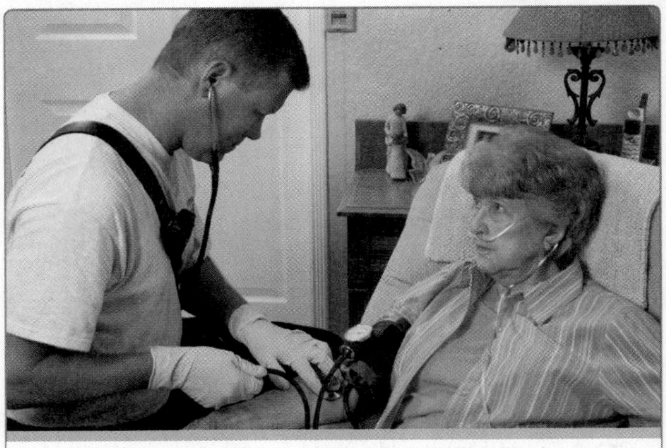

18-2-4 Reassess vital signs and chief complaint following administration.

Once you have determined that the patient is experiencing what is suspected to be cardiac-related chest pain, the following criteria must be met before you can assist the patient in taking his own nitroglycerin (Scan 18-2):

- ***The patient has his own prescription with him.*** Be sure to confirm the "five rights" and that the prescription has been issued in the name of the patient and not another family member.
- ***The prescription is current and not expired.*** In some cases the expiration date on the bottle may be missing or difficult to read. Do not administer medication that you cannot confirm as current.

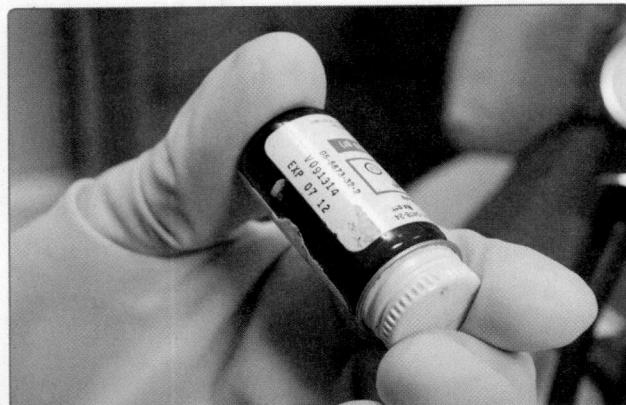

- ***The patient has not taken Viagra or a similar medication (Cialis, Levitra®) for erectile dysfunction within the past 24 to 72 hours.*** In some EMS systems the protocol is to contact medical direction prior to the administration of nitroglycerin for patients who take erectile dysfunction medications at all.
- ***The patient has a systolic blood pressure of at least 100.*** This requirement also varies from region to region and may range from 90 mmHg to 120 mmHg. Nitroglycerin may also be contraindicated in patients with very rapid or slow pulses. Always check your local protocols.

Typical instructions for the administration of nitroglycerin are to place one tablet (or one spray) beneath the tongue (sublingually) and allow it to dissolve completely. If the medication is in pill form, instruct the patient not to swallow it. If the patient does not experience an improvement in symptoms within three to five minutes, repeat the dose every five minutes up to a maximum of three doses in a 15-minute period of time. Follow local protocols.

Following each dose, you must reassess vital signs and confirm that the patient's systolic blood pressure remains above 100 mmHg. Because nitroglycerin has the potential to cause a significant drop in blood pressure, resulting in the patient becoming light-headed and possibly unresponsive, allow the administration of this medication only with the patient securely seated or lying down.

> **CLINICAL CLUE**
>
> **Nitroglycerin Safety**
>
> Always wear gloves when handling or assisting with the administration of nitroglycerin. Do not allow the tablets or spray to come in contact with your skin, because doing so may allow the medication to be absorbed into your bloodstream.

If at any point the patient's systolic blood pressure drops below 100 mmHg, or if a significant increase in pulse or decrease in responsiveness occurs, initiate transport to an appropriate receiving facility while continuing the history and physical exam and providing the indicated care en route.

The Use of Aspirin

In addition to nitroglycerin, aspirin has proven to be highly beneficial for the treatment of patients suspected of having a cardiac event. Aspirin minimizes the formation of blood clots within the circulatory system and reduces the chance of serious heart damage due to clotting by inactivating blood platelets.

Many EMS systems are adding the administration of aspirin to the list of EMT skills (Figure 18-15 ▪). *Follow local protocols.*

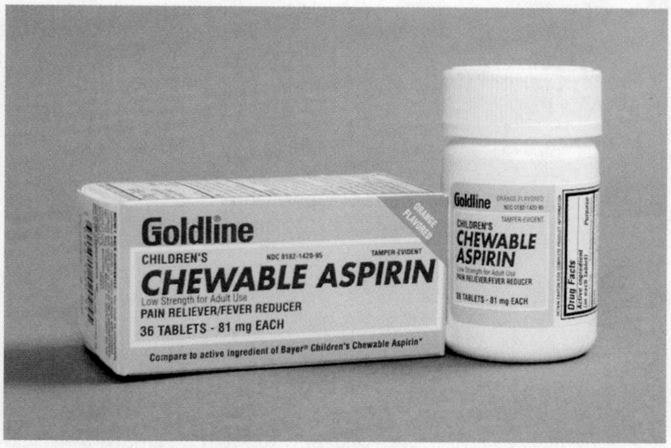

Figure 18-15 Low dose (81 mg) chewable aspirin.

STOP, REVIEW, REMEMBER!

Multiple Choice

For each question, place a check next to the correct answer.

1. Supplemental oxygen helps the cardiac patient by:

   _____ a. acting as a pain reliever.

   _____ b. increasing circulation to the heart.

   _____ c. increasing the concentration of oxygen in the blood.

   _____ d. dilating the coronary arteries.

2. Which one of the following is *not* a link in the Chain of Survival?

   _____ a. Early access

   _____ b. Early CPR

   _____ c. Early diagnosis

   _____ d. Early advanced care

(continued on next page)

(continued)

3. A common side effect of nitroglycerin is:

_____ a. nausea.

_____ b. increased blood pressure.

_____ c. dry mouth.

_____ d. headache.

4. The patient's blood pressure must be at least ____________ systolic prior to the administration of nitroglycerin.

_____ a. 80

_____ b. 100

_____ c. 110

_____ d. 120

5. Which one of the following actions should be performed after each administered dose of nitroglycerin?

_____ a. Repeat vital signs.

_____ b. Increase oxygen flow.

_____ c. Have the patient lie down.

_____ d. Contact medical direction.

Fill in the Blank

Complete each sentence to conform to properly assisting a patient with the administration of nitroglycerin.

1. Confirm that the patient has a ________________________ for nitroglycerin.

2. Confirm that the medication has not ________________________.

3. Confirm that the patient has not taken any medication for erectile dysfunction in the past ________________________ hours.

4. Confirm that the patient has a ________________________ blood pressure of at least ________________________.

Critical Thinking

1. Describe how nitroglycerin helps the patient who is experiencing cardiac-related chest pain.

____

____

____

____

2. What are the contraindications to allowing a patient to take his own nitroglycerin?

____

____

____

____

3. How does supplemental oxygen help the patient who is experiencing cardiac compromise?

____

____

____

____

Hospital-Based Emergency Interventions for Acute MIs

18-14 Discuss the indications and contraindications for fibrinolytic therapy and percutaneous transluminal coronary angiography in patients with acute myocardial infarctions.

An acute myocardial infarction (AMI) is the result of a complete blockage of one or more of the coronary arteries. Since the late 1980s, the mainstay of the emergency care of patients with acute myocardial infarction has been to open the blocked arteries as soon after arrival in the emergency department as possible. There are two general techniques used to open blocked coronary arteries in patients having an AMI—**fibrinolytic therapy** and **percutaneous transluminal coronary angiography (PTCA).**

fibrinolytic therapy the use of specialized drugs to dissolve blood clots in patients with suspected myocardial infarctions and certain types of strokes.

percutaneous transluminal coronary angiography (PTCA) a procedure in which a wire catheter is inserted through the femoral or brachial artery directly into the coronary arteries in order to visualize the status and condition of the vessels.

fibrinolytics specialized drugs used to dissolve blood clots. Also known as *thrombolytics*.

Fibrinolytic Therapy

Fibrinolytics, also known as *thrombolytics*, are drugs that can break down blood clots that have formed in the arteries of the heart. Not every patient with signs and symptoms of cardiac compromise will be a candidate for fibrinolytics. In general, only patients with acute myocardial infarction are candidates for fibrinolytic therapy. Because these drugs can make bleeding worse for some patients, they must be evaluated very carefully by a physician to identify dangerous contraindications. Current AHA guidelines recommend that fibrinolytics be administered within 30 minutes of patient arrival at the hospital to optimize the chances of minimizing the damage of an AMI. This time interval from emergency department arrival until the administration of the fibrinolytic drug is called the *door-to-needle time*.

Percutaneous Transluminal Coronary Angiography

Percutaneous transluminal coronary angiography (PTCA) is a procedure where a specially trained cardiologist inserts a wire catheter through the femoral or brachial artery directly into the coronary arteries. Once the catheter is in place, dye is introduced and the exact site of the blockage is identified with X-rays. The cardiologist will then either open the blockage with a balloon or by placing a stent to clear the blockage. Although there is a lesser risk of bleeding with PTCA than with fibrinolytics, it is a technically more difficult procedure that requires highly specialized physicians and a technologically advanced catheterization lab where the procedure is done.

Current national standards recommend that PTCA be performed within 90 minutes from the time of arrival at the emergency department to optimize the chances of minimizing the damage of an acute MI. The time interval from emergency department arrival until the opening of the coronary artery in the catheterization lab is called the "door-to-balloon time."

Not all hospital emergency departments are capable of administering fibrinolytic drugs, nor are all hospitals capable of having a catheterization lab open 24/7. As the

EMT who will be transporting the patient, it will be important for you to know the facilities in your area that can deliver these medications. Always follow local transport protocols.

Fundamentals of Early Defibrillation

18-15 Explain the importance of early defibrillation in cardiac arrest.

Depending on what source you read, anywhere from 300,000 to 450,000 people die each year in the United States from sudden cardiac arrest. It is believed that many of those people could be saved with the strengthening of the Chain of Survival.

For many years the weak link in the Chain of Survival has been early defibrillation. While many ambulances and fire departments carry and use defibrillators, there is often a significant delay in delivering the first shock due to long response times. Research has shown that the sooner a victim of sudden cardiac arrest can receive a shock, the better the likelihood of a positive outcome. Because AEDs require so little training to operate, they are being placed in more and more public places such as airports and casinos, allowing for quicker delivery of shocks following collapse.

18-17 Compare and contrast ventricular fibrillation, ventricular tachycardia, and asystole.

dysrhythmia any variation from the normal rate or rhythm of the heart. Also called *arrhythmia*.

arrhythmia any variation from the normal rate or rhythm of the heart. Also called *dysrhythmia*.

ventricular fibrillation (VF) one of the most common electrical rhythms associated with sudden cardiac arrest in which the ventricles of the heart contract spontaneously and in an uncoordinated manner, thus preventing the heart from circulating any meaningful amount of blood. Also called *V-fib*.

How AEDs Save Lives

Not all patients experiencing a heart attack (MI) go into cardiac arrest. In fact, the majority of MI patients actually remain responsive and survive the event. A number of procedures performed at the hospital can help these patients lead normal lives following a heart attack.

AEDs are designed specifically to help convert the heart rhythm of victims of sudden cardiac arrest (Figure 18-16 ■). While the term *cardiac arrest* does imply that the heart has stopped pumping blood, the heart often remains electrically active. The electrical activity that remains in the heart can be any one of a number of uncoordinated electrical rhythms called **dysrhythmia** or **arrhythmia.** One of the most common electrical rhythms associated with sudden cardiac arrest is **ventricular fibrillation** or simply **VF** or **V-fib** (Figure 18-17 ■).

VF causes the ventricles of the heart to contract spontaneously and in an uncoordinated manner, thus preventing the heart from circulating any meaningful amount of blood. A patient in VF will not have any palpable pulses and is rendered unresponsive, pulseless, and not breathing within seconds following the onset of VF.

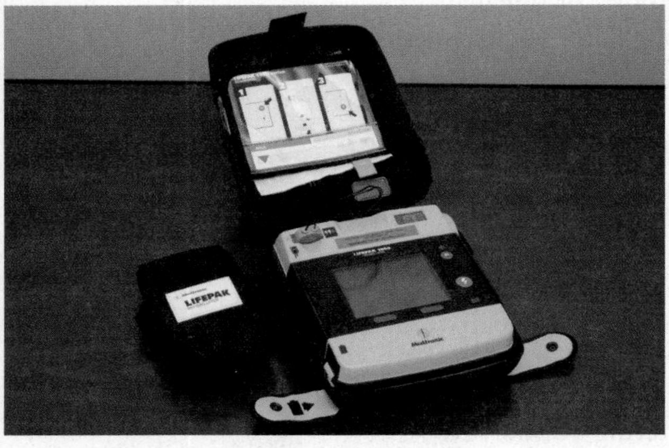
LIFEPAK

Figure 18-16 A typical AED used in EMS.

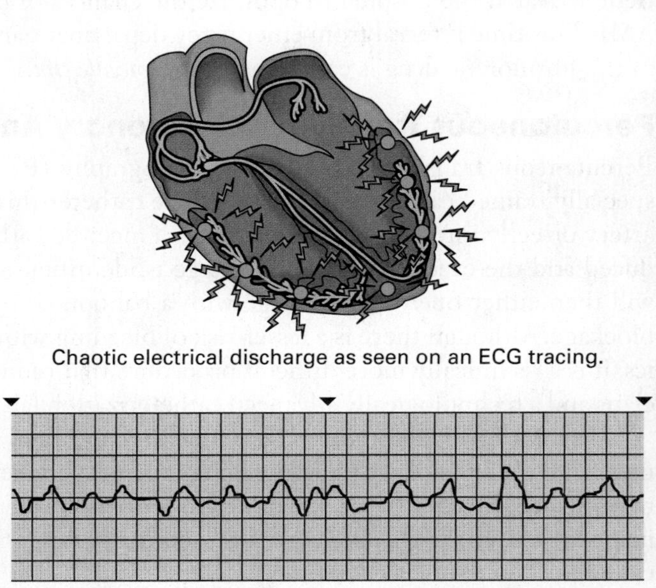
Chaotic electrical discharge as seen on an ECG tracing.

Figure 18-17 The electrical pattern of ventricular fibrillation as it is seen on a cardiac monitor.

Ventricular tachycardia (**VT** or **V-tach**) is another rhythm that may be shocked by a defibrillator. V-tach is a rapid and uncoordinated rhythm that originates in the ventricles. It is a potentially life-threatening rhythm that may or may not produce pulses. In some cases of V-tach, an AED may deliver a shock.

ventricular tachycardia (VT) a rapid and uncoordinated life-threatening electrical rhythm that originates in the ventricles. Also called *V-tach*.

Asystole, also known as *flat line*, is the absence of electrical activity in the heart. AEDs are not programmed to deliver a shock when the heart is in asystole.

asystole the state of no electrical activity within the heart; not an AED shockable rhythm. Also known as *flat line*.

The job of the AED is to automatically analyze the heart rhythm and "reboot" the heart, not unlike rebooting a computer that has locked up. In other words, the AED provides a measured dose of electricity through the heart in an attempt to convert the electrical activity to a normal perfusing rhythm.

Advantages of AEDs

AEDs offer many advantages over the traditional manual defibrillator used by both hospital and EMS personnel. Those advantages are:

18-16 Describe the features, functions, advantages, disadvantages, use, and precautions in the use of automated external defibrillators (AEDs).

- ***Ease of operation.*** It is easier to learn to operate an AED than it is to learn CPR. The newest machines provide extremely detailed instructions for the operator, which minimize confusion and costly delays in care.
- ***Speed of operation.*** The ease of operation and layperson access allow for the opportunity to deliver a shock to the patient sooner than having to wait for EMS to arrive.
- ***Safer operation.*** An AED uses adhesive electrode pads to both analyze and deliver a shock, making a hands-off operation that is safer for both the patient and the operator. Once placed, the large electrode pads allow for more consistent shocks over a larger area than most manual defibrillator paddles.
- ***Continuous monitoring.*** Once the AED pads are in place and the device is turned on, it will continually analyze the patient's rhythm at regular intervals and advise if a shock is necessary, making the job of the rescuer easier. Some devices have an LCD screen that shows a real-time moving image of the patient's heart rhythm.

Indications for the Use of an AED

Not all patients will benefit from the use of an AED. A responsive patient complaining of chest pain is clearly not in VF; therefore, the AED will not help him. A patient must meet the following criteria before an AED may be used:

- The patient must be unresponsive.
- The patient must be pulseless.
- The patient must be nonbreathing.
- The patient must be one month of age or older.

CLINICAL CLUE

AEDs and Kids

According to the 2010 American Heart Association Guidelines, you should use an AED with pediatric pads for children one to eight years old. If pediatric pads are not available, then you may use standard AED pads. For infants (patients younger than one year), a manual defibrillator is preferred. If one is not available, an AED with pediatric pads is desirable. If neither is available, a standard AED with adult pads may be used.

It is important to confirm that the patient does indeed have a clear airway before attaching the AED. Even if the patient is in VF, he cannot be successfully resuscitated until the airway is open and you are able to provide adequate ventilations during CPR.

Contraindications to the Use of an AED

Now that AED use is recommended for pediatric patients, there are essentially no contraindications for its use in unresponsive, pulseless, and nonbreathing patients. While not contraindicated, the use of AEDs for the treatment of cardiac arrest due to trauma or hypothermia has proven less effective and may not be included in treatment protocols for these specific patients. You will need to verify any contraindications for AED use with your local EMS agency.

While it is possible that an AED could deliver an inappropriate shock, it is extremely unlikely. A way to minimize the likelihood of inappropriate shocks is to place an AED only on a patient who meets all the appropriate criteria and to keep the AED in good working order by performing regularly scheduled maintenance checks.

STOP, REVIEW, REMEMBER!

Multiple Choice

1. Abnormal electrical rhythms of the heart are called:
   _____ a. anomalies or dysrhythmia.
   _____ b. aberrancies or anomalies.
   _____ c. angina.
   _____ d. dysrhythmia.

2. Rapid defibrillation is the ____________ link in the Chain of Survival.
   _____ a. first
   _____ b. second
   _____ c. third
   _____ d. fourth

3. The primary cause of cardiac arrest in adult patients is:
   _____ a. ventricular fibrillation.
   _____ b. trauma.
   _____ c. vehicle collision.
   _____ d. respiratory arrest.

4. The use of AEDs is now being encouraged for patients as young as ____________ year(s) of age.
   _____ a. one
   _____ b. three
   _____ c. five
   _____ d. eight

Fill in the Blank

1. When given to suspected myocardial infarction and angina patients, aspirin acts to ________________________ the formation of blood clots.

2. Early CPR is the ________________________ link in the Chain of Survival.

3. One of the most common electrical rhythms associated with sudden cardiac arrest is ________________________.

4. The use of AEDs for the treatment of cardiac arrest due to ________________________ and hypothermia has proven less effective and may not be included in treatment protocols for these specific patients.

Critical Thinking

1. What makes AEDs today so easy to operate?

2. Discuss the role that time plays in the successful resuscitation of a cardiac-arrest patient.

3. Discuss at least two advantages that AEDs have over the more traditional manual defibrillators.

Types of AEDS

While there are many manufacturers and models of AED on the market today, defibrillators all operate using the same principles: They analyze the heart rhythm of a patient without a pulse and based on that analysis will decide whether a shock is appropriate (Figure 18-18 ■). Initially there were two types of defibrillators—fully automated and semi-automated. The fully automated defibrillator is turned on and attached to the patient and, as the name suggests, requires minimal or no input from the EMT. Semi-automated defibrillators require constant interaction with the device including pressing the "analyze" and "shock" buttons when prompted to do so.

Most defibrillators in use today are semi-automated defibrillators. Another distinction between defibrillators is their ability to deliver energy that is monophasic vs. biphasic. Monophasic defibrillators deliver shocks at set energy levels to all patients. Biphasic defibrillators are newer and more technologically advanced. They measure the resistance of the chest and deliver more effective shocks at lower energy levels and patterns.

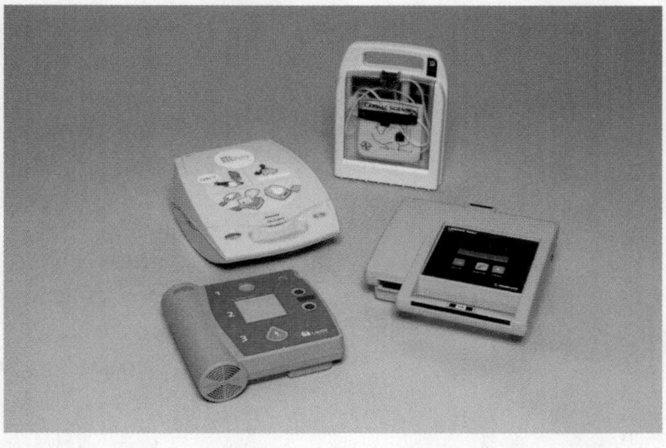

Figure 18-18 Despite the different models, AEDs all perform the same task.

The American Heart Association sets specific guidelines for the energy levels delivered by monophasic defibrillators. Biphasic defibrillators deliver shocks based on manufacturer's recommendations and measurements of the patient obtained by the defibrillator. Since AEDs are pre-programmed, you will not have to choose or specify an energy level before defibrillating a patient.

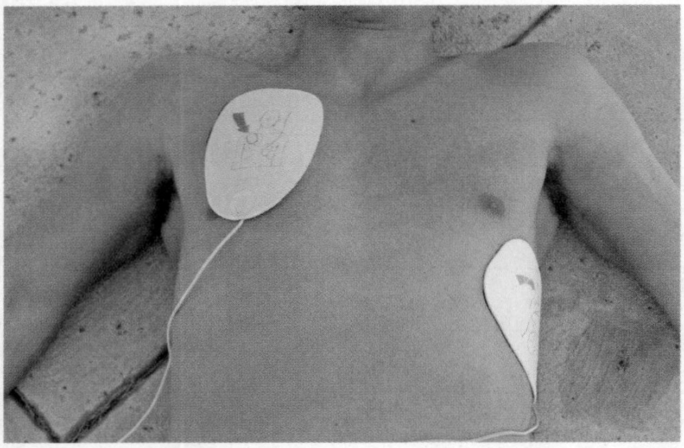

Figure 18-19 The proper placement of AED electrode pads.

Rhythm Analysis

One of the design features that make AEDs so simple to use is the sophisticated rhythm analysis software. The electrode pads capture the patient's heart rhythm and send it to a microprocessor in the main unit for interpretation (Figure 18-19 ■). The rhythm is then quickly analyzed for several criteria to ensure that it is indeed a shockable rhythm. Because of the sophistication of the analysis software, there is little chance of an inappropriate shock being delivered. The software is specifically designed to identify both shockable and nonshockable rhythms. The safety of the device is further enhanced by the activation of the shock button *only* if the software detects a shockable rhythm. This prevents the operator from inadvertently delivering an inappropriate shock.

There are two rhythms that an AED would consider shockable. The first is ventricular fibrillation (V-fib). The second is a rhythm called *rapid ventricular tachycardia*. It is not important that you know what each of these rhythms looks like, because that is the job of the AED.

The energy delivered by an AED is measured in units called *joules*. A joule is the amount of energy delivered by one watt of power in one second. For instance, a 100-watt lightbulb uses 100 joules every second. Depending on the age and model of the AED, it may deliver anywhere from 150 to 360 joules each time it delivers a shock. Some models provide shocks with increasing energy levels, while others use the same energy level for all shocks. Newer models are able to utilize lower energy settings due to biphasic technology.

Analyze/Shock Sequence

Once the AED is turned on, it will begin a set of preprogrammed voice commands designed to assist the rescuer in following the correct sequence of steps. After the electrode pads are properly placed on the patient, it will follow a preset sequence of analyze and shock phases.

If, after the first analyze phase, the AED recognizes a shockable rhythm, the voice prompt will state that a shock is advised and prompt the rescuer to press the shock button. Following delivery of each shock, the AED will advise the rescuer to perform CPR for two minutes before analyzing the heart rhythm again. This sequence of analyze, delivery of a single shock, and two minutes of CPR will repeat as appropriate.

The analyze/shock sequence is as follows:

- Single shock
- Two minutes of CPR
- Single shock
- Two minutes of CPR
- Single shock

New resuscitation guidelines are allowing local medical directors to recommend two minutes of CPR (five cycles) before attempting defibrillation when the response

SCAN 18-3 Using an AED for Cardiac Arrest

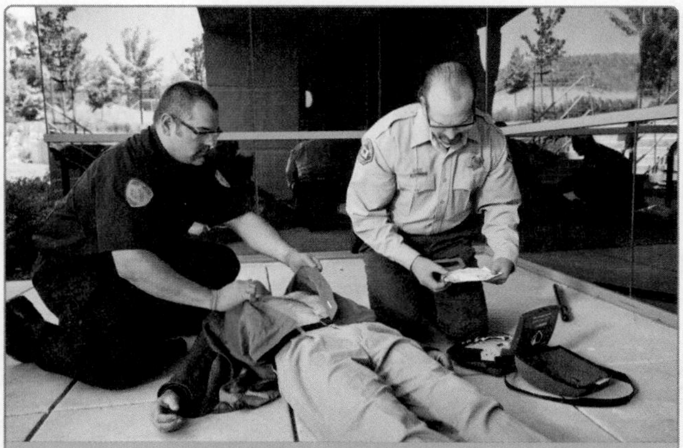
18-3-1 Once you have confirmed the patient is pulseless and apneic, expose the chest.

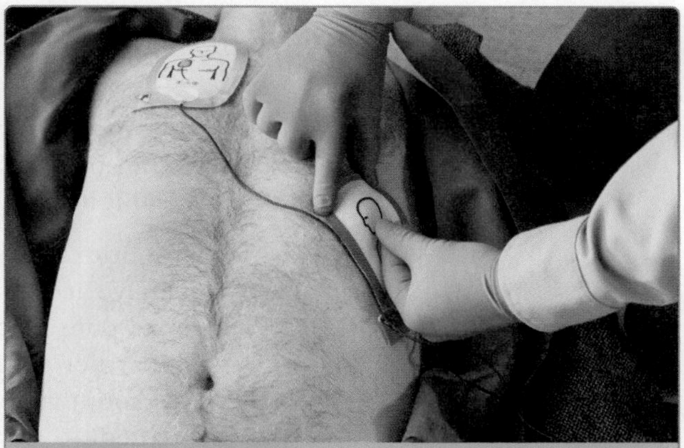
18-3-2 Place the electrode pads and connect to device if not already connected.

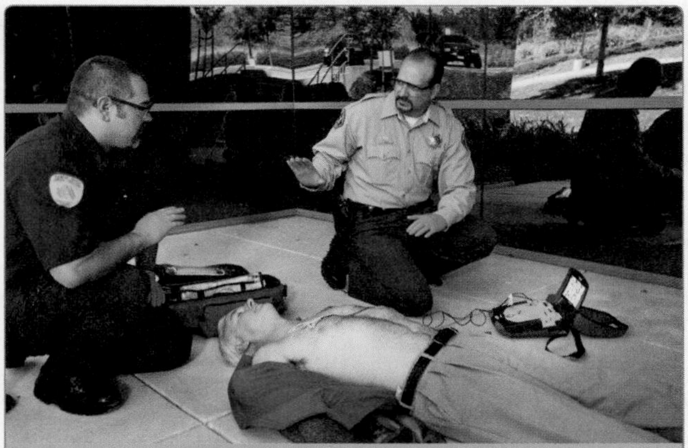
18-3-3 Analyze the rhythm and deliver a shock when indicated.

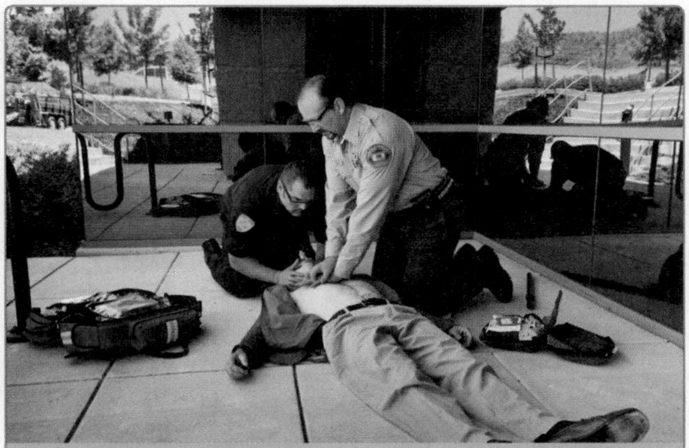
18-3-4 Immediately begin chest compressions following the shock.

time is greater than four to five minutes. This will help ensure that the heart is adequately perfused before the first shock. Always know and follow your local protocols.

If there is no return of spontaneous pulses, begin CPR.

Operating an AED

The AED should be applied and used immediately in any witnessed arrest. Follow your local protocols. Once you have confirmed that the scene is safe and your primary assessment has confirmed that your patient meets all the criteria for the application of an AED, perform the following steps (Scan 18-3):

1. Turn on the AED.
2. Position the electrode pads. (You may have to stop CPR if it is already in progress.)
3. Confirm that no one is touching the patient.

4. Initiate the analyze phase. (This may require that you press the "analyze" button depending on the type of AED.)
5. If a shock is advised, confirm everyone is clear of the patient and press the "shock" button if required. Then provide CPR for two minutes.
6. If no shock is advised, perform CPR for two minutes.
7. Follow the voice prompt of your AED. About every two minutes, you will be directed to clear the patient while the AED analyzes the rhythm. You may also be prompted to recheck the pulse.
8. Transport as soon as practical.
9. Limit interruptions during CPR.

Continue to follow the voice prompts from the AED until ALS takes over or you arrive at an appropriate receiving facility. Should you find yourself transporting a responsive patient who suddenly goes into cardiac arrest, initiate CPR while your partner stops the ambulance and climbs into the back of the ambulance to assist. You must continue CPR until your partner can properly place the AED on the patient.

Regardless of whether you are alone or working with another rescuer, the steps for using an AED are essentially the same. If you are alone, you must turn on the AED and then perform your assessment of the patient. With two rescuers, one of you will perform the assessment while the other prepares the AED for use.

CPR and the use of an AED are only two of the five links in the Chain of Survival. Whenever possible, integrate your care with advanced life support (ALS) care to maximize the likelihood of patient survival. ALS care will provide more advanced airway care as well as the necessary medications to help the patient regain a normal heart rhythm.

Recurrent Ventricular Fibrillation

Once you have regained a pulse during resuscitation, continually monitor the patient's carotid pulse during transport. A patient in cardiac arrest may regain and lose a pulse several times during a resuscitation attempt. If you are unable to palpate a carotid pulse, initiate the analyze phase of the AED.

Once you have begun transport of a cardiac-arrest patient, it may be necessary to come to a complete stop in the ambulance in order to allow the AED to properly analyze the patient's rhythm. Motion can cause the electrodes to pick up inappropriate electrical activity and the machine may advise "Check electrodes." If this occurs while in motion, stop the ambulance and press the "analyze" button to reinitiate the analyze phase.

CLINICAL CLUE

Chest Compressions

Compression quality is improved if the number and length of any interruptions in compressions is reduced. An example can be found in automobile travel. When you travel in an automobile, the number of miles you travel in a day is affected not only by the speed that you drive (your rate of travel) but also by the number and duration of any stops you make (interruptions in travel).

Interruption of CPR

Interrupting compressions severely reduces circulation of blood throughout the body. So, interruptions in CPR during AED use must be limited to analysis of the rhythm and delivering shocks to the patient. However, you may interrupt CPR for the following reasons when using an AED:

- During the analyze phase
- During the shock phase

It is important to keep CPR going as long as possible and minimize the times that CPR is interrupted during a resuscitation attempt. The sooner the patient can receive a shock, the better his chances of being successfully resuscitated. Once the AED is on the scene, do not delay the application of the device. Make every attempt to apply the pads without interrupting chest compressions.

Post-resuscitation Care

Should the cardiac-arrest patient be fortunate enough to regain a pulse following CPR and defibrillation, there is still much you must do during transport to the hospital to ensure a successful outcome. Post-resuscitation care consists of the following components:

- Rapid transport to an appropriate receiving facility
- Continuous monitoring of patient's airway, breathing, and circulatory status
- Consideration of ALS intercept for advanced care
- Use of supplemental oxygen
- Completion of a secondary exam

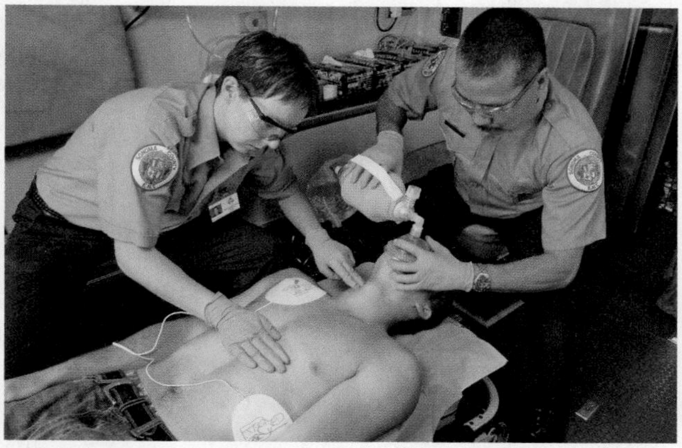

Figure 18-20 Continue to monitor the patient for both pulse and breathing during transport.

Monitor your patient continuously and carefully during transport and be prepared to initiate CPR and the AED as appropriate (Figure 18-20 ■). Consider taking an additional rescuer such as a firefighter or other emergency responder with you in the ambulance. The extra hands will become very helpful should the patient go back into cardiac arrest during transport.

AED Safety Considerations

Use of AEDs have proven to be successful in saving many lives and have an excellent safety record. However, they are not invulnerable. They must be respected and handled with care. The following safety tip regarding moisture must be followed to ensure a safe environment for everyone working with or around an AED: Ensure that the patient's chest is completely dry before placing the electrode pads. Moisture on the chest from sweat, rain, or other sources can cause the electrical energy to travel (arc) across the chest rather than through the chest. This may cause burning of the skin and will not provide proper defibrillation. It is also important to make certain the patient is not lying in a puddle of water prior to defibrillation. While simply lying on wet ground is not a problem, lying in a puddle of standing water may cause arcing and places other rescuers at risk of being shocked. Carefully move the patient out of the standing water before defibrillation. Remove the medication patch and wipe any remaining medication from the skin before placing the defibrillator pad.

Defibrillator Maintenance

Like any piece of equipment used for the care and transport of a patient, the AED has specific maintenance requirements that must be followed to ensure proper function of the device.

Self-Diagnostic Checks

Most if not all AEDs have built-in sophisticated diagnostic software that performs automated self checks at regular intervals. The self checks ensure that all internal circuitry is operating normally and require little if any work on the part of the operator. A visible indicator or audible tone will alert the operator should one of the self checks find a malfunction in the device.

Defibrillator malfunction is frequently due to a battery failure. It is important to inspect the batteries on a regular basis and confirm they are not leaking and have not expired. Batteries have a limited life and must be changed once expired. Expiration dates are clearly marked on all batteries.

Routine Inspections

In addition to the self checks, each AED manufacturer provides a detailed maintenance checklist for each device. Depending on where the AED is being used, the inspection may be performed daily, weekly, or monthly. At a minimum, all AEDs must be checked every 30 days to ensure they are ready for service.

In addition to ensuring that the device is in working order, the operator must see that the necessary supplies are stored with the AED. The following list of supplies should be stored with the AED and inspected at regular intervals:

- Extra set of electrode pads
- Extra battery
- Shaver for removal of chest hair
- Scissors for cutting away clothing
- Supply of 4 × 4 gauze pads for wiping away moisture
- Protective gloves and barrier mask

Medical Direction

In most states, AED programs must have medical oversight. This is most often provided by the EMS system's medical director. Medical directors provide oversight of the deployment of AEDs and training requirements of personnel who will be using the devices. They must also review each incident in which an AED was used. Following the use of an AED, a written report must be submitted to the medical director along with the data downloaded from the device. The medical director will review all details concerning the event and provide feedback for program quality improvement.

In addition, most AEDs require the prescription of a physician before they can be purchased. One AED manufacturer has received Federal Food and Drug Administration (FDA) approval for the sale of one specific model of AED designed for home use.

Whether as part of an EMS system or in the private sector, one of a medical director's primary goals is to ensure the continuous quality improvement (CQI) of the AED program. The goal of CQI is to ensure that local EMS systems are providing the best possible care at all times to victims of cardiac arrest. By reviewing each incident in which an AED was used, important statistical information can be gathered that will assist in making improvements to the AHA guidelines and protocols that direct how AEDs are used.

Like any skill you might use as an EMT, make sure you review procedures and practice using the AED as often as necessary to maintain proficiency. Cardiac arrest is a time-sensitive emergency, and maintaining proficiency with the AED will minimize unnecessary delays in providing care for the patient.

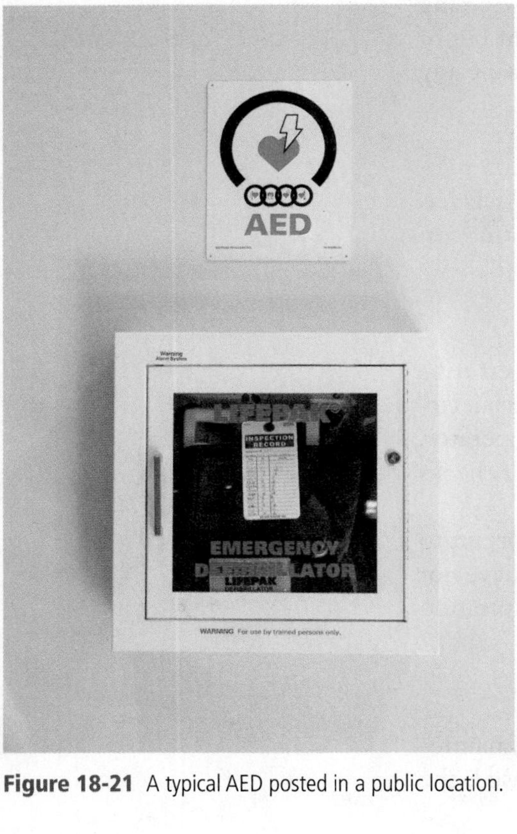

Figure 18-21 A typical AED posted in a public location.

Public Access Defibrillation

It is only a matter of time before you respond to the scene of a cardiac arrest and find an AED in use by someone from a private company or organization. Amusement parks, airports, shopping malls, and even some cities and towns are developing what are known as public access defibrillation programs, making AEDs available in public places (Figure 18-21 ■).

The American Heart Association and similar organizations have developed specific training and implementation programs for the public use of AEDs. The organizations are promoting public access defibrillation programs in an effort to decrease the time to shock following collapse from a cardiac arrest.

EMERGENCY DISPATCH SUMMARY

Once on scene, the paramedics intubated the patient, started a jugular IV, and implemented the cardiac drug protocols. Incredibly, the patient regained a pulse and a low but consistent blood pressure. She was then quickly transported to the city's heart hospital where she was transferred to their care in the same precarious condition. Whether she lived or not is unknown. Sometimes EMS personnel just do what they can and never have the opportunity to follow up or learn whether they ultimately made a difference.

Chapter Review

To the Point

- Cardiac compromise and acute coronary syndrome are conditions most often caused by ischemia of the heart muscle.
- The heart is driven by an electrical conduction system that initiates the contraction of the heart muscle, which in turn pumps the blood to the body.
- When the heart muscle does not receive an adequate supply of blood (ischemia) and oxygen (hypoxia), it can result in cardiac compromise.
- A myocardial infarction occurs when a portion of the heart dies due to an insufficient supply of oxygenated blood. Angina occurs when the heart muscle does not receive an adequate supply of oxygenated blood.
- The elderly, diabetic patients, and women may have a less typical presentation when experiencing cardiac compromise.
- Heart failure occurs due to a decrease in the efficiency of the heart's ability to pump blood. It can result in a backup in the left, right, or both sides of the heart.
- Whenever possible, ALS should be called to assist a patient with cardiac compromise.
- The assessment of a suspected cardiac patient should center on the chief complaint. You can use the SAMPLE and OPQRST tools for your assessment.
- You may assist a patient who has a prescription for nitroglycerin with taking his medication to help relieve the chest pain during an episode.
- Fibrinolytics (thrombolytics) are often used to help minimize the damage to heart tissue caused by a blood clot. These medications are most often given at the emergency department.
- The use of an AED has become an important component of the survival of sudden cardiac arrest and should be initiated as soon as it is available.

Chapter Questions

Multiple Choice

1. The primary vessels responsible for supplying the heart muscle with blood are the:

_____ a. cardiac veins.

_____ b. pulmonary arteries.

_____ c. coronary arteries.

_____ d. pulmonary veins.

2. Nitroglycerin is indicated for the treatment of:

_____ a. angina.

_____ b. pectoris.

_____ c. anxiety.

_____ d. shortness of breath.

(continued on next page)

(continued)

3. Which one of the following is *not* a side effect of nitroglycerin?

_____ a. Drop in blood pressure
_____ b. Headache
_____ c. Pulse rate changes
_____ d. Shortness of breath

4. Which one of the following is caused by a backup of fluids from the circulatory system when the heart can no longer pump blood efficiently?

_____ a. Angina
_____ b. Congestive heart failure
_____ c. Myocardial infarction
_____ d. Subcutaneous emphysema

5. Which one of the following is *not* a typical sign or symptom of cardiac compromise?

_____ a. Chest discomfort
_____ b. Low back pain
_____ c. Nausea and vomiting
_____ d. Shortness of breath

6. It is recommended that the AED inspection checklist be completed at least every _____________ to ensure readiness for an emergency.

_____ a. day
_____ b. week
_____ c. 30 days
_____ d. year

7. You are operating an AED on an adult victim of cardiac arrest. The AED has just delivered a shock. You should:

_____ a. analyze again and deliver a shock if indicated.
_____ b. check for a pulse and begin CPR if no pulse.
_____ c. resume compressions immediately.
_____ d. assess for pulse and breathing and transport.

8. Which one of the following is *not* considered a component of post-resuscitation care?

_____ a. Rapid trauma assessment
_____ b. Rapid transport
_____ c. Monitoring of ABCs
_____ d. Administration of supplemental oxygen

9. You are caring for a victim of cardiac arrest and have just completed your second round of CPR. You should:

_____ a. allow the AED to analyze the rhythm.
_____ b. deliver one shock.
_____ c. continue with another two minutes of CPR.
_____ d. remove the electrode pads.

10. You are on the scene of a cardiac arrest and the AED has given a "No shock advised" prompt. You should:

_____ a. initiate another analyze phase.
_____ b. remove the electrode pads.
_____ c. assess for pulse and breathing.
_____ d. perform CPR for two minutes.

Critical Thinking

1. Discuss the difference between a heart attack and a cardiac arrest.

____

____

____

____

2. Discuss the role of the EMT in the Chain of Survival.

____

____

____

____

3. Discuss the differences between fully automatic and semiautomatic AEDs.

4. What are the two rhythms that an AED will recognize as shockable?

5. Discuss the role of the medical director in an AED program.

Case Studies

Case Study 1

You have been dispatched to a local gym for a man down. On arrival, you find an approximately 60-year-old man unresponsive on the floor. A gym employee is performing CPR and advises that the patient collapsed about 10 minutes ago and that the employee started CPR almost immediately. You direct the employee to stop CPR while you check for a carotid pulse. You feel a pulse. The man, however, is still not breathing.

1. How will you proceed with caring for this man?

2. After a few minutes of rescue breathing, you discover that the patient no longer has a pulse. What will you do next?

(continued on next page)

(continued)

3. The AED has delivered one shock. What will you do next?

Case Study 2

While working the first aid station at the local county fair, an approximately 45-year-old man is brought to the station by some family members. The family states that he is having trouble breathing and needs some assistance. You sit the man down in the station and begin to assess him. He reveals that his primary complaint is a pressure on his chest, which seems to be causing the difficulty breathing. He states that he had a similar episode about six months ago and had a stent inserted into one of his coronary arteries. He denies any other history other than high cholesterol, for which he takes Lipitor®. His blood pressure is 106/68, pulse 88 strong and regular. He appears a little pale and sweaty.

1. How will you begin your care for this patient?

2. The man states that he has some nitroglycerin in his wife's purse and asks if he should take one. What will you want to know before you assist him in taking a nitroglycerin pill?

The Last Word

Patients with the signs and symptoms of cardiac compromise make up a large percentage of the calls you will see as an EMT. Your understanding of the cardiovascular system and the signs and symptoms that appear when it begins to malfunction is essential to the well-being of your patients. While the causes of cardiac compromise can be many and varied, the presentation is often very similar. When in doubt, provide care for the worst possible scenario and initiate transport and access to ALS care as soon as possible.

Caring for Patients with Seizures and Syncope

19

Education Standards

Medicine: Neurology

Competencies

Applies fundamental knowledge to provide basic emergency care and transportation based on assessment findings for the acutely ill patient.

Objectives

After completion of this lesson, you should be able to:

19-1 Define key terms introduced in this chapter.

19-2 Discuss the pathophysiology of seizures.

19-3 List common causes of seizures.

19-4 Differentiate primary and secondary seizures.

19-5 Describe the various types of seizures and the ways that they can present.

19-6 Explain the concerns associated with prolonged or successive seizures.

19-7 Describe the assessment and emergency medical care of patients experiencing seizures.

19-8 Describe the assessment and emergency medical care of patients in a postictal state.

19-9 Describe the assessment and emergency medical care of patients who are unresponsive, actively seizing, or in status epilepticus.

19-10 List relevant questions to ask while gathering a history of the seizure activity.

19-11 Describe common causes of syncope.

19-12 Describe the proper management of patients with syncope.

Key Terms

absence seizure p. 529
clonic p. 528
complex partial seizure p. 529
convulsion p. 526
epilepsy p. 527
febrile seizure p. 529
generalized seizure p. 528
postictal phase p. 528
primary seizures p. 527
secondary seizures p. 527
seizures p. 526
simple partial seizure p. 528
status epilepticus p. 529
syncope p. 533
tonic p. 528
tonic-clonic seizure p. 528
vasovagal response p. 534

Introduction

In this chapter two specific medical conditions known as *seizures* and *syncope* are discussed. Seizures are a potentially life-threatening medical condition. In general terms, they are episodes of abnormal brain function that cause changes in attention or behavior. They are caused by abnormally excited electrical signals in the brain.

Syncope is a partial or complete loss of consciousness with interruption of awareness of oneself and one's surroundings. Most nonmedical people refer to it as *fainting*. Whatever the exact cause, the common mechanism that causes syncope is a transient loss of adequate blood flow to the brain, resulting in a loss of normal consciousness. In syncope the loss of consciousness is temporary and there is spontaneous recovery to a normal mental status. Syncope is a common reason why EMS is called and accounts for many emergency department visits each year.

EMERGENCY DISPATCH

"Unit 93, 9-3, respond to 79656 Tropicana for a syncopal episode on the sidewalk. Showing you dispatched at 1523 hours."

EMTs Gracie Grajalva and Bernadette Fong quickly packed away their half-eaten lunches—already delayed by back-to-back calls—and acknowledged the dispatch before heading out into the thickening late afternoon traffic.

"I don't know what happened," a woman clutching numerous shopping bags rushed up to Bernie as she stepped from the truck. "Anne was walking down the sidewalk and then she just got really pale and fell over."

"Did she hit her head?" Gracie asked, pulling the stretcher from the back and eyeing the gathering crowd.

"What, before?"

"No, ma'am, when she fell."

"Oh," the woman thought for a moment. "I don't know."

Bernie approached the woman who was still lying motionless on the sidewalk and held her head in a neutral, in-line position while saying, "Anne, can you hear me?"

The woman blinked several times and then shielded her eyes with the back of one shaky hand. "What happened? Oh my, what's going on?"

Seizures

19-2 Discuss the pathophysiology of seizures.

19-5 Describe the various types of seizures and the ways that they can present.

seizure a temporary electrical disturbance in the brain that is sometimes characterized by a loss of consciousness and convulsions.

convulsion full body muscle contractions.

Seizures occur when an area or areas of the brain receive a burst of abnormal electrical signals that temporarily interrupts normal electrical brain function. Depending on the location within the brain where the seizure begins and how extensively the abnormal electrical pattern travels, the patient may experience anything from a brief lapse in awareness or uncontrolled muscle contractions of an extremity to a total loss of consciousness accompanied by full-body muscle contractions (**convulsions**) lasting up to several minutes (Figure 19-1 ■).

Seizures are often manifested by localized (focal) or body-wide contractions of muscles. In other instances, seizures may be mild and relatively unnoticeable. Most patients you will encounter who have seizures have a chronic seizure disorder. Many of them and their family members are familiar with the way seizures appear and very often will not call EMS when a typical seizure occurs. Sometimes seizures are related to a temporary condition, such as exposure to drugs, withdrawal from certain drugs, a sudden spike in fever, or abnormal levels of sodium or glucose in the blood. Once the underlying problem is corrected, the person may never experience a related seizure again.

Depending on the type, a seizure can last from a few seconds to a couple of minutes. In rare cases a seizure can last more than several minutes. A seizure lasting more than several minutes is a serious emergency and must receive more advanced care as soon as possible.

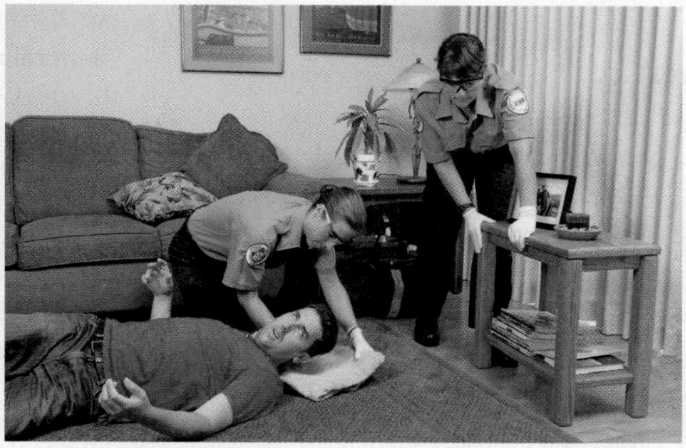

Figure 19-1 Convulsions are a common characteristic of a generalized tonic-clonic seizure.

Pathophysiology of Seizures

Seizures are not a disease, but instead a sign of some underlying problem caused by an injury, disease, or other abnormal condition. One of the most common causes of seizures in adults is a chronic medical condition called **epilepsy.** Epilepsy is a neurological disorder characterized by sudden recurring attacks of motor, sensory, or psychic malfunction with or without loss of consciousness or convulsive seizures.

There are other common causes of seizures:

- ***Alcohol withdrawal.*** Chronic alcoholics who abruptly stop drinking alcohol go through withdrawal, which often causes them to experience seizures.
- ***Traumatic injury.*** Patients who sustain an injury to the head will sometimes experience seizures following the injury.
- ***Brain tumors.*** As a tumor grows inside or around the brain, pressure on the brain can cause seizure activity.
- ***Infection.*** Generalized infections within the body and localized infections within the brain are capable of causing seizure activity, especially when fever is present.
- ***Metabolic causes.*** Changes or imbalances in the body's chemistry are frequently the cause of seizures.
- ***Hypoxia.*** Insufficient oxygen to the brain can lead to seizure activity.

19-3 List common causes of seizures.

epilepsy a neurological disorder characterized by sudden recurring attacks of motor, sensory, or psychic malfunction with or without loss of consciousness or convulsive seizures.

Seizures are categorized as primary or secondary. **Primary seizures** are those thought to be caused by a genetic disorder or some unidentified cause. An epileptic seizure is one type of primary seizure. Primary seizures can be manifested as either generalized or partial. **Secondary seizures** are those directly caused by a known source such as a medical condition or injury. Common causes of secondary seizures include trauma, fever, infection, hypoxia, diabetes, and alcohol and drug withdrawal. Secondary seizures most often manifest as generalized seizures.

You will likely encounter patients who have a history of seizures and who may be taking prescribed antiseizure medications. Become familiar with the more common antiseizure medication names. (See Table 19-1 for common seizure medications.)

19-4 Differentiate primary and secondary seizures.

primary seizures seizures that are thought to be caused by a genetic disorder or an unidentified cause.

secondary seizure a seizure that is directly caused by a known source such as a medical condition or injury.

CLINICAL CLUE

Common Cause of Seizures

In adult patients the most common cause of seizures is the failure of a seizure patient to properly take prescribed antiseizure medications. Many of these patients will outright refuse transport by ambulance, even if they have injured themselves during the seizure. If they do refuse transport, do your best to see that there is someone there to watch over them for at least an hour or two following the seizure.

Types of Seizures

There are several types of seizures that a patient may experience. The type of seizure varies, depending on the specific cause and the location in the brain at which the abnormal electrical activity is occurring.

TABLE 19-1 COMMON SEIZURE MEDICATIONS

phenytoin (Dilantin®)
phenobarbital
ethosuximide (Zarontin®)
carbamazepine (Tegretol®)
valproic acid or divalproex sodium (Depakene® or Depakote®)
primidone (Mysoline®)
clonazepam (Klonopin®)
clorazepate (Tranxene®)
felbamate (Felbatol®)
tiagabine (Gabitril®)
lamotrigine (Lamictal™)
oxcarbazepine (Trileptal®)
gabapentin (Neurontin®)
topiramate (Topamax®)
vigabatrin (Sabril®, Keppra®)

generalized seizure a seizure that involves both hemispheres of the brain and are characterized by a loss of consciousness and convulsions. Also called *grand mal seizure.*

tonic-clonic seizure a seizure that is characterized by intermittent muscle contractions and relaxation.

tonic prolonged muscle contractions as seen with generalized seizures.

clonic the contraction and relaxation of muscles during a seizure.

postictal phase the state that occurs when a seizure has stopped and the brain is attempting to recover, characterized by unconsciousness.

simple partial seizure a seizure that involves just one side of the brain and often produces a jerky spasm of a specific part of the body. Also called *focal motor seizure.*

Generalized Seizures

Generalized seizures are those seizures that affect both hemispheres of the brain. One of the most obvious and dramatic types of generalized seizure is called a **tonic-clonic seizure.** Generalized tonic-clonic seizures, also known as *grand mal seizures*, are characterized by a loss of consciousness and convulsions (full-body muscle contractions). The medical term **tonic** refers to prolonged muscle contraction. The term **clonic** refers to the contraction and relaxation of muscles during the seizure. Both can be very dramatic and frightening to watch for the first time but are usually not life threatening.

It is very possible for a person experiencing a generalized seizure to lose consciousness while standing and injure himself during the fall to the ground. You must carefully consider the need for spinal precautions when caring for a generalized seizure patient.

During a generalized tonic-clonic seizure, the patient may also experience anywhere from a partial to a complete airway obstruction. This is expected. However, no attempt should be made to insert anything into the mouth of a convulsing patient. Due to the short duration of most seizures, it is appropriate to wait until the seizure has stopped before providing airway care.

Signs and symptoms of a generalized tonic-clonic seizure include:

- Unresponsiveness
- Full-body convulsions
- Partial to full airway obstruction
- Loss of bladder or bowel control
- Fixed gaze on one side
- Noisy breathing
- Accumulation of fluids in the airway (foaming)

Many patients who have a history of seizures will describe what is called an *aura* just prior to the onset of a seizure. The aura can appear in many different ways, such as a visual disturbance, a sound, an unusual taste or smell, or an upset stomach. Auras can serve as a warning to some patients that a seizure is about to occur. This may give the patient enough time to find a safe place to lie down while the seizure takes its course.

Postictal Phase

Immediately following a generalized seizure, the patient will enter what is called the **postictal phase.** This is the phase that occurs when the electrical activity in the brain has stopped and the brain is attempting to recover. The patient will appear to be asleep and may not be responsive for several minutes (Figure 19-2 ■). It is during this phase that you can begin caring for your patient and managing the ABCs. You may need to roll the patient onto his side to help manage the airway. You should begin talking to the patient and explaining all that you are doing, even if he appears to be unresponsive. The postictal phase may last anywhere from just a few minutes to as long as a half an hour, depending on the individual. Be patient, and continue to comfort and monitor the patient as he regains consciousness.

Simple Partial Seizure

A **simple partial seizure** is also known as a *focal motor seizure*. (*Focal* means focused on one specific area, and *motor* refers to the movement of muscles.) This type of seizure involves just one side of the brain and often produces a jerky spasm of a specific part of the body. It may involve a foot, hand, arm, or muscles of the face. The patient is not able to control the movement but is typically awake and aware of the situation.

A partial seizure can move from one side of the body to the other and in some cases may progress to a full generalized seizure. Simple partial seizures typically last just a few seconds to a minute or so. In rare cases they can last from 20 to 30 minutes.

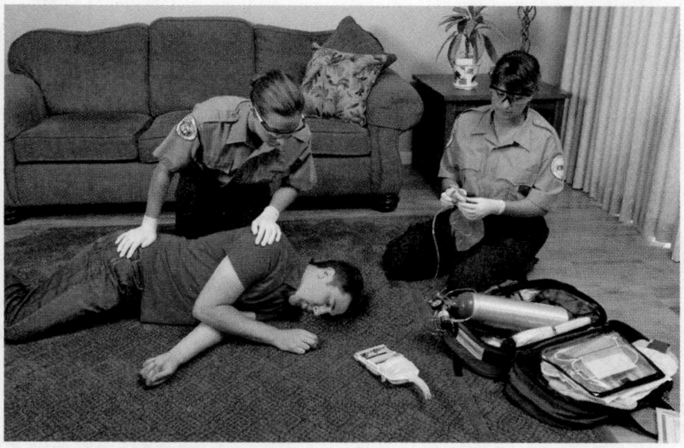

Figure 19-2 Following a generalized seizure is the postictal phase, during which the patient may remain unresponsive for several minutes.

Complex Partial Seizure

A **complex partial seizure**—also known as a *psychomotor seizure* or *temporal lobe seizure*—involves just one hemisphere of the brain and can last a few seconds to two minutes. It is different from the simple partial seizure in that the patient is not aware of the surroundings during the seizure.

complex partial seizure a seizure that involves just one hemisphere of the brain. It typically lasts a few seconds to two minutes and the patient is unaware that it is occurring. Also called *psychomotor seizure* or *temporal lobe seizure.*

This type of seizure often begins with the patient staring off into space and may involve random movements, such as hand tapping, lip smacking, or chewing. The patient will appear to be awake with eyes open, but will not respond to the environment. The patient also may make random sounds or repeat words over and over.

Care for these patients involves providing reassurance and monitoring them to make sure they do not harm themselves. It is important to monitor them throughout the episode because the seizures can progress into generalized seizures.

absence seizure a seizure common in children, characterized by a blank stare and unresponsiveness. Also called *petit mal seizure.*

Absence Seizure (Petit Mal)

Absence seizures—also known as *petit mal seizures*—are most commonly characterized by a blank stare that starts and stops suddenly. They occur most commonly in children and are often confused with daydreaming. The patient usually is unaware of his surroundings, and the episodes can occur without anyone noticing. Because these seizures affect both hemispheres of the brain and the patient does not recall them occurring, they are technically categorized as a type of generalized seizure.

CLINICAL CLUE

Petit Mal Seizure

Another type of seizure known as a *petit mal seizure* or *absence seizure* is characterized by the patient appearing to be awake but unresponsive to verbal or painful stimuli.

Febrile Seizures

The most common cause of seizures in children is a sudden spike in fever. This type of seizure is referred to as a **febrile seizure.** Attempts should be made to cool the child as soon as possible. Cool the patient by removing clothing to the underwear, sponging with tepid water, and fanning. Do not use alcohol, ice, or cold water, which can cause hypothermia.

febrile seizure a seizure common in young children, caused by a sudden spike in fever.

Status Epilepticus

19-6 Explain the concerns associated with prolonged or successive seizures.

A patient who experiences generalized seizures that last more than five minutes or that occur back-to-back without regaining consciousness is said to be in **status epilepticus.** Of all the situations related to seizures, this is the most dangerous and life threatening. These patients require advanced life support and medications that will help stop the convulsions. The danger stems from the prolonged periods of hypoxia experienced by the brain through repeated seizures. This is a serious emergency and requires quick action by the EMT. You must provide supplemental oxygen with a nonrebreather mask and rapid transport to the hospital. Do not delay transport while setting up the oxygen.

status epilepticus a condition characterized by seizures lasting more than five minutes or recurrent seizures with no period of consciousness.

CLINICAL CLUE

Status Epilepticus

In general, seizures are rarely life threatening. However, they can become life threatening if the patient has multiple seizures in a row. Repeated seizures without regaining consciousness or one continuous seizure lasting five minutes or more can result in the brain becoming hypoxic and eventually lead to brain damage and even death. This is a condition known as *status epilepticus* and is considered a serious emergency. Transport immediately, apply oxygen by nonrebreather mask, and initiate an ALS intercept if available. This condition is life threatening.

Emergency Care of the Seizure Patient

19-7 Describe the assessment and emergency medical care of patients experiencing seizures.

The following steps should be followed when caring for a person experiencing a generalized tonic-clonic seizure (Scan 19-1):

1. Take the necessary BSI precautions.
2. Protect the patient from injury by removing objects that he may strike and place something soft beneath his head.
3. Consider the use of supplemental oxygen by nonrebreather mask while he is still convulsing.
4. Have suction ready.
5. Do *not* attempt to pry open a clinched mouth or place anything inside the mouth of a seizing patient.

19-8 Describe the assessment and emergency medical care of patients in a postictal state.

Once the convulsions have stopped, continue your care by completing the following steps:

1. Perform a primary assessment and establish or maintain an open airway and suction as necessary.
2. Complete a secondary assessment, looking for possible injury. Ask bystanders if the patient has a history of seizures.
3. If there is no suspected spine injury, place the patient in the recovery position. Consider the need for supplemental oxygen, if it has not already been started (Figure 19-3 ■).
4. Perform reassessment as necessary.
5. If transportation is necessary, transport the patient in the recovery position.

19-9 Describe the assessment and emergency medical care of patients who are unresponsive, actively seizing, or in status epilepticus.

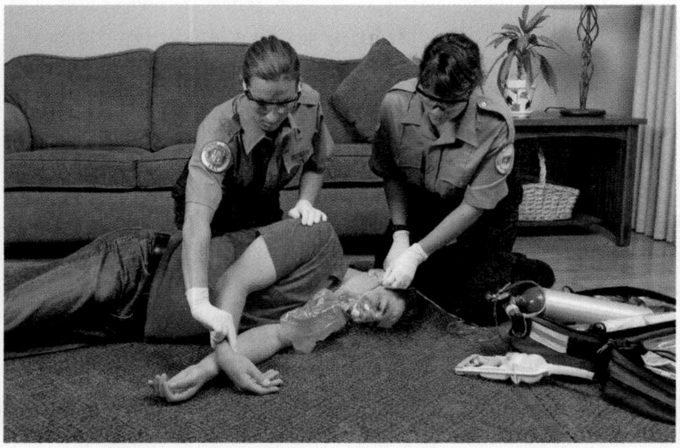

Figure 19-3 Once the convulsions have stopped, carefully place the patient in the recovery position to help maintain the airway.

A seizure patient experiencing convulsions should not be forcibly restrained. The emphasis of your care should be on protecting the patient from injury as his body seizes. Move any obstacles away from the patient and place something soft beneath the patient's head.

Following a generalized tonic-clonic seizure, the patient will remain unresponsive or may be sleepy or groggy for up to 30 minutes or so. This is quite normal and is called the postictal phase. Because the patient may have an accumulation of fluids in the airway following the convulsion, it is especially important to immediately ensure a clear airway and adequate breathing.

In most instances the patient will have stopped convulsing prior to your arrival. So, it will be important to get an account of the events from witnesses. As you gather a history of the incident, be sure to ask witnesses if they saw the patient fall, how he landed, how the patient was moving during the convulsion, and how long

SCAN 19-1 Caring for the Seizure Patient

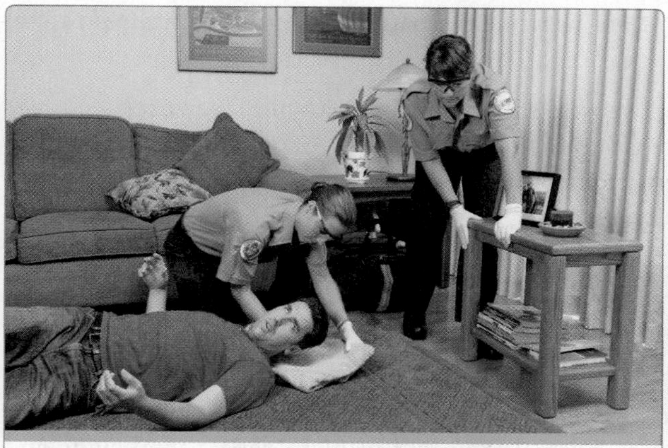

19-1-1 If the patient is actively seizing, protect him from further harm.

19-1-2 Once the convulsions have stopped, open the airway and assess breathing.

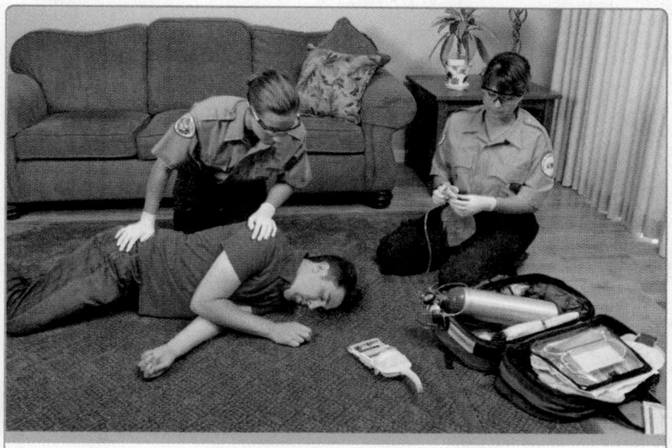

19-1-3 If you do not suspect a head or spine injury, roll the patient into the recovery position.

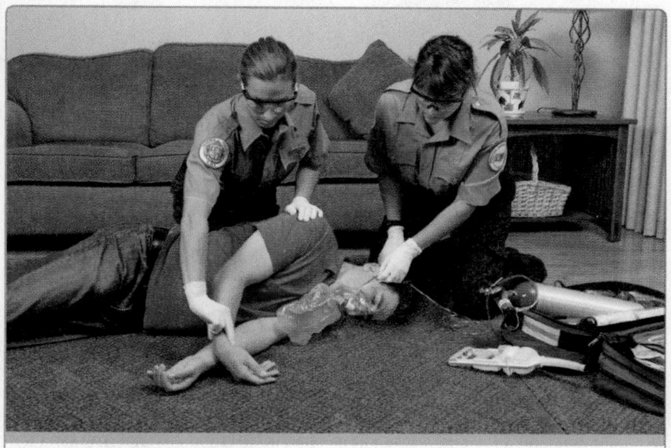

19-1-4 Initiate oxygen therapy as per local protocols.

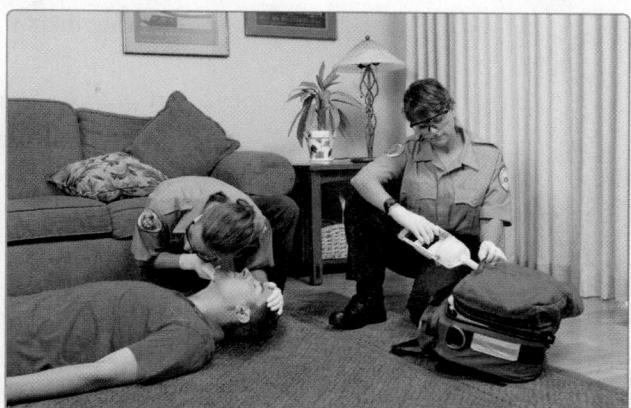

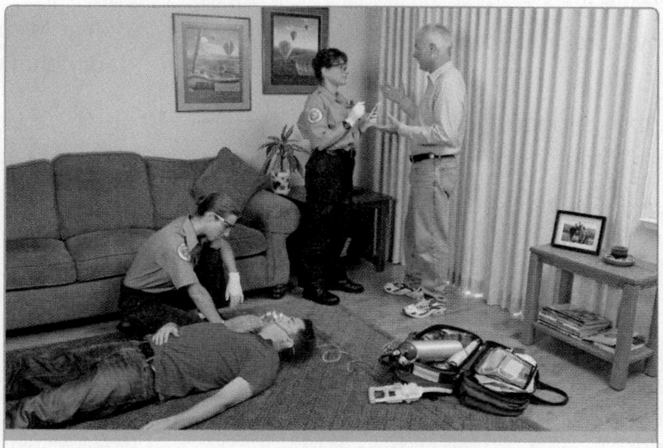

19-1-5 Complete a secondary assessment and determine if there is any past medical history related to seizures.

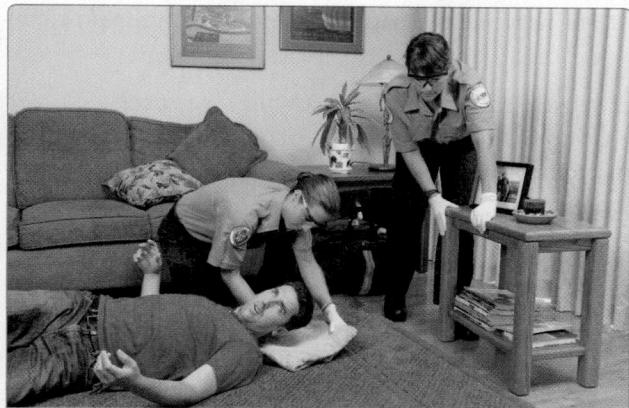

19-10 List relevant questions to ask while gathering a history of the seizure activity.

the convulsion lasted. It is common for the victim of a seizure to injure himself from a fall or during the tonic-clonic phase of the seizure by striking his head or arms against a hard surface. Be sure to perform a thorough secondary assessment on all seizure patients.

Once you are sure the patient has not been injured, consider asking witnesses or family members the following questions while the patient emerges from the postictal state:

- If the patient has a history of seizure activity, was this a typical seizure?
- When was the last time the patient had a seizure?
- Is the patient on any antiseizure medications?
- Has the patient been ill lately?

If there is no one at the scene who can answer these questions immediately, be sure to ask the patient once he regains consciousness.

Reassessment of the Seizure Patient

As with most patients, your reassessments will focus on ensuring the airway remains clear and the breathing returns to normal. You will want to repeat vital signs and should see them return to normal within 10 to 15 minutes following the seizure.

STOP, REVIEW, REMEMBER!

Multiple Choice

For each question, place a check next to the correct answer.

1. Seizures occur when one or more areas of the brain:

_____ a. receive a larger than expected volume of blood.

_____ b. receive a burst of abnormal electrical signals.

_____ c. are affected by increased blood pressure.

_____ d. become damaged by a rupture or clot.

2. Seizures lasting more than several minutes:

_____ a. are common among the elderly.

_____ b. can be caused by a prolonged fever or withdrawal from drugs.

_____ c. are serious emergencies requiring advanced levels of care.

_____ d. require a tongue depressor to be inserted into the patient's mouth.

3. A patient who experiences a secondary seizure is most likely also suffering from:

_____ a. an infection or alcohol withdrawal.

_____ b. a genetic disorder.

_____ c. epilepsy.

_____ d. petit mal syndrome.

4. When caring for the postictal patient, you should first:

_____ a. clear away bystanders.

_____ b. manage any bleeding.

_____ c. manage possible fractures.

_____ d. manage issues with the ABCs.

5. Which one of the following best represents how a patient who is having a complex partial seizure might present?

_____ a. Alert with a slight spasm of either the left or right hand

_____ b. Full body tonic-clonic convulsions

_____ c. As if he is staring into space, with repetitive movements or sounds

_____ d. As if he is daydreaming

Matching

Match the term on the left with the applicable definition on the right.

1. _____ Febrile seizure
2. _____ Generalized tonic-clonic seizure
3. _____ Complex partial seizure
4. _____ Absence seizure
5. _____ Simple partial seizure

A. Involves one hemisphere of the brain and may begin with the patient staring off into space. This patient is not aware of surroundings.

B. Typically experienced by children, and brought on by a sudden spike in fever

C. Characterized by a loss of consciousness and full body convulsions

D. Involves one hemisphere of the brain and causes shaking that may involve a hand, arm, leg, or foot. This patient is aware of what is happening.

E. Characterized by staring into space, which can be confused with daydreaming

Critical Thinking

1. Why is it important to restrict your care to protecting the patient while he seizes, instead of restraining him?

____

____

____

____

2. Describe the differences between primary and secondary seizures.

____

____

____

____

Syncope

19-11 Describe common causes of syncope.

syncope a sudden and temporary loss of consciousness; fainting.

Syncope is the medical term for fainting. It is defined as a sudden and temporary loss of consciousness. Whatever the specific cause of syncope, it is the result of inadequate blood flow to the brain, resulting in a brief loss of consciousness. In younger patients syncope is most often caused by a sudden drop in blood pressure (hypotension) secondary to a slowing of the heart rate. In these patients an episode of syncope is frequently preceded by dizziness, loss of vision (blackout), nausea, weakness, and sweating. This response is primarily caused by an overreaction by the parasympathetic

vasovagal response an exaggerated response by the parasympathetic nervous system, causing syncope.

nervous system, which causes a sudden slowing of the heart rate and drop in blood pressure. It is often called a **vasovagal response** or *vasovagal episode. (Vaso* refers to the vessels, and *vagal* refers to the vagus nerve, which is the primary pathway where these nerve impulses are transmitted.)

Heart dysrhythmias, or sudden abnormal heart rhythms, are a common cause of syncope in older adults, as are adverse reactions to medications.

PERSPECTIVE

Anne—The Patient

I've never experienced anything like that before. Julie and I had been shopping all afternoon and I started feeling a little dizzy. I figured it was the heat, or maybe the wine at lunch. But one moment I'm talking about Bob traveling to Australia on business and the next minute I was on the sidewalk looking up at some woman who wasn't letting me move my head. I was so confused and scared!

PRACTICAL PATHOPHYSIOLOGY

The parasympathetic side of the autonomic nervous system is a major culprit in cases of syncope. It is responsible for a rapid dilation of blood vessels that results in a sudden drop in blood pressure (hypotension) and thus reduced perfusion to the brain.

Types of Syncope

Syncope caused by a vasovagal episode is common enough that most teenagers and adults have experienced episodes or near episodes at some time in their lives. In most incidents, the person experiences some of the symptoms already mentioned and attempts to lie down. Lying flat improves perfusion to the brain and in most instances the person feels better almost immediately.

Not all cases of syncope are simple vasovagal episodes, and in certain cases syncope may be a sign of potentially life-threatening pathophysiology. Dangerous causes of syncope include abnormal electrical activity in the heart, resulting in too slow or too rapid a pulse rate, blockage of the blood supply to the brain, or inadequate blood volume (hypovolemia). In those cases the decrease in perfusion is so rapid and unexpected that the person has no time to react and simply falls to the ground and appears unresponsive for a few to several seconds. Clues that syncope may be from a more serious cause include syncope in older adults, no preceding warning symptoms before syncope, and obvious trauma as a result of the syncope being so sudden that the patient was unable to protect himself from the impact on the surfaces around him.

It is not uncommon for untrained bystanders to confuse a syncopal episode with a seizure due to the collapsing of the patient and the loss of consciousness.

PERSPECTIVE

Bernadette—The EMT

There's always that split second when someone wakes from syncope or a seizure when you don't know what they are going to do, you know? Some people get really scared, some start fighting, others pretend they're fine out of embarrassment or something. I've always found that talking calmly and clearly, using their name and repeating that I am there to help seems to work. Can you imagine? You're just buzzing through your day thinking about what to make for dinner and then the next second you're on the pavement with my face in yours! I always try to reassure people in that situation because that's what I'd want.

Emergency Care of the Syncope Patient

19-12 Describe the proper management of patients with syncope.

In most cases, you will care for a patient with syncope who already made it to the ground, either voluntarily or involuntarily. Make sure to rule out any possibility of injury to the head or neck. Ask if the patient hit his head, and palpate the neck for tenderness. If there is neck pain or any evidence of trauma to the head, manually stabilize the head and neck. Obtain a thorough history of events prior to the syncopal episode, as well as a thorough medical history. If the patient is lying on the ground and there is no injury to the spine, elevate the legs 8 to 12 inches to promote circulation to the brain. All patients with syncope should be transported to an emergency department for further evaluation.

You must be especially alert when you allow a patient who has been lying down for an extended period of time to sit up. Have the patient rest after each repositioning. Be sure to have someone on either side of the patient when assisting with walking. As soon as the patient begins to feel dizzy, nauseous, or light-headed, have him sit down. If he does not feel better right away, have him lie down.

Any patient who has experienced a syncopal episode for unknown reasons or who remained unconscious for more than a few seconds should be transported to an emergency department for further evaluation.

STOP, REVIEW, REMEMBER!

Multiple Choice

For each question, place a check next to the correct answer.

1. A patient suffering from syncope is most likely experiencing:

_____ a. tachycardia secondary to increased blood pressure.

_____ b. a sudden drop in blood pressure due to a slow heart rate.

_____ c. a sudden increase in blood pressure.

_____ d. traumatic brain injury.

2. When assessing a patient who has suddenly experienced an episode of syncope, it is important to first:

_____ a. move the patient into the recovery position.

_____ b. check to see if the patient has bitten his tongue.

_____ c. assess the head and neck for injury that may have resulted from a fall.

_____ d. have the patient sit up to reconnect with his surroundings.

3. Why is it important to have a patient who may be experiencing an episode of syncope lie down?

_____ a. The patient may be taking a medication that prevents him from sitting or standing for a long period of time.

_____ b. Lying down will help increase perfusion to the brain.

_____ c. Syncope can only be cured by lying down.

_____ d. It allows you to do a more thorough assessment.

4. Clues that syncope may be from a potentially life-threatening cause include episodes involving:

_____ a. older adults.

_____ b. teenagers.

_____ c. well-defined symptoms prior to the event.

_____ d. significant emotional stress.

(continued on next page)

(continued)

Short Answer

1. What is the first thing you should do with a patient who may be experiencing syncope?

2. What external factor can cause an elderly patient to experience syncope?

Critical Thinking

1. Explain the role the parasympathetic nervous system plays in syncope?

EMERGENCY DISPATCH SUMMARY

The patient was immobilized to a long backboard, given supplemental oxygen by way of a nonrebreather mask, and transported to City University Hospital for evaluation. She was released that same evening after all tests returned normal, and has had no further incidents since then.

Chapter Review

To the Point

- Seizures are a disturbance in the electrical activity within the brain and can occur without warning.
- Common causes of seizures include epilepsy, fever, brain tumors, head injury, alcohol withdrawal, and infection.
- Seizures with an unknown origin or that are caused by a genetic disorder are referred to as primary seizures.
- Seizures caused by a known source such as fever, tumor, trauma, or alcohol withdrawal are referred to as secondary seizures.
- There are several common types of seizures including generalized, simple partial, complex partial, absence, and febrile.
- Status epilepticus is a condition manifested by seizures lasting longer than five minutes or seizures that occur back-to-back. This is a serious life-threatening condition.
- Management of a patient who is actively seizing focuses on protecting him from injury.
- Management of a patient who is in the postical state involves caring for the ABCs, placing the patient in the recovery position, providing supplemental oxygen, and comfort care.
- A thorough medical history is important when assessing the patient with a first-time seizure.
- Syncope is the sudden and temporary loss of consciousness caused by inadequate blood flow to the brain.
- Although many cases of syncope are simple vasovagal episodes, in certain cases syncope may be a sign of potentially life-threatening pathophysiology.
- Management of the patient following a syncopal episode includes assessing for trauma, keeping him lying flat, and elevating the legs 8 to 12 inches.

Chapter Questions

Multiple Choice

For each question, place a check next to the correct answer.

1. Children commonly experience seizures as a result of a sudden spike in fever. How would you care for a child who has just experienced a febrile seizure?
   _____ a. Cool the child with tepid water.
   _____ b. Place the child in an ice bath prior to transport.
   _____ c. Try to warm the child to regulate his temperature.
   _____ d. Wipe the child's forehead with a cotton swap moistened with alcohol.

2. For a patient who is in status epilepticus, what is the most significant threat to life?
   _____ a. Spine injury
   _____ b. Hypoxia
   _____ c. Blood clots
   _____ d. Skull fracture

3. What might a patient suffering from syncope experience just before loss of consciousness?
   _____ a. Increased adrenaline, nausea, sense of impending doom
   _____ b. Dizziness, sweating, tingling in the left arm
   _____ c. Increased heart rate, shortness of breath, nausea
   _____ d. Loss of vision, nausea, weakness, sweating

4. Care for the postical patient includes:
   _____ a. airway management and suction if necessary.
   _____ b. a rapid secondary assessment and transport.
   _____ c. minimal cervical-spine precautions.
   _____ d. CPR immediately after the tonic-clonic phase begins.

(continued on next page)

(continued)

5. Epilepsy is a medical condition that can be characterized as:
   _____ a. induced by alcohol withdrawal or brain tumors.
   _____ b. caused by infection.
   _____ c. reoccurring convulsive or nonconvulsive seizures.
   _____ d. any seizure lasting for more than 30 minutes.

6. Syncope is characterized by a:
   _____ a. sudden, temporary loss of consciousness.
   _____ b. sudden loss of motor control, generally accompanied by convulsions.
   _____ c. sudden but temporary loss of consciousness caused by a sudden increase in blood pressure.
   _____ d. gradual loss of brain function that affects memory, motor control, and behavior.

Short Answer

1. Briefly describe the cause of a febrile seizure.

2. List four signs and/or symptoms the patient might experience just prior to a syncopal episode.

Critical Thinking

1. Describe how you would care for a postictal patient.

2. What external elements can injure a patient who suddenly experiences a seizure or episode of syncope while standing or walking? What precautions might you take while evaluating this patient?

Case Study

One night you and a group of five friends are on your way to dinner. The parking lot at the restaurant is full, so you park several blocks away. As you make your way down the sidewalk to the restaurant, one of your friends suddenly collapses to the ground and begins to convulse uncontrollably.

1. Describe how you will utilize your friends in the proper care for the friend having the seizure.

____

____

____

____

2. One in the group tries to put a pen in the patient's mouth to "prevent him from swallowing his tongue," and another reaches out to restrain the patient's arms. Is there anything wrong with the care your friends are trying to administer? Why?

____

____

____

____

3. After close to a minute, the seizure stops. What is the first thing you should check to make sure your friend recovers well and how might you treat him?

____

____

____

____

The Last Word

The majority of seizure patients you encounter will be in the postical phase of recovery. It is important that you get a history from bystanders to find out if the patient fell and to rule out any chance of head or neck injury. After that, most of your care will be supportive in nature, monitoring the ABCs and providing reassurance. Most seizure patients will recover quickly without incident. Anyone with a first-time seizure should seek further medical evaluation from a physician to rule out any life-threatening causes.

Most of us will faint or nearly faint at some point in our lives due to vasovagal syncope and fully recover without complications. Always remember that not all cases of syncope are that simple. Syncope also can be the first sign of a potentially life-threatening medical emergency.

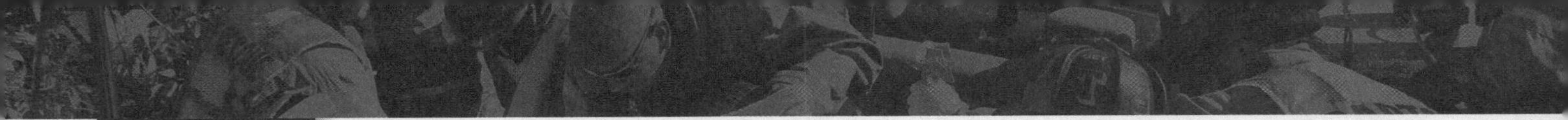

20 Caring for Patients with Altered Mental Status, Stroke, and Headache

Education Standards

Medicine: Neurology

Competencies

Applies fundamental knowledge to provide basic emergency care and transportation based on assessment findings for an acutely ill patient.

Objectives

After completion of this lesson, you should be able to:

20-1 Define key terms introduced in this chapter.

20-2 List common causes of altered mental status.

20-3 Describe the common signs and symptoms of altered mental status.

20-4 Describe an assessment-based approach to altered mental status.

20-5 Explain the reason for paying particular attention to airway assessment and management in patients with altered mental status.

20-6 Describe the emergency care of a patient with altered mental status.

20-7 List common risk factors for stroke.

20-8 Describe the pathophysiology of stroke and distinguish between ischemic stroke and hemorrhagic stroke.

20-9 Describe the signs and symptoms of stroke.

20-10 Describe the relationship between stroke and transient ischemic attack.

20-11 Describe an assessment-based approach to stroke and transient ischemic attack.

20-12 Describe the use of the Cincinnati Prehospital Stroke Scale.

20-13 Describe the elements of the Glasgow Coma Scale and how it is applied to the assessment of a patient with altered mental status.

20-14 Describe ways of communicating with patients who have difficulty speaking.

20-15 Describe the appropriate care for a patient with a suspected stroke.

20-16 Describe the common classifications of headache.

20-17 Recognize indications that a headache may have a potentially life-threatening underlying cause, such as toxic exposure, hypertension, infectious disease, or hemorrhagic stroke.

20-18 Describe the appropriate emergency medical care for a patient suffering from headache.

Key Terms

altered mental status (AMS) p. 541
aphasia p. 547
aura p. 555
basilar artery p. 548
brain tumor p. 542
cluster headaches p. 555
coma p. 542
dementia p. 542
dysphasia p. 547
embolism p. 548
Glasgow Coma Scale (GCS) p. 544
hemiparesis p. 547
hemiplegia p. 547
hemorrhagic stroke p. 548
hyperglycemia p. 542
hypoglycemia p. 542
inflammatory headache p. 555
intracerebral hemorrhage p. 548
ischemic stroke p. 548
migraine p. 555
occult p. 550
organic headache p. 555
stroke p. 546
subarachnoid hemorrhage p. 548
tension headaches p. 555
thrombus p. 548
traction headache p. 555
transient ischemic attack (TIA) p. 550

Introduction

Patients who experience a sudden illness or suffer a significant injury often become confused, violent, or slow to respond to your questions or events around them. Such patients are said to have an **altered mental status (AMS).** A patient can be described as having an altered mental status any time he is not acting normally or appears abnormally sleepy, confused, violent, or even completely unresponsive. Because there are so many possible causes, some of them life threatening, a patient who presents with an altered mental status should be considered unstable and a high priority for transport. These patients become particularly serious when the patient's level of responsiveness decreases to a point at which he may not be able to maintain his own airway.

altered mental status (AMS) a condition in which a patient appears to be abnormally sleepy, confused, violent, or even completely unresponsive.

EMERGENCY DISPATCH

EMTs Ray Dunn and Jason Toomey pulled into the small, desolate parking lot just as the police arrived, their headlights illuminating a tow truck with the driver's door hanging open and a man lying on the pavement not far from it.

"I drove by about 10 minutes ago," one of the officers told them, adjusting his duty belt after climbing from his cruiser. "He was hooking that car up and he waved at me. Seemed fine then."

Ray sized up the scene and then cautiously approached the patient—a man approximately 35–40 years old, wearing a tow-company uniform and with a messy tangle of long hair that obscured his face. The first thing that Ray noticed was blood oozing thickly from the man's scalp. A quick inspection with his gloved fingers exposed a three-centimeter laceration just above the man's right ear. The man groaned.

"We're with the ambulance," Ray said. "Can you tell us what happened?"

The man groaned louder and said something unintelligible. He was trying to sit up.

"Relax. Hold on," Ray said, trying to keep the man from moving his head or neck.

"What, what, help me!" The man shouted, pulling away from Ray and trying to get to his knees.

"We are trying to help." Jason appeared next to Ray and attempted to gently restrain the man.

"You, uh, you, uh, why are, I mean, oh no," the man stammered as he began pushing the EMT's hands away. "There's a green, a green, oh, what am I saying? Were we talking? Just now?"

"We've got to get this guy boarded," Ray said to Jason before turning to the police officers. "Can you guys help to hold him? We can't let him keep moving around like this."

The Patient with Altered Mental Status

20-2 List common causes of altered mental status.

hypoglycemia an abnormally low blood glucose level.

hyperglycemia an abnormally high blood glucose level.

coma a deep state of unconsciousness lasting more than six hours.

There are many causes of an altered mental status, including illnesses and injuries. For many patients the underlying cause is often a decrease in perfusion to the brain. Patients experiencing such medical conditions as **hypoglycemia** (low blood sugar), **hyperglycemia** (high blood sugar), seizures, strokes, and significant poisonings almost always have some degree of altered mental status. Patients experiencing a traumatic event such as blunt trauma to the head or significant blood loss also commonly present with altered mental status. If the patient cannot be aroused from a deep state of unconsciousness even with painful stimuli, he is said to be in a **coma.**

While it is not the responsibility of the EMT to always know the cause of a patient's altered mental status, becoming familiar with some of the more common causes will allow you to provide the most appropriate care. In every case, be sure to gather as thorough a history as possible. See Figure 20-1 ■ for some of the more common causes of altered mental status. A memory aid for remembering many of the common causes of altered mental status is AEIOU-TIPS (Table 20-1).

Assessment of a Patient with AMS

20-4 Describe an assessment-based approach to altered mental status.

brain tumor an abnormal growth of cells within the brain.

dementia a condition involving gradual development of memory impairment and cognitive disturbance.

Determining if a patient is actually presenting with an altered mental status is not always easy. In some patients with psychiatric disorders or certain chronic medical conditions, such as a **brain tumor** or **dementia,** an altered mental status may be their normal presentation. It is always important to refer to family members or caregivers to determine the patient's baseline mental status before forming any conclusions on your own. Look for medical identification jewelry and obtain the following history from family or caregivers if possible:

- Nature of onset (sudden or gradual)
- Prior relevant symptoms (fever, stiff neck, headache)
- Duration of altered mental status

TABLE 20-1 AEIOU-TIPS

A	Acidosis, alcohol
E	Epilepsy
I	Infection
O	Overdose
U	Uremia (kidney failure)
T	Trauma
I	Insulin-related (diabetes)
P	Psychosis
S	Stroke

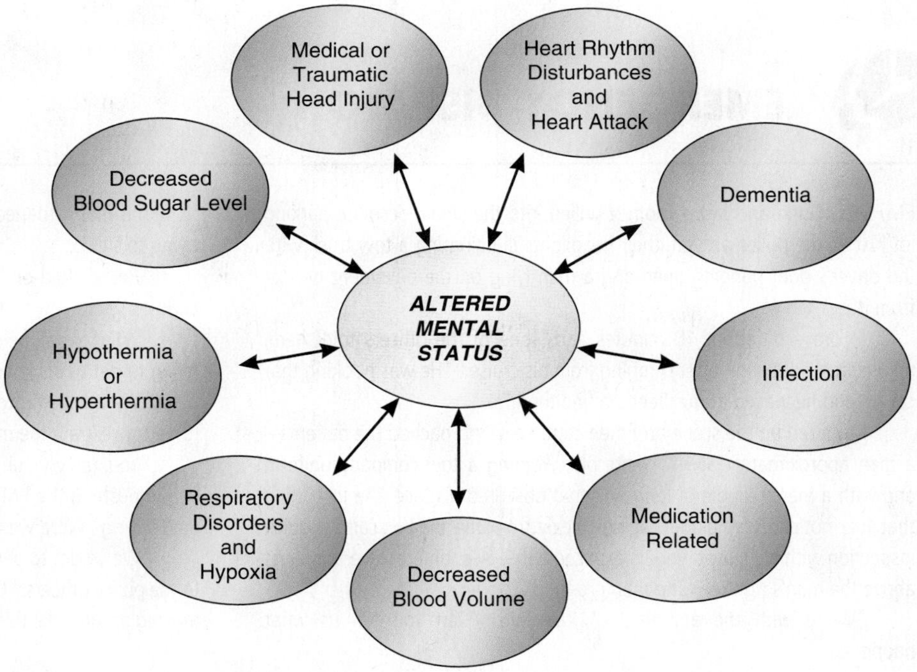

Figure 20-1 Common causes of altered mental status.

- History of recent head trauma
- Alcohol or drug abuse
- Known medical conditions (such as diabetes, stroke, dementia)

Assessment of the patient's mental status should be an ongoing process. Patients with an altered mental status often experience changing levels of responsiveness over short periods. In most cases, the best way to monitor mental status is to maintain constant verbal communication with the patient. Continually ask questions and monitor responses. Remain extra vigilant about monitoring the ABCs of any patient who is unresponsive. Recheck the vital signs as frequently as practical.

PRACTICAL PATHOPHYSIOLOGY

When the cells do not receive an adequate supply of oxygen and nutrients (perfusion), they begin to starve (hypoperfusion) and shift from aerobic to anaerobic metabolism. The root cause of metabolic acidosis is the buildup of the lactic acid that results from anaerobic metabolism. Many conditions cause acidosis in the body, resulting in changes in levels of responsiveness. They include sepsis from an overwhelming infection, diabetic ketoacidosis (high blood sugar), kidney failure, liver failure, severe diarrhea, cancer, seizures, and a prolonged lack of sufficient oxygen for any reason.

For most patients presenting with altered mental status, the primary concern is airway patency. As people become less responsive, they become less able to manage and protect their own airway. For supine patients, the tongue can easily become an airway obstruction. If patients vomit, they will be less able to clear their own airways. Monitor your patient's airway status and be prepared to intervene, if necessary.

20-5 Explain the reason for paying particular attention to airway assessment and management in patients with altered mental status.

Finally, consider your own safety. Although many patients are incapacitated by their condition, some can pose a threat to the care provider because of their unpredictability. Many EMS providers have been attacked and injured by patients presenting with altered mental status. Assess the patient for such a threat through observation and by obtaining a thorough history. It is also important to continue your scene size-up throughout the call. Hypodermic needles, toxic substances, and other hazards may still be present. Remember to assess for environmental causes of altered mental status and remain extra alert while working in close proximity to an unpredictable patient.

PERSPECTIVE

Ray—The EMT

I'm still not sure what happened. One minute this guy is just doing his job and the next he's got a head laceration and is obviously altered. The cops thought that he might have been mugged or something. We never found his wallet. But it was obvious that he didn't know what was going on. If you take a patient with a head wound who starts off unresponsive and then wakes up but is talking gibberish and resists help, it sends up all sorts of red flags.

CLINICAL CLUE

Airway Is King

Patients with an altered mental status are at risk of losing their normal protective airway reflexes. Be wary of the patient who suddenly has difficulty swallowing or managing his own oral secretions. Obese patients with altered mental status should be positioned with the head of the bed elevated to prevent airway obstruction by the tongue. The airway should be kept open manually with a head-tilt/chin-lift or a jaw-thrust maneuver, if necessary. Vomiting and secretions should be suctioned immediately to prevent their inhalation into the lungs. When breathing appears inadequate, assist ventilations with a bag-mask and supplemental oxygen. Use of an oropharyngeal airway (OPA) or nasopharyngeal airway (NPA) is recommended when bag-mask ventilation is required.

20-13 Describe the elements of the Glasgow Coma Scale and how it is applied to the assessment of a patient with altered mental status.

Glasgow Coma Scale

The **Glasgow Coma Scale (GCS)** is a widely used method of evaluating and quantifying a patient's mental status (Figure 20-2 ■). The patient is rated in three categories related to neurological function: eye opening, verbal response, and motor response. A GCS score can range from a low of 3 (bad) to a high of 15 (good). The GCS can be used as a neurological assessment tool for all patients, regardless of medical or trauma classification.

Glasgow Coma Scale (GCS) a widely used, objective scale for rating a patient's level of responsiveness.

20-3 Describe the common signs and symptoms of altered mental status.

Glasgow Coma Scale	
Eye Opening	
Spontaneous	4
To verbal command	3
To pain	2
No response	1
Verbal Response	
Oriented and converses	5
Disoriented and converses	4
Inappropriate words	3
Incomprehensible sounds	2
No response	1
Motor Response	
Obeys verbal commands	6
Localizes pain	5
Withdraws from pain (flexion)	4
Abnormal flexion in response to pain (decorticate rigidity)	3
Extension in response to pain (decerebrate rigidity)	2
No response	1

Figure 20-2 The Glasgow Coma Scale is used to evaluate the responsiveness of a patient with altered mental status.

Signs and Symptoms of AMS

In many cases, the cause of altered mental status will be readily apparent. However, you must consider that it might be due to injury by looking for outward signs of visible trauma. Remember to check for deformity, swelling of the head, and ecchymosis around the eyes and behind the ears, if head injury is suspected. Always consider the risk of secondary trauma in cases of patients with a medical cause for altered mental status, who are then injured as they collapse to the ground. It is essential to obtain a history when possible. Begin with the patient and seek additional history from family members, bystanders, and caregivers when possible. The following is a list of some of the more common signs and symptoms of an altered mental status:

- Decreased level of responsiveness
- Confusion
- Sluggish to respond
- Disorientation
- Asking repeated questions
- Unequal or abnormal pupils
- Obvious signs of injury to the head
- Agitation or unusually violent
- Loss of bowel or bladder control
- Lacerations to the tongue indicating seizure activity

Remember that altered mental status can range from slight confusion to complete unresponsiveness and can get better or worse during your care. Pay close attention to your patient and continually monitor mental status for changes.

Emergency Care of the Patient with AMS

Emergency care of the patient with altered mental status is as follows:

20-6 Describe the emergency care of a patient with altered mental status.

1. Take appropriate BSI precautions.
2. Perform an appropriate primary assessment and provide the necessary airway and breathing support.
3. Maintain spinal precautions if trauma is suspected.
4. Utilize an airway adjunct when appropriate.
5. Suction as necessary to keep the airway clear.
6. Provide oxygen as necessary to maintain SpO_2 at $\geq$94%.
7. Provide positive pressure ventilations if breathing becomes inadequate.
8. Check a blood glucose level on all patients with an altered mental status, including trauma patients, if permitted to do so by local protocols.
9. Place nontrauma patients in the recovery position for ease of airway control during transport.
10. Consider the need for ALS intercept as guided by local protocols.

STOP, REVIEW, REMEMBER!

Multiple Choice

For each question, place a check next to the correct answer.

1. The first assessment of a patient's mental status should be conducted during which segment of the patient assessment?

_____ a. Scene size-up
_____ b. Primary assessment
_____ c. SAMPLE history
_____ d. Secondary assessment

2. Which one of the following is *not* one of the characteristics measured by the Glasgow Coma Scale?

_____ a. Eye opening
_____ b. Verbal response
_____ c. Motor response
_____ d. Grip strength

3. A patient who opens his eyes only when you speak to him, appears disoriented, and withdraws from pain, would have a Glasgow Coma Scale score of:

_____ a. 11.
_____ b. 9.
_____ c. 7.
_____ d. 5.

4. Which one of the following best describes how often vital signs should be repeated on an unresponsive patient?

_____ a. Only once
_____ b. Every 15 minutes
_____ c. Every 5 minutes
_____ d. Twice

5. You are caring for a patient who responds only to painful stimuli. Respirations are 8 and shallow and the pulse is 88 strong and regular. You should:

_____ a. hold manual stabilization of the head and neck.
_____ b. provide oxygen by nasal cannula at 6 L/minute.
_____ c. provide oxygen by nonrebreather mask at 15 L/minute.
_____ d. provide ventilations with a bag-mask device.

(continued on next page)

(continued)

Fill in the GCS Score

For each of the following patient descriptions, identify the appropriate GCS score.

1. Your patient is a 22-year-old man who is awake and his eyes are open. He is confused and is only able to tell you where he hurts. ______________________________

2. Your patient is a 45-year-old woman who responds only to pain by opening her eyes, is moaning, and withdraws from your painful stimulus.
____

3. Your patient is a 76-year-old woman who appears unconscious and does not open her eyes. She offers no verbal response to your questions and offers no motor response. ______________________________

Critical Thinking

1. Describe at least six common causes of altered mental status.
____
____
____
____

2. Discuss why a patient with an altered mental status would or would not be considered a high-priority patient.
____
____
____
____

3. Discuss why the position of the patient with an altered mental status is so important during transport.
____
____
____
____

The Stroke Patient

stroke a condition that occurs when the blood supply to an area of the brain is interrupted. Also called *cerebral vascular accident* and *brain attack.*

Another patient who is seen fairly regularly in the prehospital setting and who presents with an altered mental status is the patient who has suffered a **stroke** (also called a *cerebral vascular accident* or *brain attack*). Strokes often occur with little warning. They can produce a range of effects from mild signs and symptoms lasting minutes or hours to severe signs and symptoms such as unresponsiveness and respiratory arrest. Stroke is the third leading cause of death in the United States and is the number one cause of disability.

A stroke occurs when the blood supply to an area of the brain is interrupted. The interruption can be the result of a blocked artery (ischemic stroke) or a ruptured artery (hemorrhagic stroke). Ischemic strokes are far more common than hemorrhagic strokes. Blood flow also can be interrupted from pressure on the surface of the brain caused by bleeding in the skull or from the formation of a tumor. Because of the way nerve paths from the brain cross, a stroke affecting one side of the brain will cause symptoms, such as weakness or paralysis, on the opposite side of the body.

Presenting signs and symptoms of a stroke may differ, depending on the location of the stroke within the brain, so it is helpful to recall the brain's three major components: the cerebrum, the cerebellum, and the brainstem. Most strokes occur within the cerebral hemispheres. The two cerebral hemispheres make up the largest part of the brain, while the brainstem is the lower section connected to the spinal cord. The cerebellum sits superior and posterior to the brainstem (Figure 20-3 ■).

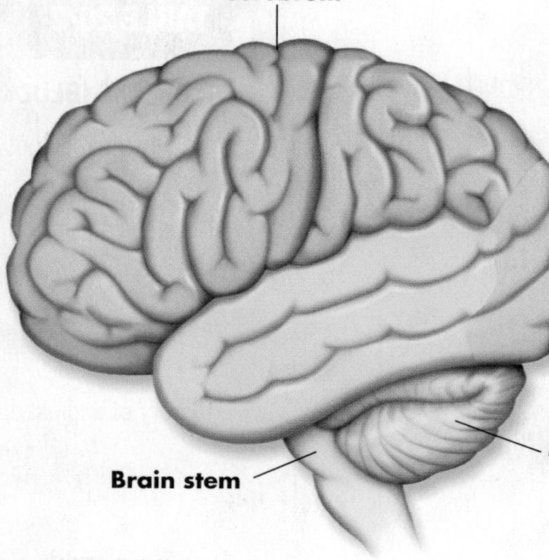

Figure 20-3 The structures of the brain and brainstem.

Risk Factors for Stroke

Several medical conditions and behaviors can be elicited from the patient history to help identify the patient with increased risk for stroke. Among them are abnormal heart rhythms, hypertension (HTN), diabetes mellitus, high red blood cell count, prior history of transient ischemic attack (TIA) or stroke, and smoking. Risk factors that cannot be controlled include gender, age, race, and heredity.

20-7 List common risk factors for stroke.

Signs and Symptoms of a Stroke

Patients who have suffered a stroke may present with some or all of the following signs and symptoms:

20-9 Describe the signs and symptoms of stroke.

- Altered mental status up to and including unresponsiveness
- **Hemiparesis** (weakness on one side of the body)
- **Hemiplegia** (paralysis of one side of the body)
- Asymmetry of facial muscles (facial droop)
- Difficulty swallowing
- **Dysphasia** (slurred or garbled speech)
- Unequal or sluggish pupils
- Blurred or double vision
- Sudden, severe headache
- **Aphasia** (difficulty understanding or expressing words)
- Nausea or vomiting
- Dizziness
- Loss of bladder or bowel control
- Unstable gait
- Seizures

hemiparesis weakness on one side of the body.

hemiplegia paralysis of one side of the body.

dysphasia a condition in which a patient is not able to generate clear and understandable speech.

aphasia a condition in which the patient loses the ability to understand or express speech.

Stroke Classification

The severity of the stroke depends on many factors, including the location within the brain, the size of the artery affected, the age of the patient, and the root cause of the stroke. Strokes are classified as either ischemic strokes or hemorrhagic strokes.

20-8 Describe the pathophysiology of stroke and distinguish between ischemic stroke and hemorrhagic stroke.

TABLE 20-2 COMPARISON OF STROKES

ISCHEMIC (BLOCKAGE) MOST COMMON	HEMORRHAGIC (RUPTURE) LESS COMMON
Usually the result of atherosclerosis	Usually the result of hypertension, cerebral aneurysm, or vessel malformation
Develops abruptly	Develops abruptly
Long history of risk factors	Commonly occurs during stress or exercise
Associated with atrial fibrillation	Associated with cocaine use and prescribed blood thinners
History of angina, previous strokes	Often shows no symptoms before rupture

Ischemic strokes are far more common than hemorrhagic strokes. Generally speaking, hemorrhagic strokes tend to produce the most severe symptoms and have the poorest outcomes for the patient (Table 20-2).

Ischemic Stroke

ischemic stroke the most common kind of stroke; caused by an interruption in the flow of blood to the brain by a blocked vessel.

embolism a clot, particle, or air bubble that travels from its original site to another location in the body.

thrombus a blood clot that forms in a vessel and remains there.

An **ischemic stroke** is usually caused by an **embolism** or **thrombus** that blocks an artery in the brain, which then prevents a portion of brain tissue from receiving oxygen and nutrients (Figure 20-4 ▪). Ischemic strokes account for 85% of all strokes. It is the only type of stroke that may be potentially treated with "clot-busting" drugs called *fibrinolytics*. Although usually caused by a thrombus (a blood clot that forms in one place), an ischemic stroke also can be caused by an embolism, which can be a clot, particle, or air bubble that travels from another part of the body to the small vessels of the brain creating a blockage.

Carotid Artery Blockage

Strokes can occur from a blockage in the carotid arteries of the neck. The carotid arteries feed the cerebral hemispheres of the brain and the retinas of the eye. Symptoms from blockage of a retinal artery include darkened vision, diminished night vision, and temporary loss of vision in one eye. When a cerebral hemisphere is affected, signs and symptoms can include speech problems, partial and temporary paralysis on one side of the body, facial droop, or numbness and tingling on one side of the body. Patients may experience difficulty speaking or understanding and occasionally exhibit seizures.

Basilar Artery Blockage

basilar artery an artery arising from the vertebral arteries of the spine at the base of the skull.

The **basilar artery** arises from the vertebral arteries of the spine at the base of the skull. Both cerebral hemispheres and the cerebellum can be affected from a basilar artery blockage and present the following range of signs and symptoms: reduced vision, nausea, vomiting, dizziness, difficulty swallowing, difficulty walking, posterior headache, and numbness and tingling of the mouth or face. Weakness of the arms and legs can sometimes cause a sudden fall. Brainstem involvement means the patient's vital functions related to heart rate, breathing, and blood pressure may be affected, even while speech and understanding remain undisturbed.

Hemorrhagic Stroke

hemorrhagic stroke stroke caused by a ruptured blood vessel.

intracerebral hemorrhage bleeding within the brain matter.

subarachnoid hemorrhage bleeding into the cerebrospinal fluid surrounding the brain.

A **hemorrhagic stroke** is caused by a ruptured blood vessel. An **intracerebral hemorrhage** occurs in the brain matter itself. A **subarachnoid hemorrhage** refers to bleeding into the cerebrospinal fluid (CSF) that surrounds the brain (Figure 20-5 ▪).

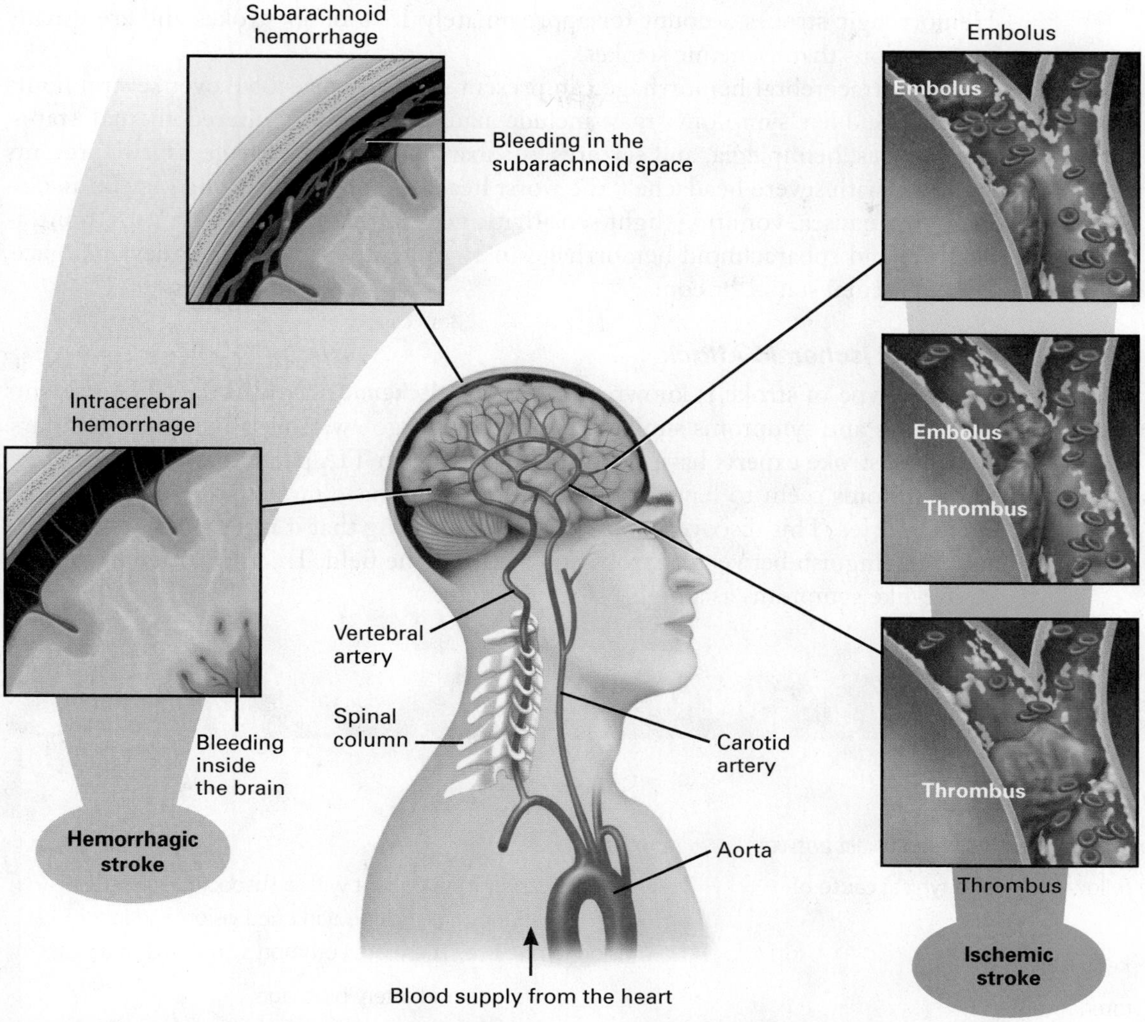

Figure 20-4 A hemorrhagic stroke occurs when a cerebral artery ruptures and spills blood into the brain or areas around the brain. An ischemic stroke occurs when a cerebral artery becomes blocked either by a thrombus or an embolism.

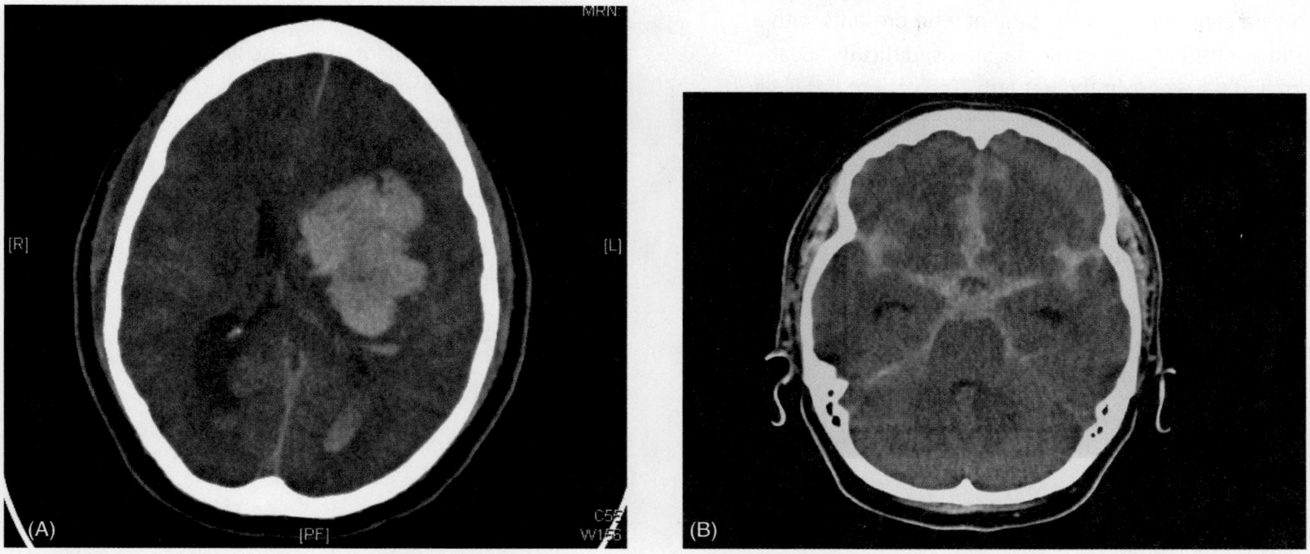

Figure 20-5 (A) An intracerebral hemorrhage as seen on a CAT scan. (© Edward T. Dickinson, MD) (B) A subarachnoid hemorrhage as seen on a CAT scan. (© Edward T. Dickinson, MD)

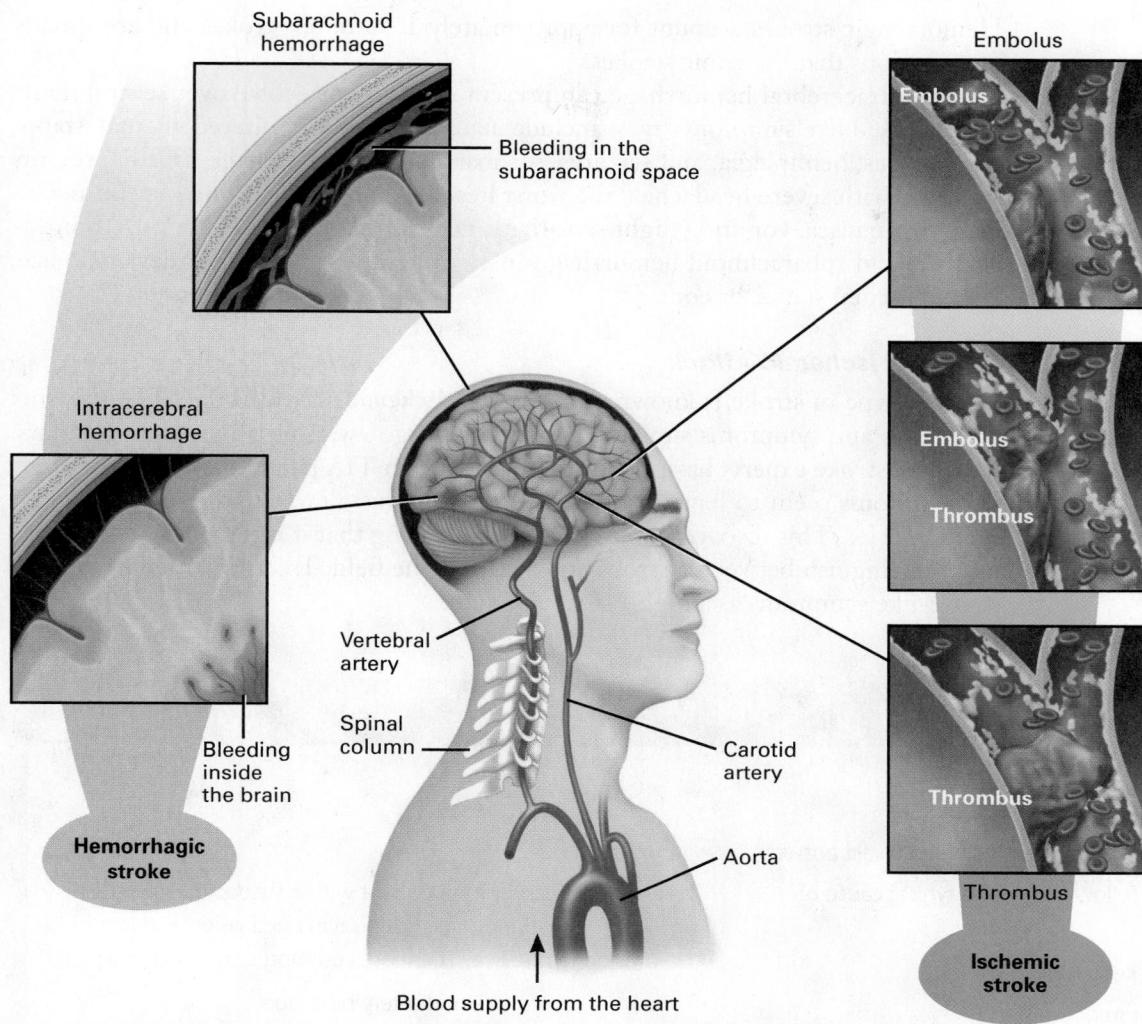

Hemorrhagic strokes account for approximately 15% of all strokes and are usually more serious than ischemic strokes.

occult refers to something that is hidden, such as bleeding within the skull.

An intracerebral hemorrhage can present suddenly or evolve over several hours (**occult**). Sudden symptoms may include nausea, vomiting, altered mental status, hemiparesis, hemiplegia, and seizures. A subarachnoid hemorrhage usually presents suddenly with severe headache ("the worst headache of my life"), and may be associated with nausea, vomiting, light sensitivity, neck stiffness, and seizures. Both intracerebral and subarachnoid hemorrhages may present with a fixed or deviated gaze, altered mental status, or coma.

Transient Ischemic Attack

20-10 Describe the relationship between stroke and transient ischemic attack.

transient ischemic attack (TIA) a condition for which signs and symptoms similar to a stroke go away, usually within 24 hours.

Another type of stroke is known as a **transient ischemic attack (TIA).** A TIA presents with signs and symptoms similar to a stroke that go away, usually within 24 hours. Recently, stroke experts have discovered that certain TIA patients whose neurological symptoms seem to have resolved within hours have in fact suffered permanent brain injuries. This discovery reinforces your training that it is not your responsibility to distinguish between a stroke and a TIA in the field. Treat all patients with any stroke-like symptoms as a high-priority patient.

STOP, REVIEW, REMEMBER!

Multiple Choice

For each question, place a check next to the correct answer.

1. Which one of the following is *not* a typical cause of stroke?

    _____ a. Blocked artery
    _____ b. Ruptured artery
    _____ c. Dilated artery
    _____ d. Pressure on an artery

2. You are caring for an adult patient who presents with a sudden onset of altered mental status, difficulty speaking, and weakness in the left arm. The patient has likely suffered a stroke to the:

    _____ a. brainstem.
    _____ b. right hemisphere.
    _____ c. left hemisphere.
    _____ d. cerebellum.

3. The majority of all strokes are the result of:

    _____ a. ischemia.
    _____ b. hemorrhage.
    _____ c. aneurysm.
    _____ d. tumor.

4. You are caring for a patient with a suspected stroke. Her signs and symptoms include darkened vision and loss of vision in one eye. These are common symptoms of a:

    _____ a. carotid artery blockage.
    _____ b. transient ischemic attack.
    _____ c. hemorrhagic stroke.
    _____ d. retinal artery blockage.

5. You are caring for a patient who describes having a temporary weakness in his left arm and leg and slurred speech that resolved within an hour. This patient likely experienced a:

    _____ a. transient stroke.
    _____ b. subarachnoid bleed.
    _____ c. minor stroke.
    _____ d. transient ischemic attack.

Critical Thinking

1. Describe the difference in pathophysiology between an ischemic and a hemorrhagic stroke.

2. Differentiate the signs and symptoms of a stroke and transient ischemic attack.

Assessment of the Stroke Patient

20-11 Describe an assessment-based approach to stroke and transient ischemic attack.

Your assessment of the suspected stroke patient will differ slightly, depending on the patient's level of responsiveness. Make every effort to obtain a thorough history directly from the patient whenever possible. If the patient is unable to communicate, obtain the history from a family member, caregiver, or bystander. Be sure to ask exactly when the symptoms began. Determining and documenting the exact time of onset of stroke symptoms is critical information that the emergency department staff will need to know. Knowing when the symptoms first appeared will determine if the patient is able to receive specialized treatment. You must perform a thorough secondary assessment looking for signs of weakness or paralysis on one side of the body.

Unresponsive Patient

Many unresponsive patients will be found lying down. If not, then have him lie down to avoid falls. Be sure to rule out any possibility of spine injury before moving the patient. If he is lying face down, carefully roll him over and begin your primary assessment.

As with any patient, focus on the adequacy of the airway and respirations. Take your time as you look, listen, and feel for breathing and carefully assess both rate and tidal volume. If there is any doubt as to the adequacy of respirations, assist the patient's respirations and provide suction as necessary.

There are typically few signs in the unresponsive stroke patient that will reveal what is going on. For this reason, the best you can do is gather as much history as you can from family members, caregivers, or bystanders. Do not waste valuable time at the scene. The patients must be considered high priority and should be transported immediately to an appropriate receiving facility.

When transporting a possible stroke patient, provide the hospital with as much advance notice as possible. They may have to activate a specialized stroke team to care for the patient upon arrival.

Responsive Patient

Strokes are sudden and quiet events that often are unnoticed or are blamed on other conditions. In many instances, the patient remains awake and somewhat alert. An example is the husband and wife who are enjoying some quiet time together watching television. The wife decides to go into the kitchen to make some lunch. When she returns a few minutes later, she finds her husband sitting just as she had left him, but he is unable to respond to her. He is able to look at her and makes attempts to speak but can only produce garbled or slurred words that do not make sense.

Upon arrival, you will likely find a somewhat alert patient with a worried or frightened look on his face. Once you are certain that the ABCs are intact, focus your attention on your secondary assessment. Begin assessing for signs of stroke. Use the Cincinnati Prehospital Stroke Scale, if appropriate (see below). Note any difference in sensation and motor function from one side to the other. A new onset of weakness may be an indication of a stroke on the opposite side of the brain. Look closely at the pupils and note any differences between them. In some victims of stroke, the affected pupil will become sluggish, unresponsive, or dilated.

20-14 Describe ways of communicating with patients who have difficulty speaking.

It is important to understand the fear and frustration that responsive stroke patients are experiencing. They know something is terribly wrong but are unable to communicate well or ask questions about what is going on. For this reason be sure to communicate continuously with your patient and explain everything that is happening. Provide lots of reassurance to both the patient and family members who are present.

20-12 Describe the use of the Cincinnati Prehospital Stroke Scale.

Speak directly to the patient and look him in the eyes as you do so. Be patient and wait for any response that he is able to generate. Acknowledge that he is having difficulty speaking and that you will keep him aware of what is going on. It can be very difficult and frustrating trying to get a history from a patient suffering a stroke, even when he appears to be responsive.

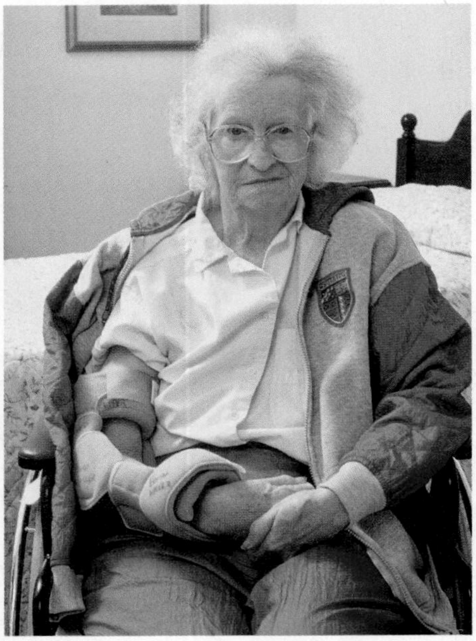

Figure 20-6 Facial droop caused by a loss of nerve stimulus to the facial muscles on one side of the face can be a sign of stroke.

Cincinnati Prehospital Stroke Scale

There are several assessment tools that can be helpful when assessing a responsive patient suspected of having a stroke. One of the most common is the Cincinnati Prehospital Stroke Scale (CPSS). The CPSS uses three assessment characteristics to evaluate for the likelihood of a stroke. They are as follows:

- ***Facial droop.*** Have the patient look directly at you and smile or show his teeth. Observe if the facial muscles do not move symmetrically or if there is drooping on one side or the other (Figure 20-6 ▪).
- ***Arm drift.*** Have the patient hold both arms straight out in front of him and close his eyes. Observe for arm drift (one arm that drops down while the other remains up). It is also significant if the patient cannot bring both arms up together (Figure 20-7 ▪).
- ***Abnormal speech.*** Ask the patient to repeat a simple phrase or recite the alphabet. Observe for slurred speech, inappropriate words, or an inability to respond verbally.

Presence of an abnormality in any one of the three areas of the CPSS indicates a strong likelihood of a stroke.

PRACTICAL PATHOPHYSIOLOGY

The brain must receive a constant supply of oxygen and glucose in order to maintain normal function. When a vessel ruptures, the area of the brain that was being fed by the vessel begins to starve for blood, oxygen, and glucose. Depending on the specific area of the brain affected, the specific signs and symptoms will vary. Remember that nerve pathways cross over from one side of the body to the other high up in the cervical spine. For this reason a stroke on the left side of the brain will affect the right side of the body.

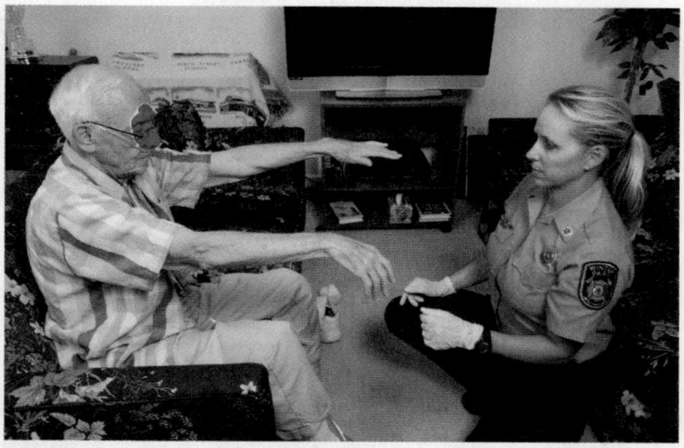

Figure 20-7 The inability to hold both arms out in front (arm drift) may be a sign of stroke.

Emergency Care of the Stroke Patient

20-15 Describe the appropriate care for a patient with a suspected stroke.

The following steps should be followed when caring for a person with a suspected stroke (Scan 20-1):

1. Take appropriate BSI precautions.
2. Perform a primary assessment and provide the necessary airway and breathing support.
3. Use the Cincinnati Stroke Scale or other approved tool to help assess the patient.
4. Provide supplemental oxygen as appropriate, and check glucose level if allowed to do so.
5. Perform an appropriate secondary assessment based on the chief complaint, including determining the time of onset of symptoms.
6. Keep the responsive patient lying flat and have suction ready to help maintain a clear airway. Place the unresponsive patient in the recovery position for airway control.
7. Initiate transport to the nearest stroke center. Provide an early alert of "stroke notification," giving the time of symptom onset.
8. Perform reassessments as necessary and focus on adequacy of airway and breathing.

CLINICAL CLUE

Fibrinolytics

Recent advances in stroke care include the development of clot-busting drugs called *fibrinolytics*. Such drugs can break up the clot that is causing the disruption of blood flow in the brain. Not all stroke patients are candidates, but one thing is certain: The sooner a suspected stroke patient gets to the hospital, the sooner he can be evaluated for the use of fibrinolytics.

The general rule is that a patient must receive these drugs within three hours following the initial onset of symptoms. However, a patient must be evaluated with a CT scan of the head to ensure that there is no hemorrhagic stroke.

There is new evidence that some patients may benefit from receiving fibrinolytics even up to four and a half hours after onset of symptoms. Eligibility will be determined by the receiving facility, so rapid transport is still indicated even outside the three-hour window.

SCAN 20-1 Assessment and Care of the Stroke Patient

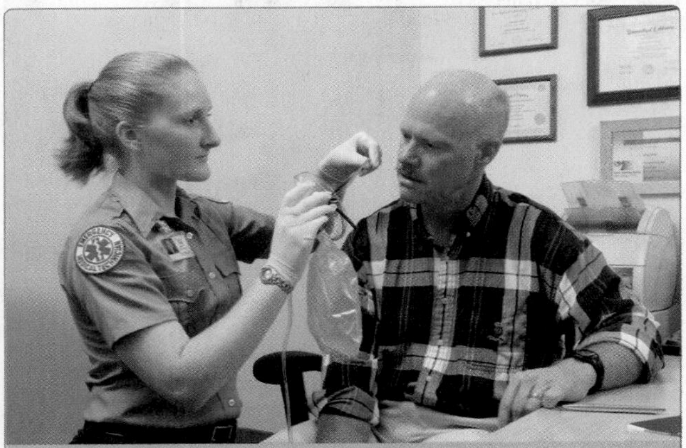

20-1-1 Maintain an oxygen saturation between 94% and 99%.

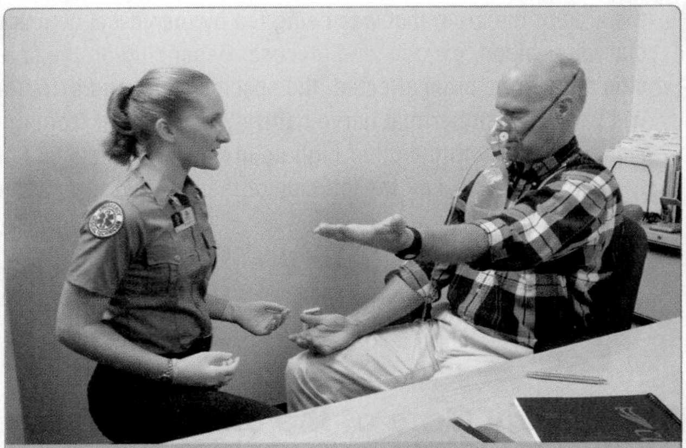

20-1-2 Perform an appropriate secondary assessment, including the Cincinnati Prehospital Stroke Scale or similar tool.

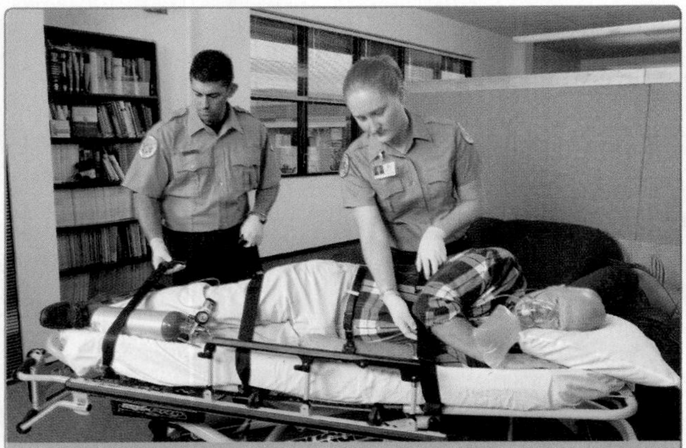

20-1-3 Place the patient in the recovery position for transport.

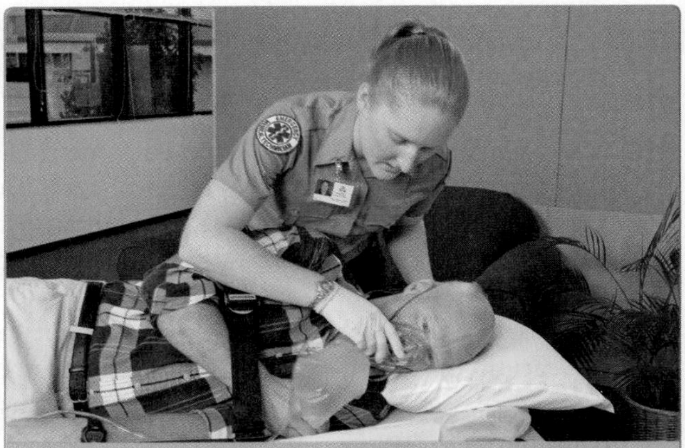

20-1-4 Reassess the ABCs continuously throughout transport.

CLINICAL CLUE

Neurointervention

A relatively new approach to stroke care is the use of catheterization procedures at a specialized stroke center known as a *neurointerventional lab*. Both ischemic and hemorrhagic strokes may be effectively treated this way. A blocked cerebral artery may be stented open in a way similar to a cardiac stent procedure in a heart catheterization lab, and a ruptured vessel may be repaired. The decision to treat stroke at a neurointerventional lab as opposed to more traditional methods is dependent on availability and physician and patient preference.

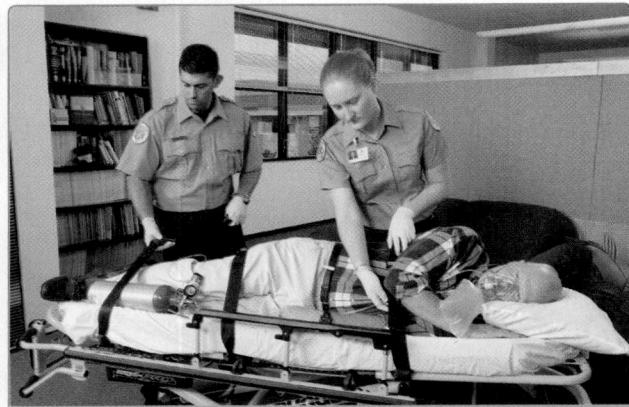

The Headache Patient

The patient with a chief complaint of headache can be challenging for the EMT. The wide variety of possible causes and presentations makes it difficult to identify an exact cause. Headaches may occur as an isolated condition or as an ominous sign of a much more serious problem such as a stroke, infection, or tumor.

20-17 Recognize indications that a headache may have a potentially life-threatening underlying cause, such as toxic exposure, hypertension, infectious disease, or hemorrhagic stroke.

Headache Classifications

20-16 Describe the common classifications of headache.

A **migraine** is a type of headache that appears to be caused by spasm of the cranial vessels and often results in a throbbing pain, sensitivity to light (photosensitivity), sweating, nausea, and vomiting. Many migraine headache sufferers report visual disturbances or other odd symptoms referred to as an **aura** just prior to the onset of the migraine. High blood pressure (hypertension) can be a cause of vascular headaches, especially when the diastolic blood pressure is elevated.

Cluster headaches also may have a vascular origin, but the intense pain is typically "clustered" to one area of the head or face, often centered behind one eye. Symptoms that may typically accompany cluster headaches are nausea, vomiting, and facial tenderness. Affected patients may exhibit runny nose, tearing, or eyelid drooping.

Tension headaches are one of the most common types of headaches. The onset is typically gradual and is caused by muscle tension, leading to aching or a squeezing pressure in the frontal, temporal, and occipital regions of the head. The pain often radiates to the neck and shoulders.

Organic headache, traction headache, or **inflammatory headache** are symptoms of an associated neurological problem such as hemorrhagic stroke, meningitis, or tumor.

Of course, as an EMT you are not expected to determine the exact cause of a patient's headache. However, knowing the pathophysiology behind some of the common causes of headaches may enhance your ability to assess patients who present with a chief complaint of headache.

migraine severe, throbbing headache often characterized initially by an aura and accompanied by sensitivity to light, sweating, nausea, and vomiting. Also called *vascular headache*.

aura a particular symptom experienced just prior to the onset of a migraine or seizure; often manifested as a strange light, unpleasant smell or taste, or strange thoughts.

cluster headache intense pain typically "clustered" or confined to one area of the head or face that may be accompanied by nausea, vomiting, and facial tenderness.

tension headaches pain that has a gradual onset caused by muscle tension that leads to a "squeezing" sensation in various regions of the head, often radiating to the neck and shoulders.

organic headache a symptom of an associated neurological problem such as hemorrhagic stroke, meningitis, or tumor.

traction headache a symptom of an associated neurological problem such as hemorrhagic stroke, meningitis, or tumor.

inflammatory headache a symptom of an associated neurological problem such as hemorrhagic stroke, meningitis, or tumor.

Assessment of the Patient with Headache

Your assessment of the patient should begin with an assessment of the surroundings that may reveal a likely cause of the headache. Conduct a thorough history and pain evaluation using the OPQRST assessment tool. Pain often increases heart rate and blood pressure, but beware that an altered mental status and other significant neurological changes could indicate a serious underlying condition. Watch for behavioral changes and assess for motor or sensory deficits, including a change in vision. Remain alert for the possibility of seizures.

Fever or stiff neck may be a sign of possible meningitis. Protect yourself in this case by donning a mask, and placing one on your patient as well. Elicit further information about others in the household who have been ill or exposed. Advise the receiving hospital of your concern for meningitis, so they can also prepare to protect their staff and other patients from possible exposure.

Emergency Care of the Headache Patient

20-18 Describe the appropriate emergency medical care for a patient suffering from headache.

Because a headache can herald the presence of a more serious condition, the patient with headache requires appropriate monitoring. Reassessments are helpful to identify a change in mental status early. Simple measures to reduce muscle tension and pain include providing a comfortable temperature en route to the hospital and offering to cover the eyes of the photosensitive patient. Emergency medical care should include the following:

1. Take appropriate BSI precautions.
2. Perform a primary assessment and provide the necessary airway and breathing support.

3. Administer oxygen as appropriate.
4. Place the patient in a position of comfort and transport.
5. Monitor airway and breathing throughout transport and provide reassurance.

EMERGENCY DISPATCH SUMMARY

The patient was secured to a long backboard, given supplemental oxygen, and transported with lights and siren to the University Trauma Center downtown. There, he was found to have a skull fracture and some intracranial bleeding. He has since made a full recovery but still has no recollection about the events of that night.

Chapter Review

To the Point

- One of the biggest challenges for the EMT is the fact that there are so many potential causes of altered mental status. Your priority will be managing the ABCs and obtaining the best possible history from the patient, family, or bystanders at the scene.
- Signs of altered mental status include a decreased level of responsiveness, confusion, slow to respond, abnormal behavior, and disorientation, just to name a few.
- Your assessment should focus on obtaining a history of the onset of symptoms and the activities that occurred prior to onset. Obtaining a thorough past medical history also may reveal clues to the cause of the problem.
- Patients with altered mental status are at greater risk for airway compromise, so it is essential that you provide airway support as needed.
- Look for clues at the scene as well as clues during your secondary assessment to the possible causes of the altered mental status.
- Speak slowly and clearly to help ensure the patient understands your questions. Continually provide reassurance.
- In the case of a suspected stroke, it will be especially important to determine the exact time of symptom onset and transport to an appropriate stroke center when possible.

Chapter Questions

Multiple Choice

1. The condition caused by interruption of blood flow to the brain from a ruptured artery is known as a(n):

_____ a. embolic stroke.
_____ b. hemorrhagic stroke.
_____ c. syncopal episode.
_____ d. transient ischemic attack.

2. Which one of the following is *not* one of the assessment findings in the Cincinnati Prehospital Stroke Scale?

_____ a. Facial droop
_____ b. Arm drift
_____ c. Headache
_____ d. Abnormal speech

3. It is essential to report the time of stroke symptom onset to the receiving facility, so that the patient can:
_____ a. be taken to surgery.
_____ b. receive fibrinolytic therapy.
_____ c. receive physical therapy.
_____ d. be intubated.

4. Fibrinolytics are most effective when they can be administered within _____________ hours following the onset of stroke symptoms.
_____ a. 3
_____ b. 6
_____ c. 9
_____ d. 12

5. Common types of classic isolated headaches include:
_____ a. migraines.
_____ b. syncopal headaches.
_____ c. hemorrhagic headaches.
_____ d. seizure headaches.

6. You arrive to find a patient who appears to have suffered a stroke. She is unresponsive with snoring respirations. You should:
_____ a. take spinal precautions.
_____ b. perform a secondary assessment.
_____ c. open the airway.
_____ d. provide oxygen.

7. A patient who experienced a sudden onset of weakness on the right side and slurred speech for a period of about an hour, has likely experienced a:
_____ a. syncopal episode.
_____ b. hemorrhagic stroke.
_____ c. temporary stroke.
_____ d. transient ischemic attack.

8. You arrive to find an approximately 50-year-old woman lying in bed, unable to speak and with gurgling respirations. You should:
_____ a. perform a Cincinnati Prehospital Stroke Scale assessment.
_____ b. suction the airway.
_____ c. apply oxygen by nasal cannula.
_____ d. obtain vital signs.

9. You are caring for a responsive patient with signs and symptoms of a stroke who has a patent airway and normal breathing. The ideal position for transport is:
_____ a. the recovery position.
_____ b. Fowler's position
_____ c. semi-Fowler's position.
_____ d. supine.

10. You have responded to an 88-year-old patient with a gradual onset of confusion over the past several hours. Which assessment finding would concern you most?
_____ a. Blood pressure of 196/106
_____ b. Blood glucose level of 82 mg/dL
_____ c. Heart rate of 72 and regular
_____ d. Pupils equal and reactive

Critical Thinking

1. Describe the assessment and care of the stroke patient.

____
____
____
____

2. Describe the care you would provide a patient who presents with signs and symptoms of a severe migraine.

____
____
____
____

Case Studies

Case Study 1

You have been dispatched to an office building for an unknown medical problem. Upon arrival, you are led to an approximately 40-year-old woman who is lying under a desk with her head supported. She grimaces with pain, saying she has a throbbing headache and the light is making it worse. A coworker tells you that she came by her friend's desk to go to lunch and found her lying down. As you speak with the patient, you learn her mother has a history of disabling migraine headaches. The patient reports she personally has never had one this bad. Her heart rate and blood pressure are elevated and she says she doesn't want to talk or move.

1. What further information will you attempt to gather from the patient or her friend?

2. The patient is alert, oriented, and has not lost consciousness. She reports seeing halos around objects right before the headache started. What is most likely this woman's problem?

3. How will you continue to care for this patient?

Case Study 2

You have responded to an assisted-living facility for a possible stroke and arrive to find an approximately 80-year-old woman sitting at a table in the recreation room. The facility manager states that one minute she was playing bridge with her friends at the table and the next she couldn't talk. The patient is awake and appears to be alert. However, she is only able to make garbled sounds as she attempts to speak. You notice that the right side of her mouth has a slight droop and she is moving her left hand but not her right.

1. You decide to assess this woman using the Cincinnati Prehospital Stroke Scale. What factors of this patient's presentation will you be assessing?

2. Based on her presentation, on which side of the brain has the stroke likely occurred?

3. How will you care for this patient?

The Last Word

There are, perhaps, almost as many causes of an altered mental status as there are patients. However, several common causes are seen in EMS, including diabetic emergencies, seizures, strokes, poisoning, and overdose emergencies. While it is not essential for you to identify the specific cause of a patient's altered mental status, it is important to gather as much history as possible before leaving the scene.

The focus of all care when dealing with a patient presenting with an altered mental status is the ABCs. The patient may not be breathing adequately and certainly will be less able to maintain his own airway, especially if he vomits. Continuously monitor the patient's airway and respiratory status, even if he is responsive. Provide supplemental oxygen as soon as is practical, and initiate transport to an appropriate receiving facility.

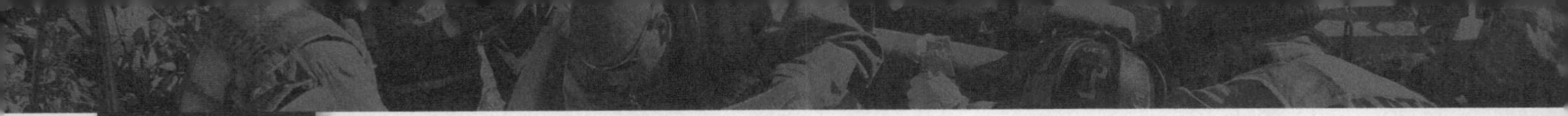

21 Toxicology

Education Standards

Medicine: Toxicology

Competencies

Applies fundamental knowledge to provide basic emergency care and transportation based on assessment findings for an acutely ill patient.

Objectives

After completion of this lesson, you should be able to:

21-1 Define key terms introduced in this chapter.

21-2 List the primary concerns of the EMT in managing toxicological emergencies.

21-3 Describe each of the four routes by which a poison can enter the body: ingestion, inhalation, injection, and absorption.

21-4 Describe the important steps in assessing and managing a poisoning patient, regardless of the specific poison or route of exposure.

21-5 Explain the importance of contacting the poison control center with as complete a patient history as possible, and list specific types of information you should include.

21-6 Explain the limited role of specific antidotes in toxicological emergencies.

21-7 Describe the general steps of assessment-based management of a patient with an ingested poison.

21-8 Describe the indications, contraindications, mechanism of action, side effects, dosage, and administration of activated charcoal.

21-9 Describe the steps of assessment-based management involving a patient who has inhaled a poison.

21-10 Describe the steps of assessment-based management involving a patient who has been exposed to an injected poison.

21-11 Describe the steps of assessment-based management involving a patient who has absorbed a poison.

21-12 Describe the steps of assessment-based management involving a patient experiencing a drug or alcohol emergency.

21-13 Describe special considerations in managing violent drug- or alcohol-abuse patients.

21-14 Describe special considerations in assessing and managing patients with carbon monoxide poisoning and exposure to nerve agents.

Key Terms

absorbed poisons p. 574
activated charcoal p. 563
adsorbs p. 567
alcohol intoxication p. 578
alcohol withdrawal syndrome p. 578
antidote p. 564
chemical asphyxiants p. 570
chronic alcoholics p. 578
delirium tremens (DTs) p. 579
ingested poisons p. 565
inhaled poisons p. 567
injected poisons p. 573
ischemia p. 570
metabolic acidosis p. 570
nerve agents p. 581
poisons p. 561
simple asphyxiants p. 569
supportive care p. 564
toxicology p. 561
toxin p. 564
withdrawal p. 578

Introduction

Poisons (also called *toxins*) are substances that can cause harm to living organisms. The study of the harmful interaction between humans and toxic substances is called **toxicology.**

poisons substances that can harm the body by altering cell function or structure.

toxicology the medical study of toxins and how they affect living organisms.

The environment is filled with thousands of substances that are potentially poisonous. Whether poisonings are accidental or intentional, they can result in a wide spectrum of signs and symptoms from mild nausea and eye irritation to respiratory and cardiac arrest. Consider the following poisoning scenarios:

- An industrial worker is rendered unconscious moments after being exposed to hydrogen sulfide that leaks from a faulty valve at a petrochemical plant.
- A confused elderly patient passes out after accidentally taking three tablets of his heart medication instead of one.
- A young man becomes violent and jumps out of a moving car after he unknowingly smokes marijuana that has been laced with PCP.
- A migrant farmer is found unconscious in the back of his van where he was using a small cooking stove to stay warm overnight.
- A toddler sustains oral burns after eating a handful of crystalline drain cleaner left out by her parents.
- A college student develops nausea, vomiting, and diarrhea two hours after eating at a roadside chicken BBQ stand.

As an EMT you will encounter many poisoning-related emergencies. Your ability to recognize, assess, and treat the patients, while maintaining your own personal safety, will be critical factors in ensuring optimal outcomes.

Poisoning Overview

21-2 List the primary concerns of the EMT in managing toxicological emergencies.

You must learn to recognize when a poisoning has occurred and be prepared to provide the appropriate emergency medical care. However, you must always ensure your own personal safety when you are called to the scene of a poisoning. The substance that made the patient ill could still be present in a quantity or form that poses a threat to you. In addition, a patient who has attempted to commit suicide through the use of a poison may become violent toward those who are attempting to help him.

When confronted with an incident involving a chemical, it may be necessary to request the hazmat team to assess the situation and render the scene safe, even before patients can be accessed and assessed by you. Always size up the scene of a suspected poisoning carefully, and remain alert at all times because they can be dynamic, ever-changing situations.

EMERGENCY DISPATCH

"Please help him!" The woman screamed, clutching at EMT Alexis Berg's arm. "You need to do something!"

"Ma'am," Alexis turned and said sternly. "We're going to do everything that we can, okay? But I need for you to calm down and let me do my job."

The woman's hands slid from Alexis's sleeve and she slumped into a nearby chair, crying.

The two-year-old boy was sobbing and coughing as Alexis and her partner Rob Morrow removed his bleach-soaked clothing and rinsed him with water. "How much do you think he drank?" Rob asked the woman.

"I don't know," she said. "I measured out about one cup and when I turned around he had it in his mouth and all over his clothes." She then dropped her face into her hands and cried, "I don't know what I'll do if he dies!"

"I don't think he's going to die," Rob said soothingly. "But we do need to get him to the hospital right away. Can you help us bring him out to the ambulance?"

"I, I think so," the boy's mother stood, took a deep breath and wiped the tears away from her cheeks.

Portals of Entry

21-3 Describe each of the four routes by which a poison can enter the body: ingestion, inhalation, injection, and absorption.

In order to do harm, a poison must make contact with and enter the body. There are four general routes through which poisons enter the body (Figure 21-1 ■). They are often referred to as *portals of entry*.

- ***Ingestion*** (swallowing). The ingestion of pills or other medications is a common cause of poisoning. Children, especially toddlers, frequently swallow medications and other household substances. Adults who are threatening suicide will intentionally overdose by ingesting multiple pills. Signs and symptoms commonly associated with a poisoning by ingestion include nausea, vomiting, diarrhea, altered mental status, abdominal pain, and possible odor of the substance on the breath. In most cases there is a known or suspected history of poisoning by ingestion reported by family or witnesses. Depending on the substance, there also may be evidence of chemical burns on the lips and mucus membranes of the mouth.
- ***Inhalation*** (breathing). The most common cause of serious inhalation poisoning is carbon monoxide. Other inhaled agents include hydrogen sulfide and cyanide gas, as well as certain chemical nerve agents such as sarin vapor. Signs and symptoms of inhaled substances include difficulty breathing, cough, hoarseness, dizziness, confusion, headache, seizures, and in some cases chest pain.
- ***Injection*** (inserting through the skin through the use of a sharp object). Intravenous drug abuse and the injection of venom by insects (by stingers) and snakes (by fangs) are common types of injection-related poisonings. Common signs and symptoms of a toxic injection include altered mental status, slow or difficulty breathing, dizziness, chills, fever, nausea, and vomiting. In some cases, such as bee stings, severe allergic reactions can occur.
- ***Absorption*** (taking in through the unbroken skin or mucous membranes including the nose, eyes, and mouth). Certain chemicals such as organophosphates, nerve agents, and solvents can be absorbed directly through intact skin and cause poisoning. Other agents cause direct chemical burns to the skin surface. Signs and symptoms include evidence of substance on the skin, redness, burning, itching, and irritation.

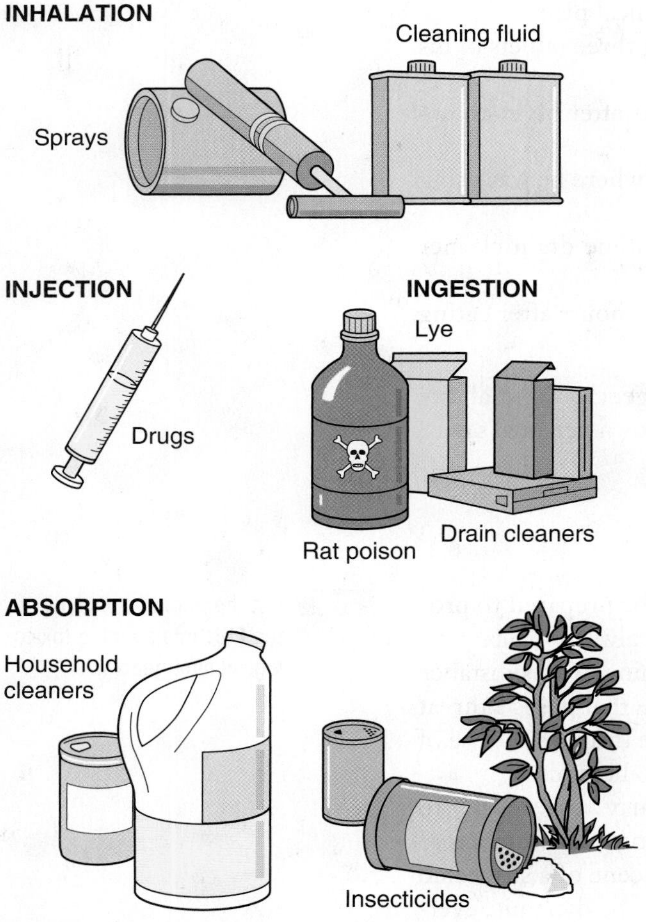

Figure 21-1 Overview of routes of poisoning.

Some substances such as insecticides can enter the body simultaneously by more than one of the routes described above.

Assessment of the Poisoning Patient

A thorough scene size-up is the first step in the assessment of a potential poisoning patient. It is also an essential step in ensuring your personal safety. Remember that inhaled and absorbed poisons that harmed the patient also can pose a risk to your safety and others at the scene. If during the scene size-up you determine the substance that rendered the patient ill is still present and poses a hazard to rescuers, then request a hazardous materials (hazmat) unit be dispatched. Similarly, if the scene appears unsafe due to illicit drug activity, summon law enforcement personnel to secure the scene prior to your entry. Do not enter a scene that you think may be unsafe unless you are properly trained and equipped.

21-4 Describe the important steps in assessing and managing a poisoning patient, regardless of the specific poison or route of exposure.

As with any patient, control of the patient's airway is the top priority during the primary assessment and subsequent care. The airway can be particularly difficult to manage during poisonings. For example, chemical burns may cause swelling of the structures of the upper airway. Poisonings also can lead to excessive secretions that may obstruct the airway. Sudden deterioration of the patient's mental status also can cause the tongue to obstruct the airway.

One of the most important things you can do when assessing a suspected poisoning patient is to obtain a thorough and accurate history. A good history can help medical direction, the poison center, and the emergency department staff make correct and timely decisions about treatment of the patient. Question the patient, family members, or bystanders and try to determine the following:

21-5 Explain the importance of contacting the poison control center with as complete a patient history as possible, and list specific types of information you should include.

- What substance was the source of the poisoning?
- When did the patient ingest or become exposed to the substance?
- How much of the substance did the patient ingest (if an ingestion)?
- Over how long a period was the patient exposed to the substance? Or over how long a period was he ingesting the substance?
- What has been done to help the patient since the poisoning? Has he washed? Has he had milk or water?
- What is the patient's estimated weight?

PERSPECTIVE

Rob—The EMT

I was actually relieved to hear that there had only been one cup of bleach. Although I know he got some in his mouth, with the amount that he had on his clothes and the puddle on the floor, I don't think much could have gone down. It always amazes me the things that kids think would be good to taste. I mean, I take one whiff of bleach and it makes my eyes water and I want to throw up, and yet this isn't the first kid we've responded to who tried drinking it!

Poison Control Centers

Many agencies have protocols that direct emergency medical personnel to contact the local poison control center for any case of suspected poisoning. In such systems, the poison control center is usually allowed to provide medical direction to the EMT, including approval of the use of **activated charcoal.** Poison control centers have been established across the United States and Canada. Most are staffed 24 hours a day and can be reached by way of a toll-free telephone number (800-222-1222). The experienced professionals at the centers have access to information on a wide variety of

activated charcoal a substance that binds with the ingested substance inside the gastrointestinal tract and reduces the amount the body can absorb.

poisons, treatment options, and even potential antidotes. They can answer almost any question about poisoning that you are likely to encounter. Be sure your local poison control center's phone number is easily accessible in your cell phone and aboard every emergency vehicle.

If you call a poison control center, be prepared to provide as much detail as possible about the patient and the circumstances of the poisoning. This will include the following: the patient's estimated age and weight; the patient's condition, including level of responsiveness, skin color, presence or absence of vomiting, and so on; and as many specifics as you can on the poison itself, including product labels or MSDS (material safety data sheet).

21-6 Explain the limited role of specific antidotes in toxicological emergencies.

antidote a substance that will neutralize a poison of its effects.

toxin a noxious or poisonous substance.

Emergency Care of Poisoning Patients

An **antidote** is an agent used to neutralize or counteract the effects of a poison. Despite the impression that may have been imparted by popular media, there are relatively few true antidotes available to the prehospital provider that dramatically reverse the effects of **toxins** in human beings.

21-7 Describe the general steps of assessment-based management of a patient with an ingested poison.

supportive care interventions in cases of poisonings or toxic exposures, such as keeping the airway clear by suctioning, providing supplemental oxygen or ventilation, and treatment for shock.

Although there are some exceptions, as an EMT you will manage most poisonings with what is referred to as **supportive care.** Supportive care means providing care to prevent any further exposure to the poison, keeping the airway open and clearing it with suctioning as needed, giving oxygen, and assisting ventilations for patients with inadequate breathing.

The specific steps in assessing and managing a poisoning or overdose patient will vary, depending in large measure on the route by which the exposure occurred.

STOP, REVIEW, REMEMBER!

Multiple Choice

For each question, place a check next to the correct answer.

1. All of the following are examples of an ingested poisoning *except*:

_____ a. a person who eats spoiled sandwich meat and becomes ill.

_____ b. a person who swallows a handful of prescription drugs.

_____ c. a person who smokes crack cocaine.

_____ d. a toddler who collapses after swallowing his mother's blood pressure pills.

2. A 12-year-old boy is stung by a bee and develops trouble breathing. This is an example of a poisoning by:

_____ a. inhalation.

_____ b. ingestion.

_____ c. absorption.

_____ d. injection.

3. The first priority in the management of the poisoned patient is:

_____ a. administrating activated charcoal.

_____ b. contacting the poison control center.

_____ c. decontamination of the patient.

_____ d. ensuring the safety of you and your crew.

4. Which one of the following is true about supportive care?

_____ a. Is based on the early administration of an antidote specific to the toxic agent encountered

_____ b. Should not be initiated until told to do so by the appropriate poison control center

_____ c. Includes ensuring an open airway, suctioning, and the provision of ventilations if needed

_____ d. Is far less common an EMT intervention than the administration of a specific antidote

Matching

Match the term on the left with the applicable definition on the right.

1. _____ Ingestion
2. _____ Injection
3. _____ Absorption
4. _____ Inhalation

A. Heroin addict uses a needle to "skin pop"
B. Furnace malfunction releases carbon monoxide
C. Suicidal patient swallows a handful of Tylenol®
D. Farmer covered with pesticide powder

Poisoning by Ingestion

Ingested poisons can enter the body accidentally (for example, a toddler eating an entire bottle of colorful, sweet-tasting children's vitamins) or intentionally (a suicidal person taking an overdose of sleeping pills, or a teenager taking illicit drugs to get "high").

ingested poisons poisons that are swallowed.

Signs and Symptoms

Specific signs and symptoms associated with poisoning by ingestion include the following:

- History of ingesting a poisonous substance (gathered from patient, family members, bystanders, or evidence on the scene)
- Nausea
- Vomiting
- Abdominal pain
- Altered mental status
- Chemical burns around and inside the mouth
- Unusual odors on the breath

Emergency Care

The emergency medical care for poisoning by ingestion includes the following steps (Scan 21-1):

1. Ensure scene safety. Take appropriate BSI precautions.
2. Perform a thorough primary assessment.
3. Provide supplemental oxygen, if signs of altered mental status or shortness of breath are present.
4. Ensure adequate breathing. If breathing is inadequate, ventilate using a bag-mask device. (Use of the pocket mask is not generally recommended for ventilating a poisoning patient.)
5. Remove any visible pills, tablets, or fragments from the patient's mouth with a gloved hand. (Do not attempt to remove material from a patient's mouth if there is a risk you will be bitten.)
6. Consult medical direction or poison control center to determine if the administration of activated charcoal is appropriate. If it is, follow the steps for administration of activated charcoal. If administration of activated charcoal is not appropriate, proceed to the next step.

SCAN 21-1 Ingested Poisons

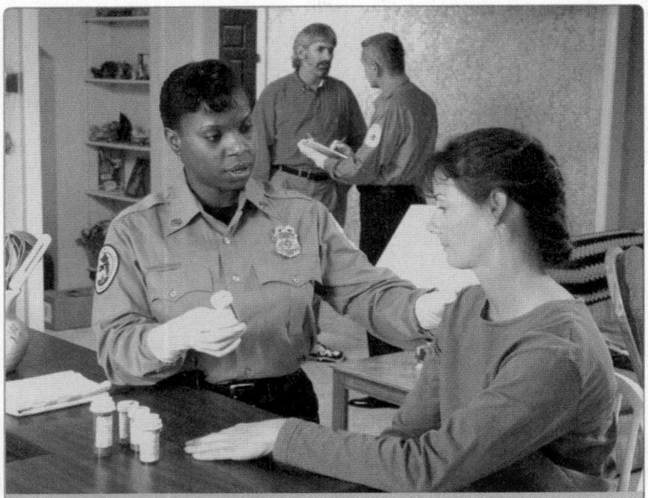

21-1-1 Quickly gather information.

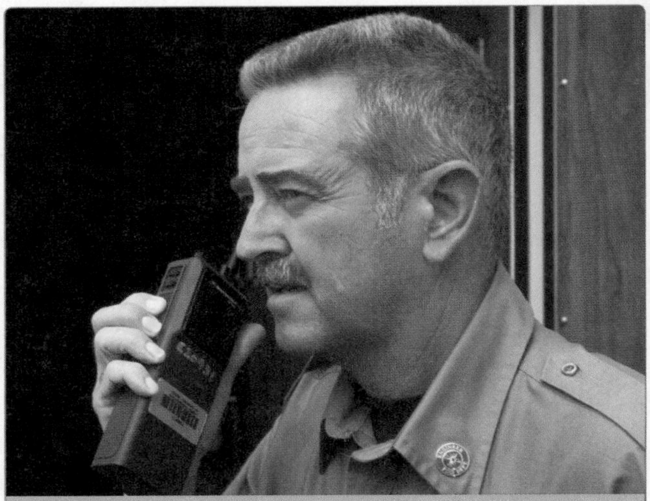

21-1-2 Call medical direction on scene or en route to the hospital.

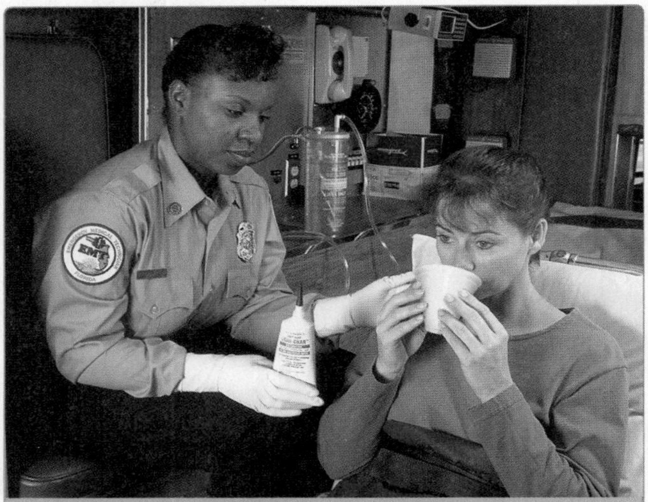

21-1-3 If directed, administer activated charcoal. You may wish to administer it in an opaque cup that has a lid with a hole for a straw.

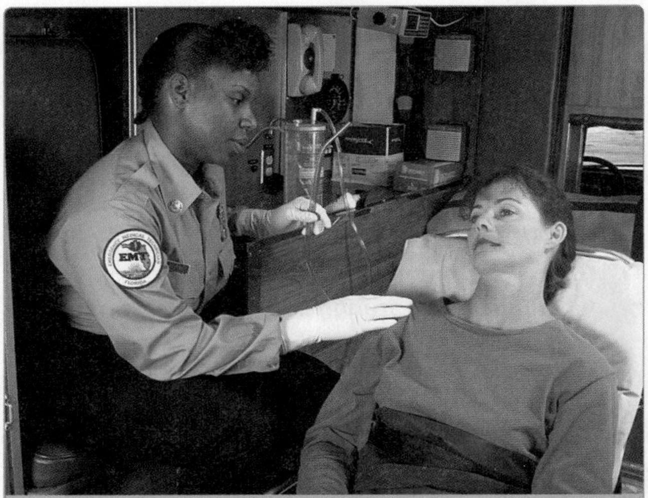

21-1-4 Position the patient for vomiting and save all vomitus. Have suction equipment ready. When a patient has ingested a poison, avoid mouth-to-mouth contact. Provide ventilations by way of a bag-mask device.

7. Complete a thorough secondary assessment as appropriate.
8. Transport the patient with all containers, bottles, and labels from the substance.
9. Perform reassessments en route. Carefully monitor the patient's airway and breathing and be prepared to suction and provide bag-mask ventilations.

PERSPECTIVE

Alexis—The EMT

Boy, sometimes the family members are more difficult to care for than the patients. I mean, I have a little girl myself and I understand the feelings of helplessness when she gets hurt or something, I really do. But I'd never get so upset that I'd make it hard for someone trying to take care of her. Then again it would probably be pretty unbearable if I was the one who accidentally caused the illness or injury, like in this case with her leaving the bleach out and taking her eye off the boy. Maybe you just never know how you're going to react until you get in the situation yourself.

Activated Charcoal

21-8 Describe the indications, contraindications, mechanism of action, side effects, dosage, and administration of activated charcoal.

adsorbs the binding of molecules to a substance such as activated charcoal.

Activated charcoal is sometimes the medication of choice for field and hospital providers for a limited number of poisonings and overdose patients whose portal of entry was ingestion (Scan 21-2). It **adsorbs** (binds) with the ingested substance inside the gastrointestinal tract and reduces the amount the body can absorb. Activated charcoal is particularly effective in binding medications that were very recently ingested in pill form. It is not very effective against most liquid ingestions such as alcohol.

The greatest risk of using activated charcoal is that the patient may vomit and aspirate the material. This is especially likely when an overdose patient who was initially alert and able to drink the charcoal has a sudden decreased mental status and can no longer protect his own airway when he vomits. It is for this reason that the decision to use activated charcoal is based on the specific toxin ingested, how long ago it was ingested, the patient's current mental status, and the likelihood that the substance ingested will result in a sudden decrease in mental status after its administration. Because of those multiple variables, the decision as to whether to use prehospital activated charcoal is usually made by either medical direction or the poison control center. Follow your local treatment protocols.

Poisoning by Inhalation

21-9 Describe the steps of assessment-based management involving a patient who has inhaled a poison.

The initial approach to any toxic inhalation situation is the same. Your safety is paramount. The rescuer is at significant risk to fall victim to the same inhaled agents as the patient. Use of appropriate hazmat resources, personal protective equipment including positive-pressure self-contained breathing apparatus (SCBA), and decontamination measures are mandatory when managing patients with toxic inhalations.

Once the patient is safely accessible to the EMT, the mainstay of patient treatment is supportive care with supplemental oxygen and ventilation assistance with a bag-mask as needed.

Types of Inhalation Poisons

inhaled poisons poisons that are breathed in.

Inhaled poisons can harm patients in a variety of ways. Some agents cause direct irritation and injury to the airway. Other inhaled agents displace oxygen and cause severe disruption at the cellular level of the body.

SCAN 21-2 Activated Charcoal

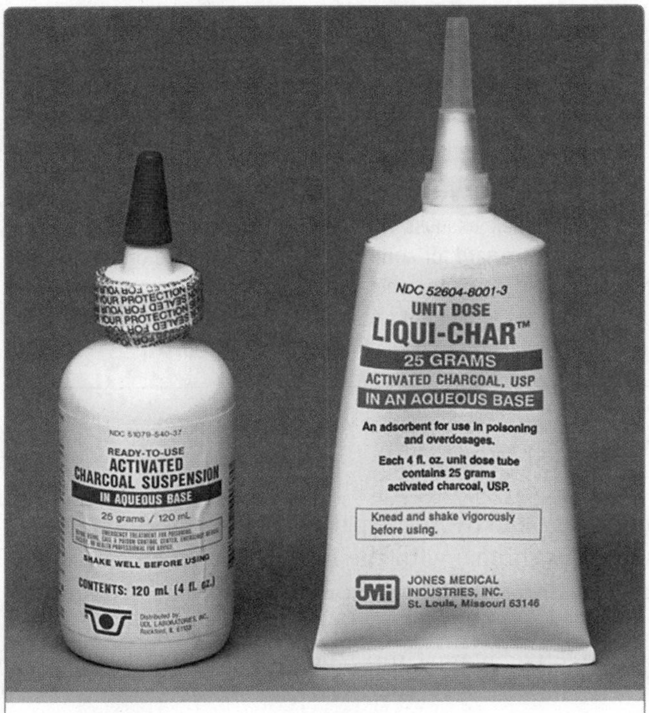

21-2-1

MEDICATION NAME

1. **Generic:** activated charcoal
2. **Trade:** SuperChar, InstaChar, Actidose, Liqui-Char, and others

INDICATIONS

Poisoning by mouth

CONTRAINDICATIONS

1. Altered mental status
2. Ingestion of acids or alkalis
3. Inability to swallow

MEDICATION FORM

1. Pre-mixed in water, frequently available in plastic bottle containing 12.5 grams of activated charcoal
2. Powder, which should be avoided in field

DOSAGE

1. **Adults and children:** 1 gram activated charcoal per kg of body weight
2. **Usual adult dose:** 25 to 50 grams
3. **Usual pediatric dose:** 12.5 to 25 grams

STEPS FOR ADMINISTRATION

1. Consult medical direction.
2. Shake container thoroughly.
3. Because the medication looks like mud, the patient may need to be persuaded to drink it. Providing a covered container and a straw will prevent the patient from seeing the medication and so may improve patient compliance.
4. If patient does not drink the medication right away, the charcoal will settle. Shake or stir it again before administering.
5. Record the name, dose, route, and time of administration of the medication.

ACTIONS

1. Activated charcoal adsorbs (binds) certain poisons in the digestive tract and prevents them from being absorbed into the body.
2. Not all brands of activated charcoal are the same: some adsorb much more than others, so consult medical direction about the brand to use.

SIDE EFFECTS

1. Black stools
2. Some patients may vomit, particularly those who have ingested poisons that cause nausea. If the patient vomits, repeat the dose once.

REASSESSMENT STRATEGIES

Be prepared for the patient to vomit or deteriorate further. If the patient worsens, provide oxygen as you have been trained to do.

CLINICAL CLUE

Staying Safe

Whenever you are called to the scene of an inhalation poisoning, remember that you, too, are at risk of becoming ill (or worse) from exposure to inhaled toxic agents. *Never* enter a scene without appropriate personal protective equipment including positive pressure self-contained breathing apparatus (SCBA) if there is any chance of coming in contact with the toxic substances that harmed the patient. If necessary, request that a hazmat unit be dispatched to the scene to secure it.

Inhaled agents manifest their toxic effects by four different mechanisms: physical particulates, simple asphyxiants, chemical irritants, and chemical asphyxiants. Additionally, if the inhalation occurs in the setting of a fire, heat can cause life-threatening upper-airway burns.

Physical Particulates

Physical particulates are small, solid particles, such as dust or combustion soot, that are carried by gases or atmospheric air into the body through inhalation. In general, they cause physical irritation to the upper airways. In some cases, extremely small particles may even be carried down to the alveolar level and cause mechanical problems, such as impairment of proper gas exchange. Physical particulates can act as vehicles that carry toxic chemicals, such as organic acids, throughout the respiratory system. This situation is encountered most commonly with cases of smoke inhalation.

The signs and symptoms of physical particulate exposure are the result of irritation of the respiratory system, which usually includes excessive coughing and some degree of shortness of breath. If the affected patient has a history of underlying pulmonary disease, such as asthma or chronic obstructive pulmonary disease (COPD), then those effects can be greatly magnified and even cause the patient to get worse, which results in severe respiratory distress.

Simple Asphyxiants

Simple asphyxiants cause injury by merely being present in an environment. These gas agents include carbon dioxide (CO_2), nitrogen, methane, and natural gas. Simple asphyxiants are encountered when the environmental atmosphere becomes abnormally loaded with one of these gases at such high concentrations that they significantly or completely push the normal oxygen out. Simple asphyxiants have no inherent toxic or metabolic effect on the body's cells, other than causing hypoxia due to lack of adequate environmental oxygen.

simple asphyxiants chemicals, such as carbon monoxide, that cause injury by their presence in an environment, rather than the presence of normal levels of atmospheric oxygen.

Chemical Irritants

Chemical irritants express their toxic effects by chemical reaction with the mucus membranes of the eyes and respiratory system. There are two general classes of chemical irritants: those that react readily with water and those that do not.

Chemical irritants that are highly reactive with water are called *hydrophilic* ("water loving") chemicals. Hydrophilic inhaled agents include hydrochloric acid and ammonia. These agents react quickly with the moist membranes of the eyes and the upper respiratory tree, causing immediate intense burning and pain.

Because nonhydrophilic agents do not readily react with the moist membranes of the upper respiratory tract, they can pass more deeply into the lungs and cause direct lung injury. Sometimes these effects are delayed, and a patient may be relatively stable for a while and then decompensate with respiratory failure due to acute lung injury. An example of a nonhydrophilic chemical irritant is phosgene gas.

Chemical Asphyxiants

chemical asphyxiants chemicals, such as carbon monoxide, that asphyxiate patients at the cellular level by massively deranging normal cellular utilization of oxygen.

ischemia an inadequate blood supply to an organ or part of the body, especially the heart muscles.

metabolic acidosis the accumulation of excess lactic acid in the bloodstream as a result of hypoperfusion of the body's cells.

Simply stated, **chemical asphyxiants** cause injury by asphyxiating patients at the cellular level by interrupting normal cellular utilization of oxygen. The most common example of a chemical asphyxiant is carbon monoxide (CO). A product of combustion, CO rapidly displaces oxygen from the hemoglobin, forming carboxyhemoglobin (COHgb). Other examples of inhaled chemical asphyxiants are cyanide gas (HCN) and hydrogen sulfide (H_2S). Both HCN and H_2S block the effective use of oxygen within the cell. This causes rapid body-wide **ischemia,** resulting in a severe **metabolic acidosis** (buildup of acid in the bloodstream).

Signs and symptoms of inhaled chemical asphyxiant exposure depend on the specific agent to which the patient has been exposed. CO poisoning often has a gradual onset of symptoms, including headache, chest pain, and decreasing mental status. Frequently, the patient progresses to coma and death. Patients exposed to H_2S and HCN tend to have a very rapid onset and progression of symptoms.

PERSPECTIVE

Terri—The Mother

How could I have been so careless? I know that he's still in that stage where everything that comes in contact with his hand has to go into his mouth, for heaven sakes. I've been so distracted lately. With Doug being deployed overseas and all of the fights we had right before he left, I just keep replaying them over and over. We fought over everything from money problems to his mom not liking how we were raising Scottie, and then he was gone and I won't see him for months. Scottie's all I've got now, and then this happens. Oh, Doug's mom is never going to let me forget this one.

Signs and Symptoms

Specific signs and symptoms associated with poisoning by inhalation include the following:

- History of inhalation of toxic substances (gathered from the patient, family members, bystanders, or evidence at the scene)
- Detection of an elevated environmental level of dangerous gases by fire-rescue or hazmat teams (Figure 21-2 ■). In suspected cases of carbon monoxide (CO) poisoning a special "co-oximeter" that detects the percentage of blood hemoglobin bound to CO may be used to assess the patient if permitted by local protocol (Figure 21-3 ■).
- Difficulty breathing
- Chest pain
- Cough
- Hoarseness
- Dizziness
- Headache
- Altered mental status
- Seizures
- Respiratory or cardiac arrest

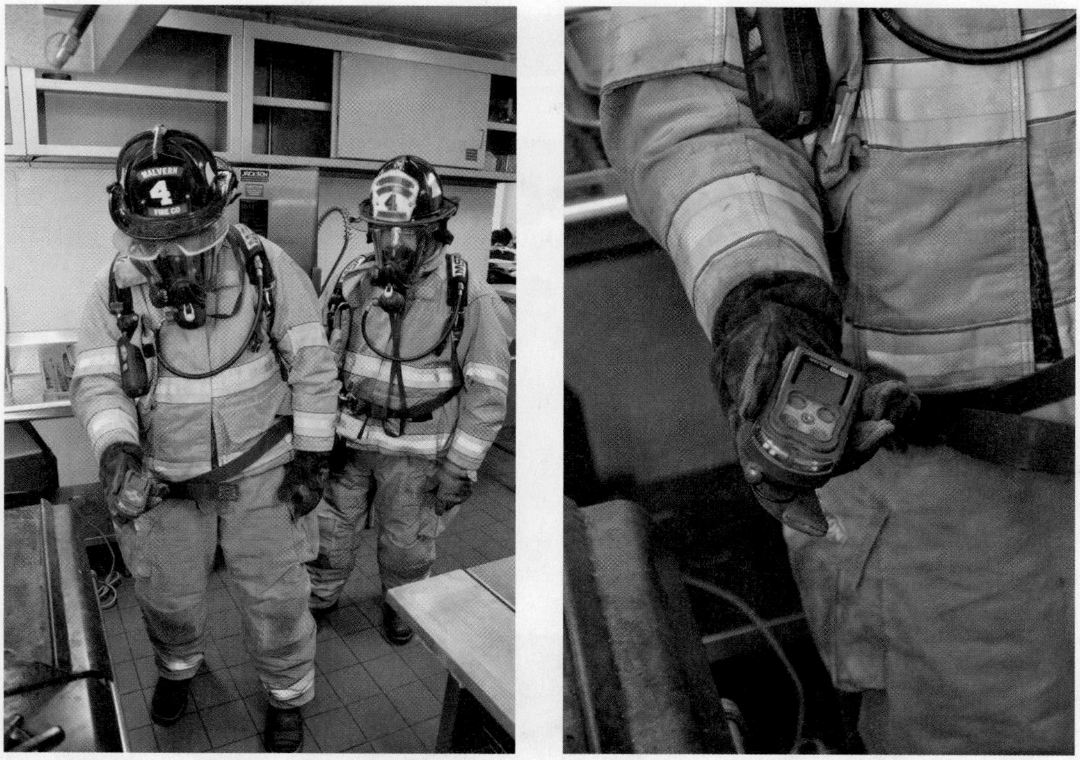

Figure 21-2 Environmental gas detector. (© Edward T. Dickinson, MD)

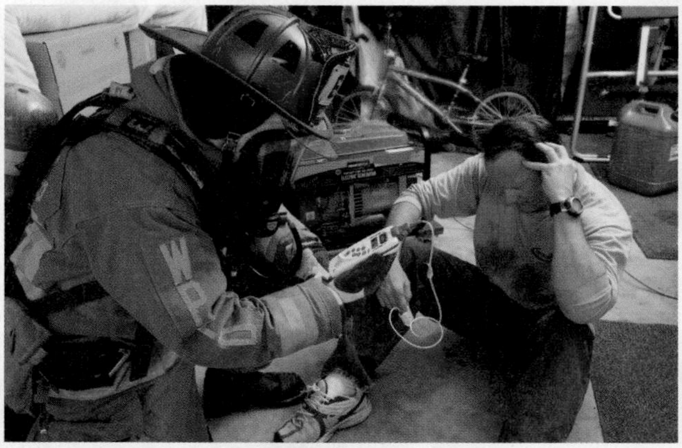

Figure 21-3 Carbon monoxide monitor.

Emergency Care

The emergency care for poisoning by inhalation includes the following steps (Scan 21-3):

1. Have appropriately trained and equipped rescuers remove the patient from the poisonous environment.
2. Ensure scene safety. Take appropriate BSI precautions.
3. Perform a thorough primary assessment.
4. Provide the patient with supplemental oxygen.
5. Be prepared to provide positive pressure ventilations with supplemental oxygen by way of bag-mask device. (Do not use a pocket mask when ventilating a patient poisoned by an inhaled agent due to the risk of self-contamination.)

SCAN 21-3 Inhaled Poisons

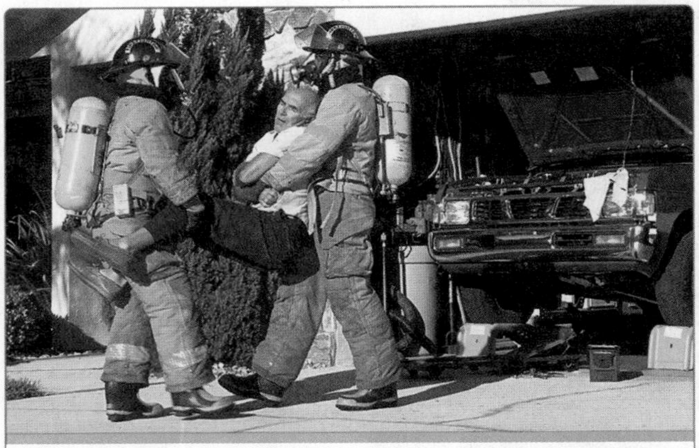

21-3-1 Remove the patient from the source of the poison.

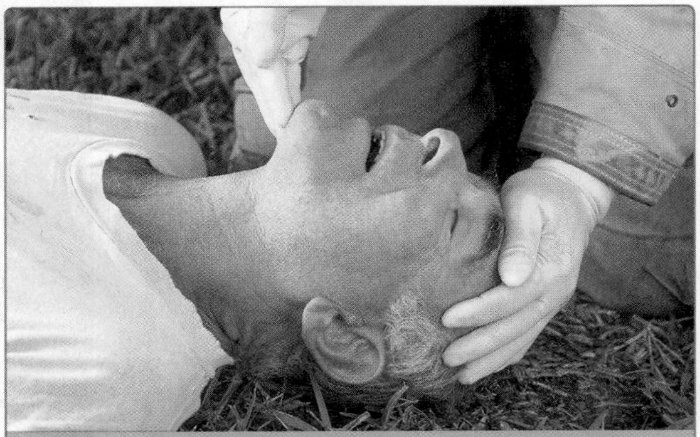

21-3-2 Establish an open airway.

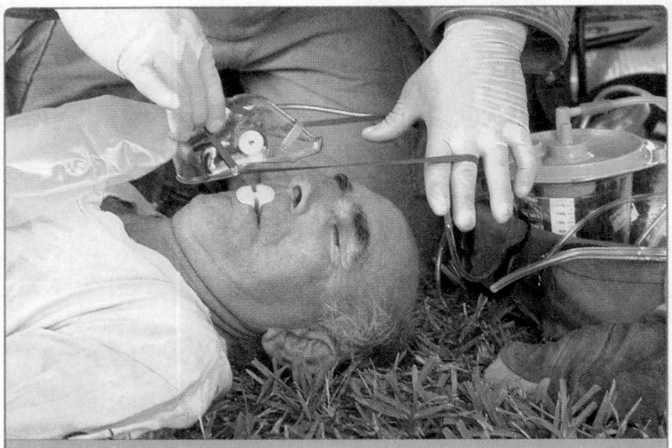

21-3-3 Insert an oropharyngeal airway and administer supplemental oxygen by nonrebreather mask.

21-3-4 Gather the patient's history, take baseline vital signs, and expose the chest for auscultation.

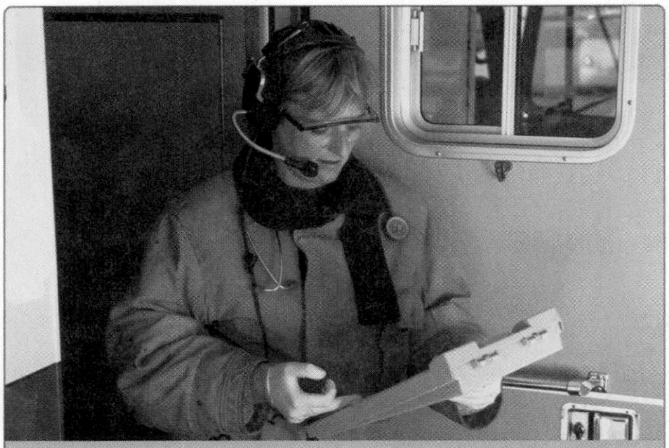

21-3-5 Contact medical direction.

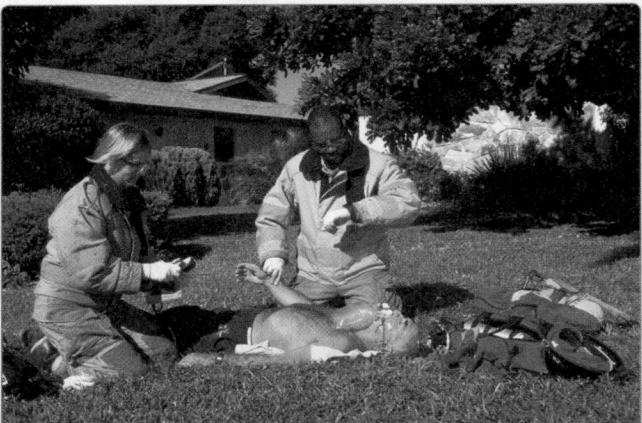

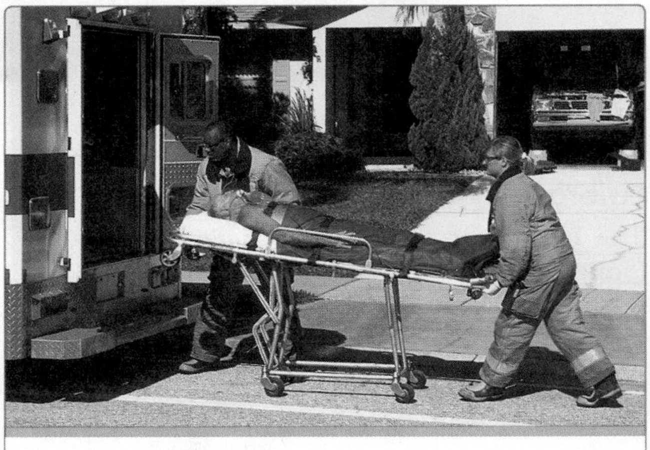

21-3-6 Transport the patient.

Note: In the presence of hazardous fumes or gases, wear the proper PPE and SCBA or wait for those who are properly trained and equipped to enter the scene and bring the patient out.

6. Perform a thorough secondary assessment as appropriate.
7. Transport the patient to the receiving facility. Bring whatever information is available on scene about the inhaled substance (bottles, labels, and so on) to the receiving facility.
8. Perform reassessments en route. Carefully monitor the patient's airway and breathing and be prepared to suction and to provide bag-mask ventilations.

CLINICAL CLUE

Hazmats and MCIs

As a first arriving EMT, it may be your responsibility to determine when a poisoning crosses a line of magnitude to become a hazardous materials (hazmat) incident or a multiple-casualty incident (MCI) requiring the use of additional resources. Most cases of ingestion and injection can be managed as simple poisonings or overdoses with a single EMS crew. Incidents in which illnesses are caused by absorbed or inhaled toxic substances are potentially more likely to involve multiple patients and require more extensive hazmat and MCI resources.

Poisoning by Injection

21-10 Describe the steps of assessment-based management involving a patient who has been exposed to an injected poison.

Among the most common forms of poisoning by injection are the stings and bites of animals such as spiders and snakes (discussed in detail in Chapters 24 and 37) and intravenous drug overdoses. The most commonly injected street drugs are cocaine and narcotic drugs, such as heroin. Narcotic overdoses can produce a classic picture of unresponsiveness, inadequate breathing, and pinpoint (very small) pupils.

Be especially careful of your own safety when called to the scene of a potential drug overdose. Some drug abusers may be calm when you first arrive, but grow more agitated as time passes. If you think there is a potential for violence at a scene, retreat and request law enforcement backup. Do not return until the scene is secure.

Also remember that drug abusers often use hypodermic needles. An accidental puncture with a used needle can transmit infectious diseases. Always take appropriate body substance isolation (BSI) precautions and watch where you put your hands.

Signs and Symptoms

Specific signs and symptoms associated with **injected poisons** include the following:

injected poisons poisons that are inserted through the skin.

- A history of injection of a harmful substance (gathered from the patient, family members, bystanders, or evidence at the scene)
- The presence of "track marks" on the arms or necks of intravenous drug users
- Weakness
- Dizziness
- Chills
- Fever
- Nausea
- Vomiting
- Pinpoint pupils
- Altered mental status
- Chest pain
- Inadequate or absent breathing

Emergency Care

Always exercise extreme caution when performing emergency medical care for a patient with poisoning by injection. Avoid punctures from contaminated needles that the patient may have on him or that are lying about the scene. Follow these steps:

1. Ensure scene safety. Take appropriate BSI precautions.
2. Perform a thorough primary assessment.
3. Provide oxygen and assist ventilations as necessary.
4. Be alert for vomiting and prepare to suction the airway.
5. Perform a thorough secondary assessment as appropriate.
6. Transport the patient to the receiving facility. Bring whatever information is available on scene about the injected substance (bottles, labels, and so on) to the receiving facility.
7. Perform reassessments en route. Carefully monitor the patient's airway and breathing and be prepared to suction or provide bag-mask ventilations.

Poisoning by Absorption

21-11 Describe the steps of assessment-based management involving a patient who has absorbed a poison.

absorbed poisons poisons taken into the body through unbroken skin.

Absorbed poisons can pose significant risks to both the patient and the EMT. Many absorbed poisons, such as organophosphate insecticides, are highly toxic and can be fatal rapidly. Other absorbed toxic agents can cause severe chemical burns. Take all necessary precautions during scene size-up. Use appropriate personal protective equipment. If the amount of poisonous material released poses a significant threat, request that a hazardous materials (hazmat) unit be dispatched to the scene.

Signs and Symptoms

Specific signs and symptoms associated with poisoning by absorption include the following:

- History of exposure (gathered from the patient, family members, bystanders, or evidence at the scene)
- Liquid or powder on the patient's skin
- Excessive saliva production
- Excessive tear production
- Uncontrolled diarrhea
- Burns
- Itching
- Skin irritation
- Redness of the skin

Emergency Care

The emergency medical care for poisoning by absorption includes the steps described below (Scan 21-4). Be sure to use all the appropriate protective equipment.

1. Ensure scene safety. Take appropriate BSI precautions.
2. Perform a thorough primary assessment.
3. Provide oxygen and assist ventilations as necessary.
4. Remove the substances from the patients in the following ways:
   - Remove contaminated clothing.
   - If the substance is a powder, carefully brush as much of it off the patient as possible. When doing so, be careful not to make the substance airborne and cause wider contamination. Irrigate the site of contamination with clean water for at least 20 minutes at the scene. Continue irrigating en route to the receiving facility if possible.

SCAN 21-4 Absorbed Poisons

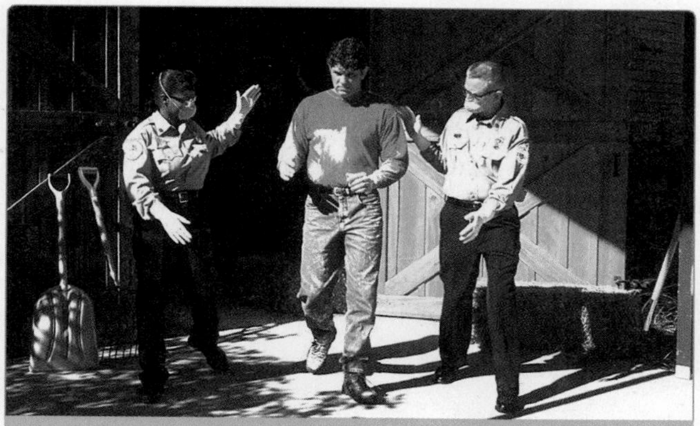

21-4-1 Remove the patient from the source or remove the source from the patient. Avoid contaminating yourself with the poison.

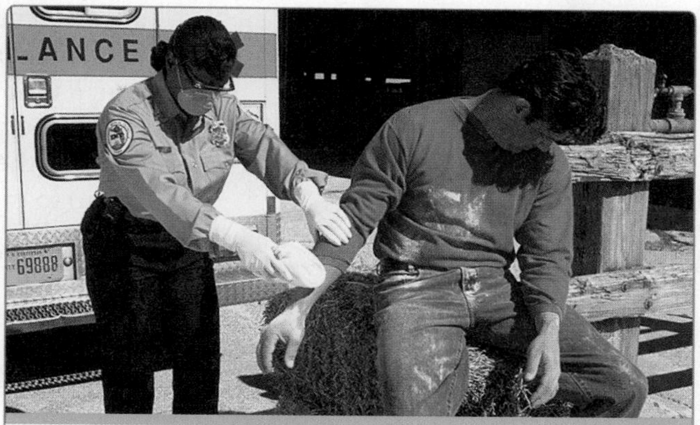

21-4-2 Brush powders from the patient. Be careful not to abrade the patient's skin.

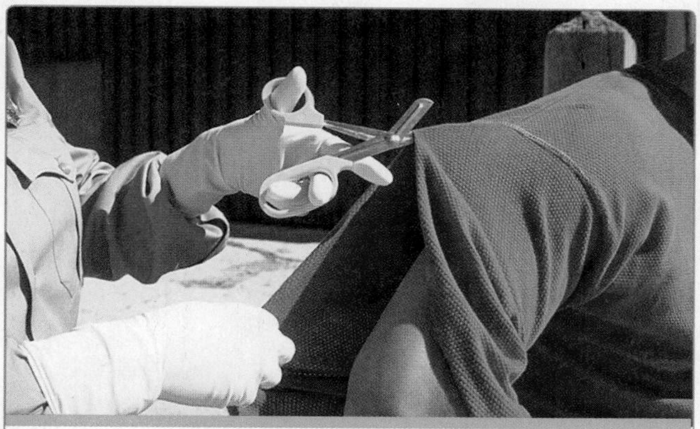

21-4-3 Remove contaminated clothing and other articles.

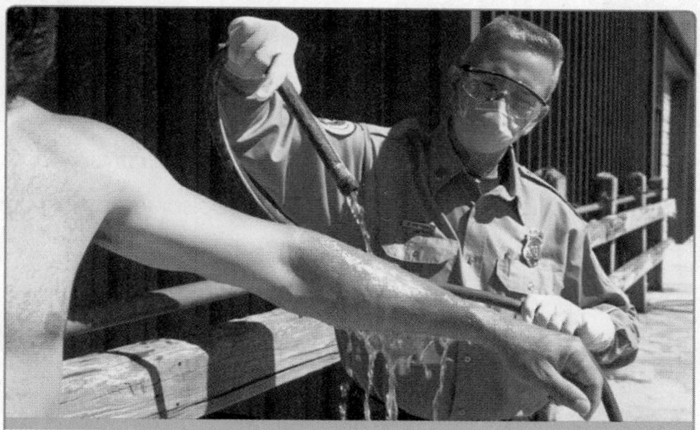

21-4-4 Irrigate with clear water for at least 20 minutes. Catch contaminated runoff and dispose of it safely.

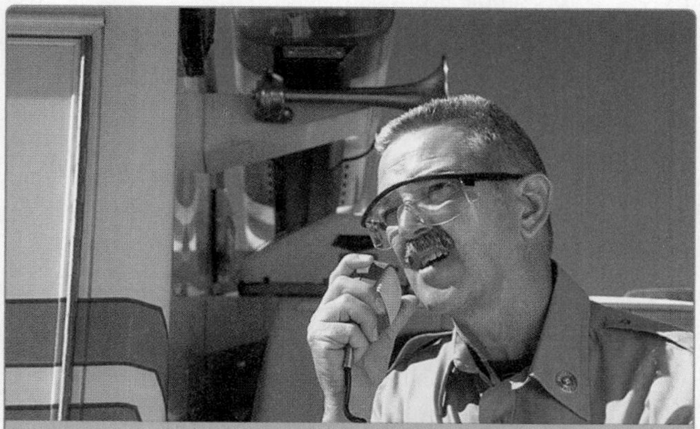

21-4-5 Contact medical direction.

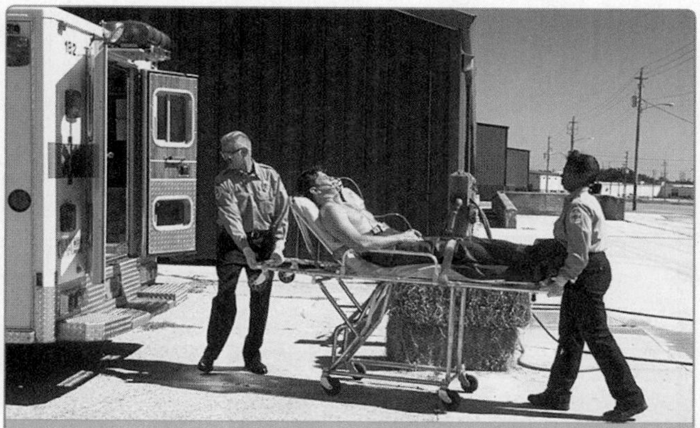

21-4-6 Transport the patient.

Take care to protect your skin from contact with poisonous substances. Wear protective clothing. If necessary, have firefighters or others who are properly protected hose off the patient before you touch him.

- If the substance is a liquid, irrigate the contaminated area with clean water for at least 20 minutes at the scene.
- If the eyes have been contaminated, irrigate them with clean water for at least 20 minutes. Position the patient so that the water drains away from the affected eye and does not wash back into it or into the other eye. Continue irrigating en route to the receiving facility if possible.

5. Perform a thorough secondary assessment as appropriate.
6. Transport the patient to the receiving facility. Bring whatever information is available on the scene about the absorbed substance (containers, bottles, labels, and so on) to the receiving facility. However, do not transport potentially hazardous materials.
7. Perform reassessments en route. Carefully monitor the patient's airway and breathing and be prepared to suction or provide bag-mask ventilations.

STOP, REVIEW, REMEMBER!

Multiple Choice

For each question, place a check next to the correct answer.

1. Toddlers are at particular risk for poisoning by:
   ____ a. inhalation.
   ____ b. ingestion.
   ____ c. absorption.
   ____ d. injection.

2. Irrigation is the most effective means of treating poisoning by:
   ____ a. inhalation.
   ____ b. ingestion.
   ____ c. absorption.
   ____ d. injection.

3. Activated charcoal is selectively used to treat patients with an ______________ poisoning.
   ____ a. inhaled
   ____ b. ingested
   ____ c. absorbed
   ____ d. injected

4. Most poisonings are managed by EMTs with:
   ____ a. specific antidotes.
   ____ b. decontamination.
   ____ c. supportive care.
   ____ d. activated charcoal.

5. Cyanide is an example of a:
   ____ a. physical particulate.
   ____ b. simple asphyxiant.
   ____ c. chemical irritant.
   ____ d. chemical asphyxiant.

6. You are caring for a six-year-old who has ingested an unknown quantity of adult daily vitamins. Your patient is alert and breathing normally. You should:
   ____ a. contact the poison control center for medical direction.
   ____ b. administer 25 grams of activated charcoal.
   ____ c. administer oxygen and transport immediately.
   ____ d. try to get the child to vomit while preparing for transport.

Short Answer

1. Define the term *toxicology*.

2. List the four portals of entry for toxins into the body.

3. List the four general mechanisms by which inhaled poisons exert their toxic effects.

Critical Thinking

1. You are the first arriving EMT at a chemical plant for an "unknown emergency." As you pull up to the plant's front gate, you can see three unresponsive workers lying on the ground just beyond the guard shack. Describe your sequence of actions based on your initial scene size-up.

2. You are dispatched to the scene at a garden supply store for a dispatch of a "fall" victim. Upon arrival, the store manager reports that your patient fell from the loading dock approximately six feet into the bed of a small pickup truck filled with 50-pound bags of dry lime. Upon approaching the patient, you see a male lying in the bed of the pickup covered in white dry lime powder that has spilled from multiple 50-pound bags of dry lime that have apparently been ruptured by his impact. He is holding his obviously deformed left lower leg and screaming for help. Describe how you would specifically manage this patient in regard to decontamination.

Additional Aspects of Toxicology

Substance Abuse

As an EMT, you will encounter many patients who purposefully use (or misuse) prescription medications, illicit drugs, or other substances to achieve a desired effect such as euphoria, excitation, or relaxation. The recurrent use of substances (both legal and illegal) for those types of effects is considered substance abuse. Sadly, over time, substance abuse patients may become psychologically dependent (addicted) and in some cases medically dependent from the chronic continuous use of the drugs. Patients who are medically dependent on certain drugs such as alcohol develop a chemical and biological need to take the drug. Suddenly stopping the prolonged use of the substances can cause significant and even life-threatening complications called **withdrawal.** Unfortunately, substance abusers can suffer from a wide variety of emergencies for which EMS is summoned, including:

withdrawal the severe physical reaction that results when a person who chronically uses drugs, such as alcohol or narcotics, is deprived of those drugs.

21-12 Describe the steps of assessment-based management involving a patient experiencing a drug or alcohol emergency.

- Acute life-threatening overdoses
- Complications from the toxic effects that the long-term use of these drugs have on the body
- Complications of withdrawal from suddenly ceasing to use substances to which they are dependent
- Trauma-related emergencies that result from the impaired judgment of patients under the influence of drugs (including alcohol)

Specific Drugs of Abuse

Ethanol

By far the most commonly abused drug is ethanol, the alcohol contained in beer, wine, and spirits. With moderate use, ethanol causes a sense of well-being, relaxation, and mild euphoria. However, patients who quickly consume excessive amounts of alcohol can develop **alcohol intoxication,** which is characterized by impaired judgment, staggering gait, vomiting, altered mental status, low blood pressure, and even death.

alcohol intoxication alteration of normal mental status as a result of ingestion of ethanol.

chronic alcoholics people who chronically ingest and are physically addicted to ethanol.

alcohol withdrawal syndrome a spectrum of physical reactions (that can include anxiousness, tremors, seizures, and even hallucinations) caused when chronic alcoholics suddenly stop their normal consumption of ethanol.

Ethanol can be very addictive. Patients who are chronic abusers of ethanol are characterized as **chronic alcoholics** (Figure 21-4 ■). Alcoholics can develop chronic illnesses such as liver disease and be at increased risk for gastrointestinal bleeding and certain types of brain hemorrhages. It is estimated that the life span of a chronic alcoholic can be 10 to 15 years shorter than those who only drink occasionally and in moderation.

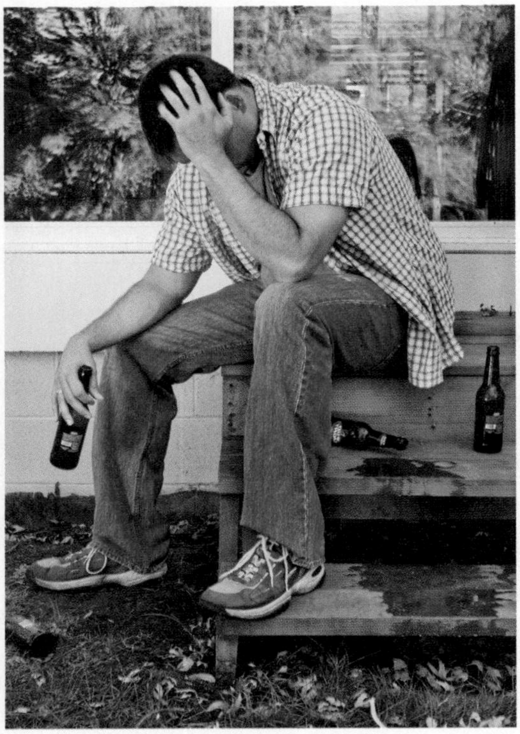

Figure 21-4 Chronic ethanol abuser.

> **CLINICAL CLUE**
>
> **Sensing Pain**
>
> Patients who are intoxicated as a result of alcohol or other drug use pose a challenge for trauma assessment. Intoxication can alter their ability to sense pain. For example, they may have a significant cervical-spine injury, yet deny any neck pain. Patients who are intoxicated and have a significant mechanism of injury should be fully immobilized even if they report no injuries.

Over time, the central nervous systems of alcoholics develop a chemical dependency to ethanol. When a chronic alcoholic suddenly stops (on purpose or due to illness) drinking his regular daily consumption of alcohol-containing beverages, **alcohol withdrawal syndrome** may result. The onset of this syndrome can occur as early as six to eight hours after the chronic alcoholic stops drinking. Initial signs and symptoms are restlessness, tremulous hands, elevated pulse, and elevated blood pressure. If left untreated, or if the person fails to consume additional alcohol, these symptoms could worsen over the next 24 to 48 hours and the patient may develop seizures.

After three to five days without ethanol, approximately 5% of alcohol withdrawal patients will go on to develop a syndrome called **delirium tremens (DTs).** This life-threatening condition is characterized by hallucinations and profound disorientation. Even with the best care, about one in 10 patients with DTs will die.

delirium tremens (DTs) the most severe type of alcohol withdrawal during which the patient experiences visual hallucinations.

Illicit Street Drugs

Illicit street drugs is a very broad category of substances that patients purposefully use to obtain desired effects such as "a high," "a buzz," to become more calm, or in some cases even to induce hallucinations (Table 21-1). Certain prescription drugs

TABLE 21-1 COMMONLY ABUSED DRUGS

UPPERS	DOWNERS	NARCOTICS	MIND-ALTERING DRUGS	VOLATILE CHEMICALS
Amphetamine (benzedrine, bennies, pep pills, ups, uppers, cartwheels)	Barbiturates (downers, dolls, barbs, rainbows) Note: barbiturates include amobarbital, pentobarbital, phenobarbital, and secobarbital.	Codeine (often in cough syrup)	*Hallucinogenic drugs:*	Amyl nitrate (snappers, poppers)
Biphetamine (bam)	Amobarbital (blue devils, downers, barbs, Amytal®)	Demerol (meperidine)	DMT LSD (acid, sunshine)	Butyl nitrate (locker room, rush)
Cocaine (coke, snow, crack)	Pentobarbital (yellow jackets, barbs, Nembutal®)	Dilaudid fentanyl (Sublimaze®)	Mescaline (peyote, mesc)	Cleaning fluid (carbon tetrachloride)
Desoxyn (black beauties)	Phenobarbital (goofballs, phennies, barbs)	Heroin ("H," horse, junk, smack, stuff)	Morning glory seeds, PCP (angel dust, hog, peace pills)	Furniture polish
Dextroamphetamine (dexies, Dexedrine®)	Secobarbital (red devils, barbs, Seconal®)	Methadone (dolly)	Psilocybin (magic mushrooms)	Gasoline
Methamphetamine (speed, crank, meth, crystal, diet pills, methedrine)	Chloral hydrate (knockout drops, Noctec®)	Morphine opium (op, poppy)	STP (serenity, tranquility, peace)	Glue
Methylphenidate (Ritalin®)	Methaqualone (Quaalude®, ludes, spoors)	Paregoric (contains opium)	*Nonhallucinogenic drugs:*	Hair spray
Preludin®	Nonbarbiturate sedatives (various tranquilizers and sleeping pills, such as Valium or diazepam, Miltown®, Equanil®, meprobamate, Thorazine®, Compazine®, Librium® or chlordiazepoxide reserpine, Tranxene or clorazepate, and other benzodiazepines)	Acetaminophen with codeine (1, 2, 3, 4)	Hash, marijuana (grass, pot, tea, wood, dope)	Nail polish remover
	Paraldehyde		THC	Paint thinner
				Typewriting correction fluid

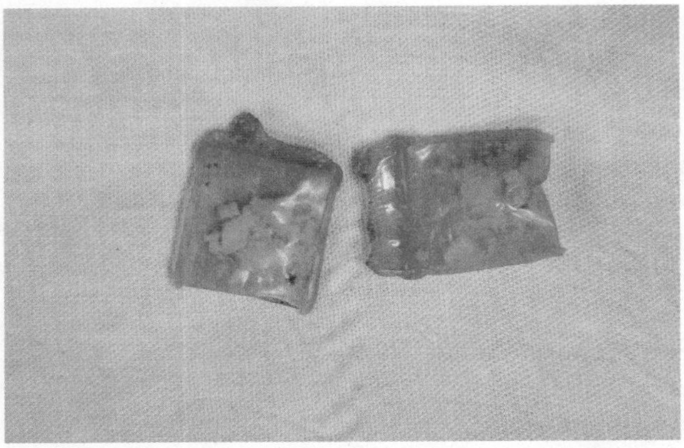

Figure 21-5 Crack cocaine in fingernail-size packages. (© Edward T. Dickinson)

that are abused or resold on the streets (such as the narcotic oxycodone) fall into the category of illicit street drugs. However, the vast majority of illicit street drugs do not have standard concentrations and dosages. Therefore, harmful overdoses of these substances are very common simply because users have no idea of how much of the drug they can "safely" take.

Depending on the specific substance being abused, illicit drugs enter the body by all portals of entry. Some drugs can be introduced in multiple ways. Cocaine, for example, can be absorbed through the nasal mucosa (snorting), smoked (in the form of crack (Figure 21-5 ■), or injected in the vein or into the skin. Heroin, a strong illicit narcotic, is also commonly injected into the skin or vein. Patients who inject illicit drugs into their veins may have evident scarring in the skin over the veins. That scarring is characteristic of intravenous drug abuse and is referred to as *track marks* (Figure 21-6 ■).

In addition to drugs that you might normally consider street drugs (e.g., PCP, marijuana, cocaine), remember that various household and industrial substances are also often abused by patients, sometimes with catastrophic consequences. The inhalation of vapors from volatile chemicals has become common and is referred to as "huffing" or "bagging" (Figure 21-7 ■). The use of these unconventional substances of abuse is ever changing, perhaps enhanced by the rapid dissemination of information by way of the Internet. Recently there have been clusters of poisoning by such things as over-the-counter bath salts or plant foods that come with benign-sounding names such as "Ivory Wave" and "Vanilla Sky," and are typically snorted, smoked, injected, and even mixed with water as a beverage. This is an example of why, as an EMT, you should keep up to date with the ever-evolving world of drugs of abuse.

21-13 Describe special considerations in managing violent drug- or alcohol-abuse patients.

Remember that the top priority in all poisoning and overdose emergencies is ensuring your own safety and the safety of your crew as part of scene size-up and throughout the call. This reality is even more heightened in situations involving illicit drugs in which needles, weapons, and unpredictable patients can complicate your care. If you determine the scene to be unsafe during scene size-up, then stage your unit a safe distance away and wait for law enforcement to render the scene safe before you enter it. If during the call you feel that conditions are deteriorating and your safety has been compromised, then retreat to a safe position and call for law enforcement backup immediately.

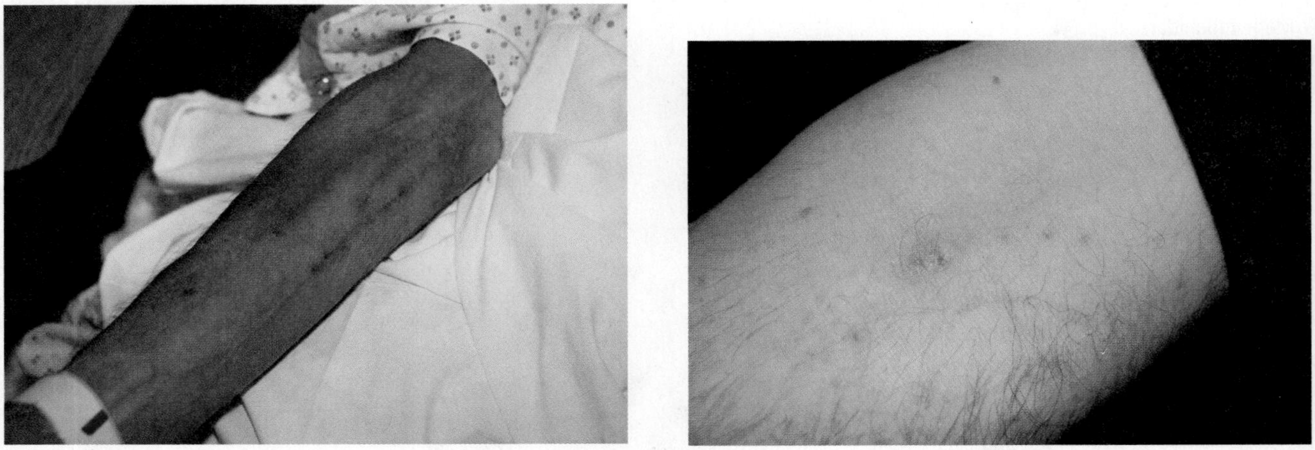

(A) (B)

Figure 21-6 (A) Track marks caused by chronic IV drug abuse. (© Edward T. Dickinson) (B) Fresh IV drug track marks on the arm. (© Edward T. Dickinson)

Specific Poisonings

Carbon Monoxide

Carbon monoxide (CO) is by far the most common cause of death in inhalation poisonings. CO poisoning can result from structural fires, malfunctioning heating systems, and accidental or intentional exposure to automotive exhaust.

The symptoms of CO poisoning can be subtle and nonspecific. They may include headache, nausea, dizziness, and slight alteration in mental status. With such nonspecific symptoms, it can be difficult to determine whether a patient has sustained a dangerous exposure to CO. The most reliable indicator of potentially serious CO poisoning is any loss of consciousness. Other signs of potentially serious CO exposure include chest pain and stroke-like symptoms. Cases of serious CO poisoning may require specialized treatment in a hyperbaric chamber.

All patients with symptoms that may be related to CO exposure based on activation of a home CO detector, a history of having been in an atmosphere that contained high levels of CO, and those patients with elevated CO levels on specialized finger probe co-oximeters should be placed on supplemental oxygen and transported to the hospital for further evaluation.

Identify any patients who are found unresponsive or who have a history of loss of consciousness and be sure this information is relayed to the emergency department staff. Identifying them is especially important when caring for multiple patients with potential CO exposure, such as in a multiple-occupancy dwelling. In those cases, vital information about high-risk patients can too easily get overlooked as a dozen or more CO-poisoning patients suddenly inundate the emergency department. Patients with CO poisoning who have a loss of consciousness, active chest pain, and those who are pregnant are often treated with oxygen delivered in a hyperbaric chamber.

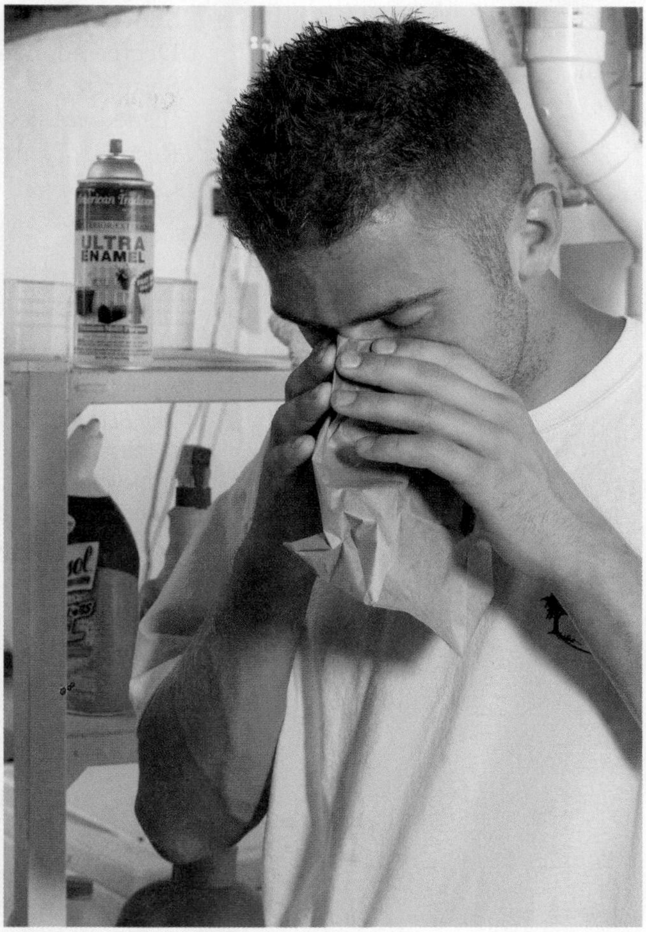

Figure 21-7 "Bagging" spray paint vapors.

21-14 Describe special considerations in assessing and managing patients with carbon monoxide poisoning and exposure to nerve agents.

Nerve Agents and Organophosphates

Military **nerve agents** and related industrial compounds called *organophosphates* are a group of profoundly toxic materials. Organophosphates are widely used in industrial insecticides. The onset and severity of symptoms vary based on the specific agent, concentration of that chemical, the duration of exposure, and the portal of entry. Onset of symptoms may be within minutes with high-dose exposure, but can be delayed up to 18 hours in some cases with lower-concentration exposures. The most common portal of entry is absorption through the skin, but inhalation and ingestion are also potential ways these chemicals get into the body.

nerve agents chemicals (often used as weapons) that incapacitate and kill by deranging normal function of the central nervous system.

Signs and symptoms of nerve agent or organophosphate exposure include:

- Rapid or slow heart rate
- High blood pressure
- Excessive sweating (diaphoresis)
- Excessive drooling (salivation)
- Excessive tearing (lacrimation)
- Uncontrolled urination
- Uncontrolled diarrhea
- Uncontrolled vomiting (emesis)
- Constricted pupils

- Shortness of breath
- Decreased mental status
- Seizures
- Inadequate respiration
- Respiratory arrest
- Cardiac arrest

CLINICAL CLUE

SLUDGE

The classic signs of nerve agent or organophosphate poisoning are best remembered by the mnemonic *SLUDGE*: salivation, lacrimation, urination, diarrhea, GI symptoms, emesis. The chemicals also cause respiratory distress by increasing bronchial secretions (bronchorrhea) and airway constriction (bronchoconstriction), and also can cause a slow heart rate (bradycardia). For this reason some toxicologists recommend using the "SLUDGE-BBB" mnemonic as the best way to remember the signs and symptoms of nerve agent or organophosphate poisoning.

The emergency care of patients with nerve agent or organophosphate poisoning includes scene safety with decontamination, supportive care with aggressive airway suctioning, and bag-mask ventilation for patients with inadequate respirations.

There are two drugs that act as specific antidotes for nerve agent or organophosphate poisoning. The two drugs are atropine and pralidoxime. Atropine is a drug universally carried by paramedic units. The combination of atropine and pralidoxime is available in the form of an auto-injector called the *Mark 1 kit*. Military personnel, hazmat team members, and some EMTs are trained to use the Mark 1 kit both for treatment of patients and for self use in cases of nerve agent exposure.

Antidotes

Antidotes are agents used to neutralize or counteract the effects of a poison. There are only a handful of toxic agents that have truly effective antidotes to counteract their effects on patients. The rest of poisoning and overdose patients receive supportive care in both the prehospital and hospital settings.

TABLE 21-2 AVAILABLE PREHOSPITAL ANTIDOTES

TOXIC AGENT	ANTIDOTE	LEVEL OF CARE
Carbon monoxide	High-concentration oxygen	BLS/ALS
	Hyperbaric oxygen	Specialized hyperbaric center
Narcotics	Naloxone (Narcan®)	ALS
Nerve Agents	Atropine	ALS
Organophosphates	Atropine and pralidoxime (Mark 1 Kit)	BLS*/ALS
Cyanide	Cyanide Kit	ALS
	Hydroxocobalamin	

*In certain EMS systems EMTs are approved to treat patients and/or themselves with Mark 1 kits. In addition, military and some hazmat personnel are trained to self-administer Mark 1 kits.

At the EMT level the most widely used antidote is supplemental oxygen for patients with CO poisoning. Supplemental oxygen speeds the rate at which carbon monoxide clears from the hemoglobin in the bloodstream.

Some antidotes are carried only by ALS personnel, while others are available only in a hospital setting. As an EMT you should be familiar with what agents are carried by prehospital ALS providers (paramedics) in your system so that they can be dispatched to begin antidote treatment as soon as possible.

STOP, REVIEW, REMEMBER!

Multiple Choice

For each question, place a check next to the correct answer.

1. The Mark 1 kit contains:

_____ a. activated charcoal.

_____ b. atropine.

_____ c. pralidoxime.

_____ d. atropine and pralidoxime.

2. Carbon monoxide (CO) poisoning is:

_____ a. best detected by its characteristic smell.

_____ b. rarely serious.

_____ c. best treated with oxygen by nasal cannula.

_____ d. the most common cause of serious inhalation poisonings.

3. A common sign of nerve agent exposure includes:

_____ a. diarrhea.

_____ b. low blood pressure.

_____ c. violent and aggressive behavior.

_____ d. large pupils.

4. The most serious complication of alcohol withdrawal syndrome is:

_____ a. seizures.

_____ b. delirium tremens.

_____ c. high blood pressure.

_____ d. suicidal thinking.

5. You and your partner are caring for a patient suffering from a suspected narcotic overdose. She is unresponsive with a respiratory rate of 6 and shallow, and a pulse of 64, weak and regular. You should:

_____ a. begin chest compression and ventilations.

_____ b. apply oxygen by nonrebreather mask.

_____ c. provide ventilations by bag-mask device.

_____ d. place her on a stretcher and transport immediately.

Short Answer

1. Write out the specific signs of organophosphate poisoning identified in the "SLUDGE" mnemonic.

____

____

____

____

(continued on next page)

(continued)

2. List the signs and symptoms that most reliably represent serious CO poisonings.

Critical Thinking

1. You have responded to the scene of an organophosphate poisoning. You find that two patients have been exposed. Once the patients are decontaminated by hazmat, they are transferred to your care. One patient is in cardiac arrest, and the other is in severe respiratory distress. Your unit has only one Mark 1 auto-injector, which you are authorized to use. On which patient should you use the auto-injector and why?

2. Of those toxic agents that have antidotes, only one is a standard medication carried by EMTs. Which medication is it, what is the proper dose, and to which patient should it be administered?

EMERGENCY DISPATCH SUMMARY

The patient was transported with his mother to the Saint Luke's Emergency Department for evaluation. While en route, Alexis had mom help by holding the oxygen mask by the boy's face and reassuring him, which helped to calm her as well as the patient. He was released later that afternoon, and according to his mother, has been his happy and playful self since the incident.

Chapter Review

To the Point

- Scenes involving poisonings and overdoses have unique risks for the EMT. Your safety and the safety of your crew are your highest priorities.
- The four portals of entry in toxicology are absorption, ingestion, inhalation, and injection.
- There are only a limited number of antidotes for poisonings.
- Most patients with poisonings and overdoses will be managed with supportive care (maintaining an open and clear airway, providing supplemental oxygen, and bag-mask ventilation for those with inadequate breathing).
- Poison control centers are excellent resources for managing poisoning and overdose patients.
- Activated charcoal is used to treat certain ingested poisons.
- Activated charcoal should *never* be given to patients with altered mental status.
- The most commonly abused drug is ethanol, the alcohol contained in beer, wine, and spirits.
- Alcohol withdrawal is a potentially life-threatening syndrome.
- Carbon monoxide poisoning is the most common serious inhalation poisoning.
- The treatment of carbon monoxide poisoning is supplemental oxygen.
- SLUDGE-BBB is a mnemonic used to remember the signs of nerve agent and organophosphate poisoning.

Chapter Questions

Multiple Choice

For each question, place a check next to the correct answer.

1. The "S" in the SLUDGE-BBB mnemonic stands for:
   _____ a. symptoms.
   _____ b. seizures.
   _____ c. salivation.
   _____ d. syndrome.

2. The most common inhalation poisoning is:
   _____ a. cyanide.
   _____ b. carbon monoxide.
   _____ c. hydrogen sulfide.
   _____ d. methane.

3. All of the following have specific antidotes *except*:
   _____ a. cyanide.
   _____ b. cocaine.
   _____ c. carbon monoxide.
   _____ d. narcotics.

4. The treatment of choice for carbon monoxide poisoning is:
   _____ a. the Mark 1 kit.
   _____ b. oxygen by nasal cannula.
   _____ c. naloxone.
   _____ d. oxygen by nonrebreather mask.

5. Which one of the following is a late sign of a serious CO poisoning?
   _____ a. Headache
   _____ b. Red skin
   _____ c. General weakness
   _____ d. Chest pain

6. Toxicology is best defined as the study of the:
   _____ a. beneficial effects of radiation on patients.
   _____ b. beneficial effects of toxins on patients.
   _____ c. harmful interactions of infectious diseases on the cardiovascular system.
   _____ d. harmful interaction between humans and toxic substances.

(continued on next page)

(continued)

7. Activated charcoal is best used to treat certain poisonings that are the result of:
   _____ a. inhalation. _____ c. absorption.
   _____ b. ingestion. _____ d. injection.

8. A firefighter develops trouble breathing after smoke exposure. This is an example of a poisoning by:
   _____ a. inhalation. _____ c. absorption.
   _____ b. ingestion. _____ d. injection.

9. A heroin addict stops breathing after injecting heroin in his vein. This is an example of a poisoning by:
   _____ a. inhalation. _____ c. absorption.
   _____ b. ingestion. _____ d. injection.

10. An infant eats several leaves from a household plant and has a seizure. This is an example of a poisoning by:
   _____ a. inhalation. _____ c. absorption.
   _____ b. ingestion. _____ d. injection.

Short Answer

1. List the hazards that are often present on the scene of emergencies involving illicit drugs.

____

____

____

____

2. List those toxic agents and poisons that do have specific prehospital antidotes available.

____

____

____

____

3. List the four portals of entry for toxins into the body.

____

____

____

____

4. Describe the signs and symptoms of delirium tremens.

____

____

____

____

5. Describe the progression of symptoms in alcohol withdrawal syndrome.

Critical Thinking

1. Compare and contrast the asphyxiation pathophysiology of carbon monoxide (CO) poisoning as opposed to a carbon dioxide (CO_2) poisoning.

2. Explain the pathophysiology of why patients with underlying COPD and asthma are specifically prone to suffer from the toxic effects of physical particulates.

Case Studies

Case Study 1

You arrive at the scene of a college fraternity party. Your patient is a 22-year-old male whom you find vomiting into the toilet. Your assessment reveals a strong odor of alcohol and vomit on his breath, and you note his speech to be slurred. He is too intoxicated to stand up, but when he turns his head, you note that he is bleeding from his mouth and several teeth appear to be missing. He tells you he did not call 911 and does not want your help. His fraternity brothers, who also have been drinking heavily, say they will "keep an eye on him."

1. In this situation are you obligated to obey the wishes of the patient and not treat him?

(continued on next page)

(continued)

2. What is your most important concern during his primary assessment?

3. How does this patient's evident intoxication affect your trauma assessment and management?

Case Study 2

You are dispatched to an abandoned building for a drug overdose. The location is well known to your department as a crack house that generates frequent calls for overdoses and drug-related violence. As your rookie partner pulls up to the front of the building, a woman runs out into the street to your passenger-side window and tells you, "He's on the second floor. Hurry, he's all messed up!"

1. Discuss the scene size-up considerations of this call.

2. Discuss the specific hazards you might encounter on the scene of this call.

3. Once the scene is secured and rendered safe by the police, what specific equipment should you bring into the building with you to be prepared to manage the patient based on the limited information provided?

The Last Word

Your powers of observation combined with a thorough history are necessary when caring for victims of a possible toxicological emergency. First and foremost, conduct a thorough scene size-up and confirm that the environment is safe for you and your partner. Toxic substances are often invisible to the eye and can pose a serious hazard to rescuers. It is critical to make certain the environment is not toxic. If necessary, you should call for additional trained rescuers who can safely enter the environment and remove the patient. Once you can safely access the patient, be careful not to come in contact with any toxic substance that may be on the patient or his clothing. Always use proper BSI precautions.

Once you have determined the scene is safe, you must perform a primary assessment and confirm the patient has an adequate airway, breathing, and circulation. As with all patients, a clear airway and adequate respirations are your first concern when beginning care. Keep a portable suction unit handy because the patient could vomit at any time. If necessary, provide assisted ventilations with a bag-mask and supplemental oxygen. Early contact with medical direction or your poison control center can often be valuable. They can provide additional guidance for specific care.

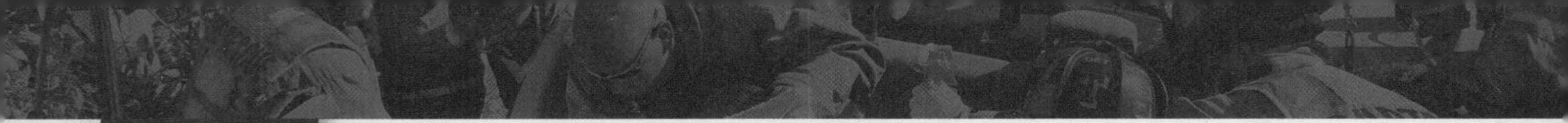

22 Caring for Patients with Acute Abdominal Emergencies

Education Standards

Medicine: Abdominal and gastrointestinal disorders, gynecology, genitourinary and renal

Competencies

Applies fundamental knowledge to provide basic emergency care and transportation based on assessment findings for an acutely ill patient.

Objectives

After completion of this lesson, you should be able to:

22-1 Define key terms introduced in this chapter.

22-2 Describe the anatomy and physiology of the structures of the abdominal cavity, including boundaries of the abdominal cavity, visceral and parietal peritoneum, intraperitoneal and retroperitoneal organs, and the relationship between the topographic anatomy of the four abdominal quadrants and the organs corresponding to them.

22-3 Compare and contrast the general characteristics of hollow and solid organs and vascular structures found in the abdominal cavity.

22-4 List the general mechanisms and types of abdominal pain.

22-5 Describe the pathophysiology and the signs and symptoms associated with common causes of acute abdomen, including abdominal aortic aneurysm, appendicitis, cholecystitis, esophageal varices, gastroenteritis, gastrointestinal bleeding, hernia, intestinal obstruction, pancreatitis, peritonitis, and ulcers.

22-6 Explain the assessment-based approach to acute abdomen, including appropriate emergency care.

22-7 Describe the basic anatomy and physiology of the female reproductive system.

22-8 Describe the pathophysiology and the signs and symptoms associated with common gynecological conditions, including endometriosis, endometritis, ovarian cyst, and pelvic inflammatory disease.

22-9 Explain the assessment-based approach to acute gynecological emergencies, including appropriate emergency care.

Key Terms

abdominal aortic aneurysm (AAA) p. 606
adhesions p. 608
appendicitis p. 606
cholecystitis p. 594
diaphragm p. 592
dysmenorrhea p. 609
endometriosis p. 609
endometritis p. 609
esophageal varices p. 604
gastroenteritis p. 607
gastrointestinal (GI) p. 593
hematemesis p. 604
hematochezia p. 605
hernia p. 608
intraperitoneal p. 593
jaundice p. 600
melena p. 605
menstrual p. 594
ovarian cyst p. 609
pancreatitis p. 598
parietal peritoneum p. 593
pelvic inflammatory disease (PID) p. 609
peritonitis p. 594
retroperitoneal p. 593
spontaneous abortion p. 609
ulcers p. 595
visceral peritoneum p. 593

Introduction

Emergencies and diseases within the abdomen can be very difficult to diagnose and treat. The abdominal cavity contains a variety of vital structures that serve several different body systems. The abdomen also has a rich blood supply, including large blood vessels that traverse its vault. An abdominal complaint is difficult to assess because these organs and vessels lay deep beneath layers of muscle and skin and, unlike a fractured arm or a lacerated scalp, cannot be visualized externally. Life-threatening conditions can present with subtle, nonspecific findings and the most important signs and symptoms can be confusing, hidden, and at best difficult to pinpoint. However, there are successful strategies for assessing and treating patients with abdominal complaints.

As a prehospital provider, you should take a generalized approach to patient assessment, identifying any signs of an immediate life threat. Although you may not know exactly what is causing the problem, your rapid identification of a condition such as shock in a patient complaining of abdominal pain could make the difference between life and death. With this understanding and a basic knowledge of abdominal anatomy, it is possible to use external signs and the patient's symptoms to recognize common patterns of dangerous abdominal disorders.

This chapter reviews the anatomy and physiology of the abdomen, as well as assessment techniques that will help you identify the critical patient. The presentation and pathophysiology of important illnesses involving the abdomen are also covered so that you can learn to recognize the patterns of common dangerous abdominal disorders.

EMERGENCY DISPATCH

EMTs Donnie Traverso and Mika Black had just finished checking the fluids and washing their ambulance when the radio buzzed. "6-2-9, 629, respond to Hollywood Skate on Commerce Boulevard for an abdominal pain."

"And so our shift begins!" Mika pushed the wash bucket into the utility shed and quickly rinsed his hands with the hose as Donnie started the truck. About eight minutes later they arrived at the parking lot of the town's lone roller skating rink, which was obviously packed on this early summer afternoon.

"He's over here," a rink employee shouted over the loud, thumping music and skated ahead of the EMTs as they moved the gurney through the crowd. "He was doubled over in the middle of the rink."

The patient, a 13-year-old boy wearing shorts and a football jersey, was pale, sweating, and curled in the fetal position on a carpeted bench next to the rink. His brightly colored skates were pulled up tightly to the backs of his thighs.

"How are you doing, buddy?" Mika squatted down to talk, and then sprang back as the boy suddenly vomited all over the bench and floor.

Anatomy and Physiology

22-2 Describe the anatomy and physiology of the structures of the abdominal cavity, including boundaries of the abdominal cavity, visceral and parietal peritoneum, intraperitoneal and retroperitoneal organs, and the relationship between the topographic anatomy of the four abdominal quadrants and the organs corresponding to them.

diaphragm the large flat muscle responsible for breathing; forms the upper border of the abdominal vault.

The abdominal vault is bordered superiorly by the **diaphragm,** the flat muscle of breathing. The cavity continues from the diaphragm to its lower border at the bottom of the pelvis. The abdomen is commonly separated into four quadrants (Figure 22-1 ▪). The right and left quadrants are divided by the midline, and the upper and lower quadrants are divided by the umbilicus (the belly button). This quadrant system provides a means to identify underlying organs as well as to describe the location of pain, tenderness, and injury. Note that the lower quadrants extend below the common waistline of most clothing.

A common mistake made when assessing the abdomen is to assess only what is visible. An accurate and thorough inspection with palpation should involve all four full quadrants, not just what is visible above the patient's clothes. (See Table 22-1 for a list of the abdominal quadrants and major organs that occupy space in them.)

Note that some organs lie along the midline. The pancreas occupies space in both the right and left upper quadrants. The liver does the same (although the majority of this organ lies in the right upper quadrant). The uterus in females is found in both the right and left lower quadrants and the urinary bladder also occupies space in both lower quadrants.

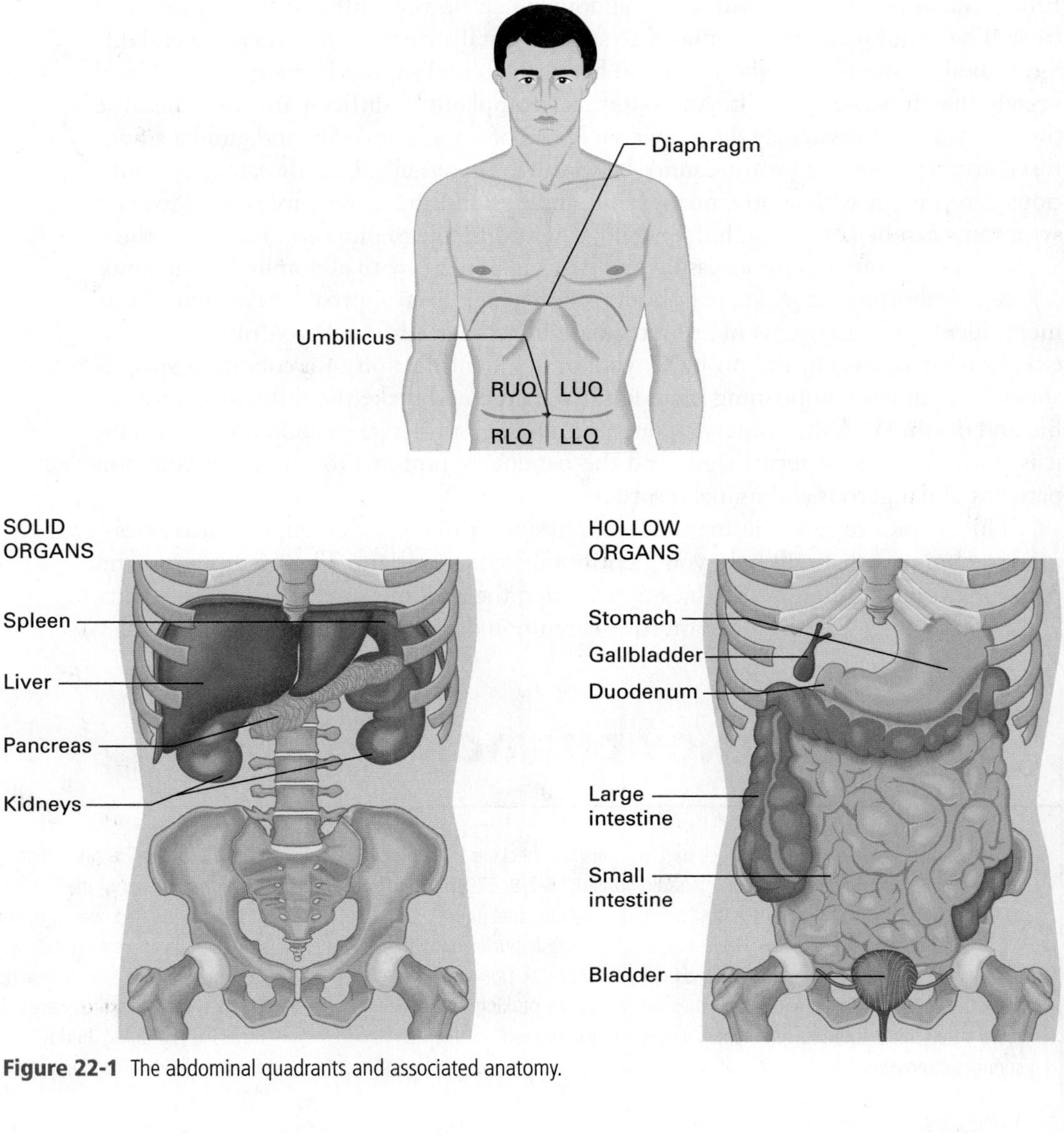

Figure 22-1 The abdominal quadrants and associated anatomy.

TABLE 22-1 ABDOMINAL QUADRANTS

RIGHT UPPER QUADRANT (RUQ)	LEFT UPPER QUADRANT (LUQ)
• Liver (in both upper quadrants) • Gall bladder • Pancreas (extends through both upper quadrants) • Large intestine (in all four quadrants) • Small intestine (in all four quadrants)	• Liver (in both upper quadrants) • Spleen • Pancreas (extends through both upper quadrants) • Stomach • Large intestine (in all four quadrants) • Small intestine (in four quadrants)
RIGHT LOWER QUADRANT (RLQ)	**LEFT LOWER QUADRANT (LLQ)**
• Appendix • Large intestine (in all four quadrants) • Small intestine (in all four quadrants) • Right ovary and fallopian tube (women only) • Ureter (in both lower quadrants)	• Large intestine (in all four quadrants) • Small intestine (in all four quadrants) • Left ovary and fallopian tube (women only) • Ureter (in both lower quadrants)

The organs of the abdomen are enclosed within a fibrous membrane that surrounds the abdominal cavity called the *peritoneum*. The outermost layer of the peritoneum is attached to the abdominal wall and is called the **parietal peritoneum.** The innermost layer is adhered to the abdominal organs and is called the **visceral peritoneum.** There is a potential space between the two layers filled only with a slight amount of lubricating *serous fluid*. Organs contained within the peritoneal space are referred to as **intraperitoneal.** Some organs, such as the kidneys, are found behind the abdominal cavity and are referred to as **retroperitoneal.** This is one reason why illness and injury involving the kidneys or aorta often present with pain in the back or flanks.

parietal peritoneum the outermost layer of the peritoneum attached to the wall of the abdomen.

visceral peritoneum innermost lining of the peritoneum adhered to the abdominal organs.

intraperitoneal within the peritoneal cavity.

retroperitoneal outside the peritoneal cavity.

gastrointestinal (GI) a term that refers to the digestive system, including the stomach and intestines.

It is also helpful to consider the body systems housed within the abdomen. Certainly the **gastrointestinal (GI)** system takes up a large amount of space within the abdominal cavity. Hollow organs, such as the stomach, colon, and small intestine, are all used to digest food and transfer key nutrients and water into the bloodstream. The stomach is generally located in the left upper quadrant. The colon traverses all four quadrants beginning in the right lower quadrant and ascending into the right upper quadrant, across to the left upper quadrant, descending to left lower quadrant, and then terminating in the rectum. The roughly 20 feet of small intestine in the average adult also occupies space in all four quadrants. The liver is used to produce bile to help digest fats and can be found in the right upper quadrant. The gall bladder is attached to the liver and stores bile. It too can be found in the right upper quadrant. The pancreas lies in the midline of both upper quadrants and produces digestive enzymes that assist in the breakdown of foods.

The endocrine system has key organs that can be found within the abdominal vault. The endocrine portion of the pancreas produces insulin and glucagon, both critical in metabolism of sugar. In the retroperitoneal space, adrenal glands that significantly contribute to the regulation of body systems sit affixed to the superior portion of each kidney.

The cardiovascular system is well represented in the abdomen. The spleen, found in the left upper quadrant, is used to regulate red blood cells and filter blood. In addition, the descending aorta and the ascending inferior vena cava travel through the abdominal space in the retroperitoneal cavity. All of these structures contain vast quantities of circulating blood and pose a risk of massive hemorrhage if damaged or diseased.

22-7 Describe the basic anatomy and physiology of the female reproductive system.

The female reproductive system is housed in the abdominal cavity. The female reproductive organs are normally present only in the lower abdominal quadrants. However, in advanced pregnancy the uterus ascends in the midline into the upper abdomen. Assessment of abdominal emergencies in women is particularly challenging because their reproductive organs lay superimposed on the gastrointestinal and urinary organs found in both genders.

menstrual pertaining to the female reproductive cycle.

It is worth taking a moment to review the specific placement and functions of the female reproductive organs. The ovaries are the organs that produce ova (the eggs). They are located on both sides in the lower abdominal quadrants. The fallopian tubes connect the ovaries to the uterus and are used to transport the ova. During the **menstrual** cycle, the egg is transported from the ovulating ovary through a fallopian tube to the uterus. If fertilization occurs, it typically happens during this transfer. The egg is then implanted in the uterus. If it has not been fertilized, it will be sloughed off along with the innermost lining of the uterus in the form of a menstrual period. If it has been fertilized, it will develop into a fetus. The uterus is a muscular, highly vascular organ designed to house the fetus. It lies in the midline between the two lower quadrants. In a nonpregnant woman the uterus is only roughly three inches long, but it will geometrically expand in a pregnant state. The vagina, or birth canal, connects the uterus to the outside world.

peritonitis inflammation of the peritoneum, typically from infection.

cholecystitis inflammation of the gall bladder.

Pain is the most common complaint that patients express about their abdomens. Understanding abdominal pain is not as simple as knowing the location of the organs. For example, pain associated with hollow organs tends to be described as "cramping" and frequently comes and goes. This is usually linked to the movement of peristalsis in the hollow organs of the digestive system. In addition, abdominal organs, including solid organs, tend to be associated with *visceral* pain. Visceral pain is often described as dull, achy, and difficult to pinpoint. Unlike the pain of a laceration or of a fracture, abdominal pain can be diffuse or even referred to a different location. The parietal peritoneum is very sensitive to irritation from blood or infections. Inflammation of the parietal peritoneum is called **peritonitis.** A patient with peritonitis will have a diffusely painful and tender abdomen. An example of referred pain would be pain from **cholecystitis** (infection of the gall bladder) presenting as right upper quadrant abdominal pain, as well as dull right shoulder pain.

22-3 Compare and contrast the general characteristics of hollow and solid organs and vascular structures found in the abdominal cavity.

Hollow organs, such as the intestines, may become obstructed, resulting in pain, nausea, and vomiting. Solid organs tend to be very vascular and typically contain a high volume of blood. That means these organs can be responsible for massive hemorrhage if damaged. (Table 22-2 classifies the different abdominal organs as either solid or hollow.)

TABLE 22-2 HOLLOW AND SOLID ABDOMINAL ORGANS

HOLLOW ORGANS	SOLID ORGANS
• Stomach	• Kidneys
• Large intestine	• Liver
• Small intestine	• Pancreas
• Gall bladder	• Spleen
• Appendix	• Ovaries
• Urinary bladder	

Pathophysiology of the Abdomen

22-4 List the general mechanisms and types of abdominal pain.

In terms of pathophysiology, the abdomen is particularly vulnerable to trauma. Key organ systems within the abdomen have rich blood supplies and are relatively exposed with regard to external forces. Chapter 33 covers abdominal injuries, but this chapter offers a review of common medical pathologies in order to provide a larger framework for discussion of abdominal assessment.

From a medical standpoint, the organs of the abdomen are at risk from a number of dangerous conditions. Because of the vascular nature of many of the organs and the large supply of blood traveling through the abdominal vault, hemorrhage is a major risk. Internal bleeding is probably the single largest risk factor for a patient with an abdominal complaint. Bleeding can certainly be caused by trauma, but also can present as a result of **ulcers,** aneurysms, and perforations.

ulcers points within the stomach where the inner lining has been worn thin or destroyed.

Infection is also a common abdominal dysfunction. Organs can be infected by bacteria, viruses, or fungi and can become inflamed and painful, and their function can be compromised. Consider hepatitis C. In this case a viral disease affects the liver. It causes inflammation, which in turn can cause abdominal pain, and if left untreated, can destroy the cells of the liver. More common infectious diseases include appendicitis and simple viral infections of the GI tract causing crampy pain, nausea, vomiting, and diarrhea.

Occasionally, acute abdominal pain can be caused by obstruction, rupture, or perforation of abdominal organs and vascular structures. In an abdominal aortic aneurysm, the descending aorta develops a weak section and can burst under the pressure of blood flow. In ectopic pregnancy, the development of a misplaced fetus in the fallopian tube can cause that tube to burst and cause severe hemorrhage. Generally, rupture of an abdominal structure poses two very dangerous problems. The first is severe and potentially life-threatening bleeding. The second is the spilling of organ contents (such as stool from the bowel) into the abdominal vault. The presence of blood or digestive contents outside the organs can lead to peritonitis.

Abdominal organ systems, like any other tissue in the body, require constant perfusion. Blood flow to abdominal organs can be interrupted by obstructions, hernias, clots, and shock states. Organ ischemia results from this hypoperfusion and, if the condition persists, can lead to cell death.

There are far too many injuries and diseases that can occur within the confines of the peritoneum and retroperitoneum to be covered in the scope of this text. The EMT is not expected to be able to diagnose the exact cause of abdominal symptoms, such as pain, gastrointestinal bleeding, nausea, vomiting, or diarrhea. However, as an EMT, the more knowledge you have of abdominal dysfunctions, the better prepared you will be for your patient assessment.

PERSPECTIVE

Donnie—The EMT

Initially, we were thinking it could be anything. I mean, some sort of trauma from crashing while skating, or a flu bug, or maybe some sort of ingested substance. Kids do sometimes make bad choices when they're out with friends, you know. But, man, with that vomiting, and his obvious fever, and the fact that the pain really seemed to be focused in his lower right quadrant, I definitely suspected appendicitis. Of course, Mika reminded me that it's not really our job to try to diagnose anything in the field. We provide emergency care and transport based on signs and symptoms, which is actually good because we don't need to always try to figure out what the problems might be.

PRACTICAL PATHOPHYSIOLOGY

Anticipating the risk of internal bleeding is exceptionally important in assessing and treating a patient with an abdominal complaint. Bleeding can occur within the GI tract, resulting in vomiting blood (an "upper GI bleed") or passing blood from the rectum (a "lower GI bleed"). In cases of GI bleeding, blood loss is usually obvious. Bleeding also can occur from solid organs, most commonly as a result of trauma. In that case the blood spills into the peritoneal cavity or fills the retroperitoneal space resulting in pain but no external blood loss. Because of the rich blood supply of the abdominal organs, any bleeding whether visible or not can be life threatening and result in hypoperfusion and the signs of shock. Rapid heart rate, pale skin, and even a fast respiratory rate are indicators that the body is responding to blood loss. Use those findings in both your primary and secondary assessments to help identify patients rapidly with this type of life-threatening problem.

STOP, REVIEW, REMEMBER!

Multiple Choice

For each question, place a check next to the correct answer.

1. Which one of the following organs is generally found in the left upper quadrant?

_____ a. Liver

_____ b. Spleen

_____ c. Gall bladder

_____ d. Appendix

2. Which one of the following organs would generally be considered retroperitoneal?

_____ a. Large intestine

_____ b. Pancreas

_____ c. Kidneys

_____ d. Stomach

3. An ectopic pregnancy would generally take place in which one of the following abdominal structures?

_____ a. Fallopian tube

_____ b. Descending aorta

_____ c. Ureter

_____ d. Kidney

4. Pain that comes and goes and is described as cramping would most likely be associated with dysfunction in which one of the following organs?

_____ a. Spleen

_____ b. Liver

_____ c. Small intestine

_____ d. Descending aorta

5. Pain associated with the liver would most likely be located in the ____________ quadrant of the abdomen.

_____ a. right upper

_____ b. left upper

_____ c. left lower

_____ d. right lower

Matching

Match the organ on the left with the description on the right.

1. _____ Spleen
2. _____ Gall bladder
3. _____ Liver
4. _____ Kidney
5. _____ Appendix

A. Hollow, right upper quadrant
B. Solid, left upper quadrant
C. Solid, right upper quadrant
D. Hollow, right lower quadrant
E. Solid, retroperitoneal

Critical Thinking

1. Describe why the pain associated with a hollow organ is often described as coming and going or cramping.

____

____

____

____

2. Describe why internal bleeding is a severe risk associated with abdominal complaints.

____

____

____

____

3. Describe what is meant by the term *referred pain*.

____

____

____

____

Assessment of the Acute Abdomen Patient

22-6 Explain the assessment-based approach to acute abdomen, including appropriate emergency care.

The assessment of the acute abdomen is a multistep approach designed first and foremost to identify immediate life threats. Once life threats are identified and emergency care is provided, a more specific examination may be conducted. EMTs should remember that identifying a particular diagnosis may never be possible and should rarely be the goal of this type of an assessment. However, with careful review, specific patterns of abdominal problems can be identified and dangerous conditions can and should be considered.

Scene Size-up

When a patient complains of abdominal pain, the scene may contain very important information. Every scene assessment must first determine safety for providers, but after ensuring this, the EMT should gather information from the patient's surroundings. Consider smells because they can indicate the foul odor of a GI bleed, the coppery smell of blood, the smell of vomit, or even the odor of a patient who is incontinent to feces or urine. Ensure appropriate personal protective equipment if faced with body fluids. Look for medications.

Frequently, patients with chronic abdominal complaints take medications such as antacids, and H2 blockers such as Pepcid or Tagamet. Dietary considerations such as fatty foods or alcohol intake also can impact and exacerbate chronic abdominal conditions such as gall bladder disease and **pancreatitis.**

pancreatitis inflammation of the pancreas.

Gather a general impression of the patient. Patients in severe abdominal pain frequently present in the fetal position (knees flexed up against the chest). Occasionally, visceral pain causes restlessness in patients. You may find them pacing and unable to sit still due to the pain. Use all these findings to inform the more specific assessments to come.

Primary Assessment

The primary assessment is used in all patients to rapidly identify life threats. This may be most important with patients who have an abdominal complaint. Because many vital organs are housed within the abdominal vault, dysfunction can be rapidly life threatening.

The primary assessment should be consistent in all patients and this is equally true in patients with an abdominal complaint. After ruling out external bleeding (rarely a problem associated with a medical abdominal disorder), the EMT must examine airway and breathing. Although abdominal problems rarely affect the airway, there can be conditions that you must address. Ruptured esophageal varices can cause major hemorrhage and vomiting of blood that spills over into the upper airway. The bleeding can cause airway compromise and frequently requires immediate suctioning and occasionally more definitive airway protection.

Mental status problems associated with shock also can affect the patient's ability to keep the airway patent. Any abdominal patient exhibiting signs of shock should be reassessed frequently to ensure the maintenance of adequate mental status to protect the airway. Establish a baseline in order to recognize changes when they occur.

Problems as simple as pain can make breathing more difficult and can impact alveolar ventilation. Life-threatening problems associated with abdominal complaints can be evident in tachypnea because it is a sign of compensation for hypoperfusion. For example, a patient with a massive GI bleed may present with rapid respirations as his body compensates for the blood loss. Rapid respiratory rates should be considered "red flags," especially when associated with clear lung sounds. These most often indicate shock. Patients found in respiratory failure require immediate intervention.

The assessment of the cardiovascular system will most likely identify the immediate abdominal life threat, which is likely to be massive hemorrhage. So recognizing the signs and symptoms of shock is extremely important when assessing the patient with an abdominal complaint. Look for signs of shock such as a rapid pulse, pale skin, delayed capillary refill time (beware of unreliability in adults), and even anxiety. Signs such as altered mental status, weak or absent peripheral pulses, and hypotension are ominous findings and point to shock.

Once the primary assessment is complete, consider the need for immediate interventions and transport. You should not waste important time with a secondary assessment if more important needs must be addressed. However, if it is reasonable to do so, obtain a baseline set of vital signs. They will give you an important starting point to help identify dangerous trends in your patient. Consider also exposing the abdomen to look for distention, bruising, or any unusual findings that might help identify the source of the problem.

Secondary Assessment

The secondary assessment should be conducted only if there are no more pressing priorities for your patient. The secondary assessment should never delay life-saving therapies or immediate transport when necessary. However, there are many cases in which no immediate life threats are found in the primary assessment. This would allow for a comprehensive secondary assessment.

In many cases of patients complaining of an abdominal complaint, the secondary assessment can be incredibly important. Not all life-threatening abdominal complaints will be obvious, and frequently more subtle, concerning signs are found only upon a more detailed and thorough examination. The secondary assessment is also the opportunity to gather information that could allow you to identify a pattern representing a common abdominal disorder. Pattern recognition frequently requires combining information from both a patient history and a physical, head-to-toe examination.

Physical Examination

The physical examination of the acute abdomen patient should focus on the abdomen itself. However, other body systems must be included. Although the head-to-toe exam is primarily associated with the trauma patient, there are vital findings for medical patients as well. As a result, providers should always consider a head-to-toe approach on all patients and adjust the level of detail to the condition at hand.

During the secondary assessment, inspect and palpate the abdomen. Expose the patient's belly and look for unusual findings such as distention (although it is worth noting that distention is often a late sign and frequently difficult to discern), bruising, edema, and anything you might consider abnormal (Figure 22-2 ▪). If the abdomen appears distended to you, ask the patient if he feels as though the abdomen is distended. You should gently palpate the abdomen feeling for tenderness, rigidity, guarding, and masses (Figure 22-3 ▪). Guarding is the flexion of the abdominal muscles in anticipation of pain. Patients with severe pain often present with guarding.

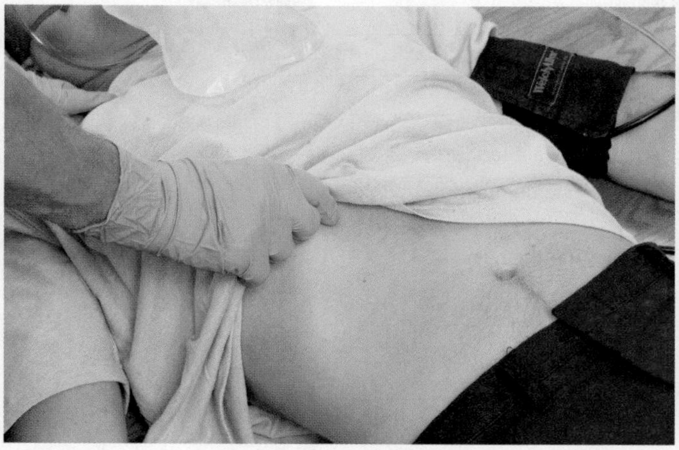

Figure 22-2 It is appropriate to expose the abdomen during assessment.

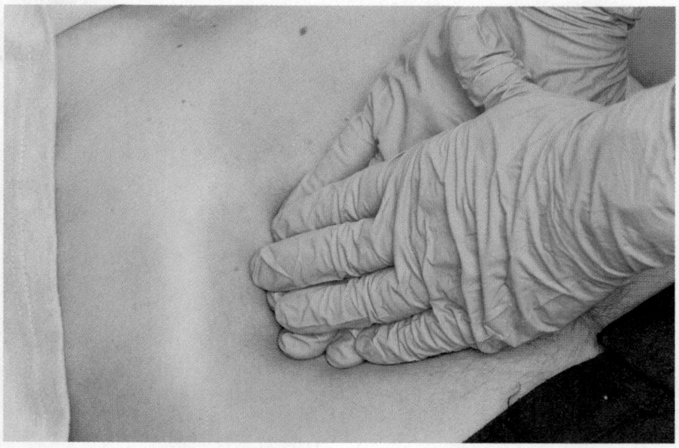

Figure 22-3 Use both hands to palpate each quadrant of the abdomen.

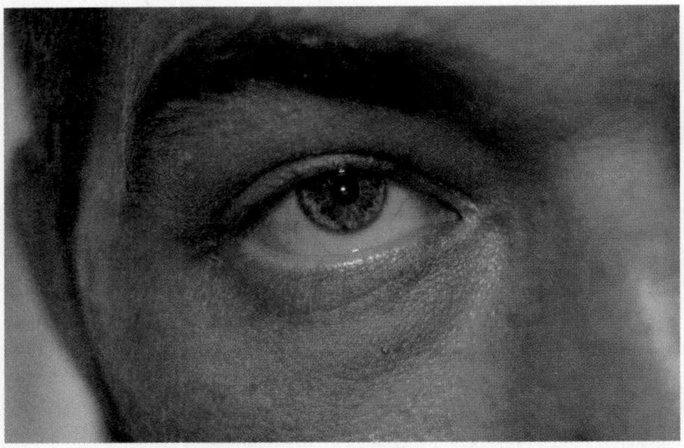

Figure 22-4 The yellow discoloration of the skin and eyes may be a sign of liver disease. (© Edward T. Dickinson, MD)

jaundice the yellowing of the skin and mucous membranes caused by a buildup of bilirubin; a condition that is commonly associated with liver failure.

Palpation of the abdomen should include all four quadrants and the area around the umbilicus. Prior to palpating the abdomen, ask the patient in what quadrant is in the most pain. That quadrant should be palpated last. Gently press and beware of eliciting pain. Often tenderness can be localized to a specific area and give you clues to the patient's problem based on the underlying anatomy.

In addition to examining the abdomen, consider the remainder of the secondary assessment. Although you may not be looking for bumps and bruises, pertinent findings abound. For example, **jaundice** or a yellowish tinge to the skin (Figure 22-4 ▪), particularly in the conjunctiva and the sclera of the eyes, fluid around the belly (called *ascites*), and venous distention on the abdominal wall can be signs of advanced liver problems. In addition, patients with abdominal complaints frequently describe referred pain (Figure 22-5 ▪). Pain in the shoulder, for example, must also be examined because it could very well represent a more serious abdominal emergency in which the diaphragm is being irritated. For example a ruptured spleen could refer pain to the left shoulder and an inflamed gall bladder could cause a complaint of right shoulder pain. Be thorough and the subtle findings will be found.

PERSPECTIVE

Mika—The EMT

Wow, talk about guarding! As soon as I touched that boy's abdomen, he yelled, smacked my hand away, and curled into an even tighter ball. He was in some serious pain, even started to cry. I looked around and saw a few kids his age in the crowd giggling. That's when I told Donnie that we needed to get him on the gurney and out to the truck. Crowds bug me sometimes. People can get surprisingly insensitive sometimes when someone is ill or injured. I see my job as an advocate for my patient extending beyond just the emergency care, you know? I try to be very conscious of a patient's feelings and surroundings, because when you're big sick, you're also very vulnerable. This boy didn't need kids laughing at him. He needed a hospital and he probably needed surgery.

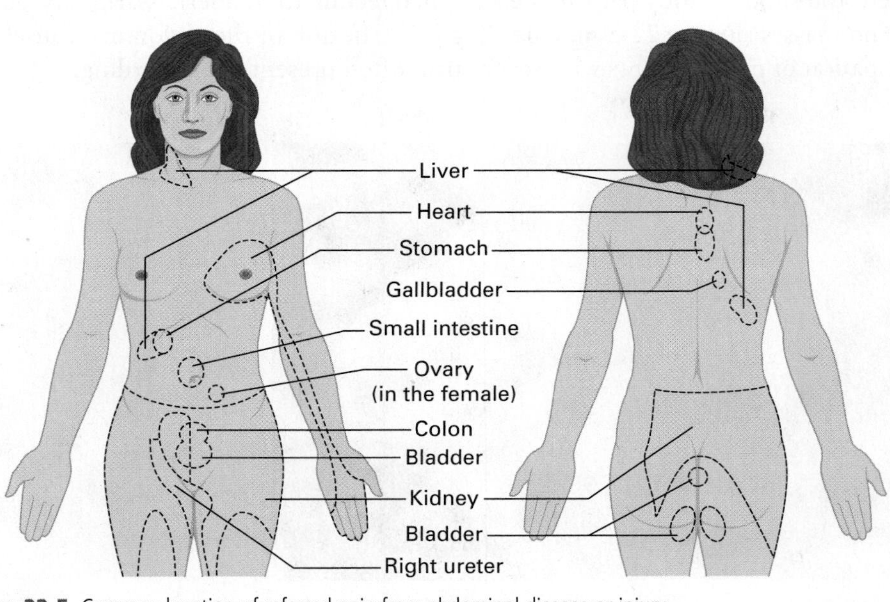

Figure 22-5 Common location of referred pain from abdominal disease or injury.

Patient History

Patient history is an extremely important element of the assessment of a patient with an abdominal complaint. Because the contents of the abdomen cannot be seen, physical examination is limited. A history and an examination of the chief complaint may be the best source of information. Furthermore, many abdominal complaints fit into a pattern and often the history of the present illness is key to identifying a likely disorder.

Obtaining the patient's chief complaint is one of the most important elements in obtaining a patient history. Ask the patient what is wrong and have him describe that complaint in his own words. It is frequently useful to ask the patient to actually point to the area where pain is present. This provides a probable indication of where the problem is likely centered. Use OPQRST to gather further information. Findings such as onset and quality of the pain can help make some conditions more or less likely. For example, problems with hollow organs tend to be described as cramping and coming and going. Aortic aneurysm pain is typically described as tearing.

A SAMPLE history is also very important. Using it as a memory aid can help make your patient interview more thorough, which may help you identify the problem of the moment. Even otherwise insignificant findings such as the patient's last meal can be very important to establishing the nature of an abdominal complaint. For example, gall bladder pain is frequently associated with recent fatty meals such as fried food. Exacerbation of chronic pancreatitis is frequently associated with alcohol intake. Of course these are not hard and fast rules, but rather they can help you establish a common pattern associated with particular disorders.

Risk factors are also important considerations that can help identify a pattern associated with certain conditions. For example, for a woman to have an ectopic pregnancy, she must be sexually active. Although this is a delicate question to ask, establishing the absence of sexual activity can help rule out ectopic pregnancy. Other risk factors include chronic hypertension and smoking (part of a pattern for aortic aneurysm), recent surgeries (for bowel obstructions), and gastroesophageal reflux disease (for ulcers and GI bleeding).

Remember that reassessment is vitally important with acute abdominal patients. In many cases life threats are difficult to identify and may only show as the patient's condition worsens. Constant reevaluation is necessary to identify these types of patients.

PRACTICAL PATHOPHYSIOLOGY

An ectopic pregnancy develops when a fertilized egg is implanted in the fallopian tube (or surrounding area) rather than in the uterus. As the fetus develops, the fragile tissue of the tube cannot stretch to accommodate growth and ruptures. The abdominal pain from ruptured ectopic pregnancies is usually sudden in onset, begins in either the left or right lower quadrants before spreading, and is often associated with vaginal bleeding. Note that sometimes the patient is unaware of her pregnancy. Any sexually active female of child-bearing age with sudden onset of lower abdominal pain should be considered at a high risk for an ectopic pregnancy. Conversely, if she is not sexually active, she cannot be experiencing an ectopic pregnancy.

STOP, REVIEW, REMEMBER!

Multiple Choice

For each question, place a check next to the correct answer.

1. Which one of the following conditions is commonly associated with airway compromise in a patient with an abdominal complaint?

_____ a. Esophageal bleeding

_____ b. Gastroesophageal reflux disease

_____ c. Pancreatitis

_____ d. Peritonitis

2. The most dangerous condition associated with tachypnea with clear lung sounds in a patient who has an abdominal complaint is:

_____ a. shock.

_____ b. pain.

_____ c. anxiety.

_____ d. nausea.

3. Which one of the following would be a specific indicator of shock in a patient with an abdominal complaint?

_____ a. Tachycardia

_____ b. Tachypnea

_____ c. Absent radial pulse

_____ d. Anxiety

4. A 77-year-old man complains of abdominal pain. He is confused and quite pale. His vital signs are pulse 122, respiration 28, and blood pressure 82/58. After completing the primary assessment, you should next:

_____ a. obtain a SAMPLE history.

_____ b. utilize OPQRST to examine the chief complaint.

_____ c. initiate transport.

_____ d. conduct a head-to-toe examination.

5. The flexion of the abdominal muscles in anticipation of pain is also known as:

_____ a. distention.

_____ b. tenderness.

_____ c. ascites.

_____ d. guarding.

Critical Thinking

1. Describe how assessment of the scene can improve your assessment of the acute abdomen patient.

____

____

____

____

2. Describe the findings that may indicate shock in a patient with an abdominal complaint.

____

____

____

____

3. Describe why establishing a baseline set of vital signs and then reassessing them is important in a patient with an abdominal complaint.

4. Describe a scenario in which you would *not* complete a secondary assessment of a patient with an abdominal complaint.

5. Describe why completing a SAMPLE history is important in a patient with an abdominal complaint.

Emergency Care of the Acute Abdomen Patient

In general, emergency care should focus on the most immediate threat to life. Given that internal bleeding and infection are the most likely critical condition in the acute abdomen patient, the EMT should take steps to provide emergency care for shock. Initiate immediate transport, maintain body temperature, and place the patient in a supine position if it can be tolerated. Supplemental oxygen should be considered. Most likely, this patient will require surgical intervention and, therefore, is similar to the multisystem trauma patient. That is, the most important element of emergency care is rapid transport. Consider ALS backup or intercept, based on the call logistics. Just as in trauma care, early communication with the receiving facility will improve the overall care for this patient.

Consider any life threat found in the primary assessment and treat accordingly. Manage airway, breathing, and circulation. Other considerations include patient position. If shock is identified, then the supine position is preferred, but a patient with abdominal pain will likely prefer a seated, lateral recumbent, or even a position with flexed knees (Figure 22-6 ■). It is likely that a patient in severe pain will choose his own most comfortable position.

Nausea and vomiting is often a side effect of a variety of abdominal complaints. You should be prepared to handle vomiting with an emesis basin and suction when

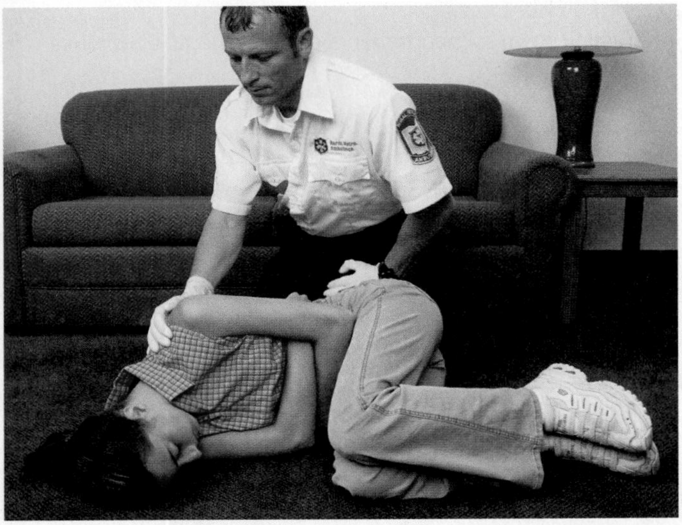

Figure 22-6 The position of comfort for a patient with abdominal pain often is the fetal position.

necessary. Beware of vomiting in a patient with an altered mental status. Be prepared to clear and manage the airway. Take appropriate BSI precautions.

Because many abdominal complaints result in surgery, patients should be given nothing by mouth and prevented from eating or drinking prior to arrival at the hospital.

As stated previously, constant reassessment is very important because the patient's condition can deteriorate rapidly. Be aware of patients exhibiting signs of shock because rapid blood loss can quickly compromise the patient. Stay alert to trends in vital signs and constantly reevaluate the patient's status.

Differential Diagnosis and Pattern Recognition

22-5 Describe the pathophysiology and the signs and symptoms associated with common causes of acute abdomen, including abdominal aortic aneurysm, appendicitis, cholecystitis, esophageal varices, gastroenteritis, gastrointestinal bleeding, hernia, intestinal obstruction, pancreatitis, peritonitis, and ulcers.

Making an exact diagnosis for the cause of an abdominal complaint is not your primary goal. Rather, you must look for, identify, and provide care for immediate life threats. In many cases, a specific diagnosis may not be possible in the field. However, there are certain conditions that are important to recognize. Those conditions are generally identified through patterns of signs and symptoms particular to the pathophysiology of the disorder.

Acute Myocardial Infarction

Although an acute myocardial infarction is not in fact an abdominal disorder, it does from time to time manifest itself as an abdominal complaint. Heart-attack patients frequently complain of upper midline abdominal pain and/or nausea. Because the heart lies close to the diaphragm and shares similar nervous pathways, cardiac pain can be referred to the abdomen. It may be very difficult to discern the true origin of this type of pain. As such, EMTs should consider a cardiac origin for patients with acute onset abdominal pain. In most cases, medical direction should be consulted as to whether cardiac treatments such as aspirin or nitroglycerin are appropriate. Access to 12-lead ECG is very important in these cases and should be obtained as soon as possible. Depending on your system, this may mean a rendezvous with advanced life support.

Gastrointestinal Bleeding

Many conditions can cause bleeding within the gastrointestinal (GI) system. Common causes include abnormal blood vessels or damaged blood vessels in the wall of the esophagus or bowel and ulcers within the stomach (Figure 22-7 ■). In those cases slow bleeding within the digestive tract may be difficult to detect. However, bleeding in the GI tract also can be massive and very evident.

hematemesis the vomiting of blood.

esophageal varices an increase in pressure and exposure of the blood vessels of the esophagus.

Traditionally, blood from a GI bleed can be seen in different forms. **Hematemesis,** or blood in vomit, often indicates profuse bleeding in the upper portions of the GI tract, indicating a condition called **esophageal varices** in which abnormally dilated veins in the esophagus become vulnerable to rupture. The condition is common in chronic alcoholics and patients with advanced liver disease, and can be made even worse when blood flow through the liver is restricted from conditions such as sclerosis. Esophageal varices can be a deadly disorder if they rupture suddenly. Profuse bleeding not only poses a risk of shock, but also a significant airway risk due to the proximity to the upper airway.

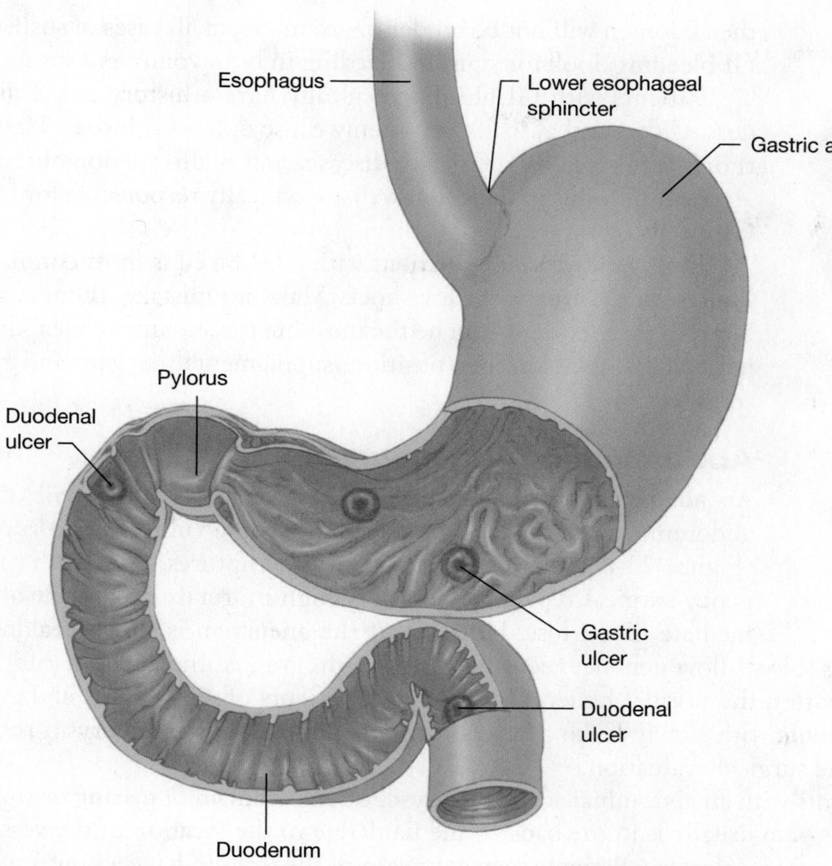

Figure 22-7 A common source of internal bleeding is stomach and intestinal ulcers.

Hematochezia, or fresh blood being passed with a bowel movement, is an indication of severe GI bleeding. Fresh blood can be a sign that there is bleeding very low in the GI tract where blood does not have time to be digested. In contrast, **melena,** or coffee ground-like tarry stool, is a sign of bleeding high in the GI tract. This foul-smelling discharge may not be recognized by the patient as blood, but it is blood that has passed through a large portion of the GI system and has been partially digested.

hematochezia the passing of blood through the feces.

melena black tarry feces associated with blood in the stool.

Patients who are bleeding in the GI tract frequently present with life-threatening signs of shock. It is important to thoroughly focus on the circulatory aspect of the primary assessment in these patients. EMTs must recognize the signs of compensated shock and intervene as soon as possible. Look for tachycardia, tachypnea (especially with clear lung sounds), pale skin, and delayed capillary refill time.

Upper abdominal pain is a frequent complaint associated with gastrointestinal bleeding. It is commonly associated with stomach ulcers (small lesions in the lining of the stomach) and gastritis (chronic inflammation of the lining of the stomach). Both conditions are typically chronic and can severely damage the stomach. If progressive enough, blood vessels in the wall of the stomach and esophagus can become eroded causing massive hemorrhage. If a perforation all the way through the stomach wall occurs, abdominal pain is typically described as sudden onset and severe in nature as the contents of the stomach spill into the peritoneal cavity, causing irritation and peritonitis.

On physical examination, patients with a GI bleed may present with signs of shock. Their abdomens may be tender, guarded, and possibly distended if the bleeding is severe. Though, interestingly, many massive lower GI bleeds are painless and

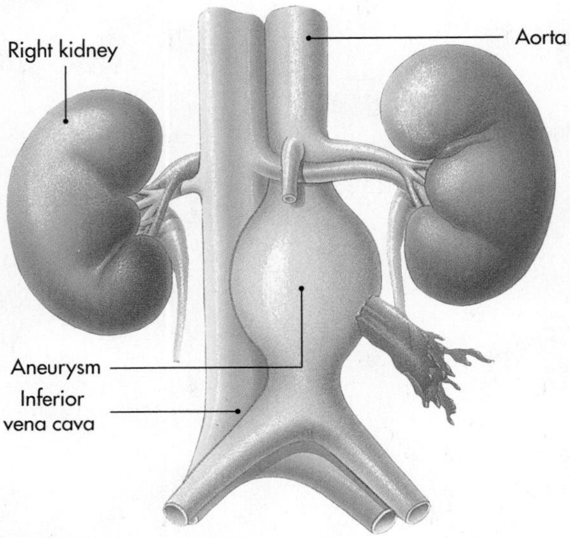

Figure 22-8 An abdominal aortic aneurysm occurs when an area of the aorta bulges and becomes thin.

the abdomen will not be tender on exam. So, in all cases of suspected GI bleeding, look for signs of bleeding in both vomit and stool.

Patients with GI bleeding typically have a history of GI disorders. Ulcers and gastritis commonly cause upper GI bleeds. Hemorrhoids, diverticulosis, Crohn's disease, and malformations between arteries and veins in the colon wall are typically responsible for lower GI bleeds.

Emergency care of a patient with a GI bleed is most commonly limited to the treatment for shock. Make no mistake, though, a GI bleed in these patients can be the most life threatening of all abdominal complaints. Consider position, supplemental oxygen, and rapid transport.

Abdominal Aortic Aneurysm

abdominal aortic aneurysm (AAA) the abnormal bulging of an artery wall.

An **abdominal aortic aneurysm (AAA)** occurs when the wall of the abdominal aorta begins to bulge and become vulnerable to rupture (Figure 22-8 ■). If the aortic aneurysm ruptures, even with emergency surgical repair, there is very high mortality as a result of immediate blood loss. However, if the aneurysm is slowly leaking or dissecting (blood flow gets between the layers in the wall of the aorta, rather than flowing within the normal lumen in the center), patients often describe abdominal pain. Patients with slowly leaking or dissecting abdominal aortic aneurysm require immediate surgical evaluation.

Patients with an abdominal aortic aneurysm often complain of tearing or ripping pain. This pain usually is in the back or the flank due to the location of the vessel in the retroperitoneal space. Patients may complain of the urge to have a bowel movement as well.

Physical findings are typically nonspecific. If a rupture has occurred, shock will rapidly progress. Other physical findings can include, in the midline of the abdomen, a mass felt on palpation that has a detectable pulse. Use caution not to be too aggressive when palpating such a finding. Depending on the location of the abdominal aortic aneurysm, you also may find different levels of perfusion from side to side in the lower extremities.

Many patients with an aneurysm are aware they have the problem. A history of a diagnosed aneurysm certainly increases the likelihood of a second event. History of hypertension and cigarette smoking are also significant risk factors.

Emergency care varies depending on the status of the patient. Signs of shock or internal bleeding require rapid transport.

Appendicitis

appendicitis inflammation of the appendix.

The appendix is a small sac located near the junction of the small and large intestines in the right lower quadrant. Its function is largely not understood and it is thought to be either a genetic remnant or possibly a storage area for bacteria. This small sac can be obstructed and become infected, causing a condition called **appendicitis.** In appendicitis, the appendix becomes inflamed, swollen, and can rupture if not corrected. Although not usually life threatening, a ruptured appendix can spill intestinal content into the peritoneal space, causing peritonitis and an infection that can indeed be life threatening.

Appendicitis typically presents as abdominal pain. The classic description of abdominal pain from appendicitis is that it begins as a vague pain in the center of the abdomen and then settles into the right lower quadrant. Appendicitis is often accompanied by fever and nausea and sometimes vomiting.

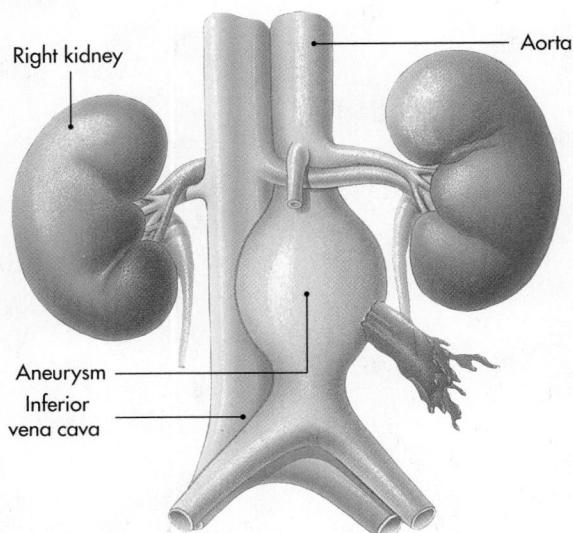

Physical examination will show fever (sometimes) and tenderness mostly in the right lower quadrant. If a rupture has occurred, signs of shock can be present, although this is rare.

Emergency care generally requires surgery, so nothing should be given to eat or drink. If shock is present, provide emergency care accordingly.

Pancreatitis

Pancreatitis refers to inflammation of the pancreas. The vast majority of pancreatitis cases are caused by chronic disorders such as alcohol abuse. In these cases the chronic insult on the pancreas results in permanent damage and continuing destruction. In acute cases, obstructions from gallstones that block the drainage of the digestive enzymes of the pancreas can cause more rapid onset of symptoms. Although typically an ongoing issue, pancreatitis patients can become acutely and severely ill over a short amount of time. If the damage to the pancreas is severe enough, hemorrhage and shock can result. More commonly, the patient presents with severe pain typically localized in the left upper quadrant or around the midline. Pancreatic pain commonly radiates through to the back and is exacerbated by drinking alcohol. Patients present with severe nausea and repetitive vomiting. They are often tender in the upper quadrants.

Risk factors for pancreatitis include a history of chronic pancreatitis and alcohol abuse (especially recent ingestion of alcohol).

Emergency care for these patients is centered around transport and supportive care. Assess and treat for shock.

Cholecystitis

Cholecystitis is an inflammation (usually an infection) of the gall bladder. The gall bladder is responsible for the storage and distribution of bile, which assists in the digestion of fats. Most cholecystitis is caused by the creation of stones within the gall bladder. The stones obstruct the common bile duct and cause severe pain and inflammation when bile cannot be excreted.

The pain of cholecystitis is typically unilateral and centered in the right upper quadrant. It often is described as cramping and coming and going as severity increases when the gall bladder contracts and pushes against the obstructed bile duct. Pain also frequently occurs after eating a greasy or fatty meal (as the gall bladder attempts to empty to help digest the fat).

Cholecystitis pain can be referred to the right shoulder and toward the midline. It is often difficult to differentiate this pain from the pain of acute myocardial infarction because it typically occurs just below the chest. Patients are also frequently diaphoretic (sweaty) and sometimes pale with this condition. Nausea and vomiting are also common.

Physical examination may reveal tenderness and agitation in the patient. This condition is not usually life threatening, but can lead to peritonitis in certain circumstances. Emergency care is mostly supportive. Place the patient in a position of comfort and transport.

Gastroenteritis

Gastroenteritis is a condition in which the mucosal lining of the stomach and the intestines become inflamed and irritated. The condition can be either acute or chronic and most commonly results in abdominal discomfort and diarrhea. Although in the United States these conditions are more of a nuisance than a life threat, in many developing nations diarrhea disorders are the leading cause of pediatric death. In gastroenteritis, the main problem is dehydration from frequent diarrhea. Because the intestinal lining is responsible for the absorption of water, this condition can

gastroenteritis an inflammation and breakdown of the lining of the stomach and intestines, resulting in diarrhea.

lead to severe fluid loss and shock, particularly in vulnerable populations such as the elderly and childen.

Gastroenteritis usually is caused by a virus or bacteria, and as a result these patients frequently show signs of infectious disease. Fever is common. Abdominal discomfort may be described as crampy pain often associated with the need to have a bowel movement. If the upper GI system is affected, nausea and vomiting is common.

Physical findings may include diarrhea. Signs of GI bleeding and shock may be present in extreme cases. Emergency care is mostly supportive. Place the patient in a position of comfort and transport.

Bowel Obstructions

adhesions internal scar tissue that connects tissues that are not normally connected.

hernia a protrusion of abdominal organs through a membranous wall such as the diaphragm.

Bowel obstructions occur when the flow through the intestine becomes blocked. This typically results from **adhesions** and scarring from previous surgeries and **hernias.** Hernias occur when abdominal contents (such as the small bowel) extend through weak spots in the normal abdominal muscles and into the subcutaneous abdominal wall (Figure 22-9 ▪). Abdominal hernias most commonly occur in the groin, around the umbilicus, or at the site of past surgeries. If the defect in the abdominal wall muscle is too tight, then the loop of bowel can become obstructed within the hernia and even have its blood supply compromised. This is called a *strangulated hernia*.

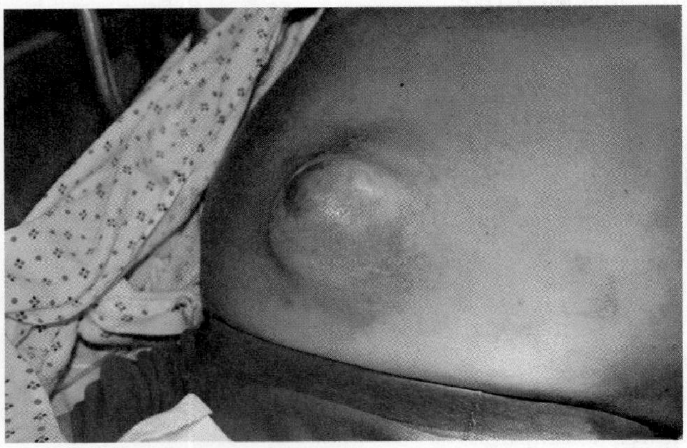

Figure 22-9 An abdominal hernia. (© Edward T. Dickinson)

Bowel obstructions can be extremely painful and life threatening if not corrected. Patients with a bowel obstruction will complain of diffuse, visceral pain. Commonly the pain comes and goes with normal movement of the intestines. Patients may also complain of severe nausea and vomiting.

Physical examination can identify previous surgical scars, palpable and tender hernias, abdominal distention, and diffuse tenderness. In extreme cases, shock from the breakdown of the intestines may be evident. Risk factors include previous bowel obstructions and recent abdominal surgeries.

Emergency care for patients with gastroenteritis or bowel obstructions is primarily supportive. Assess for shock and transport in a position of comfort.

Urinary System Causes of Abdominal Pain

The renal and urinary system is covered in more detail in Chapter 25. Common causes of abdominal pain from the urinary system include kidney stones, kidney infections (pyelonephritis), and bladder infections (cystitis). Only a portion of the urinary bladder sits within the peritoneal cavity. The rest of the organs (the kidneys and ureters) are retroperitoneal. For this reason the pain associated with these conditions is often dull and nagging with associated nausea and vomiting. In the cases of pyelonephritis and cystitis, pain upon urination, abnormally frequent urination, and fevers are often encountered. Emergency care is mostly supportive. Place the patient in a position of comfort and transport.

22-8 Describe the pathophysiology and the signs and symptoms associated with common gynecological conditions, including endometriosis, endometritis, ovarian cyst, and pelvic inflammatory disease.

22-9 Explain the assessment-based approach to acute gynecological emergencies, including appropriate emergency care.

Dysfunction in the Female Reproductive Organs

Gynecological emergencies present a unique challenge to the EMS provider. Emergencies in the female reproductive system can be vastly different in a pregnant woman compared to one who is not pregnant. A few of the more common reasons for abdominal pain follow. (Obstetrical and gynecological emergencies are discussed in detail in Chapter 27.)

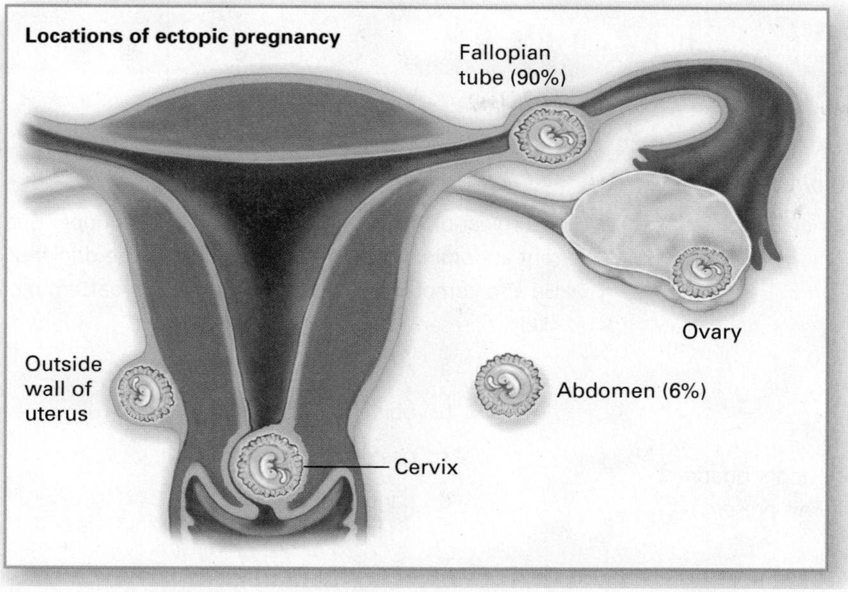

Figure 22-10 Locations of an ectopic pregnancy.

The most life-threatening pregnancy-related abdominal emergency in women is a ruptured ectopic pregnancy (Figure 22-10 ■). The most common cause of unexpected vaginal bleeding is caused by a **spontaneous abortion,** also known as a *miscarriage*. A spontaneous abortion occurs when the pregnant woman expels the developing fetus prior to full gestation. This most commonly occurs in the first three months of pregnancy.

spontaneous abortion the expulsion of the developing fetus prior to full gestation. Also called *miscarriage*.

In nonpregnant women gynecological reasons for abdominal pain include:

- ***Ruptured ovarian cysts.*** With each menstrual cycle, an egg is expelled through the wall of one of the ovaries. The site on the surface of the ovary where the egg was expelled may develop a blood blister-like cyst. If that **ovarian cyst** ruptures, it can cause sudden unilateral lower abdominal pain and even localized peritonitis as blood irritates the peritoneal lining of the lower abdominal cavity.
- ***Endometritis.*** This is the inflammation of the inside lining of the uterus. Symptoms of **endometritis** include lower abdominal pain, fever, vaginal bleeding, and abnormal vaginal discharge.
- ***Endometriosis.*** This is the seeding of the peritoneal cavity with the specialized tissue that normally lines only the uterus. **Endometriosis** pain is chronic and is often worse at the time of a woman's menstrual bleeding.
- ***Pelvic inflammatory disease (PID).*** This condition is the sexually transmitted bacterial infection of the cervix, uterus, and fallopian tubes. **Pelvic inflammatory disease (PID)** results in diffuse lower abdominal pain often associated with increased vaginal discharge.
- ***Dysmenorrhea.*** A general term, **dysmenorrhea** refers to problems with menstruation that include crampy, painful periods and abnormally heavy, irregular, or protracted vaginal bleeding.

ovarian cyst the development of a fluid-filled sac on the outside of the ovaries.

endometritis an infection of the lining of the uterus.

endometriosis development of uterine-lining cells outside the uterus; typically on the external surface of the uterus and the ovaries.

pelvic inflammatory disease (PID) general term used to describe processes (typically sexually transmitted diseases) that cause inflammation of the uterus, ovaries, and the fallopian tubes.

dysmenorrhea pain during menstruation.

Emergency care involves managing bleeding, supporting the ABCs, and placing the patient in a position of comfort. If signs of shock are present, it may be appropriate to elevate the patient's legs 12 to 18 inches.

STOP, REVIEW, REMEMBER!

Multiple Choice

For each question, place a check next to the correct answer.

1. Inflammation of the gall bladder is also known as:

   _____ a. pancreatitis.

   _____ b. peritonitis.

   _____ c. cholecystitis.

   _____ d. appendicitis.

2. A 26-year-old woman presents with right upper quadrant abdominal pain referred to her shoulder. This presentation most likely represents the pattern of:

   _____ a. cholecystitis.

   _____ b. pelvic inflammatory disease.

   _____ c. ectopic pregnancy.

   _____ d. hepatitis.

3. Protrusion of the small bowel through the abdominal wall muscle layer is also known as:

   _____ a. aortic aneurysm.

   _____ b. abdominal hernia.

   _____ c. perforated ulcers.

   _____ d. esophageal varices.

4. A 52-year-old man presents with severe left upper quadrant abdominal pain exacerbated after binge drinking. He also complains of severe vomiting. This pattern most likely represents:

   _____ a. acute myocardial infarction.

   _____ b. bowel obstruction.

   _____ c. gastroenteritis.

   _____ d. pancreatitis.

5. Development of uterine tissue on structures outside the uterus is otherwise known as:

   _____ a. endometriosis.

   _____ b. endometritis.

   _____ c. pelvic inflammatory disease.

   _____ d. ovarian cysts.

Critical Thinking

1. Describe the two major life threats associated with a ruptured esophageal varices patient.

____

____

____

____

2. Describe how the findings associated with a lower GI bleed would be different from the findings associated with an upper GI bleed.

____

____

____

____

3. Describe why the pain associated with a bowel obstruction is commonly described as coming and going.

4. Describe the common presentation of a woman experiencing an ectopic pregnancy.

5. Describe why a patient with gastroenteritis would become dehydrated.

EMERGENCY DISPATCH SUMMARY

Mika and Donnie moved the patient to the gurney, allowing him to stay curled on his side, and initiated supplemental oxygen therapy during the 10-minute drive to Community Regional Hospital. After a brief assessment in the emergency department, the patient was taken to surgery to have his appendix removed. Two days later he was released from the hospital and is expected to make a full recovery.

Chapter Review

To the Point

- The abdominal cavity extends from the diaphragm to the lower border of the pelvis. Abdominal organs are contained within the peritoneum with the exception of the retroperitoneal organs.
- Solid organs are dense and highly vascular. Hollow organs are at risk of rupture and frequently cause cramp-like pain.
- Abdominal pain has a huge array of causes. Finding the exact cause often is less important than recognizing any immediate life threats.
- Recognizing patterns of specific abdominal disorders can help you identify immediate life threats and improve your capability to diagnose abdominal problems.
- Emergency care of abdominal problems often is generalized. Recognize and treat shock, initiate transport, and support your patient.
- The female reproductive system poses specific challenges to assessment and care. Many reproductive system-specific causes can be the route of abdominal pain and bleeding.

Chapter Questions

Multiple Choice

For each question, place a check next to the correct answer.

1. The stomach would be most likely found in which one of the following abdominal quadrants?
   _____ a. Left upper quadrant
   _____ b. Right upper quadrant
   _____ c. Left lower quadrant
   _____ d. Right lower quadrant

2. Melena is most likely caused by a:
   _____ a. massive GI bleed.
   _____ b. slow GI bleed.
   _____ c. ruptured esophageal varices.
   _____ d. dissecting aortic aneurysm.

3. A 40-year-old man complains of crampy abdominal discomfort and uncontrolled diarrhea after travel to South America. He presents with a fever. He is most likely suffering from:
   _____ a. gastroenteritis.
   _____ b. peptic ulcers.
   _____ c. a bowel obstruction.
   _____ d. pancreatitis.

4. Which one of the following would best define hematochezia?
   _____ a. Blood in vomit
   _____ b. Blood in urine
   _____ c. Fresh blood in stool
   _____ d. Tarry or coffee ground-like blood in stool

5. The most common cause of vaginal bleeding is:
   _____ a. spontaneous abortion.
   _____ b. sexual assault.
   _____ c. sexually transmitted diseases.
   _____ d. ovarian cysts.

6. A 65-year-old obese woman complains of right upper quadrant abdominal pain after eating a greasy meal. This pattern most likely represents:
   _____ a. pancreatitis.
   _____ b. gastroenteritis.
   _____ c. cholecystitis.
   _____ d. endometritis.

7. The female reproductive structure responsible for the transfer of the ovum to the uterus is the:
   _____ a. ovary.
   _____ b. fallopian tube.
   _____ c. ureter.
   _____ d. vagina.

Fill in the Blank

1. The outermost layer of the peritoneum is called the ______________________ peritoneum.
2. The organ responsible for filtering the blood and managing red blood cell levels is the ______________________.
3. An infection of the inner lining of the uterus is called ______________________.

Critical Thinking

1. You are caring for a patient who complains of pain in the right upper quadrant of his abdomen. In what organs should you suspect dysfunction?

2. A 61-year-old man complains of pain along the midline of his upper two abdominal quadrants. He notes the pain had an acute onset and is now sharp and steady. Describe at least two conditions that match this pattern.

3. A 68-year-old man complains of tearing pain in his back. He notes a long history of hypertension and today the development of pain. Describe the most likely condition associated with this pattern.

4. For each of the following abdominal quadrants list an organ found within it.
   a. Right upper quadrant

   b. Left upper quadrant

   c. Right lower quadrant

   d. Left lower quadrant

(continued on next page)

(continued)

Case Study

A 55-year-old man complains today of chronic abdominal pain. He notes he has recently been vomiting blood. On arrival you note he is awake and alert. He seems slightly agitated but is ambulatory. He tells you he feels like he needs to vomit again.

1. What information is immediately important regarding this patient?

2. What immediate assessment steps would you perform?

The patient's airway is patent, but you note an elevated respiratory rate. On auscultation you note clear lung sounds. You find that this patient has a weak radial pulse and a tachycardic heart rate.

3. What, if anything, do the tachypnea and tachycardia indicate?

4. What initial care does this patient require?

5. What additional assessments would be necessary for this patient?

The Last Word

Although this chapter describes a variety of patterns associated with abdominal dysfunctions, beware becoming bogged down by diagnostics when you should be providing emergency care to the patient. Abdominal disorders can be some of the most complex medical puzzles, but more often than not, solving the puzzle is not to the immediate benefit of the patient. You should focus your attention first on identifying and treating life threats. Then, and only then, should you move on to a more detailed assessment.

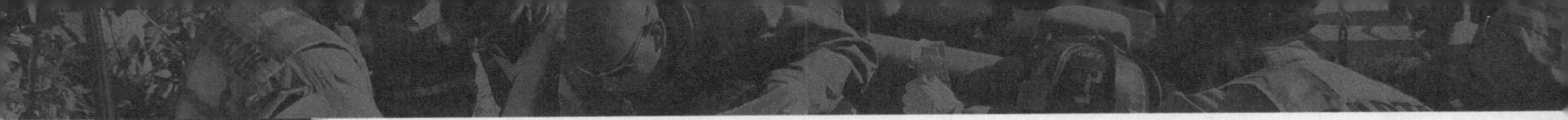

23

Caring for Patients with Acute Diabetic Emergencies

Education Standards

Medicine: Endocrine Disorders

Competencies

Applies fundamental knowledge to provide basic emergency care and transportation based on assessment findings for an acutely ill patient.

Objectives

After completion of this lesson, you should be able to:

23-1 Define key terms introduced in this chapter.

23-2 Describe the function of glucose in the body.

23-3 Describe the response of brain cells and other body cells to insufficient glucose levels.

23-4 Describe the relationship of glucose and water in the body.

23-5 Describe how glucose levels are regulated in normal metabolism.

23-6 Describe how insulin and glucagon function to control blood glucose levels.

23-7 Discuss the pathophysiology of diabetes mellitus (DM) and contrast type 1 insulin-dependent diabetes mellitus (IDDM) with type 2 noninsulin-dependent diabetes mellitus (NIDDM).

23-8 Explain the purposes and process of checking blood glucose levels.

23-9 Discuss the pathophysiology, assessment, and emergency medical care of a hypoglycemic emergency.

23-10 Discuss the pathophysiology, assessment, and emergency medical care of hyperglycemia and diabetic ketoacidosis (DKA).

23-11 Identify indications and contraindications to the administration of oral glucose.

23-12 Compare and contrast the speed of onset and the signs and symptoms of hypoglycemia and hyperglycemia.

Key Terms

diabetes mellitus (DM) p. 617
diabetic ketoacidosis (DKA) p. 623
gestational diabetes p. 619
glucagon p. 618
glucose p. 617
hyperglycemia p. 617
hypoglycemia p. 619
insulin p. 618
islets of Langerhans p. 619
polydipsia p. 618
polyuria p. 618
type 1 diabetes mellitus p. 619
type 2 diabetes mellitus p. 619

Introduction

Diabetes mellitus (DM) is a medical condition that affects approximately 25 million adults and children in the United States. Interestingly only two-thirds, or approximately 18 million, have been officially diagnosed with the disease. That leaves approximately 8 million individuals who are undiagnosed each year. According to the Web site Diabetes.org, there are approximately 79 million individuals in the United States who are defined as "prediabetic" and may go on to develop diabetes. Because diabetes affects so many of all ages, EMS responses for emergencies related to diabetes are quite common.

This chapter will introduce you to the pathophysiology of diabetes, some of the most common signs and symptoms of emergencies, and the appropriate care and management of a patient experiencing a diabetic emergency.

diabetes mellitus (DM) a group of metabolic disorders that cause patients with the disease to have an abnormally high blood-glucose level. Also known as *hyperglycemia*.

EMERGENCY DISPATCH

"Personally," the police officer nodded his head toward the woman sitting on the park bench. "I think she's drunk. But department policy says I need to let you check her out before I take her in."

EMT Renee Bollinger thanked the officer and walked over to the shabbily dressed woman, who was swaying slightly on the bench and watching the EMTs approach with heavy-lidded eyes. "Hi, ma'am, my name is Renee. I'm here to make sure you're okay. Have you been drinking or taking any drugs today?"

The woman examined Renee's face closely for a moment before sitting back, crossing her arms clumsily, and shaking her head with a flourish. "Nope," she said.

"You see what I mean?" The officer walked up and unsnapped the handcuff case on his duty belt. "Can I take her now?"

"Hold on a second," Renee said, turning to her partner Lou Calle. "Can you hand me the glucometer, please?"

As Renee turned back to the patient, she found the woman's unsteady hand bobbing right in front of her face, index finger extended toward her. Renee smiled and said, "That's what I thought."

After absorbing the drop of blood from the patient's finger, the glucometer's display window flashed 36. As Renee turned back to Lou, he was already holding out a tube of glucose gel and tongue depressor.

"Well, I'll be." The police officer shrugged and snapped the handcuff case closed.

Diabetes Mellitus

Diabetes mellitus (DM) is a group of metabolic disorders that cause patients with the disease to have an abnormally high blood glucose level known as **hyperglycemia.** **Glucose** is a simple sugar and the primary source of energy for the cells. You may remember from the discussion on cellular respiration in Chapter 6 that glucose is required for proper cell metabolism and the production of ATP. However, too much of anything can be a bad thing and this is certainly the case with abnormally high sugar levels in the bloodstream.

Proper regulation of glucose in the body is essential to maintain normal function of all body systems and processes (Figure 23-1 ▪). Many cells throughout the body can compensate for a lack of glucose by burning fats and proteins for fuel. The brain, however, does not have these as a backup source for fuel and must rely only on glucose to function. For this reason the brain is extremely sensitive to changes in the levels of available glucose in the blood. When the brain is not getting an adequate supply of glucose, normal mental function is impaired and you will see changes in the patient's mental status. (More about the signs and symptoms of low blood sugar, or hypoglycemia, appears later in this chapter.)

23-2 Describe the function of glucose in the body.

hyperglycemia abnormally high levels of blood glucose.

glucose a simple sugar that is necessary for normal cell metabolism.

23-3 Describe the response of brain cells and other body cells to insufficient glucose levels.

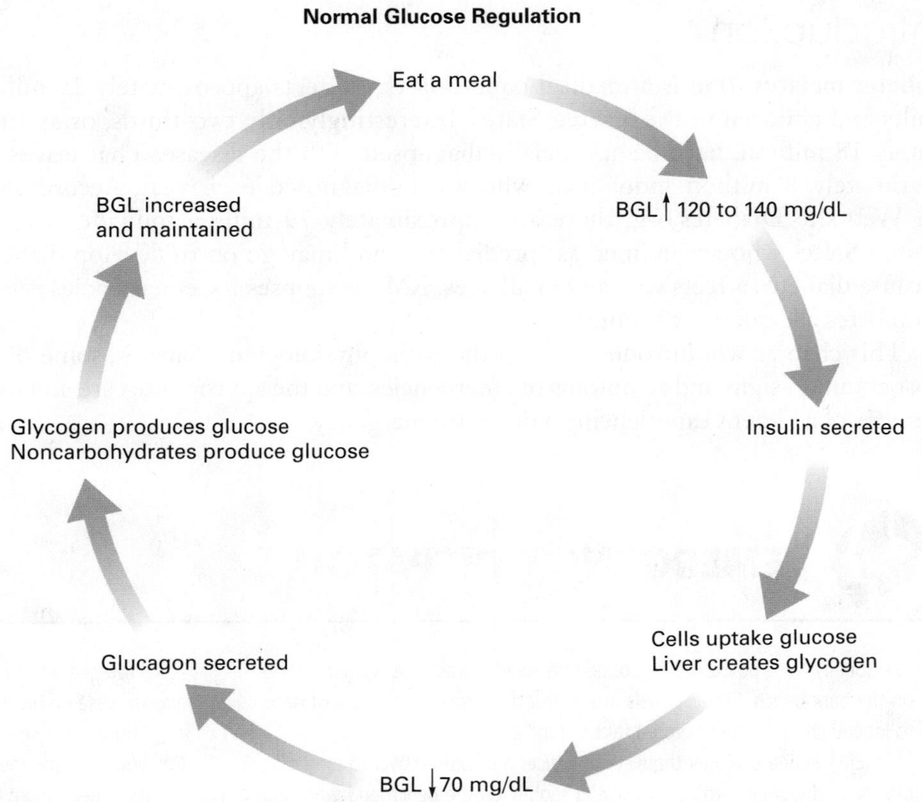

Figure 23-1 The cycle of normal glucose regulation within the body.

23-4 Describe the relationship of glucose and water in the body.

polyuria excessive urination.

polydipsia excessive thirst.

When the levels of blood glucose become abnormally high (hyperglycemia), it can result in the excess glucose being excreted by the kidneys. When this happens, the glucose tends to draw water along with it. This can lead to dangerous levels of dehydration because the body loses too much fluid volume. The frequent urination that is associated with diabetes is referred to as **polyuria** and is the reason why these patients often complain of being abnormally thirsty. Excessive thirst and increased oral intake of liquids is known as **polydipsia.**

PRACTICAL PATHOPHYSIOLOGY

As glucose moves across the cell membrane, it has a tendency to draw water with it. When the blood glucose gets abnormally high, the kidneys dump the excess glucose into the urine. As the glucose spills into the urine, it draws with it water causing mild to severe dehydration. For this reason the patient will become abnormally thirsty in an effort to replace the water being lost through frequent urination.

23-5 Describe how glucose levels are regulated in normal metabolism.

insulin a hormone produced by the pancreas.

glucagon a hormone produced by the pancreas.

Glucose Regulation

The pancreas functions as both a gland and an organ. As a gland of the endocrine system, it excretes important hormones, such as **insulin** and **glucagon,** that play an important role in the regulation of glucose (Figure 23-2 ■). As an organ of the digestive system, the pancreas produces digestive enzymes that aid in the digestion of food in the small intestine.

An area of the pancreas called the **islets of Langerhans** is responsible for monitoring the levels of glucose in the blood. When the cells in this area detect an abnormally low blood glucose level, also known as **hypoglycemia,** they begin to produce the hormone glucagon. The release of glucagon causes the liver to produce glucose, which is then released into the bloodstream.

When the cells of the islets of Langerhans detect levels of blood glucose that are too high, the pancreas produces another hormone called *insulin*. Simply stated, insulin allows the glucose to transfer out of the blood and into the cells where it can be utilized for fuel, thus lowering the levels of glucose in the blood.

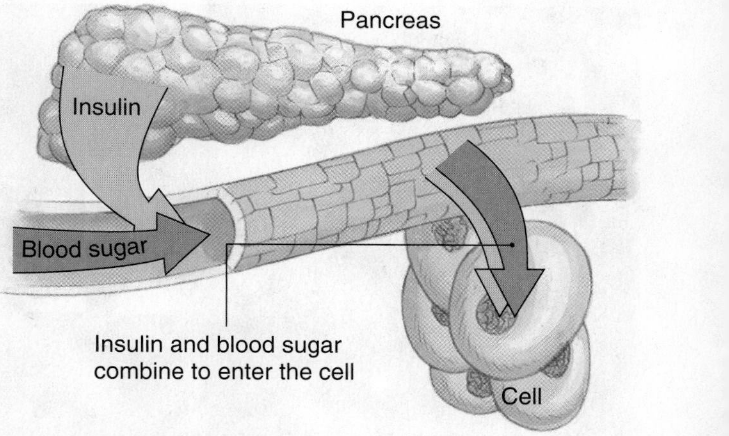

Figure 23-2 The pancreas produces insulin, which is required for the transfer of glucose from the blood to the cells.

Diabetes Mellitus—Type 1

Type 1 diabetes mellitus, also known as *insulin-dependent diabetes mellitus (IDDM)*, is an autoimmune disorder that causes destruction of the insulin-producing beta cells within the pancreas. Type 1 diabetes accounts for approximately 10% of all diabetic patients. The onset of type 1 diabetes most often occurs in childhood but can occur far into adulthood as well. Factors such as diet, obesity, and genetics all play a part in the cause of diabetes.

The signs and symptoms of a new onset of type 1 diabetes include:

- Polyuria (frequent urination)
- Polydipsia (increased thirst)
- Polyphagia (increased hunger)
- Fatigue
- Weight loss

Diabetes Mellitus—Type 2

Type 2 diabetes mellitus, also known as *noninsulin dependent diabetes mellitus (NIDDM)* is caused by both genetic and lifestyle factors. Genetic causes can be from a decrease in the amount of insulin produced by the pancreas or a resistance by the body to utilize insulin appropriately. Lifestyle factors include diet, obesity, stress, and lack of exercise. Type 2 diabetes occurs most often in adulthood, which is why it is sometimes known as *adult onset diabetes*. Type 2 diabetes accounts for 90% of all diabetic patients. The signs and symptoms of type 2 diabetes are much the same as type 1, with polydipsia and polyuria being the most common.

Gestational Diabetes

Another form of diabetes that affects between 3% and 10% of all pregnant women is called **gestational diabetes.** It is characterized by abnormally high glucose levels and most often presents in the third trimester of pregnancy. Glucose levels almost always return to normal following delivery.

Blood Glucose Monitoring

A diabetic patient must carefully manage and monitor the level of glucose in his bloodstream. Diabetics can manage their glucose levels in several ways. Some are able to control glucose levels simply by eating properly and minimizing the intake of sugar and starchy foods that the body converts to sugar. Others must take oral medications to help stimulate the cells to better utilize what insulin the pancreas does produce. Many diabetics must take injections of insulin several times a day in order to control the level of glucose in the blood. Regardless of the method, diabetics are constantly walking a fine line between too much and too little sugar in the blood.

23-6 Describe how insulin and glucagon function to control blood glucose levels.

islets of Langerhans the region of the pancreas responsible for monitoring blood glucose and producing hormones such as glucagon and insulin.

hypoglycemia abnormally low levels of blood glucose.

23-7 Discuss the pathophysiology of diabetes mellitus (DM) and contrast type 1 insulin-dependent diabetes mellitus (IDDM) with type 2 noninsulin-dependent diabetes mellitus (NIDDM).

type 1 diabetes mellitus a type of diabetes mellitus that results from an insufficiency of insulin production.

type 2 diabetes mellitus a type of noninsulin dependent diabetes mellitus.

gestational diabetes a temporary condition that results in abnormally high glucose levels during pregnancy.

23-8 Explain the purposes and process of checking blood glucose levels.

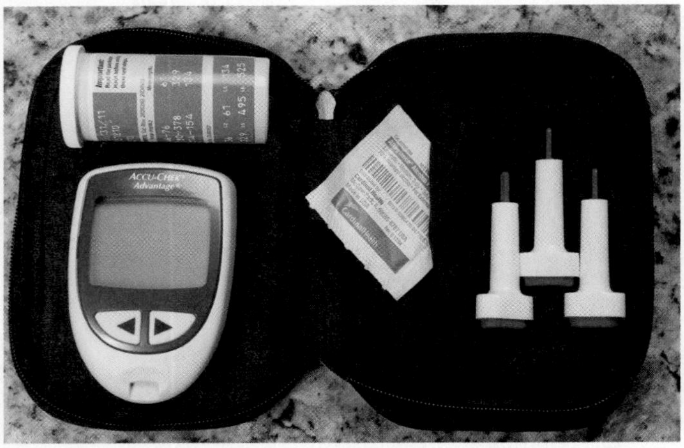

Figure 23-3 Blood glucose can be easily monitored by the patient with a device called a *glucometer*.

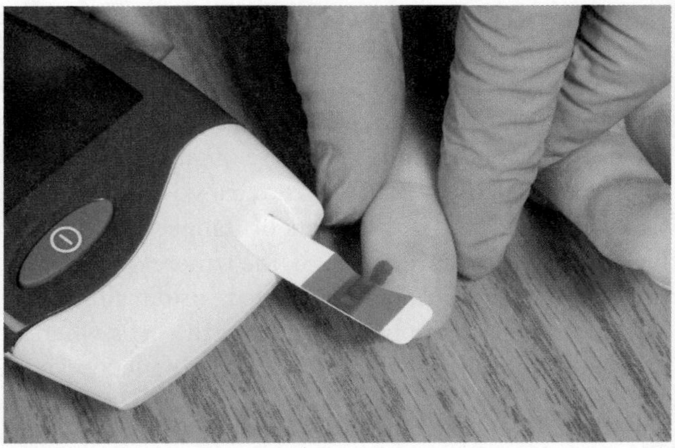

Figure 23-4 A small amount of blood is placed onto a test strip, which is inserted into the device. The results are given within a few seconds.

The most common method a diabetic patient uses to monitor blood glucose level is through a device called a *glucometer* (Figure 23-3 ■). It is a small device that quickly analyzes a tiny sample of the patient's blood and provides a readout of the current blood glucose level (Figure 23-4 ■).

Blood glucose levels are measured in milligrams per 100 milliliters of blood (deciliters) and are expressed as mg/dL. For most diabetic patients, the normal values for blood glucose range between 80 and 120 mg/dL. A patient who is experiencing the symptoms of hypoglycemia with a blood glucose level of less than 80 mg/dL is said to be hypoglycemic. Typically, symptoms of hypoglycemia are not evident until the levels of glucose drop to 50 mg/dL or less. A patient with a value greater than 120 mg/dL is said to be hyperglycemic. Symptoms of hyperglycemia usually do not develop until blood levels are in excess of 200 mg/dL.

Blood glucometers are small, simple to use, and provide accurate results. For that reason, most diabetic patients use them to monitor their blood glucose levels occasionally or up to several times each day. Knowing the results helps them determine how much to eat or how much medication they may need at any given time. By keeping their glucose levels stable, they will experience fewer complications, both in the short and long term.

Because glucometers are so common and easy to use, you are likely to encounter them in the field while caring for a diabetic patient. Some EMS systems are now allowing EMTs to carry and use glucometers as a matter of protocol for managing the diabetic patient. They provide definitive results when the patient cannot provide an appropriate history or is unresponsive.

Not all glucometers are created equal. While similar, each has specific instructions for use and requires calibration with compatible test strips. For those reasons, it is not advised that you use the patient's own glucometer if you are going to obtain a glucose reading. If your system does not allow EMTs to obtain glucose readings, have the patient or appropriate caregiver obtain a reading using the patient's own device. If you are allowed by protocol to obtain glucose readings, only do so with the device provided by your agency. Follow these steps when using a glucometer to obtain blood glucose readings (Scan 23-1):

1. Take the proper BSI precautions.
2. Pull out the device, a test strip, a lancet, and some small gauze pads.

CLINICAL CLUE

Glucometers

Specific directions for obtaining a blood glucose sample may differ, depending on the device being used. Always follow the manufacturer's directions. Glucometers provide just one small piece of the total patient assessment puzzle. Focus on basic assessment skills first, and use the glucometer to confirm your assessment findings. Some EMS systems using glucometers recommend that glucose levels be checked during transport to the hospital only.

SCAN 23-1 Using a Glucometer

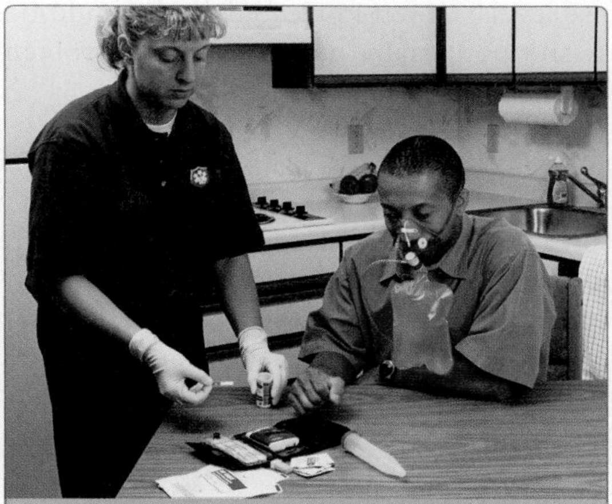

23-1-1 Prepare the glucometer by placing the test strip into the device.

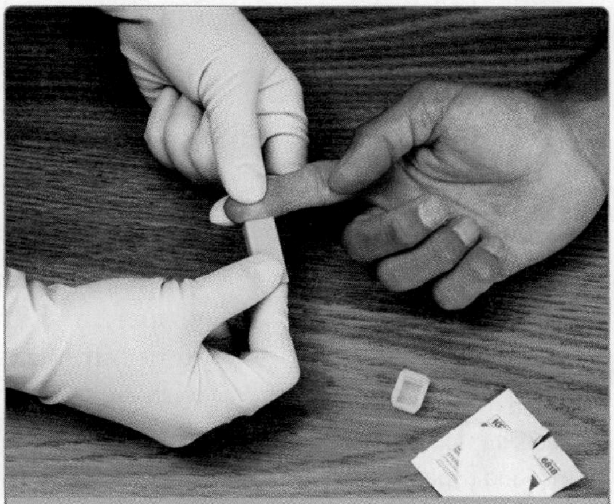

23-1-2 Clean the site and perform a stick.

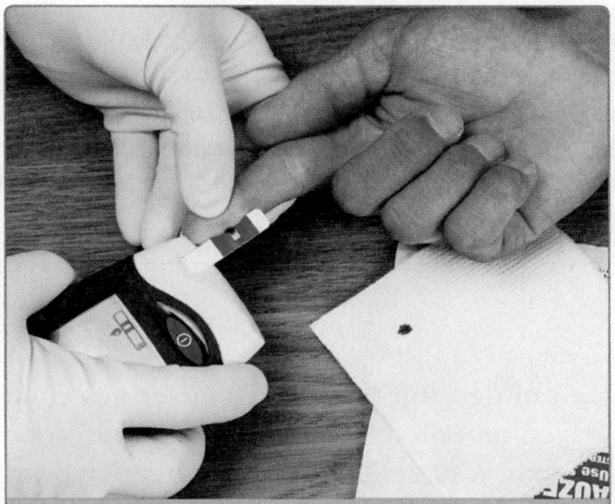

23-1-3 Wipe the first drop away with clean gauze, and then place the second drop onto the test strip.

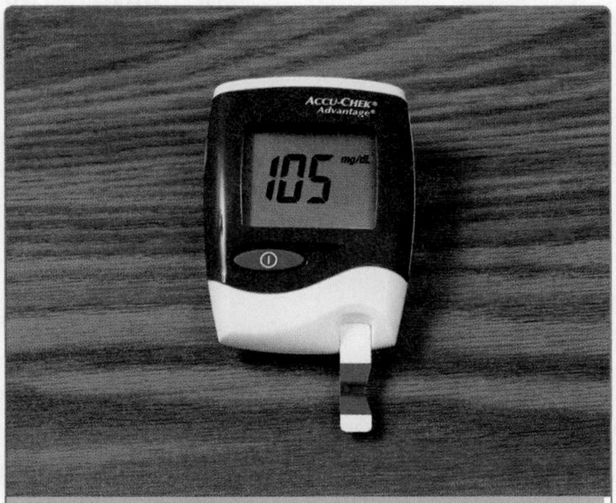

23-1-4 Wait a few seconds and then record the reading.

3. Confirm that the test strips have been calibrated to the device and, if appropriate, place the strip in the device.
4. Prepare the patient by cleaning the tip of one finger with an alcohol wipe.
5. Once the alcohol has dried, stick the finger using the lancet. Wipe away the first drop of blood that appears. It may be necessary to squeeze the finger to produce a second drop.
6. Apply one drop of blood to the test strip.
7. Read and record the value given by the device. This may take 15 to 60 seconds.
8. Assess the puncture site and provide pressure to control bleeding if necessary.

Acute Diabetic Emergencies

There are essentially two types of diabetic emergencies you will encounter in the field—hyperglycemia (abnormally high blood-glucose levels) and hypoglycemia (abnormally low blood-glucose levels). If left untreated, both conditions will result in an altered mental status and potentially life-threatening problems for the patient.

Hypoglycemia

23-9 Discuss the pathophysiology, assessment, and emergency medical care of a hypoglycemic emergency.

23-12 Compare and contrast the speed of onset and the signs and symptoms of hypoglycemia and hyperglycemia.

When glucose levels get too low, hypoglycemia will result. The signs and symptoms of hypoglycemia can develop quickly (30 minutes to two hours) and most often are caused by the patient taking a routine dose of insulin without balancing it with a proper meal. Hypoglycemia also can develop in the patient who does everything right but burns off the calories too quickly through exercise. A diabetic who is sick with certain illnesses can sometimes become hypoglycemic when he takes his normal dose of insulin but is unable to eat or keep the food down.

PERSPECTIVE

Tanya—The Patient

Heck, I've been diabetic for so many years it just gets old. I know I know better. My friends lecture me all the time, usually when they see how I eat! Hey, at least this time wasn't as bad as last May. I passed out on the subway and rode the city for a couple of hours before a transit cop checked on me. My problem is that I take my insulin habitually because I've been doing it most of my life, but I just eat when I remember to. Obviously, sometimes too late or too little. I need to get it together though. One of these days.

If left untreated, hypoglycemia can develop rapidly into a serious condition. For years, severe hypoglycemia was commonly referred to as *insulin shock* due to the shock-like symptoms that can result. A patient with severe hypoglycemia will display many of the signs that mimic shock due to the response of the sympathetic nervous system. As the glucose levels drop, the sympathetic nervous system responds by releasing epinephrine in an attempt to shut down insulin production and stimulate production of glucagon. Signs and symptoms of hypoglycemia include:

- Rapid onset of altered mental status, including the appearance of intoxication, confusion, and unresponsiveness
- Blurred vision
- Hunger
- Irritability
- Slurred speech
- Cool, moist skin
- Elevated heart rate (tachycardia)
- Seizures
- Dizziness
- Headache

Hyperglycemia

When glucose levels get too high, hyperglycemia will result. If left untreated, hyperglycemia can develop into a severe condition called **diabetic ketoacidosis (DKA).** If the patient with hyperglycemia does not receive the appropriate care, he may become unresponsive and critically ill, requiring admission to an intensive care unit. Hyperglycemia can take many hours (24 to 72) to develop to a point where the patient begins showing obvious signs and symptoms. In general, hyperglycemia occurs when the patient does not take his medication as prescribed and continues to eat, or increases the amount of food intake without adjusting his insulin intake.

23-10 Discuss the pathophysiology, assessment, and emergency medical care of hyperglycemia and diabetic ketoacidosis (DKA).

diabetic ketoacidosis (DKA) a potentially life-threatening condition in which the body begins to burn fat for energy rather than glucose, causing high acid levels in the blood.

The development of DKA also can be associated with infections such as pneumonia. In some cases, especially those involving children, profound hyperglycemia with an altered mental status may be the initial presentation that ultimately results in the diagnosis of diabetes. Signs and symptoms of hyperglycemia include:

- Altered mental status, including unresponsiveness
- Headache
- Frequent urination
- Fruity odor to breath
- Extreme thirst
- Hot dry skin
- Abdominal cramping
- Nausea and vomiting
- Rapid, deep respirations

Diabetic ketoacidosis (DKA) is a potentially life-threatening condition that can occur in patients with diabetes when there is an insufficient supply of insulin in the body. It is most common in patients with type 1 diabetes but can occur in patients with type 2. With a shortage of insulin, the body does not have access to the glucose that is building up in the bloodstream. Without a supply of glucose for energy, the body switches to burning fatty acids for energy. This burning of body fats instead of glucose produces a by-product called *ketones*. The buildup of ketones causes the blood to become acidic. The body attempts to correct the acid buildup by blowing off excess carbon dioxide through rapid deep respirations (Kussmaul breathing).

CLINICAL CLUE

Kussmaul's Respirations

Respirations that are both rapid and deep are frequently seen in patients with extreme hyperglycemia (diabetic ketoacidosis) and are called Kussmaul's respirations.

PERSPECTIVE

Renee—The EMT

It's sad but I see this so often with some long-term diabetics. What starts out as an almost religious conviction about insulin and proper diet sort of deteriorates into an "I'll take care of myself when I get around to it" sort of attitude. I wish they understood how much damage they were doing to their bodies every time they let their sugar get too high or too low. And I see many of these folks refuse to be evaluated at the hospital once we get them stabilized. I admit I've never been in their shoes, but if I ever develop diabetes I would really do everything I could to stay healthy and keep my sugar balanced.

STOP, REVIEW, REMEMBER!

Multiple Choice

For each question, place a check next to the correct answer.

1. A diabetic who has taken his insulin as prescribed but has not balanced it with appropriate food intake will likely experience:

_____ a. hypoglycemia.

_____ b. hyperglycemia.

_____ c. insulin coma.

_____ d. diabetic coma.

2. You are caring for a patient who is a known diabetic with an altered mental status. She is able to tell you that she has eaten both breakfast and lunch today, but has not taken her normal injection of insulin. She is most likely suffering from:

_____ a. insulin shock.

_____ b. hypoglycemia.

_____ c. diabetic shock.

_____ d. hyperglycemia.

3. A diabetic who is experiencing a shortage of insulin will begin burning ____________ for energy.

_____ a. oxygen

_____ b. glucagon

_____ c. fatty tissue

_____ d. insulin

4. The ____________ does not require insulin in order to utilize glucose for energy.

_____ a. liver

_____ b. brain

_____ c. pancreas

_____ d. stomach

5. Excess glucose in the blood is excreted by the kidneys and results in a loss of:

_____ a. fluid volume.

_____ b. mental status.

_____ c. insulin.

_____ d. polyuria.

Matching

Match the definition on the left with the applicable term on the right.

1. _____ A medical condition that results when a person's pancreas will no longer produce an adequate supply of insulin
2. _____ It is required to facilitate the transfer of glucose (sugar) from the blood to the tissues and cells where it can be used as fuel.
3. _____ If left untreated, this condition can develop into a condition known as *diabetic ketoacidosis*.
4. _____ If left untreated, this condition can develop rapidly and produce shock-like signs.
5. _____ A device used to measure the blood glucose level in patients.

A. Hypoglycemia

B. Hyperglycemia

C. Glucometer

D. Diabetes

E. Insulin

Critical Thinking

1. Describe the relationship between blood glucose and insulin.

2. Describe how you would differentiate a patient experiencing hypoglycemia versus hyperglycemia.

3. Describe how insulin and glucagon help regulate blood glucose levels in the body.

Assessment of the Diabetic Patient

When assessing a patient who presents with an altered mental status you must complete a thorough history, including asking if the patient has a history of diabetes. In some instances the patient, family members, or other caregivers can provide you with this information. When no one is available to provide this information, look for medical identification jewelry on the patient's neck, wrists, and ankles. Also inspect the scene for evidence of diabetes medications (Figure 23-5 ■). Insulin comes in a liquid form and must be kept refrigerated. So be sure to look in the refrigerator for insulin vials. Common diabetes medications include:

- Insulin (for injection)
- Glucophage® (pill form)
- Diabinese® (pill form)
- Oral glucose (paste or tablet form)
- Orinase® (pill form)
- Glucagon (for injection)
- Micronase® (pill form)

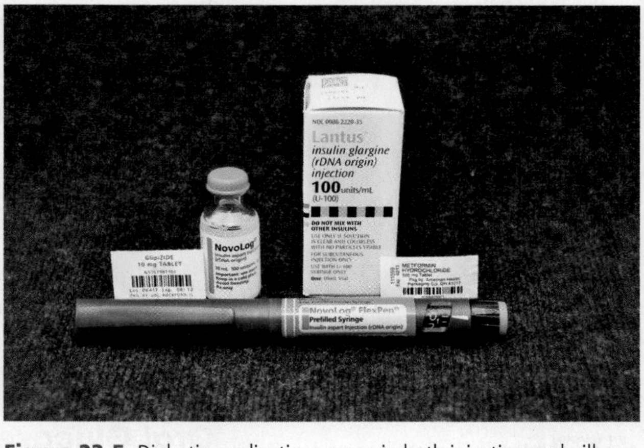

Figure 23-5 Diabetic medications come in both injection and pill form. (© Edward T. Dickinson, MD)

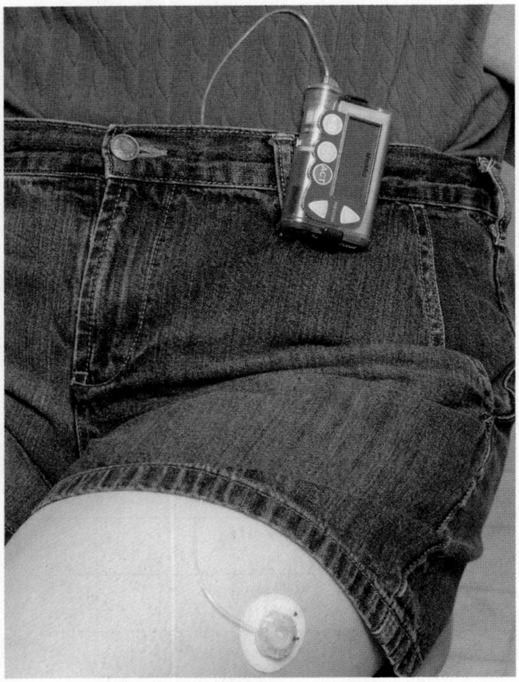

Figure 23-6 A typical insulin pump.

Some diabetics receive injections of insulin by way of an insulin pump (Figure 23-6 ■). An insulin pump is a small, cell-phone size, battery-operated pump that is connected to a catheter. The end of the catheter is inserted through the wall of the lower abdomen. The pump is programmed to automatically deliver small injections of insulin throughout the day. The patient also can manually activate the pump to deliver insulin as needed.

When gathering a SAMPLE history on a known diabetic patient, in addition to the usual questions, you will want to determine the answers to the following:

- *When did you last eat?* You will want to know when and what the patient had last to eat.
- *Do you take diabetes medications?* This will help determine the type of diabetic he is. Type 1 diabetics require insulin injections, often for life. Type 2 diabetics often control their glucose levels by diet or oral medications or a combination of the two.
- *Have you taken your medication today as prescribed?* This will help the hospital staff determine the cause of the patient's problem and provide the most appropriate care.

> **CLINICAL CLUE**
>
> **Insulin Pumps**
>
> One of the newest technologies being used by patients with insulin-dependent diabetes is an insulin pump. The size of a cell phone and usually worn on the belt, these small pumps inject insulin directly into the patient by way of a catheter placed in the lower abdomen. Always check patients with altered mental status and those with known diabetes for the presence of an insulin pump.

Emergency Care of the Diabetic Patient

It is not essential that you know for certain which condition the patient may be suffering—hyperglycemia or hypoglycemia. The focus of your care will be to manage the patient's ABCs and obtain a thorough history. When you are uncertain as to which condition it may be, it is appropriate to treat the problem as hypoglycemia and provide oral glucose if indicated and allowed by protocol or medical direction.

Providing glucose to the hypoglycemic patient is likely to improve his condition within a few minutes. If he happens to be hyperglycemic already, the small dose you provide will not make a significant difference in his condition. When in doubt, and depending on the system in which you are working, contact medical direction before administering oral glucose to any patient. *Follow local protocols.*

Management of the airway and breathing status are of the utmost importance with patients presenting with an altered mental status. If the use of oral glucose is indicated and your local treatment protocols allow for its use, you must be very certain the patient is capable of protecting his own airway. One way to determine this is by asking the patient to swallow. If he can follow your directions and is able to swallow easily, he is likely to be responsive enough for you to administer oral glucose safely.

Perform the following steps when caring for a patient presenting with an altered mental status and a history of diabetes:

1. Conduct an appropriate scene size-up and take the necessary BSI precautions.
2. Perform a primary assessment and consider the need for supplemental oxygen.
3. Complete a SAMPLE history and secondary assessment and confirm a prior history of diabetes, last oral intake, and last time and dose of medication taken.
4. If responsive, confirm that the patient can swallow without difficulty.
5. Consider the administration of oral glucose in accordance with local protocols or medical direction.
6. Perform reassessments as necessary.
7. Transport in the recovery position.

Oral Glucose

23-11 Identify indications and contraindications to the administration of oral glucose.

Oral glucose is an over-the-counter (OTC) medication that is carried on most ambulances and is within the scope of care of the EMT (Scan 23-2). Indications for its

SCAN 23-2 Oral Glucose

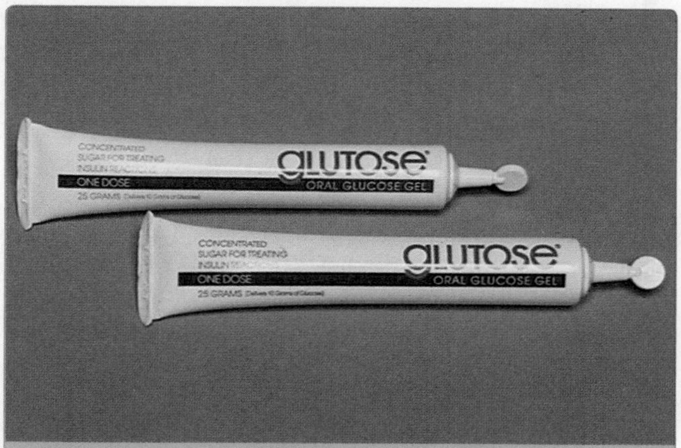

23-2-1 Oral glucose comes in dosages ranging in concentrations from 15 to 45 grams. (Shown are 25 gram tubes.)

MEDICATION NAME

1. **Generic:** glucose, oral.
2. **Trade:** Glutose, Insta-glucose, BD Glucose Tablets.

INDICATIONS

1. Patients with altered mental status with a known history of diabetes.
2. Patient has taken insulin but no food recently and may have been very physically active.

CONTRAINDICATIONS

1. Unresponsiveness or unable to swallow or otherwise manage own airway.
2. Known diabetic who has not taken insulin for days.

MEDICATION FORM

Gel, in toothpaste-type tubes; chewable tablets.

DOSAGE

One tube; three 5.0 gram chewable tablets. This dose can be used for both adults and children. Tubes can come in 15 to 45 mg dosages.

STEPS FOR ADMINISTRATION

1. Ensure signs and symptoms of altered mental status with a known history of diabetes.
2. Ensure patient is alert enough to swallow.
3. Administer glucose.
   a. Self-administered into mouth and swallowed.
   b. Place on tongue depressor between cheek and gum.
   OR
   c. Have patient chew one to three tablets.
4. Perform reassessment.

ACTIONS

Increases blood sugar levels.

SIDE EFFECTS

None when given properly.

use are any patient presenting with an altered mental status who has a known history of diabetes.

Oral glucose is a simple sugar that is metabolized relatively quickly. So once you have administered the oral glucose to a patient, you might see an improvement in his condition within a few minutes. Continue to monitor his mental status and ABCs throughout transport. It may be necessary to administer multiple doses to maintain responsiveness. If the patient becomes unresponsive, remove any material from his mouth, if possible, and suction as necessary, place him in the recovery position, and provide the indicated care. Remember that oral glucose is absorbed rapidly through the digestive tract and it must be ingested to be most effective.

CLINICAL CLUE

Did Your Patient Eat?

If a patient has eaten but has not taken his diabetic medications, there is a strong possibility he may be experiencing an episode of hyperglycemia. If the patient has not eaten and has taken his diabetic medications, the probability of hypoglycemia is high.

STOP, REVIEW, REMEMBER!

Multiple Choice

For each question, place a check next to the correct answer.

1. You are caring for a patient who must take daily injections of insulin to regulate blood glucose levels. This patient is categorized as a(n):

_____ a. type 2 diabetic.

_____ b. type 1 diabetic.

_____ c. diabetic acidotic.

_____ d. adult diabetic.

2. Your patient just completed a blood glucose check on herself prior to your arrival. The reading came back at 104. You would describe this as:

_____ a. hyperglycemic.

_____ b. hypoglycemic.

_____ c. abnormal.

_____ d. within normal limits.

3. A diabetic patient who has not eaten in the past several hours but has taken his medication will most likely develop:

_____ a. hypoglycemia.

_____ b. hyperglycemia.

_____ c. an insulin reaction.

_____ d. diabetic shock.

4. Which one of the following is a contraindication for administering oral glucose to a known diabetic patient?

_____ a. Low blood glucose readings

_____ b. Unresponsiveness

_____ c. Inability to swallow easily

_____ d. Insulin was administered recently

5. A typical adult dose of oral glucose would be:

_____ a. 5 mg.

_____ b. 10 mg.

_____ c. one tube.

_____ d. two tubes.

Fill in the Blank

1. A normal blood glucose level for an adult patient is between ____________________ mg/dL.

2. The three common symptoms of a new onset diabetic are ____________________, ____________________, and ____________________.

3. ____________________ can take many hours to develop, while ____________________ can develop in several minutes to an hour or so.

Critical Thinking

1. Describe the physiology behind the shock-like signs that can develop with hypoglycemia.

2. Describe the difference between hyperglycemia and diabetic ketoacidosis.

3. Describe your care of a patient with an altered mental status and a history of diabetes.

EMERGENCY DISPATCH SUMMARY

A few minutes after being given the glucose gel, the patient became much more lucid and steady. She apologized to the police officer and the two EMTs for taking their time and refused to be transported to the emergency department, and instead opted to walk home. Several months later, while working with a paramedic on an ALS ambulance, Renee encountered the same patient, this time she was unresponsive behind the wheel of her car in a bank parking lot. After receiving IV dextrose and regaining consciousness, she did agree to be transported to the hospital and admitted to Renee that she was finally ready to start managing her condition properly.

Chapter Review

To the Point

- Glucose is the primary source of energy for the cell of the body.
- While all other cells in the body require insulin to aid in the metabolism of glucose, the brain can utilize glucose without insulin.
- When there is an excess of glucose in the blood, the body attempts to eliminate it through the kidneys. When this happens, it also eliminates large amounts of fluid causing dehydration.
- During normal metabolism, blood glucose is regulated by two hormones produced by the pancreas called *insulin* and *glucagon*.
- Insulin is produced when glucose levels become elevated. It helps facilitate the transfer of glucose from the blood into the cells where it is used for fuel.
- Glucagon is produced when glucose levels become low. It helps the liver create more glucose to raise the levels of glucose in the blood.
- Type 1 diabetes is also known as *insulin-dependent diabetes mellitus (IDDM)* and most often comes on early in life. Type 2 diabetes is known as *noninsulin dependent diabetes mellitus (NIDDM)* and most often comes on in adulthood.
- Diabetics must monitor their blood glucose levels regularly through the use of a device called a *glucometer*.
- Hypoglycemia commonly occurs when the patient has taken his medication but has not eaten enough food to balance it. Signs and symptoms can come on quickly, beginning with an altered mental status. Care for a conscious patient with hypoglycemia is oral glucose or other source of sugar.
- Hyperglycemia commonly occurs when the patient has not taken his medication but has eaten food. Signs and symptoms typically come on slowly over a period of 24 to 72 hours. Care for a patient with hyperglycemia is supportive care and transport.
- Nothing should be given orally to the diabetic patient who has a significant decrease in mental status. He must be able to swallow normally and follow simple commands in order to receive oral glucose or other form of sugar.

Chapter Questions

Multiple Choice

For each question, place a check next to the correct answer.

1. Without ______________, a patient's blood sugar levels can become dangerously elevated.

_____ a. potassium
_____ b. sodium
_____ c. insulin
_____ d. glucose

2. All of the following are potential causes of hypoglycemia *except*:

_____ a. excessive blood sugar.
_____ b. excessive exercise.
_____ c. skipping meals.
_____ d. excess insulin.

3. You have arrived on the scene of a 54-year-old diabetic patient. She is in bed and you can hear snoring respirations. You should:

_____ a. check her blood glucose.
_____ b. obtain a medical history.
_____ c. obtain vital signs.
_____ d. open her airway.

4. You are caring for a responsive diabetic patient with an altered mental status. Your protocols call for the administration of one dose of oral glucose. You should:
_____ a. give the patient one half of a tube of glucose.
_____ b. call medical direction to confirm the protocol.
_____ c. have the patient ingest the full tube of glucose.
_____ d. have the patient take small amounts every five minutes.

5. Which one of the following is the best means by which hypoglycemia can be differentiated from hyperglycemia?
_____ a. Ask how fast the signs and symptoms appeared.
_____ b. Assess the patient's mental status.
_____ c. Evaluate the vital signs.
_____ d. Obtain a blood glucose reading.

6. Prior to the administration of oral glucose, a patient's blood glucose level was 35 mg/dL. Which one of the following blood glucose readings would you expect to find following the administration of a full dose of oral glucose?
_____ a. 25 mg/dL
_____ b. 35 mg/dL
_____ c. 88 mg/dL
_____ d. 300 mg/dL

7. You have been dispatched to a possible diabetic emergency. During your assessment, you find a medical bracelet that indicates the patient has a history of type 1 diabetes. Based on this information, you would expect that:
_____ a. the patient takes daily injections of insulin.
_____ b. she manages her condition with diet and exercise only.
_____ c. has a chronically low blood-glucose level.
_____ d. must take oral medications to control her condition.

8. During your assessment of a diabetic patient, you obtain a blood glucose reading of 320 mg/dL. This would be an indication of:
_____ a. DKA.
_____ b. hyperglycemia.
_____ c. hypoglycemia.
_____ d. diabetic shock.

9. A diabetic patient presents as alert but irritable and confused. His airway is patent and breathing is adequate. You have no way to obtain a blood glucose level and are not sure if his blood sugar is high or low. You should:
_____ a. provide oxygen and transport.
_____ b. have the patient self-administer his insulin.
_____ c. administer oral glucose and transport.
_____ d. call medical direction.

10. Which one of the following patients is most likely experiencing a diabetic emergency?
_____ a. Diabetic patient with chest pain.
_____ b. Patient with an altered mental status and a glucose of 44 mg/dL.
_____ c. Patient with an altered mental status and a glucose of 122 mg/dL.
_____ d. Patient with difficulty breathing and a glucose of 88 mg/dL.

Critical Thinking

1. Explain the pathophysiology of frequent urination and excessive thirst in the diabetic patient.

____

____

____

____

(continued on next page)

(continued)

2. What is your primary concern when caring for a diabetic patient with an altered mental status?

Case Studies

Case Study 1

You have been dispatched to an office building for an unknown medical problem. Upon arrival, you are led over to an approximately 60-year-old man who is seated at his desk and appears awake but is staring straight ahead. A coworker tells you that he came by his friend's desk to go to lunch and found him acting strangely and difficult to understand. You discover a medical bracelet that states the man is an insulin-dependent diabetic. As you begin to ask the man questions, he responds by looking at you and speaking. However, his words are difficult to understand. He has a rapid pulse and his skin appears pale and moist.

1. What information will you attempt to gather from the patient or his friend?

2. You are able to determine that the man did indeed take his normal dose of morning insulin but has had nothing to eat since. What is most likely this man's problem?

3. How will you care for this patient?

Case Study 2

You have been dispatched to a residence for a 17-year-old patient. Upon arrival, you are led to an upstairs bedroom and find her unresponsive and lying supine in bed with rapid deep snoring respirations.

1. How will you initially manage this patient?

2. You are told by a family member that the patient is a type 1 diabetic and spent the night at a sleepover with some friends. What information will you attempt to gather from family members?

3. What is this patient's most likely underlying medical problem?

The Last Word

The most common presentation for diabetic patients who are experiencing an emergency related to their condition is a change in mental status. They often become agitated, irritable, and confused. It is not essential that you determine the exact cause of their problem. Your priorities will be to manage the ABCs and provide transport to the hospital. For patients with a known history of diabetes and who are able to manage their own airway, the administration of oral glucose is often indicated. Always follow local protocol.

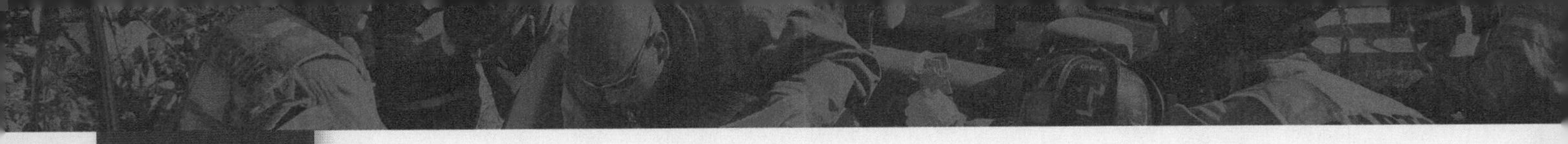

24 Caring for Patients with Allergy-Related Emergencies

Education Standards

Medicine: Immunology

Competencies

Applies fundamental knowledge to provide basic emergency care and transportation based on assessment findings for an acutely ill patient.

Objectives

After completion of this lesson, you should be able to:

24-1 Define key terms introduced in this chapter.

24-2 Describe the physiology of a normal immune response.

24-3 List common allergens and the ways they can be introduced into the body.

24-4 Differentiate the physiology of a mild allergic reaction and anaphylaxis.

24-5 Differentiate the signs and symptoms of a mild allergic reaction and an anaphylactic reaction.

24-6 Describe the life-threatening mechanisms of anaphylaxis, including airway compromise, impaired ventilation and oxygenation, and impaired perfusion.

24-7 Describe the two physiological responses that indicate a severe anaphylactic reaction.

24-8 Describe the assessment of a person with a suspected allergic reaction.

24-9 Describe the appropriate care of a person with a suspected allergic reaction.

24-10 Describe the role of epinephrine in the treatment of anaphylaxis and the criteria and procedure for administration of epinephrine.

Key Terms

allergens p. 635
allergic reaction p. 635
anaphylactic shock p. 638
anaphylaxis p. 638
angioedema p. 637
antibodies p. 635
antigen p. 635
contact dermatitis p. 638
epinephrine p. 643
erythema p. 638
histamine p. 636
hives p. 637
immunoglobulin E (IgE) p. 636
lacrimation p. 638
pruritus p. 638
rhinitis p. 638
sensitization p. 636
urticaria p. 638

Introduction

Allergies affect some 50 million people in the United States. Allergies are the fifth leading chronic disease in the United States and the third leading chronic disease among children. More than 40 million people have indoor/outdoor allergies as their primary allergy and greater than 17 million people visit their doctor for allergies annually. Food allergies account for 50,000 visits to hospital emergency departments annually.

While most allergic reactions are mild, some reactions can be very severe and become life threatening if not treated promptly. This chapter offers you a description of what happens to the body during an **allergic reaction** and ways to distinguish between a mild reaction and a more severe life-threatening reaction.

allergic reaction the body's exaggerated response when exposed to specific substances to which it has been sensitized.

EMERGENCY DISPATCH

Harold and his wife Shannon, EMT partners for the city's ambulance service, pulled into the parking lot of The Ice Cream Station and stopped near a frantically waving woman.

"Quick! He's on the floor!" The woman shouted as the pair quickly stacked their equipment on the stretcher and followed her. "The after-school crowd came in a little while ago, and this one boy just started acting really, really, oh I don't know. He's just really sick!"

The patient, a 13-year-old boy, was unresponsive, cyanotic, and obviously swollen around his face and neck. The shop employees were trying to keep the area clear as a sea of faces jostled for better views and talked in forced whispers.

"He's not breathing," Shannon knelt next to the boy. "Give me an OPA and call for ALS."

A young girl stepped from the crowd and burst into loud sobs, holding her shaking hands over her mouth. "Oh my God. I'm so sorry! This is all my fault."

"What do you mean, honey?" Shannon was struggling to get the airway adjunct into the boy's airway—and losing the battle. She finally tossed it aside, and Harold attempted to ventilate the boy with the bag-mask. No luck.

"He kept making this big deal about him and peanuts." The girl was sobbing harder now. "And we didn't believe it . . . and we . . . I tricked him into eating them."

Harold looked from the crying girl to the crowd of students. "Does he have an auto-injector? Have you ever seen him with a thing that looks like a really fat pen, maybe with a plastic cap on one end?" Their blank stares answered his question.

"Let's just go, Harold! We can't wait for the ALS unit to get here. We're going to have to meet up with them on the road somewhere. This isn't looking good."

The Body's Immune Response

24-2 Describe the physiology of a normal immune response.

An allergic reaction is the body's way of responding to an "invader." When the body senses an **antigen** (a foreign substance), the immune system is triggered to respond. Immune system responses are normally protective. However, they can become exaggerated or be directed toward harmless antigens to which we often are exposed. When that occurs, the response is termed *allergic*. An antigen that causes an allergic response is called an **allergen.**

antigen a substance that when introduced into the body stimulates the production of antibodies.

allergens a substance that when introduced into the body causes an allergic reaction.

Allergens enter the body through various paths: *absorption* through the skin, *inhalation* into the lungs, *ingestion* into the digestive tract, or *injection* (a puncture through the skin from a needle, for example, or an insect sting).

24-3 List common allergens and the ways they can be introduced into the body.

Allergens can cause an exaggerated response by the immune system. In the body, white blood cells produce **antibodies** as part of a normally functioning immune system. Antibodies are protein molecules that are capable of identifying and neutralizing foreign bodies such as allergens, viruses, and bacteria. When the body is exposed to an allergen, a series of reactions begins.

antibodies protein molecules used by the immune system to identify and neutralize foreign bodies such as viruses and bacteria.

CLINICAL CLUE

Intolerance to Food

Food intolerance is not the same as a food allergy. Allergies are an immune system response. Food intolerance is a digestive system response in which a person is unable to properly digest or break down a particular food.

sensitization the production of antibodies to a specific allergen.

immunoglobulin E (IgE) a class of antibody that is responsible for causing the most severe allergic reactions.

histamine a chemical mediator that triggers an inflammatory response by the immune system.

The white blood cells produce an antibody specific to an allergen in a process called **sensitization.** Antibodies are assigned the task of detecting and destroying substances that cause diseases and illness. In allergic reactions, a class of antibody called **immunoglobulin E (IgE)** is most often responsible for the release of **histamine.** Histamine is the chemical (neuro-transmitter) your body produces when you are having an allergic reaction. It is a vasodilator (causes flushing) and contributes to an inflammatory response. It also causes the constriction of smooth muscle (located in the respiratory system), which can cause shortness of breath and wheezing.

Histamine has an effect on local tissue and organs in addition to activating more white blood cell defenders. Histamine is responsible for many of the signs and symptoms characteristic of an allergic response such as inflammation, pain, heat, redness, and itching.

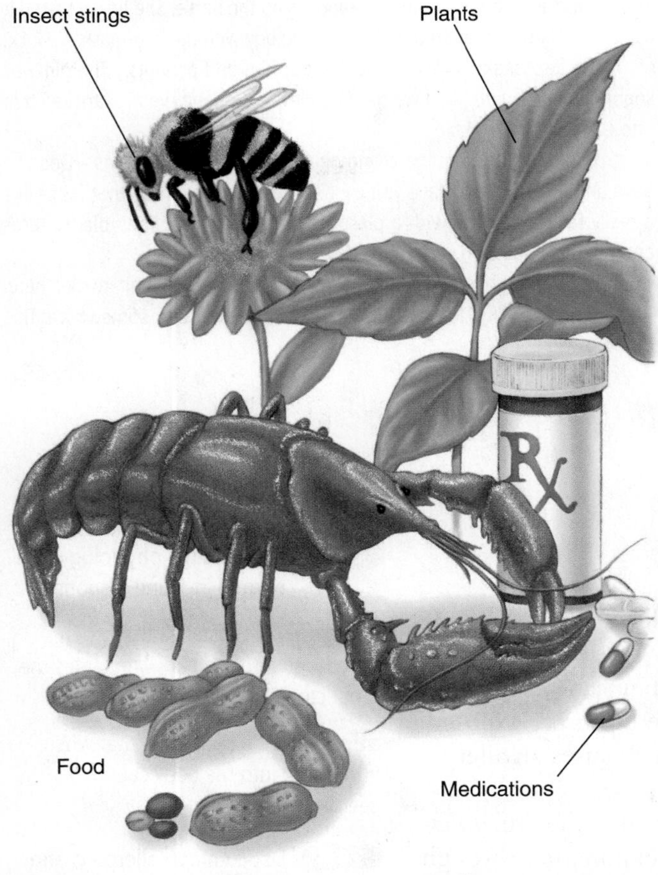

Figure 24-1 Common substances that can cause allergic reactions.

Allergic reactions normally have slow onsets, but if the release of histamines is sudden and extreme, the reaction by the body may be sudden and severe.

Common allergens include (Figure 24-1 ▪):

- Insect bites and stings (wasps, bees, fire ants)
- Food (milk, eggs, nuts, shellfish such as shrimp, strawberries, wheat, soy, food additives, and vaccines)
- Plants (poison oak, poison ivy, pollen)
- Medications (penicillin, sulfa drugs, codeine, iodine, ibuprofen)
- Others, such as latex, mold, dust, animal dander, chemicals

Allergies tend to be genetically based with members of families sharing the same or similar allergy responses. Likewise, people with certain health conditions such as asthma, skin sensitivity, or sinus disorders are often predisposed for allergies.

While a first-time exposure can produce only a mild reaction, repeated exposures could lead to more serious reactions. Once a person has had a previous exposure and sensitization, even a very small amount of allergen can trigger a severe reaction.

Allergic reactions can vary from very mild localized reactions confined to a small area of the body to severe and life-threatening systemic reactions that affect the entire body. Severe reactions are called *anaphylaxis*.

24-4 Differentiate the physiology of a mild allergic reaction and anaphylaxis.

Mild and Moderate Allergic Reactions

Mild allergic reactions are often confined to a specific area of the body, such as the swelling around the area of a bee sting or the localized reaction from exposure

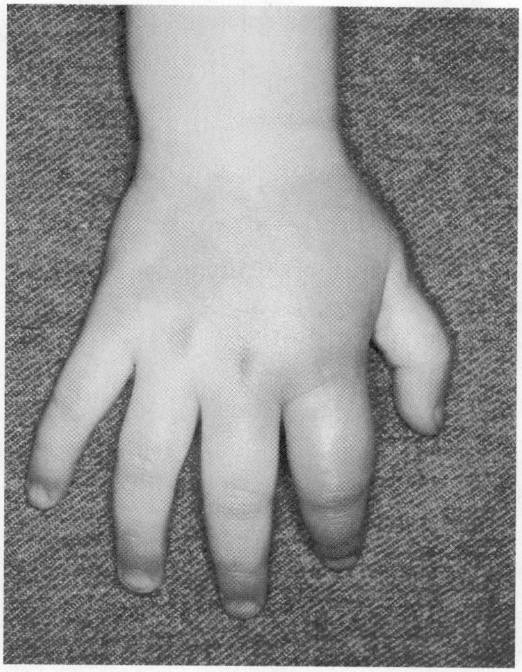

(A)

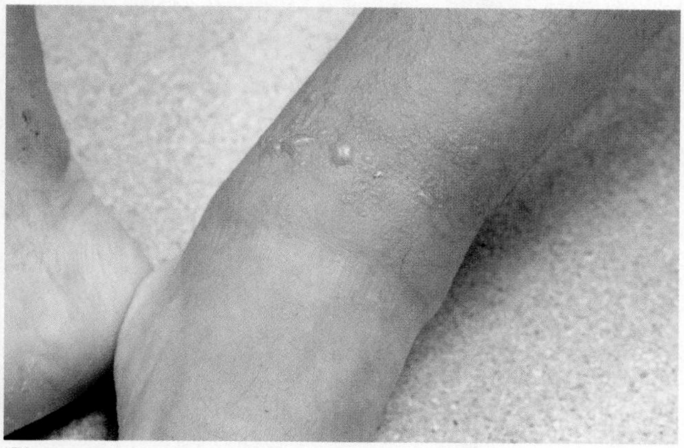

(B)

Figure 24-2 (A) Localized reaction from a bee sting. (Scott Camazine/Photo Researchers, Inc.) (B) Localized reaction from exposure to poison oak. (© Christopher J. Le Baudour)

to poison oak (Figure 24-2 ▪). Moderate allergic reactions can also involve a more generalized body response such as **hives** (urticaria) (Figure 24-3 ▪), itching, or wheezing. Swelling that occurs in the dermis and subcutaneous layers of the skin and the mucus membranes is called **angioedema** (Figure 24-4 ▪). It most commonly appears in the face and tissues of the mouth and throat. It differs from hives in that the swelling is deeper within the tissues, and hives appear as raised areas on top of the skin. Angioedema that is mild or moderate may last for several hours. Angioedema that is severe can cause dangerous swelling of the airways and must be cared for quickly.

24-5 Differentiate the signs and symptoms of a mild allergic reaction and an anaphylactic reaction.

hives red, itchy, possibly raised blotches on the skin; can be from insect bites or food allergy.

angioedema swelling that occurs in the dermis and subcutaneous layers of the skin and the mucus membranes following an allergic response.

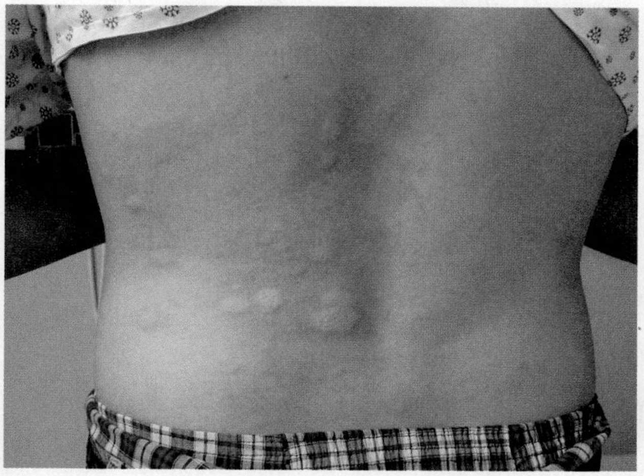

Figure 24-3 Hives caused by an allergic reaction.
(© Charles Stewart, MPH, EMDM)

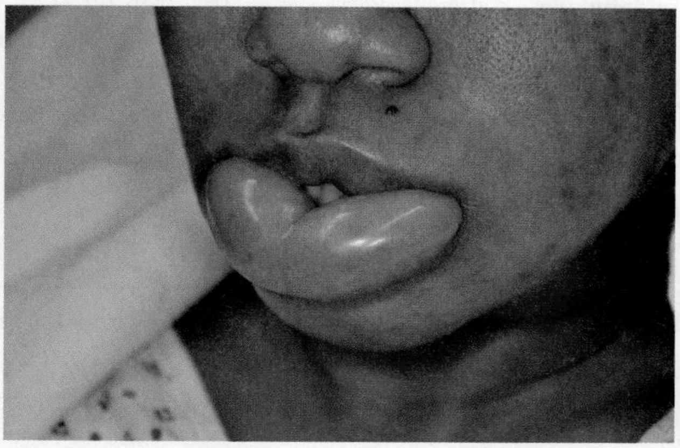

Figure 24-4 Angioedema of the face and lips.
(© Edward T. Dickinson, MD)

Common signs and symptoms of a mild or moderate allergic reaction include:

pruritus itching of the skin.

urticaria hives.

erythema redness of the skin.

lacrimation the secretion of tears.

rhinitis nasal irritation or inflammation.

contact dermatitis localized rash or irritation of the skin.

- **Pruritus** (itching)
- **Urticaria** (hives)
- **Erythema** (redness of the skin)
- Angioedema (swelling of the dermis, subcutaneous tissue, or mucosal tissues)
- **Lacrimation** (the secretion of tears)
- Wheezing
- Conjunctivitis (inflammation or infection of the membrane lining the eyelids)
- **Rhinitis** (nasal irritation or inflammation)
- **Contact dermatitis** (localized rash or irritation of the skin)
- Tachycardia (increased heart rate)

An important characteristic of mild and moderate allergic reactions is that they reach a point at which they do not continue to get worse. Signs and symptoms can persist for several hours but are not progressive and do not pose a threat to life.

CLINICAL CLUE

Latex Allergy

Allergies to latex are becoming more common in the EMS profession. It is now known that frequent exposure to latex, such as when an EMT wears latex gloves while providing patient care, can cause a latex sensitivity. If you now use latex gloves and have noticed your hands becoming dry, red, swollen, and itchy following glove use, you may be developing a sensitivity to latex. Try switching to a nonlatex-style glove to see if your symptoms go away. It is important to know that some patients you will be caring for also might have an allergy to latex. Caring for a patient who is sensitive to latex while wearing latex gloves can cause a reaction in the patient. It is becoming common practice to include this question as part of the history gathering.

Severe Allergic Reactions

24-6 Describe the life-threatening mechanisms of anaphylaxis, including airway compromise, impaired ventilation and oxygenation, and impaired perfusion.

anaphylaxis sudden, severe allergic reaction.

anaphylactic shock progression of a severe allergic reaction; may result in death.

24-7 Describe the two physiological responses that indicate a severe anaphylactic reaction.

A sudden and severe allergic reaction, **anaphylaxis,** occurs usually within minutes of exposure to an allergen. Anaphylactic reactions progress rapidly and can lead to a life-threatening condition known as **anaphylactic shock.** If left untreated or if treatment is delayed, death can occur within minutes.

A severe reaction is characterized by many of the same signs and symptoms as a moderate reaction, except in a severe reaction they quickly worsen and become life threatening. The patient experiencing anaphylaxis may present with any combination of the signs and symptoms listed in Table 24-1.

There are two primary mechanisms at work in the patient experiencing severe anaphylaxis. The exaggerated immune response causes the blood vessels to dilate while

PERSPECTIVE

Shannon—The EMT

That was just a bad call. It was the worst allergic reaction that I've ever seen. We couldn't get an airway and what kid with such a severe peanut allergy doesn't have an auto-injector? We even searched his backpack. If only he had an epinephrine auto-injector, we would have at least had a shot at slowing down his reaction.

TABLE 24-1 SIGNS AND SYMPTOMS OF ANAPHYLAXIS

UPPER AIRWAY	LOWER AIRWAY
Hoarseness	Bronchospasm
Stridor	Increased mucus production
Laryngeal or epiglottic edema	Accessory muscle use
Rhinorrhea (runny nose)	Wheezing
	Decreased breath sounds
CARDIOVASCULAR SYSTEM	**GASTROINTESTINAL SYSTEM**
Tachycardia	Nausea
Hypotension	Vomiting
Dysrhythmia (abnormal cardiac rhythm)	Abdominal cramps
Chest tightness	Diarrhea
NEUROLOGICAL SYSTEM	**SKIN RESPONSES**
Anxiety	Angioedema
Dizziness	Urticaria
Syncope (loss of consciousness)	Pruritus
Weakness	Erythema
Headache	Edema
	Lacrimation

causing the airway passages to constrict. Blood vessel dilation causes the blood pressure to drop, which decreases the perfusion to the brain and other vital organs. Additionally, the air passages begin to swell, progressively getting smaller. Breathing becomes much more difficult as the body begins to struggle to bring in an adequate supply of oxygen.

For these reasons, the allergic patient who presents with signs of shock (hypoperfusion) *or* respiratory distress must be considered to be experiencing anaphylaxis and *must* receive the appropriate care *immediately!*

PRACTICAL PATHOPHYSIOLOGY

During anaphylaxis there is an exaggerated response by the immune system that causes the release of large amounts of histamine. Histamine is the chemical mediator that triggers bronchoconstriction, vasodilation, and increased permeability of the capillaries. Bronchoconstriction results in an increased work of breathing while vasodilation causes a decrease in blood pressure. The increased permeability of the capillaries results in swelling of the soft tissues.

STOP, REVIEW, REMEMBER!

Multiple Choice

For each question, place a check next to the correct answer.

1. What is caused when the body becomes exposed to specific substances for which it has been sensitized?

_____ a. Allergen

_____ b. Allergic reaction

_____ c. Anaphylaxis

_____ d. Altered mental status

2. Which one of the following is *not* a common allergen?

_____ a. Bee stings

_____ b. Shellfish

_____ c. Vinyl gloves

_____ d. Medications

(continued on next page)

(continued)

3. All of the following are common signs and symptoms of an allergic reaction *except*:

_____ a. decreased pulse rate.

_____ b. difficulty breathing.

_____ c. urticaria.

_____ d. lacrimation.

4. Two clinical findings that indicate the progression of a mild allergic reaction into anaphylaxis are:

_____ a. difficulty breathing and decreased heart rate.

_____ b. altered mental status and hypertension.

_____ c. increased heart rate and increased blood pressure.

_____ d. difficulty breathing and hypoperfusion.

5. Signs and symptoms of which type of reaction can last for several hours but typically do not progress to a life-threatening emergency?

_____ a. Mild

_____ b. Severe

_____ c. Anaphylaxis

_____ d. Allergen defense

Fill in the Blank

1. ____________________ are caused when the body becomes exposed to specific substances for which it has sensitivities.

2. Substances that cause sensitivities are called ____________________ and can be just about anything.

3. ____________________ are often confined to a specific area of the body, such as the swelling around the area of a bee sting.

4. A sudden and severe allergic reaction that occurs within minutes of exposure is called ____________________.

5. If left untreated or if treatment is delayed, a severe reaction will develop into ____________________ and death can occur within minutes.

Critical Thinking

1. Describe the role that allergens play in an allergic reaction.

____

____

____

____

2. Describe the differences between a mild and a severe allergic reaction.

____

____

____

____

3. Describe how the body responds during a severe allergic reaction.

____

____

____

____

Assessment of the Patient

A quick assessment of the scene and the patient is especially important with patients experiencing allergic reactions. These reactions can progress rapidly and require prompt care to ensure a successful outcome.

Scene Size-up

24-8 Describe the assessment of a person with a suspected allergic reaction.

Your assessment must begin with an appropriate scene size-up. You will want to confirm that the information received from dispatch is consistent with what you find as you arrive on scene. Because an allergic reaction can present with so many signs and symptoms, there are many possible ways the call could be described by those on scene. For instance the call might come in as difficulty breathing, choking, or even as an unresponsive person. You may not get any information during the dispatch that lets you know an allergy is causing the patient's problems.

There are causes of an allergic reaction (such as to toxic exposures and insect stings) that pose a hazard to EMS personnel. So be sure you know what you are walking into. For example, the swarm of bees that stung the patient could pose a hazard for the EMTs, who can be stung as well. If possible, move the patient to a safe place, such as indoors or the back of the ambulance, before initiating emergency care.

Primary Assessment

Pay particular attention to the patient's mental status and breathing effort as you approach the patient. Note his position. Is he sitting or standing upright and interacting with others around him? Or is he lying unresponsive on the ground? This information will help determine how aggressive you will need to be in managing the patient.

Remember that the most likely threat to the patient in a severe allergic reaction will be airway compromise and breathing difficulty as the airways become more constricted. Be sure to listen to lung sounds early and repeat lung sounds frequently. You can expect to hear wheezing as the bronchioles become constricted.

PRACTICAL PATHOPHYSIOLOGY

As the body reacts to the allergen, the airways become constricted, the soft tissues of the mouth and throat begin to swell, and the blood vessels become dilated. Work of breathing will increase as the body demands more oxygen. The patient may become altered, even unresponsive, as the blood pressure drops in response to the vessels dilating.

If possible, try to determine the most likely cause of the reaction. Evaluate the environment. (Was the patient indoors or out when the situation began?) Ask about activities just prior to the onset of signs and symptoms, as well as any food or chemical exposures. Do not delay care to determine the exact cause. Provide any indicated emergency medical care as soon as possible.

Anticipate the need to provide positive pressure ventilations should you determine that the patient is not breathing adequately. Verify the presence of a pulse at the carotid artery. The radial pulse may be difficult to palpate if the blood pressure is abnormally low. If the patient is responsive, allow him to remain in a position of comfort. If he is unresponsive, place him in a recovery or supine position, depending on the care needed.

Obtain a set of baseline vitals as soon as practical. Your partner can be doing this while you complete your primary assessment.

Secondary Assessment

Once you have confirmed that any issues relating to the primary assessment have been properly dealt with, you may move on to your secondary assessment. Remember that a severe allergic reaction is a serious emergency and transport should begin as soon as possible. Do not delay transport to perform a secondary assessment on scene.

Perform an appropriate physical exam if time and the patient's condition allow it. Look for any signs such as redness, swelling, bite or sting marks, and so on. Assuming your patient is responsive, perform a focused secondary assessment. In addition to the typical SAMPLE history, obtain the answers to the following questions:

- Any previous history of allergies or similar reactions?
- What was the patient exposed to?
- How was he exposed?
- When did the signs and symptoms begin?
- How have the signs and symptoms progressed?
- What interventions have been used so far?
- Does the patient have a prescription for and carry an epinephrine auto-injector?
- Has he self-administered the epinephrine yet?

PRACTICAL PATHOPHYSIOLOGY

Many of the symptoms of both moderate and severe allergic reactions are the result of the body's response to histamines that are released from specialized cells when the body is exposed to an allergen. Patients with a history of previous allergic reactions will often take a dose of an oral antihistamine, such as Benadryl® (diphenhydramine) in an attempt to self-medicate and stop the allergic reaction prior to calling EMS. Paramedic units also carry injectable diphenhydramine that can be used to treat serious allergic reactions.

Reassessment

Nearly all allergic reactions are progressive. In other words, they begin with somewhat mild symptoms that progressively get worse. Mild reactions may progress only to a point of mild swelling and itching. Severe reactions can progress to respiratory failure and cardiac arrest. You simply cannot know when the reaction will stop. For this reason, frequent reassessment is necessary. Constantly monitor the patient's ABCs, focusing on both respiratory status and mental status. Repeat vital signs as often as the patient's condition will allow.

Emergency Care of the Patient

While most allergic reactions will not require life-saving measures, it is important to initiate care as quickly as possible. Some reactions may have a slow onset, and it is best to begin care sooner rather than later.

Caring for Mild or Moderate Allergic Reactions

24-9 Describe the appropriate care of a person with a suspected allergic reaction.

Most mild or moderate reactions will take care of themselves with time, but there are some things you should do regardless of the reaction. If the allergic reaction was caused by an insect bite or sting, place a cool gauze or washcloth over the sting site. It could help with the pain, swelling, and itching. If the patient refuses to be transported, be sure to inform him of the signs and symptoms of anaphylaxis and instruct him to call EMS should his condition worsen. Be sure to stay with him long enough to determine that the signs and symptoms are not getting worse.

Patients presenting with signs and symptoms of only a mild or moderate reaction are not candidates for **epinephrine.**

epinephrine a hormone produced by the body. As a medication, it constricts blood vessels and dilates respiratory passages and is used to relieve severe allergic reactions. Also known as *adrenaline*.

Caring for a Severe Reaction

Focus your attention on the adequacy of the airway and breathing. Administer supplemental oxygen by nonrebreather mask. Airway compromise is likely to occur in a severe allergic reaction, so be prepared to provide ventilations if either the patient's respiratory rate or tidal volume falls below acceptable minimums. Proper airway management is critical.

PERSPECTIVE

Harold—The EMT

There are those cases—and luckily they seem to be few and far between—where EMTs just don't really have a chance. I think this was one. This kid had no airway, and as anyone who's been in an EMT course for two minutes knows, no "A" makes "B" and "C" pretty insignificant. On that entire call, we never moved beyond care for the airway, forget about the medical exam and history.

If the patient has a prescription for an epinephrine auto-injector and has the medication with him, instruct him to self-administer or assist him in doing so. Follow local protocols. Contact medical direction as appropriate.

Whether or not the patient has an epinephrine auto-injector available, if the patient is experiencing a severe allergic reaction, transport immediately. You can help the patient self-administer the epinephrine while en route.

It will be important to watch your patient closely for signs of improvement and reassess vitals shortly after administration of the medication. Document the patient response to the medication. If the patient experiencing a severe allergic reaction does not have an epinephrine auto-injector available, transport immediately.

Constant monitoring of the patient is essential, because his condition is progressive and you may need to assist his breathing at any moment. In addition to the typical elements of the reassessment, you will want to assess and document any changes in the patient's condition following the administration of the epinephrine.

Follow these steps when caring for the patient with anaphylaxis:

1. Perform a scene size-up to ensure you will not be exposed to whatever the patient was exposed to.
2. Take appropriate BSI precautions.

3. Perform a primary assessment and initiate supplemental oxygen by nonrebreather mask.
4. Assist with the administration of an epinephrine auto-injector, if available. Follow local protocols and contact medical direction as appropriate.
5. Perform an appropriate secondary assessment if patient condition allows.
6. Transport to the closest appropriate facility and/or initiate an ALS intercept, if available.
7. Perform frequent reassessments as appropriate.
8. Document all assessment findings, care provided, and any responses to care by the patient.

If at any time your patient becomes unresponsive or you determine that respirations are not adequate, begin providing assisted ventilations by way of a bag-mask device with supplemental oxygen. Do not wait for the patient to stop breathing completely before assisting ventilations. Place the patient in a supine position, attempt to insert an airway adjunct, and provide assisted ventilations as necessary. Have suction at the ready should the patient vomit. Transport immediately and request an ALS intercept if available.

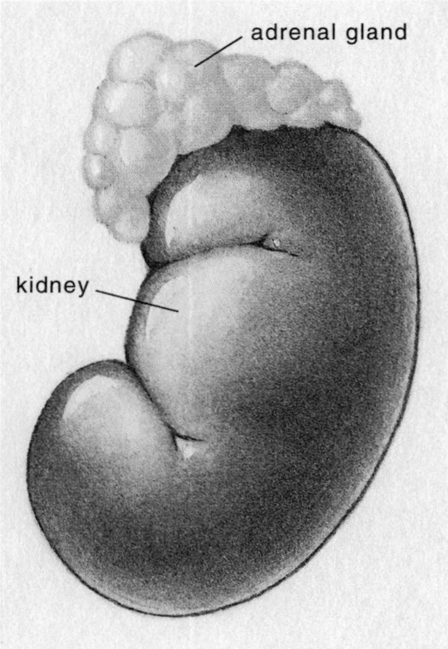

Figure 24-5 The adrenal gland is located on the top of each kidney.

Epinephrine

24-10 Describe the role of epinephrine in the treatment of anaphylaxis and the criteria and procedure for administration of epinephrine.

Epinephrine has already been mentioned several times. Also known as *adrenaline*, epinephrine is a hormone produced by the adrenal glands, which are located above the kidneys (Figure 24-5 ▪). Epinephrine is a very potent stimulant that primarily affects the sympathetic nervous system. When it is released into the bloodstream, it quickly causes an increase in heart rate, constriction of the blood vessels, and dilation of the air passages. For those reasons, epinephrine is the ideal medication for the patient experiencing anaphylaxis (Figure 24-6 ▪).

On the down side, the body's supply of epinephrine is limited and its effects last for only a few minutes. Because the symptoms of anaphylaxis progress beyond the effects of the body's own supply of epinephrine, another source of epinephrine is needed to control the life-threatening reaction (Scans 24-1 and 24-2).

Epinephrine can be manufactured in the laboratory and has been for many years. It has been available as a treatment for anaphylaxis for decades in the form of ANA-Kits® and Epi-Kits®, which sometimes required the manual drawing up of the solution and injection into the patient. Today, a tool called an *epinephrine auto-injector* (such as an Epi-Pen) makes the delivery of the medication much simpler.

PERSPECTIVE

The Patient's Mother

Eric should have had his Epi-Pen, but this was the one day he forgot it at home. He usually keeps it in his backpack. But he was running late today and couldn't find one of his shoes. And, you know, he hadn't had an attack in a couple of years. You know the worst part? When I came home from the hospital, I put Eric's stuff up in his room, and his Epi-Pen was just sitting there on his dresser. I picked it up and haven't been able to put it down since.

Epinephrine auto-injectors come in single and double dose injectors for both adult and pediatric patients. The adult dose is 0.3 mg, recommended for patients greater than 66 pounds and carries a bright yellow label. The pediatric dose is 0.15 mg

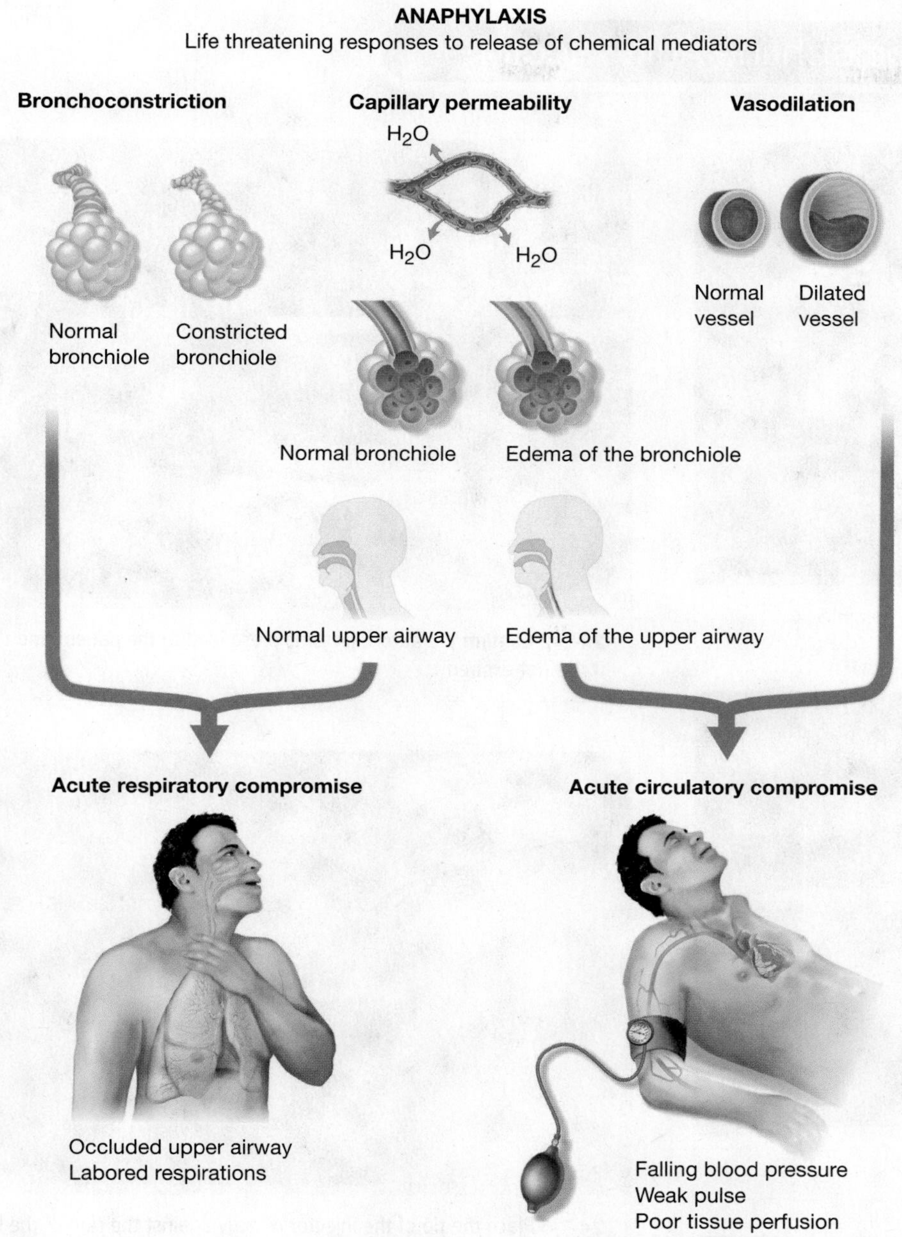

Figure 24-6 An anaphylactic reaction causes life-threatening reactions within the body.

and carries a white label. It is recommended for children weighing between 33 and 66 pounds. Sometimes a single dose of epinephrine may not be enough to completely reverse the effects of an anaphylactic reaction. For that reason, the patient's physician may have prescribed more than one auto-injector or a double dose injector, which requires a separate administration.

The beneficial effects of epinephrine occur within minutes following administration. However, the effects of the epinephrine may only last between 10 and 20 minutes. It is important that you initiate transport and/or an ALS interface as soon as possible. Continue to seek more advanced medical care even if the patient states that he feels better. Complete all necessary documentation.

Bring the used auto-injector with you to the hospital. Handle the auto-injector carefully following the injection. The needle may remain exposed from the end of the device and you must prevent yourself or anyone else from getting stuck. When

CLINICAL CLUE

Patient Communication and Epinephrine

To minimize patient anxiety, prepare the patient for how he is going to feel after administration of the epinephrine. Tell him that he will feel his heart rate begin to increase and he may feel jittery and get a headache. If the patient is prepared for what is about to happen, he is less likely to be surprised and scared, which would only make things worse.

SCAN 24-1 Using an Epinephrine Auto-Injector

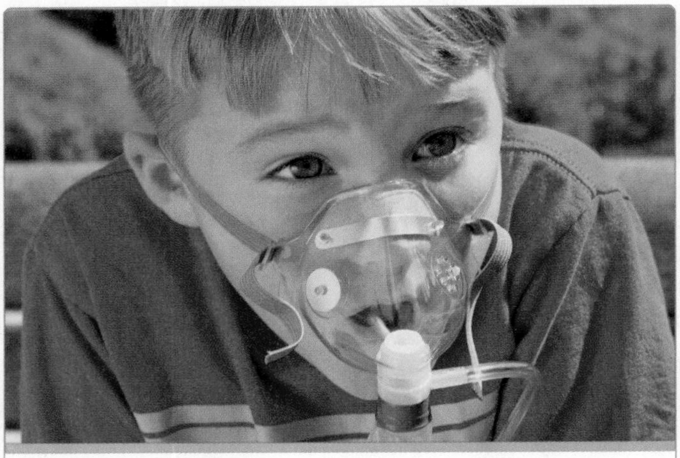

24-1-1 Provide supplemental oxygen as soon as possible.

24-1-2 Confirm the auto-injector is prescribed to the patient and that it has not expired.

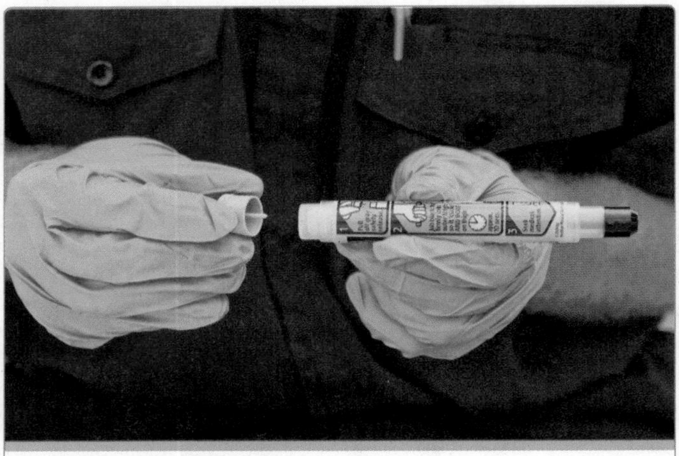

24-1-3 Remove the safety cap.

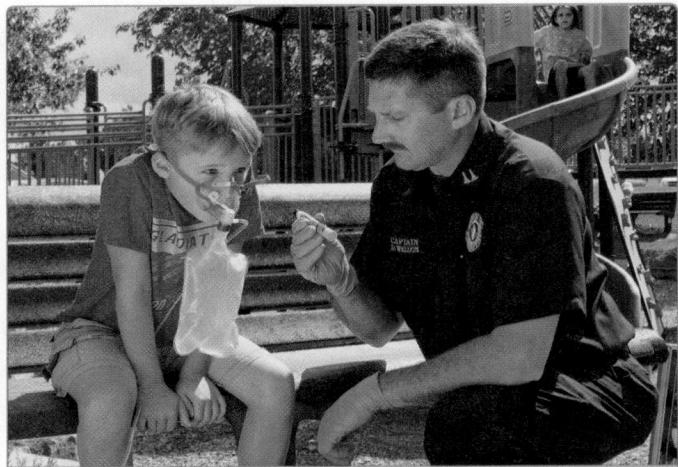

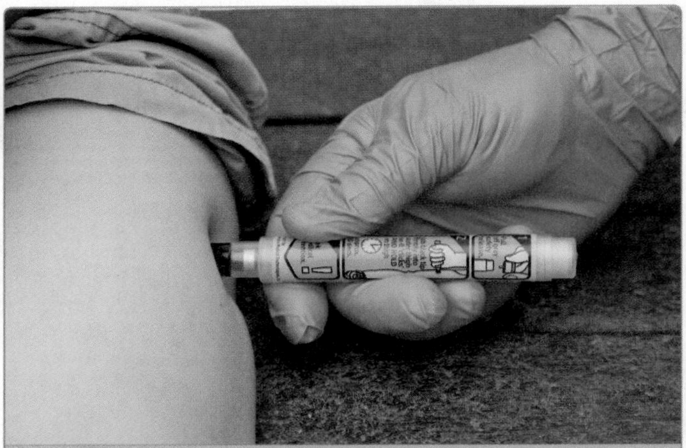

24-1-4 Place the tip of the injector directly against the skin of the lateral thigh and push in firmly. Hold in place for 10 seconds.

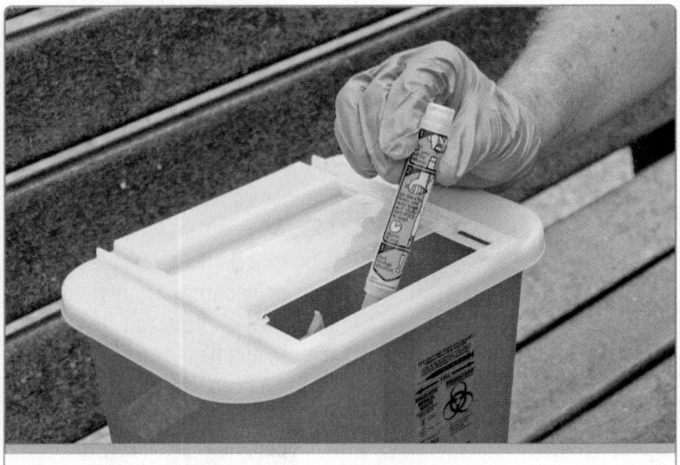

24-1-5 Dispose of the auto-injector appropriately.

SCAN 24-2 Epinephrine Auto-Injectors

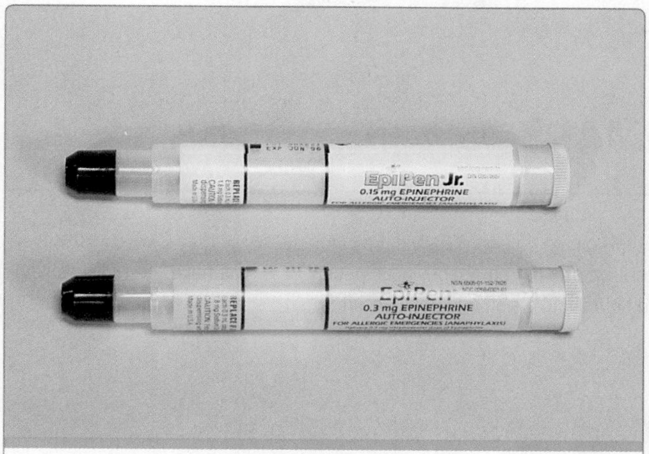

24-2-1 Epi-Pen auto-injectors are available in both adult (0.3 mg) and pediatric (0.15 mg) dosages.

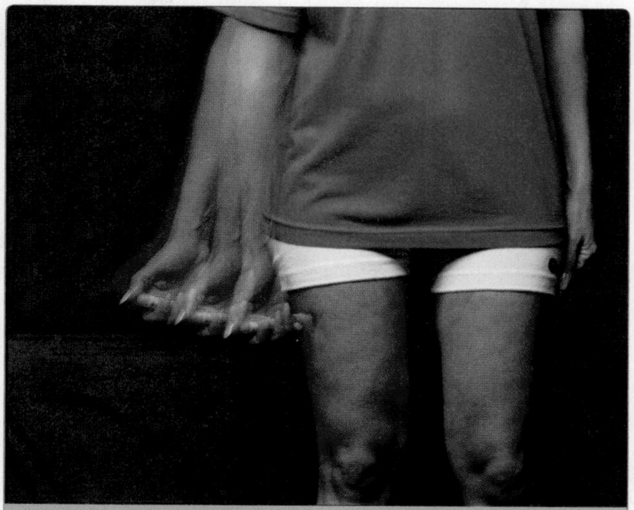

24-2-2 The auto-injector is ideally suited for self injection at the lateral thigh.

MEDICATION NAME

1. **Generic:** epinephrine
2. **Trade:** Adrenalin, Epi-Pen

INDICATIONS

Must meet the following three criteria:

1. Patient exhibits signs of a severe allergic reaction, including either respiratory distress or shock.
2. Medication is prescribed for this patient.
3. Medical direction authorizes the use for this patient.

CONTRAINDICATIONS

There are no contraindications when used in a life-threatening situation.

MEDICATION FORM

Liquid form of 1:1,000 concentration. Administered by an automatically injectable needle-and-syringe system.

DOSAGE

Adults: one adult auto-injector (0.3 mg)
Infant and child: one infant/child auto-injector (0.15 mg)
Adult has a yellow label and the pediatric has a white label.

STEPS FOR ASSISTING PATIENT

1. Obtain patient's prescribed auto-injector. Ensure right medication, right dose, right route, right patient, and right time. Note that most auto-injectors have a two-year shelf life. Medication will discolor (yellowish) when expired.
2. Obtain order from medical direction.
3. Remove cap from auto-injector. Then grasp the auto-injector barrel, avoiding placing your thumb over the end of the device.
4. Place tip of auto-injector against patient's lateral thigh, midway between hip and knee. You may inject through clothing if necessary.
5. Push the injector firmly against the thigh until the injector activates.
6. Hold the injector in place until the medication is injected (at least 10 seconds).
7. Document the time and any response to the medication.
8. Dispose of injector in biohazard container.

ACTIONS

Dilates the bronchioles.
Constricts blood vessels.

SIDE EFFECTS

1. Increased heart rate.
2. Dizziness.
3. Chest pain.
4. Headache.
5. Nausea.
6. Vomiting.
7. Excitability, anxiety.
8. Pale skin.

REASSESSMENT STRATEGIES

1. Initiate transport to an appropriate receiving facility as soon as practical.
2. Continue assessment of airway, breathing, and circulatory status. If patient's condition continues to worsen (decreasing mental status, increasing breathing difficulty, decreasing blood pressure):
   a. Obtain medical direction for an additional dose of epinephrine.
   b. Provide care for shock, including administration of oxygen per local protocols.
   c. Prepare to initiate basic life support (CPR, AED).
3. If patient's condition improves, provide supportive care:
   a. Continue oxygen.
   b. Provide care for shock.

exposed, the manufacturer recommends pressing the exposed needle against a hard surface and bending it over. Then place the injector *needle first* into the plastic storage tube. A small amount of fluid will remain in the device following injection. *Do not attempt to use the same device a second time.*

EMERGENCY DISPATCH SUMMARY

The boy never regained consciousness and was pronounced dead in the emergency department of the Palm Harbor Regional Hospital. The medical director has since authorized the city's EMS system to stock all of the ambulances with epinephrine auto-injectors and train the crews in their use. The next time that Harold, Shannon, or any of their EMT coworkers are confronted with an anaphylactic patient, they will have the tools available to help avoid a similarly tragic result.

Chapter Review

To the Point

- An antigen is a foreign substance that triggers an immune response in the body. In a normal response, the immune system is triggered and sends white blood cells to attack the invader. This response results in a mild to moderate allergic reaction.
- Common allergens include pollen, peanuts, insect bites and stings, shellfish, poison oak and poison ivy, and many medications.
- Allergens can enter the body in one of four ways: ingestion, injection, absorption, or inhalation.
- A milder allergic reaction is characterized by localized swelling, hives, itching, watery eyes, and runny nose.
- A mild reaction quickly can develop into a life-threatening response known as *anaphylaxis*. Anaphylaxis must be recognized early and care provided immediately to minimize impact on the patient.
- Signs and symptoms of anaphylaxis include swelling of the airway, difficulty breathing, drop in blood pressure, altered mental status, wheezing, and anxiety.
- The primary mechanisms at work during an anaphylactic reaction are a constricting of the bronchioles, making breathing very difficult, and dilation of the blood vessels, resulting in a drop in blood pressure and decreased perfusion.
- Two signs that differentiate a mild reaction from a severe reaction are increased difficulty breathing and a decreasing blood pressure.
- The care for a mild reaction is generally supportive and includes placing a cool gauze over the area of redness or itching.
- Care for anaphylaxis must be immediate and includes ensuring a patent airway and adequacy of breathing.
- If the patient with signs and symptoms of anaphylaxis has a prescribed Epi-Pen, assist with the administration of the device. Follow local protocols.
- Support the ABCs and initiate transport as soon as possible. Reassess the patient frequently.

Chapter Questions

Multiple Choice

For each question, place a check next to the correct answer.

1. The care for anaphylaxis should focus on:
   _____ a. maintaining responsiveness.
   _____ b. patient comfort.
   _____ c. obtaining a thorough history.
   _____ d. airway and breathing adequacy.

2. Which one of the following would *not* be an appropriate history question for the patient experiencing an allergic reaction?
   _____ a. When did your symptoms begin?
   _____ b. Is there a history of cardiac disease in your family?
   _____ c. Do you have a prescription for epinephrine?
   _____ d. Have you had similar reactions in the past?

3. When should supplemental oxygen be initiated in the emergency care of a patient with an allergic reaction?
   _____ a. Immediately
   _____ b. After the scene size-up
   _____ c. During the primary assessment
   _____ d. After the secondary assessment

4. The adult dose of epinephrine is:
   _____ a. 0.15 mg.
   _____ b. 1.5 mg.
   _____ c. 3.0 mg.
   _____ d. 0.3 mg.

5. The effects of epinephrine last as little as _____________ minutes.
   _____ a. 5 to 10
   _____ b. 10 to 20
   _____ c. 20 to 30
   _____ d. 30 to 60

6. Anaphylaxis is commonly associated with _____________ compromise.
   _____ a. neurogenic
   _____ b. airway
   _____ c. mental status
   _____ d. cerebrovascular

7. Which one of the following is *not* a sign or symptom of anaphylaxis?
   _____ a. Itching
   _____ b. Difficulty breathing
   _____ c. Decreased pulse rate
   _____ d. Swelling of the throat

8. A pediatric Epi-Pen contains which one of the following doses of epinephrine?
   _____ a. 1.5 mg
   _____ b. 0.15 mg
   _____ c. 3.0 mg
   _____ d. 0.3 mg

9. A common cause of allergic reaction in an increasing number of EMS professionals is:
   _____ a. latex gloves.
   _____ b. vinyl gloves.
   _____ c. paper face masks.
   _____ d. cleaning solution.

10. A severe allergic reaction will cause the blood vessels to _____________ while at the same time causing the airways to _____________.
    _____ a. constrict, dilate
    _____ b. dilate, constrict
    _____ c. constrict, constrict
    _____ d. dilate, dilate

(continued on next page)

(continued)

Critical Thinking

1. Describe how emergency care might differ between a patient with a mild allergic reaction and one with a severe allergic reaction.

2. Describe how epinephrine affects the body when given to a victim of anaphylaxis.

3. Discuss the critical elements of your patient reassessment following the administration of epinephrine.

Case Studies

Case Study 1

You have been dispatched to a campground for a person with difficulty breathing. Upon your arrival, a park aide escorts you to a campsite where several people are surrounding what appears to be an approximately 40-year-old woman lying on a picnic table. A man who identifies himself as the woman's husband tells you that they were just breaking down the tent when his wife suddenly screamed and shouted that she had just been bitten by something under her right arm near the armpit. When you attempt to get a history from the patient, she appears to be sleepy and confused and is unable to provide any valuable information.

1. What will be your first priority for this patient in terms of assessment and care?

2. Your primary assessment reveals that she has an open airway with a respiratory rate of 10 and shallow. Her pulse is rapid and weak. Does this patient require further care pertaining to her respiratory status? If so, what care will you provide?

3. What questions will you want to ask the husband regarding her medical history?

Case Study 2

You have responded to a local park for a possible allergic reaction and are met in the parking lot by a pair of frantic parents holding what appears to be an approximately three-year-old boy. The father states that his son was stung twice by bees and is concerned that he may be having an allergic reaction to the stings. You begin to assess the child while he is being held by his father and see one sting mark on his hand and another on his shoulder. Both are small red dots similar to mosquito bites. The child appears calm, considering the circumstances. His mother states that he was stung about 15 minutes ago.

1. What will you look for to determine the extent of this boy's reaction to the bee stings?

2. The boy appears to be breathing adequately and his level of alertness seems appropriate for his age. His hand appears to be getting more swollen just in the 10 minutes that you have been on scene. What type of reaction is this boy likely experiencing?

3. The patient's parents are insisting that you get him to the hospital before he has a severe reaction. How will you handle this request? What care will you provide for the child?

The Last Word

Nearly everyone experiences at least a mild allergic reaction sometime in his life. While most reactions do not represent a threat to life, severe reactions known as *anaphylaxis* progress rapidly and can be deadly. Anaphylaxis is differentiated from mild and moderate reactions by the fact that it causes difficulty breathing and can include signs and symptoms of shock (hypoperfusion). Rapid assessment, care, and transport are essential for the survival of victims of anaphylaxis.

Epinephrine can be life saving if given in time. It may only be administered to patients with a prescription who happen to be carrying their own medication. Follow local protocols when administering or assisting with the administration of epinephrine and consult medical direction as appropriate.

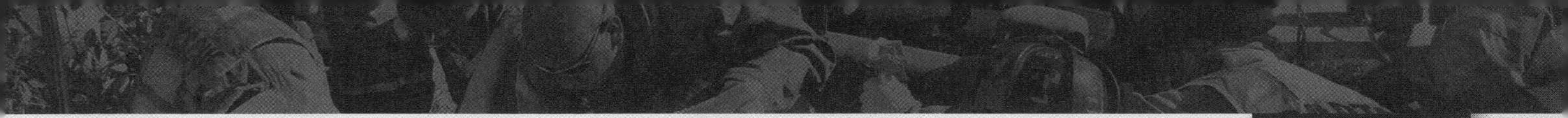

Caring for Patients with Hematologic and Renal Emergencies

25

Education Standards

Medicine: Hematology, Genitourinary, Renal

Competencies

Applies fundamental knowledge to provide basic emergency care and transportation based on assessment findings for an acutely ill patient.

Objectives

After completion of this lesson, you should be able to:

25-1 Define the key terms introduced in this chapter.

25-2 Describe the components of the blood system.

25-3 Describe the physiology by which the body forms clots when hemorrhage occurs.

25-4 List diseases and medications that can interfere with normal clotting.

25-5 Describe the potential consequences for a patient who cannot clot normally.

25-6 Describe the assessment and management of a person who cannot clot normally.

25-7 Describe the pathophysiology of sickle cell disease.

25-8 Describe the assessment of a person with sickle cell disease.

25-9 Describe the management of a patient with complications of sickle cell disease.

25-10 Describe the anatomy and physiology of the renal/urinary system.

25-11 List common diseases associated with the urinary system.

25-12 Describe the complications related to urinary catheters.

25-13 Describe the causes and consequences of acute and chronic renal failure.

25-14 Describe the complications related to renal dialysis.

25-15 Describe the management of a patient with complications of renal dialysis.

Key Terms

anemia p. 657
clotting factors p. 655
coagulopathy p. 655
dialysis p. 663
end-stage renal disease (ESRD) p. 663
hemodialysis p. 663
kidney stones p. 661
peritoneal dialysis p. 663
peritonitis p. 666
pyelonephritis p. 661
renal failure p. 661
sickle cell anemia (SCA) p. 657
thrill p. 663
urinary catheter p. 661

Introduction

Good health depends on the human body's multiple organ systems working seamlessly together. As an EMT, you will focus much of your medical attention on acute emergencies that can be attributed to the cardiovascular and respiratory systems. However, there will be emergencies involving patients who have diseases or problems with their *hematologic system* (pertaining to blood) or *renal system* (pertaining to the kidneys). *Hematology* is the medical specialty concerned with blood disorders. *Nephrology* is the medical specialty concerned with renal/kidney diseases. Dozens of medical conditions can arise from diseases involving those two body systems.

EMERGENCY DISPATCH

"There is just nothing on television tonight," EMT Hossein Najafi clicked off the flat screen in the Station 6 lounge, leaned back on the couch, and looked over at his partner, Lauren Canfield. "What are you reading?"

"My paramedic textbook."

"Quiz me," he smiled. "Ask me anything."

"Alright," she flipped dramatically to a chapter in the middle of the large book. "What is the titration rate for . . . ."

Loud dispatch tones interrupted her question and Hossein shrugged, "Oh darn. I was totally going to get that one right, too!"

"Station 6 EMS, respond to the Pizza Palace restaurant at 19113 Old Canyon Highway for a generalized pain. Showing you dispatched at 2309 hours."

Several minutes later, the EMTs arrived at the nearly empty parking lot of the restaurant, which had a "Closed" sign prominently displayed in the window. As they rolled the gurney up to the door, they were met by a small man wearing a white apron smeared with pizza sauce and flour.

"He's in the last stall in the men's bathroom," the man said as he held the door for them. "Seems to be in real bad shape."

As the EMTs entered the dark, musty bathroom they could hear groans and heavy breathing echoing from the row of stalls. "We're from the ambulance service," Hossein said loudly. "Here to help you."

"I need a hospital, man," a voice boomed back at them. "I'm having a sickle cell crisis."

The Hematologic System

25-2 Describe the components of the blood system.

Although central to the function of the cardiovascular system, blood actually represents its own organ system. As you learned in Chapter 5, each component of the blood has specific functions that, when working properly, are critical to a patient's health and survival, such as:

- Control of bleeding by clotting
- Delivery of oxygen to the cells
- Removal of carbon dioxide from the cells
- Removal and delivery of other waste products to organs that provide filtration and removal such as the kidneys and liver

Blood is made up of solid components (including red blood cells, white blood cells, and platelets) suspended in a liquid called *plasma*. The solid components of blood are created in the bone marrow, which forms the specialized core of many of the body's bones. Red blood cells, white blood cells, and platelets survive in the circulation for only a finite period of time, and are then removed from circulation by means such as the filtration of the spleen.

Each component of the blood has specialized functions. They are:

- ***Red blood cells (RBCs).*** RBCs make up the majority of the cells in the circulation and give blood its characteristic red color. These cells contain specialized molecules called *hemoglobin* that bind to oxygen and are responsible for oxygen delivery to the cells.

- ***White blood cells (WBCs).*** WBCs are critical body cells that respond to infection and are mediators of the body's immune response. (See Chapter 24.)
- ***Platelets.*** Platelets are actually fragments of larger cells that are crucial to the initial formation of clots.
- ***Plasma.*** Plasma is the liquid in which the blood cells and platelets are suspended. Plasma contains dissolved nutrients and also carries certain crucial proteins known as **clotting factors.** The clotting factors form the most stable clots, replacing the initial efforts of the platelets to stop bleeding.

clotting factors proteins made in the liver that form clots through the activation of clotting cascades.

Blood Clotting

25-3 Describe the physiology by which the body forms clots when hemorrhage occurs.

When internal or external bleeding occurs as a result of a medical condition or injury, the body must mobilize its clotting system to control the bleeding or the patient could literally bleed to death. There are two major components within the blood that are responsible for clotting: platelets and clotting factors. Clumping (called *aggregation*) of platelets is the body's most rapid and initial response to stop bleeding at a site of injury.

PRACTICAL PATHOPHYSIOLOGY

Although platelets play a crucial role in stopping hemorrhage, in some situations the clumping of platelets is not desirable, such as when a plaque in a coronary artery ruptures. In this situation, the rapid clumping of platelets can cause a clot that then completely blocks the coronary artery causing a heart attack (myocardial infarction). One of the most effective and widely available drugs to prevent the aggregation of platelets is aspirin. That is why patients who are having an acute heart attack, or a potential heart attack, are routinely given an aspirin as part of emergency care.

Clotting factors are a group of proteins that are produced in the liver and released into the bloodstream. Clotting factors circulate in the blood in inactive forms, but are activated to initiate clotting when damage occurs to the lining of damaged blood vessels. Once activated, clotting factors form clots through specific steps that are described as *clotting cascades*.

Coagulopathies

The term **coagulopathy** is defined as abnormal clotting of the blood. Coagulopathy can occur when the body forms clots too readily, or (and most relevant to the EMT) when the patient clots too slowly, resulting in uncontrolled bleeding. Coagulopathies that result in abnormally slow clotting can occur because of problems with the clotting cascades as a result of too few platelets or due to platelets that are not functioning correctly. Some patients may even be coagulopathic for more than one of those reasons.

coagulopathy lack of normal clotting.

25-4 List diseases and medications that can interfere with normal clotting.

Certain diseases make patients prone to poor clotting. Because the clotting factors are manufactured in the liver, patients with advanced liver diseases, such as cirrhosis, may not make adequate amounts of clotting factors to form stable clots. There are also certain inherited genetic disorders that result in coagulopathy. Hemophiliacs, for example, have inherited disorders that prevent them from producing certain clotting factors. Similarly, von Willebrand's disease is the most common inherited bleeding disorder occurring in about one in 1,000 persons. In this common disease, although the patient has a normal number of platelets circulating in the blood, the patient's platelets are functionally defective, thus allowing for excessive bleeding when injury occurs.

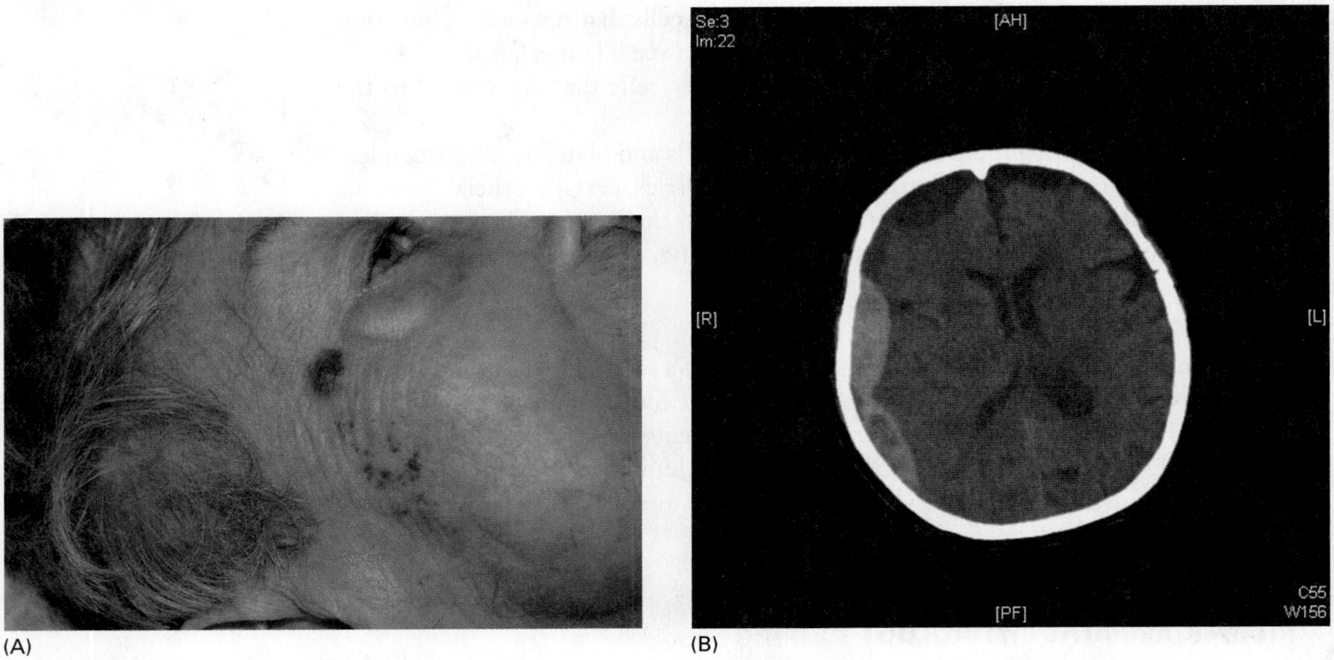

Figure 25-1 (A) A patient on Plavix® with a minor head injury. (© Edward T. Dickinson, MD) (B) The CT scan of this patient's intracranial hemorrhage. (© Edward T. Dickinson, MD)

There are certain medical conditions in which the normal ability to form clots can worsen the patient's disease, such as in those at risk for heart attacks or strokes or those with abnormal cardiac rhythms, such as atrial fibrillation. For this reason, hundreds of thousands of patients are on prescription drugs commonly referred to as *blood thinners*. Drugs such as Coumadin® (warfarin), Pradaxa® (dabigatran), and Lovenox® (enoxaparin) inhibit certain clotting factors. Other drugs, such as aspirin and Plavix (clopidogrel), inhibit platelet aggregation.

25-5 Describe the potential consequences for a patient who cannot clot normally.

Patients with diseases that prevent normal clotting, or those on medications that prevent normal clotting, are more prone to have life-threatening bleeding when they are injured than patients who are not on those medications. In some EMS systems, injured patients taking those medications are frequently transported to a trauma center, even with apparently minor injuries. This is due to their increased risk of uncontrolled bleeding. Patients with head injuries are at particular risk for catastrophic bleeding complications. Follow your local trauma triage protocols when managing patients on blood thinners (Figure 25-1 ▪).

Patients with Clotting Disorders

A thorough patient history becomes most important when assessing patients with suspected clotting disorders. Be sure to gather as much history from the patient or caregivers while managing all immediate life threats. When the patient's condition permits, you also should complete a thorough secondary assessment.

Patient Assessment

25-6 Describe the assessment and management of a person who cannot clot normally.

A critical aspect of being able to manage patients with potential coagulopathies is identifying that the patient is in fact at risk for abnormal bleeding based on his past medical history and the medications he is taking. Although EMS providers have traditionally focused less on medications when obtaining a SAMPLE history in trauma patients, the increasing number of patients on these medications mandates that every trauma patient should be specifically asked if they are taking any medications that thin their blood. Additional historical and physical clues that a patient may be having an underlying coagulopathy include:

- History of atrial fibrillation (one of the most common chronic medical conditions for which patients are placed on blood thinners)
- Abnormally severe bleeding from what seem like minor wounds
- Adult patient with extensive bruising that appears to be in various stages of resolving

Emergency Care

Emergency treatment of a patient with a potential clotting disorder is as follows:

1. Take appropriate BSI precautions.
2. Perform a primary assessment and care for any immediate life threats.
3. Obtain a history of the patient at risk for a coagulopathy.
4. If the patient is on blood-thinning medications, specifically identify which ones the patient is taking and convey this information to hospital staff so they can optimally manage the specific cause of the patient's bleeding disorder.
5. Monitor the patient carefully for the development of signs of shock or decreasing mental status
6. Administer supplemental oxygen if the patient appears to be in shock or has a decreased mental status
7. Transport to an appropriate receiving hospital. The patient may require large amounts of blood products not available in smaller hospitals. Follow local protocols.

Anemia

Lack of a normal number of red blood cells in the circulation is called **anemia.** There are many reasons why a patient becomes anemic. *Acute anemia* may be the result of trauma or sudden massive bleeding from the gastrointestinal tract. These patients may rapidly exhibit classic signs of shock (hypoperfusion) such as tachycardia, cool moist skin, and eventual hypotension. *Chronic anemia* occurs over time and can be caused by conditions such as recurrent heavy menstrual periods, slow gastrointestinal blood loss, or diseases that affect the bone marrow or the structure of the hemoglobin molecule itself. Patients with chronic anemia often appear more pale than normal (from a lack of circulating red blood cells) and often complain of fatigue and shortness of breath with exertion (because of a lack of adequate oxygen being delivered to the body's cells). Only after a very prolonged period of time will these patients potentially begin to show signs of shock.

anemia lack of a normal number of red blood cells in the circulation.

Sickle Cell Anemia

Sickle cell anemia (SCA) is an inherited disease in which patients have a genetic defect in their hemoglobin that results in an abnormal structure of the red blood cells. Sickle cell anemia can occur in patients of African, Middle Eastern, or Indian descent but is most common in patients of African descent.

sickle cell anemia (SCA) an inherited disease in which a genetic defect in the hemoglobin results in abnormal structure of the red blood cells.

25-7 Describe the pathophysiology of sickle cell disease.

A normal red blood cell is doughnut-shaped with a depression rather than a hole in the center. Normal red blood cells can be compressed as they move and squeeze through small capillaries to deliver oxygen to the cells of the body's organs. Patients with sickle cell disease have red blood cells composed of defective hemoglobin that causes them to lose their ability to be compressed. Their shape resembles that of a sickle when observed under a microscope (Figure 25-2 ■). Because of that abnormal shape, the RBCs do not survive in the circulation as long as normal RBCs, which results in chronic anemia.

25-8 Describe the assessment of a person with sickle cell disease.

The complications of sickle cell anemia are generally attributed to the sludging of the abnormally shaped red blood cells, which causes blockages within the body's small blood vessels. The complications of sickle cell anemia include:

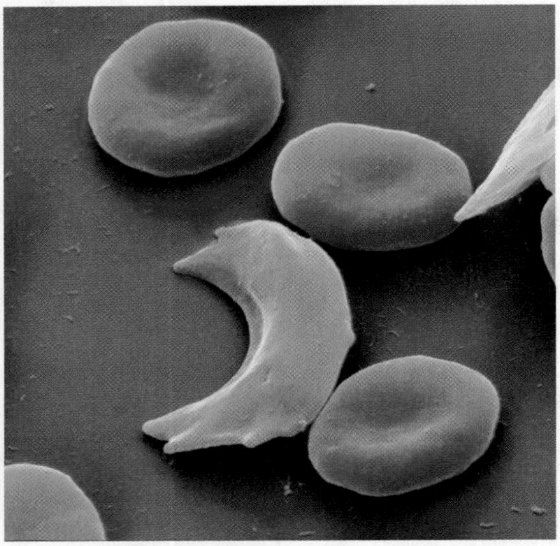

Figure 25-2 Scanning electron photomicrograph of normal red blood cells contrasted with a sickle cell. (Eye of Science/Photo Researchers, Inc.)

- ***Destruction of the spleen.*** The spleen, as it filters the blood, becomes blocked by the abnormal RBCs. Because the spleen is important in fighting infections, its loss places patients with sickle cell anemia at higher risk for severe, life-threatening infections.
- ***Sickle cell pain crisis.*** Sickle cell crisis is caused by the sludging of sickled RBCs in capillaries, which results in severe pain in the arms, legs, chest, and abdomen. This is referred to as a *vaso-occlusive crisis.*
- ***Acute chest syndrome.*** Chest syndrome is characterized by shortness of breath and chest pain associated with hypoxia when blood vessels in the lungs become blocked.
- ***Priapism.*** Painful prolonged erections in men occur because sludging RBCs prevent normal blood drainage from the erect penis.
- ***Stroke.*** Stroke can occur when sludging RBCs block blood vessels that supply the brain.
- ***Jaundice.*** The liver becomes overwhelmed by the breakdown in red blood cells, resulting in yellowish pigmentation of body tissues.

PERSPECTIVE

Lauren—The EMT

I've never encountered a sickle cell patient before. That's got to be just horrible! I've read that the pain is incredible when the blood cells get caught up in the capillaries, and this guy definitely confirmed that. I mean, the pain on his face. His teeth were clenched the entire time we were with him. I just wished that I could have given something other than oxygen, you know? I realize that as EMTs, rapid transport is sometimes the most effective care we can provide, but I'm in this business because I want to make people feel better and there was just nothing that we could do to make it better for that guy until he got to the hospital.

25-9 Describe the management of a patient with complications of sickle cell disease.

PRACTICAL PATHOPHYSIOLOGY

Some patients may tell you that they have "sickle cell trait" as part of their past medical history. These patients carry the gene for sickle cell disease but do not have the disease. Therefore, they do not suffer the complications of sickle cell anemia and have normal life spans. It is estimated that one in 12 African Americans have sickle cell trait.

Despite advances in modern medical care, patients with sickle cell anemia still have an abnormally short life span. In addition, some sickle cell patients suffer so persistently from painful vaso-occlusive crises that they become dependent on narcotic pain medications.

Emergency care of a patient with sickle cell anemia is as follows:

1. Take appropriate BSI precautions.
2. Perform an appropriate primary assessment and care for issues related to airway and breathing.
3. Administer supplemental oxygen.
4. Monitor patients with acute chest syndrome for signs of inadequate respiration and provide bag-mask ventilation as necessary.
5. Perform a thorough secondary assessment.
6. Monitor patients with high fever for signs of shock. Treat for shock as necessary.
7. Transport patients with acute stroke symptoms to a designated stroke center, if available. Follow local protocols.

STOP, REVIEW, REMEMBER!

Multiple Choice

1. Patients with sickle cell anemia (SCA):

_____ a. have a longer life-span than the general population.

_____ b. are usually of South and Central American decent.

_____ c. are at lesser risk of serious infections than the general population.

_____ d. are at greater risk of stroke than the general population.

2. Which one of the following patients is most likely to be on a prescription blood thinner?

_____ a. 27-year-old man with sickle cell trait

_____ b. 82-year-old man with atrial fibrillation

_____ c. 57-year-old woman with type 2 diabetes

_____ d. 43-year-old woman with sickle cell disease

3. All of the following medications are considered a "blood thinner" *except*:

_____ a. Pradaxa (dabigatran)

_____ b. Plavix (clopidogrel)

_____ c. Humulin® (insulin)

_____ d. Coumadin (warfarin)

4. Patients with sickle cell trait:

_____ a. represent approximately one in two of all African Americans.

_____ b. represent approximately one in 200 of all African Americans.

_____ c. develop sickle cell anemia as a result of recurrent infections of their spleen and lungs.

_____ d. carry a gene for sickle cell, but do not suffer the same complications as those with sickle cell anemia.

5. Which one of the following is most likely to cause acute anemia?

_____ a. Heat exhaustion

_____ b. Ruptured spleen

_____ c. Acute pneumonia

_____ d. Sickle cell trait

Short Answer

1. List three complications of sickle cell disease.

____

____

____

____

2. List two medical conditions (not medications) that place patients at risk for a coagulopathy.

____

____

____

____

(continued on next page)

(continued)

3. List two causes of chronic anemia other than sickle cell disease.

Critical Thinking

1. Explain why patients with sickle cell disease are more prone to serious infections than patients who do not suffer from it.

2. Explain why a patient who is awaiting a liver transplant due to severe cirrhosis from hepatitis B would have a coagulopathy.

The Renal System

25-10 Describe the anatomy and physiology of the renal/urinary system.

The renal system is made up of two kidneys, two ureters (to carry urine from each kidney to the bladder), the urinary bladder, and a single urethra (to carry urine from the bladder to the outside of the body) (Figure 25-3 ■).

As you learned in Chapter 5, the kidneys are responsible for the filtration of the blood and the removal of certain waste products, excessive salts, and excessive fluid from the body. In addition, in times of dehydration the kidneys also help the body retain needed fluid. Because they perform those critical functions, the kidneys are essential to life.

Diseases of the Renal System

25-11 List common diseases associated with the urinary system.

There are many diseases that involve the urinary and renal system. They affect different parts of the system and can range from minor problems that are easily treated to life-threatening conditions.

Urinary Tract Infections

Urinary tract infections (UTIs) are perhaps the most common disease process that afflicts the renal and urinary system. Most UTIs are limited to the bladder and cause symptoms of painful urination and frequent urination. If left untreated, an infection in the bladder can ascend up into the ureters and infect the kidney, a condition known as **pyelonephritis.** Patients with pyelonephritis generally appear much more ill than those with simple UTIs. They can exhibit high fevers, severe one-sided flank pain, nausea, and vomiting.

Urinary tract infections can be a serious and life-threatening disease (especially in the elderly), if the bacteria spread into the bloodstream.

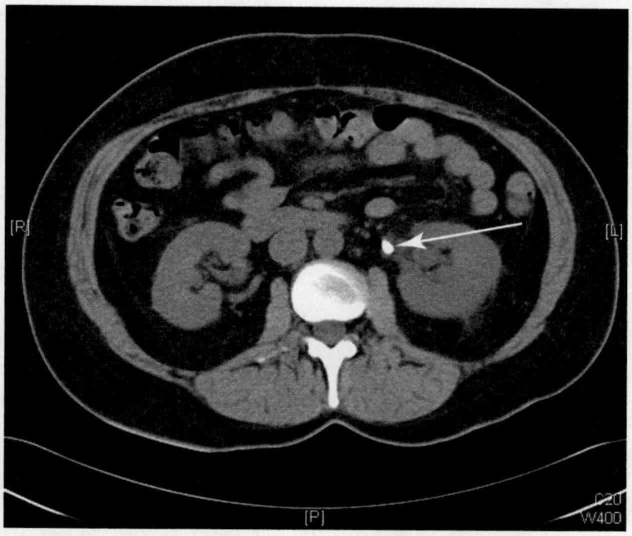

Figure 25-3 CT scan showing a kidney stone (see arrow) lodged in the proximal left ureter. (© Edward T. Dickinson, MD)

pyelonephritis an infection of the kidney.

PRACTICAL PATHOPHYSIOLOGY

In children and young adults, UTIs are much more common in women than in men. This is largely because of the relatively short length of the female urethra as compared to the male urethra, which extends the length of the penis. The short length of the female urethra allows bacteria to enter the bladder more easily and cause infection.

Kidney Stones

Kidney stones are a painful and common condition related to the renal system. Usually made of calcium, if these stones remain within the kidney, they usually cause no symptoms and the patient is unaware of their presence. However, when a kidney stone drops out of the kidney and becomes lodged in the ureter (Figure 25-4 ■), the patient will suddenly develop unilateral flank and groin pain associated with nausea and often vomiting.

kidney stones small rock-like structures formed in the kidneys of certain patients; cause symptoms of flank pain when they become lodged in the ureter.

Patients with Urinary Catheters

25-12 Describe the complications related to urinary catheters.

As an EMT, you will encounter certain patients who have lost the ability to urinate normally. This can be a result of obstruction of out-flow from the bladder (such as a tumor or large prostate) or because a neurological disorder has caused them to lose the ability to initiate urination. These patients commonly use a **urinary catheter** to drain their bladder.

urinary catheter a device usually placed in the urethra of patients who have lost the ability to drain their bladder either due to obstruction or loss of necessary neurological control of the bladder.

Some urinary catheters are left in place for the long term, while other patients actually place a catheter into their own urethra each time they urinate ("self-cathers").

The most common complication of having a urinary catheter is developing a urinary tract infection. Other complications of urinary catheters include local trauma to the urethra and the development of a less common type of kidney stone due to recurrent infections.

Renal Failure

The most serious disease of the kidneys is called **renal failure.** Renal failure occurs when the kidneys lose their ability to adequately filter the blood and remove toxins and excess fluid from the body.

renal failure loss of the kidneys' ability to filter the blood and remove toxins and excess fluid from the body.

25-13 Describe the causes and consequences of acute and chronic renal failure.

There are many reasons why patients develop renal failure. Some causes for renal failure are sudden (acute) and some develop gradually over time (chronic). *Acute renal failure* can occur as a result of shock, toxic ingestions, and other causes. Some patients who experience acute renal failure can recover normal kidney function if the underlying cause of the insult to the kidneys is rapidly identified and corrected. An example

Renal System

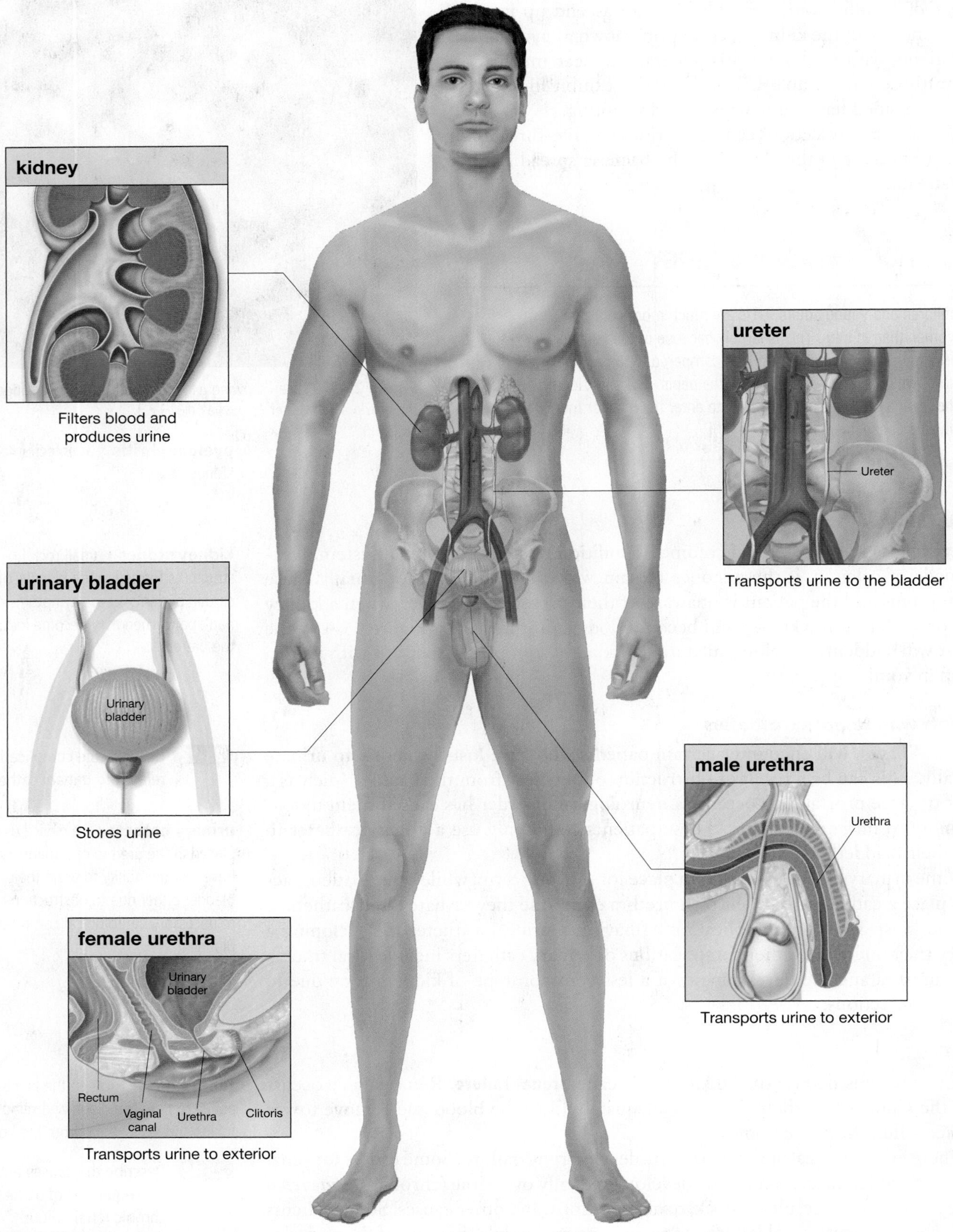

Figure 25-4 The renal system.

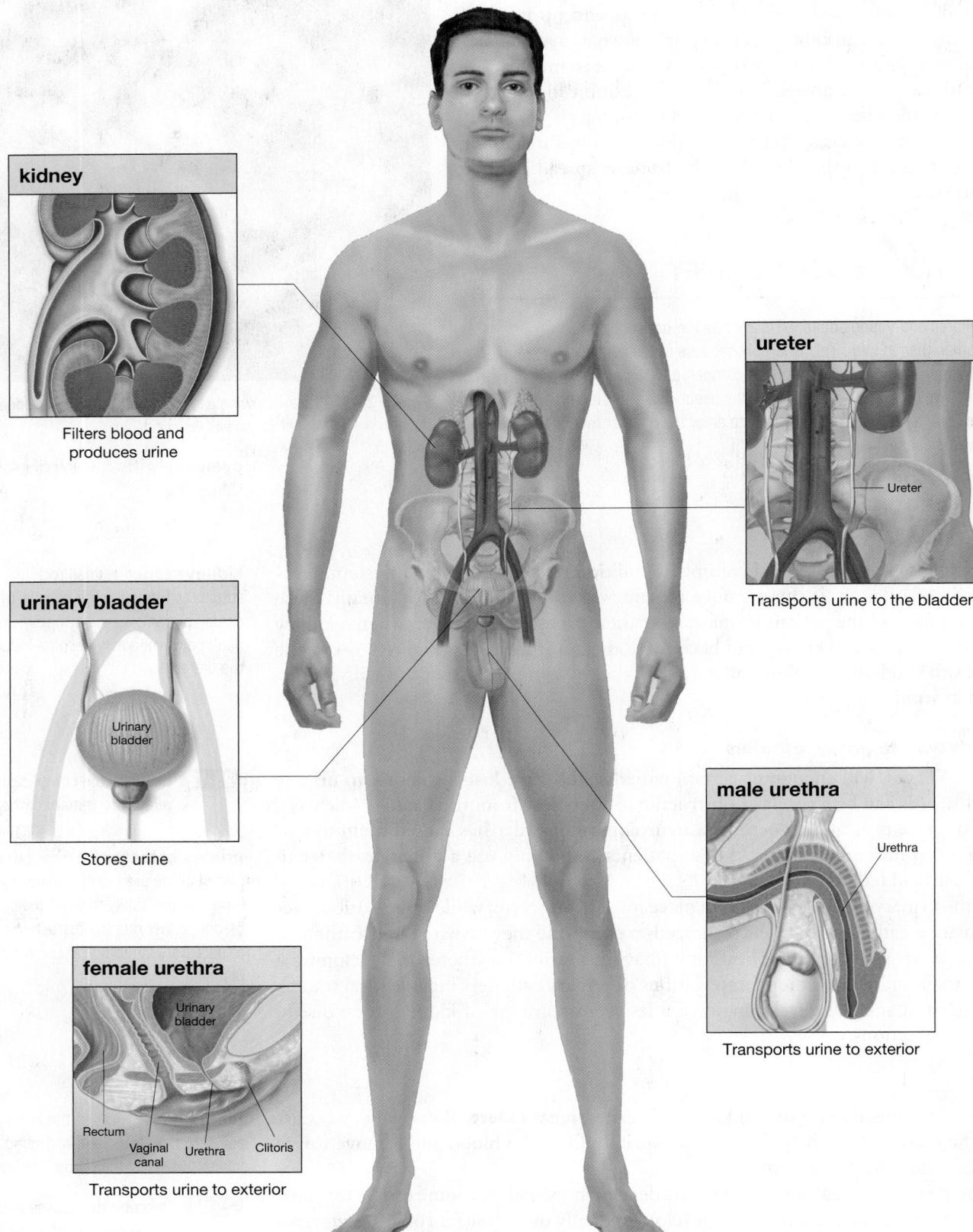

of this would be severe dehydration in a patient trapped in a building collapse for several days who, with aggressive treatment with intravenous fluids, can recover normal renal function over time. However, others who suffer acute renal failure never recover normal kidney function. Causes of *chronic renal failure* can include inherited diseases such as polycystic kidney disease. More commonly, however, the long-term damage is caused by poorly controlled diabetes or high blood pressure that results in the loss of normal renal function.

Patients who go on to develop irreversible renal failure—to the extent that their kidneys can no longer provide adequate filtration and fluid balance to sustain life—are defined as patients with **end-stage renal disease (ESRD).** Patients with ESRD usually require **dialysis** to survive. More than half a million people in the United States have ESRD, and more than 350,000 of them are on chronic dialysis.

end-stage renal disease (ESRD) irreversible renal failure to the extent that the kidneys can no longer provide adequate filtration and fluid balance to sustain life; survival with ESRD usually requires dialysis.

dialysis the process by which toxins and excess fluid are removed from the body by a medical system independent of the kidneys.

hemodialysis the clearing of blood toxins and waste products in patients with renal failure by placing the patient on a machine that filters the blood externally and then returns the filtered blood to the body.

peritoneal dialysis the clearing of blood toxins and waste products in patients with renal failure by placing specialized dialysis fluid into the peritoneal cavity by way of a specialized catheter and then draining the fluid out in an exchange.

Dialysis is the process by which an external medical system independent of the kidneys is used to remove toxins and excess fluid from the body. There are two general types of dialysis: **hemodialysis** and **peritoneal dialysis.** Over 90% of ESRD patients who require dialysis get hemodialysis in specialized outpatient dialysis centers rather than peritoneal dialysis. Only 8% of U.S. dialysis patients treat themselves at home with home hemodialysis or peritoneal dialysis. The vast majority of the more than 350,000 people on dialysis who are treated in dialysis centers undergo three treatments a week, each lasting three or four hours. Although some patients get to their dialysis appointments by their own means, many others use medical transport to get to and from dialysis. This need for medical transport has created a frequent interface between EMTs and patients with ESRD.

Hemodialysis

In hemodialysis (HD), the most common form of dialysis, a patient is connected to a dialysis machine that pumps his blood through specialized filters to remove toxins and excess fluid (Figure 25-5 ▪). A patient is connected to a dialysis machine by two large catheters. One catheter allows blood to flow out of the body into the dialysis machine and the other catheter returns blood to the body after filtration. This creates a circuit by which the blood is removed from the body, filtered, and returned to the body continuously over several hours while the patient is connected to the machine.

Because hemodialysis requires a large blood flow from the body, ESRD patients on this type of chronic dialysis have specialized means of access to the body's blood circulation. Hemodialysis patients will have either a specialized two-port catheter that is inserted in one of the major veins of the torso (Figure 25-6 ▪) or have a special surgically created fistula in one of their extremities that connects arterial and venous blood flow (Figure 25-7 ▪). Because a fistula contains turbulent flow between a surgically connected artery and vein (A-V), a properly functioning A-V fistula will have a characteristic vibration, called a **thrill** when gently palpated. ESRD patients are very protective of their fistulas and will insist that you use another extremity to obtain a blood pressure. This is appropriate, given the importance and vulnerability of the fistula.

thrill a vibration felt on gentle palpation, such as that which typically occurs within an arterial-venous fistula.

Peritoneal Dialysis

Patients who manage their ESRD on peritoneal dialysis (PD) usually do so in their own home. Peritoneal dialysis is a slower process than hemodialysis and requires multiple treatments every day for most patients. Despite requiring more frequent treatments, many patients prefer peritoneal dialysis because it allows them to be treated at home. Outside the United States and Canada, peritoneal dialysis is the most common form of dialysis.

Peritoneal dialysis works by utilizing the large surface area inside the peritoneal cavity that surrounds the abdominal organs as a means of removing toxins and

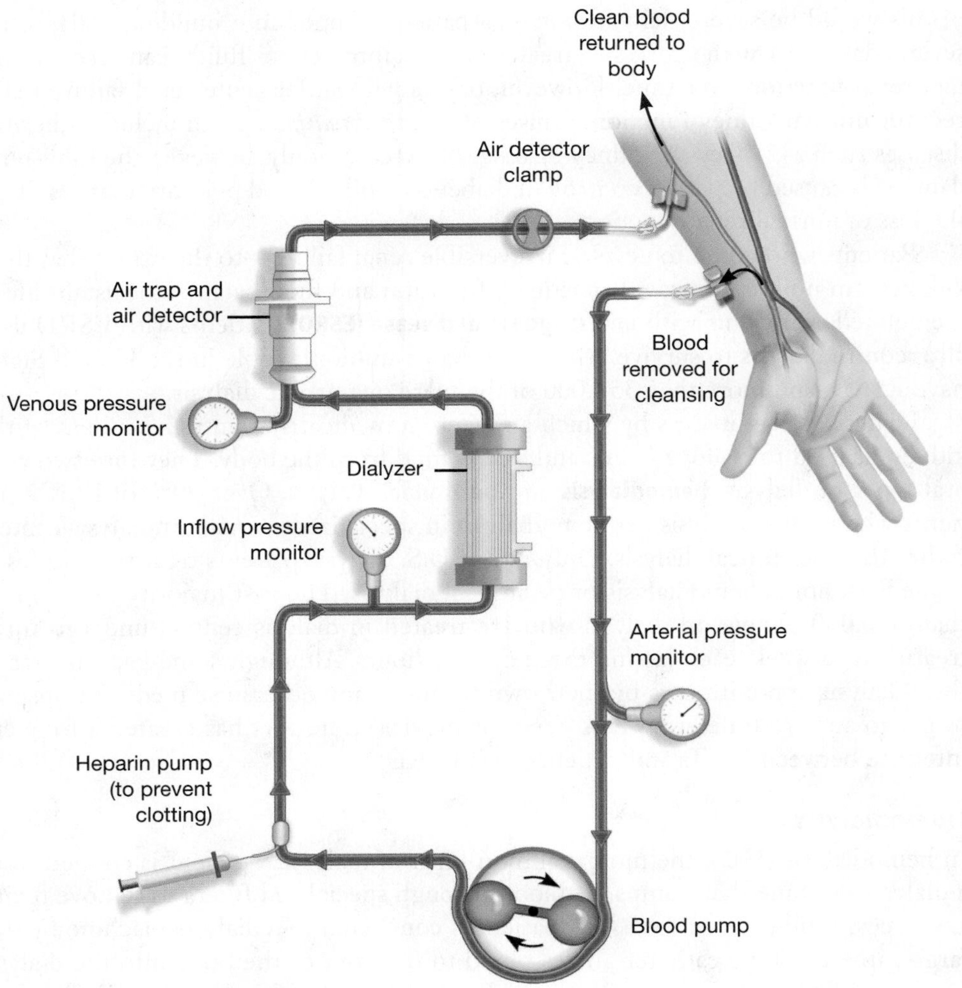

Figure 25-5 How hemodialysis works. (Adapted from Treatment Methods for Kidney Failure, National Institute of Diabetes and Digestive and Kidney Diseases; U.S. Centers for Disease Control and Prevention (CDC).

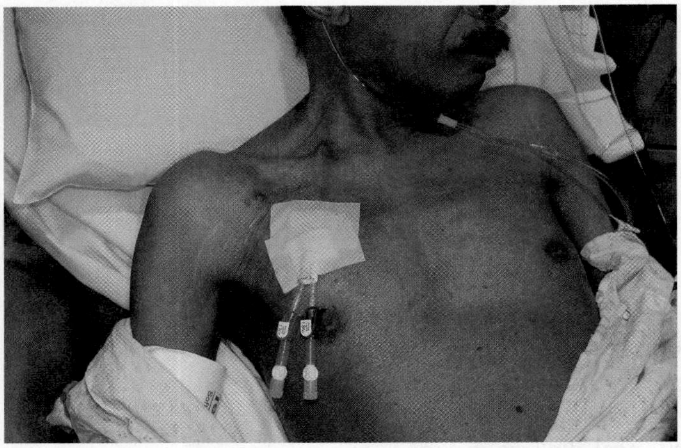

Figure 25-6 A two-port catheter for hemodialysis inserted into a major vein of the torso. (© Edward T. Dickinson, MD)

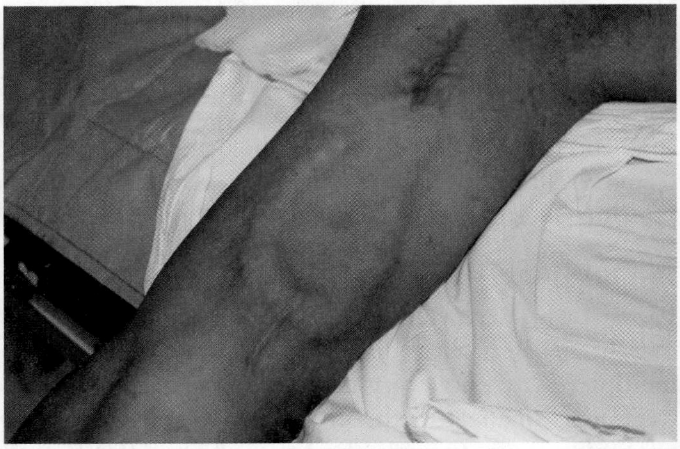

Figure 25-7 A fistula surgically connects an artery and a vein in an extremity. (© Edward T. Dickinson, MD)

excess fluid from the body (Figure 25-8 ■). ESRD patients on peritoneal dialysis have a permanent catheter that is implanted through their abdominal wall and into the peritoneal cavity. Several liters of a specially formulated dialysis solution are run into the abdominal cavity and left in place for several hours, where it absorbs waste material and excess fluid. Then the fluid is drained back out into the bag and is discarded.

The peritoneal dialysis fluid setup looks much like a large IV bag and tubing. Each cycle of filling and draining the peritoneal cavity is called an *exchange*.

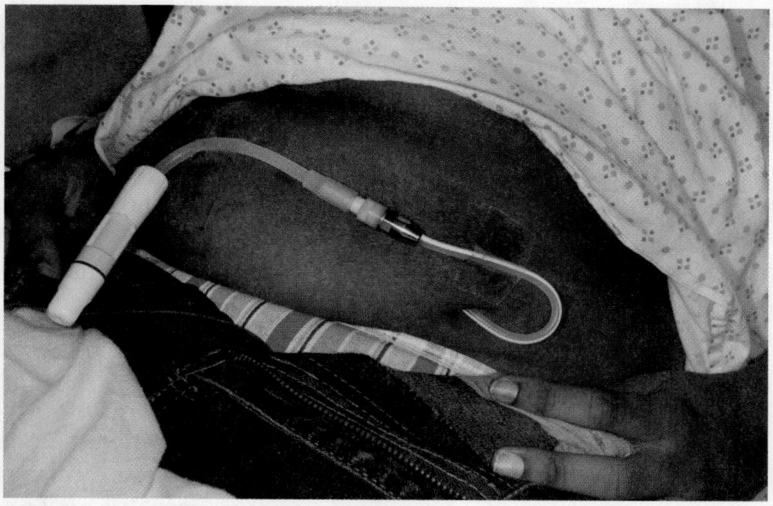

Figure 25-8 Peritoneal dialysis catheter. (© Edward T. Dickinson, MD)

Medical Emergencies with End-Stage Renal Disease

Medical emergencies encountered in patients with ESRD can be broadly divided into two groups: those that arise from the loss of normal kidney function and those that are complications of their dialysis treatments. In addition, never forget that the vast majority of dialysis patients have other underlying diseases such as diabetes and high blood pressure, so they are at risk for medical emergencies related to those diseases as well, independent of renal failure.

Complications of ESRD

The most serious complications of ESRD seen by the EMT occur when patients fail to be dialyzed. Bad weather, illness, and poor compliance are all common reasons why patients with ESRD miss their dialysis appointments.

> **CLINICAL CLUE**
>
> **Hemodialysis**
>
> When natural disasters occur, patients who require hemodialysis will be unable to obtain necessary treatments due to disruptions in the normal transportation infrastructure. During the recovery phase of such disasters, expect to see increased numbers of emergencies in ESRD patients who have missed their dialysis appointments.

Because they lack the ability to rid the body of excess fluid, patients who have missed dialysis often present with signs and symptoms similar to those seen in congestive heart failure. (See Chapter 18.) These include shortness of breath because of fluid buildup in the lungs and the accumulation of fluids elsewhere, such as the ankles, hands, and face. In addition, because patients with ESRD can no longer balance and clear excess electrolytes as well as other toxins, those who have missed dialysis may suffer from electrical disturbances of the heart (dysrhythmia). This is because the proper functioning of the heart's electrical system requires that the balance of electrolytes in the bloodstream be kept within a certain tight range. Elevated levels of the electrolyte potassium are particularly dangerous, and can result in patient death from heart dysrhythmias.

Patients Who Missed Dialysis

When encountering an ESRD patient who has missed dialysis and is experiencing problems, follow these steps:

1. Take appropriate BSI precautions.
2. Perform a primary assessment and care for issues related to the airway and breathing.
3. When you obtain vital signs, obtain a blood pressure on an arm that does not have a fistula.
4. Place the patient in a position of comfort. This is usually sitting upright on the stretcher.
5. Administer supplemental oxygen.
6. Perform a secondary assessment as appropriate.
7. Monitor the patient's vital signs carefully and be prepared to attach and use the AED if the patient becomes unresponsive and pulseless. Be aware that ESRD patients who suffer cardiac arrest may not respond to defibrillation. Paramedics carry certain drugs that can be administered in the field to help stabilize ESRD-induced dysrhythmia. Consider ALS backup, but do not delay transport to the hospital.
8. Transport the patient to a hospital that has renal dialysis capabilities.

Complications of Dialysis

25-14 Describe the complications related to renal dialysis.

The major complications for patients on hemodialysis have to do with the fact that they must frequently have large blood vessels accessed multiple times each week for their dialysis. Other complications include:

- Bleeding from the site of the A-V fistula when the dialysis needles are removed
- Clotting and loss of function of the A-V fistula. This results in the fistula feeling hard to the touch and loss of the normal thrill felt on palpation.
- Bacterial infection of the blood due to contamination at the A-V fistula or dialysis catheter site during machine connection and disconnection

peritonitis bacterial infection within the peritoneal cavity.

The most common serious complication of ESRD patients on peritoneal dialysis is acute **peritonitis,** a bacterial infection within the peritoneal cavity. Patients on peritoneal dialysis who develop peritonitis may develop abdominal pain, fever, and the tell-tale sign that their dialysis fluid appears cloudy when it is drained from the peritoneal cavity rather than its normal clear appearance. Infected peritoneal dialysis fluid is much like chicken broth in color and turbidity.

Emergency Care

25-15 Describe the management of a patient with complications of renal dialysis.

When encountering an ESRD patient who is experiencing complications of dialysis, follow these steps:

1. Take appropriate BSI precautions.
2. Perform a primary assessment and care for immediate life threats as appropriate. Immediately control any serious bleeding from the site of the A-V fistula. Use direct pressure, elevation, and hemostatic dressings as needed. Generally, a tourniquet should be avoided in this situation because it may damage the A-V fistula. Contact medical direction if bleeding remains uncontrolled.
3. Administer supplemental oxygen.
4. Perform a secondary assessment as appropriate.
5. Be aware that ESRD patients with peritonitis or a bacterial infection in their blood may present with signs of shock. Treat for shock by keeping the patient supine and warm.
6. If peritonitis is suspected in a patient on peritoneal dialysis, transport the bag of exchanged dialysis fluid with the patient so it may be tested for bacteria at the hospital to confirm the diagnosis.

Finally, never forget that the vast majority of dialysis patients have other underlying diseases such as diabetes and high blood pressure, so they are at increased risk for medical emergencies related to those diseases as well, independent of their renal failure.

Kidney Transplant Patients

Kidneys are the most commonly transplanted organs. Patients with end-stage renal disease may be candidates for renal transplant, which, if successful, can provide the patient with a normally functioning kidney and end his need for dialysis.

There are approximately 16,000 kidney transplants performed by specialized surgeons in the United States each year. Thanks to the kindness of organ donors, a renal transplant places a single healthy kidney in the lower abdomen of the patient with ESRD. The surgeon then connects a blood supply and a ureter to the transplanted kidney, allowing the patient the opportunity to regain normal renal function.

Patients with kidney transplants spend the rest of their lives on a special class of drugs that prevent organ rejection by suppressing the body's immune system. However, those same drugs also make the patients more susceptible to serious infections.

STOP, REVIEW, REMEMBER!

Multiple Choice

For each question, place a check next to the correct answer.

1. Which one of the following is associated with patients on hemodialysis?

_____ a. Peritonitis

_____ b. A-V fistula

_____ c. Continuous ambulatory peritoneal dialysis

_____ d. Continuous cycler-assisted peritoneal dialysis

2. Most kidney stones are made up of:

_____ a. potassium.

_____ b. magnesium.

_____ c. calcium.

_____ d. uric acid.

3. Most urinary tract infections (UTIs) occur in the:

_____ a. ureter.

_____ b. kidney.

_____ c. bladder.

_____ d. urethra.

4. When a patient misses several dialysis appointments, the electrolyte that can become elevated in the blood and cause irregular electrical activity in the heart is:

_____ a. potassium.

_____ b. magnesium.

_____ c. calcium.

_____ d. uric acid.

5. Which one of the following is true about peritoneal dialysis?

_____ a. It is more common in the United States than hemodialysis.

_____ b. It only has to be done on an average of three times each week.

_____ c. It can be done at home more easily than hemodialysis.

_____ d. It is rarely used outside the Unites States.

(continued on next page)

(continued)

Matching

Match the term on the left with the applicable definition on the right.

1. _____ Thrill		A. Missed dialysis
2. _____ Pyelonephritis		B. Dialysis access
3. _____ Peritonitis		C. Vibration
4. _____ A-V fistula		D. Serious UTI
5. _____ Elevated potassium		E. Peritoneal dialysis

Fill in the Blank

1. An infection in the kidney is called ______________________________.

2. The most common complication of a urinary catheter is a(n) ______________________________.

Short Answer

1. What does infected peritoneal dialysis fluid look like?

____

____

____

____

2. What is a *thrill*?

____

____

____

____

Critical Thinking

1. Which gender is more prone to urinary tract infections? Why?

____

____

____

____

2. What is the difference between chronic and acute renal failure?

____

____

____

____

3. What are the complications that may be seen if a patient misses a dialysis appointment? What signs and symptoms will the patient potentially display?

____

____

____

____

EMERGENCY DISPATCH SUMMARY

Hossein and Lauren helped the patient onto the gurney, moved him to the ambulance, and transported him to Highland Grove Hospital. While en route, Lauren continued supplemental oxygen therapy, monitored the patient's vital signs, and encouraged him through the obvious discomfort. Once at the emergency department, after receiving intravenous pain medication, the patient thanked both EMTs profusely for transporting him quickly, and he thanked Lauren specifically for her encouragement and caring demeanor. And as the EMTs walked back out into the warm night, they were both smiling broadly.

Chapter Review

To the Point

- Blood consists of red blood cells, white blood cells, and plasma.
- Blood delivers oxygen to the cells, removes carbon dioxide from the cells, and controls bleeding by clotting.
- Patients may lose their normal ability to form clots due to both chronic diseases and prescribed medications.
- Anemia is a lack of red blood cells in circulation.
- Sickle cell anemia is an inherited disease in which a defect in the hemoglobin results in a sickle shape to red blood cells. This misshapen form inhibits movement of the red blood cells through capillaries, causing sludging and blockages in smaller blood vessels.
- The renal system is composed of the kidneys, the ureters, and the urethra.

- The kidneys perform a vital filtering of the blood to remove waste products. They also help maintain a water balance within the body.
- Problems with the renal system include infection, kidney stones, and renal failure.
- Renal failure is a condition in which the kidneys are unable to filter waste and provide a balance of fluids in the body.
- In dialysis, an external system filters the blood and removes excess fluid from the body. Dialysis may be performed in either of two ways: hemodialysis or peritoneal dialysis. Dialysis at dialysis centers is generally performed three times per week.
- The main complications with patients in end-stage renal disease generally occur after the patient has missed a dialysis appointment.

Chapter Questions

Multiple Choice

For each question, place a check next to the correct answer.

1. The primary function of red blood cells is:
   _____ a. part of the immune response.
   _____ b. carrying oxygen.
   _____ c. initial or early clotting.
   _____ d. cascade or later clotting.

2. The primary function of white blood cells is:
   _____ a. part of the immune response.
   _____ b. carrying oxygen.
   _____ c. initial or early clotting.
   _____ d. cascade or later clotting.

3. Patients on peritoneal dialysis:
   _____ a. receive dialysis three times a week.
   _____ b. receive dialysis once a week.
   _____ c. use the body's own membranes to filter out toxins in the blood.
   _____ d. use an external filter system to filter out toxins in the blood.

4. The primary function of platelets is:
   _____ a. part of the immune response.
   _____ b. carrying oxygen.
   _____ c. initial or early clotting.
   _____ d. cascade or later clotting.

5. A patient with _____________ is most likely to present with painful priapism.
   _____ a. sickle cell disease
   _____ b. liver cirrhosis
   _____ c. sickle cell trait
   _____ d. acute renal failure

6. A patient with _____________ is most likely to have abnormal blood clotting.
   _____ a. sickle cell disease
   _____ b. liver cirrhosis
   _____ c. sickle cell trait
   _____ d. acute renal failure

7. A patient with _____________ is most likely to have a normal life span without medical complications.
   _____ a. sickle cell disease
   _____ b. liver cirrhosis
   _____ c. sickle cell trait
   _____ d. acute renal failure

8. A patient with _____________ is most likely to have sludging of the red blood cells.
   _____ a. sickle cell disease
   _____ b. liver cirrhosis
   _____ c. sickle cell trait
   _____ d. acute renal failure

9. Patients on hemodialysis:
   _____ a. receive dialysis on a daily basis.
   _____ b. receive dialysis once a week.
   _____ c. use the body's own membranes to filter out toxins in the blood.
   _____ d. use an external filter system to filter out toxins in the blood.

10. A patient who goes into shock after being pinned in a building collapse for 18 hours is most likely to develop:
   _____ a. von Willebrand's disease.
   _____ b. chronic renal failure.
   _____ c. acute renal failure.
   _____ d. kidney stones.

Short Answer

1. What is sickle cell anemia?

____

____

____

2. What is sludging in a patient with sickle cell anemia?

____

____

____

____

3. What is anemia?

____

____

____

____

4. What is a kidney stone?

____

____

____

____

5. What ethnic group is most likely to carry the gene for sickle cell anemia?

____

____

____

____

(continued on next page)

(continued)

Critical Thinking

1. You are treating a patient who has missed dialysis. Because of a fluid buildup, the patient has signs and symptoms similar to congestive heart failure. What are these signs and symptoms?

2. You are evaluating a patient involved in a motor-vehicle crash. The patient lost consciousness briefly when her head hit the windshield and you note a bruise on her forehead. Her mental status is completely normal at this time. Does the fact that the patient is taking Plavix alter your care for the patient? Why?

3. You are treating a patient who is complaining of stroke symptoms. He has a history of sickle cell disease. Does sickle cell disease make the diagnosis of a stroke more likely or less likely in this patient? Why?

4. A patient with sickle cell anemia tells you of severe, recurring infections. Why would a sickle cell anemia patient have this problem?

Case Studies

Case Study 1

You have a patient with a history of sickle cell crisis who is complaining of severe pain in his legs. The patient refuses to move because it hurts so much. Your partner thinks the patient is being overdramatic and falsely complaining of pain to get drugs from the hospital.

1. Do you agree with your partner? Why or why not?

2. What should you do for the patient?

Case Study 2

You are sent to a "routine transfer" nonemergency call to transport a 64-year-old patient from a long-term care facility to a dialysis appointment. You arrive to find the patient with an altered mental status and "not feeling well." You note the patient has poor color, which the staff tells you is normal for the patient. The patient is somewhat anxious and her skin is warm to the touch.

1. What are your initial steps in assessing this patient?

2. How does the dialysis history fit into the patient picture at this point?

(continued on next page)

(continued)

You complete a primary assessment and find the patient is breathing somewhat rapidly but adequately at 28/minute. The patient has peripheral pulses and no obvious external bleeding. Pulse oximetry reveals a saturation of 94%. The patient will respond to questions but is sleepy and a little confused. The staff says this is a new development in the patient, who is usually quite oriented.

3. What assessments should you perform next?

4. What patient care interventions would be appropriate at this time?

The patient's pulse and respirations are slightly elevated. Her blood pressure is 108/58, her skin is warm and dry, and her pupils are equal and reactive to light. The patient has slight difficulty breathing and some fluid is noticeable around her ankles. Her lungs show some mild crackles (also known as *rales*) in the bases. Blood glucose is 102. Even though the patient cannot follow instructions for the stroke scale, she does not have facial droop or slurred speech. The staff says she seemed fine when she went to bed last night.

5. The staff asks you to take the patient to her dialysis appointment and says they think "she'll be fine by the time she gets back." Should you transport her to dialysis or to a hospital?

The Last Word

People with diseases and dysfunctions of the hematologic and renal systems represent an important patient population. Whether they suffer from inherited diseases (such as sickle cell anemia), the consequences of an acquired disease (such as cirrhosis from hepatitis B), or as a complications of prescription medications (such as blood thinners), having a basic understanding of the challenges these patients face will enhance your ability as an EMT to care for these patients.

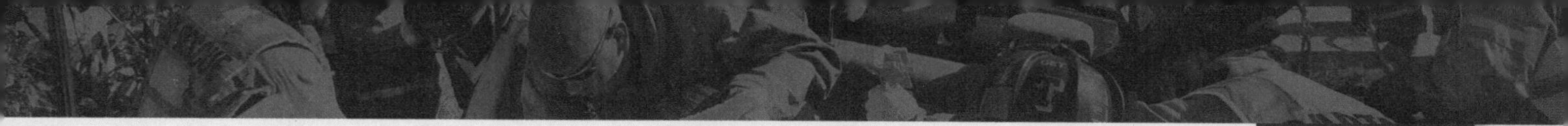

Caring for Patients with Behavioral Emergencies

26

Education Standards

Medicine: Psychiatric

Competencies

Applies fundamental knowledge to provide emergency care and transportation based on assessment findings for an acutely ill patient.

Objectives

After completion of this lesson, you should be able to:

26-1 Define key terms introduced in this chapter.

26-2 Explain the importance of recognizing and responding to patients suffering from behavioral emergencies.

26-3 Describe indications of danger associated with a response to a behavioral emergency.

26-4 Discuss common underlying physical and psychological causes of behavioral emergencies.

26-5 Describe the behavioral characteristics of the following conditions: agitated delirium, anxiety, bipolar disorder, depression, paranoia, phobias, psychosis, and schizophrenia.

26-6 Describe risk factors associated with suicide and violence toward others.

26-7 Discuss basic principles related to the assessment and management of patients with behavioral emergencies.

26-8 Identify signs of attempted suicide during scene size-up and patient assessment.

26-9 Prioritize patient care needs in terms of managing physical and behavioral problems.

26-10 Discuss the indications for physical restraint of a patient and follow principles of safe physical restraint of patients.

26-11 Evaluate the need for law enforcement and medical direction involvement in a behavioral emergency.

26-12 Discuss the role of documentation for calls involving behavioral emergencies and patient restraint.

Key Terms

agitated delirium p. 679
altered mental status p. 677
anxiety p. 678
attempted suicide p. 680
behavioral emergency p. 677
bipolar disorder p. 679
delusions p. 679
depression p. 679
hallucinations p. 679
organic p. 677
panic attack p. 679
paranoia p. 679
phobia p. 678
positional asphyxia p. 688
psychosis p. 679
schizophrenia p. 679
suicide p. 680

Introduction

26-2 Explain the importance of recognizing and responding to patients suffering from behavioral emergencies.

According to the World Health Organization (WHO), as many as one in three people worldwide report symptoms with sufficient basis to diagnose a mental disorder. Although the vast majority of people live normal and productive lives, this statistic shows just how widespread psychiatric disorders are. From a prehospital standpoint, psychiatric emergencies impact patients on a variety of levels. Patients in acute psychiatric crisis can be depressed, anxious, or even acting in unusual and potentially dangerous ways. Psychiatric disorders also can confound or worsen concurrent medical conditions. Underlying medical issues can be present with psychiatric issues, making assessment of medical patients more difficult.

EMERGENCY DISPATCH

"You're always talking down to me, Judy!" the man yelled, spittle flying from his lips. "You know how much I hate that!"

"Sir, you need to calm down. My name is Theresa. There's no Judy here," EMT Theresa Hoagland said, feeling fear creeping up from her stomach. The patient had just suddenly—and for no apparent reason—become angry. "We're here to help you. Just relax on the cot." Theresa glanced out the back window of the ambulance as it bounced along the dark city streets. Thank God, she thought, only about three minutes to the hospital.

"You know what, Judy?" the patient shouted. He was a homeless man and ambulance regular with a history of delusional but nonviolent behavior. "I'm so done dealing with you!" He then began to unbuckle the cot straps and stand up. Theresa's partner, Jerry, saw this in the rearview mirror and quickly pulled the ambulance to the curb and activated the hazard lights.

"Headquarters, 4-54," he said into the radio as he climbed out of the driver's seat. "We're pulled over at Fifth and Walker for an uncooperative patient. I've got to get Theresa out of the back."

"Copy, 54," the dispatcher responded. "PD is rolling to your location."

Several minutes later when city police officer Dan Tomlinson arrived, he found Jerry holding an ice pack to Theresa's swollen left eye. "Where's your patient?" The officer peered into the back of the disheveled ambulance.

"Oh, probably about Fifteenth Street by now," Jerry said, pointing down Walker Avenue. "He shouldn't be too hard to find, though. He was taking his clothes off as he ran."

Types of Behavioral Emergencies

Major psychiatric disorders are the third leading cause of disability in the world and the leading cause of disability under the age of 30. Many of these patients' underlying mental problems cause very real physiological issues. In fact, a patient with a serious psychiatric diagnosis has a significantly shorter life span than a person without such a disorder. As an EMS provider, you should understand that behavioral emergencies are serious medical emergencies with physiological and potentially life-threatening consequences.

As health care professionals, EMTs need to avoid assigning stereotypes and stigmas to psychiatric disorders and treat these patients with care and respect. Understand that although the behaviors such patients may be exhibiting are difficult to handle, those behaviors are frequently a sign of a harmful disease and not a personal attack. An EMT must see the behaviors as they would symptoms such as chest pain or shortness of breath. Furthermore, an EMT must remember that not all unusual behavior is attributed to psychiatric disorders. Acute mental status changes can be caused by a wide variety of medical and traumatic conditions that must be ruled out before arriving at a psychiatric diagnosis.

Behavioral emergencies can be both difficult and potentially dangerous for the EMT. Ensuring your own personal safety and the safety of your crew will be an essential part of your management of behavioral emergencies. Understanding some basic concepts about mental illness will help to prepare you. This chapter addresses some key psychiatric disorders as well as the assessment and management of the patient who has an acute behavioral disorder.

A **behavioral emergency** is defined as a situation where a patient's behavior becomes intolerable, dangerous, or bizarre enough to cause the concern of family, bystanders, or the patient (Figure 26-1 ■). Note that this definition does not include the term *normal*. Normal behavior is extremely difficult to define and really is based on the day-to-day expectations of the patient and the patient's family. It would be unfair to label or require behavior that is based only on your personal expectations.

behavioral emergency a situation in which a patient's behavior becomes intolerable, dangerous, or bizarre enough to cause the concern of family, bystanders, or the patient; a situation in which emotional issues interrupt normal life activities.

CLINICAL CLUE

Behavior

Your patients respond to their environment based on the events that they encounter through the course of their daily lives. Those responses can vary greatly, depending on the nature of their experiences. For example, it is natural to have an emotional response to a difficult or traumatic event. It is important to remember that responses can vary from person to person and what prompts a dramatic or emotional response in one person may not elicit the same behavior in another.

Cultural differences also can change the way a person interacts with the environment and be at the root of different behavioral responses. Consider body language, such as eye contact, communication skills, or the relationship to personal space. For example, in some cultures women are expected to have a shy and reserved outward appearance. Although this may not be the typical American expectation, it is not always abnormal.

As an EMT you will encounter a wide range of patients experiencing psychiatric problems. They will include people from every part of society, every race, every culture, and both genders. Some patients will be withdrawn and depressed, while others may exhibit behavior that is considered bizarre or dangerous to themselves or others.

When you receive a call for a psychiatric patient, safety will be a primary concern from the outset of the call. In most areas, it will be the police who make initial contact with the patient and ensure scene safety. Not all psychiatric patients are dangerous, but some can be, so caution is prudent.

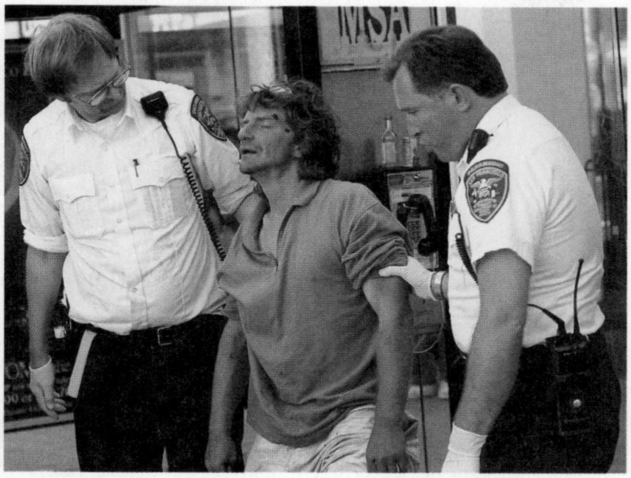

Figure 26-1 Many patients experiencing a behavioral emergency will have an altered mental status. (© Craig Jackson/In the Dark Photography)

You must consider all patients experiencing behavioral emergencies as having an **altered mental status** caused by a medical condition or trauma until proven otherwise. Altered mental status caused by an illness or injury is referred to as **organic** in nature. Organic causes of altered mental status must always be ruled out first. If you assume that all patients who are acting strangely are behavioral emergencies, you may cause harm to your patient by missing some treatable physical problem.

26-4 Discuss common underlying physical and psychological causes of behavioral emergencies.

As you will recall from prior chapters, many medical conditions can present much like a behavioral emergency (Figure 26-2 ■). Diabetic patients, patients who are hypoxic, hypo- or hyperglycemic, or intoxicated and those experiencing strokes and some types of seizures may present with unusual behavior. You also must understand that patients who have suffered trauma, such as a head injury, can display similar abnormal behaviors (Figure 26-3 ■).

altered mental status change in alertness and awareness.

organic caused by medical or traumatic etiology, as opposed to a psychiatric origin.

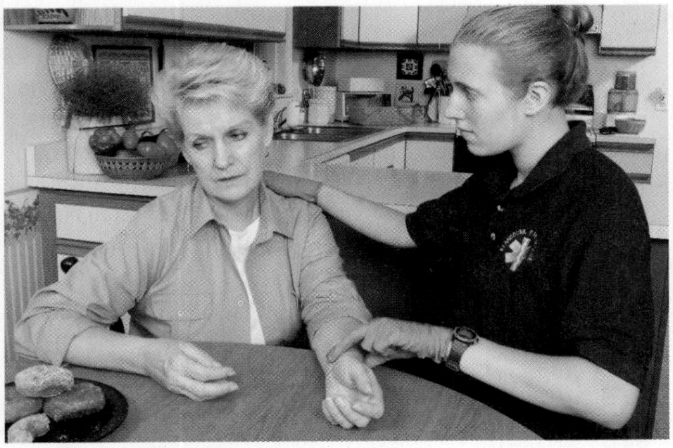

Figure 26-2 Medical conditions such as diabetes can present much like a behavioral emergency.

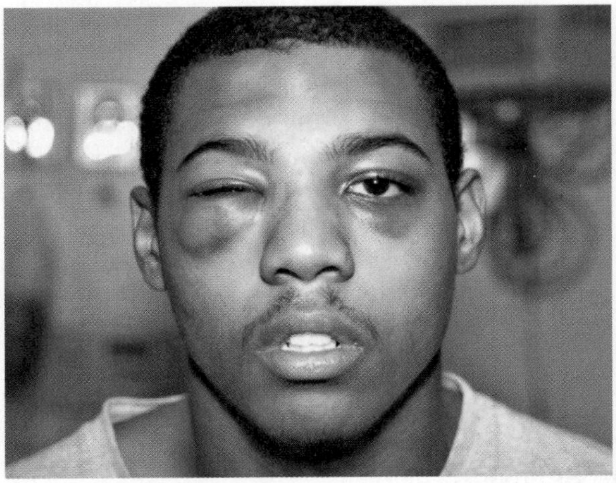

Figure 26-3 Patients who have suffered a head injury may present much like a patient experiencing a behavioral emergency.
(© Edward T. Dickinson, MD)

CLINICAL CLUE

Altered Mental Status

Never assume a patient with an altered mental status is a psychiatric emergency or is simply intoxicated until other medical conditions have been ruled out.

Of course, psychiatric conditions can cause those behaviors, too. Your thorough patient assessment and history will help you care for all patients who appear to be having an altered mental status, including those who are experiencing behavioral emergencies.

PRACTICAL PATHOPHYSIOLOGY

Mental status is controlled in the brain by the reticular activating system. This series of structures controls alertness and the ability to maintain consciousness. A wide range of problems can disrupt that function. From trauma to infection and clots to toxins, any condition that creates a harmful environment for the brain can interfere with the reticular activating system and alter the level of responsiveness. It is reasonable, therefore, to look for likely organic causes first when altered mental status is identified.

Psychiatric Disorders

26-5 Describe the behavioral characteristics of the following conditions: agitated delirium, anxiety, bipolar disorder, depression, paranoia, phobias, psychosis, and schizophrenia.

There are many types of psychiatric disorders that can lead to a behavioral emergency. As with many other emergencies, your primary role will be to provide emergency care for the patient and transport him safely to the hospital. Making a specific diagnosis may not be necessary.

You may, however, hear the patient or a family member relay a history to you that includes a type of psychiatric problem the patient has and the specific medications he takes. For this reason, it is helpful to understand some of the more common behavioral, emotional, and psychiatric conditions you may encounter in the field. Some of them include:

anxiety a state characterized by excess worry or fears.

phobia an unfounded or intense fear of an object or situation.

- *Anxiety.* A very common condition, **anxiety** is characterized by excess worry or fears. While everyone has occasional fears, patients with this condition are fearful for a prolonged time in a way that interferes with daily activities and functioning. A **phobia** is a specific type of anxiety disorder related to a fear of an object or situation that causes the patient distress. A phobia patient goes to great lengths to avoid exposure to the root of this fear. For example, agoraphobia is the fear of leaving the home and an agoraphobia patient would have great distress when removed from his primary residence.

- ***Panic attack.*** A sudden onset of a fear or discomfort, a **panic attack** includes signs and symptoms such as sweating, trembling, feelings of shortness of breath or chest tightness, nausea and vomiting, and fears of dying or loss of control. It generally occurs for a short period of time but is quite profound to the patient experiencing it. Panic attacks are common symptoms of underlying anxiety disorders.
- ***Depression.*** Everyone at some point or another feels depressed. **Depression** becomes a problem and is diagnosed as a disorder when it persists for a long time, affects major portions of life (such as work or relationships) and involves weight loss or gain, a constant desire to sleep or the inability to sleep, feelings of worthlessness and guilt, and occasionally the desire to die. You will read later that depression is a risk factor for suicide.
- ***Bipolar disorder.*** A **bipolar disorder** (previously referred to as a *manic/depressive disorder*) is a condition in which the patient experiences episodes of high energy levels, increased cognition, and improved mood, and in contrast at different times displays signs of depressive downturns (although depression does not always have to be present to diagnose a bipolar disorder).
- ***Schizophrenia.*** A serious condition, **schizophrenia** involves unusual or bizarre thoughts, behaviors, and speech, including **delusions, paranoia, psychosis,** and **hallucinations.** The onset of schizophrenia is typically in the late teens and early twenties. Patients may be very quiet or catatonic in some presentations of the disease. Some conditions seen in schizophrenia include:
  - Delusions, which are false beliefs (for example, believing one is a famous person or religious figure).
  - Psychosis, which is unusual or bizarre behavior indicating a lack of being in touch with reality.
  - Paranoia, which is a delusion in which the patient believes he is being followed, persecuted, or harmed.
  - Hallucinations, which are sensory perceptions without an external stimulus. Hallucinations associated with schizophrenia are most commonly auditory. Visual hallucinations are rare and usually indicate a co-existing organic cause such as alcohol withdrawal.
- ***Agitated delirium.*** Also known as *excited delirium*, **agitated delirium** is a highly dangerous condition to providers and a life threat to patients. A severe anxiety state, it is frequently caused by drug use, and results in highly combative, psychotic, and delirious behavior in the patient. As a consequence, these patients must be approached very carefully. In addition, this agitated condition causes severe stress to the patient's physiology with literally every system operating at its highest output state. Such severe stress puts patients at risk for sudden death, especially when restrained. In most cases patients require both physical restraints to control violent behavior and chemical sedation (by ALS personnel or emergency department staff) to slow the stress on the body.

PERSPECTIVE

Theresa—The EMT

He hit me! I really don't know what his problem was. I have personally transported that guy at least 10 times. I know he's kind of wacky, but I'd never in a million years guess that he'd get violent. Maybe it goes to show you that you always have to stay alert. I mean, patients can turn on you in an instant. I'm probably lucky that he just used his fist.

panic attack sudden onset of a fear or discomfort including symptoms such as sweating, trembling, palpitations, feelings of shortness of breath or chest tightness, nausea and vomiting, and fears of dying or loss of control.

depression profound sadness or feeling of melancholy; may affect major portions of the patient's life including work, relationships, weight changes, sleeping difficulties, feeling of worthlessness and guilt, and occasionally the desire to die.

bipolar disorder a behavioral condition characterized by extreme increases in mood and activity contrasted by periods of depression.

schizophrenia a serious condition that involves unusual or bizarre thoughts, behaviors, speech, and auditory hallucinations. The patient may be very quiet or catatonic in some presentations of the disease.

delusions false beliefs.

paranoia a delusion in which the patient believes he is being followed, persecuted, or harmed.

psychosis unusual or bizarre behavior indicating a lack of touch with reality.

hallucinations sensory perceptions without an external stimulus.

agitated delirium a dangerous condition of extreme anxiety and agitation usually associated with drug use.

CLINICAL CLUE

Panic Attacks

Because patients having panic attacks often complain of chest pain and shortness of breath, it is particularly difficult to determine if the cause is from a psychiatric emergency or from an organic cardiopulmonary source. When in doubt, presume the cause of chest pain and shortness of breath are due to a respiratory or cardiac emergency and treat accordingly.

Suicide

26-6 Describe risk factors associated with suicide and violence toward others.

suicide the taking of one's own life.

attempted suicide attempting or threatening to take one's own life.

Some may say that **suicide** is an epidemic. The facts about suicide are somewhat shocking. According to the Centers for Disease Control and Prevention (CDC), suicide is the third leading cause of death in the 15- to 24-year-old age group (first is accidental trauma, second is murder) and eighth in the overall population. A dramatic increase in suicide also has been noted in the geriatric population.

Statistically speaking, it is likely that you will be called to a suicide and too many more patients who have attempted or threatened to take their own lives or harm themselves in some way, known as **attempted suicide.** Those calls will pose very specific safety risks and challenges to patient care.

Several risk factors for suicide have been identified. They include patients who:

- Are single, widowed, or divorced
- Are depressed
- Abuse alcohol or other substances
- Have formed a detailed suicide plan (such as giving away possessions or purchasing or gathering items to use in the suicide attempt)
- Have experienced the prior suicide of a loved one (especially a same-sex parent)
- Have made prior suicide attempts

While patients who commit suicide may have one or many of the risk factors, the individual situations will vary from patient to patient. It is usually the role of the EMT to transport a patient to a professional who can formally evaluate the patient and provide appropriate immediate and long-term treatment. In virtually all jurisdictions, a patient who expresses the intent to kill himself may not legally refuse medical care. If you are in doubt about the intentions of the patient or if a potentially suicidal patient refuses care, utilize law enforcement, medical direction, or community crisis response teams to assist you.

There are many misconceptions about risk factors for suicide. Many experienced EMS personnel may tell you that a patient who is threatening suicide but has threatened many times before may simply be "looking for attention." This is a dangerous attitude, because patients who have attempted suicide before are statistically more likely to commit suicide. Take all threats of suicide seriously, even if they appear minor or half-hearted.

Remember that there is an increasing rate of suicide and depression in the geriatric population. The recent loss of a spouse or close friends, a decrease in mobility, isolation, and related depression, as well as the diagnosis or worsening of a medical condition are additional risk factors for suicide in this age group.

Responding to the Suicidal Patient

26-8 Identify signs of attempted suicide during scene size-up and patient assessment.

When responding to calls for a patient who may have attempted harm to himself, you should use an extra level of awareness in your scene size-up. When possible, the police should make initial contact and secure the scene prior to your entry. In these situations, EMS will usually stage their vehicles a safe distance (for example, out of gun range) from the scene until advised by law enforcement that it is safe to proceed into the scene. While most patients expressing suicidal thoughts are not looking to harm you, some may wish to lash out at others. Also, any time a potentially lethal mechanism has been employed (for example, firearms or carbon monoxide) a hazard exists for you.

In some cases suicide may be done by proxy. That means the person wishing to commit suicide will arrange a situation in which someone else will perform a lethal act. One scenario is "suicide by cop," where a person confronts a police officer with a gun (often a toy gun) or other weapon, causing the officer to shoot him. In other cases patients will walk in front of vehicles or trains.

As part of your size-up, look for mechanisms that can cause harm to you or your patient. Do this not only for safety, but also because such mechanisms will be important to the patient history and documentation of the suicide or attempted suicide. You may also see suicide notes or hear statements that will be part of your history and documentation.

Remember that you will bring the patient to the hospital where the mental health professionals will have no knowledge of the scene. It is important that you document and explain pertinent facts, such as the means used in the attempt, whether there was a note, dynamics of family and friends present, and other facts that will help the patient's immediate and long-term care.

Another confounding factor is the complex nature of psychological and suicide emergencies compared to other kinds of emergencies to which you usually respond. For example, if a patient is bleeding, you have been trained to stop it. If the patient has chest pain, you have been taught many possible causes, and you can administer oxygen and assist with medications. Many such emergencies are surprisingly cut and dried compared to psychological emergencies and suicide.

When dealing with a patient who has attempted suicide, you should provide emergency care for medical conditions as you would for any patient. Emergencies such as overdose, bleeding, carbon monoxide exposure, falls, and others should be treated according to the guidelines for care discussed throughout this text. In addition, psychological care of the suicidal patient includes the following:

- Position yourself so that you have a clear path of exit should the situation deteriorate and you need to retreat. (Do not position yourself in a way that could allow the patient to block your exit.)
- Be sure to identify yourself and your role.
- Be prepared to spend some time with the patient in order to develop a rapport. The patient in emotional distress of any type may not open up to you immediately.
- Listen.
- Get down to the patient's level, if it is safe to do so.
- Use appropriate body language.
- Be calm, regardless of the level of excitement or agitation of the patient.
- Do not speak or act in a judgmental manner.

When you communicate with the suicidal patient, be polite and somewhat direct. It will be part of your assessment to determine the patient's complaint (what he did, why, and his intent). So, even if you find it uncomfortable, it is crucial that you ask, "Why did you try to kill (or harm) yourself?" It may seem too direct or insulting. Do it anyway. Experienced EMTs realize that being direct, yet respectful, is often appreciated by the patient (Figure 26-4 ▪). Consider this exchange in which an EMT approaches a patient, introduces himself, and tries to identify the chief complaint:

EMT: My name is Dan. I'm an EMT, and I'd like to help you today. Okay?

Patient: Sure. Whatever.

EMT: I can see you've got some cuts there on your wrist. Are you hurt anywhere else?

Patient: No.

EMT: Can you tell me what happened?

Patient: (pause) I got really pissed off and just wanted to end it all. Just end it.

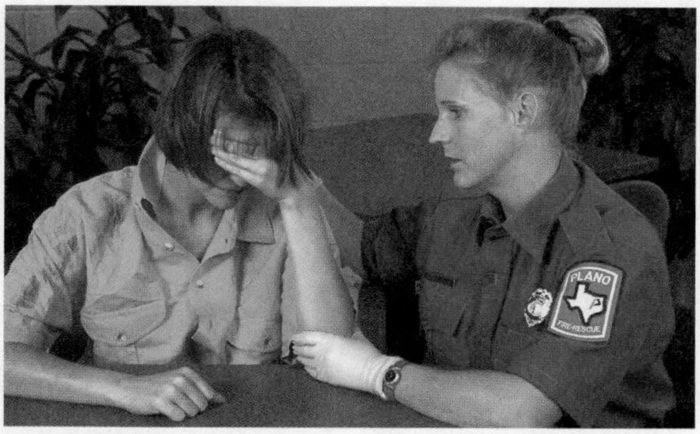

Figure 26-4 Get down at eye level and use body language that expresses concern and compassion.

The patient in the example above has given you the opportunity to use his terminology. You can now determine his history and use the phrase "end it all" because the patient volunteered it first. You can then say, "While I take care of your wrist, can you tell me about your wanting to end it all?"

Even though the police may have told you what happened, getting some sort of statement from the patient begins the process of talking. And recall from the assessment chapters that open-ended questions such as "Can you tell me what happened?" are good to ask rather than yes-or-no statements or questions such as "The police say you cut your wrist. Is that true?"

Of course some patients may be angry, others silent, both posing challenges in communication. However, the communications guidelines just discussed, along with some sensitivity and patience, will go far in dealing with your patients.

STOP, REVIEW, REMEMBER!

Multiple Choice

For each question, place a check next to the correct answer.

1. An unfounded or intense fear that causes distress and avoidance behaviors in a patient is referred to as a:

_____ a. psychosis.

_____ b. paranoia.

_____ c. phobia.

_____ d. philia.

2. Depression is considered a disorder when it:

_____ a. causes feelings of sadness in the patient.

_____ b. interferes with the patient's ability to conduct normal interactions.

_____ c. causes physiological responses such as nausea.

_____ d. persists for more than two days.

3. A patient with unusual behavior should be considered to have a(n) _____________ until proven otherwise.

_____ a. psychiatric problem

_____ b. medical problem

_____ c. overdose

_____ d. unusual personality

4. Which one of the following would be considered an organic cause of altered mental status?

_____ a. Acute anxiety disorder

_____ b. Bipolar disorder

_____ c. Agitated delirium

_____ d. Hypoxia

5. A 16-year-old man has threatened to cut his wrist with a razor blade. Law enforcement has secured the scene and removed the knife. You should next:

_____ a. introduce yourself and ask permission to care for the patient.

_____ b. determine if the cutting was an attempt at suicide.

_____ c. restrain the patient to prevent further suicidal attempts.

_____ d. transport the patient while creating a nonjudgmental environment.

Short Answer

1. Define behavioral emergency without using the words "normal" or "abnormal."

2. List five medical conditions that can appear to be a psychiatric emergency.

3. List five risk factors for suicide.

Critical Thinking

1. How would your assessment help you determine the difference between a psychiatric crisis and a medical emergency that causes unusual behavior? List three examples.

2. You are treating a patient who has attempted suicide. You introduce yourself and ask if you can help. The patient says, "I just took 14 antihistamines because I couldn't take it any more. I don't know, can you help me?" What do you say?

Behavioral Crises

Attempted suicide is just one type of behavioral crisis. Consider the following situations, which are all behavioral emergencies you may encounter:

- You are called to a naked man standing in an intersection yelling at cars.
- You are called to a school for children with emotional problems for a 12-year-old child who has been withdrawn and unwilling to speak to teachers for two days.
- You are called to a residence where a man's elderly mother seems depressed and he is very worried about her.

The assessment and care of all behavioral emergency patients is essentially the same, even though the patients may present in dramatically different ways. While each of the situations described above is different, each should be considered altered mental status until common causes such as diabetes, injury, overdose, and so on are ruled out.

Scene Safety and the Behavioral Patient

26-3 Describe indications of danger associated with a response to a behavioral emergency.

26-11 Evaluate the need for law enforcement and medical direction involvement in a behavioral emergency.

Not all behavioral emergency patients are violent, but because some are, EMS providers should have an increased level of alertness prior to entering such a situation. Behavioral emergencies can be dynamic and unstable and because behavior can rapidly turn to violence, EMTs should be hypervigilant. Suicidal ideations often involve harming others, and even simple hallucinations or delusions can lead to harmful actions. Providers should always assess their own safety prior to entering a scene. It may be most appropriate to allow law enforcement to enter a scene before you do. If your size-up indicates any threat of violence, the police should be requested immediately.

Remember that all human behavior is inherently unpredictable, but it is even more so in a psychiatric crisis state. Although behavior is impossible to predict, there are signs of imminent physical violence and signs that indicate a higher risk of physical violence. EMTs should be especially aware of the following findings:

- Presence of a weapon and/or closed fists
- Actual threats of physical harm
- Previous acts of physical violence
- The patient positioning himself in a fighting stance
- Cursing
- Scene clues indicating physically violent acts such as broken glass or furniture
- Intoxication or the presence of intoxicating substances

When dealing with a patient with altered mental status (of any origin), be prepared for potentially harmful actions. Your preparations should include a plan for emergency egress, maintenance of appropriate and safe personal space, and a plan for restraint if necessary. More importantly, providers should employ these preparations for every patient, not just on those deemed behavioral emergencies.

Assessment of Behavioral Emergency Patients

You may feel that assessing behavioral emergency patients is different because you cannot see the condition as you can a broken leg. In reality, though, you cannot see chest pain either. You must rely on your observations, assessment, and what the patient, family, and bystanders tell you.

Your size-up should ensure that there are no immediate or potential dangers before you enter the scene.

Your assessment of the patient begins with your approach and introduction. Identify yourself and your role, and be sure to let the patient know what you are doing. Use a calm, reassuring voice with your patient, and remember to listen.

Then gather information from a number of sources. Key information you should obtain is sometimes referred to as a "mental status examination." It could actually be considered the secondary assessment for the mind. Components of the mental status exam include:

- ***Orientation.*** You perform this exam on all your patients. It includes determining if the patient is oriented to person, place, time, and event.
- ***Appearance.*** The patient's appearance is unusually telling. Observe him to determine if he is disheveled or neat. Is his clothing appropriate for the weather conditions? Does his hygiene indicate that he can take care of himself properly?
- ***Activity.*** What is the patient doing? Does it match the environment? Is he active, hyperactive, or catatonic? Does he show aggressive movements or is he withdrawn?
- ***Speech.*** While most patients will be talking to some extent, the volume, urgency, and content of their speech tell quite a bit about their condition and status. Even the fact that a patient will say nothing can indicate anything from depression to anger. Another speech pattern you might see is called *pressured speech*. This patient talks almost constantly. It seems that when his mouth opens, words come out as if they are under pressure and often do not make sense. One more speech pattern you might encounter is called *disorganized speech*. When someone without a behavioral emergency speaks, the sentences and paragraphs have a logical link and flow. Not so with disorganized speech, which is sometimes seen in patients with psychosis or schizophrenia.
- ***History.*** The patient's medical history will help you identify other potential causes for the patient's behavior (for example, a diabetic emergency) as well as identify any prior psychiatric conditions the patient may have been diagnosed with. Medications taken by the patient also provide a clue to his history. (See Table 26-1 for common medications taken by patients with psychiatric conditions.)

The patient's actions, speech, orientation, and appearance will help you identify and document specific signs and symptoms (the "S" in SAMPLE history) you find in the psychiatric patient. Continue to gather an appropriate medical history, using other parts of the SAMPLE history to help you as you would for any patient.

TABLE 26-1 COMMON PRESCRIPTION MEDICATIONS TAKEN BY PATIENTS WITH PSYCHIATRIC CONDITIONS

ANTIPSYCHOTIC MEDICATIONS	ANTIDEPRESSANT MEDICATIONS
fluphenazine (Prolixin®)	fluoxetine (Prozac®)
risperidone (Risperdal®)	sertraline (Zoloft®)
quetiapine (Seroquel®)	paroxetine (Paxil®)
chlorpromazine (Thorazine®)	nortriptyline (Pamelor®)
haloperidol (Haldol®)	imipramine (Tofranil®)
lithium (Lithobid®)	amitriptyline (Elavil®)
ziprasidone (Geodon®)	desipramine (Norpramin®)

PERSPECTIVE

Jerry—The EMT

I've never dealt with that particular guy before, but my first indication that he was a little off was how he looked. I mean, not to be judgmental or anything, but he had this long stringy hair, he smelled, and was wearing a lady's silk robe type-of-thing over his clothes. When he was first talking to us, he was actually kind of funny, the kind of patient who you try your best not to laugh at, but you just can't help yourself. I never would have thought that he'd get violent.

As always, take vital signs as part of your assessment. This is possible for most behavioral emergency patients, if you explain what you are going to do. Occasionally, patients may be violent or potentially violent and you will be hesitant to take vital signs. Remember that vitals are a critically important part of the assessment process and they must be taken whenever possible. However, never endanger yourself to obtain vitals if the patient is violent or very uncooperative. You may be able to obtain some vital signs from a safe distance, including respirations, skin color, and level of responsiveness. Be sure to document the reasons for not obtaining the other vitals.

When dealing with patients who are exhibiting extremes of behavior (Figure 26-5 ■), your goal is to get the patient to where he is calm, communicative, and cooperative. The following may help you communicate with your patient and gain cooperation:

- Observe your patient's reactions to you and his surroundings. If he becomes more agitated with something you are discussing, talk about something else. If a family member or another person in the patient's presence seems to be agitating the patient, removing this person from the patient's sight may help.
- If you discuss something with your patient and the patient seems to respond (for example, he increases eye contact or improves body language), continue along that course. Similarly, if a patient responds to one person on a call better than another, that other person should continue talking with the patient.

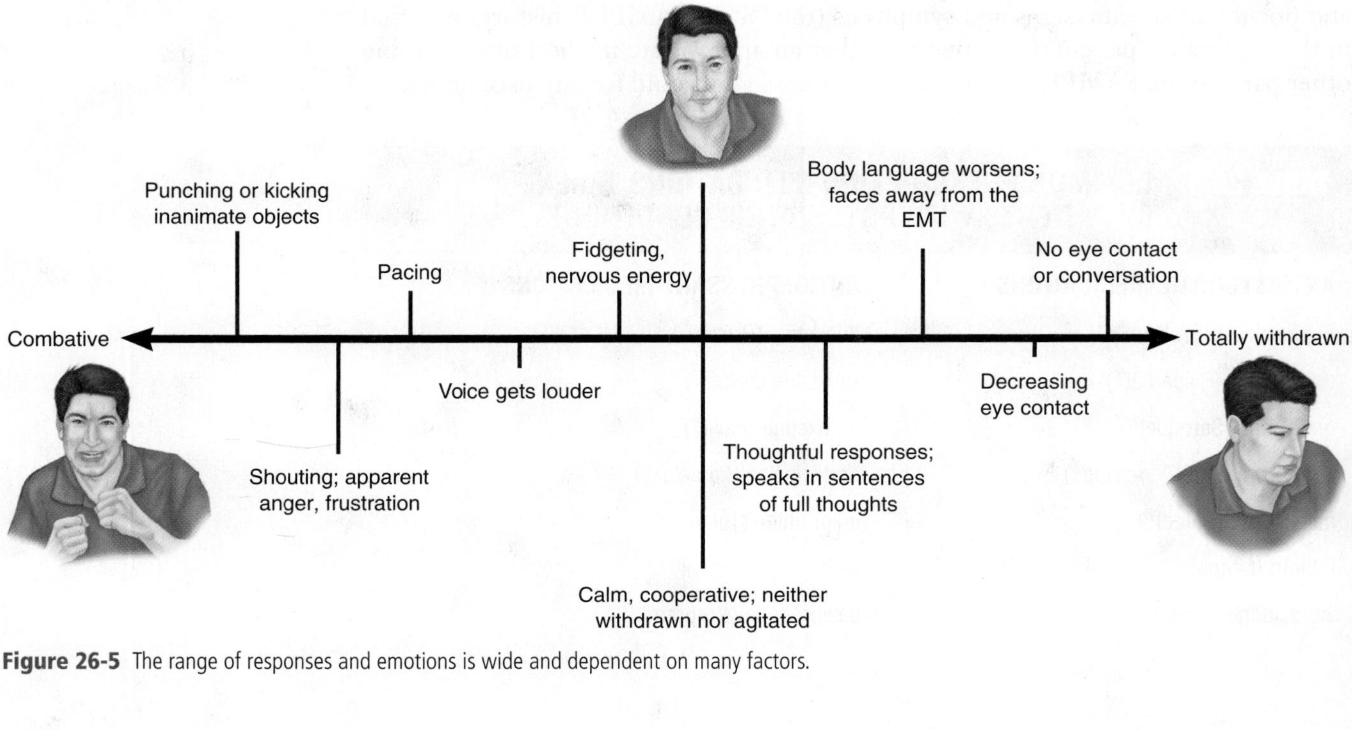

Figure 26-5 The range of responses and emotions is wide and dependent on many factors.

- Watch for signs of escalation to behavior that is increasingly agitated or violent. Use the warning signs of a louder voice and increasing activity (for example, pacing, violent hand movements) as signs you should retreat and let the police deal with the situation.

Care for Behavioral Emergency Patients

Your care for behavioral emergency patients will cover two areas:

- ***Care for injuries or medical problems.*** You may be called for a suicidal patient who has been pulled from a garage filled with carbon monoxide or a patient with wrist lacerations. You may be called for a patient exhibiting bizarre behavior and find him to have low blood sugar. Emergency medical care, including life-saving interventions performed during the primary assessment (for example, airway care and oxygen), is vital. Medical conditions must have the same priority for behavioral emergency patients as for patients who are not exhibiting behavioral signs.
- ***Care for behavioral issues.*** Once care for injuries or medical problems has been provided and medical causes for the behavioral emergency have been ruled out, your care for the behavioral emergency patient is largely supportive. Calming the patient, protecting him from harm, and transporting him to an appropriate facility are the key components of behavioral care.

26-7 Discuss basic principles related to the assessment and management of patients with behavioral emergencies.

26-9 Prioritize patient care needs in terms of managing physical and behavioral problems.

26-12 Discuss the role of documentation for calls involving behavioral emergencies and patient restraint.

PERSPECTIVE

The Dispatcher

I always send for law enforcement for uncooperative patients. Always. Even if the crews say they don't need them. If you tell me that your patient has deteriorated to the point that you have to pull the rig over, then you need backup. About 11 years ago I was new in dispatch and one of my crews had to pull over for a patient who was going off. The EMT was this ex-football player who competed in judo and stuff, and he told me not to worry the cops about this "little guy." So me, being green, I didn't send anybody. Well, that ex-football player is still out on disability. Now, I always send the police.

Refusal of Care

You will encounter patients who are violent and beyond reason or a danger to themselves or others and wish to refuse care. In those cases you may be asked by the police to transport a patient against his will. Remember that for a patient to refuse care he must have the capacity to make an informed decision. Many behavioral emergency patients, as well as those who are intoxicated or drugged, will not have the mental capacity to fully understand their situation or the potential consequences of their refusal, and therefore may not legally refuse. In most areas, the police are given the authority to force someone to go to the hospital against his will.

Judging a patient's capacity is not always clear cut. A person who has cut his wrists is a danger to himself and should be transported. The same is true for a person who has ingested a quantity of pills. However, there will be other cases that are less clear. A patient who is disoriented and does not know to stay out of traffic can be a harm to himself. A patient who insists on going out on a bitter winter day for a long walk without a coat may also be a harm to himself. To evaluate those patients, you may wish to call a mobile crisis outreach team if one is available in your area. These teams assist in assessment and care of patients experiencing behavioral emergencies. If a team is not available, seek additional help from the police and medical direction.

Not all patients who wish to refuse care will be violent, and a firm but respectful attitude is often successful. Patients in crisis often respond positively to structure. For example: "The police have told me that you are going to the hospital. They also told me that you don't want to go. We're going to take you and treat you very well. Now I need you to get on my stretcher."

You will have greater success with firmness than if you send a mixed message about what you are going to do. It may feel uncomfortable or awkward to speak decisively, and you might worry that something you say will cause the patient to act out. However, if you speak with conviction *and* compassion, you will have the best results.

If the police call you and have the legal authority to force a patient to go to the hospital, avoid asking questions such as "Would you like to go to the hospital?" because in that case there really is not a choice. If the patient will not cooperate, restraint will be necessary.

Restraint

26-10 Discuss the indications for physical restraint of a patient and follow principles of safe physical restraint of patients.

Restraint is the process of restricting motion, which allows an unwilling or combative patient to be transported to the hospital. There are many different methods of restraint, and there are some dangers associated with restraint.

Before restraint is initiated, be sure to have the legal authority to do so and enough personnel to perform the restraint effectively and safely. The main principle of restraint is to restrain the patient with a minimal amount of force and without injury to the patient or emergency personnel on scene.

The process of restraining a violent patient should be handled by the police. Yet there are times when you may be called on to assist in the restraint process. Follow these guidelines (Scan 26-1):

- Be sure you have adequate help. Too few people may result in excessive force being used, which may cause injury. Too many rescuers can cause confusion. Generally, five people is ideal. Each of the first four can take an extremity and the fifth can secure the patient.
- Avoid being directly in the path of danger (patient's feet, fists, and mouth) to prevent injury.
- Develop a plan. Once the plan is implemented, act quickly. Indecision can cause injury.
- Use only the amount of force necessary to effect the restraint. Restraint is never punitive.
- Communicate with the patient while you are restraining him.
- Use only soft restraints (such as gauze).
- Restrain the patient in a face-up position.
- Never hog-tie the patient or restrict expansion of the chest cavity in any way.
- Reassess the patient frequently during transport.

Problems can occur during restraint. If the patient remains violent and struggling, you will find it best to position the restraints so they prevent the use of major muscle groups. Place a surgical or oxygen mask (with oxygen flowing) over the face of a patient who is spitting at you.

positional asphyxia death of a patient who has been restrained; a condition often associated with extreme exertion (long foot chases or struggling against restraints), drug or alcohol use, and hog-tie or hobble restraints.

Do not restrain a patient face down. Many will argue it is more efficient, but it prevents you from properly assessing the patient throughout transport.

There is a condition known as **positional asphyxia.** It involves the death of patients who have been improperly restrained. This condition is often associated with extreme exertion (long foot chases or struggling against restraints), drug or alcohol

SCAN 26-1 Restraining a Patient

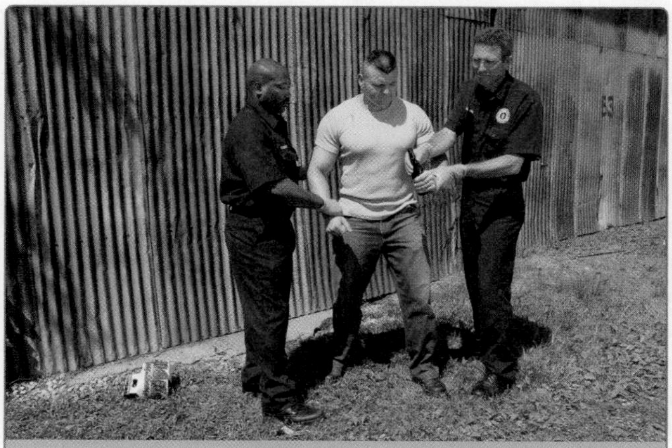

26-1-1 Make sure you have enough help, and approach the patient at the same time.

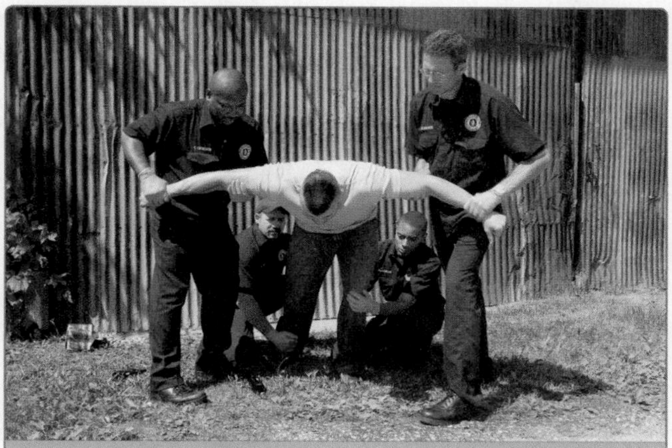

26-1-2 Each rescuer should attempt to control a limb.

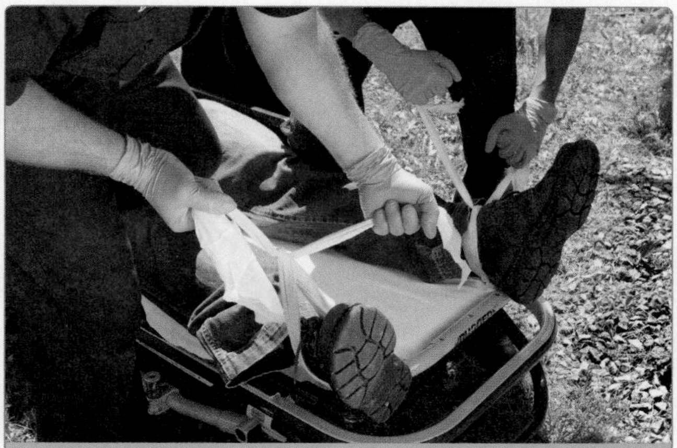

26-1-3 If possible, place the patient in a supine position on the stretcher.

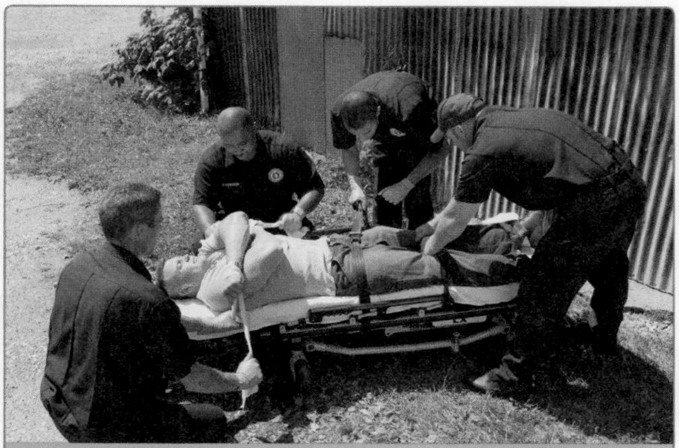

26-1-4 Use approved restraints to secure the patient to the stretcher.

use, and being hog-tied (face down with arms and legs secured behind). A common scenario is that during transport and upon arrival at the hospital, the patient who was loud and combative appears to have calmed down, when in fact he is dead. When such a tragic death occurs, there is also significant liability for EMS providers. To prevent positional asphyxia:

- Never restrain a patient face down (hog-tied).
- Recognize situations where positional asphyxia is likely.
- Monitor your restrained patient continuously, and focus especially on the ABCs.
- Be alert for sudden changes in mental status, especially changes from argumentative and struggling to suddenly becoming quiet.

Agitated delirium patients are at high risk for sudden death during physical restraint. Remember that although their motion is restricted, the high anxiety state may continue in the body. Although their extremities are not moving, their heart, lungs, and other body systems may remain in overdrive. Because of this risk, it is often advisable to consider the need for sedation with medications (chemical restraint). Although this is not a likely option at an EMT level, advanced providers may be able to initiate such treatments if local protocols allow. When dealing with a person in suspected agitated delirium, consider contacting ALS for the possibility of prehospital sedation.

Documentation

Documentation is exceptionally important with regard to behavioral emergencies. Care should be taken to objectively document your findings and treatments in a nonjudgmental manner. In addition to providing a record of patient care, this information is important for recognizing trends in behavior and may be evidentiary if physical violence has occurred. Be sure to document scene clues and information given to you by bystanders and family.

Most important is documenting the events surrounding patient restraint. Because injury is not uncommon, it is important to not only include how restraint was utilized but also why the decision to restrain was made. Objectively note the factors that went into making a decision to restrain. Some systems require contact with medical direction prior to restraint. When possible, discussing this decision with medical direction is never a bad idea. Careful documentation of your constant monitoring of the patient's respiratory status and perfusion while in restraints is also essential. Always follow local protocol.

PERSPECTIVE

Theresa—The EMT

At first the cop was angry that we let the guy run away. But, come on! There was no way that we were going to get that guy under control. Just the two of us, trying to restrain him while he was swinging his fists and yelling at people who weren't there? Now that's just plain stupid. It isn't safe, and quite frankly it is the job of the police.

STOP, REVIEW, REMEMBER!

Multiple Choice

For each question, place a check next to the correct answer.

1. Constant talking about nonsensical topics is referred to as:

_____ a. pressured speech.

_____ b. catatonic speech.

_____ c. expressive aphasia.

_____ d. disorientation.

2. You are called to the scene of a 56-year-old man who is exhibiting unusual behavior. As you approach, you should first:

_____ a. assess the orientation of the patient.

_____ b. make sure there are no threats to providers.

_____ c. determine the location of the patient.

_____ d. examine the appearance of the patient.

3. A patient who dies during or as a result of restraint may have experienced:

_____ a. terminal psychosis.

_____ b. psychotic asphyxia.

_____ c. positional asphyxia.

_____ d. myocardial infarction.

4. A 29-year-old man has an altered mental status and is making threatening gestures toward you and your partner. Law enforcement is en route but has not yet arrived on scene. You should:

_____ a. await the arrival of law enforcement before approaching the patient.

_____ b. attempt to physically restrain the patient to enable a more thorough examination.

_____ c. approach the patient using calm tones in an attempt to deescalate the situation.

_____ d. use forceful tones to intimidate the patient into calming down.

5. You are caring for a patient who is exhibiting bizarre behavior. Which action is least likely to help calm the patient?

_____ a. Introducing yourself and explaining you are there to help

_____ b. Ordering the patient to calm down

_____ c. Using positive body language

_____ d. Listening

Short Answer

Write the definition of each of the following terms.

1. Capacity

____

____

2. Psychosis

____

____

3. Soft restraints

____

____

(continued on next page)

(continued)

Critical Thinking

1. You are transporting a violent patient to the psychiatric center at the request of the police. The patient begins spitting at you. He has been fighting, so he has a bloody lip. List two things you could do to minimize exposure to his blood.

____

____

____

____

2. Why is it important to communicate with the patient while you are restraining him?

____

____

____

____

3. Define positional asphyxia and explain how to prevent it.

____

____

____

____

EMERGENCY DISPATCH SUMMARY

The patient was apprehended, completely naked, on 17th Street, trying to break the window of a parked car with his shoe. He was restrained by law enforcement and transported to St. Luther Hospital, home of the county's mental health unit. Theresa recovered fully from the assault but now does not hesitate to call for police assistance if her patient is acting unusual in any way.

Chapter Review

To the Point

- As many as one in three people encountered by EMTs may have some degree of mental disorder. It is important to recognize the signs of a behavior so that you can provide the most appropriate care.
- A behavioral emergency is defined as a situation in which a patient's behavior becomes intolerable, dangerous, or bizarre enough to cause the concern of family, bystanders, or the patient.
- Patients experiencing a behavioral emergency may pose a safety risk to themselves as well as to those around them, including rescue personnel.
- Behavioral emergencies can be caused by illness or injury. Always consider possible medical and traumatic causes and treat the patient accordingly.
- Patients experiencing a behavioral emergency may be experiencing such things as anxiety, phobias, depression, bipolar disorder, paranoia, psychosis, schizophrenia, or agitated delirium.
- Some of the risk factors associated with violence and suicide include a history of depression, recent divorce, history of alcohol or drug abuse, previous suicide attempts, and loss of a loved one.
- Strategies for a successful encounter with a patient experiencing a behavioral emergency include clearly identifying yourself, being patient, listening well, getting down to patient's eye level, and remaining calm and nonjudgmental.
- If a patient becomes violent, immediately retreat from the scene and call law enforcement if they are not already en route.
- On rare occasions it may be necessary to physically restrain a patient to avoid injury to EMS personnel or to the patient. If possible, always wait for law enforcement. Make a plan, act quickly, and only use the minimum necessary force to achieve your objective.
- Calls involving restraint are at very high risk for litigation. It is especially important to document all aspects of the call and include the accounts of other EMS or rescue personnel in your report.

Chapter Questions

Multiple Choice

For each question, place a check next to the correct answer.

1. The condition that can lead to a patient dying while restrained is called:

_____ a. positional asphyxia.
_____ b. psychotic asphyxia.
_____ c. terminal asphyxia.
_____ d. myocardial asphyxia.

2. Unusual or bizarre behavior, indicating a lack of touch with reality, is referred to as:

_____ a. delusions.
_____ b. psychosis.
_____ c. paranoia.
_____ d. hallucinations.

3. A 22-year-old woman has displayed behavior her family believes indicates a suicidal tendency. Which one of the following findings would demonstrate the highest risk of suicide?

_____ a. Her gender
_____ b. The fact that she has been treated for depression in the past.
_____ c. Her age
_____ d. Her detailed plan to take pills

(continued on next page)

(continued)

4. A 30-year-old man is reporting paranoid delusions and auditory hallucinations. Which one of the following disorders would best describe this type of behavior?

_____ a. Bipolar disorder
_____ b. Anxiety disorder
_____ c. Schizophrenia
_____ d. Severe depression

5. Which one of the following would be the best way to prevent positional asphyxia?

_____ a. Restrain the patient face down.
_____ b. Hobble the patient by tying his legs and arms behind his back.
_____ c. Use multiple straps across the patient's chest.
_____ d. Restrain the patient face up.

Matching

Match the condition or behavior on the left with the correct description on the right.

1. _____ Phobia
2. _____ Psychosis
3. _____ Delusion
4. _____ Depression
5. _____ Panic
6. _____ Paranoia

A. Unusual or bizarre behavior
B. Sudden onset of fear or discomfort
C. False belief one is being followed or persecuted
D. Alteration of mood with feelings of worthlessness, fatigue, guilt, and lack of interest in daily activities
E. False belief
F. Unfounded or intense fear

Critical Thinking

1. Some say that behavioral emergency patients just need restraint and there is nothing you can do to prevent the need. Defend or agree with this statement.

____

____

____

____

2. You are called to a patient with an altered mental status who has both a diabetic history and a psychiatric history. How might you determine the patient's problem and the care you should give?

____

____

____

____

3. You are called to a residence for a behavioral emergency. You are met at the curb by a parent who states that her son, who has a history of schizophrenia, has thrown some furniture around. He is calm now. The police are not on scene. Should you enter the residence? Why or why not?

Case Study

Your ambulance is called to the corner of Main and Emmons Streets for a "subject acting strangely." You arrive to find a man talking with a police officer. As you approach, you hear the man tell the officer that he was at the Last Supper and is spreading the word as the Lord told him to. The officer asks for identification to which the man replies, "I am from Heaven. Disciples of God do not need identification."

1. List three ways you would determine if a medical problem is causing this patient's behavior.

2. Why would this man's belief that he was at the Last Supper and is from heaven be considered a delusion?

3. The patient is calm until the police tell him he must go to the hospital. What signs might you see that indicate increased agitation?

4. What verbal or interpersonal techniques might you perform to counteract this agitation?

The Last Word

Patients who are experiencing behavioral emergencies pose unique challenges for the EMT. Instead of having a list of steps to follow, like the ones you will learn for controlling bleeding, you will have to rely on communication, observation, and some interpersonal skills while treating your patient. Using courtesy and respect will go a long way with these or any patients you encounter.

Just because you cannot see this patient's condition, as you might a laceration or a skin rash, does not mean that it is not real. A significant percentage of the population has some sort of psychological condition ranging from depression and anxiety (as much as 10% of the population) to schizophrenia (less common). Suicide is the third leading cause of death in the 15- to 24-year-old age group and increasing rapidly in our geriatric population. So, yes, before long you will certainly deal with patients who have some sort of behavioral emergency.

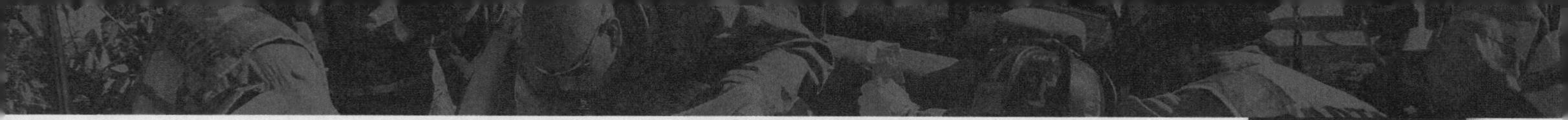

Obstetrics and Care of the Newborn

27

Education Standards

Special Patient Populations: Obstetrics, Neonatal Care

Competencies

Applies fundamental knowledge of growth, development, aging, and assessment findings to provide basic emergency care and transportation for a patient with special needs.

Objectives

After completion of this lesson, you should be able to:

27-1 Define key terms introduced in this chapter.

27-2 Describe the anatomy of pregnancy, the menstrual cycle, and the prenatal period.

27-3 Describe physiological changes in pregnancy, including changes to the reproductive, respiratory, cardiovascular, gastrointestinal, urinary, and musculoskeletal systems.

27-4 Describe the pathophysiology, assessment, and emergency care of patients with predelivery emergencies, including abruptio placentae, ectopic pregnancy, placenta previa, preeclampsia/eclampsia, pregnancy-induced hypertension, ruptured uterus, spontaneous abortion, and supine hypotensive syndrome.

27-5 Describe the assessment-based approach to predelivery emergencies.

27-6 Describe the stages of labor.

27-7 Describe the assessment-based approach to a patient in active labor with normal delivery.

27-8 Describe the steps of assisting with a normal prehospital delivery.

27-9 Discuss reassessment of the postpartum patient.

27-10 Describe the assessment-based approach to a patient in active labor with abnormal delivery.

27-11 Describe the management of abnormal prehospital obstetric deliveries, including breech and limb presentations, meconium staining, multiple births, post-term pregnancy, precipitous delivery, premature birth, premature rupture of membranes, preterm labor, prolapsed umbilical cord, and shoulder dystocia.

27-12 Describe the management of postpartum complications, including postpartum hemorrhage and embolism.

27-13 Demonstrate the steps of assessing and managing the newborn, including initial care (drying, wrapping, suctioning, and positioning) and Apgar scoring.

27-14 Describe the signs that indicate the need for neonatal resuscitation.

27-15 Apply the concepts of the neonatal resuscitation pyramid to the care of neonates in need of resuscitative measures.

Key Terms

Introduction

Childbirth is a wondrous and amazing event that in most cases occurs without the need for significant intervention. However, when EMS becomes involved, the underlying implication is that something unusual has happened. EMS is called when a complication occurs or the plan for delivery is taking a very different pathway. The limited resources of prehospital childbirth present unique challenges and threats to both the mother and baby, which can increase the likelihood of potentially dangerous complications. As an EMT, you must be prepared to face those difficulties in a very high-stress situation.

It is not particularly shocking to say that men and women are different, but this is a very important concept to keep in mind when dealing with emergency obstetrics. The female reproductive system consists of organs and structures different from a male's and can present unique and life-threatening emergencies when disrupted. Although in most deliveries your care will be primarily supportive, in some situations, your immediate actions mean the difference between life and death for the newborn and even for the mother.

This chapter discusses emergency childbirth. It begins with a review of female reproductive anatomy and physiology, and goes on to help prepare you for assisting in uncomplicated deliveries and for the significant challenges of complicated deliveries. Also covered are the assessment and care of a newborn, including resuscitation.

ovary female organ that produces ova (eggs).

fallopian tube structure that extends from the ovary to the uterus.

ovum an unfertilized egg. Plural, *ova*.

embryo the stage of fetal development between the zygote and the fetus.

fetus the clinical term for an unborn baby.

EMERGENCY DISPATCH

"Why did the dispatcher say it was an OB as in baby call?" Mark asked. He was a new EMT in his second week of field training. "Isn't it kind of obvious that an OB emergency will have something to do with babies?"

"Because sometimes over the radio it can sound like OD, as in overdose," Mark's trainer, Ling, said as she deftly maneuvered the ambulance around cars on the rain-slick roadway. "You obviously don't want to confuse those two calls."

"True."

The patient was a 17-year-old who was in the passenger seat of her boyfriend's pickup truck. A highway patrolman had pulled them over for speeding on the interstate and quickly realized what the rush was, so he radioed for an ambulance.

The patrolman approached Ling and Mark as they stepped from their truck and explained why he had called. "Oh, and another thing," he said. "She's deaf and the boyfriend doesn't know sign language."

"Okay, thanks. Mark, pull out your notepad and get a pen," Ling said as she walked up to the truck and peered into the cab. "Oh, hey, never mind! Open the OB kit now!"

Female Reproductive Anatomy and Physiology

27-2 Describe the anatomy of pregnancy, the menstrual cycle, and the prenatal period.

27-3 Describe physiological changes in pregnancy, including changes to the reproductive, respiratory, cardiovascular, gastrointestinal, urinary, and musculoskeletal systems.

The two **ovaries** are the organs responsible for producing ova (eggs) for conception. They are small, round organs and are located bilaterally in the lower abdominal quadrants of a woman (Figure 27-1 ▪). The ovaries also produce many of the hormones necessary for the process of reproduction.

Ovaries are connected to the uterus by the **fallopian tubes.** The fallopian tubes are small, highly vascular tubes designed to transport the **ovum** to the uterus. If the ovum is fertilized by a man's sperm, it then becomes an **embryo** that will implant in the lining of the uterus and develop into a **fetus.** When **fertilization** of the ovum occurs, it typically happens in the fallopian tubes and then the fertilized ovum travels into the uterus.

Occasionally, a fertilized ovum will implant in the fallopian tubes. If it begins to develop into a fetus there, a dangerous condition called **ectopic pregnancy** occurs. Because the fallopian tube cannot stretch significantly, the growing fetus can rupture

fertilization the union of an ovum (egg) and sperm.

ectopic pregnancy a pregnancy in which the fetus develops in an area other than the uterus.

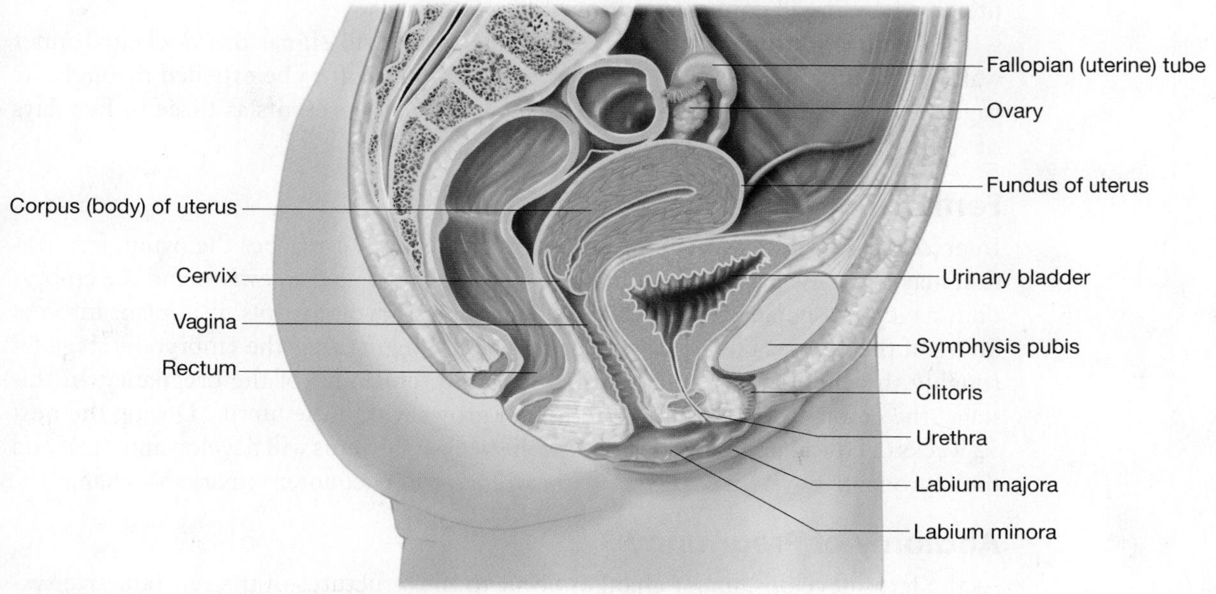

Figure 27-1 Anatomy of the female reproductive system.

the tube and cause massive internal bleeding. (Ectopic pregnancy is described in greater detail later in this chapter.)

uterus the muscular organ that contains the developing fetus.

The **uterus** (also known as the *womb*) is a hollow, muscular organ located along the midline in the lower abdominal quadrants. A fetus, the clinical term for an unborn baby, develops inside the uterus during the course of a pregnancy. Unlike the fallopian tubes, the uterus has the capability to stretch and grow as the fetus increases in size. The uterus is generally located in the lower quadrants but its top, also known as the *fundus*, can be pushed as high as the xiphoid process in a late-term pregnancy.

birth canal passageway that extends from the cervix to the vaginal opening through which the baby is born. Also called the *vagina*.

cervix the opening of the uterus.

vagina the birth canal.

menstrual cycle monthly recurrent changes in the female reproductive system.

labia soft tissues that protect the exterior entrance to the vagina.

perineum the skin between the vagina and the anus.

The uterus connects to the vagina to form the **birth canal.** The **cervix** is a muscular ring that forms the lower border of the uterus and serves as the gate between the uterus and vagina. During pregnancy, the cervix closes off the uterus to allow the fetus to develop. The **vagina** is a passageway made up of smooth muscle and connects the uterus to the outside world. It has the capability to stretch to allow transportation of the fetus and it also serves as the passageway for menstrual waste products leaving the uterus at the conclusion of the **menstrual cycle.**

The **labia** are the soft tissues that protect the exterior entrance to the birth canal. The urethral opening and the clitoris, located in a position superior to the vagina, are also protected by the labia. These tissues are nerve rich and highly vascular and bleed heavily as a result of trauma.

The **perineum** is the soft tissue and muscle found between the vaginal opening and the anus. This tissue is also highly vascular and can tear during childbirth.

The Reproductive Cycle

Once a woman reaches puberty, a biological cycle that lasts approximately 28 days occurs within her reproductive system to allow for the possibility of pregnancy. Hormones such as estrogen and progesterone chemically direct these events. First, ovulation occurs, during which the ovaries are stimulated to release an ovum (egg). Simultaneously the walls of the uterus thicken to prepare for implantation of the egg if fertilization occurs.

Next, the fallopian tubes slowly transport the ovum to the uterus. If fertilization occurs, it typically happens during this transportation process. With successful fertilization, the ovum (now considered an embryo) is implanted into the wall of the uterus where it will continue to grow into a fetus.

If fertilization does not occur, hormone levels will signal the thickened inner walls of the uterus to break down and begin to slough off to be expelled through the vagina. This process is called *menstruation* and usually presents as three to five days of vaginal bleeding.

Fertilization

Intercourse introduces sperm into the birth canal and if it reaches the ovum, fertilization may occur. As previously noted, a fertilized egg is called an *embryo* and the embryonic stage of pregnancy lasts eight weeks as the embryo attempts to implant into the lining of the uterus. The fetal stage of pregnancy begins after the embryonic stage (at roughly the eighth week) and continues for the remainder of the pregnancy. In this stage, the embryo develops into a fetus and grows within the uterus. During the next 32 weeks (a typical pregnancy lasts about 40 weeks), the fetus will develop and grow and the reproductive system of the pregnant woman will encounter remarkable changes.

Anatomy of Pregnancy

As the fetus develops, major changes occur to the structures of the reproductive system and to the pregnant woman's body in general (Figure 27-2 ■). First and foremost,

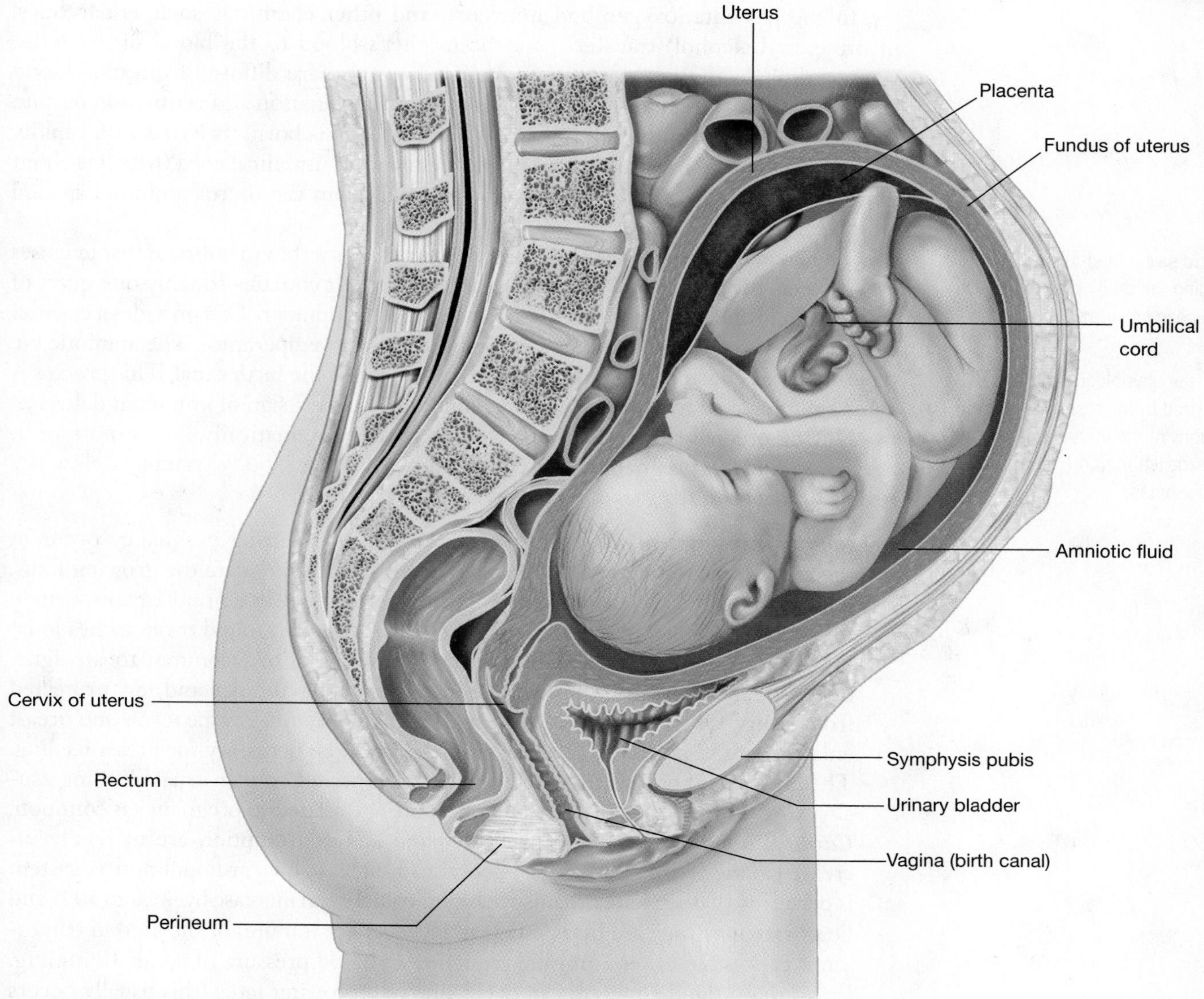

Figure 27-2 Anatomy of pregnancy.

the body must accommodate a growing fetus that occupies more and more space over time. As the fetus grows, the uterus stretches and becomes more thin-walled and less protected by the pelvis. As the uterus expands, it becomes more vulnerable to injury.

The 40 weeks (roughly nine months) of pregnancy are divided into three three-month periods called *trimesters*. The fetus is being formed and remains quite small during the first **trimester,** so there is little uterine growth during this period. Once the second trimester begins, the uterus grows rapidly, reaching the height of the umbilicus (navel) by the fifth month (20 weeks) and height of the epigastrium (upper abdomen) by the seventh month.

trimester division of the pregnancy period, usually 13 weeks, or about one-third of the pregnancy.

As the fetus develops, it receives oxygen and nutrients and disposes of waste products through an organ called the **placenta.** The placenta is a highly vascular organ that develops in the uterus along with the fetus. The placenta brings maternal blood vessels into close proximity to fetal blood vessels and this allows the process of diffusion to occur in a manner similar to the process that occurs in the alveoli. The mother's blood does not flow directly through the fetus's body. Rather, fetal blood is transported to and from the placenta through the blood vessels of the **umbilical cord.**

placenta anatomical structure that provides nutrition to the fetus and eliminates fetal waste.

umbilical cord an anatomical structure that connects the fetus to the placenta.

In the placenta, oxygen and nutrients (and other chemicals such as narcotics, nicotine, and alcohol) transfer from the mother's blood to the blood of the fetus. Carbon dioxide and certain other waste products also are diffused from fetal blood back to maternal circulation. This process allows oxygenation and ventilation despite the fact the fetus is not breathing air. When the baby is born, its circulation rapidly changes to adapt to breathing air. The placenta and its umbilical cord (which is about one inch in diameter and 22 inches long) detach from the uterus and are expelled after the birth of the baby.

amniotic sac fluid-filled sac surrounding the developing fetus. Also called the *bag of waters*.

labor the physiological process characterized by increasingly intense contractions of the uterus, whereby the fetus is expelled from the uterus of a pregnant woman.

The **amniotic sac,** also known as the *bag of waters*, is a thin membrane that encloses and protects the fetus while it develops in the uterus. It contains roughly one quart of amniotic fluid and allows the fetus to float during development. This provides a cushion against injury and helps maintain a constant fetal body temperature. The amniotic sac typically breaks during **labor** and the fluid exits through the birth canal. This process is commonly referred to as "the water breaking" and can be a sign of imminent delivery.

During pregnancy, the body of a woman changes dramatically. It is important to keep in mind how pregnancy impacts the most significant body systems. Below is a review of key changes:

- ***Reproductive system.*** The most profound changes during pregnancy occur in the reproductive system. Most changes occur to accommodate the growing fetus. The most significant change occurs to the uterus itself. In a nonpregnant woman the uterus is a small oval or pear-shaped organ, usually around three inches long. However, as the fetus grows, this small organ stretches to accommodate an eight- to ten-pound fetus. As it grows, the uterus becomes thinner and less protected from injury. Other changes include markedly different hormone levels and breast enlargement in preparation for lactation that will be necessary for breast feeding. The presence of pregnancy ends the menstrual period, so menstrual bleeding usually stops. However, slight bleeding or "spotting" related to pregnancy is common.
- ***Cardiopulmonary system.*** Oxygen demand and consumption are markedly increased in the pregnant woman. Theoretically at least, her cardiopulmonary system is perfusing two separate organisms. Blood volume can increase by 40% to 50% and heart rate may increase by as much as 15 beats per minute. In the second trimester, it is possible to see a normal reduction in blood pressure of about 10 mmHg. Pressure on the diaphragm can occur due to a growing fetus (this usually occurs in the later stages of pregnancy). The volume of air in a woman's lungs decreases and she may find it more difficult to breathe. She also may have decreased oxygen reserves and less of an ability to compensate in the event of illness or injury.
- ***Gastrointestinal system.*** In the GI system, a growing fetus puts pressure on the stomach and intestines and can slow digestion. Hormone levels can affect stomach acid levels. Nausea and vomiting are therefore very common complaints of pregnant women especially in their first trimester.
- ***Musculoskeletal system.*** In the musculoskeletal system, the ligaments of a pregnant woman become more elastic and therefore become more vulnerable to injury. With stretched ligaments, dislocations often pose a higher risk than fractures. The additional weight gained during pregnancy can also affect posture and lead to back pain as well as affect balance.

Pregnancy also may impact preexisting medical conditions in the mother. Diseases such as asthma, high blood pressure, seizures, and diabetes can all be exacerbated by pregnancy.

Assessment of the Female Patient

A female patient should be assessed in the same manner as a male patient. The primary and secondary assessments include the same elements. However, specific anatomical differences require special considerations. There are injuries and disorders that are uniquely female. Assessment of any female patient must consider such possibilities. Later in this chapter many of the life-threatening gynecological and obstetrical emergencies are described in further detail, but it is important to remember that those problems must be considered when assessing a woman.

Pregnancy is a consideration that must be accounted for during the assessment of a female patient in her child-bearing years. In many cases, a woman will tell you that she is pregnant, but in other situations, you may have to look to the findings that indicate this condition. In late stages of pregnancy, the woman's abdomen will become enlarged to accommodate the growing uterus. Sometimes this is quite obvious, but other times it is less easy to see. The menstrual period typically ceases during pregnancy, so missed or delayed menstruation can be a sign indicating the possibility of pregnancy. It is important to remember that many women have irregular menstrual periods, so often this is an unreliable sign.

Discretion and professionalism are very important elements of any assessment of any patient's reproductive system. "Is there any chance you could be pregnant?" is not always an easy question to answer in a crowded room or when surrounded by coworkers. Examination and specific questioning can be embarrassing, intrusive, and awkward. You must do your best to consider the environment you are in, the risk versus the value of exposing specific anatomy, and the emotional condition of the patient before assessing elements of the reproductive system and reproductive history.

Specific Gynecological Emergencies

27-5 Describe the assessment-based approach to predelivery emergencies.

Many gynecological emergencies are not related to childbirth. In fact, there are numerous other emergencies related to a women's reproductive system that will require you to consider her unique anatomy and physiology.

Vaginal Bleeding

Vaginal bleeding is a common gynecological emergency. Bleeding can be minor or severe and in certain circumstances it can even lead to shock and death. It will be very difficult to distinguish the actual cause of vaginal bleeding given limited prehospital diagnostic resources, but it is very important to recognize that it can be an indication of a number of life-threatening conditions.

Vaginal bleeding (unless it results from external trauma) results from internal bleeding. In most cases a component or part of the reproductive system is hemorrhaging. It can result from damage to other abdominal organs and can represent an important clue that a severe condition exists. In some cases, vaginal bleeding results from a pregnancy-related emergency (described later in this chapter).

It is not common for an EMT to examine the vaginal area. However, if a woman has direct trauma and resultant significant bleeding to her vagina or perineum, it will be necessary to examine the area and control any external bleeding.

Examine the vagina by observation only. Look for trauma and determine the rate of blood loss. If the patient is bleeding from her vagina due to an internal source of hemorrhage, then the rate of bleeding prior to your arrival can be assessed by asking the patient how many absorbent pads she has had to use. Never do any type of internal examination or place anything inside the vagina to stop the bleeding. Absorbent materials should be placed outside the vaginal opening to absorb the fluid and blood. The dressings can be changed as needed during transport and to make the patient comfortable.

Treat vaginal bleeding as you would any other sign of internal bleeding. Assess for the symptoms of shock and treat accordingly. Consider supplemental oxygen.

PRACTICAL PATHOPHYSIOLOGY

Vaginal bleeding can originate from a variety of sources. Some etiologies are very benign. For example, a woman will typically lose approximately 80 to 100 mL of blood during her normal menstrual period. Some women suffer from hormone-related complications of menstrual periods by which they bleed far more heavily and for many days longer than normal periods. This group of vaginal bleeding disorders is referred to as *dysfunctional uterine bleeding.*

Potentially life-threatening pregnancy-related conditions that result in abnormal vaginal bleeding include ectopic pregnancy (in the first trimester) and placenta previa and abruptio placentae (in the third trimester).

Sexual Assault

The care for male or female sexual assault patients differs slightly from that of other trauma patients. While the care for soft-tissue injuries is the same, there are evidentiary concerns as well as emotional concerns that must be addressed. To care for sexual assault patients, consider the following points:

- A sexual assault is a crime scene. Ensure that the scene is safe prior to entering. It may be necessary to stage your unit near the scene until the scene is rendered safe by police.
- The patient has just been assaulted and will require gentle, nonjudgmental compassionate care. Having a same-sex EMT deal with the patient can be beneficial. If this is not possible, it is even more important that the care be compassionate and nonjudgmental.
- Remember that there may be injuries to other parts of the body from the assault. Be sure to do a complete assessment.
- Recognizing that an assault victim has experienced loss of control is vital to proper care. Provide a renewed sense of control to the patient. Be conscious of personal space. Explain your examinations and treatments beforehand. Be sensitive to the patient's fears and embarrassment and ask her permission to look, to touch, and to provide care.
- Avoid saying things like, "It will be okay," or "He'll definitely go to jail."
- Try to prevent the patient from bathing, showering, going to the bathroom, douching, or otherwise cleaning up. They could destroy evidence.
- Do not allow the patient to wash hands until instructed to do so by an evidence technician. This is because important DNA evidence from a sexual assault incident may be found under the fingernails of the victim.
- Learn what social service resources are available in your area. Consider providing referrals.
- Your local protocols may have specific legal requirements for reporting a sexual assault. Learn your specific local regulations and be sure to document your report objectively and thoroughly.

27-4 Describe the pathophysiology, assessment, and emergency care of patients with predelivery emergencies, including abruptio placentae, ectopic pregnancy, placenta previa, preeclampsia/eclampsia, pregnancy-induced hypertension, ruptured uterus, spontaneous abortion, and supine hypotensive syndrome.

Obstetrical Emergencies

There are several emergencies related specifically to pregnancy. Emergency childbirth and complications associated with delivery are described later in this chapter. The following offers a review of specific life threats that may occur to pregnant women *before* they give birth.

Ectopic Pregnancy

An ectopic pregnancy is a potentially life-threatening condition. It is a pregnancy that implants and develops in an area other than the uterus (Figure 27-3 ■). This is almost exclusively observed in the first trimester of pregnancy, sometimes before the patient is even aware that she is pregnant.

Approximately every 28 days, an ovum (egg) is released from an ovary and is guided into a fallopian tube by fingerlike projections called **fimbriae.** Fertilization of the egg typically occurs in the fallopian tube, and several days later the fertilized egg implants into the uterine wall. Occasionally, the egg will implant somewhere other than the wall of the uterus, such as in the fallopian tube, cervix, or abdomen. When this happens, the pregnancy is called an *ectopic pregnancy*. Because those other locations are not designed to grow and stretch with the developing fetus, a potentially life-threatening condition can occur.

fimbriae fingerlike projections that propel ova into the fallopian tubes.

It is common for a patient experiencing an ectopic pregnancy to report a missed or delayed menstrual period (indicating pregnancy). As a rule, you should consider any woman of childbearing age who complains of abdominal pain and vaginal bleeding to have an ectopic pregnancy until proven otherwise.

The chief complaint of a patient with an ectopic pregnancy will commonly be abdominal pain. The pain can occur with or without vaginal bleeding. Abdominal pain is usually sharp and unilateral in nature (one sided). Occasionally, the pain of ectopic pregnancy can be referred to the shoulder, but this is a late sign (usually associated with shock) when bleeding in the abdomen from the ectopic pregnancy is so extensive that the blood causes irritation of the diaphragm.

Ectopic pregnancies can lead to severe hemorrhage and shock and as such, should be treated as a serious emergency. Care for the patient with abdominal pain and vaginal bleeding from this or any cause includes supplemental oxygen and prompt transport to an appropriate hospital.

Spontaneous Abortion

There are times when the embryo or fetus does not survive and delivers very prematurely. This is called a **spontaneous abortion.** It is also commonly referred to

spontaneous abortion the natural delivery of the embryo or fetus before it is able to survive on its own. Also called a *miscarriage*.

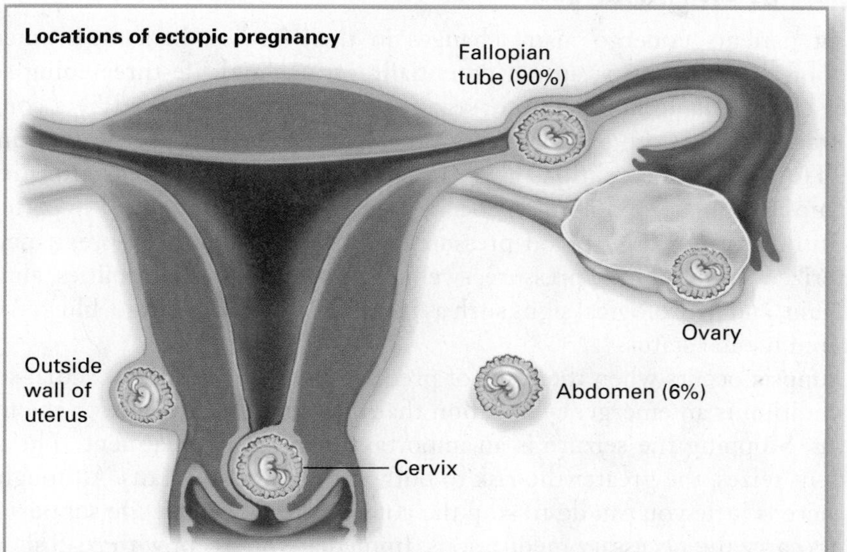

Figure 27-3 Various locations of an ectopic pregnancy.

as a miscarriage. Women who are having a spontaneous abortion often experience cramps, abdominal pain, vaginal bleeding, and possibly the expulsion of fetal tissue from the vagina.

Sometimes miscarriages are preceded by problems with the pregnancy, such as slight bleeding, and other times the mother may have a history of miscarriages. A significant number of pregnancies end in first-trimester miscarriages, so it is not a tremendously unusual situation. However, it is as painful emotionally to the parents as any other complication of childbirth that results in a nonliving baby. Compassion and caring on the part of the EMT can make this situation much less debilitating for the family. Remember that for couples who experience miscarriage, the words, "You can always have another baby" are not well received at this time.

Bleeding can be severe and potentially life threatening in a miscarriage. Assess for the signs and symptoms of shock and treat accordingly. If it is evident that a fetus or other tissue materials (usually whitish in color) are contained within the vaginal bleeding, they should be collected and transported with the patient to the hospital so they can be examined. Transport the patient and any expelled fetal tissue to the hospital promptly.

Supine Hypotensive Syndrome

In the third trimester of the pregnancy, the growing fetus takes up considerable space in the pelvic and abdominal cavities. One potential negative effect on the mother's body is **supine hypotensive syndrome.** This occurs when the pregnant patient lies flat and the fetus compresses the inferior vena cava. The compression reduces blood flow back to the heart and causes significant hypotension (low blood pressure). This is observed by low blood pressure measurements, dizziness, diaphoresis, and other signs of shock when the patient is supine.

supine hypotensive syndrome a condition that occurs when the pregnant patient lies flat and the fetus compresses the inferior vena cava. This compression reduces blood flow back to the heart and causes significant hypotension (low blood pressure).

The condition can be corrected by having the patient roll onto or lean toward her left side. If the patient is immobilized on a backboard, the board may be tilted by propping up the right side. Leaning the supine patient to the left will relieve the pressure on the inferior vena cava and allow normal blood return to the heart.

Any time you transport a third-trimester pregnant patient in the ambulance, you should position the patient to prevent supine hypotensive syndrome.

Seizures in Pregnancy

Pregnant patients undergo many changes in their bodies. In some women, the changes of pregnancy can cause a potentially serious and life-threatening seizure disorder called **eclampsia.** Eclamptic seizures are typically preceded by a condition called **preeclampsia.** Both preeclampsia and eclampsia usually occur in the third trimester. However, the conditions also can occur up to several weeks after delivery. Preeclampsia is most commonly associated with pregnancy-induced hypertension, even if no history of high blood pressure was present before the pregnancy. It is characterized by high blood pressure, swelling in the face and extremities, abnormal weight gain, and neurological signs such as ringing in the ears, vertigo, blurred vision, and altered mental status.

eclampsia pregnancy complication characterized by severe hypertension (high blood pressure), convulsions, and coma.

preeclampsia pregnancy complication characterized by hypertension (high blood pressure) and edema.

Eclampsia occurs when the signs of preeclampsia progress to an actual seizure. This condition is an emergency situation that threatens the life of both the mother and fetus. Stopping the seizure is an important element of treatment. The longer the patient seizes, the greater the risk to both the mother and fetus. Although as an EMT there is little you can do to stop the convulsions, advanced life support (ALS) providers carry the necessary medications. Immediate intercept with ALS should be arranged.

Your initial treatment involves protecting the patient from harm during the seizure, administering oxygen, and transporting promptly. Transport the patient on her left side while carefully monitoring the airway.

Preterm Labor

Occasionally, labor will begin prior to the patient's expected due date. In some cases, the baby will actually be delivered. (Premature delivery is described in the next section.) However, more often, the mother experiences **contractions** that do not lead to an actual delivery.

contractions repeated tightening of the uterus to expel the baby.

As the uterus prepares for delivery, it begins contracting frequently. Those contractions are called *Braxton Hicks contractions* (also known as *false labor*) and are occasional and typically not sustained. Many mothers, however, can mistake them for actual labor. Until the contractions stop, it is impossible to discern Braxton Hicks contractions from actual labor in the field. In most cases, you must treat the woman as if she is actually in labor.

Premature Rupture of Membranes

Amniotic fluid surrounds and protects the fetus while it develops in the uterus. The amniotic sac usually stays intact until delivery is imminent. However, in some cases, it can rupture prematurely and lead to fetal difficulties. Loss of amniotic fluid can increase the risk of infection for the fetus and needs to be taken seriously. The earlier the fluid is lost in pregnancy, the more concerning the event.

EMS care in this situation is purely supportive. Although it is a serious condition, premature rupture of membranes is not typically immediately life threatening to either mother or fetus. Initiate transport to an appropriate facility where obstetrical services are available.

Abruptio Placentae and Placenta Previa

Abruptio placentae and **placenta previa,** as their names indicate, involve the placenta. Both occur late in pregnancy (second and third trimesters), can cause significant bleeding, and are serious emergencies for both the mother and the fetus.

abruptio placentae a condition in which the placenta prematurely separates from the uterine wall and causes pain and bleeding.

placenta previa a condition in which the placenta is attached to the uterine wall over the opening of the cervix, but in the wrong position.

In abruptio placentae (Figure 27-4 ■) the placenta prematurely separates from the uterine wall. In this condition, the placenta may partially or fully detach. Because the placenta is a highly vascular organ and contains blood vessels from both the mother and fetus, massive hemorrhage can occur. Abruptio placentae is typically characterized by sharp, tearing abdominal pain and vaginal bleeding and should be considered a major life threat.

Placenta previa (Figure 27-5 ■) is a condition in which the placenta is attached to the uterine wall but has attached near the cervix and is in the way of delivery. In placenta previa, the placenta can fully or partially obstruct the entrance to the birth canal. As the fetus begins to move down into position for birth and the cervix begins to dilate, the placenta tears and begins to bleed. Women who have had routine **prenatal** care often know that they have placenta previa, but bleeding may be the only sign in other cases.

prenatal refers to a time before birth.

Care for both conditions includes oxygen, treating for shock, and prompt transport to an appropriate hospital where obstetrical services are available.

Uterine Rupture

A related condition can occur if the integrity of the uterus is violated. In **uterine rupture,** the uterus itself tears and potentially spills its contents into the abdominal cavity (Figure 27-6 ■). This is frequently caused by trauma, but can occur as a result of

uterine rupture a tearing of the muscular wall of the uterus.

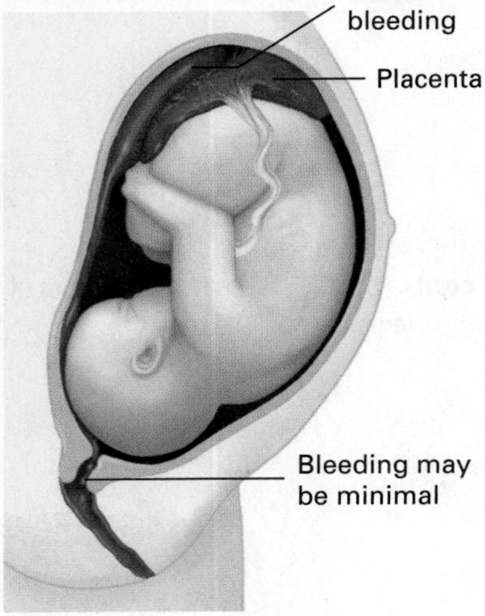

Figure 27-4 Abruptio placentae.

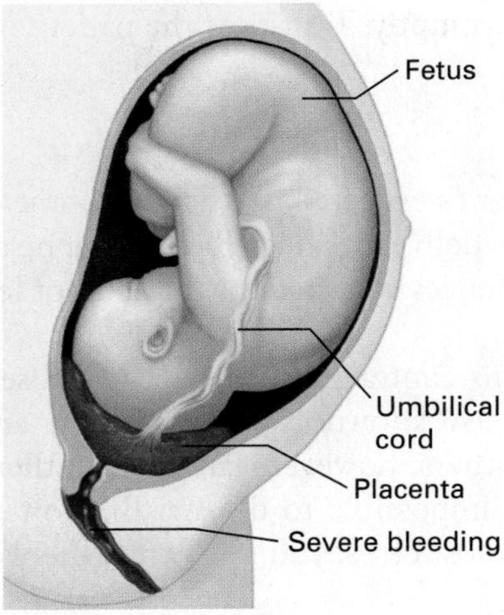

Figure 27-5 Placenta previa.

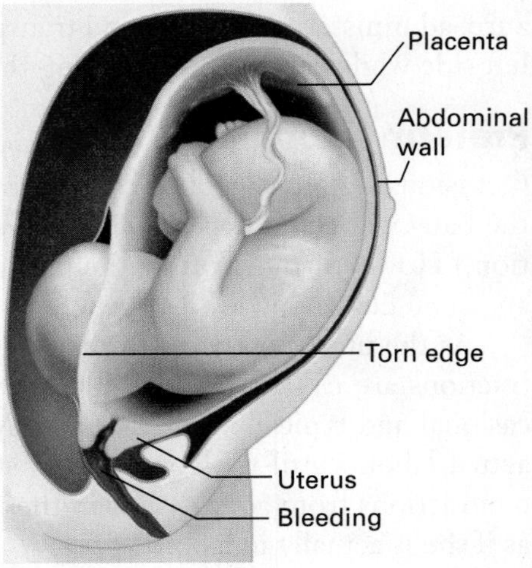

Figure 27-6 Uterine rupture.

childbirth. Signs of this condition include tearing pain, changes to the pregnant abdomen, and shock as a result of hemorrhage. The uterus is an incredibly vascular organ and when it is ruptured, bleeding is severe and life threatening. Prehospital care is generally limited to treating for shock and initiating immediate appropriate transport.

Trauma During Pregnancy

If you are called to a situation in which a pregnant patient has been injured, assess and treat the patient the same as you would any other trauma patient. However, you also must keep in mind some considerations that are unique to a pregnant patient. When the expectant mother has internal bleeding from trauma, she will cut off supply to the baby first as she begins to shunt blood to her own vital organs. The baby will be in distress long before the mother's vital signs will show distress.

Do not transport a third-trimester pregnant patient flat on her back. As mentioned in a prior section on supine hypotensive syndrome, this could cause a serious drop in blood pressure. Roll the breathing, non-spine-injured patient to her left side. If the patient is secured to a backboard, place a pillow under the right side of the backboard to displace the patient slightly to the left.

In the event of unstable injuries, or when resuscitation is futile, you may decide to perform CPR to provide some blood to the fetus on the way to the hospital where a **cesarean section** (C-section) may be performed to surgically remove the baby from the uterus.

cesarean section procedure that surgically removes the baby from the uterus. Also called a *C-section*.

PERSPECTIVE

The Boyfriend

I didn't know what to do. I mean, she never told me she was pregnant when we started going out. Then all of a sudden tonight, she starts acting like she's sick or hurt. She kept saying that she was fine. And then I thought she like wet herself or something. Then she said I needed to take her to a doctor right away. Man, I freaked out! All I could think of was getting her over to Rogers County Hospital. Now that I think about it, it probably wasn't the closest. But that's where I had my appendix out and I knew how to get there.

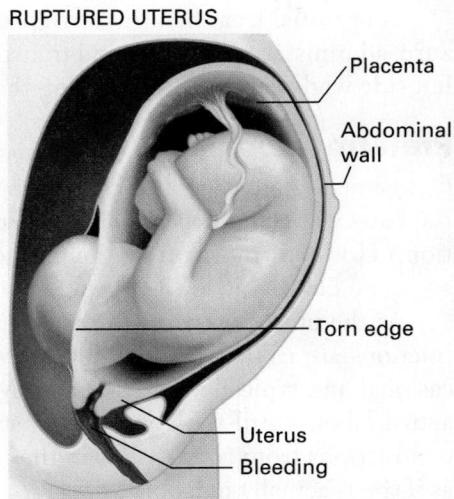

STOP, REVIEW, REMEMBER!

Multiple Choice

For each question, place a check next to the correct answer.

1. Which one of the following would be an expected change in a woman's body as a result of pregnancy?
   _____ a. Increased oxygen consumption
   _____ b. Increased capacity for air in her chest
   _____ c. Decreased blood volume
   _____ d. Decreased pulse rate

2. The female reproductive organ responsible for the production of the egg is called the:
   _____ a. uterus.
   _____ b. ovary.
   _____ c. fallopian tube.
   _____ d. cervix.

3. A 22-year-old woman presents with severe vaginal bleeding. You should:
   _____ a. insert a tampon into the vagina to stop the bleeding.
   _____ b. use an absorbent pad to collect the blood and then treat for shock.
   _____ c. perform an internal examination to determine the source of bleeding.
   _____ d. not cover the vagina but instead suggest a visit to a physician.

4. The condition in which the placenta prematurely pulls away from the wall of the uterus is called:
   _____ a. abruptio placentae.
   _____ b. placenta previa.
   _____ c. uterine rupture.
   _____ d. ectopic pregnancy.

5. A 29-year-old woman complains of acute onset lower right abdominal pain. She notes pain in her right shoulder also. She is awake and her vital signs are respiration 28, pulse 140, and blood pressure 86/60. These findings would most likely indicate:
   _____ a. abruptio placentae.
   _____ b. placenta previa.
   _____ c. uterine rupture.
   _____ d. ectopic pregnancy.

Short Answer

1. What is the EMT's emergency care for vaginal bleeding?

____

____

____

____

(continued on next page)

(continued)

2. Describe the changes in the reproductive system that occur during pregnancy.

3. Describe what happens in a spontaneous abortion.

Critical Thinking

1. You are caring for a woman who has been raped. She wishes to use the bathroom. What would you tell her?

2. Does care for trauma to the genitalia differ from soft-tissue injuries in other parts of the body? Why or why not?

Childbirth

27-6 Describe the stages of labor.

27-7 Describe the assessment-based approach to a patient in active labor with normal delivery.

27-8 Describe the steps of assisting with a normal prehospital delivery.

Labor is a term used to describe the process of childbirth. It is characterized by contractions of the uterus that cause pain and a sensation of pushing as the baby is delivered. This section of the chapter concentrates on normal, uncomplicated childbirth, including the stages of labor and the process of delivering a baby. Subsequent sections will explain complications you may see before, during, and after childbirth.

For the patient about to experience childbirth, it is important for you to consider the emotional needs of the patient and family. This is critical when a baby may be delivered in a location far from the planned hospital. If the mother or father is concerned about complications, or if the baby is a first delivery, or if previous pregnancies have ended tragically, the anxiety level will likely be exceptionally high. You must learn to remain calm, reassuring, and confident as you manage the birth of the child and care of the mother.

Because you will examine the mother for **crowning,** palpate the abdomen, and complete other tasks that are very personal, always consider the privacy of the mother during all phases of care. This is an emotional time for both mother and father. They need to be treated compassionately. Maintain a high level of professionalism as you complete the tasks associated with this situation. Carefully explain to both mother and father everything you do before you do it.

crowning refers to the baby's head becoming visible at the vaginal opening.

Childbirth is a natural process. In an uncomplicated delivery you will be there to assist the mother and other family members in delivering a new family member.

Stages of Labor

There are three stages of labor. The **first stage of labor** begins with the onset of contractions. The sensation (and pain) of contractions is felt as the uterus prepares for delivery. Typically, mild contractions begin well before birth and progress to more frequent, aggressive, and painful contractions as the delivery progresses. This process helps to dilate the cervix, preparing it to accommodate the large head of a newborn as it passes through. The first stage of labor continues until the cervix is fully dilated and ready for birth.

first stage of labor refers to the time of the beginning of uterine contractions until full dilation of the cervix.

The **second stage of labor** begins with full dilation of the cervix and continues through delivery of the baby (Figure 27-7 ■). Once the cervix is dilated, the contractions will intensify to move the baby through the birth canal. As this begins, the mother may report a feeling of having to push or to move her bowels. These sensations often indicate birth is imminent.

second stage of labor refers to the time of full dilation of the cervix until delivery of the baby.

Shortly after the baby is born, contractions will begin again. These contractions are to deliver the placenta. Resumption of contractions signals the start of the **third stage of labor** (Figure 27-8 ■), which will continue until the delivery of the placenta. This stage takes much less time than childbirth, often only 10 to 15 minutes and generally should not delay transport of the patient.

third stage of labor refers to the time from the birth of the baby until delivery of the placenta.

Assessment of a Woman in Labor

Assessment is a valuable tool when faced with a woman in labor. Not only will a thorough assessment help you identify potential life threats such as abruptio placentae and placenta previa, but it also will help you determine the most appropriate strategies to best treat your patient.

Stay or Go—The Transport Decision

Most patients make it to the hospital to deliver their baby. There are times when this does not happen. Some are related to logistics—anything from not having a ride to

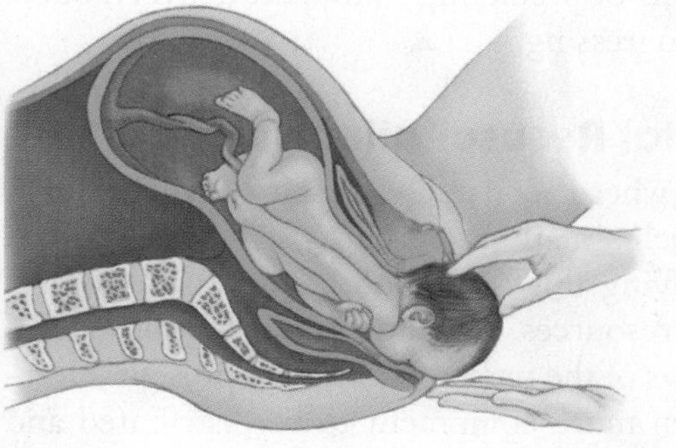

Figure 27-7 The second stage of labor involves the delivery of the baby.

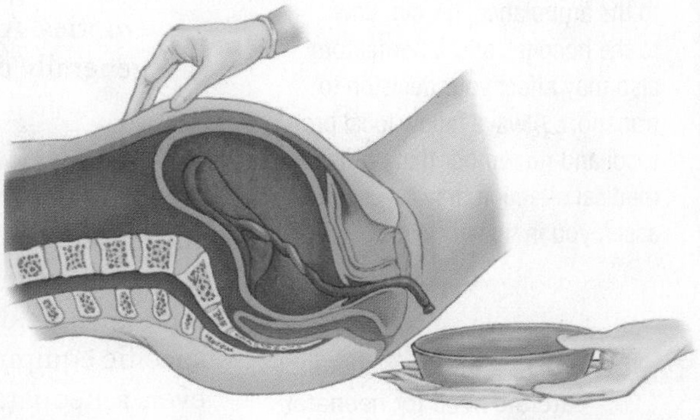

Figure 27-8 The third stage of labor involves the delivery of the placenta.

being stranded in a storm; others are caught by surprise when labor begins and progresses rapidly. A first delivery usually is a prolonged event. In subsequent pregnancies, labor will often be much shorter than a woman's first delivery. It is often women with their second, third, or fourth deliveries that are caught off guard by the speed at which their labor progresses and end up needing EMS assistance.

When possible, it is always best to deliver a baby in a hospital, but if you must deliver a baby in the field, it is probably better not to be in the back of an ambulance. There are times when you must make a decision as to whether you will have time to reach the hospital or whether you should stay in the house and deliver on scene. This decision must be based on any number of factors including distance, timing, and method of transport. Patient assessment and history can help you make this decision. Assessment can be used to help identify an imminent delivery and can point out those situations where staying in the house and preparing for delivery would be the best course of action. Assessment can identify life-threatening situations where immediate transport is indicated, regardless of when the baby will be delivered.

The following assessment elements will help you make an appropriate transport decision:

breech presentation refers to the buttocks or both lower extremities as the presenting part at the vaginal opening. Also called a *breech birth*.

presenting part the part of the baby that first becomes visible at the vaginal opening.

- Are there any known complications? Problems such as placenta previa and a **breech presentation** should not be handled in the field. Anticipation of such issues indicates immediate transport.
- Is the fetus crowning? Crowning is an absolute sign of imminent delivery. It occurs as the **presenting part** of the baby becomes visible at the vaginal opening. The patient also may note that she feels the baby has "dropped" or feels the baby's head. In a vast majority of cases the presenting part is the head (crowning will show the top of the scalp first), but it may be the buttocks (breech presentation) or an extremity (limb presentation). Breech and limb presentations are complications (discussed later in the chapter) that generally require immediate transport to a hospital where obstetrical services are available.
- Does the mother feel the urge to push? Does she feel like she needs to move her bowels? Either of those findings can indicate an imminent delivery.
- Is the patient having contractions or pain? Contractions generally grow in intensity and frequency as delivery becomes imminent. Measuring the time between contractions to predict delivery is frequently inaccurate, but can be helpful because generally the timing between contractions shortens as delivery draws near.
- How many times previously has the patient given birth? Although this is not always true, typically each successive delivery will take less time. Was the previous delivery fast? This can help predict how long the current delivery will take.
- Did the water break? The breaking of the amniotic sac (also known as the *rupture of membranes*) generally occurs close to delivery. The mother will often identify a discharge of sometimes bloody fluid and often feels a trickle or gush as the sac empties. Again, this is not exact in terms of predicting imminent delivery, but it generally does indicate that labor is progressing.

CLINICAL CLUE

Stay or Go?

The best tactic in an imminent delivery is to stay in place and deliver on scene. Although there are some situations such as breech presentations that indicate immediate transport, it is far easier to handle a delivery (and in the worst case scenario a neonatal resuscitation) on scene than in the back of an ambulance. Distance to the ambulance, terrain, time to the hospital, and other factors also may affect your decision to transport. Always follow local protocol and remember that on-line medical direction may be used to assist you in this decision.

Predicting the Need for Neonatal Resuscitation

27-14 Describe the signs that indicate the need for neonatal resuscitation.

Assessment can help you identify situations where neonatal resuscitation will be likely. Although it is impossible to identify all such situations, certain assessment findings make resuscitation more probable. Identifying this likelihood helps you make better transport decisions and better allocate resources. Usually, childbirth will require specific equipment and will tap the resources of the personnel who are present. However, a neonatal resuscitation requires even more equipment to be distributed and ready and will likely require additional personnel to be called to the scene.

The following assessment findings can indicate a likely resuscitation:

- ***Premature birth.*** Always ask a woman how long she has been pregnant. Pregnancy is considered to begin at the time of the patient's last menstrual period. The earlier the delivery, the more likely a resuscitation will need to occur. Depending on your local resources, a pregnancy is considered viable (that is, developed to a point where the baby can survive outside the womb) after around 20 to 23 weeks.
- ***Lack of prenatal care.*** Pregnant patients generally see an obstetrician for a series of appointments prior to giving birth. This prenatal care identifies a great deal of important information, from the presence of multiple babies to complications such as breech presentations and placenta previa. A lack of prenatal care creates an unknown environment. Therefore, resuscitation should be anticipated.
- ***Multiple birth.*** Twins, triplets, or more (also known as *multiple gestations*) make resuscitation far more likely. The potential of a **multiple birth** indicates a serious consideration for resuscitation preparation.
- ***Known complications.*** You should ask your patient if she is aware of any complications to her pregnancy. Complications can include actual problems with the pregnancy such as placenta previa or breech presentation, but may include associated complications such as pregnancy-induced hypertension, diabetes, or even preeclampsia. Complications increase the likelihood of resuscitation.
- ***Trauma.*** Labor induced by trauma or medical conditions affecting the mother make the likelihood of resuscitation very high.

multiple birth delivery of more than one baby. Also called *multiple gestations.*

Resuscitation can never be fully predicted and you should always be ready. However, when assessment indicates a high likelihood, you should take appropriate steps to prepare before the baby comes. Consider readying equipment and requesting additional personnel. A likelihood of resuscitation may impact your transport decision. Stay-or-go and destination decisions can all be affected by the probability of resuscitation.

Preparation for Delivery

There are several things to do to prepare for a delivery in the field. The first is to use appropriate personal protective equipment. That includes gloves, face protection, and protection for your clothes (gown). Childbirth can expose you to a variety of potentially infectious fluids including amniotic fluid and blood.

The mother will likely choose to lie on her back with her knees drawn up and spread apart. Using materials from your obstetrics (OB) kit (Figure 27-9 ■), cover or drape the mother's legs and place a towel or clean cloth under her buttocks. This setting will create a sterile (or clean) field in which you will deliver the baby. (Table 27-1 lists the contents of a typical OB kit.)

Also prepare a bag-mask device of an appropriate neonatal size in case resuscitation is necessary. Consider a means to keep the **neonate** warm. Ask yourself: Do you have enough blankets or towels to dry and then wrap the newborn baby? Think of the ambient temperature. The warmer you can make the environment, the less likely the neonate will lose heat after birth.

neonate newborn infant up to one month of age.

Remember the stress the mother will feel in an unexpected home or other non-hospital delivery. She and her family may have wanted a birth with their obstetrician in a planned setting. The delivery at home is stressful, and may be frightening and frustrating. Be sure to continuously reassure and communicate calmly with the mother and any other family present throughout the preparation, delivery, and transport after delivery. While you do not want to frighten the family or render medical

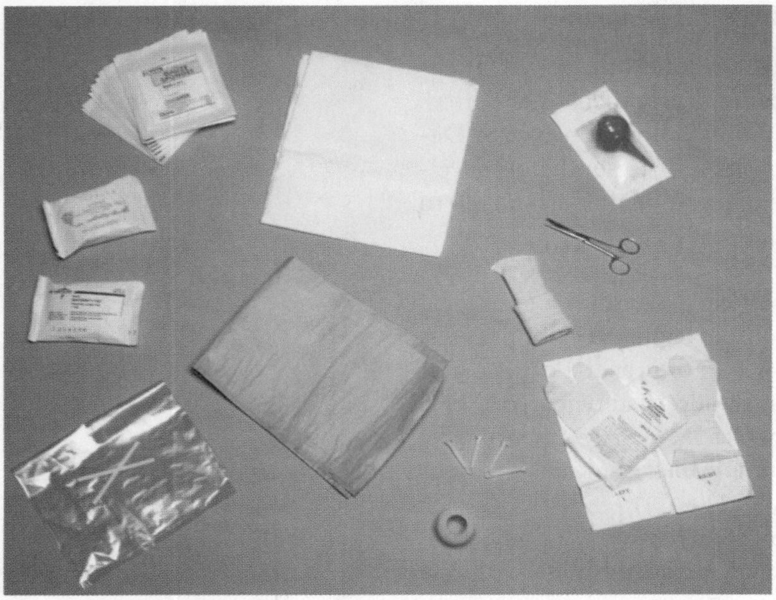

Figure 27-9 The contents of a typical field obstetrics (OB) kit.

TABLE 27-1	TYPICAL CONTENTS OF THE OBSTETRICS (OB) KIT

- Sterile gloves
- Towels or drapes
- Scissors (to cut the cord)
- Clamps for the umbilical cord
- Large gauze pads or sponges
- Bulb syringe (for suction)
- A blanket for the baby
- Sanitary napkins
- Plastic bag (for transportation of the placenta)

decisions, if the birth is not progressing well, refrain from promising that the baby will be all right. Say nothing you cannot guarantee to be true, and do not unnecessarily predict problems.

CLINICAL CLUE

Warm Is Good

The most common complication of prehospital delivery is that the neonate becomes cold (hypothermia). When preparing for delivery in the ambulance, a critical step is to turn up the patient compartment heat to provide a warm environment for the coming delivery. After the baby is delivered, drying the neonate, placing him in a dry wrap, and placing a cap on his head will be additional steps to take to prevent hypothermia.

Delivery

Complete the preparation described in this chapter when possible. However, sometimes that is not possible. You could be called to a woman who is delivering at the moment you arrive on scene. In that situation, you will be required to deliver the baby without the drapes and positioning discussed earlier. The following steps will guide you through the principles of most delivery situations (Scan 27-1):

1. Take the appropriate BSI precautions, including a gown if available.
2. Place the patient in a position lying on her back with her knees drawn up and spread apart.
3. Observe the vaginal area. Do not touch this area or do any sort of physical exam of the external or internal **genitalia.**
4. When the head becomes visible (crowning), delivery is imminent. Place gentle pressure with your gloved hand on the infant's head to prevent an explosive birth. Avoid placing pressure on the infant's **anterior fontanels** and face (Figure 27-10 ■).

genitalia male or female reproductive organs.

anterior fontanels soft spots lying between the cranial bones.

SCAN 27-1 Assisting with a Normal Delivery

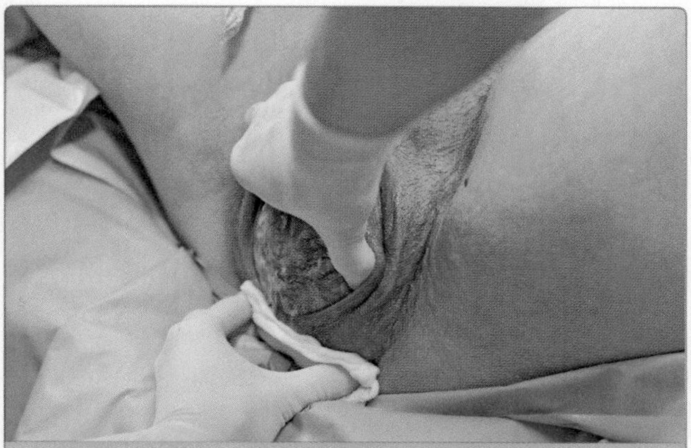

27-1-1 Crowning is evident as the head emerges from the vagina.

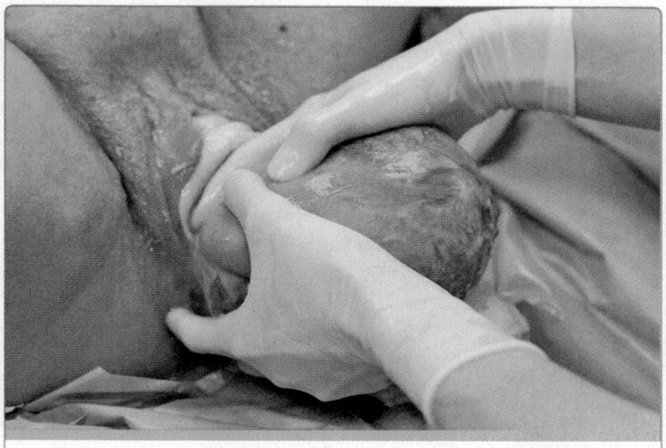

27-1-2 Support the head with both hands as it is delivered and check the neck for the presence of the umbilical cord (nuchal cord).

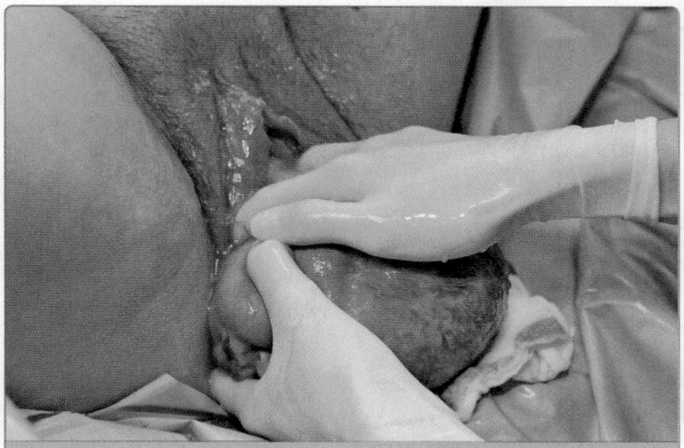

27-1-3 Guide the baby's head downward to facilitate the delivery of the upper shoulder.

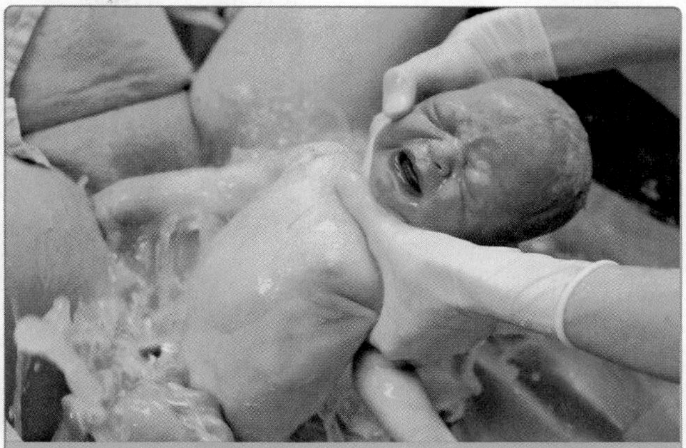

27-1-4 Use both hands to support the baby following delivery.

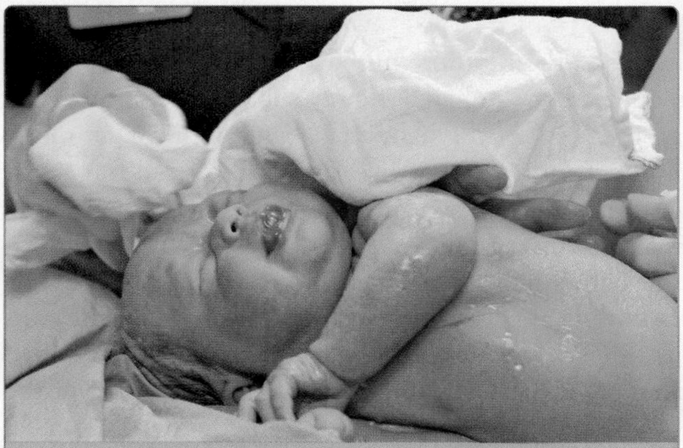

27-1-5 Carefully dry the baby and cover him to conserve heat.

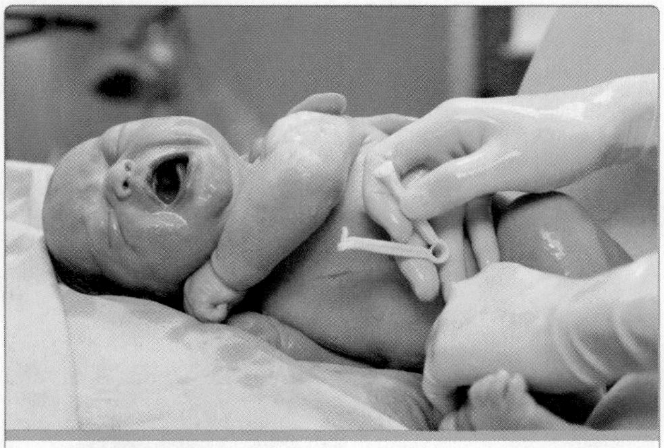

27-1-6 Wait at least one minute before clamping the cord.

(Continued)

SCAN 27-1 Assisting with a Normal Delivery (*Cont.*)

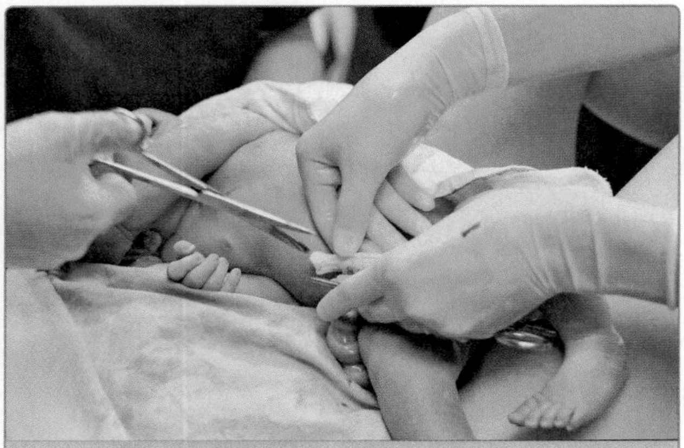

27-1-7 Cut the cord between the clamps.

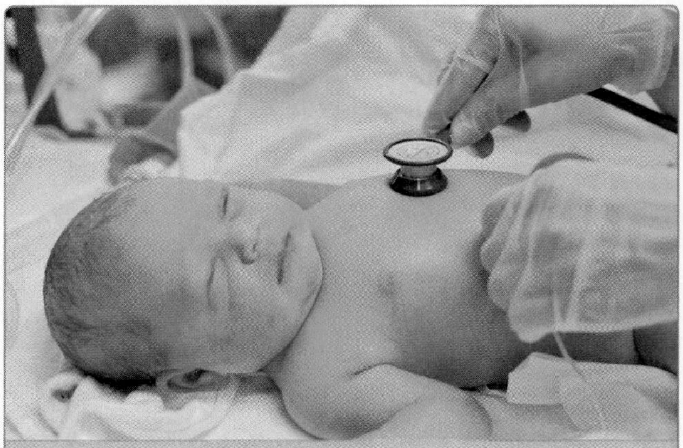

27-1-8 Assess breathing and pulse rate to ensure they are within normal limits.

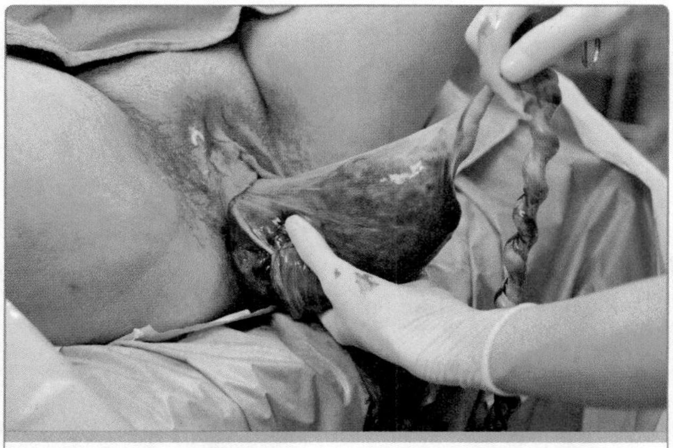

27-1-9 Expect delivery of the placenta within 20 to 30 minutes following the delivery of the baby.

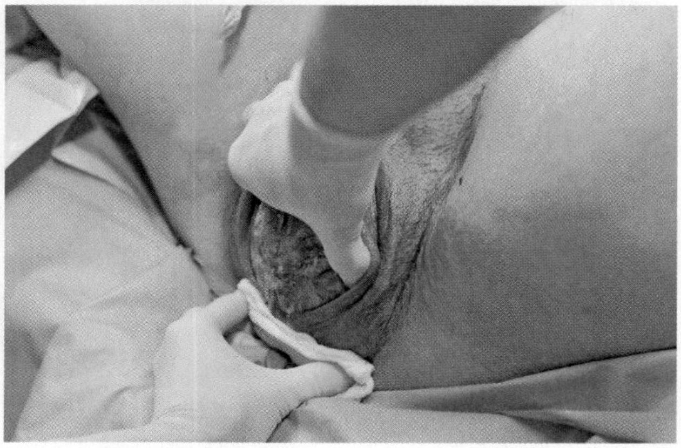

Figure 27-10 Use a gloved hand to place gentle pressure on the top of the baby's head to help control the delivery.

5. In many cases, the mother will have reported that her "water broke" or that she had a **bloody show.** Other times, you will find the head of the baby delivering with the amniotic sac still intact. In the latter case, use your gloved fingers or a clamp to rupture the sac and pull it way from the infant's face. Expect a rush of fluid.
6. After the baby's head is delivered, observe the neck to be sure the umbilical cord is not wrapped around it. This condition is called *nuchal cord*, and if it is present there are two options. First, if there is enough cord, gently slip it over the baby's head. (That will be the easiest remedy to most nuchal cords.) Second, if the cord is not long enough to slip over the head and threatens to tighten around the neck, carefully clamp the cord by placing two clamps three to four inches apart. Then cut the cord between the clamps.

7. The shoulders, torso, and remainder of the baby will come out a bit more rapidly than the head. Be prepared to support the infant. Hold him or her carefully and securely. Remember, the infant will be very slippery.
8. Once the neonate is born, assess the airway. Although most active babies will not require suctioning, for some it will be necessary. Suctioning will be important if positive pressure ventilations are necessary or if secretions threaten the airway or obstruct normal breathing.

   To suction, hold the baby's head slightly lower than the torso to allow drainage with gravity. Compress the syringe and then carefully insert the tip of the syringe into the baby's mouth. Then release the bulb to allow fluids to be drawn into the syringe. Control the release with your fingers. Withdraw the tip and discharge the syringe's contents onto a towel. Suction the mouth first, then the nostrils and repeat the procedure as necessary. The tip of the syringe should not be inserted more than one-half inch into the baby's nostril.
9. Document the time of birth. Hospitals consider this important information for birth records. Do not stop caring for the child while you make note of the time.
10. Keep the neonate warm. Heat loss is a significant issue to the health of the baby. Turn up the heat in the room or in the ambulance. Dry the infant to prevent heat loss and wrap the infant in dry blankets. Do not use the wet blankets to wrap the neonate. Be sure the baby's head is covered. One member of your crew should be responsible for your second patient, the mother.
11. Monitor both patients after the birth for changes in condition.
12. Transport. If the mother will hold the newborn, have her hold the neonate on her upper abdomen and encourage the mother to begin breast feeding. This will help the neonate retain body heat and promote contraction of the uterus in the mother. Know your local protocols for transporting a neonate. Always follow local guidelines.
13. At some point after delivery of the infant, often in a half hour or less, the placenta will deliver. Watch for it while preparing for and during transport.
14. When the placenta delivers, wrap it in a towel and place it in a plastic bag from your OB kit.
15. Place a sterile pad over the mother's vagina and have her lower her legs.

bloody show refers to the amniotic sac rupturing early in labor; an initial discharge of blood and mucus at the beginning of labor.

Cutting the Umbilical Cord

In most cases cutting the umbilical cord should be a relatively low priority and there is no rush to complete this task. The need for resuscitation or a cord wrapped around the neck may require immediate cutting, but in general there is little urgent need to do so. In a normal birth, the infant must be breathing on his own before you clamp and cut the cord. Additionally, there is increasing evidence that you should wait at least one minute after birth before clamping and cutting the cord unless there is a need for resuscitation.

Before clamping and cutting the cord, palpate the cord with your fingers to make sure it is no longer pulsating. Pulsation typically stops shortly after delivery. *Do not tie, clamp, or cut the cord of a baby who is not breathing on his own unless you have to do so to remove the cord from around the baby's neck during birth, or unless you have to perform CPR on the infant. Do not cut or clamp a cord that is still pulsating.*

If you need to cut the cord, use the sterile clamps or umbilical tape found in the OB kit. Apply one clamp or tie to the cord about six inches from the baby (Figure 27-11 ■). This leaves enough cord for an intravenous line to be placed by hospital staff, if it is needed. Place a second clamp or tie about two inches from the first. The proximal clamp should be about the width of four fingers from the distal clamp.

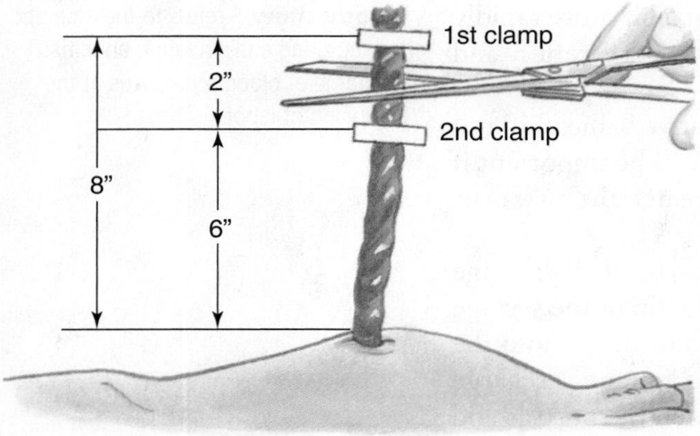

Figure 27-11 Cutting the umbilical cord.

Cut the cord between the clamps or knots using sterile scissors or a scalpel from the OB kit. Use caution and protect your eyes when cutting the cord because a spurt of blood is very common. Never untie or unclamp a cord once it is cut. Examine the fetal end of the cord for bleeding. Do not attempt to adjust the clamp or retie the knot. If bleeding continues, apply another tie or clamp as close to the original as possible. Be careful when moving the baby so that no trauma is brought to the clamped cord. If the cord does not remain closed off completely, the baby may bleed to death from seemingly little blood loss. In most cases, the cord vessels will collapse and seal themselves.

If an OB kit is not available, most of the items needed to cut a cord can be improvised. If no clamps or tying devices are on hand, use clean shoelaces or similar soft, clean ties. Use standard scissors soaked in alcohol or boiling water to cut the cord. Remember that in most cases there is no absolute need to cut the cord.

STOP, REVIEW, REMEMBER!

Multiple Choice

For each question, place a check next to the correct answer.

1. Which one of the following would most likely indicate an imminent birth?

_____ a. Contractions less than five minutes apart

_____ b. The mother stating an urge to push

_____ c. A first pregnancy or delivery

_____ d. Multiple gestations

2. The average pregnancy lasts about _____________ weeks.

_____ a. 25–27

_____ b. 30–32

_____ c. 34–36

_____ d. 38–42

3. The second stage of labor is best defined as:

_____ a. conception to the time actual contractions begin.

_____ b. from the time contractions begin until full dilation of the cervix.

_____ c. from full dilation of the cervix to delivery of the baby.

_____ d. delivery of the baby until expulsion of the placenta.

4. The term *crowning* is defined as:

_____ a. the unusual shape of the head seen in newborns immediately after delivery.

_____ b. the soft spot on the baby's head.

_____ c. when the head becomes visible at the vagina.

_____ d. suctioning the mouth and nose before the baby's shoulder delivers.

5. A 35-year-old pregnant woman states that she is in labor. She notes that she feels the urge to push and that she feels like she needs to move her bowels. You should:

_____ a. initiate immediate transport and leave evaluation to the hospital staff.

_____ b. initiate immediate transport and evaluate the perineum en route.

_____ c. delay transport and prepare for an imminent delivery.

_____ d. allow the patient to use the bathroom and then complete your assessment.

Sorting

Write a 1, 2, or 3 by each of the following events to represent the correct stage of labor.

1. ______________ Uterine contractions have begun.
2. ______________ The placenta is being delivered.
3. ______________ The mother has a feeling of having to move her bowels.
4. ______________ The baby is being delivered.
5. ______________ Contractions intensify as the baby moves through the birth canal.
6. ______________ The cervix is partially dilated.

Critical Thinking

1. You are questioning your pregnant patient, who is in labor. List five questions that can influence your care or decision making regarding transport or predicting complications.

____

____

____

____

____

2. List three things to do in preparation for delivery.

____

____

____

____

PERSPECTIVE

Mark—The EMT

Holy Toledo! I can't believe we delivered a baby! That was amazing. Wow! At first I was really scared though. You know, one thing they never told me in school is that newborns look kind of dead. I mean, that baby came out and it was gray and purple and just covered with blood and stuff. And it didn't move. It just looked like a rubber doll in Ling's hands. But once she started stimulating it—him—he just came alive, crying and turning pink. That was amazing. Just amazing.

Post-Delivery Care

Emergency childbirth requires the care of two patients. Most births are exciting but do not pose critical problems for the mother or neonate. If there are complications with mother or baby, you will find yourself and your crew busy with two patients. This is why it is so important to evaluate the need for additional resources early. Use assessment to help you predict the need for resuscitation and get resources moving before you need them. If there are no problems or complications, the mother and baby can be transported together. In the event of complications or when resuscitation is necessary, a second crew (ALS if available) will transport one patient separately.

Care of the Neonate

27-13 Demonstrate the steps of assessing and managing the newborn, including initial care (drying, wrapping, suctioning, and positioning) and Apgar scoring.

A newborn infant, also called a *neonate*, requires immediate care after birth. This care is centered around clearing the airway if necessary, drying, and warming the newborn. Heat loss is very dangerous to neonates. Their thermoregulatory systems have not fully developed and as a result, they have a great deal of difficulty maintaining normal body temperature. Hypothermia is a great risk. Since heat can be lost very quickly in the exposed, wet neonate, it takes only a few minutes for hypothermia to develop. Prevent evaporative heat loss by drying the baby and wrapping him in dry blankets. Heat loss can occur at an accelerated pace from the head, so it is important to keep the top of the baby's head lightly covered.

As you examine the neonate, reassess the airway. If fluids pose a risk to breathing due to obstruction of the airway, suction may be important.

After assessing and suctioning the airway, drying, and warming, evaluate the neonate. Many EMS systems have adopted a specific evaluation protocol, so always follow local guidelines. A general evaluation usually assesses the neonate's breathing, heart rate, crying, movement, and skin color. A normal neonate should have a pulse greater than 100 per minute and be breathing easily, crying (vigorous crying is a good sign), moving his extremities (the more active, the better), and showing blue coloration only at the hands and feet. Five minutes later, these signs should still be apparent, with breathing becoming more relaxed. The blue coloration may linger, but it should not spread to other parts of the body.

Apgar score system for evaluating a newborn's physical condition.

The **Apgar score** is a specific evaluation tool that many EMS systems use. An Apgar score assigns a number value to the neonate's assessment findings. However, it does not guide resuscitation efforts, and efforts to determine the Apgar score must never interfere with more important resuscitation efforts. The Apgar score is the total of five values, and ranges from 0 to 10 (Table 27-2). It is usually determined one minute after birth and then again five minutes after birth.

If your assessment of the newborn reveals inadequate breathing or pulse, you must immediately provide the indicated care. Fortunately, this is rare. In the case of

TABLE 27-2 THE APGAR SCORING SYSTEM

SIGN	0	1	2
Heart rate	Absent	Slow; less than 100 beats/min	Greater than 100 beats/min
Respiration	Absent	Slow; irregular	Good breathing with crying
Muscle tone	Flaccid	Some flexion of extremities	Active movement of extremities
Reflex response	Absent	Grimace; noticeable facial movement	Vigorous cry; coughs; sneezes; pulls away when touched
Skin color	Pale or blue	Pink body, blue extremities	Pink body and extremities

Source: Data from Apgar, V. (1966). The newborn (Apgar) scoring system, reflections and advice. http://profiles.nlm.nih.gov/ps/access/CPBBJY.pdf

inadequate breathing, the simplest actions (such as drying and warming) typically are enough to stimulate active breathing. Of course this is not always the case, and in some situations you will need to move to more aggressive actions such as ventilations with an appropriate bag-mask device.

Neonatal Resuscitation

The steps of neonatal resuscitation are guided by the **inverted pyramid** (Figure 27-12 ▪). The most common and least invasive techniques are listed at the wide top of the diagram. As you move down the steps in the pyramid, more invasive steps to resuscitate the newborn are presented. Some of these steps are ALS procedures. If needed, be sure to request ALS early to the scene or as an intercept.

27-15 Apply the concepts of the neonatal resuscitation pyramid to the care of neonates in need of resuscitative measures.

inverted pyramid a graphic that illustrates the types and frequency of care given to the neonate at birth.

If a neonate is not breathing, your first step is to stimulate him. You can do this by gently flicking the soles of his feet or by rubbing his back (Figure 27-13 ▪). Many times just drying and warming the baby will be enough to stimulate him to breathe. If that does not work, you must move on to the next step of resuscitation.

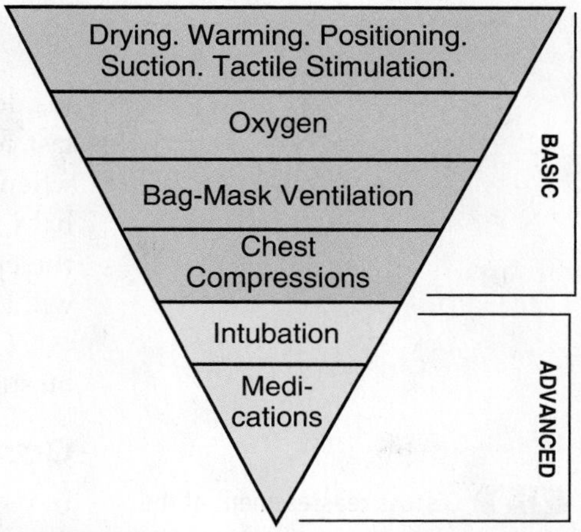

Figure 27-12 The inverted pyramid of neonatal resuscitation.

If breathing has not begun or if breathing appears slow or shallow, begin ventilating the newborn. Use a neonatal bag-mask device with small volumes of air at a rate of 40 to 60 per minute. *Ventilate the neonate only enough to gain chest rise.* Overinflation or ventilations that are too fast will cause air to enter the newborn's stomach and actually interfere with breathing. Reassess the infant's respiratory efforts after 30 seconds. If there is no change in the effort of breathing, continue with ventilations and reassessment. It is not necessary to attach supplemental oxygen to the bag-mask device during neonatal resuscitation. Use room air to deliver the initial ventilations. Consider supplemental oxygen only if oxygen saturations remain low following the resuscitation.

Next, evaluate the pulse. Listen to the heart with a stethoscope placed near the left nipple. If the heart rate is less than 100 beats per minute, then continue to provide artificial ventilations at a rate of 40 to 60 per minute. If the heart rate is less than 60 beats per minute, regardless of the breathing status, then initiate chest compressions. The two-thumb-encircling-hands method is recommended in CPR for neonates.

Chest compressions should be applied with two thumbs over the lower third of the sternum and should be delivered at a rate of at least 100 compressions per minute. Use the fingers to support the neonate's back. The depth of compression is one-third of the anterior-posterior depth of the chest. Breaths should be delivered at a ratio of 30:2 for a single rescuer and 15:2 for two rescuers. Care should be taken to allow full recoil of the chest following compression.

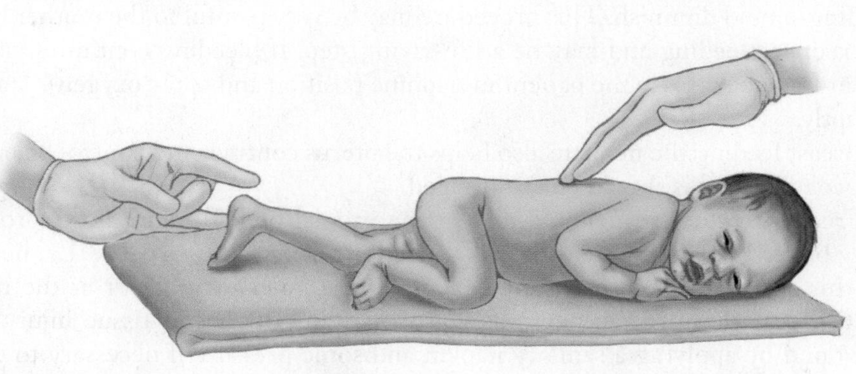

Figure 27-13 Stimulate the baby to breathe by rubbing the back or flicking the bottoms of the feet.

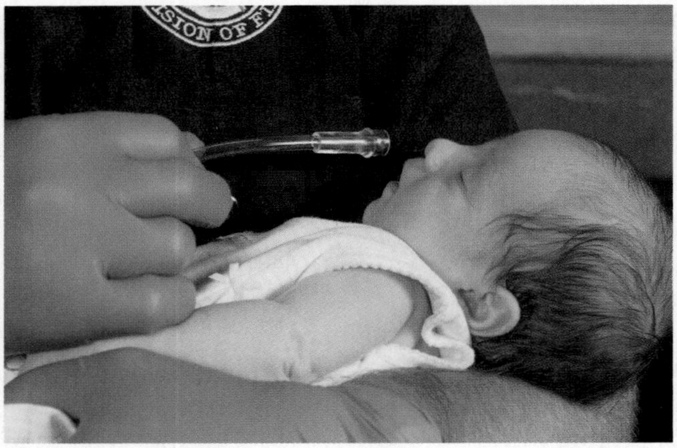

Figure 27-14 Use the end of oxygen tubing to provide blow-by oxygen if the baby shows signs of hypoxia.

After 30 seconds, reevaluate the neonate. If the newborn begins to have more rapid, adequate breathing and a pulse above 100, you should stop compressions. If there is no response to your previous steps, continue chest compressions and ventilations.

Suction the airway if needed and consider oxygen administration. Supplemental oxygen should be administered if cyanosis persists or if oxygen saturation remains low more than 10 minutes after birth. Oxygen is best delivered by placing the end of an oxygen tube close to, but not directly into the infant's face (Figure 27-14 ■). This will ensure a more "blended" mixture of air and oxygen.

When a baby is born, it may take up to 30 seconds for breathing to begin as he adjusts to his non-fluid-filled world. It is also common for a baby to have a pink torso but pale or blue extremities initially. For dark-skinned infants observe the inside of the mouth, palms of the hands, and nail beds for color changes. This should last for only a few minutes. Remember that the extremities will become pink only when oxygenated blood reaches them, and that takes a few moments to occur. The baby should gradually become pink from its core body outward to the extremities. If the cyanosis does not clear up or if it spreads, ventilations and possibly compressions will be required.

Consider heat loss when resuscitating a neonate. To prevent loss to a cold surface, be sure to place blankets or towels under the infant.

Care of the Mother

27-9 Discuss reassessment of the postpartum patient.

27-12 Describe the management of postpartum complications, including postpartum hemorrhage and embolism.

In most cases, mothers who have just given birth need only supportive care. However, dangerous complications can develop, such as serious bleeding, infection, and emboli.

Post-Delivery Bleeding

One of the most common problems with the post-delivery mother is excessive bleeding. Some bleeding after birth is common and may seem excessive the first time you observe a delivery. As much as 500 mL is considered normal. This may look like quite a bit, especially in conjunction with amniotic fluid that also will be present. Usually, bleeding ceases shortly after delivery but sometimes bleeding continues, causing hypovolemia and shock.

If blood loss is excessive, massage the mother's uterus. To do so, first open your hand and fingers. Place your hand around the uterus. It will likely feel like a pronounced grapefruit-size area on the mother's abdomen above the pubic bone. Use a kneading motion over this area. The uterus should contract and become firm, and the bleeding should diminish. This procedure may be very painful to the mother but will help reduce bleeding and may be a life-saving step. If bleeding continues, treat the patient for shock (place the patient in a supine position and apply oxygen). Transport promptly.

Breast feeding the neonate also helps the uterus contract and control bleeding. If protocol allows, this should be encouraged.

Frequently, the perineum is torn at the vaginal opening during the process of giving birth. The mother may feel the discomfort from this torn tissue. Let her know that this is normal and that the problem will be quickly cared for at the medical facility. Treat the torn perineum as you would any other soft-tissue injury. Dress the wound by applying a sanitary napkin and some pressure if necessary to control bleeding.

Post-Delivery Embolism

An embolism occurs when air or a solid object is transported in the bloodstream and eventually obstructs blood flow. The post-delivery state creates a period of high risk for embolisms. Hypercoagulation occurs in the body, causing enhanced clotting. Amniotic fluid also can mix with maternal blood vessels as the placenta separates from the uterus. Both of these factors create a risk for developing emboli.

Emboli become very dangerous when they obstruct vessels in the lungs (pulmonary embolism) or in the brain (stroke). Although pulmonary emboli are rare in **postpartum** women (it is estimated that about 1 in 1,000 deliveries will develop an embolism and most will be asymptomatic), they can cause a life-threatening condition. Your evaluation of the postpartum woman must recognize signs and symptoms that indicate this condition. In a pulmonary embolism, blood is obstructed in a portion of the lung. As blood can no longer reach the alveoli, gas exchange is affected. Therefore, the key symptom is acute onset shortness of breath. As lung tissue becomes ischemic, chest pain usually develops as well. In severe cases you may see profound hypoxia and shock.

postpartum refers to the mother and the period of time beginning immediately following the birth of the child.

Pulmonary emboli require immediate transport. Supplemental oxygen is appropriate as well.

PERSPECTIVE

The Highway Patrolman

It's surprising how many people will fake an illness or a pregnancy or something to try to get out of a speeding ticket. The stories that I got after 15 years on the job are unbelievable! But sometimes they're for real. Like that girl today. I was at the births of three of my five kids, and while you'll never catch me claiming to be some sort of medical expert, I just knew that poor kid in the pickup was in serious trouble.

Complications During Delivery

Complications during delivery can be serious, life-threatening emergencies and may require immediate intervention to preserve the lives of both the mother and the baby. Often these complications cannot be managed in the field and may require rapid transport to an appropriate facility.

27-10 Describe the assessment-based approach to a patient in active labor with abnormal delivery.

27-11 Describe the management of abnormal prehospital obstetric deliveries, including breech and limb presentations, meconium staining, multiple births, post-term pregnancy, precipitous delivery, premature birth, premature rupture of membranes, preterm labor, prolapsed umbilical cord, and shoulder dystocia.

Precipitous Delivery

Precipitous delivery occurs when birth progresses too rapidly. Although precipitous delivery is not really a complication, risks to the mother do exist. Abnormally fast delivery can lead to tearing of the perineum and damage to the birth canal. This type of delivery is common in women who have had multiple other children, but it can occur in any delivery. EMS providers can prevent explosive deliveries by placing a gloved hand on the presenting scalp of the neonate as it emerges from the birth canal. Although you should not attempt to impede progress, gentle pressure can help prevent tearing.

Prolapsed Cord

Prolapsed cord (Figure 27-15 ■) is a presentation in which the umbilical cord enters the birth canal before the baby's head. This creates an extremely serious condition in which the baby's head (or other presenting part) blocks blood flow through the cord, which cuts off the baby's supply of oxygen and nutrients.

prolapsed cord refers to the umbilical cord entering the birth canal before the baby's head.

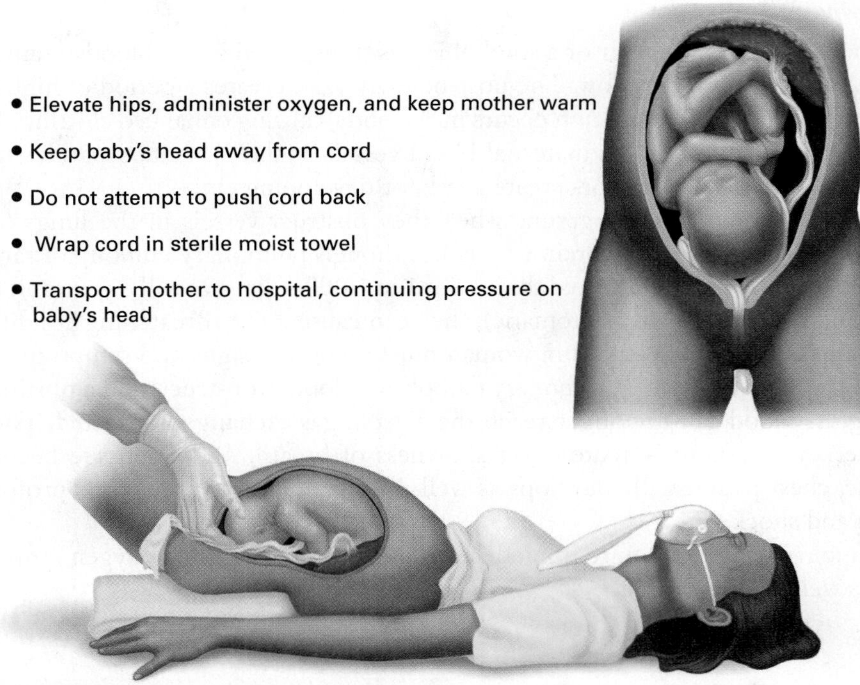
• Elevate hips, administer oxygen, and keep mother warm
• Keep baby's head away from cord
• Do not attempt to push cord back
• Wrap cord in sterile moist towel
• Transport mother to hospital, continuing pressure on baby's head

Figure 27-15 Prolapsed cord.

In addition to your normal scene size-up, assessments, and vital signs, you should observe the vagina of a woman in labor. With a prolapsed cord, you will note that the umbilical cord is visible.

Emergency care for prolapsed cord will include placing the mother in a position in which gravity helps to take pressure off the umbilical cord. Frequently this is a supine position with her head lower than her hips or the mother on her hands and knees. You will need to insert your gloved hand into the vagina to gently push the baby's head back away from the cord. This is the only exception to the rule that you never insert your hand or any item into the vagina. If possible, insert fingers on each side of the neonate's mouth and nose and split your fingers into a "V" shape to create an opening.

When you insert your gloved hand into the vagina and move the head off the umbilical cord, you should feel pulsations return to the cord. You must maintain this position throughout your care and transport until you arrive at the hospital. Monitor the cord frequently to ensure that pulsations are present.

PRACTICAL PATHOPHYSIOLOGY

Although it is a fairly rare complication (less than 1% of deliveries), a prolapsed umbilical cord is the cause of many neonatal deaths each year. It is important to understand the pathophysiology behind this complication.

In the uterus, the fetus relies on the umbilical cord for a supply of oxygen, nutrients, and for removal of waste products such as carbon dioxide. In certain delivery situations the cord can emerge prior to the baby, causing impingement and obstruction of blood flow. This can be a disastrous complication for the fetus because if blood flow is truly obstructed, no oxygen can reach the baby's system. Hypoxia ensues and death will occur if not rapidly corrected. There are many risk factors for this complication including prematurity, excessive amniotic fluid, and breech presentations. Providers should be vigilant to guard against this issue and rapid in their response to it if found.

Breech Presentation

Breech presentation, or breech birth (Figure 27-16 ■), occurs when the buttocks or both lower extremities are the presenting part. If the mother has received prenatal care and **ultrasound** imaging during her pregnancy, she may be aware that this is expected.

If you observe a breech presentation, prepare for transportation immediately. Place the mother in a position in which the hips are higher than her head. Administer supplemental oxygen. Do not wait for delivery.

The mother is at a higher risk of prolapsed cord in a breech presentation. If a prolapsed cord is observed, insert your gloved hand into the vagina and lift the baby off the cord until pulsations of the cord resume.

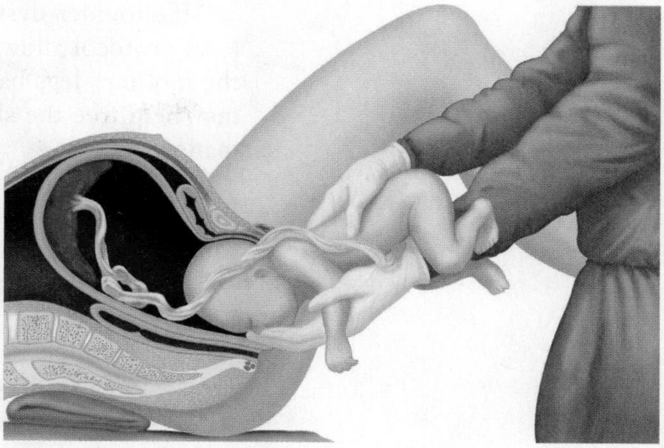

Figure 27-16 Breech presentation.

If delivery does occur—and it may—use the steps listed earlier for a normal delivery, and guide the baby's body as it delivers. Remember that in this case the head will be last. Support the torso while awaiting delivery of the head. Care for the baby as you would in a normal delivery. Never pull on the legs to stimulate delivery.

ultrasound an examination technique that uses sound to produce a visual image.

Limb Presentation

A **limb presentation** (Figure 27-17 ■) occurs when a single limb presents first from the birth canal. This condition is more serious than when two legs or feet are visible. It is not likely that the baby will deliver, and prompt transportation to the hospital is necessary, preferably one that can handle complications of pregnancy and delivery.

limb presentation refers to a single limb presenting at the vaginal opening.

As with other complications of delivery, place the mother in a Trendelenburg position and administer supplemental oxygen. Never pull on an exposed limb to facilitate delivery or for any other reason.

Shoulder Dystocia

Shoulder dystocia occurs when the shoulder of the neonate is obstructed by the mother's pelvis. Effectively, progress is stopped as the shoulder is pinned. This will be evident when you see the head partially delivered but further delivery does not progress. You may note the "turtle sign" in that the baby's head will partially emerge during contractions and then withdraw back into the birth canal upon relaxation. This condition can be extremely dangerous to the baby because often the umbilical cord is impinged by the baby's body in the birth canal. Hypoxia can develop rapidly.

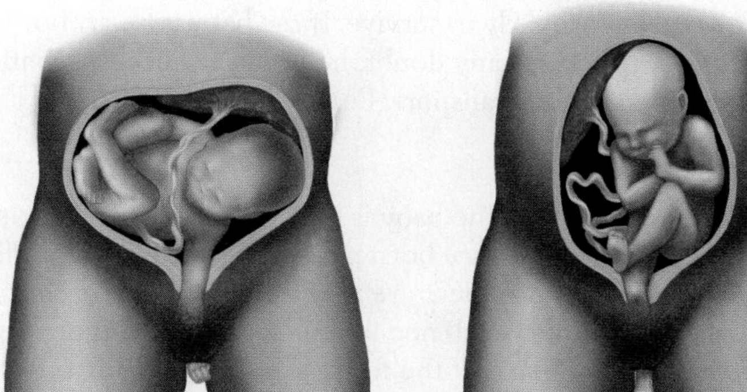

(A) (B)

Figure 27-17 Limb presentations.

If shoulder dystocia is identified, rapid transport is immediately indicated. If local protocol allows, it may be possible to assist in this type of delivery by flexing the mother's legs back toward her abdomen. This essentially widens the pelvis and may help free the shoulder. Always initiate transport before attempting resolution maneuvers.

Multiple Births

Multiple births are not necessarily a physical complication. In many cases, twins are delivered in a series of two normal births. Multiple births do have some potential problems, including premature delivery and taxing the resources of rescuers on the scene. Remember that you have two patients with a normal delivery in the field; with twins you will have three, with triplets you will have four, and so on.

Ask the mother if she has received prenatal care. In most cases, when the mother has received prenatal care, she is aware of the fact that she is carrying more than one baby. Without prenatal care, be alert for an unusually large abdomen that does not reduce significantly in size after a first birth.

Twins may share a single placenta or have separate placentas. Proceed with cord clamping and cutting as you would with a normal, single gestation delivery.

Be sure to call for help early if you expect multiple births. Something as simple as twins will quickly take you from one patient to three. If one or more patients need continued care or resuscitation, this is even more demanding of resources. When triplets or more babies are expected, risks are substantially higher for premature birth and complications.

Premature Births

premature birth birth before the baby has fully developed that occurs prior to a 38-week gestation.

gestation length of time from conception to birth.

Premature birth may progress like any other birth. The potential for problems begins when the baby is born. Depending on the length of **gestation** achieved, the baby may require resuscitation. In fact, the earlier the baby arrives, the more likely it is you will have to provide resuscitation. As noted earlier, pregnancy normally lasts approximately 38 to 42 weeks or about nine months. Babies born after about 36 or 37 weeks have much of the development required to thrive after birth. Babies born before this time are more prone to problems. Modern medicine and new technology have been able to stabilize and support babies born after only 20 to 23 weeks, but even then, survival is not guaranteed. These babies can weigh only about one pound.

The general rule is to deliver, suction, and keep the baby warm and dry. Provide resuscitation according to the inverted pyramid as necessary.

You may find that a baby has delivered long before it is viable to survive outside the uterus. Or you may find that a baby has developed for a significant time in the uterus but failed to develop properly to survive. If the baby is *clearly* born dead, resuscitation is not required. If there is any doubt, however, begin resuscitative measures immediately and provide prompt transport. Follow local protocols.

Post-Term Pregnancy

Post-term pregnancy occurs when the baby is delivered after the forty-second week of gestation. Although many babies are born past their due date (typically as a result of inaccurate due date estimation), there are risks associated with this complication. The rate of stillborn (babies born dead) neonates is statistically higher in this population. Also because of the larger size of the fetus, dystocia and difficult deliveries are more common. There is little that EMS can do to diminish these risks, but EMTs should be aware that post-term deliveries can pose a risk for resuscitation and for a complicated birth.

Meconium

Meconium is fecal matter excreted by the baby while he is still in the uterus. It is often a sign of fetal distress before birth. It appears as a dark, possibly green or yellow-brown substance on the baby or in the amniotic fluid, which normally should be clear. When meconium is evident, you should always be ready to begin neonatal resuscitation.

meconium fecal matter excreted by the baby while still in the uterus.

Meconium is a concern in that it can indicate fetal distress, but in a neonate who is born active and breathing, its presence is no problem at all. If the neonate requires resuscitation (that is, he is born not breathing), meconium presents a more significant issue.

When meconium is present in a neonate that requires resuscitation, do not stimulate the baby before suctioning the oropharynx. Suction the mouth and then the neonate's nose. Resuscitate as indicated and transport as soon as possible. Monitor the airway carefully during transport, and notify the receiving hospital that meconium was observed.

PERSPECTIVE

Ling—The EMT

It's kind of weird delivering a baby. It's really great but such a contrast, I guess. How do I explain it? It's like 95% of my job is dealing with sick and dying people. I've honestly lost count of the number of people that I've seen die. I couldn't even guess anymore. And yet today I held a brand new life in my hands. I was the first human being that little boy encountered in this world. That probably sounds odd, huh? I don't know. Maybe I'm just overly philosophical right now, or maybe you just have to be in that situation to understand what I mean.

STOP, REVIEW, REMEMBER!

Multiple Choice

For each question, place a check next to the correct answer.

1. Fetal defecation during the birthing process is commonly a sign of:
   _____ a. fetal distress.
   _____ b. preterm delivery.
   _____ c. post-term pregnancy.
   _____ d. placenta previa.

2. During the assessment of a woman in labor, you note a prolapsed umbilical cord. You should:
   _____ a. tug on the cord to speed delivery.
   _____ b. reinsert the cord back into the birth canal.
   _____ c. instruct the mother to push during contractions.
   _____ d. apply a moist dressing and initiate rapid transport.

3. The one condition in which an EMT must insert a gloved hand into the vagina is:
   _____ a. placenta previa.
   _____ b. breech presentation.
   _____ c. prolapsed cord.
   _____ d. multiple births.

4. Which one of the following describes the condition in which development of the placenta obstructs the birth canal?
   _____ a. Placenta previa
   _____ b. Breech presentation
   _____ c. Prolapsed cord
   _____ d. Abruptio placentae

(continued on next page)

(continued)

5. During an emergency delivery, you note that the baby's head emerges but then withdraws as the contraction ends. You should suspect:

_____ a. nuchal cord.

_____ b. prolapsed cord.

_____ c. placenta previa.

_____ d. shoulder dystocia.

Short Answer

For each of the following history statements by a mother in labor, explain any concerns or actions you would take to prepare for delivery.

1. "My doctor told me I am having twins."

___

___

___

___

2. "I think I am only 32 weeks pregnant."

___

___

___

___

3. "At my last ultrasound the doctor told me the baby was breech. We were hoping he would turn around. They were going to do a C-section next week."

___

___

___

___

4. "I don't believe in prenatal visits. I believe childbirth should be totally natural and I haven't seen a doctor."

___

___

___

___

Critical Thinking

1. What should you assess in the newborn? List an example of each. (Hint: Apgar)

2. Draw the inverted pyramid representing the steps of neonatal resuscitation. Label the BLS steps in the triangle.

EMERGENCY DISPATCH SUMMARY

Ling and Mark delivered a healthy 6 lb 8 oz baby boy named Nathan Ray in the cab of the pickup truck and then transported both mother and child to Fleischmann's Hospital on Old County Road. Two months later, both EMTs were surprised to receive invitations to the wedding of Nathan Ray's mother and her boyfriend. Both medics plan to attend.

Chapter Review

To the Point

- Understanding female reproductive anatomy is vital to the thorough assessment of a woman.
- Use anatomy and physiology to recognize the patterns of female reproductive emergencies.
- A woman's body changes dramatically during pregnancy. Understanding how this process affects body systems will improve your ability to assess your patient and help you better predict injury and illness.
- Ectopic pregnancy should be considered a potential diagnosis in all women of childbearing age who present with abdominal pain.
- Vaginal bleeding should elicit suspicions of sexual assault. Consider the possibility of a crime scene.
- Vaginal bleeding is controlled externally. Never insert anything into the patient's vagina.
- Suspect abruptio placentae in late-term pregnant women with abdominal pain and/or vaginal bleeding.
- In addition to recognizing life threats, the assessment of the pregnant woman in labor should focus on when to transport and the likelihood of neonatal resuscitation.
- Most deliveries will not require intervention, but preparation is key for the unusual circumstance. Ensure proper equipment and resource readiness before untoward circumstances emerge.
- Following delivery, assess the neonate for the need of suctioning and keep the baby warm and dry.
- Neonatal resuscitation must be initiated in any depressed neonate.
- Use the inverted pyramid to progress through the "assess-treat" steps of neonatal resuscitation.
- Start CPR on neonates who have heart rates less than 60 beats per minute.
- Assess the postpartum mother for the risk of hemorrhage and emboli.
- Complicated deliveries often require immediate appropriate transport to preserve the life of the baby.
- In a prolapsed cord, you must insert a gloved hand to take pressure off the impinged cord.
- The pulse oximeter should be utilized for all patients as a basic vital sign tool. It will reveal the oxygen saturation of the peripheral blood supply. A measurement between 95% and 100% is considered normal.
- Breech presentations often can be delivered normally. However, this finding should be an indicator for immediate transport just in case the delivery is complicated.

Chapter Questions

Multiple Choice

1. A fontanel is:
   _____ a. a soft spot on a baby's head.
   _____ b. a twist in the umbilical cord.
   _____ c. an airway obstruction in the newborn caused by fluid or tissue during delivery.
   _____ d. the name for the part of the baby that is visible first at the vaginal opening.

2. When a patient reports "breaking her water," she is referring to:
   _____ a. becoming incontinent of urine due to the late stage of pregnancy.
   _____ b. rupture of the amniotic sac.
   _____ c. delivery of the placenta.
   _____ d. vaginal bleeding.

3. You have a patient who has given birth but has consistent vaginal bleeding that does not stop. To help control this you should:
_____ a. pack the vagina with absorbent dressings.
_____ b. apply direct pressure to the vaginal opening.
_____ c. massage the uterus.
_____ d. clamp the umbilical cord.

4. When suctioning a newborn, you should suction the:
_____ a. mouth first, and then the nose.
_____ b. nose first, and then the mouth.
_____ c. nose only.
_____ d. mouth only.

5. Which one of the following statements is most correct in regard to limb presentation?
_____ a. The delivery will be relatively normal, so prepare to deliver the baby on scene.
_____ b. You should gently but firmly manipulate the uterus to get the other limb to present.
_____ c. Your treatments include transportation of the patient in a head-down position with oxygen.
_____ d. Transportation of the patient in this condition is too dangerous, so prepare for delivery when the other limb appears.

Matching

Match the term on the left with the applicable definition on the right.

1. _____	Meconium	A.	The umbilical cord protruding from the vagina
2. _____	Breech presentation	B.	More than one fetus
3. _____	Placenta previa	C.	A fetus born at 32 weeks gestation
4. _____	Premature birth	D.	Fetal fecal matter in the amniotic fluid
5. _____	Multiple birth	E.	Both legs as the presenting part
6. _____	Prolapsed cord	F.	One arm as the presenting part
7. _____	Limb presentation	G.	Vaginal bleeding
8. _____	Abruptio placentae	H.	Premature separation of the placenta from the uterine wall
		I.	Positioning of the placenta near the cervix
		J.	Ruptured uterus

Critical Thinking

1. Why are most mothers aware that they may have multiple births or potential complications? How will this affect your history taking?

____

____

____

____

2. Why is it important to dry a newborn and maintain warmth?

____

____

____

____

(continued on next page)

(continued)

3. List five components of an OB kit and what each listed item is used for.

Case Study

You are called to a "woman in labor" in an apartment building. You walk the three flights of stairs because there is no elevator. Entering the apartment, you find a woman lying on the floor breathing heavily. She is obviously near full term, based on the size of her abdomen. "Hi. We're from the fire department. We're going to help you out." The woman's name is Maria. She is there with her husband, George, in their new apartment.

You determine answers to a few key questions and find that this is Maria's first baby. Labor started only about an hour ago, but the contractions are very intense, long, and close together. She feels the urge to move her bowels. You explain to Maria that you are going to look to see if the baby is coming. You see crowning.

When you ask Maria if she knew of any problems from her doctor visits and ultrasounds, she looks at George who replies, "We have no money. We couldn't afford any doctor visits. None." He looks sad, and to you for help.

1. What does the fact that the patient had no prenatal care mean to your care and decision making at the scene?

2. How would you handle the fact that you are on a third floor with no elevator?

3. How would you tell if the patient was having more than one baby?

4. What resources, if any, would you call for? Why?

____

____

____

____

The Last Word

This chapter covered a wide range of situations. Some "natural" emergencies like childbirth are things that you will not see often in the field. Many EMTs will go for an entire career and not deliver a baby. Although not commonly encountered, you could come in contact with patients who have a critical need for your assistance. Most parents plan a pregnancy to end at the hospital in a controlled medical setting. When those plans go awry, the calmness, professionalism, and experience you bring to the patient and her family will be remembered long after mother and baby come home from the hospital.

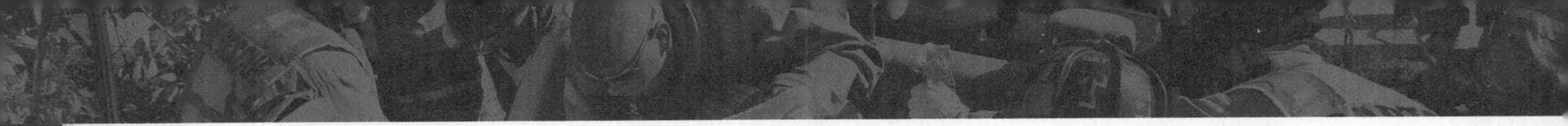

Module 3: Review and Practice Examination for Chapters 15–27

DIRECTIONS: *Assess what you have learned in this module by placing a check mark in the blank beside the best answer for each multiple-choice question. When you are done, check your answers against the Answer Key at the back of the book.*

1. The name of a drug listed in the *United States Pharmacopoeia* is its ______________ name.
   ____ a. trade ____ c. proprietary
   ____ b. chemical ____ d. generic

2. The name given to a drug by the pharmaceutical company for marketing purposes is its ______________ name.
   ____ a. trade
   ____ b. chemical
   ____ c. pharmaceutical
   ____ d. generic

3. Which one of the following medication routes would take the longest to have its effect?
   ____ a. Injection of epinephrine
   ____ b. Oral glucose gel
   ____ c. Tylenol tablet
   ____ d. Puff of albuterol

4. The reason a medication is given is its:
   ____ a. action.
   ____ b. indication.
   ____ c. contraindication.
   ____ d. incentive.

5. Undesirable consequences of a medication are known as:
   ____ a. contraindications.
   ____ b. actions.
   ____ c. side effects.
   ____ d. mis-actions.

6. Once you receive an order to administer medication to a patient, you should first:
   ____ a. repeat the order to the physician.
   ____ b. confirm the order with the family.
   ____ c. confirm the order with the patient.
   ____ d. ask the patient to repeat the order.

7. You are caring for an adult patient who is having a severe allergic reaction. You would be most likely to receive an order for which one of the following medications?
   ____ a. 0.3 mg of epinephrine
   ____ b. 0.3 mg of nitroglycerin
   ____ c. 0.15 mg of epinephrine
   ____ d. Activated charcoal

8. Bronchodilators are given to treat patients presenting with which one of the following problems?
   ____ a. Chest pain
   ____ b. Poisoning or overdose
   ____ c. Difficulty breathing
   ____ d. Diabetes

9. Which one of the following is an acceptable way to measure a patient's respiratory distress?
   ____ a. How many stairs he can climb without difficulty
   ____ b. How long he can hold his breath
   ____ c. How much oxygen the patient uses at home
   ____ d. Number of words he can speak between breaths

10. Abnormal breathing patterns are commonly caused by:
    ____ a. liver disease.
    ____ b. open fractures.
    ____ c. altered mental status.
    ____ d. brain injury.

11. Which one of the following is a respiratory illness in which the walls of the alveoli break down, allowing air to become trapped in the lungs?
    ____ a. Asthma ____ c. Emphysema
    ____ b. Bronchitis ____ d. Tuberculosis

12. Which one of the following psychological conditions may be caused by hypoxia?
    ____ a. Psychosis ____ c. Amnesia
    ____ b. Paranoia ____ d. Anxiety

13. Which one of the following devices delivers aerosolized respiratory medication through a mask or mouthpiece over an extended period of time?
____ a. Small-volume nebulizer
____ b. Metered-dose inhaler
____ c. Spacer
____ d. Steam vaporizer

14. Hearing crackles when listening to the lungs with a stethoscope is an indication of:
____ a. poor technique of listening to breath sounds.
____ b. lower airway constriction.
____ c. partial upper airway obstruction.
____ d. fluid in the alveoli.

15. In dark-skinned individuals skin color changes can best be detected by observing the:
____ a. inside of the lower lip.
____ b. back of the hand.
____ c. nape of the neck.
____ d. medial (inside aspect) of the arm.

16. The ability of the heart to generate its own electrical impulses is called:
____ a. conductivity. ____ c. automaticity.
____ b. contractility. ____ d. propensity.

17. Which one of the following is *not* one of the links in the chain of survival for cardiac arrest?
____ a. Early CPR
____ b. Early aspirin
____ c. Early defibrillation
____ d. Early advanced life support

18. The general term applied to patients who present with an emergency related to the heart is:
____ a. cardiac compromise.
____ b. cardiac arrest.
____ c. angina.
____ d. myocardial infarction.

19. Another name for a heart attack is:
____ a. congestive heart failure.
____ b. dysrhythmia.
____ c. myocardial infarction.
____ d. angina.

20. Your 50-year-old male patient has no previous cardiac history. He began having pain in his chest and left arm along with some nausea while watching television. Over the next hour, his symptoms worsened and he began to feel short of breath. These symptoms are most consistent with:
____ a. congestive heart failure.
____ b. myocardial infarction.
____ c. angina.
____ d. asystole.

21. Jugular vein distention is most commonly associated with:
____ a. congestive heart failure.
____ b. cardiac arrest.
____ c. myocardial infarction.
____ d. ventricular fibrillation.

22. Which one of the following is *not* a contraindication for the administration of nitroglycerin to a patient with chest pain?
____ a. The patient took Cialis earlier in the day.
____ b. The blood pressure is 88/50.
____ c. The patient does not have his own prescription for nitroglycerin.
____ d. The patient rates his pain less than a "7" on a scale from 1 to 10.

23. When a diabetic patient takes too much insulin and eats too little food, he will experience:
____ a. hyperglycemia.
____ b. hypoglycemia.
____ c. diabetic coma.
____ d. insulin effect.

24. A normal blood glucose reading is between ____________ and ____________ mg/dL.
____ a. 40, 80 ____ c. 100, 120
____ b. 80, 120 ____ d. 120, 150

25. An abnormal surge of electrical signals in the brain is known as a(n):
____ a. convulsion. ____ c. seizure.
____ b. coma. ____ d. epileptic fit.

26. The period of time in which a patient remains altered following a seizure is known as the ____________ period or phase.
____ a. grand mal ____ c. postictal
____ b. petit mal ____ d. generalized

27. Which one of the following is a common cause of stroke?
____ a. Hematoma ____ c. Seizure
____ b. Overdose ____ d. Embolism

28. Your patient is a 70-year-old man who experienced a sudden onset of paralysis on his right side and difficulty expressing himself. He is quite frustrated because he cannot make you understand what he wants to say. Which one of the following is the best response?
____ a. There are new cures for strokes. You'll be good as new in no time.
____ b. Don't try to say anything. I know just how you feel.
____ c. With physical and speech therapy you may be able to regain a useful life.
____ d. Let's get you to the hospital and see what they can do to make you better.

29. The EMT's primary concern in caring for any patient with an altered mental status is:
____ a. finding the cause of altered mental status.
____ b. getting a good history.
____ c. anticipating airway and breathing problems.
____ d. stabilizing the cervical spine.

30. When managing a scene that may be contaminated by dangerous gases or substances, what might an EMT consider doing before entering?
____ a. Check for scene safety a second time.
____ b. Ensure that proper BSI precautions have been taken.
____ c. Request a hazmat crew to assess the scene.
____ d. Remove easily removable toxic substances.

31. Hydrogen sulfide, which can cause difficulty breathing and eye irritation, is an example of a toxin that enters the body through:
____ a. injection.
____ b. inhalation.
____ c. ingestion.
____ d. absorption.

32. Which part of your assessment is most important when treating a patient who has potentially been poisoned?
____ a. Airway
____ b. Pulse
____ c. Chief complaint
____ d. Vital signs

33. It is important to contact a poison control center when you suspect a patient may have been poisoned. Why is it important to provide the center with as much information about the patient and the potential contaminate as possible?
____ a. For data collection and research purposes
____ b. The poison control center may be authorized to provide medical direction.
____ c. A report will be generated and sent to the receiving emergency department.
____ d. There is a possibility of future litigation.

34. How does activated charcoal work in the body after a toxin or poison has been ingested?
____ a. It causes the patient to vomit, thus removing the substance from the body.
____ b. It neutralizes the substance rendering it harmless.
____ c. It adsorbs the substance and reduces the amount the body can absorb.
____ d. It coats the intestine, allowing the toxin to pass through the body.

35. You are caring for a 32-year-old male patient who has come into contact with a toxic liquid. How would you attempt to remove the substance?
____ a. Irrigate the site for at least 20 minutes with clean water.
____ b. Brush the liquid off with a shirt or clean cloth.
____ c. Allow the substance to dry, and then rinse off.
____ d. Cover the site with protective sheeting and transport. The emergency department will remove the substance.

36. You are caring for a patient who is a heavy drug user. During your primary assessment he is cooperative. However, after several minutes he becomes violent and combative and exhibits signs that he may be hallucinating. How would you manage this patient?
____ a. Talk calmly to the patient and remind him that you are there to help.
____ b. Use the straps of your gurney to attempt to restrain him.
____ c. Forcibly move him to the ground and wait for law enforcement to arrive.
____ d. Immediately back away from the scene and only reenter after law enforcement has secured it.

37. Conscious patients whom you suspect may have been exposed to high levels of carbon monoxide should be treated with supplemental oxygen by way of:
____ a. pocket mask.
____ b. nasal cannula.
____ c. nonrebreather.
____ d. bag-mask device.

38. Which one of the following organs is typically found only in the right upper quadrant of the abdomen?
____ a. Appendix ____ c. Gall bladder
____ b. Pancreas ____ d. Colon

39. For a patient complaining of acute abdominal pain, what is the most notable risk factor?
____ a. Infection
____ b. Internal bleeding
____ c. Bruising of the liver
____ d. Inflammation

40. The large intestine is an example of which kind of organ?
____ a. Smooth ____ c. Vascular
____ b. Hollow ____ d. Solid

41. For which condition should an EMT provide emergency care when treating a patient experiencing acute abdominal pain?
____ a. Shock
____ b. Myocardial infarction
____ c. Hypertension
____ d. Anemia

42. A patient with bleeding within the GI tract may present with which one of the following signs?
____ a. Bradycardia
____ b. Accelerated capillary refill time
____ c. Decreased respirations
____ d. Tachycardia

43. For a nonpregnant woman, a sudden and severe onset of lower abdominal pain would most likely be caused by:
____ a. ruptured ovarian cyst.
____ b. endometriosis.
____ c. dysmenorrhea.
____ d. endometritis.

44. A patient who is experiencing appendicitis may describe the condition as:
____ a. pulsating sensation in the upper left quadrant that turned into stinging pain.
____ b. pain that increases with lying down.
____ c. pain that increased over time in the center of the abdomen then finally settled in the lower right quadrant.
____ d. tingling sensation that started in the lower left quadrant and now resides in the upper left quadrant.

45. Which one of the following is associated with anaphylaxis, but not with mild or moderate allergic reactions?
____ a. Airway obstruction
____ b. Rash
____ c. Hives
____ d. Increased heart rate

46. You have just assisted a patient with a severe shellfish allergy in using her Epi-Pen. As you are loading her into the ambulance, she becomes anxious and her heart rate increases from 100 to 140. In addition, she tells you she feels like she is going to throw up. Which one of the following should you consider?
____ a. Giving a second dose of epinephrine because the patient is getting worse
____ b. Reassessing the patient
____ c. Reassuring the patient that what she is experiencing is a normal reaction to epinephrine
____ d. b and c

47. The purpose of white blood cells is to:
____ a. carry proteins known as clotting factors.
____ b. respond to infections and regulate immune response.
____ c. transport hemoglobin to red blood cells.
____ d. initially form clots.

48. What function does the spleen play in the circulation of blood?
____ a. Remove contaminates as well as hemoglobin
____ b. Create plasma
____ c. Create platelets
____ d. Store bacteria that are later distributed to the appendix

49. What might a person suffering from advanced liver disease experience when a blood vessel becomes damaged?
____ a. Excessive bleeding due to reduced clotting factor being produced
____ b. Shock due to weakened immune system
____ c. Excessive bleeding due to increased red blood cells
____ d. Limited bleeding as a result of reduced blood volume

50. Which one of the following is the appropriate care for a trauma patient with a history of difficulty clotting?
____ a. The patient should be transported to a stroke center for care.
____ b. The rescuers will spend more time on scene to discover all potential injuries.
____ c. The patient should be transported to a trauma center.
____ d. Before completing a thorough assessment, the patient should be transported to minimize time on scene.

51. During the primary assessment of a patient, how might an EMT discover that the patient has a condition or is taking a medication that makes clotting more difficult?
____ a. This may not be known until the patient is admitted to an emergency department.
____ b. Observation of excessive bleeding
____ c. During the SAMPLE history
____ d. OPQRST line of questioning

52. Why do red blood cells affected by sickle cell anemia not last as long in circulation as healthy red blood cells?
____ a. Their shape causes them to bunch together and be removed by the spleen in greater quantities.
____ b. They are composed of defective hemoglobin, which prevents them from compressing and moving around the circulatory system effectively.
____ c. The cells end up being smaller in size and are absorbed into the body.
____ d. White blood cells react to the abnormal shape and trigger an immune response.

53. A patient suffering from a vaso-occlusive crisis may experience severe pain in the:
____ a. arms and legs.
____ b. fingers and toes.
____ c. ears and nose.
____ d. left arm and leg.

54. Which of the following is one of the primary responsibilities of the kidneys?
____ a. Removal of waste and filtration of the blood
____ b. Store bacteria
____ c. Produce bile and regulate blood glucose levels
____ d. Manufacture proteins responsible for clotting

55. Urinary tract infections are caused by a(n):
____ a. virus.
____ b. contact infection.
____ c. overactive immune system.
____ d. bacterial infection.

56. Patients who require the use of urinary catheters are more likely to develop:
____ a. renal failure.
____ b. urinary tract infection.
____ c. blood clots.
____ d. heart failure.

57. When the kidneys can no longer properly filter and balance fluid in the body, they are said to be suffering from:
____ a. renal malfunction.
____ b. end-stage renal disease (ESRD).
____ c. end-stage kidney disease (ESKD).
____ d. hemodialysis.

58. A patient experiencing complications with dialysis may present with signs of:
____ a. myocardial infarction.
____ b. flu-like symptoms.
____ c. shock.
____ d. stroke.

59. A patient who has missed a dialysis treatment may present with signs of:
____ a. congestive heart failure (CHF).
____ b. stroke.
____ c. chronic obstructive pulmonary disease (COPD).
____ d. anaphylaxis.

60. Characteristics of schizophrenia may include all of the following *except*:
____ a. paranoia.
____ b. multiple personalities.
____ c. psychosis.
____ d. delusions.

61. Which one of the following guidelines applies to the patient who is threatening or has attempted suicide?
____ a. Always have law enforcement restrain the patient.
____ b. Be prepared to transport immediately.
____ c. Do not confront the patient directly.
____ d. Directly ask about suicidal thoughts and intentions.

62. Your patient is a 22-year-old woman who is breathing rapidly, clutching her chest, and begging you not to let her die. Her roommate tells you that the patient has a history of panic attacks. Which one of the following is an appropriate approach to the patient?
____ a. Looking the patient directly in the eye and stating, "You need to get a hold of yourself. There's no reason for you to be panicked."
____ b. Standing back from the patient and asking whether or not she wants to go to the hospital.
____ c. Getting on the patient's level and stating, "I'm an EMT with the ambulance service. Let's see what we can do to help you."
____ d. Placing your hand on the patient's shoulder and letting her know that EMTs are not trained to handle psychiatric problems and that she should contact her psychiatrist.

63. In a pregnant patient, indications of imminent delivery include all of the following *except*:
____ a. contractions are two minutes apart or less.
____ b. the mother states she needs to have a bowel movement.
____ c. crowning is present.
____ d. the mother has delivered at least one child previously.

64. In a normal delivery, the first part to present is the:
____ a. placenta.
____ b. buttocks.
____ c. head.
____ d. feet.

65. You have just assisted with the delivery of a full-term infant. You have clamped and cut the cord, but the infant is not breathing. Which one of the following should you do first?
____ a. Insert an oropharyngeal airway and ventilate the patient with a bag-mask device.
____ b. Stimulate the baby by rubbing his back.
____ c. Perform mouth-to-mask ventilations.
____ d. Administer supplemental oxygen.

66. When the placenta separates prematurely from the uterine wall, this is known as:
____ a. placenta previa.
____ b. ectopic placentae.
____ c. preeclampsia.
____ d. abruptio placentae.

67. AEDs are designed to help which one of the following types of patients?
____ a. All patients having a myocardial infarction
____ b. All patients in cardiac arrest
____ c. Patients in ventricular fibrillation
____ d. Patients with no electrical activity in the heart

68. Which one of the following is *not* a contraindication to the use of an AED?
____ a. Patient experiencing chest pain
____ b. 10-year-old patient in cardiac arrest
____ c. Patient not breathing but has a pulse
____ d. Unresponsive diabetic

69. For a patient who remains in a shockable rhythm, an AED will deliver ____________ shock(s) between prompts to perform CPR.
____ a. 1 ____ c. 6
____ b. 3 ____ d. 9

70. In a normal pregnancy, where will the embryo implant itself in a woman's reproductive system?
____ a. Uterine lining
____ b. Fallopian tube
____ c. Ovum
____ d. Cervix

71. What organ allows for the transport of oxygen and nutrients from the mother's blood to that of the developing fetus?
____ a. Amniotic sac ____ c. Placenta
____ b. Cervix ____ d. Uvula

72. During pregnancy the total volume of the mother's blood can increase as much as:
____ a. 20% to 25%. ____ c. 55% to 65%.
____ b. 30% to 40%. ____ d. 45% to 50%.

73. As pregnancy progresses, the pressure on the diaphragm causes:
____ a. the respiratory drive to diminish.
____ b. decreased lung volume.
____ c. increased lung volume.
____ d. inability to completely exhale.

74. Severe vaginal bleeding in a pregnant patient may indicate:
____ a. imminent delivery of the baby.
____ b. a life-threatening emergency.
____ c. trauma.
____ d. initiation of contractions.

75. What is the purpose of contractions in the first stage of labor?
____ a. To dilate the cervix
____ b. To move the baby through the birth canal
____ c. To deliver the placenta
____ d. To align the baby for delivery

76. After the baby is born, what signals the third stage of labor?
____ a. Cutting of the umbilical cord
____ b. Conclusion of contractions
____ c. Delivery of the placenta
____ d. Baby latching

77. A baby presenting in the breech position will require:
____ a. immediate transport.
____ b. assistance to rotate position.
____ c. more time on scene to assess.
____ d. immediate suctioning when delivered.

78. Massaging the uterus may be helpful to:
____ a. deliver the baby.
____ b. stop postpartum blood loss.
____ c. reorient a baby with limb presentation.
____ d. deliver the placenta.

79. An emergency involving a prolapsed cord may be resolved by:
____ a. placing the mother in a position where her hips are higher than her shoulders.
____ b. placing the mother in a left lateral position.
____ c. placing the mother in a position of comfort to alleviate contractions.
____ d. placing the mother in a sitting position.

80. Shoulder dystocia may be observed by the:
____ a. lack of crowning, even as the mother pushes.
____ b. umbilical cord being wrapped around the baby's shoulder.
____ c. presentation of the baby's shoulder at the vaginal opening.
____ d. baby's head presenting during contractions and withdrawing on relaxation.

81. Once a baby is fully born, you should:
____ a. dry the baby.
____ b. suction the baby.
____ c. cut the umbilical cord.
____ d. warm the baby.

82. What is the normal respiratory rate for a neonate?
____ a. 30 to 40 per minute
____ b. 20 to 30 per minute
____ c. 40 to 60 per minute
____ d. 50 to 60 per minute

83. Compression should be initiated if the neonate's heart rate falls below ______________ beats per minute.
____ a. 60 ____ c. 40
____ b. 100 ____ d. 70

84. If cyanosis persists, oxygen should be administered after ______________ minutes.
____ a. 5 ____ c. 2
____ b. 15 ____ d. 10

85. If compressions need to be administered, what should the anterior-posterior chest compression depth be?
____ a. One-fifth the depth of the chest
____ b. One-third the depth of the chest
____ c. Half the depth of the chest
____ d. Two-thirds the depth of the chest

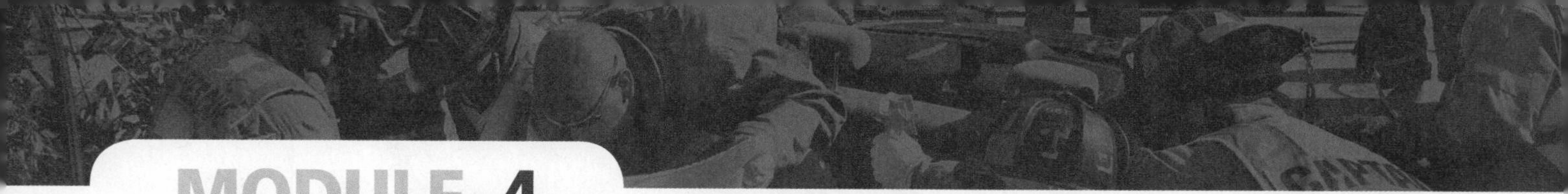

MODULE 4

Trauma Emergencies

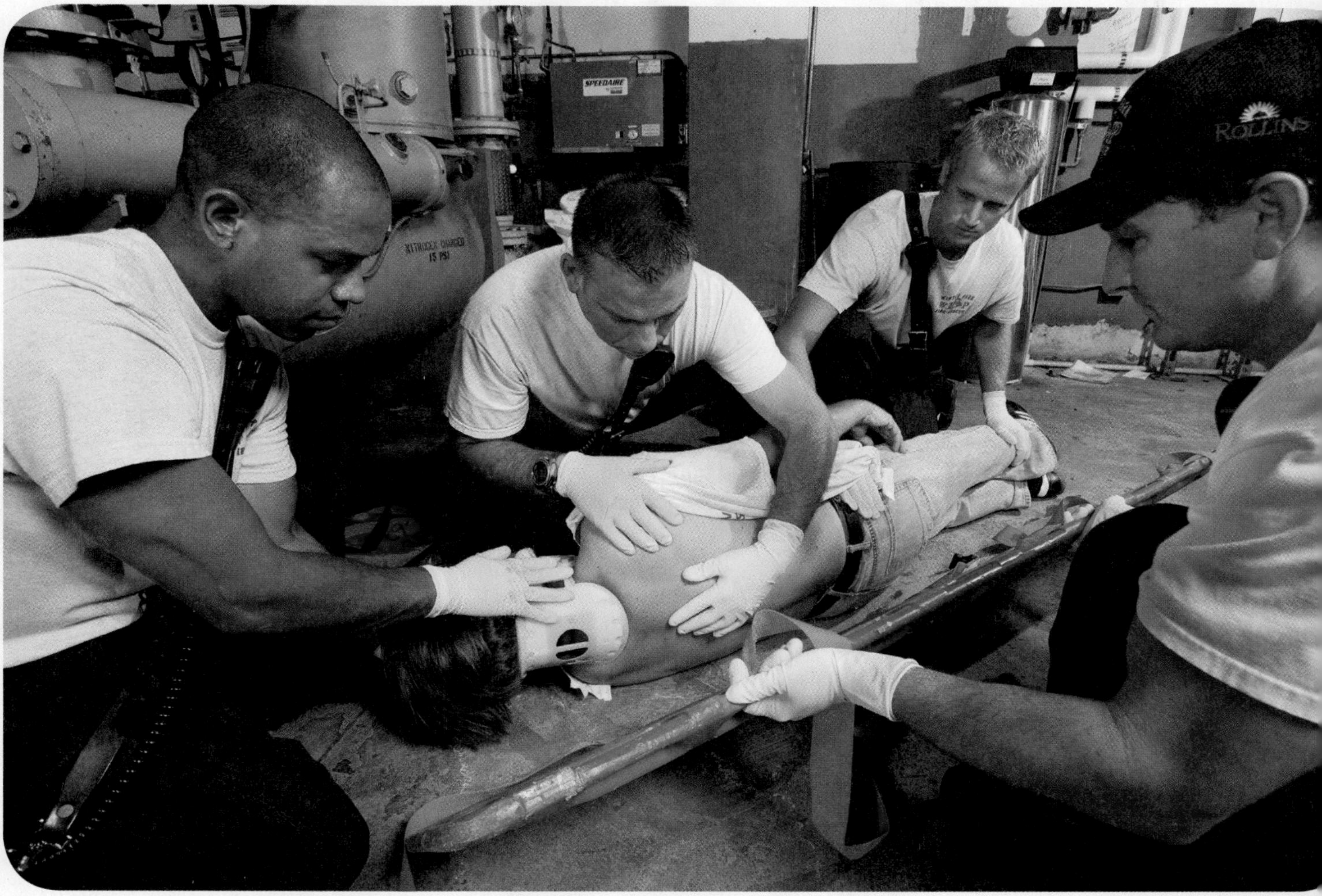

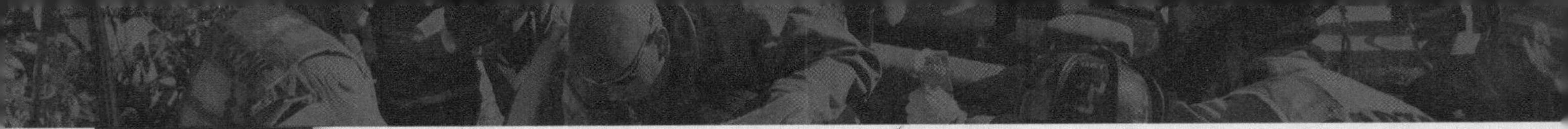

28 Your Approach to the Trauma Patient

Education Standards

Assessment: Secondary assessment, monitoring devices, reassessment

Competencies

Applies scene information and patient assessment findings to guide emergency management.

Objectives

After completion of this lesson, you should be able to:

28-1 Define key terms introduced in this chapter.

28-2 Differentiate a medical patient from a trauma patient.

28-3 Discuss the importance of differentiating the medical patient from the trauma patient.

28-4 Discuss the importance of the general impression.

28-5 Discuss the importance of vital signs and the anatomy of injury when assessing the trauma patient.

28-6 Discuss the significance of the mechanism of injury when assessing the trauma patient.

28-7 Differentiate between significant and nonsignificant mechanism of injury.

28-8 Discuss the role of time on scene with the trauma patient.

28-9 Discuss the importance of choosing the appropriate receiving facility when caring for trauma patients.

Key Terms

anatomy of injury p. 744
focused secondary assessment p. 748
mechanism of injury p. 746
medical patient p. 743
mentation p. 744
nonsignificant mechanism of injury p. 747
on-scene time p. 748
rapid secondary assessment p. 747
significant mechanism of injury p. 747
trauma centers p. 748
trauma patient p. 743

Introduction

As discussed in Chapter 15, in emergency care there are two general categories of patients—those who have an illness (the **medical patient**) and those who have an injury (the **trauma patient**). Your assessment approach to the two general types of patients will differ in both subtle and obvious ways. This chapter describes your approach to the assessment and management of a trauma patient who has experienced a sudden injury.

28-2 Differentiate a medical patient from a trauma patient.

medical patient a patient whose chief complaint is related to an acute illness or disease process.

trauma patient a patient whose chief complaint is related to a sudden injury.

As you will see, this chapter differs from other chapters in this textbook in that it is meant to provide only a broad philosophical framework within which you should consider each of the topics in this module, Module 5 "Trauma Emergencies."

Medical Patient or Trauma Patient?

You must identify a trauma patient as soon as possible because many life-threatening injuries can only be corrected by rapid surgical intervention at a hospital. In contrast, many important interventions required for a medical patient may be provided at the scene.

Your assessment of any patient begins with the information you receive from dispatch. Typical dispatches that you might receive for a trauma patient might sound like this:

Dispatch 1: "Unit 2760, respond code 3 for a victim of an assault."

Dispatch 2: "Rescue 13, priority response for an unconscious woman."

Dispatch 3: "Engine 1730, respond code 3 for motor-vehicle collision."

Dispatch 4: "Unit 113, respond priority 2 for a man down."

As you can see, you have very little to go on given just the information provided by the dispatch. In most cases, dispatchers are well trained and experienced at staying calm, calming the reporting party, and doing the best they can at getting credible information from frightened and upset family and friends who are faced with an emergency. That is not an easy task. With most of the dispatches listed above, the information is highly suggestive of an incident involving injuries. While you cannot always be certain, you can begin to think about what you will do if the situation does indeed involve injuries.

So Why Does It Matter?

Why all the discussion? Aren't we going to care for all patients the same anyway? Well, yes and no. *Yes*, you will care for all patients in the most appropriate, compassionate, and respectful manner regardless of the underlying problem. *No*, you will not manage medical and trauma patients in the same exact way.

28-3 Discuss the importance of differentiating the medical patient from the trauma patient.

First and foremost when you suspect the emergency is a medical one, your approach will be to center on a complete and thorough patient history. To accomplish that, you must become an expert detective and hone your interviewing skills like a well-sharpened knife. In contrast, your approach to a trauma patient will center on your evaluation of the mechanism of injury and your physical assessment of the injured body part or area.

The Trauma Patient

The General Impression

The general impression is your gut feeling of how critical your patient is. It is a very important step in determining how critical the patient's condition is and how urgently you will need to transport. Some EMS folks call this the "doorway diagnosis"

28-4 Discuss the importance of the general impression.

or the "big sick, little sick" decision. While it may be referred to as a "gut" decision or some sort of intuition, it really is more objective than that in most cases. For your general impression and help in defining what type of patient you have, you combine the information from dispatch, your observations at the scene, and your first visual contact with the patient. As you approach the patient, ask yourself:

mentation the mental activity of a patient.

- ***Mentation.*** Simply put, **mentation** addresses the question, "Is the patient awake or unresponsive?" If he is awake, how is he responding to the environment? Is he alert and interacting with those around him, or sluggish and confused with little interaction? Position plays a part in this as well. A person who is sitting up will likely be more responsive than someone who is lying supine.
- ***Skin color.*** Look at the patient's face if he is light-skinned, or inspect the oral mucosa, nail beds, and palms of the hands of the dark-skinned patient. Check specifically for color. Is it pink as it should be? Or is it pale indicating poor perfusion?
- ***Level of distress.*** Patients are most commonly in distress for two reasons—pain and difficulty breathing. Does the patient appear to be in immediate distress for either one of those reasons or both? An unresponsive patient is always considered critical and thus is a high priority for transport.

So, your "gut" is actually responding to a few very important observations or findings that help form your "big sick, little sick" decision.

National Trauma Triage Protocol

In order to quickly differentiate those patients who have suffered a significant injury, the Centers for Disease Control and Prevention (CDC) has developed the "Field Triage Decision Scheme: The National Trauma Triage Protocol" (Figure 28-1 ▪). This resource has been created to help EMS systems develop a consistent method for identifying patients who are at high risk of life-threatening injury from trauma. EMS systems around the country have the option to develop their own guidelines or use the CDC model for trauma triage.

The premise of the CDC recommendations is that the most reliable indicators of serious injury in patients are abnormal vital signs and visible injuries that you will identify during your assessments. In addition, a number of mechanisms of injury (MOI) have been identified as those that place trauma patients at high risk for serious injury.

Vital Signs

28-5 Discuss the importance of vital signs and the anatomy of injury when assessing the trauma patient.

Based on the data collected from thousands of trauma patients, certain vital sign abnormalities have been identified as reliable indicators to objectively identify the most severely injured trauma patients. Vital sign abnormalities that identify high priority trauma patients are as follows:

- Glasgow Coma Scale score of less than 14, or
- Systolic blood pressure of less than 90 mmHg in adults, or
- Respiratory rate of <10 or >29 breaths per minute (<20 in infants younger than one year).

If during your assessment you identify a patient who meets any one of these vital sign criteria, he should be considered a high-priority trauma patient.

anatomy of injury the term used in the National Trauma Triage Protocol to identify life-threatening injuries, which require the highest level of transport priority and emergency care.

Anatomy of Injury

The National Trauma Triage Protocol uses the term **anatomy of injury** as a way to identify those evident injuries that require the highest level of transport priority and

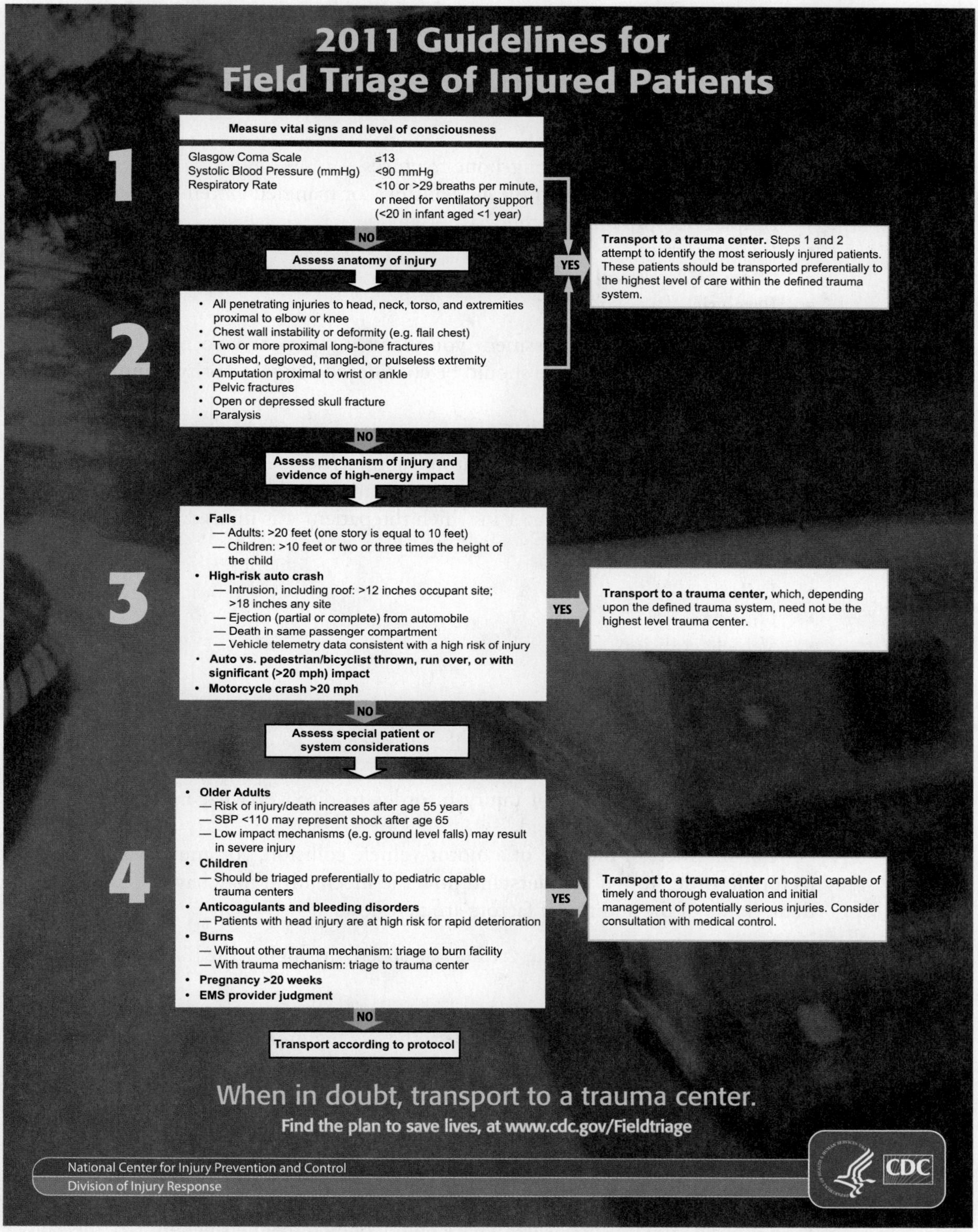

Figure 28-1 National Trauma Triage Decision Scheme: The National Trauma Triage Protocol. (Centers for Disease Control and Prevention (CDC))

trauma care because they present a potentially life-threatening risk. The following are considered significant anatomy of injury findings:

- All penetrating injuries to the head, neck, torso, and extremities proximal to the elbow or knee
- Flail chest
- Two or more proximal long-bone fractures
- Crushed, degloved (a significant avulsion), or mangled extremity
- Amputation proximal to the wrist or ankle
- Pelvic fractures
- Open or depressed skull fracture
- Paralysis

When during your assessment you identify a patient who meets any of these anatomy of injury criteria, he should be considered a high-priority trauma patient.

The Mechanism of Injury

28-6 Discuss the significance of the mechanism of injury when assessing the trauma patient.

mechanism of injury (MOI) the forces involved in causing an injury.

Beyond abnormal vital signs and anatomical injuries, one of the most important factors in determining the priority of a trauma patient is the **mechanism of injury (MOI).** The MOI describes the manner in which the patient was injured. Common mechanisms of injury include:

- Fall
- Gunshot
- Vehicle collision
- Blunt trauma
- Amputation

While the mechanisms of injury listed above can be significant and result in life-threatening injuries, usually they do not. In fact you must dig much deeper when evaluating the mechanism of injury in order to discover what injuries the patient most likely may have sustained.

For instance, in the case of a motor-vehicle collision, you must evaluate several factors in order to truly understand how the mechanism may have affected the patient. Some of the additional factors are as follows:

- ***Speed of the vehicles.*** The greater the speed, the higher the likelihood of significant injury.
- ***Location of impact.*** Where the vehicle was struck in relation to where the patient was positioned within the vehicle can have a big impact on the extent of injury.
- ***Use of restraints and air bags.*** Whether or not the patient was properly restrained and air bags deployed will greatly determine extent of injury.

Similar factors must be evaluated with each mechanism of injury. Among them are:

- ***Fall.*** Consider such factors as height of the fall, surface the patient landed on, and the position he was in when he landed.
- ***Gunshot.*** You must consider where on the body the bullets penetrated, the caliber of the weapon, and the number of injuries sustained.
- ***Blunt trauma.*** You must consider where on the body the patient sustained trauma, the type of instrument used, and the approximate force applied.
- ***Amputation.*** The first thing to consider is how far up (proximal) did the amputation occur on the limb. The closer to the torso, the larger the arteries affected, and the more bleeding.

Each situation you encounter will be different and require the evaluation of the specific factors involved.

It is important to understand that not all mechanisms of injury represent a threat to life. For instance, the warehouse worker who gets his foot run over by a forklift is not likely to be in danger of dying as a result of his injury. He will certainly be in a significant amount of pain and may even lose his foot, but the injury is not one that threatens his life. On the other hand, the bar patron who gets stabbed in the chest during a brawl is at great risk for loss of life given the potential for damage to vital organs contained within the chest cavity.

28-7 Differentiate between significant and nonsignificant mechanism of injury.

In order to more efficiently care for victims of trauma using the National Trauma Triage Decision Scheme, categorize them into one of two categories: **significant mechanism of injury** or **nonsignificant mechanism of injury.** Should it ever be unclear as to which category a patient falls in, it is best to consider the MOI significant and provide care accordingly.

significant mechanism of injury a mechanism of injury that results in a high likelihood of life-threatening injury.

nonsignificant mechanism of injury a mechanism of injury that does not result in a high likelihood of life-threatening injury.

The following mechanisms of injury that identify patients at significant risk for serious injury are contained in the National Trauma Triage Protocol. These patients should all be considered to have a significant MOI:

- Falls
  - Adults: more than 20 feet (one story is equal to 10 feet)
  - Children: more than 10 feet or two to three times the height of the child
- High-risk auto crash
  - Intrusion: more than 12 inches at occupant site; more than 18 inches at any site
  - Ejection from vehicle (partial or complete)
  - Death in same passenger compartment
  - Vehicle telemetry data consistent with high risk of injury
- Auto vs. pedestrian/bicyclist thrown, run over, or with significant impact (more than 20 mph)
- Motorcycle crash at more than 20 mph

The Assessment Path

There are two basic assessment paths you can follow when assessing the trauma patient. (Review Chapter 14.) They are the focused secondary assessment and the rapid secondary assessment. Keep in mind that all assessments must begin with a complete primary assessment. You must identify and care for any identified immediate life threats before moving on to a secondary assessment.

rapid secondary assessment a variation of the secondary assessment that is performed on unstable patients and on patients who have sustained a significant mechanism of injury.

Rapid Secondary Assessment

The **rapid secondary assessment** is the preferred path when you are caring for a trauma patient who meets major trauma criteria based on vital signs or the anatomy of injury, or who has suffered a significant MOI. This rapid assessment takes approximately 60 to 90 seconds and involves a quick visual and hands-on assessment of the patient from the head to the knees. This area of the body is sometimes referred to as the *kill zone* because it contains all of the vital organs and major structures that can result in life-threatening bleeding or other dysfunction when injured (Figure 28-2 ■). The patient's clothing should be removed in order to reveal any evidence of an injury during the rapid assessment. You are exposing the body and assessing for any evidence of trauma such as bleeding, tenderness, deformity, open wounds, and crepitus.

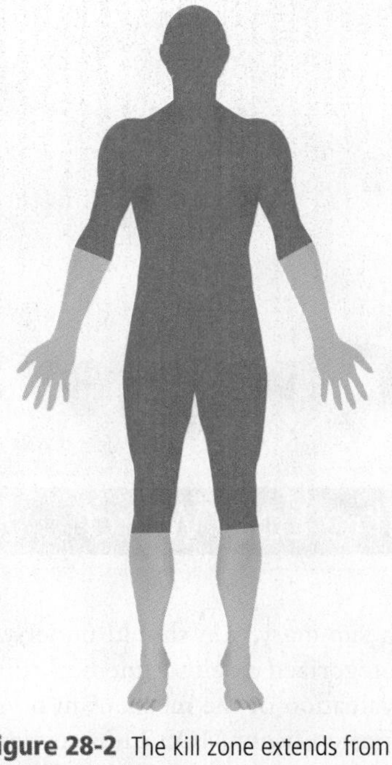

Figure 28-2 The kill zone extends from the top of the head to the knees.

Focused Secondary Assessment

The alternative assessment path after the primary assessment is called the **focused secondary assessment** and is recommended only for any trauma patient who has normal vital signs, no significant anatomy of injury, and has been subjected to an MOI considered as nonsignificant. The focused assessment will allow you to zero in on the specific injury and perform a thorough exam of the specific body part or region affected.

focused secondary assessment a variation of the secondary assessment during which the EMT focuses on the specific body part or region affected; performed on stable medical and trauma patients.

On-Scene Time

28-8 Discuss the role of time on scene with the trauma patient.

on-scene time the time spent on scene assessing, caring for, and preparing the patient for transport.

The time spent assessing and caring for a patient at the scene of the emergency is often referred to as the **on-scene time** or just *scene time*. When caring for victims of significant trauma, scene time must be kept to a minimum. Often the only intervention that is going to save the patient from life-threatening injuries is surgery. The sooner you can get the patient to the most appropriate receiving hospital, the greater his chances of survival.

Unless access to the patient is restricted or extrication is required, it is usually best to limit scene time to no more than 10 minutes. Once you have determined your patient has been injured as a result of a significant MOI, your assessment and care should be provided as you move toward the hospital.

Determining Your Destination

28-9 Discuss the importance of choosing the appropriate receiving facility when caring for trauma patients.

trauma centers specially designated trauma receiving hospitals that are staffed and equipped to manage victims of trauma.

There are specially designated trauma hospitals that are staffed and equipped to manage victims of trauma. These facilities are referred to as **trauma centers.** Studies have shown that patients who have suffered serious injuries are more likely to survive when they are transported to a trauma center rather than to a hospital that is not. A hospital can achieve trauma center designation by passing a rigorous site inspection and by meeting very specific requirements established by individual states or by the American College of Surgeons (ACS). The ACS recognizes three levels of trauma center designation with Level I being the most capable. Some states have as many as five levels of trauma center designation. There are approximately 200 Level I trauma centers in the United States.

When deciding to which hospital to take a patient, you must understand and follow local protocols in your area or region. In some instances, it may be appropriate to bypass one hospital for the services of a trauma center. Your instructor should be able to tell you about the trauma centers in your area and the protocol for deciding which patients should go where.

Chapter Review

The Last Word

In summary, you should understand that in the medical world, especially the world of EMS, patients are categorized as either medical (illness) patients or trauma (injury) patients. Trauma patients require careful evaluation of the mechanism of injury and a clear understanding of the differences between significant and nonsignificant MOI. Those patients who have suffered a significant MOI require rapid assessment and transport to an appropriate receiving hospital, preferably a trauma center.

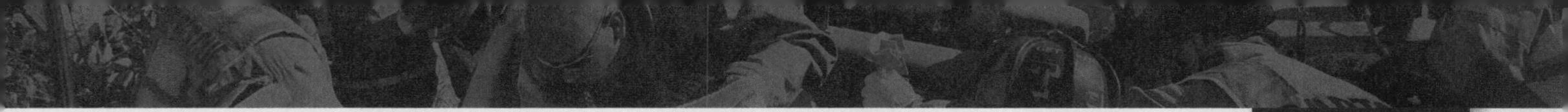

Recognition and Care of the Shock Patient

29

Education Standards

Shock and Resuscitation

Competencies

Applies fundamental knowledge of the causes, pathophysiology, and management of shock.

Objectives

After completion of this lesson, you should be able to:

29-1 Define key terms introduced in this chapter.

29-2 Describe the physiology of maintaining adequate perfusion.

29-3 Explain the pathophysiology of shock (hypoperfusion).

29-4 Describe how inadequate vascular volume, inadequate heart function, and decreased peripheral vascular resistance can lead to shock.

29-5 Explain the mechanisms and pathophysiology of each of the following categories and types of shock: cardiogenic, distributive (anaphylactic, septic, and neurogenic), hypovolemic (hemorrhagic and nonhemorrhagic), metabolic or respiratory, and obstructive.

29-6 Differentiate between early (compensated) and late (decompensated/irreversible) signs of shock.

29-7 Explain how compensatory mechanisms to shock are maintained through direct nerve stimulation and release of hormones.

29-8 Describe the progression of shock through the compensated, decompensated (progressive), and irreversible stages.

29-9 Explain the influence of age on the assessment and management of patients with shock.

29-10 Explain how to identify the patient who is in a shock state and demonstrate the assessment of patients to identify shock.

29-11 Discuss the prehospital management of patients with shock.

Key Terms

anaphylactic shock p. 753
cardiogenic shock p. 753
compensated shock p. 760
decompensated shock p. 760
hemorrhagic shock p. 753
hypoperfusion p. 751
hypovolemic shock p. 753
neurogenic shock p. 753
obstructive shock p. 753
perfusion p. 751
psychogenic shock p. 753
respiratory/metabolic shock p. 753
septic shock p. 753
shock p. 751

Introduction

Ours is a very active and mobile society, so it is no surprise that trauma is the leading cause of death among all people in the United States between the ages of 1 and 44. In most EMS systems nearly half of all requests for an ambulance are for some type of injury. Injury can result in uncontrolled internal and external bleeding, which if left untreated, can lead to life-threatening shock. This chapter will help you learn to identify the signs and symptoms of shock (hypoperfusion) and to care for a patient with suspected internal bleeding. Chapter 30 addresses how to control external bleeding that can result in shock.

EMERGENCY DISPATCH

EMT Johnny Franklin and his partner Greg Stone had just finished washing their ambulance when the emergency radio crackled to life. "Hey guys, I need you to head out to County Line Road. There's been an injury there at the tire factory."

"We're on our way, Becky," Johnny replied as he climbed behind the steering wheel and started the engine.

"Man," Greg said as he shut off the hose and got into the passenger seat. "I hope it's not like the last call we had there. That guy with the amputated leg. Remember?"

"Yup," Johnny frowned. The road dust that the tires were kicking up was already settling on the glistening truck.

When they arrived on scene and determined it was safe to enter, they found the patient was a 53-year-old machinist who was holding a blood-soaked towel tightly around his right forearm. Johnny immediately noticed that the man's pants were covered with blood and that he was very pale.

"What happened?" Greg asked as he helped the man onto the stretcher.

"It was, um, I was working a hydraulic punch and, and . . ." the man's voice trailed off and sweat began to accumulate on his forehead.

"Quick," Johnny said. "Lay him down. Someone get me a blanket or some jackets."

Protecting Yourself with BSI Precautions

Because of the potential for exposure to blood, you must be especially diligent about taking BSI precautions when you care for victims of trauma. A patient with an open wound may be thrashing about in pain, which poses a serious risk of exposure as you attempt to care for him. A patient with facial trauma may splatter blood as he coughs, sneezes, or simply tries to answer your questions. Just because the patient is not actively bleeding when you get on scene does not mean you will not be exposed to the patient's blood.

Remember that the areas of your body most susceptible to exposure are:

- Hands
- Eyes
- Mucous membranes (nose and mouth)
- Open wounds or sores

Use great caution and don the appropriate personal protective equipment (PPE) prior to making contact with any trauma patient. There might be times when goggles or a face shield is necessary. Other times a gown will be required to protect your clothing. You must anticipate the level of protection that will be necessary prior to making contact with your patient.

It is also important to properly clean and decontaminate the ambulance and all equipment following each call. And even though you were wearing gloves, do not forget to wash your hands following their removal.

Perfusion

Perfusion is the adequate flow of well-oxygenated blood throughout the entire body, especially the vital organs. When the circulatory system is functioning properly, a patient is said to be perfusing well.

The cells of the body require a constant supply of oxygen and glucose in order for aerobic metabolism to take place. Aerobic metabolism ensures the production of adenosine triphosphate (ATP), which is necessary for normal cell function and for proper maintenance of the sodium/potassium pump.

In addition to an adequate supply of oxygen and glucose, good perfusion requires a minimum of three components: an adequate volume of blood, a properly functioning heart, and an intact system of blood vessels (Figure 29-1 ■). Should any one of these components fail, **hypoperfusion** eventually will result.

Signs of adequate perfusion include:

- Normal skin signs
- Normal mental status
- Normal vital signs

When a person is not perfusing well, it is frequently due to a malfunction of one or more of the components of the circulatory system: the heart, the blood, or the blood vessels. A patient who is not perfusing well is said to be suffering from hypoperfusion. Most of the time, the terms *shock* and *hypoperfusion* are used interchangeably as they are in this textbook.

Signs and symptoms of inadequate perfusion include:

- Abnormal skin signs (pale, cool, and moist)
- Altered mental status (agitation, restlessness, sluggishness, confusion, or decreased responsiveness)
- Abnormal vital signs (increased pulse and respiratory rate, decreased blood pressure)

For the most part, the type of shock described in this chapter results from an excessive amount of blood loss and is called *hemorrhagic shock*.

29-2 Describe the physiology of maintaining adequate perfusion.

perfusion the supply of oxygen to and removal of wastes from the cells and tissues of the body as a result of the flow of blood through the capillaries.

hypoperfusion inadequate perfusion of blood to an organ or organs. Also called *shock*.

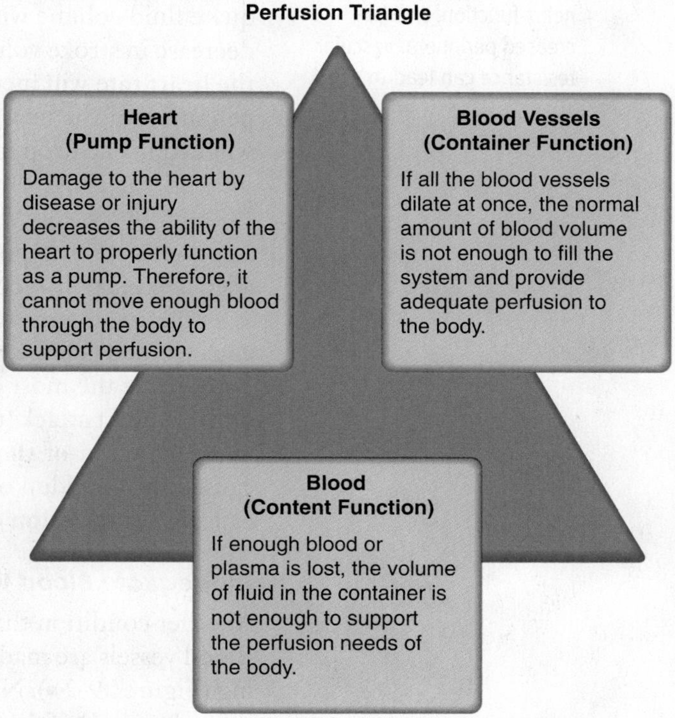

Figure 29-1 The three primary components related to perfusion.

PERSPECTIVE

Jason—The Patient

That was weird. I thought that I was doing okay. I've hurt myself before but this time I got tunnel vision and started feeling really nervous, like something bad was about to happen but I couldn't really put my finger on it. That's definitely the strangest feeling that I've ever had.

Shock

29-3 Explain the pathophysiology of shock (hypoperfusion).

Shock is a progressive condition that occurs when a patient does *not* receive an adequate supply of well-oxygenated blood to all organs of the body. It can occur for several reasons, including damage to the heart, loss of blood, and abnormal dilation of the vessels.

shock inadequate perfusion of blood to an organ or organs. Also called *hypoperfusion*.

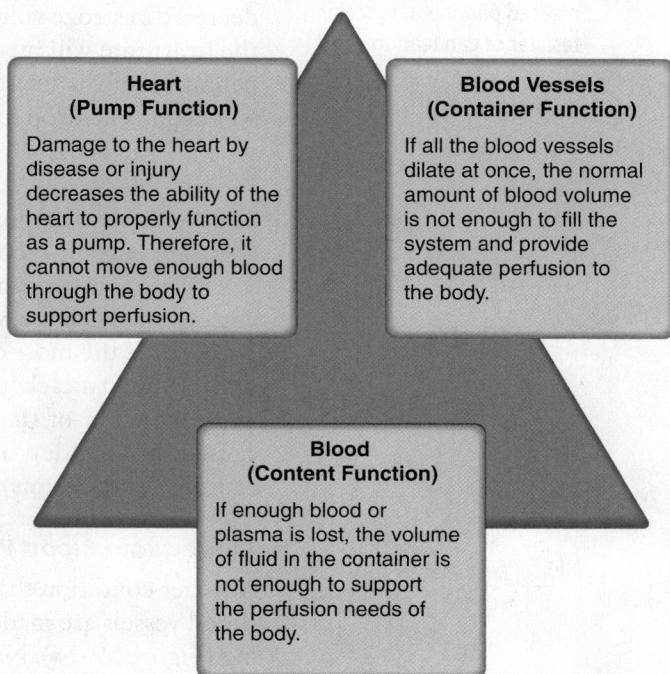

As a direct result of poor perfusion, the cells of the various organs (liver, kidneys, brain, heart, lungs) begin to starve for oxygen and suffer from the effects of accumulating wastes. When enough cells within a particular organ have failed, the entire organ or organ system begins to malfunction and eventually shuts down. Without prompt recognition in the field and treatment at a hospital, patients in shock die.

Causes of Shock

Inadequate vascular volume, inadequate heart function, and decreased peripheral vascular resistance can lead to shock.

Inadequate Volume

29-4 Describe how inadequate vascular volume, inadequate heart function, and decreased peripheral vascular resistance can lead to shock.

A patient can have an inadequate amount of blood or plasma or both depending on whether they are bleeding uncontrollably or dehydrated. In either case, an inadequate fluid volume will result in a decrease in cardiac preload that will in turn cause a decrease in stroke volume. In an effort to compensate for a decrease in stroke volume, the heart rate will increase in order to maintain a normal cardiac output. If the compensation of the heart rate cannot keep up with the volume loss, the cardiac output will drop. The drop in cardiac output results in a decrease in systolic blood pressure.

Pump Failure

Another cause of hypoperfusion is the failure of the heart to pump with enough force to adequately supply blood to the body. The body depends on the heart to maintain a constant minimum pressure as it pumps blood throughout the body. Even if there is an adequate blood volume, when the pump weakens (fails), the result is inadequate perfusion.

One of the most common causes of pump failure is damage to the heart muscle due to a heart attack (myocardial infarction). Other causes of pump failure are trauma and restriction of the ability of the heart to contract and expand properly. This is caused by a buildup of blood or fluid in the pericardial sac that surrounds the heart, causing compression of the heart (pericardial tamponade).

Inadequate Blood Vessel Tone

Another condition that results in poor perfusion is poor blood vessel tone or control. Blood vessels are made up of smooth muscle that is capable of dilating and constricting (Figure 29-2 ▪). Normally, the body automatically controls vessel tone and adjusts it for the needs of the body. This is also referred to as *systemic vascular resistance (SVR)*.

A minimum amount of SVR is required to maintain an adequate blood pressure. When vessel tone is lost, the vessels are allowed to dilate abnormally causing a drop

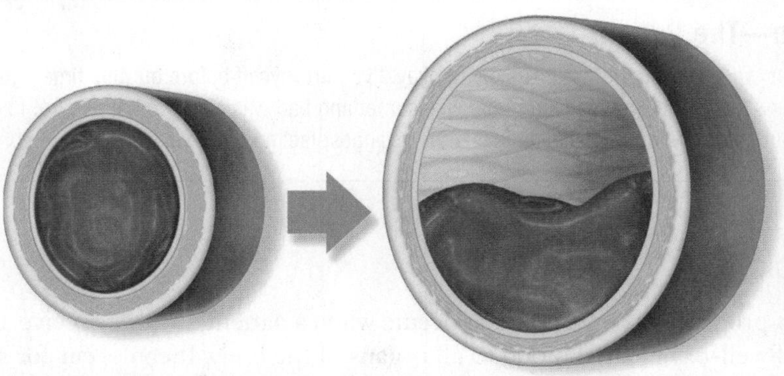
Normal-sized vessel full of blood.
Dilated vessel only partially filled with blood.

Figure 29-2 The sympathetic nervous system controls vessel tone.

in SVR. When faced with a falling SVR, the heart will try to compensate and increase its cardiac output by increasing the heart rate. Because blood pressure is determined by SVR and cardiac output, when the heart can no longer compensate by raising heart rate, a drop in systolic blood pressure will occur, resulting in hypoperfusion. SVR can suddenly drop as a result of injury, overwhelming infections, and damage to the spinal cord.

PRACTICAL PATHOPHYSIOLOGY

The sympathetic nervous system controls the dilation and constriction of the blood vessels. When the spinal cord becomes injured and damaged, it can no longer stimulate the sympathetic nervous system and vessel tone is lost, causing a decrease in systemic vascular resistance.

29-5 Explain the mechanisms and pathophysiology of each of the following categories and types of shock: cardiogenic, distributive (anaphylactic, septic, and neurogenic), hypovolemic (hemorrhagic and nonhemorrhagic), metabolic or respiratory, and obstructive.

Types of Shock

Not all incidences of shock are caused by bleeding. The following list describes several other types of shock and their root causes:

- ***Anaphylactic shock.*** An overreaction of the immune system when exposed to an allergen, **anaphylactic shock** occurs when the blood vessels dilate, resulting in a decrease in blood pressure and a corresponding decrease in perfusion. (Refer to Chapter 24 for more information.)
- ***Cardiogenic shock.*** **Cardiogenic shock** is caused when the heart can no longer pump blood adequately, resulting in a decrease in cardiac output and thus a decrease in perfusion.
- ***Hemorrhagic shock.*** Loss of blood causes **hemorrhagic shock.**
- ***Hypovolemic shock.*** **Hypovolemic shock** is caused by a sudden decrease in body fluids (blood or other fluids such as severe diarrhea). That decrease in fluid volume causes a decrease in stroke volume and a corresponding decrease in perfusion.
- ***Neurogenic shock.*** A response to injury to the spinal cord, **neurogenic shock** is the abnormal dilation of the blood vessels, resulting in a decrease in blood pressure and a corresponding decrease in perfusion.
- ***Septic shock.*** This type of shock typically is caused by a severe infection that abnormally dilates the blood vessels. In **septic shock** there is a decrease in systemic vascular resistance with a corresponding decrease in perfusion.
- ***Psychogenic shock.*** **Psychogenic shock** is caused by a sudden and temporary dilation of the blood vessels from psychological causes, resulting in a decrease in blood pressure and a corresponding decrease in perfusion.
- ***Obstructive shock.*** This form of shock results when forward movement of blood flow is obstructed. Conditions such as pulmonary embolism, tension pneumothorax, and pericardial tamponade can cause **obstructive shock.**
- ***Respiratory/metabolic shock.*** This form of shock is caused by a disruption in the ability of cells to utilize oxygen effectively. Certain poisons such as cyanide and carbon monoxide can cause the development of **respiratory/metabolic shock.**

anaphylactic shock type of shock caused by an overreaction of the immune system when exposed to an allergen.

cardiogenic shock type of shock caused when the heart can no longer pump blood adequately, resulting in a decrease in cardiac output and thus a decrease in perfusion.

hemorrhagic shock type of shock caused by loss of blood.

hypovolemic shock type of shock caused by a sudden decrease in body fluids (blood or other body fluids).

neurogenic shock type of shock caused when the vessels dilate abnormally in response to injury to the spinal cord.

septic shock type of shock caused by severe infections that abnormally dilate the blood vessels.

psychogenic shock type of shock caused by a sudden and temporary dilation of the blood vessels from psychological causes.

obstructive shock a form of shock that blocks the forward movement of blood within the circulatory system.

respiratory/metabolic shock a form of shock caused by a disruption in the ability of cells to utilize oxygen effectively.

Internal Bleeding

A sudden loss of a significant quantity of blood is dangerous and, if left untreated, life threatening (Table 29-1). It is relatively uncommon for a patient to die from external bleeding if there are people at the scene who can assist. Because most external bleeding is obvious, it usually gets the attention of bystanders or rescuers and attempts are quickly made to control the bleeding.

TABLE 29-1 APPROXIMATE BLOOD VOLUME BY SIZE

ADULT	CHILD	INFANT
70 mL/kg of blood	80 mL/kg of blood	80 mL/kg of blood
An average-size adult weighing 70 kg (154 lb) would have approximately 4,900 mL of blood.	A child weighing 30 kg (66 lb) would have approximately 2,400 mL of blood.	An infant weighing 10 kg (22 lb) would have approximately 800 mL of blood.

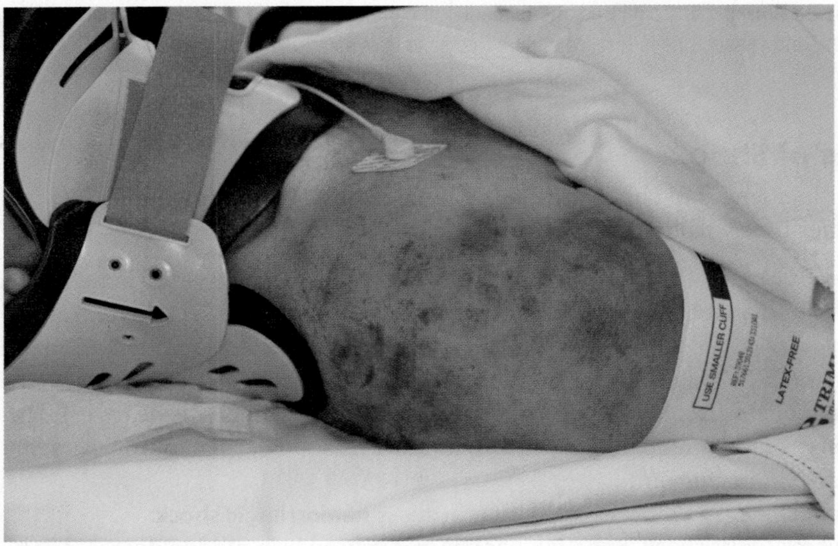

Figure 29-3 Bruising is a common sign of internal bleeding. (© Edward T. Dickinson, MD)

In the case of internal bleeding (Figure 29-3 ■), the blood being lost from the circulatory system is contained within the body and cannot be easily detected by rescuers. Even when internal bleeding is suspected, there is little that can be done to stop the bleeding in the field. Patients with internal bleeding generally require surgical intervention to repair the damage and control the bleeding. For this reason, early recognition and rapid transport are essential.

Severity of Blood Loss

The numerous organs contained within the torso and the many vessels that supply them with blood present a great potential for life-threatening internal bleeding. The areas of greatest concern for internal blood loss are the:

- Chest
- Abdomen
- Pelvis

The volume of blood loss from internal bleeding can exceed several liters. In some larger patients, even injuries to the extremities can conceal enough blood to cause shock (Table 29-2).

Predicting Internal Bleeding

Because internal bleeding cannot be seen, you must use other means to predict the likelihood that it exists. In trauma, an important initial tool used to predict the

TABLE 29-2 APPROXIMATE INTERNAL BLOOD LOSS ASSOCIATED WITH UNDERLYING FRACTURES

BONE	APPROXIMATE BLOOD LOSS
Rib	125 cc
Radius/ulna	250–500 cc
Humerus	500–750 cc
Tibia/fibula	500–1,000 cc
Femur	1,000–2,000 cc
Pelvis	1,000–3,000 cc

potential for internal bleeding is the mechanism of injury (MOI). Any significant mechanism, such as penetrating trauma, rapid deceleration, blunt trauma, or crushing injury that affects the chest, abdomen, or pelvis has the potential for causing life-threatening internal bleeding. You must maintain a high index of suspicion for internal bleeding with any of the following mechanisms:

- Falls from a height (Figure 29-4 ■)
- Motorcycle collisions
- Vehicle vs. pedestrian impacts
- Automobile collisions
- Blast injuries
- Penetrating trauma to the chest, abdomen, pelvis, or proximal limbs
- Significant blunt trauma
- Rapid deceleration
- Blunt trauma

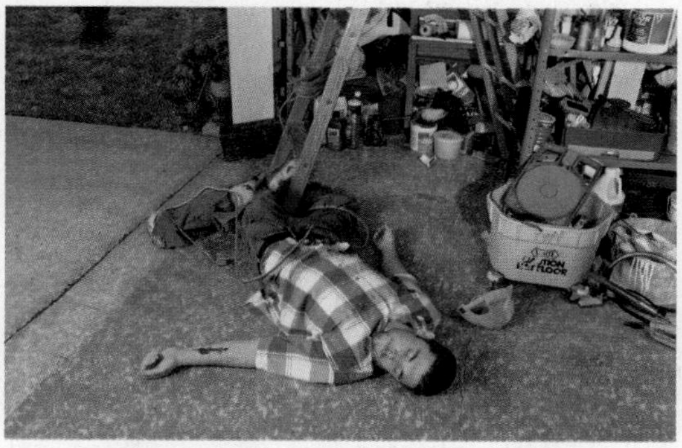

Figure 29-4 Maintain a high index of suspicion for internal bleeding with any patient who has suffered a significant mechanism of injury such as a fall from a height.

When you link the mechanism of injury to physical findings consistent with shock (rapid pulse, cool moist skin, decreased blood pressure), often you will be able to identify patients who are suffering from significant internal bleeding.

In addition to trauma, certain medical conditions can cause sudden internal bleeding. Leakage or rupture of an aortic aneurysm as well as bleeding from the stomach and intestines can be other causes of serious internal bleeding.

Signs and Symptoms of Internal Bleeding

In addition to evaluating the mechanism of injury, you must carefully assess the patient and identify any signs or symptoms that might indicate the presence of internal bleeding. The following is a list of some of the more common signs and symptoms of internal bleeding:

- Rigid or distended abdomen or pelvic region
- Pain, tenderness, swelling, or discoloration on or near the suspected site of injury
- Bleeding from the mouth, rectum, or vagina
- Vomiting bright red blood or dark coffee-ground-colored blood (digested blood)
- Bleeding during a bowel movement or stools that are bloody or dark and tarry in color
- Signs and symptoms of shock without external bleeding: rapid pulse; cool, moist, pale skin; decreased mental status; and low systolic blood pressure

PERSPECTIVE

Johnny—The EMT

That guy lost quite a bit of blood. There was a good amount on and around the machine that he was using, who knows how much had soaked into his clothing, and that white towel was all red. I knew right away that shock was going to be an issue in this call, so I started planning for it. You know, going over in my head the steps to follow. Being that Greg and I are EMTs, we can't give IV fluids or anything like that to counter the blood loss, but we can definitely help.

STOP, REVIEW, REMEMBER!

Multiple Choice

For each question, place a check next to the correct answer.

1. Which one of the following is *not* a sign of good perfusion?

_____ a. Pink, warm, and dry skin
_____ b. Confused mental status
_____ c. Alert and normal mental status
_____ d. Vital signs within normal limits

2. If left untreated, _______________ can lead to shock.

_____ a. bleeding
_____ b. high blood pressure
_____ c. a rapid respiration
_____ d. an altered mental status

3. In many cases, patients with internal bleeding will require _______________ in order to survive.

_____ a. late detection of shock
_____ b. surgical intervention
_____ c. ongoing assessments
_____ d. a rapid trauma assessment

4. The type of shock that develops when too much blood is lost is known as _______________ shock.

_____ a. psychogenic
_____ b. metabolic
_____ c. hemorrhagic
_____ d. anaphylactic

5. What type of shock is caused when the vessels dilate abnormally in response to injury to the spinal cord?

_____ a. Anaphylactic
_____ b. Hemorrhagic
_____ c. Cardiogenic
_____ d. Neurogenic

Fill in the Blank

1. _____________________________ is the leading cause of death among all persons between the ages of 1 and 44.

2. Perfusion is the adequate flow of _____________________________ blood throughout the entire body, especially the vital organs.

3. A patient with adequate perfusion will have normal skin signs, normal _____________________________, and normal vital signs.

4. A patient who is not perfusing well is said to be suffering from _____________________________.

5. The areas of greatest concern for internal blood loss are the _____________________________, abdomen, and pelvis.

Critical Thinking

1. Describe the relationship between mechanism of injury and the likelihood of internal bleeding.

2. Explain why internal bleeding is frequently more deadly than external bleeding.

3. List as many signs and symptoms of internal bleeding as you can.

Signs and Symptoms of Shock

The signs and symptoms of shock are progressive and develop over time. The speed at which they develop will depend on the extent of bleeding and the care the patient receives. The following is a list of signs and symptoms of shock:

- Increased pulse rate (tachycardia)
- Altered mental status, including restlessness and anxiety
- Increased respiratory rate (tachypnea)
- Increased capillary refill time
- Weak peripheral pulses
- Pale, cool, and clammy skin
- Thirst
- Sluggish and dilated pupils
- Nausea or vomiting
- Decreasing blood pressure (late sign)

PERSPECTIVE

Greg—The EMT

As soon as the patient started to go out, I called for the ALS truck, but Becky told us that there had been a rollover collision out on the interstate and Tom wasn't available. So we did what we could. Do you know what the most effective treatment for shock is on a BLS ambulance with no ALS help available? I call it "diesel therapy." It goes something like this: Control any bleeding that you can see, load the patient in the ambulance, and get to the hospital as quickly and safely as possible!

The signs and symptoms of shock tell us that the body is attempting to compensate for the loss of blood—or heart malfunction, vessel dilation, or other causes—and the inadequate perfusion that results. It is working properly to try and save itself, and making every attempt to compensate for the decrease in perfusion.

Richard: A Case Study for the Progression of Shock

29-8 Describe the progression of shock through the compensated, decompensated (progressive), and irreversible stages.

Richard is a 44-year-old man who was ejected from a minivan rollover. He has suffered significant injury to his abdomen and is bleeding internally. He is responsive and is lying supine on the ground in pain. During your rapid trauma assessment, you discover that Richard was not restrained during the incident and he is complaining of severe abdominal pain on palpation of both upper quadrants. There is no evidence of external trauma or bleeding, and Richard is alert and oriented × 4.

Richard's vital signs prior to the incident are as follows:

Time	Respirations	Pulse	BP	Skin	Pupils	Mental
1100	16, good tidal volume, unlabored	76, strong, regular	118/76	pink, warm, dry	PERRL	A&O × 4

Ten minutes following the incident there is a loss of approximately 500 cc of blood and vital signs are as follows:

Time	Respirations	Pulse	BP	Skin	Pupils	Mental
1110	18, good tidal volume, unlabored	94, strong, regular	126/86	pink, warm, dry	PERRL	A&O × 3

Ten minutes following the incident, Richard is still shaken up and experiencing the effects of the adrenaline that was released as a result of the psychological and physical stress of the crash. The rush of adrenaline has caused his respirations, pulse, and blood pressure to increase slightly for the time being. His circulatory system is damaged, and blood is spilling into his abdomen. The increase in pulse rate from the initial rush of adrenaline has managed to compensate for the blood loss—at least for now.

Twenty minutes following the incident, there is a loss of approximately 1,000 cc of blood and vital signs are as follows:

Time	Respirations	Pulse	BP	Skin	Pupils	Mental
1120	22, good tidal volume, labored	120, strong, regular	118/84	pale, warm, dry	PERRL	A&O × 3 anxious

Richard has lost a full liter of blood into his abdomen, and the adrenaline rush from the incident has completely worn off. His body must now work extra hard in an attempt to maintain adequate perfusion. His respiratory and pulse rates are up slightly. Considering what he has been through, the EMT finding Richard with these vital signs might not think the situation is that bad. Anyone who has just survived a rollover collision and is in pain could have these vital signs.

But unlike the EMT at the scene, you have the luxury of knowing his vitals both before the incident and 10 minutes following. This begins to illustrate just how easy it is to think your patient is doing okay, when in reality he has already begun to spiral into shock.

Also notice that Richard's mental status and skin signs have changed slightly. The brain is the organ most susceptible to changes in perfusion, and his change in mental status reflects it. His skin is pale now, too, because the vessels in the skin have constricted in an effort to redirect more blood to the core of the body. This decrease in blood flow to the skin causes changes in both color and temperature.

Thirty minutes following the incident, there is a loss of approximately 2,000 cc of blood and vital signs are as follows:

Time	Respirations	Pulse	BP	Skin	Pupils	Mental
1130	26, shallow, and labored	140, weak, regular	108/88	pale, cool, clammy	dilated, sluggish	A&O × 2 restless and confused

The most obvious change in Richard's condition at 30 minutes is his altered mental status. He can be aroused only by verbal stimuli and knows his name but cannot provide any other meaningful details. His pulse has increased significantly in an attempt to maintain blood pressure, and his respirations have increased in response to the tissues demanding more oxygen. The vessels in the skin and extremities have all constricted as far as they can, causing his pale and cool skin signs. His clammy skin is due to the enormous stress his body is under, trying to save itself. His blood pressure is falling now and is the reason for weak or absent peripheral pulses. The loss of adequate perfusion also is causing his pupils to dilate and to respond sluggishly to light.

Up until this point, Richard's body has been able to compensate for the loss of blood and poor perfusion. Eventually, even the mechanisms that are trying to sustain his life will fail due to poor perfusion.

Forty minutes into the incident, there is a loss of approximately 2,500 cc of blood and vital signs are as follows:

Time	Respirations	Pulse	BP	Skin	Pupils	Mental
1140	8, shallow, labored	130, weak, regular	60/palpation	pale, cool, clammy	dilated, nonresponsive	unresponsive

After 40 minutes and a blood loss of 2,500 cc, Richard's body has now lost the ability to compensate and all body systems are beginning to fail. His blood pressure is falling rapidly. Soon he will be in cardiac arrest, and the likelihood of survival from a blunt trauma cardiac arrest will be almost nonexistent.

PRACTICAL PATHOPHYSIOLOGY

One of the major factors in determining good perfusion is adequate blood volume. A typical adult has approximately 70 mL of blood for every kilogram of body weight. A patient weighing 82 kg (180 lb) will have approximately 5,700 mL of blood. Blood volume is a factor of body mass. A loss of 1 liter of blood for a 50 kg patient is much more dangerous than for a 100 kg patient.

Compensated vs. Decompensated Shock

29-6 Differentiate between early (compensated) and late (decompensated/irreversible) signs of shock.

One of the points in using a case study as an example of how shock progresses is to show you that sometimes the early signs of poor perfusion are there, and you may not see them. They are hidden behind the pain and stress that are so much a part of most trauma calls. Therefore, you must anticipate shock and maintain a high index of suspicion when the mechanism of injury suggests it. Remember that an increased pulse rate is an early sign, and a decreasing blood pressure is a late sign. Do *not* wait for signs and symptoms of shock to be obvious to initiate care and transport.

29-7 Explain how compensatory mechanisms to shock are maintained through direct nerve stimulation and release of hormones.

The body compensates for shock with two primary responses: first, direct nerve stimulation and second, through the release of hormones. When shock occurs, the sympathetic nervous system is activated and sends signals to the heart and blood vessels in an attempt to maintain an adequate blood pressure. The early effects of the sympathetic nervous system are:

- Increased heart rate
- Increase in the force of heart contractions
- Constriction of the blood vessels (increased SVR)

During shock, the adrenal glands release the hormones epinephrine and norepinephrine. Their release produces a more sustained sympathetic effect. The release of epinephrine causes stimulation of both alpha and beta receptors, while the release of norepinephrine affects mostly alpha receptors. The stimulation of $beta_1$ receptors affects the heart and causes an increase in rate and strength of contractions. The stimulation of alpha receptors causes a constriction of the blood vessels.

compensated shock when the patient is developing shock but the body is still able to maintain perfusion.

decompensated shock when the body can no longer compensate for low blood volume or lack of perfusion. Late signs, such as decreasing blood pressure, become evident.

Early signs of shock, such as increased pulse, increased breathing rates, and pale skin, are indications that the body is working to compensate for blood loss. This is known as **compensated shock.** If the blood loss is allowed to continue, the body's own compensatory mechanisms will begin to shut down due to poor perfusion, and the patient will enter a state referred to as **decompensated shock.** A major indication that the patient has entered the decompensated shock state is a significant drop in blood pressure. In addition to the drop in blood pressure, the patient will present with a significant decrease in mental status. During this phase, the pulse will become very weak until it finally goes away and the patient experiences cardiac arrest (Table 29-3).

Shock in Pediatric and Geriatric Patients

29-9 Explain the influence of age on the assessment and management of patients with shock.

Pediatric patients have an excellent ability to compensate for blood loss. Some pediatric patients are capable of maintaining what appears to be a normal blood pressure until nearly half of their blood volume is lost. Once the child's body can no longer compensate, his condition quickly deteriorates and death may be sudden. It is

TABLE 29-3 COMPENSATED VS. DECOMPENSATED SHOCK

VITAL SIGN	COMPENSATED SHOCK	DECOMPENSATED SHOCK
Respirations	Increased rate	Decreasing rate
Pulse	Increasing rate	Becomes weaker
Blood pressure	Normal to low systolic Normal to elevated diastolic	Decreasing to absent
Skin	Pale, cool, moist	Pale, cool, moist
Pupils	Sluggish but responsive	Sluggish to fixed and dilated
Mental status	Slightly altered	Very altered to unresponsive

especially important to anticipate shock with pediatric patients and initiate care and transport as soon as possible.

Geriatric patients may show signs of shock more readily than younger patients. This can be due to changes of age such as blood vessels that are stiffer and less responsive to the sympathetic stimulus to contract. In addition, older patients may be on medications such as beta blockers that prevent the heart rate from increasing in response to blood loss. Patients on beta blockers can be difficult to assess for shock, because they will not be as tachycardic as you would expect and at the same time may progress to decompensated shock more quickly because of the inability to raise heart rate and constrict blood vessels.

Assessment of the Shock Patient

Use a standard approach to your patient assessment as you would with any patient, beginning with the scene size-up and primary assessment.

29-10 Explain how to identify the patient who is in a shock state and demonstrate the assessment of patients to identify shock.

Scene Size-up

Once you have taken the appropriate BSI precautions, you must confirm that the scene is safe. Make sure that there are no hazards, such as downed power lines, that pose a threat to you and others. As you approach the scene, begin evaluating the mechanism of injury. Do your best to determine the exact mechanism or mechanisms the patient may have suffered. For instance, if the MOI is a motor-vehicle collision, how much damage is there to the outside of the vehicle? How about the inside of the vehicle? Does it appear that the patient was restrained? Did an air bag deploy? Did the vehicle roll over?

If the MOI was a fall, how far did the patient fall? What type of surface did he land on? What position was he in when he hit the ground?

Your evaluation of the MOI does not end when you discover the patient. It must continue throughout the time you are with the patient, and you must attempt to gather as many details as possible without compromising patient care.

Maintain appropriate spinal precautions for all victims of trauma.

Primary Assessment

Confirm that the patient's ABCs are all intact and that breathing is adequate. Just because the patient looks okay does not mean he will not get worse. Monitor the ABCs carefully, and initiate supplemental oxygen by nonrebreather mask as soon as possible.

If you have enough help at the scene, baseline vital signs should be obtained simultaneously during the primary assessment. Be sure to obtain and document a complete set of baseline vitals that can be used for trending later. Be sure to document them in a place where you can easily see them. This will help you spot trends that would otherwise be difficult to identify. Since this information can be critical to saving a life, it is important to pay attention to the previous sets of vitals each time you take new ones.

Secondary Assessment

All patients with signs of shock or those who have sustained a significant mechanism of injury must receive a rapid secondary assessment. This is a quick head-to-toe exam looking for all obvious injuries and points of pain. It can be done in about 90 seconds and is almost always completed while on scene.

Gather as much history from the trauma patient and bystanders as possible as you perform your rapid assessment. You should already be planning transport, and one of the simplest ways to transport these patients is on a long backboard.

Continuously monitor the patient's ABCs and repeat the vital signs at least every five minutes if the patient is unstable. Consider increasing the oxygen flow, if appropriate, and confirm that all external bleeding is controlled.

Emergency Care of the Shock Patient

29-11 Discuss the prehospital management of patients with shock.

Perform the following steps when caring for a patient whom you suspect may have internal bleeding or who is presenting with the signs and symptoms of shock (Scan 29-1):

1. Conduct an appropriate scene size-up and take the necessary BSI precautions.
2. Manually stabilize the spine as appropriate for the MOI.
3. Perform a primary assessment and initiate supplemental oxygen.
4. Control any external bleeding.
5. Keep the patient supine. If the cause of shock is due to illness, you may elevate the legs 8 to 12 inches.
6. Conserve body heat by covering the patient with a blanket when appropriate.
7. Place the patient on a long backboard as appropriate for the MOI.
8. Initiate transport and request an ALS intercept if available.
9. Perform reassessments as appropriate and be alert for changing vital signs (trending).

Remember that victims of trauma may have suffered a spine injury. Evaluate the MOI and take the appropriate spinal precautions with all victims of trauma. If the patient is unresponsive and spine injury is suspected, use the jaw-thrust maneuver to open the airway. If you are unable to establish an appropriate airway, perform a head-tilt/chin-lift maneuver.

Pneumatic Anti-Shock Garment

The pneumatic anti-shock garment (PASG) is a pair of inflatable trousers designed for patients who have suffered specific types of injuries (Figure 29-5 ■). Originally developed by the military for the treatment of shock, they were once known as military anti-shock trousers (MAST). Indications for the use of PASG vary, so check your local protocols to determine if and when it should be used. Indications for the PASG may include:

- Suspected lower extremity fracture(s). In this case, you may use only the leg compartments as a splint.
- Suspected pelvic fracture(s) with signs of shock.

As for use with suspected extremity and pelvic fractures, it is thought that the inflated garment acts as a splint, allowing a more stable fracture, which in turn means less soft tissue damage, less bleeding, and less pain.

The use of PASG and its relative value is controversial, and protocols for its use will vary considerably from system to system. In many areas it is no longer used at all.

There are a few instances when the use of the PASG is contraindicated. They are as follows:

- Cases of known pulmonary edema or increased respiratory difficulty following application
- Cardiogenic shock

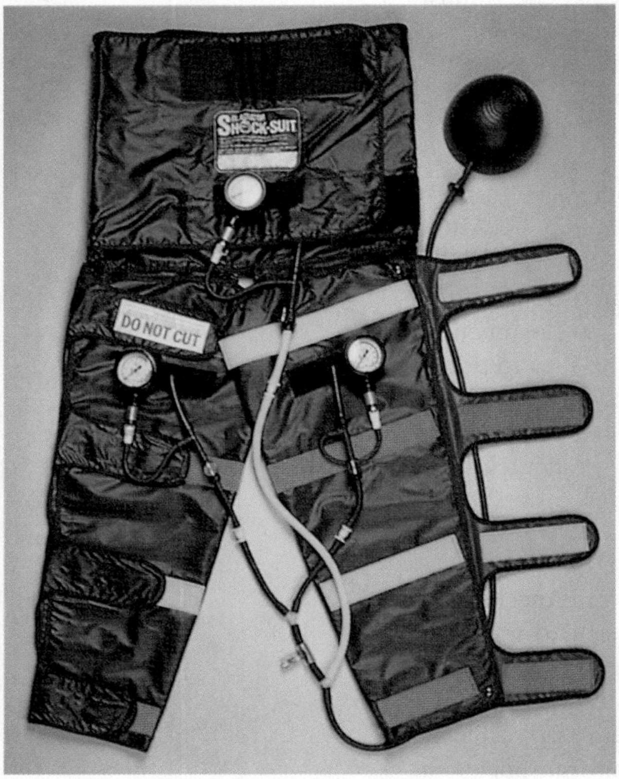

Figure 29-5 A pneumatic anti-shock garment (PASG).

SCAN 29-1 Management of a Shock Patient

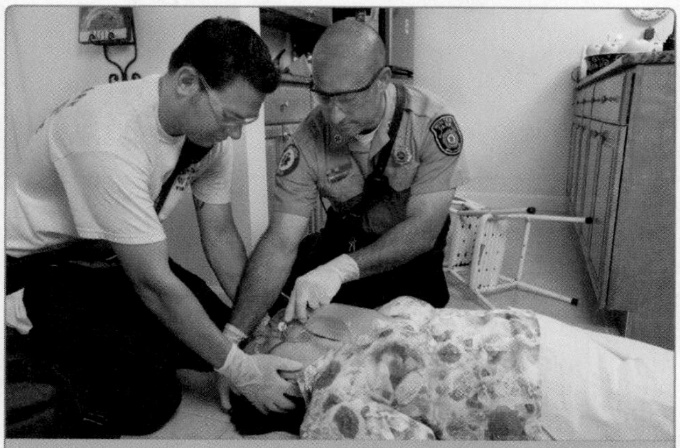

29-1-1 Perform a primary assessment and provide supplemental oxygen.

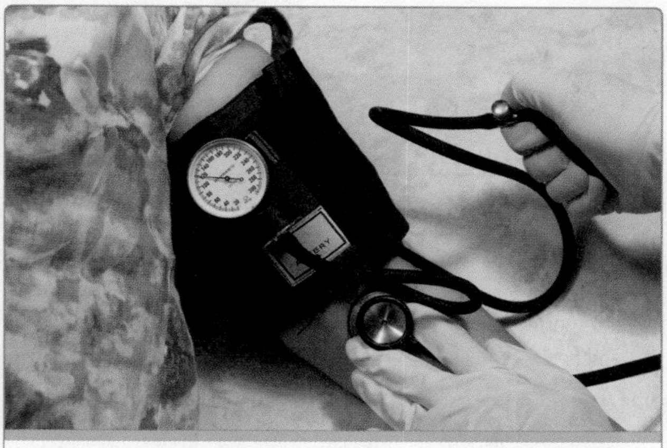

29-1-2 Obtain a baseline set of vitals and monitor vitals every five minutes.

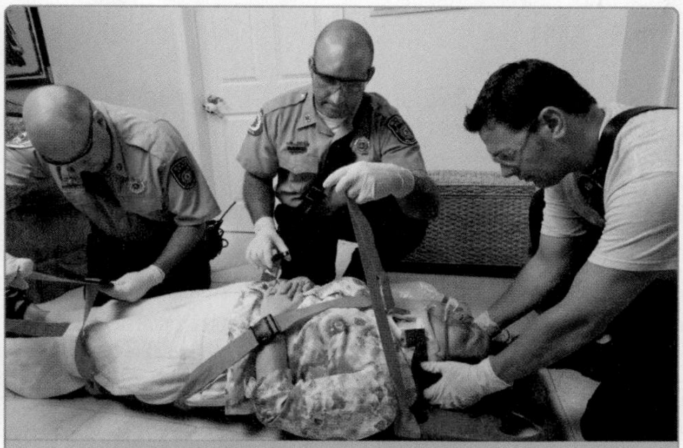

29-1-3 If appropriate, immobilize the patient for transport.

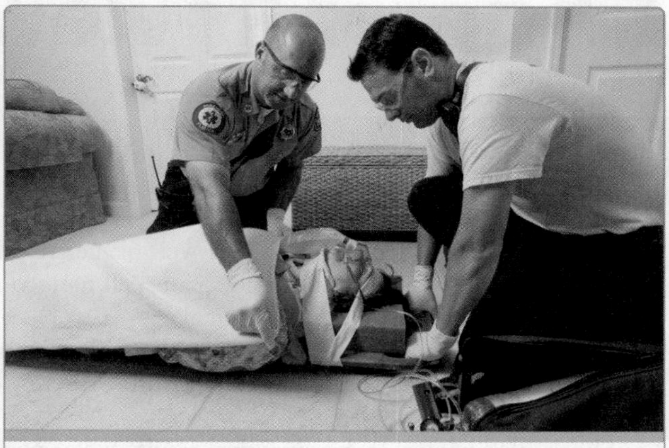

29-1-4 Monitor body temperature and minimize heat loss.

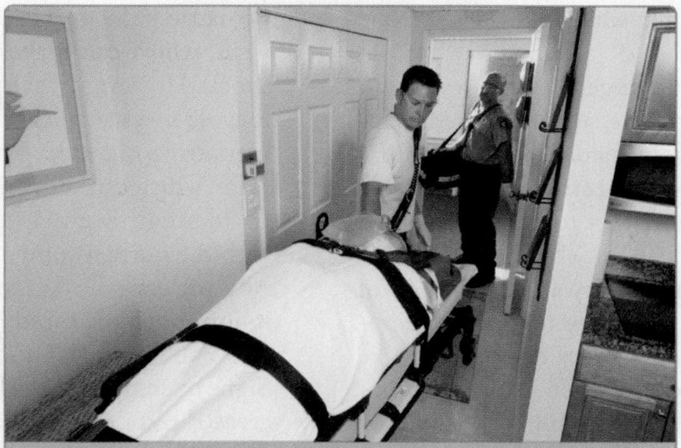

29-1-5 Transport immediately to an appropriate hospital.

- Internal bleeding of the chest
- Impaled objects in the abdomen
- Third trimester of pregnancy
- Evisceration

EMERGENCY DISPATCH SUMMARY

The patient was secured on the stretcher, covered with a blanket, and placed on 15 L/min of oxygen with a nonrebreather mask. His bleeding was controlled with direct pressure and elevation of the limb. He was then rapidly transported to Farmer's Hospital where he was treated for shock, blood loss, and two seven-centimeter lacerations on his right forearm.

The patient was released two days later and, except for some numbness in two fingers, he has recovered fully. He has since returned to work and has joined the factory's emergency response team.

Chapter Review

To the Point

- Perfusion is the adequate supply of well-oxygenated blood to the cells. When perfusion is adequate, cell metabolism is allowed to occur aerobically as normal.
- When perfusion becomes inadequate, cell metabolism becomes anaerobic and the production of ATP drops significantly.
- Shock, also known as *hypoperfusion*, results when perfusion is compromised. There are three broad categories of shock: volume loss, pump failure, and loss of vessel tone.
- Hypovolemic (hemorrhagic and nonhemorrhagic) shock occurs as a result of fluid loss, which results in a drop in systolic blood pressure.
- Distributive (anaphylactic, septic, neurogenic) shock results in a disruption of the sympathetic nervous system to properly control vessel tone, resulting in a drop in systolic blood pressure.
- Cardiogenic shock results when the heart is no longer able to pump efficiently, and the cells begin to starve for blood and oxygen.
- Obstructive shock occurs when the forward movement of blood is restricted. This can be caused by tension pneumothorax, cardiac tamponade, and pulmonary embolism.
- Respiratory/metabolic shock occurs when oxygen cannot be effectively utilized by the cells. It is commonly caused by poisons such as carbon monoxide and cyanide.
- During shock, the body attempts to compensate for a lack of adequate perfusion by initiating specific responses driven by the sympathetic nervous system. Direct nerve stimulation and the release of hormones causes the heart to beat faster and stronger and the blood vessels to constrict among other responses.
- The body will continue its attempts to compensate for the lack of adequate perfusion until the body systems responsible for compensation also begin to fail. This is called *decompensated shock* and is characterized by an altered mental status, significant drop in blood pressure, narrow pulse pressure, and other signs.
- Pediatric patients have a very strong compensatory mechanism, which can make it appear as though they are not in shock. However, when the compensatory mechanisms fail, they do so very quickly and death will soon follow.
- Geriatric patients have a much weaker compensatory mechanism, which can cause them to get worse much more rapidly. In addition they may be taking medications that interfere with the normal compensatory mechanisms.
- Any patient who has sustained a significant mechanism of injury should be cared for with a high index of suspicion for internal bleeding and shock.
- Signs of compensated shock include increased pulse rate; increased respiratory rate; normal to low blood pressure; nausea; and pale, cool, and sometimes moist skin.
- The best way to manage any patient who may be in shock is to manage the ABCs, provide oxygen, and transport rapidly.

Chapter Questions

Multiple Choice

For each question, place a check next to the correct answer.

1. All of the following are signs of shock *except*:

_____ a. increased pulse rate.
_____ b. decreasing blood pressure.
_____ c. pink, warm, moist skin.
_____ d. altered mental status.

2. The most appropriate method for opening the airway of an unresponsive trauma patient is the _____________ maneuver.

_____ a. jaw-thrust
_____ b. chin-lift
_____ c. head-tilt
_____ d. jaw-tilt

3. Some pediatric patients are capable of maintaining what appears to be a normal blood pressure until _____________ of their blood volume is lost.

_____ a. one-third
_____ b. nearly half
_____ c. two-thirds
_____ d. nearly one-quarter

4. When used for the treatment of suspected pelvic fractures, the PASG helps by:

_____ a. pushing blood out of the area of the fracture.
_____ b. redirecting blood back into the area of the fracture.
_____ c. stabilizing the suspected fracture site.
_____ d. increasing the patient's heart rate.

5. All of the following are contraindications for the use of the PASG *except*:

_____ a. suspected pelvic fracture.
_____ b. internal bleeding of the chest.
_____ c. late stage pregnancy.
_____ d. cardiogenic shock.

6. An adult weighing 70 kg has approximately _____________ mL of blood volume.

_____ a. 2,400
_____ b. 3,900
_____ c. 4,200
_____ d. 4,900

7. Signs of internal bleeding may include all of the following *except*:

_____ a. rigid abdomen.
_____ b. an elevated blood pressure.
_____ c. tenderness on palpation.
_____ d. signs of shock without external bleeding.

8. Shock that results when the heart is damaged and can no longer pump an adequate amount of blood to the body is called _____________ shock.

_____ a. septic
_____ b. anaphylactic
_____ c. neurogenic
_____ d. cardiogenic

9. Which one of the following is *not* a sign of hemorrhagic shock?

_____ a. Decreased pulse rate
_____ b. Increased breathing rate
_____ c. Decreased blood pressure
_____ d. Pale, cool, and clammy skin

10. When the body can no longer compensate for the blood loss, the pulse _____________ and the blood pressure _____________.

_____ a. increases, increases
_____ b. decreases, decreases
_____ c. decreases, increases
_____ d. increases, decreases

(continued on next page)

(continued)

Matching

Match the type of shock on the left with the applicable definition on the right.

1. _____ Decompensated shock
2. _____ Cardiogenic shock
3. _____ Anaphylactic shock
4. _____ Hypovolemic shock
5. _____ Neurogenic shock
6. _____ Compensated shock

A. Type of shock caused by an overreaction of the immune system when exposed to an allergen

B. When the patient is developing shock but the body is still able to maintain perfusion

C. Type of shock caused when the heart can no longer pump blood adequately, resulting in a decrease in cardiac output and thus a decrease in perfusion

D. Type of shock caused by a sudden decrease in body fluids (blood or other fluids)

E. Type of shock caused when the vessels dilate abnormally in response to injury to the spinal cord

F. Occurs when the body can no longer compensate for low blood volume or lack of perfusion. Late signs such as decreasing blood pressure become evident.

Critical Thinking

1. What is the actual cause of death in a patient who is said to have died from shock?

____

____

____

____

2. Discuss why a low blood pressure is a late sign of shock in a trauma patient.

____

____

____

____

3. Discuss the difference in the signs and symptoms of internal bleeding and those of shock.

____

____

____

____

Case Studies

Case Study 1

You have responded to a baseball field for an unknown injury. Upon arrival, you are escorted into one of the dugouts where you find an approximately 35-year-old man. He is dressed in an umpire uniform, and one of the coaches states that the umpire took a direct blow to the chest with a bat as one of the players was warming up. This happened about 45 minutes ago and, after recovering from getting the wind knocked out of him, he decided to go on with the game. At the last break between innings, the man had come into the dugout to rest and get some water when he nearly passed out. He appears a little confused, his skin is pale, cool, and moist, and his pulse is rapid and weak.

1. What are the significant elements of this man's history and current presentation?

2. How will you care for this patient?

3. How often will you want to perform reassessments on this patient?

Case Study 2

You are caring for a 12-year-old boy who, while being pulled behind a ski boat on a flotation device, struck something floating in the water. The incident happened just under an hour ago, and the boy is now complaining of increased pain in the left upper and lower quadrants of his abdomen. The only obvious sign of injury is a bright red abrasion down his left side. He is tender to the touch and his vital signs are pulse 120 weak and regular, respirations 24 with good tidal volume and slightly labored, and blood pressure 90/60. His skin appears normal and his pupils are PERRL. He has vomited twice in the past 15 minutes prior to your arrival.

1. What are the signs that this boy could be bleeding internally?

(continued on next page)

(continued)

2. Is this patient showing signs of compensated shock or decompensated shock? Explain your answer.

3. This boy has pain and abrasions over his left abdomen. What internal structures lie under the skin on the left side of the abdomen that may have been damaged?

The Last Word

The human body depends on a constant supply of well-oxygenated blood flowing to all tissues. This flow of well-oxygenated blood is known as *perfusion*. In addition, this flow of blood permits the body to rid itself of the waste products of normal cell metabolism. When the body senses a decrease in perfusion, it begins to compensate by increasing the pulse rate and decreasing blood flow to less vital areas, such as the skin and extremities. If left untreated, poor perfusion will eventually lead to shock, and the patient will eventually die due to inadequate perfusion to the vital organs.

Early detection based on the mechanism of injury, your patient assessment, and trending of vital signs will lead to early care and rapid transport to an appropriate receiving facility. Many patients with internal bleeding will require surgical intervention to control the bleeding and save their lives. Always document all appropriate information in your prehospital care report.

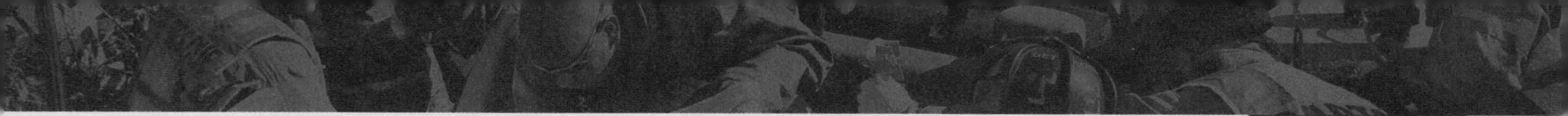

Controlling Bleeding

30

Education Standards

Trauma: Bleeding

Competencies

Applies fundamental knowledge to provide basic emergency care and transportation based on assessment findings for an acutely injured patient.

Objectives

After completion of this lesson, you should be able to:

30-1 Define key terms introduced in this chapter.

30-2 Review the components and function of the cardiovascular system.

30-3 Explain the importance of recognizing uncontrolled bleeding.

30-4 Describe the factors that influence the severity of bleeding.

30-5 Describe the body's own response to controlling bleeding.

30-6 Differentiate the types of external bleeding.

30-7 Describe methods of controlling external bleeding.

30-8 Discuss the precautions when using a tourniquet for bleeding control.

30-9 Describe the use of hemostatic dressings for bleeding control.

30-10 Explain special considerations and appropriate care for chest injuries, abdominal injuries, impaled objects, amputations, and large neck injuries.

30-11 Explain why bleeding from the nose, ears, or mouth is of special concern, and describe the appropriate care for bleeding from the nose, ears, or mouth.

Key Terms

aorta p. 771
bleeding out p. 773
brachial artery p. 771
carotid artery p. 771
direct pressure p. 778
elevation p. 778
epistaxis p. 788
femoral artery p. 771
hemostatic dressing p. 782
plasma p. 773
platelets p. 773
pressure dressing p. 778
radial artery p. 771
red blood cells p. 773
tourniquet p. 778
white blood cells p. 773

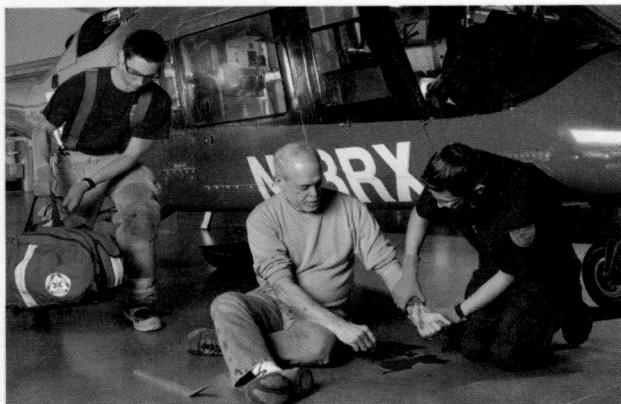

Figure 30-1 Controlling bleeding from a traumatic injury.

Introduction

Bleeding control is one of the most basic of skills that must be mastered by all EMTs. While everyone has experience managing minor cuts and scrapes, as an EMT you will encounter major wounds with severe bleeding. You must be able to distinguish between minor and severe bleeding and provide the appropriate care as quickly as possible. Uncontrolled bleeding will lead to shock and even death if not rapidly controlled. This chapter offers a review of the importance of good perfusion as well as instruction on how to identify and care for all types of external bleeding (Figure 30-1 ■).

EMERGENCY DISPATCH

"Ouch! Son of a gun!" EMT Olin Barger pulled his arm from the rear compartment of the ambulance and took a stumbling step backward. Blood poured down the front of his uniform and began pooling on the concrete floor of the ambulance bay.

"What the heck happened, Olin?" His partner, Ken, left the equipment that he had been inventorying and hurried over.

"I don't know." Olin held his forearm tightly with a blood-slick hand. "That backboard was stuck on something, and it wouldn't go in, so I just shoved it."

"Let me see your arm." Ken grabbed a jump bag from a nearby stretcher and fished out a handful of gauze packages while donning a pair of exam gloves.

Olin turned his arm toward the other EMT and slowly released his grip. A 15-centimeter laceration, extending from Olin's wrist to mid-forearm, burst open and blood jetted into the air.

"Oh, geez!" Ken quickly covered the wound with wads of gauze and yelled toward the other side of the ambulance bay. "Mark! Mark, get out here, quick! I need you to drive!"

"Oh, wow!" The color began fading from Olin's face. "I don't feel so well."

Review of the Cardiovascular System

30-2 Review the components and function of the cardiovascular system.

Before continuing on with this chapter, it will be helpful to review some of the basic anatomy and physiology of the cardiovascular system. Also known as the *circulatory system*, the cardiovascular system has three components: the heart, the blood, and the vessels that carry the blood throughout the body. Certain injuries can affect one or all of those vital components, thereby reducing the effectiveness of the circulation.

Perfusion

As discussed in detail in Chapter 29, perfusion is the flow of well-oxygenated blood throughout the entire body, including the vital organs and other tissues. When the circulatory system is functioning properly, a patient is said to be perfusing well. Signs of adequate perfusion include normal skin signs, normal mental status, and normal vital signs.

When a person is not perfusing well, it is frequently but not always due to a malfunction of one or more of the components of the circulatory system. Signs and symptoms of inadequate perfusion include:

- Abnormal skin signs (pale color, cool temperature)
- Altered mental status (sluggishness, confusion, or decreased responsiveness)
- Abnormal vital signs (increased pulse and respiratory rate, and eventually, decreased blood pressure)

A properly functioning circulatory system, including an adequate blood pressure, is essential for good perfusion.

The Heart

The heart is the pump in the system and is responsible for the continuous flow of blood throughout the body. The heart is made up of four interconnected chambers: the top two chambers are the atria and the bottom two are the ventricles. Deoxygenated blood (blood with little or no oxygen) enters the heart at the right atrium and then flows down into the right ventricle. The right ventricle then pumps the blood into the pulmonary arteries for transport to the lungs where it can pick up oxygen. Upon leaving the lungs by way of the pulmonary veins, the blood reenters the heart at the left atrium, then flows down into the left ventricle. The left ventricle is the largest chamber of the heart, because it must then pump blood out to the entire body. Blood leaves the left ventricle, entering the aorta for transport to the body.

PRACTICAL PATHOPHYSIOLOGY

Good blood pressure is the foundation for good perfusion. Systolic blood pressure is an indicator of cardiac output, while diastolic pressure is an indicator of systemic vascular resistance (SVR).

The Blood Vessels

The blood vessels are the "plumbing" or "hoses" of the circulatory system (Figure 30-2 ■). They are often described by their function, location, and whether they carry blood to or from the heart. All vessels that carry blood away from the heart are called *arteries*, while vessels that carry blood to the heart are called *veins*.

Arteries begin as larger vessels, branch into smaller ones, and eventually terminate in tiny vessels called *arterioles*. Conversely, veins begin as tiny venules and eventually merge into large vessels before entering the heart. The tiny vessels that connect arterioles and venules and where oxygen and nutrients are exchanged for waste products from the body's cells are called *capillaries*.

Following is a list of some of the major vessels of the body, along with their location and function:

- ***Aorta.*** The largest artery in the body, the **aorta** is attached directly to the left ventricle. It is responsible for carrying oxygenated blood directly from the heart to all the areas of the body.
- ***Venae cavae.*** These are the two major veins that carry oxygen-poor blood from the body to the right atrium. The superior vena cava carries blood from the head. The inferior vena cava carries blood from the lower body. Plural *venae cavae*.
- ***Coronary arteries.*** The small coronary arteries carry oxygenated blood to the heart muscle (myocardium) itself. A disruption in flow through these arteries can cause chest pain and damage to the heart muscle.
- ***Pulmonary artery.*** The pulmonary artery carries oxygen-poor blood from the heart to the lungs.
- ***Pulmonary vein.*** The pulmonary vein carries oxygen-rich blood from the lungs to the heart.
- ***Carotid artery.*** The **carotid artery** is the major artery of the neck and a primary supplier of blood to the head. There are two carotid arteries, one on each side of the neck. It is the artery most often used to check for a pulse in patients who are unresponsive.
- ***Brachial artery.*** Artery of the upper arm that is palpated to obtain a pulse in infants and to control bleeding from the arm in all age groups. Found near the elbow, the **brachial artery** is the artery you auscultate when obtaining a blood pressure.
- ***Radial artery.*** The **radial artery** supplies blood to the forearm and hand. It is palpated on the lateral aspect of the anterior wrist.
- ***Femoral artery.*** The **femoral artery** is the major supplier of blood to the leg. It is palpated near the crease formed by the abdomen, leg, and groin.

aorta the largest artery in the body, which transports blood from the left ventricle to begin systemic circulation.

carotid artery a large neck artery that carries blood from the heart to the head; one on each side of the neck.

brachial artery the major artery of the upper arm.

radial artery artery of the forearm; felt when taking the pulse at the wrist.

femoral artery an artery located in the anterior groin area; these arteries supply blood to the lower extremities.

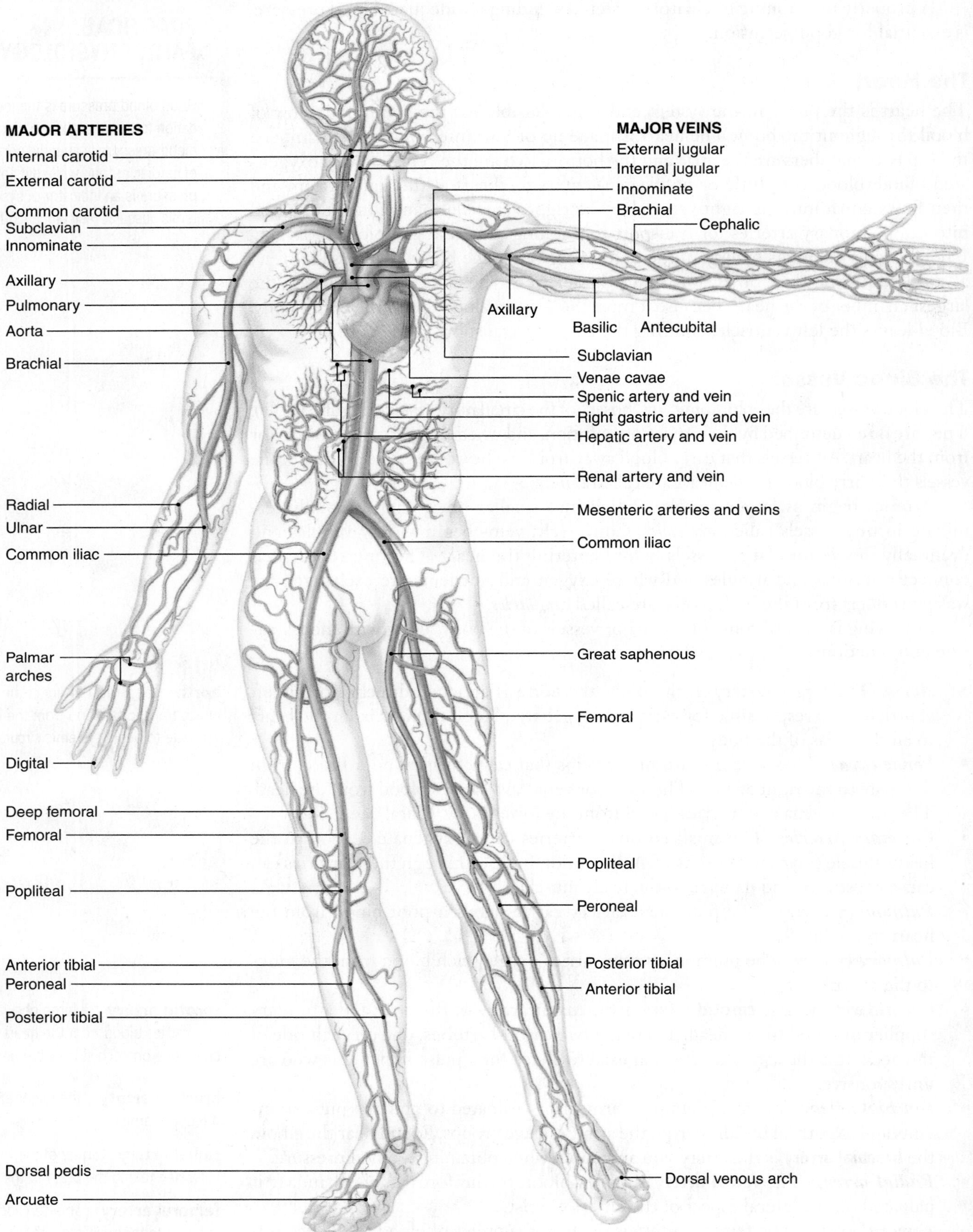

Figure 30-2 The major arteries and veins of the body.

The Function of Blood

Blood serves many essential functions as it is carried by the circulatory system throughout the body. Its most fundamental duty is to carry oxygen and nutrients to the cells and to carry away waste products generated by cellular metabolism.

Blood is made up of several components, each with a specialized function or functions. The major components of blood are as follows:

- ***Plasma.*** **Plasma** is the clear, yellowish fluid in which the other components of blood are suspended.
- ***Red blood cells.*** The disk-shaped **red blood cells** are responsible for transporting oxygen and carbon dioxide to and from the tissues.
- ***White blood cells.*** **White blood cells** help protect the body from infection and disease.
- ***Platelets.*** Irregularly shaped cell fragments, **platelets** are responsible for promoting blood clotting.

plasma the fluid portion of the blood.

red blood cells specialized blood cells containing hemoglobin.

white blood cells specialized blood cells that produce substances that help the body fight infection.

platelets components of the blood; membrane-enclosed fragments of specialized cells involved in clotting. Also called *thrombocytes*.

In addition to the functions of each of its components, blood must be present in a sufficient quantity to sustain life. There is a direct connection between the volume of blood within the circulatory system, blood pressure, and perfusion. When a patient loses blood from within the circulatory system, blood pressure will eventually fall and perfusion will become inadequate to sustain life.

PERSPECTIVE

Ken—The EMT

We were getting ready to start our shift and Olin had to put in a new long backboard. Honestly, the crew that had the rig last should've done it. It goes that way sometimes, I guess. You should have seen that laceration! Even as an EMT I don't see lacerations that bad very often. In the moment before I got it covered with gauze, I could see muscle and tendons, and there was obviously an artery damaged in there somewhere. Man, oh, man. We just couldn't get that bleeding to stop completely. I tried applying direct pressure on the wound with a trauma dressing. And then there was shock. I've never run a gnarly trauma call before my shift even started!

Blood Loss

30-3 Explain the importance of recognizing uncontrolled bleeding.

Whether it is the mechanic who is forever scraping a knuckle, the five-year-old girl who skins her knee learning to roller skate, or the shipping clerk who cuts his hand opening some boxes, bleeding and blood loss are common. The vast majority of instances are not life threatening. For example, the average blood loss from a woman's menstrual cycle is 40 to 60 cc (only 8 to 12 teaspoonfuls). Some women can lose up to 400 cc (500 cc is about a pint) and not become symptomatic. And each day there are people all across the world who donate a pint of blood and shortly after are allowed to drive home.

Most bleeding occurs to the outside of the body (external) and in most cases is easily controlled with simple first-aid measures. In other instances, bleeding can occur deep within the body (internal) and go unnoticed by patients and those around them. This type of bleeding has the most potential to be life threatening because it is difficult to detect and difficult to care for in the field. You may hear the term **bleeding out** used in describing a trauma patient. It simply means that the patient is losing a significant amount of blood from within the circulatory system and is not specific to internal or external blood loss.

bleeding out term that refers to the loss of blood and is not specific to internal or external blood loss.

Classes of Hemorrhage

Patient Signs Associated with Classes of Hemorrhage							
Class	Blood Loss	Vasoconstriction	Pulse Rate	Pulse Strength	Blood Pressure	Respiratory Rate	Respiratory Volume
I	<15%	↑	↑	Adequate	Adequate	↑	Adequate
II	15% to 30%	↑	↑	↓	Adequate	↑	↑
III	30% to 40%	↑	↑	↓	↓	↑	↓
IV	>40%	↓	Variable	↓	↓	Variable	Variable

Classes of Hemorrhage

Hemorrhage can be categorized in four progressive classes:

- ***Class I.*** Blood loss of up to 15%. The patient may display some nervousness and marginally cool skin with slight pallor. In the 70 kg adult that is up to 750 mL of blood loss, slightly more than you might give during a blood drive. The healthy patient can easily compensate for such a blood volume loss by way of vascular constriction and an increased heart rate. Blood pressure remains stable as does respiratory rate.
- ***Class II.*** Blood loss of 15% to 30%. The patient will be thirsty, show some anxiety and restlessness, have cool, moist skin, and an increased respiratory rate. In an adult, blood loss would be from 750 to 1,500 mL. The body's first-line compensatory responses can no longer maintain perfusion and secondary mechanisms begin to be employed. The patient becomes tachycardic, pulses may become weak, and respiratory rate increases. Blood pressure may still be within normal limits but will likely have dropped below the patient's baseline pressure.
- ***Class III.*** Blood loss between 30% to 40%. The patient will become increasingly short of breath and experience severe thirst, anxiety, and restlessness. Because blood loss is 1,500 to 2,000 mL, the body's compensatory mechanisms are unable to cope. Tachycardia is more pronounced and blood pressure begins to fall. The peripheral pulses may be absent or barely palpable. The level of responsiveness decreases, and the patient becomes very pale, cool, and moist. This patient is still compensating for the blood loss but that compensation is becoming more and more ineffective. Survival is unlikely without rapid intervention.
- ***Class IV.*** Blood loss is greater than 40%. In an adult, that blood loss is greater than 2,000 mL. The patient's central pulses become barely palpable, respirations are ineffective and the rate begins to decline, and the patient is extremely lethargic, confused, and may be unresponsive. The skin is very cool, moist, and extremely pale. Even with aggressive fluid resuscitation and blood transfusions, patient survival is unlikely.

NOTE: These descriptions of the classes of hemorrhage presume that the patient is a normally healthy adult. Certain patients react differently to blood loss. The expectant mother is somewhat protected from the effects of serious hemorrhage (in late pregnancy she has about 50% more blood volume than normal), but the fetus may be deprived of adequate circulation early in the blood loss and is more susceptible to harm. A well-conditioned athlete may move more slowly through the early classes of blood loss with greater loss percentages needed to advance from one class to another. Infants and children show few signs of blood loss until they move quickly into shock's later stages. In obese patients only a small blood loss may have a more serious effect than in other patients. An alcoholic's compensation is slow and less effective. The elderly are likewise more adversely affected by blood loss than average adults.

Bleeding Severity

Blood loss becomes dangerous when it is sudden and rapid and large enough volumes are involved. Blood loss becomes even more dangerous when it is complicated by other medical or traumatic problems, such as respiratory compromise or organ damage. Two factors that have a major influence on the severity of blood loss are time and quantity.

The sudden loss of the following quantities of blood can be life threatening to their respective age groups:

- One liter (1,000 cc) of blood in the adult patient
- One-half liter (500 cc) of blood in the child (one to eight years)
- 100 cc to 200 cc of blood in an infant (younger than one year)

Your assessment of the severity of blood loss is based on several factors, including your general impression of the patient, the patient's signs and symptoms, the mechanism of injury, and visible evidence of external blood. A trauma patient who is presenting with the signs and symptoms of shock, despite the lack of any external bleeding, should be considered a high priority for transport due to the high likelihood of internal bleeding.

The natural response of the body to bleeding is to control the blood loss as quickly as possible. Two mechanisms are automatically triggered whenever there is damage to soft tissues resulting in blood loss: Injured vessels constrict (get smaller) in an attempt to slow the loss of blood, and a clot forms at the site of injury.

The vessels constrict as components in the blood bind together and harden in an attempt to create a dam (clot) to stop the blood loss. Of course, the injury may be so significant that those mechanisms are not adequate to control the blood loss. In those instances, the EMT will have to provide specific care to help control the bleeding. (Emergency care is discussed later in this chapter.) The bottom line is this: Uncontrolled bleeding, no matter how slow, can eventually lead to shock and death.

PRACTICAL PATHOPHYSIOLOGY

Internal blood loss is easily hidden in many areas of the body and difficult to estimate. The chest, abdomen, and pelvic area are especially good at hiding significant blood loss. The thigh of an adult is capable of concealing as much as 1,500 mL of blood.

30-4 Describe the factors that influence the severity of bleeding.

30-5 Describe the body's own response to controlling bleeding.

STOP, REVIEW, REMEMBER!

Multiple Choice

For each question, place a check next to the correct answer.

1. The largest artery of the body is the:
   _____ a. vena cava.
   _____ b. aorta.
   _____ c. pulmonary artery.
   _____ d. femoral artery.

2. Which one of the following is responsible for transporting oxygen within the blood?
   _____ a. Red blood cells
   _____ b. White blood cells
   _____ c. Plasma
   _____ d. Platelets

3. Which chamber of the heart is responsible for pumping blood to the body?
   _____ a. Left atrium
   _____ b. Right atrium
   _____ c. Left ventricle
   _____ d. Right ventricle

4. All of the following are factors that will help your assessment of the severity of blood loss *except*:
   _____ a. your general impression of the patient.
   _____ b. the patient's signs and symptoms.
   _____ c. the mechanism of injury.
   _____ d. the patient's past medical history.

(continued on next page)

(continued)

5. The sudden loss of ____________ cc of blood in a child between one and eight years of age is considered significant.

_____ a. 250
_____ b. 300
_____ c. 500
_____ d. 1,000

Fill in the Blank

1. ____________________________ is the flow of well-oxygenated blood throughout the entire body, including the vital organs and other tissues.

2. Signs of good perfusion include normal skin signs, normal mental status, and normal ____________________________.

3. A patient who is in shock will have skin that is pale, cool, and ____________________________.

4. The ____________________________ is the largest chamber of the heart and pumps blood out to the entire body.

5. Bleeding that is ____________________________ has the most potential to be life threatening because it is difficult to detect and difficult to care for in the field.

Critical Thinking

1. Discuss the relationship between perfusion and blood pressure.

2. Describe how a patient might present who is not perfusing well.

3. Discuss why it might be important to be able to estimate blood loss in a patient who is bleeding externally.

External Bleeding

Bleeding that occurs through an opening in the body such as a puncture or laceration is referred to as *external bleeding*. The amount of blood loss can vary significantly, depending on the mechanism of injury, and range anywhere from very minor (a scrape) to severe and difficult to control. Bleeding is further classified by the types of vessels that are involved. The larger the vessel, the greater the chance that there will be significant blood loss and the greater the likelihood that the bleeding will be difficult to control. Certain areas of the body tend to bleed more because of their rich blood supply. For example, even a small laceration to the face or scalp can produce heavy external bleeding.

30-6 Differentiate the types of external bleeding.

All three types of vessels—arteries, veins, and capillaries—can be damaged and cause bleeding from an open wound. While each may have its own characteristics when damaged, it is often difficult and unnecessary to distinguish between them. In the case of a large wound, you are likely to encounter damage to all three types of vessels.

PRACTICAL PATHOPHYSIOLOGY

Blood pressure is regulated by both baroreceptors and chemoreceptors located throughout the body. Baroreceptors are sensitive to stretch caused by changes in blood pressure. Chemoreceptors detect changes in oxygen, carbon dioxide, and the pH level of the blood. The receptors send messages to the brain, endocrine system, and nervous system that can change heart rate and vessel size as necessary.

Bleeding from Arteries

Arteries are the vessels that carry blood from the heart and to the tissues and organs of the body. They are under higher pressure than other vessels and for that reason can allow for the loss of a large quantity of blood in a relatively short amount of time. Blood from arteries is generally bright red, due to higher oxygen content, and often can be seen spurting from an open wound with each beat of the heart. Because of the pressure inside arteries, arterial bleeding can be difficult to control. You will not always see arterial blood spurting from a wound, because as a patient loses blood, his blood pressure decreases and so will the amount and intensity of spurting from an injured artery.

Bleeding from Veins

Veins are the vessels that carry blood back to the heart. Venous flow is under much less pressure than arterial flow and, for this reason, does not spurt from the wound but instead flows steadily (Figure 30-3 ■). The steady, flowing blood from veins may appear darker in color than arterial blood. While it is possible to die from external venous blood loss, it is less likely because the lower pressures make it easier to control than arterial bleeding.

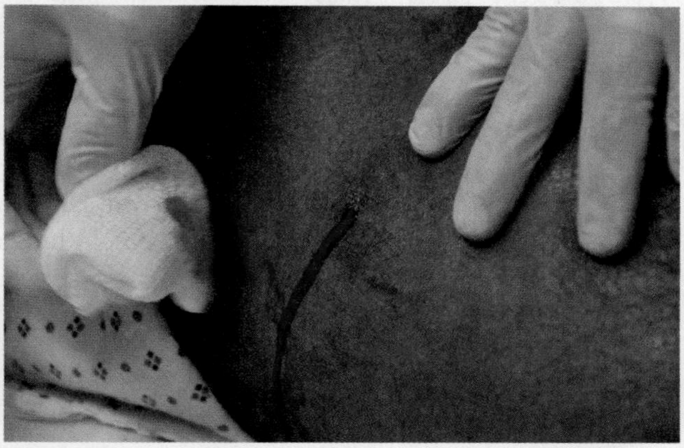

Figure 30-3 Venous bleeding is slow and steady and appears dark red in color. (© Edward T. Dickinson, MD)

PERSPECTIVE

Olin—The Patient

I'm still not sure exactly how or on what I cut myself. I was trying to get that backboard in the slot, and it kept getting hung up on something. I just got mad, I guess, and jammed it in. I remember that it felt like I got punched in the forearm, like a dull pain, you know? It wasn't until I pulled my arm out of the compartment that I saw how bad it really was. You know what's kind of goofy though? The first thought that went through my mind when I saw this huge gash on my forearm was that once it scarred up people would think that I tried to commit suicide. Isn't it odd what goes through our heads during those times? Of course, then I passed out.

CLINICAL CLUE

Body Substance Isolation

Always use appropriate personal protective equipment (PPE) such as disposable gloves and eye protection while controlling bleeding. If you were to have a small cut or puncture on your hand, the patient's blood could enter your body through this opening in the skin.

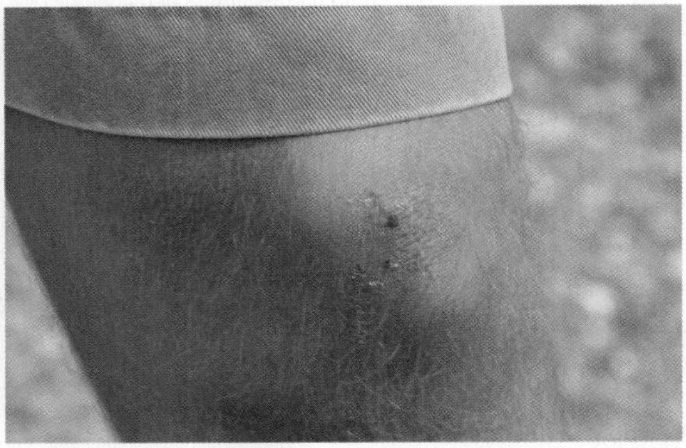

Figure 30-4 Capillary bleeding comes from tiny vessels near the surface of the skin and appears bright red and oozing. (© Edward T. Dickinson, MD)

Bleeding from Capillaries

Capillaries are the tiny vessels that connect arterioles and venules. The most common causes of capillary bleeding are scrapes, abrasions, or the classic skinned-knee injury (Figure 30-4 ■). Capillary bleeding will almost always stop spontaneously and is not life threatening.

Controlling Bleeding

One of the most basic skills an EMT can perform is bleeding control. When bleeding is severe enough, a patient can bleed out in a matter of minutes. The steps of controlling severe bleeding are direct pressure, elevation (if possible), application of a pressure dressing (optional), and application of a tourniquet (only for life-threatening bleeding).

30-7 Describe methods of controlling external bleeding.

direct pressure pressure applied using the fingers, palm, or entire surface of one hand to help control bleeding.

pressure dressing a dressing that applies pressure to control bleeding from a wound to an extremity that is still actively bleeding. Also called a *pressure bandage*.

tourniquet method designed to stop all blood flow past the point at which it is applied.

It is important to understand that those steps represent a progressive approach to bleeding control. In other words, you do not stop one to begin another. You must begin with **direct pressure** and continue to hold pressure while elevating the injured limb. You can apply a **pressure dressing,** while your partner maintains pressure and elevation. While applying the **tourniquet,** you may have another EMT—or even the patient—continue to hold pressure and elevation.

Direct Pressure

Depending on the size of the wound, direct pressure can be applied by the EMT using fingers, palm, or the entire surface of one hand (Figures 30-5 ■). Larger wounds require a larger surface area of pressure and usually more pressure as well. If dressing material is not immediately available, use your gloved hand to initiate direct pressure. As soon as practical, place a sterile or clean dressing between your hand and the wound. For larger wounds, you may have to use several dressings to help absorb the blood while you attempt to control bleeding.

Elevation

elevation elevating the injury site above the level of the patient's heart to reduce the amount of pressure at the site and make it easier for bleeding to be controlled.

Elevation can be used to assist in controlling bleeding in the arms and legs (Figure 30-6 ■). The combination of direct pressure and elevation can control most of the bleeding you might see in the field. Of course, elevation should be used only if it can be performed without causing more harm to the patient. For instance, elevation would not be indicated for a wound to the forearm that is associated with a suspected fracture. Elevating an arm that could be fractured will cause severe pain and likely increase the bleeding from the surrounding soft tissues. In most cases, placing the patient in a supine position will make it easier to elevate an injured extremity.

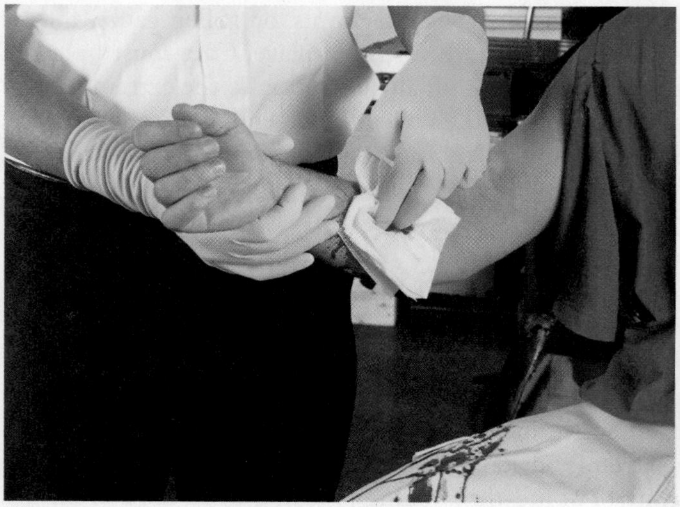
(A)

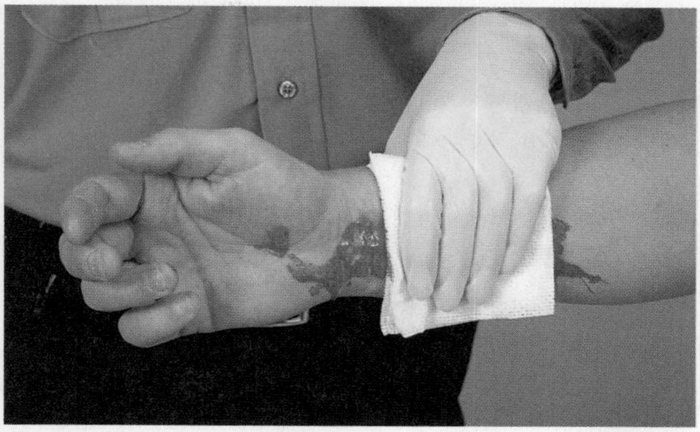
(B)

Figure 30-5 (A) Smaller wounds may require fingertip pressure to control bleeding. (B) Larger wounds may require pressure from a larger area in order to control bleeding.

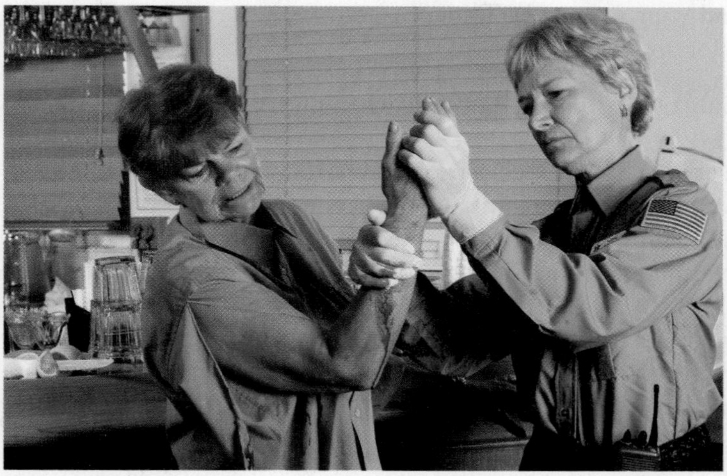
(A)

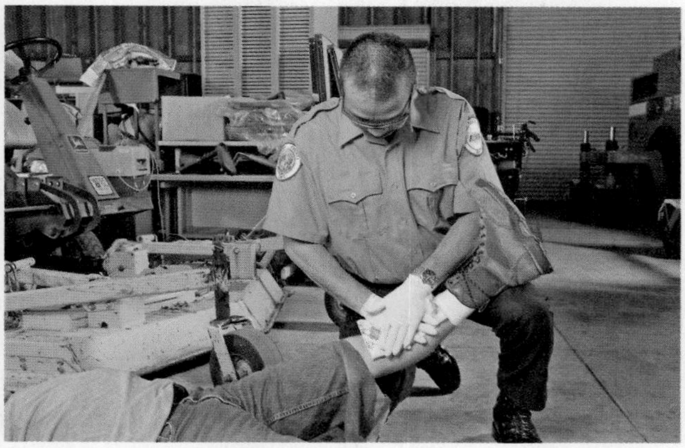
(B)

Figure 30-6 (A) Elevating the arm can help control bleeding. (Follow local protocol.) (B) Elevate the lower extremity only if there is no underlying skeletal injury or excessive pain. (Follow local protocol.)

PERSPECTIVE

Dr. Sanjay—The Trauma Surgeon

Mr. Barger is a very, very fortunate man to have survived. He managed to dissect the artery lengthwise, preventing it from sealing itself. All in all, I guess if you're going to accidentally almost kill yourself with a traumatic injury, doing it next to a staffed ambulance is probably ideal.

Pressure Dressing

A pressure dressing is used to help control bleeding from a wound on an extremity. If you are working with another EMT or rescuer, one of you can maintain direct pressure and elevation while the other applies a pressure dressing. It should be applied early in case you need to release direct pressure to apply a tourniquet.

The pressure dressing is composed of either cravats or roller gauze that is wrapped tightly around a wound, securing a dressing in place. Care must be taken not to secure the bandage too tightly and cut off all circulation to the extremity. The objective of the pressure dressing is to slow the flow of blood enough to allow for the formation of a clot at the site of the injury. It is *not* designed to cut off all circulation, as with a tourniquet.

Tourniquets

The use of tourniquets has long been suggested as a last-resort measure to control severe bleeding from an extremity. While they have a reputation as being dangerous and difficult to apply, recent innovations and experience have changed our understanding of the value of tourniquets. Experience in the military setting has shown that tourniquets are effective in stopping severe bleeding quickly with no or minimal damage to the extremity distal to the tourniquet. Tourniquets are now a mainstay of care for the control of life-threatening bleeding from the extremities (Figure 30-7 ▪).

A properly applied tourniquet is designed to stop all blood flow past the point at which it is applied. On your ambulance you may use commercially available tourniquets (Figure 30-8 ▪). They are applied and used according to the recommendations of the manufacturer and your protocols. Though there are several varieties on the market, the guidelines for application are generally the same. They are as follows:

- Use a tourniquet only on extremities and only when direct pressure has failed to control bleeding.
- Apply the tourniquet at least two inches proximal to the wound.
- Do not place the tourniquet over a joint.
- Tighten the tourniquet until bleeding stops. Secure it so pressure is maintained.
- Document the time of application and provide this information to the hospital staff upon arrival.
- Reassess the tourniquet intermittently to make sure bleeding remains controlled.
- Notify other EMS providers and hospital personnel who assume patient care that a tourniquet has been applied.

An additional benefit of commercial tourniquets is that many models may be applied with one hand. This makes the tourniquet useful for self-care in tactical or combat situations.

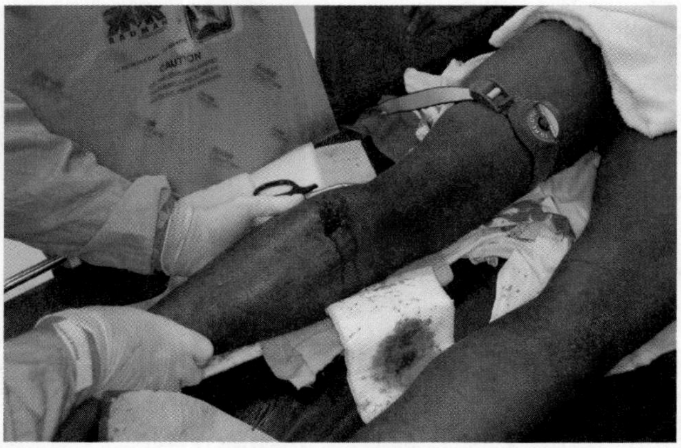

Figure 30-7 If direct pressure is unable to control bleeding, a tourniquet must be applied. (© Edward T. Dickinson, MD)

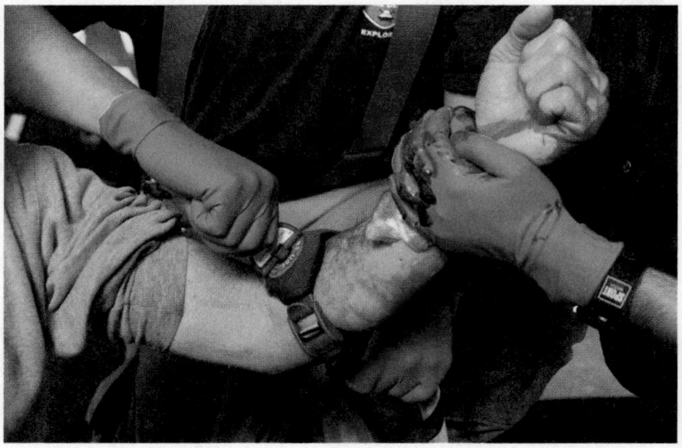

Figure 30-8 Application of a commercial tourniquet.

CLINICAL CLUE

Indications for a Tourniquet

It is important to know the difference between bleeding and life-threatening bleeding. Your care will depend on it. Life-threatening bleeding is that which is likely to cause shock or death in a short period of time if not immediately controlled. Examples include blood that is spurting or flowing heavily, or blood that is flowing but, because of other vital issues such as airway compromise or multiple patients, you cannot spend time controlling it. The overwhelming majority of bleeding cases can be controlled by direct pressure and elevation. Life-threatening bleeding, however, would require a tourniquet if it could not be controlled by direct pressure and elevation.

If a commercial tourniquet is not immediately available, you may use a cravat or similar material to fashion an improvised tourniquet. Follow these steps to apply an improvised tourniquet (Figure 30-9 ■):

1. Take appropriate BSI precautions.
2. Have your partner maintain direct pressure and elevation while you apply a pressure dressing or prepare for the application of the tourniquet.
3. Fold a triangular bandage several times until you have a long bandage approximately two to four inches wide.
4. Place the center of the bandage just above the injury site and wrap it firmly around the limb twice. Tie a half knot.
5. Place a stick or similar device over the half knot and tie a full knot over the stick.
6. If possible, locate the distal pulse in the extremity and rotate the stick until the distal pulse goes away.
7. Secure the stick in place using another triangular bandage or similar tie.
8. Confirm that bleeding has been controlled, document the time the tourniquet was applied, and transport immediately.

It is true that if the tourniquet remains in place for several hours, chances are increased that the limb may suffer damage to nerves, vessels, and soft tissue. The bottom line, however, is that tourniquets are a valuable life-saving tool when all other methods of controlling bleeding have failed.

An alternative method for applying a tourniquet is to place a blood pressure cuff just above the injury site (Figure 30-10 ■). Palpate the distal pulse and inflate the cuff until the pulse goes away. Confirm through observation that the bleeding appears

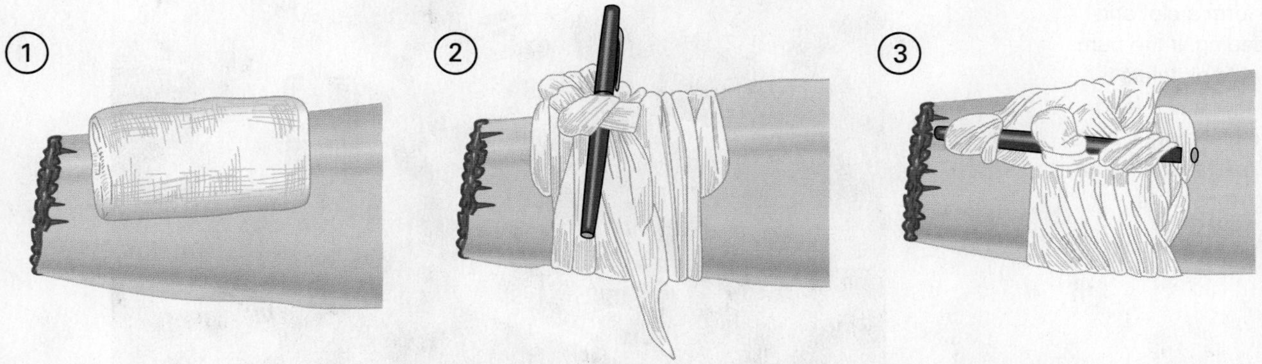

Figure 30-9 Application of an improvised tourniquet includes the following: (1) Apply a roller gauze or similar pad over the center of the limb. (2) Wrap a cravat or similar material around the limb as tightly as possible and secure with a half knot. Place a stick over the half knot and tie a full knot over it. (3) Twist the stick until bleeding is controlled and secure it with the remaining ends of the cravat.

controlled. Monitor the cuff to ensure that it does not deflate and that the Velcro remains affixed.

Though a tourniquet can certainly be life saving, if applied improperly, it can cause unnecessary pain and tissue damage. Keep the following principles in mind when using tourniquets:

- Use a wide bandage (two to four inches) and secure tightly.
- Do not use wire, rope, string, or any other material that could cut into the skin and underlying tissue.
- Do not remove or loosen the tourniquet once it is applied unless directed to do so by protocol or medical direction.
- Leave the tourniquet in open view so hospital personnel will see it.
- Do not apply a tourniquet directly on a joint.

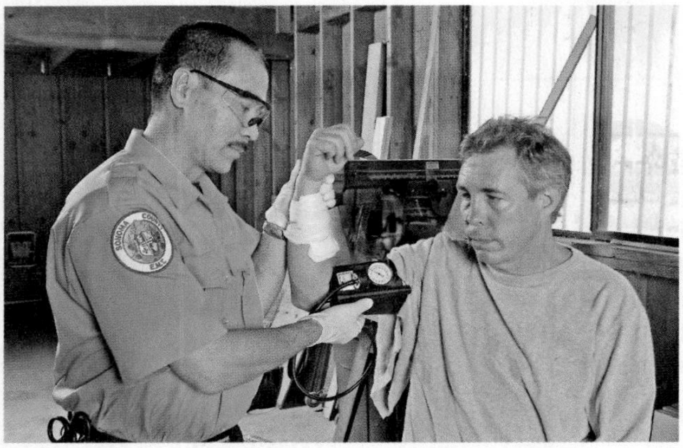

Figure 30-10 A blood pressure cuff can be used as a tourniquet when a commercial tourniquet is not available.

30-8 Discuss the precautions when using a tourniquet for bleeding control.

30-9 Describe the use of hemostatic dressings for bleeding control.

hemostatic dressing a specialized gauze dressing treated with a chemical agent that promotes clotting.

Hemostatic Dressings

Hemostatic dressings have been used in the military for many years. They contain an organic material that helps to rapidly form clots and stop severe bleeding (Figure 30-11 ■). Hemostatic dressings are ideal when a tourniquet cannot be used. Some systems allow the use of these dressings before or in combination with a tourniquet. Always follow manufacturer recommendations and local protocols for application. General guidelines, however, are as follows:

- Open the hemostatic dressing packet or pouch.
- Remove any non-hemostatic gauze from the wound.
- Apply the hemostatic dressing into and over the wound. Large wounds may require more than one dressing.
- Press the dressing into the wound with your fingers.

Early hemostatic dressings commonly caused a heat reaction when placed onto an open wound. This reaction caused considerable heat at the wound site and could be uncomfortable for the patient. Newer generation hemostatic dressings are formulated to minimize this reaction.

PRACTICAL PATHOPHYSIOLOGY

Components of the blood called *platelets* (thrombocytes) are responsible for the clotting function of blood. When bleeding occurs anywhere on or in the body, platelets rush to the site of bleeding to form a clot and stop the bleeding. If the number of available platelets is abnormally low, it can lead to excessive bleeding. If too high, it can lead to the formation of dangerous clots.

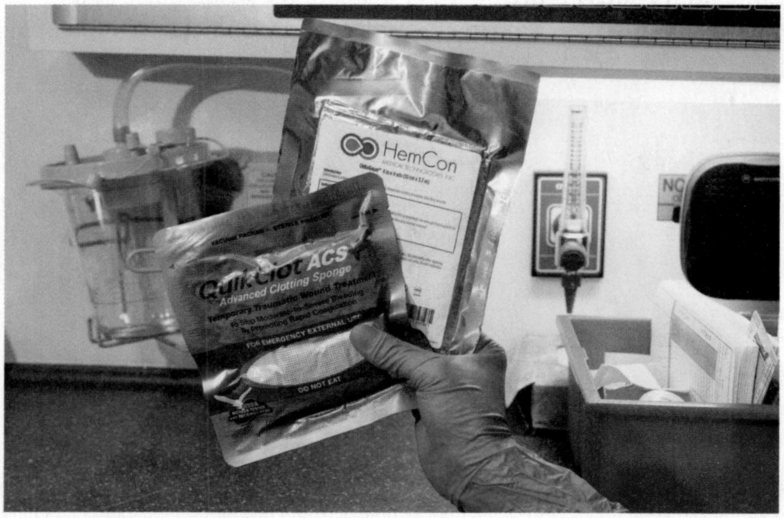

Figure 30-11 Two brands of hemostatic dressings.

SCAN 30-1 Controlling Severe Bleeding

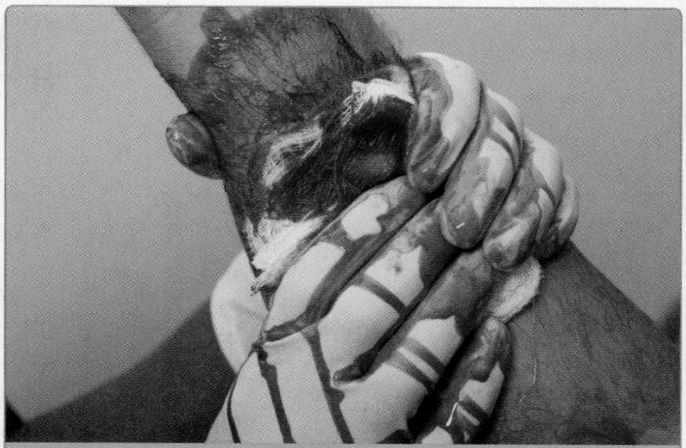

30-1-1 Take appropriate BSI precautions and apply direct pressure to the wound with a clean gauze.

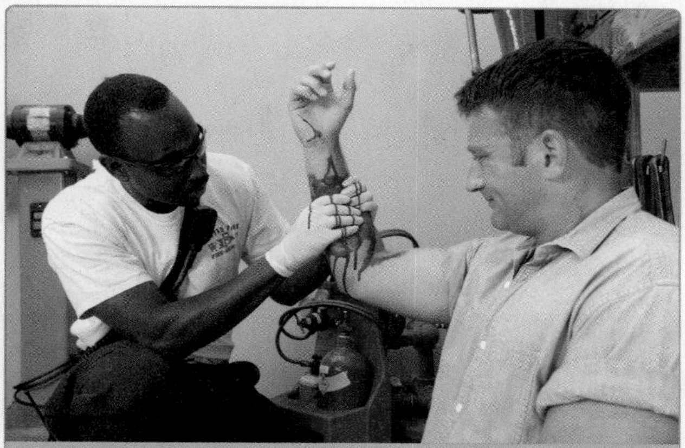

30-1-2 If there are no contraindications, elevate the limb while maintaining direct pressure.

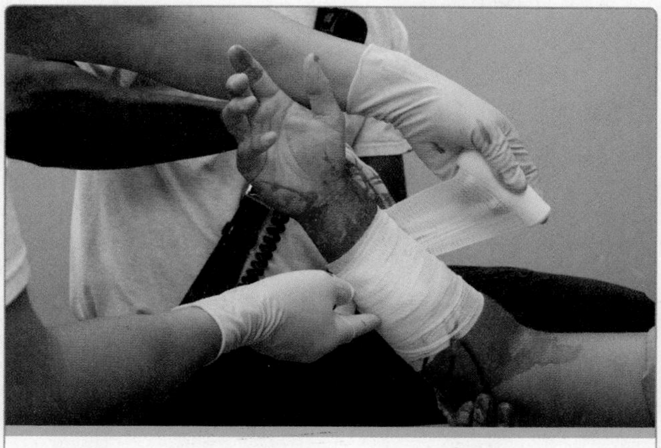

30-1-3 Apply a pressure dressing.

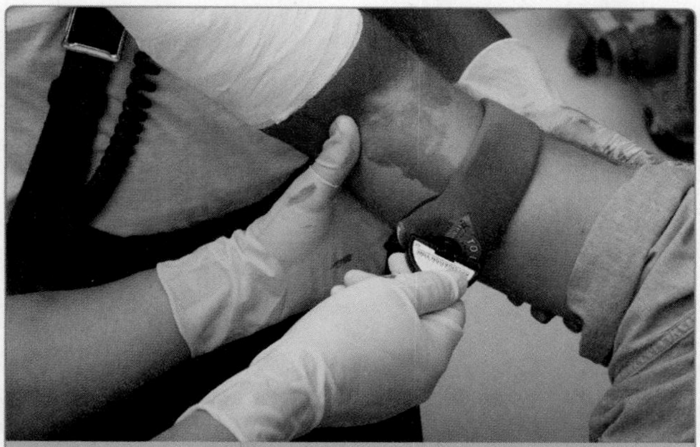

30-1-4 If bleeding cannot be controlled by direct pressure, apply a tourniquet.

Perform the following steps when caring for a patient with external bleeding (Scans 30-1 and 30-2):

1. Take the appropriate BSI precautions and perform a scene size-up.
2. Perform a primary assessment.
3. Attempt to control severe bleeding using direct pressure first, elevation, pressure dressing, and finally a tourniquet as needed. Note that a hemostatic dressing may be used in place of a tourniquet or in places where a tourniquet cannot be applied. Follow your local protocols in this decision.
4. Initiate oxygen therapy.
5. Perform a secondary assessment as appropriate.
6. Immobilize the injured extremity as appropriate.

SCAN 30-2 Application of a Hemostatic Dressing

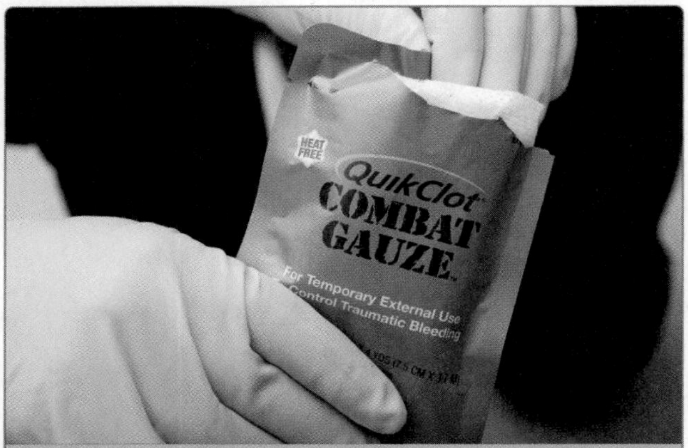

30-2-1 Commercial hemostatic dressing.

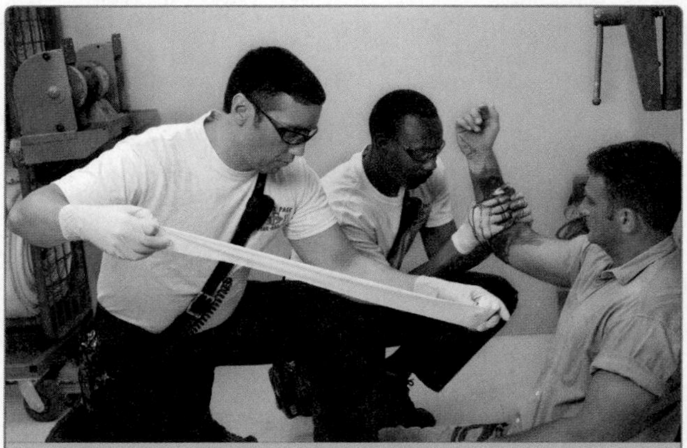

30-2-2 Open the package and remove a generous amount of dressing material.

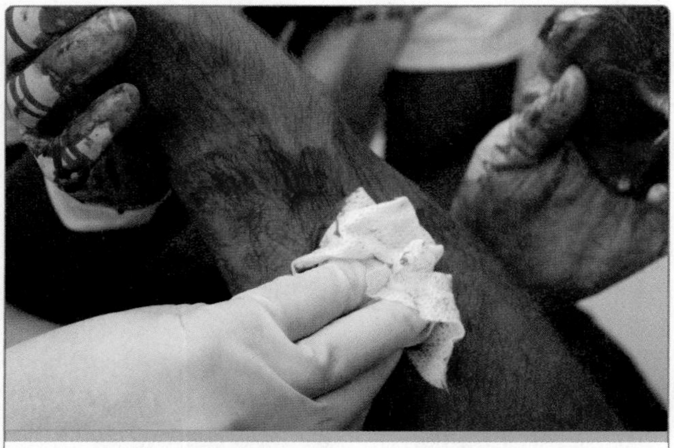

30-2-3 Pack the open wound with a generous amount of the dressing material.

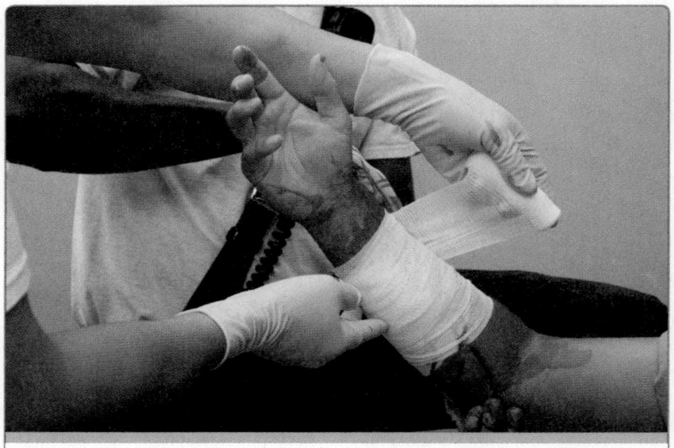

30-2-4 Use a bandage to secure the dressing in place. If bleeding is not controlled, apply a tourniquet.

7. Initiate transport.
8. Perform reassessments.
9. Watch for signs and symptoms of shock and expedite transport if necessary.

PERSPECTIVE

Mark—The EMT

So there I am, having a cup of coffee and watching the weather channel, and all of a sudden Ken's yelling at me from the garage. You gotta understand how suspicious that made me. Last time somebody did that, it was a fellow EMT named Jerry, and when I ran out of the break room, he hit me with a rubber glove completely filled with saline. Oh yeah, real funny. That was a hoot. Not. But once I saw all the blood and the look on Olin's face, I knew that something had really hit the fan.

CLINICAL CLUE

Hemostatic Dressings

A new classification of dressing now available is called a *hemostatic dressing*. They contain agents that promote more rapid and aggressive clotting of the blood and thus better control of bleeding. They may be used in places other than extremities and, depending on your protocols, also may be used before tourniquet application for uncontrolled bleeding. These dressings are commonly used in tactical and combat situations.

STOP, REVIEW, REMEMBER!

Multiple Choice

For each question, place a check next to the correct answer.

1. The vessel most likely to cause severe bleeding if compromised is a(n):

_____ a. artery.

_____ b. vein.

_____ c. capillary.

_____ d. arteriole.

2. Bleeding from arteries is often seen as:

_____ a. bright red and flowing.

_____ b. dark red and flowing.

_____ c. bright red and spurting.

_____ d. dark red and spurting.

3. Isolated bleeding from capillaries is most often caused by:

_____ a. lacerations.

_____ b. abrasions.

_____ c. contusions.

_____ d. avulsions.

4. The correct order of the steps used to control bleeding is:

_____ a. direct pressure, pressure dressing, and tourniquet, elevation.

_____ b. pressure dressing, tourniquet, direct pressure, and elevation.

_____ c. elevation, pressure dressing, direct pressure, and tourniquet.

_____ d. direct pressure, elevation, pressure dressing, and tourniquet.

5. Wounds to the head and torso are best controlled using which method?

_____ a. Tourniquet

_____ b. Elevation

_____ c. Direct pressure

_____ d. Pressure point

Fill in the Blank

1. _____________________ are under higher pressure than other vessels and, for that reason, can allow for the loss of a large quantity of blood in a relatively short amount of time.

2. Arterioles and venules are connected by tiny vessels called _____________________.

3. Bleeding from veins is often steady and flowing and appears to be _____________________ in color.

4. It is thought that _____________________ the injury site to a position above the level of the patient's heart will reduce the amount of pressure at the site and therefore make it easier for the bleeding to be controlled.

5. The ideal placement for a tourniquet that is used to control bleeding in an extremity is just _____________________ to the wound.

(continued on next page)

(continued)

Critical Thinking

1. Explain why bleeding from arteries is often more difficult to control than bleeding from veins or capillaries.

____

____

____

____

2. Describe how the use of a pressure dressing helps to control bleeding.

____

____

____

____

3. Explain the dangers of securing a pressure dressing too tightly around an extremity in an attempt to control severe bleeding.

____

____

____

____

Immobilization

Splints can be helpful in the management of certain wounds, especially if there is a possibility of an underlying fracture (Figure 30-12 ▪). It may be necessary to straighten an angulated extremity injury in order to immobilize it properly. While it may cause more pain initially, straightening an angulated long bone fracture will make it easier to immobilize and therefore reduce pain and soft-tissue damage during transport. If the injury involves a joint and the patient is unable to move the limb, do not attempt to straighten it. Doing so may cause further damage to the joint. In this case, you must get creative and do your best to immobilize the injury in the position you found it. (Refer to Chapter 34 for more information on straightening an angulated limb.)

Air splints (Figure 30-13 ▪) may help control bleeding because they can maintain a constant pressure when applied properly. Monitor the wound carefully, because it may be difficult to determine if bleeding has stopped with an air splint in place.

The majority of fatalities from pelvic fractures are associated with internal bleeding. Early recognition of a suspected pelvic fracture and appropriate stabilization will

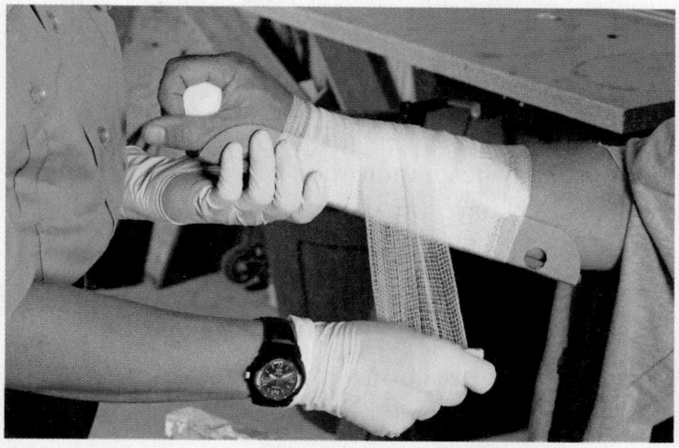

Figure 30-12 Immobilization of an injury using a cardboard splint.

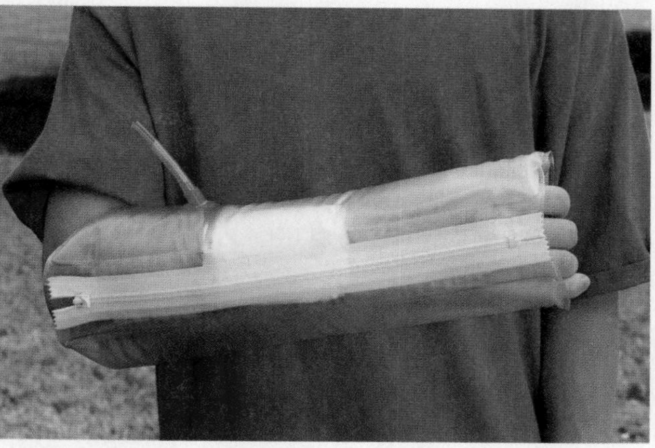

Figure 30-13 Immobilization of an injury using an air splint.

help to minimize blood loss. While the PASG can be used to help stabilize suspected pelvic fractures, specialized devices such as the traumatic pelvic orthopedic device (TPOD) and other pelvic stabilization devices have been developed specifically for this purpose (Figure 30-14 ■). Once in place, pelvic stabilization devices maintain circumferential stabilization of the pelvis, reducing pain and minimizing internal blood loss. Check your local protocols regarding recommended devices.

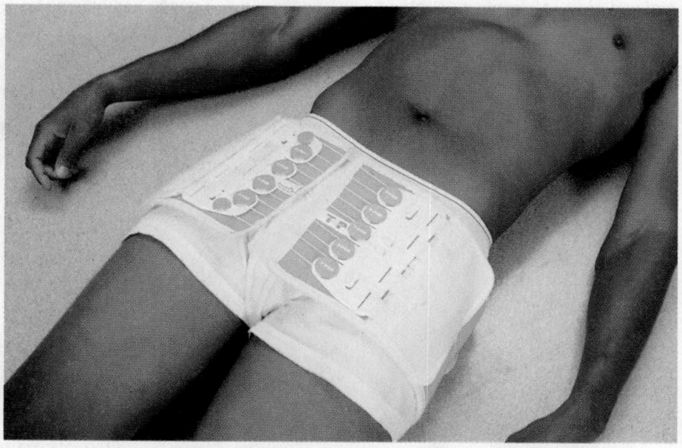

Figure 30-14 The application of a commercial pelvic splint.

Special Considerations in Bleeding Control

The way to control bleeding varies depending on many factors. One is location. Tourniquets may be used on extremities but not on the torso, head, or neck. Different parts of the body are more vascular (contain more blood vessels), so they bleed more vigorously. Some bleeding, such as that from the nose, will not be directly accessible. Finally, each area of the body will have special considerations because of the particular function of that area, the underlying structures and organs, and any potential to compromise the airway.

Wounds to the Head, Neck, and Torso

30-10 Explain special considerations and appropriate care for chest injuries, abdominal injuries, impaled objects, amputations, and large neck injuries.

For injuries to the head, neck, and torso you will have to resort to direct pressure as the primary means of controlling bleeding. The key is to be patient and carefully monitor the flow of blood from the wound. For open wounds to the neck or torso, apply an occlusive dressing first and then an absorbent dressing on top. In cases of severe bleeding that cannot be controlled with direct pressure, you may have to expose the wound and use fingertip pressure directly on the bleeding vessel. Your protocols may allow the use of hemostatic dressings for severe bleeding to the torso or neck. (More about caring for specific types of wounds may be found in Chapter 31.)

Remember that a victim of trauma could have suffered a spine injury. Evaluate the mechanism of injury and take the appropriate spinal precautions with all victims of trauma. If the patient is unresponsive and spine injury is suspected, use the jaw-thrust maneuver to open the airway.

Bleeding from the Nose, Ears, and Mouth

30-11 Explain why bleeding from the nose, ears, or mouth is of special concern, and describe the appropriate care for bleeding from the nose, ears, or mouth.

Bleeding from the nose, ears, and mouth may be an indication of more severe underlying trauma. Bleeding from these areas may have any of numerous causes, such as:

- Head trauma
- Facial trauma
- Digital trauma (nose picking)
- Sinusitis and other upper respiratory tract infections
- Hypertension (high blood pressure)
- Coagulation disorders

Bleeding from the ears or nose may be an indication of an underlying skull fracture. If the bleeding is the result of trauma, do not attempt to stop the blood flow. Instead, cover the areas with a loose dressing.

epistaxis a simple nosebleed.

Epistaxis (nosebleed) is a common occurrence and rarely life threatening. Follow these basic steps when caring for a nontraumatic nosebleed (Figure 30-15 ■):

1. Be sure to don appropriate personal protective equipment because these patients may be coughing and spitting up blood.
2. Place the patient in a sitting position and have him lean forward.
3. Use a gloved hand to apply direct continuous pressure by pinching the fleshy portion of the nostrils together.
4. Reassure the patient and keep him calm and quiet.

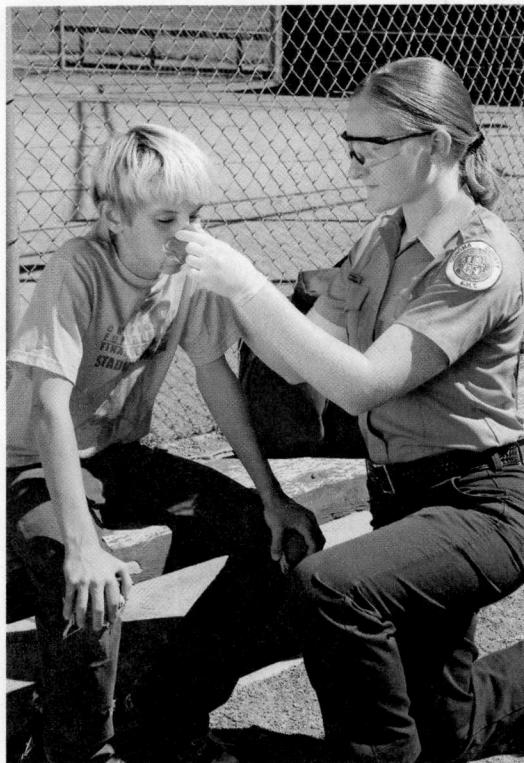

Figure 30-15 Have the patient with a simple nosebleed lean forward while you hold pressure with clean gauze.

Many people think that leaning back is the appropriate position for controlling a nosebleed. In fact, this position directs much of the blood to the back of the airway, where it may cause the patient to gag or obstruct the airway. This position also directs the flow of blood to the stomach, which can cause nausea and vomiting and likely make the bleeding worse. These risks may be minimized by having the patient lean forward.

PRACTICAL PATHOPHYSIOLOGY

Blood is irritating to the stomach lining and in sufficient quantities will cause nausea and vomiting. For this reason it is best to keep the patient with a nosebleed leaning forward to direct blood flow out the nose and minimize the amount of blood that flows down the esophagus and into the stomach.

Similar to nosebleeds, bleeding from the mouth is generally easy to control and rarely life threatening. The biggest concern with bleeding from the mouth is the possibility that the patient's airway could become blocked. Responsive patients may assume a position of comfort and hold clean dressings inside the mouth until the bleeding is controlled. Unresponsive patients can be managed by placing them in the recovery position, if injury permits. It may be necessary to suction the mouth frequently to minimize the chances of an airway obstruction.

PERSPECTIVE

Olin—The EMT

Shock. I can't remember ever going into shock before! It was like my stomach started knotting up, and I got really panicky, like I had to do *something* but I couldn't think of what it was. Then my vision started closing in and I got cold all over . . . and nauseous. I could actually feel each drop of sweat popping out on my forehead. Man, that was weird. And right before I blacked out, I remember thinking that I was actually dying . . . and I was disappointed that there was absolutely nothing peaceful about it! Talk about anxiety. When I came to, I was totally confused and riding in the back of the ambulance with a nonrebreather mask on my face. Now that I look back on that whole thing, though, I'm really glad that it happened. It helped my patient care skills so much. I mean, now I truly know what my patients are going through.

Signs and Symptoms of Shock

A patient who has suffered an injury and is presenting with the signs and symptoms of shock should be considered a high priority for transport. This patient may have lost a significant amount of blood and his body is attempting to compensate. Remember that not all blood loss is obvious, and victims of trauma can have internal as well as external bleeding. (Review Chapter 29.)

A patient who has signs and symptoms of shock may be in need of surgical intervention. Perform the necessary steps for controlling all obvious bleeding and transport immediately.

Signs and symptoms of shock include:

- Increased pulse rate (tachycardia)
- Altered mental status, including restlessness and anxiety
- Increased respiratory rate (tachypnea)
- Increased capillary refill time
- Weak peripheral pulses
- Pale, cool, and moist skin
- Thirst
- Sluggish and dilated pupils
- Nausea and/or vomiting
- Decreasing blood pressure (late sign)

CLINICAL CLUE

Shock

Not all patients who are bleeding internally will show signs of shock right away. Do not wait for signs to appear before transporting. Carefully evaluate the mechanism of injury, assess the patient, and initiate care for shock before signs and symptoms appear.

EMERGENCY DISPATCH SUMMARY

Olin made a complete recovery from his injury, although he is admittedly still somewhat self-conscious of the scar. Both he and his partner, Ken, realized more than ever that transport time for bleeding patients can be so critical to their survival.

Chapter Review

To the Point

- Uncontrolled bleeding is one of the most life-threatening problems any patient can have. It is important to assess every patient thoroughly for external bleeding and attempt to control it immediately.
- There are several factors that can influence the severity of blood loss, such as the type of vessels involved, the amount of blood loss, underlying medical conditions, and additional organ damage.
- The body initiates two primary responses that are triggered by the sympathetic nervous system in response to bleeding. They are increased clotting at the site of injury and a decrease in vessel size.
- Most wounds have the potential to cause all three types of bleeding—arterial, venous, and capillary. Arterial bleeding is the most serious and is characterized by bright red blood that is spurting from the wound. Venous bleeding also can be serious but is characterized by darker red blood that flows from the wound. Capillary bleeding is very superficial and will almost always stop on its own.
- Most external bleeding is easily controlled by direct pressure, using your hands and a pressure dressing. The steps for controlling bleeding are direct pressure, elevation, pressure dressing, and tourniquet.
- When using a tourniquet for bleeding control, you must use a material that is two to four inches wide. It must be placed proximal to the wound and as close to the wound as possible. The tourniquet should be tightened just enough to control bleeding.
- Hemostatic dressings are specially treated with a clot-promoting agent and should be packed into an open wound and bandaged in place. The chemical in the bandages helps promote clotting.
- Bleeding from the nose and mouth poses an extra risk because bleeding can contribute to an airway obstruction. Proper positioning of the patient is necessary when caring for bleeding from the nose and mouth.

Chapter Questions

Multiple Choice

For each question, place a check next to the correct answer.

1. Bleeding from ______________ is under high pressure and sometimes is found to be spurting from the wound.

   _____ a. the venae cavae
   _____ b. capillaries
   _____ c. veins
   _____ d. arteries

2. What technique involves placing a dressing firmly over the injury site in an attempt to slow the bleeding at the wound?

   _____ a. Direct pressure
   _____ b. Pressure point
   _____ c. Pressure dressing
   _____ d. Elevation

3. The purpose of a tourniquet is to:

   _____ a. put pressure directly on the wound.
   _____ b. slow blood flow to the injury site.
   _____ c. stop all blood flow to the injury site.
   _____ d. stop all venous blood flow only.

4. Which one of the following represents the most appropriate method for controlling a simple nosebleed?

   _____ a. Pinch the nose and have the patient lean back.
   _____ b. Allow the nose to bleed freely while the patient leans forward.
   _____ c. Allow the nose to bleed freely while the patient leans back.
   _____ d. Pinch the nose and have the patient lean forward.

5. All of the following are signs and symptoms of hemorrhagic shock *except:*

_____ a. increased pulse rate.
_____ b. increased respirations.
_____ c. decreased blood pressure.
_____ d. decreased pulse rate.

6. The two factors that contribute most to the severity of blood loss are:

_____ a. time and quantity.
_____ b. time and injury.
_____ c. body size and weight.
_____ d. body size and injury.

7. The sudden loss of _____________ cc of blood in the adult patient can be life threatening.

_____ a. 100
_____ b. 500
_____ c. 1,000
_____ d. 2,000

8. Bleeding from _____________ is often steady and flowing and appears dark in color.

_____ a. veins
_____ b. arteries
_____ c. capillaries
_____ d. venules

9. An abrasion will most likely have which type of bleeding?

_____ a. Arterial
_____ b. Capillary
_____ c. Venous
_____ d. Severe

10. The most appropriate placement of a tourniquet is _____________ the wound.

_____ a. over
_____ b. just below
_____ c. just above
_____ d. above the joint proximal to

Matching

Match the term on the left with the applicable definition on the right.

1. _____ Plasma
2. _____ Red blood cells
3. _____ White blood cells
4. _____ Platelets
5. _____ Bleeding out
6. _____ Direct pressure
7. _____ Elevation

A. Irregularly shaped cell fragments that are responsible for promoting blood clotting
B. Pressure applied to the surface of a wound to help control bleeding
C. Disk-shaped cells responsible for transporting oxygen and carbon dioxide to and from the tissues
D. Raising the injury site above the level of the patient's heart to reduce the amount of pressure at the site and make it easier for the bleeding to be controlled
E. Any of the colorless or white cells in the blood that help protect the body from infection and disease
F. The clear, yellowish fluid portion in which the other components of blood are suspended
G. Term meaning the patient is losing blood from within the circulatory system; not specific to internal or external blood loss

Critical Thinking

1. Describe the type of bleeding you might see from a large wound and the methods you would use in an attempt to control the bleeding.

____

____

____

____

(continued on next page)

(continued)

2. Describe why bleeding from arteries is generally more difficult to control than bleeding from other vessels.

3. List at least three signs and symptoms of shock and their causes.

Case Studies

Case Study 1

You have responded to a business park for a possible amputation. Upon arrival, you are escorted into one of the warehouses where you find an approximately 20-year-old woman who is bleeding from the right hand. You can see a large towel that has been completely soaked with blood wrapped around her right hand. One of the workers tells you that they were performing routine maintenance on one of the conveyor belts, when it suddenly started and Monique got her hand stuck in the belt. Monique is lying on her back and in severe pain. She is crying and saying something in Spanish that you cannot understand. One of the workers tells you that Monique is saying that she cannot feel her hand. You can see blood flowing down her arm and onto the cement floor beneath her.

1. What is your priority of care for this patient?

2. You have removed the bloody towel and see that Monique's hand appears to have been crushed. There are several breaks in the skin on both sides of her hand and between the fingers. There is blood spurting from an open wound on her palm. What type of bleeding is present, and how will you manage it?

3. What can you do to treat Monique for shock?

Case Study 2

You have been dispatched to the local hardware store for a possible head injury. Upon arrival, you are met by one of the employees who escorts you to the supply room at the back of the store. There you find an approximately 70-year-old man who is bleeding from the scalp. One of the employees is holding a dressing on the wound, but blood continues to flow down the side of his head. You are told that the man was removing a box from a shelf, when a piece of metal fell, hitting him on the head.

1. Other than the bleeding wound, what must you be concerned about with this patient?

2. How will you control bleeding from this wound?

3. Once bleeding has been controlled, what other care will you provide for this patient?

The Last Word

Blood loss due to injury is lost through arteries, veins, and capillaries. The more blood that is lost, the lower the blood pressure eventually falls, resulting in a condition known as *shock* (hypoperfusion).

Most external bleeding that you encounter in the field is likely to be minor and therefore easily controlled with direct pressure, elevation, pressure dressing, and in rare cases, the use of tourniquets. Do not be concerned about completing a thorough patient assessment until all severe bleeding is controlled. Remember that the primary ways to control external bleeding are direct pressure, elevation, pressure dressing (optional), and use of tourniquets in that order.

Apply supplemental oxygen to the patient as soon as practical and watch for the development signs and symptoms of shock. Expedite transport to an appropriate receiving hospital or request an ALS intercept as appropriate. Document all appropriate information in your prehospital care report.

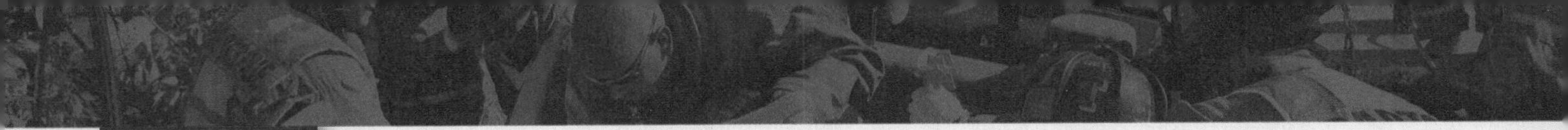

31 Caring for Patients with Soft-Tissue Injuries

Education Standards

Trauma: Bleeding and soft-tissue trauma

Competencies

Applies fundamental knowledge to provide basic emergency care and transportation based on assessment findings for an acutely injured patient.

Objectives

After completion of this lesson, you should be able to:

31-1 Define key terms introduced in this chapter.

31-2 Differentiate the layers of the skin.

31-3 Describe the different functions of the skin.

31-4 Discuss the role that proper PPE plays when caring for patients with soft-tissue injuries.

31-5 Explain the importance of recognizing and providing emergency medical care to patients with soft-tissue injuries to control bleeding, minimize shock, and prevent the contamination of wounds.

31-6 List types of closed soft-tissue injuries and describe the assessment-based approach to closed soft-tissue injuries, including emergency medical care.

31-7 List types of open soft-tissue injuries.

31-8 Describe the assessment-based approach to open soft-tissue injuries, including emergency medical care.

31-9 Explain special considerations and appropriate care for impaled objects, amputations, and large neck injuries.

31-10 Describe various types of dressings and bandages, including the purpose and methods of applying pressure dressings, and the general principles of dressing and bandaging.

Key Terms

abrasions p. 799
air embolism p. 808
amputation p. 805
avulsions p. 799
compartment syndrome p. 797
contusions p. 797
crush injuries p. 797
dermis p. 795
dressings p. 811
epidermis p. 795
hematomas p. 797
impaled object p. 805
lacerations p. 799
occlusive dressing p. 808
penetration injuries p. 800
position of function p. 814
pressure dressing p. 813
subcutaneous p. 795

Introduction

Soft-tissue injuries can be some of the most visually disturbing images an EMT will encounter in the field. They also can be life threatening to the patient, depending on the extent of the damage and amount of blood loss. While these wounds will certainly require care, it is important not to let the visual impact of an open wound distract you from your priorities. Ensuring an open airway, adequate breathing, and adequate circulation are your first priorities. Once they are cared for, you will then control all external bleeding and apply the appropriate dressings and bandages. This chapter describes the various types of wounds you are likely to see, along with the appropriate emergency care for each.

EMERGENCY DISPATCH

"Am I going to die?" The nine-year-old girl named Cassie looked up at EMT Moe Brenner, tears streaming down her cheeks.

"Honey," Moe said gently. "We are here to help you." Moe and his partner, Keenan, had been dispatched to the Running Water Fun Park for some sort of "leg injury" and had arrived to find a young girl with a blood-soaked towel wrapped around her left lower leg. According to witnesses, the girl had struck her leg on an exposed bolt while on one of the water slides.

The girl fought to control her sobs. "Is my leg going to look weird when it heals?"

Moe slowly removed the towel, and gasps erupted from the surrounding crowd as a large section of flesh slowly slid away from the girl's leg. The flap was still connected by a two-inch area of skin and ended up hanging limply above the ground, blood falling to the concrete in bright red drops.

"I imagine you'll probably end up with a scar," Moe said softly as he replaced the avulsed piece with a gloved hand. "Please try not to worry about that too much right now. Just keep being brave while we wrap this up and get you to the doctor, okay?"

The girl sniffed a little and nodded as Keenan handed Moe a trauma dressing and several rolls of gauze.

A Review of Skin Function

31-2 Differentiate the layers of the skin.

31-3 Describe the different functions of the skin.

The skin is the largest organ of the body. As you may remember from your study of anatomy in Chapter 5, the skin serves many important functions including the following:

- ***Protection.*** The skin protects the inner body from a hostile outside environment, which includes extreme temperatures, life-threatening pathogens (bacteria and viruses), and impacts from outside forces (blunt trauma).
- ***Temperature regulation.*** The skin helps the body maintain a consistent core temperature.
- ***Sensation.*** The skin houses the important sensory nerves that allow us to feel heat, cold, and pain.
- ***Fluid balance.*** The skin serves as a barrier against fluid loss and helps maintain a proper fluid balance by controlling evaporation.

The skin is composed of three layers (Figure 31-1 ■). They are:

- ***Epidermis.*** The **epidermis** is the outermost layer of skin.
- ***Dermis.*** The layer just below the epidermis, the **dermis** contains many of the blood vessels and nerve endings.
- ***Subcutaneous.*** Located below the dermis, the **subcutaneous** layer contains most of the fat and soft tissues of the skin. It helps with temperature regulation, as well as shock absorption.

epidermis the outer layer of the skin.

dermis the inner (second) layer of the skin found beneath the epidermis. It is rich in blood vessels and nerves.

subcutaneous the deepest layer of the skin. It is made mostly of fatty tissue and provides shock absorption and insulation for the body.

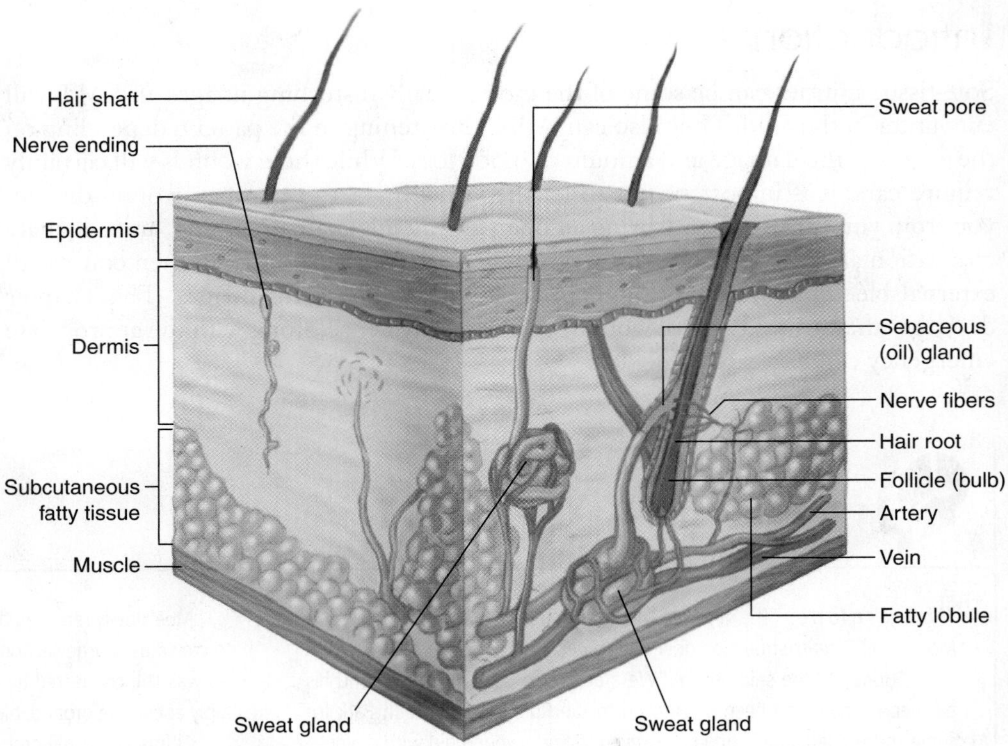

Figure 31-1 A cross section of the skin showing detailed anatomy.

PRACTICAL PATHOPHYSIOLOGY

The epidermis is a very important layer of protection for the body. If this layer becomes damaged, it can allow the entry of pathogens, which could result in infection. In addition, if the damaged area is large enough, evaporation of significant amounts of fluid could occur, causing dehydration.

BSI Precautions

31-4 Discuss the role that proper PPE plays when caring for patients with soft-tissue injuries.

One of the greatest risks to the EMT when caring for victims of trauma with open injuries is the exposure to blood. As you have already learned, blood is capable of carrying life-threatening pathogens, such as viral hepatitis and HIV. It is always important to take appropriate BSI precautions and don the necessary personal protective equipment—such as gloves, facemask, eye protection, and a gown—when caring for patients with open wounds.

Injuries to Soft Tissues

31-5 Explain the importance of recognizing and providing emergency medical care to patients with soft-tissue injuries to control bleeding, minimize shock, and prevent the contamination of wounds.

Injuries to soft tissues can include damage to the skin, muscles, and in some cases the underlying organs. Soft-tissue injuries are classified as either open or closed. A closed injury occurs when the underlying tissues are damaged without a break in the surface of the skin. Open injuries result when the skin is broken, exposing the lower layers or, in cases of severe injury, the soft tissues and organs that lie below.

Remember your priorities of care when dealing with injuries such as major chest trauma, burns, or penetrating injuries. The sight of such injuries can easily distract you from identifying life-threatening problems with the airway, breathing, or circulation. As with all patients, begin with ensuring an open and clear airway and adequate breathing before attempting to address less immediate life-threatening problems.

Closed Injuries

31-6 List types of closed soft-tissue injuries and describe the assessment-based approach to closed soft-tissue injuries, including emergency medical care.

Closed injuries to soft tissues can range from very minor to severe and life threatening. The difference often depends on the amount of tissue damage, how much bleeding there is, and what organs may be affected. The two mechanisms primarily associated with closed soft-tissue injuries are blunt force and crush force.

Blunt Force Trauma

Blunt force trauma is typically caused when the body is struck with a blunt surface, such as the ground following a fall or the dashboard of a car in a collision (Figure 31-2 ■). Blunt force trauma also can be caused when an object strikes the body, such as a baseball bat or blows from a fist during an assault. The force of the impact is transferred to the underlying tissues and organs. The outside skin remains intact but may show evidence of the impact, such as discoloration and bruising. Blunt force trauma can easily cause severe damage to underlying soft tissue and organs, resulting in blood loss, shock, and even death.

Figure 31-2 Blunt force injuries are common in falls from a height.

Crush Force Trauma

Crush injuries, also called *crush force trauma*, are typically caused when a part of the body becomes trapped between two surfaces and the pressure from both sides causes damage to the soft tissues. For example, this can occur when someone is pinned between a wall and a vehicle, when he is run over by a vehicle, or when an extremity gets trapped in a piece of machinery. There are many causes of crush injuries and these are just a few examples. While breakage of the skin is common with crush injuries, they also can occur without damage to the outer layers of the skin. Crush injuries to the torso can cause significant organ damage and blood loss, resulting in shock and death in extreme cases.

A condition called **compartment syndrome** can occur following a crush injury, as well as with burns and fractures. Compartment syndrome is the compression of blood vessels, nerves, and muscles inside a closed space within the body following an injury. The most common location for compartment syndrome to develop is in the extremities where muscle groups can become crushed by blunt trauma. The pressure increases with swelling within the closed muscle compartment, cutting off blood flow to the affected tissues and preventing blood from flowing distally in the extremity. If not identified and corrected, it can lead to loss of function and may eventually require amputation of the limb.

crush injuries injuries typically caused when a patient or a part of the patient's body becomes trapped between two surfaces and the pressure from both sides causes damage to the soft tissues and/or internal organs.

compartment syndrome damage to tissues due to the buildup of pressure within a confined space within an injured limb.

contusions injuries resulting when the tissues below the epidermis are damaged and cause bleeding into the surrounding tissues following a blunt trauma or crushing force. Also called *bruises*.

hematomas areas of localized swelling caused by the accumulation of blood and other fluids beneath the skin.

Signs of Closed Injuries

Aside from pain, there are at least two significant signs of closed soft-tissue injury: **contusions** (Figure 31-3 ■) and **hematomas** (Figure 31-4 ■). Contusions, also known as *bruises*, appear as reddish blue discoloration of the skin and may be painful. They are caused when blood vessels beneath the skin become ruptured secondary to trauma. Some reddening of the skin at the injury site may be all you see at the emergency scene. Greater discoloration usually does not appear for several hours after the injury occurs. A simple contusion is rarely life threatening by itself, but it may be the only sign of more significant underlying injury.

A hematoma is an area of swelling beneath the skin caused by an accumulation of blood. One of the most common types of hematoma is the classic "goose egg" that often results from a blow to the head. The presence of a hematoma may indicate a more significant injury involving larger vessels. Depending on the location, a patient can lose up to a liter or more of blood with a hematoma (Table 31-1).

Both contusions and hematomas are indicative of bleeding beneath the surface of the skin. They can occur alone or together, depending on the amount of tissue damage.

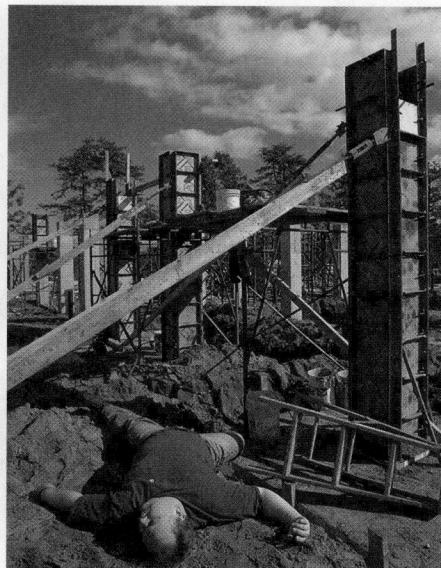

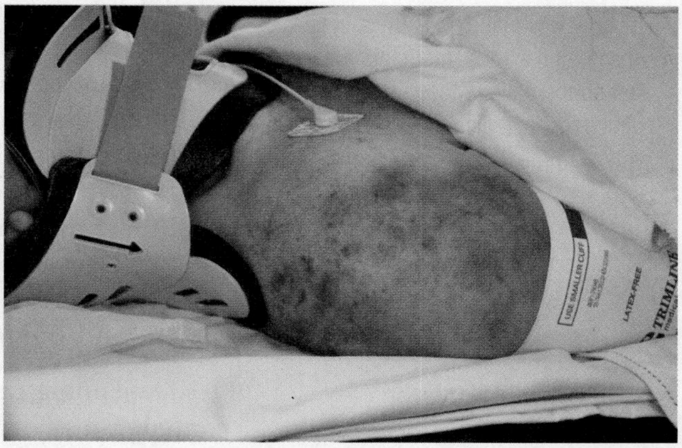

Figure 31-3 Contusions to the shoulder. (© Edward T. Dickinson, MD)

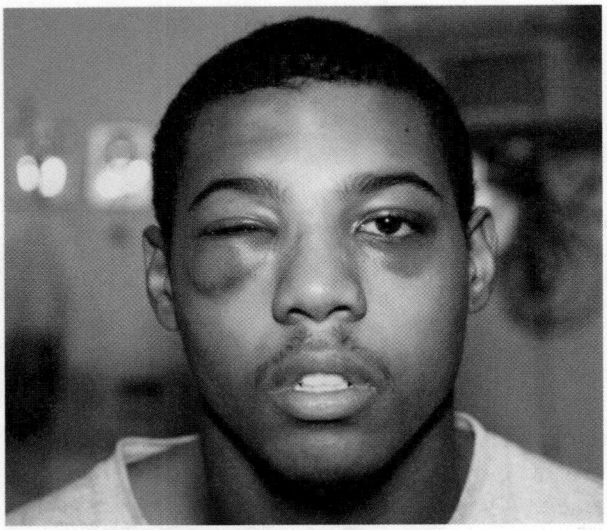

Figure 31-4 Hematoma below the right eye. (© Edward T. Dickinson, MD)

TABLE 31-1 CONTUSIONS AND HEMATOMAS

SIGN	INDICATION
Discoloration/bruising of the skin	Tissue damage below the skin. If over the chest, abdomen, or pelvis, suspect injury to underlying organs.
Swelling or deformity at the site of injury	The presence of a hematoma or possible fracture. Consider proper immobilization of injury.
Bruising behind the ears or around the eyes	Trauma to the head and possible skull fracture. Assess for fluid or blood coming from the nose, mouth, or ears. Take proper spinal precautions.

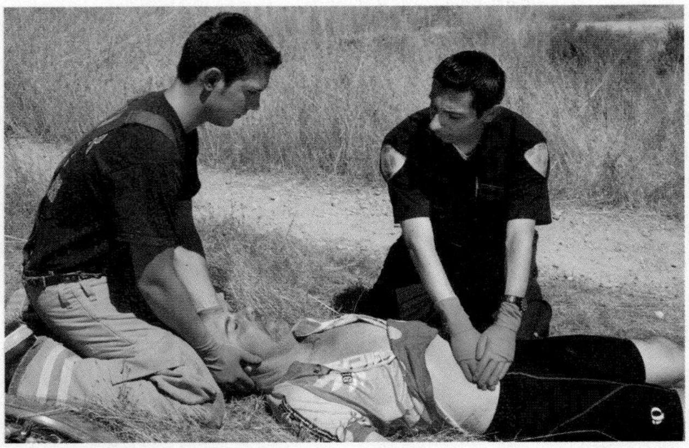

Figure 31-5 Use both hands when assessing the chest, abdomen, and pelvis. Watch the patient's facial expressions as you palpate.

Assessment of Closed Injuries

Your assessment of the patient must begin with an evaluation of the mechanism of injury (MOI). This will be especially helpful in patients who are unresponsive and unable to provide any history or offer a response to pain. Maintain a high index of suspicion for internal injuries when the MOI suggests it, even in the absence of obvious signs and symptoms such as contusions, hematomas, or pain.

Your physical exam must be thorough. Use both hands when palpating the chest, abdomen, and pelvis. Expose and examine each area thoroughly (Figure 31-5 ■). As you palpate, watch the patient's face for grimacing, which usually indicates tenderness and possible underlying injury. Expose all areas of pain and tenderness, as appropriate, and observe for evidence of injury. Not all internal injuries will present with external signs.

> **CLINICAL CLUE**
>
> **Palpation and Pain**
>
> If you know that pain is present in a certain area, palpate that area last so the patient does not experience residual discomfort when you examine uninjured areas.

Emergency Care for Closed Injuries

Follow these steps when caring for a patient who presents with the signs and symptoms of a closed soft-tissue injury:

1. Take the appropriate BSI precautions and perform a scene size-up.
2. Perform a primary assessment.
3. Attempt to control any external bleeding, using direct pressure, elevation, pressure dressing (optional), and tourniquets as needed.
4. Initiate oxygen therapy as appropriate.
5. Perform a secondary assessment as appropriate.
6. Immobilize the injured extremities as appropriate.
7. Initiate transport.
8. Perform reassessments.
9. Watch for signs and symptoms of shock and expedite transport if necessary.

Depending on the nature and extent of the injury and the presentation of the patient, it may be necessary to initiate transport and conduct a secondary assessment while en route to the hospital.

Open Injuries

31-7 List types of open soft-tissue injuries.

Open soft-tissue injuries occur when the mechanism of injury causes a break in the integrity of the skin and the underlying tissue becomes exposed. Bleeding from open wounds is usually obvious and must be controlled as soon as possible. Infection is a serious concern. Therefore, you must take care to minimize contamination of the wound during your care. (This will be discussed in more detail later in this chapter.)

There are several types of open wounds commonly seen in the field. Some of them represent minor injuries with minimal bleeding, while others involve major arteries and significant bleeding that is difficult to control. The following are descriptions of the most common types of open soft-tissue injuries:

abrasions injuries to the skin that involve the wearing down or removal of the superficial layers of the skin.

lacerations open wounds that can have jagged or straight edges.

avulsions injuries in which the skin and/or underlying tissue is forcibly torn away.

- *Abrasions.* **Abrasions** involve the wearing down or removal of the superficial layers of the skin (Figure 31-6 ■). Scraped elbows and skinned knees are common examples of abrasion injuries. Everyone has had them, so you know how painful they can be, but they rarely, if ever, pose a serious threat to life. Bleeding from abrasions is typically minimal and easy to control, because blood slowly oozes from the wound. Infection is a big concern with abrasions, especially large abrasions, so they must be covered with a clean dressing as soon as possible.
- *Lacerations.* These are open wounds that typically have jagged edges, although they can have straight, even edges as well (Figure 31-7 ■). They can be caused by many things, but most often are caused by sharp objects or forceful impact. Their depth will vary, depending on the mechanism. **Lacerations** have the potential to cause severe bleeding, depending on the vessels or organs that are affected.
- *Avulsions.* These injuries occur when the skin and/or underlying tissue is forcibly torn away by the mechanism of injury (Figure 31-8 ■). In some cases the injury causes a loose flap of skin, but it also can result in skin being torn completely off. Injuries caused when a piece of nose or an ear is torn away and even when an eye is torn from its socket are all described as **avulsions.** Depending on the involvement of vessels, bleeding from avulsions will vary.
- *Penetration injuries.* These injuries are caused when an object penetrates the skin and underlying soft tissues or organs

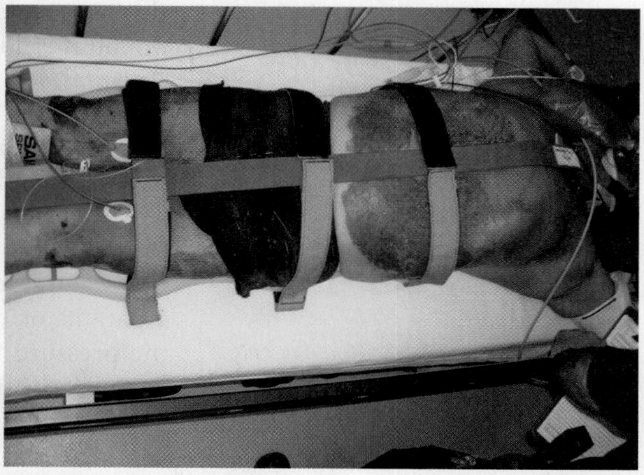

Figure 31-6 Major abrasions over the entire body. (© Pat Songer)

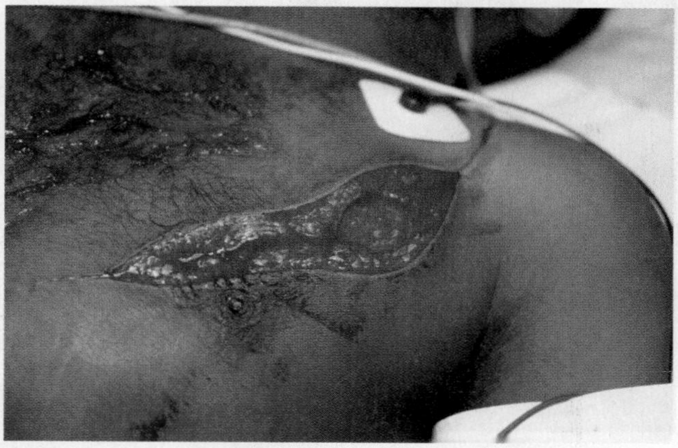

Figure 31-7a Large laceration to the chest. (© Edward T. Dickinson, MD)

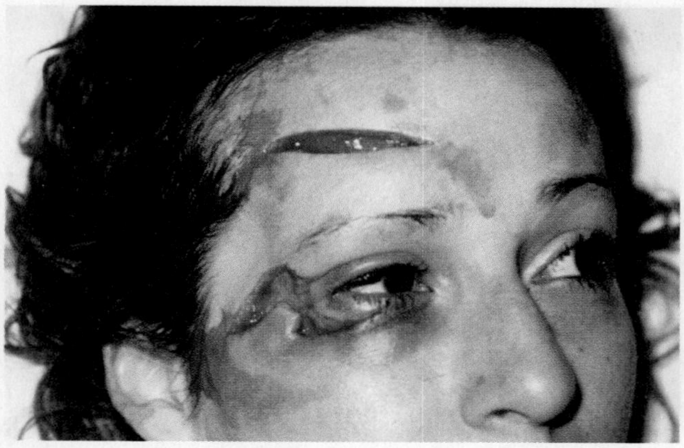

Figure 31-7b Lacerations to the face. (© Edward T. Dickinson, MD)

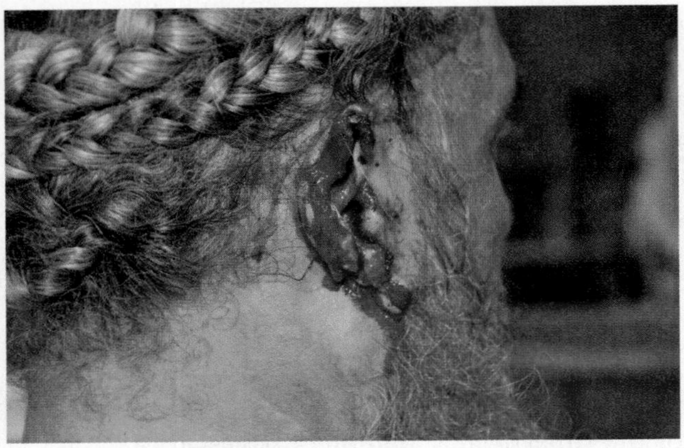

Figure 31-8 Avulsion injury to the ear. (© Edward T. Dickinson, MD)

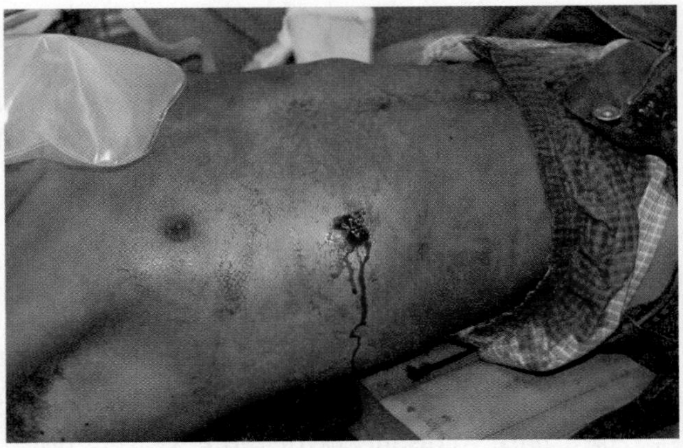

Figure 31-9 Penetration injury to the chest caused by a bullet. (© Edward T. Dickinson, MD)

penetration injuries injuries caused by an object that passes through the skin or other body tissues.

(Figure 31-9 ■). While typically caused by sharp objects, such as a knife, some **penetration injuries** are caused by bullets and large blunt objects. Depending on the mechanism of injury, penetrating injuries may have little or no external bleeding. Most of the damage is deep within the body and can result in severe internal bleeding. Penetration injuries always have at least an entry site and could also have an exit site. An object that has penetrated the skin and remains in the wound is called an *impaled object*.

- ***Amputations.*** These injuries occur when the mechanism of injury causes a loss of a limb or part of a limb (Figure 31-10 ■). Depending on the mechanism of injury, the bleeding associated with an amputation will vary. With traumatic amputations, where there is a significant tearing mechanism, the tissues and vessels are pulled to the point of failure. For this reason, the blood vessels have a tendency to retract into the wound and bleeding may be minimal.
- ***Crush injuries.*** As described earlier, these injuries are typically caused when a patient or a part of his body becomes trapped between two surfaces and the pressure from both sides causes damage to the soft tissues and possibly internal organs (Figure 31-11 ■). When they involve the extremities, crush injuries frequently cause fractures. Depending on the mechanism and area affected, crush injuries may have minimal external bleeding and major internal bleeding.

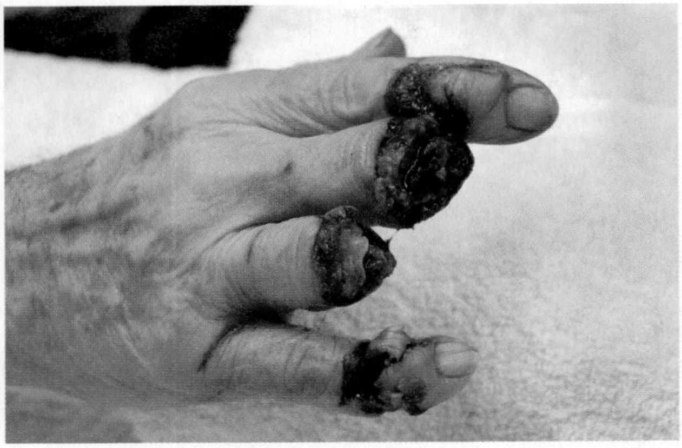

Figure 31-10 Amputation injury to the fingers. (© Edward T. Dickinson, MD)

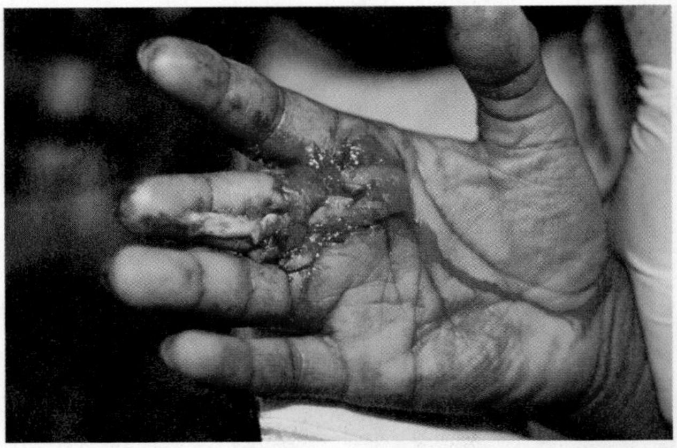

Figure 31-11 Open crush injury to the hand. (© Edward T. Dickinson, MD)

STOP, REVIEW, REMEMBER!

Multiple Choice

For each question, place a check next to the correct answer.

1. The ______________ is the outermost layer of skin.
   _____ a. epidermis
   _____ b. dermis
   _____ c. subdermis
   _____ d. subcutaneous

2. Which one of the following would *not* be considered a normal function of the skin?
   _____ a. Protection from infection
   _____ b. Temperature regulation
   _____ c. Fluid balance
   _____ d. Fluid filtration

3. A patient who has fallen 12 feet onto a hard surface has suffered what is referred to as ______________ force trauma.
   _____ a. crush
   _____ b. mild
   _____ c. blunt
   _____ d. severe

4. An injury caused when a patient's leg is run over by a vehicle is an example of ______________ force trauma.
   _____ a. crush
   _____ b. mild
   _____ c. blunt
   _____ d. severe

5. An injury that results in the tearing away of skin and other soft tissue is described as a(n):
   _____ a. laceration.
   _____ b. amputation.
   _____ c. avulsion.
   _____ d. abrasion.

Matching

Match the definition on the left with the applicable term on the right.

1. _____ The outermost layer of skin
2. _____ The layer just below the epidermis, which contains many of the blood vessels and nerve endings
3. _____ Contains most of the fat and soft tissue of the skin and helps with temperature regulation
4. _____ Result when the skin is broken, exposing the lower layers
5. _____ Caused when the body is struck with a blunt surface
6. _____ Caused when a patient or a part of his body becomes trapped between two surfaces
7. _____ Results when bleeding occurs below the skin, causing discoloration
8. _____ Areas of localized swelling caused by the accumulation of blood beneath the skin

A. Subcutaneous
B. Epidermis
C. Dermis
D. Crush injury
E. Blunt trauma
F. Contusion
G. Open injuries
H. Hematoma

(continued on next page)

(continued)

Critical Thinking

1. Describe each of the functions of the skin.

2. Explain why closed soft-tissue injuries can be more deadly than open soft-tissue injuries.

3. Describe the difference between a contusion and a hematoma and how each may present during a patient assessment.

PERSPECTIVE

Moe—The EMT

It was kind of weird, actually. I mean that was probably the worst avulsion that I've ever seen. But there really wasn't much bleeding. Man, when I unwrapped that towel and the skin just, sort of, came off, it caught me off guard! But that little girl was so scared. I really hope I hid my reaction well enough. I wanted her to feel like the whole thing was routine and that she was going to be perfectly fine. No big deal, you know? But inside I was a little uneasy.

31-8 Describe the assessment-based approach to open soft-tissue injuries, including emergency medical care.

Open soft-tissue injuries are some of the most common injuries you will encounter. Use your standard approach, beginning with the scene size-up and primary assessment. Do not let the sight of the injury distract you from your priorities of care.

Scene Size-up

Many injuries involving open wounds are caused by a mechanism of injury that could still pose a threat as you approach the scene. Motor-vehicle collisions, assaults, and unsecured machinery are just a few examples. Obtain as much information from dispatch as possible prior to arrival, and use extra caution when approaching the scene. If necessary, request additional resources, such as law enforcement, fire department, or utility company to manage any hazards that may exist.

Primary Assessment

Once you have determined that the scene is safe, approach the patient and begin your primary assessment. Do not let the unpleasant site of an open wound distract you from properly addressing the ABCs. Once airway and breathing have been addressed, control all external bleeding. If the patient does not have an adequate airway or breathing and uncontrolled bleeding is present, work with your partner to manage both problems at the same time. One of you must address the airway and breathing, while the other controls bleeding. Provide supplemental oxygen as soon as practical.

Secondary Assessment

After the ABCs have been properly addressed, gather a patient history and perform a physical exam. Once again, the specific assessment path will depend on the mechanism of injury. A rapid secondary assessment is required for the patient who has sustained a significant MOI. For the patient with a nonsignificant MOI, perform a focused secondary assessment.

It may be necessary to remove or cut away clothing to expose the wound for assessment and care. Whenever possible, use sterile dressings to minimize further contamination of the wound. Once bleeding has been controlled, apply an appropriate dressing and bandage. Calm and reassure the patient as necessary. Monitor the patient closely for signs and symptoms of shock and expedite transport.

PERSPECTIVE

Cassie—The Patient

I was going down the water slide and at this one part I saw this thing sticking up. I think it's supposed to have some plastic thingy on it, but it didn't. And I just slid over it because I couldn't stop or anything. It hurt, but I didn't know how bad until I got to the bottom. At first it didn't feel nearly as bad as it looked. I wanted my Dad! I got really worried that I could die or that my leg would end up looking all deformed and that everyone would laugh at me when I wore shorts and stuff. The ambulance guys were nice, but I just couldn't stop crying. It hurt so much, and I was really scared!

Follow these steps when caring for a patient with an open soft-tissue injury:

1. Take the appropriate BSI precautions and perform a scene size-up.
2. Perform a primary assessment.
3. Attempt to control any external bleeding, using a sterile dressing with direct pressure, elevation, pressure dressing (optional), and tourniquet as needed.
4. Administer supplemental oxygen as appropriate.
5. Perform a secondary assessment as appropriate.
6. Immobilize the injured extremities as appropriate.
7. Initiate transport.
8. Perform reassessments.
9. Watch for signs and symptoms of shock and expedite transport if necessary.

Depending on the nature and extent of the injury and the presentation of the patient, it may be necessary to initiate transport and conduct a secondary assessment while en route to the hospital.

STOP, REVIEW, REMEMBER!

Multiple Choice

For each question, place a check next to the correct answer.

1. In addition to blood loss, ____________ is a major concern when caring for open wounds.

_____ a. CHF
_____ b. disfigurement
_____ c. infection
_____ d. function

2. What type of injury occurs when the skin and underlying tissues are forcibly torn away by the mechanism of injury?

_____ a. Crush injury
_____ b. Avulsion
_____ c. Laceration
_____ d. Penetration

3. Your patient is unresponsive with gurgling respirations and is bleeding profusely from an open wound to the right femur. You should:

_____ a. suction the airway.
_____ b. hold manual stabilization of the leg.
_____ c. administer supplemental oxygen.
_____ d. apply a tourniquet.

4. The first step in the control of external bleeding is:

_____ a. elevation.
_____ b. pressure dressing.
_____ c. direct pressure.
_____ d. application of a tourniquet.

5. A patient who has sustained a significant MOI should receive which type of assessment?

_____ a. Focused secondary
_____ b. Rapid physical
_____ c. Focused physical
_____ d. Rapid secondary

Sorting

Write the letters A through I in the blanks to show the correct order in which emergency care should be provided to a patient with an open soft-tissue injury.

1. _____ Perform a primary assessment.
2. _____ Make transport decision.
3. _____ Immobilize the injured extremities as appropriate.
4. _____ Administer supplemental oxygen.
5. _____ Take the appropriate BSI precautions and perform a scene size-up.
6. _____ Perform reassessments.
7. _____ Perform a secondary assessment as appropriate.
8. _____ Watch for signs and symptoms of shock and expedite transport if necessary.
9. _____ Attempt to control any external bleeding, using a sterile dressing with direct pressure, elevation, pressure dressing, and a tourniquet as needed.

Emergency Care for Specific Wounds

Certain injuries may require additional care beyond what has been described. They include impaled objects, amputations, and open injuries to the neck. Information on the assessment and care for abdominal and chest wounds will be discussed in Chapter 33.

31-9 Explain special considerations and appropriate care for impaled objects, amputations, and large neck injuries.

Impaled Objects

An object that has penetrated the skin and remains embedded in the wound is referred to as an **impaled object** (Figure 31-12 ■). It is typically a sharp, piercing object such as a knife, steel rod, sharp stick, or piece of glass. In most cases, a portion of the object remains visible outside the wound.

impaled object penetrating trauma in which the object remains in the body.

In almost all situations involving an impaled object, you are to leave it in the wound and stabilize it prior to transport (Scans 31-1 and 31-2). Removing it will likely result in an increase in both internal and external bleeding. This is especially true if the object has penetrated an organ or major blood vessel.

Do your best to manually stabilize the object with your gloved hands while your partner cuts away clothing to expose the area around the wound. Use sterile dressings and direct pressure to control any external bleeding. You must then attempt to stabilize the object with material such as large bulky dressings, roller gauze, or triangular bandages.

In rare cases, the object may be too long to allow for proper transport, or its position may prevent you from performing appropriate airway management or chest compressions. In those cases, you may attempt to shorten the object or, if that does not work, remove it completely. Contact medical direction and follow local protocols, if you should need to remove an impaled object.

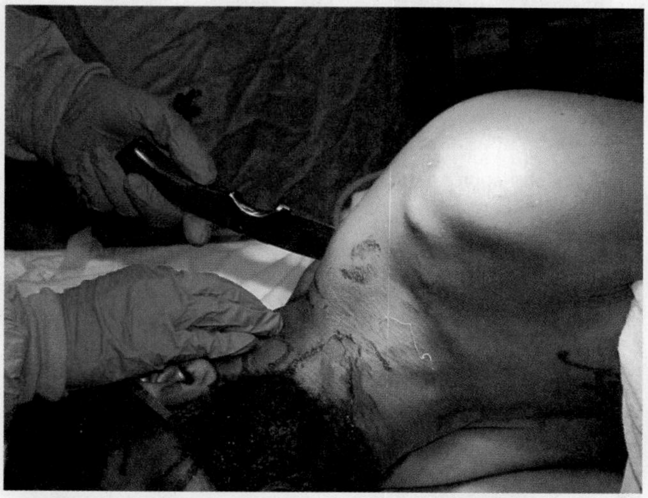

Figure 31-12 Impaled knife into the back. (© Edward T. Dickinson, MD)

An object impaled only in the cheek may be safely removed in the field, especially if leaving it in place could compromise the patient's airway. Objects that have impaled the trachea or are otherwise causing an airway obstruction may be removed as well. Follow local protocols. Have suction ready prior to removal and be prepared to suction the airway to keep it clear.

When caring for a patient with an impaled object, follow these steps:

1. Manage the ABCs as appropriate.
2. Administer supplemental oxygen.
3. Manually stabilize the object to minimize movement.
4. Have your partner cut away clothing to expose the wound and help control any external bleeding.
5. Attempt to stabilize the object for transport by securing it with bulky dressings.
6. Care for shock and transport the patient immediately.
7. Initiate an ALS intercept if available.

Amputations

An **amputation** is the traumatic loss of a limb, organ, or part of the body (Figure 31-13 ■). Amputations commonly seen by EMS include fingers, hands, arms, feet, and legs. Amputations can present special challenges to the EMT because, while your primary concern is for the well-being of the patient, you must remember to provide appropriate care for the amputated part. The way you manage the amputated part can significantly influence the possibility of reattachment.

amputation injury resulting in the loss of a limb or part of a limb.

SCAN 31-1 Stabilizing an Impaled Object

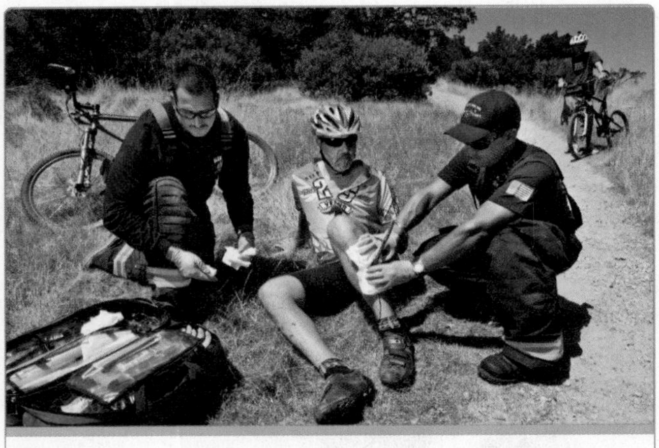

31-1-1 Take appropriate BSI precautions and control bleeding with clean dressings.

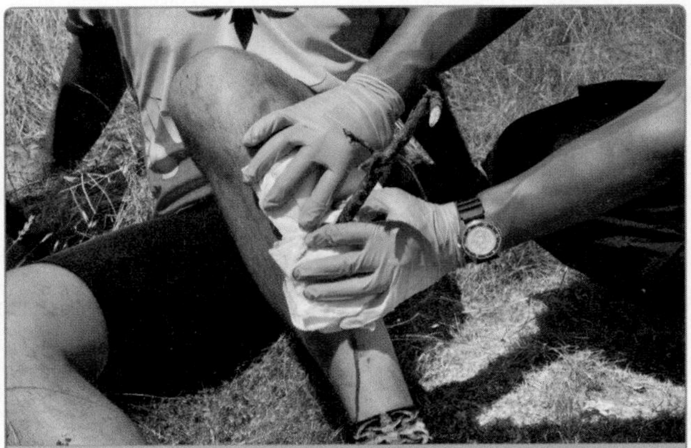

31-1-2 Carefully stabilize the object in place with your hands.

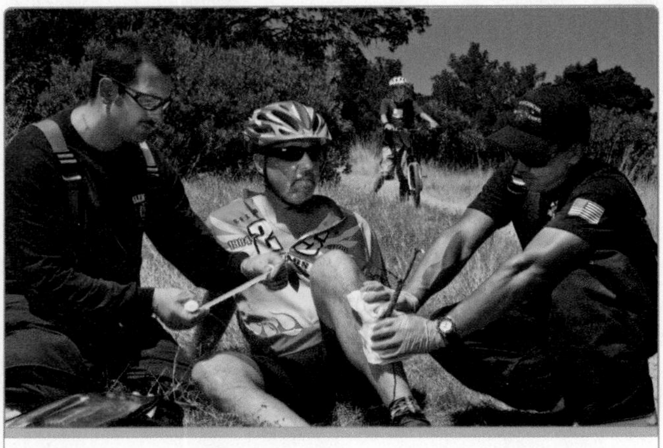

31-1-3 Apply bulky dressings around the object to help stabilize it.

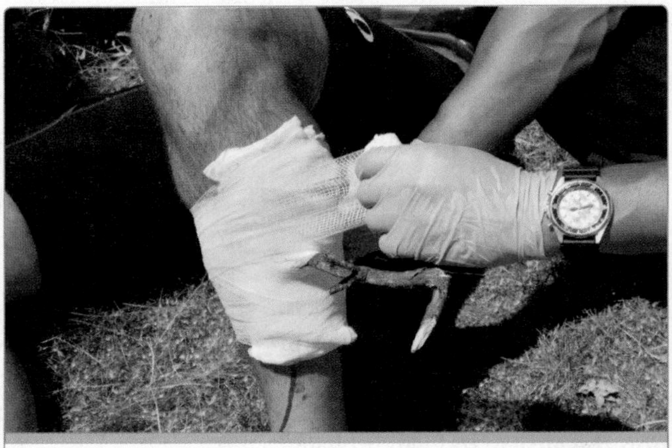

31-1-4 Secure the bulky dressings with roller gauze to stabilize the object.

Once you have addressed all immediate life threats to the patient, direct your attention to the amputated part (Scan 31-3). If necessary, enlist the help of other rescuers to locate the part and provide the indicated care. Follow these steps:

1. Wrap the amputated part in sterile dressings. If the part is large, such as a leg, cover the damaged open tissue with sterile dressings. Moisten the dressings with sterile saline. Follow your local protocols. *Do not immerse the part in water.*
2. For a smaller part, place it in a plastic bag or cover the area with plastic to conserve moisture. The common red biohazard bags work well. Properly label the bag with the patient's name so that it does not get thrown away by mistake.

SCAN 31-2 Stabilizing an Impaled Object in the Eye

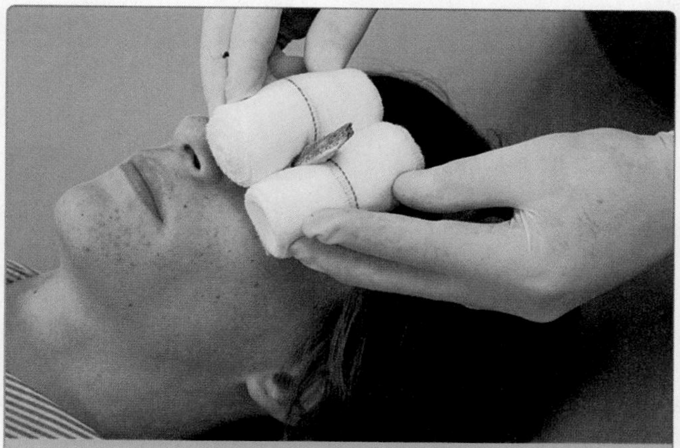

31-2-1 Stabilize the object with bulky dressings.

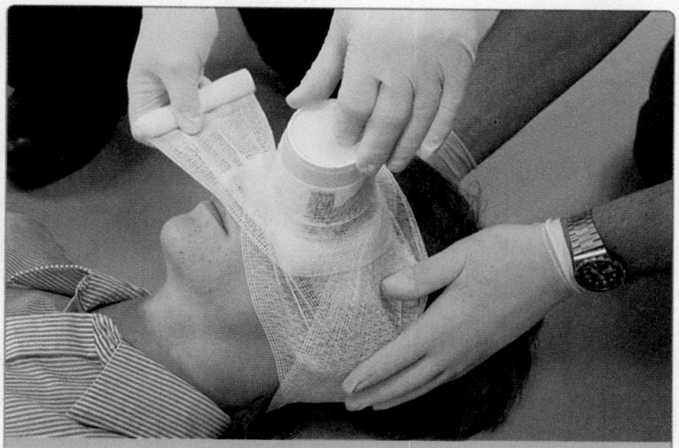

31-2-2 Secure a cup or similar object over the impaled object for protection.

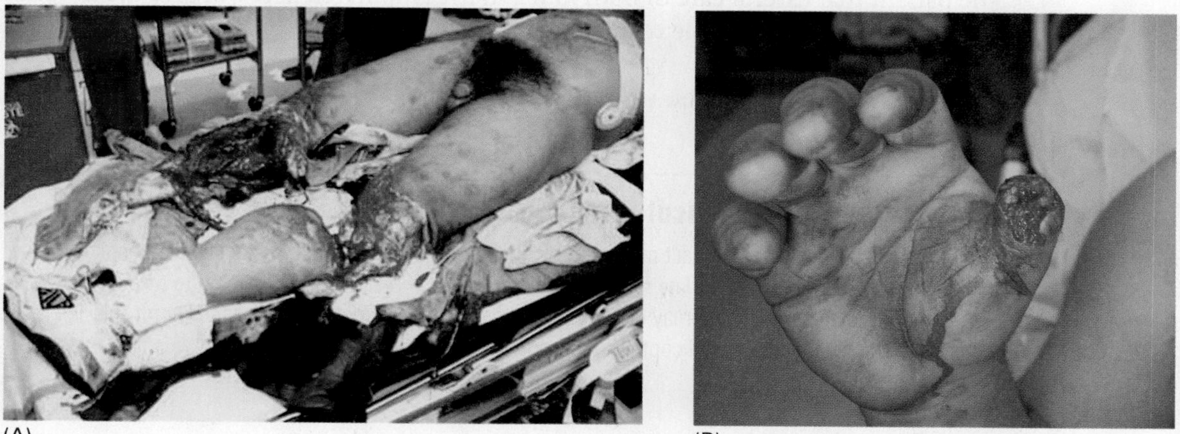

(A) (B)

Figure 31-13 (A) Amputation of the legs. (B) Amputation of the thumb. (© Edward T. Dickinson, MD)

3. Keep the part cool by using cool packs and placing them side by side with the bagged part. Use caution not to overcool or freeze the part. Do *not* place the amputated body part in ice or directly on ice.
4. If possible, always transport the amputated part with the patient to minimize the chances of its becoming lost or getting sent to the wrong hospital. Do not delay transport of a patient in order to locate and care for an amputated part.

Partial or incomplete amputations can present more of a challenge for the EMT. Do *not* attempt to complete the amputation by cutting or tearing away the last pieces of tissue. They may be providing valuable blood supply to the damaged part. Instead, carefully immobilize the entire limb and transport immediately.

Many amputations cannot be reattached because of the extent of tissue injury, but that decision must be made by highly trained surgeons at the hospital. Treat all

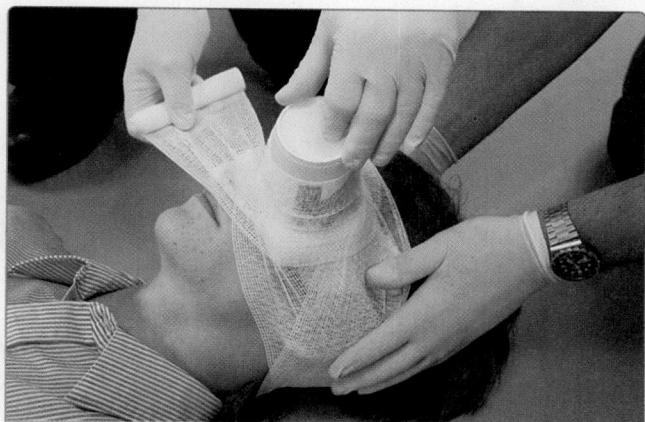

SCAN 31-3 Caring for an Amputated Part

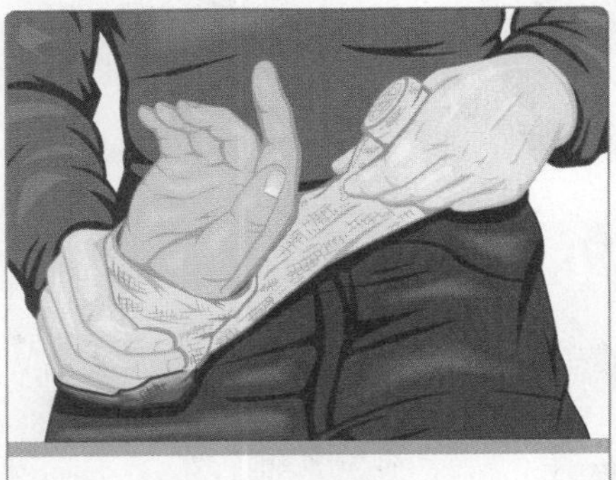

31-3-1 Wrap the amputated part in sterile gauze.

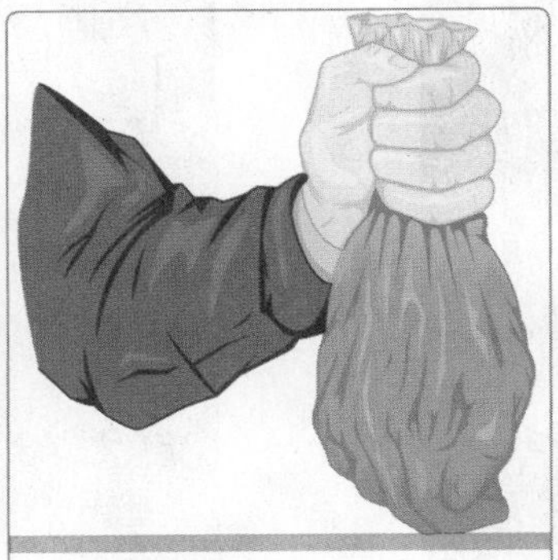

31-3-2 Place the part in a plastic bag.

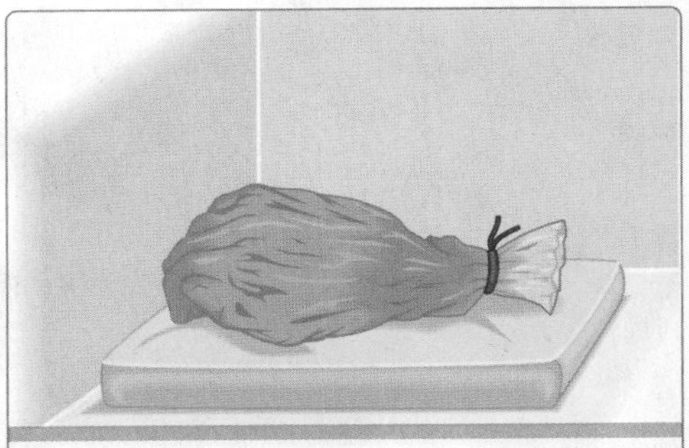

31-3-3 Apply cool packs during transport.

amputated parts carefully as described above. However, because reattachment is not always possible, be careful not to raise false expectations with the patient. Reassure the patient that careful care of both him and the amputated part will give the hospital the best chance for possible reattachment.

CLINICAL CLUE

Amputation and Medical Direction

It may be appropriate to contact medical direction in cases of amputation. The closest hospital may not be the most appropriate resource for this patient if reattachment is going to be attempted. Medical direction may direct you to the most appropriate receiving facility for this patient. Consider calling a helicopter if transport times will be extended.

Open Wounds to the Neck

air embolism a bubble of air that enters the circulatory system.

occlusive dressing a type of dressing that will not allow air to pass through; typically used to cover wounds on the chest and neck to prevent air from entering the wound.

Aside from the risk of severe bleeding and airway compromise, open injuries to the neck can result in an **air embolism.** This can occur when a major vessel in the neck becomes damaged and air is allowed to enter the vessel. The air, in the form of a bubble, can cause an obstruction of blood flow within the brain, heart, or lungs. This is a potentially life-threatening event. Open wounds to the neck should be covered as soon as possible with a gloved hand or **occlusive dressing** in order to minimize the chances of air entering the circulatory system (Figure 31-14 ■).

Any significant open wound to the neck should be considered a risk for an air embolism. To minimize that risk, follow these steps when caring for a patient with an open neck wound:

1. Cover the wound with an occlusive dressing as soon as possible. Use a gloved hand, if necessary, until an appropriate dressing can be applied. Make certain that the dressing covers the wound on all sides.

2. Add an additional absorbent dressing over the occlusive dressing to help with bleeding control.
3. Use fingertip pressure to control bleeding and minimize pressure on the airway. Compress the carotid artery only if it is necessary to control bleeding. Never compress both carotid arteries at the same time.
4. Monitor the patient's airway and breathing status closely, provide supplemental oxygen, and transport.

Remember that injuries to the neck are often associated with spine injury. Carefully evaluate the mechanism of injury as you begin your care and take the necessary spinal precautions as appropriate.

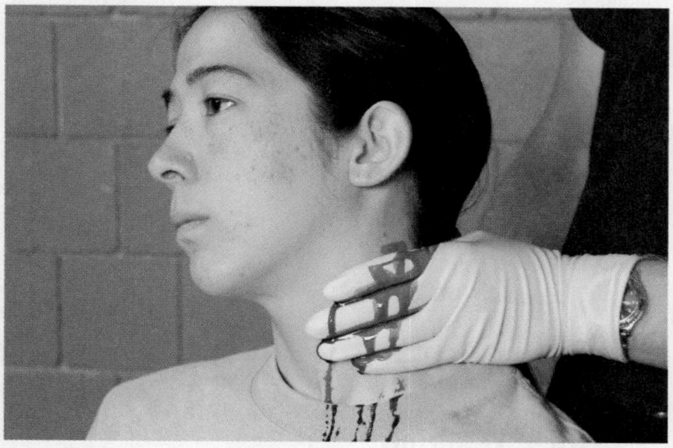

Figure 31-14 Cover an open wound to the neck with a gloved hand and an occlusive dressing.

STOP, REVIEW, REMEMBER!

Multiple Choice

For each question, place a check next to the correct answer.

1. Impaled objects in the ______________ may be removed by the EMT in the field.

_____ a. neck

_____ b. chest

_____ c. abdomen

_____ d. cheek

2. The first step in caring for an amputated part is to:

_____ a. wrap it with a sterile dressing.

_____ b. cool the part.

_____ c. control bleeding from the part.

_____ d. elevate the part.

3. In general you are not to remove an impaled object in the field, because removing it could cause:

_____ a. more contamination.

_____ b. more damage to soft tissues.

_____ c. increased internal and external bleeding.

_____ d. a decrease in pulse.

4. A potentially dangerous complication that can result from an open wound to the neck is a(n):

_____ a. thrombosis.

_____ b. air embolism.

_____ c. pneumothorax.

_____ d. hemothorax.

5. Remove an impaled object in the field for all of the following reasons *except* when the object interferes with:

_____ a. transport.

_____ b. chest compressions.

_____ c. proper care of the airway.

_____ d. rolling the patient.

(continued on next page)

(continued)

Matching

Match the term on the left with the applicable definition on the right.

1. _____ Amputation
2. _____ Impaled object
3. _____ Crush injuries

A. Injury typically caused when a patient or a part of his body becomes trapped between two surfaces and the pressure from both sides causes damage to the soft tissues and internal organs

B. Injury resulting in the loss of a limb or part of a limb

C. Penetrating trauma in which the object remains in the body

Critical Thinking

1. Describe the unique challenges the EMT faces in the emergency care of a patient with an impaled object.

____

____

____

____

2. Describe the complications that can result from an open wound to the neck.

____

____

____

____

3. Describe how you would care for a partial amputation of the hand.

____

____

____

____

31-10 Describe various types of dressings and bandages, including the purpose and methods of applying pressure dressings, and the general principles of dressing and bandaging.

Dressing and Bandaging

An important skill that every EMT must learn is the proper way to dress and bandage each of the many types of wounds encountered in the field. There are two main purposes for the application of a dressing and bandage to an open wound. First and foremost is bleeding control. The second purpose is to minimize further contamination of the wound. This section describes the various types of dressings and bandages, and the techniques used to apply them.

Dressings

Dressings are typically made of absorbent gauze and are available in many shapes and sizes and in both sterile and nonsterile applications. In general, sterile dressings are preferred in wound care. When placed directly over an open wound, dressings help control bleeding by aiding in the formation of a clot. They also help protect against the introduction of contaminants that might cause infection.

dressings sterile or nonsterile material placed directly over an open wound.

Dressings come in a wide variety of shapes and sizes, depending on their intended purpose. The following are examples of some of the more common dressings used in EMS and their intended use:

- ***Adhesive dressing.*** The brand of dressing most familiar to everyone is Band-Aid®. Self-adhering dressings are also available in a variety of sizes and shapes and are ideal for small cuts and scrapes.
- ***Gauze pads.*** Used with small to medium-size wounds, these are layered pads that come in a variety of sizes, such as 2″ × 2″, 4″ × 4″, 5″ × 9″, and 8″ × 10″ (Figure 31-15 ▪). Most are available as individually wrapped sterile dressings. However, some (such as the 4″ × 4″ and 2″ × 2″) come in bulk, nonsterile packages.
- ***Trauma/abdominal dressings.*** These are similar to the smaller gauze pads just listed but they are bigger (10″ × 30″ and larger) and thicker and are designed for large open wounds. Sometimes called *abdominal pads* or *ABD pads*, these dressings are well suited for large, open wounds to the chest and abdomen (Figure 31-16 ▪).
- ***Occlusive dressings.*** These dressings are typically thin pads of sterile gauze that have been saturated with petroleum jelly or a similar material to occlude, or prevent, air from passing through. They are available in a variety of sizes (Figure 31-17 ▪).

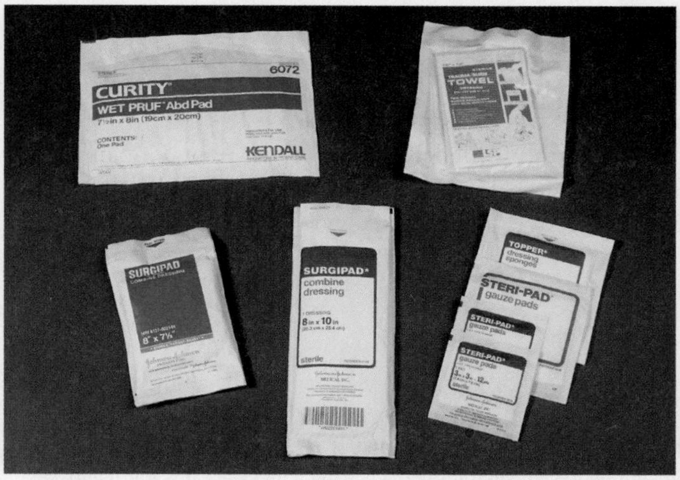

Figure 31-15 Small and medium-size sterile dressings.

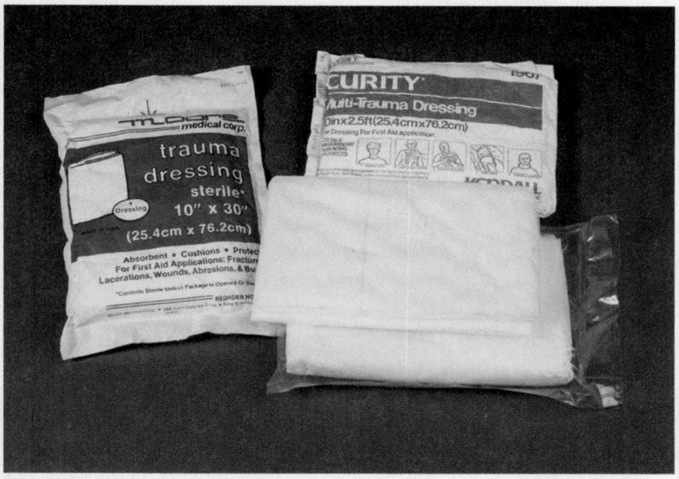

Figure 31-16 Large sterile trauma dressings.

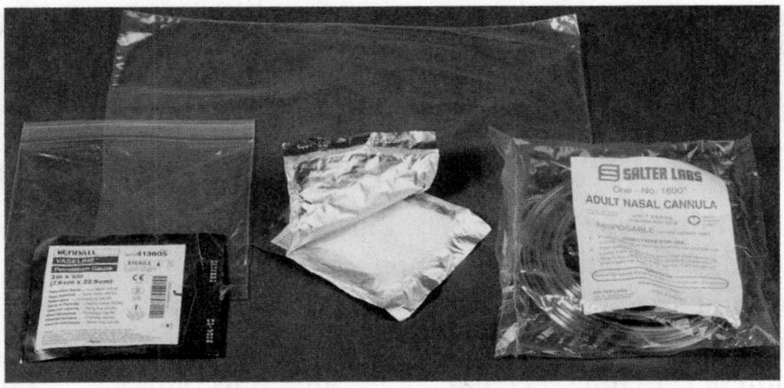

Figure 31-17 Commercial and improvised occlusive dressings.

PERSPECTIVE

Moe—The EMT

Although it wasn't bleeding that much, I knew that I had to get her leg bandaged right away. Since she had been swimming and sliding at a public water park all day and the injury was caused by what sounded like an old rusty bolt, I just didn't want to risk any further contamination. I'd hate to have this poor girl lose her leg, or worse, because of infection. I just can't imagine that, you know? Taking a school field trip to a water park to have fun with your friends, and then ending up injured and to have it deteriorate to the point where one of your limbs, or even your life, is in danger. I hope that she recovers okay. I really do.

Bandages

Bandages are typically made of strips of gauze or thin cloth material and are available in both sterile and nonsterile applications. The primary function of a bandage is to hold a dressing or dressings in place over a wound.

Much like dressings, bandages come in a wide variety of shapes and sizes, depending on their intended purpose. The following are examples of some of the more common bandages used in EMS and their intended use:

- ***Gauze rolls.*** Available in both sterile and nonsterile applications, these are rolls of thin gauze that come in a variety of widths (1″, 2″, 3″, 4″, and 6″) (Figure 31-18 ■).
- ***Triangular.*** Most commonly thought of as slings, triangular bandages are among the bandages most universally available. They provide a fast and easy way to secure dressings to extremities and the head. When folded like a cravat, triangular bandages are ideal for use as pressure dressings (Figure 31-19 ■).
- ***Self-adhering bandage.*** Commonly called Kling®, Kerlix™, or Coban™, this type of bandage comes in a variety of widths and adheres to itself when overlapped, eliminating the need for tape.

CLINICAL CLUE

Adhesive Tape Allergy

Some patients are allergic to the adhesive on many types of tape. If you are going to use tape directly on the skin, ask the patient if he has an allergy to tape or tape adhesive. Consider using hypoallergenic tape if it is available.

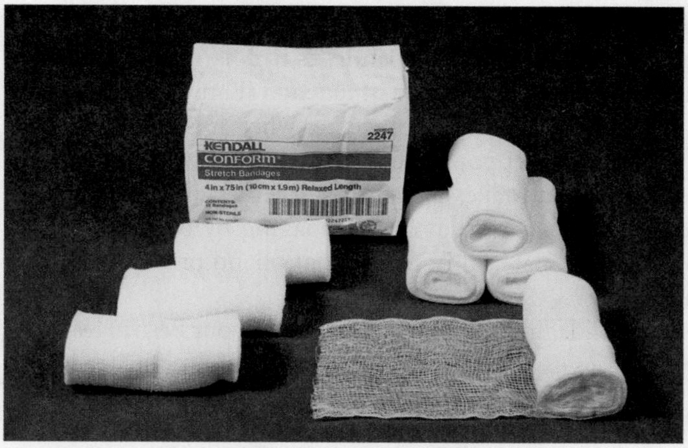

Figure 31-18 Roller-style bandages made of gauze.

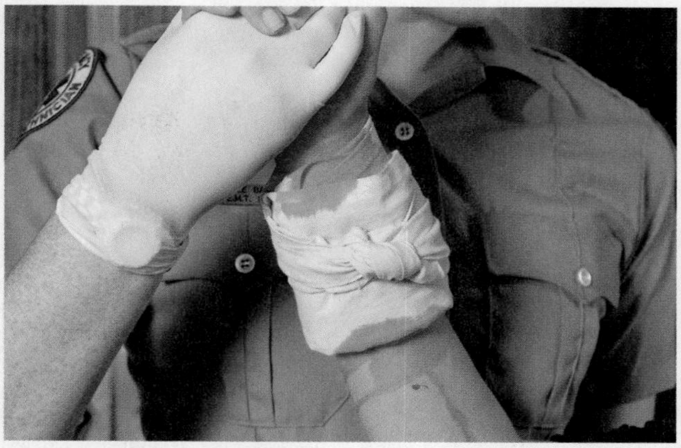

Figure 31-19 A cravat is a fast and efficient tool for applying a pressure dressing.

Application of Dressings and Bandages

Simply put, there is more than one way to dress and bandage wounds. While there are a few simple guidelines that you can follow to ensure the proper application of a dressing and bandage, among your most valuable assets will be your ability to improvise and adapt to the situation at hand.

First and foremost, you need to assess the wound to determine the immediate needs. Is the wound still actively bleeding?—in which case you may need to apply a specific type of dressing called a **pressure dressing.** This will be discussed later. If the bleeding is already controlled, the primary purpose will be to protect the wound from contamination.

pressure dressing dressing that applies pressure to control bleeding from a wound to an extremity that is still actively bleeding. Also called a *pressure bandage*.

Use the following guidelines when applying dressings and bandages:

- Remove any jewelry that might get in the way, especially rings that may be difficult to remove once the finger has become swollen.
- Choose an appropriate-size sterile dressing and apply it to the wound. If sterile dressings are not available, select the cleanest material available. The dressing should be large enough to extend beyond the wound on all sides. If necessary, apply additional dressings to adequately cover the wound.
- If dressings become blood soaked, replace them with fresh dressings. However, *do not* remove the first dressing that is covering the wound. That dressing is helping with the formation of a clot.
- Select the most appropriate means to secure the dressing in place. Tape may be appropriate for small wounds or wounds to the torso. For wounds on the head or extremities, roller gauze or triangular bandages work best.
- When using a roller bandage, start at the narrowest part of the limb and work your way up from there. To begin the bandage, make two or three wraps directly over one another to ensure a firm foundation for the bandage. Then overlap each spiral by approximately one-third to one-half to ensure adequate coverage of the dressing.
- The bandage should extend beyond the dressing on all sides. Secure the bandage with tape or by tying it off.
- Once the bandage is secured, continuously monitor distal circulation, sensation, and motor function to ensure that the bandage is not too tight.
- If appropriate, immobilize the injured limb and elevate. Watch to see that the bleeding remains controlled during transport.

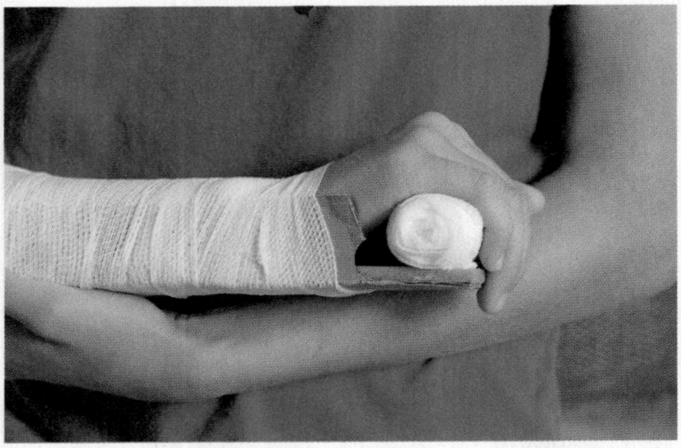

Figure 31-20 When bandaging or splinting an extremity, place the hand in the position of function.

Position of Function

When applying dressings and bandages to a hand, it is important to keep the hand in the **position of function** (Figure 31-20 ▪). This is the position the hand normally takes when it is at rest. You can see this when you let your hands fall relaxed at your sides. Notice how your hand takes a slightly curved shape. You can help to maintain this position during bandaging by placing a roll of gauze or similar material in the patient's hand prior to applying the bandage.

When bandaging the hands and feet, do your best to leave the fingers and toes exposed so that you can monitor circulation, sensation, and motor function following application of the bandage.

Practice the dressing and bandaging of specific types of wounds, including scalp, eye, hand, elbow, arm, foot or ankle, and knee (Scan 31-4).

position of function the slightly curved position the hand normally takes when it is at rest.

Pressure Dressing

A pressure dressing, sometimes called a *pressure bandage*, is used to help control bleeding from a wound to an extremity that is still actively bleeding. There is less concern for contamination and more focus on establishing a constant force of direct pressure to control the bleeding. By quickly applying a pressure dressing, the EMT is free to deal with other priorities, such as managing the airway or controlling bleeding from other injuries.

A pressure dressing differs from other types of dressings in these ways:

- It is used on wounds that are actively bleeding.
- More pressure is required.
- It is applied quickly.

You can use either roller gauze or cravats to secure a pressure dressing to a wound. Cravats are preferred because they are faster and easier to secure tightly. Use caution when tying any bandage around a limb. Do not secure it so tightly that it cuts off all blood flow to the limb. After applying the bandage to an extremity, recheck distal circulation, sensation, and motor function. If circulation or sensation are compromised, check to see that your bandage is not too tight.

Follow these steps when applying a pressure dressing:

1. Place several layers of an appropriate dressing directly on the wound and hold direct pressure while elevating the limb. Use caution when elevating the limb because it may have an underlying fracture.
2. Using a cravat or roller gauze, have your partner begin wrapping the dressing to the wound as tightly as possible without cutting off distal circulation to the limb. Secure the dressing with tape or tie it off.
3. If possible, keep the wound above the level of the heart and maintain direct pressure if you are not needed elsewhere.
4. Monitor the wound closely and add additional dressings and bandages if needed to control the bleeding. Consider the use of a tourniquet only as a last resort.

Following the application of any bandage, tourniquet, or splint to an extremity, it is important to monitor distal circulation, sensation, and motor function continuously. This is to ensure that you have not inadvertently tied something too tightly and are cutting off distal circulation to the limb. Bandages and splints that are applied improperly can cause unnecessary pain as well as tissue, nerve, and vessel damage. Monitor the dressing, bandage, and distal extremity throughout transport, and make adjustments as necessary.

SCAN 31-4 Dressing and Bandaging

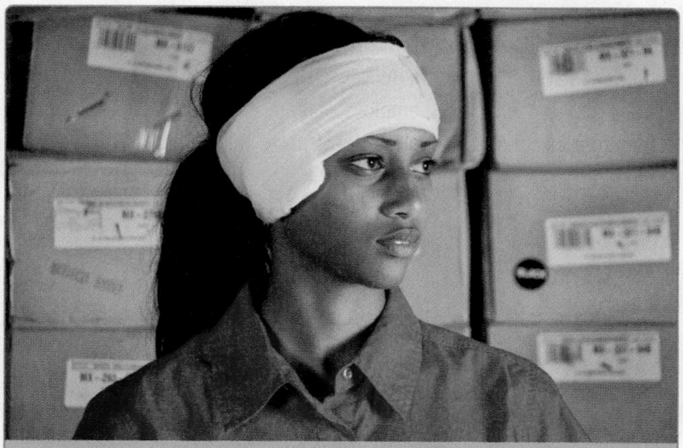

31-4-1 A roller bandage used to secure a dressing to the scalp.

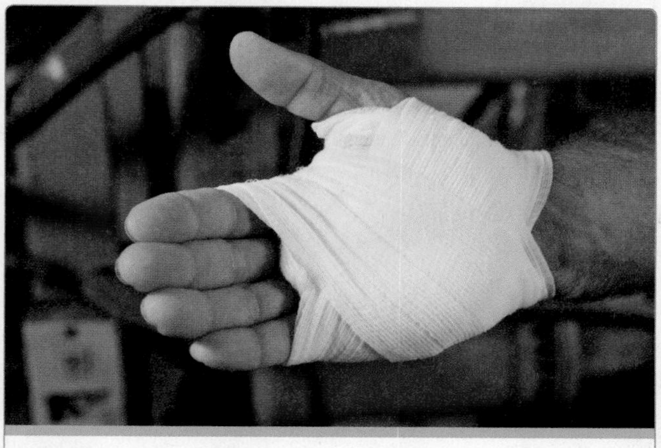

31-4-2 Hand injury.

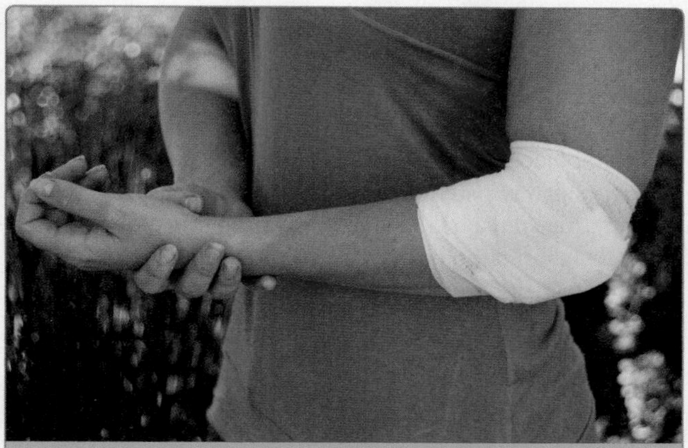

31-4-3 Elbow injury.

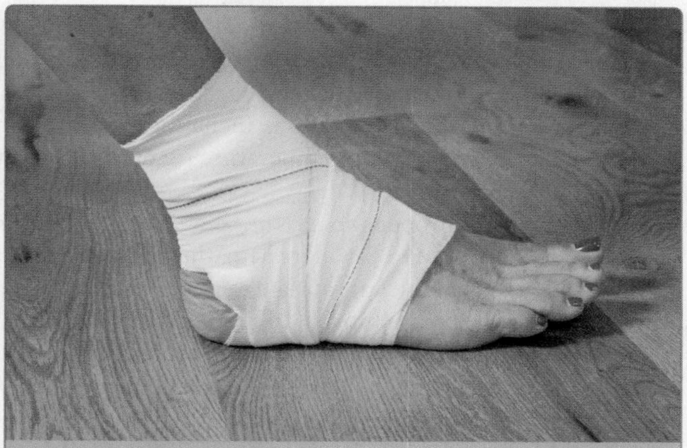

31-4-4 Foot and ankle injury.

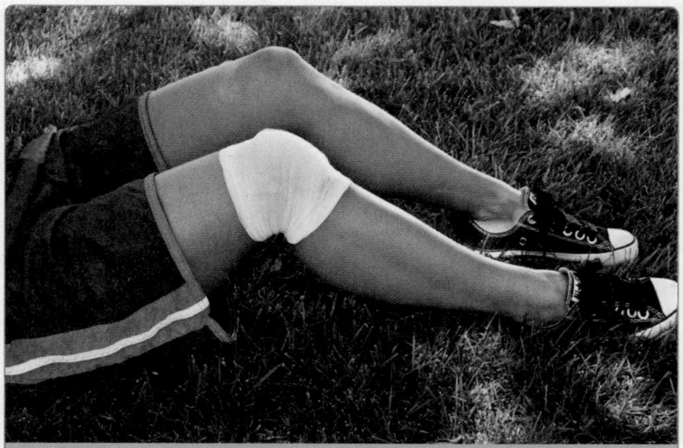

31-4-5 Knee injury.

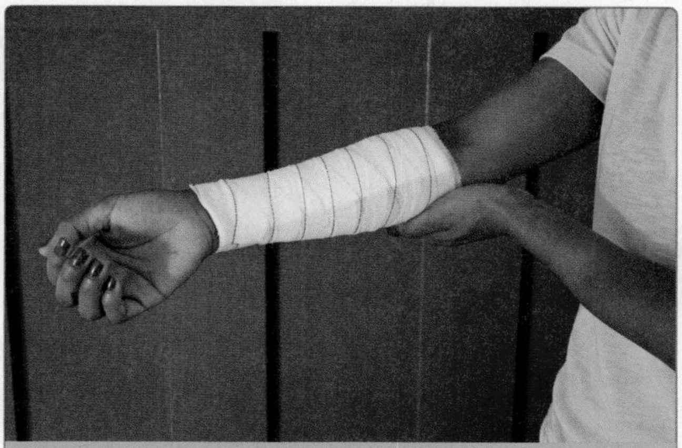

31-4-6 Forearm injury.

EMERGENCY DISPATCH SUMMARY

The patient was transported to the emergency department at Physician's Hospital where the avulsion was repaired. After several complications caused by postoperative infections, the patient was discharged and sent home with her parents. The wound has since healed to a very thin V-shaped scar that, according to the patient's doctor, will become even less noticeable as she grows older. City health inspectors blamed the incident on poor maintenance at the water park. All seven of its water slides have since been replaced and the park now employs a team of off-duty EMTs, including Keenan, to appropriately respond to any future incidents.

Chapter Review

To the Point

- The skin is made up of three primary layers that include the epidermis, dermis, and subcutaneous layers.
- The skin serves many functions including protection from the outside environment, temperature regulation, sensation, and fluid maintenance.
- All patients with open wounds pose a potential risk to the EMT for exposure to bloodborne pathogens. It is especially important to don the appropriate personal protective equipment prior to approaching all injured patients.
- Early recognition and management of soft-tissue injuries is important to minimize blood loss, infection, and the effects of shock from excessive blood loss.
- Closed soft-tissue injuries are most often caused by blunt trauma. Evidence of such trauma is often seen in the form of contusions and hematomas at the site of injury. Bleeding from damaged tissue, vessels, and organs can lead to significant blood loss, shock, and even death.
- Evaluation of the mechanism of injury and the presenting signs and symptoms should reveal the likelihood of internal bleeding.
- There are several common types of open soft-tissue injuries including abrasions, lacerations, avulsions, penetrating injuries, amputations, and crush injuries.
- Impaled objects must be stabilized in place unless they interfere with airway patency.
- Amputations must be managed by controlling bleeding, covering the amputated part with a sterile dressing, putting it in a plastic bag, and then gently cooling it during transport.
- Open neck injuries should be managed by covering with an occlusive dressing to minimize the chances of an air embolism.
- Dressings are generally made of absorbent gauze material and come in both sterile and nonsterile applications. Dressings range in size from very small (2″ × 2″) to very large (10″ × 30″) to address the many wounds encountered by EMS.
- A dressing should extend beyond the wound on all sides. A bandage should secure the dressing to the wound and extend beyond the edges of the dressing.

Chapter Questions

Multiple Choice

For each question, place a check next to the correct answer.

1. When placed directly over an open wound, ____________ help control bleeding by aiding in the formation of a clot.
   _____ a. bandages
   _____ b. dressings
   _____ c. cravats
   _____ d. tourniquets

2. Which one of the following is *not* a common type of dressing used by an EMT?
    _____ a. Occlusive
    _____ b. Surgical
    _____ c. Trauma
    _____ d. Adhesive
3. The primary function of a pressure dressing is to:
    _____ a. minimize contamination.
    _____ b. stop all blood flow to the wound.
    _____ c. control active bleeding.
    _____ d. act as a tourniquet.
4. All of the following are commonly used as bandages *except*:
    _____ a. traction splints.
    _____ b. roller gauze.
    _____ c. tape.
    _____ d. triangular bandages.
5. Signs or symptoms of an improperly applied dressing and bandage include all of the following *except:*
    _____ a. excessive pain following application.
    _____ b. loss of distal circulation.
    _____ c. numbness and tingling of the extremity.
    _____ d. good distal circulation.
6. The functions of the skin are protection, temperature regulation, fluid balance, and:
    _____ a. sensation.
    _____ b. excretion.
    _____ c. motor function.
    _____ d. vessel dilation.
7. The layer of skin that consists mainly of fat and connective tissue is the:
    _____ a. epidermis.
    _____ b. dermis.
    _____ c. subcutaneous.
    _____ d. cutaneous.
8. Swelling caused by an accumulation of blood beneath the skin is known as a:
    _____ a. contusion.
    _____ b. bruise.
    _____ c. dermis.
    _____ d. hematoma.
9. A wound that has a linear cut in the skin is described as a(n):
    _____ a. abrasion.
    _____ b. laceration.
    _____ c. avulsion.
    _____ d. contusion.
10. Aside from capillary bleeding, abrasions have a strong likelihood for developing a(n):
    _____ a. infection.
    _____ b. hematoma.
    _____ c. contusion.
    _____ d. arterial bleeding.

Fill in the Blank

1. The two main reasons to dress and bandage a wound are to control ____________________ and minimize ____________________.
2. When placed directly over an open wound, a ____________________ helps control bleeding by aiding in the formation of a clot.
3. ____________________ dressings are ideal for small cuts and scrapes.
4. ____________________ dressings consist of thin pads of sterile gauze that have been saturated with petroleum jelly to prevent air from passing through.
5. The primary function of a ____________________ is to hold a dressing or dressings in place over a wound.
6. The ____________________ is the position the hand normally takes when it is at rest.

(continued on next page)

(continued)

Critical Thinking

1. Describe the purposes of a dressing and a bandage.

2. Explain the reasons for learning to properly apply dressings and bandages.

3. Describe how a pressure dressing differs from other types of dressings or bandages.

Case Studies

Case Study 1

You have been dispatched to a construction site for a "man down." Upon arrival, you are directed to an adult male lying face up on a concrete slab. Bystanders advise that the man slipped and fell from the roof approximately 12 feet above and landed on a bucket. The patient denies any loss of consciousness and is complaining of severe pain to his right abdomen. Upon examination, you find redness to the right side of his abdomen and severe pain on palpation.

1. Describe your treatment priorities and how you will care for this patient.

2. What type of MOI has this man likely sustained?

Case Study 2

You are caring for an adult male patient who was driving a water-tank truck when it rolled and he was ejected. As the truck rolled, he was caught underneath and sustained significant injury to both legs. His right leg appears to be completely severed above the knee, and the left leg appears to be partially amputated below the knee. He suffered no other injuries to his torso, neck, or head.

1. What will be your treatment priorities for this man's injuries?

____

____

____

____

2. Bleeding from the left leg proves difficult to control with direct pressure and a pressure dressing. What will you do next to control the bleeding?

____

____

____

____

3. How will you care for the injury to the right leg?

____

____

____

The Last Word

Soft-tissue injuries can be both internal and external, depending on the mechanism of injury. Most of the bleeding from open wounds can be managed easily by applying direct pressure. If direct pressure alone does not control the bleeding, it is appropriate to combine direct pressure with pressure dressings and elevation. Tourniquets should be used when necessary. Remember to carefully evaluate the MOI and maintain a high index of suspicion for internal bleeding if the mechanism is significant. All patients with open or closed wounds must be monitored closely for evidence of shock.

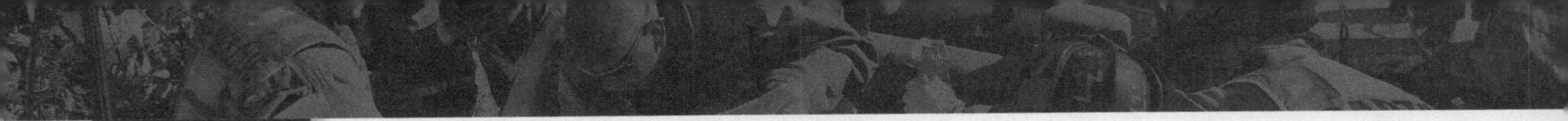

32 Caring for Patients with Burn Injuries

Education Standards

Trauma: Soft-tissue trauma

Competencies

Applies fundamental knowledge to provide basic emergency care and transportation based on assessment findings for an acutely injured patient.

Objectives

After completion of this lesson, you should be able to:

32-1 Define key terms introduced in this chapter.

32-2 Discuss each of the following sources of burns: chemical, electrical, radiation, and thermal.

32-3 Discuss each of the following mechanisms of burn injuries: contact, electrical, flame, flash, inhalation, scald, and steam.

32-4 Describe the effects of burns on the following body systems: skin, cardiovascular, respiratory, renal, nervous, musculoskeletal, and gastrointestinal.

32-5 Explain the classification of burns by depth.

32-6 Explain the system used to estimate the body surface area involved in burns for both adult and pediatric patients.

32-7 Discuss considerations of burn depth, location, body surface area involved, the patient's age, and any preexisting medical conditions in determining the severity of burn injuries.

32-8 Describe the assessment-based approach to burns.

32-9 Describe special considerations in the scene size-up when responding to calls involving burned patients.

32-10 Explain the concept of stopping the burning process.

32-11 Identify indications of inhalation injury.

32-12 Discuss special considerations for dressing burns, including burns to specific anatomical areas.

32-13 Describe special considerations in responding to, assessing, and managing chemical and electrical burns.

Key Terms

body surface area (BSA) p. 828
chemical burn p. 821
circumferential burn p. 835
electrical burn p. 822
full-thickness burn p. 824
light burn p. 822
partial-thickness burn p. 824
radiation p. 822
rule of nines p. 828
rule of palm p. 829
superficial burn p. 824
thermal burn p. 821

Introduction

Severe burns can be among the most traumatic of all injuries. Burns not only affect the skin, they also affect many of the body's organ systems and the patient's emotional well-being. Aside from the obvious disfigurement, burns can result in severe infection and loss of function to the extremities. Caring for a patient with severe burns can be a traumatic event for the members of the EMS team.

This chapter describes care for patients with all kinds of burns. You will learn about the different sources of burns (what causes them) and how burns are classified both by depth of injury (how deep the burn is) and by body surface area (BSA) affected. By assessing those three elements, you will be able to determine the most appropriate care for the burn patient.

EMERGENCY DISPATCH

"Are we just doing a standby then?" Brianna, an EMT with the city ambulance service, asked her partner as they rolled to a stop about two blocks from a fully engulfed house fire.

"I don't know." Shane rolled the truck to a stop and peered through the windshield at the dark smoke that rose high into the night sky. "But this is as far as we go with the ambulance." The road ahead of them was blocked by a mass of unoccupied fire and police vehicles, all parked helter-skelter across both lanes, their emergency lights pale in comparison to the fire. Brianna and Shane climbed out, got the cot from the back, and loaded it with their equipment.

"This is for a fire stand-by, right?" Shane asked into the portable radio.

"Affirmative," the dispatcher responded through static. "At least I think so. Report to the incident commander."

Brianna and Shane rolled the cot cautiously up the street, straining against the smoke and the intermittent darkness to find the command post.

"Medics!" The shout came from off to their left, toward the rear of the house. "Over here quick!"

There was a small group of firefighters—just silhouettes against the raging house fire—waving their arms and shouting. The EMTs hurried over, struggling to get the cot over the web of hoses that criss-crossed the pavement. As they approached, they saw that the firefighters were standing over a naked man who was lying on the sidewalk.

"I just pulled him out of the house," a firefighter shouted breathlessly. "He's alive, but I think I broke his arm!"

The wild-eyed man was severely burned from his scalp down to the bottoms of his feet. Brianna could see the top layers of his skin beginning to slough off in large sheets, exposing the raw, bleeding tissue underneath. The EMTs looked at each other with wide, questioning eyes.

"Get him on the cot and get him out of here!" an older firefighter shouted as the group hastily picked the now screaming man up and set him on the gurney. "Now go! Go!"

Common Sources and Mechanisms of Burns

Burns can be caused by a variety of sources and the emergency care you provide to the patient will be determined by the exact one. The following are the most common sources and mechanisms of burns:

- ***Thermal (heat) burn.*** Most commonly caused by exposure to fire and flames (Figure 32-1 ■), **thermal burns** also can occur through contact with a heated object, hot liquids (scalds, Figure 32-2 ■), and exposure to steam. Heated and superheated gases can cause burns to the upper and lower respiratory systems when the patient breathes them in (inhalation burns). Finally, thermal flash burns are burns that result from a sudden very brief exposure to intense heat. Patients subjected to a flash burn often scorch off their hair, but have relatively superficial burns to the skin (Figure 32-3 ■). The extent of injury from flash and other types of thermal burns is largely dependent on how long the patient was in contact with the heat source.
- ***Chemical burn.*** When the skin is exposed to substances such as acids, bases, corrosives, and caustics, **chemical burns** are the result (Figure 32-4 ■).

32-2 Discuss each of the following sources of burns: chemical, electrical, radiation, and thermal.

32-3 Discuss each of the following mechanisms of burn injuries: contact, electrical, flame, flash, inhalation, scald, and steam.

thermal burn a type of burn most commonly caused by exposure to fire, steam, hot objects, and hot liquids. Also called a *heat burn.*

chemical burn a type of burn caused when the skin is exposed to substances such as acids, bases, and caustics.

Figure 32-1 Fire is a common source of thermal (heat) burns. (© Edward T. Dickinson, MD)

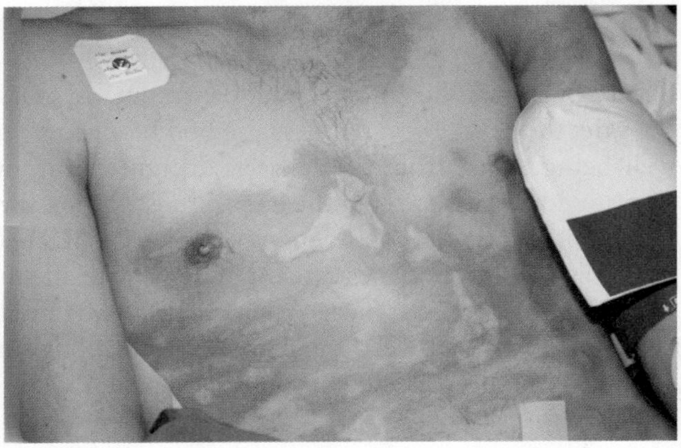

Figure 32-2 Scald burn to the chest from hot radiator fluid. (© Edward T. Dickinson, MD)

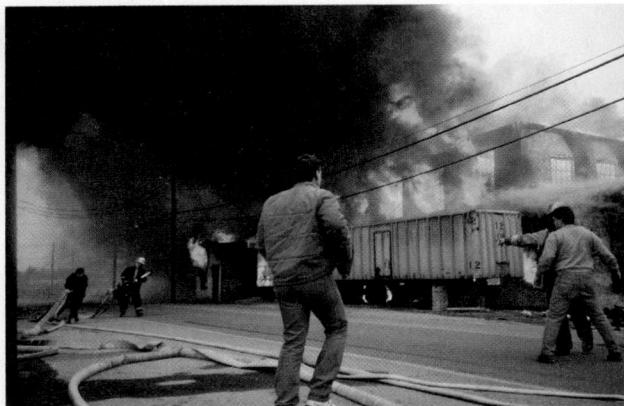

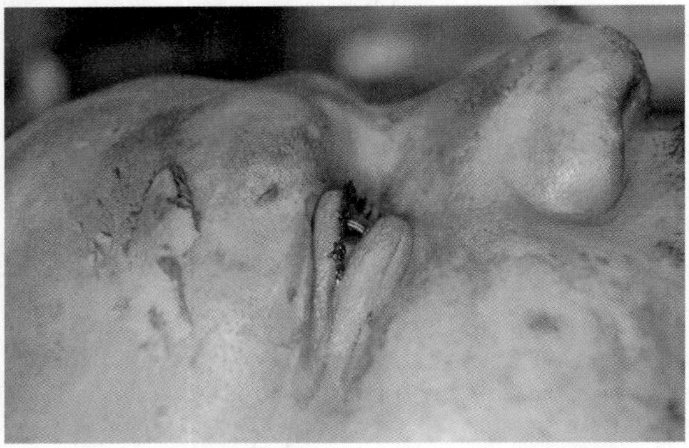

Figure 32-3 Flash burn to the face. (© Edward T. Dickinson, MD)

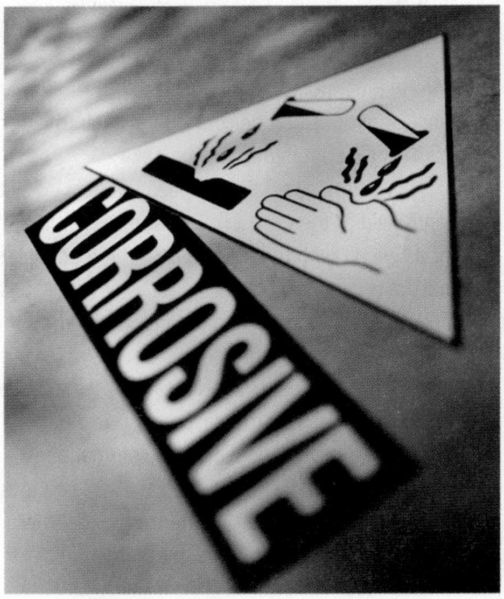

Figure 32-4 Corrosives placard. (Getty Images/Steve Cole)

electrical burn burn caused when the body becomes exposed to an electrical current as it passes through the body.

radiation a type of burn from sources of radiation such as nuclear fallout or radioactive materials used in medicine.

light burn burn caused by high-intensity light sources including the sun and lasers.

- ***Electrical burn.*** When the body becomes exposed to an electrical current and that current passes through the body, it can cause burns along its path (Figure 32-5 ▪). **Electrical burn** will vary, depending on the amount of electricity involved, which can cause both entrance and exit wounds as it passes through the body. Electrical sources can be household current, downed power lines, and even lightning. Electrical flash burns also can occur when the patient is caught in the path of an electrical arch, an intense momentary blue flash of electrical energy. The majority of damage caused by electrical burns occurs deep inside the body and cannot be seen by the EMT.
- ***Radiation.*** Though somewhat rare, burns from sources of **radiation,** such as nuclear fallout or the radioactive materials used in medicine, may be seen in the field (Figure 32-6 ▪).
- ***Light burn.*** Light is a form of energy. High-intensity light sources can cause significant burns. The most common source of **light burn** is the sun. High-intensity lasers and welding also are common sources of intense light that can damage the eyes and skin if exposed (Figure 32-7 ▪).

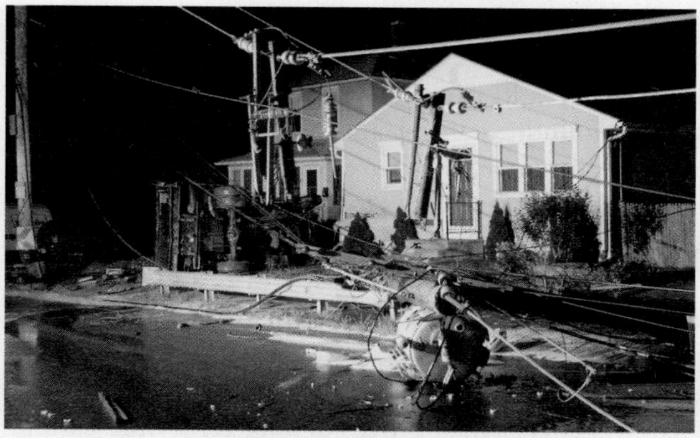

Figure 32-5 Downed electrical lines are hazardous and can be a cause of electrical burns. (© Mark C. Ide)

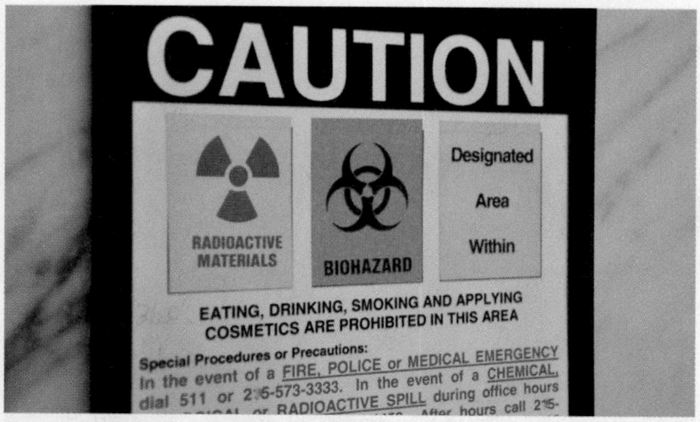

Figure 32-6 Radiation hazard placard. (© Edward T. Dickinson, MD)

CLINICAL CLUE

Safety Concerns

Most sources of burns can present a serious safety risk for the rescuer. Make certain that the scene is safe before attempting to care for the patient. In cases of chemical and radiation burns, caring for the patient can expose the rescuer to the same source that injured the patient. Know your training limitations and the limitations of your PPE before providing care. Request additional resources such as the fire department and a hazmat team as appropriate.

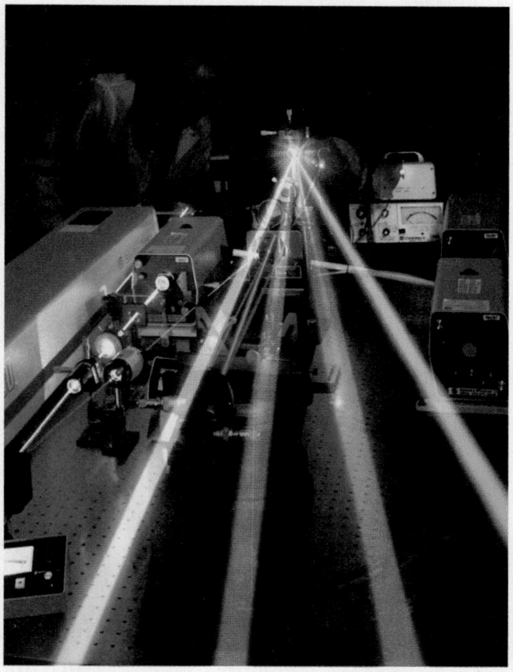

Figure 32-7 High-energy lasers. (Lawrence Livermore National Laboratory)

Burn Pathophysiology

32-4 Describe the effects of burns on the following body systems: skin, cardiovascular, respiratory, renal, nervous, musculoskeletal, and gastrointestinal.

Burns render damage to the human body in many ways. Multiple organ systems are potentially affected by burns, including the following:

- ***Skin system.*** The most common organ system affected by thermal burns is the skin. The depth of burn into the layers of the skin and the amount of surface area affected will determine how seriously damaged the skin's normal functions will be.
- ***Cardiovascular system.*** Major burns can result in significant external fluid loss as well as loss of fluid from the normal vascular spaces in muscle and skin. Fluid loss can result in hypovolemic shock. In addition, electrical current resulting in burns can induce irregular electrical activity in the heart (dysrhythmia) that can result in cardiac arrest.
- ***Respiratory system.*** Airway burns are the most immediately life-threatening respiratory complication. They can quickly result in loss of the airway because the tissue in the mouth and pharynx swells and prevents air passage. Inhalation of heated gases and steam also result in damage to the deeper lung structures, which will prevent effective oxygen exchange.
- ***Renal system.*** Major burns can go through the layers of skin and penetrate muscle. Burn patients are at risk for acute renal failure because of the resulting dehydration combined with the potential damage done to the kidneys by the products of muscle and tissue breakdown. The breakdown of muscle (rhabdomyolysis) can result in turning the patient's urine a characteristic brick red or cranberry color (Figure 32-8 ■).

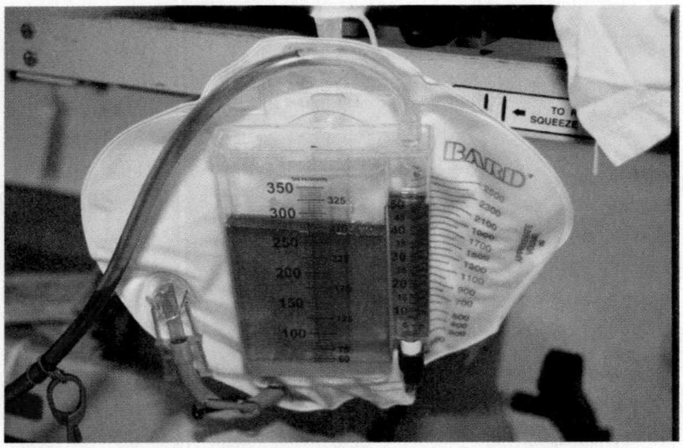

Figure 32-8 Products of muscle breakdown in urine of major burn victim. (© Edward T. Dickinson, MD)

- ***Nervous system.*** By far the greatest impact burns have on the nervous system is the damage they cause to the peripheral sensory nerves in the skin. Thermal burns to the skin are often profoundly painful and the specific reason that EMS is called for emergency care of the patient.
- ***Musculoskeletal system.*** Injuries to the musculoskeletal system can occur during high-voltage electrical burns. The intensity of the current either throws the patient, resulting in blunt trauma, or the current causes direct damage to bones and muscles. Deep thermal burns can affect muscles, tendons, and bones. In the long term, recovery of the function of the musculoskeletal system is a major focus of long-term burn care.
- ***Gastrointestinal system.*** Burns to the esophagus are a serious complication from ingested caustic agents. Over several days, radiation poisoning can result in the loss of the normal lining of the intestines, resulting in dehydration and bleeding.

PRACTICAL PATHOPHYSIOLOGY

An example of an immediately life-threatening situation involving the interaction of multiple organ systems occurs when a patient suffers a full-thickness burn to his entire torso. Because the skin is deeply burned, it loses its normal elasticity and becomes as rigid as dried animal hide. Normal respiratory function requires the chest to expand inward to allow air flow, but a rigid burned chest can make normal breathing, and even assisted ventilations with a bag-mask device, impossible, leading rapidly to death.

Classification of Burns by Depth

32-5 Explain the classification of burns by depth.

superficial burn a burn that affects the outermost layer of skin, the epidermis.

partial-thickness burn burn that extends down beyond the epidermis and into the dermis.

full-thickness burn burn that extends beyond all layers of the skin, causing damage to underlying muscle, bone, nerves, and vital organs.

Regardless of the source or cause of the burn, burns are classified based on the depth of injury, or how deep into the tissues the burn has reached (Figure 32-9 ■). A burn that affects only the outer layer of skin (epidermis) is referred to as a **superficial burn.** A burn that reaches down to the dermis is referred to as a **partial-thickness burn.** Any burn that reaches down to or past the subcutaneous layer, even potentially reaching the muscle, bone, and organs, is referred to as a **full-thickness burn.**

Rarely are burns of a single depth. For example, it is common to have an area of full-thickness burn surrounded or mixed in with areas of partial-thickness burns.

CLINICAL CLUE

Burn Classification

You may remember that at one time burns were classified as first-, second-, or third-degree burns, depending on the depth of injury. The reference to degree is still seen in the medical literature today. However, the terms *superficial, partial-thickness,* and *full-thickness burns* are more descriptive of the type of injury and should be used as much as possible.

Superficial Burns

Superficial burns are burns that affect the outermost layer of skin, the epidermis. They most often present with redness and mild to moderate stinging pain (Figure 32-10 ■). In extreme cases there may be mild swelling. The most common cause of superficial

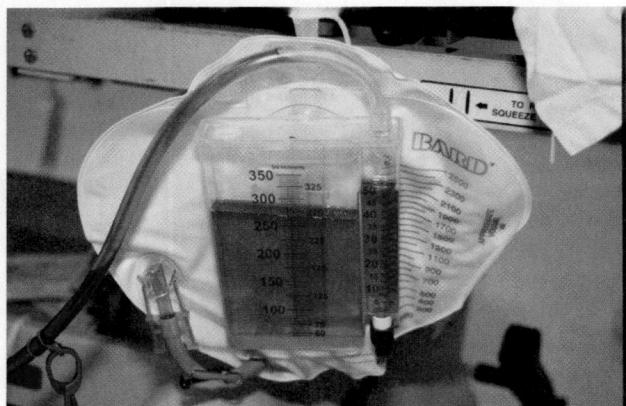

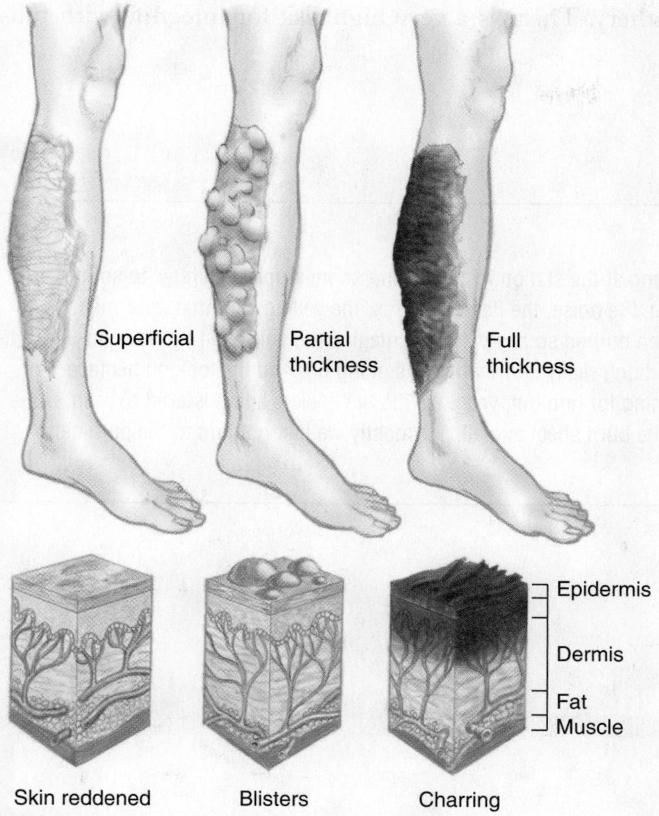

Figure 32-9 Classification of burns by depth.

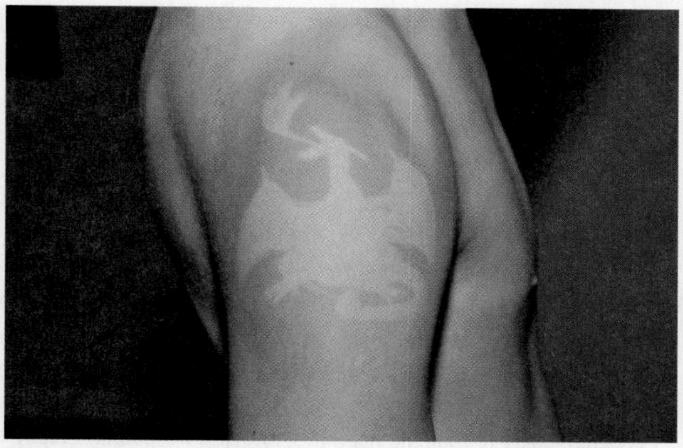
Figure 32-10 A patient with a superficial burn surrounding normal skin that had been protected from the sun by skin paint. (© Edward T. Dickinson, MD)

burns is the sun. Superficial burns require no immediate emergency care and will heal completely on their own. Cooling the burn with tap water or a moistened towel can help to ease the pain considerably.

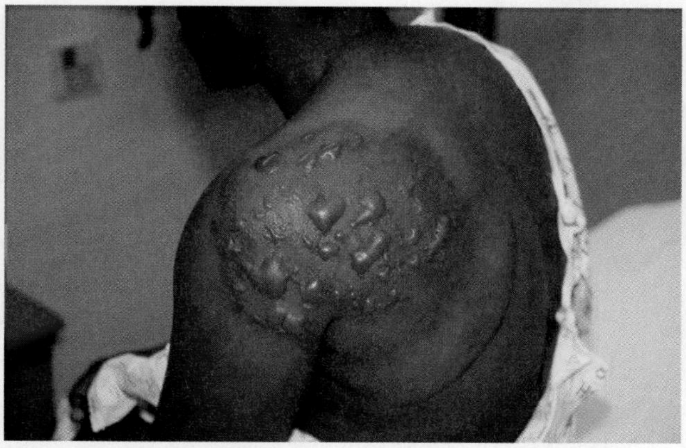
Figure 32-11 Characteristic blisters of a partial-thickness burn. (© Edward T. Dickinson, MD)

Partial-Thickness Burns

Partial-thickness burns are burns that extend down beyond the epidermis and into the dermis. Partial-thickness burns are characterized by pain, mottled skin color, and the presence of blisters (Figure 32-11 ■). Blisters are formed by the accumulation of fluids that are released from damaged cells and may take several hours to appear. It is important to note that there are likely to be areas of superficial burns around the perimeter of the partial-thickness burns, adding to the patient's pain and discomfort. Providing that the blisters remain intact during the healing process, there is little that needs to be done in the way of emergency care. If blisters break, the risk of infection is great. Provide care for open blisters just as you would for any other open soft-tissue injury.

Full-Thickness Burns

Full-thickness burns extend beyond all layers of the skin and can even cause damage to underlying muscle, bone, and vital organs (Figure 32-12 ■). While there may be little to no pain associated directly with the full-thickness burn due to the destruction of the nerves, there will be areas of partial-thickness and superficial burns around the perimeter causing severe pain. Full-thickness burns are characterized by a white, dark brown, or charred color

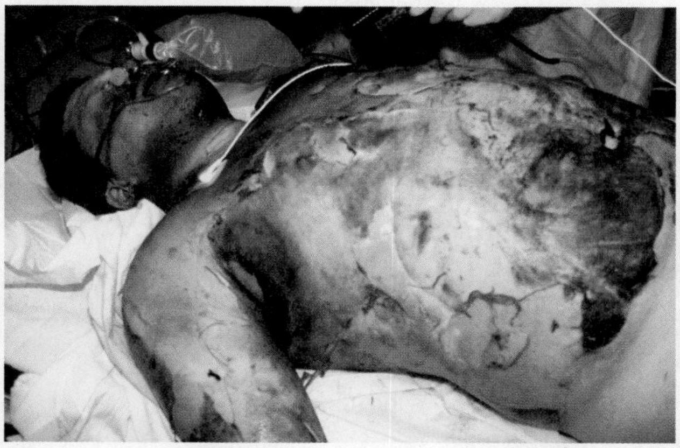
Figure 32-12 Full-thickness burns. (© Edward T. Dickinson, MD)

and may appear dry and leathery. There is a very high risk for infection with full-thickness burns.

CLINICAL CLUE

Body Temperature

You must manage the body temperature of a burn patient carefully. This patient is much more susceptible to becoming hypothermic due to the skin's decreased ability to regulate heat. If necessary, cover the patient with a blanket to conserve body heat.

PERSPECTIVE

Shane—The EMT

That was unreal. To go from sitting at the station just watching some stupid TV show, to something like a war zone. The smoke, the noise, the flashing lights, the yelling, and that poor man. I've never in my life seen a person burned so badly. I can't imagine the pain. And he was conscious and looking at us like he didn't really know what was going on. And the look on his face. We couldn't really even do anything for him but, yeah, we did the basics: administered oxygen, tried to keep him covered with the burn sheet and all, but mostly we just got him to the burn center as fast as we could.

STOP, REVIEW, REMEMBER!

Multiple Choice

For each question, place a check next to the correct answer.

1. A burn affecting the outermost layer of skin and producing only a reddish color is described as a ______________ burn.

_____ a. full-thickness
_____ b. partial-thickness
_____ c. superficial
_____ d. subcutaneous

2. In which type of burn is the majority of soft-tissue damage internal and cannot be seen by the EMT?

_____ a. Electrical
_____ b. Radiation
_____ c. Thermal
_____ d. Chemical

3. A burn that appears mottled in color and has developed blisters is described as a ______________ burn.

_____ a. full-thickness
_____ b. partial-thickness
_____ c. superficial
_____ d. subcutaneous

4. What type of burn is most often caused by fire, steam, hot objects, and hot liquids?

_____ a. Chemical
_____ b. Radiation
_____ c. Electrical
_____ d. Thermal

5. A burn that is black and charred and produces a leathery appearance to the skin is described as a:

_____ a. full-thickness burn.
_____ b. partial-thickness burn.
_____ c. superficial burn.
_____ d. subcutaneous burn.

Fill in the Blank

1. The appropriate care of all burn patients must include a thorough assessment of the ______________________, ______________________, and ______________________ of the burn.

2. A ______________________ burn is most commonly caused by exposure to fire, steam, hot objects, and hot liquids.

3. ______________________ burns are caused when the skin is exposed to substances such as acids, bases, and caustics.

4. A burn that affects only the outer layer of skin (epidermis) is referred to as a ______________________ burn.

5. A burn that reaches down to the layers of the ______________________ is referred to as a partial-thickness burn.

6. A burn that reaches down to or past the subcutaneous layers is commonly referred to as a ______________________ burn.

Critical Thinking

1. Using your current work environment, list as many potential sources of burns as you can.

____

____

____

____

2. In reference to your workplace, what safeguards are in place to prevent employees from becoming burned while on the job?

____

____

____

____

3. Discuss why patients with full-thickness burns are frequently in severe pain, even though the nerve endings have been damaged.

____

____

____

____

Assessment of the Burn Patient

As an EMT you must learn to quickly assess a burn patient to determine the overall severity of the burns as well as the patient's general condition. An appropriate assessment assists in the determination of the most appropriate care. In some situations, it may be determined that the patient should be transported directly to a burn center for definitive care rather than to the closest facility.

The assessment of a burn patient includes an evaluation of the following factors:

- Airway patency and adequacy of breathing
- Depth of injury
- Percentage of **body surface area (BSA)** affected
- Location of the injury
- Patient's age
- Preexisting medical conditions

body surface area (BSA) the amount of body surface area affected by burns.

Depth of Injury

You have already learned the way that burns are classified based on depth of injury. This determination can be difficult at best and requires a careful visual assessment. In many instances, it can be difficult to distinguish between partial-thickness and full-thickness burns. When in doubt, assume the worst and classify uncertain areas as full-thickness.

PERSPECTIVE

Ed Rhome—The Rescue Firefighter

A neighbor told me he saw all three occupants run out of the house, but when I got into that back bedroom, the smoke cleared for just a second and I thought I saw a person under a burning bedsheet. Well, the sheet wasn't on fire, like full-on flames or anything, but it was black and the edges were glowing and, you know, moving toward the center. Like when you watch newspaper burn. I felt around until I touched a hand, and then I just yanked the guy over my shoulder and took off. I hope I found him quick enough. I really do.

Percentage of BSA Affected

32-6 Explain the system used to estimate the body surface area involved in burns for both adult and pediatric patients.

rule of nines a method of determining the body surface area (BSA) burned based on dividing the adult body into areas of approximately 9% each.

When assessing the burn patient, one of the most important factors that must be established is an estimate of body surface area (BSA) affected. The method most commonly used in EMS to estimate BSA is the **rule of nines** (Figure 32-13 ▪). The rule of nines is based on dividing the adult body into areas of approximately 9% (or multiples of 9%) each. This method allows the EMT to quickly arrive at an estimate of BSA affected. A modified version of this method can be applied to infants and children.

The rule of nines for adults is as follows:

- Head and neck, 9%
- Each upper extremity, 9%
- Anterior trunk, 18%
- Posterior trunk, 18%
- Each lower extremity, $9\% \times 2 = 18\%$
- Genitals, 1%

For infants and children the only adjustment is that the lower extremities represent 14% instead of 18% and the head represents 18% instead of 9%.

The rule of nines is simply a guideline and not expected to determine the exact percentage of BSA affected. You must learn to use the rule of nines as a tool and

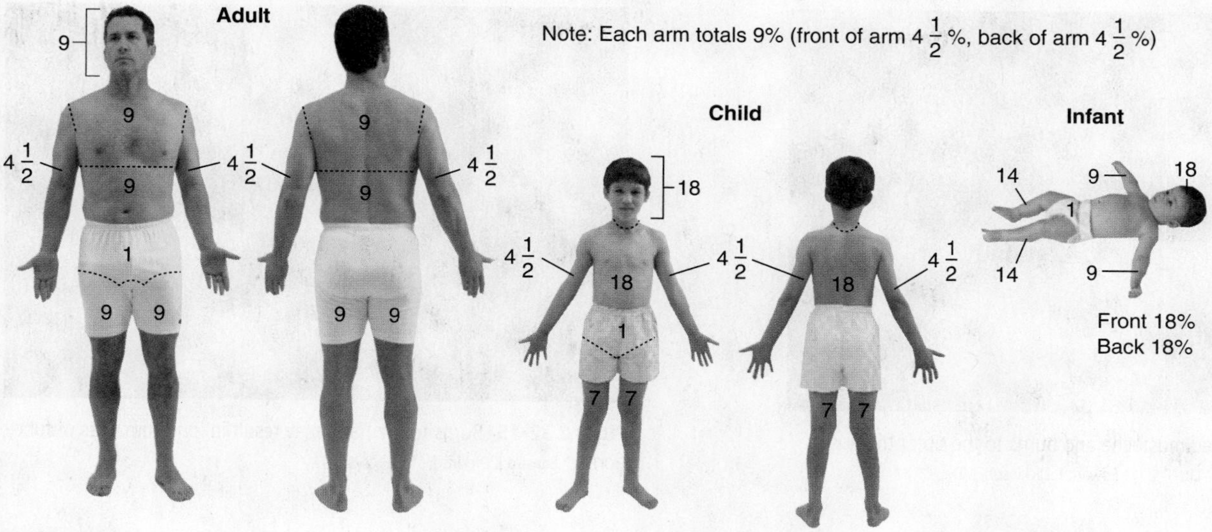

Figure 32-13 The rule of nines.

understand that it may be necessary to adjust the percentage, depending on the area affected. For instance, if only a portion of an arm or a portion of the chest were affected, you would adjust the estimate accordingly.

Another tool that can be used by the EMT to assess BSA is sometimes called the **rule of palm.** It is based on the principle that the area of a patient's palm is equal to approximately 1% of his BSA. This can be helpful when trying to assess small burns or multiple areas of injury spread over the entire body.

rule of palm method of estimating the body surface area (BSA) burned based on the principle that a patient's palm is equal to approximately 1% of his BSA.

> **CLINICAL CLUE**
>
> **Rule of Nines**
>
> The rule of nines and similar methods are used only to provide close estimates of BSA burned. The percentages may not always equal exactly 100% when totaled.

Location of Burns

Specific areas of the body are considered more significant than others when affected by burns. Burns to the following areas should be considered serious, requiring further care at an appropriate facility:

- *Face.* Burns to the face can affect the eyes and air passages (Figure 32-14 ▪). If the airways become exposed to heated smoke, steam, or flames, they can begin to swell, causing increased respiratory difficulty. Observe the areas around the mouth and nose for evidence of smoke, soot, or singed hairs that indicate exposure to heat. In addition, the patient may be coughing up soot-laden sputum evident at the mouth. When these findings are identified, it should be presumed that an inhalation injury has occurred.
- *Hands and feet.* Burns to the hands and feet are considered serious due to the potential for long-term loss of function if not cared for properly (Figure 32-15 ▪).
- *Genitalia.* Burns to the genitals are considered serious, because they can affect both form and function if not cared for properly. Burns to the inner thighs and buttocks are more prone to infection.

32-7 Discuss considerations of burn depth, location, body surface area involved, the patient's age, and any preexisting medical conditions in determining the severity of burn injuries.

32-11 Identify indications of inhalation injury.

> **PERSPECTIVE**
>
> **Warren Souther, MD—The Emergency Physician**
>
> That poor guy isn't going to survive. I did an RSI, uh, rapid sequence intubation, and when I got the blade in there, his airway was just black. There was soot and burns as far as I could see. I got the endotracheal tube placed and everything, but I'll be surprised if he makes it past two days, four at the outside. Even though everybody did their jobs perfectly, from the firefighters to the ambulance crew to my staff, sometimes nothing is enough. I truly feel for the guy.

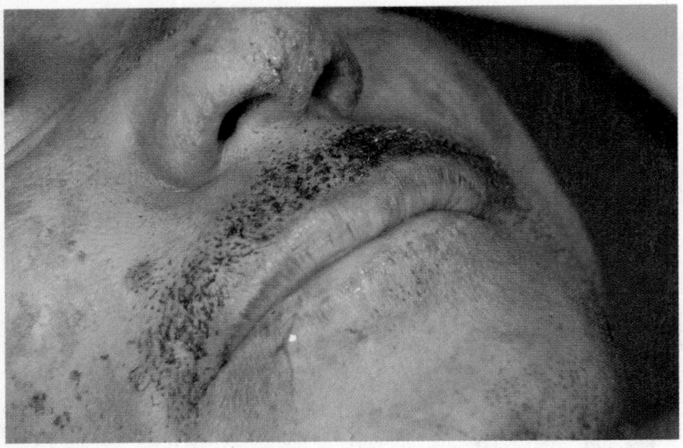

Figure 32-14 A singed mustache and burns to the tip of the nose signal danger of airway burns. (© Edward T. Dickinson, MD)

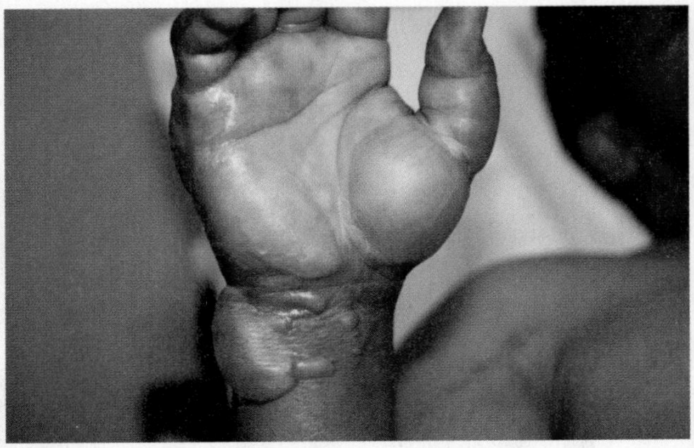

Figure 32-15 Burns to the hand may result in long-term loss of function. (© Edward T. Dickinson, MD)

The Patient's Age

The age of the patient can play a significant role in the way he responds to an injury caused by burns. The very young (younger than five years old) and patients over the age of 55 have more difficulty combating the effects of severe burns.

In children, the body surface area is greater in relation to their total body size. This results in greater fluid loss than in adults. Infants have a higher risk of shock, airway problems, and hypothermia.

In late adulthood, the ability of tissues to heal from any injury is lessened and the time of healing is increased. The body's ability to cope with any injury is reduced by aging tissues and failing body systems.

Preexisting Medical Conditions

When possible, obtain a thorough medical history of your patient. The history may reveal preexisting medical conditions that can complicate the treatment and recovery process. Preexisting respiratory conditions can result in an exaggerated response, causing severe respiratory distress. The stress of being burned can cause a patient with a cardiac history to suffer angina or a heart attack. Patients with kidney or immune problems also have greater difficulty during the recovery process due to the extreme stress on the body. Diabetic patients may have increased problems related to proper healing of burn wounds.

Establishing Patient Priority

32-8 Describe the assessment-based approach to burns.

Your rapid assessment of the patient with burns will help to quickly determine both treatment and transport priorities. Not all burns are life threatening, requiring the care of a specialized burn center. In fact, many burns are considered minor and can be managed appropriately by most hospital emergency departments. Table 32-1 will help you identify the priority of patients with burn injuries.

Your EMS system may have its own burn care protocols that specify the severity of burns and what type of receiving hospital is most appropriate for a given burn injury. In some regions where designated burn centers are available, EMS may be directed to bypass their usual destination hospital and go directly to the burn center.

32-9 Describe special considerations in the scene size-up when responding to calls involving burned patients.

Scene Size-up

As always, your safety and the safety of other rescuers and bystanders on the scene is your top priority. Scenes that involve a burn mechanism may present both obvious

TABLE 32-1 DETERMINING BURN PATIENT PRIORITY

HIGH PRIORITY (SEVERE)

- Full-thickness burns involving the hands, feet, face, or genitalia
- Burns associated with airway or respiratory injury
- Full-thickness burns affecting more than 10% of BSA
- Partial-thickness burns affecting more than 30% of BSA
- Burns complicated by an extremity injury such as a fracture
- Moderate burns in young children or elderly patients
- Circumferential burns to the arm, leg, or chest

MEDIUM PRIORITY (MODERATE)

- Full-thickness burns affecting 2% to 10% of BSA, excluding hands, feet, face, genitalia, and upper airway
- Partial-thickness burns affecting 15% to 30% of BSA
- Superficial burns affecting more than 50% of BSA

LOW PRIORITY (MILD)

- Full-thickness burns affecting less than 2% of BSA
- Partial-thickness burns affecting less than 15% of BSA
- Superficial burns affecting less than 50% of BSA

and unseen hazards. Keep your eyes and ears open as you approach the scene, and take in as much of it as you can. If necessary, stop and remain at a safe distance until the appropriate resources can mitigate the hazards. Whenever possible, coordinate your activities with the incident commander.

If the mechanism causing the burn is still active (fire, steam, chemicals, electricity), you must do what you can to safely stop the burning process. But do *not* put yourself at unreasonable risk. Be aware that metal objects such as jewelry, belt buckles, and buttons can remain hot and continue to burn soft tissue long after the heat source has been eliminated. Those objects also can pose a hazard to the rescuer. In most instances involving thermal or chemical burns, water may be used to stop the burning process.

Primary Assessment

32-10 Explain the concept of stopping the burning process.

Once you have determined that the scene is safe and the burning process has been stopped, approach the patient and begin the primary assessment. It is not uncommon for the clothing of seriously burned patients to continue to be on fire or smolder as they are handed off to EMS personnel. It is essential that you extinguish any remaining burning garments as you begin your assessment. Pay particular attention to the patient's back because it can harbor burning cloth not immediately evident to the EMT. Whenever possible, use available water or saline solution rather than a dry chemical extinguisher to put out smoldering material. If possible, use additional rescuers for this purpose.

Your assessment should focus on the patient's airway and ability to breathe adequately. Carefully assess the nose and mouth for evidence of soot or singed hair. They can be an indication the patient has inhaled superheated air that may cause swelling of the airway. A hoarse-sounding voice and coughing also may be an indication of a burned airway. A patient who dies early as a result of a burn mechanism does so because of airway swelling and compromise. Do not let the presence of severe burns distract you from managing the patient's ABCs.

Complete the primary assessment by confirming the presence of an adequate pulse and initiating supplemental oxygen. Then make a decision regarding priority for transport.

Secondary Assessment

Once you have completed your primary assessment and managed any immediate issues relating to the ABCs, complete an appropriate history and physical exam. As with any victim of trauma, the specific assessment path you take will depend on the significance of the burns (mechanism of injury). Any patient suffering moderate to severe burns should receive a rapid trauma assessment. Patients with mild burns should receive a focused trauma assessment. When deciding which assessment path is most appropriate, you must consider all aspects of the patient's condition and not only the burns.

Take time during transport to expose as much of the patient as possible and reassess the extent and depth of the burns. When appropriate, based on the patient's condition, obtain a thorough medical history.

Remember that infection will be a serious concern during the healing process. Use appropriate BSI precautions and sterile dressings whenever possible.

Emergency Care of the Burn Patient

Emergency care for the burn patient is not unlike most care for victims of trauma (Scan 32-1). In the case of the burn patient, it is important to confirm that all burning has stopped before beginning emergency care. Once the burning has stopped, complete the following steps:

1. Ensure the scene is safe to enter.
2. Take appropriate BSI precautions.
3. Perform an appropriate primary assessment.
4. Carefully extinguish smoldering clothing with water and remove hot metallic items.
5. Initiate oxygen therapy once you have ensured that all smoldering has been extinguished.
6. Assess burned areas to estimate BSA affected and depth of injury.
7. Cover burned areas with dry sterile dressings to minimize contamination and heat loss. Some EMS systems recommend moistening the dressings with sterile saline if less than 10% BSA.
8. Perform an appropriate secondary assessment.
9. Continually monitor the airway for evidence of compromise.
10. Transport to an appropriate receiving facility.

PERSPECTIVE

Shane—The EMT

One positive thing that this guy had going for him was where he lived. His house is literally six miles from Baptist Hospital, which is the top burn center in the entire state. We notified them that we were en route, and by the time we wheeled him through the doors, there was a team of people that just descended on him. It was actually pretty amazing to watch. I just hope it'll make a difference.

SCAN 32-1 Care of a Burn Patient

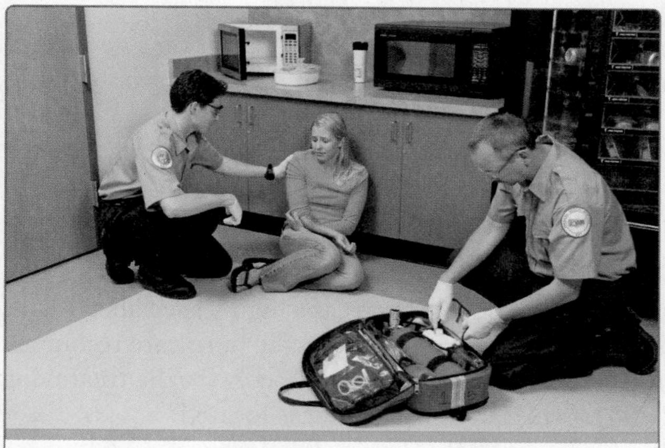

32-1-1 Make sure the scene is safe to enter and take BSI precautions.

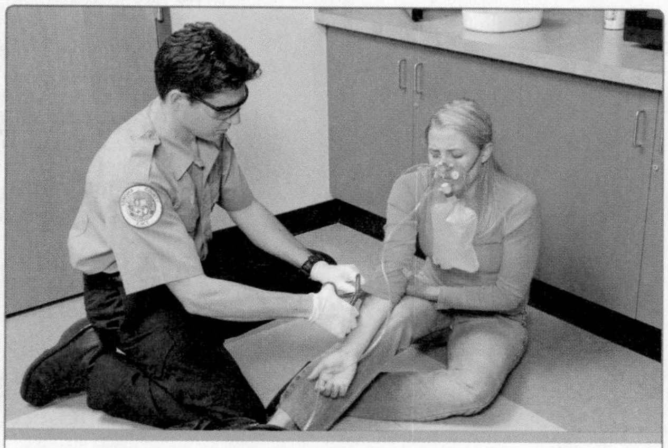

32-1-2 Place the patient on oxygen (if indicated) while your partner cuts away the clothing around the burn.

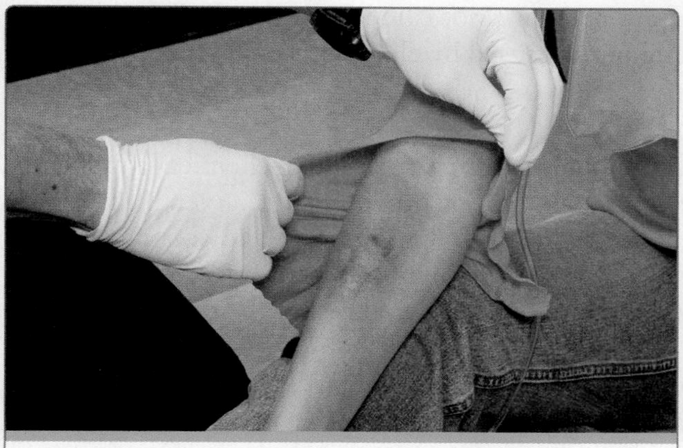

32-1-3 Expose the burned area.

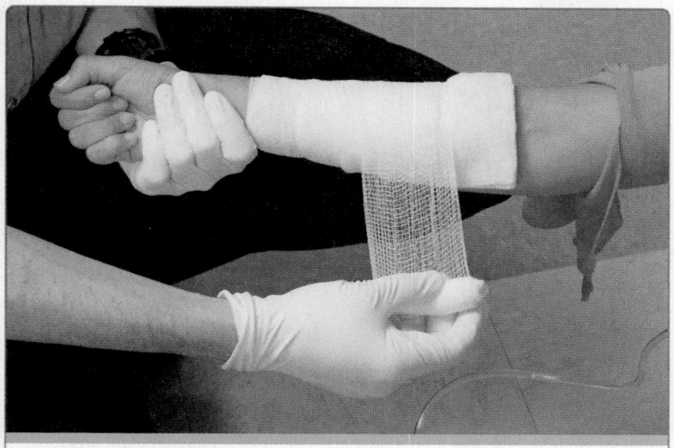

32-1-4 Cover the burns with sterile dressings.

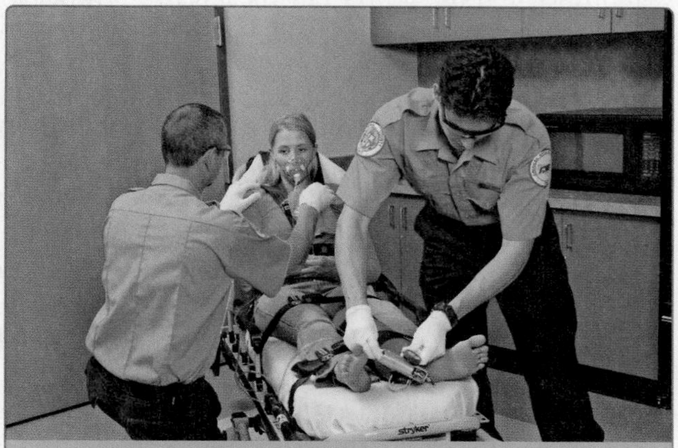

32-1-5 Load the patient onto the stretcher and prepare for transport.

There are several things that should be mentioned as "what *not* to do" when caring for burns. Despite the fact that some of the following "don'ts" pertain to home remedies handed down from generation to generation, they have no place in prehospital care. They are:

- Do *not* use any type of burn cream, ointment, lotion, or antiseptic on a new burn. They serve as insulators and cause heat to be retained in the wound, potentially making the burn worse.
- Do *not* intentionally break blisters that form over a burn. Doing so only creates an open wound and greatly increases the risk of infection.
- If possible, avoid the use of a dry chemical or a CO_2 fire extinguisher directly on the patient. Both can further worsen soft-tissue injury.

The emergency care of burns, especially severe burns, is a highly specialized skill. One of the best things you can do for your patient is to know the burn care resources within your EMS system. Become familiar with the local protocols for the treatment of burn patients and where the nearest specialty burn center is located.

Special Considerations

Certain types of burns require special consideration because they can present unique hazards to both the rescuer and the patient if not cared for properly. Two examples are burns caused by chemicals and burns caused by electricity.

Chemical Burns

32-13 Describe special considerations in responding to, assessing, and managing chemical and electrical burns.

Caring for a patient who has suffered burns from some type of chemical almost certainly presents a hazard to the rescuers who will be providing care. Even if the source of exposure has been controlled, there will likely be some residual chemical on the patient that poses a risk to the EMT. Be sure to conduct a careful and thorough scene size-up before entering the scene and call for additional resources, such as a hazmat team, if necessary.

Note that the typical BSI precautions taken by most EMTs may not be adequate when caring for the victim of a chemical burn. If you are not certain, call for additional resources. You will certainly want to wear appropriate gloves and eye protection at a minimum, and you may want to consider donning a protective gown as well. A face mask or even a positive pressure self-contained breathing apparatus may be appropriate if the source chemical is in a powder form.

Follow these simple guidelines when caring for patients who have been exposed to dangerous chemicals:

- Unless the skin was moist at the time of exposure, dry powders should be carefully brushed off the skin prior to flushing with water.
- When you are able, immediately begin flushing the affected areas with clean water and continue flushing during transport.
- When flushing, be careful not to let the runoff contaminate other areas of the body.
- If possible, have the patient remove contaminated clothing to minimize the risk of continued contact with the chemical as well as the risk of rescuer exposure.

Electrical Burns

One of the most dangerous characteristics of electricity is its invisibility. You cannot see the very thing that has injured the patient, and therefore it is a significant risk to rescuers on scene. When approaching the scene, you and your partner must look up, down, and all around for any evidence of an electrical source. Downed high-power electrical lines can jump around on the ground. Stay well clear of them at all times. Electricity can also jump a considerable distance as it seeks to find a ground. Keeping a safe distance from any electrical source is your best defense.

Do *not* attempt to approach or touch a patient until you are absolutely certain that the electrical source has been shut off. In most instances involving high-power lines, you must wait for the utility company to shut off the power before you can approach the patient. Follow these additional guidelines when caring for patients with electrical injuries:

- Monitor the patient's respiratory and circulatory status closely. Depending on the path the electricity takes through the body, it can cause either respiratory or cardiac arrest and in some cases both.
- In the majority of cases most of the damage is internal, following the path the electricity took as it passed through the body. There may be little or no evidence of injury on the outside.
- Some electrical injuries will have an entrance and an exit wound (Figure 32-16 ■). A thorough assessment should be conducted on all victims of electrical injuries to look for both wounds.
- There may be little or no bleeding at the site of entrance and exit wounds. However, they should be cared for in the same way you would care for any soft-tissue injury.

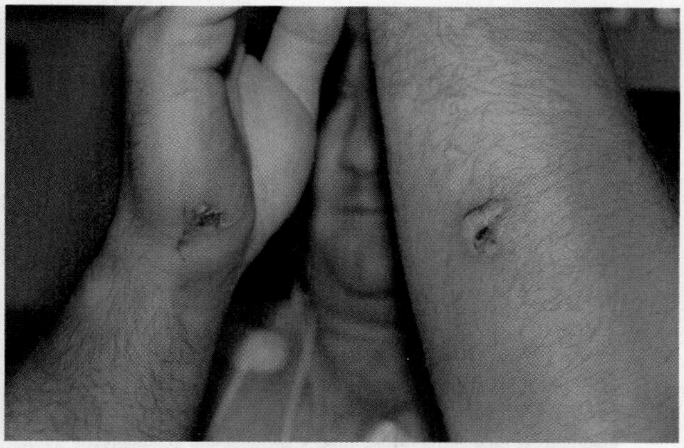

Figure 32-16 Entrance (right hand) and exit (left forearm) wounds from an electrical burn. (© Edward T. Dickinson, MD)

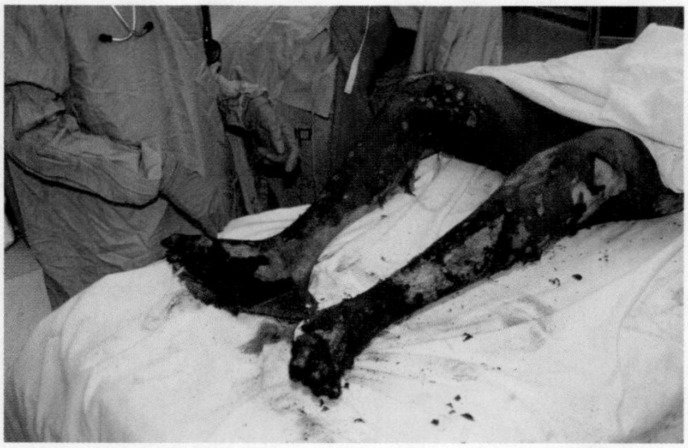

Figure 32-17 Full-thickness circumferential burns to both legs. (© Edward T. Dickinson, MD)

Circumferential Burns

Circumferential burns are burns that completely surround a body part such as a finger, arm, leg, and the chest (Figure 32-17 ■). Burns that completely encircle a part of the body can cause swelling, especially with partial- and full-thickness burns. This swelling can cause pressure similar to that of a tourniquet and restrict blood flow to an extremity. Circumferential burns that affect the chest can severely restrict a patient's ability to breathe adequately. The presence of circumferential burns will not necessarily change the way you care for the patient, but they will make the patient a high priority for transport.

circumferential burns burns that completely surround a body part such as a finger, arm, leg, and chest.

Burns to the Hands and Feet

32-12 Discuss special considerations for dressing burns, including burns to specific anatomical areas.

Special care should be provided for burns to the hands and feet. Be sure to remove any jewelry, such as rings and bracelets, which can restrict blood flow should the area become swollen. When bandaging burns to the hands and feet, place sterile dressings between each of the digits before covering the entire area with dressings and bandage (Figure 32-18 ■).

PERSPECTIVE

Brianna—The EMT

So as soon as the doctor intubated that guy, he shouts that he needs a scalpel and then just sliced right down his chest from his armpits to the bottom of his ribs. Oh man, that was nasty! I turned to this nurse I know and asked why he did that. She tells me that the guy had a circumferential burn of the chest and the doctor had to reduce the pressure around the chest so he could effectively ventilate the patient. I feel so badly for that man, and I hope to never be burned like that. It's got to be the worst.

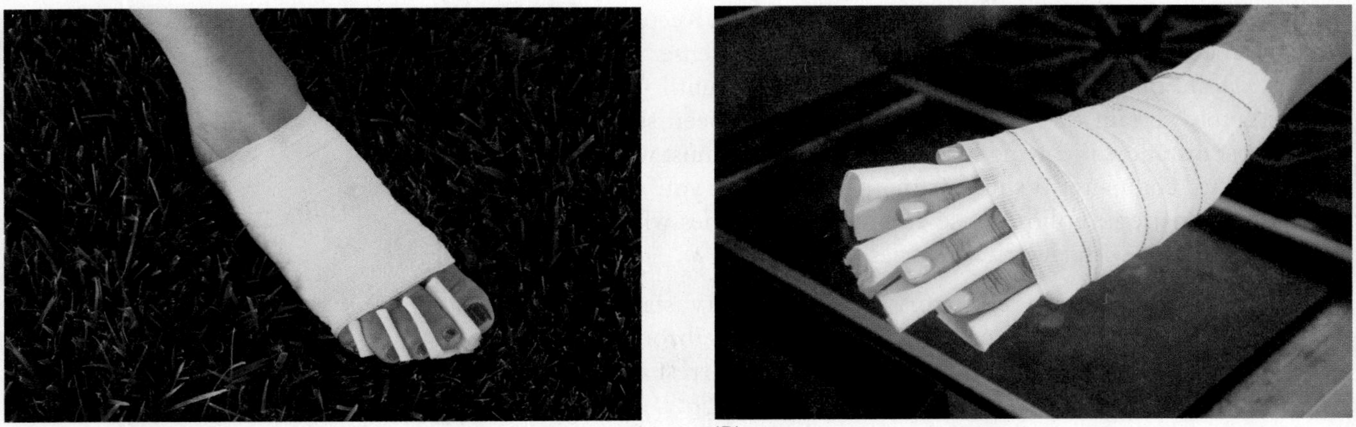

(A) (B)

Figure 32-18 Separate burned toes and fingers with dry sterile gauze.

Pediatric Considerations

Infants and children are particularly susceptible to the effects of burns, even mild burns. Due to their greater skin surface area relative to their overall size, they are much more prone to the effects of heat loss and fluid loss. This makes them more susceptible to hypothermia and shock. Burns are also a common form of abuse by adults, and you should always be alert for signs of neglect and abuse when caring for children suffering from burns.

STOP, REVIEW, REMEMBER!

Multiple Choice

For each question, place a check next to the correct answer.

1. A burn affecting the entire right arm and the anterior torso of an adult patient would amount to an approximate BSA of:

_____ a. 12.5%.

_____ b. 18%.

_____ c. 22.5%.

_____ d. 27%.

2. Which one of the following is *not* routinely considered a special critical area for burns?

_____ a. Face

_____ b. Hands

_____ c. Chest

_____ d. Genitals

3. Which one of the following best describes the appropriate priorities when caring for a burn patient?

_____ a. ABCs, stop the burning, cover wounds, transport

_____ b. ABCs, cover wounds, stop the burning, transport

_____ c. stop the burning, cover wounds, ABCs, transport

_____ d. stop the burning, ABCs, cover wounds, transport

4. Which one of the following would be considered the highest priority for care and transport?

_____ a. Partial-thickness burns affecting more than 30% of BSA

_____ b. Full-thickness burns affecting 2% to 10% of BSA

_____ c. Partial-thickness burns affecting 15% to 30% of BSA

_____ d. Superficial burns affecting more than 50% of BSA

5. Which one of the following most accurately represents the amount of BSA affected in a pediatric patient with burns to the front of one leg, the entire back, and half of one arm?

_____ a. 14%

_____ b. 25%

_____ c. 29.5%

_____ d. 33%

Matching

Match the term on the left with the applicable definition on the right.

1. _____ Depth of injury
2. _____ Rule of nines
3. _____ High priority
4. _____ Medium priority
5. _____ Low priority

A. Partial-thickness burns affecting less than 15% BSA

B. Full-thickness burns involving the hands, feet, or genitalia

C. The method used to classify burns

D. Common method used to estimate body surface area

E. Partial-thickness burns affecting 15% to 30% BSA

Critical Thinking

1. List the six factors that must be assessed when determining the overall condition of a burn patient.

____

____

____

____

2. Describe the role that each of the above factors plays in determining the overall condition of the patient.

____

____

____

____

3. Identify at least two potential hazards that could exist at the scene of a burn patient and how you might mitigate those hazards before caring for the patient.

____

____

____

____

EMERGENCY DISPATCH SUMMARY

The patient, who remained conscious and able to maintain his own airway, was transported on supplemental oxygen to the Baptist Hospital Burn Center. He died four days later due to complications from airway burns and injury to his lungs from inhaling superheated smoke and gases. The incident has been added as a case study to the ambulance company's continuing education program.

Chapter Review

To the Point

- Burns can occur as a result of exposure to thermal, electrical, chemical, and radiation sources.
- Single or multiple organ systems can be affected by burn injuries.
- In thermal burns the severity of the injury is largely determined by the depth and body surface area of the burn.
- The rule of nines and the rule of palm are methods used to estimate the body surface area that has been burned.
- The depth of a burn is described as superficial, partial-thickness, or full-thickness.
- Burns that involve the upper airway can be rapidly fatal due to swelling and the blockage of air flow.
- The depth and extent of burns, along with other factors such as the patient's age, the presence of co-existing chronic illness, and the specific location of the burn are combined to determine the priority and transport destination of the burn victim.
- Electrical burns can be very serious even with only minimal visible evidence of a burn present.

Chapter Questions

Multiple Choice

For each question, place a check next to the correct answer.

1. Thermal burns are most commonly classified by:
   _____ a. open or closed injury.
   _____ b. cause of injury.
   _____ c. depth of injury.
   _____ d. degree.

2. A superficial burn is best described as a burn that affects the:
   _____ a. epidermis only.
   _____ b. dermis.
   _____ c. subcutaneous layers.
   _____ d. epidural only.

3. Superficial burns are characterized by:
   _____ a. dark charred skin.
   _____ b. a leathery appearance.
   _____ c. blisters.
   _____ d. redness and pain.

4. A partial-thickness burn is best described as a burn that affects the:
   _____ a. epidermis only.
   _____ b. dermis.
   _____ c. subcutaneous layers.
   _____ d. epidural only.

5. Partial-thickness burns are characterized by:
   _____ a. dark charred skin.
   _____ b. a leathery appearance.
   _____ c. blisters.
   _____ d. redness and pain.

6. A full-thickness burn is best described as a burn that affects the:
   _____ a. epidermis only.
   _____ b. dermis.
   _____ c. subcutaneous layers.
   _____ d. epidural only.

7. Full-thickness burns are characterized by:
   _____ a. dark or brown charred skin.
   _____ b. a mottled appearance.
   _____ c. blisters.
   _____ d. redness and pain.

8. Care for most chemical burns should include:
   _____ a. flushing the area with water.
   _____ b. flushing the area with lemon juice.
   _____ c. wrapping the area with moist dressings.
   _____ d. covering the area with nonsterile dressings.

9. Circumferential burns are burns that:
   _____ a. cover the anterior chest.
   _____ b. affect the face.
   _____ c. involve a foot.
   _____ d. encircle a body part.

10. What is the approximate BSA of a burn to the entire right arm of an adult patient?
   _____ a. 4.5%
   _____ b. 9%
   _____ c. 13.5%
   _____ d. 8%

Matching

Match the term on the left with the applicable definition on the right.

1. _____ Thermal burn
2. _____ Chemical burn
3. _____ Electrical burn
4. _____ Radiation burn
5. _____ Light burn

A. Burns caused when the skin is exposed to substances such as acids, bases, and caustics

B. Burns caused by exposure to fire, steam, hot objects, and hot liquids

C. Burns from sources such as nuclear fallout

D. High-intensity lasers and welders are common sources of these types of burns

E. When the body becomes exposed to an electrical current that passes through the body

Critical Thinking

1. Describe how you would care for a patient with full-thickness burns to both hands and arms.

____

____

____

____

(continued on next page)

(continued)

2. Explain the complications caused by a circumferential burn to the chest and to one of the extremities.

Case Studies

Case Study 1

You have responded to a residence for a burn victim. Upon arrival you are met by a family member and directed to the backyard. There you find an approximately 11-year-old boy lying on the ground with his arms and face over the edge of a pool. His mother tells you that he was attempting to light the barbecue when the can of fluid exploded in his hands. You observe what appears to be both partial-thickness and some full-thickness burns to the entire hand and forearm of both arms. You also observe some redness and swelling to his face.

1. What would you estimate the affected BSA to be for this patient?

2. Describe how you will bandage this patient's injuries.

3. What complications could arise as a result of the burns to this patient's face?

Case Study 2

Using the rule of nines, estimate the BSA affected for each of the following patients.

1. A 55-year-old man with burns over the fronts of both legs and half of his anterior torso

2. A four-year-old patient with burns over her entire head and entire right arm

3. A three-month-old infant with burns over the entire back and the backs of both arms.

The Last Word

Responding to the scene of a burn patient can present a variety of risks to the EMT. Be extra cautious and perform a thorough scene size-up prior to making patient contact. In most cases, the burn patient who is critical will need airway and ventilatory care on scene and en route to the hospital. Do not let the sight of severe burns distract you from the ABCs. Infection is a major concern with burn patients, so whenever possible use sterile dressings and sterile saline when caring for burns.

Know the capabilities of the receiving hospitals in your area and the location of the nearest specialty burn center. When in doubt, contact medical direction for transport instructions. Always document all appropriate information in your prehospital care report.

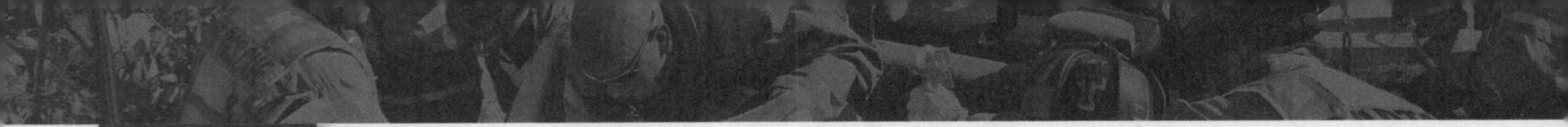

33 Caring for Patients with Chest, Abdominal, and Genital Trauma

Education Standards

Trauma: Chest Trauma

Competencies

Applies fundamental knowledge to provide basic emergency care and transportation based on assessment findings for an acutely injured patient.

Objectives

After completion of this lesson, you should be able to:

33-1 Define key terms introduced in this chapter.

33-2 List the major structures of the thoracic cavity.

33-3 Define and list specific types of open chest injury.

33-4 Define and list specific types of closed chest injury.

33-5 Explain the pathophysiology of each of the following injuries: cardiac contusion, flail segment, hemothorax, open pneumothorax, tension pneumothorax, pericardial tamponade, pulmonary contusion, rib injury, and traumatic asphyxia.

33-6 Discuss an assessment-based approach to manage patients with chest trauma.

33-7 Discuss the following aspects of chest trauma care: general emergency care for chest trauma and specific emergency care for an open chest wound.

33-8 Describe the anatomy of the abdominal cavity and its contents.

33-9 Differentiate hollow and solid organs and vascular structures in the abdomen.

33-10 Give examples of both blunt and penetrating mechanisms of abdominal trauma and discuss the potential for severe internal bleeding.

33-11 Discuss an assessment-based approach to management of the patient with open and closed abdominal injury, including evisceration and impaled objects.

33-12 Describe signs and symptoms associated with injuries to the abdomen.

33-13 Explain the general emergency care for abdominal trauma.

33-14 Explain the special considerations in management of trauma to the male and female genitalia.

Key Terms

cardiac contusions p. 849
commotio cordis p. 849
diaphragm p. 844
evisceration p. 860
flail chest p. 847
floating ribs p. 847
hemothorax p. 849
occlusive dressings p. 853
open pneumothorax p. 851
paradoxical motion p. 847
pericardial tamponade p. 852
peritoneum p. 856
pleura p. 845
pleural space p. 845
pneumonia p. 846
pneumothorax p. 848
pulmonary contusions p. 849
retroperitoneal p. 856
rib fracture p. 846
spontaneous pneumothorax p. 849
tension pneumothorax p. 848
thoracic cavity p. 844
traumatic asphyxia p. 849

Introduction

The chest and abdomen house and protect the body's most important organ systems. Both the cardiovascular and respiratory systems primarily reside within the chest cavity. Massive blood vessels cross through the chest as the heart pumps blood to the cells of the body. The lungs occupy most of the space within the chest cavity, and the diaphragm and intercostal muscles power the respiratory system. The abdomen houses vital structures of the digestive, endocrine, and reproductive systems. Those highly vascular organs are fed by a rich and constant blood supply.

The combination of vital organs and the dense network of large blood vessels make the chest and abdomen—collectively known as the *torso*—a very vulnerable area for trauma. Loss of function due to injury in the respiratory or circulatory system and the threat of internal bleeding mean there is no such thing as a simple injury to these areas. Damage can create rapidly developing, life-threatening problems.

To effectively treat chest and abdominal emergencies, you must develop a strong understanding of the internal anatomy. Injuries frequently occur beneath the surface and may not be evident on visual inspection. Knowing what lies underneath can help you anticipate and prioritize emergencies and improve your assessment capabilities.

Even with a strong sense of anatomy and physiology, the chest and abdomen present many complicated challenges to obtaining a specific diagnosis. As an EMT, always remember that identifying a specific diagnosis is less important than recognizing a general life threat. For example, it is vitally important that you recognize the signs of internal bleeding. You may never be able to narrow down the specific damaged organ, but that is not necessary because emergency care is generally the same regardless of the cause. In most cases, EMT care of chest and abdominal injuries focus on recognizing and treating the major life threat first and then initiating high-priority transport to an appropriate receiving facility (a trauma center, if available) that can definitively manage the injury.

EMERGENCY DISPATCH

Nancy's heart was racing just a little bit as she and her partner Brandi responded to a reported stabbing. She calmed herself by visualizing a plan of action that she later reviewed out loud with Brandi. "If this is the real deal, we need to get an occlusive dressing on the wound, if it's anywhere near the chest, and be off the scene quickly. You get the oxygen on and I'll take care of the assessment."

As they neared the address, dispatch relayed that law enforcement was on scene and it was safe to proceed. As the ambulance turned onto Justice Avenue, Nancy and Brandi saw a variety of police cars and a crowd of people surrounding the front of a pizza restaurant.

Nancy grabbed the trauma bag and Brandi went around to retrieve the stretcher. As the crowd parted, Nancy saw a young man lying on the ground with a wound to his abdomen that appeared to have intestines hanging out of it. "What happened?" Nancy asked a police officer.

The officer responded, "He tried to hold up the pizza place. The owner stabbed him in the belly. He ran out but collapsed when he got here." As Brandi and Nancy looked at the patient, Brandi said, "Nancy, I don't think he is breathing."

The Chest

You already know the importance of proper respiration and circulation. The chest is the home of both of those functions. The ribs, sternum, and muscles of the chest protect the heart and the many great vessels of the circulatory system and allow for their normal function. The chest also houses the organs of the respiratory system. The trachea, bronchiole tubes, and lungs are located there. The muscles of the chest, combined with the diaphragm, serve as the mechanism to move air into and out of the body. So, an intact and functioning chest is essential to a properly functioning respiratory system.

Injuries and illnesses to the structures of the chest threaten the operation of both the respiratory and circulatory systems. Understanding the basic physiology of these systems will help you comprehend how injuries can impair their function.

Anatomy and Physiology of the Chest

33-2 List the major structures of the thoracic cavity.

thoracic cavity the area that lies inferior to the clavicles and superior to the diaphragm.

The chest, or **thoracic cavity,** comprises roughly the upper half of the torso (Figure 33-1 ▪). The thoracic cavity is the area that lies superior to the diaphragm. The anterior of the upper torso (commonly called the *chest*) and posterior portion of the upper torso (commonly called the *back*) are the exterior walls of the thoracic cavity. The contents of this cavity are protected by the 12 pairs of ribs, the sternum, and the spine.

The mediastinum can be found at the center of the chest. It is a group of structures that includes the heart, trachea, esophagus, and several large blood vessels. It begins in the neck, but continues into the chest and down to the diaphragm. The heart lies in the center of the chest and is surrounded by large blood vessels. The aorta is the largest artery in the body and arches off the top of the heart and branches through the chest and abdomen. The vena cava also travels through both the superior and inferior chest and connects to the right atrium.

The lungs fill the remainder of the chest. Lung tissue can be found as high as above the clavicles and as low as the diaphragm. The lungs are divided into lobes. The right lung has three lobes and the left lung has two. Lung tissue is elastic and adheres at least in theory to the moving chest wall to allow for expansion and contraction as the chest moves in and out. The movement of the chest and the elasticity of lung tissue move air in and out of the lungs.

diaphragm the large, flat muscle that forms the lower border of the thoracic cavity and is used as an important element of the respiratory system.

The inferior border of the chest is formed by a large flat muscle called the **diaphragm.** The diaphragm moves down when it contracts, causing an increase in

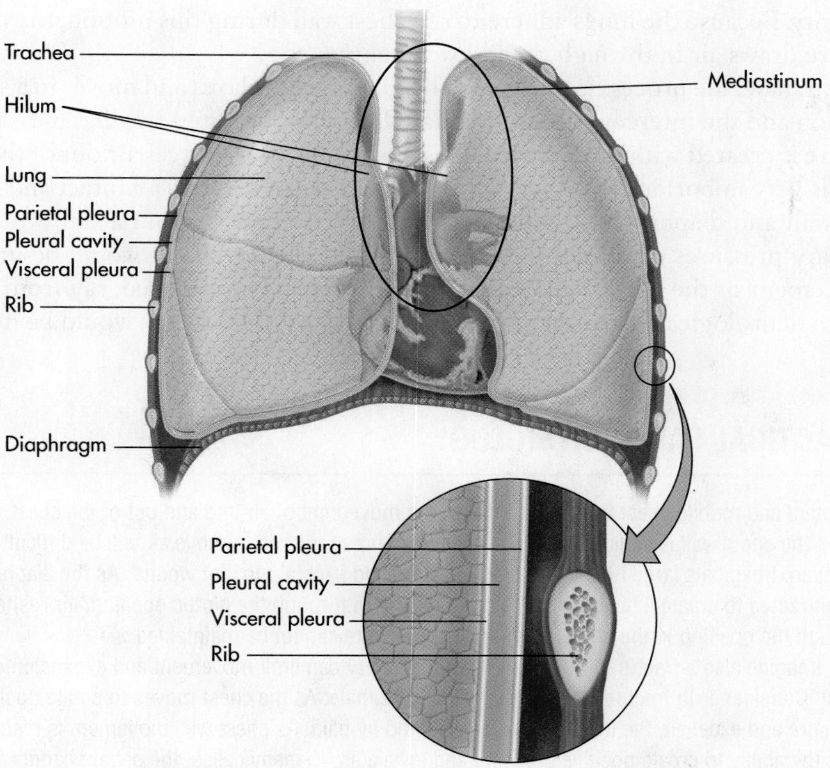

Figure 33-1 The anatomy of the thoracic cavity.

pressure in the thoracic cavity. It is an essential component of breathing. During a deep exhalation, the diaphragm rises to about nipple-level (the fourth or fifth rib) and during a deep inhalation, it drops to just above the level of the umbilicus. This means that open wounds from the nipple line to the navel could involve the contents of the chest or the abdomen or both, depending on when the wound occurred in the respiratory cycle.

The thoracic cavity is lined with two layers of tissue called **pleura.** The *parietal pleura* lines the chest wall, while the *visceral pleura* covers the lungs. There is a very small amount of fluid between these layers that lubricates and reduces friction during breathing. The pleural layers also help the lungs adhere to the chest wall during breathing. The space between the parietal and visceral pleura is called the **pleural space.** The pleural space is not really a space, but rather a potential space. Under normal circumstances the lung adheres directly to the chest wall with only a small amount of fluid in between. In some cases, however, air or blood can get into this space and push the lung tissue away from the chest wall.

pleura two tissue layers that line the chest wall and cover the lungs.

pleural space potential space between the two tissue layers that line the chest wall and cover the lungs.

An example of the relationship between the pleural layers can be seen with a drinking glass on a table. If the table is dry, the glass can be picked up easily. If the table is wet, the glass will stick to the table a bit. It will feel as if there is some suction holding it to the table. This is similar to the relationship of the pleura and the fluid between them.

The Physiology of Breathing

Air is moved in and out of the chest by changing pressure within the thoracic cavity. To inhale, the diaphragm contracts and moves in an inferior direction. The muscles between the ribs (called the *intercostal muscles*) are used to expand the chest wall. These actions cause the chest to increase in size, creating a negative pressure within the cavity. Because the lungs adhere to the chest wall during this motion, the negative pressure draws air in through the glottic opening.

To exhale, the process is reversed. The diaphragm relaxes and moves in a superior direction and the intercostal muscles relax. The chest becomes smaller and a positive pressure is created within the cavity. This positive pressure forces air out of the lungs.

It is very important to remember that this process requires an intact and moving chest wall and diaphragm. If a hole were to be created, say from a stab wound, the necessary pressures could not be maintained and air movement would be impaired. If movement of the chest wall or diaphragm were to be restricted, say from trauma or from neurological impairment from a spine injury, the process would be defeated.

PRACTICAL PATHOPHYSIOLOGY

An intact and mobile chest wall is essential to the movement of air into and out of the chest. When the chest wall is violated or injured, the pressures required to move air will be difficult to maintain. Imagine a large hole in the chest wall created from a gunshot wound. As the diaphragm is contracted to create a negative pressure to pull air in through the glottic opening, air rushes in through the opening in the chest. The negative pressure cannot be maintained.

Imagine also a fractured rib. The pain of this injury can limit movement and expansion of the chest. Consider a rib fracture patient attempting to exhale. As the chest moves to create positive pressure and expel air, the movement is interrupted by pain. As chest wall movement is restricted, so is the ability to create positive pressure and exhale air. In many cases, the patient cannot fully empty the lungs.

Consider any injury to the chest not just dangerous because of underlying organs, but also because it threatens the mechanism of breathing.

Closed Chest Injuries

33-4 Define and list specific types of closed chest injury.

33-5 Explain the pathophysiology of each of the following injuries: cardiac contusion, flail segment, hemothorax, open pneumothorax, tension pneumothorax, pericardial tamponade, pulmonary contusion, rib injury, and traumatic asphyxia.

A closed chest injury is an injury to the chest that does not penetrate the chest wall. Closed chest injuries are usually the result of blunt trauma, such as from a fall or a vehicle collision. Although the chest cavity remains intact, internal structures may be severely damaged. With enough force, blunt trauma can cause major damage to the internal organs and vessels of the chest and significantly damage the structure of the chest wall itself. In closed chest injuries, knowledge of anatomy and physiology is used to predict the possible underlying damage and a thorough patient assessment is used to confirm suspicions.

Closed chest injuries can occur from a variety of mechanisms. Underlying organs can be damaged, such as shearing of the aorta in a rapid deceleration injury, or the structure of the chest itself can be damaged. Consider how even a minor injury to the chest wall can impact the respiratory system: Bruising can cause pain that limits the expansion of the chest wall, thereby preventing air from moving completely in and out of the chest. This can cause decreased oxygenation (hypoxia) and an increase in retained carbon dioxide (hypercapnia). A lung that does not expand normally for a longer period of time is at risk for developing **pneumonia,** or infection of the lung tissue.

pneumonia infection of the lung.

Rib Fracture

rib fracture any break in a rib.

Rib fracture is a common type of closed chest injury and is frequently caused by blunt trauma (Figure 33-2 ▪). Every rib is connected posteriorly to a thoracic vertebra. The first 10 pairs of ribs are connected anteriorly to the sternum, either directly

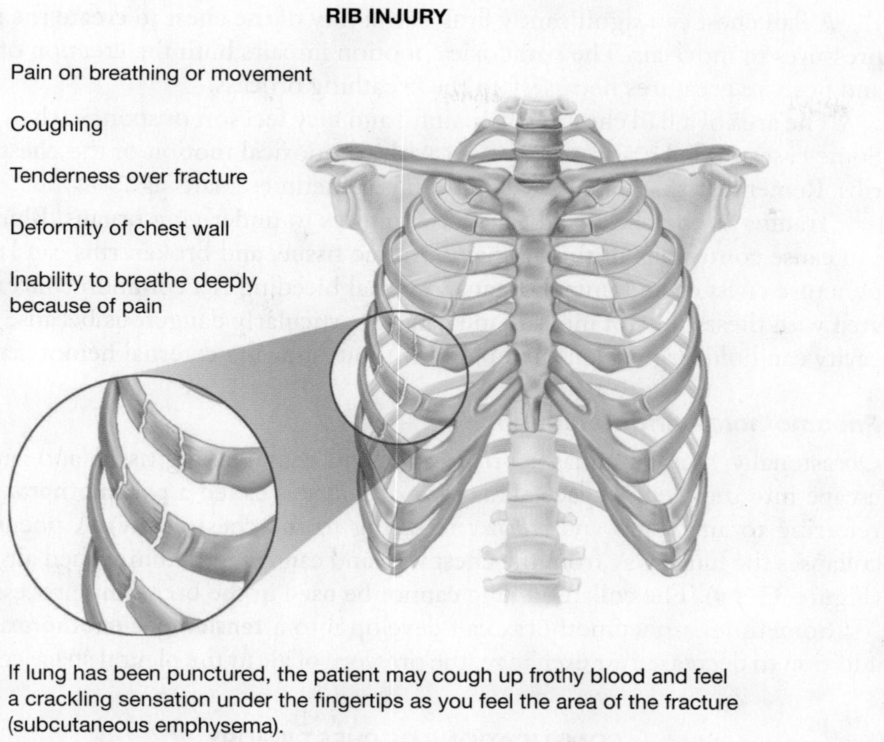
RIB INJURY
Pain on breathing or movement
Coughing
Tenderness over fracture
Deformity of chest wall
Inability to breathe deeply because of pain
If lung has been punctured, the patient may cough up frothy blood and feel a crackling sensation under the fingertips as you feel the area of the fracture (subcutaneous emphysema).

Figure 33-2 Injury to the ribs can affect normal breathing by causing a decrease in tidal volume due to pain.

floating ribs the two ribs that are connected to vertebrae but not to the sternum.

flail chest two or more ribs broken in two or more places.

paradoxical motion movement of a flail segment opposite to the motion of the nonfractured ribs.

or by cartilage. The last two pairs are called **floating ribs** because they are connected to vertebrae but not to the sternum. Ribs that are connected anteriorly to the sternum are more likely to fracture. Fractures to the sternum and to the clavicles can have a similar effect as rib fractures. Sternal fractures are very concerning because the heart lies directly underneath and frequently is damaged in this type of an injury. Clavicle fractures can also damage underlying lung tissue.

Signs and symptoms of rib fracture include pain made worse by breathing, deformity (although this is somewhat rare), crepitus, and tenderness to palpation.

One of the most concerning problems associated with rib injuries (including fractures) is poor ventilation. A rib fracture is a very painful injury and commonly the patient is unable to take a normal breath. The impaired chest wall movement can lead to hypoxia and hypercapnia and can be particularly dangerous in patients who have underlying lung illnesses such as COPD. Advanced life support will be important when dealing with these patients because pain management is a very important part of successful treatment.

Flail Chest

A **flail chest** occurs when two or more ribs have been broken in two or more places (Figure 33-3 ■). It results in an unstable segment that may appear as **paradoxical motion** of the chest wall. On inhalation the floating segment is drawn in as the rest of the chest expands, and on exhalation the floating segment is pushed out. Because of the force necessary to create a flail chest, underlying lung injury is very common.

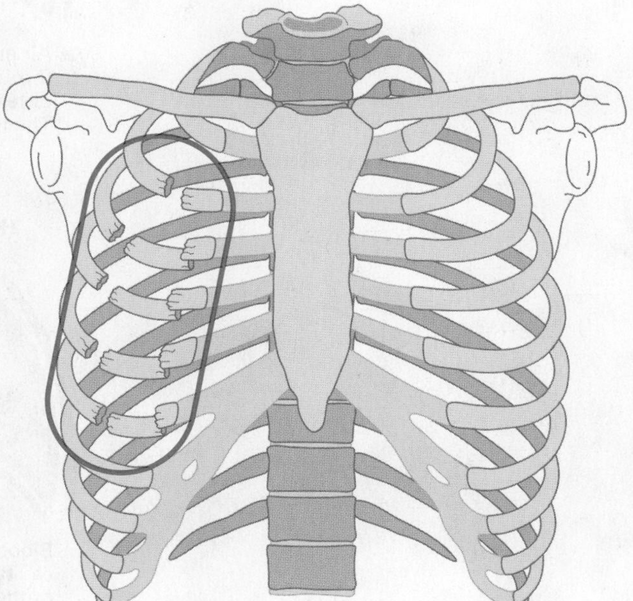

Figure 33-3 A flail chest can occur when two or more ribs are broken in two or more places. It is often caused by blunt trauma.

A flail chest can significantly limit the ability of the chest to create the necessary pressures to move air. The paradoxical motion impairs both the creation of negative and positive pressures necessary to the breathing process.

The area of a flail chest is very painful and may feel soft or spongy when palpated. Some cases of flail chest may present with paradoxical motion of the chest wall and ribs. Remember that paradoxical motion is sometimes a late sign.

Trauma to the chest wall can cause injuries to underlying organs. Blunt trauma can cause contusions of the lung and cardiac tissue, and broken ribs can lacerate or puncture chest or abdominal organs. Internal bleeding is a common concern associated with these types of injuries and can be particularly dangerous because the chest cavity can hold large volumes of blood without showing external hemorrhage.

Pneumothorax and Hemothorax

pneumothorax air within the pleural space.

tension pneumothorax buildup of air under pressure within the thorax, resulting in compression of the lung, which severely reduces the effectiveness of respirations.

Occasionally, blunt trauma or broken ribs will damage lung tissue and cause air to escape into the pleural space. This type of injury is called a **pneumothorax** (*pneumo-* referring to air or gas and *-thorax* referring to the chest cavity). A pneumothorax collapses the lung away from the chest wall and can result in diminished air exchange (Figure 33-4 ■). The collapsed lung cannot be used in the breathing process.

Sometimes a pneumothorax can develop into a **tension pneumothorax.** Here, in addition to decreased air exchange, the pressure of air in the pleural space compresses

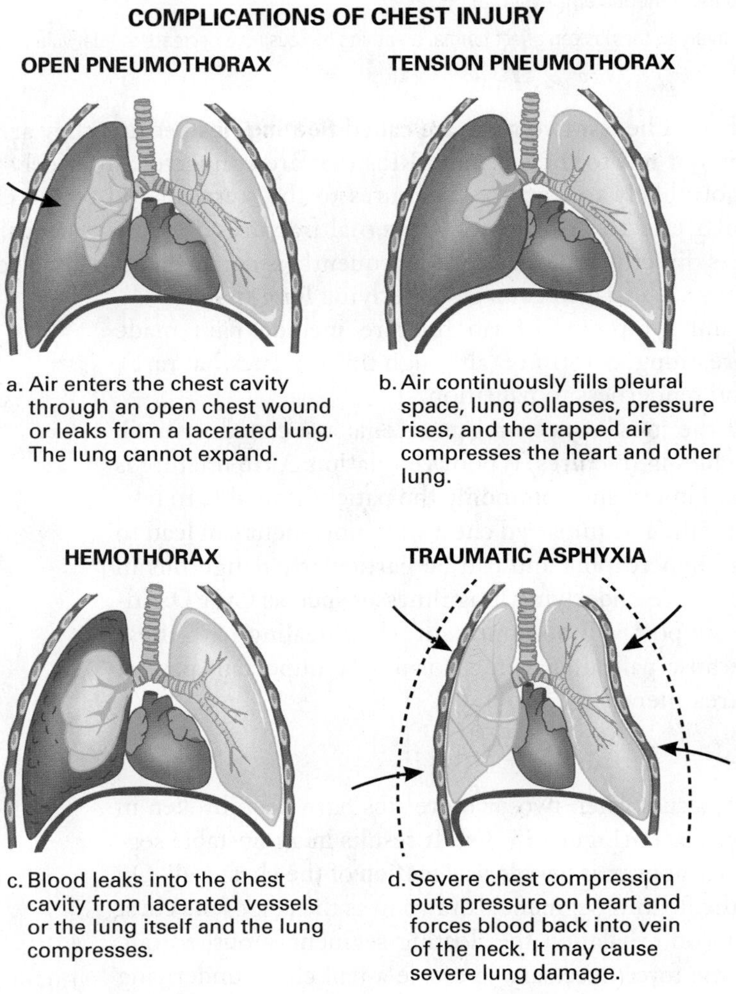
COMPLICATIONS OF CHEST INJURY
OPEN PNEUMOTHORAX
TENSION PNEUMOTHORAX
a. Air enters the chest cavity through an open chest wound or leaks from a lacerated lung. The lung cannot expand.
b. Air continuously fills pleural space, lung collapses, pressure rises, and the trapped air compresses the heart and other lung.
HEMOTHORAX
TRAUMATIC ASPHYXIA
c. Blood leaks into the chest cavity from lacerated vessels or the lung itself and the lung compresses.
d. Severe chest compression puts pressure on heart and forces blood back into vein of the neck. It may cause severe lung damage.

Figure 33-4 Pathophysiology of common chest injuries.

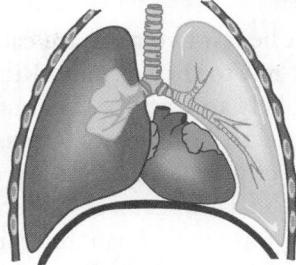

the heart and great vessels and prevents the normal filling of the heart with blood. This decrease in *preload* (the amount of blood that fills the heart prior to systolic ejection) results in a decrease in cardiac output. This problem rapidly causes shock and death of the patient, if not promptly corrected.

A **spontaneous pneumothorax** is a condition where a pneumothorax develops without a traumatic cause. It can happen when a disease such as COPD has damaged the lung or in some cases without any obvious cause. This happens with some frequency in tall, thin individuals during exertion such as running. These patients often present with a sudden onset of one-sided sharp chest pain and increasing shortness of breath. It is important to remember that any pneumothorax, whether caused by trauma or medical reasons, can develop into a tension pneumothorax and be life threatening.

spontaneous pneumothorax a condition in which a pneumothorax develops without a traumatic cause.

Blood also can accumulate in the pleural space. This is caused most commonly by trauma and is referred to as a **hemothorax** (*hemo-* referring to blood). In many cases both blood and air can occupy space.

hemothorax a condition in which blood accumulates within the pleural space.

Traumatic Asphyxia

Traumatic asphyxia is a condition in which a severe blunt compressive force or weight is placed on the chest, stopping ventilation and forcing blood from the right atrium up into the circulation of the head and neck (Figure 33-5 ■). In this type of injury, you often see respiratory failure, and bilateral pneumothoraces are possible. Bulging neck veins, dark red or purple discoloration of the head and neck, swelling and discoloration of the lips and tongue, deformity of the chest, and bulging eyes are common findings. Respiratory or cardiac arrest often develops.

traumatic asphyxia a condition in which a severe blunt force or weight is placed on the chest, forcing blood from the right atrium up into the circulation of the head and neck.

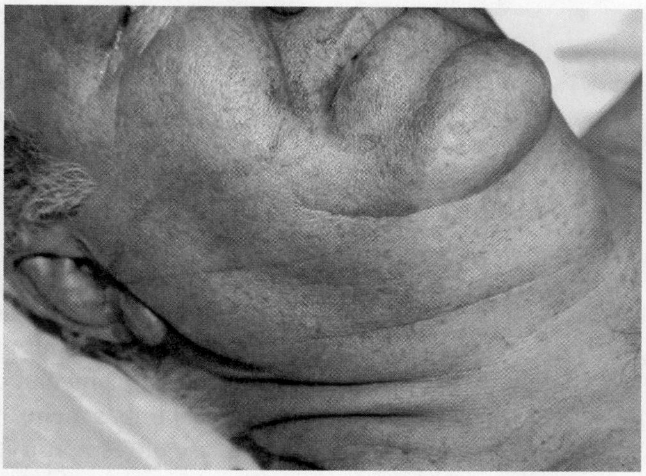

Figure 33-5 Signs of traumatic asphyxia. (© Edward T. Dickinson, MD)

Pulmonary and Cardiac Contusions

Underlying organs such as the heart and lungs can be bruised in blunt trauma-related injuries. In **pulmonary contusions** (bruised lung), damaged lung tissue can no longer be used in gas exchange. This injury can occur immediately or hours after the injury as lung tissue becomes swollen secondary to the trauma.

The heart also can be damaged by blunt force trauma. **Cardiac contusions** occur in a similar fashion to pulmonary contusions. Blunt force causes both immediate and delayed injuries to underlying heart tissue. The physical damage, bruising, and secondary swelling to the muscle used to pump blood can significantly affect cardiac output.

Commotio Cordis

Commotio cordis occurs when blunt trauma to the chest affects the electrical function of the heart. Here blunt force depolarizes the heart electrically and causes cardiac arrest. This is most commonly seen in sport-related injuries such as a baseball player being struck in the chest with a baseball.

pulmonary contusions bruising of the lung tissue typically as the result of blunt trauma.

cardiac contusions bruising of the heart tissue typically as the result of blunt trauma.

commotio cordis cardiac arrest caused by bunt force trauma to the chest.

PRACTICAL PATHOPHYSIOLOGY

In a pulmonary contusion, lung tissue is damaged by blunt force trauma and begins to bleed, disrupting the exchange of gases. Swelling of lung tissue and blood that fills the alveoli also will interfere with the normal exchange of gases. Decompensation due to pulmonary contusion can occur hours after the injury.

33-6 Discuss an assessment-based approach to manage patients with chest trauma.

33-7 Discuss the following aspects of chest trauma care: general emergency care for chest trauma and specific emergency care for an open chest wound.

Assessment of Closed Chest Injuries

The breathing portion of the primary assessment should focus on the chest. After ensuring a patent airway, adequacy of breathing must be assessed. Look for signs of respiratory distress or respiratory failure. If breathing is inadequate, positive pressure ventilations must be initiated.

In many closed chest injuries, the patient will complain of difficulty breathing. Dyspnea can be caused by pain or by damage to underlying structures that affect the exchange of gas (or by both). The patient may be able to localize pain or tenderness and therefore help pinpoint your assessment to a specific area or underlying organ.

Your primary assessment also must assess circulation and identify any signs and symptoms of shock. Frequently with chest injuries, signs of shock will indicate bleeding associated with internal injuries.

Use inspection to visualize the chest wall. Expose the chest and look for bruising, paradoxical movement, and deformity. Occasionally, injuries such as a flail chest may present as external deformity to the chest wall.

Listen to lung sounds. Auscultation helps to identify impaired air movement from conditions such as a pneumothorax or hemothorax. In a pneumothorax, traditionally the patient complains of shortness of breath and displays unequal lung sounds. As air develops in the pleural space on one side, air movement will sound different when auscultated. Unequal lung sounds must make you immediately consider a pneumo- or hemothorax. Unequal lung sounds with shock should make you immediately assume a tension pneumothorax (a life-threatening emergency).

Palpation will help identify tenderness, crepitus (subcutaneous emphysema), and paradoxical motion. Be careful touching the chest of a patient with a chest injury because your palpation could cause severe pain.

Other important assessment findings in the case of a closed chest injury include mental status (particularly as it applies to oxygenation and ventilation) and the presence of jugular vein distention (which might indicate pneumothorax or traumatic asphyxia).

Emergency Care of Closed Chest Injuries

To treat closed chest injuries, consider the underlying problem. Closed chest injuries commonly result in poor gas exchange; therefore, supplemental oxygen can be helpful. Supplemental oxygen should be applied to any patient showing signs of respiratory impairment or hypoxia. Positive pressure ventilation may be necessary in the case of respiratory failure, and it may improve gas exchange in situations where the mechanism of breathing has been disrupted. For example, when two or more ribs are broken in two or more places, causing what is referred to as a *flail chest*, positive pressure ventilation can help stabilize the movement of the flail segment during inhalation (although it should be applied only in situations of respiratory failure).

Some rib fracture patients benefit from being allowed to hold a pillow against their chest while breathing. The pressure of the pillow splints the ribs and soothes the pain, making breathing easier. Although passive measures like a pillow may help, you should never splint rib fractures or flail segments externally because restriction of the chest wall is often far worse for the patient than the fracture itself.

In many cases the best treatment for a closed chest injury is prompt transport to an appropriate facility. As most life-threatening injuries occur beneath the chest wall, prehospital care is generally limited. In many situations, surgery will be required.

Maintain a high index of suspicion with regard to mechanisms of injury that affect the chest. Remember that these injuries can be immediate, but worsen over time. If a mechanism of injury linked with the physical examination indicates the possibility of an underlying chest injury, transport and further evaluation are high priorities.

As stated previously, advanced life support resources can play an important role in the treatment of closed chest injuries. Paramedics have the ability to relieve the pressure that may be building up in the chest and they can help manage the pain.

PERSPECTIVE

Nancy—The EMT

I wasn't expecting a pneumothorax with an abdominal injury. I mean it looked bad, but I didn't anticipate that it would have affected the lungs. When I listened to his chest, I knew it was a pneumothorax and I knew that guy was in trouble. I remembered learning about tension pneumothorax and thinking that we needed ALS. At the time I wasn't even thinking about the hospital. Luckily, Brandi reminded me that Porter General Hospital was right down the street.

Open Chest Injuries

33-3 Define and list specific types of open chest injury.

When an injury penetrates the chest wall, it is considered an open chest injury. Open chest injuries are caused by penetrating trauma such as a knife, bullet, or any mechanism that pierces the rib cage.

Open chest injuries can cause a variety of problems in the chest. First and foremost, the penetrating object can damage both the chest wall and underlying organs (depending on the depth of penetration). Organ and blood vessel damage as a result of penetrating trauma can lead to severe internal bleeding and shock. The chest cavity can hold several liters of blood and it is possible to bleed to death from internal injuries to the chest without ever presenting with external hemorrhage.

Signs and symptoms of open chest wounds include:

- A mechanism of injury that indicates penetration of the chest cavity such as a gunshot wound or stab wound (Figure 33-6 ■). Consider also abdominal and shoulder injuries.
- An open wound to the anterior, posterior, or lateral area of the chest wall. Remember that these injuries may be small and difficult to notice without careful inspection. Some of them may bubble or make a sucking noise.
- Difficulty breathing
- Signs of shock, including rapid pulse and respirations, restlessness and anxiety, and decreased blood pressure (late sign)
- A narrowing pulse pressure (the difference between the systolic and diastolic blood pressures)
- Diminished or absent breath sounds over one or more areas of the chest

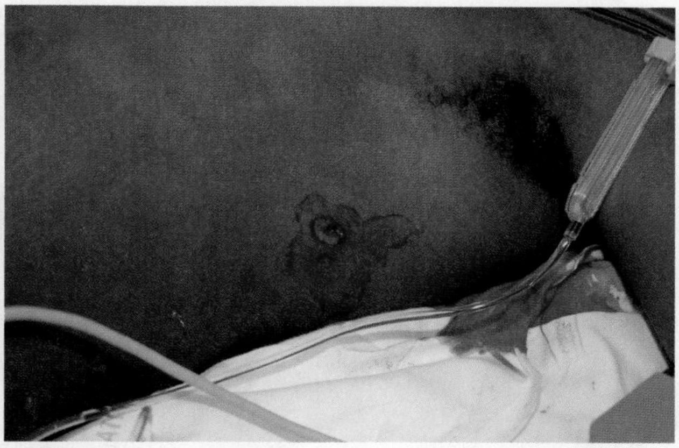

Figure 33-6 A gunshot wound to the left lateral chest.
(© Edward T. Dickinson, MD)

Open Pneumothorax

When the chest wall is penetrated, the ability to create the necessary pressures for adequate breathing can be disrupted. If air is entering a hole in the chest wall, the negative pressure used to pull air into the lungs cannot be maintained. At times, this type of an injury can present externally with air bubbling from a wound on inhalation and exhalation. This is called an **open pneumothorax,** also known as a *sucking chest wound*.

open pneumothorax air within the pleural space that is accumulating due to a penetration of the chest wall.

Holes in the chest wall or lung (or both) can allow air or blood (or both) to accumulate in the pleural space. If enough air or blood accumulates, the lung will collapse away from the chest wall, creating a pneumo- or hemothorax. If pressure builds up and compresses the heart, a tension pneumothorax will be created.

In both pneumothorax and hemothorax, you may auscultate the chest and note decreased or absent breath sounds on one side when compared to the other. In smaller pneumothoraces, air accumulation is seen first in the upper areas of the lungs and will be hard to detect by auscultation. Auscultation will provide some information, but the clinical picture of the patient (respiratory distress, shock, and so on) is the best indicator of serious internal thoracic injury.

Penetrating chest injuries do not always involve just the chest. Consider the dynamic nature of the size of the chest cavity and movement of the diaphragm. During a deep inhalation, the thoracic cavity may extend well into the abdomen. Remember also that lung tissue extends as high as the clavicles. You should assume that any penetrating trauma to the chest, shoulder, and abdomen could include damage to the lungs.

Pericardial Tamponade

pericardial tamponade collection of blood in the sac surrounding the heart.

Pericardial tamponade is a condition often caused by open and closed chest injuries. In the case of an open chest injury, a penetrating object such as a knife or bullet damages the heart and causes blood to accumulate in the surrounding pericardial sac. Because this sac is fibrous and does not stretch well, the buildup of blood compresses against the heart and prevents the filling of the chambers (Figure 33-7 ■). As a result, cardiac output can be significantly impaired.

Signs of pericardial tamponade are referred to as *Beck's triad* and include narrowing pulse pressure, jugular vein distention (as a result of venous backup), and muffled heart sounds (although heart sounds can be difficult to assess even under optimal conditions). In many cases, pericardial tamponade will be considered based on the mechanism of injury and anatomical location of the injury. Always assess the complete picture to include both the mechanism and assessment findings.

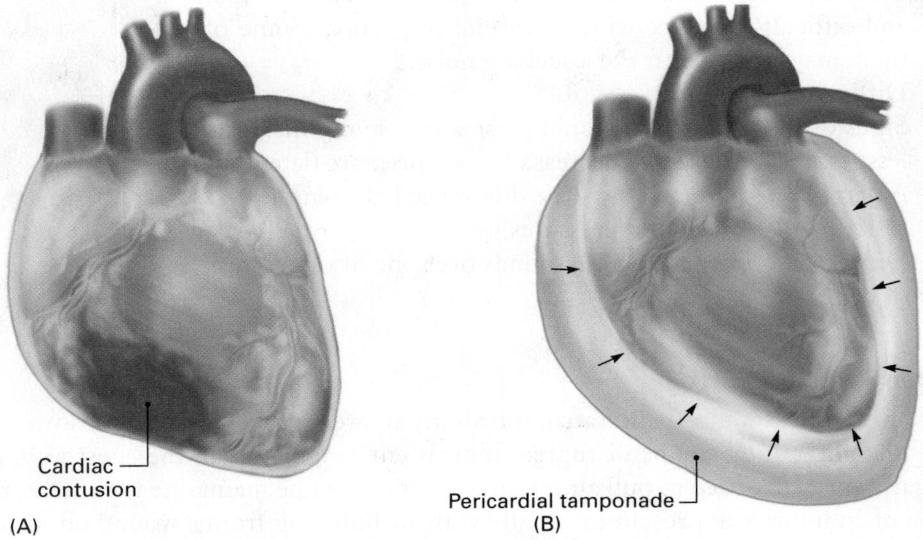

Figure 33-7 Traumatic cardiac injuries. (A) Bleeding into the pericardial sac from contusion to the myocardium. (B) Accumulation of fluid in the pericardial sac.

PRACTICAL PATHOPHYSIOLOGY

Many injuries to the chest can impact the return of venous blood to the heart. When this occurs, cardiac output drops. Cardiac output (the amount of blood pumped by the heart in one minute) is a function of both heart rate and stroke volume. Stroke volume (the amount of blood pumped in one contraction) is a function of contractility, afterload (the amount of pressure the heart has to pump against), and preload. When an injury impacts the return of blood, preload is reduced.

In a tension pneumothorax, air trapped in the pleural space puts pressure on the great vessels, including the vena cava. This pressure diminishes the amount of blood that can travel through it. When less blood travels through the vena cava, less blood returns to the heart.

In pericardial tamponade, blood between the outside of the heart and the pericardial sac actually squeezes the heart itself. This external pressure decreases the size of the heart's chambers and therefore limits filling volume.

When preload is decreased, cardiac output is decreased. This drop in the function of the heart can greatly impact perfusion of body tissues. If less blood is being pumped, less blood reaches vital organs.

Assessment of Open Chest Injuries

Open wounds to the chest must be considered life threatening and cared for promptly. Consider any penetrating injury to the chest serious and initiate rapid transport. In addition, consider the need to support breathing.

In the primary assessment ensure a patent airway and adequate breathing. Use positive pressure ventilation if breathing becomes inadequate. Because chest wounds can interfere with gas exchange, consider supplemental oxygen to treat hypoxia.

Expose and assess the chest. Remember that penetrating trauma can affect lung tissue in areas as low as the umbilicus and in areas as high as the clavicles. Look, listen, and feel. Visually inspect for punctures and open wounds. Remember that small holes can cause large underlying problems. Be sure to expose the chest and look at four sides of any trauma patient (front, back, and both sides). Often punctures can be small and difficult to notice, but finding them is very important. Palpate the chest and assess for bleeding, paradoxical motion, and tenderness. Listen with a stethoscope to ensure equal air movement on both sides.

Open chest wounds must be sealed off to prevent air from entering. Remember that when air is pulled in, negative pressure cannot be maintained. **Occlusive dressings** (also known as *nonporous dressings*) do not allow air to pass through them. There are a variety of commercially available occlusive dressings, but impervious items, such as a rubber glove, plastic bag, or defibrillator pads could be used if commercially available occlusive dressings are not on hand.

occlusive dressings a dressing that does not allow air to move through it; an airtight dressing. Also called a *nonporous dressing.*

To place an occlusive dressing, follow these steps:

1. Select a commercially available occlusive dressing or other clean impervious item. Be sure the dressing is large enough to prevent it from being sucked into the wound.
2. Ideally the dressing should be placed at the end of exhalation, but this should not delay the placement of the dressing.
3. Tape the dressing on three sides (Figure 33-8 ■). The untaped side will seal shut during inhalation but will open and allow air to escape during exhalation.

It should be noted that the evidence to support a three-sided dressing is unclear. It may or may not be effective in relieving the buildup of pressure. The most important element is sealing off the open chest wound, and your first and most

CLINICAL CLUE

Sealing a Chest Wound

Seal any chest wound you believe may have penetrated into the thoracic cavity, whether it is actually bubbling or not.

important efforts should be designed to get the dressing in place. However, if you have time, taping three sides remains the standard of care in applying an occlusive dressing.

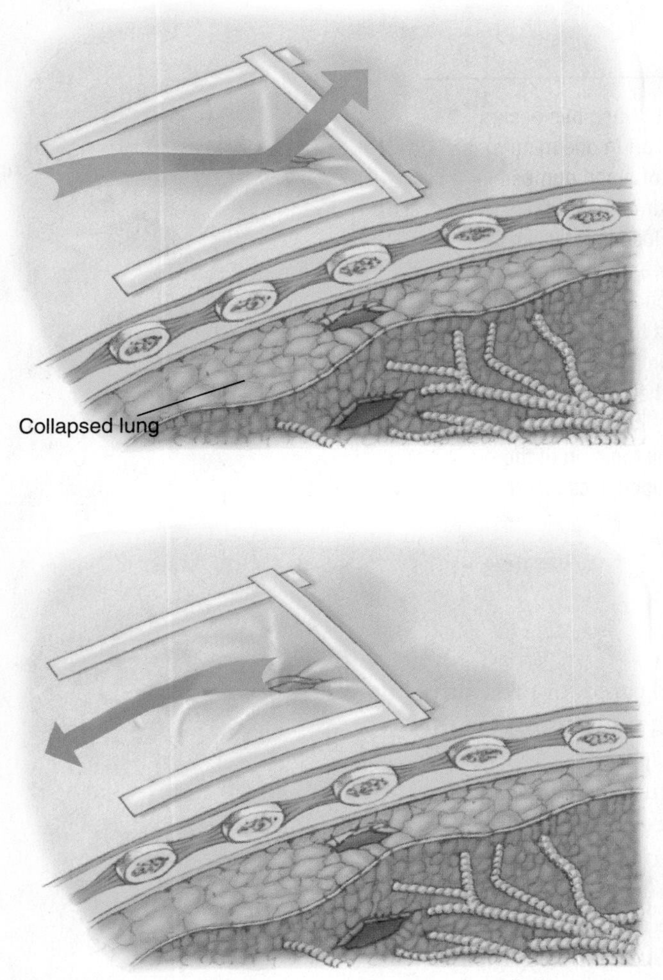

Figure 33-8 An occlusive dressing placed over an open chest wound and taped on three sides will prevent air from entering the opening but still allow air to escape.

> **CLINICAL CLUE**
>
> **Tension Pneumothorax**
>
> Monitor all patients with open chest injuries very carefully for adequacy of respiratory rate and tidal volume. Just because you have an occlusive dressing in place does not mean pressure cannot build inside the chest. If the patient's respiratory status becomes worse, consider the possibility of a tension pneumothorax. Immediate ALS intercept may be life saving in this circumstance.
>
> You may consider removing the occlusive dressing temporarily to allow pressure to escape if you may have inadvertently induced a tension pneumothorax by sealing the wound. Lift the dressing briefly as the patient breathes out, and then place it back down as he begins to inhale. Try this a few times to see if air escapes from the wound. In some cases a tension pneumothorax will develop regardless of your best efforts.

Internal bleeding is a serious threat in an open chest wound. Always assess for the signs and symptoms of shock and assume internal bleeding when any of those findings are present. Treat for shock as appropriate.

Remember that penetrating trauma to the chest can result in injuries that develop over time. A tension pneumothorax or pericardial tamponade will not necessarily develop immediately. Those complications will be seen on reassessment of the injured patient.

In many cases, the most appropriate treatment for an open chest injury is rapid transport. For example, there is little that can be done for a pericardial tamponade in the field. This patient requires immediate surgical intervention. If your assessment identifies this type of injury, initiate transport immediately and consider an appropriate trauma center destination.

Emergency Care of an Open Chest Injury

Follow these general steps when caring for an open chest injury:

1. Take appropriate BSI precautions.
2. Manage the ABCs as appropriate.
3. Cover the wound with an occlusive dressing that is sealed on three sides or, as permitted in some protocols, sealed on four sides with one corner left untaped to serve as a "flutter valve." If necessary, use a gloved hand to seal the wound until an appropriate occlusive dressing can be obtained. Make sure the dressing extends well beyond the wound on all sides and allows air to escape from the chest cavity. Follow local protocols regarding the use of occlusive dressings.
4. Initiate supplemental oxygen.
5. Treat for shock and transport immediately.
6. Initiate an ALS intercept if available.

STOP, REVIEW, REMEMBER!

Multiple Choice

For each question, place a check next to the correct answer.

1. Which one of the following is *not* located in the thoracic cavity?

_____ a. Larynx

_____ b. Bronchi

_____ c. Alveoli

_____ d. Mitral valve

2. A 22-year-old patient complains of chest pain and difficulty breathing after striking his chest on a steering wheel during a motor-vehicle collision. He tells you that he is okay, however, and does not wish to be transported. You should:

_____ a. force the patient to allow transport because he cannot refuse. He clearly has an altered mental status.

_____ b. sign the patient off and document the situation carefully.

_____ c. have law enforcement place the patient in protective custody.

_____ d. discuss your concerns about pulmonary and cardiac contusions with the patient in an attempt to convince him to be transported.

3. A common complication from an open chest injury is a(n):

_____ a. evisceration.

_____ b. perforated ulcer.

_____ c. pneumothorax.

_____ d. ruptured aorta.

4. Occlusive dressings taped on three sides are most appropriate for which type of injuries?

_____ a. Closed abdominal wounds

_____ b. Open abdominal wounds

_____ c. Closed chest wounds

_____ d. Open chest wounds

5. A 25-year-old man has been shot in the chest. On examination of your patient's chest, you hear unequal lung sounds. His vital signs are respiration 40, pulse 130, and blood pressure 70/55. These findings most likely indicate:

_____ a. a tension pneumothorax.

_____ b. commotio cordis.

_____ c. pericardial tamponade.

_____ d. pulmonary contusion.

Matching

Match the condition on the left with the correct definition on the right.

1. _____ Pneumothorax
2. _____ Hemothorax
3. _____ Tension pneumothorax
4. _____ Pericardial tamponade
5. _____ Flail chest

A. Collection of blood in the thoracic cavity

B. Two or more ribs broken in two or more places

C. Increasing pressure in the thoracic cavity, placing pressure on lungs, the heart, and great vessels

D. Air in the thoracic cavity

E. Collection of blood in the sac that surrounds the heart

(continued on next page)

(continued)

Critical Thinking

1. What are the differences in care between open and closed chest wounds?

____

____

____

____

2. Why is an occlusive dressing for an open chest wound sealed on only three sides?

____

____

____

____

The Abdomen

Just like the chest, the abdomen is a cavity that holds many vital organs and blood vessels. Unlike the chest, however, the abdomen contains a large number of different organs that impact a wide range of body systems. As a result, abdominal injuries can be a complex diagnostic dilemma. In most cases reaching a conclusive diagnosis is less important than recognizing the possibility of an immediate life threat, such as internal bleeding. Anatomy and physiology will help focus your abdominal assessment and may help you recognize common characteristics of life-threatening disorders, but in many cases it may be more appropriate to address general symptoms and treat broad life threats first.

Anatomy and Physiology of the Abdomen

33-8 Describe the anatomy of the abdominal cavity and its contents.

33-9 Differentiate hollow and solid organs and vascular structures in the abdomen.

Chapter 22 described the anatomy and physiology of the abdomen. For more depth on the topic, please reference that chapter. With trauma in mind, it is important to review the anatomical locations of key abdominal structures.

The abdomen is commonly separated into four quadrants, divided at the umbilicus (Figure 33-9 ■). When assessing a trauma patient, it is exceptionally important to recall that the lower quadrants extend below the common waistline of most pants. Be sure to remove clothing as necessary to allow for full inspection and assessment of the lower quadrants.

When considering a mechanism of injury, it is helpful to understand the organs that lie beneath the surface. Table 33-1 is a list of the major abdominal quadrants and the organs that occupy space in them.

Recall also the role of the fibrous membrane that lines the abdominal cavity. It is called the **peritoneum.** Remember that organs such as the descending aorta and the kidneys are found behind the peritoneum (**retroperitoneal** space).

peritoneum the membrane of connective tissue that lines and separates the abdominal cavity.

retroperitoneal behind the abdominal cavity.

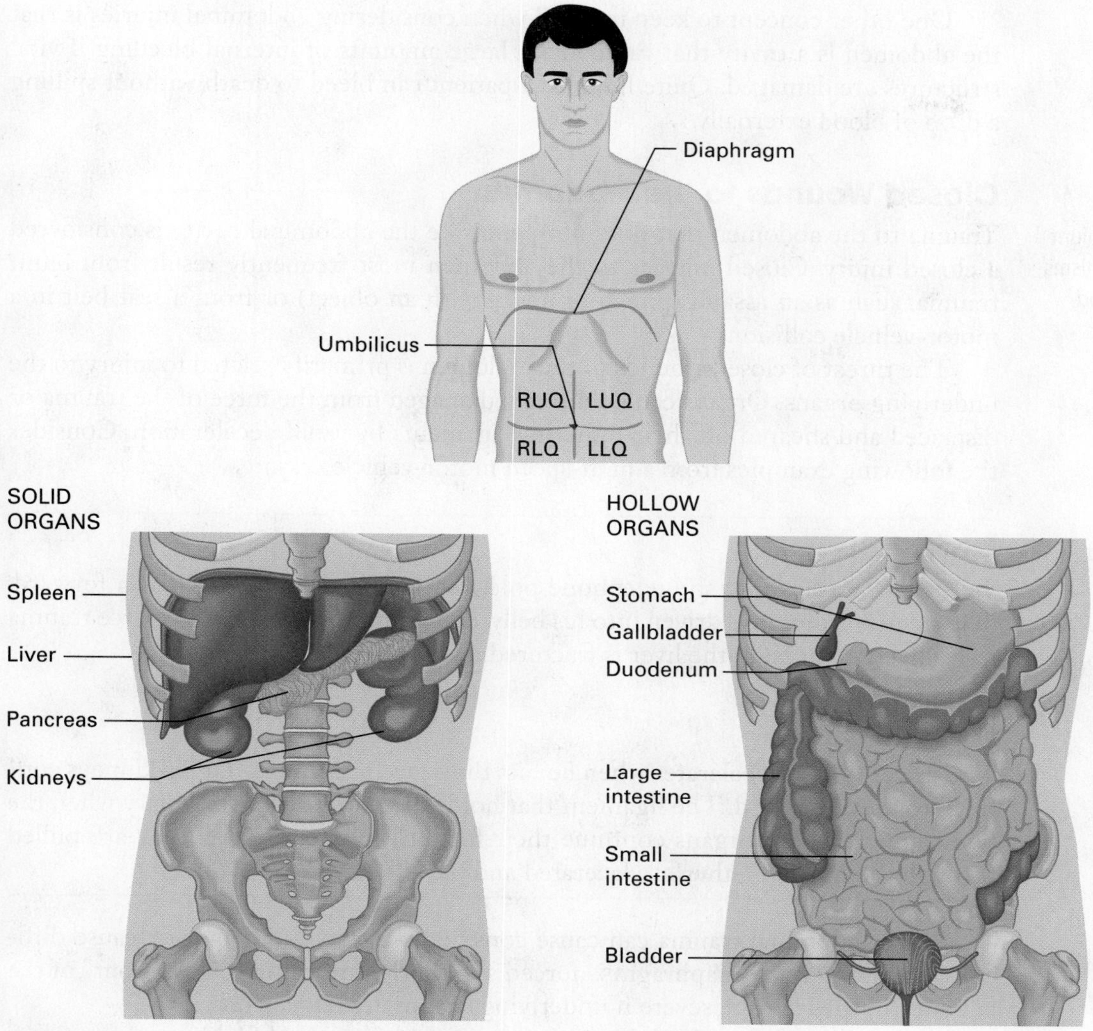

Figure 33-9 The structures and organs of the abdomen.

TABLE 33-1 ABDOMINAL QUADRANTS

RIGHT UPPER QUADRANT (RUQ)	LEFT UPPER QUADRANT (LUQ)
• Liver (in both upper quadrants) • Gall bladder • Pancreas (extends through both upper quadrants) • Large intestine (in all four quadrants) • Small intestine (in all four quadrants)	• Liver (in both upper quadrants) • Spleen • Pancreas (extends through both upper quadrants) • Stomach • Large intestine (in all four quadrants) • Small intestine (in four quadrants)
RIGHT LOWER QUADRANT (RLQ)	**LEFT LOWER QUADRANT (LLQ)**
• Appendix • Large intestine (in all four quadrants) • Small intestine (in all four quadrants) • Right ovary and fallopian tube (women only) • Ureter (in both lower quadrants)	• Large intestine (in all four quadrants) • Small intestine (in all four quadrants) • Left ovary and fallopian tube (women only) • Ureter (in both lower quadrants)

One other concept to keep in mind when considering abdominal injuries is that the abdomen is a cavity that can contain large amounts of internal bleeding if vital structures are damaged. Quite literally, a patient can bleed to death without spilling a drop of blood externally.

Closed Wounds to the Abdomen

33-10 Give examples of both blunt and penetrating mechanisms of abdominal trauma and discuss the potential for severe internal bleeding.

Trauma to the abdomen that does not penetrate the abdominal cavity is considered a closed injury. Closed injuries to the abdomen most frequently result from blunt trauma, such as an assault (punch or strike with an object) or from a seat belt in a motor-vehicle collision.

The threat of closed wounds to the abdomen is primarily related to injury to the underlying organs. Organs can be directly damaged from the force of the trauma or displaced and sheared off their tethering ligaments by rapid deceleration. Consider the following examples from a high-speed motor-vehicle crash:

Example 1:

As the car crashes into the telephone pole, the unbelted driver is thrown forward. The steering column is driven into his belly, delivering significant blunt force trauma to his liver. As a result, the liver is fractured and is now bleeding.

Example 2:

The driver's body decelerates when he hits the steering column, but his kidneys continue to move forward. The ligament that holds them in place is stationary when the body stops, but the organs continue their forward momentum. As they are pulled through the ligament, they are lacerated and bleed heavily.

Blunt abdominal trauma can cause considerable pain and may even cause difficulty breathing if the diaphragm is forced superiorly, "knocking the wind out" of the patient. Injuries may be severe if underlying organs are damaged.

Certain abdominal organs are more vulnerable than others. Some organs—such as the spleen—are less protected by ribs, and other organs—such as the liver—are more fragile due to their role in the body.

Abdominal organs can be either hollow or solid (Table 33-2). Solid organs tend to be rich in blood supply and susceptible to damage due to their density and lack of elasticity. The liver is a solid organ used to filter blood. When solid organs such as the liver are damaged, internal bleeding can be severe. Hollow organs, such as the lungs, stomach, and intestine are more flexible, but also can rupture.

TABLE 33-2 HOLLOW AND SOLID ABDOMINAL ORGANS

HOLLOW ORGANS	SOLID ORGANS
• Stomach	• Kidneys
• Large intestine	• Liver
• Small intestine	• Pancreas
• Gall bladder	• Spleen
• Appendix	• Ovaries
• Urinary bladder	

Rupture can occur due to any blunt force trauma including falls, blast injuries, and motor-vehicle collisions. Rupture of a hollow organ can spill contents into the abdomen, causing irritation, pain, and infection.

Some organs, like the spleen, are highly vascular and have a tremendous amount of blood flowing to them. Damage to these organs can cause severe, life-threatening bleeding. Large, high-pressure blood vessels, such as the descending aorta, also traverse the abdominal cavity. Damage to them can result in rapid blood loss and death.

33-11 Discuss an assessment-based approach to management of the patient with open and closed abdominal injury, including evisceration and impaled objects.

Assessment of Closed Abdominal Injuries

Closed abdominal injuries are extremely dangerous. Not only are they often overlooked in a multisystem trauma patient, the extent of the blunt force trauma is often difficult to identify from an external assessment. In most cases, an examination of the mechanism of injury will help identify possible blunt forces affecting the abdomen. Use those findings to predict injury and to focus your assessment. Remember also to communicate the mechanism of injury to hospital staff. Your findings are important to the ongoing care of the patient.

33-12 Describe signs and symptoms associated with injuries to the abdomen.

33-13 Explain the general emergency care for abdominal trauma.

In a closed abdominal injury, the primary assessment will help you rapidly identify life threats. Remember that any abdominal injury could include injuries to organs of the chest. For example, lower rib fractures frequently affect the upper quadrants of the abdomen. Ensure a patent airway and check for adequate breathing. Look for signs and symptoms of shock. Often these findings (in context with a blunt force mechanism of injury) may be your only indication of internal bleeding and the extent of a closed abdominal injury. Assess distal pulses and skin color. Check mental status. Treat for shock if necessary.

Expose and inspect the abdomen. Look for bruising, distention, discoloration, or any abnormal findings that might indicate blunt force trauma. Distention can be seen by recognizing a rise in the abdomen between the pubis and xiphoid process. Although this may be difficult to discern, it can indicate the presence of blood or fluid. Remember that inspection of the abdomen must include the front, back, and two sides.

Palpate all four quadrants of the abdomen. Notice any tenderness, guarding (the tensing of muscles due to pain), and rigidity. As stated previously, be sure to assess the lower quadrants and pubis as well. Remember to assess the retroperitoneal areas. You also can recognize abdominal bleeding by seeing blood in vomit or stool.

Consider the position of the patient. Patients with abdominal pain will frequently draw their legs up toward their chest. Straightening them may increase the pain.

The most common complaint associated with an abdominal injury is pain. In many cases the pain will be localized and can assist in focusing your assessment in a specific area. Remember that pain from abdominal injuries can be referred. Referred pain is identified in areas far away from the actual organ. For example, a patient with a ruptured spleen might complain of shoulder pain.

Signs and symptoms of closed abdominal injuries include the following:

- Mechanism of injury associated with blunt force trauma
- Pain, spontaneous or on palpation
- Bruising, redness, or discoloration
- Swelling or distention
- Rigidity on palpation of the abdominal wall
- Referred pain to the area of the shoulder
- Signs and symptoms of shock, including rapid pulse and breathing, cool and clammy skin, restlessness or anxiety, and decreasing blood pressure (late sign)

Assessment of closed abdominal injuries often relies on assuming the worst. Because of the high risk of vital organs lying beneath the skin, many times a closed abdominal injury should be assumed to be life threatening until proven otherwise.

Emergency Care of Closed Abdominal Injuries

Care for closed abdominal injuries is best accomplished by treating life threats first. Support airway and ventilations and treat for shock. Consider the mechanism of injury and recognize the signs and symptoms of shock. If you suspect serious injuries, treat for shock and promptly transport the patient to an appropriate facility.

To care for the patient with a closed abdominal injury follow these steps:

1. Take appropriate BSI precautions.
2. Perform a primary assessment and manage life threats as appropriate.

3. Take spinal precautions, if the mechanism of injury suggests spine injuries are possible.
4. If you do not suspect spine injury, place the patient in a position of comfort. This is commonly a recumbent or laterally recumbent position with the knees flexed.
5. Administer supplemental oxygen by nonrebreather mask, especially if you find respiratory impairment or hypoxia.
6. Transport promptly.

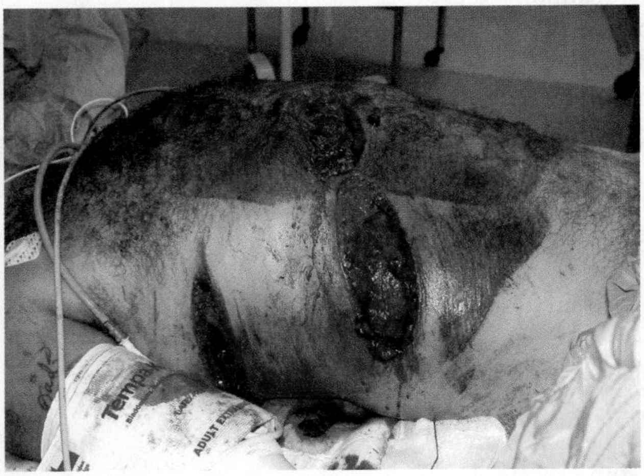

Figure 33-10 Significant open wounds to the abdomen and chest require immediate attention. (© Edward T. Dickinson, MD)

Open Wounds to the Abdomen

An abdominal wound is considered open when it penetrates the abdominal cavity (Figure 33-10 ■). Common open abdominal wounds include gunshots and stabbings. In a stabbing, hand-driven force inflicts damage and is limited to the pathway of the knife. In gunshot wounds, medium- and high-velocity forces are applied. Handguns and shotguns typically deliver medium-velocity energy. Rifles and explosion fragments deliver high-velocity energy. In medium- and high-velocity penetrations the damage includes not just the direct pathway wound, but also the expansion of the cavity as air creates pressure in the wake of the bullet. Open abdominal injuries are particularly dangerous because they directly threaten the organ systems that lie in the pathway of the offending object. Knowledge of anatomy and physiology will help you identify the potential damage in any given pathway.

In open injuries, just as with closed injuries, internal bleeding is a serious risk. Damaged organs can hemorrhage blood into the abdominal cavity. Ruptured hollow organs can bleed and spill their contents, causing shock and later infection. Small holes can create massive internal damage. Damage can be immediate, but also prolonged because later developing infections are frequently life threatening.

evisceration an injury to the abdomen resulting in the protrusion of the intestinal organs through the abdominal wall.

Occasionally, an open abdominal injury results in an abdominal **evisceration.** This type of injury occurs when intestinal organs or the fat that surrounds them protrude through the abdominal wall (Figure 33-11 ■). An evisceration is a dramatic injury. Though for all its drama, it may be the least concerning part of that particular injury. Although an evisceration must be handled carefully to prevent further damage, you should recognize that injuries to underlying organs and internal bleeding can be far more dangerous than the evisceration itself.

Do *not* attempt to insert protruding organs back into the abdomen. Instead, the eviscerated organs should be covered with a sterile dressing moistened with sterile saline. All eviscerations require prompt surgical intervention when the patient arrives at the hospital.

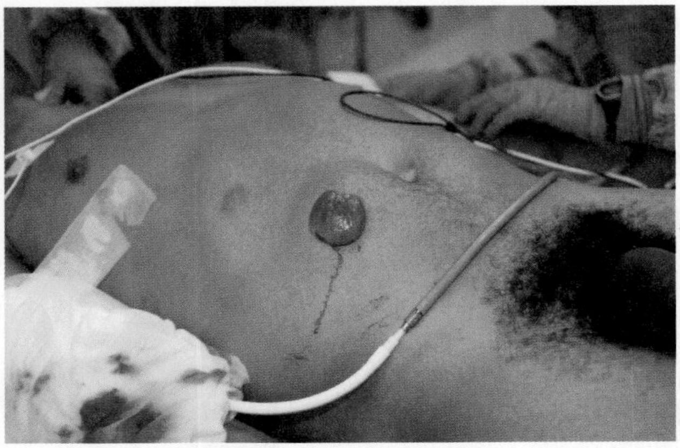

Figure 33-11 A small abdominal evisceration caused by a stab wound. (© Edward T. Dickinson, MD)

Assessment of Open Abdominal Injuries

As with any patient, your assessment should begin with ensuring a patent airway and adequate breathing. Supplemental oxygen should be applied, especially if the patient has respiratory impairment or signs and symptoms of hypoxia. The chief life threat associated with an open abdominal injury is internal bleeding. Use the primary assessment to rapidly identify signs and symptoms of shock and treat accordingly.

Just as with closed abdominal injuries, you should inspect and palpate the four quadrants of the abdomen to assess for injury. Inspection is incredibly important with this type of injury. Abdominal penetrations can be tiny but create massive underlying damage. Be sure to expose four sides of the trauma patient in your search for holes. Identify puncture wounds and consider their pathways. Ask yourself: What structures lie in the way? Is there an exit wound (or is it just another hole)?

CLINICAL CLUE

Not All Damage Can Be Seen

Bullets often enter the body, cause damage as they traverse through tissue, and then exit the body. The terms entry wound and exit wound are commonly used to describe this pattern of injury. However, as an EMT you should never speculate and never document wounds as either "entry" or "exit." You should simply note the locations of the wounds. Because gunshot wounds are always subject to investigation by law enforcement, your documentation of a wound as "entry" or "exit" could contradict the subsequent expert determination by a forensic specialist and complicate legal proceedings.

Emergency Care of Open Abdominal Injuries

Most bleeding in an abdominal injury will be internal. Usually, direct pressure does little to stop it, and the most important treatment is getting your patient to an operating room. Remember that abdominal wounds can frequently impact the chest cavity as well. You should consider an occlusive dressing for any abdominal injury that could include a threat to the integrity of the chest. In the event of an evisceration, treat the wound carefully to prevent further damage (again, remember that this may be the least life-threatening problem associated with the injury).

Follow these steps when caring for an abdominal evisceration (Scan 33-1):

1. Take appropriate BSI precautions.
2. Manage the ABCs as appropriate.
3. Administer supplemental oxygen.
4. Protect the organs by covering them with a large sterile dressing moistened with sterile saline. Do not touch the protruding organs with your hands, if it can be avoided. Do not attempt to reinsert the organs into the abdomen.
5. Place plastic over the moistened dressings to seal in the moisture.
6. Control external bleeding as appropriate.
7. When possible, place the patient in a supine position with his knees bent. This will reduce pressure on the abdominal muscles.
8. Care for shock and transport immediately.
9. Initiate an ALS intercept if available.

Occasionally, penetrating abdominal injury will include an impaled object such as a knife. Do not remove impaled objects from the abdomen or chest because they may actually be preventing internal bleeding. Removal could open previously occluded holes and lead to rapid blood loss. In most cases the removal of an impaled object requires surgical intervention. Rapid transport to an appropriate destination is therefore essential. Stabilize the impaled object to prevent movement. This can be accomplished by placing bulky dressings on either side of the object and securing it with tape.

As with other abdominal injuries, assume the worst. It is very difficult to assess the extent of an open abdominal injury by looking at the exterior. Assume internal bleeding. Initiate rapid transport and reassess frequently.

SCAN 33-1 Dressing an Abdominal Evisceration

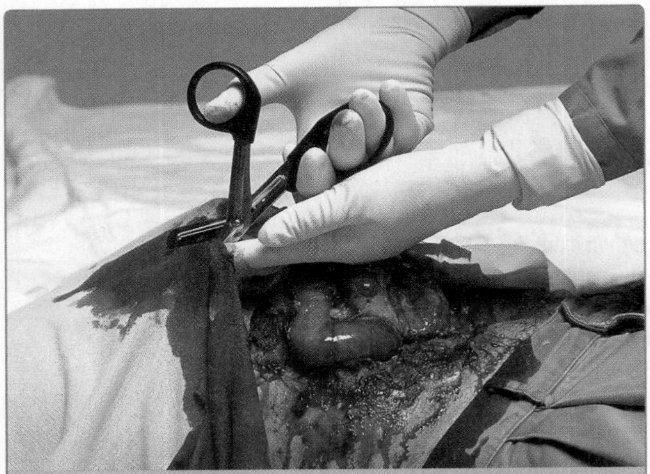

33-1-1 Expose the evisceration.

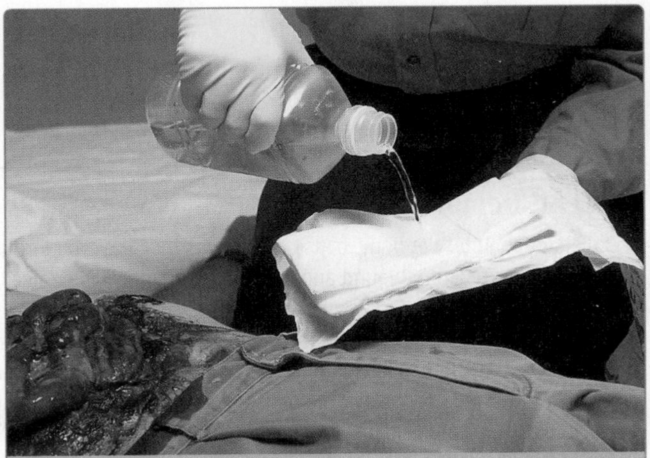

33-1-2 Moisten a large sterile dressing.

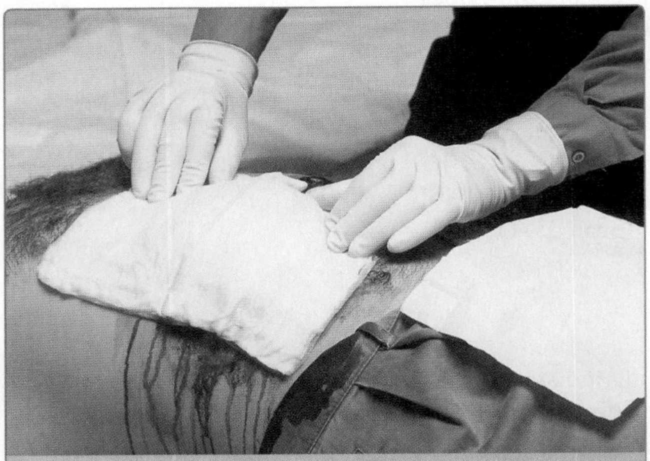

33-1-3 Place the moist dressing over the exposed abdominal contents.

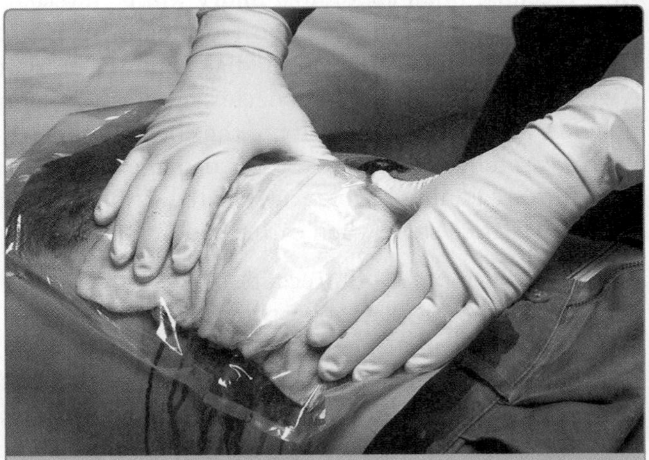

33-1-4 Place a plastic cover over the dressing to contain the moisture.

External Genitalia Trauma

33-14 Explain the special considerations in management of trauma to the male and female genitalia.

Injury to the external genitalia, both male and female, is rarely life threatening but considered significant nonetheless. Such injuries are painful, embarrassing, and potentially life altering. Care should be taken to address both the physical and emotional issues surrounding them.

Both female and male external genitalia are rich in blood supply and can bleed heavily when damaged. Always consider hemorrhage as your most immediate physical concern. If necessary, use direct pressure and absorbent dressings to control blood loss.

A major concern regarding external genitalia trauma is sexual assault. Each year there are nearly 200,000 rapes and sexual assaults reported in the United States and, unfortunately, it is estimated that more that 50% of them go unreported to authorities. The statistics suggest that as an EMS provider you will likely encounter such a situation in your career. Because of the prevalence of sexual violence, one must consider sexual assault when dealing with external genitalia trauma. Of course, not all will be related to violence. There are myriad other causes. However, as an EMS provider, you should be suspicious as part of your professional responsibility.

If sexual assault is suspected, law enforcement should be requested. Remember, in these cases there are evidentiary concerns. As a health care provider, your first responsibility is treatment of the patient but, when possible, you should respect the integrity of the crime scene. That means, if possible, do not allow the victim to wash or change clothes. Do not disturb the setting of the crime scene more than necessary. Be sure to document thoroughly and objectively.

A victim of sexual assault may have both physical and emotional injuries. Be sensitive and nonjudgmental. Again, offer medical assistance first, but also be prepared to offer psychosocial referrals as well. At a minimum, transport will typically offer hospital-based psychosocial resources, but also keep in mind the support resources in your community. Many advocacy groups offer EMS training and can help you offer referrals to victims. Each case presents unique challenges and you should know your own limitations.

When deciding who will obtain a history and physical exam from a suspected sexual assault victim, consider using a same gender EMT for this purpose. A female patient is likely going to be more receptive to a female EMT. You must also carefully consider cultural differences when it becomes necessary to assess and care for injuries to the genitalia.

Know the laws in your state for reporting crimes. You may be legally obligated to report suspected sexual assault and certainly crimes of abuse involving minors.

Vaginal Bleeding

Vaginal bleeding can occur from injury to external genitalia or as a result of internal injuries. Providers should recognize this type of hemorrhage as a concerning indicator of internal bleeding. In trauma, vaginal bleeding can be a sign of a ruptured pregnant uterus or the result of bony fragments from a severe pelvic fracture lacerating the inside wall of the vagina. Providers should consider the mechanism of injury as well as other findings when assessing vaginal bleeding. If bleeding is suspected to be the result of internal injuries, immediate and appropriate transport is vital.

External vaginal bleeding can be the result of sexual assault or a variety of other traumatic mechanisms. The classic mechanism that results in external bleeding from the vaginal area is a "straddle" injury. For example, a straddle injury occurs when a child runs on a pool edge and slips with one leg going into the pool and the other staying on the deck, resulting in direct impact to the vaginal area.

If bleeding is severe, consider using an absorbent pad to contain hemorrhage. Direct pressure may be applied, if necessary. Providers should never insert anything into the vagina itself.

STOP, REVIEW, REMEMBER!

Multiple Choice

For each question, place a check next to the correct answer.

1. An open wound to the abdomen that results in the abdominal contents protruding through the wound is known as a(n):
   _____ a. pneumothorax.
   _____ b. hemothorax.
   _____ c. dissection.
   _____ d. evisceration.

2. A 19-year-old man presents with a loop of intestine protruding through a large stab wound to his abdomen. After assessing and treating the ABCs, you should:
   _____ a. push the intestine back into the abdominal cavity.
   _____ b. apply dry sterile dressings over the intestine.
   _____ c. apply moistened dressings over the intestine.
   _____ d. not apply a dressing over the intestine.

3. The structure that separates the thoracic cavity from the abdomen is the:
   _____ a. lung.
   _____ b. heart.
   _____ c. diaphragm.
   _____ d. stomach.

4. The organs of the abdomen are enclosed in the:
   _____ a. pleura.
   _____ b. perineum.
   _____ c. peritoneum.
   _____ d. retroperitoneal space.

5. A 22-year-old man complains of shoulder pain after being struck in the upper left quadrant of his abdomen with a hockey stick. Which one of the following best explains this patient's shoulder pain?
   _____ a. Referred pain from an injury to his spleen
   _____ b. Referred pain from an injury to his ovary
   _____ c. Secondary shoulder injury after the initial hit
   _____ d. Chronic shoulder injury exacerbated by the hit

Matching

Match the abdominal organ on the left with the function on the right.

1. _____ Stomach	A. Stores bile and aids in fat digestion
2. _____ Gall bladder	B. Removes water from waste and moves waste to the rectum
3. _____ Liver	C. Has no known function
4. _____ Pancreas	D. Removes nutrients from waste
5. _____ Spleen	E. Detoxifies
6. _____ Large intestine	F. Filters red blood cells
7. _____ Small intestine	G. Secretes insulin
	H. Collects food from the esophagus; acid-secreting organ

Critical Thinking

1. Why is there a difference in care between an open and a closed abdominal wound?

____

____

____

____

2. For each abdominal quadrant, list an organ found within it.

   a. Right upper quadrant: ______________________

   b. Left upper quadrant: ______________________

   c. Right lower quadrant: ______________________

   d. Left lower quadrant: ______________________

EMERGENCY DISPATCH SUMMARY

Nancy and Brandi quickly covered the protruding intestine with moistened dressings and the wound with an occlusive dressing. The patient was rapidly transferred to the ambulance for transport. A police officer came along to help out in the back. As the police officer ventilated the patient, Nancy called the hospital. She wanted to give the trauma team as much notice as possible. On reassessment, Nancy recognized that they had lost the patient's pulse. She began chest compressions while the police officer continued to ventilate. The hospital trauma team met them in the ambulance bay and the patient was swiftly moved to the trauma room. Although the team worked valiantly in a resuscitation effort, the injuries were just too significant. The trauma coordinator came in to the EMS room as Nancy and Brandi were finishing their documentation of the call. He thanked them for the work they had done and noted that the stab wound had severed a large blood vessel in the abdomen as well as causing a tension pneumothorax after apparently piercing the diaphragm. The two EMTs discussed the call and recognized that even though their care was appropriate, there was little that could have been done to save this patient.

Chapter Review

To the Point

- The chest and abdomen contain many vital structures necessary to sustain life.
- Injury to the vital structures of the chest and abdomen can rapidly lead to life-threatening problems.
- Understanding anatomy and physiology will improve your assessment of patients with chest and abdominal injuries.
- When assessing the mechanism of injury, use the anatomical location of underlying chest and abdominal structures to help focus your assessment and predict injuries.
- A closed chest or abdominal injury suggests that the force has not penetrated the outer walls.

- An open chest or abdominal injury suggests penetrating trauma.
- With chest injuries, always assess impact on breathing. Guard against respiratory failure.
- Remember that certain injuries to the heart and lungs, such as contusions, pneumothorax, and pericardial tamponade develop over time. Understand their common presentations and use reassessment to identify them.
- With abdominal injuries, the largest risk factor is internal bleeding. Use your primary assessment to rule out shock in all patients with an abdominal mechanism of injury.
- In many cases of both chest and abdominal injury, prehospital treatment is very limited. Anticipate the need for surgical intervention and initiate rapid and appropriate transport.

Chapter Questions

Multiple Choice

For each question, place a check next to the correct answer.

1. The left lung has ____________lobe(s).

_____ a. one
_____ b. two
_____ c. three
_____ d. four

2. A 35-year-old man has been stabbed in the chest. Your assessment reveals narrowing pulse pressure, jugular vein distention, and muffled heart sounds. You should suspect:

_____ a. pericardial tamponade.
_____ b. cardiac contusion.
_____ c. spontaneous pneumothorax.
_____ d. abdominal evisceration.

3. A 17-year-old has been stabbed in the chest. He is alert and complaining of pain and shortness of breath. You note no lung sounds on the right side and his vital signs are pulse 120, respiration 36, and blood pressure 110/68. You should:

_____ a. apply direct pressure over the stab wound.
_____ b. insert bulky dressings into the stab wound.
_____ c. apply an occlusive dressing over the stab wound.
_____ d. leave the stab wound open.

4. A patient with a closed abdominal injury may wish to be placed:

_____ a. in a sitting position.
_____ b. in a supine position.
_____ c. recumbent with knees drawn toward the chest.
_____ d. sitting or supine with legs extended.

5. A 44-year-old man has fallen from a tree and is complaining of pain in his chest. On inspection, you note deformity and paradoxical movement on his right side. You should:

_____ a. apply a sandbag to the patient's right chest to splint the fractures.
_____ b. apply supplemental oxygen and initiate rapid transport.
_____ c. use tape to stabilize the ribs.
_____ d. apply a bulky dressing and exert direct pressure on the flail segment.

Fill in the Blank

1. Blood in the sac surrounding the heart is called pericardial ____________.
2. Dressings used to cover abdominal eviscerations are moistened with sterile ____________.
3. The abdominal aorta and kidneys are located in the ____________space.

Critical Thinking

1. You are caring for a patient who has received a stab wound to the upper right quadrant of the abdomen. In what organs should you suspect injury? What are the implications?

2. You are caring for an adult patient who while jogging developed a sudden onset of difficulty breathing. If this patient developed a spontaneous pneumothorax, what signs and symptoms would you expect to see?

3. What is the pulse pressure? Would you expect it to widen or narrow in cases of tension pneumothorax?

Case Study

You are called to a patient who has been involved in a motor-vehicle collision. He was thrown from the vehicle and found about 20 feet from the car. Your scene size-up reveals damage to the steering wheel. There was no air bag deployment.

The patient is unresponsive. After opening and suctioning the airway, while manual stabilization of the spine is maintained, you note that the patient is using accessory muscles to breathe. He appears to have respiratory distress with very rapid, shallow respirations. You observe a depression on the anterior chest that involves the third through seventh ribs on the left side and extends from the anterior axillary line to the sternum.

1. What airway and breathing care would this patient receive?

(continued on next page)

(continued)

2. How would you determine if this patient had a flail segment?

____

____

____

____

3. What injuries could occur within the chest if a broken rib were to cause damage?

____

____

____

____

The Last Word

This chapter covered injuries to two of the most significant regions of the body, the chest and abdomen. When you find a trauma patient in shock with no open injuries, it is highly likely that there are injuries to one or both of those regions. They contain organs that are vital to breathing and circulation. They are also very vascular, meaning they have a rich blood supply and will cause profound internal bleeding when damaged. Your recognition of injuries to the chest and abdomen combined with appropriate emergency care and prompt transportation can make the difference between life and death.

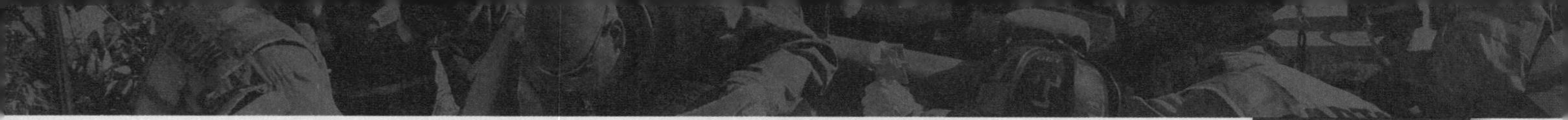

Caring for Patients with Musculoskeletal Injuries

34

Education Standards

Trauma: Orthopedic trauma

Competencies

Applies fundamental knowledge to provide basic emergency care and transportation based on assessment findings for an acutely injured patient.

Objectives

After completion of this lesson, you should be able to:

34-1 Define key terms introduced in this chapter.

34-2 Describe the structures and functions of the musculoskeletal system, including bones, skeletal muscle, tendons, ligaments, cartilage, and joints.

34-3 Give examples of direct, indirect, and twisting forces that can produce musculoskeletal injuries.

34-4 Describe each of the following types of injuries and their associated signs and symptoms: fractures, strains, sprains, and dislocations.

34-5 Describe the assessment-based approach to bone and joint injuries.

34-6 Establish the priority for assessing and treating musculoskeletal injuries with respect to a patient's overall condition.

34-7 Discuss the significance of assessing a musculoskeletal injury for each of the following findings: pain, pallor, paralysis, paresthesia, and pulses.

34-8 Explain the rationale for splinting musculoskeletal injuries.

34-9 Describe the term *position of function* and the role that it plays during immobilization.

34-10 Describe the characteristics and uses of various types of splints, including the air (pneumatic) splint, long backboard, rigid splint, sling and swathe, traction splint, and vacuum splint.

34-11 Discuss special considerations in splinting pelvic fractures.

34-12 Discuss hazards of improper splinting.

34-13 Describe the basic pathophysiology of compartment syndrome.

Key Terms

cartilage p. 870
closed skeletal injury p. 875
compartment syndrome p. 896
direct force p. 871
dislocation p. 875
fracture p. 875
indirect force p. 872
ligaments p. 870
open skeletal injury p. 875
parasthesia p. 878
position of function p. 883
sprain p. 873
strain p. 873
tendons p. 870
twisting force p. 873

Introduction

Injuries to muscles and bones are some of the most commonly seen injuries encountered by EMTs. While certainly painful, isolated injuries to muscles and bones are rarely an immediate life threat. Because many patients will require further medical care, it will be necessary to prepare them properly for transport to an appropriate receiving facility. That includes an appropriate assessment and careful immobilization of the injury to minimize pain and further injury. This chapter describes some of the more common types of musculoskeletal injuries and how they occur, and offers guidelines for proper immobilization.

EMERGENCY DISPATCH

"Do you think it's broken?" The young man, still sweating and out of breath, was sitting on the living room floor in obvious pain. "I felt it pop, but it could just be dislocated, right?"

EMTs Jeri Turner and Pat Shipley had been dispatched to a residence for a leg injury. It turned out to be a painfully small apartment crowded with teens, all trying to hide alcohol bottles as the firefighters, EMTs, and police officers squeezed in. One of the teens had wisely called 911.

"So what happened exactly?" Pat asked as he pulled scissors from his belt and began cutting the patient's pant leg to better expose the injury site.

"David, uh, was showing us some new dance moves," a girl said as she tried to hide a smile behind her hand.

"This damn carpet caught my shoe." The patient pointed down angrily. "And it ain't funny!" Some in the crowd started to laugh and one young man began to lurch around the cramped room, imitating the patient's dance moves. By the time he grabbed his knee and dramatically fell to the floor, everyone, including the patient and many of the emergency personnel, were laughing.

"Okay, okay," the injured teen nodded. "So, it was stupid. But is it bad? Could it just be a sprain or something?"

"Well," Pat palpated the patient's knee. "It is certainly swollen, but that doesn't always mean anything. Let's get you to the hospital so you can get an X-ray. The police officer will give your parents a call to let them know we are on the way to the hospital."

Review of the Musculoskeletal System

34-2 Describe the structures and functions of the musculoskeletal system, including bones, skeletal muscle, tendons, ligaments, cartilage, and joints.

Now is a good time to review the musculoskeletal system (Figure 34-1 ■) in this section and in Chapter 5 for more details. Though it is not essential for you to know the name of each and every bone in the body, it is important to become familiar with all the major bones and their functions. That knowledge will allow you to better assess, describe, and document the injuries you manage.

The musculoskeletal system is made up of the bones and the muscles of the body. Muscles are attached to bone, and together both give us our basic form. The skeletal system consists of all 206 bones as well as the **ligaments** that help hold the bones of the skeleton together. **Cartilage,** another component of the skeletal system, is a tough elastic connective tissue found in various parts of the body such as the joints, ears, nose, and larynx. **Tendons** connect muscle to bone, allowing for movement (Figure 34-2 ■).

ligaments tissues that connect the bones of the skeleton.

cartilage tough elastic connective tissue found in various parts of the body such as the joints, ears, nose, and larynx.

tendons tissues that connect muscle to the skeleton.

Bones are made up of dense, semirigid living tissue and serve many purposes other than just structure and support. They come in many shapes and sizes. Some bones are long and thin (extremities), while others are short and wide (vertebrae). Each has a specific purpose such as movement, protection, or support, based on its specific location and structure.

Ligaments are the tough fibrous tissues that connect two or more bones at a joint (Figure 34-3 ■). When joints become injured, ligaments can become stretched or torn, making the joint unstable. An injury to a ligament is commonly referred to as a *sprain*.

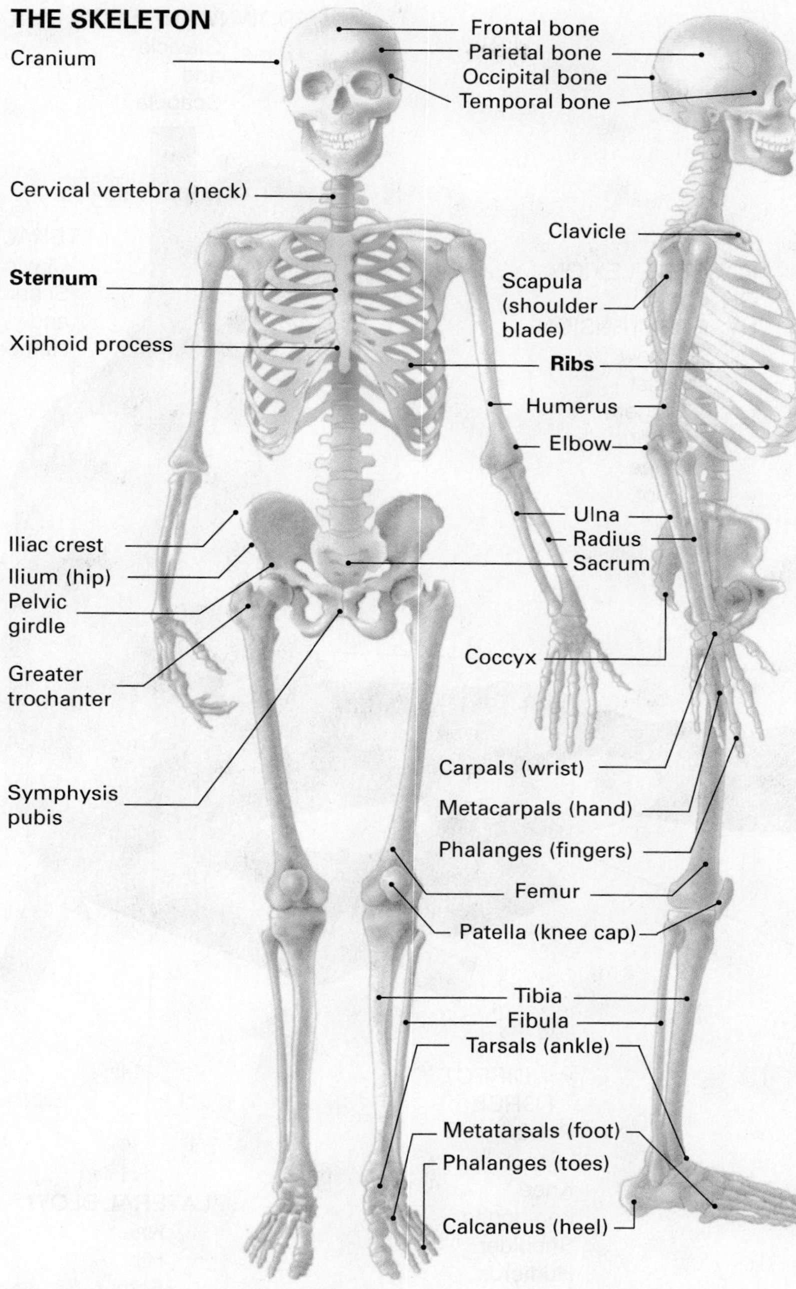

Figure 34-1 Major bones of the human skeleton.

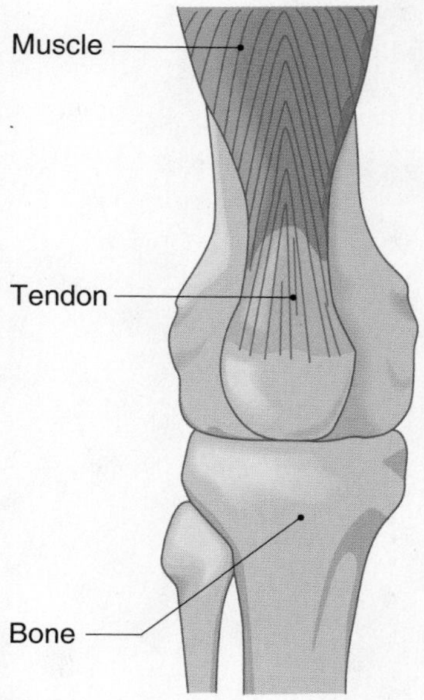

Figure 34-2 Tendons are the structures that connect muscle to bone.

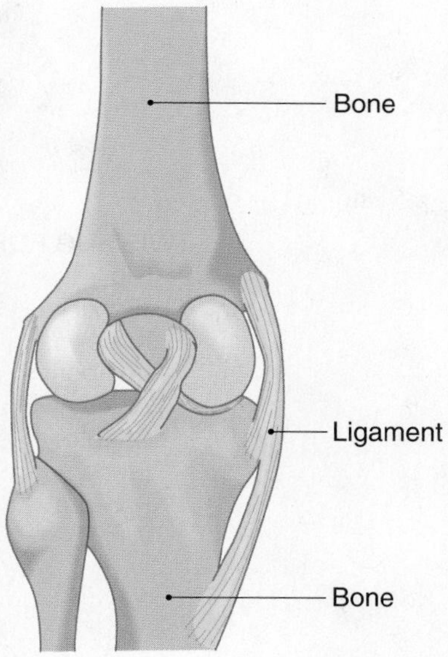

Figure 34-3 Ligaments are the structures that connect bones together at a joint.

Musculoskeletal Injuries

Injuries to the musculoskeletal system involve damage to soft tissues, bones, and joints in any combination.

34-4 Describe each of the following types of injuries and their associated signs and symptoms: fractures, strains, sprains, and dislocations.

Common Mechanisms of Injury

In most cases, the type and extent of a musculoskeletal injury depends on the mechanism and forces involved. The most common forces responsible for musculoskeletal injuries are direct, indirect, and twisting (Figure 34-4 ■).

34-3 Give examples of direct, indirect, and twisting forces that can produce musculoskeletal injuries.

Direct force is caused by a direct blow to an area of the body. Most blunt trauma is caused by direct force of some kind. An arm struck by a baseball bat and a leg struck by the bumper of a car are examples of direct-force mechanisms. The extent of injury

direct force the force caused by a direct blow to an area of the body.

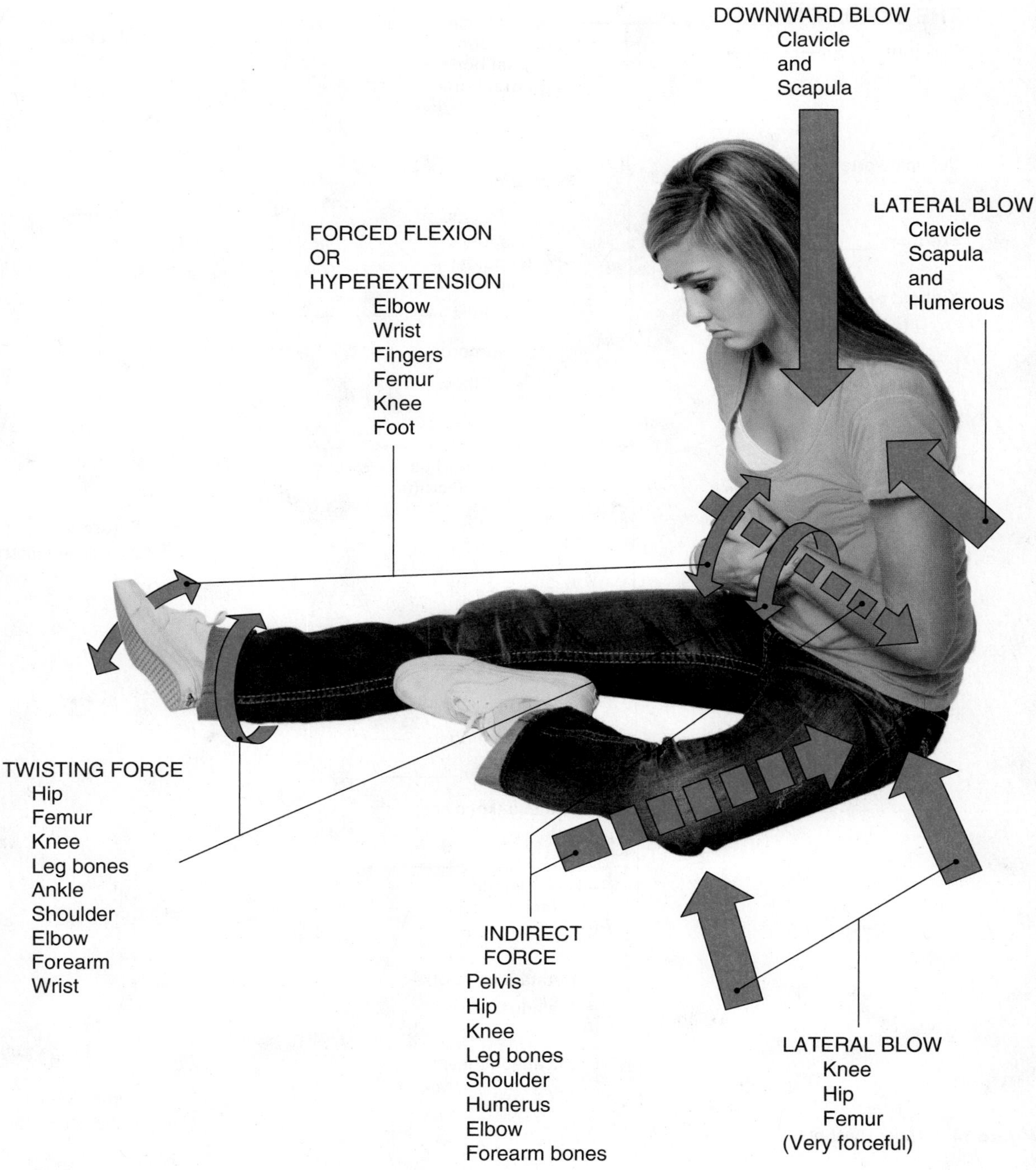

Figure 34-4 Common mechanisms of musculoskeletal injury. (© Edward T. Dickinson, MD)

depends on the amount of force. If the force is significant enough, damage to the bone underlying the point of impact is likely.

indirect force the force that occurs when energy is transferred along a bone, usually proximal to the site of impact.

An injury caused by **indirect force** occurs when the energy of the force is transferred along a bone, usually proximal to the site of impact. One of the most common causes of indirect-force injury is a person falling on outstretched hands in an attempt to break his fall. This kind of fall can cause a direct-force injury to the wrist. In some cases, it also causes indirect-force injury to the elbow, clavicle, or shoulder because the energy from the impact is transferred along the arm to the elbow or shoulder. Another common cause of indirect-force injury is the knees of an unrestrained occupant in a vehicle collision striking the dashboard. The knees take the direct force, but the energy is transferred along the femur, frequently causing injury to the hip.

Among the most common **twisting force** injuries is the twisted ankle or twisted neck. The force is applied as the foot, for example, stays firmly planted while the rest of the body twists around the foot, causing damage to the foot, the ankle, and the lower leg.

twisting force the force that occurs when one end of a limb is stationary and the other end moves in a circle.

PERSPECTIVE

David—The Patient

Oh, man, that hurt! I was just messing around, and I tried to do this spin move, but my sneaker had a better grip on the carpet than I thought. Everything above my knee spun. Everything below it didn't. For a split second I actually thought I broke my leg off! And of course it doesn't help when all of your friends are laughing at you too hard to help.

Soft-Tissue Injuries

A **strain** occurs when a muscle is pulled or torn. This is likely to cause moderate to severe pain. However, isolated muscle injuries of this kind generally are not justification for calling an ambulance. A **sprain** is another injury that involves soft tissues. Sprains can occur anywhere there is a joint, resulting in the stretching or tearing of the ligaments that support the joint. A sprained ankle is a good example of this type of injury.

strain injury caused when a muscle is pulled or torn, causing severe pain.

sprain injury caused by the stretching or tearing of the ligaments and tendons that support the joint.

Most victims of injuries that involve the soft tissues of the musculoskeletal system self-treat their injuries, using elevation and ice to help reduce the pain and swelling. In some cases, the pain is so great that there is no way to tell if it is a soft-tissue injury or a bone injury. In situations such as this, you must assume the worst and provide care for a suspected fracture. (This will be discussed a little later in this chapter.)

PERSPECTIVE

Pat—The EMT

There was definitely swelling around the guy's knee, but I didn't notice crepitus or any glaring instability or deformity. Who knows what he did to it. It's hard to respond when patients want a diagnosis. I do not diagnose. Or what's even worse is when you're sure it's a fracture and you say that in your verbal report to the emergency department, but you turn out to be wrong. Nowadays, unless I can see the end of a bone sticking through the patient's skin, all I ever say is that the injury has "swelling, pain, and deformity."

STOP, REVIEW, REMEMBER!

Multiple Choice

For each question, place a check next to the correct answer.

1. Which one of the following structures is made of a tough fibrous tissue that surrounds a joint and connects two or more bones together?

_____ a. Cartilage

_____ b. Tendon

_____ c. Ligament

_____ d. Metacarpal

2. Which one of the following connects each muscle to the skeleton and allows for movement?

_____ a. Cartilage

_____ b. Tendons

_____ c. Ligaments

_____ d. Metatarsals

(continued on next page)

(continued)

3. An injury to the wrist as a result of a fall onto outstretched hands is caused by which type of force?

_____ a. Direct force

_____ b. Indirect force

_____ c. Twisting force

_____ d. Straight force

4. When a muscle is stretched and torn, the injury is described as a:

_____ a. sprain.

_____ b. fracture.

_____ c. pull.

_____ d. strain.

5. Which one of the following injuries occurs anywhere there is a joint and often results in the stretching or tearing of the ligaments that support the joint?

_____ a. Sprains

_____ b. Fractures

_____ c. Pulls

_____ d. Strains

Labeling

Using the illustration, correctly label all the major bones of the human skeleton.

THE SKELETON

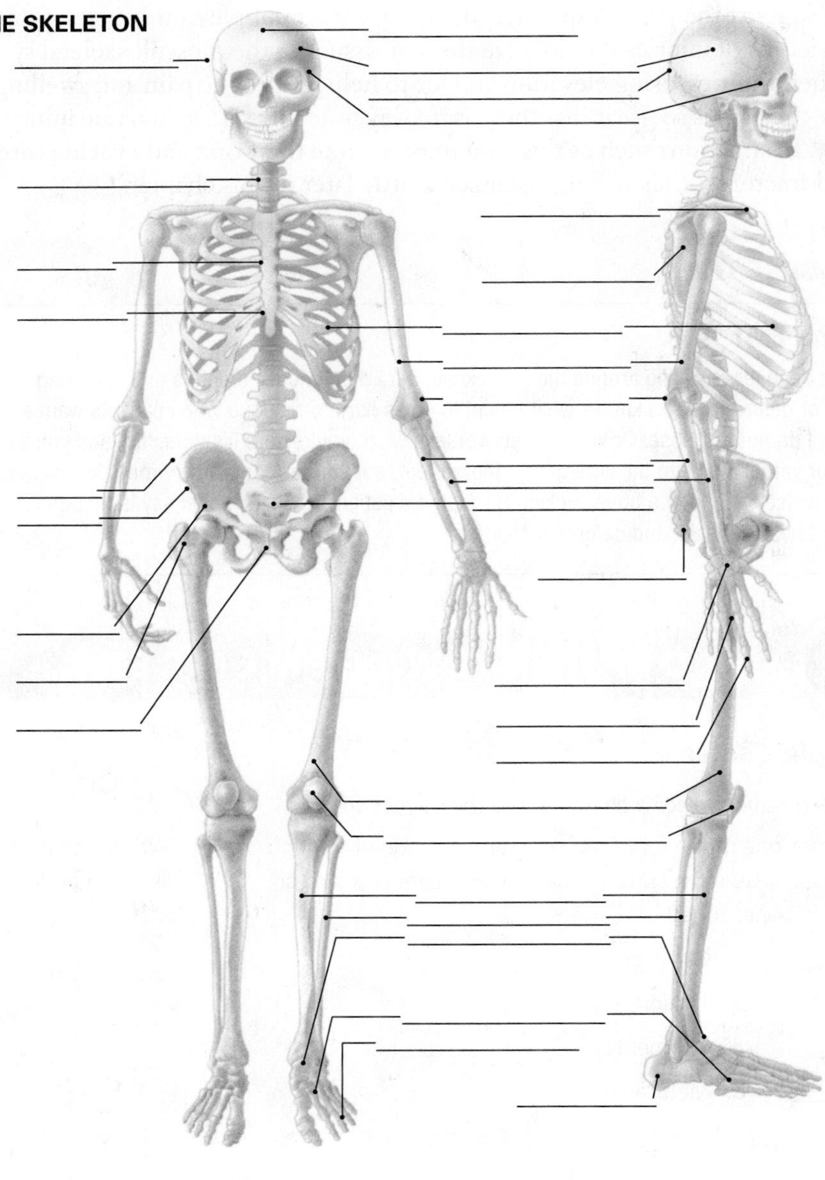

Critical Thinking

1. Describe the difference between a strain and a sprain.

____

____

____

____

Skeletal Injuries

Skeletal injuries are most commonly **fractures** or **dislocations.** Fractures are broken bones and can be as minor as a hairline crack to a badly shattered and deformed extremity. The most common symptom of a skeletal fracture is pain. For this reason, you should consider all complaints of skeletal pain to be suspected fractures and provide the appropriate care. Dislocations are displacements of the bones that make up a joint, such as the finger, elbow, shoulder, knee, or hip (Figure 34-5 ■).

Injuries involving joints can result in sprains, fractures, dislocations, or any combination. Injured joints require special attention and care because of the unique function of the joint and the fact that most joints are surrounded by a large supply of vessels and nerves. Damage to joints places those vessels and nerves at great risk of injury as well.

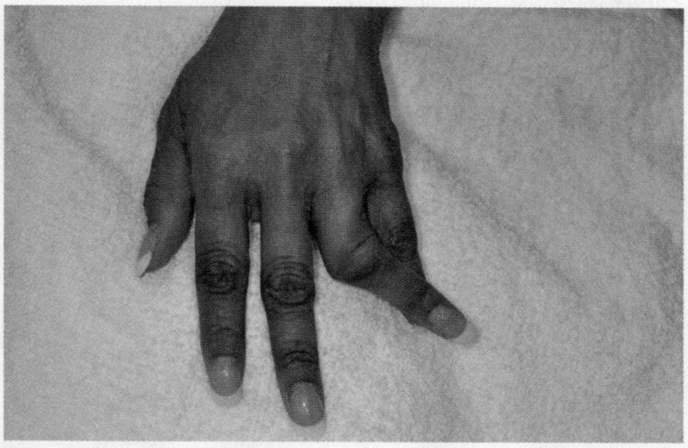

Figure 34-5 Deformity caused by a dislocated finger joint. (© Edward T. Dickinson, MD)

fracture broken bone; can be as minor as a hairline crack all the way to a badly shattered bone that appears deformed.

dislocation displacement of the bones that make up a joint, such as the elbow, shoulder, knee, or hip.

PRACTICAL PATHOPHYSIOLOGY

Large bones such as the femurs and pelvis have large arteries and veins required for perfusion of the bone tissue. When those structures are damaged, bleeding can be quite severe and even life threatening. Maintain a high index of suspicion for internal bleeding and carefully manage injuries to minimize movement during transport.

Skeletal injuries are further classified as open or closed (Figure 34-6 ■). A **closed skeletal injury** is one that is not associated with any break in the overlying skin (Figure 34-7 ■). An **open skeletal injury** occurs when the skin is damaged, causing an open soft-tissue wound in connection with the skeletal injury (Figure 34-8 ■). For instance, the force of the injury can break a bone end, which can then penetrate the skin, causing an open wound in close proximity to the fracture. Open skeletal injuries also can be caused when a projectile such as a bullet penetrates the skin and the underlying bone. The risk of complication due to infection is very high with open skeletal injuries. It will be important to immediately control any severe bleeding with sterile dressings.

closed skeletal injury skeletal injury not associated with any break in the overlying skin.

open skeletal injury skeletal injury in which the skin is damaged causing an open soft-tissue wound in connection with the injury.

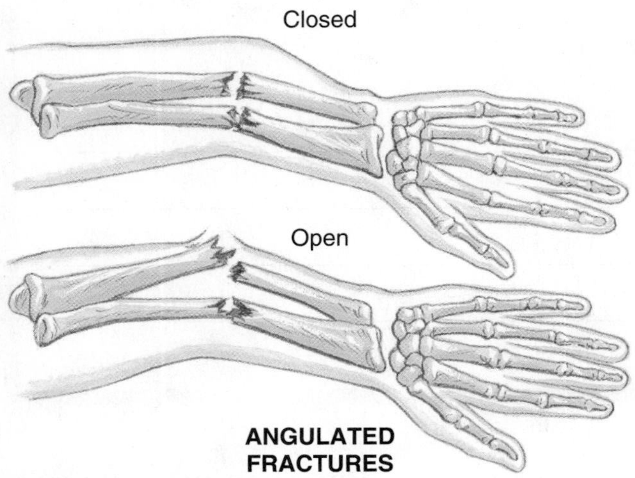

Figure 34-6 Skeletal injuries may be open or closed.

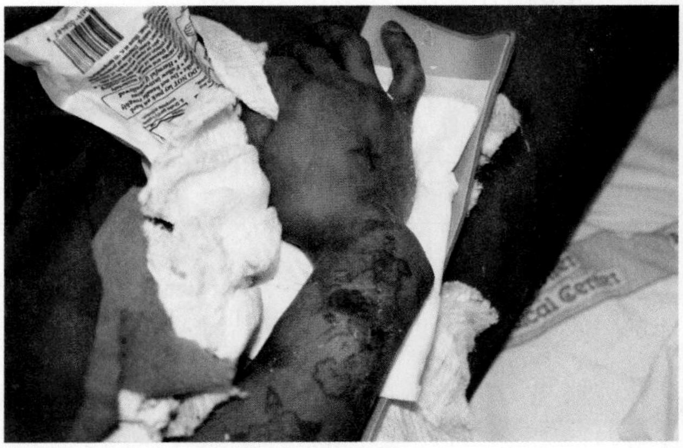

Figure 34-7 Deformity caused by a closed fracture of the wrist. (© Edward T. Dickinson, MD)

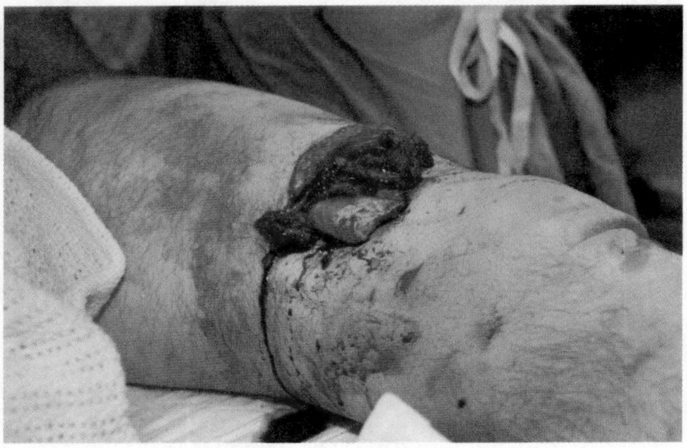

Figure 34-8 An open fracture of the femur. (© Edward T. Dickinson, MD)

CLINICAL CLUE

Suspected Fracture

The term *suspected fracture* is used to describe an injury involving the skeletal system. Because, EMTs do not diagnose, you must use terminology that clearly describes your findings without the appearance of a diagnosis. Even when caring for injuries that present as deformed and angulated, describe and document them as such and refrain from using the word *fracture*, which is a diagnostic term. A possible exception may be an obvious open fracture with bone ends protruding through the wound.

Assessment of Musculoskeletal Injuries

34-5 Describe the assessment-based approach to bone and joint injuries.

34-6 Establish the priority for assessing and treating musculoskeletal injuries with respect to a patient's overall condition.

The assessment of a patient with a suspected musculoskeletal injury begins with an evaluation of the mechanism of injury. As you approach the scene, look for evidence that might suggest the mechanism involved. If it is a vehicle collision, assess the extent of damage to both the inside and outside of the vehicle. If the patient is a victim of a fall, do your best to determine how far he fell, how he may have landed, and what type of surface he landed on. All of those factors will help determine the overall mechanism of injury. Remember to consider the need for spinal immobilization if the mechanism of injury suggests it, even if the chief complaint is simply an extremity injury.

Although musculoskeletal injuries can sometimes be grotesque, do not allow them to distract you from the more important assessment and management of the patient's ABCs. Once you have completed your primary assessment and there are no other immediate life threats to the patient, you must focus your assessment on the chief complaint. Remember to perform an appropriate rapid secondary assessment for any patient who has suffered a significant mechanism of injury. A patient with a low-energy mechanism of injury with a resultant isolated injury to an extremity should receive a focused secondary assessment of the affected extremity.

PERSPECTIVE

Jeri—The EMT

The patient and his friends told us that he just sat down on the floor after twisting his knee, so there was really no need to worry about spinal immobilization. With most falls, though, I usually use the backboard. I had a patient a few years ago who was hanging a picture in his den, was just standing on his tiptoes, and then lost his balance and fell. He denied any back or neck pain, and we all got a little too focused on this open fracture of his wrist. It wasn't until we were transferring him to the bed in the emergency department that his extremities started going numb. It turned out that he had actually fractured his neck. He came out of it okay, but I never take chances now.

CLINICAL CLUE

Skeletal Injury

Do not let the sight of serious skeletal injuries distract you from your priorities of care. Regardless of the injuries, you must always begin with the primary assessment and confirm the adequacy of the ABCs.

34-7 Discuss the significance of assessing a musculoskeletal injury for each of the following findings: pain, pallor, paralysis, paresthesia, and pulses.

When performing a focused assessment of an injured area, begin by attempting to determine where the pain is centered. To do this, ask the patient to point with one finger to where it hurts the most. Next, you must expose the area and observe for any signs of possible skeletal injury. Signs and symptoms of a musculoskeletal injury include the following:

- Pain and tenderness
- Deformity (swelling or angulation)
- Discoloration (redness, pallor, or bruising)
- Open wounds and external bleeding
- Exposed bone
- Crepitation (grating sound)
- Locked joint (unable to move)

Palpate the area gently to pinpoint the suspected injury site. Palpate distal and proximal to the injury site, assessing for additional injury that may have been caused by indirect force. Be sure to assess any joint that may be distal or proximal to the injury site. A joint that is injured may be stuck in a fixed position and unable to move freely. Ask the patient if he can move the joint on his own. Do *not* force an injured joint that is painful or difficult to move. Severe and permanent damage could result. If the patient is unable to move the joint, immobilize it in the position in which it is found. (More will be discussed on immobilization later in this chapter.)

PRACTICAL PATHOPHYSIOLOGY

Long bones, such as the femur and humerus, have a neurovascular bundle made up of a nerve, an artery, and a vein that run parallel closely along the surface of the bone. Because of this close proximity, fractures can readily damage those structures. Extremity injuries can present with paresthesia (numbness and decreased sensation) secondary to direct nerve damage as well as circulatory compromise due to damaged blood vessels. However, the presence of paresthesia can indicate a possible spinal-cord injury. Carefully evaluate the MOI when caring for patients with musculoskeletal injuries.

Assessing the Distal Extremity

When assessing extremity injuries, you must always check the distal extremity for the presence of adequate circulation, sensation, and motor function (CSM). This can be accomplished by assessing for the presence of a radial pulse in the wrists or the

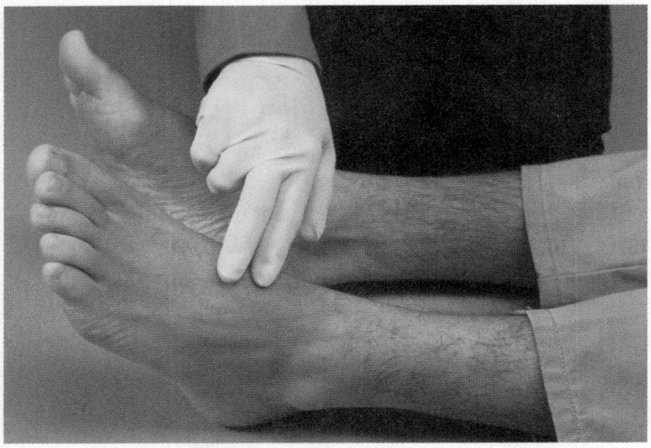

Figure 34-9 Checking distal pulses to ensure adequate circulation.

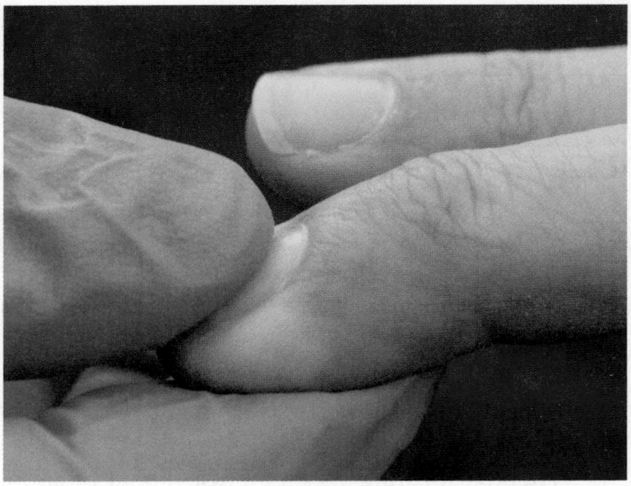

Figure 34-10 Capillary refill is another way to assess distal circulation in an extremity.

pedal pulse in the feet (Figure 34-9 ■). In some patients it may be difficult to find a distal pulse in the foot. In such cases, it is a good idea to also check capillary refill as a backup to the pulses (Figure 34-10 ■). The presence of capillary refill, even in the absence of a pulse, is an indication that the limb has some degree of circulation. Pallor or pale skin may be an indication of inadequate circulation.

If the injury is angulated and you cannot confirm the presence of circulation either by palpating a pulse or seeing capillary refill, you may have to straighten the extremity. Advise the patient of what you are planning to do before moving the limb. Support the extremity with both hands and carefully straighten the limb while pulling gentle traction. Reassess CSM after the extremity has been straightened. Follow local protocols regarding the straightening of an angulated extremity.

You will then assess sensation by asking the patient if, without looking, he can feel you touching his fingers or toes. A change in sensation such as numbness, burning, or tingling is known as **paresthesia.** Have him identify the specific toe or finger you are touching. Ask him if he has normal feeling or if he feels numbness or tingling as you palpate the fingers and toes.

paresthesia a sensation of tingling, burning, pricking, or numbness in an extremity.

CLINICAL CLUE

Distal Foot Pulse

It is a good idea to mark with a pen the location where the distal pulse in the foot is found. This will be a reminder to keep that area accessible as you splint. It also will make it easier to locate during your reassessment of CSM.

PERSPECTIVE

Pat—The EMT

The first thing I did after looking at his knee was to check for a pedal pulse. I tell you, sometimes those are really difficult to find. It can take such a light touch, and just when you think you've got it, it rolls away. I've started drawing a little "X" on the top of the patient's foot where I found the pulse. It makes it easier to find again during reassessment and it seems that the emergency department docs appreciate it, too.

Check motor function of the feet by having the patient push down against your hands simultaneously with both feet (Figure 34-11 ■). Then have them pull up against your hands. This must be done with both sides at the same time in order to detect slight differences in strength. When assessing the hands, have the patient grip the thumbs or fingers of both your hands simultaneously (Figure 34-12 ■). You should be

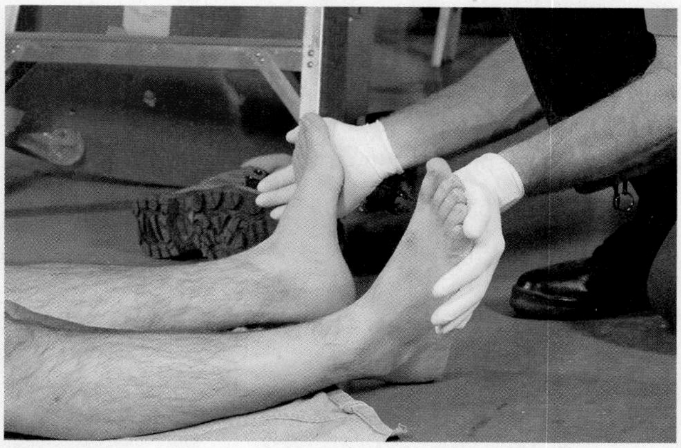

Figure 34-11 Assess motor function of the feet by having the patient push and pull against your hands.

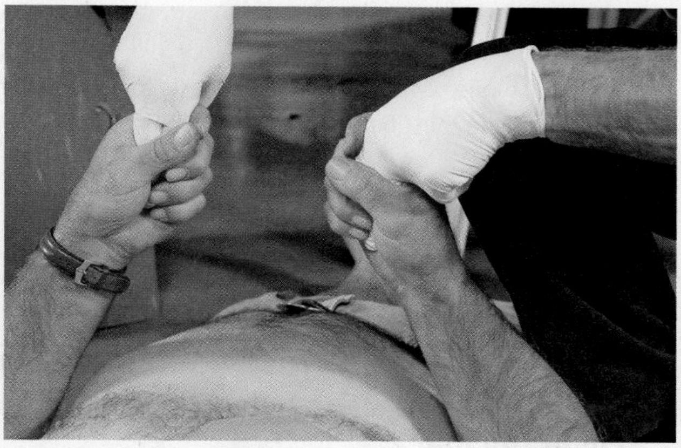

Figure 34-12 Assess motor function of the hands by having the patient squeeze your hands.

aware that many times the ability to move the hands and feet on the injured side will be less than the noninjured side. This is commonly due to the pain involved and not always an indication of nerve damage or spine injury.

CLINICAL CLUE

Assessing Sensation

While most patients can easily tell which finger you are touching without looking, they may have difficulty differentiating which toe is being touched. This is common and normal. When assessing sensation in the feet, choose either the big or little toe when asking the patient which toe you are touching.

STOP, REVIEW, REMEMBER!

Multiple Choice

For each question, place a check next to the correct answer.

1. An injury to the bones of the forearm that was caused by a gunshot would be an example of a(n):

_____ a. closed skeletal injury.

_____ b. open skeletal injury.

_____ c. dislocation.

_____ d. strain.

2. The risk of complication due to infection is very high with:

_____ a. long-bone splint injuries.

_____ b. joint and ligament injuries.

_____ c. open skeletal injuries.

_____ d. closed skeletal injuries.

3. The assessment of a patient with a suspected musculoskeletal injury begins with a(n):

_____ a. evaluation of the mechanism of injury.

_____ b. evaluation of the distal extremity.

_____ c. detailed secondary assessment.

_____ d. rapid trauma assessment.

(continued on next page)

(continued)

4. Which one of the following is specific to an extremity injury and must be assessed *prior to* immobilizing the extremity?

_____ a. ABCs

_____ b. Distal temperature

_____ c. Mental status

_____ d. Circulation, sensation, and motor function

5. Which one of the injuries that follow can occur anywhere there is a joint and often result in the stretching or tearing of the ligaments that support the joint?

_____ a. Sprains

_____ b. Fractures

_____ c. Pulls

_____ d. Strains

Fill in the Blank

1. The most common symptom of a skeletal fracture is ____________________.

2. Injuries involving ____________________ can result in sprains, fractures, dislocations, or any combination.

3. A(n) ____________________ skeletal injury is one that is not associated with any break in the overlying skin.

4. An open skeletal injury occurs when the ____________________ is damaged, causing an open soft-tissue wound in connection with the skeletal injury.

5. The assessment of a patient with a suspected musculoskeletal injury begins with an evaluation of the ____________________.

Critical Thinking

1. How does the care for a suspected joint injury differ from that of a long-bone injury?

____

____

____

____

2. Describe your priorities of care for an open skeletal injury.

____

____

____

____

3. What might it mean if a patient with a suspected fracture has abnormal distal circulation, sensation, or motor function (CSM) findings?

____

____

____

____

Emergency Care for Musculoskeletal Injuries

34-8 Explain the rationale for splinting musculoskeletal injuries.

As noted earlier, it is not the role of the EMT to determine for certain whether a patient has sustained a fracture or simply a sprain or strain. An evaluation of the mechanism of injury along with an appropriate assessment of the injury site should determine the most appropriate care. In most cases, the injury should be treated as a suspected fracture and immobilized accordingly. Once you have conducted an appropriate scene size-up and primary assessment and care for any immediate life threats, you must focus your attention on managing the specific injury. It is important to properly manage all musculoskeletal injuries so you can minimize movement during transport. By immobilizing the injury, you will minimize pain, movement, additional soft-tissue damage, and bleeding.

Follow these steps when caring for a suspected fracture:

1. Take the appropriate BSI precautions.
2. Perform a primary assessment.
3. Expose and assess the injury site and surrounding area.
4. Assess distal circulation, sensation, and motor function (CSM).
5. Immobilize the injury as appropriate.
6. Reassess distal circulation, sensation, and motor function (CSM).
7. Administer oxygen as appropriate.
8. Elevate the extremity if appropriate.
9. Apply a cold pack to the injury site.

The injured extremity should be elevated only after it has been properly immobilized and only if it does not cause further pain for the patient. Gently place a cold pack over or near the injury site to help minimize swelling.

Immobilizing Extremity Injuries

Most patients with skeletal injuries will need more advanced care than can be provided in the field. A thorough evaluation of the injury by a physician and most likely an X-ray will be the minimum care necessary to identify the extent of the injury. For that reason, patients must be transported to an appropriate receiving facility. Transporting patients by ambulance, of course, means subjecting them to movement. Any movement of a patient with skeletal injuries may result in movement of the injury site, which can result in more damage and certainly more pain for the patient. That is why immobilizing the injury is an essential element of proper care for these patients.

Within a few seconds following the injury, a patient will find a position that is most comfortable for his injury. This does *not* mean he is pain free. He is typically self-splinting the injury and has simply found a position that is least painful.

As you approach the patient to begin your assessment, provide care, load him into the ambulance, and transport him to the hospital, you will subject him to movement he cannot control. To minimize complications caused by movement, immobilize the injury prior to transport. The following is a list of complications that can be minimized through proper immobilization of an injury prior to transport:

- Unnecessary pain
- Additional bleeding
- Additional swelling
- Further damage to soft tissues, nerves, and blood vessels
- Creation of an open injury from an existing closed injury
- Paralysis caused from a damaged spinal column

Immobilization can be accomplished using one of two methods—manual stabilization or splinting. Manual stabilization is accomplished by using your gloved hands to stabilize the injury site. This is typically used as an initial step until enough help and supplies are available to properly splint the injury. Splinting involves the application of external devices such as cardboard, wood, or plastic to aid in stabilizing the injury site so that the patient does not have to continue to stabilize it himself.

Splinting does not have to be a complicated process. By following a few simple guidelines, you will be able to quickly and effectively immobilize an injury and minimize discomfort for the patient.

PERSPECTIVE

David—The Patient

At first I thought that they were going to hurt me with that splint. It was just this big, floppy orange thing that they started wrapping around my leg. I didn't know how it would help to hold my leg still. By that time I was in so much pain I really, really needed to keep it still. But then they used this bicycle-pump-looking thing to suck the air out of the splint and, man, it hardened right up and my leg didn't move again until we got to the hospital. My leg was still hurting, but not nearly as much as it had been.

Splinting

The following guidelines should be followed when splinting a suspected skeletal injury:

- Properly assess the injury site by exposing it as appropriate.
- Control any bleeding and cover open wounds with sterile dressings.
- Assess distal circulation, sensation, and motor function before and after splinting, and document any changes.
- Immobilize the injury site.
- Immobilize the joint above and below the injury site.
- Pad all splinting material as appropriate for patient comfort.
- If there is a severe deformity or if the distal extremity is cyanotic or lacks pulses, align to the normal anatomical position with gentle traction before splinting.
- Do not intentionally replace any protruding bones.

As a rule, an injured joint with compromised distal circulation, sensation, or motor function should not be moved in an attempt to restore CSM. If the patient is able to move the limb without too much pain, then allow him to do so and recheck CSM status. Otherwise, immobilize the joint in the position found and transport immediately. For injuries involving long bones, such as the radius, ulna, tibia, or fibula, with compromised CSM, it is appropriate to attempt to straighten the limb into its normal anatomical position.

CLINICAL CLUE

Splint or Not?

When caring for a patient who has sustained a significant mechanism of injury, it is important not to waste valuable time attempting to splint all extremity injuries. Patients who have sustained multisystem trauma or who are presenting with the signs and symptoms of shock should be immobilized on a long backboard and transported as quickly as possible.

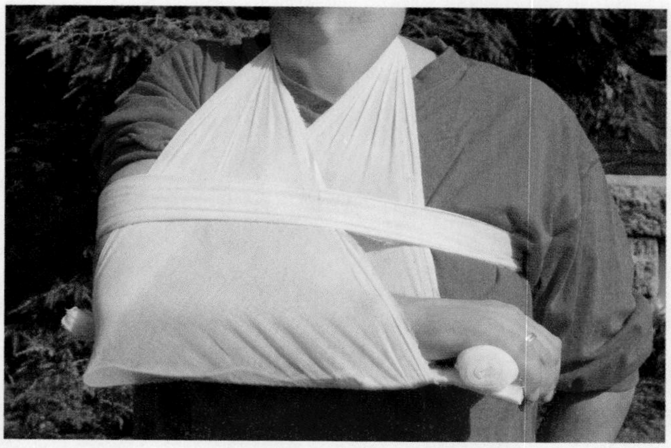

Figure 34-13 The hand immobilized in the position of function.

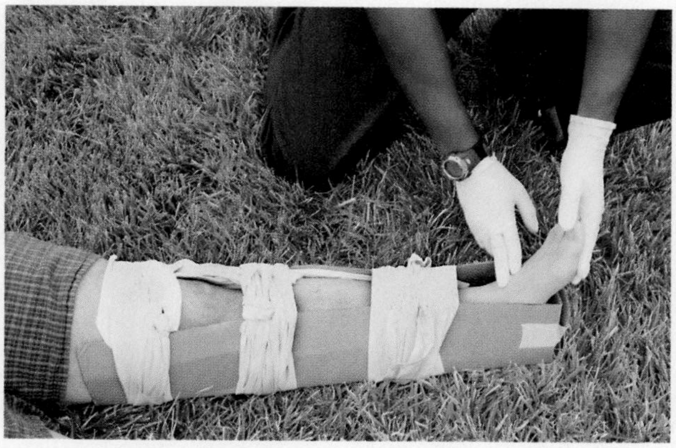

Figure 34-14 A leg immobilized with the foot in the position of function.

Position of Function

The term **position of function** refers to the position of the hands and feet when they are at rest and not under any type of force. When you are placing a splint, it is important for the patient's comfort to maintain the affected hand and foot in the position of function. That can easily be accomplished by placing a four-inch roller bandage or similar item in the hand prior to splinting or by allowing the fingers to curl naturally over the end of the splint (Figure 34-13 ▪). The foot should simply be allowed to rest in the most natural position, not forced into a flexed or extended position (Figure 34-14 ▪).

34-9 Describe the term *position of function* and the role that it plays during immobilization.

position of function position of the hands and feet when they are at rest without any type of force.

Materials Used for Splinting

Just about anything can be used to splint an injury or suspected fracture. The important thing is that you become familiar with the specific tools that will be available to you. By applying the guidelines just outlined, you should be able to utilize any piece of equipment or material at your disposal to properly splint a patient's injuries.

34-10 Describe the characteristics and uses of various types of splints, including air (pneumatic) splint, long backboard, rigid splint, sling and swathe, traction splint, and vacuum splint.

Rigid Splints

As the name suggests, rigid splints are made of rigid material such as wood, cardboard, metal, or plastic (Figure 34-15 ▪). Because they are generally made of a hard material, it is especially important to pad them prior to applying them to a patient.

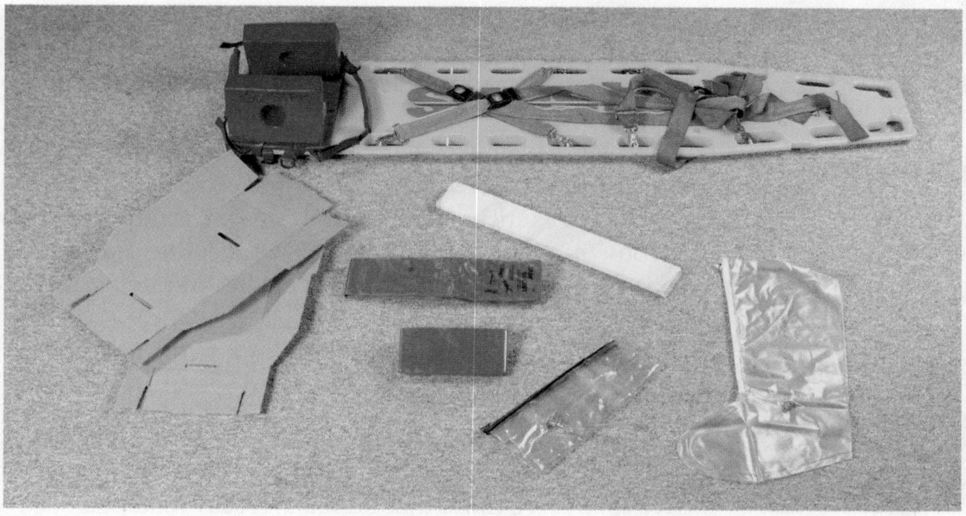

Figure 34-15 Several examples of rigid and pneumatic splints.

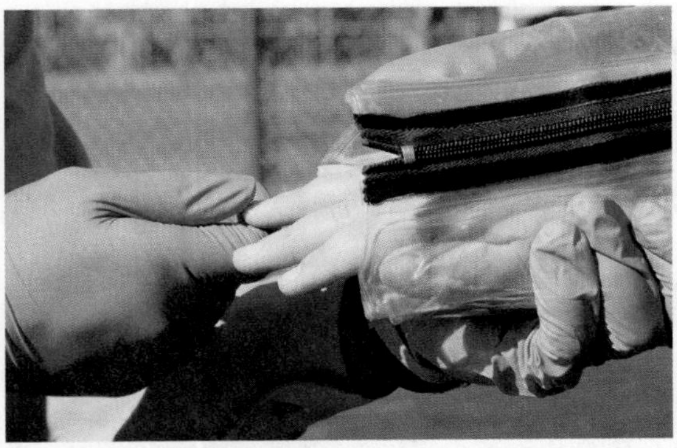

Figure 34-16 A pneumatic splint applied to the arm to immobilize the wrist.

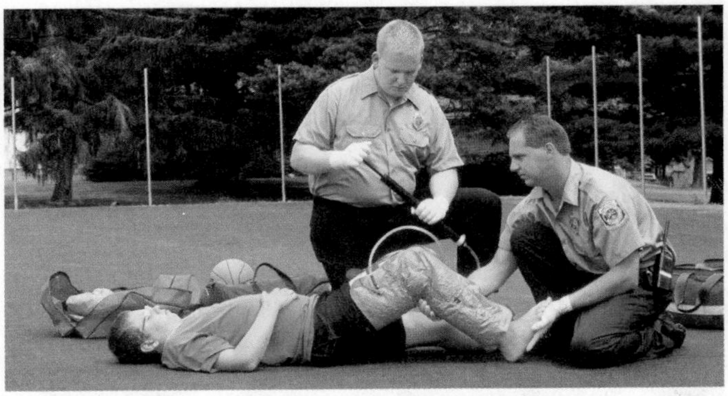

Figure 34-17 A vacuum splint applied to an injured knee.

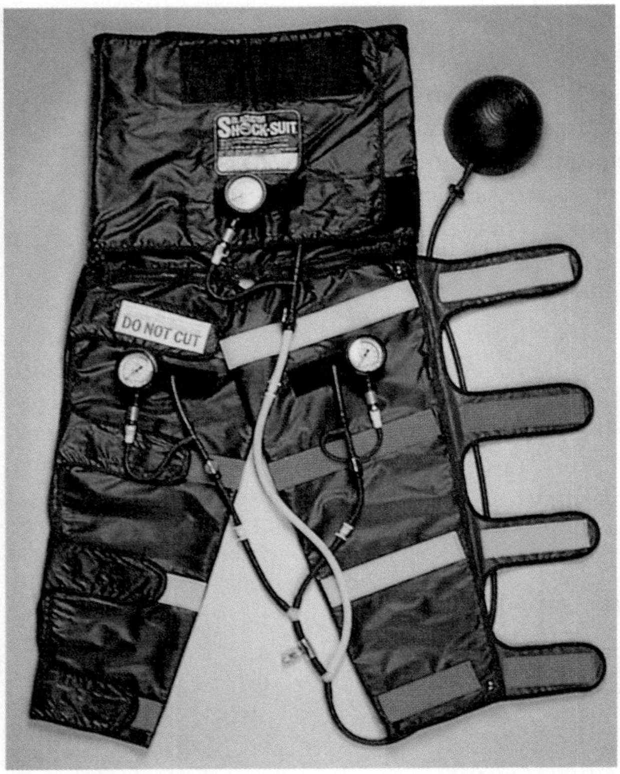

Figure 34-18 A pneumatic antishock garment (PASG) can be used for immobilizing pelvic and lower extremity fractures.

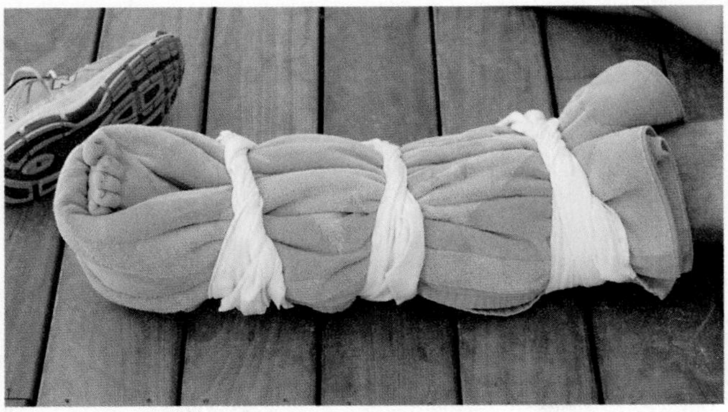

Figure 34-19 A towel makes a good improvised splint.

Some rigid splints are commercially manufactured and designed for specific injuries. Some have integrated padding and Velcro-style closures, making them easier to apply.

Pneumatic Splints

The air splint is one type of pneumatic splint. It is composed of a bladder that can be placed completely around an injured extremity and inflated to provide stability to the area that it covers (Figure 34-16 ■). Air splints are easy to apply. However, they do not allow for further assessment of the injury site because they cover the majority of the limb. Like balloons, air splints are subject to leaks and pressure changes such as altitude changes. This is especially important if the patient is transported by air ambulance.

Vacuum splints are another type of pneumatic splint. They operate on the opposite principle of air splints. They consist of a specially shaped bag filled with tiny beads. When the bag is placed around an injured extremity, a suction pump is used to remove all the air inside the bag. When the air is removed, the bag becomes a rigid splint that conforms to the extremity, much like a mold (Figure 34-17 ■). The same disadvantages that apply to the air splint apply here as well. The effectiveness of the splint relies on the bag's ability to remain airtight, and the splint greatly reduces access to the injured extremity for further assessment.

Another pneumatic device that is occasionally used for patients with suspected pelvic or lower-extremity fractures is the pneumatic antishock garment (PASG). You must follow local protocols when using the PASG as a splint, and in some instances you may have to contact medical direction prior to applying it (Figure 34-18 ■).

Soft and Improvised Splints

Not every splint you apply must be a commercially manufactured splint designed for that purpose. Some of the most effective splints are those that utilize everyday materials such as pillows, blankets, newspapers, and magazines (Figure 34-19 ■).

SCAN 34-1 Application of a Sling and Swathe

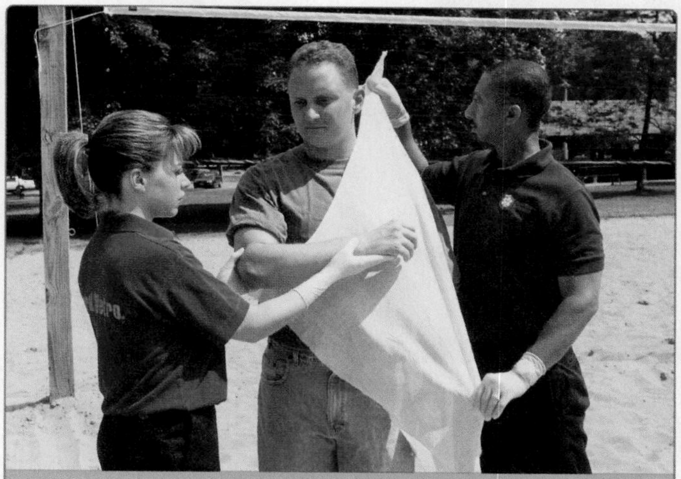

34-1-1 Place one end of the triangular bandage over the top of the uninjured shoulder. Make sure the apex of the triangle is pointing toward the injured elbow.

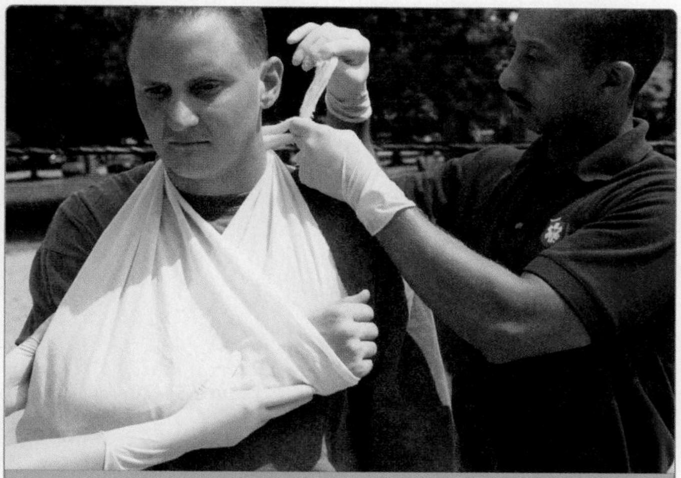

34-1-2 Bring the lower end of the bandage up and over the injured shoulder. Tie a knot at the side of the neck.

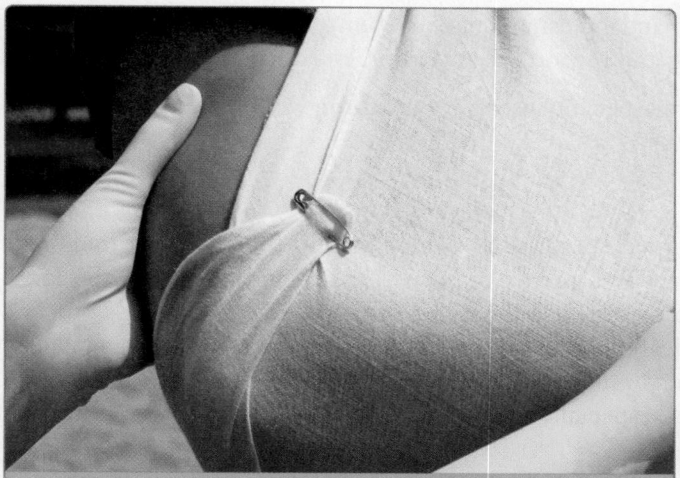

34-1-3 Tape or pin the apex of the bandage to form a pocket for the elbow.

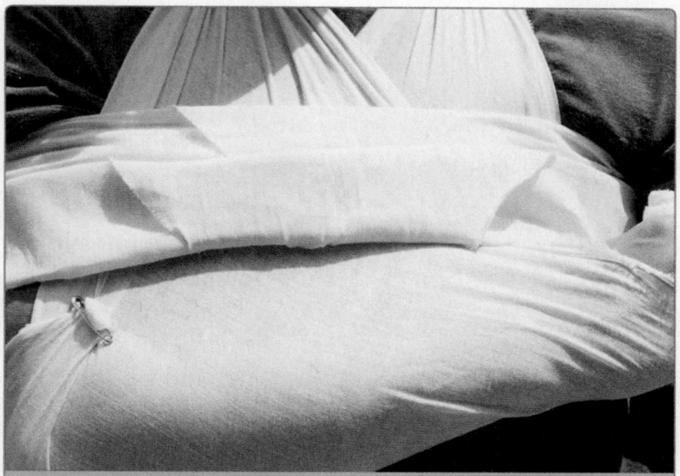

34-1-4 Place a swathe as low and tight as possible to restrict movement of the shoulder.

One of the most effective devices used to immobilize a shoulder, elbow, or forearm injury is the sling. All by itself, a properly applied sling does an excellent job of immobilizing a bent elbow. When combined with a swathe, it becomes an excellent tool for immobilizing both the elbow and the shoulder. Follow these steps for the proper application of a sling and swathe (Scan 34-1):

1. Place one end of the base of an open triangular bandage up and over the uninjured shoulder. Make sure that the apex of the triangle is behind the injured elbow and pointing in the same direction as the injured elbow.

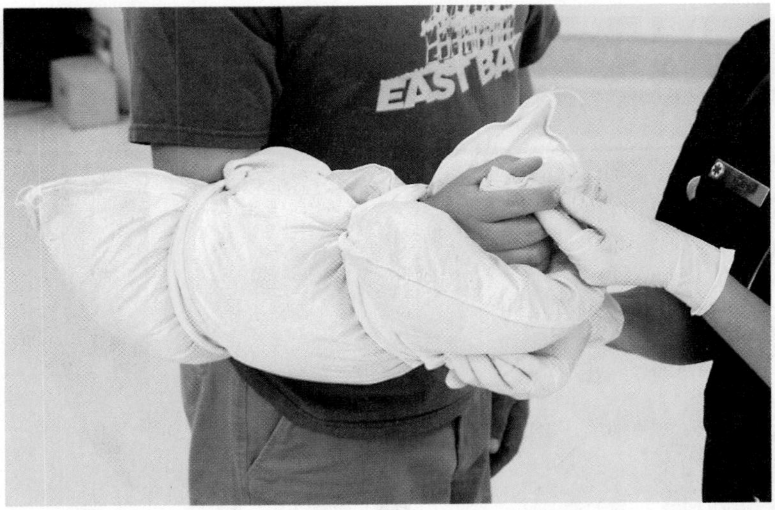

Figure 34-20 A pillow makes for a good improvised splint for a forearm.

2. Now bring the bottom tip of the triangle up and over the shoulder of the injured arm. Be sure the hand of the injured arm is at or above the level of the elbow on the same side.
3. Tie both ends of the bandage at the side of the neck and pad behind the knot as necessary.
4. Secure the apex of the bandage using a pin, tape, or tying in a knot.
5. Secure a swathe as snug and low on the arm as practical.

Pillows and blankets are especially useful for splinting wrist, forearm, elbow, and ankle injuries (Figure 34-20 ■).

Traction Splints

The traction splint is designed specifically to help stabilize a suspected mid-shaft femur fracture (Figure 34-21 ■). When a femur is broken and displaced, the large muscles of the thigh begin to spasm, pulling the broken bone ends across one another. This causes a great deal of pain as well as increased soft-tissue damage, bleeding, and swelling. Traction splints are contraindicated for patients with pelvic, hip, knee, and lower leg injuries, especially injuries that might involve a partial amputation of the extremity.

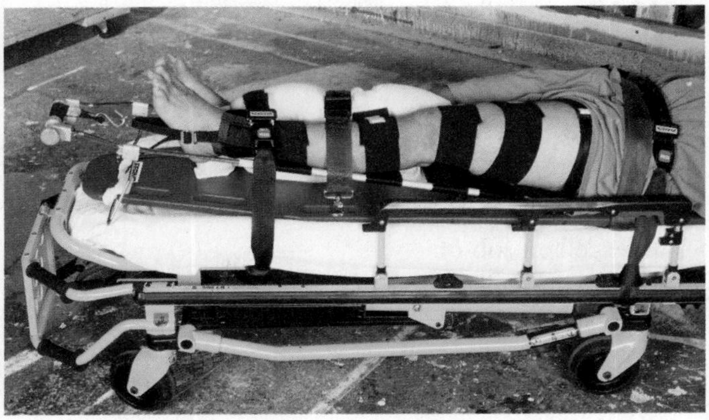
Figure 34-21 A traction splint is indicated for immobilization of some suspected femur fractures.

Once applied, gentle traction should be maintained throughout transport. The rule of thumb is to apply traction force equal to approximately 10% of the patient's total body weight up to a maximum of 15 pounds of traction. Some devices (Sager) have a gauge that will indicate the amount of traction being applied. With others, you must estimate the correct amount of traction. Initially, the patient may experience increased pain as the muscles feel the pressure and the bones begin to move. Within a minute or so, the patient will begin to experience some relief as the muscle spasms begin to relax.

Long Backboard

In some instances when a significant mechanism of injury is involved and rapid transport is required, it may be more appropriate to use a long backboard to immobilize the entire body of the patient. In those situations, do not waste valuable time attempting to manage each and every skeletal injury. Instead, carefully secure the patient on a long backboard and initiate transport.

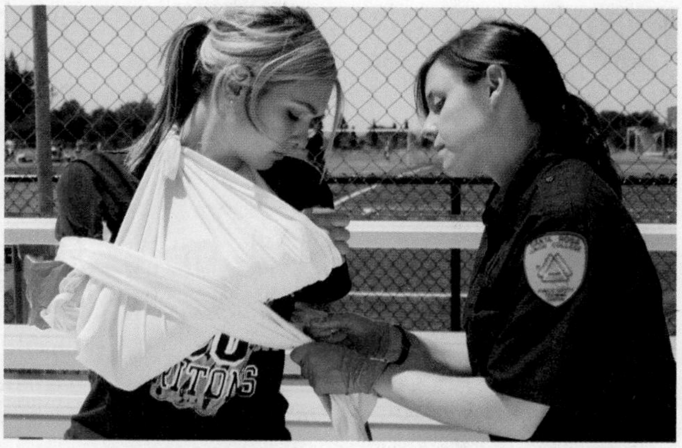

Figure 34-22 Place the swathe as low across the arm as possible to restrict movement of the shoulder.

Splinting Specific Injuries

The following section provides guidelines for splinting specific injuries.

Shoulder

Injuries to the shoulder may involve the shoulder joint or the clavicle and can be splinted the same way regardless of which one is involved. The sling and swathe are the main components required. Be sure the swathe is placed as low and tight across the arm as possible to minimize movement of the shoulder (Figure 34-22 ■).

Upper Arm

Depending on the extent of injury and position, an injury to the upper arm (humerus) can sometimes be managed easily with a sling and swathe. For additional support and protection, a short rigid splint may be applied to the outer (lateral) side of the upper arm and secured with a pair of cravats.

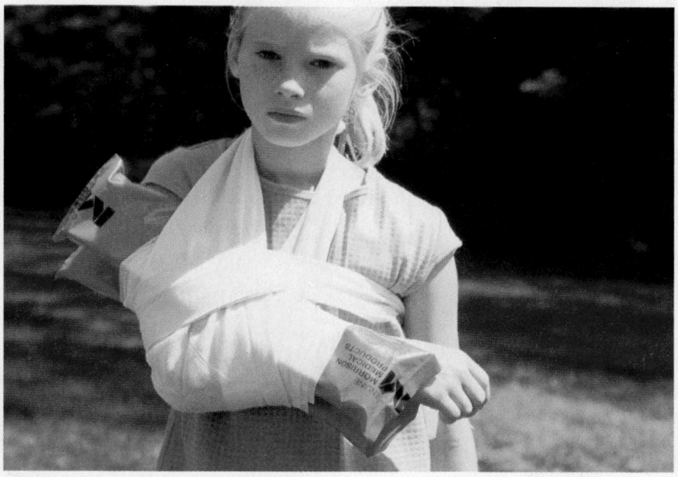

Figure 34-23 Two rigid splints placed across the arm can help immobilize an elbow injury.

Bent Elbow

An elbow found in the bent position is one of the easiest to splint and is ultimately in the most comfortable position for the patient. If the elbow is not found in the bent position, you can ask the patient if he can move it into that position. Do not move the elbow yourself. You must allow the patient to move it. If he is unable to move it, immobilize it in the position in which it is found.

At least two methods can be used to immobilize an elbow injury. The first is a rigid splint in conjunction with the sling and swathe, and the second is a method that uses two short, rigid splints secured to the arm at 45-degree angles (Figure 34-23 ■). If possible, always incorporate the wrist into one of the splints because it represents the joint below the injury site and must be immobilized.

PRACTICAL PATHOPHYSIOLOGY

An extremity injury that results in pallor and the loss of distal pulse and capillary refill may indicate circulatory compromise to the distal extremity. In those situations it is appropriate to attempt to reposition the extremity in an attempt to restore circulation. Always follow local protocol.

Straight Elbow

An elbow that is injured and found in the straight position must be managed differently than a bent elbow. First confirm that the patient cannot move the elbow

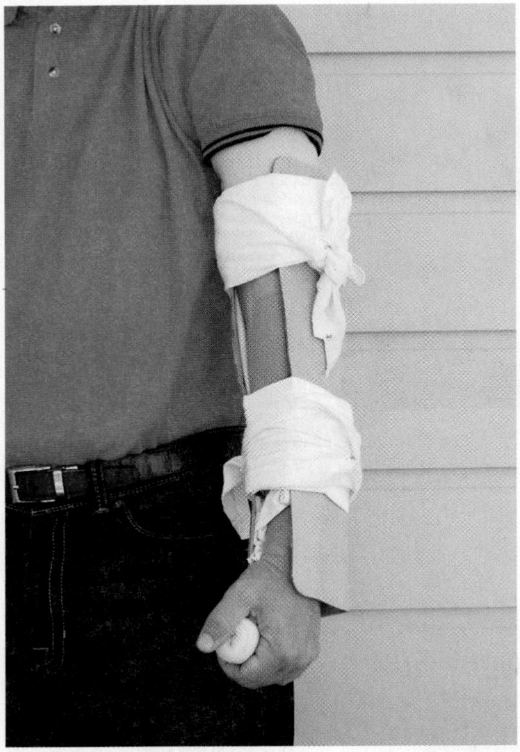

Figure 34-24 Immobilization of an elbow injury in the straight position.

into the bent position. If he cannot, then you must immobilize it in the straight position. Immobilize the joint using a rigid splint, and then secure the entire upper extremity to the body (Figure 34-24 ■). (See Scan 34-2 for steps for immobilizing an elbow injury.)

Forearm, Wrist, and Hand

Injuries to the forearm, wrist, and hand are among the most common. A simple rigid or pneumatic splint that extends from the elbow past the wrist will usually suffice. Once the splint is applied, the injured extremity should be placed in a sling and swathe. Whenever possible, it is important to maintain the hand on the injured arm at or above the level of the elbow. This will minimize pain caused by throbbing.

Finger

Injured fingers are not typically a reason to be transported by ambulance but can be associated with other injuries and need attention. One of the simplest splints for an injured finger is the tongue blade or bite stick. Pad the splint with gauze and tape or wrap the finger(s) to the splint. Securing the injured finger to an adjacent finger is helpful for additional support (Figure 34-25 ■), and is commonly referred to as "buddy taping."

Pelvis

34-11 Discuss special considerations in splinting pelvic fractures.

The potential for life-threatening blood loss from a pelvic injury is high. Ongoing movement of the unstable pelvic fracture results in increased bleeding from damaged pelvic blood vessels. Treatment of suspected unstable pelvic fractures once called for use of the PASG to minimize movement of the pelvis during transport. Today, there are several devices designed specifically for the stabilization of pelvic fractures in the field. One is the trauma pelvic orthopedic device (TPOD) (Figure 34-26 ■). Devices such as the TPOD are easy to use and have been proven effective in maximizing pelvic stability during transport.

Femur

Fractured femurs are significant injuries best managed using a traction device such as those manufactured by Hare (bipolar device) or by Sager or Kendrick (single-pole

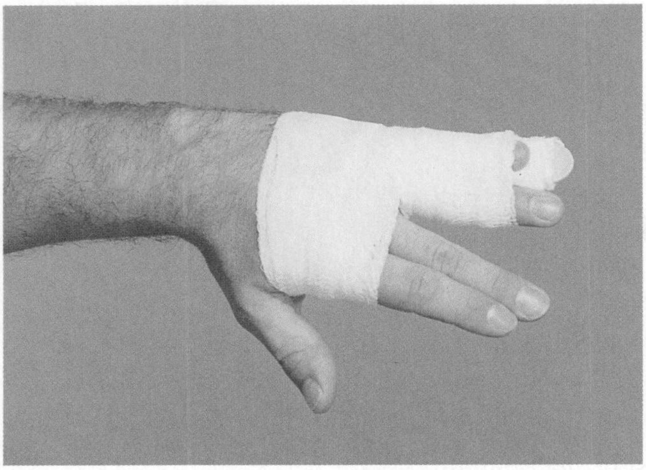

Figure 34-25 An injured finger can be secured to an adjacent finger for stabilization.

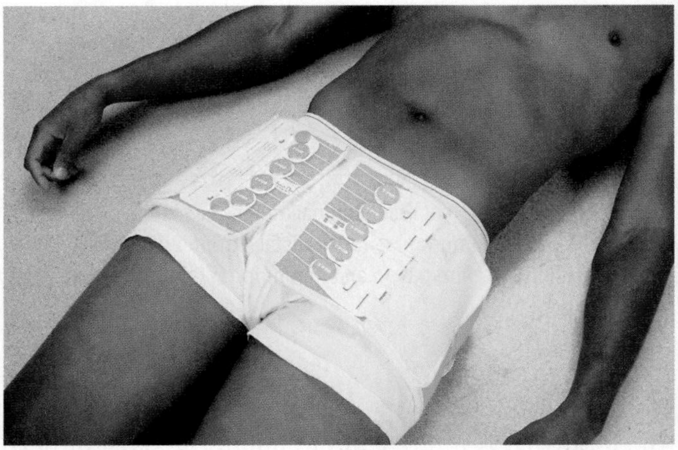

Figure 34-26 Immobilization of a suspected pelvic fracture using a commercial pelvic splint.

SCAN 34-2 Immobilizing an Elbow Injury

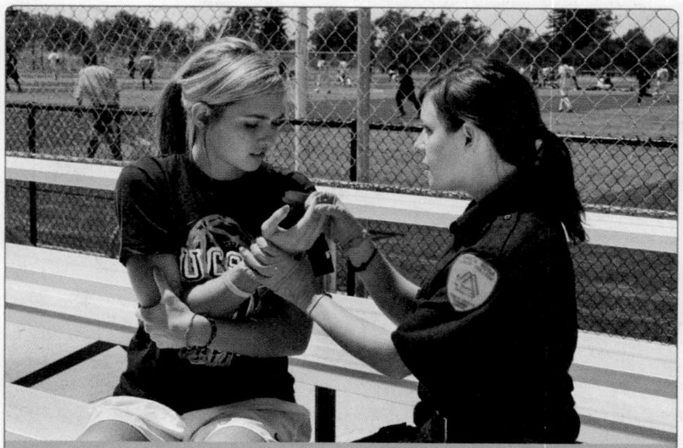

34-2-1 Check circulation, sensation, and motor function prior to splinting.

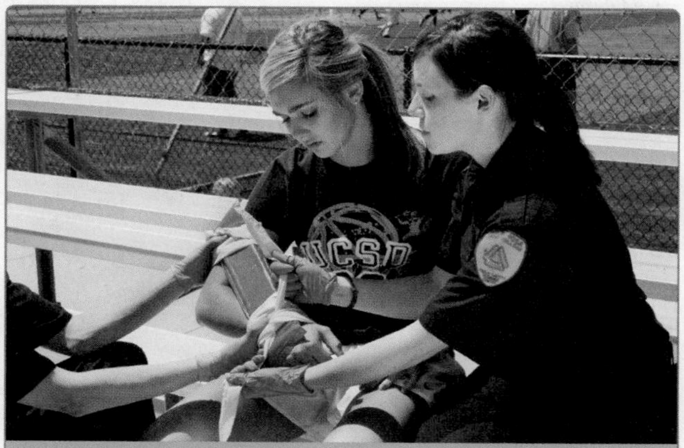

34-2-2 Secure a rigid splint to the arm. Be sure to pad the splint.

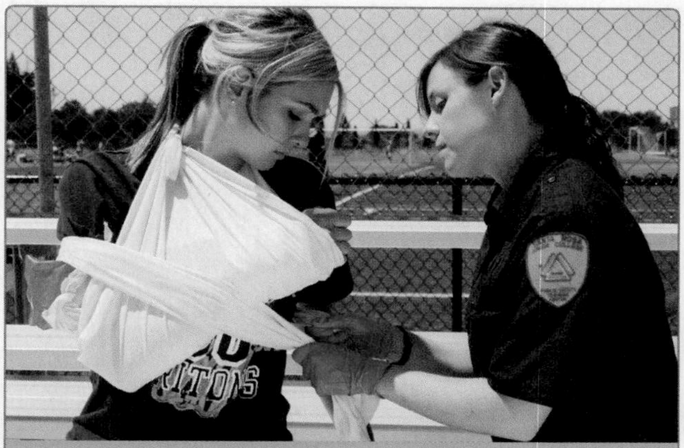

34-2-3 Apply a sling and swathe.

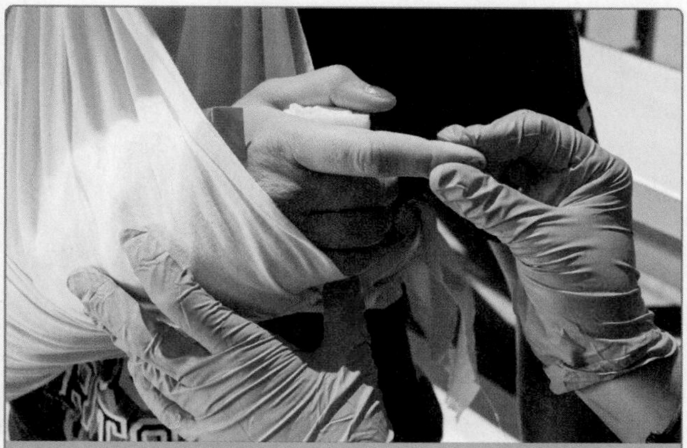

34-2-4 Recheck circulation, sensation, and motor function.

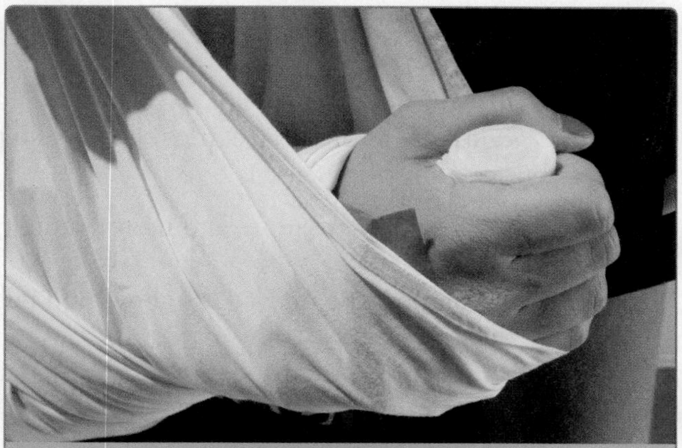

34-2-5 Ensure that the hand is in the position of function.

SCAN 34-3 Application of a Hare Traction Splint

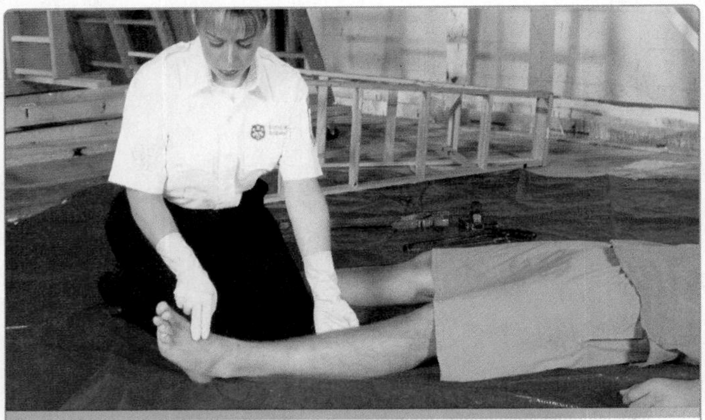

34-3-1 Check circulation, sensation, and motor function prior to splinting.

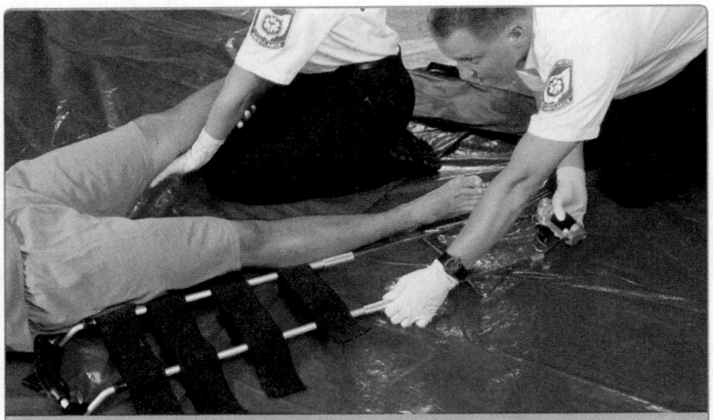

34-3-2 Measure the splint using the uninjured leg.

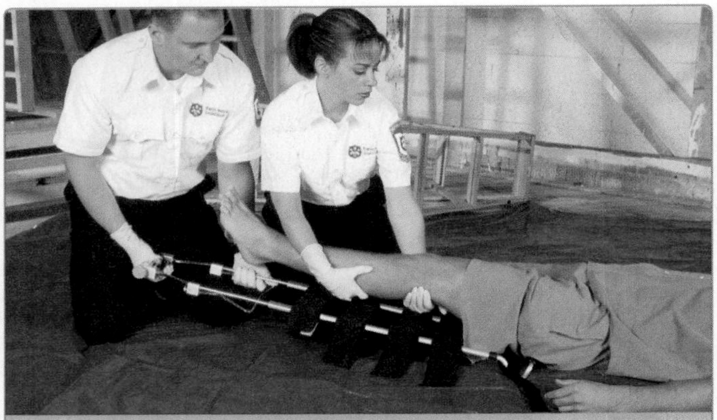

34-3-3 Apply manual traction while placing the splint under the injured leg.

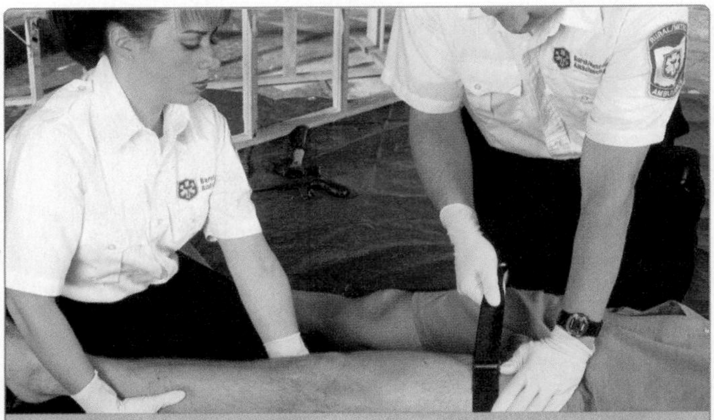

34-3-4 Secure the thigh/groin strap.

devices). Regardless of the device, the following steps should be followed when placing a traction splint (Scan 34-3):

1. Assess circulation, sensation, and motor function (CSM) distal to the injury and record.
2. Manually support the injured leg above and below the suspected fracture site.
3. Apply the ankle hitch.
4. Adjust the splint to the proper length using the uninjured leg and position the splint on the injured leg.
5. Carefully apply the ankle hitch.
6. Apply manual traction using the ankle hitch.
7. Apply the proximal securing device (groin strap).
8. Engage the ankle hitch in the distal splint mechanism.

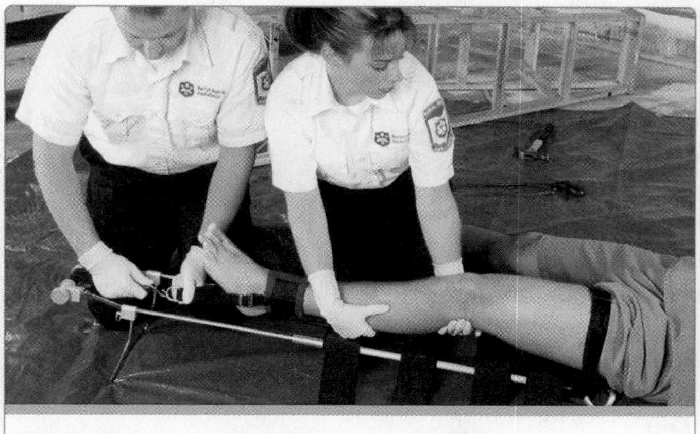

34-3-5 Connect the ankle strap and initiate traction.

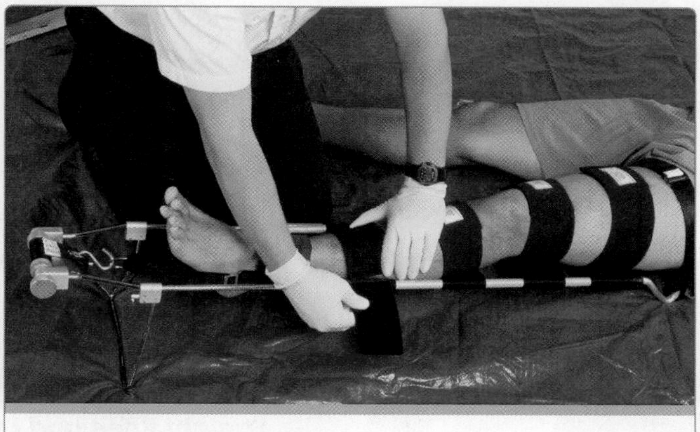

34-3-6 Secure the support straps.

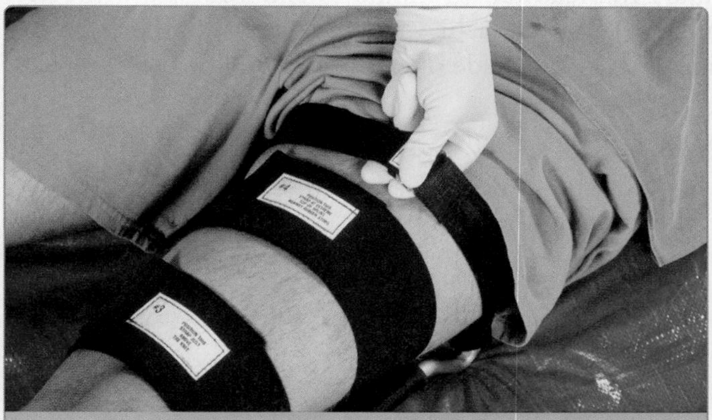

34-3-7 Recheck the thigh/groin strap and ankle hitch for tightness.

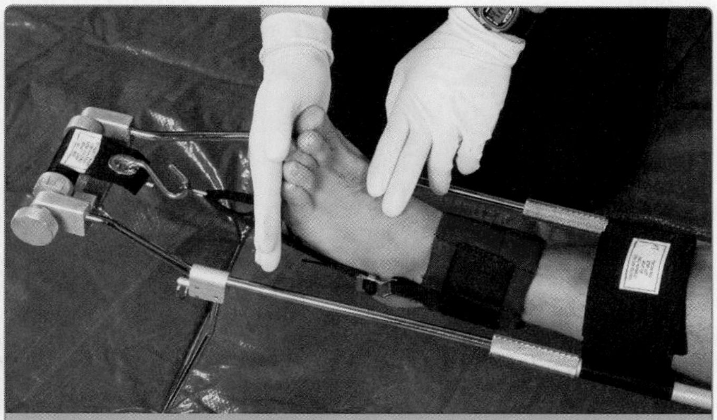

34-3-8 Reevaluate distal circulation, sensation, and motor function.

9. Apply mechanical traction.
10. Position and secure the support straps.
11. Reevaluate the proximal and distal securing devices.
12. Reassess distal CSM.

Once the splint has been properly applied to the injured extremity, the patient should be secured to a long backboard for transport. If using a bipolar device, be sure to secure the device to the backboard with tape so that it does not slide around during transport.

Application of a Hare-style traction splint should follow these steps:

1. Assess distal CSM.
2. Manually stabilize the injury.
3. Attach the ankle strap.

4. Prepare and measure the splint.
5. Apply manual traction and place the splint under the leg and secure the groin strap.
6. Initiate mechanical traction.
7. Reassess CSM.
8. Secure the patient and device to the long backboard.

To apply a Sager traction splint, use the following steps (Scan 34-4):

1. Assess distal CSM.
2. Manually stabilize the injury.
3. Attach the ankle strap.
4. Prepare and measure the splint and place it along the leg.
5. Attach the groin and ankle strap and initiate traction.
6. Reassess CSM.
7. Secure the patient and device to the long backboard.

Straight Knee and Lower Leg

Injuries to the lower extremities that involve a straight knee or a lower leg can be splinted using the same basic techniques. At the very least, a splint used to immobilize a straight knee should be long enough to extend well beyond the knee in both directions. A splint used for an injury to the lower leg should extend from below the heel to well above the knee (Scan 34-5). You will achieve better support of the extremity if you use a three-sided splint, such as one made of cardboard. Follow these steps:

1. Check CSM.
2. Manually stabilize the leg.
3. Slide cravats under the leg (two above the knee and two below).
4. Measure the splint and slide it under the leg.
5. Secure the splint with ties.
6. Reassess CSM.

Bent Knee Injury

A knee that is injured and found in the bent position can be a challenge to properly splint. One option for splinting uses two rigid splints, one on either side of the leg to create a triangle. The second uses the uninjured leg as an anchor point for the injured leg. To use the two-splint technique, follow these steps (Scan 34-6):

1. Check CSM.
2. Pad and secure the splints just below the injured knee.
3. Secure the ankle on the injured side to the uninjured leg.
4. Recheck CSM.

To use the anchor point technique, follow these steps:

1. Check CSM.
2. Secure the ankle on the injured side to the uninjured leg using a cravat.
3. Use a pillow or blanket to support under the injured knee.
4. Recheck CSM.

Ankle and Foot Injuries

Ankle and foot injuries can be a challenge to splint, because there are few premanufactured splints for these injuries. One of the best devices for immobilizing the ankle and foot is the folded blanket or pillow. The trick is to fold the blanket in a long narrow fashion and place it under the bottom of the foot and up along both

SCAN 34-4 Application of a Sager Traction Splint

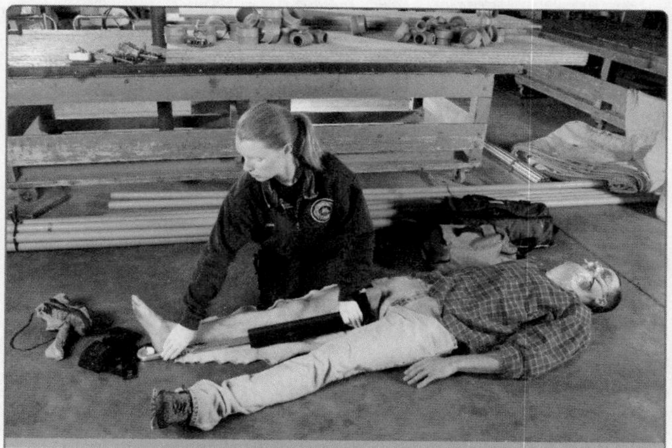

34-4-1 After checking circulation, sensation, and motor function, place the splint between the legs.

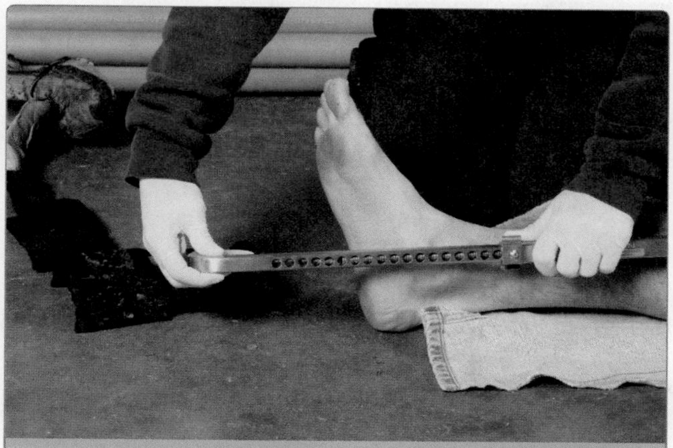

34-4-2 Extend the splint to just beyond the end of the injured leg.

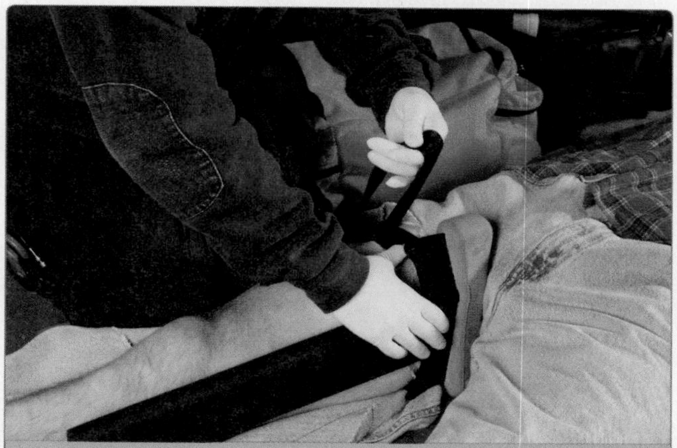

34-4-3 Secure the thigh/groin strap.

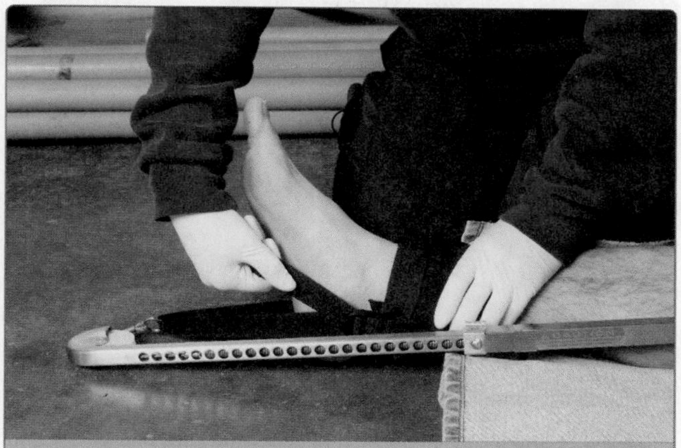

34-4-4 Secure the ankle strap.

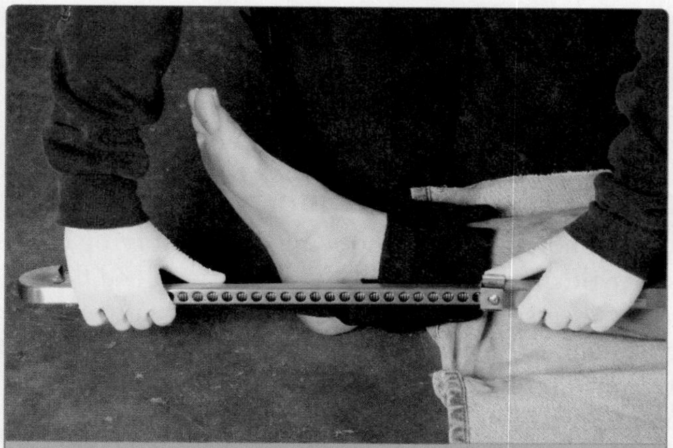

34-4-5 Initiate traction.

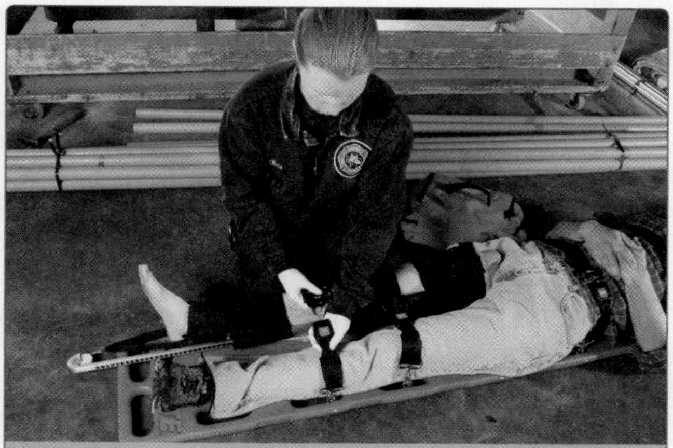

34-4-6 Prepare the patient for transport.

SCAN 34-5 Immobilizing a Lower Extremity

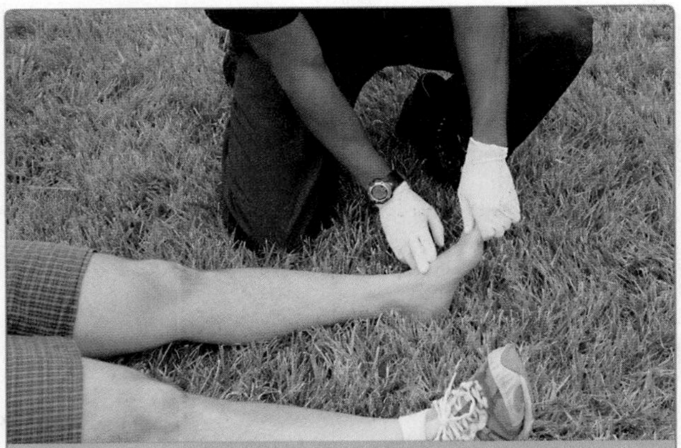

34-5-1 Assess circulation, sensation, and motor function prior to splinting.

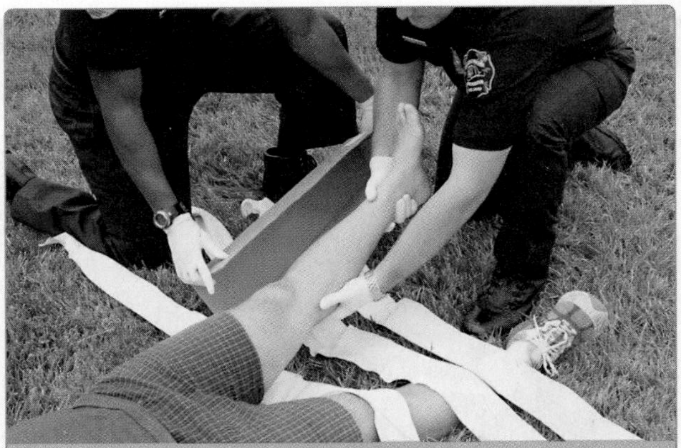

34-5-2 Choose a splint that extends from the heel to well above the knee.

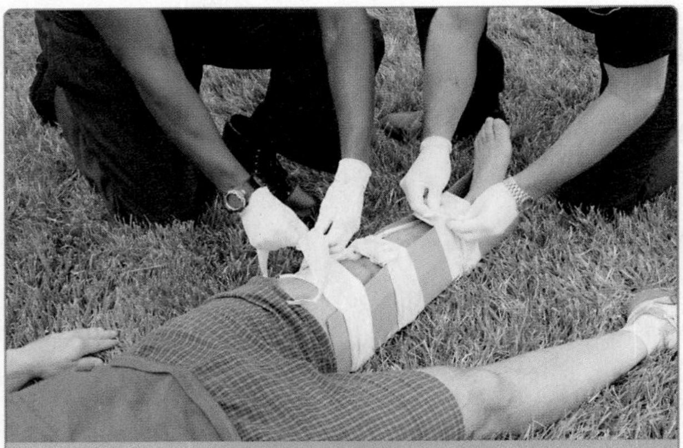

34-5-3 Secure the splint above and below the knee and at the ankle.

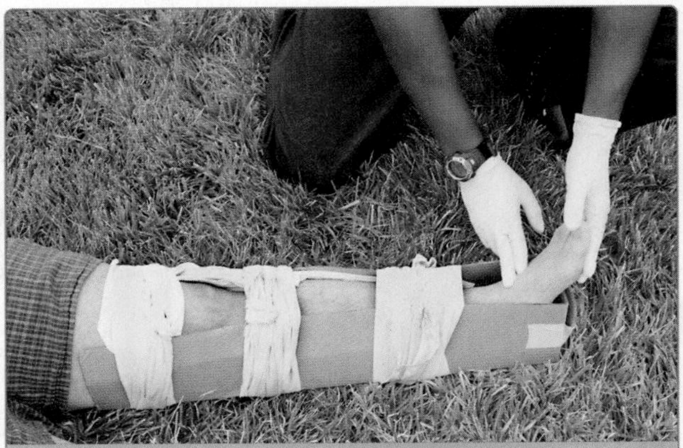

34-5-4 Reassess circulation, sensation, and motor function after the splint is secure.

sides of the lower leg for support. Use cravats to secure the blanket or pillow to the extremity. Be sure to keep the toes exposed for easy assessment of CSM.

Complications Caused by Improper Splinting

34-12 Discuss hazards of improper splinting.

An improperly applied splint can do more harm than no splint at all. If it is too tight, splints can cause painful pressure points, compress nerves, and restrict blood flow. If it is too loose, the splint will allow excessive movement of the injury that will cause unnecessary pain, bleeding, and swelling.

Valuable time can be wasted attempting to splint low-priority extremity injuries when the patient may have suffered a more serious injury that needs immediate attention. Before attempting to splint an isolated extremity injury, carefully evaluate the overall mechanism of injury and the patient for signs of more potentially serious injuries. In some situations it may be best to secure the patient to a long backboard

SCAN 34-6 Immobilizing a Bent Knee

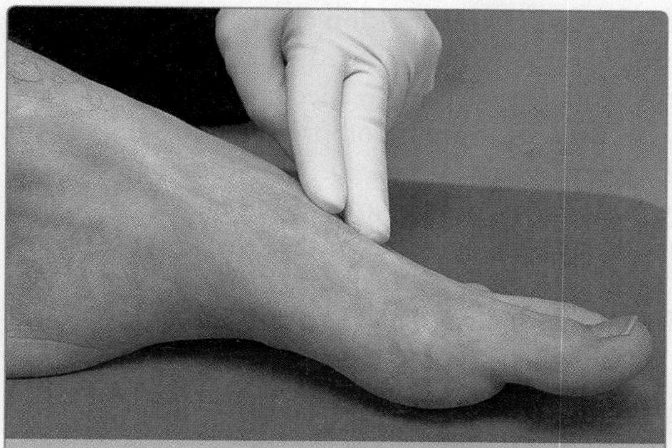

34-6-1 Check circulation, sensation, and motor function prior to splinting.

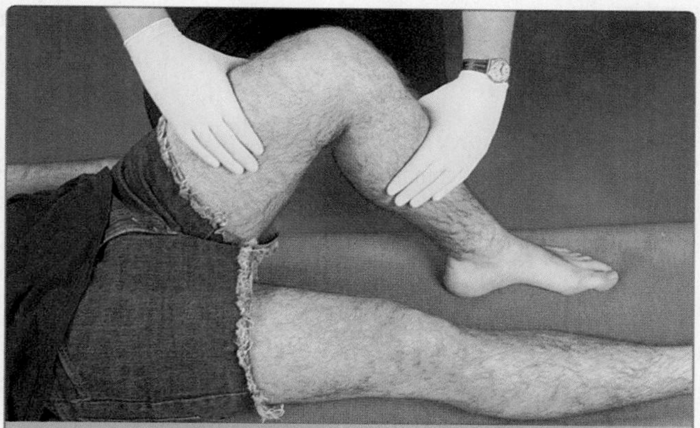

34-6-2 Manually stabilize the injured knee.

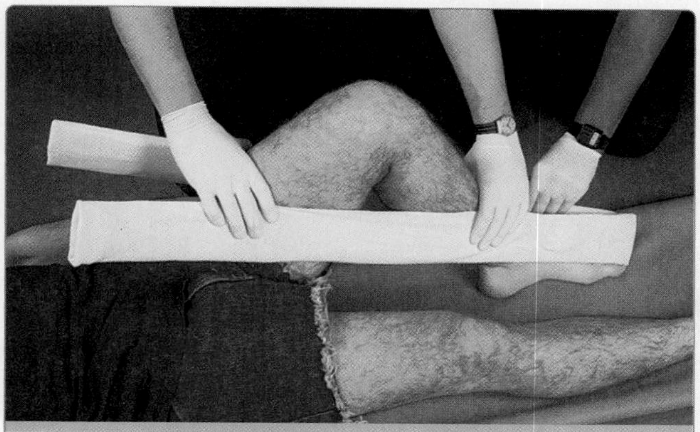

34-6-3 Place padded splints on either side of the leg at an angle.

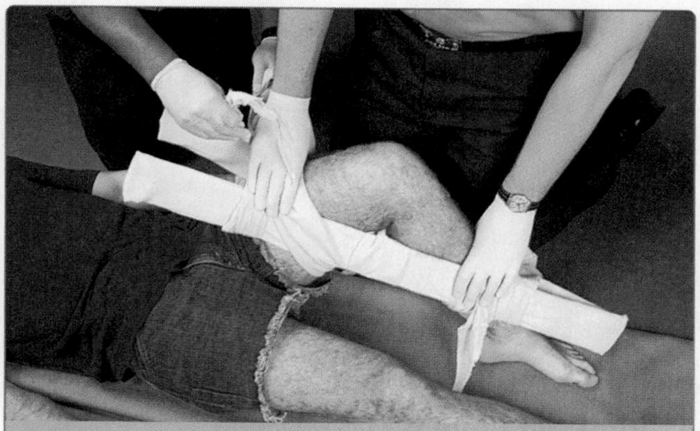

34-6-4 Secure the splints to the leg.

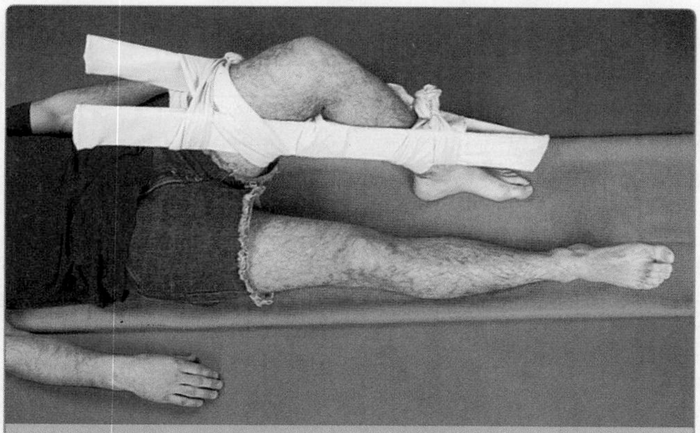

34-6-5 Recheck circulation, sensation, and motor function following splinting.

as a unit and not try to splint isolated injuries. Be sure to document all appropriate information in your prehospital care report.

Compartment Syndrome

34-13 Describe the basic pathophysiology of compartment syndrome.

compartment syndrome a condition caused by the compression of nerves, vessels, and other soft tissue within a closed space within the body.

Compartment syndrome is a potentially dangerous condition caused by the compression of nerves, vessels, and other soft tissues within a closed space within the body following an injury. The uncontrolled pressure caused by bleeding and swelling can lead to tissue death as blood supply within the space is compromised. Compartment syndrome most commonly affects the arms and lower legs. It can occur in the setting of fractured bones or simply due to crush injury of the muscles surrounding the bones. Swelling and bleeding increases pressure within the closed muscle compartment, cutting off blood flow to the affected tissues and preventing blood from flowing distally in the extremity. If not identified and corrected, it can lead to loss of function and possible amputation of the limb.

Compartment syndrome is characterized by what are known as the "Five Ps." They are:

- Pain that is extreme for the evident injury ("pain out of proportion")
- Paresthesia
- Pallor
- Paralysis (a late sign)
- Pulselessness (a late sign)

There is little the EMT can do for compartment syndrome beyond recognition of the signs and symptoms and traditional immobilization techniques.

STOP, REVIEW, REMEMBER!

Multiple Choice

For each question, place a check next to the correct answer.

1. All of the following examples are reasons to immobilize a skeletal injury *except* to:

_____ a. minimize movement.

_____ b. minimize pain.

_____ c. minimize bleeding and swelling.

_____ d. reduce blood flow to the injury site.

2. Immobilization of a suspected skeletal injury can be accomplished by _____________ stabilization and splinting.

_____ a. manual

_____ b. lateral

_____ c. distal

_____ d. proximal

3. All of the following rules should be followed when immobilizing a suspected skeletal injury *except:*

_____ a. expose the injury site.

_____ b. assess CSM before and after splinting.

_____ c. immediately straighten angulated injuries.

_____ d. immobilize the injury site.

4. When caring for a patient with a suspected fracture of the femur, what is the best way to immobilize the joint above the injury (hip)?

_____ a. Place the patient in the recovery position.

_____ b. Secure the patient to a long backboard.

_____ c. Tie both legs together.

_____ d. Ask the patient to remain still.

5. Which one of the following best describes the term *position of function*?

_____ a. Position of comfort

_____ b. Position in which you find the patient

_____ c. Position in which the patient is sitting

_____ d. Position of a hand or foot at rest

Fill in the Blank

1. In most cases, a musculoskeletal injury should be treated as a suspected ______________________________ and immobilized accordingly.

2. The injured extremity should be ______________________________ only after it has been properly immobilized and only if it does not cause further pain for the patient.

3. To minimize complications caused by ______________________________, it will be necessary to immobilize the injury prior to transport.

4. Immobilization can be accomplished using one of two methods: ______________________________ and splinting.

5. The ______________________________ refers to the position of the hands and feet when they are at rest and not under any type of force.

Critical Thinking

1. List the most common signs and symptoms of a closed skeletal injury.

____

____

____

____

2. Describe how you would care for a suspected fracture of the knee if it were locked in a bent position.

____

____

____

____

3. What is the value of immobilizing the joint above and below a suspected fracture site?

____

____

____

____

EMERGENCY DISPATCH SUMMARY

David was transported to University Hospital where he was found to have a dislocated knee. Several attempts by the physician to manually reposition it proved unsuccessful, and the joint had to be realigned in surgery. David was released two days later and is currently undergoing physical therapy.

Chapter Review

To the Point

- The musculoskeletal system is made up of all the muscles, bones, and connective tissues such as tendons, ligaments, and cartilage.
- Musculoskeletal injuries are some of the most common injuries encountered by EMS. Injuries result from forces such as direct, indirect, and twisting.
- Common musculoskeletal injuries include muscle strains, joint sprains, fractures, and dislocations.
- Careful assessment is necessary to properly assess for and manage musculoskeletal injuries. Assessment begins with evaluating the site of injury and then moving both distally and proximally to determine the extent of the injury.
- Signs and symptoms of a musculoskeletal injury include pain, tenderness, deformity such as swelling and angulation, pallor, inability to move the extremity, and paresthesia.
- It is important to prioritize musculoskeletal injuries with other injuries or complaints the patient may have. You must not allow the unsightly nature of some injuries to distract you from addressing issues related to the ABCs.
- Proper splinting will minimize pain, movement, swelling, and tissue damage during transport.
- When immobilizing an injured extremity, it is important to try to keep the hand and foot in the position of function for maximum comfort.
- There are many options for immobilizing musculoskeletal injuries, including both commercial and improvised splints. Common splints used in EMS are cardboard splints, wooden splints, moldable splints, traction, and pelvic splints.
- Injuries to the femurs and pelvis are particularly dangerous due to the significant internal bleeding that can occur when these bones are damaged.
- You must always evaluate a splint after application to ensure it is not causing more pain. An improperly applied splint can cause pain and swelling, and cut off normal circulation to the extremity.
- Compartment syndrome can occur following an injury to an extremity. It results when bleeding and swelling inside a closed space within the limb put pressure on nerves and blood vessels.

Chapter Questions

Multiple Choice

For each question, place a check next to the correct answer.

1. All of the following are examples of rigid splints *except:*

_____ a. cardboard.
_____ b. wood.
_____ c. air splint.
_____ d. aluminum.

2. There are two basic types of pneumatic splints, air and:

_____ a. vacuum.
_____ b. pressure.
_____ c. ladder.
_____ d. balloon.

3. The pneumatic antishock garment may be used to immobilize a suspected fracture of the:
   _____ a. femur. _____ c. spine.
   _____ b. pelvis. _____ d. ankle.
4. When caring for a patient with a suspected fracture of the wrist, what is the best way to immobilize the joint above the injury (elbow)?
   _____ a. Rigid splint _____ c. Air splint
   _____ b. Sling _____ d. Vacuum splint
5. Which one of the following would be the simplest way to immobilize an injured elbow that is found in the bent position?
   _____ a. Air splint _____ c. Vacuum splint
   _____ b. Traction splint _____ d. Sling and swathe
6. Which one of the following would best immobilize an injured shoulder?
   _____ a. Air splint _____ c. Sling and swathe
   _____ b. Vacuum splint _____ d. Rigid splint
7. The bone in the upper arm is called the:
   _____ a. femur. _____ c. ulna.
   _____ b. radius. _____ d. humerus.
8. Which one of the following statements is most accurate regarding the proper care for joint injuries?
   _____ a. Immobilize in the position found. _____ c. Treat with manual traction.
   _____ b. Straighten prior to splinting. _____ d. Elevate prior to splinting.
9. It is recommended that you should leave the _____________ exposed when splinting a foot injury.
   _____ a. ankle _____ c. toes
   _____ b. heel _____ d. injury site
10. Which one of the following is *not* a complication that can result from improper splinting?
   _____ a. Increased circulation _____ c. Decreased circulation
   _____ b. Increased bleeding _____ d. Increased swelling

Matching

Match the splinting device on the left with the practical applications on the right.

1. _____	Long rigid splint	A. Forearm, upper arm, lower extremity, bent arm (triangle)
2. _____	Short rigid splint	B. Foot, ankle
3. _____	Sling	C. Shoulder
4. _____	Swathe	D. Bent elbow
5. _____	Blanket	E. Straight knee, straight arm, bent knee (triangle)
6. _____	Pillow	F. Hand, wrist, forearm

Critical Thinking

1. List the most common signs and symptoms of an open skeletal injury.

____

____

____

____

(continued on next page)

(continued)

2. Describe how you would care for a suspected closed fracture of the shoulder.

3. In most cases there is a weakness on the side of injury when you compare both extremities. What is likely the most common cause for this difference?

Case Studies

Case Study 1

You respond to a dispatch for a vehicle collision a few miles outside of town. Upon arrival, you are directed down an embankment by a police officer at the scene. He states that the only patient is the driver of a motorcycle that appears to have hit the guardrail before exiting the roadway. As you approach the patient, you find a bystander holding a bloody towel on the patient's head. The bystander states that he is a trained emergency medical responder and that the patient is unresponsive but appears to have a good airway and is breathing. Your primary assessment finds this to be accurate, and your rapid trauma assessment reveals deformity to the lower right leg, upper left leg, and right forearm.

1. Now that you know the patient's ABCs are okay, what will be your priority for emergency care?

2. How will you care for this man's extremity injuries?

3. Is this patient a candidate for a traction splint? If so, for which leg?

Case Study 2

You are caring for a 14-year-old girl who fell while roller blading and has pain and deformity in her right forearm. She was wearing a helmet and denies hitting her head or any loss of consciousness. She states that she hit her arm on the curb as she fell. Your assessment of the distal extremity reveals numbness, tingling, the absence of a pulse, and delayed capillary refill. The girl's mother is on scene and has provided consent for treatment.

1. What is your primary concern as you care for this patient?

2. How will you manage the fact that there appears to be no circulation in the distal extremity?

3. Describe exactly how you will immobilize this injury.

The Last Word

Injuries to muscles and bones, while painful, are rarely life threatening. They can be as simple as a sprained ankle and as severe as an open fracture of the femur. It is essential to identify and manage all immediate life threats before attempting to splint a skeletal injury.

The basics of splinting are centered around the core steps of assessing distal circulation, sensation, and motor function before and after splinting; immobilizing the injury site; immobilizing the joints above and below the injury site; and making the patient as comfortable as possible. Be sure to document all appropriate information in your prehospital care report.

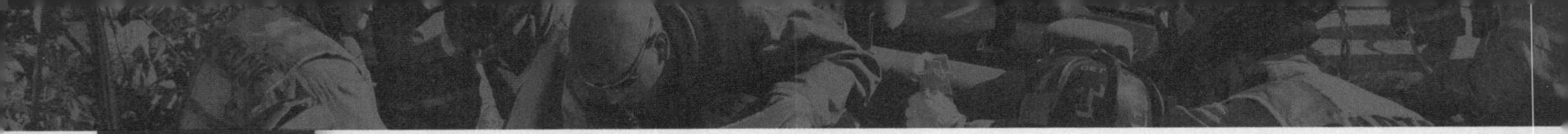

35 Caring for Patients with Head Injuries

Education Standards

Trauma: Head, face, neck, and spine trauma

Competencies

Applies fundamental knowledge to provide basic emergency care and transportation based on assessment findings for an acutely injured patient.

Objectives

After completion of this lesson, you should be able to:

35-1 Define key terms introduced in the chapter.

35-2 Explain the importance of recognizing and providing emergency medical care to patients with injuries to the head.

35-3 Identify the anatomy of the skull.

35-4 Identify the meningeal layers and the spaces into which intracranial bleeding can occur.

35-5 Associate each of the major anatomical portions of the brain with its functions.

35-6 Explain the pathophysiology and key signs and symptoms of injuries to the scalp, skull, and brain, including scalp lacerations, skull fractures, cerebral concussion, cerebral contusion, and intracranial hematomas.

35-7 Discuss factors that can worsen traumatic brain injuries, including hypoxia, hypocarbia, hypercarbia, and hypotension.

35-8 Describe the goals of emergency treatment of patients with traumatic brain injuries.

35-9 Describe the pathophysiology and key signs of increased intracranial pressure and brain herniation.

35-10 Describe the neurological assessment of patients with suspected traumatic brain injury.

35-11 Discuss the focus of history taking and assessment for patients with injuries to the head.

35-12 Explain the importance of reassessment of the patient with an injury to the head.

Key Terms

arachnoid membrane p. 905
ataxic (Biot's) respirations p. 919
basilar skull p. 904
Battle's sign p. 916
brainstem p. 905
central nervous system p. 904
central neurogenic hyperventilation p. 919
cerebellum p. 905
cerebrospinal fluid p. 905
cerebrum p. 905
Cheyne-Stokes respirations p. 919
closed head injury p. 908
concussion p. 909
contusion p. 909
cranial vault p. 904
Cushing's triad p. 912
decerebrate p. 910
decorticate p. 910
dura mater p. 905
epidural hematoma p. 912
Glasgow Coma Scale (GCS) p. 917
herniation p. 910
hypercarbia p. 909
hypocarbia p. 909
intracranial pressure p. 909
mandible p. 904
maxilla p. 904
medulla oblongata p. 906
meninges p. 905
nasal bones p. 904
open head injury p. 908
orbits p. 904
pia mater p. 905
raccoon eyes p. 916
subdural hematoma p. 912
temporal bones p. 904
temporomandibular joint p. 904
zygomatic bone p. 904

Introduction

35-2 Explain the importance of recognizing and providing emergency medical care to patients with injuries to the head.

Head injuries can range from minor to fatal and occur in a wide range of circumstances. The skull is a closed container with little cushioning or room for expansion. Because of this, any trauma to the outside of the head can cause serious injury to the brain within. And because you cannot see inside, the assessment, decision-making, and care you provide will be critical. Even with recent advances in understanding and treatment of traumatic brain injury, injuries to the head remain one of the most potentially devastating situations you will encounter as an EMT. Your accurate assessment and proper care of these patients will optimize their chances for survival and a meaningful recovery.

Head injuries are frequently associated with spine injuries, because of the forces that cause them. Although spine injuries are always a concern when assessing and managing patients with head injuries, they are specifically covered in the next chapter, Chapter 36. This chapter will detail head injuries only.

EMERGENCY DISPATCH

"Hold on! We're gonna get hit!" EMT Ron Hyde shouted back into the patient compartment as he spun the steering wheel away from the headlights that were rapidly descending toward the ambulance's windshield. The large truck's tires squealed, lost traction, and bounced violently across the pavement toward the freeway median.

The evasive maneuver was enough to prevent the airborne Volkswagen from hitting them head on. Instead, it impacted the passenger side of the cab, collapsing it almost right up to where Ron was sitting. The force of the hit tilted the ambulance up onto the left-side tires for a moment before it righted itself with a thundering crash. For a long moment after the ambulance scraped to a halt on the edge of the median, there was silence, broken only by the hissing of something in the truck's damaged engine.

"What happened?" Ron's partner, Barry Luden, called from the patient compartment.

"I'm, uh, not exactly sure," Ron said, taking off his seat belt. "How's the patient?"

"I'm okay," Mrs. Lawson, their geriatric patient with shortness of breath said. Her voice was muffled by the nonrebreather mask.

"Dispatch, Medical 9." Ron waited for the dispatcher's response before continuing. "We're on, uh, 53, just east of the Merrimac exit. I think I need help." Ron then pushed his door open and fell, unconscious, onto the pavement.

Anatomy and Physiology of the Head

35-3 Identify the anatomy of the skull.

cranial vault portion of the skull containing the brain and composed of the temporal, frontal, parietal, and occipital bones. Also called the *cranial skull*.

basilar skull portion of the skull that forms the floor of the skull.

temporal bones bones that form part of the side of the skull. There is a right and a left temporal bone.

maxilla the upper jaw bone, which is formed by two bones fused together.

mandible the lower jaw bone.

nasal bones the bones that form the upper third, or bridge, of the nose.

temporomandibular joint the movable joint formed between the mandible and the temporal bone. Also called the *TM joint*.

zygomatic bone the facial bone that forms the cheek.

orbits the bony structures around the eyes; the eye sockets.

central nervous system part of the nervous system composed of the brain and spinal cord.

The bony structure called the *head* is actually a series of bones that are joined. Together they are called the *cranium* or *skull*. The skull itself can be divided into the **cranial vault** (or *cranial skull*) and the facial bones. The cranial vault's primary function is to protect and support the brain.

The cranial vault is composed of a series of fused bones including the temporal, frontal, parietal, and occipital bones (Figure 35-1 ■). The **basilar skull** forms the floor of the skull. There are many small protrusions or ridges that rise from the basilar skull that can injure the brain when it is moved or compressed. The basilar skull and the **temporal bones** are the weakest areas of the skull, and more prone to fracture and subsequent damage to areas adjacent to the brain.

The facial bones include the **maxilla, mandible,** zygomatic, and **nasal bones.** The temporal bone of the skull and the mandible form the **temporomandibular joint,** which allows for the opening and closing of the mouth. The **zygomatic bone** of the face and the zygomatic process of the temporal bone connect to form the zygomatic arch, which is what gives structure to the cheek. The **orbits** are the bony structures around the eyes.

Inside the skull is the brain, one part of the **central nervous system.** The central nervous system consists of the brain and the spinal cord. It is responsible for involuntary functions of the body such as heartbeat, breathing, and temperature regulation, as well as functions such as thought, reasoning, sensation, and movement throughout the body.

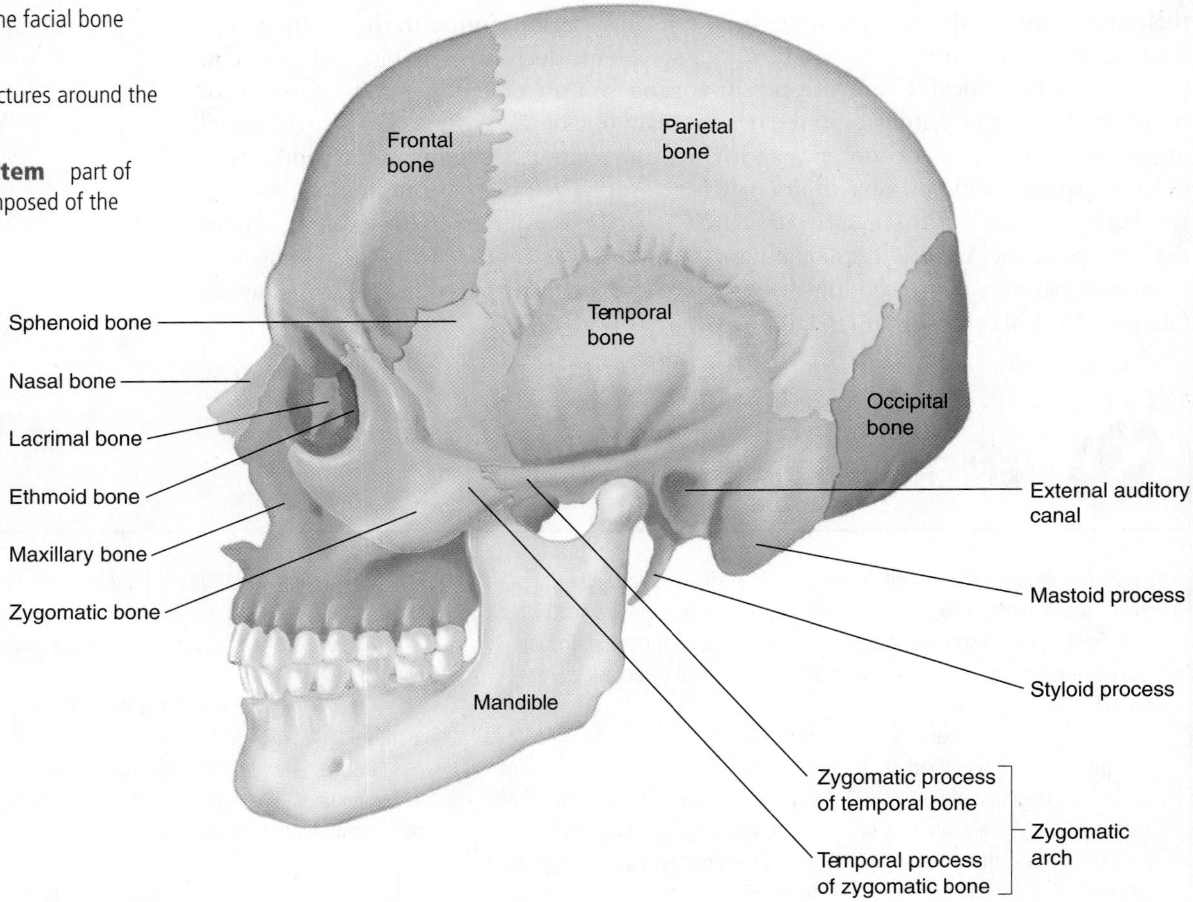

Figure 35-1 The bones of the human skull.

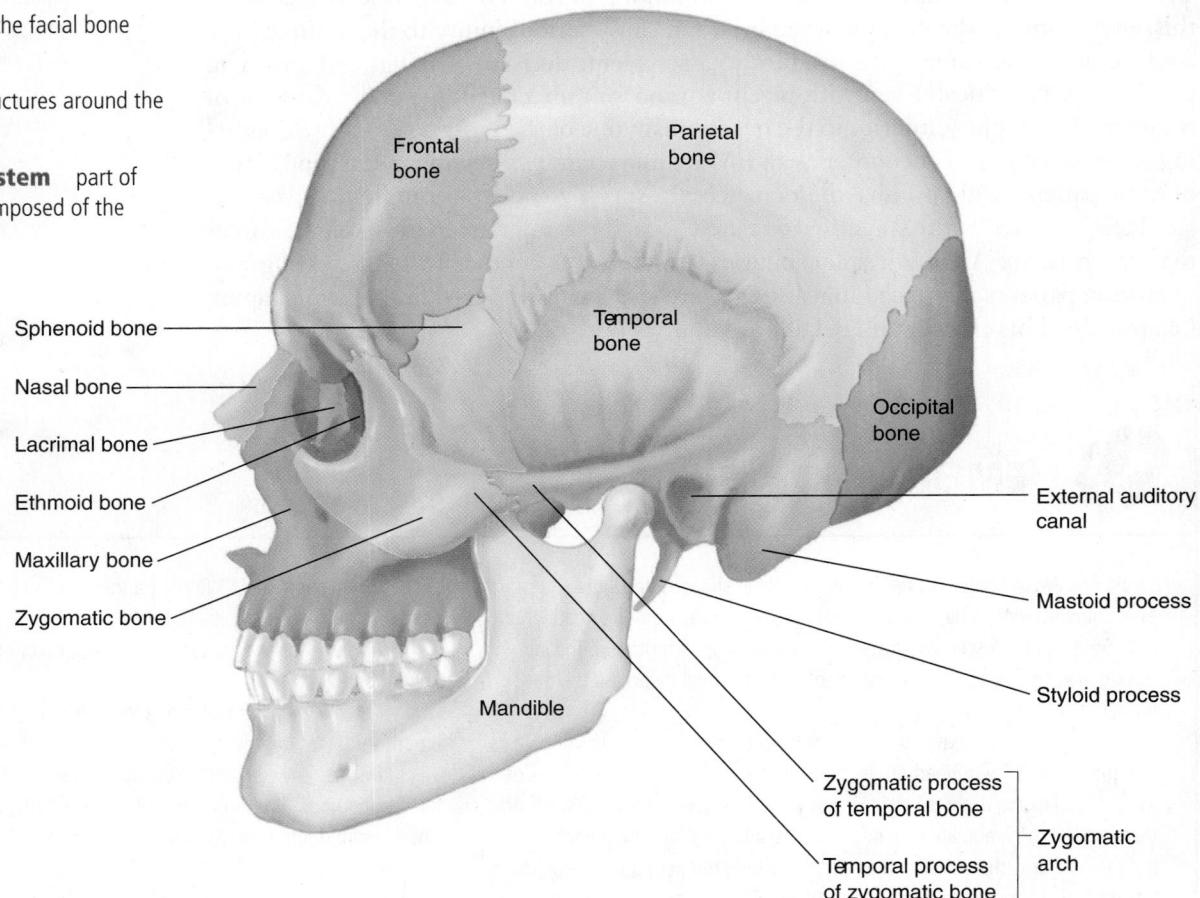

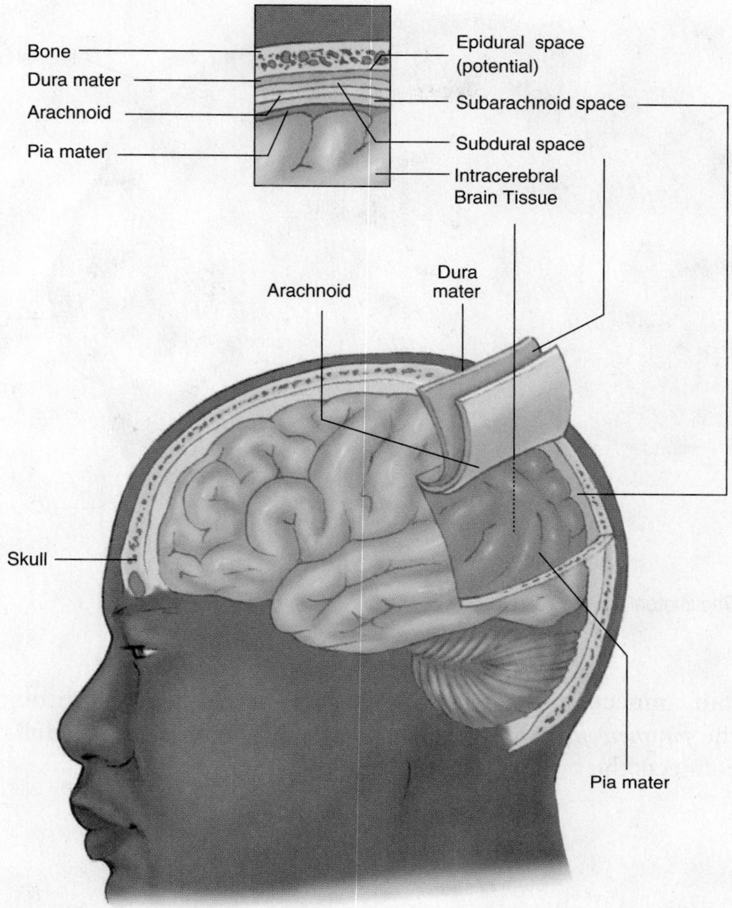

Figure 35-2 Meninges of the brain.

The brain is covered with three membranes or layers (Figure 35-2 ▪). The **dura mater** is a fibrous layer that lines the inside of the cranial vault. The **pia mater** lies directly over the brain tissue. Between the two layers is a very thin, weblike layer called the **arachnoid membrane.** The three layers are called the **meninges,** and also cover the spine.

Cerebrospinal fluid is produced within the brain and resides in the subarachnoid space. Cerebrospinal fluid is found around both the brain and spinal cord. It acts as a cushion to the brain in the event of trauma. You will see later in this chapter that a clear fluid (cerebrospinal fluid) coming from the nose or ears may indicate a serious head injury.

The brain, which takes up the vast majority of the cranial vault, is composed of several regions, each with a specific function (Figure 35-3 ▪). They include:

- ***Cerebrum.*** The largest portion of the brain, the **cerebrum** is divided into four sections or lobes and is responsible for conscious activities, personality, and sensory input. Emotions, speech, and motor functions are associated with its frontal lobe. Sensory functions lie within the parietal lobe. Memory and some components of speech lie in the temporal lobe, and vision is in the occipital lobe.
- ***Cerebellum.*** The **cerebellum** sits behind and under the cerebrum. It is responsible for coordination, posture, and equilibrium.
- ***Brainstem.*** Located at the base of the brain, the **brainstem** controls vital activities such as respiration, cardiac function, and blood pressure. There are several parts of the brainstem including the midbrain, pons, and medulla.

35-4 Identify the meningeal layers and the spaces into which intracranial bleeding can occur.

dura mater fibrous layer of tissue lining the inside of the cranial vault.

pia mater layer of tissue directly covering the brain.

arachnoid membrane weblike layer of tissue located between the dura mater and the pia mater.

meninges three membranes that surround and protect the brain and spinal cord: the dura mater, the pia mater, and the arachnoid membrane.

cerebrospinal fluid liquid found around the brain and spinal cord that helps cushion them.

35-5 Associate each of the major anatomical portions of the brain with its functions.

cerebrum largest portion of the brain, responsible for conscious activities, personality, and sensory input.

cerebellum portion of the brain that lies behind and under the cerebrum; responsible for coordination, posture, and equilibrium.

brainstem portion of the brain located at the base, responsible for vital activities such as respiration, cardiac function, and blood pressure.

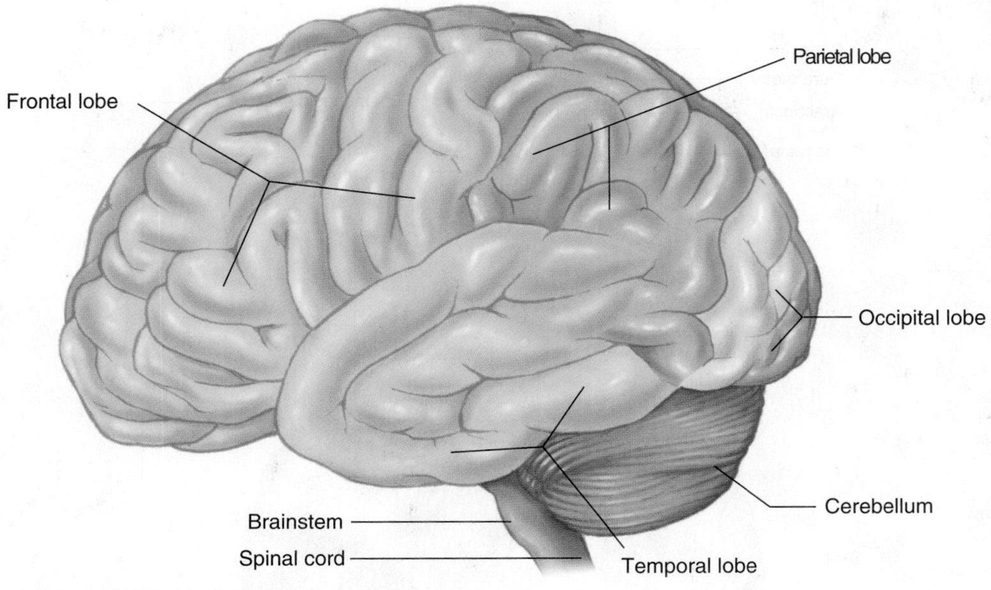

Figure 35-3 The anatomy of the brain.

medulla oblongata portion of the brain that directly connects to the spinal cord. Also called the *medulla*.

The brain connects to the spinal cord at the base of the skull through an opening called the *foramen magnum*. The medulla, also known as the **medulla oblongata,** physically connects the brain to the spinal cord.

STOP, REVIEW, REMEMBER!

Multiple Choice

For each question, place a check next to the correct answer.

1. The weakest areas of the skull are the ______________ bones.

_____ a. temporal and occipital
_____ b. parietal and occipital
_____ c. frontal and temporal
_____ d. basilar and temporal

2. The layers of the meninges in order from skull to brain are:

_____ a. dura, arachnoid, pia.
_____ b. arachnoid, pia, dura.
_____ c. pia, arachnoid, dura.
_____ d. dura, pia, arachnoid.

3. Which one of the following is *not* a facial bone?

_____ a. Maxilla
_____ b. Mandible
_____ c. Zygomatic
_____ d. Axis

4. Which one of the following statements in reference to cerebrospinal fluid is *false?*

_____ a. Cerebrospinal fluid covers the brain and spinal cord.
_____ b. Cerebrospinal fluid coming from the ears or nose may indicate serious head injury.
_____ c. Cerebrospinal fluid coming from the mouth indicates minor head injury.
_____ d. Cerebrospinal fluid is clear in color.

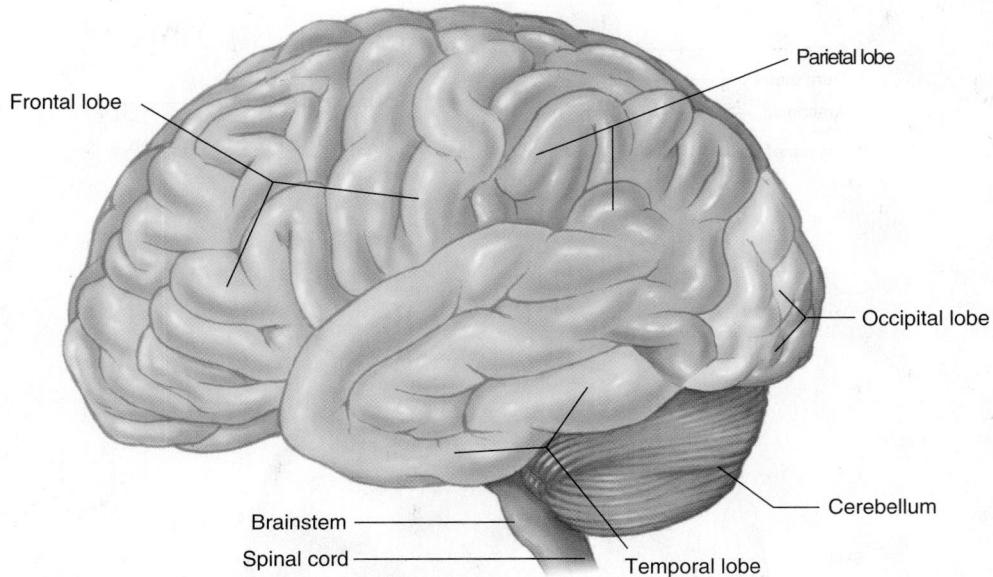

5. The portion of the brain responsible for vital functions, such as respiration and cardiac activity, is the:

_____ a. cerebrum.

_____ b. cerebellum.

_____ c. brainstem.

_____ d. spinal cord.

Matching

Match the function on the left with the portion of the brain responsible for that function on the right.

1. _____	Coordination	A. Cerebrum (frontal)
2. _____	Vision	B. Cerebrum (parietal)
3. _____	Speech	C. Cerebrum (temporal)
4. _____	Emotions	D. Cerebrum (occipital)
5. _____	Respiration	E. Cerebellum
6. _____	Memory	F. Brainstem
7. _____	Sensory	
8. _____	Equilibrium	

Critical Thinking

1. Why is the skull also called the *cranial vault*?

____

____

____

2. Explain the dura mater's connection to the other layers of the brain.

____

____

____

____

Head Injury Classifications

There are two types of head injury—open head injury and closed head injury. Within these two broad classifications, there are many types of injuries, some minor and some very serious.

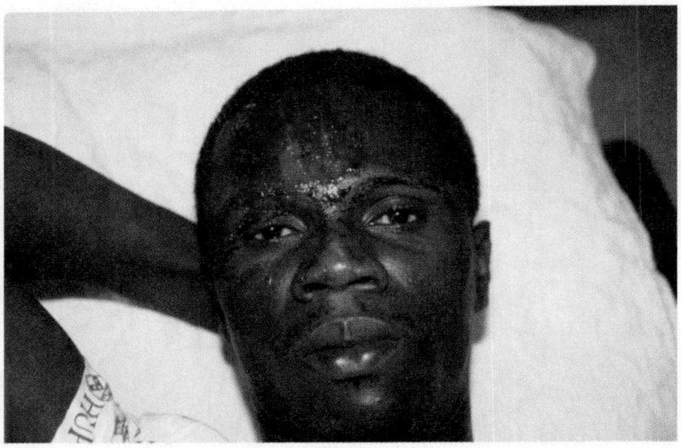

(A)

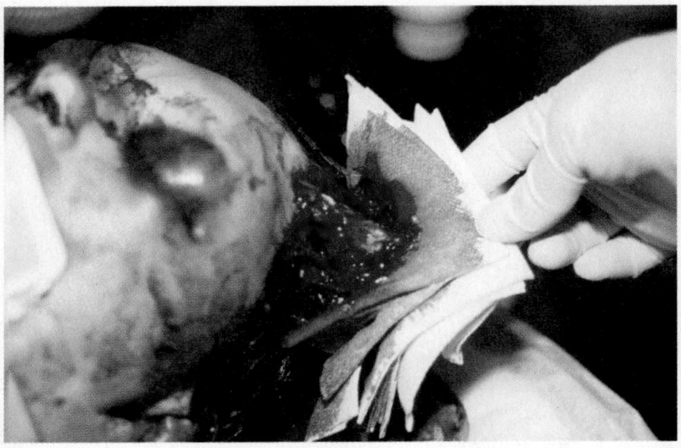

(B)

Figure 35-4 (A) Evidence of a closed head injury involving forehead abrasions from windshield impact. (© Edward T. Dickinson, MD) (B) A serious open head wound involving a gunshot wound to the head with brain exposed. (© Edward T. Dickinson, MD)

35-6 Explain the pathophysiology and key signs and symptoms of injuries to the scalp, skull, and brain, including scalp lacerations, skull fractures, cerebral concussion, cerebral contusion, and intracranial hematomas

open head injury head injury in which there is a break in the skin and cranium.

closed head injury head injury that involves damage to the skull or brain by a traumatic force that does not cause an open injury of the skin or cranium.

An **open head injury** is one in which there has been a break in the skin and the cranium. The injury can range from relatively minor, such as a laceration or abrasion to serious or even fatal, such as a crush injury or gunshot wound that exposes brain tissue through a fractured skull (Figure 35-4 ■).

A **closed head injury** involves damage to the skull or brain by a traumatic force that does not cause an open injury of the skin or cranium (Figure 35-5 ■). Do not be fooled into thinking that an injury is not serious simply because there is no bleeding or an open wound. Dangerously high pressures can develop within the skull in a closed head injury, pressures that can cause death if left untreated.

In addition to the open and closed classifications, head injuries can be described by the structure that is injured. For example, trauma to the scalp may involve an open head injury caused by the head striking the windshield in a motor-vehicle collision. An injury to the skull might involve damage to the bony structure housing the brain and the bones of the face. Even though the skull is quite durable, it can be fractured (Figure 35-6 ■). Skull fractures may range from undetectable cracks to areas that can be palpated and identified as depressed to major trauma in which brain tissue is exposed.

The brain itself may be injured, whether the head injury is open or closed. In severe skull fractures, brain tissue could be crushed, lacerated, or even exposed in an open injury. Head trauma can cause bleeding and swelling within the skull, creating pressure on the brain that will compress it and alter its function. Excessive bleeding or swelling (discussed in greater detail later in this chapter) within the skull will cause serious injury and often death.

PERSPECTIVE

Barry—The EMT

In my head I just keep hearing those really irregular snoring respirations that Ron had. And the sound of tires crunching on broken glass as other cars were driving slowly past the crash scene on their way to wherever they were going, you know? I kept seeing their eyes darting around as they rolled past. The passersby are always curious but not always concerned. It seemed to go on forever. I put a nonrebreather mask on Ron and now I was trying to care for two patients, you know? I didn't know what else to do.

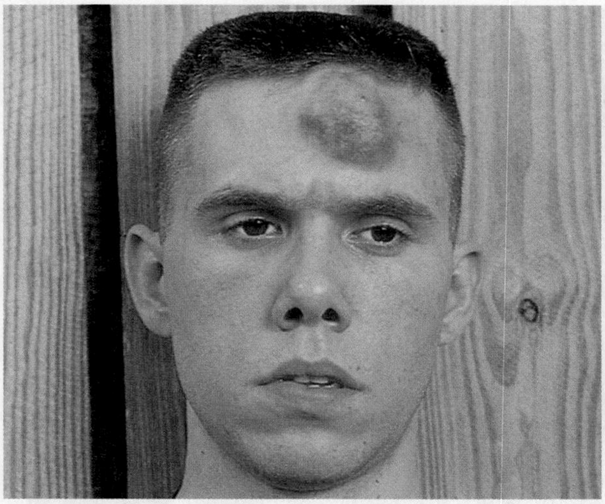

Figure 35-5 A closed head injury.

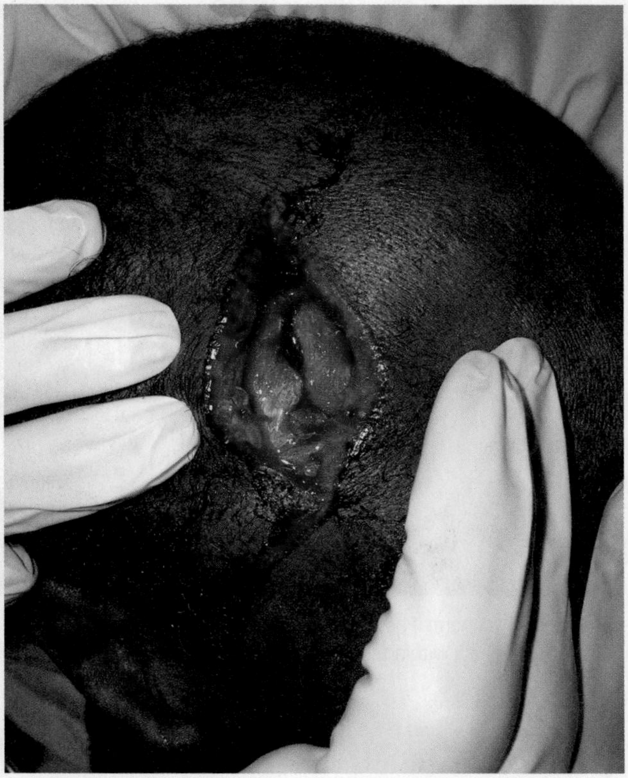

Figure 35-6 An open skull fracture. (© Edward T. Dickinson, MD)

You may also hear the terms *concussion* and *contusion* in reference to a head injury. A **concussion** is defined as a temporary alteration in normal brain function after head impact. It is caused by a jarring of the brain, resulting in temporary signs and symptoms. It can cause a loss of consciousness immediately after the injury as well as other forms of altered brain function, including loss of memory about the incident, visual problems, confusion, and headache. A concussion is not visible on specialized tests, such as a CT scan or MRI. There is usually no permanent damage from a concussion, although signs and symptoms may appear serious at first and persist for some time (called *post-concussion syndrome*). Repeated concussions can lead to permanent injury and long-term disability. This is common among athletes who participate in contact sports.

concussion type of injury causing a jarring to the brain and temporary signs and symptoms including loss of memory about the incident and confusion.

contusion bruising of the brain tissue.

A **contusion** is a bruising of brain tissue itself. The bleeding in this type of injury is usually limited but significant enough to cause altered mental status and other signs and symptoms that last longer than those of a concussion. Brain contusions are injuries that are visible on imaging tests such as CT scans.

35-7 Discuss factors that can worsen traumatic brain injuries, including hypoxia, hypocarbia, hypercarbia, and hypotension.

In the field it will not be possible to distinguish one type of brain injury from another. Most importantly, remember that all patients with signs of head trauma of any type should receive hospital-based evaluation and care.

Finally, keep in mind that damage to the brain may be due to either primary or secondary factors. The most common primary factor is trauma. Secondary factors may be conditions such as hypoxia, hypoperfusion, **hypercarbia, hypocarbia,** and others that can damage the brain as a result of a problem elsewhere in the body.

hypercarbia abnormally high carbon dioxide level in the blood that leads to dilation of the cerebral blood vessels.

hypocarbia abnormally low carbon dioxide level in the blood that leads to constriction of the cerebral blood vessels

As an EMT, there is little you can do about primary brain injuries other than identify that they have likely occurred. However, your treatment can make a real impact in reducing secondary brain injury by attending to the ABCs. That will help prevent further insults to the brain, such as hypoxia and hypoperfusion.

35-8 Describe the goals of emergency treatment of patients with traumatic brain injuries.

35-9 Describe the pathophysiology and key signs of increased intracranial pressure and brain herniation.

Intracranial Pressure

Perhaps the most serious problem associated with a head injury is the development of increasing **intracranial pressure.** The soft brain fits very tightly within the rigid skull as is evident in a CT scan of a normal brain (Figure 35-7 ■). When a blow to the head causes injury to the brain or surrounding tissues, bleeding and swelling develop. Because the soft brain is within the fixed rigid confines of the skull, it has no space

intracranial pressure increasing pressure within the cranial vault due to bleeding or swelling.

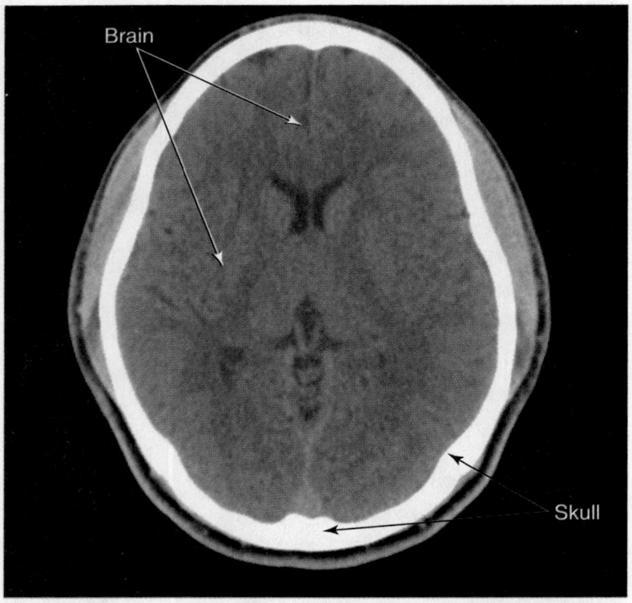

Figure 35-7 A normal head CT that shows how snugly the soft, normal brain (grey) fits within the rigid skull (white). (© Edward T. Dickinson, MD)

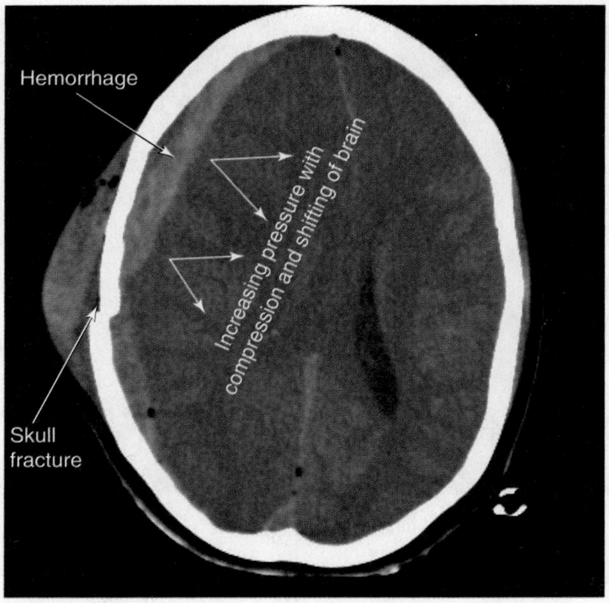

Figure 35-8 Skull fracture with hemorrhage, causing increasing pressure with compression and shifting of the brain. (© Edward T. Dickinson, MD)

in which to expand, so as intracranial pressure increases, compressing and shifting of the brain within the skull occurs (Figures 35-8 ■ and 35-9 ■). As little as 20–30 mL of blood can begin to cause intracranial pressure.

As intracranial pressure increases, so too do the signs and symptoms that the patient will display. As the pressure continues to rise, the brain is compressed more and more. Eventually, the brain begins to shift downward (**herniation**), compressing the brainstem, the part of the brain that controls the most vital bodily functions. Signs and symptoms of increased intracranial pressure include the following:

herniation tissue protrusion outside the area in which it is normally contained.

- Decreasing mental status
- Vomiting
- Headache

The patient also will exhibit some or all of the following, depending on the amount of pressure inside the cranium:

- Seizures
- Weakness or paralysis on one side of the body
- Abnormal posturing (**decorticate** or **decerebrate**) (Figure 35-10 ■)
- Abnormal breathing patterns
- Decreased pulse rate
- Increased blood pressure
- Nonreactive, dilated, or unequal pupils
- Decreasing Glasgow Coma Score

decorticate patient posture characterized by stiff flexed arms at the elbows, clenched fists, and extended legs.

decerebrate patient posture characterized by stiff extended arms at the elbows and pronated forearms.

CLINICAL CLUE

Head Injuries

Not all head injuries cause intracranial pressure. As a matter of fact, most do not. There are a wide range of bumps, scrapes, and lacerations that will cause no permanent damage. The problem is that in the field an EMT cannot see inside the skull to look for hidden damage.

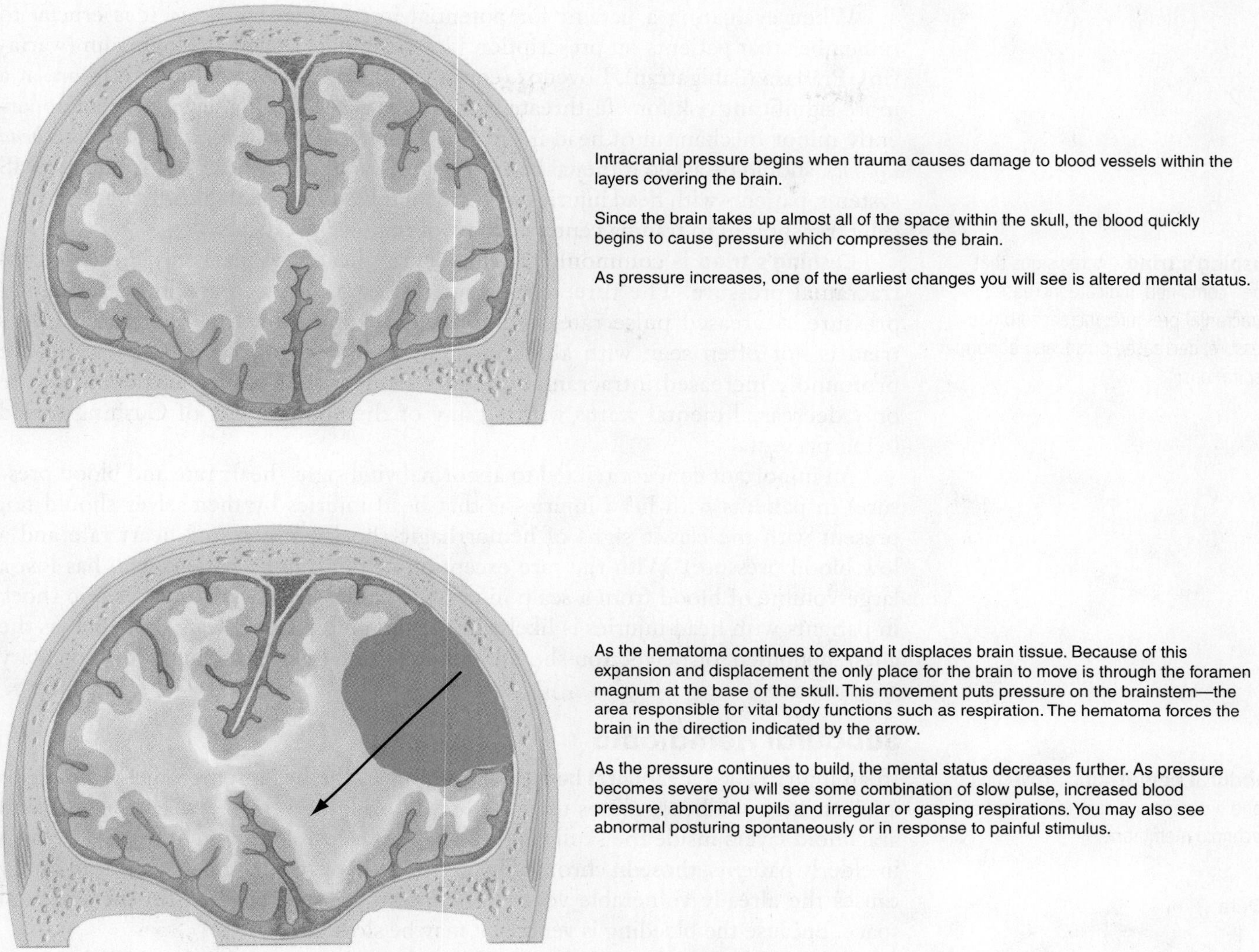
Intracranial pressure begins when trauma causes damage to blood vessels within the layers covering the brain.
Since the brain takes up almost all of the space within the skull, the blood quickly begins to cause pressure which compresses the brain.
As pressure increases, one of the earliest changes you will see is altered mental status.
As the hematoma continues to expand it displaces brain tissue. Because of this expansion and displacement the only place for the brain to move is through the foramen magnum at the base of the skull. This movement puts pressure on the brainstem—the area responsible for vital body functions such as respiration. The hematoma forces the brain in the direction indicated by the arrow.
As the pressure continues to build, the mental status decreases further. As pressure becomes severe you will see some combination of slow pulse, increased blood pressure, abnormal pupils and irregular or gasping respirations. You may also see abnormal posturing spontaneously or in response to painful stimulus.

Figure 35-9 Hemorrhage, causing shift of brain tissue as intracranial pressure increases.

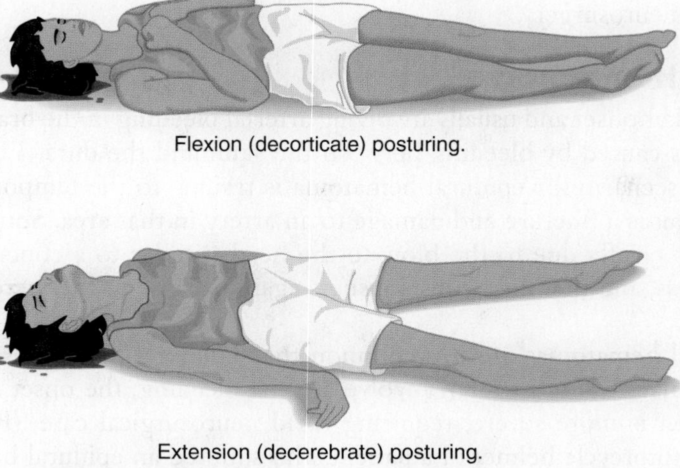
Flexion (decorticate) posturing.
Extension (decerebrate) posturing.

Figure 35-10 Decorticate and decerebrate posturing.

When evaluating a patient for potential intracranial bleeding, it is crucial to remember that patients on prescription blood thinners—such as Coumadin (warfarin), Pradaxa (dabigatran), Lovenox (enoxaparin), and Plavix (clopidogrel)—are at a more significant risk for life-threatening intracranial bleeding, even with an apparently minor mechanism of head injury. All trauma patients, *especially those with head injuries*, should be asked if they take any of these types of medications. In many EMS systems, patients with head injuries who are on these types of medications are specifically transported to trauma centers as part of regional protocols.

Cushing's triad three signs that, when combined, indicate increased intracranial pressure: increased blood pressure, decreased pulse, and abnormal respirations.

Cushing's triad is commonly taught as an indicator of markedly increased intracranial pressure. The three signs that make up the triad are increased blood pressure, decreased pulse rate, and abnormal respirations. In reality, Cushing's triad is not often seen with all three signs together. Indeed, patients can have profoundly increased intracranial pressure from a brain injury and demonstrate only decreased mental status without any of the components of Cushing's triad being present.

An important concept related to abnormal vital signs (heart rate and blood pressure) in patients with head injuries is that head injuries by themselves should not present with the classic signs of hemorrhagic shock (an elevated heart rate and a low blood pressure). With the rare exception of the trauma patient who has lost a large volume of blood from a scalp injury, the cause of signs of hypovolemic shock in patients with head injuries is likely due to blood loss from other sites such as the chest, abdomen, or pelvis. You should look for those injuries during your secondary assessment.

Subdural Hematoma

subdural hematoma collection of blood between the dura mater and the arachnoid membrane.

In an injury called a **subdural hematoma,** a blow to the head, sometimes as simple as a fall striking the head, causes tearing of small bridging veins between the dura and arachnoid layers inside the skull (Figure 35-11 ▪). Most commonly this may be seen in elderly patients, those in chronically poor health, or in alcoholics. The head injury causes the already vulnerable vessels to rupture, causing bleeding in the subdural space. Because the bleeding is venous, it may be slow.

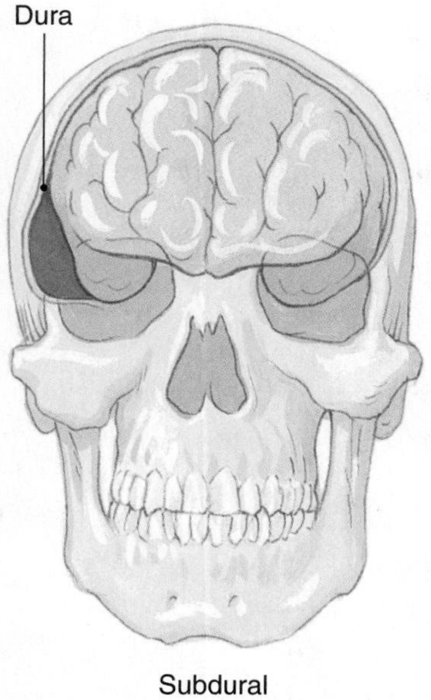

Figure 35-11 Subdural hematoma.

Subdural hematomas can begin without symptoms and develop over hours to days. In some cases, very slow bleeding may result, producing few or no symptoms for several days or even weeks. Subdural hematomas are the most common type of serious, intracranial hemorrhage associated with head injury. Its slow onset should help you to understand why all patients with head injury should go to the hospital, even if the patient seems "okay" at the scene. Most patients with acute subdural hematomas will require neurosurgery.

Epidural Hematoma

epidural hematoma collection of blood between the dura mater and the skull.

With a quicker onset and usually involving arterial bleeding in the brain, an **epidural hematoma** is caused by bleeding between the skull and the dura (Figure 35-12 ▪). A common scenario for epidural hematoma is trauma to the temporal area of the skull that causes a fracture and damage to an artery in that area. Some patients are unconscious briefly due to the blow to the head (similar to a concussion), regain consciousness, and then lose consciousness again because of the increased pressure in the brain.

Epidural hematomas are less common than subdural hematomas, but because epidural hematomas most often involve arterial bleeding, the onset is quicker and the condition is more severe, requiring rapid neurosurgical care. (Figure 35-13 ▪ shows the motorcycle helmet of a patient who suffered an epidural hematoma after an impact to the temporal skull.)

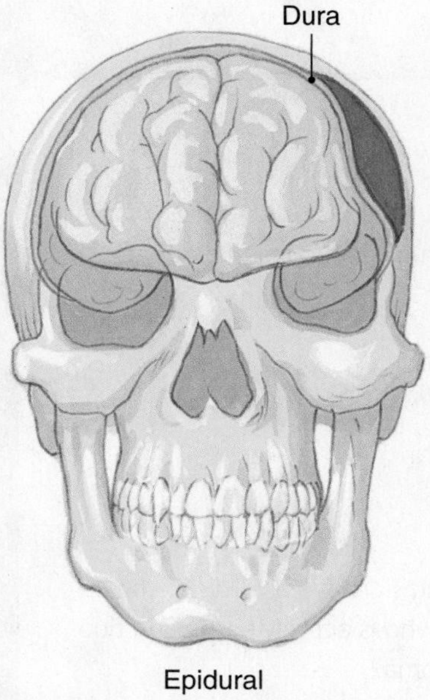

Figure 35-12 Epidural hematoma.

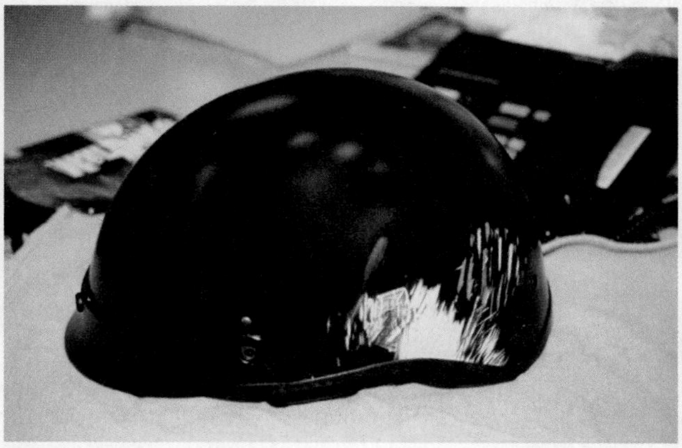

Figure 35-13 Helmet showing the temporal skull impact of a patient with an epidural hematoma. (© Edward T. Dickinson, MD)

PRACTICAL PATHOPHYSIOLOGY

Patients who suffer blunt trauma to the temporal region of the skull are at particular risk for developing epidural hematomas for two reasons. First, the temporal bone is relatively thin and more prone to fracture. Second, the middle meningeal artery lies on the inside of the temporal bone in a grooved channel. Thus when the temporal bone is fractured, the middle meningeal artery is easily torn, resulting in sudden arterial bleeding in the epidural space.

If large enough and left untreated, both subdural and epidural hematomas (as well as other types of intracranial bleeding) can result in pressure inside the cranium sufficient to cause portions of the brain to herniate. If pressure continues, the cerebrum and cerebellum are pushed into the brainstem. Then, when the brainstem is compressed, it is forced out of the skull toward the foramen magnum, and vital functions such as respiration are compromised. A herniation as a result of head injury will cause the patient to have a rapidly and profoundly decreased mental status, to exhibit abnormal breathing patterns, and often to display unequal pupils.

CLINICAL CLUE

Head Injury

It will never be your job as an EMT to determine what type of head injury a patient has sustained (epidural or subdural, for example). What is important is that you recognize a significant mechanism of injury and signs and symptoms of head injury. Any patient with a head injury should be encouraged to accept your transport to an emergency department for a complete evaluation.

PERSPECTIVE

Dr. Mendelez—Emergency Department Physician

We obviously care for all our patients, but when they bring in somebody in uniform, it somehow just changes the mood in the emergency department. And then I saw it was Ron. I had just talked to him on the phone about 20 minutes before about the patient they were bringing in. That's really tough. And as soon as they came through the doors, I could see he was posturing and, oh my heart just sank. Ron's a good guy and he doesn't deserve this kind of thing. He just doesn't. It feels different when I know the person.

STOP, REVIEW, REMEMBER!

Multiple Choice

For each question, place a check next to the correct answer.

1. Which one of the following is *not* a component of Cushing's triad?

_____ a. Increased blood pressure
_____ b. Decreased pulse rate
_____ c. Fixed pupils
_____ d. Abnormal respirations

2. Tissue forced out of an area in which it is normally contained is called:

_____ a. infarction.
_____ b. impalement.
_____ c. compression.
_____ d. herniation.

3. Subdural hematomas form between the:

_____ a. dura and arachnoid layers.
_____ b. arachnoid and pia mater.
_____ c. arachnoid layer and the brain.
_____ d. skull and the dura.

4. The most posterior portion of the brain is called the _____________ lobe.

_____ a. temporal
_____ b. frontal
_____ c. occipital
_____ d. parietal

5. Which one of the following signs is least likely to be encountered in a patient who is actively herniating due to a large epidural hematoma?

_____ a. Unequal pupils
_____ b. Mildly decreased mental status
_____ c. Irregular breathing pattern
_____ d. Significant mechanism of injury

Labeling

Label the regions and bones of the human skull on the diagram.

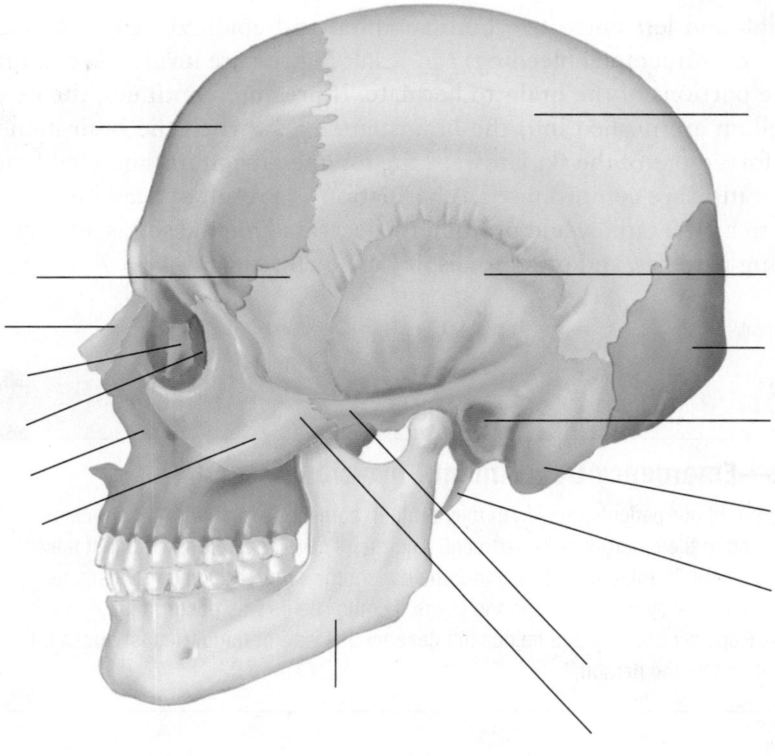

Critical Thinking

1. What is the significance of a patient with a closed head injury who is taking Coumadin for a preexisting heart condition?

2. You are treating a patient who appears to have struck his head on the windshield in a motor-vehicle crash. You observe a large hematoma on the patient's forehead. He is unresponsive, with pulse at 140, respirations 28, and blood pressure 88/52. Are these vital signs likely caused by his head injury? Why or why not?

Patient Assessment and Care

Head injuries are not only very serious, but they also can pose a significant problem for EMTs. That is because in the field it is difficult to distinguish the less serious head injuries from the life-threatening ones. For this reason, you should presume all head injuries to be potentially serious and the patient treated and transported accordingly.

Patient Assessment

As an EMT there is little you can do about primary brain injuries in the field, other than identifying that they have likely occurred based on your assessment of the mechanism of injury and of the patient. Where your patient care will make a real impact is in reducing secondary brain injury. By your attention to the ABCs, you will help prevent further insults to the brain such as hypoxia, hypocarbia, hypercarbia, and hypoperfusion.

Scene Size-up

During the scene size-up, safety is always a primary concern. Be sure you are not injured by the same trauma mechanism that injured your patient. Be alert for the mechanism of injury as you approach the scene and the patient. Remember that some patients may seem fine, but have hidden injuries. The mechanism of injury will be an important indicator to detect them.

All injuries to the head and face tend to bleed excessively due to the rich blood supply of the head. Injuries to the mouth and nose can cause blood to be sprayed when the patient speaks or shouts. Unresponsive patients with such injuries often require suction of blood or other secretions that threaten the airway.

For all these reasons, when managing patients with head injuries, use appropriate personal protective equipment, including full face protection as you determine BSI precautions.

Primary Assessment

Form a general impression as you approach the patient. Combined with the mechanism of injury, this should give you a good starting point for determining the seriousness of the patient's condition. Observe the patient's level of consciousness. An altered mental status or seizures indicate that the patient has a serious injury. Often patients with head injuries are intoxicated with alcohol or other drugs that produce altered mental status. Those situations are particularly difficult because it is nearly impossible to determine if the altered mental status is due to the drug effect, the injury, or a mixture of both. Always presume that these patients are altered because of head injury primarily and treat them as such.

Remember that injuries to the face and head have the potential for significant bleeding. Be prepared to suction the airway continuously, if necessary. This will require someone stationed at the airway for the entire call. That person also can administer oxygen and ventilate as needed.

Be sure to control severe bleeding. Check the pulse and the skin color, temperature, and condition. Remember that a very slow pulse in a patient with an altered mental status and a closed head injury might be the result of increased intracranial pressure.

CLINICAL CLUE

About Consent

Head-injured patients with an altered mental status may not refuse medical care or treatment, because they have lost the capacity to fully understand their condition and the consequences of refusal of care. You also will encounter head-injured patients who do not have altered mental status and who refuse care. Although they have the right to do so, you should make extra efforts (including asking medical direction to speak with them) to try to convince them to go to the hospital due to the significant risks associated with head injuries.

Secondary Assessment

Patients with a significant mechanism of injury should receive a rapid trauma assessment. When examining the head, feel the cranium for any signs of injury, including deformity, depression, swelling, or open injury (Figure 35-14 ▪). Examine the face, including the nose and ears for clear or blood-tinged (cerebrospinal) fluid, which may indicate a basilar skull fracture. Also observe for **raccoon eyes** (bruising around the eyes) (Figure 35-15 ▪) or **Battle's sign** (Figure 35-16 ▪), which are late signs of significant head injury.

raccoon eyes bruising around the eyes indicative of a basilar skull fracture.

Battle's sign bruising behind the ears (over the mastoid process) indicative of a basilar skull fracture.

35-11 Discuss the focus of history taking and assessment for patients with injuries to the head.

Vital Signs and History

As with any patient, trends in vital signs over time paint the best picture. Remember that mental status is the most important indicator in head-injured patients. Patients with a concussion may start with unconsciousness or confusion. In many cases they will gradually regain memory and become less confused. Patients with rising intracranial pressure have a persistent altered mental status or a gradually decreased mental status.

When possible, obtain a medical history from the patient or a family member. Be alert for other conditions that can cause an altered mental status. For example, a

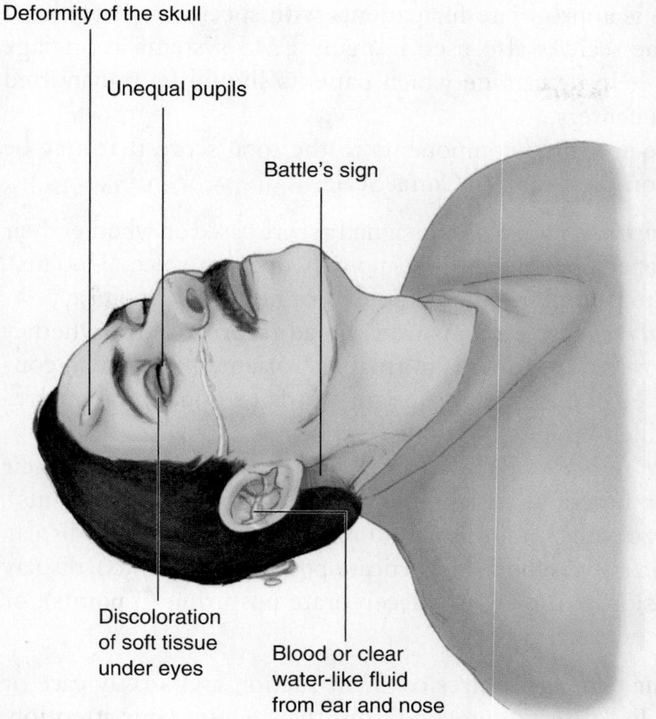

Figure 35-14 Signs of skull fracture or brain injury.

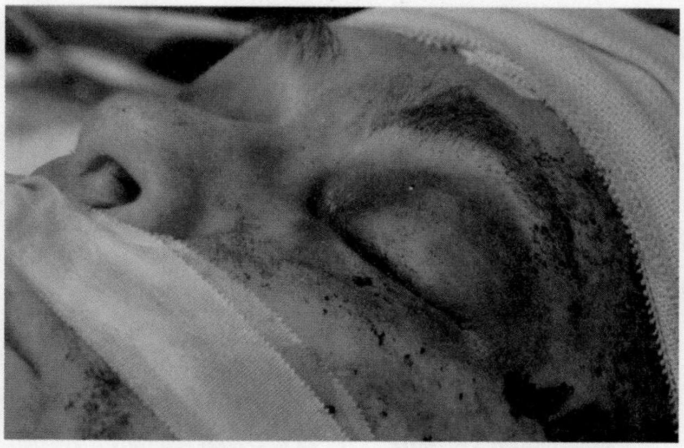

Figure 35-15 Bilateral periorbital ecchymosis (raccoon eyes). (© Edward T. Dickinson, MD)

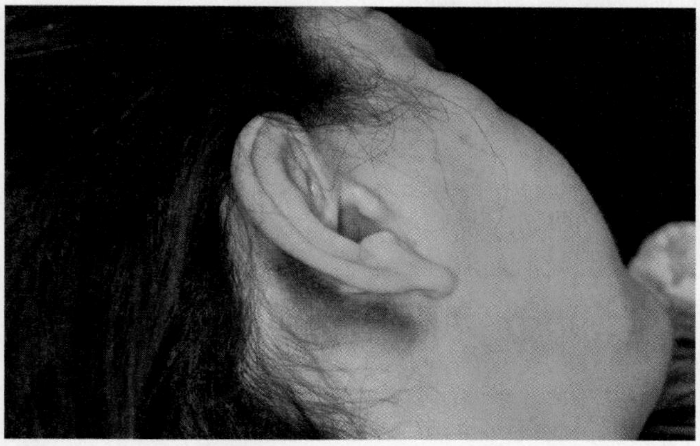

Figure 35-16 Retroauricular ecchymosis (Battle's sign). (© Edward T. Dickinson, MD)

patient in a collision may exhibit an altered mental status and appear to have a head injury but may in fact be diabetic or have suffered a seizure. Remember that medical and trauma complaints can occur at the same time in the same patient (such as a seizure that causes a fall resulting in head injury).

PERSPECTIVE

Dayna Ridge—The Paramedic

I can't believe I was responding to Ron. I mean he's Ron! He's been here longer than anyone I know. He was my first partner after I got out of EMT school and he actually came to my goofy little graduation ceremony when I got my paramedic cert. And there I was tonight, assessing him on the side of the freeway. That's the first time I've ever actually seen Cushing's in real life. That whole call was just wrong. It keeps kind of glossing over in my mind, like it's not real. And then it just jumps back into my face, you know? I don't know what to do right now.

Glasgow Coma Scale

Just as you trend vital signs, including blood pressure and pulse, you will need to trend the level of consciousness of patients who have a head injury. The most widely accepted system of trending mental status in patients with a head injury is the Glasgow Coma Scale. The **Glasgow Coma Scale (GCS)** (Figure 35-17 ■) is a numerical scale that rates patients' mental status based on eye opening, speech, and motor function. (This was covered briefly in Chapter 20. More detail is offered here.)

This scale and its scores, which range from 3 to 15, are valuable in monitoring and documenting trends in the patient's neurological status and in determining

35-10 Describe the neurological assessment of patients with suspected traumatic brain injury.

Glasgow Coma Scale (GCS) an assessment tool that provides a numerical score for rating patients on eye opening, speech, and motor function.

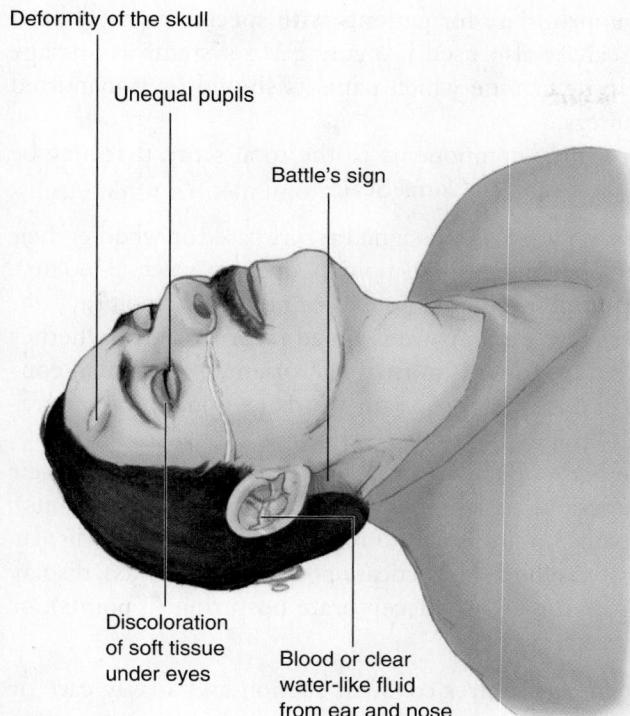

Glasgow Coma Scale	
Eye Opening	
Spontaneous	4
To verbal command	3
To pain	2
No response	1
Verbal Response	
Oriented and converses	5
Disoriented and converses	4
Inappropriate words	3
Incomprehensible sounds	2
No response	1
Motor Response	
Obeys verbal commands	6
Localizes pain	5
Withdraws from pain (flexion)	4
Abnormal flexion in response to pain (decorticate rigidity)	3
Extension in response to pain (decerebrate rigidity)	2
No response	1

Figure 35-17 Glasgow Coma Scale.

what care is appropriate for patients with specific types of head injury. The scale is also used in many EMS systems as a triage device to help determine which patients should be transported to trauma centers.

There are three components to the total score that may be obtained on the Glasgow Coma Scale:

- ***Eye opening.*** Patients are assigned a score based on whether their eyes open spontaneously (4 points), open to voice (3 points), open to painful stimulus (2 points), or not at all (1 point).
- ***Verbal response.*** Patients are assigned a score based on whether their verbal response is normal and oriented (5 points), confused (4 points), inappropriate words (3 points), incomprehensible (2 points), or none (1 point).
- ***Motor response.*** Patients are assigned a score based on their motor function: patients who follow commands (6 points), localize pain (5 points), withdraw from pain (4 points), display flexion at the elbows/decorticate posturing (3 points), display extension at the elbows/decerebrate posturing (2 points), or no response (1 point).

If your patient requires constant suction and airway care or has other life-threatening conditions that require your attention, do not spend time obtaining a GCS score. This patient already has a high priority for transport and the GCS score can be determined en route to the hospital. One of the most critical uses of the GCS is that it is not only a very good way to objectively document your initial findings, but it also is a critical part of ongoing reassessment of head-injured patients. Knowing whether a patient's GCS score is increasing or decreasing over the course of prehospital care is essential information for the receiving hospital.

35-12 Explain the importance of reassessment of the patient with an injury to the head.

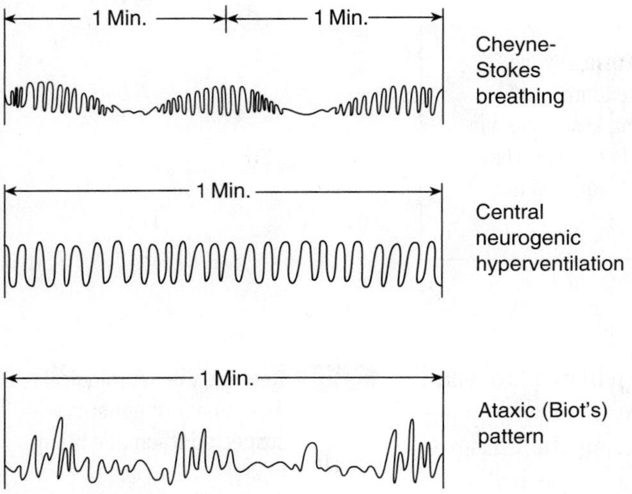

Figure 35-18 Abnormal breathing patterns associated with severe head injuries.

CLINICAL CLUE

Glasgow Coma Scale

The National Trauma Triage Protocol identifies that a GCS score of less than 14 is by itself an indication to transport a trauma patient to the highest level of care within a trauma system because it is a reliable indicator of a serious head injury.

Abnormal Breathing Patterns

Certain abnormal breathing patterns may be observed in head-injured patients with rising intracranial pressure (Figure 35-18 ■). The patterns indicate serious conditions affecting the brain, including lack of perfusion and oxygen and increasing pressure on brain tissue. It is not critical to memorize or recognize each pattern. What is most important is that irregular patterns such as these generally indicate significant injury.

Abnormal breathing patterns include:

- The **Cheyne-Stokes respirations** pattern is characterized by gradually increasing and then decreasing tidal volume with a period of apnea.
- Caused by damage or injury to the brainstem such as may be seen in herniation syndrome, the **central neurogenic hyperventilation** breathing pattern is made up of deep, rapid respirations (as indicated by the term *hyperventilation*).
- The breathing pattern of **ataxic (Biot's) respirations** is characterized by deep, gasping breaths separated by periods of apnea.

Cheyne-Stokes respirations pattern of respirations characterized by gradually increasing and then decreasing tidal volumes with a period of apnea.

central neurogenic hyperventilation pattern of respirations characterized by deep, rapid respirations; condition caused by damage or injury to the brainstem such as may be seen in herniation syndrome.

ataxic (Biot's) respirations pattern of respirations characterized by deep, gasping breaths separated by periods of apnea.

CLINICAL CLUE

Avoiding Hypoxia and Low Blood Pressure

Brain injury experts have determined the two things that most negatively affect the recovery of head-injured patients are allowing hypoxia or low blood pressure to develop after the initial injury. Prevention, early recognition, and aggressive treatment of airway problems, breathing difficulties, and hypoperfusion are the most important prehospital interventions that can be made for the head-injured patient.

Patient Care

Your care for the head-injured patient will depend on your assessment. Care for a head injury begins during the scene size-up when you take BSI precautions and observe the mechanism of injury. If you suspect spine injury, take spinal stabilization maneuvers as you begin your primary assessment. Be alert for airway problems. Open head injuries can bleed profusely. If blood is near or flows into the patient's airway, constant monitoring and frequent suction will be required. Also during the primary assessment, you are to observe the patient's mental status. An altered mental status is one of the most significant signs of head injury. Note the patient's mental status initially and throughout the call. Decreasing mental status is a serious sign. Time and priorities permitting, track changes in the patient during your care with GCS scores.

PERSPECTIVE

Barry—The EMT

I heard him open the driver's door and thought that he was either checking on the other driver or was going to open the back doors. But then I heard him hit the ground and he didn't respond to my yelling. I got worried. My immediate fear was that it might be some kind of head injury, you know? He seemed a little confused on the radio. But, holy Toledo, that was a big, big crash. That other car was actually imbedded in the cab of our truck. I'm surprised that none of us were killed. He better be okay. I'd better call his wife.

Oxygenation and Ventilation

Head-injured patients require oxygen. Patients with head injuries who have altered mental status and who are breathing adequately should receive oxygen by nonrebreather mask. Those who are breathing inadequately should receive assisted ventilation with a pocket mask or bag-mask device.

For head-injured patients, there is one additional and very important consideration: the rate of assisted ventilations or artificial ventilation. In the past, EMTs were instructed to hyperventilate all head-injured patients to help reduce intracranial swelling and pressure. Research has demonstrated that ventilating too fast was actually harmful. Ventilating a head-injured patient too quickly can cause excessive hypocarbia that decreases blood flow to the brain. In this case, more is not better. Normal ventilations at the rate of 10 to 12 per minute are appropriate in most cases of head-injured patients who require ventilation due to inadequate breathing.

However, if the patient is experiencing the most severe form of head injury, cerebral herniation, ventilating at a slightly faster rate has been recommended. Signs of herniation that would cause you to ventilate at a faster rate include:

- Evidence of a head injury or history indicating head involvement, such as headache before losing consciousness
- Unresponsiveness
- Pupillary changes including unilateral (one-sided) dilation, nonreactive, or asymmetrical pupils
- Decerebrate (extension) posturing
- Rapidly decreasing Glasgow Coma Scale scores

Ventilation rates for patients experiencing signs of herniation are 20 per minute for adults, 30 per minute for children, and 35 per minute for infants.

Ventilate the patient with slow, full breaths as you would for artificial ventilation. The patient may have some respiratory effort or be exhibiting an abnormal breathing pattern (for example, Cheyne-Stokes or ataxic respirations). If so, ventilate during an inspiration ("assisting" the patient's own breath), and do not exceed the recommended number of ventilations.

Other emergency care for head injuries includes:

- Ensuring that the airway is open and clear. Be prepared for vomiting. Suction as needed.
- Providing cervical-spine stabilization
- Administering oxygen to the patient
- Controlling bleeding. Avoid pressure over depressed areas or unstable areas where the skull fracture is suspected.
- *Not* stopping the flow of cerebrospinal fluid from the nose or ears
- Stabilizing any objects impaled in the head
- Preventing the patient from moving or exerting himself
- Transporting the patient in a supine position (head neither elevated nor lower than the body)
- Treating for shock

STOP, REVIEW, REMEMBER!

Multiple Choice

For each question, place a check next to the correct answer.

1. A reliable early sign of a serious closed head injury in a patient with a significant mechanism of injury is:

_____ a. raccoon eyes and a GCS of 12.

_____ b. unequal pupils and a GCS of 15.

_____ c. Battle's sign and a GCS of 12.

_____ d. scalp swelling and a GCS of 12.

2. Battle's sign is observed:

_____ a. around the eyes.

_____ b. in the cheek.

_____ c. at the temples.

_____ d. behind the ears.

3. Patients with a concussion usually:

_____ a. are unconscious, wake, and then go unconscious again.

_____ b. are unconscious and never regain consciousness.

_____ c. have a gradually improving mental status.

_____ d. have a gradually decreasing mental status.

4. The breathing pattern that involves gradually increasing volume followed by decreasing volume and apnea is called:

_____ a. Kussmaul's respirations.

_____ b. Cheyne-Stokes respirations.

_____ c. Biot's respirations.

_____ d. central neurogenic hyperventilation.

5. The lowest score on the Glasgow Coma Scale is:

_____ a. 0.

_____ b. 1.

_____ c. 3.

_____ d. 5.

Fill in the Blank

For each of the following patients, determine the appropriate Glasgow Coma Scale score.

1. Patient opens his eyes when you talk to him, appears confused, and follows commands.

____

2. Patient does not open his eyes, moans briefly and occasionally, and has decorticate/flexion posturing to pain.

____

3. Patient is awake and alert. He appears oriented and follows commands. _______________

4. Patient does not respond to any stimulus at all. There is no motor response. _______________

5. Patient opens eyes to painful stimulus, mutters sounds you do not understand, and pulls away when you apply the painful stimulus. _______________

Critical Thinking

1. You have two hospitals in your area. One is a community hospital that is 20 minutes away. The other is a trauma center that is 35 minutes away. What factors would your protocols likely take into consideration in making a transport decision for a patient with a serious head injury?

____

____

____

____

(continued on next page)

(continued)

2. Your 27-year-old male patient has been involved in a motor-vehicle collision. His head struck the "B" post between the driver's and rear passenger door when his car was "t-boned" by a truck into his door. He is awake but somewhat agitated and has the following vital signs: pulse 120, respirations 28 rapid and a bit shallow, blood pressure 94/62, skin cool and moist, and GCS 15. Is this patient's presentation caused by a head injury?

____

____

____

____

EMERGENCY DISPATCH SUMMARY

The collision investigation determined that the Volkswagen had been traveling southbound on Highway 53 when it was struck from behind by a tractor-trailer whose driver had fallen asleep. The small car was launched over a three-foot-high concrete barrier, into the northbound lanes, and into the ambulance driven by Ron Hyde. The car's driver was killed during the initial collision. EMT Ron Hyde suffered an epidural hematoma following the impact and required surgery to repair a damaged artery and to release some of the pressure. He still requires a wheelchair and struggles with aphasia, but continues to make positive steps toward recovery, thanks to an intensive traumatic brain injury rehabilitation program.

Chapter Review

To the Point

- Injuries to the head remain one of the most potentially devastating situations you will encounter as an EMT.
- Accurate assessment and proper care of head-injury patients will optimize their chances for survival and a meaningful recovery.
- The brain is well protected by the skull, but the fixed space in which the brain sits does not allow for expansion when bleeding and swelling occur. This leads to increased intracranial pressure.
- The most reliable sign of a brain injury is altered mental status.
- Patients on "blood thinners" are at particular risk for catastrophic brain injuries.
- A critical role of the EMT is to prevent secondary brain injury by aggressively treating hypoxia and hypoperfusion.
- The Glasgow Coma Scale is an objective measure of brain function that should be used whenever possible for assessment of the head-injured patient.
- The most devastating consequence of a closed head injury is herniation of portions of the brain.
- All patients with altered mental status should receive supplemental oxygen.
- Patients with signs of acute brain herniation should be ventilated at an increased but controlled rate.

Chapter Questions

Multiple-Choice

For each question, place a check next to the correct answer.

1. Meninges are layers:
   _____ a. that cover the brain.
   _____ b. that cover the skull (or cranium).
   _____ c. of the cerebrum.
   _____ d. (components) of the brainstem.

2. The medulla oblongata is part of the:
   _____ a. cerebrum.
   _____ b. cerebellum.
   _____ c. parietal lobe.
   _____ d. brainstem.

3. Increased blood pressure, decreased pulse, and abnormal respirations are collectively called:
   _____ a. Battle's sign.
   _____ b. Cushing's triad.
   _____ c. Starling's law.
   _____ d. Beck's triad.

4. As little as _____________ of blood can begin to cause intracranial pressure.
   _____ a. 20–30 mL
   _____ b. 100–150 mL
   _____ c. 200–300 mL
   _____ d. 2–3 liters

5. The three components of the Glasgow Coma Scale are:
   _____ a. pulse, respirations, and blood pressure.
   _____ b. appearance, pulse, and grimace.
   _____ c. speech, facial asymmetry, and motor function.
   _____ d. eye opening, speech, and motor function.

6. All of the following medications increase the risk of bleeding in patients with head injuries *except:*
   _____ a. Coumadin.
   _____ b. Albuterol.
   _____ c. Plavix.
   _____ d. Pradaxa.

7. According to the National Trauma Triage Protocol, what has been identified as a determination of the need for transport to a trauma center?
   _____ a. Heart rate <60
   _____ b. Systolic blood pressure greater than 190 mmHg
   _____ c. Glasgow Coma Scale score of >14
   _____ d. Glasgow Coma Scale score of <14

8. The most likely site of skull impact that will result in an epidural hematoma is the _____________ skull.
   _____ a. occipital
   _____ b. frontal
   _____ c. temporal
   _____ d. parietal

9. If an adult patient suddenly exhibits signs of likely herniation, the appropriate rate to ventilate the patient is _____________ per minute.
   _____ a. 10
   _____ b. 20
   _____ c. 30
   _____ d. 40

10. Components of the Glasgow Coma Scale include all of the following *except*:
   _____ a. verbal response.
   _____ b. pupil response.
   _____ c. motor response.
   _____ d. eye opening.

(continued on next page)

(continued)

Labeling

Label the following layers of the brain.

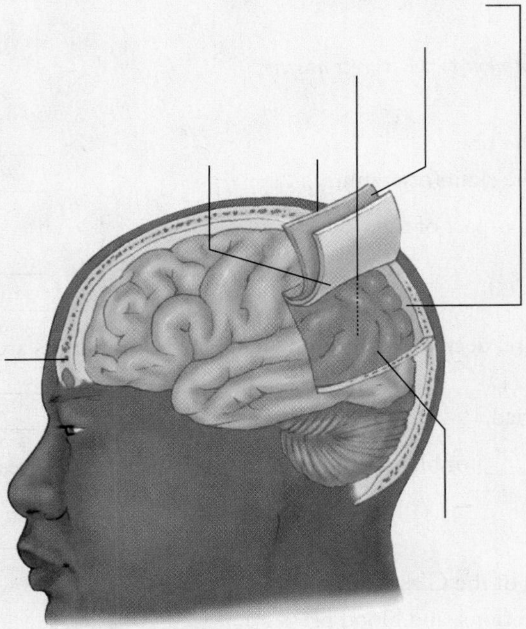

Critical Thinking

1. Explain how to determine the difference between a concussion and a cerebral contusion injury in the field.

2. What is the most significant indication of head injury you will observe in the field? Why?

Case Study

You are called to a patient who is "weak and vomiting." You arrive to find the 56-year-old male patient sitting on the closed lid of the toilet, slumped over the sink, and vomiting frequently into a waste basket. The vomitus is light brown and contains obvious food. The patient is sweaty. His daughter who just came home tells you that her father was supposed to walk a three-mile benefit walk that morning and, by the looks of the kitchen, had lunch a short time ago. The patient is unable to lift his head, but you believe you hear him mumble "headache" before he vomits again. You ask, "Have you fallen or did you hit your head?" He nods his head, indicating he did.

The daughter explains that your patient has a history of high blood pressure and takes medication for that and also some sort of blood thinner. You obtain a pulse and respirations and find that his pulse is 62 and respirations are 14 and labored. The vomiting ceases, and you are able to place the patient on a nonrebreather mask at 15 L/minute. You identify this patient as a high priority and place him on a Reeves stretcher for transport to the ambulance.

En route to the hospital, the patient loses consciousness. His vital signs in the ambulance are pulse 56 strong and regular, respirations 24 and shallow, and blood pressure 182/98. After five minutes vitals are pulse 48 and regular, respirations about 18 per minute, irregular and gasping, and blood pressure 210/105. Pupils do not respond. The patient has begun decerebrate posturing.

1. What indications did the patient give that his condition was serious in the first minute of the call?

2. En route to the hospital, the patient's condition worsened. Based on the vital signs and other observations, what do you believe the patient's problem is?

3. What should your care for this patient be?

The Last Word

Care for head injuries is about three things: suspicion, setting priorities, and decision making. You should suspect that all patients who have evidence of head trauma have a potentially serious head injury. You will set priorities such as minimizing scene time, airway care, determining which is the best receiving hospital for a given patient, and whether you have adequate time and resources to do sequential Glasgow Coma Scale determinations. Finally, your decision making will involve determining the rate at which your patient should be ventilated and which hospital is best for your patient. Remember to document all appropriate information in your prehospital care report.

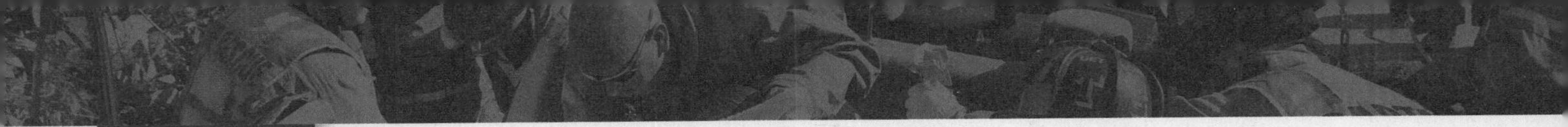

36 Caring for Patients with Spine Injuries

Education Standards

Trauma: Head, face, neck, and spine trauma

Competencies

Applies fundamental knowledge to provide basic emergency care and transportation based on assessment findings for an acutely injured patient.

Objectives

After completion of this lesson, you should be able to:

36-1 Define key terms introduced in this chapter.

36-2 Describe the structure and function of the spinal column, spinal cord, and tracts within the spinal column.

36-3 Describe common mechanisms of spine injury.

36-4 Differentiate spinal-column injury from spinal-cord injury.

36-5 Differentiate between spinal shock and neurogenic hypotension.

36-6 Describe the assessment of circulation, sensation, and motor function (CSM) in the extremities of a patient who is suspected of having an injury to the spine.

36-7 Describe signs and symptoms of injury to the spinal column and spinal cord.

36-8 Explain how complications of spine injury can result in inadequate breathing, paralysis, and inadequate circulation.

36-9 Describe appropriate emergency care for the patient with suspected spine injury.

36-10 Describe proper immobilization techniques for suspected spine injury patients who are supine, seated, and standing.

36-11 Describe the indications and correct procedures for rapid extrication.

36-12 Explain special handling and immobilization considerations when spine injury is suspected for helmet removal; football injuries, including removal of face mask and immobilization; and in infants and children, including extrication from a car seat.

Key Terms

central nervous system (CNS) p. 928
cervical vertebrae p. 929
coccygeal vertebrae p. 929
compression p. 932
displaced fracture p. 931
distraction p. 934
extension p. 932
flexion p. 932
lumbar vertebrae p. 929
manual stabilization p. 937
neurogenic hypotension p. 930
nondisplaced fracture p. 931
occipital p. 953
paralysis p. 927
peripheral nervous system (PNS) p. 928
priapism p. 935
rapid extrication p. 954
sacrum p. 929
spinal column p. 928
spinal cord p. 928
spinal shock p. 930
thoracic vertebrae p. 929
transection p. 931

Introduction

The spinal cord is the center of communication for the body. Every day literally millions of messages travel to and from the brain through the complex network of nerve tissue that makes up the spinal cord. This pathway of communication is essential for sustaining everyday functions. Tasks ranging from simple movement of the fingers to vital regulation of breathing and heart rate rely on a constant and efficient transfer of messages through the spinal cord.

36-4 Differentiate spinal-column injury from spinal-cord injury.

As an organ, the spinal cord is composed of delicate nerve tissue that is fragile and easily damaged. However, layers of bone, ligament, and muscle stand guard against trauma and form a protective barrier for this vulnerable organ system. In fact, despite the spinal cord's fragile nature, most injuries to the spine do not involve the spinal cord, but rather are limited to the bones, ligaments, and muscles that make up the spinal column.

Despite how well protected, no organ system is completely safe from the forces caused by high-energy trauma. With enough force, the spinal cord can be directly damaged or damaged by broken bone ends during movement after the injury. Regardless, the outcome of a significant spinal-cord injury can be devastating. Trauma that actually damages the cord can result in permanent neurological injuries that result in **paralysis.** As such, EMTs must be vigilant in the assessment and care of victims of spinal trauma.

paralysis suffering temporary or permanent loss of muscular power or sensation.

In this chapter the anatomy of the spinal column including the spinal cord, common mechanisms of injury, and the proper assessment and management of common spinal-cord injuries are discussed.

EMERGENCY DISPATCH

"How's that look now?" Gary balanced on the top step of the aluminum ladder, trying to hold a satellite dish in place.

"That's perfectly clear, Gary!" His wife called through the open kitchen window. "Leave it right there."

"Okay," he said. "But can I get you to come out for a second? I dropped the wrench."

Dena walked out into the backyard, drying her hands with a dish towel. "Where is it?"

"Down there." Gary motioned with his head, sweat dripping from the tip of his nose.

She saw the wrench glinting in the dark green of the lawn, picked it up, and held it high above her head. As Gary reached for it, the ladder began to wobble beneath his feet. He let go of the satellite dish, which crashed down to the patio, and tried to grab the edge of the roof to steady himself. The ladder slowed its sway for a second and then suddenly toppled over, sending Gary, arms pinwheeling crazily, to the grass below.

Dena screamed as Gary hit the lawn face first and then flipped over, landing on his back. He quickly climbed to his feet and stood, dazed.

"Where'd my hat go?" he said, looking around.

"Are you okay, honey?" Dena rushed up to him. "You really hit the ground hard."

"I'm fine, Baby," he said, shaking his head. "Just a little surprised, I guess. Oh, there it is." Gary took a couple of shaky steps toward his baseball cap and then slowly began to slump to the ground, coming to rest in a tangle of arms and legs.

"Oh my gosh, Gary! What's wrong?" Dena ran over and dropped to her knees next to him.

"Please! Call somebody, quick," he said into the grass. "I, I can't feel my legs."

The Spine and Nervous System

36-2 Describe the structure and function of the spinal column, spinal cord, and tracts within the spinal column.

36-8 Explain how complications of spine injury can result in inadequate breathing, paralysis, and inadequate circulation.

Anatomy

The nervous system is composed of the brain and spinal cord and an elaborate network of fibers called *nerves* that thread throughout the body. The nervous system is the control center for the entire body and coordinates all of the body's actions and reactions by sending impulses between the brain and the nerve endings.

central nervous system (CNS) the brain and spinal cord.

spinal cord the central nervous system (CNS) pathway responsible for transmitting sensory input from the body to the brain and for conducting motor impulses from the brain to the body muscles and organs.

peripheral nervous system (PNS) the nerves that enter and leave the spinal cord and those that extend from brain to organs without passing through the spinal cord.

The **central nervous system (CNS)** consists of the brain and **spinal cord.** The spinal cord is an organ made up of nervous tissue that is roughly the diameter of the thumb. It begins at the brainstem (the medulla oblongata) and extends roughly 18 inches down through the spinal column to the lumbar region of the back. The cord itself consists of a combination of both motor and sensory tissue designed to transmit messages back and forth from the brain.

Certain regions within the spinal cord are predominately sensory in nature, in that they move messages to the brain. Other areas are primarily motor in nature, in that they move messages from the brain out to the body. All along the length of the spinal cord, spinal nerves exit forming the basis for the complex network called the **peripheral nervous system (PNS).**

The PNS is made up of all the sensory and motor nerves that extend from the brain and spinal cord and travel to all parts of the body (Figure 36-1 ■). These nerves, and the spinal cord itself, allow for the exchange of information between the brain and the outside environment and for response from the brain to external stimuli. The warm feeling you get as you hold your hands by a fire is made possible by nervous tissue transmitting the sensation from your hands through your spinal cord to your brain. Your ability to pull your hands away when they become too warm is afforded to you by motor messages transmitted from your brain, through your spinal cord, and to your arms and hands.

Because the spinal cord is such an important message pathway, injuries to this tissue can be life threatening. Not only are peripheral sensation and motor function threatened, but also vital signaling to autonomic systems like the heart and lungs. When those pathways are interrupted, important bodily functions are affected. The higher up on the cord the injury occurs, the more bodily functions that may be affected. Furthermore, the nervous system has far less regenerative abilities than other tissues of the body; therefore, damage is more likely to be permanent.

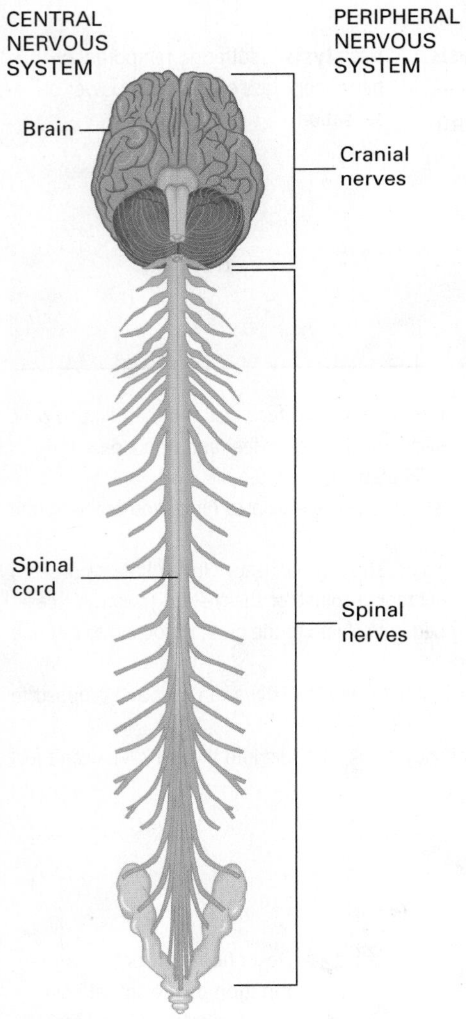

Figure 36-1 Components of the central and peripheral nervous system.

PRACTICAL PATHOPHYSIOLOGY

In many ways the spinal cord is similar to the telephone wires that deliver phone service to your house. Consider a telephone line that runs between the switching station and the end of the street. There is a central wire that carries messages strung from telephone pole to telephone pole, and then there are a series of smaller lines that run from the telephone poles to houses along the street. This telephone system can be damaged anywhere along its span. If a wire is cut at its very end, only the last few houses will go without service. On the other hand, if the wire is damaged as it leaves the switching station, all the houses along its span will lose service.

In the same way, the spinal cord carries messages from the brain to the terminal ends of the nerve fibers. Nerve pathways branch off the cord all along its length and carry messages to different areas of the body. As in the telephone wire analogy, damage to the cord can cause varying levels of neurological deficit, depending on where the damage occurs. If the injury transects the spine at lower levels, fewer nervous pathways are affected. If the damage occurs high in the spine, more neurological deficits will be present.

spinal column the 33 stacked bones that extend from the base of the skull to the pelvis and contain the spinal cord.

To protect against injury, the nervous system is housed within a pair of protective bony structures known as the *skull* and **spinal column.** The skull protects the brain, and the spinal column provides protection for the delicate spinal cord.

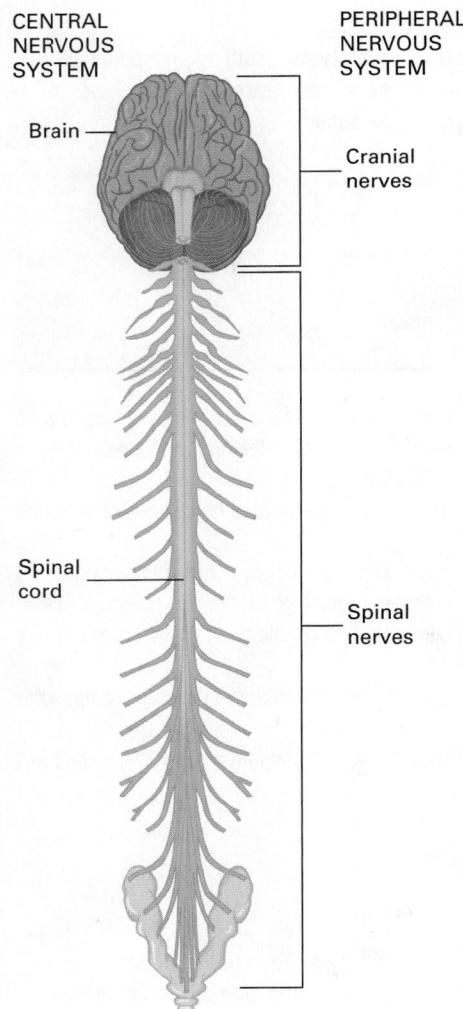

The spinal column is made up of 33 irregularly shaped bones stacked or fused together. They extend from the base of the skull to the coccyx (tail bone). The spinal column serves as both a support mechanism for the upper body and a protective structure that surrounds the spinal cord (Figure 36-2 ■).

The spinal column is divided into five sections, beginning at the top. The first seven vertebrae, which are located in the neck, are known as the **cervical vertebrae.** The next section comprises 12 vertebrae called the **thoracic vertebrae.** Each of the 12 thoracic vertebrae is attached directly to one of the 12 pairs of ribs that form the rib cage.

Next are the five **lumbar vertebrae.** Below the lumbar region is the triangular-shaped bone known as the **sacrum** or *sacral vertebrae*. The sacrum begins as four or five bones during childhood that eventually become completely fused around age 26. The sacrum helps form the posterior wall of the pelvis.

Finally, the **coccygeal vertebrae,** more commonly known as the *coccyx*, begin life as four or five bones that eventually fuse together in adulthood. The coccyx is an important attachment point for many muscles in the lower back and pelvis.

cervical vertebrae the seven vertebrae that begin at the head and meet the thoracic vertebrae.

thoracic vertebrae the 12 vertebrae that help form the thoracic cage. A pair of ribs is attached to each thoracic vertebra.

lumbar vertebrae the five vertebrae that form the lower back area.

sacrum fused vertebrae that help to form the pelvis. Also called *sacral vertebrae*.

coccygeal vertebrae fused vertebrae making up the coccyx or tailbone.

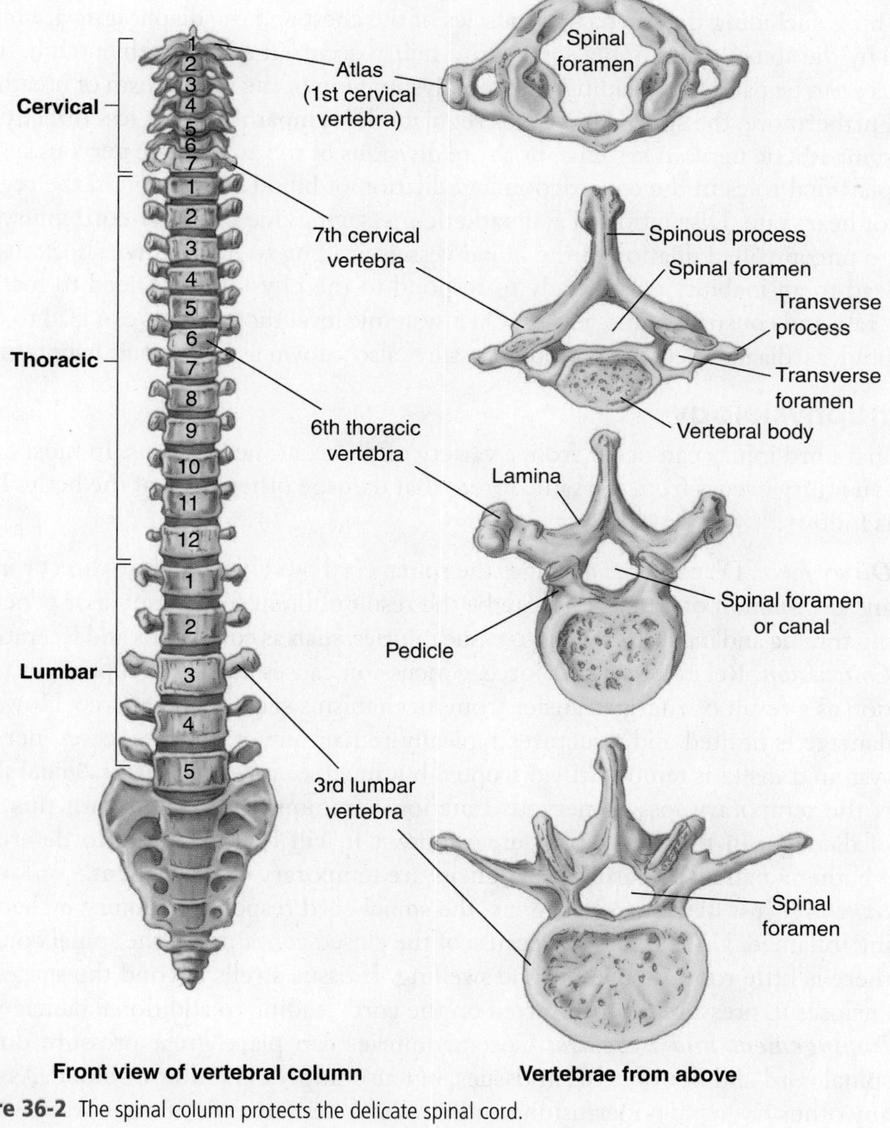

Figure 36-2 The spinal column protects the delicate spinal cord.

As noted earlier, injury at any point along the spinal column that causes damage to the spinal cord can result in the loss of sensation and function below (or distal to) the site of injury. It will be essential to carefully assess patients with suspected spine injury and minimize any movement of the spine during care and transport.

PRACTICAL PATHOPHYSIOLOGY

The diaphragm muscle accounts for approximately 60% of the respiratory effort for normal breathing. When an injury occurs high in the spinal column, affecting C5, C4, or C3, there is a possibility that the nerves controlling the diaphragm will be affected. The primary nerve that controls the diaphragm is called the phrenic nerve and originates mainly from the fourth cervical nerve (C4). You must anticipate that patients with cervical injuries may need ventilator assistance if those nerves are affected.

36-5 Differentiate between spinal shock and neurogenic hypotension.

In addition to transmitting sensory and motor messages to the arms and the legs, the spinal cord plays a vital role in regulating breathing and circulation. The muscles of breathing, including the intercostal muscles of the chest and the diaphragm, are innervated by the spinal column. If a spinal-cord injury occurs at a level high enough, those muscles can be paralyzed, leading to severe dysfunction of the mechanism of breathing.

Furthermore, the spinal cord helps regulate the sympathetic and, less directly, the parasympathetic nervous systems. Both are divisions of the autonomic nervous system and play vital roles in the constriction and dilation of blood vessels and in the regulation of heart rate. Disruption of sympathetic messaging due to spinal-cord injury can lead to uncontrolled dilation of the blood vessels, leading to distributive shock. It also can lead to an inability of the body to respond to the physiological need to increase heart rate and constrict blood vessels. On a systemic level those events can lead to relative bradycardia and decreased blood pressure, also known as **neurogenic hypotension.**

neurogenic hypotension bradycardia and decreased blood pressure secondary to a disruption of sympathetic nervous system messaging; usually results from a spinal-cord injury.

Pathophysiology

A spinal-cord injury can occur from a variety of different mechanisms. In most cases, such an injury occurs from the same forces that damage other areas of the body. They are as follows:

- ***Direct force.*** Direct force damages the spinal cord by subjecting it to direct trauma and destruction of tissue. This can be the result of blunt force trauma or penetrating trauma and include other soft-tissue injuries, such as contusions and lacerations.
- ***Concussion.*** Related to direct force, concussion causes a brief disruption in function as a result of energy transfer from mechanisms such as blunt force. However, damage is limited and structures typically remain intact. In these cases, nervous system transfer is temporarily disrupted but function is restored later. **Spinal shock** is the temporary loss of nervous function commonly associated with this type of damage. In the prehospital environment it will be impossible to determine whether a patient's neurological deficits are temporary or permanent.
- ***Swelling.*** Just like any other tissue, the spinal cord responds to injury by becoming inflamed. Unfortunately, because of the closed container of the spinal column, there is little room to contain the swelling. If tissue swells beyond the space that encloses it, pressure can be exerted on the cord, leading to additional damage.
- ***Impingement and ischemia.*** Certain injuries can place great pressure on the spinal cord and not only harm tissues, but also impede the flow of blood. As with any other tissue, hypoperfusion can injure and destroy cells, if not corrected.

spinal shock a temporary, concussion-like injury to the spinal cord.

Damage to the spinal cord can be devastating. An injury that completely severs the spinal cord is referred to as a **transection.** This type of injury interrupts all nervous transmission below it and most commonly results in permanent paralysis. Although this type of injury is typically instantaneous, other injuries can develop over time and result from the effects of swelling and ischemia, which can be equally devastating.

transection a complete severing of the spinal cord.

Incomplete injuries also can occur. In those cases the spinal cord is only partially severed and affects only a specific anatomical region. An incomplete injury can lead to nerve dysfunction, but frequently leaves certain pathways intact.

Primary and Secondary Injuries

Spinal-cord injuries pose enormous risks to the patient. They can permanently affect sensory and motor function throughout the body. In many cases, this damage has occurred long before prehospital providers arrive on the scene, but occasionally, spinal-cord injury is worsened after the immediate insult.

Primary injury is the injury that occurs immediately as a direct result of the trauma. These are the injuries that EMTs must assess and care for. *Secondary injuries* develop after the original insult and pose an additional risk that prehospital providers must consider. Most secondary spinal-cord injuries are the result of swelling and ischemia. As the injured area becomes inflamed, increased pressure in the spinal column can lead to damage of the cord. Furthermore, as pressure increases, blood flow to the spinal cord is often impeded, leaving areas of hypoxic tissue. Although EMTs can do little to stop secondary events, appropriate care of the patient can help minimize their effects. Prevention of hypoxia through supplemental oxygen and caring for shock are two ways to reduce the damage associated with secondary injuries.

Other secondary injuries can be caused by the movement of displaced bone ends into the delicate spinal-cord tissue. Because the bones of the spinal cord are connected to each other with muscle and ligaments, it is thought that improper movement of the patient poses a risk of manipulating jagged bone ends into fragile nervous tissue. It is unclear exactly how high this risk is or exactly how much EMS personnel can do to prevent it, but it is best to guard against secondary injuries resulting from excessive movement.

One way to prevent excessive movement is to keep the patient's head, neck, and spine in an in-line neutral position for immobilization and during coordinated movements (both of which will be discussed in the next section). Therefore, it is essential that during a thorough patient assessment, EMTs identify the circumstances for which movement and immobilization devices are necessary.

Displaced vs. Nondisplaced Injuries

It is common for a patient to suffer a fracture to one or more vertebrae without direct injury to the spinal cord itself. This can occur when the fracture remains in place. It is referred to as a **nondisplaced fracture,** such as a bone that is cracked but not deformed. A **displaced fracture** is one that has some deformity associated with it, and the pieces of bone are separated from one another. The likelihood of spinal-cord injury is greater with displaced injuries than with nondisplaced ones.

nondisplaced fracture a fracture of the spinal column that results in no displacement of the broken bones.

displaced fracture a fracture of the spinal column that results in displacement of the broken bones.

It is not your job to try to diagnose a displaced injury in the field. In fact, without an X-ray, the task is virtually impossible. This is, however, the rationale for minimizing movement of the spine during assessment and utilizing an in-line neutral position during immobilization. Your careful handling of the patient will minimize the chances of a nondisplaced injury becoming displaced or a displaced injury penetrating the spinal cord.

Assessment of the Patient with a Spinal-Cord Injury

Assessment of the patient with a suspected spine injury is very important. Many injuries are subtle in their presentation. Missing a spine injury can have devastating effects. EMTs should maintain a high index of suspicion for spinal-cord injury any time the forces of trauma suggest injury to the torso, neck, or back. Furthermore, even when those forces are questionable, a thorough patient assessment should be used to guard against the risk of missing an injury.

Scene Size-up

As an EMT you will have the unique opportunity to gather information about the patient from clues they encounter on the scene. This is especially important when assessing a potential spine-injured patient. You should anticipate potential injuries based on the information contained in the initial dispatch. For instance, if you have been dispatched to a vehicle collision, anticipate head and neck injuries and the need for spinal immobilization. You will confirm this when you evaluate the actual mechanism of injury. Ensure that the scene is safe and, if possible, request the appropriate additional resources prior to making patient contact.

Once on scene, look at factors such as the angle of impact, the amount of damage to the vehicle and intrusion into the passenger compartment, and whether or not the patient was wearing a seat belt. Maintain manual stabilization of the spine until the patient can be properly immobilized.

Common Mechanisms of Injury

36-3 Describe common mechanisms of spine injury.

One of the most important factors that helps determine the presence of a suspected spine injury is the mechanism of injury (MOI). Even in the absence of obvious signs and symptoms, it is important to maintain a high index of suspicion for spine injury when the mechanism suggests it.

The following is a partial list of situations that would suggest an injury to the spine:

- Motor-vehicle crashes
- Pedestrian versus vehicle collisions
- Falls
- Blunt trauma to head, neck, or torso
- Penetrating trauma to head, neck, or torso
- Motorcycle crashes
- Hangings
- Diving into shallow water
- Unresponsive patients with an unknown mechanism
- Soft-tissue injuries to the head, neck, back, shoulders, or abdomen associated with trauma

The spinal column can be subjected to a wide variety of injuries, depending on the MOI. The following describes the most common MOIs associated with injury to the spine (Figure 36-3 ■):

compression mechanism of injury caused by direct force from the top or the bottom, causing vertebrae to jam together.

flexion mechanism of injury caused by thrusting the head forward into a flexed position.

extension mechanism of injury caused by thrusting the head back.

- ***Compression.*** Any force that impacts the spine from the top or bottom has the potential to cause what is referred to as a **compression** injury or axial load injury. In this kind of injury, the stack of vertebrae compress against one another, causing damage (fracture) to one or more of the vertebrae. Common causes of compression injuries are diving into shallow water and falling from a height.
- ***Flexion, extension, rotation, and lateral bending.*** Any mechanism that causes an exaggerated movement of the head in any position can cause a **flexion, extension,**

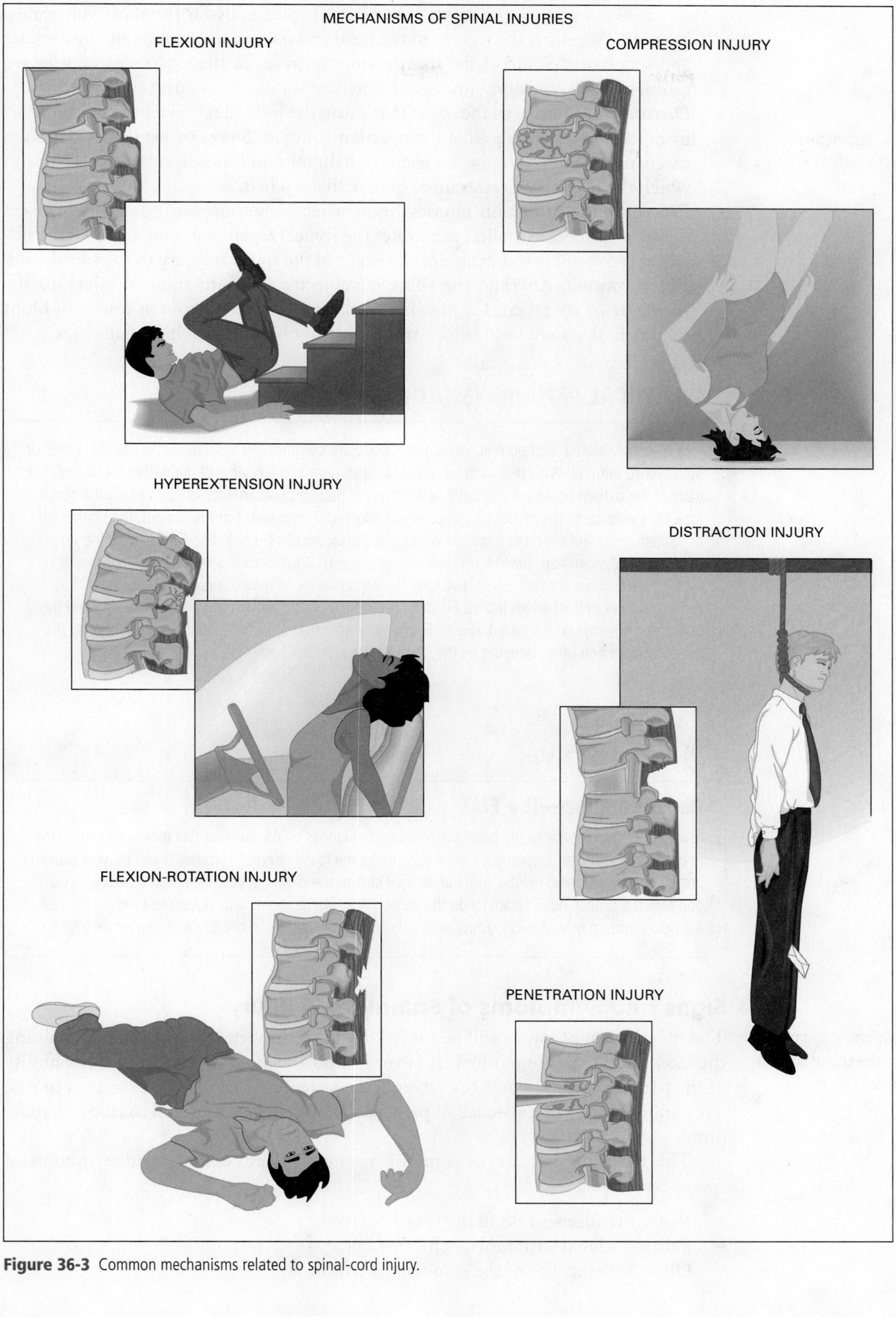

Figure 36-3 Common mechanisms related to spinal-cord injury.

or rotation injury to the spine. The cervical spine is by far the most vulnerable, because it supports the weight of the head and itself is supported only by muscles and soft tissue. Some of the most common causes of these types of injuries are motor-vehicle collisions, diving into shallow water, and blunt trauma.

- ***Distraction.*** Injuries to the spine that cause the individual vertebrae to pull apart from one another are called **distraction** injuries. Some of the most common mechanisms of distraction injuries are hangings and motor-vehicle collisions in which the occupant is restrained only with a lap belt.
- ***Penetration.*** Penetration injuries result when something such as a sharp object (knife) or projectile (bullet) penetrates the spine. Depending on the path of the object, it can result in either an open fracture of the spine or injury to the spinal cord.
- ***Blunt trauma.*** Anytime the spine is subjected to blunt trauma, injury to the vertebrae or spinal cord is possible. Some of the more common causes of blunt trauma injuries are falls, being struck with an object, and vehicle collisions.

distraction mechanism of injury caused by pulling forces such as in a hanging.

PRACTICAL PATHOPHYSIOLOGY

As previously stated, certain mechanisms of injury are commonly associated with specific types of spinal-cord injuries. With this in mind, scene assessment and a review of the particular forces that caused the patient harm are essential to a thorough patient assessment. As you review the scene, look for evidence of the forces of compression. Consider movement of the patient, the shattering of windshields, and even the depth of water in a diving accident. Look also for the bending forces (the forces of extension, flexion, and lateral movement). Consider the speeds and movements involved in a motor-vehicle crash. Evaluate the potential for whiplash forces, and consider the position of the patient when found. Finally, consider the possibility of penetrating trauma and the potential pathways of the penetrations. Remember also that objects like bullets and shrapnel are unpredictable and often ricochet as they tumble through the body.

PERSPECTIVE

Racer Ramirez—The EMT

Man, as soon as I got into the backyard and saw the ladder on its side and this guy in a heap on the grass, my stomach tightened up. Spinal calls make me really nervous. I mean, if you move a broken arm, it causes pain and maybe some additional soft-tissue damage, you know, but a neck? If you don't keep a broken neck steady, then the person that you're above, whose scared eyes you're looking down into, may be driving around in a wheelchair for the rest of his life. And that's heavy.

Signs and Symptoms of Spinal-Cord Injury

36-7 Describe signs and symptoms of injury to the spinal column and spinal cord.

The mechanism of injury will be one of the most important factors in determining the likelihood of a spine injury. It is very important to understand that the ability of the patient to walk, move his extremities, or feel sensation is not a reason to rule out a spine injury. The absence of pain also should not be a reason to rule out spine injury.

The following is a list of some of the more common signs and symptoms of spinal-cord injury:

- Pain or tenderness along the spine
- Pain associated with movement
- Obvious deformity of the spine on palpation

- Numbness, weakness, or tingling in the extremities
- Loss of sensation on the torso
- Loss of sensation or paralysis in the extremities
- Incontinence (loss of bowel or bladder control)
- **Priapism** (persistent erection of the penis)

priapism persistent erection of the penis that may result from spine injury and some medical problems.

In addition to the above signs and symptoms, another serious complication of spinal-cord injury is the disruption of normal breathing. Injury to the spinal cord at or above the third cervical vertebra can affect the diaphragm, which is the primary muscle of respiration. As with all patients, closely monitor respiratory status and assist with ventilations if necessary.

STOP, REVIEW, REMEMBER!

Multiple Choice

For each question, place a check next to the correct answer.

1. Which one of the following mechanisms of injury would most likely be associated with a patient who hung himself?

_____ a. Distraction
_____ b. Compression
_____ c. Flexion
_____ d. Extension

2. The spinal column is made up of approximately how many bones?

_____ a. 7
_____ b. 12
_____ c. 22
_____ d. 33

3. The region of the spine that is located in the neck and contains seven vertebrae is called the _____________ region.

_____ a. cervical
_____ b. thoracic
_____ c. lumbar
_____ d. sacral

4. Each vertebra of the _____________ spine is connected to a pair of ribs that wrap around to form the rib cage.

_____ a. cervical
_____ b. thoracic
_____ c. lumbar
_____ d. sacral

5. Which one of the following best describes how a spine injury can cause neurogenic hypotension?

_____ a. Blood loss from other associated injuries
_____ b. Arterial bleeding from the spinal blood vessels
_____ c. Loss of fluid due to edema at the injury site
_____ d. Loss of control over blood vessel dilation

(continued on next page)

(continued)

Labeling

Label the following sections of the spinal column: coccyx, cervical spine, lumbar spine, thoracic spine, and sacral spine.

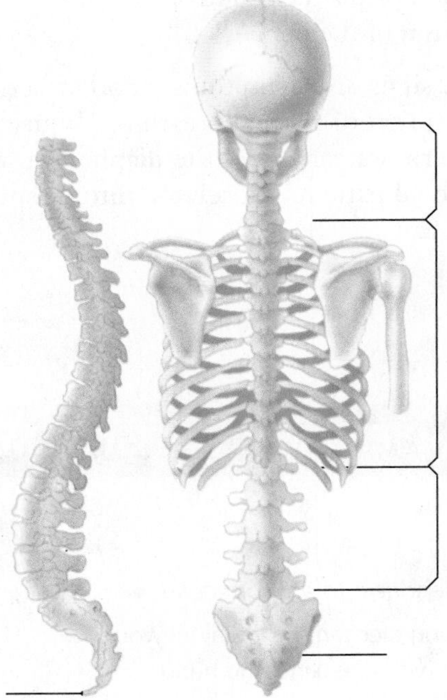

Critical Thinking

1. Discuss the role the mechanism of injury plays in the assessment and care of the patient with a suspected spine injury.

2. How do the central and peripheral nervous systems differ in function?

3. Explain why it is so important to minimize the movement of a patient with a suspected spinal-cord injury.

PERSPECTIVE

Dena—The Patient's Wife

I was so scared that my husband was going to die or something. I just can't believe it. One minute he's putting up our new satellite dish and the next he's getting strapped to a plastic board and he can't feel me holding his hand. He hit so hard, though. I mean, just bam! Like a spear or something, right into the ground. And then as they were getting him on the stretcher, he wet himself and he didn't even notice. I didn't say anything. Oh, my gosh, he would've just died of embarrassment.

Manual Stabilization

Although emergency care usually follows assessment, patients with a suspected spine injury present an exception to this rule. Before beginning a physical examination, you should take steps to secure the patient's head from moving. Although it will be part of a larger immobilization strategy, this should be initiated at first contact with the patient. Start by advising the patient to remain as still as possible. Then immobilize the patient's head and neck by using a technique called **manual stabilization** (Figure 36-4 ■). Firmly grasp the patient's head with both hands and attempt to keep it from moving while another EMT assesses and cares for the patient.

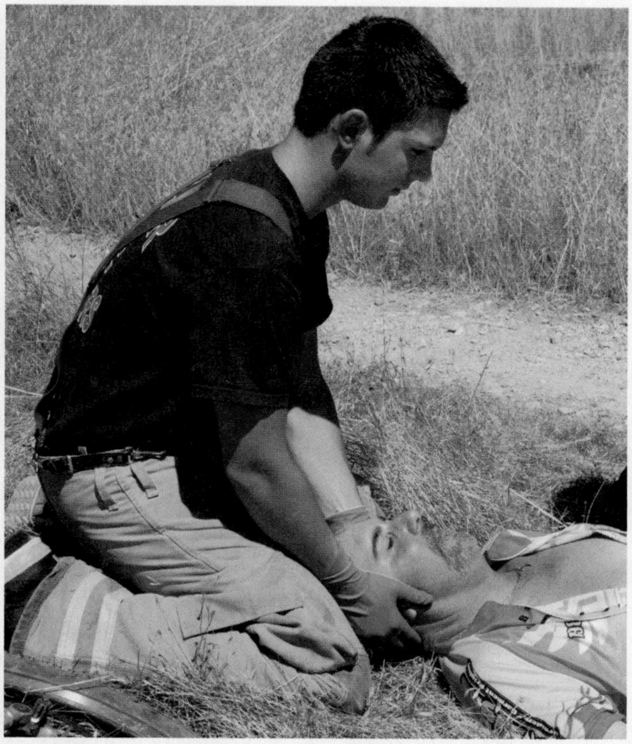

Figure 36-4 Use both hands to manually stabilize the head and neck prior to beginning your assessment.

If that is impossible due to limited resources (you are by yourself, for example), stabilize the head yourself and wait for additional resources, or at least instruct the patient to not move his neck. Stabilize the patient's head and neck as resources become available. If the patient has problems with the ABCs that need immediate attention, you must address them, while being mindful of the potential for neck injury.

Whenever possible, place the patient's head in alignment with the spine and the rest of the body. Usually that involves grasping the head with both hands and gently rotating it in line with the spine. Use caution when realigning the head with the rest of the body and stop immediately if resistance or pain is felt.

As you proceed with the assessment, instruct the responsive patient to answer your questions with a verbal response only and not to shake or nod his head. You also will want to be gentler when handling the extremities. Do not move the patient in an attempt to elicit a painful response.

manual stabilization method of stabilization in which the EMT firmly grasps the patient's head with both hands and attempts to keep it from moving.

Primary Assessment

While maintaining appropriate stabilization of the spine, ensure that the patient's ABCs are intact and manage any uncontrolled bleeding. Management of the airway of an unresponsive patient should be accomplished using the jaw-thrust maneuver, not the head-tilt/chin-lift maneuver, which moves the head and neck significantly. Whenever possible consider the insertion of an appropriate airway adjunct. Maintain the patient's airway and provide manual ventilations with as little movement of the head and neck as possible.

Although not every spine injury will cause respiratory or circulatory compromise, there is a direct link between your management of the ABCs and the ultimate outcome of the spine-injured patient. It is now known that hypoxia and shock play a major role in secondary spine injuries and furthermore the ability to control and mitigate those issues in the field can reduce the incidence of secondary injuries. Be very aware that your actions during the primary assessment can play a vital role in the long-term recovery of your patient.

Secondary Assessment

36-6 Describe the assessment of circulation, sensation, and motor function (CSM) in the extremities of a patient who is suspected of having an injury to the spine.

As you continue your assessment, try to pinpoint any pain or tenderness along the spine as best as you can. To accomplish this simply ask the patient if he has pain and palpate the entire spine. Do the latter when the patient is on his side during a log-roll onto a long backboard by a team of rescuers. Be sure to spend a little more time assessing all four distal extremities for adequate circulation, sensation, and motor function (Figure 36-5 ■).

If the patient is unresponsive, your assessment will rely mostly on the MOI and any obvious signs of trauma. Do your best to obtain additional information from others at the scene who may have seen the event or were with the patient prior to your arrival. Try to determine if the patient was responsive at all before you arrived.

Your secondary assessment must include a patient history and a physical examination because both can provide clues about the spine injury. Look for pain, tenderness, and deformity especially around the spine. Any finding of this nature would indicate a probability of spine injury. Remember to use the BP-DOC or similar assessment tool and look for anything out of the ordinary including penetrations and other signs of injuries that likely pose a risk for spine injury. As you begin your assessment, have your partner obtain a baseline set of vital signs. The trending of vital signs can help you identify signs of shock.

Pay special attention to the circulation, sensation, and motor function (CSM) status of each extremity. Identify any disruption of sensory or motor function. While poor motor function can be a result of pain and not necessarily spine injury, any amount of decreased function, numbness, or tingling should be investigated further. Be aware that any abnormality is an important finding that must be documented. Move up the arms or legs beginning at the feet to determine how far the numbness or tingling goes.

A thorough neurological examination will include an assessment of the patient's ability to sense both sharp and dull contact. Use a pen or a cotton applicator to assess both types of sensation. Make a mark on the patient's extremity using a pen to signify the point at which normal sensation begins. Remember also that not every spine-injured patient will have motor loss or paralysis. A loss of only sensation or only motor function can absolutely indicate a significant injury.

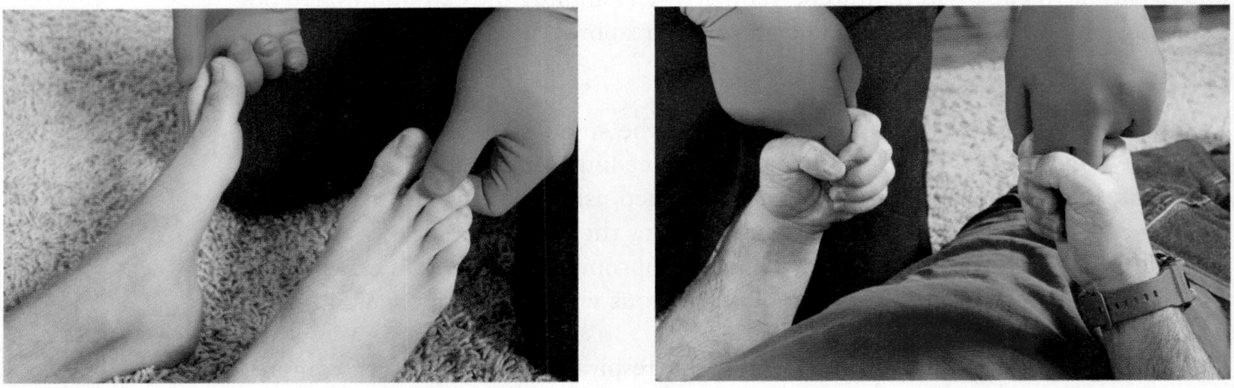

(A) (B)

Figure 36-5 Assess for normal circulation, sensation, and motor function (A) in the feet and (B) in the hands.

Other injuries, such as a long-bone fracture, can complicate your physical assessment. Occasionally, severe pain from such an injury can mask pain from a less painful injury to the spine. Be aware of this fact and maintain a high index of suspicion in patients with those types of injuries.

Patient history is an equally important component of the assessment. Patients with significant injuries frequently will be able to pinpoint pain and localize the injury site. Their description of the mechanism of injury may be invaluable to your overall understanding of the forces that were in play. Some underlying conditions such as osteoporosis (a chronic softening of the bones) can make spine injuries more likely. It is also important to understand that intoxicants such as alcohol or drugs can make your physical assessment and neurological examination less reliable. Treat these patients also with a high degree of suspicion for spine injury.

Note that not every spinal-cord injury completely transects the spinal cord. In many cases, trauma can cause injury to only a portion of the spinal cord. Such injuries present unique assessment challenges.

A cross section of the spinal cord can identify very specific tracts of nerve tissue, each with individual functions. For example, some nerve pathways located toward the sides of the spinal cord carry messages regarding the sensation of pain and temperature. Those pathways are best tested by assessing the patient's ability to feel sharp sensation such as pain or a pinprick. In addition, nerve pathways located in the anterior portions of the spinal cord control motor function. It is feasible in an incomplete spinal-cord injury that one tract could be damaged while another remains intact. For example, injuries to the central portion of the spinal cord from a hyperextension MOI can result in upper extremity weakness with intact strength in the lower extremities.

Overall, what is most concerning about these types of incomplete spinal-cord injuries is their ability to preserve sensation and function in one area while losing them in another. Despite a very serious injury, this patient may appear normal on many levels. A poor or incomplete assessment will miss dangerous and concerning findings.

PERSPECTIVE

Gary—The Patient

I knew better than to stand on that top step. You know, the one that says "not a step" on it. But nothing bad has ever really happened to me before, so I figured what the heck! I don't remember much. I remember a surge of adrenaline as the ladder started to rock back and forth and then this big, bright flash. And then all I could think of was finding my stupid hat. Everything after that's pretty much a blur. Isn't it odd how a quick decision like which step do I stand on can have such far-reaching effects? I am very grateful for the ambulance personnel though. The doctor told me that if they hadn't done their jobs right, I might have been much worse off than I am.

Emergency Care of the Patient with Suspected Spine Injury

36-9 Describe appropriate emergency care for the patient with suspected spine injury.

Once the ABCs have been properly managed, care will shift to immobilizing the injury and preventing further damage. Immobilization of the spinal column embraces the same concepts as splinting long bones. That is, splinting is meant to prevent movement by fixating the bones to a rigid device. The dilemma you face with spine injuries though is rather than immobilizing one bone, you must immobilize all 33 bones of the spinal column.

For the purposes of immobilization, think of the spinal column as one long bone. Just like any other bone, splint it in a position of function. In spinal immobilization, this is an in-line neutral position. In this position, the natural curve of the spinal column is accounted for and each of the 33 vertebrae is aligned as it would be naturally in the spinal column. Spinal immobilization utilizes specialized equipment designed to allow movement of the patient while at the same time maintaining this position.

In the following sections specific techniques and devices used to accomplish the goal of spinal immobilization are described. However, the common theme is the maintenance of the in-line neutral position. Because all bones of the spinal column are connected, you must limit movement by restricting motion of the entire thorax (again, considering the spinal column to be one long bone). All immobilization will be designed to preserve this natural position, and all movements will only move the body as a single unit and avoid moving individual parts. The following are key principles of spinal immobilization you should remember regardless of the device or technique you use:

- ***In-line neutral position.*** As best as possible, the immobilization and movement of a spine-injured patient should maintain the alignment and natural position of all 33 bones of the spinal column. No bone should be allowed to move independently and vertebrae should always be aligned where they naturally are positioned.
- ***Securing the three centers of mass.*** In the human body there are three areas where weight is primarily distributed. They are the head, the chest (torso), and the pelvis. If you intend to immobilize your patient, these three areas must be secured and restricted from independent movement.
- ***Coordinated movements.*** Any movement that is made with a spine-injured patient must be coordinated. The spinal column should be thought of as a single long bone. Therefore, if a move must be made, the body (especially the head, chest, and pelvis) should be moved only as a single unit.

As a general approach, use the following steps when caring for a patient with suspected spine injury:

1. Take appropriate BSI precautions.
2. Establish and maintain manual in-line stabilization of the spine.
3. Perform a primary assessment and initiate oxygen therapy when necessary.
4. Perform a rapid secondary assessment including a thorough assessment of distal CSM in all extremities.
5. Apply an appropriate cervical stabilization device (collar).
6. Place the patient on an appropriate stabilization device, depending on the position found (lying, sitting, standing).
7. Initiate transport.
8. Perform a more detailed secondary assessment as appropriate.
9. Reassess the patient throughout transport.

36-10 Describe proper immobilization techniques for suspected spine injury patients who are supine, seated, and standing.

Note that not all patients with spine injuries will present with obvious trauma. Any patient who is found unresponsive when you are not able to accurately determine the exact cause of his condition should be treated as though he has a spine injury.

36-12 Explain special handling and immobilization considerations when spine injury is suspected for helmet removal; football injuries, including removal of face mask and immobilization; and in infants and children, including extrication from a car seat.

Immobilization of the Patient with Suspected Spine Injury

Patients will be found in one of three possible positions: lying, sitting, or standing. Regardless of the position, carefully assess the patient's need for spinal immobilization and secure the patient to an appropriate device. Several devices are used to properly immobilize a patient. They include cervical collars, head immobilizers, and both long and short spinal immobilization devices.

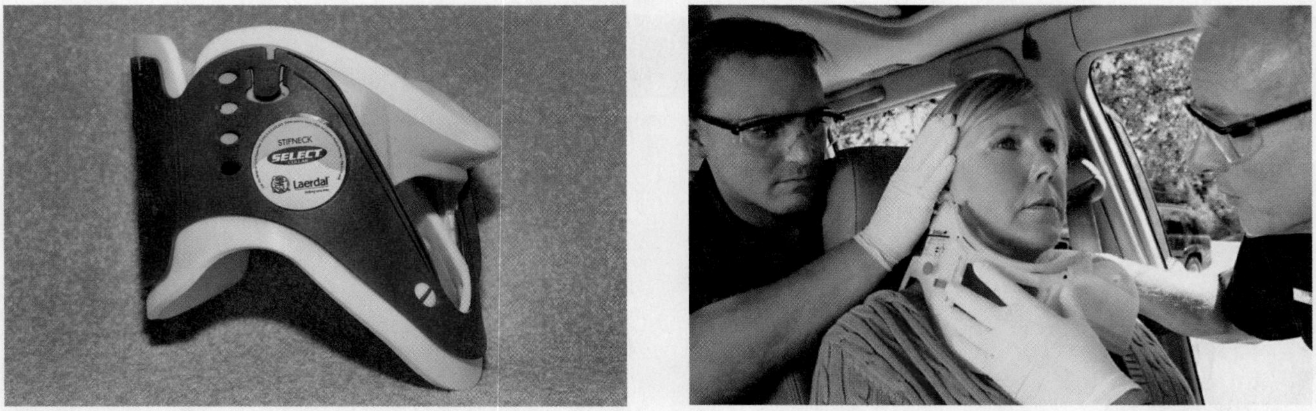

(A) (B)

Figure 36-6 (A) Typical adjustable cervical collar. (© Edward T. Dickinson, MD) (B) A cervical collar being placed on a seated patient.

Cervical-Spine Immobilization

One of the biggest challenges faced by EMTs is the proper immobilization of a patient's head and neck. The head is a large freely moving unit that has great range of motion and thus a great ability to move cervical vertebrae. Any spinal immobilization must account for the positioning and the immobilization of the head and neck.

In the previous section, the need to maintain manual stabilization of the head during assessment is discussed. Of course, limiting movement by using your hands is important, but as you begin the process of extrication, a more comprehensive system to immobilize the head and neck should be used.

Proper immobilization can be improved by using a device known as a *cervical collar* (Figure 36-6 ■). A cervical collar is indicated for any patient who is suspected of having a spine injury based on the assessment of the mechanism of injury and signs and symptoms. Cervical collars are just one piece of the overall immobilization package and *do not* by themselves ensure proper immobilization of a patient's neck.

PERSPECTIVE

Allyson—The EMT

Back in training, we always practiced holding manual stabilization on patients who were either sitting perfectly upright or lying flat on their backs. I've got to be honest, though, that in three years on this ambulance, I have yet to have a spinal call be that simple. Like this guy today. He's in a big heap on the ground and, of course, he's face down. It can be a real challenge to straighten a person's body out and turn him over so you can board him, all while maintaining effective immobilization. It takes planning and a lot of direct communication with the people helping you. All in all I think this call went well though.

To be maximally effective, a cervical collar must fit properly. A collar that is too small can restrict the airway. A collar that is too large will allow excess movement of the head and neck, increasing the potential for further injury. Each cervical collar manufacturer has specific guidelines for properly sizing the collar to the patient. Follow the guidelines for the specific device you will be using. Scan 36-1 illustrates the steps used to apply an adjustable collar to a seated patient. Scan 36-2 demonstrates how to apply a collar to a supine patient.

SCAN 36-1 Applying a Cervical Collar to a Seated Patient

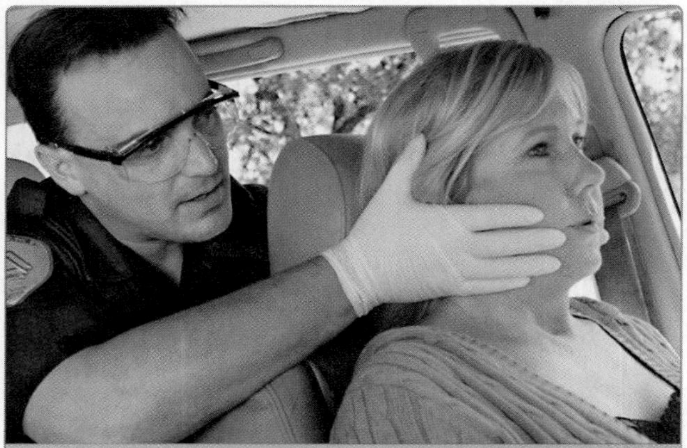

36-1-1 Establish manual stabilization of the head while your partner completes an assessment and selects a collar.

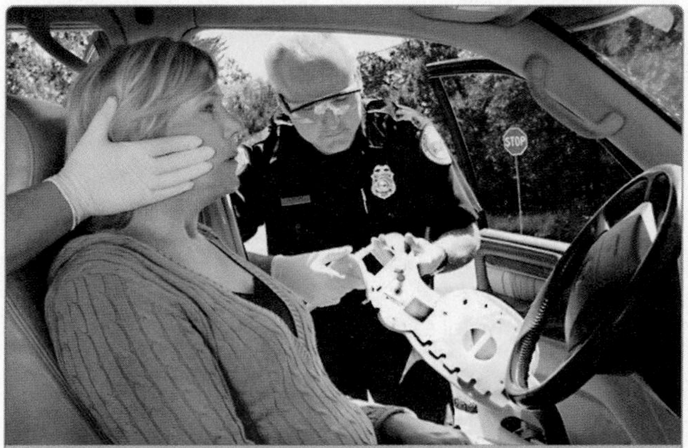

36-1-2 Properly size and adjust the collar according to the manufacturer's recommendations.

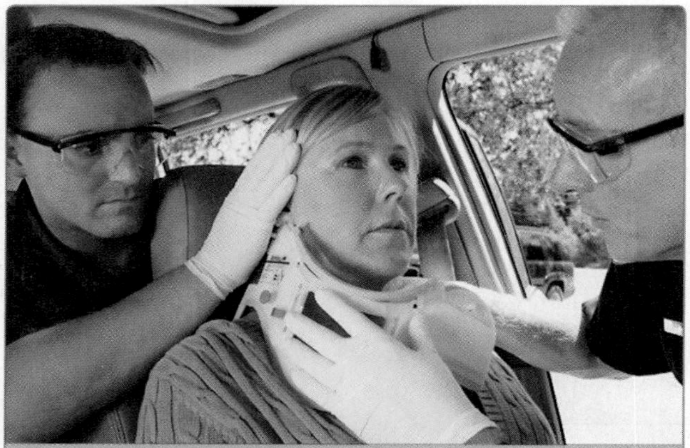

36-1-3 Place the collar beneath the patient's chin and firmly against the lower jaw. The chin should fit well within the saddle of the collar.

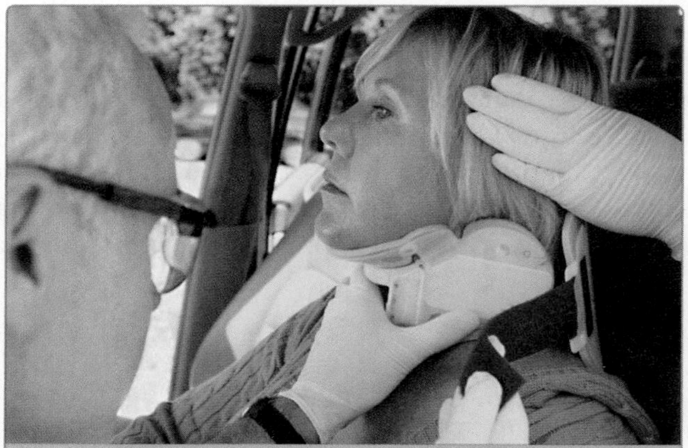

36-1-4 Secure the collar and inspect for a proper fit.

CLINICAL CLUE

Manual Stabilization

Manual stabilization of the head and spine *must* be maintained throughout the assessment process, even after the application of a cervical collar. A cervical collar only serves to "remind" the responsive patient not to move his neck. Some patients will forget and move anyway. That is why you must maintain manual stabilization until the patient is completely secured to an appropriate spinal immobilization device.

SCAN 36-2 Applying a Cervical Collar to a Supine Patient

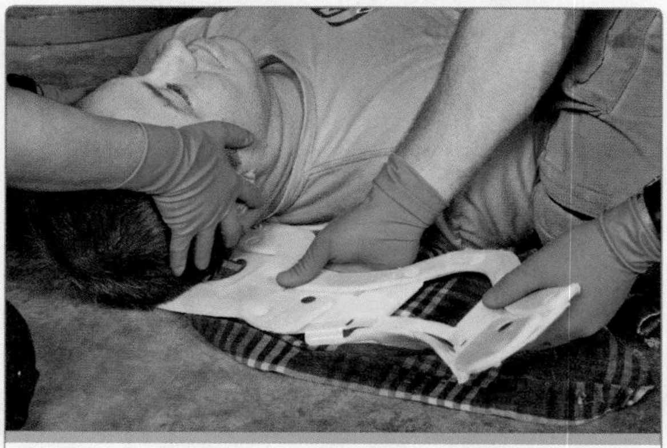

36-2-1 Establish manual stabilization of the head while your partner slides the back portion of the collar behind the patient's neck.

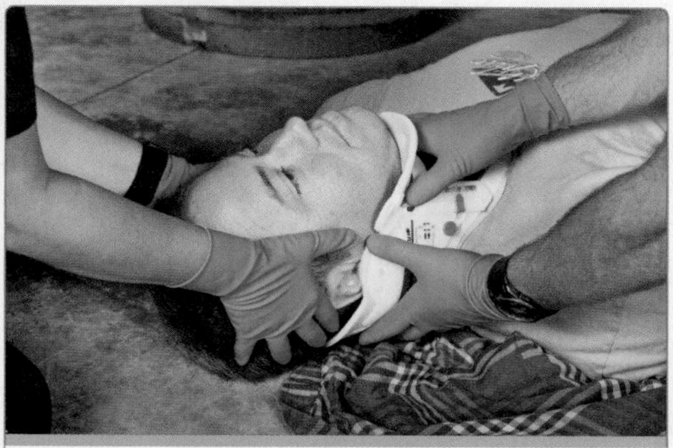

36-2-2 Secure the collar and inspect for a proper fit.

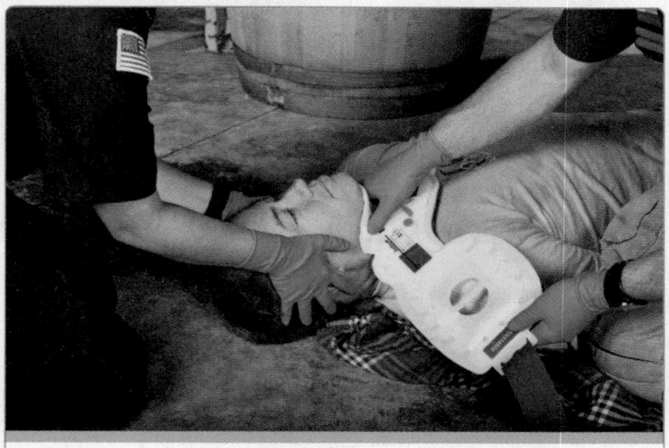

36-2-3 An alternative method is to place the collar below the chin and gently slide it upward until the chin rests firmly within the saddle of the collar.

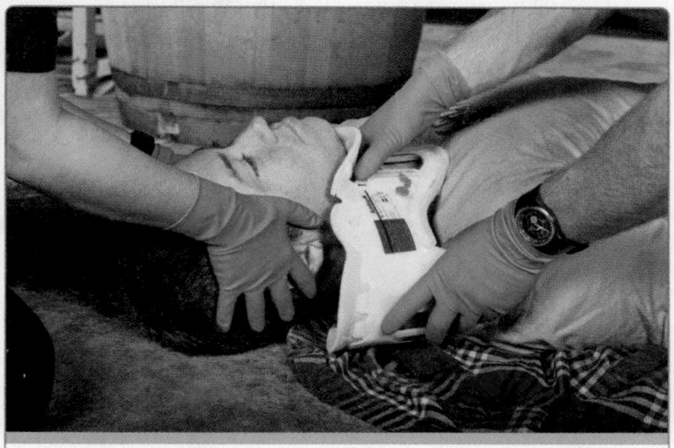

36-2-4 Hold the front of the collar in place while sliding the back portion behind the neck. Secure in place.

Even though cervical collars come in a variety of sizes, some patients may still not fit into one. An alternative is to secure the head to the board with adequate stabilization on both sides and tape across the forehead and chin.

Head Immobilizers

Head immobilizers are simple devices that are used to minimize the side-to-side motion of the head of a patient who is secured to a long backboard (Figure 36-7 ■). They can be purchased as premanufactured devices or they may be improvised by using rolled up towels or blankets (Figure 36-8 ■) or, when other options are unavailable, even the patient's own shoes. Head immobilizers are an important component of the overall spinal package, because they fill the void on either side of the patient's head and minimize side-to-side movement during transport.

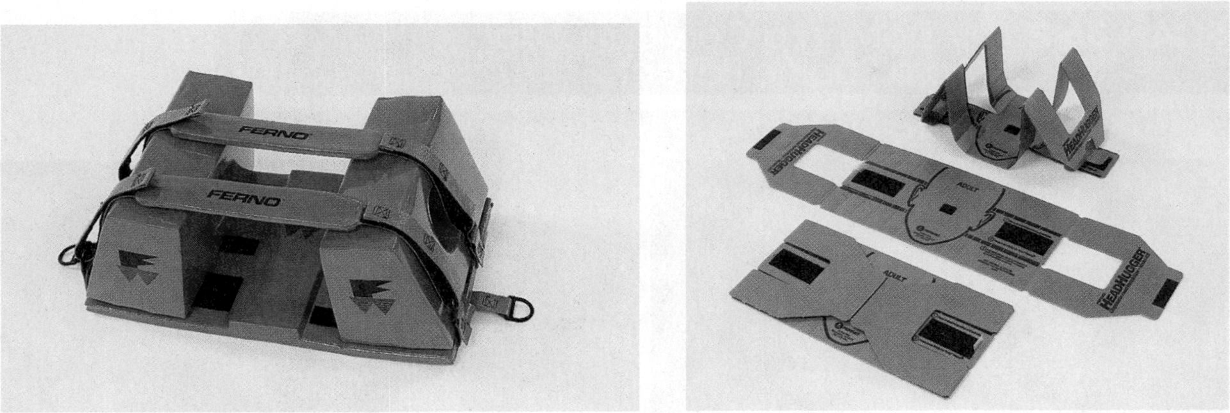

(A) (B)

Figure 36-7 (A) Reusable commercial head immobilizer. (FERNO) (B) Disposable commercial head immobilizer. (FERNO)

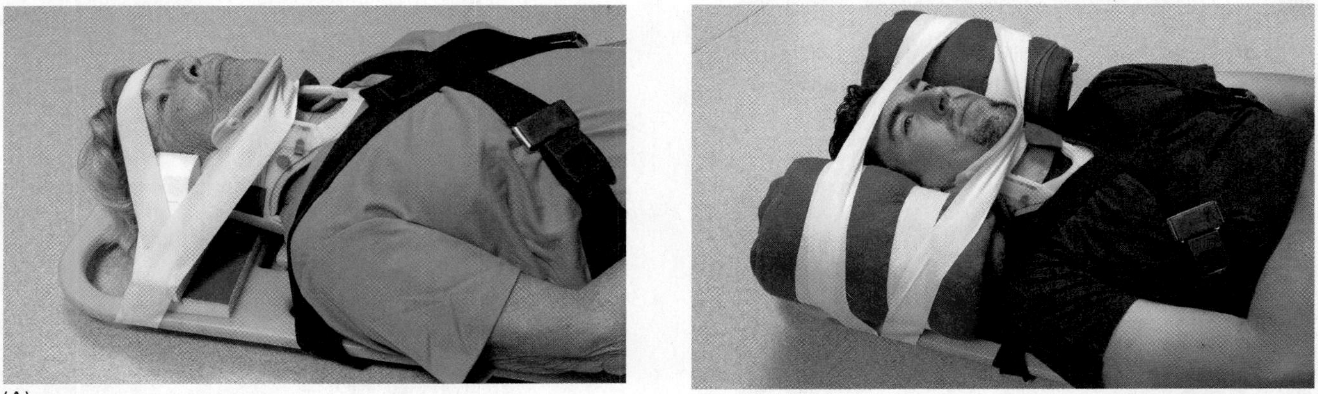

(A) (B)

Figure 36-8 (A) The patient's head secured to a long backboard, using a commercial head immobilizer. (B) Towels and blankets can serve as excellent head immobilizers when necessary.

PRACTICAL PATHOPHYSIOLOGY

The cervical spine is the most vulnerable area of the spinal column. A large center of mass (the head) sits atop a relatively poorly protected stack of vertebrae. As a result, this area of the spinal column accounts for the largest portion of spine injuries. Have a high index of suspicion with mechanisms of injury that apply dynamic force to the head. Motor-vehicle crashes and falls are notorious for damaging the cervical spine. When providing emergency care to these patients, pay particular attention to neutral alignment and coordinate all movements so that the cervical vertebrae remain in their normal position of function.

Long Backboards

The long backboard is also known as a long board or a long spine board. It is a device approximately six feet by two feet. It is made of wood, aluminum, or a plastic material (Figure 36-9 ■) and provides stabilization and immobilization to the head, neck, torso, pelvis, and extremities. Long backboards are used to immobilize patients suspected of having a spine injury who are found in a lying or standing position.

To secure a supine patient to a long backboard, follow the steps listed below (Scan 36-3). Three rescuers should perform the move, if possible.

1. One rescuer should maintain manual stabilization of the head the entire time.
2. Check CSM of all extremities and apply an appropriate cervical collar.

SCAN 36-3 Securing a Supine Patient to a Long Backboard

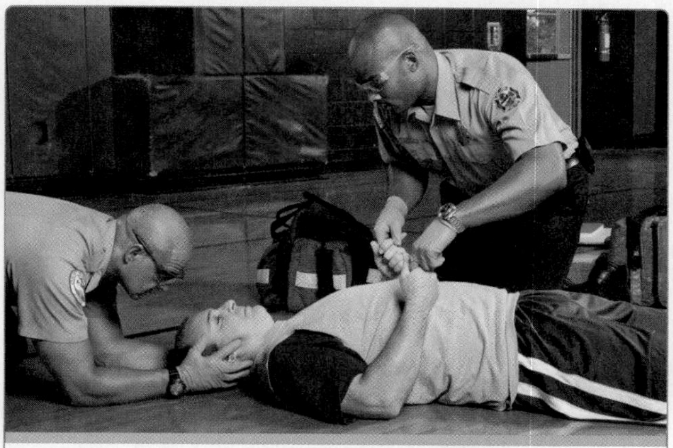

36-3-1 Initiate manual stabilization of the head and complete a primary and rapid secondary assessment.

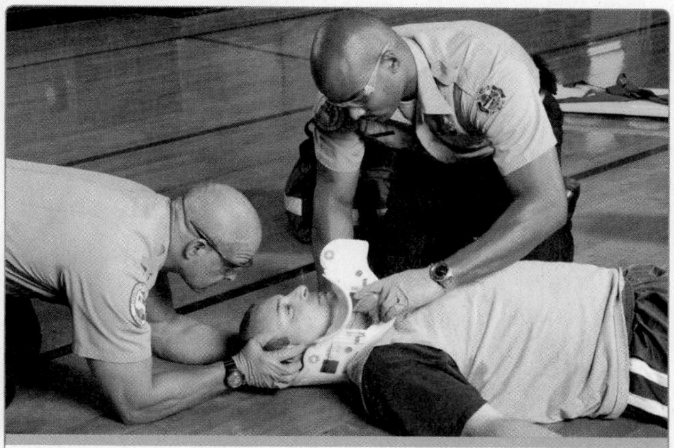

36-3-2 Place a cervical collar.

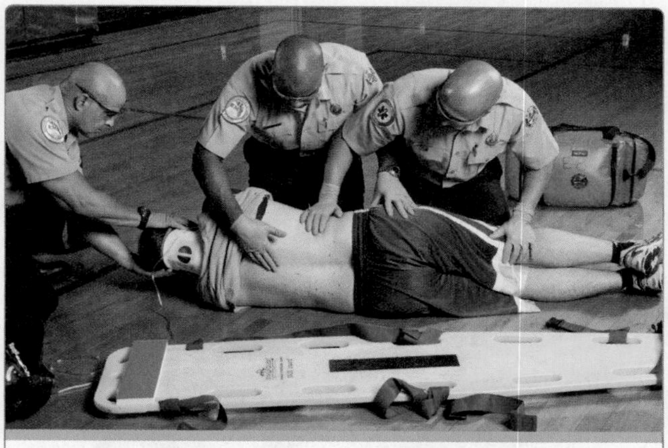

36-3-3 Carefully log roll the patient and inspect the back and spine.

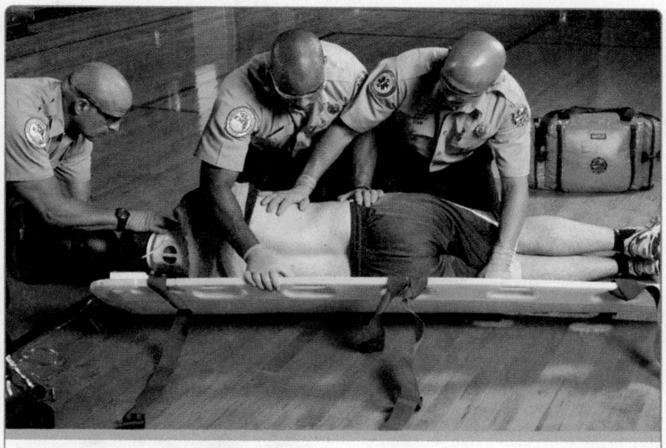

36-3-4 Place the patient onto the board.

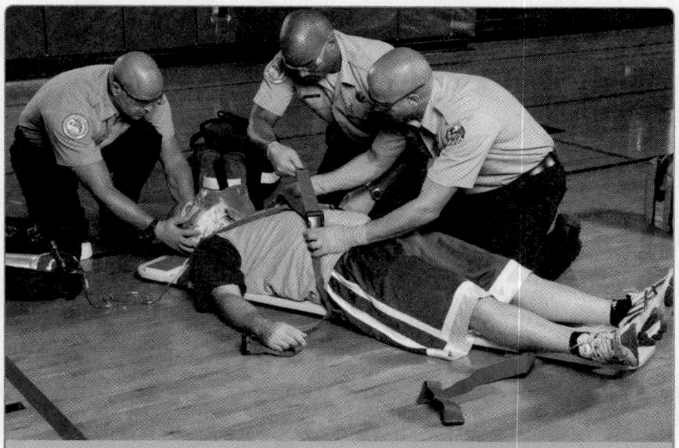

36-3-5 Next, secure the torso and legs to the board.

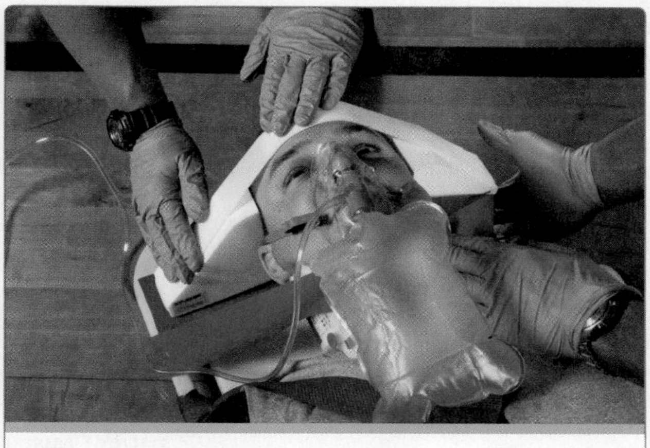

36-3-6 Then secure the head to the board.

(Continued)

SCAN 36-3 Securing a Supine Patient to a Long Backboard (*Cont.*)

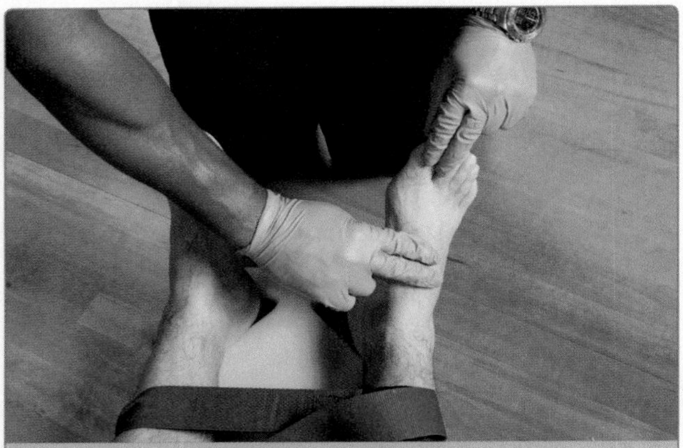

36-3-7 Reassess distal CSM in all four extremities.

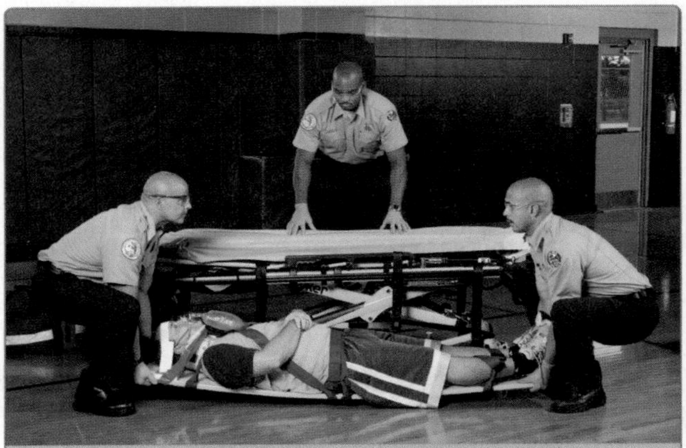

36-3-8 Place the patient onto the stretcher for transport.

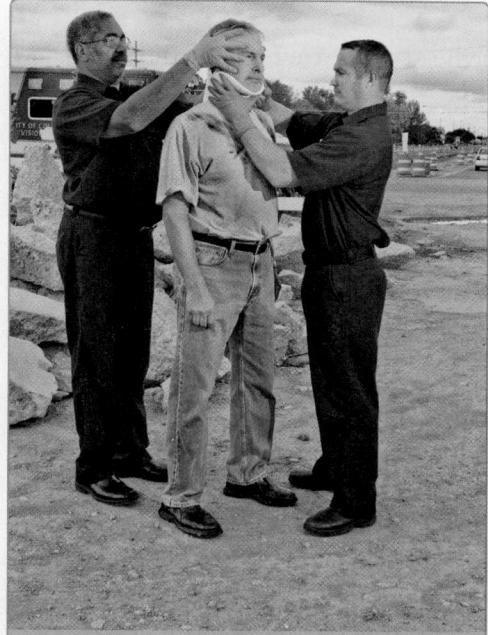

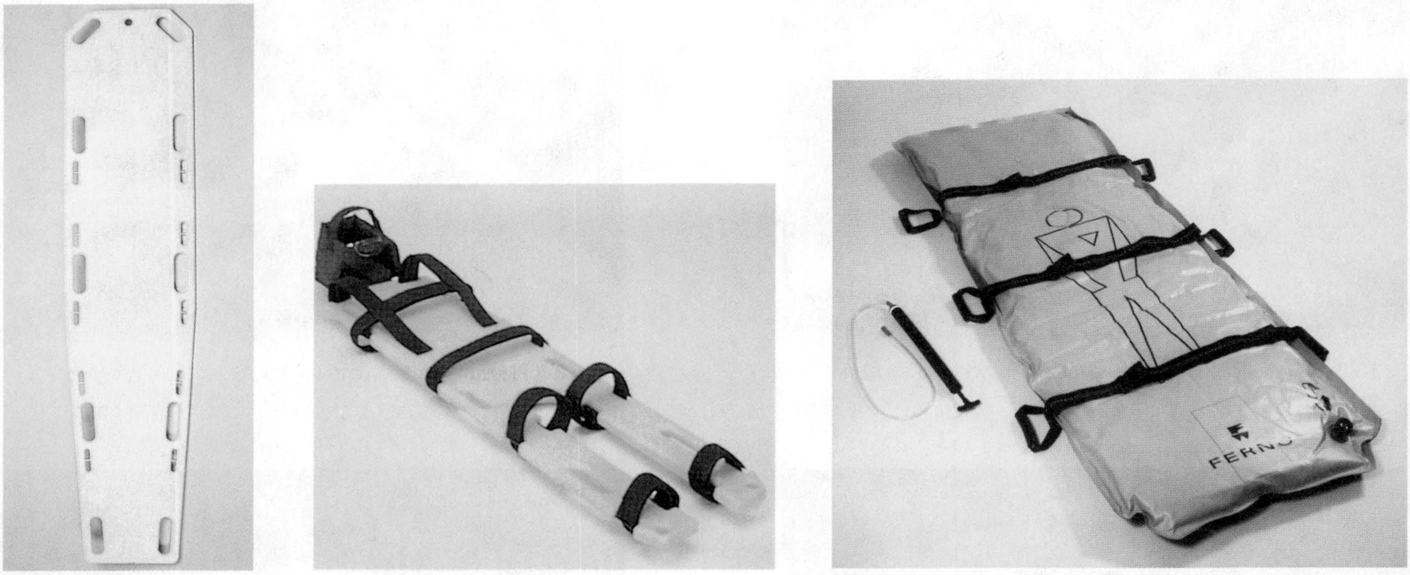

(A) (B) (C)

Figure 36-9 (A) Typical long backboard made of composite plastic. (B) Miller-style backboard. (C) Full-body vacuum splint. (FERNO)

3. Position the device at the patient's side, ensuring that it is high enough so the patient's head will be on the board once it is placed beneath him.
4. The other rescuers should position themselves on the side of the patient, opposite the board.
5. At the direction of the rescuer holding the head, all rescuers then carefully roll the patient onto his side (toward the rescuers). If possible, it is best to have the patient raise the arm that he will be rolling onto above his head.
6. Quickly inspect and palpate the patient's posterior side.
7. One rescuer should reach across the patient and position the board appropriately.

SCAN 36-4 Securing a Standing Patient to a Long Backboard

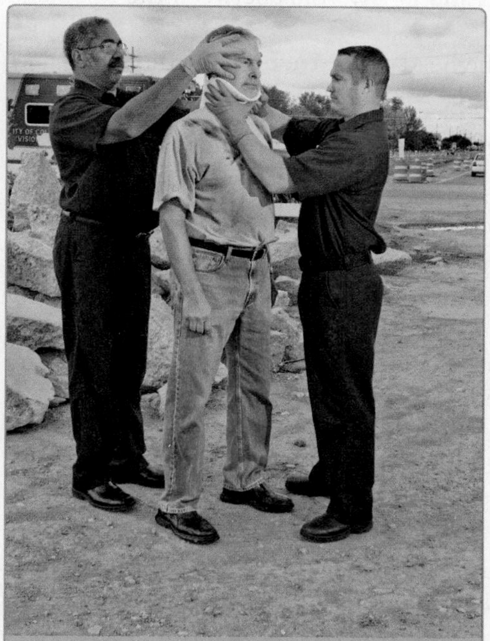

36-4-1 Initiate manual stabilization of the head and place a cervical collar.

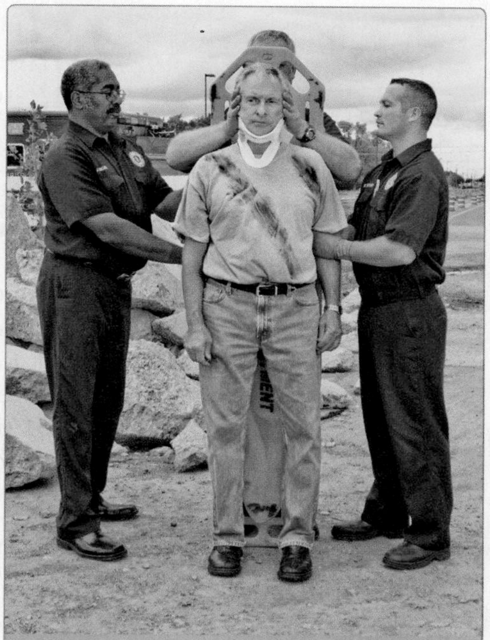

36-4-2 Position the backboard behind the patient.

36-4-3 With an EMT on each side, they reach under the patient's arms and grasp the board.

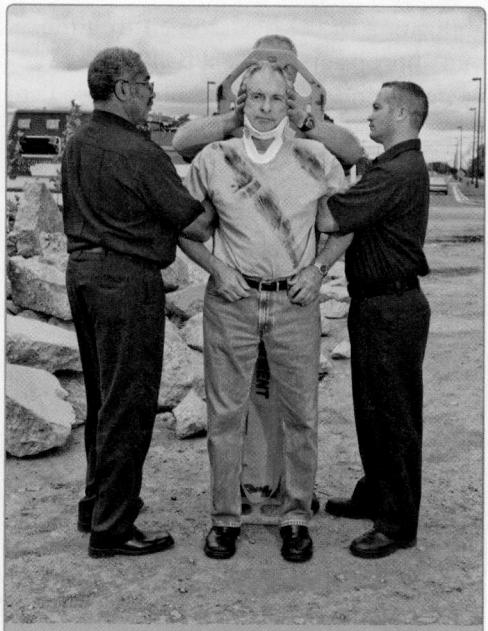

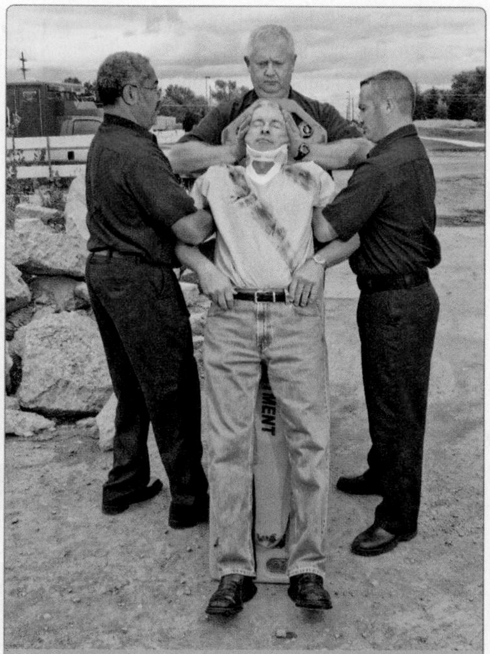

36-4-4 Carefully lower the board backward, allowing the patient to lie on the board.

8. At the direction of the rescuer holding the head, all rescuers then carefully roll the patient onto the board.
9. If necessary, the patient can be centered on the board using a coordinated up and down movement by all rescuers.
10. Place soft pads under the patient's head and in any voids between the torso and the board.
11. Secure the torso and pelvis first, then the head and extremities to the board.
12. Reassess CSM after securing to the board.

Follow these steps for securing a standing patient to a long backboard (Scan 36-4):

1. One rescuer should maintain manual stabilization of the patient's head the entire time.
2. Check CSM of all extremities and apply an appropriate cervical collar.
3. Position the device behind the patient through the arms of the rescuer holding the head.
4. Rescuers 2 and 3 should position themselves at either side of the patient and reach with the hand closest to the patient under the arm to grasp the board.
5. At the direction of the rescuer holding the head, all three should lay the board down with the patient on it. The patient can then be secured to the board as usual.

Short Immobilization Devices

A short immobilization device is used to immobilize the spine of a noncritical patient found in the seated position, such as on a seat of a vehicle. There are essentially two types of short-board immobilization devices: the vest-type device (Figure 36-10 ■) and the rigid short backboard (Figure 36-11 ■). Both devices provide immobilization of the head, neck, and torso during extrication and transport.

Follow these steps to secure a seated patient to a short immobilization device (Scan 36-5):

1. One rescuer should maintain manual stabilization of the head the entire time.
2. Check CSM of all extremities and apply an appropriate cervical collar.
3. A second rescuer should position the device behind the patient and secure it to the patient's torso.
4. The second rescuer should secure the head to the device, using appropriate padding behind the head to maintain proper alignment.
5. Reassess CSM of all extremities.

CLINICAL CLUE

Exception to Short Spine Immobilization

An exception to the application of the short spine immobilization device is for the patient who must be moved due to immediate life threats. In this case, *do not* waste valuable time applying this device to the patient. Instead, you must use a rapid extrication technique to move him to a long backboard.

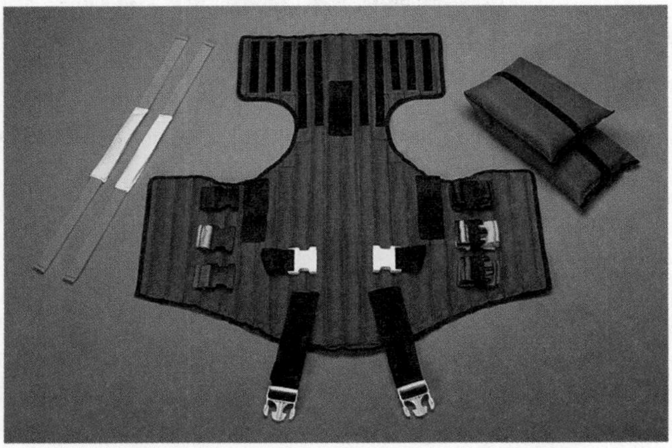

Figure 36-10 The Kendrick vest-type extrication device (KED).
(© Ferno Corporation)

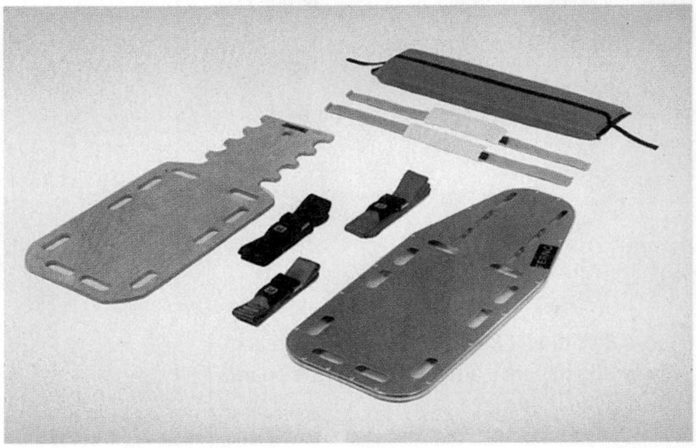

Figure 36-11 Short backboards.

SCAN 36-5 Placing a Vest-Type Extrication Device (KED) on a Seated Patient

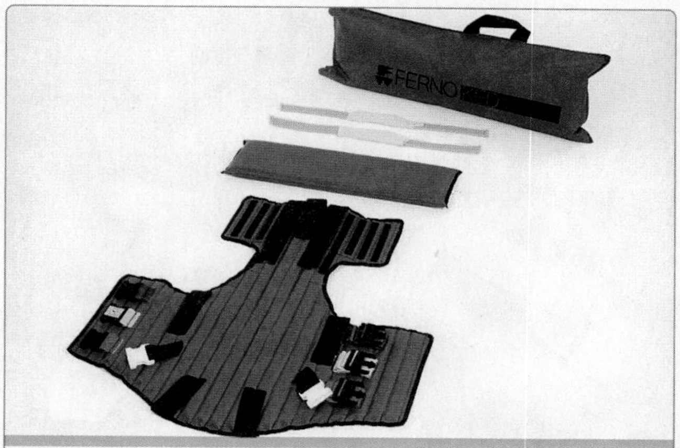

36-5-1 The Kendrick Extrication Device (KED).

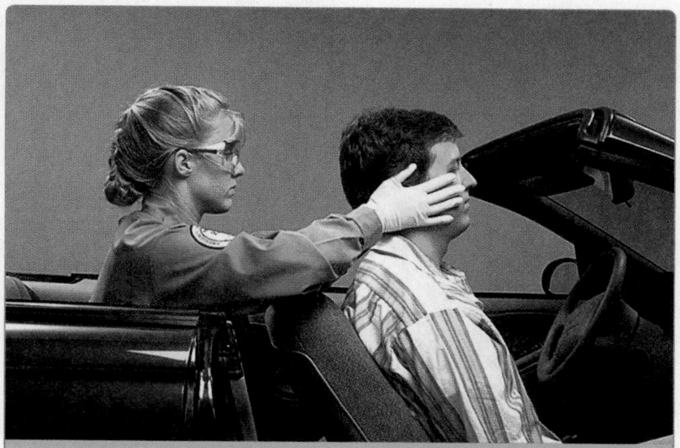

36-5-2 Initiate manual stabilization of the head and neck.

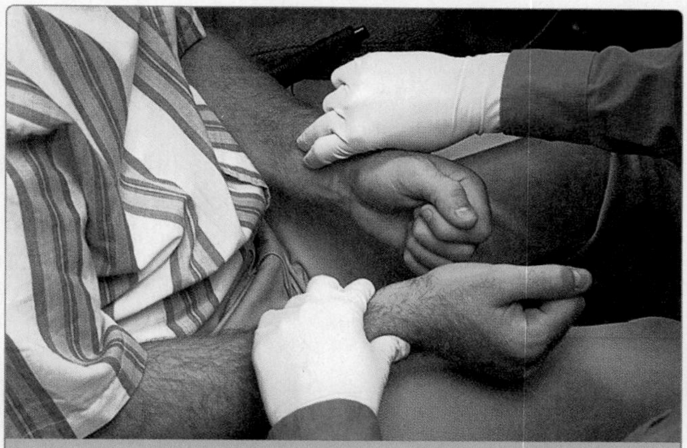

36-5-3 Next, assess CSM in all extremities.

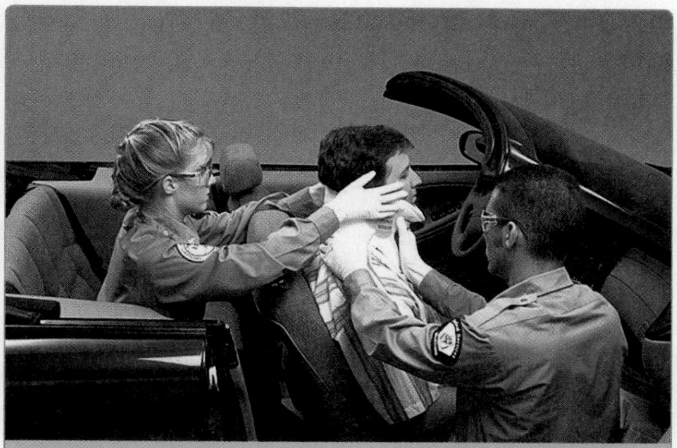

36-5-4 Then place a cervical collar on the patient.

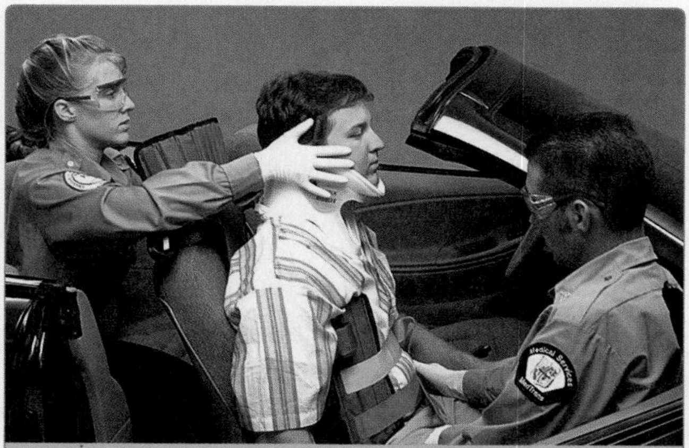

36-5-5 Next, slide the device behind the seated patient, ensure the device is snug against the patient's armpits, and secure the middle and bottom torso straps.

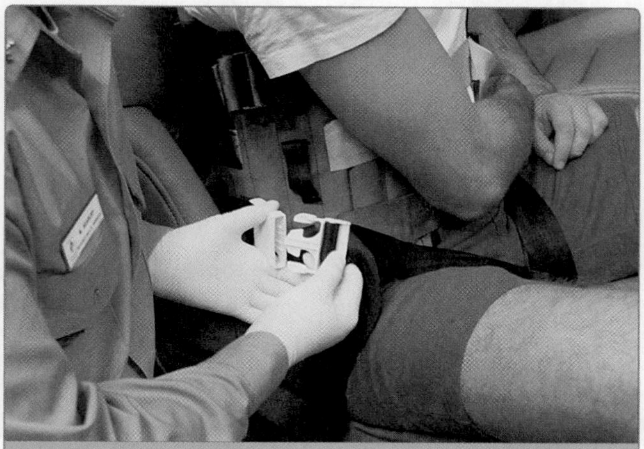

36-5-6 Secure both leg straps.

(Continued)

SCAN 36-5 Placing a Vest-Type Extrication Device (KED) on a Seated Patient (*Cont.*)

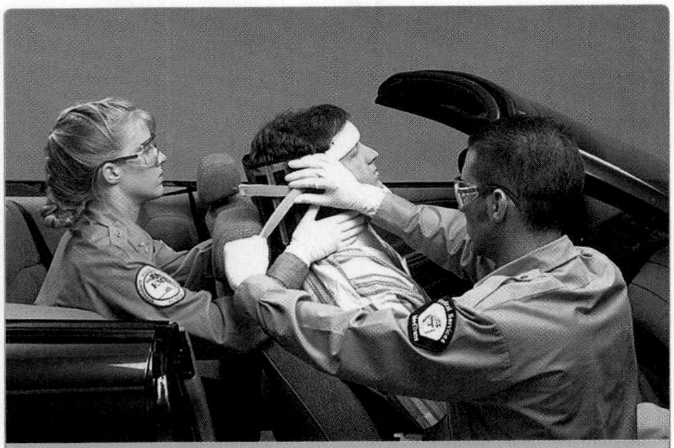

36-5-7 Then secure the head to the device.

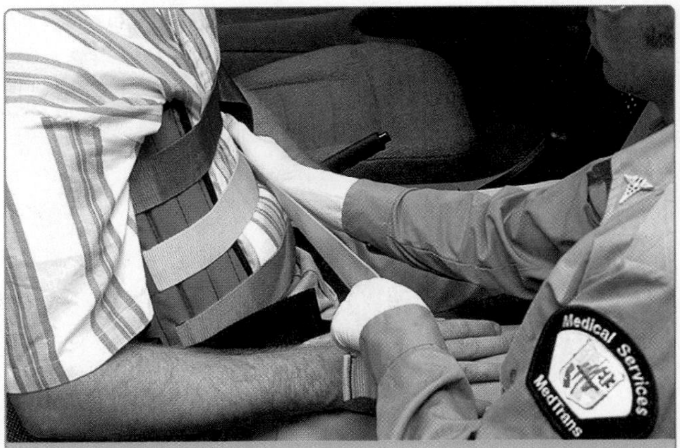

36-5-8 Tighten all the straps and carefully extricate the patient from the vehicle.

In many cases, once a patient has been properly secured to a short immobilization device, he will be moved to a long backboard for transport to the hospital. That can be accomplished by placing a long backboard under the buttocks of the patient and carefully lowering him onto the board for transport in the supine position.

STOP, REVIEW, REMEMBER!

Multiple Choice

For each question, place a check next to the correct answer.

1. The most appropriate method for opening the airway of a patient with suspected spine injury is the:

_____ a. head-tilt/chin-lift maneuver.

_____ b. jaw-thrust maneuver.

_____ c. sniffing position.

_____ d. neutral position.

2. A 22-year-old man has a suspected spine injury after a motor-vehicle collision. Your primary assessment reveals he is in respiratory failure. You should immediately:

_____ a. apply a cervical collar.

_____ b. perform a log roll.

_____ c. initiate positive pressure ventilations.

_____ d. apply a short extrication device.

3. Once the ABCs have been properly managed, emergency care of a patient with a suspected spine injury will focus on:

_____ a. vital signs.

_____ b. proper immobilization.

_____ c. oxygen therapy.

_____ d. rapid transport.

4. Which one of the following statements best describes the purpose of a cervical collar?

_____ a. It reminds the cooperative patient not to move.

_____ b. Once in place, it prevents the neck from moving.

_____ c. One collar size will fit all patients.

_____ d. It is not needed unless the patient has pain.

5. The rescuer at the _____ should be the one to direct all movement of a patient with a suspected spine injury.

_____ a. feet

_____ b. legs

_____ c. torso

_____ d. head

Labeling

Label each photo for the type of mechanism of injury.

1. Flexion
2. Compression
3. Extension
4. Distraction

____

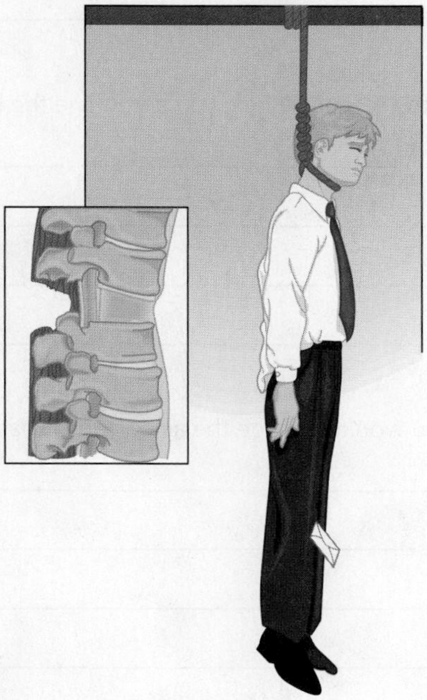

____

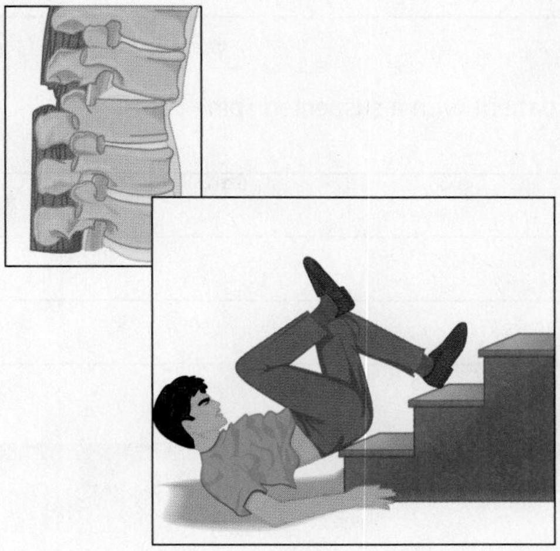

____

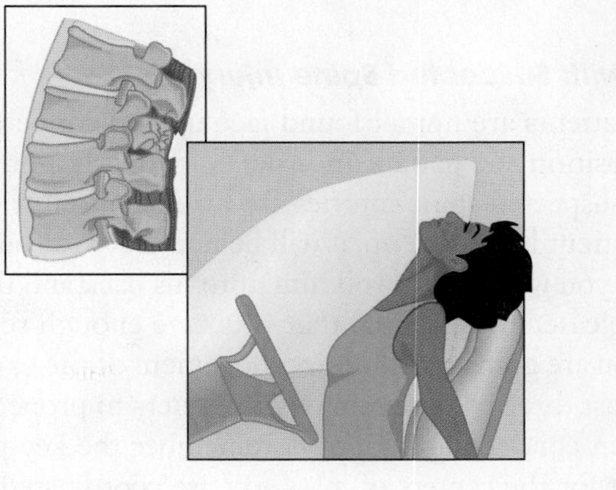

____

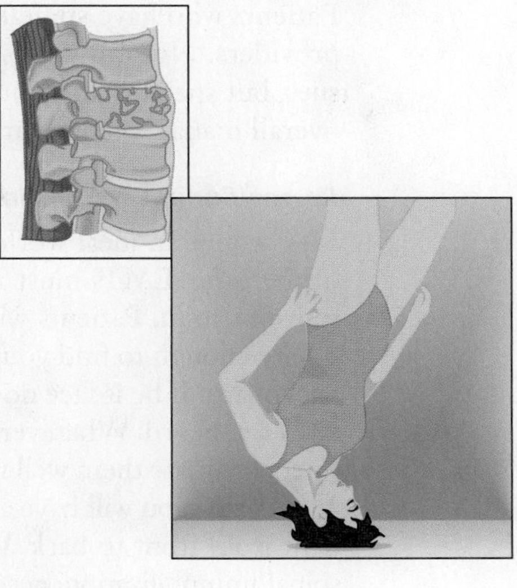

(continued on next page)

(continued)

Critical Thinking

1. Describe how you would go about determining if a patient may have suffered a spine injury.

____

____

____

____

2. What factors at the scene will help you determine the likelihood of a spine injury?

____

____

____

____

3. Describe how you would manage the airway and breathing of a patient with a suspected spine injury.

____

____

____

____

Special Considerations

Patients who have spine injuries can present a variety of specific challenges to EMS providers. Not only does the nature of the injury pose very difficult movement issues, but specific situations with individual patients must be considered as part of an overall management strategy.

Repositioning the Patient with Suspected Spine Injury

EMS is not an ideal world. Patients are not all found face up and cooperative. Much of the time, EMTs must reposition the patient in order to properly immobilize and transport him. Patients with suspected spine injuries are no exception. If you are fortunate enough to find your patient lying face up, it will be necessary to roll him onto a backboard. If he is face down, you will have to roll him onto his back and then get him onto the board. Whatever the case, it is essential that you have enough resources and can coordinate them well if you are going to minimize movement of the patient's spine.

Ideally, you will have at least three or preferably four rescuers to properly roll a patient from front to back. When conducting a log roll, remember the key principles of spinal immobilization: account for the centers of mass and use coordinated movement. One rescuer should be at the head, one at the torso, and one at the pelvis and legs. To keep the roll coordinated, all movements should be directed by the rescuer holding the head. This will help make sure the head stays aligned with the rest of the body in every move.

One of the most critical elements of a coordinated roll from the prone position to the supine position is the initial placement of the hands on the patient's head. The rescuer holding the head must place his hands in such a way that they are not upside down at the end of the roll. He must place his hands, and then envision the roll and where his hands will be at the end. It is important for all rescuers to remain balanced and stable throughout the roll to avoid any unexpected movement of the patient.

Follow the steps below to properly roll a patient from the prone to the supine position using three rescuers:

1. Rescuer 1 should kneel at the top of the patient and firmly grasp the head with both hands, making certain that his arms will not become twisted during the roll.
2. Rescuer 2 should kneel beside the patient's torso and, if possible, move the patient's arm closest to the rescuer straight up over his head.
3. Rescuer 3 should kneel beside the patient's hips and legs.
4. On the direction of rescuer 1, everyone then carefully rolls the patient in the direction of rescuer 2 and 3 and stops once the patient is on his side.
5. All rescuers should reposition themselves slightly to accommodate the rest of the roll.
6. On the direction of rescuer 1, the patient is then carefully rolled down onto his back.

If a backboard is available, place it in such a way that the patient is rolled directly onto the board, eliminating the need for an additional roll. Be sure to stop briefly to assess the patient's back while he is on his side.

In situations where you are alone or have fewer than three but perhaps two rescuers, you may have to roll the patient as best you can. This should occur only if there are immediate life threats to the patient and moving him is necessary to address one or more of the life threats.

Pediatric Patients with Suspected Spine Injury

Consider using a short spine board for a small child or infant who needs full spinal precautions. Because of the large **occipital** region (back) of the skull, pediatric patients may need additional padding placed from shoulders to feet. This will allow the head to remain in a neutral position when secured to a spinal immobilization device.

occipital posterior (back) region of the skull.

There are specialized immobilization devices designed to accommodate the pediatric patient. One such device is a properly sized backboard with the head segment lower than the body segment to accommodate the large occipital region in most pediatric patients (Figure 36-12 ▪). Other devices address the need for adequate restraint and have built in Velcro closures for securing the uncooperative patient to the device (Figure 36-13 ▪). Also, consider securing the patient to a board without a cervical collar should you not have the correct size. Using a collar that does not fit properly can cause more harm than good.

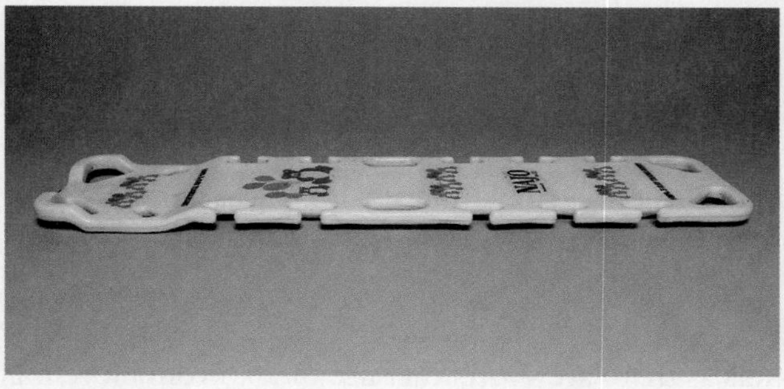

Figure 36-12 A pediatric backboard. Note the step down at the head end.

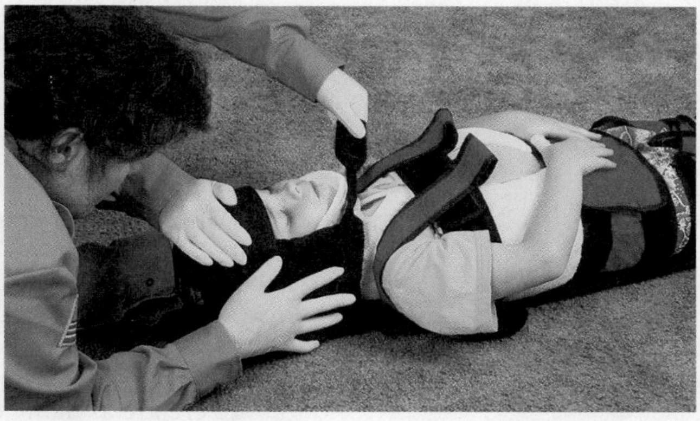

Figure 36-13 Utilizing a specialized pediatric immobilization device on a small child.

Small children often are found in car seats after a motor-vehicle collision and may require spinal immobilization. Removing a child from a car seat is not always a simple task and should be weighed carefully against the potential risks. If it is deemed necessary, remove the car seat from the vehicle. Lay the car seat back and using coordinated movements slide the child out of the seat and onto an appropriate immobilization device. The child can then be immobilized.

Some experts would argue that a child can be immobilized in a car seat as long as the seat is intact. Most car seats are rigid and have five point restraints that limit movement of the three centers of mass. If the child is left in the seat, however, you must consider the following:

- Immobilize the head and neck. The head should be secured to the seat so as to limit lateral and flexion/extension movement.
- Use small towels to fill voids around the head if necessary.
- Consider transporting the seat in a reclined position to limit the effects of compression (axial loading on the patient's neck).

Local protocols may dictate the decision for children in car seats. Always be aware of your local rules and guidelines on pediatric immobilization.

Rapid Extrication

36-11 Describe the indications and correct procedures for rapid extrication.

rapid extrication the removal of a patient from a car or other location as rapidly as possible, while remaining mindful that a potential spine injury exists.

Rapid extrication is the removal of a patient from a car or other location as rapidly as possible while remaining mindful that a potential spine injury exists. Rapid extrication may be indicated in the following situations:

- The scene becomes unsafe.
- The patient has immediate life threats that must be addressed.
- One patient is blocking access to another, more seriously injured patient.

Rapid extrication involves moving the patient when there is not enough time to properly stabilize the head, neck, and spine, such as in the case of a compromised airway or severe bleeding. It should be used only as a last resort, and the decision to use this technique should be based on the patient's condition and time.

Follow these steps to perform a rapid extrication of a seated patient from a vehicle:

1. Rescuer 1 should maintain manual stabilization of the head from behind while rescuer 2 places a cervical collar.
2. Rescuer 3 can then place a long backboard on the seat, with one end beneath the patient's buttocks and the other end on the stretcher.
3. Together rescuer 1 and 2 should carefully pivot the patient so his back faces the door opening.
4. As the patient turns, rescuer 2 should assume control of the head while rescuer 1 and 3 assist in laying the patient down on the backboard.
5. Properly secure the patient to the board and transport.

Dealing with Helmets

The use of protective helmets is becoming more and more common in many sports. This may be because of state laws and just plain common sense. In any case, you are likely to encounter a patient with a suspected spine injury who is wearing a helmet, and you will need to know how to deal with it.

TYPES OF HELMETS

There are as many types of helmets as there are sports that use them. From bicycling to kayaking to field hockey to skiing, helmets come in many shapes and sizes. Most helmets come in two basic varieties: the sports-style helmet that has an open face and opens anteriorly, and the full-face motorcycle style that slips on over the top of the head and encloses the entire face.

As you might expect, the open-face helmets provide easier access to the face and therefore make it easier to both assess and manage the airway without having to remove the helmet. Full-face helmets make assessment and management of the patient's airway and breathing much more difficult.

Depending on the situation, you may choose to leave the helmet in place or remove it. The driving factor in deciding to remove the helmet or leave it in place is the adequacy of the patient's airway and breathing. If you are able to assess the airway and breathing and find that it is adequate, look at the fit of the helmet. Does it fit snugly against the patient's head minimizing movement within the helmet? If so, then consider the patient's position. Is the helmet forcing the head into a hyperflexed position, putting pressure on the neck? The last factor you must consider is your ability to adequately immobilize the patient with the helmet in place. If the helmet will prevent you from properly securing the patient to an immobilization device, then you may have to remove it.

Leave the helmet in place when:

- There are no immediate or impending airway or breathing problems.
- It does not interfere with ongoing assessment of airway and breathing.
- It provides a snug fit with little movement of head.
- Removal would cause further injury.

Remove the helmet when:

- There is inability to assess or reassess airway and breathing.
- It prevents adequate management of the airway or breathing.
- Excessive patient head movement is possible within the helmet.
- Proper spinal immobilization cannot be performed due to the helmet.
- Cardiac or respiratory arrest occurs.

Remember that it may be possible to simply remove the face mask from the helmet to access the airway. Often face masks are secured with plastic fittings that are easily removed with simple tools or cutters. It is common for athletic trainers to have these tools on the field. This option may offer a far faster access in an emergency than even helmet removal.

GENERAL GUIDELINES FOR HELMET REMOVAL

Helmet removal will differ slightly, depending on the type of helmet encountered. The primary objective is to minimize any side-to-side motion and to remove the helmet by pulling in the direction of the spine.

The following is a sequence of steps that can be followed for the proper removal of a helmet. The specific technique that you use will depend somewhat on the actual helmet and may be modified as necessary. Remove the patient's eyeglasses prior to attempting to remove a helmet.

Follow these steps for removal of a helmet (Scan 36-6):

1. Rescuer 1 should stabilize the helmet by placing his hands on each side of the helmet with the fingers on the mandible to prevent movement.
2. Have rescuer 2 loosen, cut, or remove the chin strap, if present.
3. Rescuer 2 then should place one hand on the mandible to stabilize the chin and the other hand posteriorly at the occipital region.
4. Rescuer 1 should pull the sides of the helmet apart and gently slip the helmet halfway off the patient's head and then stop.

SCAN 36-6 Helmet Removal

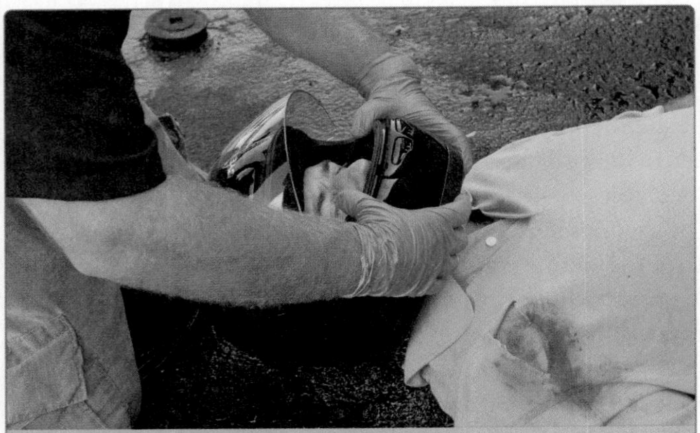

36-6-1 Rescuer 1 uses both hands to stabilize the helmet and head.

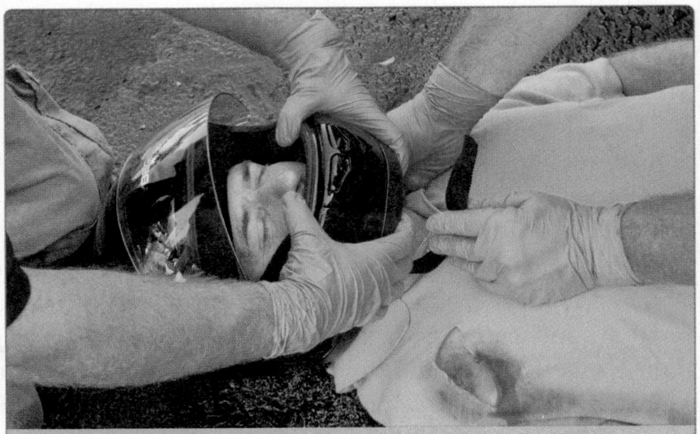

36-6-2 Rescuer 2 loosens or cuts the chin strap.

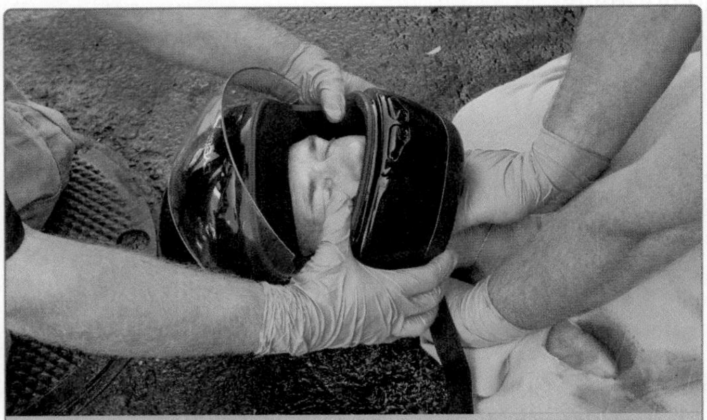

36-6-3 Next, rescuer 2 places both hands around the neck and jaw to stabilize the patient's head.

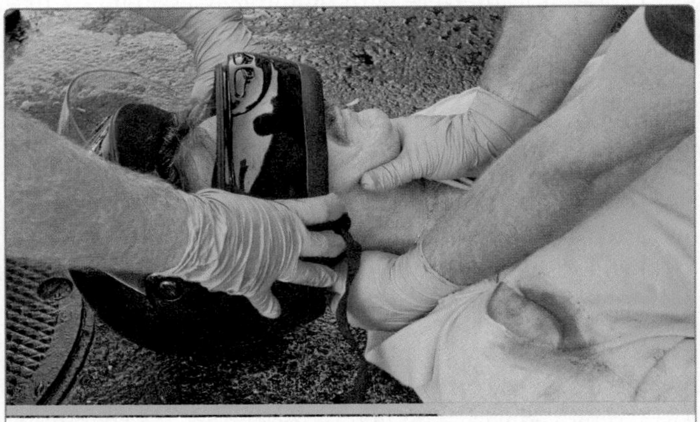

36-6-4 Then rescuer 1 gently pulls the helmet straight off the patient's head.

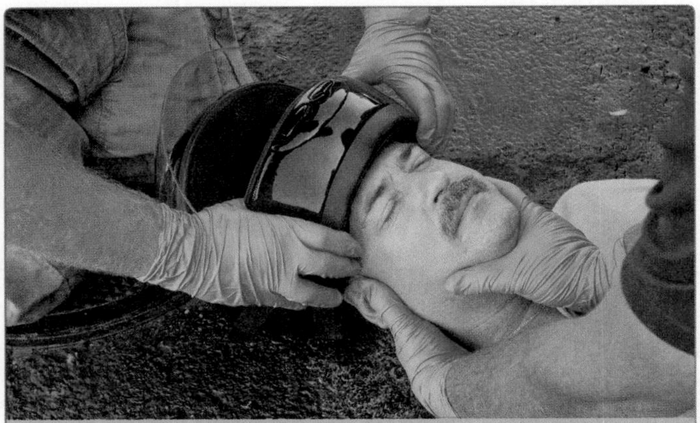

36-6-5 As the helmet is removed, rescuer 2 moves his hands upward on the patient's head.

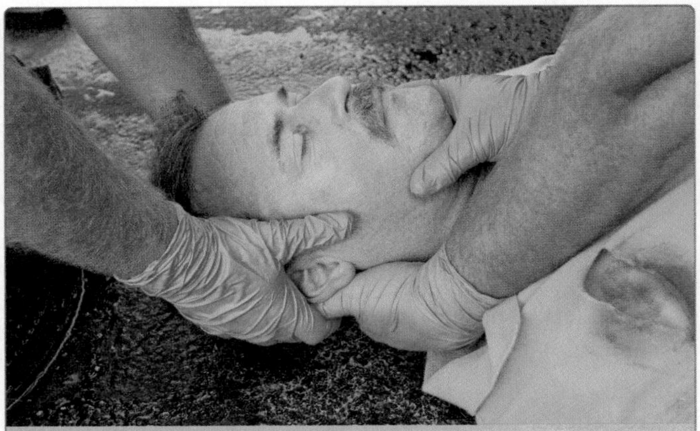

36-6-6 Once the helmet is completely removed, the patient's head is gently lowered to the ground.

5. Rescuer 2 then slides the posterior hand along the back of the patient's head to support the head as the helmet is removed.
6. Following removal of the helmet, rescuer 2 should assume normal manual stabilization of the head until full spinal immobilization is complete.

As the helmet is removed, be certain to support the head so that it does not drop suddenly. After removal of the helmet, gently lower the head onto the board. It is also appropriate to place a thin pad beneath the patient's head for comfort.

FOOTBALL HELMETS AND EQUIPMENT

Removing the helmet of a player who is wearing shoulder pads will cause the patient's head to fall into a hyperextended position. This can be prevented by leaving the helmet in place and removing the face guard of the helmet, should access to the airway be necessary. In extreme cases, in which the helmet must be removed, it will be helpful to also remove the shoulder pads.

> **CLINICAL CLUE**
>
> **Removing Football Equipment**
>
> Removing only the helmet and not the shoulder pads, or vice versa, will cause the patient's neck to hyperextend or hyperflex. It is recommended that if you must remove the helmet, you also should remove the shoulder pads in order to keep the cervical spine in correct alignment.

Negative Effects of Spinal Immobilization

Spinal immobilization is not without downsides. Immobilizing the patient on a rigid long board for prolonged periods of time can actually cause patient harm. It has been shown that even after 30 minutes of immobilization, tissue damage can begin. Now certainly the standard of care for potential spine injuries is immobilization, but given the potential negative side effects, there are a few things to consider.

If protocol allows, consider using some form of padding to soften the rigid long backboard and prevent tissue damage. Slight padding, such as a blanket applied to the board prior to application can soften the surface and make it much more comfortable for the patient. Some systems allow for the use of full body vacuum splints as both immobilization and as padding. The key is to provide padding, but yet still account for rigid immobilization.

Also, consider the need for immobilization altogether. Some EMS systems allow for the clearing of spine injury based on very specific assessment processes and findings. In those cases the need for spinal immobilization, even with a positive mechanism of injury, is assessed using a standardized protocol designed to identify situations where immobilization is not necessary. Local protocol will dictate, but common rule-out protocols examine patient reliability and then look for pain or tenderness along the spinal column and deficits after a comprehensive neurological examination. If the rule-out criteria are met, no immobilization is used. Note that rule-out or "clearing" protocols require specific training and proper application to be used safely. That said, prevention of unnecessary immobilization is certainly beneficial to your patient. As always, follow local protocol.

EMERGENCY DISPATCH SUMMARY

Gary Vandel was secured to a long backboard, given supplemental oxygen, and transported to the Northeast Medical Center on Green River Parkway. X-rays showed fractures to the C3 and C4 vertebrae, with bone fragments impacting the spinal cord in three places. Several days after surgery, Gary regained limited use of his arms and some feeling in his lower legs. Gary's doctor anticipates that he will walk again, with the assistance of a cane, but will probably always suffer from numbness and weakness in his extremities.

Chapter Review

To the Point

- The spinal cord is the message center of the nervous system. Both sensory and motor nervous transmissions use this pathway to go to and from the brain.
- An injury to the spinal cord risks interrupting this nervous pathway, thereby disrupting critical body functions.
- The spinal column is composed of 33 bones, ligaments, and muscles designed to protect the spinal cord.
- The spine is damaged in the same fashion as any other tissue in trauma. Direct force, concussion, swelling, and ischemia all pose significant risks to the delicate tissue.
- Injury to the spinal column may or may not result in damage to the cord.
- Damage to the spinal cord can be immediate or delayed and can be complete or incomplete.
- Mechanism of injury and scene clues can identify the likelihood of spine injury.
- Assessment of the spinal patient should focus on the primary assessment first and then utilize the primary and secondary assessments to identify the subtle spine injury.
- Immobilization focuses on an in-line neutral position and must account for three centers of body mass.
- All movements of spinal patients must be coordinated so as to move the body as a single unit.
- Rapid extrication should be considered when an immediate move is necessary.
- Special challenges abound in spinal immobilization. Providers should remain flexible in their thinking and decision making and be capable of adapting to unique situations.

Chapter Questions

Multiple Choice

For each question, place a check next to the correct answer.

1. The brain and spinal cord are the components of the ________ system.

_____ a. autonomic nervous
_____ b. skeletal
_____ c. central nervous
_____ d. peripheral nervous

2. The network of sensory and motor nerves that extend from the brain and spinal cord make up the ____________ system.

_____ a. autonomic
_____ b. skeletal
_____ c. central nervous
_____ d. peripheral nervous

3. You are caring for a young man who was injured during a football game. He is complaining of numbness and tingling to both legs. You should:

_____ a. manually stabilize him with his helmet in place.
_____ b. remove the helmet.
_____ c. move him off the field before placing on a backboard.
_____ d. remove both the helmet and pads.

4. Extreme twisting of the spine is an example of which type of mechanism of injury?

_____ a. Flexion
_____ b. Extension
_____ c. Rotation
_____ d. Distraction

5. A patient who has fallen from a height and landed in a seated position is likely to experience what type of spine injury?

_____ a. Flexion
_____ b. Extension
_____ c. Compression
_____ d. Rotation

6. A football player has been injured in a head-first collision and is now choking. You should:
   _____ a. remove his helmet immediately.
   _____ b. remove only his face mask.
   _____ c. remove his shoulder pads first, and then his helmet.
   _____ d. leave his helmet in place and transport.
7. Which one of the following is the most serious complication of spine injury encountered in the field?
   _____ a. Priapism
   _____ b. Incontinence
   _____ c. Inadequate breathing
   _____ d. Loss of consciousness
8. It is important to assess circulation, sensation, and motor function of all four extremities:
   _____ a. before immobilization.
   _____ b. before and after immobilization.
   _____ c. after immobilization.
   _____ d. only during the rapid trauma assessment.
9. When securing a patient with suspected spine injury to a long backboard, the head must be secured:
   _____ a. first.
   _____ b. before the torso.
   _____ c. before the legs.
   _____ d. after the torso.
10. Which one of the following best describes the function of a cervical collar?
    _____ a. It prevents movement of the neck.
    _____ b. It reminds the patient not to move his neck.
    _____ c. It provides adequate immobilization of the neck.
    _____ d. It must be placed regardless of fit.
11. Which one of the following situations is most appropriate for rapid extrication?
    _____ a. Patient with inadequate breathing
    _____ b. Responsive patient
    _____ c. Patient complaining of neck pain
    _____ d. None of the above
12. When rolling a patient who may have a spine injury, the rescuer at the _____________ should direct all movements.
    _____ a. head
    _____ b. torso
    _____ c. hips
    _____ d. legs
13. Which one of the following patients would be best suited for a vest-type immobilization device?
    _____ a. Supine patient on the ground
    _____ b. Seated patient in a vehicle
    _____ c. Prone patient on the ground
    _____ d. Standing patient
14. The first step in caring for a patient who has a suspected spine injury is to:
    _____ a. roll the patient.
    _____ b. place a cervical collar.
    _____ c. place him on an appropriate device.
    _____ d. manually stabilize the head and neck.

Fill in the Blank

1. The central nervous system includes the brain and _____________________.
2. The _____________________ nervous system is made up of all the sensory and motor nerves that extend from the brain and spinal cord to all parts of the body.
3. The first seven vertebrae located in the neck are known as the _____________________.
4. There are _____________________ vertebrae that make up the thoracic spine.
5. The _____________________ spine is located in the lower back and is composed of five vertebrae.
6. Injury at any point along the spinal column that causes damage to the spinal cord can result in the loss of sensation and function _____________________ the site of injury.
7. Any force that impacts the spine from the top or bottom has the potential to cause what is referred to as a _____________________ injury.
8. Injury to the spinal cord above the _____________________ cervical vertebra can prevent the diaphragm from assisting with spontaneous respiration.

(continued on next page)

(continued)

Critical Thinking

1. Describe at least two circumstances in which rapid extrication would be necessary.

2. Discuss the priority for proper spinal immobilization in patients needing rapid extrication.

3. Describe how you would manage an unresponsive football player with a suspected spine injury.

Case Studies

Case Study 1

You have been dispatched to a vehicle collision at a busy intersection in the center of town known for its daily occurrence of collisions. On arrival, you find two vehicles, each with substantial damage to the front end. The fire department is on scene and is caring for the patient in the first vehicle. You approach the second vehicle and see no one inside. Just then a police officer calls you over to the curb. He is taking information from a man standing beside him. The man is holding a bloody towel against his forehead and seems to be bleeding from the mouth as well. The officer informs you that this man was the driver of the second vehicle. When asked, the patient denies any neck pain but states only that his head hurts because he hit it on the windshield.

1. Is this patient a candidate for spinal immobilization? Why or why not?

2. What additional information will you want to know about this patient?

3. How will you care for this patient?

4. What device is most appropriate for immobilizing this patient?

Case Study 2

You have responded to a motorcycle versus vehicle collision. On arrival, you find the rider of the motorcycle lying motionless on his side in the intersection. A passerby is kneeling beside the patient, attempting to get a response. Your assessment reveals that the patient does not appear to be breathing and radial pulses are absent. He has a full-face helmet still in place, and it shows significant damage to the right side. A quick inspection also reveals severe deformity to his left lower leg.

1. What is your first priority for this patient?

2. Will you roll him onto his back? If so, how will you accomplish this with just the bystander as an assistant?

3. Will you want to remove this man's helmet? If so, how will you do it?

4. What would be most appropriate for immobilizing this patient?

The Last Word

Injuries to the spinal cord can result in permanent paralysis and loss of function below the injury site. Proper assessment and management of the patient is essential to minimize further damage and long-term paralysis.

Spinal immobilization is not a higher priority than the ABCs, but proper management of the ABCs can be accomplished while being mindful of a suspected spine injury.

In some situations it may be necessary, based on scene safety or patient condition, to move or extricate the patient without first providing full spinal immobilization. This is called *rapid extrication* and should be used as a last resort. Remember to complete your prehospital care report with all appropriate information.

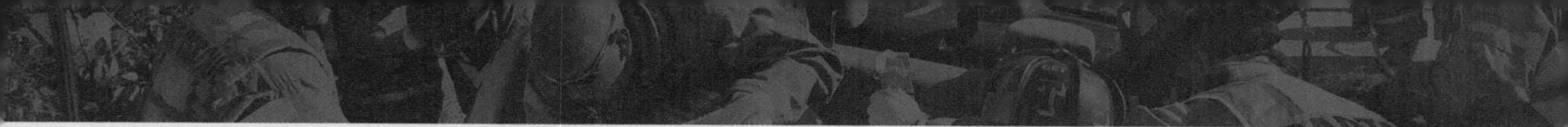

Caring for Patients with Environmental Emergencies

37

Education Standards

Trauma: Environmental emergencies

Competencies

Applies fundamental knowledge to provide basic emergency care and transportation based on assessment findings for an acutely injured patient.

Objectives

After completion of this lesson, you should be able to:

37-1 Define key terms introduced in this chapter.

37-2 Explain the importance of recognizing and providing emergency medical care to patients with environmental emergencies.

37-3 Describe the process by which the body maintains normal temperature.

37-4 Explain the mechanisms by which the body loses heat.

37-5 Explain the mechanisms by which the body gains heat.

37-6 Describe the pathophysiology of generalized hypothermia.

37-7 Recognize factors that contribute to a patient's risk for hypothermia.

37-8 Describe the pathophysiology of local cold injury.

37-9 Discuss the assessment-based approach to cold-related emergencies.

37-10 Describe the emergency medical care for local cold injury.

37-11 Describe the signs and symptoms of generalized hypothermia.

37-12 Describe the emergency medical care for generalized hypothermia.

37-13 Describe the pathophysiology of immersion/submersion injuries.

37-14 Describe the indications for spinal immobilization in drowning victims.

37-15 Describe the emergency care for the victim of an immersion/submersion injury.

37-16 Describe the pathophysiology of heat-related emergencies.

37-17 Recognize factors that contribute to a patient's risk for hyperthermia.

37-18 Differentiate the three types of heat-related emergencies.

37-19 Discuss the assessment-based approach to heat-related emergencies.

37-20 Describe the emergency medical care for suspected heat cramps and heat exhaustion.

37-21 Describe the emergency medical care for suspected heat stroke.

37-22 Describe the signs and symptoms associated with bites or stings of black widow spiders, brown recluse spiders, scorpions, and fire ants.

37-23 Describe the characteristics of common venomous snakes and factors that affect the severity of a snakebite.

37-24 Describe the emergency medical care for a bite or sting.

37-25 Describe the signs, symptoms, and patient history associated with the bite or sting of a marine animal and the emergency medical care for marine-life poisoning.

37-26 Explain the pathophysiology of lightning-strike injuries.

37-27 Describe the emergency medical care for a patient who has been struck by lightning.

37-28 Explain the pathophysiology of decompression sickness.

37-29 Recognize the signs, symptoms, and patient history associated with Type I and Type II decompression sickness.

37-30 Describe the emergency medical care of patients suffering from air embolism and decompression sickness.

Key Terms

active external rewarming p. 973
decompression sickness p. 993
drowning p. 974
electrolytes p. 981
frostbite p. 967
frostnip p. 967
heat cramps p. 982
heat exhaustion p. 982
heat stroke p. 983
hyperthermia p. 965
hypothermia p. 965
normothermic p. 965
passive rewarming p. 973
temperature regulation p. 965

Introduction

37-2 Explain the importance of recognizing and providing emergency medical care to patients with environmental emergencies.

When patients call EMS, they are most often dealing with a problem from some internal disease process or a traumatic event in which some external force has acted on the body (the patient was struck by a car, for example). Either way, the cause of the illness or injury is usually straightforward. In contrast, when the forces of Mother Nature act on the human body to produce harmful, even life-threatening effects, those forces tend to be infrequent and sometimes less recognizable than the more usual pathophysiologies. As a result, they are more difficult to identify and often confound patient assessment. As an EMT, you must understand how the environment can impact your patient. You must understand how environmental forces can cause harm and also how those same forces can worsen existing medical problems.

This chapter provides a review of common environmental problems ranging from heat and cold emergencies to poisonous bites and stings. Proper assessment and patient care for a wide array of issues are described as well. However, it is important that you continue to hone your knowledge by researching and examining further environmental threats that are specific to your own region of responsibility.

EMERGENCY DISPATCH

"You're headed to an oil field out on County Road 23," Heather, the midday dispatcher, said. "You're supposed to look for a small white sign on the south side of the road that says, Rig number 119."

"Okay, and do we have a nature yet?" EMT Jay Collins asked, turning the ambulance's air conditioner up to high. He was still sweating.

"They think it's heat stroke," Heather responded. "And now they're telling us that they'll have someone on the county road to wave you in."

"Copy," Jay responded and turned to his partner, Al Brackin. "Heat stroke? Imagine that. Heck, it's only 108 degrees."

The patient, a middle-aged man clad in a fire-retardant jumpsuit, was sitting in a shady spot at the foot of a towering oil derrick. One of his coworkers was fanning him with a rag.

"How are you feeling, sir?" Al approached the patient and peeled his exam glove from the back of his hand in order to touch the man's skin. It was hot and dry.

"There's a, um, I'm not." The man blinked his eyes several times and shook his head as if to clear it. "I'm kind of sick, I think."

"Let's get this guy into the ambulance now." Al said to Jay as he slid his hands under the man's arms to lift him.

Cold and Heat Emergencies

Cold and heat emergencies can happen in a wide range of environments and conditions. Hunting, skiing, hiking, and ice fishing are common activities that expose people to emergencies related to cold. People who work outside for prolonged times in the summer, people working in hot industrial settings, and firefighters are among those who commonly experience heat-related emergencies.

Of course, each person handles extremes of temperature differently. A geriatric patient who has fallen and remains on a cool tile floor for a relatively short time may experience the same level of **hypothermia** that a teenager experiences after many hours outside in very cold weather. Likewise, an infant outside in August for a short time may experience **hyperthermia** at the levels an adult experiences after strenuous exertion or many hours in the same environment. Pay careful attention to factors such as the temperature where the patient is found, clothing worn, age, condition of the patient prior to the exposure, and contact with any surfaces that could be contributing to the patient's condition.

hypothermia abnormally low core body temperature.

hyperthermia abnormally elevated core body temperature.

PERSPECTIVE

Al—The EMT

Man, what a classic case of hyperthermia! The guy's out working in temperatures over a hundred degrees in a jumpsuit. He starts getting faint, his skin is hot and dry, and it was pretty obvious that he has an altered mental status. That was just an absolute textbook example of heat stroke.

Temperature and the Body

37-3 Describe the process by which the body maintains normal temperature.

Temperature regulation in the body is a constant balancing act between hot and cold. The body functions best in a very narrow range of temperatures. In fact, the point at which a patient is considered **normothermic** exists only between 97.7°F and 99.5°F (36.5°C and 37.5°C). This narrow range is maintained through constant adjustments regulated in the brain by the hypothalamus.

temperature regulation the body's ability to maintain a stable core temperature.

normothermic normal body temperature.

Body heat is generated constantly by basic cellular metabolism. It is further increased by strenuous activity and through active processes such as shivering. The body can take steps to preserve heat by constricting (narrowing) blood vessels in the periphery, thereby limiting the blood's exposure to external cold. To get rid of heat, the body dilates (expands) blood vessels to bring blood close to the skin. Sweat also is produced to help the body lose heat through evaporation. The hypothalamus continually monitors body heat and makes adjustments to regulate and maintain a normal core temperature.

Ordinarily, the body is quite efficient at this regulation process. Normal health, activity, hydration, and intake of food allow the human body to tolerate a wide range of environmental conditions. However, there are many factors that can challenge the body's ability to compensate. The following are a few examples:

- ***Extremes of age.*** The very young and the very old can have difficulty adapting to temperature. For the elderly, the reason usually is poor circulation and limited body fat. In children, the ability to regulate temperature efficiently is not yet fully developed.
- ***Underlying medical conditions.*** Diseases such as diabetes and thyroid problems and injuries to the central nervous system can lead to difficulties in managing temperature.

- ***Medications.*** Certain medications, such as beta blockers, can limit the body's ability to compensate for the challenges of temperature. Patients taking these medications are often more vulnerable to becoming too hot or too cold.
- ***Shock and circulatory problems.*** The cardiovascular system is one of the body's chief means of thermoregulation. When circulation is compromised, as in traumatic injury and shock, the ability to thermoregulate is greatly challenged.

Despite the body's regulatory abilities, extremes of cold and heat can easily overwhelm it. Although the body can certainly survive beyond the two-degree difference of the thermoneutral zone, body functions suffer when core temperature is pushed to extremes. If pushed beyond the ability to compensate for prolonged periods, severe injury and death can result.

Hypothermia and hyperthermia occur when the body's ability to regulate temperature fails. Hypothermia is the result when heat loss exceeds heat produced. Hyperthermia occurs when heat gained (from metabolism and environment) exceeds heat lost.

Cold Emergencies

37-4 Explain the mechanisms by which the body loses heat.

37-7 Recognize factors that contribute to a patient's risk for hypothermia.

Most humans live in an environment that is typically cooler than the core of the body. As a result, hypothermia is a constant risk. Although you might think of hypothermia occurring in the back woods of Maine in January, remember it can occur even on a warm summer day. Any time the body is exposed to cooler temperatures without the capability to compensate, hypothermia is a risk. Consider the following example:

> It is a warm July day. You are caring for a victim of multisystem trauma in the back of your ambulance. Because you are warm, the air conditioner is running, making the interior temperature 68°F. The patient's clothes have been removed during the process of patient assessment and he is sweaty as a result of sympathetic nervous system stimulation. Now he lies in shock, moist, on a cool backboard, and his body is having difficulty regulating temperature. All of a sudden, 68 degrees seems rather cold.

Heat escapes the body through a number of means (Figure 37-1 ■). Consider them when you are treating patients with emergencies related to heat or cold. They include:

- ***Radiation.*** Body heat is lost directly into the surrounding air.
- ***Conduction.*** Body heat is transferred to an object with which the body is in contact.
- ***Convection.*** Body heat is lost to surrounding air that becomes warmer, rises or is displaced by the wind, and is replaced with cooler air.
- ***Evaporation.*** Body heat is lost when perspiration is changed from liquid to vapor.
- ***Respiration.*** Heat leaves the body with each breath.

Immersion in cold water is a specific type of conductive heat loss. It is important to consider it specifically because heat loss in this circumstance is approximately 30 times faster than radiation or convection. (Immersion is described in more detail later in the chapter.)

If you have a patient with hypothermia, emergency care should be geared toward preventing heat loss. This can be accomplished by covering the patient with blankets to minimize heat loss through radiation and convection and placing blankets under the patient to prevent conductive loss. You also may add heat to the patient by placing heat packs in his armpits and groin (adds heat through conduction).

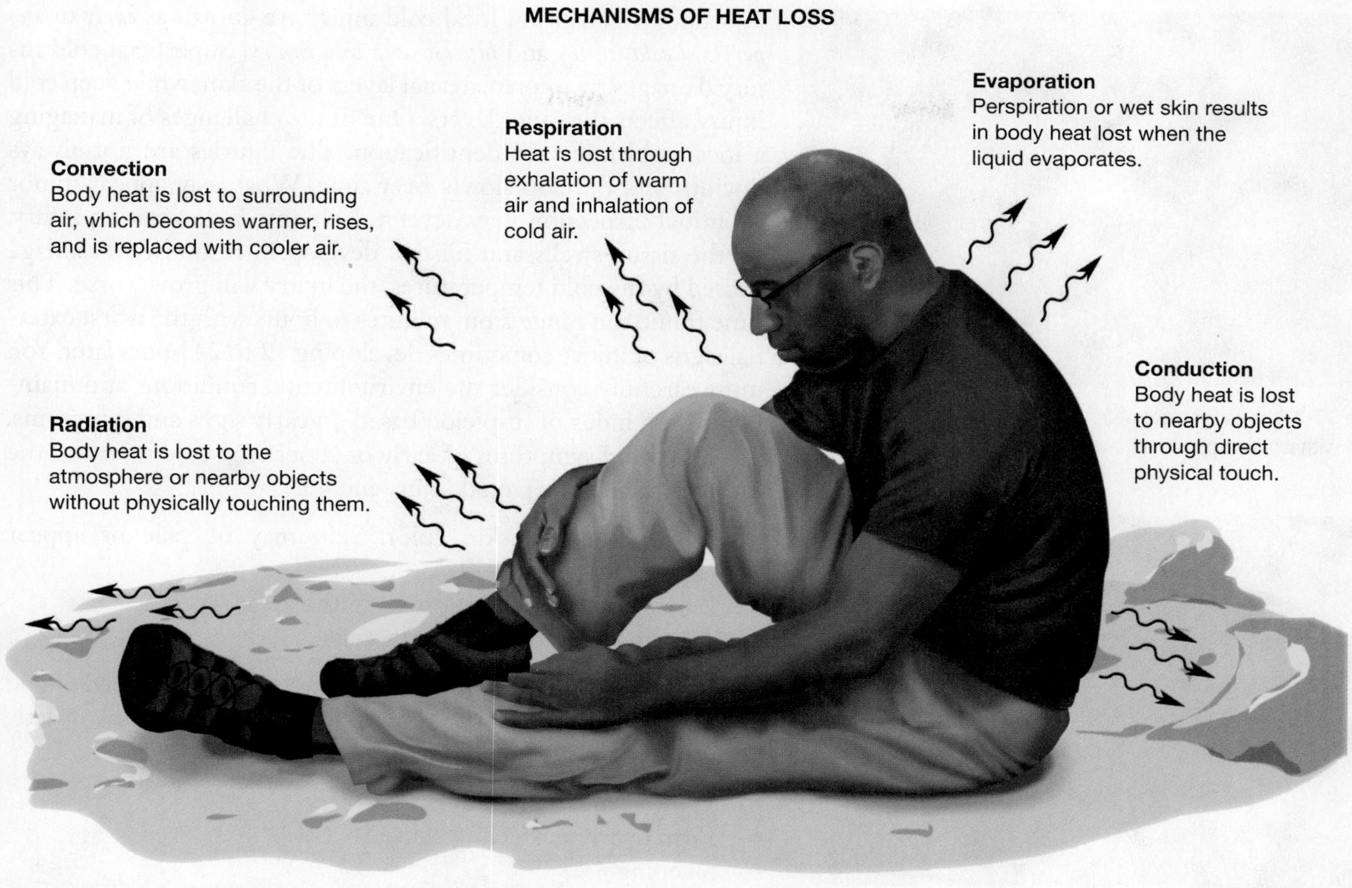

Figure 37-1 The common mechanisms that contribute to heat loss.

With hyperthermia, those principles apply in reverse. Remove the patient's clothes and fan him. Fanning fosters heat loss through conduction, convection, and evaporation of perspiration. You also may use cool packs and sometimes water to cool the patient's skin.

Overall, cold emergencies can be divided into two general categories: generalized and localized. Hypothermia is a generalized emergency; that is, it affects the whole body. A localized cold emergency (for example, frostbite) affects one specific area.

Local Cold Injury

Local cold injuries, also known as **frostbite** or **frostnip**, involve extreme cooling to local tissues of one or more parts of the body, but do not necessarily involve a generalized lowering of the body temperature as seen in hypothermia. It should be noted, however, that hypothermia may be present in the patient who has a local cold injury.

In many ways, local cold injuries are similar to burns in that cells of a particular area are damaged or destroyed by extremes of temperature (Figure 37-2 ▪). The cells are frozen and damaged by the expansion of ice crystals that form as the tissue freezes and by the subsequent reduction of blood flow to the affected area. Just as in a burn, this type of injury can affect a very small area or can be spread over a larger region of tissue. It also can be superficial or deep (Figure 37-3 ▪).

Patients with predisposing risk factors for the extremes of temperature (such as age and medical conditions) are at highest risk for severe injury. The extremities (especially the toes and fingers) and exposed areas of the head (especially the nose, cheeks, and ears) are most susceptible to local cold injury, but any tissue exposed to freezing temperatures can be at risk.

37-8 Describe the pathophysiology of local cold injury.

37-9 Discuss the assessment-based approach to cold-related emergencies.

37-10 Describe the emergency medical care for local cold injury.

frostbite local cold injury; damage to local tissues from exposure to cold temperatures.

frostnip early or superficial frostbite.

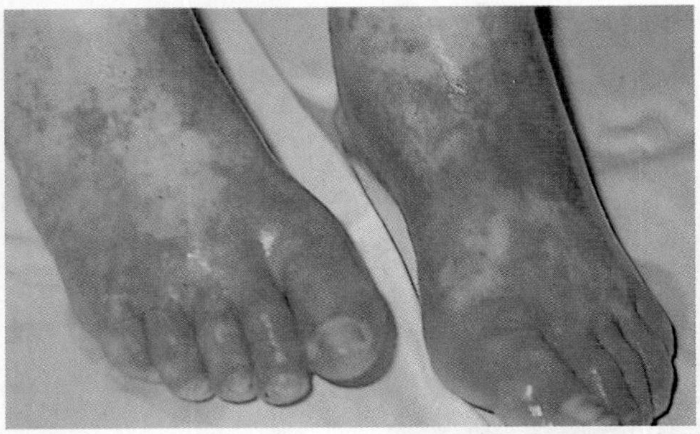

Figure 37-2 The early stages of frostbite may appear as blotchy or mottled with white to purple color variations.

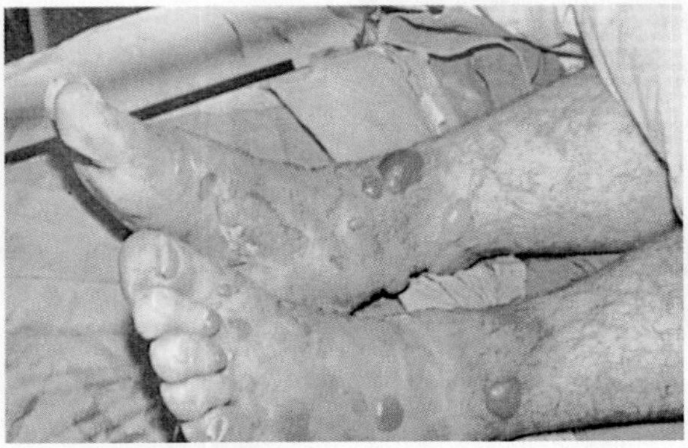

Figure 37-3 Severe frostbite is a form of local cold injury and can present with blisters much like a burn injury.

The two stages of local cold injury are known as *early* or *superficial cold injury* and *late* or *deep cold injury*. Superficial cold injury damages the more external layers of the skin, while deep cold injury affects the inner layers. One of the challenges of managing a local cold injury is identification. The injuries are not always obvious and develop slowly over time. What may appear minor on initial inspection may develop later into a devastating injury. As the tissue swells and blisters develop in response to damage caused by the cold temperatures, the injury will grow worse. This time frame can range from minutes to hours with the worst external signs of injury sometimes developing 12 to 24 hours later. You must carefully consider the environmental conditions and maintain a high index of suspicion based on early signs and symptoms.

Signs and symptoms of early or superficial cold injury or the early stages of a deep cold injury include:

- Loss of normal skin color. Skin may be pale or appear "blanched."
- Loss of feeling and sensation in the area
- Tingling sensation when rewarmed

Late or deep cold injuries typically develop after prolonged exposure and affect deeper tissues. Signs and symptoms of late, deep cold injury include:

- White, pale, waxy skin
- Firm or frozen-feeling skin
- Swelling
- Blisters
- Upon thawing, the skin may appear mottled, flushed, or cyanotic.

Emergency care for local cold injuries is based on the depth of the injury. Remember that in many cases, the local injury may not be the most significant concern. Many patients will be suffering from more generalized hypothermia as well as the local injury.

All patients with local cold injuries should be removed from the cold environment and have wet or restrictive clothing removed. Treat more generalized concerns such as airway or breathing problems first and local injuries only after more immediate life threats are addressed.

If the injury appears to be early or superficial, remove the patient's jewelry from the affected extremity, splint the extremity, and cover it to preserve warmth. Avoid rubbing or massaging the area, and do not reexpose it to cold. Perform the same steps if the injury appears to be deep or as a result of prolonged exposure to the cold. However, do not rewarm the patient or apply heat, do not break any blisters that may appear, and do not allow the patient to walk on the affected extremity.

Cold injuries often occur in remote locations, resulting in delays accessing and transporting the patient to the hospital. If a delay in transport or a long transport time is anticipated, rewarming may be performed. (Follow your local protocols.)

To rewarm a local cold injury, place the affected part in warm (not hot) water (Scan 37-1). Water should be slightly warmer than normal body temperature but should not exceed 105°F to 108°F. You may need to add additional warm water or change the water, depending on transport time.

SCAN 37-1 Management of a Local Cold Injury (Frostbite)

CONDITION	SKIN SURFACE	TISSUE UNDER SKIN	SKIN COLOR
Early, superficial	Soft	Soft	White
Late, deep	Hard	Initially soft, progressing to hard	White and waxy, progressing to blotchy white, then to yellow-gray to blue-gray

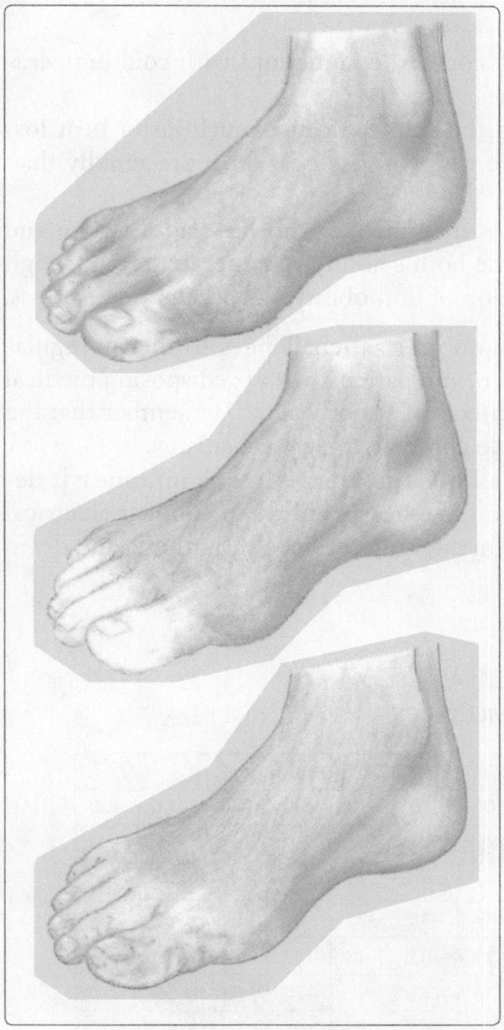

EARLY, SUPERFICIAL

Slow onset with numbing of affected part. Have the patient rewarm the part with his own body heat. Tingling and burning sensations are common during rewarming.

LATE, DEEP

Tissues below the surface initially will have their normal bounce. Protect the entire limb. Handle gently. Keep the patient at rest and provide external warmth to injury site. Untreated, this will progress to where the tissue below the surface will feel hard. Provide the same care you would for early superficial cooling. Immediate EMS transport is recommended.

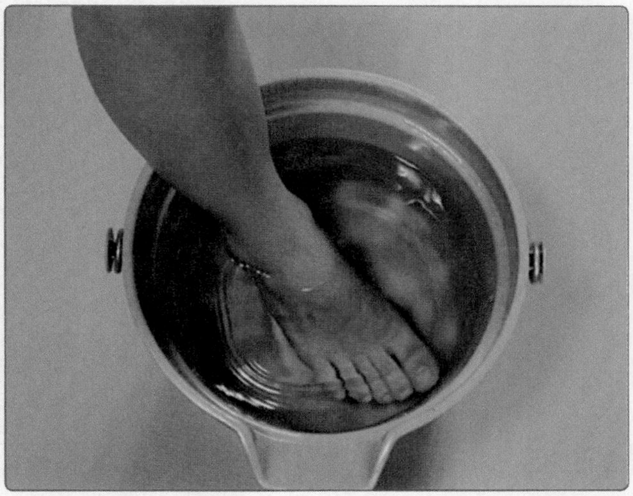

REWARMING

Only if transport is delayed in case of late or deep local cooling and if medical direction allows, rewarm the affected part by immersing it in warm water (100°F to 105°F [37.7°C to 40.5°C]). Do not allow the body part to touch the container bottom or side. After re-warming, gently dry the part and pad between fingers or toes. Dress the affected area, cover and elevate the limb, and keep the patient warm. Do not rewarm if there is any chance that the tissue may refreeze, usually due to extended exposure.

Thaw until color and sensation return and the body part is soft. This process can cause significant pain for the patient as sensation returns. Once thawed, it is critical to dry the part and maintain warmth for the patient and the affected part to prevent refreezing or hypothermia. Only rewarm the part if you can be sure that it will not refreeze.

Generalized Hypothermia

37-6 Describe the pathophysiology of generalized hypothermia.

37-11 Describe the signs and symptoms of generalized hypothermia.

Hypothermia occurs when the body loses more heat than it can generate. This is typically caused by exposure to a cold environment, but can be accelerated through a number of factors, including:

- ***Wind-chill*** (Figure 37-4 ■). This type of heat loss is caused by the convection of moving air.
- ***Submersion.*** Cold water creates more contact (conduction) with cold temperatures and vastly increases the rate of heat loss.
- ***Moisture.*** Wet clothing and water on the skin can cause much faster heat loss through evaporation. Patients who are wet will lose heat far more rapidly than those who are dry.
- ***Inability to move.*** Immobility, such as in someone who has had a stroke and cannot get up from the floor, limits the body's ability to generate heat through activity and body movements. A situation of immobility will accelerate heat loss.

Consider also the previous discussion on internal challenges to thermoregulation. Geriatric patients, very young children, and patients with predisposing medical conditions are all more vulnerable to the effects of hypothermia. Remember that the effects of drugs and alcohol also can impede compensatory mechanisms.

Hypothermia is dangerous to almost all body systems. Most significantly it depresses the central nervous system and alters the heart's ability to conduct electrical impulses. These problems can lead to life-threatening cardiac dysrhythmia and death if not managed properly.

WIND-CHILL INDEX

WIND SPEED (MPH)	WHAT THE THERMOMETER READS (degree °F.)											
	50	40	30	20	10	0	−10	−20	−30	−40	−50	−60
	WHAT IT EQUALS IN ITS EFFECT ON EXPOSED FLESH											
CALM	50	40	30	20	10	0	−10	−20	−30	−40	−50	−60
5	48	37	27	16	6	−5	−15	−26	−36	−47	−57	−68
10	40	28	16	4	−9	−21	−33	−46	−58	−70	−83	−95
15	36	22	9	−5	−18	−36	−45	−58	−72	−85	−99	−112
20	32	18	4	−10	−25	−39	−53	−67	−82	−96	−110	−121
25	30	16	0	−15	−29	−44	−59	−74	−88	−104	−118	−133
30	28	13	−2	−18	−33	−48	−63	−79	−94	−109	−125	−140
35	27	11	−4	−20	−35	−49	−67	−82	−98	−113	−129	−145
40	26	10	−6	−21	−37	−53	−69	−85	−100	−116	−132	−148

Little danger if properly clothed | Danger of freezing exposed flesh | Great danger of freezing exposed flesh

Source: U.S. Army

Figure 37-4 Wind has a dramatic effect on heat loss.

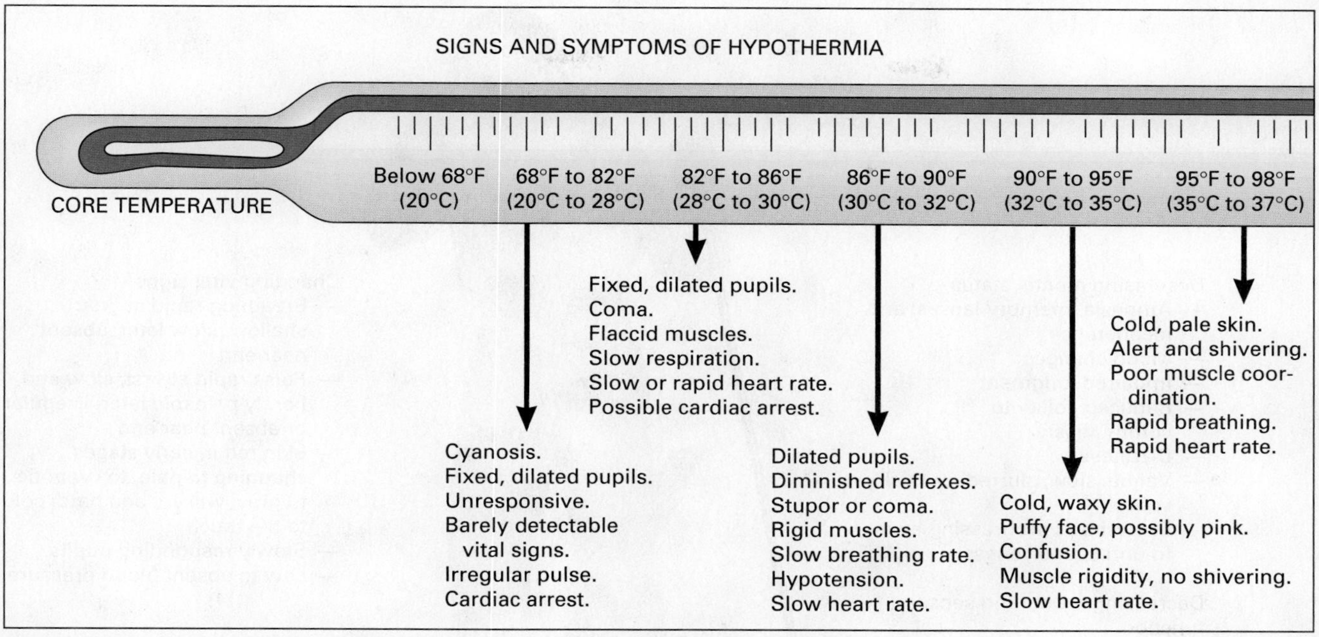

Figure 37-5 The signs and symptoms of hypothermia are progressive as core temperature drops.

The effects of hypothermia worsen as body temperature drops (Figure 37-5 ■). A dropping temperature engages the body's compensatory mechanisms in an attempt to prevent heat loss and maintain a normal core temperature. Blood vessels constrict and move blood away from the surface of the skin. This can be seen externally as pale skin and delayed capillary refill time. Shivering also begins (an early sign). This involuntary contraction of the muscles helps to generate internal heat and counteract the cold challenge. It should be known, however, that as hypothermia progresses, shivering will eventually stop, leading to a dramatic drop in temperature.

It is very common for hypothermic patients to display signs of central nervous system depression. Frequently, as hypothermia sets in, subtle signs such as impaired fine motor dexterity and diminished decision making capability are observed. It is not uncommon for hypothermic patients to become lost, cast aside important gear, or remove warm clothing as their core body temperature drops. Other signs and symptoms of generalized hypothermia include (Figure 37-6 ■):

- Altered mental status, including confusion, mood changes, and speech difficulty
- Decreased motor function, including poor coordination
- Diminished sense of cold sensation
- Pupils that respond slowly or sluggishly

Generalized hypothermia is frequently categorized as mild, moderate, or severe. These stages are associated with ranges of core body temperature. Although measuring core body temperature is the most precise way to classify the patient's condition, there are less specific findings you may use to identify the more progressive stages. They are:

- ***Mild hypothermia.*** This stage of hypothermia occurs when the patient's core body temperature drops to a range between 95°F and 90°F (35°C to 32.2°C). Although there are no absolutes and each patient can respond to hypothermia in a slightly different manner, patients with mild hypothermia typically complain of the sensation of feeling cold, display shivering, and have begun to demonstrate the signs of a depressed central nervous system. At this level, loss of fine motor dexterity and confusion are common.

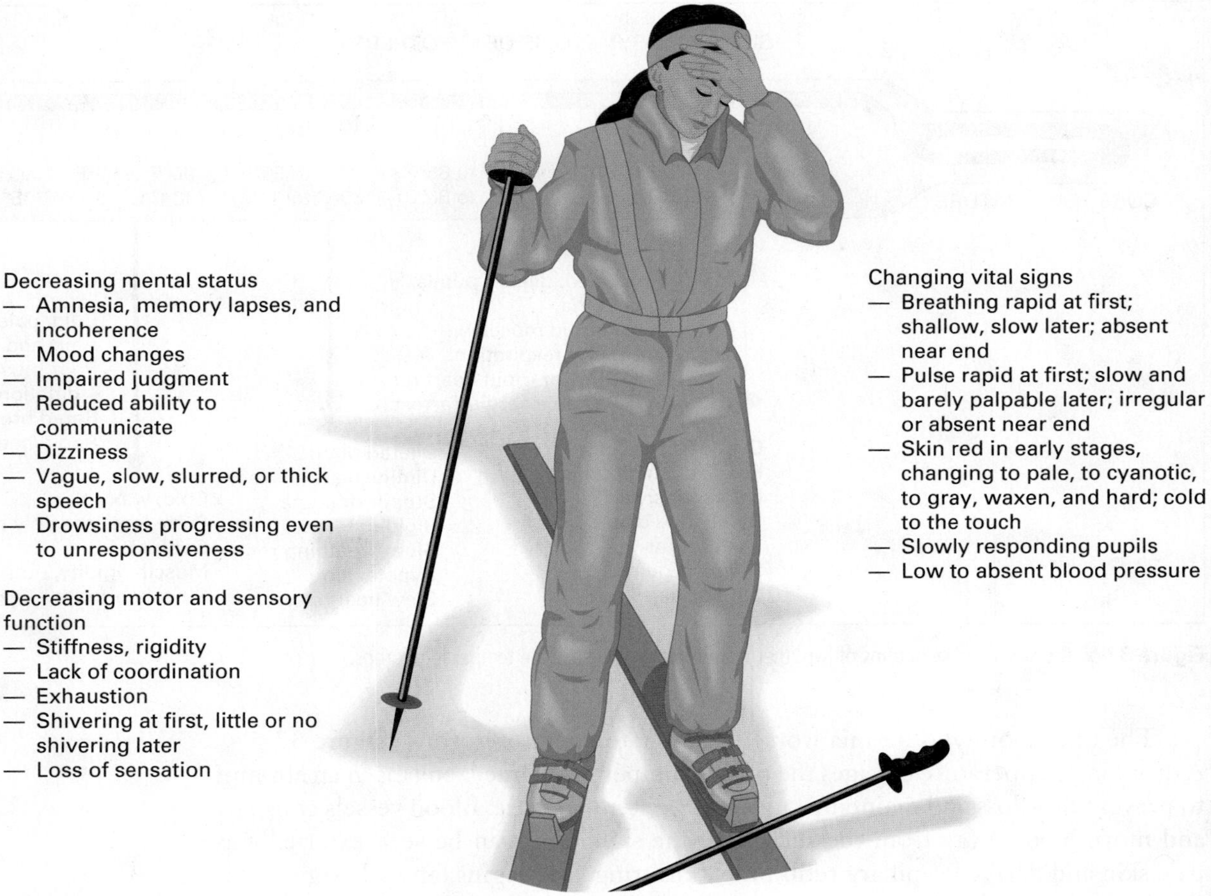

Figure 37-6 Additional signs and symptoms of hypothermia.

- ***Moderate hypothermia.*** This stage of hypothermia occurs when the patient's core temperature falls to between 90°F and 82°F (32.2°C to 27.7°C). At temperatures around 90°F, shivering can stop and the sensation of feeling cold is dulled. More profound mental status changes also occur at this stage.
- ***Severe hypothermia.*** At this stage, temperature drops below 82°F (27.7°C). Tissue is actually freezing and significant physiological effects can be seen. Severe altered mental status and unconsciousness are common. Vital sign depression, including slow respiratory rate and bradycardia, is common. In fact, vital signs may be very difficult to detect at this stage of hypothermia, so longer pulse checks should be used on unresponsive patients. At this stage, cardiac cells become electrically unstable and the patient is at high risk for ventricular fibrillation. Externally, the patient's extremities may be stiff and soft tissue may be cold or frozen.

Assessment of the Hypothermic Patient

When called to an emergency involving exposure to cold, begin by identifying situations that could have led to exposure as well as any of the factors that could have accelerated hypothermia. Remember that hypothermia can occur in warm climates and not just when the ambient temperature is cold. Perform a thorough scene size-up and remember that hypothermia may not be the most immediate problem, but it may be making that problem worse.

During your primary and secondary assessments, note the exterior skin temperature. Be sure to feel an area beneath the patient's clothing (rather than an exposed surface) to get a better idea of the patient's skin temperature. Use the back of your hand to get the most accurate reading of the patient's temperature without interference from your own. If possible, feel the skin over the abdomen to make this determination.

There are also signs and symptoms that can vary based on the severity of the hypothermia (how low the body temperature has dropped). It is critical to identify them early before they become more severe. Early assessment also should include an evaluation of risk factors (age, alcohol or drug use, and submersion).

Signs and symptoms of hypothermia that vary with severity include:

- ***Shivering.*** Present (early) or absent (late)
- ***Breathing.*** Rapid (early) or slow, shallow, and eventually absent (late)
- ***Pulse.*** Rapid (early) or slow, difficult to palpate, irregular, and eventually absent (late).
- ***Blood pressure.*** Low to absent blood pressure (late).
- ***Skin.*** Red (early) or pale, becoming cyanotic (blue or gray), and then hard (late)
- ***Musculoskeletal.*** Loss of coordination (early) or joint and muscle stiffness or rigidity (late)

Remember that severe hypothermia patients may present as if they were in cardiac arrest or they actually may be in cardiac arrest. Be sure to assess vital signs carefully and allow extra time when checking for what may be a very slow pulse rate.

Some systems measure temperature using either oral or rectal thermometers and base treatment decisions on this measurement. As always, follow local protocol, but recognize that measurement of core temperature adds precision to your assessment and can help demonstrate the true severity of the cold challenge facing your patient.

PRACTICAL PATHOPHYSIOLOGY

Patients with severe hypothermia may have a profoundly slow pulse (bradycardia). A prolonged pulse check should always be done on hypothermic patients because unnecessary CPR can actually trigger ventricular fibrillation and cardiac arrest in hypothermic bradycardic patients.

Emergency Care of the Hypothermic Patient

37-12 Describe the emergency medical care for generalized hypothermia.

The most immediate priority for any hypothermic patient (not in cardiac arrest) is to remove the cold. **Passive rewarming** should be initiated immediately. The patient should be carefully moved to a warm environment and further heat loss should be prevented. Consider increasing the ambient temperature of the ambulance. Wet clothing should be removed and replaced with dry, insulating layers and the patient's head and feet should be covered.

passive rewarming covering a hypothermic patient and taking other steps to prevent further heat loss and help the body rewarm itself.

active external rewarming application of an external heat source to rewarm the body of a hypothermic patient.

Active external rewarming can be initiated by wrapping the patient in warm blankets, using a heating wrap or placing heat packs to highly vascular areas such as the axillae (the armpits), the neck, and the groin (Figure 37-7 ▪). If heat packs are used, they should be wrapped with gauze or similar material to prevent inadvertent skin burns resulting from contact with the heat source.

Some systems allow for the use of oral replacement of calories to help treat the mild hypothermic patient. In such cases, the patient would be encouraged to drink warm, high-sugar beverages. (Do not use beverages containing caffeine or alcohol.) The beverages will not only aid in the rewarming process, but also replace valuable caloric stores necessary to help the body generate heat. You should *not* give anything by mouth to a patient in moderate to severe hypothermia or to any patient with questionable airway control.

Hypothermic patients may require *active core rewarming* to increase body temperature. It is typically initiated at the hospital and includes the administration of warmed IV fluids, instilling warmed fluids into body areas such as the bladder

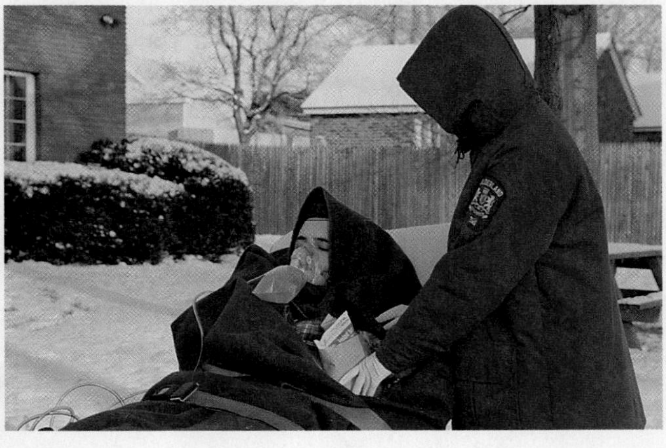

Figure 37-7 Active rewarming includes placing a heat source such as heat packs at the patient's neck, armpits, and groin.

and the peritoneal space. Some EMS systems allow providers to initiate active core rewarming by utilizing heated oxygen. In those cases a special heating device is used to warm oxygen before it is inhaled. Follow local protocol when attempting to rewarm a victim of hypothermia.

Treatment of moderate and severe hypothermia patients requires some very special considerations. In most cases the patients will require specialized active rewarming in an appropriate hospital setting. Early notification of the receiving facility will allow many of the specialized therapies to be readied before your arrival.

Moderate and severe hypothermia patients commonly present with significantly altered mental status, so no fluids should be administered by mouth. Finally, in moderate and severe hypothermia the cells of the heart become extremely unstable and aggressive movement can lead to life-threatening dysrhythmia. EMTs should be very gentle in handling and moving these patients and efforts to increase temperature should be limited to passive and active external rewarming. Patients in this category should not be allowed to walk or moved roughly.

If an unresponsive patient is hypothermic, be sure to spend 30 to 60 seconds checking for a pulse before starting CPR. In some cases, a pulse may be present, but it may be very slow and difficult to palpate.

An old adage you may hear, "A patient isn't dead until he is warm and dead," favors resuscitation of patients submerged in cold water and others found pulseless in the cold. Research in this area is ongoing. Current beliefs are that patients found within a short time after cold water submersion may in fact be resuscitated past the 5 to 10 minutes that is often fatal in normothermic patients. When the patient has been submerged for a longer period of time (more than 30 minutes) or when the patient's body has undergone significant freezing, successful resuscitation is less likely. Follow your local protocols in reference to performing CPR on hypothermic patients.

37-13 Describe the pathophysiology of immersion/submersion injuries.

Immersion/Submersion Injuries

Drowning is a term commonly used to describe those immersed or submerged in water or other liquids. The medical definition of drowning established by the World Health Organization (WHO) is the process of experiencing respiratory impairment after submersion or immersion in a liquid (Figure 37-8 ■). Patients who drown have three potential outcomes: death, full recovery, or partial recovery in which there is permanent (often neurological) damage.

drowning the process of experiencing respiratory impairment after submersion or immersion in a liquid.

There are roughly 3,500 fatal drowning incidents in the United States each year and countless other incidents involving immersion injury where the patients survive. Although these types of injuries can be associated with a variety of recreational scenarios, including boating, swimming, and other water activities, many are caused by unintentional immersion such as a child falling into an unprotected pool. Children are statistically the highest risk group and mortality increases in the younger age groups.

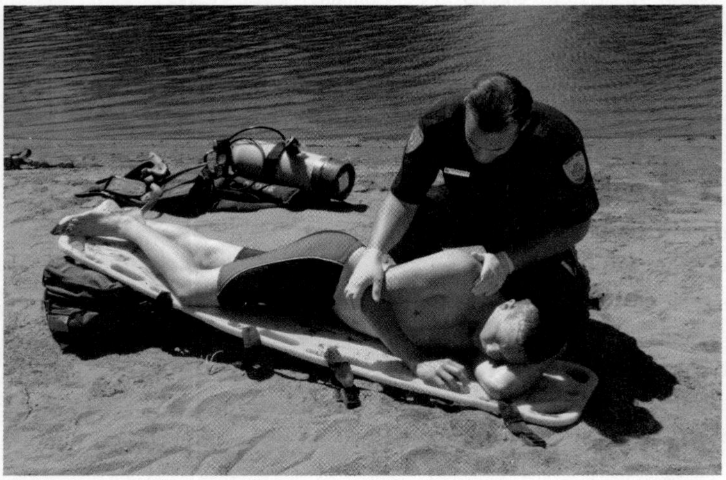

Figure 37-8 Drowning occurs when a patient becomes submersed in a liquid and respiratory compromise results.

A drowning occurs when a liquid impairs normal gas exchange in the lungs. The primary cause of injury in these types of situations is hypoxia. Although this is the most common cause of death, submersion also can be associated with a variety of other body system dysfunctions including hypothermia, trauma, and infection.

In a classic drowning there are three major events that occur in sequence. First, sudden unexpected submersion triggers breath holding, panic, and a struggle to get to the surface. Next, as the patient becomes deprived of oxygen, hypoxia develops and the patient begins to swallow water. Finally, as the central nervous system begins to fail, breath holding is overcome and involuntary gasps result in aspiration of water into the lungs. Once water enters the lungs, there is significant damage that impairs normal gas exchange. The primary damage that water causes within the lungs is washing away a chemical called *surfactant*. It is surfactant that helps keep the grape-like alveoli expanded and capable of capillary gas exchange in the lungs. If the patient is rescued, the loss of surfactant at the alveolar level will make reversal of hypoxia and return to normal gas exchange very difficult. In all cases of drowning the most important priority is immediate restoration of oxygenation and ventilation.

Interestingly enough, water temperature can play a vital role in survival. Cold water (typically defined as water temperature below 68°F) can cause apnea and trigger the *mammalian diving reflex*, which causes bradycardia and profound vasoconstriction. Although the evidence is not conclusive, there seems to be a higher survival rate in patients submerged in colder water. That said, submersion hypothermia poses a great risk for any survivor. The lower the body temperature of drowning victims at the time of rescue, the less likely they are to be successfully resuscitated.

Trauma in the Setting of Drowning

37-14 Describe the indications for spinal immobilization in drowning victims.

In addition to pulmonary complications, immersion injuries can also be associated with trauma. Although it was once thought that cervical-spine injuries were common in drownings, it turns out that cervical-spine injuries occur in less than 1% of drownings. For this reason cervical-spine immobilization should *not* be routinely performed on drowning victims unless there is a clear MOI for potential spine injury (such as a diving mechanism or a watercraft crash) or physical signs of trauma. It is believed that time spent trying to immobilize patients who do not have a spine injury only further delays initiation of oxygenation and ventilation of the patient.

Responding to an Immersion/Submersion Injury

37-15 Describe the emergency care for the victim of an immersion/submersion injury.

Safety is an enormous concern in drowning and immersion emergencies (Figure 37-9 ■). Frequently, rescue will require specialized training and equipment. Without that equipment, providers are at high risk of becoming victims themselves. When responding to such an event, you must use situational awareness and perform a thorough scene size-up to ensure it is safe to approach the patient and effect a rescue. If it is unsafe, wait for more qualified personnel.

Use the primary assessment to recognize cardiac arrest. Many submersion patients will present first in cardiac arrest due to sustained hypoxia. If this is the case, begin CPR. Some patients will present only in respiratory arrest due to severe central nervous system depression and pulmonary injury. If the patient is not breathing or breathing only with agonal respirations, begin positive pressure ventilations immediately.

If the patient is not in arrest, he may have severe difficulty breathing. Water that has entered the lungs can cause gas exchange problems and other dysfunctions including the collapse of alveoli (also known as *atelectasis*) and pulmonary edema. Supplemental oxygen will be helpful in these situations. Oxygen saturation measurement would be helpful, too, but it is often difficult to obtain due to cold skin and the associated vasoconstriction. In this case, it is better to apply oxygen if saturations are unavailable or unreliable. If you are trained and allowed by local protocol to do so, consider the use of noninvasive positive

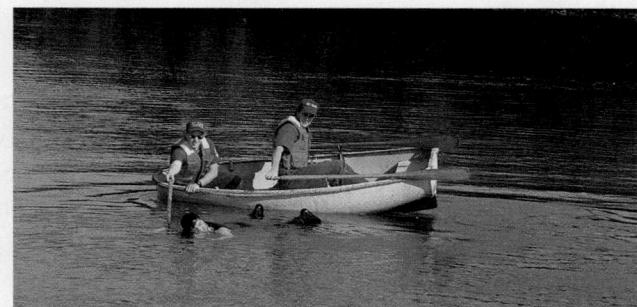

Figure 37-9 Your safety is primary when responding to victims of drowning.

pressure ventilation (NIPPV), such as continuous positive airway pressure (CPAP), when caring for immersion victims with significant respiratory distress.

PRACTICAL PATHOPHYSIOLOGY

The use of NIPPV (such as CPAP) is effective in treating drowning victims with respiratory distress because the continuous airway pressures obtained with this technology reverses atelectasis and can re-expand collapsed alveoli.

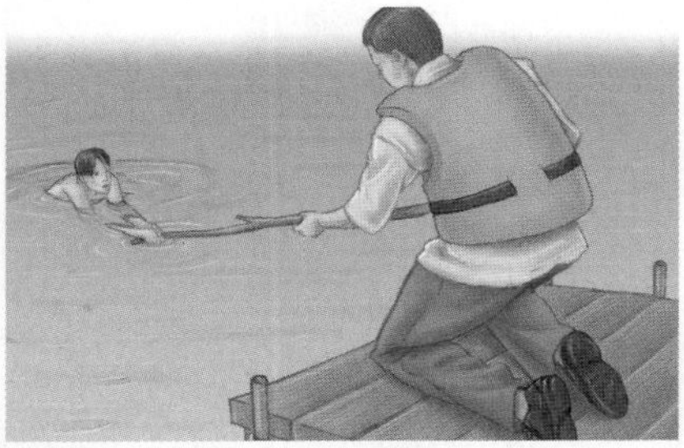

Reach

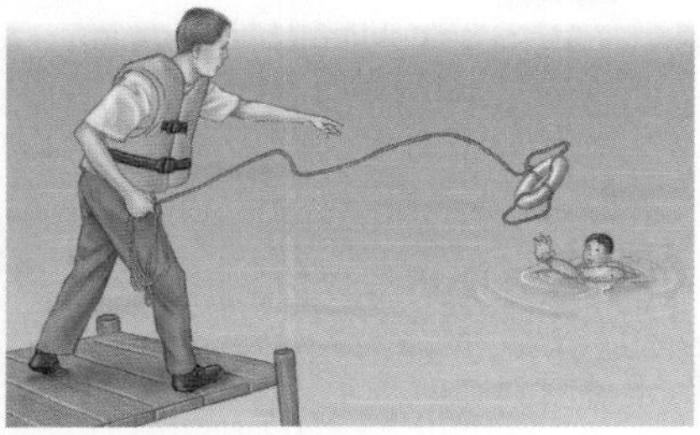

Throw and tow

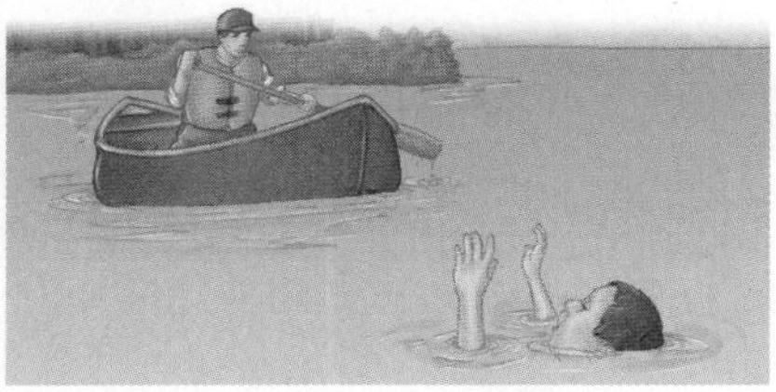

Row

Figure 37-10 Consider the safest option when attempting to help a drowning victim.

Hypothermia is an extreme risk because the conduction of water in submersion cools the body 30 times faster than radiation or convection in air. Assess for the risk of hypothermia and treat according to the guidelines outlined earlier in this chapter. Remember to remove wet clothing and dry the patient's skin as soon as possible to prevent further heat loss.

When a rescue is attempted in or around water, safety is the first concern. Emotion can cause rescuers to jump in and become victims themselves. Entering the water to rescue a drowning victim exposes the rescuer to several potential hazards. Very cold water, fast currents, and a potentially panicked patient can be dangerous to even the strongest of swimmers.

There are ways to help without entering the water. One way to remember safer methods of rescue without swimming are the terms *reach*, *throw and tow*, and *row* (Figure 37-10 ■). When close to shore or the edge of a pool, try to reach the patient with a stick or pole. If that fails, throw an item that will float tied to a rope and then tow (pull) the patient to safety. If that fails, row to the patient in a boat. While rowing to the patient is generally safer than trying to swim to him, there are still risks involved, such as capsizing the boat or falling overboard during the rescue.

Emergency care for the drowning patient includes the following:

1. Remove the patient from the water on a backboard with stabilization of the head and neck if spine injuries are suspected. If no backboard is available and the patient is in respiratory or cardiac arrest or if you are unable to maintain the patient's airway, remove him from the water immediately by the safest method.
2. Provide a prompt primary assessment including evaluation of breathing and the need for suction. Vomiting is extremely common. Suction, ventilate, and provide oxygen as needed.
3. If the patient is in respiratory or cardiac arrest, provide resuscitation.
4. Perform a secondary assessment.
5. Initiate prompt transport to an appropriate facility.

CLINICAL CLUE

Prepare to Suction

It has been reported that as many as 60% of drowning victims will vomit during emergency care. Be prepared for this eventuality. Always take a portable suction unit to the water's edge, boat dock, or pool when responding to the scene of a drowning call.

Water Extrication

Removing patients from the water must be done safely, efficiently, and with the proper priorities. Spine injuries are possible in many water emergencies, such as diving accidents and rough-current injuries. However, the need for spinal care must be balanced with the need for resuscitation. The ability to do adequate and prolonged ventilations in the water is severely limited, and chest compressions in the water are ineffective. Getting a patient to shore and to the hospital are your priorities.

Several methods of immobilization are available for use on patients in the water who have suspected spine injuries. One- and two-rescuer techniques for deep and shallow water are shown in Scans 37-2 and 37-3.

SCAN 37-2 Rescue Technique for Shallow Water

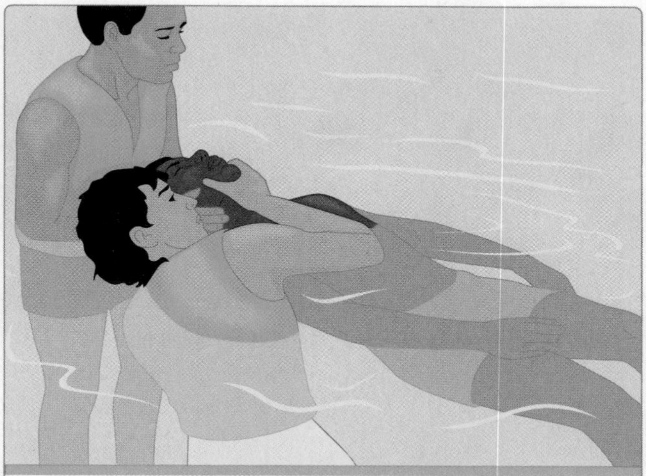

37-2-1 When there are two rescuers present, perform the head-chin support technique to provide in-line stabilization of a patient in shallow water.

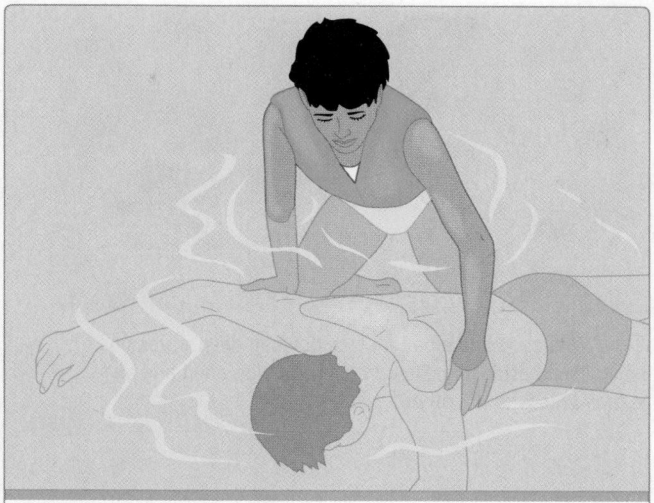

37-2-2 When you find a patient face down in shallow water, position yourself alongside the patient.

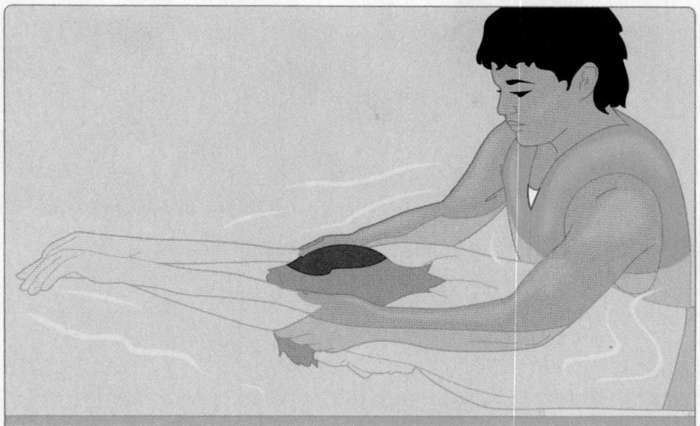

37-2-3 Extend the patient's arms straight up alongside his head to create a splint.

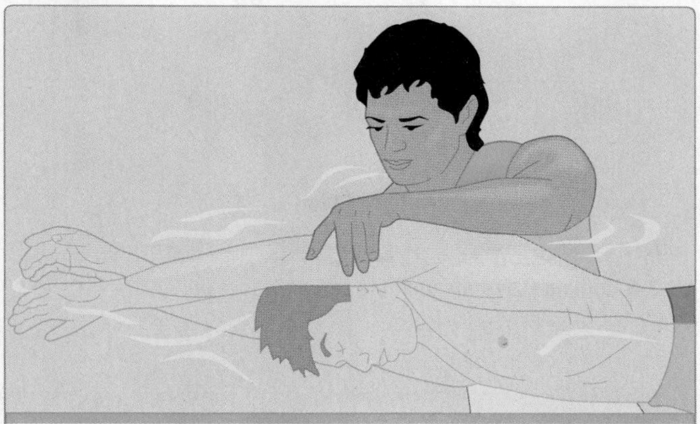

37-2-4 Begin to rotate the torso toward you.

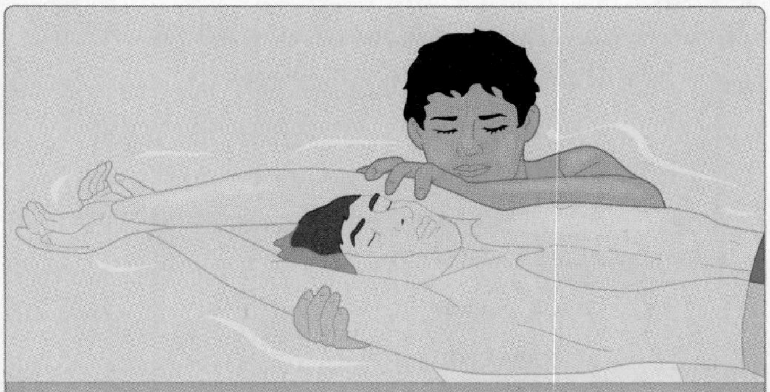

37-2-5 As you rotate the patient, lower yourself into the water.

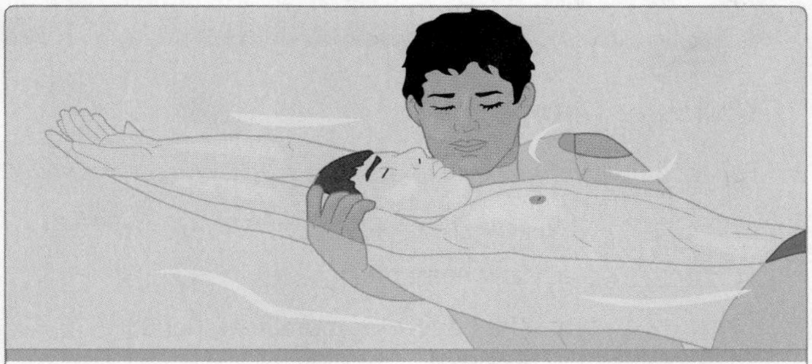

37-2-6 Maintain manual stabilization by holding the patient's head between his arms.

SCAN 37-3 Rescue Technique for Deep Water

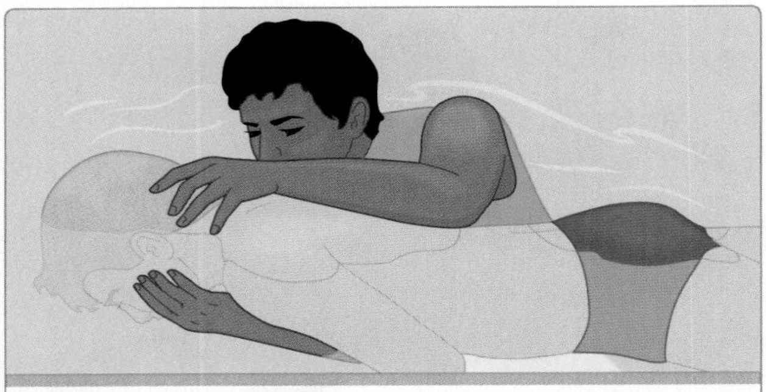

37-3-1 When you find a patient face down in deep water, position yourself beside him. Support his head with one hand and the mandible with the other.

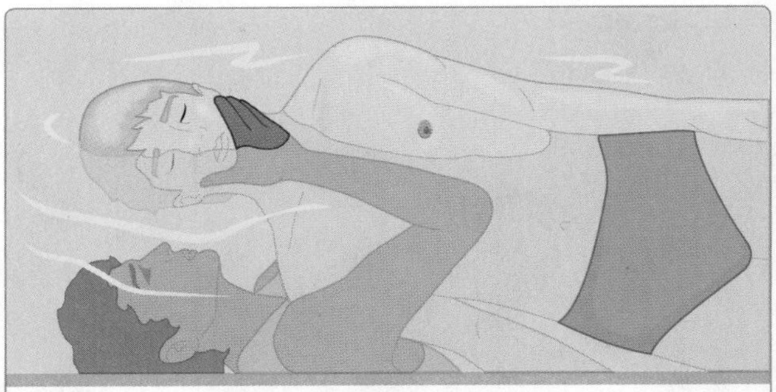

37-3-2 Then rotate the patient by ducking under him.

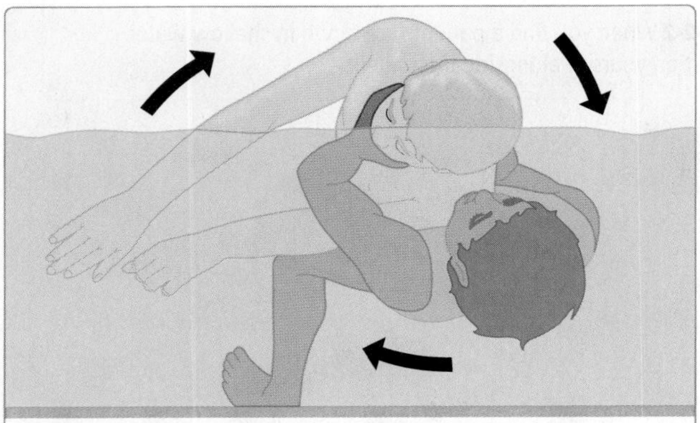

37-3-3 Continue to rotate until the patient is face up.

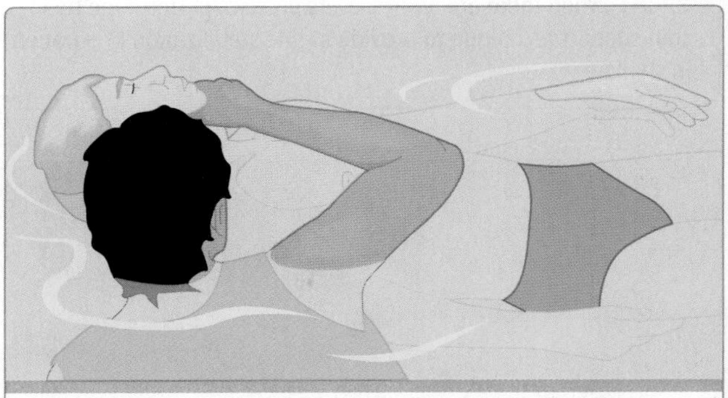

37-3-4 Maintain in-line stabilization until a backboard is used to immobilize the patient's spine.

STOP, REVIEW, REMEMBER!

Multiple Choice

For each question, place a check next to the correct answer.

1. Which one of the following best defines hypothermia?

_____ a. Low heart rate

_____ b. The body loses more heat than it generates.

_____ c. The body generates more heat than it loses.

_____ d. The body is unable to moderate temperature.

2. Applying cold packs to a patient's armpits is an example of temperature regulation by:

_____ a. conduction.

_____ b. convection.

_____ c. radiation.

_____ d. evaporation.

3. You are assessing a 22-year-old hiker suspected of being hypothermic. Which one of the following factors would make hypothermia more likely in this patient?
   _____ a. Her age
   _____ b. Tachycardic heart rate
   _____ c. Increased respiratory rate
   _____ d. Wet clothing

4. The process by which the body retains or releases heat in normal situations is called:
   _____ a. hypothermia.
   _____ b. hyperthermia.
   _____ c. temperature regulation.
   _____ d. convection/conduction reaction (CCR).

5. You are caring for a 16-year-old victim of a personal watercraft accident. She is immobilized on a backboard after being pulled from the water. The ambient temperature is 90°F. Which one of the following best describes the relative risk of hypothermia in this patient?
   _____ a. High risk due to conductive and evaporative heat loss
   _____ b. Only a risk if the water temperature is below 80°F
   _____ c. No risk because the ambient temperature is above 90°F
   _____ d. Only a risk if the wind produces convective heat loss

Matching

Match the situations on the left with the method of heat loss or gain on the right.

1. _____ A patient is lying on the floor of his patio in the winter.
2. _____ A patient has cold packs placed in his armpits and groin.
3. _____ The patient breathes rapidly.
4. _____ You cover the top of a patient with blankets.
5. _____ You remove a patient's wet clothing.
6. _____ You administer warm, humidified oxygen.

A. Radiation
B. Conduction
C. Convection
D. Evaporation
E. Respiration

Critical Thinking

1. Explain the difference between hyperthermia and hypothermia.

____

____

____

____

2. You are called to a patient who is experiencing hyperthermia. He is outside on baseball bleachers. Using what you know about heat loss methods, how could you cool this patient?

____

____

____

____

37-5 Explain the mechanisms by which the body gains heat.

37-16 Describe the pathophysiology of heat-related emergencies.

37-17 Recognize factors that contribute to a patient's risk for hyperthermia.

Heat Emergencies

In addition to heat that is generated by normal body functions such as metabolism, our bodies are exposed to many environmental heat sources. Heat can be radiated, from the sun's energy or off a hot object, for example, it can be conducted through touch, and it can be convected through warm air. In order for the body to function properly, it must constantly adjust for all those factors. Heat must be produced in sufficient quantity, but also dissipated when necessary to maintain the preferred narrow range of temperature.

The body gives off body heat by dilating blood vessels, increasing respiration, and by sweating. Sweat glands produce sweat to promote evaporative heat loss on the surface of the skin. Ordinarily, these regulatory mechanisms are efficient in dissipating heat and maintaining core temperature.

Occasionally, heat retention can exceed the body's ability to dissipate heat and a condition called hyperthermia occurs. The most serious increases in body temperature occur when the environmental temperature is so high that it prevents the body from losing heat by radiation. High humidity also reduces the ability of the body to lose heat through sweating and evaporation because the atmospheric air already has a high water content. The presence of one or both of these conditions often sets the stage for a heat emergency (Figure 37-11 ▪).

A variety of other factors besides environmental temperature and humidity can contribute to the body's ability to regulate temperature. The elderly often experience heat emergencies as a result of poor temperature-control mechanisms in the body. Certain medications also can reduce a patient's ability to regulate temperature. In those who are bedridden or who have limited mobility, it may not be possible to leave a hot environment or shed unneeded clothing.

Newborns and infants also have heat regulation problems. In these patients, the ability to regulate heat has not been fully developed. Making things worse is the fact that infants are not able to remove their own clothes as the environment becomes hot.

Strenuous work and high activity levels increase heat production in the body by as much as tenfold. Often the combination of a hot environment and increased activity quickly overwhelms the body's ability to effectively compensate.

Acclimatization is another factor that plays a role in the body's ability to deal with heat challenges. In hot environments the body adapts its responses to heat challenges.

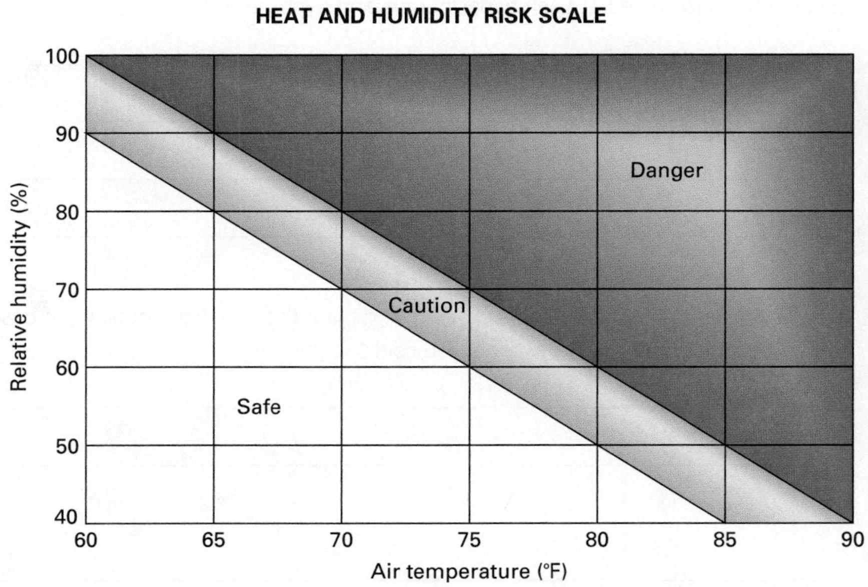

Figure 37-11 The risk for hyperthermia is increased when the relative humidity increases.

As it adjusts, responses such as sweating occur earlier and more efficiently. This adjustment process, however, can take seven to ten days to occur. People who are new to a hot or humid environment frequently find themselves maladapted to the new heat challenges. These unacclimatized patients are particularly vulnerable to heat emergencies.

Preexisting medical conditions can predispose a patient to heat emergencies. Some of those predisposing conditions are:

- Psychiatric disorders (both because of the medications taken and the patient's poor judgment)
- Heart disease
- Diabetes
- Fever
- Fatigue
- Obesity
- Dehydration

Dehydration can be caused by reduced fluid intake or from excessive perspiration. It is estimated that exercise or hard labor can cause a loss of up to one liter in an hour. This also causes a loss of important **electrolytes,** such as sodium. Electrolyte balance is critical to many body functions.

electrolytes a substance that, in water, separates into electrically charged particles.

Types of Heat Emergencies

37-18 Differentiate the three types of heat-related emergencies.

37-19 Discuss the assessment-based approach to heat-related emergencies.

As previously stated, hyperthermia occurs when the heat challenge overwhelms the body's ability to compensate. High temperatures can literally destroy cells. As the temperature increases, proteins break down, cell membranes dissolve, and cell death occurs. If allowed to go unchecked, hyperthermia can lead to cell death and eventually organ system failure (Figure 37-12 ■).

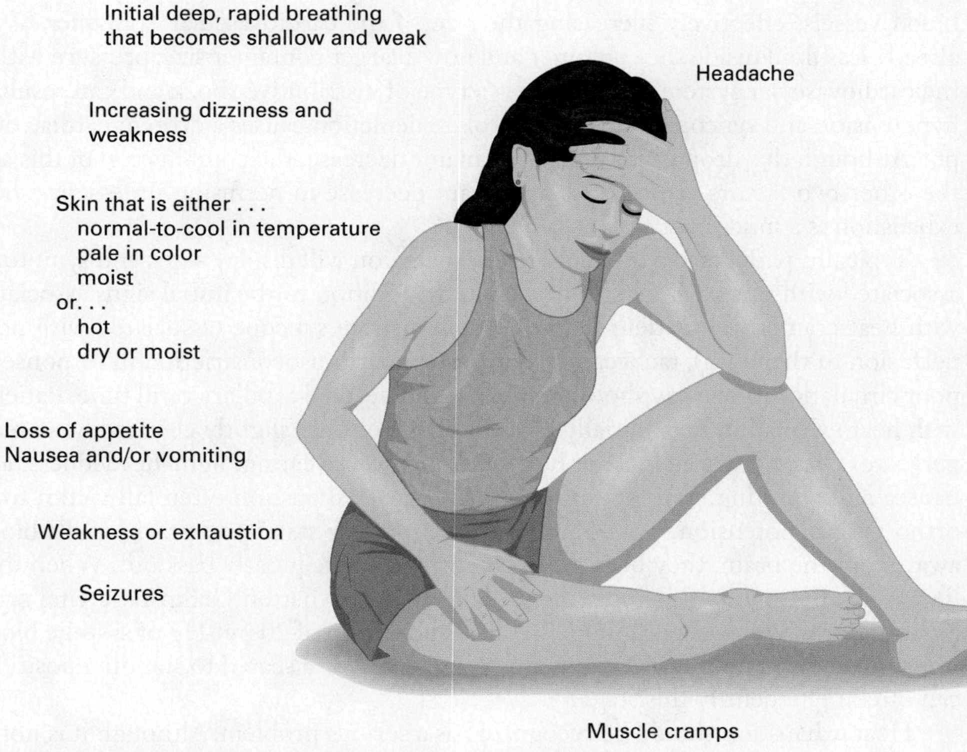

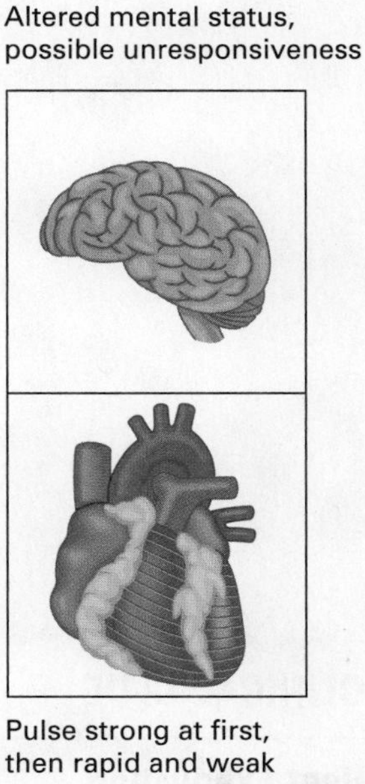

Figure 37-12 Common signs and symptoms of heat-related emergencies.

heat cramps a progressive heat injury caused by dehydration and electrolyte depletion; characterized by pain in large muscle groups.

Heat emergencies are categorized based on severity. The most common heat emergency is **heat cramps.** Heat cramps result from increasing temperature, dehydration (from increased sweating), and electrolyte imbalances (due to the loss of sodium in sweat). These conditions lead to painful contractions of the muscles and sharp pain in large muscle groups. As a patient deals with increasing environmental temperature, you may note the signs of compensation. The patient may complain of being hot, skin may appear flushed as blood vessels dilate in an attempt to dissipate heat, and profuse sweating is common.

Although heat cramps are relatively minor concerns, it is very important to recognize that they are a significant warning sign of a more serious impending heat emergency. The most appropriate treatment is to *remove the patient from the hot environment.* Continued activity in a hot environment will surely lead to more progressive injury. Remove insulating clothing from the patient, decrease the activity level, and if protocol allows, consider oral rehydration.

Rehydration of a patient with heat cramps should include both water and electrolyte replacement if available. Water replaces fluid lost in the sweating process and electrolyte solutions combine water and electrolytes such as sodium and potassium to replace depleted stores. Sports drinks typically are used for electrolyte replacement, but in their absence, the World Health Organization recommends the following formula: 1 teaspoon of salt and 8 teaspoons of sugar per 1 liter of water. Oral rehydration should never be attempted in patients with severe altered mental status or questionable control of the airway. Again, always follow local protocol.

heat exhaustion a progressive heat injury characterized by cool skin, syncope, and fatigue.

If the conditions causing the heat cramps are not corrected, they may lead to a condition called **heat exhaustion.** In this case the rising temperature and the progressive dehydration and electrolyte depletion are more than the body can handle efficiently. A combination of three factors can cause serious problems in this stage. First, the body is generally volume depleted. Sweating has physically removed fluid from the intravascular space. This causes relative hypovolemia and in some cases hypovolemic shock. Secondly, in an attempt to regulate heat, the body has dilated blood vessels, effectively increasing the size of the cardiovascular container. With already less fluid inside the container and now a larger container size, pressure within the cardiovascular system drops. This is a type of distributive shock and can result in hypotension and syncope. Finally, electrolyte depletion causes a drop in cardiac output. Although this drop is not typically a major decrease, the combination of this and the other two factors can cause a significant decrease in perfusion. In essence, heat exhaustion is a mild form of shock.

Typically, patients experiencing heat exhaustion will display signs and symptoms associated with this challenge to perfusion. In addition to the initial signs associated with heat cramps, the patient may now demonstrate syncope (associated with poor perfusion to the brain), tachycardia, and a secondary vasoconstriction in response to poor circulation. This may show as pale skin and delayed capillary refill time. Patients with heat exhaustion may initially have a normal or only slightly elevated body temperature. Other findings include headache, profuse sweating, light-headedness, and nausea and vomiting. Patients suffering from heat exhaustion often fall victim from orthostatic hypotension. That is, when they sit up or stand and gravity pulls blood away from the brain, they become hypotensive and frequently pass out. When they lie flat again, the blood is redistributed and they feel better. Orthostatic vital signs (an increase of 20 beats per minute in pulse and a drop of 20 mmHg of systolic blood pressure as the patient moves from a lying to seated or a seated to standing position) can often help identify this stage.

> **CLINICAL CLUE**
>
> **Heat Exhaustion**
>
> If the patient with heat exhaustion has already had syncope, do not test for orthostatic vital signs because it will just further subject the brain to additional hypoperfusion.

Heat exhaustion should be recognized as a serious problem. Although it is not as dangerous as heat stroke, if not corrected immediately it will progress to a much more dangerous level. Treatment of heat exhaustion includes much of the same treatment as applied to heat cramps. Remove the heat challenge and if tolerated (and allowed by local protocol) initiate oral rehydration (Figure 37-13 ▪). Because this condition is associated with shock-like pathophysiology, consider placing the patient in a supine position. Consider also passive cooling techniques such as splashing with cool water. If signs of hypoxia are present, apply supplemental oxygen.

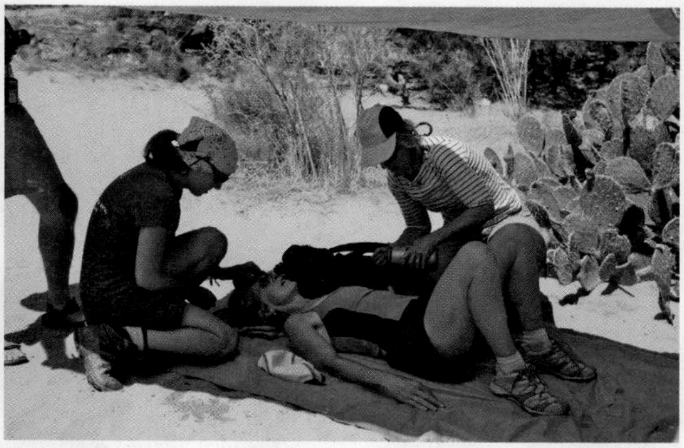

Figure 37-13 Care for heat exhaustion includes lying down in a cool place and drinking fluids.

If heat exhaustion is not corrected and the body temperature continues to rise, **heat stroke** can occur. Heat stroke is a dire emergency that occurs when body temperature reaches a point at which circulatory collapse and major organs begin to fail. Heat stroke is defined by a high body temperature and central nervous system dysfunction (such as altered mental status and/or seizures). It is characterized by dehydration, electrolyte imbalance, and profound shock and circulatory compromise. Because of poor perfusion and high core temperature, organ systems such as the brain and liver are at immediate risk. Additionally, at severely high temperature the muscle cells can actually begin to break down in a process called *rhabdomyolysis*. This process can lead to more severe injury due to the release of toxins into the bloodstream.

heat stroke a progressive heat injury characterized by altered mental status, hot skin, and shock.

Classically, heat stroke has been differentiated from heat exhaustion by the cessation of sweating. As body temperatures climb and fluid volume reserves are depleted, sweating can cease and although this can be a clear hallmark of heat stroke, *it is certainly not a reliable sign*. You should not wait for the cessation of sweating to begin your care. Some conditions such as heat stroke from exertion will not be associated with the cessation of sweating. Furthermore, profuse sweating in the prior stages of the heat emergency can make detection of the cessation of sweating very difficult.

Key findings to indicate heat stroke include hot skin (because temperature has exceeded the body's ability to compensate) and altered mental status. Any patient with a suspected heat-related emergency who presents with hot skin and altered mental status should be assumed to have heat stroke until proven otherwise. Other findings include low blood pressure, tachycardia, signs of shock, and elevated core temperature. Temperatures greater than 105°F are considered by definition heat stroke.

PERSPECTIVE

The Oil Rig Supervisor

Sometimes it's so hard to prevent heat emergencies out here on the job. It's tough physical work and, on days like today, it's not like we can just shut down so everyone can take a break. I try to make them drink water, but as the old saying goes, you can lead a horse to water. . . .

Emergency Care for Heat Emergencies

Care for heat emergencies is based on patient presentation and the severity of the emergency. Heat cramps and heat exhaustion are treated similarly. The first and most immediate priority should be to remove the patient to a cooler environment. This might be a shady area out of the sun, but preferably would be a climate-controlled setting such as an air-conditioned ambulance. Outer layers of clothing should be removed and passive cooling, such as fanning or moistening the skin with cool water, should be initiated. If the patient has a normal mental status and is capable of protecting his airway, consider oral rehydration as well. Heat exhaustion patients who have

37-20 Describe the emergency medical care for suspected heat cramps and heat exhaustion.

37-21 Describe the emergency medical care for suspected heat stroke.

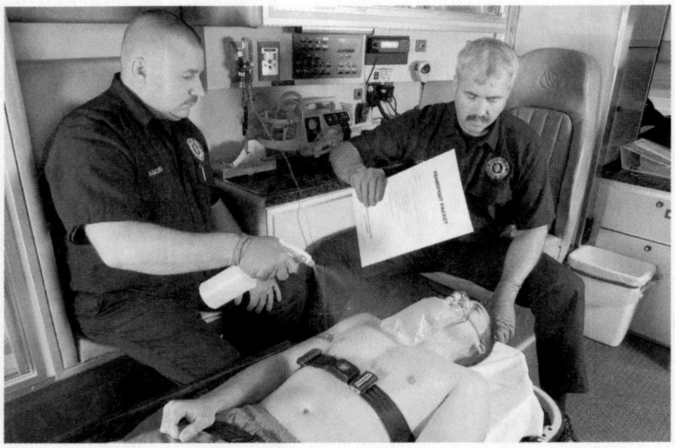

Figure 37-14 Victims of heat stroke should be cooled aggressively during transport to the hospital.

experienced syncope or a near-syncopal episode may benefit from being placed in a supine position. Most importantly, both heat exhaustion and heat cramps should be considered warning signs, and despite patient improvement, care should be taken to avoid allowing reentry into the hot environment.

In heat stroke, high body temperature has caused an immediately life-threatening situation and must be aggressively treated by actively decreasing the body's temperature.

All patients suffering from heat-related emergencies will benefit from being removed from the hot environment. The most practical location for this is the back of the air conditioned ambulance. Not only can you begin transport but you can use the air conditioning as a means of cooling the patient (Figure 37-14 ■). If you know you are responding to a heat emergency, turn on the air conditioner in the back of the ambulance before you go to the patient's side so it will be cool when you return.

Although assessment of a heat-injured patient is not quite this simple, it may be helpful to classify two categories of treatment. In the first category warm or cool skin in your patient indicates heat cramps and heat exhaustion. In the second category hot skin in your patient indicates heat stroke.

For patients with warm or cool skin (may be dry or moist):

1. Move the patient to a cooler environment.
2. Place him in a supine position.
3. Remove the outer layers of the patient's clothing.
4. Fan the patient to provide extra cooling, and consider dowsing him with cool water.
5. Consider the administration of supplemental oxygen.
6. Consider oral rehydration. (Follow local protocols.)

For patients with hot skin (may be dry or moist):

1. Move the patient to a cooler environment.
2. Place him in a supine position.
3. Remove the outer layers of the patient's clothing.
4. Apply cool packs to the neck, armpits, and groin (active cooling).
5. Wet the skin and fan the patient aggressively to promote cooling.
6. Consider the administration of supplemental oxygen.
7. Transport immediately.

Remember that altered mental status in the setting of a heat-related emergency should be considered an indication of heat stroke. Such patients should be actively cooled and transported rapidly to the hospital. Always follow local protocol.

PERSPECTIVE

Jay—The EMT

I couldn't even guess what that guy's temperature was, but he was way overheated. So we got him in the truck, turned the A/C on high, cut off his jumpsuit, and packed him with cool packs. And our service just bought us these cool little fans, the kind with the squirt bottles attached to them. Have you seen those? They work great on patients. Some of us, not mentioning any names, but some of us have been known to use them between calls on hot afternoons.

STOP, REVIEW, REMEMBER!

Multiple Choice

For each question, place a check next to the correct answer.

1. Patients experiencing a more serious heat emergency will have which skin characteristics?

_____ a. Cool, moist

_____ b. Pale, moist

_____ c. Hot, moist

_____ d. Cool, pale

2. A 65-year-old woman has been found in heat stroke. She is confused and displaying signs of shock. After ensuring a patent airway and adequate breathing, you should:

_____ a. immerse her in an ice bath.

_____ b. wet her down and begin fanning her.

_____ c. initiate oral rehydration with an electrolyte solution.

_____ d. place the patient in the recovery position and transport.

3. A 50-year-old man has just arrived in equatorial South America for a mountain climb. The ambient temperature is 88°F with 90% humidity. Which one of the following factors explains best why this patient is at a higher risk for hyperthermia than his local counterparts?

_____ a. At 50, his age makes him more vulnerable.

_____ b. He may be taking medications that diminish his abilities to compensate.

_____ c. His body has not yet acclimatized to the environment.

_____ d. High altitude can make him more vulnerable.

4. Increased core temperature as a result of lying in the sun would be considered an example of the _____________ method of heat transfer.

_____ a. radiation

_____ b. convection

_____ c. evaporative

_____ d. conduction

5. Which one of the following is the best example of a passive cooling technique?

_____ a. Immersion in ice water

_____ b. Cold packs in the groin, neck, and armpits

_____ c. Decreasing the temperature in the ambulance by using the air conditioning

_____ d. Wetting the patient down and fanning

Fill in the Blank

For each of the following signs and symptoms of heat-related emergencies, write "cramps," "exhaustion," or "stroke" to best describe the condition the finding indicates.

1. No sweating _______________
2. Hot skin _______________
3. Pale, cool skin _______________
4. Muscle contraction _______________
5. Altered mental status _______________
6. Profuse sweating _______________
7. Low blood pressure _______________

(continued on next page)

(continued)

Critical Thinking

1. What are the differences between heat exhaustion and heat stroke?

2. Describe the differences in treatment of a heat exhaustion patient compared to the treatment of a heat stroke patient.

PERSPECTIVE

Al—The EMT

There was one important thing we almost forgot. We got the guy in the ambulance, cut off his clothes, and put cool packs in some very personal places, if you know what I mean. Yet I didn't know his name. Sometimes we get into a serious call like this and forget the most basic thing. We had his medical care right. He trusted us and let us do it. But knowing someone's name from the beginning seems to make the call go better. So we introduced ourselves and kept going and finally asked his name. John, he said. When all is done, he won't remember that we may have saved his life, or even the cold packs in the groin. But he will remember that we took good care of him. And a big part of that is knowing and using his name when addressing him.

Other Environmental Emergencies

Spending time outdoors can expose a person to emergencies unrelated to heat and cold. Environmental emergencies can result from the bites and stings of animals and also from the environment itself, such as lightning strikes and the effects of altitude. Most of the situations described in the following section are relatively rare emergencies. However, there are providers whose service area would be considered high risk (especially when considering certain poisonous species). Because there is a wide range of local protocols, it would be beneficial for those providers to seek further information regarding their particular environmental challenges.

Animal Bites and Stings

Bites and stings can range from an annoyance to a life-threatening emergency. Although relatively rare, the bites of particular venomous species can lead to serious consequences if not treated appropriately (Figure 37-15 ▪).

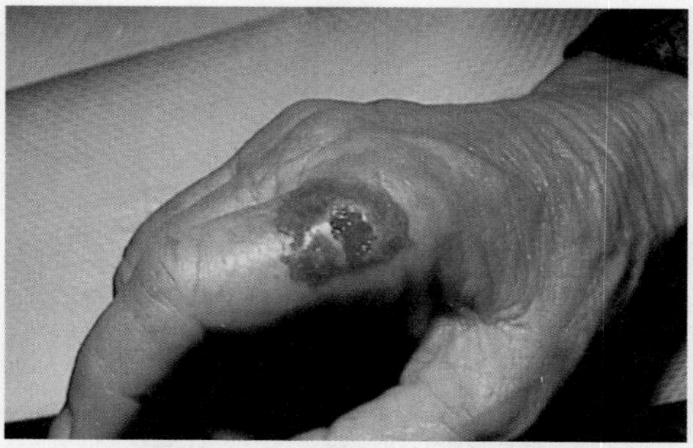

Figure 37-15 A bite from a brown recluse spider.

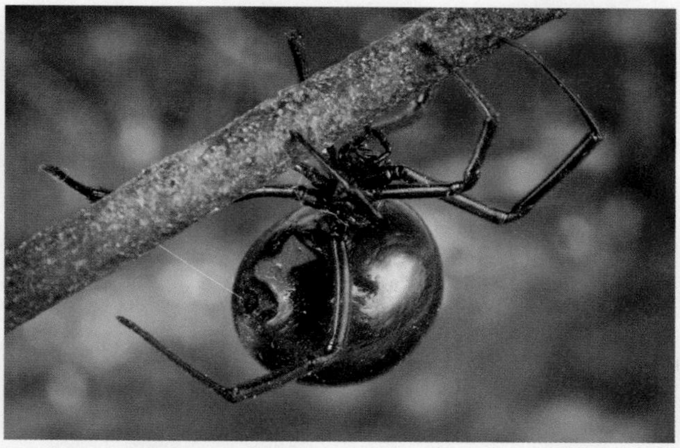

Figure 37-16 A black widow spider. (Centers for Disease Control/Paula Smith)

Bites and stings can have either local or systemic effects (and sometimes both). The local injury is the damage done by the actual sting or bite. Typically, the injury is minor, but at times certain venoms and toxins can cause systemic changes that are life threatening. Although most venoms or toxins are usually either local or systemic in nature, some poisonous animals deploy venoms that have both properties.

Patients can develop systemic effects by an exaggerated immune response to the venom or toxin. Although the bite may be limited to local damage, if an anaphylactic reaction occurs, dangerous systemic effects will be present. In fact, anaphylaxis may be the most deadly effect of all.

There are many poisonous animals in the world. In the United States, providers are exposed to relatively few species that are particularly harmful. Although it is certainly possible to encounter an exotic or rare poisonous snake or other animal, the following sections discuss only those that are most common.

Black Widow and Brown Recluse Spiders

Of the thousands of species of spiders in the United States, there are very few that are considered harmful. In fact only the black widow and brown recluse spiders pose any real threat.

37-22 Describe the signs and symptoms associated with bites or stings of black widow spiders, brown recluse spiders, scorpions, and fire ants.

Black widow spiders are dispersed throughout the United States (Figure 37-16 ■). Although they are venomous, bites are actually rare and usually occur only if the spider is provoked. The black widow is a small spider. Its body is roughly one-half inch long and is usually jet black in color. Only female black widows are dangerous to humans and they can be identified by their characteristic hourglass shape red-orange coloration on the underside of their body. The bite of a black widow spider contains a systemic neurotoxin but it rarely injects enough venom to be deadly. In fact, no deaths from black widow spiders have been reported in the United States since 1983.

In extreme cases, black widow venom can lead to systemic dysfunction secondary to failure of the central nervous system. This venom is most dangerous to the more vulnerable populations, such as the very young and older patients. The bite itself is not very painful. In fact, most patients who are bitten by a black widow spider will never know they were bitten. If envenomation has occurred, systemic symptoms can occur within one to two hours. The site of the bite may become red and slightly swollen. Symptoms include abdominal pain, cramping in large muscle groups such as the back and thighs, and nausea. Sometimes the patients will display tremors. Most symptoms will subside within five to seven days. In rare cases, neurological dysfunction can affect heart and lungs.

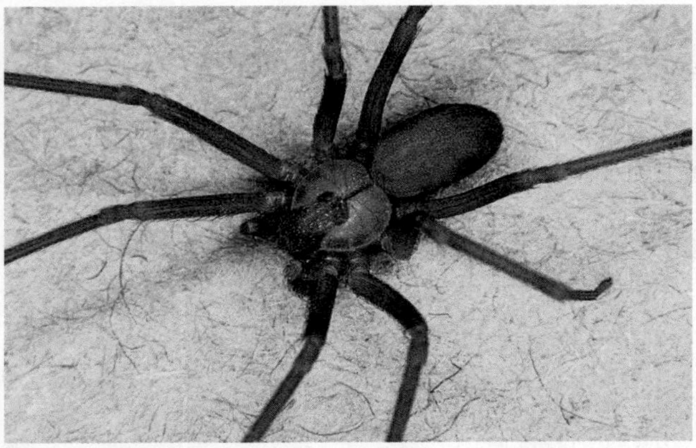

Figure 37-17 A brown recluse spider. (Centers for Disease Control)

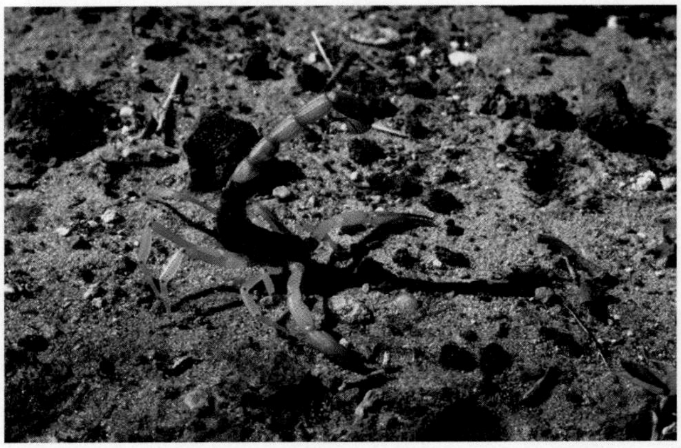

Figure 37-18 A common scorpion. (U.S. Fish and Wildlife Service/Gary M. Stolz)

Brown recluse spiders are also distributed throughout the United States but are more common to the Southern and Midwestern states (Figure 37-17 ▪). This small, one-quarter to one-half inch brown spider is particularly shy and lives in cracks, crevices, and spaces within human structures. As with the black widow, bites are very rare and fatalities are not at all common. The venom of a brown recluse is both cytotoxic and hemotoxic. This means that it affects local tissue and also the cells of the blood. As a result, brown recluse bites typically result in localized damage as opposed to the systemic effects of a black widow.

Typically, the initial bite of the brown recluse is not felt. The bite is only noticed when pain increases as a result of local toxins taking effect. The most common signs and symptoms include pain at the site of the bite as well as swelling, discoloration, and local tissue death resulting in a wound-like lesion. The characteristic tissue death (necrosis) will not appear immediately, but over hours and days.

Emergency care for both black widow and brown recluse spider bites is primarily supportive. All jewelry should be removed before swelling occurs. Known bites of the black widow can be cleaned with soap and water and a cool pack should be applied. Patients should be transported and evaluated at an appropriate facility. In rare cases, in which the effects become systemic, support airway and breathing as necessary.

Scorpions

Scorpions are small creatures common to the Southwestern United States and Mexico (Figure 37-18 ▪). Although there are well over a thousand species of scorpions, only one species in the United States is harmful to humans. The genus of scorpions known as *centruroides* inhabits the Southern states and injects a powerful neurotoxin that can create systemic effects. Central nervous system dysfunction is the main risk associated with this creature.

Scorpion bites are generally painful and can cause local tissue damage. Neurological effects typically set in within minutes but can develop hours later. Common signs of the neurotoxic venom include altered mental status, blurred vision, vertigo, and poor balance. If the effects are severe, cardiac and respiratory compromise may be present. As with spider bites, treatment is primarily supportive. However, if cardiac or respiratory failure is present, treat accordingly.

Identification of the scorpion can be helpful. However, safety should not be compromised in order to recover the animal. Always proceed with caution when dealing with any potentially dangerous creature.

An exaggerated allergic reaction is relatively common in scorpion envenomations. Chapter 24 describes how the immune system responds in a hypersensitive manner to

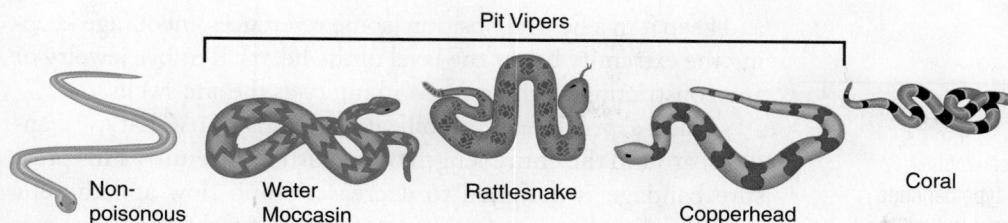

Figure 37-19 Common venomous snakes found in the United States.

foreign invaders. The hypersensitivity response leads to the release of toxins such as histamines and this can lead to systemic effects (anaphylaxis). The dangers of an anaphylactic reaction are highest when the airway and bronchial tubes become swollen, leading to poor air movement or when blood vessels dilate leading to severe hypotension.

As described in Chapter 24, the most important treatment for anaphylaxis is the use of an auto-injector to administer epinephrine. Epinephrine is a potent bronchodilator and vasoconstrictor and essentially reverses the effects of the anaphylactic reaction. If a patient who has been stung by a scorpion exhibits signs of anaphylaxis, you must aggressively treat based on those guidelines.

Snakebites

According to the American Association of Poison Control Centers, there are just over 6,000 snakebites reported each year in the United States and less than one in one thousand results in death. Although there are several poisonous snakes that inhabit the United States, by far the most common is the rattlesnake (Figure 37-19 ■). Rattlesnakes belong to the family of pit vipers and are characterized by the classic rattle on their tail and the sensory "pit" on the snake's head. Pit vipers deliver a cytotoxic venom that destroys the local tissue around the bite. Some rattlesnake species also have a venom with neurotoxic properties and can cause severe systemic reactions.

37-23 Describe the characteristics of common venomous snakes and factors that affect the severity of a snakebite.

It is important to note that not all rattlesnake bites transfer venom (Figure 37-20 ■). Some statistics note that as many as 50% result in a nonvenomous bite. That said, the severity of the effects of a rattlesnake bite is directly proportional to the amount of venom injected. As with other venoms and toxins, very young and very old patients are most susceptible to the effects and account for the majority of fatalities associated with snakebites in the United States.

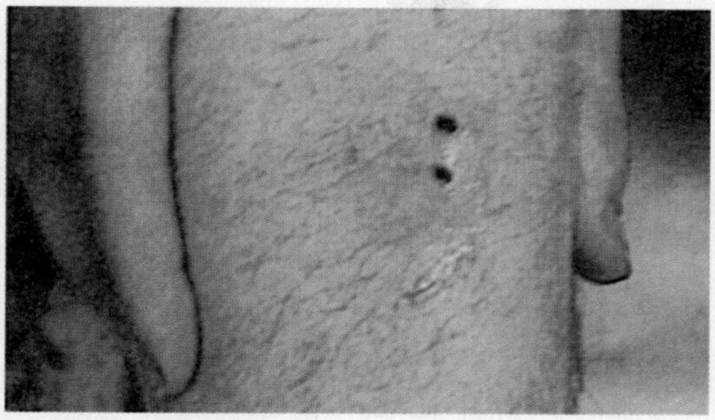

Figure 37-20 A typical rattlesnake bite.

Signs and symptoms associated with a rattlesnake bite include the following:

- Pain at the site
- Progressive weakness
- Nausea and vomiting
- Seizures
- Vision problems
- Altered mental status

In most cases, the majority of damage will occur at the location of the bite, but systemic dysfunction of the central nervous system is possible. The successful treatment of a rattlesnake bite relies a great deal on timing. The sooner the antivenom is administered, the better the prognosis for the patient. That means, as an EMT, you should not only document the time of the bite but also initiate rapid transport as soon as possible.

In addition to rapid transport, you should take steps to minimize the distribution of venom. Clean the bite with soap and water if possible. Keep the patient calm and minimize the patient's movement and activity. Consider immobilizing the bitten extremity

37-24 Describe the emergency medical care for a bite or sting.

> **CLINICAL CLUE**
>
> **AHA Guidelines**
>
> The 2010 AHA guidelines for the care of snakebites recommend the placement of a pressure-type bandage around the extremity. This bandage is meant to limit the flow through the lymph system back to the core of the body. The recommended pressure should be between 40 and 70 mmHg in the upper extremity and between 55 and 70 mmHg in the lower extremity. This pressure is difficult if not impossible to measure in the field so you must use your best guess as to tightness. Be sure to allow for a finger to be slipped beneath the bandage after it is applied. This will help ensure it is not too tight.

and keep it in a neutral position (some references encourage keeping the extremity below the level of the heart). Remove jewelry or any constricting clothing to avoid injury as the site swells.

Place a pressure immobilization bandage (ACE-type bandage) around the entire length of the bitten extremity. This pressure bandage is designed to decrease lymph flow and thereby slow the distribution of venom. Consider it tight enough if it is snug but allows a finger to be slipped under it.

As with scorpions, identification of the snake can be helpful, but also can be very dangerous to rescuers. Exercise extreme caution when dealing with a venomous snake.

There are other venomous snakes in the United States. Coral snakes deploy a very potent neurotoxin similar to that of a cobra. However, coral snake bites are very rare.

You should know what, if any, poisonous animals inhabit your response area and learn the specifics of local treatment protocol.

Other Venomous and Stinging Animals

There are a variety of other dangerous animals worthy of discussion. Although not commonly considered as dangerous as snakes and scorpions, hymenoptera, otherwise known as bees, hornets, wasps, and ants, account for more deaths in the United States than all other native poisonous species combined (Figure 37-21 ■).

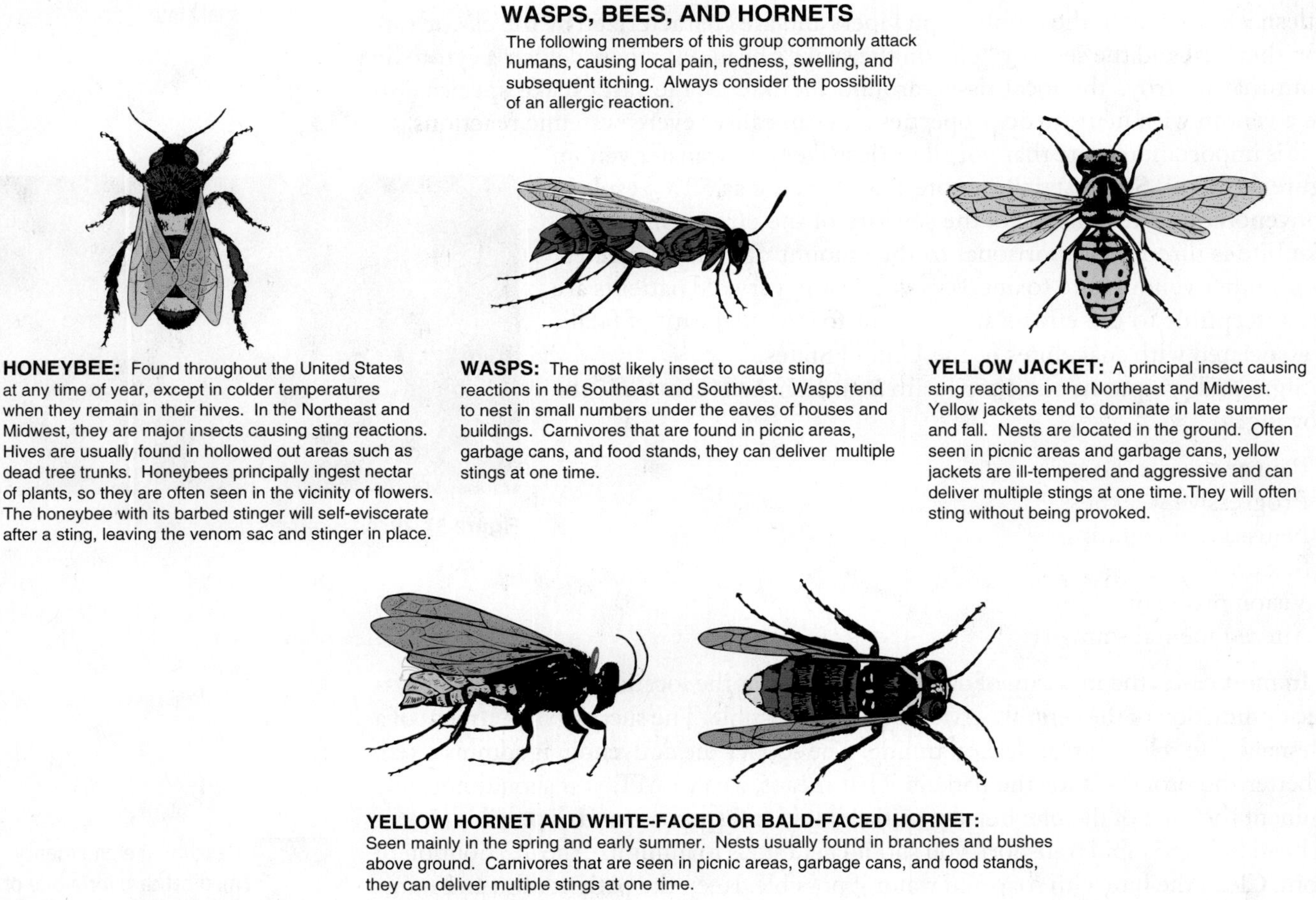
WASPS, BEES, AND HORNETS
The following members of this group commonly attack humans, causing local pain, redness, swelling, and subsequent itching. Always consider the possibility of an allergic reaction.
HONEYBEE: Found throughout the United States at any time of year, except in colder temperatures when they remain in their hives. In the Northeast and Midwest, they are major insects causing sting reactions. Hives are usually found in hollowed out areas such as dead tree trunks. Honeybees principally ingest nectar of plants, so they are often seen in the vicinity of flowers. The honeybee with its barbed stinger will self-eviscerate after a sting, leaving the venom sac and stinger in place.
WASPS: The most likely insect to cause sting reactions in the Southeast and Southwest. Wasps tend to nest in small numbers under the eaves of houses and buildings. Carnivores that are found in picnic areas, garbage cans, and food stands, they can deliver multiple stings at one time.
YELLOW JACKET: A principal insect causing sting reactions in the Northeast and Midwest. Yellow jackets tend to dominate in late summer and fall. Nests are located in the ground. Often seen in picnic areas and garbage cans, yellow jackets are ill-tempered and aggressive and can deliver multiple stings at one time.They will often sting without being provoked.
YELLOW HORNET AND WHITE-FACED OR BALD-FACED HORNET:
Seen mainly in the spring and early summer. Nests usually found in branches and bushes above ground. Carnivores that are seen in picnic areas, garbage cans, and food stands, they can deliver multiple stings at one time.

Figure 37-21 Common types of wasps, bees, and hornets.

Each year roughly 500 Americans die from the sting of bees and ants. Unlike snakes and scorpions, however, the vast majority of those deaths are attributed to severe anaphylaxis and not to the direct effect of the venom alone.

Best estimates point out that about 5% of the population is allergic to bees. This certainly does not mean that each person stung will develop an anaphylactic reaction. However, it does demonstrate the pervasiveness of this type of allergy. Because hymenoptera inhabit all areas of the United States, the risk is relatively high.

Fire ants are a particularly dangerous form of hymenoptera. The small red ants live in large colonies in the Southwest and when provoked, bite and sting. Their venom causes a painful reaction and in many cases can lead to an allergic response. Because fire ants typically are encountered in colonies, it is rare to suffer a single bite. More commonly, hundreds of bites occur over wide areas of the body. This wide dispersal of venom is a leading factor contributing to the risk of anaphylaxis.

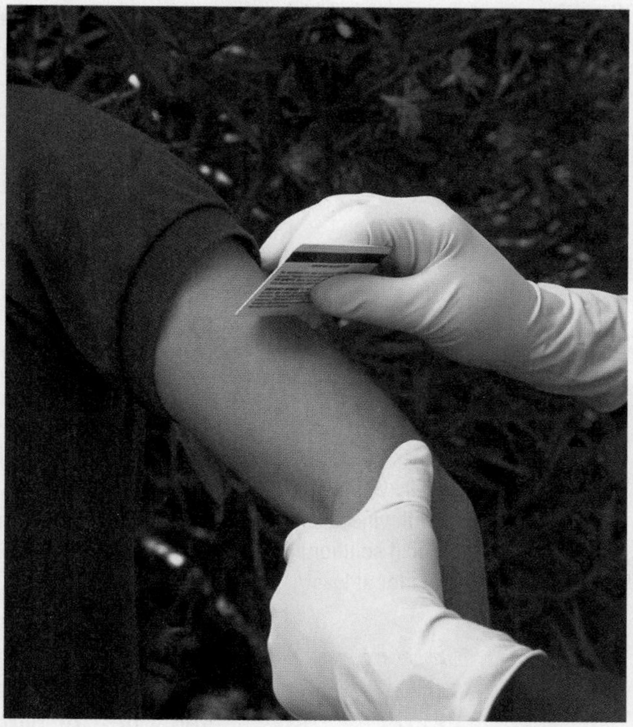

Figure 37-22 Use an object such as a credit card to scrape away the stinger. This will prevent squeezing of the venom sac and injection of more venom.

Not everyone who is stung by an ant or a bee is allergic. In fact, most are not. In the nonallergic person, the stings are still painful and can cause local swelling. To care for this patient, first consider scene safety. Are there stinging insects still present? Treatment in a non-anaphylactic scenario will focus on the site of the sting and the local damage. In some cases, hymenoptera leave a stinger in place at the site of the sting. If the stinger has been left in the patient, it should be removed. Remove the stinger by scraping it away with the edge of a credit card (Figure 37-22 ■). Do not use tweezers because they might inadvertently squeeze more venom into your patient. Remove all jewelry before swelling occurs. Wash the area with soap and water and consider applying a cool pack to help soothe the pain and decrease local swelling.

Inspect the site of the sting for redness and swelling. The patient will usually report feeling pain in the area. If you observe the area of redness expanding, involving hives or increased swelling—especially involving the face, neck, and chest—the patient may be developing anaphylaxis. Be alert for other indications of anaphylaxis such as hoarseness, a feeling of swelling or a lump in the throat, wheezing, and signs of shock.

It will be important to determine if the patient has a history of past reactions to similar stings. In the event the patient has had an allergic reaction to a specific type of bee, remain alert for anaphylaxis even if you are unsure of the type of bee involved in the sting. Since venom may be injected into the patient, other signs and symptoms may develop. They include:

- Chills
- Weakness
- Dizziness
- Fever
- Nausea
- Vomiting

The most deadly scenarios resulting from hymenoptera stings involve anaphylaxis. If the signs of severe allergic reaction are present, you must treat aggressively according to the guidelines discussed in Chapter 24.

37-25 Describe the signs, symptoms, and patient history associated with the bite or sting of a marine animal and the emergency medical care for marine-life poisoning.

Certain marine animals also can produce venomous stings. Species of jellyfish, such as the Portuguese man of war, have tentacles containing venomous nematocysts that can sting and produce harmful effects. Although deaths in the United States are rare, the stings can be very painful.

When a jellyfish stings, it attaches many nematocysts to the affected area. The venom sacs will continue to release their toxins as long as they are attached. Unfortunately, it is not simple to remove them. Simply rinsing or wiping away will not remove the poison.

One effective method of treating jellyfish stings is to use vinegar to neutralize the toxin and aid in the removal of nematocysts. The vinegar halts the release of toxins from the nematocysts and can make removal easier. If vinegar is not available, consider using a baking soda slurry to wash the area of the sting. Once the poison is neutralized by the vinegar or baking soda, the nematocysts can be gently scraped away.

Stings of jellyfish can be very painful. After removing the nematocysts, pain can be treated with hot water (a hot shower or immersion of the sting site in hot water) for 20 minutes. If hot water is not available, heat packs may be used as a substitute.

Ticks are another biting insect that can cause harm. Although ticks are not venomous, they are responsible for the spread of Lyme disease and Rocky Mountain spotted fever. If ticks are encountered, they should be removed with tweezers. Do not apply heat or petroleum jelly. Simply pull the tick straight out. The site of the tick bite should be washed and monitored. Although symptoms of infectious disease will present days and even weeks later, a characteristic bull's eye-like rash is a concerning finding and should be evaluated.

> **CLINICAL CLUE**
>
> **AHA Guidelines**
>
> In its 2010 Guidelines the AHA recommends liberally washing the affected area with vinegar (4% to 6% acetic acid solution) as soon as possible for at least 30 seconds.

Lightning Injuries

37-26 Explain the pathophysiology of lightning-strike injuries.

Lightning is a natural phenomenon that occurs every day, but when its massive energy is directed toward a human being, the results can be devastating. A single bolt of lightning can contain 50,000 volts of electricity and increase the temperature of the object it strikes up to 40,000°F. When lightning hits the body, it can cause massive damage (Figure 37-23 ■). Most prominently, lightning damages the central nervous system. As vast quantities of energy are passed through the body, nervous pathways are damaged and nervous function can shut down, temporarily or permanently.

The most dangerous event associated with a lightning strike injury is cardiac arrest. In some cases, the heart will be stopped immediately by the massive electrical depolarization. In other cases, nervous system shutdown can lead to abrupt respiratory arrest, which can then lead to cardiac arrest due to hypoxia if not immediately corrected.

Trauma is a significant concern in lightning strikes. Patients struck by lightning experience massive muscular contractions that can lead to injury, and the changing air pressure at the time of the strike can lead to blunt force trauma. Patients are frequently thrown several feet in the process of being struck.

Safety is the most important factor to consider when responding to a lightning strike situation. Be aware that as you approach, you are at risk of being struck as well. If the situation is deemed dangerous, move the patient rapidly into the ambulance or at least to a sheltered location.

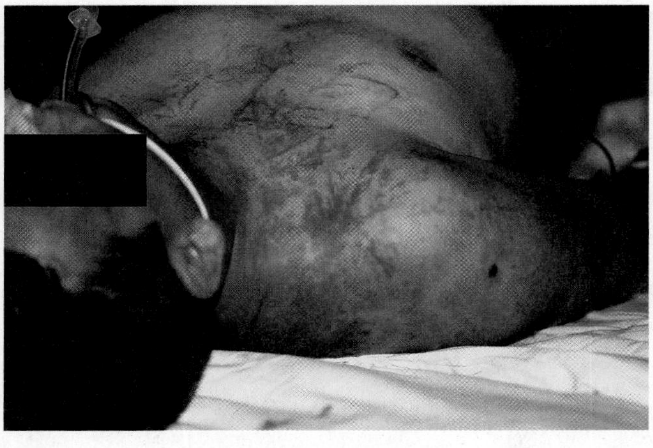

Figure 37-23 A lightning strike appears with a "feathering" pattern on the skin. (© David Effron, MD)

CLINICAL CLUE

Lightning Strike-Related Cardiac Arrest

Because of associated outdoor activities, such as summer sporting events, there are often multiple patients who are simultaneously injured by lightning at the same location. Unlike the usual emergency care standards for multiple patient incidents (where cardiac arrest patients are the lowest treatment priority group), patients in cardiac arrest from lightning strikes should be the highest priority treatment group. Rapid defibrillation using AEDs is essential to optimize survival from lightning strike-related cardiac arrest.

Because of the risk of injury, consider the need for spinal immobilization. Complete an immediate primary assessment because this will rapidly identify the need for CPR or assisted ventilations. Initiate AED use, chest compressions, and positive pressure ventilation when necessary.

37-27 Describe the emergency medical care for a patient who has been struck by lightning.

If the patient is hypoxic, administer supplemental oxygen. Provide emergency care for associated injuries and transport. The patient may have entrance and exit wounds as a result of the lightning. Remember that burns and external injuries may be the least concerning problems facing this patient. Although they should be addressed, there may be far more significant internal injuries present. Consider the need for advanced life support and cardiac monitoring capabilities. As always, follow local protocol.

Dive Injuries

Although scuba diving is relatively safe, there are hazards and injuries associated with the changing atmospheric pressure and the use of compressed gases. A small portion of diving excursions will result in decompression-related injuries and air emboli.

37-28 Explain the pathophysiology of decompression sickness.

A variety of different types of emergencies can occur in the diving environment, but generally they result from changing pressures. Dysbarism, or **decompression sickness,** results from the rapid change in pressure between diving depths and the surface. Divers who ascend too rapidly are at risk of developing nitrogen bubbles and rapid gas expansion in their bodies.

decompression sickness a condition that arises when dissolved gases come out of solution inside the body during depressurization. Also called *dysbarism* or *the bends.*

Free-floating nitrogen bubbles typically cause two types of problems. *Type I decompression sickness* occurs when nitrogen bubbles occupy space in the joints and in the soft tissues. Pain can be caused as these bubbles expand or as blood flow is restricted. This condition is often referred to as *the bends* and the pain is typically dull, achy, and worse at major joints. Skin rash and irritation are also common complaints.

37-29 Recognize the signs, symptoms, and patient history associated with Type I and Type II decompression sickness.

Type II decompression sickness occurs when nitrogen bubbles obstruct major blood flow and can affect a number of body systems:

- ***Respiratory system.*** Pulmonary emboli occur when blood flow through the lungs is obstructed. Symptoms include respiratory distress, bloody sputum, and acute-onset chest pain. This condition is commonly referred to as *the chokes* and it can be life threatening. The symptoms can be immediate or delayed 12 to 48 hours and include a burning sensation on inhalation and a nonproductive cough. Nonspecific symptoms also include pallor, cyanosis, low oxygen saturations, and accessory muscle use.
- ***Circulatory system.*** Decompression sickness can cause fluid to shift out of the blood vessels and cause hypovolemia. This disorder is characterized by the signs and symptoms of shock, including tachycardia and low blood pressure. Coagulation disorders also can lead to clot formation and perfusion-related problems.

- ***Nervous system.*** The brain and spinal cord can be affected by nitrogen bubbles and small emboli. Nitrogen narcosis, compression damage, and perfusion problems can cause neurological symptoms such as altered mental status, vision disturbance, weakness, numbness, and tingling, and even loss of bowel and bladder control. Air emboli can cause stroke-like problems and include similar symptoms, including seizures, motor and sensory deficits, and pupil changes.

In addition, arterial emboli can be caused by rupture of lung tissue. Free air then can travel into the arterial bloodstream and cause obstruction in key areas. Emboli can obstruct the flow of blood and cause perfusion deficits to tissue. In the extreme, this can cause a pulmonary embolism, but it can also cause more local signs and symptoms.

Certain conditions can predispose a patient to decompression sickness. They include:

- Flying too soon after diving (typically sooner than 12 to 24 hours)
- Diving at extreme depths (or prolonged exposure to extreme depths)
- Manual exertion (work) while diving
- Cold water
- Obesity
- Age
- Dehydration
- Prior cardiovascular conditions

A dive injury may include a variety of different injuries including both decompression sickness and trauma. Always consider spinal precautions and the likelihood of additional injuries when assessing this type of patient. Treat immediate life threats based on the findings of your primary assessment. Ensure adequacy of breathing and treat for shock. Supplemental oxygen is exceptionally important because it diminishes the effects of nitrogen.

37-30 Describe the emergency medical care of patients suffering from air embolism and decompression sickness.

When treating decompression sickness, consider the position of the patient. When spine injury is not a consideration, place the patient in the recovery position. Do not place the patient in a Trendelenburg or head-down position.

Rapid transport may be the most important therapy in a dive emergency. When making a transport decision, remember that the treatment of severe decompression sickness often requires the use of a decompression chamber. It may be advisable to facilitate transport to a facility with this type of capability. That may mean alternative transport methods, such as air medical transport. Always follow local protocol.

PERSPECTIVE

John—The Patient

I don't even know what hit me. It seemed to come on so quickly. The next thing I knew there were rescue guys there. I could barely talk. Later they told me at the hospital that I was close to dying. I'm healthy and young. Didn't think this could happen to me. Maybe I should look for work somewhere air-conditioned.

STOP, REVIEW, REMEMBER!

Multiple Choice

For each question, place a check next to the correct answer.

1. A six-year-old female patient has been bitten by a black widow spider. After ensuring a patent airway and adequate breathing, you should:
   _____ a. apply a constrictive band.
   _____ b. rinse the bite with vinegar.
   _____ c. apply cool pack to the bite wound.
   _____ d. immobilize the extremity.

2. Which one of the following is a correct way to remove a bee stinger from a patient's arm?
   _____ a. Remove it with your fingers.
   _____ b. Have the patient remove it with his fingers to prevent contamination.
   _____ c. Remove it with tweezers.
   _____ d. Scrape it out with a plastic card.

3. A 44-year-old man has been stung by a scorpion. He now complains of difficulty breathing, vertigo, and pain at the site of the sting. You note he has hives developing on his chest and his vital signs are pulse 116, respirations 24, and blood pressure 82/60. You should:
   _____ a. apply a constricting band to limit spread of the venom.
   _____ b. attempt to capture the scorpion so it may be identified.
   _____ c. administer an auto-injector of epinephrine if allowed.
   _____ d. scrape out the stinger with a plastic card.

4. A seven-year-old female patient was bitten by a rattlesnake. The bite just occurred and the patient is alert and oriented and has stable vital signs. You should immediately:
   _____ a. initiate transport.
   _____ b. apply a tourniquet to the wound.
   _____ c. apply a cold pack to the area of the bite.
   _____ d. apply suction to the bite area to extract the venom.

5. Of the animals in the following list, which one kills the most people in the United States each year?
   _____ a. Bees
   _____ b. Rattlesnakes
   _____ c. Scorpions
   _____ d. Jellyfish

Fill in the Blank

For each of the following animals, list whether the most dangerous element of their bite or sting is a cytotoxin, a neurotoxin, or anaphylaxis.

1. Wasps ____________________________
2. Rattlesnake ____________________________
3. Fire ants ____________________________
4. Brown recluse spider ____________________________
5. Black widow spider ____________________________

(continued on next page)

(continued)

Critical Thinking

1. Explain the difference in the effects of a black widow spider bite and the bite of a brown recluse spider.

2. Explain why fire ant encounters are often more severe and dangerous compared to encounters with other insects.

3. Describe the process of treating a jellyfish sting.

EMERGENCY DISPATCH SUMMARY

The patient was sufficiently cooled during transport to Atlas Memorial Hospital and was released soon after with orders to rest for two days. Based on this and similar events, the oil company began providing air-conditioned trailers at the drilling sites, with orders that the workers be rotated into them for adequate rest periods. Heat-related emergency calls in Covington County have since dropped by nearly 45%.

Chapter Review

To the Point

- Environmental injuries span a broad spectrum of causes. Although expertise in all areas is difficult to obtain, an EMT should be familiar with the most common emergencies.
- The regulation of temperature is a constant balancing act between the manufacture of heat and its dissipation.
- The body creates heat through metabolism and loses heat to the environment. Conduction, radiation, convection, and evaporation all are methods of temperature transfer.
- The body functions in a narrow range of temperature. Heat or cold insults that throw off this range can rapidly lead to system dysfunction.
- Certain conditions, medications, and disease processes can impair the body's capabilities of thermoregulation.
- Cold injuries can be generalized or localized. Local injuries destroy tissue in a process similar to burns.
- Generalized hypothermia can be mild, moderate, or severe. Overall treatment depends on the severity.
- Hyperthermia occurs when the heat challenge overwhelms the body's ability to compensate. It too can occur with varying severity.
- Providers must differentiate heat exhaustion from heat stroke and engage active cooling when heat stroke is identified.
- A variety of animals can deliver poisonous bites and stings in the United States. EMTs should be familiar with the basic characteristics of the most common venomous species.
- Safety is a major concern when dealing with an emergency involving a poisonous animal.
- Not all bites from poisonous animals deliver harmful venom. Care is based on thorough patient assessment and cautious suspicion.
- Lightning is a dangerous situation for both rescuer and patient. Assessment must focus on recognizing cardiac arrest immediately.

Chapter Questions

Multiple-Choice

For each question, place a check next to the correct answer.

1. A 30-year-old female marathon runner complains of severe pain in her legs and abdomen. She is alert and oriented and you note she is flushed and very sweaty. You should most likely suspect:

    _____ a. heat cramps.
    _____ b. heat exhaustion.
    _____ c. heat stroke.
    _____ d. fatigue from running.

2. You are assessing a patient found in the snow. Her skin is very cold and she is not responsive. After a 10-second pulse check, you cannot obtain a pulse. You should next:

    _____ a. continue checking for a pulse for an additional 20–50 seconds.
    _____ b. contact the medical examiner's office.
    _____ c. immediately begin chest compressions.
    _____ d. immediately begin positive pressure ventilations.

3. A 30-year-old woman has been bitten by a brown recluse spider. Which one of the following should you most expect?

    _____ a. Local tissue damage around the area of the bite
    _____ b. Systemic effects including respiratory paralysis
    _____ c. A combination of local and systemic effects
    _____ d. No effects because envenomation rarely occurs

(continued on next page)

(continued)

4. Which one of the following best describes why an elderly patient would be more susceptible to hypothermia than a middle-aged patient?
   _____ a. Less body fat, worsening circulation
   _____ b. Increased cardiac output and higher metabolic rate
   _____ c. Less likelihood of taking medications that would impair compensation
   _____ d. Poor hepatic function and decreased renal perfusion

5. The diving injury referred to as *the bends* is caused by:
   _____ a. nitrogen bubbles occupying space in the tissue and joints.
   _____ b. nitrogen bubbles causing an obstruction in the brain.
   _____ c. nitrogen bubbles causing an obstruction in the lungs.
   _____ d. an arterial gas embolism as a result of barotraumas in the lungs.

6. The most significant emergency care for a person suffering from an anaphylactic reaction would be:
   _____ a. oxygen.
   _____ b. epinephrine.
   _____ c. rapid transport.
   _____ d. removal of the stinger.

Critical Thinking

1. In what situation would you actively warm a deep local cold injury? How would you do it?

____

____

____

____

2. List three non-weather-related factors that might put a person at an increased risk of hyperthermia.

____

____

____

____

3. What are the differences in radiation, conduction, and convection?

____

____

____

____

Case Study

You are out with a group of friends staying in a cabin near the lake. Because it is winter, it is about 20 minutes into the camp by snowmobile and another two hours into town. You and some friends decide to go snowshoeing. While out on what you thought was a field, your friend Thom breaks through the surface of a small pond. His snowshoe gets stuck. By the time he gets his foot out of the water, it is soaked. During the trek back to the cabin, Thom tells you that he has lost sensation in his foot. You get back to the cabin and remove his boot. The boot is frozen solid. Thom's foot is white and hard. He tells you he can't feel it. His toes barely move. Thom says they are "stiff."

1. Is this a superficial or deep local cold injury? Why or why not?

2. What emergency care would you provide for Thom?

3. Would you rewarm the foot? Why or why not?

The Last Word

In environmental emergencies there is a significant chance that whatever happened to the patient may happen to you. Dangers from water, exposure to heat or cold, or meeting the same insect or animal that stung or bit your patient are risks for you. Safety must always be your first priority.

Environmental emergency patients also are often found in a position that is not safe. They may be out in the cold or heat, in the water, or far away from a road. This poses unique challenges to the EMT.

Finally, the extremes in ages (infants and the elderly) can be more seriously affected by extremes in heat and cold. Remember this information as you assess your patient and then document all appropriate information. The amount of heat or cold that you can tolerate is much more than can be tolerated by patients with limited ability for temperature regulation.

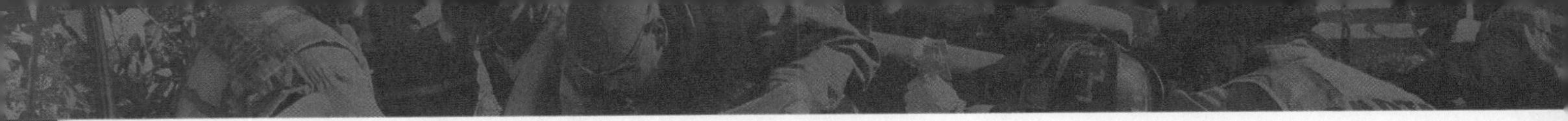

Module 4: Review and Practice Examination for Chapters 28–37

DIRECTIONS: *Assess what you have learned in this module by placing a check mark in the blank beside the best answer for each multiple-choice question. When you are done, check your answers against the Answer Key at the back of the book.*

1. The term *hypoperfusion* is often used to mean:
   ____ a. shock.
   ____ b. bleeding.
   ____ c. internal hemorrhage.
   ____ d. adequate circulation.

2. In adults, injury to which area is *least* likely to lead to hypovolemia due to blood loss?
   ____ a. pelvis
   ____ b. abdomen
   ____ c. head
   ____ d. chest

3. Which one of the following is *not* a typical indication of internal hemorrhage?
   ____ a. Vomiting material with a coffee grounds appearance
   ____ b. Slow pulse with warm skin and low blood pressure
   ____ c. Abdominal pain
   ____ d. Bruising or discoloration of the abdominal wall

4. Which one of the following statements about shock is true?
   ____ a. Once a patient is in shock, death is inevitable.
   ____ b. Shock is progressive without intervention.
   ____ c. Definitive treatment for the patient in shock is supplemental oxygen.
   ____ d. All blood loss leads to shock.

5. The largest artery in the body is the:
   ____ a. vena cava.
   ____ b. carotid.
   ____ c. jugular.
   ____ d. aorta.

6. The femoral artery is found in the:
   ____ a. neck.
   ____ b. groin.
   ____ c. arm.
   ____ d. heart.

7. The blood component responsible for carrying oxygen to the cells of the body is:
   ____ a. red blood cells.
   ____ b. white blood cells.
   ____ c. plasma.
   ____ d. platelets.

8. Which one of the following factors has the most influence on the severity of a bleeding patient?
   ____ a. Type of vessels involved
   ____ b. Amount of blood loss
   ____ c. Size of the patient
   ____ d. Mechanism of injury

9. The body's first response to an injured blood vessel is:
   ____ a. forming a blood clot.
   ____ b. decreasing the blood pressure.
   ____ c. dilation of the blood vessel.
   ____ d. increasing the heart rate.

10. Your patient has cut her hand with a knife and has bright red bleeding that is spurting. This is most likely ____________ bleeding.
    ____ a. venous
    ____ b. capillary
    ____ c. arterial
    ____ d. mixed venous and capillary

11. The first attempt to control bleeding is always:
    ____ a. applying a tourniquet.
    ____ b. elevation of the affected part.
    ____ c. application of ice to the affected part.
    ____ d. the use of direct pressure.

12. Your patient has a severe laceration to the forearm with uncontrolled bleeding. You should first:

____ a. elevate the arm.
____ b. apply oxygen.
____ c. apply a tourniquet.
____ d. apply direct pressure.

13. Your patient has a gunshot wound to the thigh with severe bleeding. You have tried direct pressure without success. You should:

____ a. apply a tourniquet.
____ b. transport immediately.
____ c. provide supplemental oxygen.
____ d. place pressure on the femoral artery

14. Which one of the following would be the best choice for improvising a tourniquet?

____ a. Electrical extension cord
____ b. Oxygen tubing
____ c. Belt
____ d. Yarn

15. Your patient is a 78-year-old woman complaining of a nosebleed that has lasted one hour. Which one of the following is the most appropriate treatment for this patient?

____ a. Have her assume a comfortable position on the stretcher and tilt her head back.
____ b. Have the patient sit down and lean forward.
____ c. Ask the patient to gently blow her nose.
____ d. Apply an ice pack to the back of her neck.

16. Major functions of the skin include all of the following *except:*

____ a. energy production.
____ b. protection from the environment.
____ c. temperature regulation.
____ d. prevention of fluid loss.

17. The blood vessels and nerve endings of the skin are located in the:

____ a. subcutaneous layer.
____ b. epidermis.
____ c. dermis.
____ d. percutaneous layer.

18. Your patient is a dockworker who is pinned underneath a forklift. This is an example of which type of soft-tissue injury?

____ a. Blunt force trauma
____ b. Crush force trauma
____ c. Penetrating trauma
____ d. Puncturing trauma

19. Which one of the following is a closed soft-tissue injury?

____ a. Laceration ____ c. Puncture
____ b. Abrasion ____ d. Hematoma

20. Which one of the following best explains the significance of a contusion to the thigh after a high-speed motor-vehicle collision?

____ a. Contusions are permanently disfiguring.
____ b. Contusions are associated with massive blood loss.
____ c. The contusion may be an indication of a femur fracture.
____ d. There is a high risk of infection associated with contusions.

21. Your patient is a 12-year-old boy who was not wearing a shirt when he fell off his skateboard while going down a steep incline. As he slid down the incline on his chest, the concrete rubbed off portions of his skin. This type of injury is best described as a(n):

____ a. hematoma.
____ b. abrasion.
____ c. laceration.
____ d. avulsion.

22. Your patient is a 35-year-old man who was stabbed in the back with a large knife. When you arrived on the scene, the knife was still embedded in the wound. Which one of the following statements regarding this situation is true?

____ a. Once airway, breathing, and circulation are assessed and appropriate interventions are performed, the object must be stabilized in place prior to transporting the patient.
____ b. It will be necessary to remove the knife in this case because the patient must be placed supine (on his back) in order to care for and transport him.
____ c. Impaled objects to the chest must always be removed to prevent a collapsed lung.
____ d. The knife should be stabilized with fluffy pillows so that he can be placed supine (on his back) for transport without placing additional pressure on the knife.

23. You are caring for a 44-year-old woman who suffered an amputation just below the knee. The wound is bleeding uncontrollably. You should:

____ a. apply a tourniquet and wait on the scene for the leg to be found.
____ b. immediately transport the patient and direct the police to bring the leg to the hospital.
____ c. ask the patient if she wants to stay and wait for the leg to be found or go ahead to the hospital.
____ d. attempt to control the bleeding and transport the patient immediately.

24. Absorbent gauze that is placed directly over a wound is best described as a:

____ a. bandage. ____ c. splint.
____ b. dressing. ____ d. plaster.

25. You have successfully controlled the bleeding from a leg wound with direct pressure. Your patient is showing signs of shock. You should:

____ a. bandage the wound and place the patient in the recovery position.
____ b. apply a tourniquet just in case it begins to bleed again.
____ c. place the patient in a supine position and administer oxygen.
____ d. place the patient in the shock position and transport.

26. A burn caused by exposure to hot liquid is classified as a(n) ____________ burn.

____ a. chemical ____ c. electrical
____ b. thermal ____ d. radiation

27. A burn that includes the epidermis and dermis is called a ____________ burn.

____ a. superficial
____ b. partial-thickness
____ c. full-thickness
____ d. deep

28. Blisters are associated with ____________ burns.

____ a. full-thickness
____ b. superficial
____ c. third-degree
____ d. partial-thickness

29. Which one of the following is *not* a consideration in determining appropriate care for a burn patient?

____ a. Depth of the burn
____ b. Anatomical location of the burn
____ c. Patient's gender
____ d. Patient's age

30. Your patient is a 16-year-old with burns to the anterior side of both legs and her entire right arm. The body surface area involved is:

____ a. 45%. ____ c. 27%.
____ b. 36%. ____ d. 18%.

31. Your patient is a 15-month-old with burns to his entire head, face, and neck. The body surface area involved is:

____ a. 9%. ____ c. 24%.
____ b. 18%. ____ d. 27%.

32. Your patient is a 68-year-old woman with burns to her anterior thigh that are about twice the size of her palm. The approximate body surface area involved is:

____ a. 18%. ____ c. 5%.
____ b. 9%. ____ d. 2%.

33. Burns are considered more serious if they affect which one of the following body parts?

____ a. Chest ____ c. Hand
____ b. Arm ____ d. Leg

34. Your patient is a 25-year-old man who has suffered a full-thickness burn about the size of a quarter on his forearm. This burn would be considered:

____ a. severe. ____ c. moderate.
____ b. intense. ____ d. mild.

35. Your patient is a 38-year-old man with a dry chemical powder on his face and hands. Which one of the following is most appropriate?

____ a. Transport him to the hospital for proper decontamination.
____ b. Brush the powder away before flushing with large amounts of water.
____ c. Wipe the powder away with a damp cloth.
____ d. Find an antidote to the chemical and apply it to the affected areas.

36. Which one of the following statements concerning electrical burns is *false*?

____ a. The greatest risk with electrical burns is thermal burns to a large percentage of body surface area.
____ b. Electrical burns can be associated with cardiac and respiratory problems.
____ c. Exposure to electrical current may cause burns both at the site where the current entered the body and where it exited the body.
____ d. Electricity generally travels internally through the body, rather than along its surface.

37. Which one of the following is generally *not* a complication of severe burns?

____ a. Infection ____ c. Hypothermia
____ b. Fluid loss ____ d. Blood loss

38. The pleural layers and the fluid between them are important in providing:

____ a. lubrication between the chest wall and lungs.
____ b. friction between the chest wall and lungs.
____ c. trapped air in the thorax.
____ d. protection from blunt trauma.

39. The EMT should consider a penetrating injury at the level of the eighth rib to be:
    ____ a. a chest injury.
    ____ b. both a chest and abdominal injury.
    ____ c. unlikely to cause serious chest or abdominal injury.
    ____ d. unlikely to cause serious chest injury.

40. Chest trauma may include injury to any of the following *except* the:
    ____ a. aorta. ____ c. heart.
    ____ b. pancreas. ____ d. bronchi.

41. When two or more consecutive ribs are each fractured in two or more places, this is called:
    ____ a. floating ribs.
    ____ b. a paradoxical segment.
    ____ c. a pneumothorax.
    ____ d. a flail chest.

42. Your patient is a nine-year-old boy who was run over by a tractor. His head and neck are purple in color, his neck veins are distended, and his eyes are bulging. This condition can best be described as:
    ____ a. paradoxical motion.
    ____ b. flail chest.
    ____ c. traumatic asphyxia.
    ____ d. hemothorax.

43. Your patient is a 22-year-old man with a gunshot wound to his right side, just below his armpit. In addition to oxygen and transport, which one of the following is required in the care of this patient?
    ____ a. Soft, bulky dressing over the site to splint the injury and reduce pain
    ____ b. Circumferential bandage around the chest
    ____ c. Dressing packed tightly into the wound to prevent an air leak
    ____ d. Occlusive dressing taped on three sides

44. The kidneys are located in the:
    ____ a. retroperitoneal cavity.
    ____ b. abdominal cavity.
    ____ c. thorax.
    ____ d. pleural space.

45. The primary concerns with damage to solid organs of the abdomen are:
    ____ a. irritation of the peritoneum and infection.
    ____ b. bleeding and hemorrhagic shock.
    ____ c. swelling and pain.
    ____ d. vomiting and diarrhea.

46. Which one of the following is the appropriate management for an evisceration?
    ____ a. Cover the site with Vaseline®-impregnated gauze taped on three sides.
    ____ b. Pack the wound with gauze.
    ____ c. Cover the site with a large sterile dressing moistened with sterile saline.
    ____ d. Rinse exposed organs with sterile saline and place them gently back inside the wound.

47. Bones are connected to one another at joints by:
    ____ a. tendons. ____ c. ligaments.
    ____ b. muscles. ____ d. marrow.

48. Mrs. Quinn fell forward onto her hands and broke her clavicle. This is an example of an injury caused by ______________ force.
    ____ a. pathological ____ c. direct
    ____ b. shearing ____ d. indirect

49. A strain is an injury to a:
    ____ a. bone. ____ c. ligament.
    ____ b. joint. ____ d. muscle.

50. Your patient is a 17-year-old skater who fell onto the ice and injured her wrist. The most appropriate approach to this patient is a:
    ____ a. detailed history and physical examination.
    ____ b. rapid trauma exam.
    ____ c. rapid history and assessment.
    ____ d. focused secondary assessment.

51. For which one of the following patients would a rapid secondary assessment be appropriate?
    ____ a. 40-year-old who stepped off a curb, twisted her ankle, and fell to her knees
    ____ b. Nine-year-old who fell 15 feet and has a deformed right arm
    ____ c. 75-year-old who stood up from her chair, felt a "snap" in her hip, and fell back into the chair
    ____ d. Seven-year-old who has a deformed forearm after performing a cartwheel in gymnastics class

52. Your patient is a cyclist who was thrown over the handlebars and has a badly deformed left forearm and no distal pulses. You have a 20-minute transport time. You should:
    ____ a. Straighten the extremity with gentle traction and splint at the point where pulses return prior to transport.
    ____ b. Splint the extremity in the position found and transport without delay.
    ____ c. Immediately call for an ALS unit.
    ____ d. Place the extremity in a sling but without using a rigid splint, apply ice, transport.

53. All of the following are reasons for splinting an injured extremity *except:*

____ a. prevent unnecessary pain.

____ b. prevent the patient from seeing how badly the extremity is injured.

____ c. minimize further bleeding.

____ d. prevent further damage to nerves, soft tissue, and blood vessels.

54. Your patient has a swollen, deformed ankle. A properly applied splint should extend from the ____________ to ____________.

____ a. ankle; the knee

____ b. toes; just above the ankle

____ c. toes; just below the knee

____ d. foot; the mid-thigh

55. A traction splint is designed to be used for which one of the following injuries?

____ a. Open fractures of the tibia

____ b. Deformed midshaft humerus fractures

____ c. Injuries to the knee

____ d. Suspected femur fractures

56. A swathe is most useful for which one of the following injuries?

____ a. Dislocated shoulder

____ b. Fractured pelvis

____ c. Suspected femur fracture

____ d. Swollen, deformed, painful finger

57. After the primary assessment, the next step in managing the patient with a musculoskeletal injury is:

____ a. checking the distal circulation, sensation, and motor function.

____ b. immobilizing the injured part.

____ c. minimizing the patient's pain.

____ d. assessing for strength.

58. The basilar skull best describes which portion of the skull?

____ a. Forehead area

____ b. Back of the head

____ c. Floor of the cranial vault

____ d. Facial bones

59. The weakest area of the skull is the ____________ area.

____ a. maxillary

____ b. temporal

____ c. parietal

____ d. occipital

60. The tough, fibrous membrane that lines the inside of the cranial vault is the:

____ a. dura mater.

____ b. pia mater.

____ c. arachnoid membrane.

____ d. middle meningeal layer.

61. The largest portion of the brain is the:

____ a. medulla oblongata.

____ b. cerebellum.

____ c. cerebrum.

____ d. frontal lobe.

62. The most immediate life-threat in a closed head injury is:

____ a. infection.

____ b. blood loss.

____ c. exposed brain tissue.

____ d. increased pressure on the brain.

63. An injury that causes a jarring of the brain with temporary signs and symptoms such as confusion and memory loss is best described as a:

____ a. cerebral contusion.

____ b. concussion.

____ c. subdural hematoma.

____ d. herniation.

64. Signs of increasing intracranial pressure typically include all of the following *except*:

____ a. increased blood pressure.

____ b. decreased heart rate.

____ c. pinpoint pupils.

____ d. seizures.

65. Which one of the following is *not* consistent with an isolated closed head injury?

____ a. Abnormal breathing pattern

____ b. Shock

____ c. Vomiting

____ d. Abnormal posturing in response to pain

66. Of the following, the highest priority in the care of the trauma patient is:

____ a. controlling bleeding.

____ b. maintaining an open airway.

____ c. providing supplemental oxygen.

____ d. taking vital signs.

67. In most cases the proper rate of assisted ventilations for an adult patient with a suspected brain herniation is ____________ per minute.

____ a. 8 to 10

____ b. 10 to 12

____ c. 20

____ d. 35

68. Which one of the following is *not* a sign of brain herniation?
___ a. Unequal pupils
___ b. Decerebrate posturing
___ c. Unresponsiveness
___ d. Increased heart rate

69. The spinal cord is part of the __________ nervous system.
___ a. accessory ___ c. peripheral
___ b. primary ___ d. central

70. The seven vertebrae of the neck are known as the __________ vertebrae.
___ a. cervical ___ c. lumbar
___ b. thoracic ___ d. sacral

71. A 30-year-old skydiver landed hard on his feet when his parachute malfunctioned. The mechanism by which he may have suffered a spine injury is:
___ a. flexion.
___ b. rotation.
___ c. distraction.
___ d. compression.

72. The most important consideration in determining the need for spinal immobilization is:
___ a. the presence of spinal deformity.
___ b. pain on palpation of the spine.
___ c. the patient's complaint of numbness or inability to move.
___ d. the mechanism of injury.

73. The first step in proper spinal immobilization is:
___ a. manual stabilization of the head and neck.
___ b. placing a properly sized cervical collar.
___ c. using a short spinal immobilization device.
___ d. logrolling the patient onto a long backboard.

74. Which one of the following is a consideration in spinal immobilization of small children?
___ a. Cervical collars are not made in pediatric sizes and must be improvised.
___ b. Children should never be immobilized unless there are signs and symptoms of spinal cord injury.
___ c. It is necessary to pad under the shoulders to prevent flexion of the neck.
___ d. It is best to use a cervical collar without a long spine board when immobilizing small children.

75. Which one of the following is a reason for rapid extrication of a patient with a possible spine injury from a vehicle collision?
___ a. The patient is in pain and complaining that it is taking too long to get her out of the car.
___ b. The patient is preventing you from accessing another occupant who is more seriously injured.
___ c. The patient does not have signs or symptoms of spine injury and a short immobilization device seems unnecessary.
___ d. None of the above

76. Which one of the following is an indication for removing the helmet of a patient who requires spinal immobilization?
___ a. Inability to assess and/or manage the airway
___ b. Snug fit of the helmet
___ c. Patient is stable
___ d. All of the above

77. You have just assisted a patient with her EpiPen in response to a severe bee sting allergy. As you are loading her into the ambulance, she becomes anxious and her heart rate increases from 100 initially to 112. In addition, she tells you she feels like she is going to throw up. You should:
___ a. give a second dose of epinephrine.
___ b. turn down the oxygen.
___ c. reassure the patient that what she is experiencing is a normal.
___ d. place her in the recovery position.

78. Which one of the following is not a significant risk factor for heat- and cold-related emergencies?
___ a. Old age
___ b. Female gender
___ c. Circulatory problems
___ d. Very young age

79. In which one of the following situations is the patient losing body heat primarily by convection?
___ a. A 55-year-old man is found lying on the frozen ground without a coat.
___ b. A 24-year-old man is wearing wet clothing after falling out of his boat while fishing.
___ c. A 32-year-old woman is outside in cool, windy weather.
___ d. A vapor cloud is created every time your 80-year-old female patient breathes into the cool night air.

80. Which one of the following is categorized as a generalized cold emergency?
____ a. Hyperthermia ____ c. Hypothermia
____ b. Frostbite ____ d. Frostnip

81. Your patient is a 30-year-old male hiker who was lost outside overnight in below-freezing temperatures. He is shivering uncontrollably and has decreased coordination. Which one of the following actions is appropriate?
____ a. Give him plenty of hot coffee.
____ b. Briskly rub his arms and legs to increase circulation.
____ c. Have the patient move around as much as possible to generate body heat.
____ d. Remove any wet clothing and cover him with blankets.

82. Which one of the following is used only during active rewarming?
____ a. Giving hot tea, cocoa, or coffee to drink
____ b. Placing hot packs at the patient's neck, armpits, and groin
____ c. Covering the patient with a blanket
____ d. Turning up the heat in the patient compartment of the ambulance

83. Care of a frostbitten extremity includes:
____ a. splinting the affected area.
____ b. breaking any blisters that form.
____ c. applying hot packs to the affected area.
____ d. gently rubbing the affected area between your hands.

84. More serious heat-related injuries should be suspected when the patient presents with:
____ a. feeling faint.
____ b. muscle cramps.
____ c. hot, dry skin.
____ d. weakness.

85. Your patient is a 25-year-old man who has been working outside in a hot, humid climate. He is alert and oriented, complaining of feeling weak and dizzy. His skin is cool and moist, and he has a heart rate of 104, a blood pressure of 110/70, and respirations of 16. You should:
____ a. place cold packs at the groin, armpits, and neck.
____ b. give the patient some cool water to drink.
____ c. offer the patient some salt tablets.
____ d. move him to a cool place and vigorously fan him.

86. Your patient was hiking in the desert and was bitten on the ankle by a rattlesnake. You should:
____ a. keep the foot lower than the level of the patient's heart.
____ b. elevate the foot on pillows.
____ c. apply a tourniquet above the bite.
____ d. apply ice to the area of the bite.

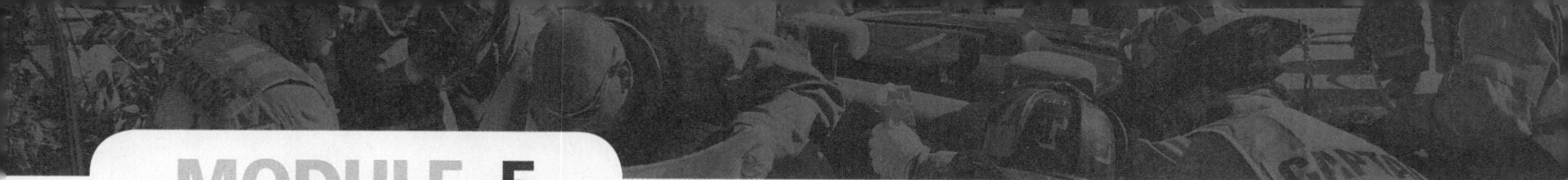

MODULE 5

Special Populations

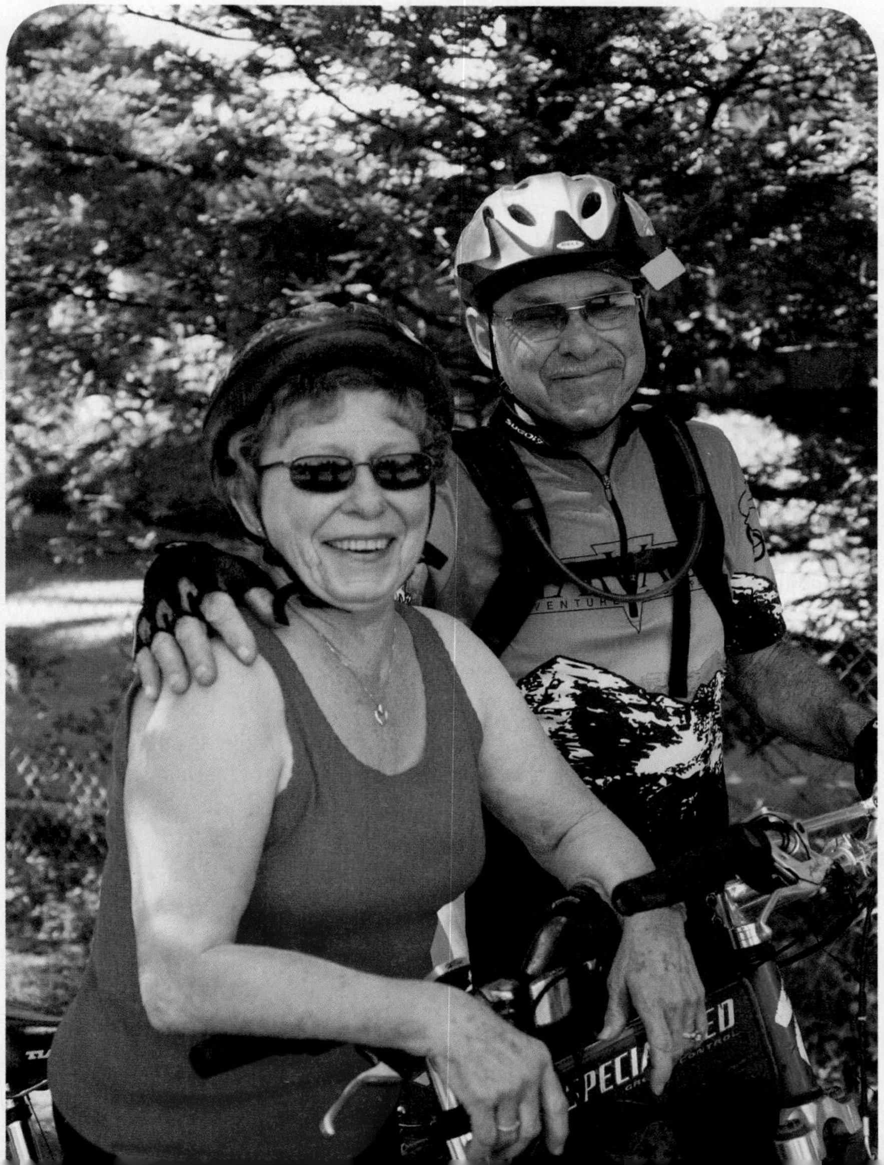

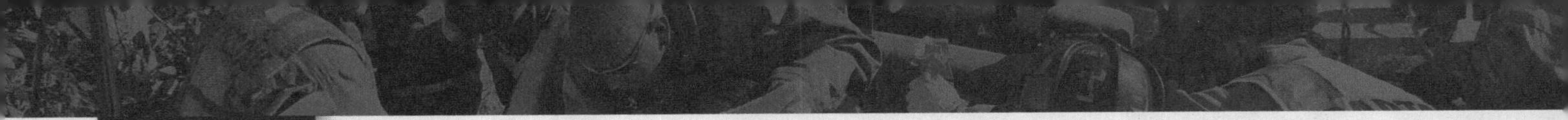

38 Caring for Pediatric Patients

Education Standards

Special Patient Populations: Pediatrics

Competencies

Applies fundamental knowledge of growth, development, aging, and assessment findings to provide basic emergency care and transportation for a patient with special needs.

Objectives

After completion of this lesson, you should be able to:

38-1 Define key terms introduced in this chapter.

38-2 Describe the major developmental characteristics and modifications of patient assessment and management techniques recommended for patients in each of the following age groups: neonates, infants, toddlers, preschoolers, school-age children, and adolescents.

38-3 Describe the major anatomical and physiological differences in children with regard to the following: airway, head, chest, lungs, respiratory system, cardiovascular system, abdomen, extremities, metabolic rate, and skin and body surface area.

38-4 Discuss the normal vital signs for children in various age groups.

38-5 Describe the use of the pediatric assessment triangle (PAT) to determine a pediatric patient's status.

38-6 Discuss special considerations for the following elements of the pediatric secondary assessment: physical exam, vital sign assessment, and history taking.

38-7 Describe signs of respiratory distress, respiratory failure, and respiratory arrest in pediatric patients.

38-8 Discuss the guidelines for emergency care of respiratory emergencies and foreign body airway obstruction.

38-9 Describe the presentation and emergency medical care for pediatric patients with the following conditions: asthma, bronchiolitis, cardiac arrest, congenital heart disease, epiglottitis, pneumonia, and shock (hypoperfusion).

38-10 Explain the assessment steps and emergency care protocol for a respiratory or cardiopulmonary emergency in the pediatric patient.

38-11 Describe the presentation and emergency medical care for pediatric patients with the following conditions: altered mental status, apparent life-threatening emergencies (ALTE), drowning, fever, gastrointestinal disorders, poisoning, seizures including status epilepticus, and sudden infant death syndrome (SIDS).

38-12 Describe special considerations in the scene size-up, emergency medical care, and assisting family members in case of suspected SIDS and the importance of the presence of parents during pediatric resuscitation.

38-13 Describe special considerations in the scene size-up, emergency medical care, and reporting of suspected child abuse or neglect.

38-14 Integrate consideration of a pediatric patient's size and anatomy into the assessment of mechanisms of injury.

38-15 Explain the importance of injury prevention programs to reduce pediatric injuries and deaths.

Key Terms

apnea p. 1031
apparent life-threatening event (ALTE) p. 1031
blow-by technique p. 1011
capillary refill time p. 1015
central perfusion p. 1016
central venous line p. 1032
compensate p. 1016
cyanosis p. 1018
decompensate p. 1016
dependent lividity p. 1031
flexion p. 1019
gastrostomy tube (G-tube) p. 1033
home ventilator p. 1032
hyperextension p. 1019
mottling p. 1015
nares p. 1019
nasal flaring p. 1014
peripheral pulses p. 1016
postictal p. 1029
respiratory arrest p. 1018
respiratory distress p. 1018
respiratory failure p. 1018
retraction p. 1014
rigor mortis p. 1031
status epilepticus p. 1029
stridor p. 1014
sudden infant death syndrome (SIDS) p. 1031
tracheostomy tube p. 1032
ventriculoperitoneal (VP) shunt p. 1033
wheezing p. 1015

Introduction

Calls involving infants and children can be both intimidating and frustrating for the EMS provider. The patient's small size, limited communication skills, and fear of strangers are just some of the reasons. An additional factor that often adds to the frustration is that quite often the patient is surrounded by highly emotional or distraught parents or caregivers. You must attend to them, too.

Understanding the differences between age groups as well as behaviors common to most young children will help you interact more successfully with pediatric patients and their families. The care they require varies enormously, because a newborn baby is as different from a 12-year-old as a 7-year-old is from an adult. As pediatric patients grow up, they progress through different stages of psychological, anatomical, and physiological development. In this chapter those differences are discussed along with effective strategies for managing many of the most common emergencies.

EMERGENCY DISPATCH

"Four-fifty-three, four-five-three, I need you to respond to an emergency at the Grand Hotel downtown. Room, uh, two-twenty. This is an infant in respiratory distress."

"Show us en route." Jake, an EMT, dropped the microphone into the holder. "Oh man, why a peds call? The shift had been going so well."

"It'll be fine," Jake's partner, Jason, said. "Just stay focused."

"They're just so little, and everything's different," Jake blasted the air horn at a car that wasn't pulling off to the right. "I just don't want a little kid to die on me. I don't know how I would handle that."

Jason sighed and looked out the window as they drove through the glass canyons downtown. He occasionally caught a glimpse of his own somber face, framed by red and blue flashes, reflected from the darkened windows of shops and office buildings. Sometimes kids don't make it, though, he thought. But after a while, you do learn how to cope. That's what he's been told anyway.

The Grand Hotel was a towering structure of mirrored windows and bright lights with a marble driveway leading to a bank of huge glass entry doors. Jason and Jake rolled the cot into the lobby and were directed to a large service elevator. On the second floor, a security guard led them down a long, carpeted hall and into an open hotel room.

"Oh, thank goodness." An older woman greeted them. "My granddaughter seems to be doing better, but she was having trouble breathing and was vomiting. She was born six weeks prematurely, so we got really nervous."

A second woman in the room, the infant's mother, held the infant up so Jake could see her. The baby was tiny, maybe four pounds, and was attached to a portable monitor that beeped quietly. A feeding tube protruded from the infant's left nostril and was taped to her cheek.

"Was she just released from the hospital?" he asked.

"They released her and showed us how to feed her and kind of what to watch for on the monitor. We were afraid that something bad would happen. That's why we stayed in town at this hotel instead of heading back home."

"Well," Jake said as he prepared the car seat. "Let's get her over to Children's Hospital and find out what's going on."

TABLE 38-1 AVERAGE PEDIATRIC WEIGHTS

AGE	WEIGHT IN KILOGRAMS	WEIGHT IN POUNDS
Newborn	3.5 kg	7.7 lb
6 months	7 kg	15.4 lb
1 year	10 kg	22.0 lb
18 months	12 kg	26.4 lb
2 years	13 kg	28.6 lb
4 years	16 kg	35.2 lb
6 years	20 kg	44.0 lb
8 years	25 kg	55.0 lb
10 years	32 kg	70.4 lb
12 years	40 kg	88.0 lb
14 years	48 kg	105.6 lb

Pediatric Development

The pediatric population ranges from birth through adolescence. Generally, children are divided into five developmental categories according to age. They are:

- Newborn/infant (birth to one year old)
- Toddler (1–3 years old)
- Preschooler (3–6 years old)
- School-age (6–12 years old)
- Adolescent (12–18 years old)

The ability to estimate age and weight is important, because many of your treatment decisions will depend on those factors. Also, definitions of pediatric age categories vary depending on the context of the emergency, such as the need for CPR and an AED. Procedures will differ according to the child's anatomy. A guide to average weights commonly associated with children is offered in Table 38-1.

The kilogram is the unit of measure used to calculate the weight of the pediatric patient. Learning to estimate age and weight (and translating that weight from pounds into kilograms) will help you improve your pediatric assessment skills. To convert pounds to kilograms, divide the patient's weight in pounds by a factor of 2.2. To estimate the patient's weight in kilograms, divide the patient's weight in pounds in half and then subtract 10%.

38-4 Discuss the normal vital signs for children in various age groups.

You will find that the normal ranges for vital signs in pediatric patients are different from an adult's. That is because children are not just miniature adults. Their bodies are actively growing and developing. Children have higher metabolic rates than adults because of a hormone that stimulates growth. For normal ranges of pediatric vital signs, please refer to Table 38-2.

TABLE 38-2 RANGE OF NORMAL PEDIATRIC VITAL SIGNS

AGE	PULSE RATE (BEATS/MIN)	RESPIRATION RATE (BREATHS/MIN)	LOWER LIMIT SYSTOLIC BLOOD PRESSURE (mmHg)*
Newborn	100–160	30–60	70
6 months	110–160	24–38	71
1 year	90–150	22–30	72
3 years	80–125	22–30	76
5 years	70–115	20–24	80
10 years	60–100	16–22	90
12 years	60–100	16–22	90
14 years	60–100	14–20	90

*Upper limit systolic blood pressures and diastolic blood pressure ranges vary depending on the weight and gender of the child.

Developmental Characteristics

Children behave differently at different ages, so it is useful to know something about the stages of child development and how you may need to tailor your patient assessment for them.

38-2 Describe the major developmental characteristics and modifications of patient assessment and management techniques recommended for patients in each of the following age groups: neonates, infants, toddlers, preschoolers, school-age children, and adolescents.

38-6 Discuss special considerations for the following elements of the pediatric secondary assessment: physical exam, vital sign assessment, and history taking.

Newborns and Infants (Birth to One Year)

When approaching the newborn or infant, it is important to keep two important considerations in mind: The infant does not like to be cold, and he does not like to be separated from his parents or primary caregivers. If an infant is crying from discomfort or anxiety, your assessment will become much more difficult to perform (Figure 38-1 ▪).

It is a good idea to look at the baby closely while he is being held by a familiar caregiver. You can evaluate level of alertness, chest movement, respiratory rate, and skin color. To preserve warmth, the infant does not need to be completely undressed. Ask the caregiver to undress the infant enough to give you a good view of the chest. Warm the head of the stethoscope before applying it to the patient's chest to listen to breath sounds. If the baby is crying, allow the caregiver to attempt to comfort him with a pacifier or similar object. You also might try distracting the baby with a toy or your penlight.

If the baby needs oxygen, try having the caregiver hold the mask in front of the baby's face rather than trying to strap it on. This form of oxygen delivery is called the **blow-by technique.** It works because the oxygen flowing freely from the mask creates an oxygen-rich environment around the infant's face, allowing him to inhale the oxygen-rich air.

Lastly, be sure to run your hand over the newborn's head to check the fontanels. These are open areas in the skull where the bones have yet to fuse together. Bulging or depressed fontanels may be an indication of the patient's fluid status. Bulging fontanels indicate possible increased intracranial pressure. Sunken fontanels indicate possible dehydration.

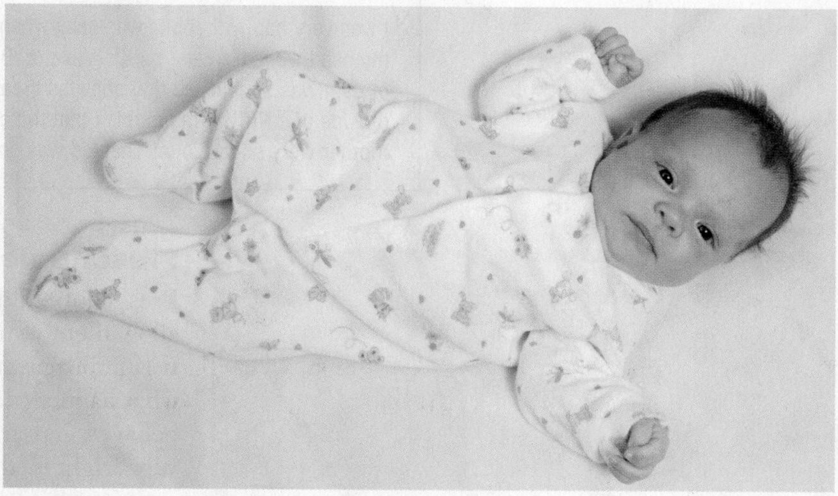

Figure 38-1 An infant.

blow-by technique providing supplemental oxygen by holding the mask or tubing near the infant or child's face if he cannot tolerate wearing a mask.

PRACTICAL PATHOPHYSIOLOGY

When an infant is born, the skull bones are not fused together, but instead are connected by fibrous membranes called *fontanels*. The fontanels allow for the newborn's head to be compressed slightly during birth. The name *fontanel* means "little fountain" because an infant's pulse can be felt flowing beneath the fontanels. Most of the smaller fontanels ossify into bone by the time the infant is one year old. However, the largest anterior fontanel is sometimes palpable up until the second birthday.

Toddlers (1–3 Years)

Typically, a toddler has developed a healthy sense of independence through walking and talking but is still unable to reason well or communicate complex ideas

Figure 38-2 A toddler.

(Figure 38-2 ■). The toddler does not like to be touched by strangers or separated from his parents. As with the infant, a good part of the assessment can be done visually while you are taking the history from the parent or caregiver. The alert child will be watching you closely.

Rather than trying to undress the toddler, listen to heart and lung sounds by pulling up his shirt and placing the head of your stethoscope underneath it. Examine the chest before the head. Use a quiet, confident, soothing voice and allow him to hold a toy or favorite object while being examined. When using a stethoscope, it may be helpful to first place it on a parent or favorite stuffed animal to show the child that it does not hurt.

The alert toddler will not tolerate an oxygen mask well, while the toddler who does not resist the mask may be seriously ill.

The toddler may interpret injury, illness, or separation from family as punishment, so he will need lots of reassurance that he is not to blame and that his parents or caregivers are with him or know where the ambulance is taking him.

PERSPECTIVE

Jake—The EMT

I was very happy that she was okay when we got there. I had all sorts of horrible scenarios in my head while we were on the elevator. But when I saw that little alert baby looking around at all of us, I was so relieved that she was breathing. It's the first time I've ever seen such a tiny baby outside of a NICU. I'm just glad that the call turned out okay. I can see why the mother and grandmother were so nervous! That kid was so cute, and so little! You should've seen her.

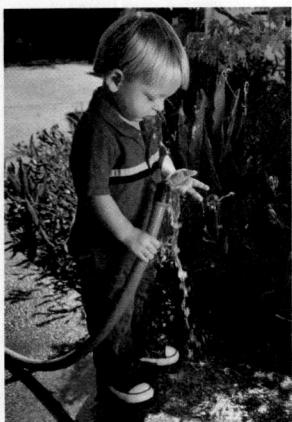

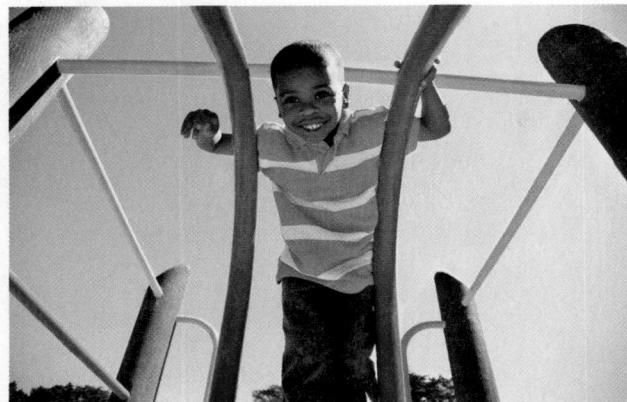

Figure 38-3 A preschooler.

Preschoolers (3–6 Years)

Preschool children have developed concrete thinking skills that allow them to understand and follow instructions (Figure 38-3 ■). It is important to ask them for their version of how they feel and what happened. Like toddlers, preschoolers may believe they misbehaved and are being punished with illness or injury. They are very frightened of potential pain, the sight of blood, and permanent injury. They need lots of reassurance and respond well to simple explanations that avoid medical or complicated terminology.

Separation causes preschoolers anxiety, so allow the parent or caregiver to hold or sit near the child as you begin your examination. In an effort to build trust, begin your examination with the extremities and then the trunk, followed by the head. The preschooler is typically quite modest, so replace items of clothing after taking them off, or allow the child to help you by having him pull up his own shirt or expose the area of injury.

School-Age Children (6–12 Years)

By the time children reach school age, they have a basic understanding of the body and its functions, and will usually try to cooperate with the physical exam (Figure 38-4 ■). They are able to communicate and understand more complex ideas. However, school-age children are very literal, so avoid using confusing language and be aware that they are listening to every word you say, even if you are not talking to them. School-age children, just like adults, are aware of and afraid of dying, pain, deformity, blood, and permanent injury. These children benefit from reassurance as well as being included in discussions involving their care.

CLINICAL CLUE

Behavior

Pay close attention to the way the child behaves and responds to your presence. A child responding inappropriately to his environment may be seriously ill. For instance, a normal six-year-old likely would be very frightened with several EMS responders showing up to care for him. A child this age who does not appear frightened or worried, but instead appears distant and disengaged from what is going on may be very ill.

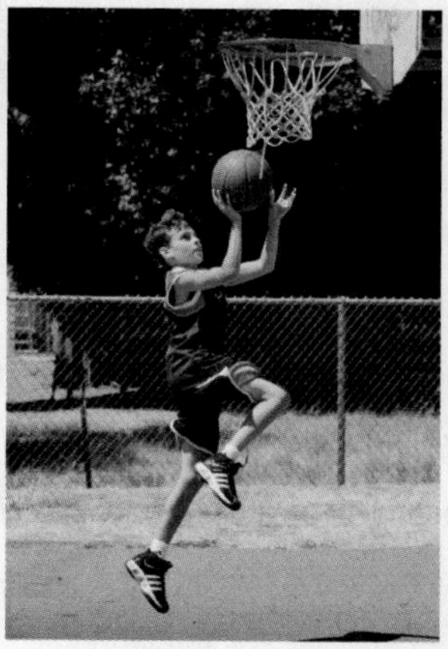

Figure 38-4 A school-age child.

Adolescents (12–18 Years)

The adolescent child has a more thorough understanding of anatomy and physiology and is able to process and express complex ideas (Figure 38-5 ■). Though adolescents are afraid of disfigurement and permanent injury, the prefrontal cortex in their brain has not fully developed, so they often believe that they are immortal or indestructible. This can lead to poor judgment and risk-taking behaviors with severe consequences.

Adolescents want to be treated as adults, but they may need the same level of support and reassurance as a younger child. By speaking to the adolescent respectfully and nonjudgmentally, you will improve your ability to obtain an accurate history. Protecting their privacy and modesty will help gain their trust. It may be helpful to interview or examine them away from parents or caregivers.

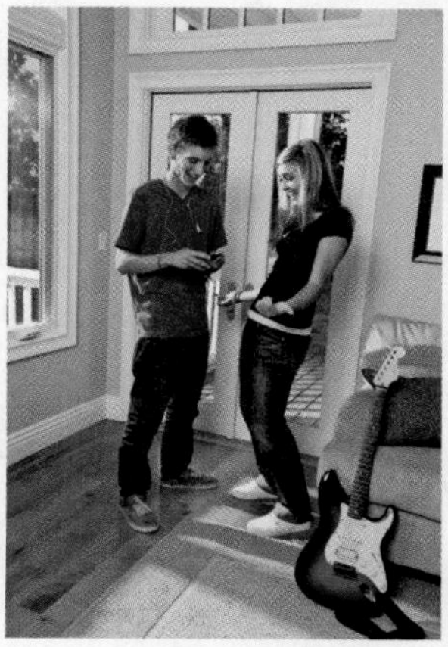

Figure 38-5 Adolescents.

PRACTICAL PATHOPHYSIOLOGY

The prefrontal cortex coordinates all the activities of the brain and allows individuals to think logically and exercise good judgment. The prefrontal cortex is often not fully developed until age 25. This means that adolescents are more likely to rely on the limbic system of their brain to make decisions. The limbic system is a more primitive emotional center linked with the flight-or-fight response, and species survival mechanisms based on pleasure such as eating and sex.

The Pediatric Airway

The most important focus of prehospital care for infants and children is airway, breathing, and oxygenation. A cardiac event in an infant or child is almost always preceded by a respiratory event such as an obstructed airway or inadequate breathing.

38-3 Describe the major anatomical and physiological differences in children with regard to the following: airway, head, chest, lungs, respiratory system, cardiovascular system, abdomen, extremities, metabolic rate, and skin and body surface area.

The head of the child is proportionately larger and heavier relative to the child's body than that of an adult, and the neck muscles are less developed. Because of those factors, the head of a supine child will likely tilt forward, possibly occluding the airway. The tongue is also larger in proportion to the lower jaw than an adult's and often falls into the oropharynx, blocking the airway. The trachea is thinner and more elastic, and can close off more easily with hyperextension of the head. Infants primarily breathe through their noses, which are easily blocked with secretions. Also, the infant and child have a higher respiratory rate and breathe mainly with their abdominal muscles, which tire quickly when stressed. All of these factors contribute to the difficulty of obtaining and maintaining an open airway and adequate breathing in the pediatric patient. Refer to Table 38-3 for additional anatomical characteristics of children.

TABLE 38-3 SPECIFIC ANATOMICAL CHARACTERISTICS OF CHILDREN

CHARACTERISTICS	SIGNIFICANCE
Infants breathe through their noses.	Secretions can cause airway obstruction.
The head is large in proportion to the body.	When the child is supine the head is flexed forward.
The tongue is large in proportion to the mouth.	The tongue can easily obstruct the airway when the child is supine.
Muscles between the ribs are immature.	Children experiencing respiratory distress tire quickly.
Abdominal breathing is common in children.	Excess gas in the stomach can impede chest expansion.
The trachea is thin and flexible.	The airway is more likely to collapse if the neck is flexed or extended.
Neck muscles are immature.	The head is more likely to flop forward.
The nose does not have much supporting cartilage.	Nasal flaring is an early indicator of respiratory distress.

Assessment of the Pediatric Patient

Environment

38-5 Describe the use of the pediatric assessment triangle (PAT) to determine a pediatric patient's status.

When responding to the scene of a pediatric emergency, carefully observe the general surroundings. Ask yourself: Is the scene safe? Is there an obvious mechanism of injury? Does the environment appear safe for a child? After ensuring your own safety and the safety of your crew, remember your role as an advocate for your patient. You have the unique opportunity to observe the child and his caregivers in the home environment and your observations can be extremely valuable to the child's physicians at the hospital and the child's future well-being.

Developed by the American Academy of Pediatrics the pediatric assessment triangle (PAT) is an important tool used to quickly prioritize and evaluate the pediatric patient. The PAT involves observing the appearance, work of breathing, and circulation to the skin of the child. Observe the child's overall appearance as you approach him. Your impression will be of a well or a sick child (Table 38-4).

Appearance

When you observe the child's appearance, ask yourself: Is the child active and attentive? Can he make eye contact? Does he respond to his parent's voice? Is he consolable or inconsolable? How is he responding to you, the stranger? How is he positioned, and how is his muscle tone? All this information gives you valuable clues about the child's mental status, possible chief complaint, and the priority of your patient (Figure 38-6 ■).

Work of Breathing

Look for symmetrical chest movement and notice if the respiratory rate appears normal, too fast, or too slow (Figure 38-7 ■). Noisy breathing, **stridor,** barking, and grunting sounds during exhalation are signs of increased work of breathing. **Retractions,** caused by immature chest wall muscles, will appear as muscles pulling in between the ribs and above the sternum with inspiration. Infants breathe mainly through their noses, and **nasal flaring** indicates increased respiratory effort. If the child is talking or crying, listen for the quality of those sounds.

stridor a harsh high-pitched sound that can occur during inhalation or exhalation, indicative of partial upper airway obstruction.

retraction muscles pulling in between the ribs and above the sternum upon inspiration.

nasal flaring the extended opening or flaring of nostrils.

TABLE 38-4 QUICK PEDIATRIC ASSESSMENT CLUES

APPEARANCE		*WORK OF BREATHING*		*CIRCULATION TO THE SKIN*	
ASSESSMENT	**INDICATION**	**ASSESSMENT**	**INDICATION**	**ASSESSMENT**	**INDICATION**
Does the child make eye contact?	Poor eye contact can indicate respiratory distress and/or shock.	Is the respiratory rate too fast?	Rapid breathing is a sign of respiratory distress.	Is the skin pink?	Pale or mottled skin can indicate shock.
Is the child afraid of strangers?	Lack of stranger anxiety is unusual in the healthy child.	Are the child's respirations noisy?	Noisy respirations indicate lower or upper respiratory obstruction.	Are the mucous membranes moist and pink?	Pale, dry mucous membranes indicate shock.
Can the child hold up his head?	Decreased muscle tone can be the result of respiratory distress and/or shock.	Is the child using accessory muscles to breathe?	Retractions and nasal flaring indicate respiratory distress.	Is the child crying tears?	Absence of tears indicates dehydration, which can lead to shock.

Begin your hands-on assessment with the chest, listening with the stethoscope for the presence or absence of breath sounds, stridor, and **wheezing.** Determine if the breath sounds are equal on both sides of the chest. Note the quality of a cough, if present, and the amount of secretions in the airway. Remember that respiratory problems are the primary cause of cardiac arrest in children.

wheezing high-pitched sounds created by air moving through narrowed air passages in the lungs.

Circulation (to the Skin)

Observe the color of the skin for paleness or **mottling,** which indicates poor circulation (Figure 38-8 ▪). Assess **capillary refill time** by squeezing the forearm or kneecap or end of a finger, fingernail, or toe until the nail bed blanches. Expect the capillary refill time to be less than two seconds centrally and peripherally in the well child. Any delay may indicate poor perfusion. At this time, you can also assess the skin temperature, color, and moisture. Capillary refill times may be delayed when the patient is cold. It also becomes a less accurate vital sign as a child ages and is considered reliable only in children younger than six years old.

mottling uneven coloration or spotting of the skin; commonly caused by poor perfusion to the skin.

capillary refill time how long it takes for the normal pink color to return after pressing on the fingernail and releasing it; normally, this takes no more than two seconds.

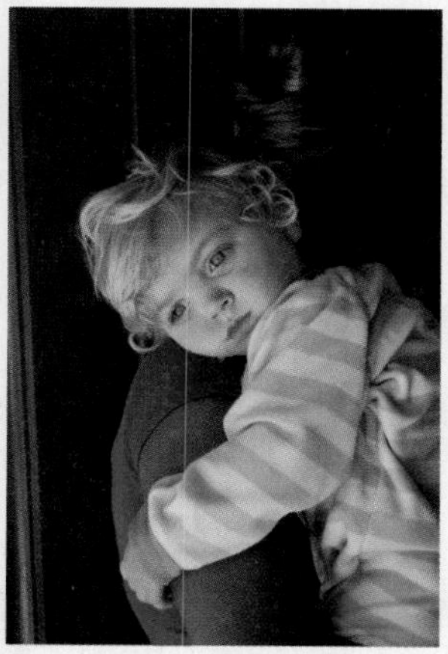

Figure 38-6 A child who is not interacting normally with his environment.

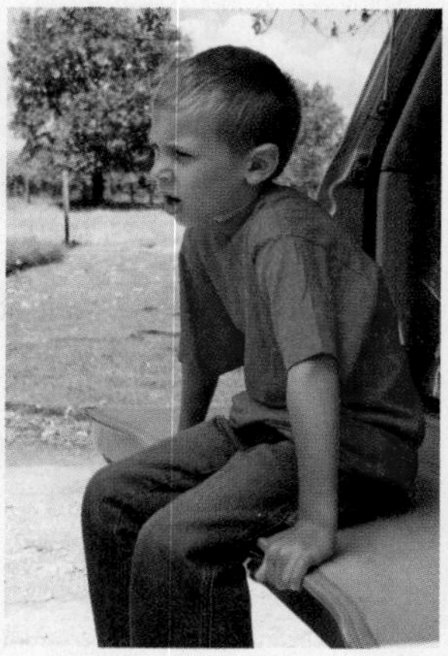

Figure 38-7 A child with an increased work of breathing.

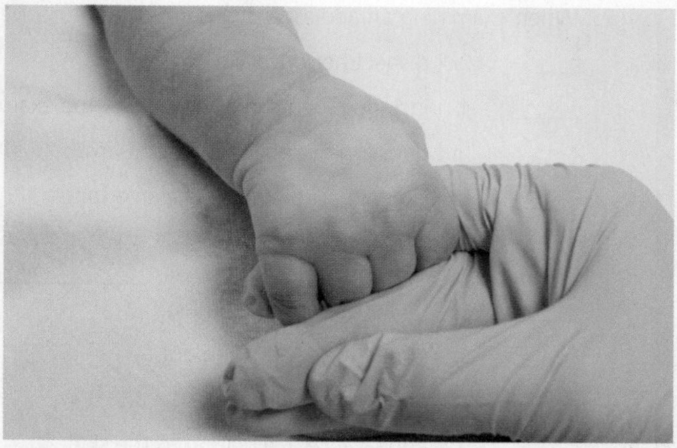

Figure 38-8 Poor capillary refill is a sign of poor perfusion.

central perfusion the supply of oxygen to and removal of wastes from central circulation, which may be assessed by palpating brachial and femoral pulses in infants and children.

peripheral pulses pulses in the distal circulation such as the radial pulse and the pedal pulse.

Assess **central perfusion** by palpating brachial and femoral pulses. In the smaller child and infant, **peripheral pulses** are more difficult to palpate. If the radial pulse is hard to find, the dorsalis pedal pulse on the top of the foot is usually easier to feel.

> **CLINICAL CLUE**
>
> **Retractions**
>
> Expose the child's bare chest to observe for retractions. The presence of retractions is a sign of increased work of breathing and may indicate significant respiratory distress.

compensate make up for a deficiency; maintain perfusion while developing shock.

decompensate become unable to compensate for low blood volume or lack of perfusion.

Blood pressures are often difficult to obtain in children under the age of three, especially if the child is fussy or crying. Therefore, your assessment of circulation must rely on mental status, the quality of pulses, and capillary refill. In children over three, be sure to use a correctly sized blood pressure cuff for the patient. It should cover approximately two-thirds of the upper arm.

Recognize that vital signs vary with age, weight, and gender in pediatric populations. It is also very important to understand that children can **compensate** for poor respirations and circulation, and vital signs may remain normal until they suddenly **decompensate** and deteriorate very quickly.

STOP, REVIEW, REMEMBER!

Multiple Choice

For each question, place a check next to the correct answer.

1. Toddlers may be intimidated if the physical exam starts with the:

_____ a. head.
_____ b. feet.
_____ c. arms.
_____ d. chest.

2. When examining an adolescent, it is important to:

_____ a. respect her privacy.
_____ b. include parents in all aspects of the exam.
_____ c. question her ability to tell the truth.
_____ d. expect her to behave like an adult.

3. The pediatric assessment triangle includes _____________, _____________, and work of breathing.

_____ a. appearance, environment
_____ b. appearance, airway
_____ c. appearance, circulation to the skin
_____ d. airway, circulation

4. If you have trouble listening to respiratory sounds because the child is talking or crying, you should:

_____ a. tell the child to be quiet.
_____ b. tell the parent to quiet the child.
_____ c. try distracting the child with a favorite toy or sound.
_____ d. place the child on your gurney, away from caregivers.

5. Children experiencing respiratory distress tire easily because they:

_____ a. eat less.
_____ b. use their abdominal muscles to breathe.
_____ c. do not sleep well.
_____ d. have a more rigid trachea.

Fill in the Blank

1. The most important focus of prehospital care for infants and children is on ______________________, ______________________, and oxygenation.

2. Brachial and femoral pulses are examples of ______________________.

3. A child's vital signs may remain within normal limits until he ______________________ and deteriorates very quickly.

Critical Thinking

1. At what age would you expect a pediatric patient to be able to give a reliable history?

____

____

____

2. How can you assess the level of responsiveness and respiratory status before you begin a hands-on exam of an infant? Of an eight-year-old?

____

____

____

____

3. How is the pediatric airway different from the adult airway?

____

____

____

____

Common Problems in Infants and Children

Respiratory Illnesses and Emergencies

Respiratory illnesses are common among pediatric patients. One of the most common causes among pediatric patients is upper respiratory infection. However, other causes include asthma, pneumonia, airway obstruction, croup, foreign body aspiration, and bronchiolitis. *The most frequent cause of cardiac arrest in children, other than trauma, is respiratory failure.* Early identification of respiratory distress and prompt treatment can avert decompensation, respiratory failure, and respiratory arrest.

TABLE 38-5 SIGNS OF RESPIRATORY DISTRESS IN CHILDREN

- Altered mental status
- Flared nostrils
- Pale or cyanotic lips or mouth
- Noisy respirations (stridor, grunting, gasping, wheezing)
- Respiratory rate greater than 60
- Retractions
- Use of abdominal muscles for breathing (seesaw breathing)
- Poor peripheral perfusion
- Decreased heart rate (a late sign of near respiratory/cardiac arrest)

38-7 Describe signs of respiratory distress, respiratory failure, and respiratory arrest in pediatric patients.

respiratory distress an abnormal physiological process (airway obstruction, asthma, pneumonia) that prevents adequate gas exchange.

respiratory failure the inability of respirations to maintain adequate oxygenation and ventilation.

respiratory arrest the absence of breathing.

cyanosis a blue or gray color resulting from lack of oxygen in the body.

Respiratory distress occurs when a child experiences an abnormal physiological process (airway obstruction, asthma, pneumonia) that prevents adequate oxygen or carbon dioxide gas exchange. That child will show signs of increased work of breathing. The increased work of breathing compensates for the inadequate gas exchange. However, as the child becomes fatigued, he will no longer be able to compensate and respiratory failure will begin very quickly (Table 38-5).

Respiratory failure occurs when the child can no longer maintain adequate oxygenation and ventilation. This may be caused by exhausted chest wall muscles or from failure of the central respiratory drive, as seen in head injury and coma patients. Successful intervention before respiratory distress develops into respiratory failure prevents respiratory arrest.

Respiratory arrest is the absence of breathing. If adequate ventilation and oxygenation are not restored, respiratory arrest will rapidly progress to full cardiopulmonary arrest. Survival rates following a full cardiac arrest in children are very low.

It is very important to differentiate between respiratory distress caused by airway disease and respiratory distress caused by airway obstruction, because management priorities are different. The patient with an upper airway obstruction may have stridor on inspiration or, in the case of complete obstruction, **cyanosis** plus no crying, speaking, or coughing. The patient with lower airway disease may have wheezing and prolonged, labored exhalations with a rapid respiratory rate and no stridor.

The child experiencing respiratory distress will be breathing rapidly and have increased work of breathing. The child may have obvious retractions in the chest wall and above the sternum, or in younger children, may be using the diaphragm to assist chest expansion. If the child is compensating well, the skin may still be pink, and the child is alert but not active. The child may have assumed a position that best supports his respiratory efforts, such as the tripod position (leaning forward, hands on knees) or the sniffing position (chin raised or thrust forward).

As respiratory distress progresses to respiratory failure, the child's mental status will decrease and he will seem distant, making poor eye contact with parents or caregivers, and will eventually stop responding to voice. The child will become pale, cyanotic, and floppy, with a delayed capillary refill time and weak pulses. You may hear audible grunting with exhalation. The child will appear visibly fatigued, and the infant may have a pronounced head bobbing with respiration. Without immediate intervention, this patient will progress to respiratory failure, become unresponsive and limp, and his heart rate will begin to decrease. Without immediate support of ventilations, he eventually will slip into cardiac arrest.

CLINICAL CLUE

From the Door

It is said you can assess a pediatric patient "from the door" as you approach. Observe whether the child is active or limp, how he responds to parents and strangers, and whether or not he has an increased work of breathing. The patient's color can tell you that he is unstable before you get to him. If you see signs the pediatric patient is unstable, prepare to provide aggressive airway care and oxygenation, transport promptly, and call ALS if available.

It is critical to ensure an open airway and adequate breathing because respiratory failure can rapidly lead to cardiac arrest in pediatric patients. Techniques for opening airways include manually opening the airway, suctioning fluid from the airway, using airway adjuncts to maintain an open airway, and maneuvers for clearing a foreign body airway obstruction. Procedures for ensuring adequate breathing include administering oxygen and assisting with or artificially ventilating the patient. Children are also more prone to specific respiratory emergencies such as asthma, pneumonia, croup, bronchiolitis, and epiglottitis.

38-8 Discuss the guidelines for emergency care of respiratory emergencies and foreign body airway obstruction.

Airway Management

The first priority of airway management is maintaining an open airway. For infants and children, the head-tilt/chin-lift maneuver should be modified slightly so that the airway can be neutrally aligned. Because of the relatively soft and collapsible larynx and trachea, the modified maneuver will avoid **hyperextension** or **flexion** of the neck. The position can be maintained by placing a small folded towel under the patient's shoulders. As the age of the child increases, slight extension of the neck may be helpful. (Note the difference in the child's position with and without the towel in Figure 38-9 ■.)

hyperextension extreme or abnormal extension or increase in the angle between bones of a joint; tilting the head backward.

flexion decrease in the angle between the bones forming a joint; tilting the head forward.

If there are secretions or vomit in the airway, the patient needs to be suctioned. A flexible bulb-type suction device is preferred when suctioning the nose and mouth of an infant. To suction, deflate the bulb prior to inserting it into the infant's nose. Once inserted, release the bulb to initiate gentle suction. For larger children, use a thin flexible plastic catheter to suction thin secretions in the nose, inserting the catheter tip just inside the **nares.** A large-bore, rigid plastic catheter is better for removing thick secretions such as vomit from the mouth. Administer supplemental oxygen prior to suctioning and only suction as long as necessary to clear the airway and no longer than 10 seconds before reapplying oxygen. Do not allow the tip of the suction catheter to touch the back of the throat, because it can stimulate the vagus nerve and slow the heart rate or cause soft-tissue injury.

nares external openings in the nasal cavity; nostrils.

When the airway becomes partially obstructed by foreign material or secretions, some air can move past the obstruction, making respirations noisy. The child also may demonstrate increased work of breathing, including retractions around the ribs and sternum, but still be alert with pink mucous membranes and skin. This child should be allowed to assume a position of comfort, which will likely be sitting up. Try not to upset the child, because anxiety and crying can worsen the airway obstruction. Allow the child to sit with a parent or familiar care provider

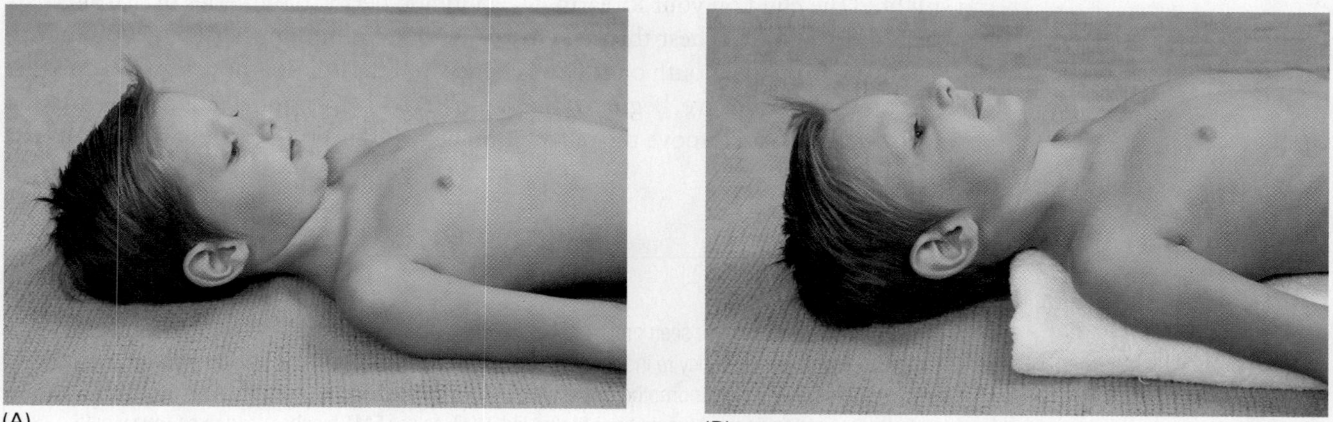

(A) (B)

Figure 38-9 (A) When an infant or young child is placed in a supine position, the head will naturally flex forward contributing to airway compromise. (B) Place a folded towel or similar object under the shoulders to maintain a neutral airway.

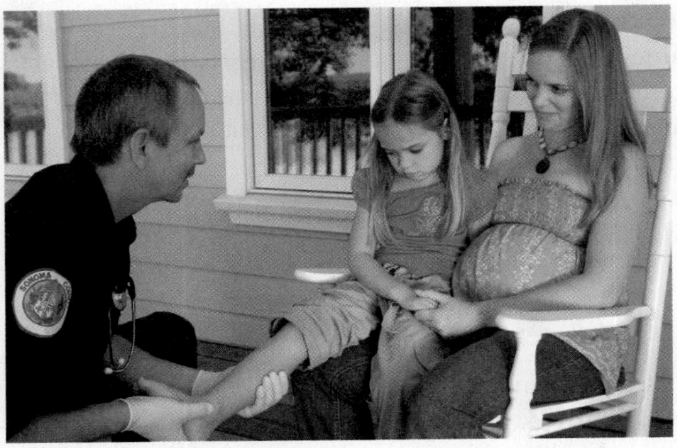

Figure 38-10 If practical, allow the child to remain in a parent's arms during the assessment.

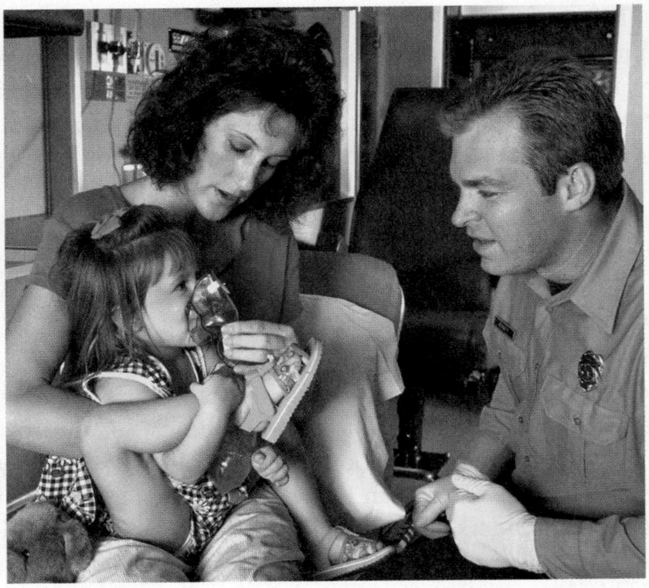

Figure 38-11 When practical, allow the parent to assist with care of a child.

(Figure 38-10 ▪). Provide supplemental oxygen with a nonrebreather mask or by using the blow-by technique. When possible, allow the parent or caregiver to hold the oxygen device (Figure 38-11 ▪).

In the event of partial or complete obstruction of the airway and the patient is not speaking or crying, or has an ineffective cough, altered mental status, or respiratory arrest, the obstruction must be removed. If after opening the airway, ventilation is ineffective or impossible, you must take action to clear the airway.

In responsive infants clearing the airway is done by delivering five back slaps followed by five chest thrusts. If a foreign object is visible, a finger sweep may be used to remove it, but do not perform blind finger sweeps because they could force an object further into the airway. The back slaps are alternated with the chest thrusts, five times each, until the object is cleared. If the object is not cleared before the infant becomes unresponsive, begin to perform CPR with one modification: look into the airway to see if you can remove the obstruction before delivering each set of ventilations.

In responsive children age one year to adolescence, position appropriately according to their size and perform airway clearing techniques similar to the adult. Perform abdominal thrusts as you would on an adult if the child is large enough. Otherwise, if you can still hold the child on your forearm like an infant, perform the series of five alternating back blows and five chest thrusts. Do not perform blind finger sweeps. Attempt to clear an object from the mouth only if you can see it. If the object is not cleared before the child becomes unresponsive, begin to perform CPR with one modification: look into the airway to see if you can remove the obstruction before delivering each set of ventilations.

PERSPECTIVE

Jason—The EMT

Man, that was a tiny baby! I've seen preemies before when we transfer them from the helicopter to the emergency department and they're in those big traveling incubators. I've never seen one out of the medical setting. That mom and grandmother must have been so scared. Heck, I was scared. I don't think that any of our neonate equipment would have fit that kid. Well, as my EMT teacher used to say, we would have had to "improvise, adapt, and overcome." Working on an ambulance makes you good at that.

Airway Adjuncts

An oropharyngeal airway (OPA) or nasopharyngeal airway (NPA) helps maintain an open airway in the child who has adequate respiratory drive but is unable to maintain his own airway. As in adults, an OPA is used for the child who is unresponsive and has no gag reflex. Unlike the method used for adults, the pediatric OPA is inserted without rotation. To choose the correct size, measure from the corner of the mouth to the tip of the earlobe. A tongue depressor inserted to the back of the tongue with downward pressure may be used to control the tongue while inserting the airway.

The nasopharyngeal airway (NPA) may be used in the responsive child who cannot maintain an open airway. Choose an NPA whose lumen diameter is slightly smaller than the child's nares. The child who is developmentally appropriate for his age and who tolerates an NPA is a very sick child. Follow these steps for insertion of an OPA:

1. Take appropriate BSI precautions.
2. Measure the OPA for the appropriate size (corner of mouth to tip of earlobe).
3. Using a tongue depressor or similar tool, place downward pressure on the tongue while directly inserting the OPA.
4. Make certain that the flange of the OPA remains visible outside the patient's lips.

Follow these steps for insertion of an NPA:

1. Take appropriate BSI precautions.
2. Measure the NPA for the appropriate size (tip of the nose to the tip of the earlobe). Also confirm that the diameter is appropriate.
3. Lubricate the NPA before gently inserting it into the child's nose.
4. Make certain that the bevel faces medially and the flange of the NPA remains visible outside the patient's nose.

Remember that NPAs should not be used if the patient has sustained severe facial trauma. In addition, ensure a properly sized adjunct. An adjunct that is too small may not provide an open airway and one that is too large may become an obstruction. An NPA can easily become obstructed by secretions. Be prepared to suction it as needed if secretions are present.

Oxygen Therapy

Hypoxia can quickly lead to a slowed heart rate (bradycardia) or altered mental status in the pediatric patient. Any infant or child showing signs of respiratory distress, inadequate respirations, or is exhibiting signs of shock should receive supplemental oxygen. Any infant or child with bradycardia should also receive supplemental oxygen. This can be delivered by way of a nonrebreather mask, using the blow-by technique, or by nasal cannula.

Remember that infants breathe primarily through their noses. Placing a nasal cannula without oxygen flowing will severely restrict the flow of air breathed in by the patient. Oxygen should be administered at 2 to 6 liters per minute through the nasal cannula (Figure 38-12 ■).

The nonrebreather mask provides a higher concentration of oxygen than the cannula. If he will tolerate it, it should be used for the infant or child who is showing signs of respiratory distress. Oxygen should be administered at 10 to 15 liters per minute. Unfortunately, most babies and young children are afraid or intolerant of the mask. As noted earlier, they can receive oxygen by way of the blow-by technique. Use oxygen tubing and hold the end of the tubing close to the patient's face (about two inches) or disguise the end of the tubing with a favorite toy or by running it through the bottom of a paper cup. Have the caregiver or parent hold the object and follow the face as it turns so the child gets as much oxygen as possible.

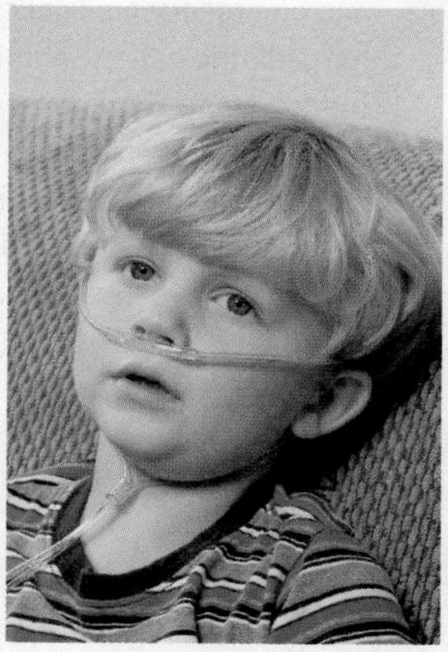

Figure 38-12 A child receiving supplemental oxygen by way of a nasal cannula.

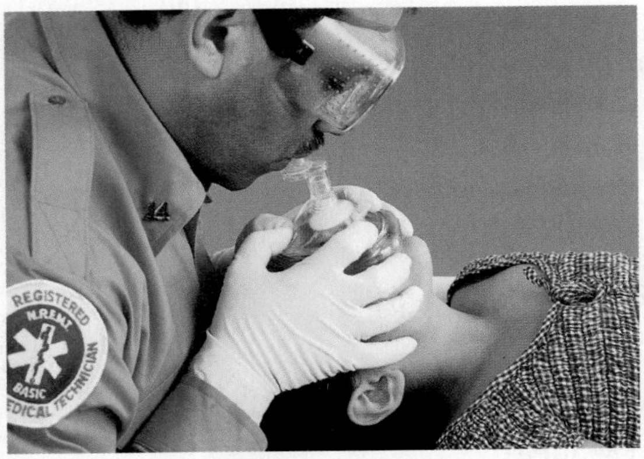

Figure 38-13 When assisting with ventilations, ensure a good mask seal and keep the head in a neutral position. Watch the chest for rise with each breath.

If the patient is receiving supplemental oxygen and remains cyanotic with an altered mental status, has poor muscle tone, or an inadequate respiratory rate, you will need to assist ventilations.

Assisted Ventilations

The presence of cyanosis, altered mental status, severe respiratory distress, respiratory failure, or respiratory arrest in an infant or child means that assisted ventilations are required. Remember, prior to beginning ventilations for infants and children, make sure the airway remains in a relatively neutral position by not flexing or hyperextending the neck. An older child may require some extension of the neck for optimal ventilation. Choose a mask for the patient that will seal well over the mouth and nose. Use a pediatric-size resuscitation bag for smaller children (younger than eight years of age) to avoid overinflating the lungs. If the patient is a victim of trauma, maintain cervical-spine precautions.

One or two hands may be used to maintain an airtight seal of the mask on the child's face (Figure 38-13 ■). Using two hands will seal the mask more tightly but requires a second person to deliver ventilations. The one-hand technique can be used by a single rescuer. In either case, avoid pressing on the neck with your fingers, which can occlude the airway. Squeeze the bag-mask device slowly and evenly over one second, so the chest rises adequately, but avoid hyperinflation. The best rate of ventilation is one breath every three to five seconds (20/min for infants and 12/min for children). Younger children require more frequent ventilations and older children can be ventilated less frequently. Whenever possible, use a bag-mask device with a reservoir that can be attached to supplemental oxygen.

You also can deliver ventilations by way of a pocket face mask with a one-way valve. Maintain a good seal with the mask and use enough air to make the chest rise adequately.

PRACTICAL PATHOPHYSIOLOGY

Children have high metabolic rates because of the hormones that stimulate growth. Their cells, compared to an adult's, demand more oxygen, which depletes the oxygen bound to hemoglobin much faster and they begin to suffer from hypoxia much sooner. This makes children especially susceptible to oxygen deprivation.

Specific Respiratory Emergencies

38-9 Describe the presentation and emergency medical care for pediatric patients with the following conditions: asthma, bronchiolitis, cardiac arrest, congenital heart disease, epiglottitis, pneumonia, and shock (hyperperfusion).

ASTHMA

Asthma is a disease characterized by chronic swelling and inflammation of the airways. Asthmatic triggers can lead to acute attacks characterized by bronchospasms that narrow the airways, causing respiratory distress. Asthma in children is frequently associated with allergic triggers. Other triggers include changes in weather, chemicals, exercise, strong emotions, smoke, and the common cold. Asthma is so common in children that it is the leading cause of school absences and pediatric hospitalizations. The most common symptom of asthma is shortness of breath, but other signs and symptoms may include tightness in the chest, wheezing, and coughing, especially at night.

PNEUMONIA

Pneumonia is an inflammation of the lungs most commonly caused by an infection. Viruses are the most common cause of pneumonia in infants and children. Signs and symptoms include fever, cough (which can produce green, yellow, or bloody mucus), respiratory distress, and sharp, stabbing chest pain with each breath. Lung sounds may be diminished on the affected side and crackles are common.

CROUP

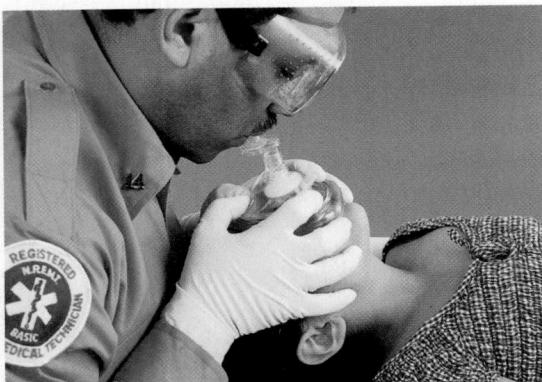

Croup is an inflammation of the throat caused by a viral infection. It is characterized by the classic "barking seal" noises the child makes while coughing. The illness tends to affect younger children under the age of five and occur during winter months. Croup is caused when an underlying viral infection causes the trachea just beneath the larynx to swell.

BRONCHIOLITIS

Bronchiolitis is the swelling and mucus buildup in the bronchioles of children under two years of age. It is most common in infants under the age of six months. Respiratory syncytial virus (RSV) is the most common cause. The illness occurs more frequently during the winter months and in premature infants or infants who are not breastfed. Bronchiolitis is characterized by a tight wheezy cough. Severe signs include cyanosis, tachypnea, nasal flaring, retractions, and fever.

EPIGLOTTITIS

Epiglottitis is an acute life-threatening disease that is characterized by the swelling and inflammation of the epiglottis. The epiglottis is the cartilage that covers the trachea when a person swallows to prevent food and liquids from entering the lungs. Epiglottitis is life threatening because the swelling of the epiglottis can be so severe that it blocks the airway completely. The disease tends to affect younger children between the ages of two and six. Initial symptoms are a high fever and sore throat. Symptoms progress to drooling, difficulty swallowing, and respiratory distress. Childhood immunizations against *Haemophilus influenza* Type B, the bacteria that causes most cases of epiglottitis, have significantly reduced the incidence of this disease, making pediatric epiglottitis now a rare disease in the United States.

Emergency Medical Care

Follow these general guidelines when caring for a pediatric patient with a respiratory emergency:

1. Take appropriate BSI precautions.
2. Perform an immediate primary assessment and ensure that the ABCs are adequate.
3. Provide supplemental oxygen as appropriate. Remember that the patient may be frightened of the device, so have a familiar caregiver hold it or consider blow-by oxygen.
4. Suction as necessary to maintain a patent airway.
5. If epiglottitis is suspected, do not insert anything into the mouth that may irritate soft tissue and cause more swelling.
6. Perform a secondary assessment.
7. Allow the patient to maintain a position of comfort.
8. Expedite transport and consider the need for an ALS intercept.

Cardiac Illnesses and Emergencies

The cardiovascular system of infants and children is extremely sensitive to hypoxia. As an infant or child becomes hypoxic, the heart rate will slow (bradycardia) and eventually stop. Infants and children who are bradycardic due to hypoxia are very responsive to interventions to improve their oxygenation and have a high survival rate. Infants and children who progress into cardiac arrest have a very poor prognosis, so it is imperative that interventions to improve oxygenation are administered before the patient's condition deteriorates into cardiac arrest.

Congenital Heart Disease

Congenital heart disease is a type of birth defect involving the structure or functioning of the heart. There are two types of congenital heart disease: cyanotic and noncyanotic. Congenital heart disease causes more deaths in infants than any other birth defect.

Signs vary widely depending on the particular condition, but may include shortness of breath, tachypnea, tachycardia, syncope, cyanosis, lethargy, or poor feeding habits. It is important to keep in mind that many infants born with congenital heart disease lead a long and healthy life, if provided with proper care and treatment early in life.

If you suspect or are informed that an infant or child has congenital heart disease, expedite transport and consider an ALS rendezvous. Include the caregiver in the treatment of the patient, because they likely are an expert on their child's condition and should know what is normal and what symptoms are of particular concern. Do not delay transport to complete a secondary assessment on scene, but complete the exam on the way to the hospital. Deliver supplemental oxygen by nonrebreather mask and be prepared to assist respirations or perform cardiopulmonary resuscitation.

Shock

38-10 Explain the assessment steps and emergency care protocol for a respiratory or cardiopulmonary emergency in the pediatric patient.

It is critical to ensure that children who are exhibiting signs and symptoms of shock are treated aggressively. Once children progress from compensated shock into decompensated shock, they are likely to progress into irreversible shock and then cardiac arrest. Pediatric survival rates from cardiac arrest are low, whereas survival rates from successful interventions during compensated shock are high.

Some of the common causes of shock or hypoperfusion in children are vomiting and diarrhea, infection, trauma, and blood loss. Less often, shock may be caused by allergic reactions or poisoning. In infants and children the presence of shock is very rarely cardiac in origin. On occasion, you may encounter children born with congenital heart disease who present with the signs and symptoms of shock.

The signs and symptoms of shock in infants and children are similar to those of adults (Table 38-6). Some of the most important questions to ask the caregivers of the infant or child are whether the child has had vomiting or diarrhea and how frequently they have changed wet diapers. In the early stages of shock, the child is inactive and floppy, or loses muscle tone. The child may have no tears when he cries and appears pale. As shock progresses, the child's mental status further deteriorates. The skin becomes cool and moist, and it may be pale or mottled. The child has a rapid heart rate, peripheral pulses are difficult to palpate and may be absent, and capillary refill is delayed.

TABLE 38-6 SIGNS AND SYMPTOMS OF SHOCK

- Rapid heart rate
- Rapid respiratory rate
- Cool extremities
- Pale skin, dry mucous membranes
- Delayed capillary refill time
- Weak central pulses
- Weak or absent distal pulses
- Altered mental status

The child who has deteriorated to late shock is a very sick child and needs to be transported immediately. Children compensate in the early stages of shock by maintaining their heart rate and blood pressure. If shock is allowed to progress without intervention, children can deteriorate very quickly.

PRACTICAL PATHOPHYSIOLOGY

In response to shock, the body activates several compensatory mechanisms, such as the sympathetic nervous system increasing the heart rate and systemic vascular resistance. Children are especially effective at maintaining vascular resistance despite low blood volumes. Often children are able to maintain a normal systolic blood pressure well into severe shock. In children it is important to look for other signs of shock such as cold and mottled extremities, delayed capillary refill, and tachycardia.

If you suspect shock in an infant or child, expedite transport and consider an ALS rendezvous. Do not delay to complete a secondary assessment on scene. Instead complete the exam on the way to the hospital. Control any obvious bleeding. Deliver supplemental oxygen by nonrebreather mask and be prepared to assist respirations. Keep the patient warm by turning up the heat in the ambulance and using blankets.

Cardiac Arrest

When you encounter an unresponsive infant or child, first check to see if the patient has a pulse. Check for 5 to 10 seconds on the brachial artery in infants and younger children and on the carotid artery in older children. If you do not feel a pulse or are unsure, then you must begin chest compressions immediately while your partner attaches the AED to the patient. As soon as the AED pads are attached to the patient, turn the AED on and initiate the analysis sequence. Follow the AED's instructions as to whether or not to shock the patient. Then resume chest compressions immediately.

When the patient is under eight years of age, a pediatric-capable AED should be used if at all possible. If a pediatric-capable AED is not available, adult AED pads can be used on an infant or child, but should be placed on the front and back of the torso to avoid short-circuiting between the pads.

When only one rescuer is available for infant CPR, the rescuer should use two fingers to administer chest compressions in the center of the chest, just below the nipple line. When two rescuers are available, one of the rescuers can wrap fingers around the back of the infant's torso and use both thumbs to deliver chest compressions. For child CPR, most rescuers use only one hand to perform chest compressions on the lower half of the sternum. For both infants and children, chest compressions should achieve a depth of approximately one-third of the patient's chest thickness.

Cardiac arrest in infants and children is usually secondary to respiratory failure, so it is important to ensure that an adequate airway is established and that properly oxygenated breaths are delivered during CPR. Due to the importance of oxygenation, when two rescuers are available, the ratio of compressions to breaths changes from 30:2 to 15:2 for both infants and children up until the age of puberty.

STOP, REVIEW, REMEMBER!

Multiple Choice

For each question, place a check next to the correct answer.

1. The first priority of care for the child in respiratory distress is:

____ a. maintaining an open airway.

____ b. oxygen by way of nasal cannula.

____ c. removing the child from the caregiver.

____ d. keeping the child warm.

2. Signs of compensated shock in an infant or child include:

____ a. slow respiratory rate.

____ b. slow heart rate.

____ c. normal mental status.

____ d. increased heart rate.

3. Which one of the following children is in shock?

____ a. Child who clings to her mother and cries tears

____ b. Child with a high fever who is sucking on his bottle

____ c. Child who is limp and pale with mottled extremities

____ d. Screaming child with a laceration to the forehead

4. The nasal cannula should be used when:

____ a. the blow-by technique is used.

____ b. a nonrebreather mask is not available.

____ c. the pediatric patient will not tolerate a mask.

____ d. the pediatric patient will not breathe through his mouth.

(continued on next page)

(continued)

Critical Thinking

1. How can you assess the respiratory rate of a crying child?

2. What kinds of distracting techniques could you use to calm the crying child in order to assess breath sounds?

3. Determine the best mode of oxygen delivery for each of the following patients:

   a. Alert one-month-old with retractions but good perfusion

   b. Wheezing eight-year-old who can only speak in short sentences

   c. Six-year-old who fell out of a tree and is not breathing, after the airway is opened while the spine is immobilized

   d. Quiet toddler with decreased lung sounds, fever, and coughing

Trauma

38-14 Integrate consideration of a pediatric patient's size and anatomy into the assessment of mechanisms of injury.

Traumatic injury is the number-one cause of death for infants and children. Most of those deaths are the result of blunt trauma. Motor-vehicle collisions are the most common cause of blunt trauma in children. Some aspects of motor-vehicle collisions are different for infants and children than they are for adults. Children are always passengers, and they may or may not be properly restrained. The unrestrained child will most likely sustain head and neck injuries because of the relative heaviness of the head and weakness of the neck muscles. The restrained child may sustain injury to the abdomen and lower spine, because their abdominal musculature is weak and underdeveloped.

Another common cause of traumatic injury in children is in a motor-vehicle versus bicycle incident, resulting in head, spine, and abdominal injuries (Figure 38-14 ■). In addition, children may be unaware of oncoming traffic and are difficult to see because of their size, resulting in pedestrian versus vehicle collisions. Usually, the bumper of the car will impact the legs of the older child, who will then be thrown onto the hood or windshield, striking the chest or abdomen, and then off the car onto the roadway, often striking the head on the ground. In toddlers, the bumper will likely impact the chest, head, or neck area. Abdominal, head, upper leg, and pelvic injuries occur frequently in these scenarios. Children who are struck by a moving vehicle are more likely to be forced downward and beneath the vehicle, causing additional injuries.

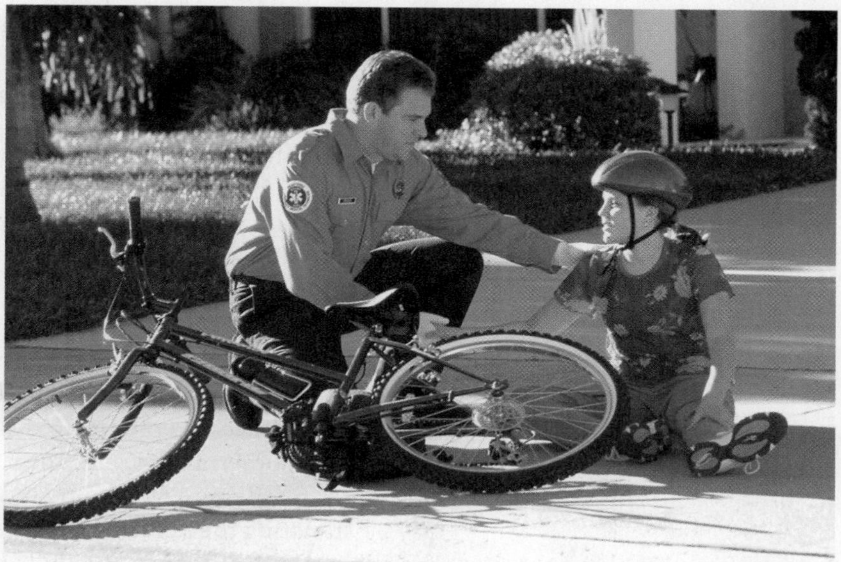

Figure 38-14 Incidents involving bicycles account for a large number of injuries in children.

Other causes of traumatic injury in infants and children include falls from a height or diving into shallow water, burns, sports injuries, and abuse.

Head Injuries

Children have proportionally larger and heavier heads than those of adults. Their neck muscles are weaker, too, which makes these areas of the body extremely vulnerable to traumatic injury. Care of the child who has sustained a head injury starts with securing an open airway. The most common cause of hypoxia in the head-injured patient is the tongue obstructing the airway. Injury to the head can result in respiratory failure and respiratory arrest that may be delayed and occur during transport. Nausea and vomiting are common signs of head injury. If the child has sustained significant blunt force to the head, other injuries are often present, including cervical-spine and internal injuries that could result in shock. Secondary injuries should always be considered in the child presenting with head injury and shock.

Chest Injuries

The ribs of children are less developed and more pliable, meaning they can bend farther than the ribs of an adult can before breaking. Because of this, there may be significant internal injury without obvious external signs, such as bruising or deformity.

Abdominal Injuries

Abdominal injuries are more common in infants and children than in adults. The abdominal muscles of infants and children are weaker, and the internal abdominal organs are less securely anchored. It may be very difficult to detect abdominal injury, especially in the crying child, but abdominal injury must be suspected in the trauma patient who is deteriorating without outward signs of injury.

It is important to remember that air can accumulate in the stomach during assisted ventilation, and air in the stomach can restrict normal ventilations. This can be avoided by maintaining an open airway, using a properly sized bag-mask device, and administering each ventilation slowly over one second.

Extremity Injuries

Isolated limb injuries may occur more frequently in the pediatric population because younger children are still developing their motor skills and older children participate in sporting activities. Isolated extremity injuries are rarely life threatening and should be managed in the same manner as for adults.

Burn Injuries

Your first priority in a pediatric burn patient is to establish an open airway and ensure adequate respirations are present. The burn patient of any age is always at risk for hypothermia because of impaired skin integrity and exposure. Children are more at risk for hypothermia because they have a larger exposed body surface area to body weight ratio. Be sure to keep them warm.

Estimating the percent of body surface area (BSA) burned in children and infants is slightly different than in adults because of their relatively large head and chest. Burns should be loosely covered with dry sterile gauze or a sterile sheet, preferably a nonsticking burn sheet. Candidates for burn centers should be identified according to local protocol.

38-15 Explain the importance of injury prevention programs to reduce pediatric injuries and deaths.

38-11 Describe the presentation and emergency medical care for pediatric patients with the following conditions: altered mental status, apparent life-threatening emergencies (ALTE), drowning, fever, gastrointestinal disorders, poisoning, seizures including status epilepticus, and sudden infant death syndrome (SIDS).

Emergency Medical Care

As with every patient, the traumatically injured infant or child requires an open and protected airway. Open the airway while maintaining cervical-spine immobilization. Be prepared to assist in protecting the airway by suctioning. Provide oxygen and use the bag-mask device to assist ventilations in the patient experiencing respiratory distress, respiratory failure, or respiratory arrest. Secure the patient to a backboard for spinal immobilization. Transport immediately to the most appropriate facility.

Pediatric Injury Prevention Programs

Countless children are severely injured in preventable accidents each year. The major cause is motor-vehicle collisions. Often children are not properly restrained in a correctly sized and secured child safety or booster seat. Educational programs can teach parents how to properly restrain children in motor vehicles and reduce the chances of injury. This is just one example of how injury prevention programs can save children's lives.

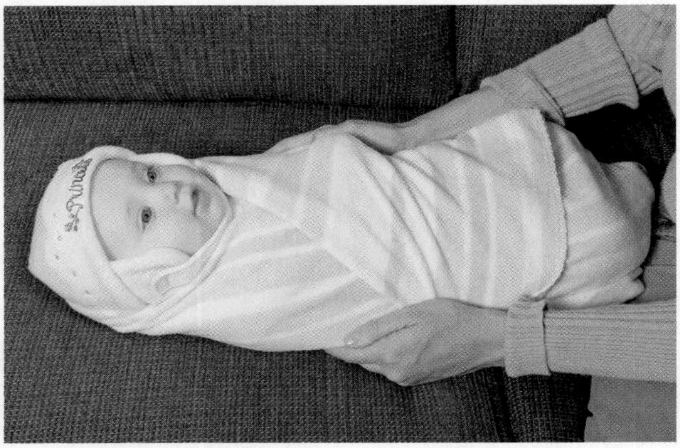

Figure 38-15 Standard care for an infant or small child includes keeping them warm.

Other Pediatric Emergencies

Hypothermia

The pediatric patient has a larger exposed body surface area to body weight ratio than that of an adult. Infants lack the kind of fat the adult body uses for insulation. Infants and children also have smaller stores of glucose in their bodies. Because of these differences, pediatric patients are more affected by environmental conditions, especially cold. Hypothermia decreases perfusion and increases glucose consumption, resulting in decreased blood sugar. It is always important to keep these patients warm (Figure 38-15 ■).

For infants, much of their heat is lost through the head, so using a cap or a blanket around the top of the head will help keep them warm. Exposing each area of the body such as the chest or a limb one at a time and replacing clothing or covering before exposing another area also can conserve heat. In the ambulance, turning on the heater will improve ambient temperatures. The child with a fever should not be subjected to aggressive cooling techniques that will cause further physiological stress and increased glucose consumption, but instead should be passively cooled by removing excess blankets and warm clothing.

Seizures

Seizures may be caused by infections, poisoning, hypoglycemia, hypoxia, or head trauma. By far the most common cause of seizures in infants and children is a sudden rise in core temperature associated with a viral illness. These are commonly referred to as *febrile seizures.* Many other children suffer from chronic seizure disorders controlled by medications that need to be constantly adjusted as they grow. When these children have seizures, it is rarely life threatening. Nonetheless, seizures in children, including febrile seizures and seizures in the chronic seizure patient, should be taken seriously.

Usually, the seizure will have stopped by the time the EMT arrives, and the patient may show typical **postictal** signs, such as decreased respiratory rate and altered mental status. Sometimes the seizures will not have stopped when you arrive on the scene and the patient may be in a state of prolonged or clustered seizures known as **status epilepticus.**

postictal recovery period after a seizure during which the patient may exhibit decreased respirations and altered mental status.

status epilepticus a prolonged seizure or cluster of seizures usually lasting longer than five minutes.

As you approach the patient, ask the caregiver how many seizures the child had, how long each lasted, and what part of the body, if any, was convulsing. Ask the caregiver if the child has a recent history of fever. If the child has a chronic seizure disorder, ask what medications the child takes. Assess the child for the presence of injuries that may have occurred during a seizure.

Treatment of the seizure patient is similar in adults and children: Maintain a patent airway, protect the cervical spine as necessary, provide oxygen and, if needed, provide assisted ventilations once the convulsions have ended. Be prepared with suction in case the child vomits. All infants and children who have had a seizure with no prior history require medical evaluation and should be transported to an appropriate facility.

Altered Mental Status

Many conditions, including hypoglycemia, poisoning, seizure, infection, head trauma, hypoxia, shock, and fatigue can result in an altered mental status in the infant or child. It is very important to try to discover the underlying cause. However, this should not delay the prompt delivery of appropriate care.

Position the patient to optimize airway management and provide supplemental oxygen. Be prepared to suction and provide assisted ventilations as necessary. Perform a thorough secondary assessment and obtain a complete medical history. It is important to determine what the child's normal mental status is in order to understand how altered he may be. Any child with an altered mental status should be transported to the hospital.

Poisoning

Accidental ingestion of a poison is a common reason for ambulance calls for infants and children (Figure 38-16 ■). Children are notoriously poor historians, but you may be able to discover the suspected substance and its container, which you should bring to the receiving facility whenever possible.

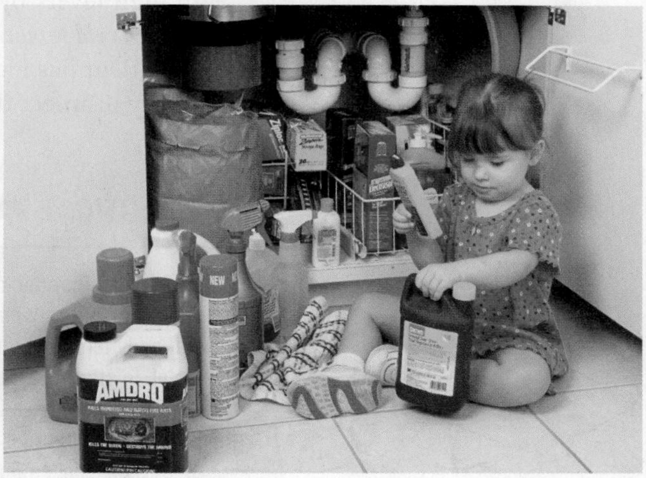

Figure 38-16 Keep potential sources of poisoning out of reach of small children.

Position the patient to optimize airway management and provide supplemental oxygen. Administer oxygen and transport while continuing to observe the patient closely for changes. Your EMS system may require you to contact a poison control center or medical direction when treating poisoned patients. If the patient is unresponsive, maintain a patent airway, provide oxygen, be prepared to suction and provide assisted ventilations, and attempt to rule out the possibility of trauma. Perform a thorough secondary assessment and obtain a complete medical history en route to the hospital.

Gastrointestinal Disorders

One of the most serious gastrointestinal problems you will encounter with infants and children is vomiting and diarrhea, which if not treated promptly will lead to dehydration and more serious complications such as shock. Gastroesophageal reflux disease (GERD) can occur in both infants and children. Signs and symptoms include abdominal pain, chest pain, or even asthma-like respiratory problems. Constipation is another problem that can occur in both infants and children. The major symptom is usually abdominal pain.

Emergency medical care consists of maintaining a patent airway, being prepared to suction and provide assisted ventilations, and transporting any infant or child presenting with signs or symptoms of gastrointestinal disorders for further evaluation.

Fever

Another common reason for ambulance calls in the pediatric population is complaint of fever. This is very seldom life threatening, although the underlying disease process causing the fever could be serious. Serious pediatric infections that cause fevers include pneumonia, kidney infections, and the most serious of all, meningitis. Meningitis is an infection of the brain and spinal cord that presents as fever, stiff neck, severe headache, nausea and vomiting, altered mental status, and photophobia (increased sensitivity to light). Most often, the underlying cause is infection by a bacterium or virus.

The numerical value of the child's temperature does not reflect the severity of the disease process, but instead the severity of the immune system's response to the pathogen. Febrile seizures can occur when the child's temperature increases rapidly. Children between the ages of six months and five years are most commonly affected by febrile seizures.

Emergency medical care consists of transporting and being alert for seizures, especially in patients under five years of age. To prevent seizures, passively cool patients with high fevers by removing warm clothing and blankets. *Do not expose the child to extremely cold temperatures because this can be just as harmful as the fever.* If you suspect your patient has meningitis, as with all patients, take BSI precautions and be sure to properly disinfect the ambulance after transporting the patient.

PRACTICAL PATHOPHYSIOLOGY

Fever is an immunological response of the body to infection. Pyrogens (fever-inducing chemicals) are produced by white blood cells in response to an infectious agent. The pyrogens raise the pre-set body temperature of the thermoregulatory system in the hypothalamus of the brain. The fever helps to stimulate the body's immune responses against the infection. Increased body temperature also stimulates the liver and spleen to sequester iron and zinc, nutrients that many infectious agents need in order to grow. Low to moderate fevers also speed up the metabolic rate of the body's tissues, so that cellular damage can be repaired faster. High fevers, however, denature proteins and enzymes, which can cause cell death and lead to failure of organ systems.

Drowning

Drowning may be defined as submersion in a liquid that prevents a person from breathing air and results in a primary respiratory impairment. Drowning incidents involving children most commonly involve prolonged submersion in the bathtub or swimming pool. Neck and head trauma from falling or diving may be a factor in some drownings. In older children and adolescents, alcohol ingestion may have contributed to the incident. The child may be in severe distress or pulseless and apneic. The child may have swallowed a lot of water and may vomit during assisted ventilations and require suctioning. All patients who have been submerged, even those who appear to be well upon EMS arrival, need to be transported to the hospital for observation because some drowning patients have delayed presentations of respiratory compromise.

All children who have experienced submersion in drowning episodes should be transported to a hospital. Providing artificial ventilation in apneic children or assisted ventilations in children with inadequate breathing is the first priority. If there is a history of or signs of trauma (such as a diving mechanism), maintain cervical-spine immobilization at all times. Provide supplemental oxygen to patients with adequate breathing. Be prepared to suction to protect the airway. Keep the child warm.

Sudden Infant Death Syndrome

The sudden unexplained death of an otherwise healthy infant in the first year of life is called **sudden infant death syndrome (SIDS).** While there are many theories, the causes of this syndrome are poorly understood. The infant is often discovered by the caregiver in the morning or after an ordinary nap period. The infant is apneic when found. The caregiver is often hysterical from extreme emotional distress, guilt, and remorse.

You must provide CPR unless the child is stiff with **rigor mortis** or shows **dependent lividity.** Maintain the airway, assist ventilations, and transport rapidly to the nearest hospital. It is important to remember that the parent or caregiver has now become a patient as well and must be treated appropriately.

Consider the psychological needs of the caregivers and recommend that they accompany the child to the hospital. Communicate clearly the patient care that you are providing for their child. Do not speculate or predict outcomes. Never leave the caregivers alone. It is not appropriate to suggest neglect or blame the caregivers.

sudden infant death syndrome (SIDS) the sudden death of healthy infants in the first year of life.

rigor mortis body stiffness or rigidity that occurs after a person has been dead for a period of time.

dependent lividity pooling of blood in the lower parts of the body after death.

38-12 Describe special considerations in the scene size-up, emergency medical care, and assisting family members in case of suspected SIDS and the importance of the presence of parents during pediatric resuscitation.

Apparent Life-Threatening Event

An **apparent life-threatening event (ALTE)** occurs in children younger than two years of age when they have an episode of **apnea,** skin color change (cyanotic, pale, or redness), loss of muscle tone, or choking or gagging not associated with feeding or a foreign body aspiration. The episodes are terrifying for the caregiver, but often the problem has completely resolved prior to EMS arrival.

All children who have experienced an ALTE should be transported to the hospital. The episode the caregiver witnessed was real and must be acknowledged as such. ALTE episodes are sometimes indications of serious underlying medical conditions and the child must undergo thorough testing at a children's specialty center. The infant or young child should be monitored closely in transport and receive supplemental oxygen or ventilations as indicated.

apparent life-threatening event (ALTE) episode in which an infant or child younger than two years of age has an episode of apnea, skin color change (cyanotic, pale, or redness), loss of muscle tone, or choking or gagging not associated with feeding or a foreign body aspiration.

apnea absence of breathing

Child Abuse and Neglect

Child abuse is defined as the use of excessive or improper action so as to cause injury or harm to a child. Child neglect is defined as failing to give sufficient attention or respect to a child who has a right to that attention. Being aware of the conditions of neglect and abuse is important for the EMT, who should learn to develop an

38-13 Describe special considerations in the scene size-up, emergency medical care, and reporting of suspected child abuse or neglect.

index of suspicion of neglect or abuse in the presence of certain signs or symptoms during the assessment of the infant or child.

Signs and symptoms of abuse include fresh burns or bruises in multiple stages of healing. Infants who have been violently shaken (shaken baby syndrome) may have a high-pitched cry or be unresponsive because of undetected brain injury. The story describing the mechanism of injury may not match with the injuries themselves, and different caregivers may tell different stories. There may have been many previous requests for emergency response from the same address. Caregivers may appear unconcerned or otherwise behave inappropriately. The child who is old enough to talk may avoid discussing how the injury occurred.

Signs and symptoms of neglect often are less obvious. There may be an apparent lack of adult supervision of the infant or child. The living environment may appear unkempt and unsanitary. The infant or child may appear malnourished. Children with chronic illnesses such as diabetes or asthma may have no medication.

Do not delay transport to accuse or confront a suspected negligent or abusive caregiver. Provide whatever emergency medical care is indicated for the injuries or illness you identify. Be sure to alert the receiving facility of your suspicions and provide them with objective information. State laws require reporting suspected abuse or neglect, and the EMT should be familiar with local regulations. Remember to report objectively, identifying specific things you saw or heard, not what you think might have happened.

Infants and Children with Special Needs

Advances in medical technology have allowed many infants and children with different types of chronic disease not only to survive, but also to live at home. Often these patients are dependent on specific supportive equipment, including tracheostomies, ventilators, central intravenous lines, feeding tubes and pumps, or cerebral spinal fluid shunts. It is important to be educated about basic complications that can occur with these devices.

tracheostomy tube tube placed through a surgical opening in the neck to provide an airway.

home ventilator a mechanical device that moves air in and out of the lungs.

central venous line intravenous catheter placed close to the heart for long-term fluid or medication administration.

Always include the caregiver of the chronically ill infant or child in your assessment and care of the patient. The caregiver will be familiar with the patient's unique medical needs, medications, and devices.

Tracheostomy tubes, for example, come in a variety of types and are usually secured around the neck with twill tape (Figure 38-17 ■). The caregiver will know the type and size. The tube may become obstructed, dislodged, or infected. Other complications include bleeding or air leaking around the cuff of a cuffed tracheostomy tube. Emergency medical care includes maintaining an open airway, providing oxygen, and suctioning as needed to improve respiratory effort. Transport the patient in a position of comfort to minimize stress.

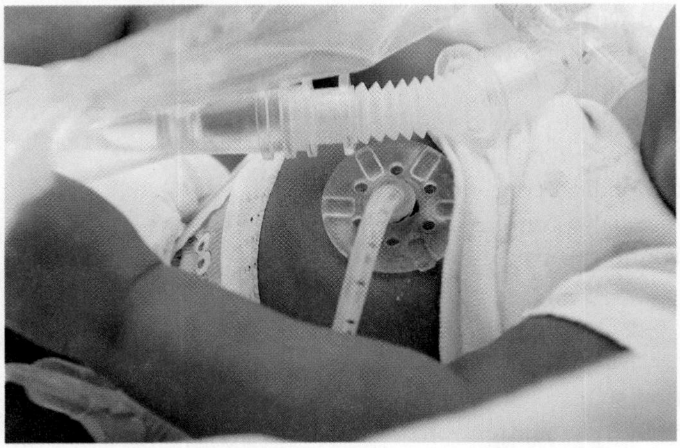

Figure 38-17 Some children require special therapies and technology with which the EMT should be familiar.

Home ventilators also come in a wide variety of types. The caregiver will be familiar with operating the device. Emergency care includes ensuring that the airway is open and that the ventilator is providing adequate ventilations, or providing assisted ventilations by way of bag-mask device directly to the patient's ventilator tube in the event of ventilator failure. Transport the ventilator with the patient.

Central venous lines are intravenous catheters placed close to the heart for long-term fluid or medication administration. Complications of the IV lines include cracking or leaking of the line, clotting of the line, bleeding from the line or around it, or infection at the insertion site and along the line. Emergency medical care includes applying pressure to stop bleeding, if present, and transporting the patient.

Gastrostomy tubes (G-tubes) are placed directly into the stomach or upper small intestine through the abdominal wall to provide nutrition to those patients who cannot eat or swallow. The tubes come in many shapes and sizes and can become dislodged or infected. Patients with feeding tubes are at risk for vomiting and aspiration. Emergency medical care includes maintaining the airway, providing oxygen, suctioning as necessary, and transporting with the head up and lying on the right side, if possible, to minimize further risk of aspiration.

gastrostomy tube (G-tube) tube placed directly into the stomach or upper small intestine through the abdominal wall to provide nutrition to a patient who cannot eat or swallow.

A **ventriculoperitoneal (VP) shunt** is a device that drains excess cerebral spinal fluid from the brain to the abdominal cavity by way of tubing that is under the skin. The shunt line is often visible or palpable on the side of the skull. Shunts may become occluded or infected. The patients may present with an altered mental status, and it is important to remember that they are prone to respiratory arrest. Emergency medical care includes maintaining an open airway, assisting with ventilations as needed, and transporting the patient.

ventriculoperitoneal (VP) shunt a device that drains excess cerebrospinal fluid from the brain to the abdomen.

Family Response

Emergency care of the infant or child does not occur in isolation from the family, and the family or caregivers may feel anxious, helpless, and afraid for the well-being of the child. They may react to the EMTs with anger or other intense emotions. If the caregiver is anxious and upset, the infant or child is more likely to respond in the same way. Calm, supportive interaction with the family often improves interactions with the patient. Allowing parents or caregivers to remain with the child, unless the child is unaware or seriously unstable, will increase trust and feelings of usefulness.

The parents or caregivers should be instructed to calm the child. They can assist in maintaining a position of comfort for the child or by holding the blow-by oxygen. Most parents have no medical training, but they are the experts on what is normal or abnormal for their child, and they know best what will be calming and comforting. Listen to their concerns and explain your interventions.

Provider Response

Many emergency medical care providers are intimidated by their perceived or actual lack of experience in the care of infants and children. They may be intimidated by a fear of failure or distracted and distressed by identifying the patient with a child of their own. However, emergency medical skills can be learned and applied to children. Much of what the provider learns about adults can be applied to children, but it is important to remember the differences. Exposure to the care of children in all settings, getting as much practice as possible with assessing the infant and child, and becoming familiar with the equipment used in their care, will improve provider confidence.

PERSPECTIVE

The Mother

It was the apnea alarm on the portable monitor that actually woke us up. And when I saw that Adrianna was struggling to breathe, I just panicked and called 911. The nurse had given us so many directions when we left the hospital that I couldn't remember what to do, so I just picked her up and she vomited and started crying. I did remember that crying was good, since it meant that she was breathing again. I'm so angry and scared right now. I really wanted Adrianna to stay in the hospital like her twin sister Alexis did. I just shudder when I think of what might have happened if that monitor alarm didn't wake up me or my mom. What a nightmare. I just want my babies to be healthy and at home with me and Mike.

STOP, REVIEW, REMEMBER!

Multiple Choice

For each question, place a check next to the correct answer.

1. You have just arrived at the side of an unresponsive pediatric patient suspected of ingesting his parent's medication. You should:

_____ a. ensure a patent airway.

_____ b. obtain a history.

_____ c. contact poison control for treatment advice.

_____ d. provide supplemental oxygen.

2. You are caring for a child who has just been pulled from a backyard swimming pool. He is pulseless and apneic. You should:

_____ a. roll him to the rescue position.

_____ b. begin chest compressions.

_____ c. begin with rescue breaths.

_____ d. perform the abdominal thrusts to remove water.

3. Which one of the following pediatric patients is mostly likely to be suffering from abuse or neglect?

_____ a. School child who develops lice

_____ b. Withdrawn, emaciated child

_____ c. Ventilator-dependent, chronically ill child

_____ d. Child from a poor neighborhood

4. The best way to interact with the infant or child's caregiver is to:

_____ a. gently take the child away to be examined.

_____ b. ask him to step outside while you examine the young child.

_____ c. listen carefully to what he thinks is wrong.

_____ d. ask him to write down his questions.

Fill in the Blank

1. A child with a rapid heart and respiratory rates with decreased responsiveness could be in ____________________.

2. The ____________________ is the most common cause of airway obstruction in the ill or injured child.

3. The first priority of care in the traumatically injured child includes maintaining ____________________ while also maintaining ____________________.

4. A rapid rise in core temperature could result in a ____________________ seizure.

Critical Thinking

1. How are hypothermia and hypoglycemia related? How can you help avoid them for your pediatric patient?

____

____

____

____

2. How will you respond when you are assessing a child you believe has been abused?

____

____

____

3. What opportunities do you have to practice your assessment of infants and children?

____

____

____

____

EMERGENCY DISPATCH SUMMARY

Adrianna was transported with her mother to Children's Hospital, where she was admitted for observation. About three weeks later, both Adrianna and her twin sister Alexis were sent home, where they have continued to develop normally with no further incidents. EMTs Jake and Jason used this call to convince their ambulance service to provide more continuing education and training scenarios focused on pediatric patients. As a result, the service's overall comfort with pediatric patients has increased and many of the EMTs and medics have expressed much less anxiety when confronted with sick or injured children.

Chapter Review

To the Point

- Pediatric patients require a different approach than adults. Appropriate assessment and treatment strategies will vary significantly, depending on the child's age and development.
- The head is proportionately larger in pediatric patients, who have weak neck muscles, so it is easy for an infant or child's head to tilt forward or backwards, occluding the airway.
- The tongue is proportionately larger in pediatric patients, so it is easy for an infant or child's tongue to block the oropharynx and occlude the airway.
- The pediatric assessment triangle (PAT) is useful for the primary assessment of pediatric patients. It includes assessing the patient's appearance, work of breathing, and circulation to the skin.
- Respiratory distress occurs when a pediatric patient experiences an abnormal physiological condition that prevents adequate exchange of oxygen and carbon dioxide.
- Respiratory failure occurs when a pediatric patient can no longer maintain adequate oxygenation and ventilation.

(continued on next page)

(continued)

- Respiratory arrest occurs when a pediatric patient becomes apneic and normal breathing ceases.
- Maintaining an open airway, administering oxygen, and assisting with or artificially ventilating the patient can manage pediatric respiratory emergencies such as asthma, pneumonia, croup, bronchiolitis, and epiglottitis.
- Infants and children are especially sensitive to hypoxia and, without proper oxygenation, their heart rate will become bradycardic.
- Prompt recognition of the signs of congenital heart disease is critical so that it can be treated effectively. Congenital heart disease is the most common form of birth defect and caregivers can be a great resource for caring for the wide variety of patients who have it.
- Rapidly recognizing the signs and symptoms of shock in pediatric patients is critical because they will compensate for a while and then suddenly decompensate into irreversible shock.
- Pediatric cardiac arrests are almost always secondary to respiratory complications, so modifications to infant and child CPR focus more on oxygenating the patient.
- Traumatic injuries are the number-one cause of death in infants and children, with motor-vehicle collisions the most common cause.
- Children are not miniature adults and proportionately have a larger head, weaker neck and abdominal muscles, and more body surface area to body weight. All of these factors affect their susceptibility to severe injuries and burns.
- Infants and children are especially sensitive to hypothermia because they do not have enough fatty insulation and glucose reserves to preserve body heat.
- There are many causes of seizures in infants and children, but one unique cause in young children is the sudden increase in body temperature from a fever.
- Poisonings are common in young children and sometimes you must act as a detective to attempt to determine the source of the poisoning.
- All drowning episodes in infants and children must be treated very seriously. Transport to the hospital even when the child appears to have recovered.
- Sudden infant death syndrome (SIDS) can be devastating to the caregivers of an infant, so all efforts must be put forth to professionally care for both the infant and the infant's family.
- Apparent life-threatening events (ALTEs) are real even though most often the patient will appear completely fine by the time you have arrived on the scene. ALTEs can indicate more serious underlying conditions, so all infants and children who have presented with an ALTE must be transported to a children's specialty center for further evaluation.
- If you suspect that an infant or child is being abused or neglected, treat and transport the patient as indicated and then report objective observations to the receiving facility and local authorities per state law.
- Many infants and children have special medical needs such as tracheostomies, home ventilators, central venous lines, gastronomy tubes, or ventriculoperitoneal shunts. While it is helpful for you to be familiar with these devices, the patient's caregivers will likely be experts on the devices and can serve as a helpful resource.
- Sick and injured infants and children are stressful for caregivers, just as they are for EMTs. Remember to act professionally and reassure the caregiver, who will in turn reassure the patient.

Chapter Questions

Multiple Choice

For each question, place a check next to the correct answer.

1. When assessing the infant or child, it is important to keep him:

_____ a. quiet.
_____ b. warm.
_____ c. undressed.
_____ d. well fed.

2. The child with nasal flaring, retractions, and decreased responsiveness is experiencing:

_____ a. respiratory distress.
_____ b. an asthma attack.
_____ c. respiratory failure.
_____ d. a choking episode.

3. If you suspect there is a foreign body in the airway of a child who is younger than one year old, you should:
   _____ a. perform a blind finger sweep.
   _____ b. try to ventilate with a bag-mask device.
   _____ c. perform five back blows followed by five chest thrusts.
   _____ d. assist the child into a position of comfort.
4. The first interventions for a child with a slow heart rate are:
   _____ a. open the airway and give supplemental oxygen.
   _____ b. ask the parents about any allergies.
   _____ c. roll the child to the rescue position.
   _____ d. apply the AED.
5. The child in shock will likely:
   _____ a. have warm extremities.
   _____ b. have a slow heart rate.
   _____ c. have an increased heart rate.
   _____ d. be drooling and crying tears.

Matching

Match the definition on the left with the applicable term on the right.

1. _____	Retractions	A. Absence of respiration
2. _____	Stridor	B. Barky or noisy breathing
3. _____	Wheezing	C. Whistling breath sound
4. _____	Cyanosis	D. Deteriorate rapidly
5. _____	Apnea	E. Pale, bluish skin
6. _____	Decompensate	F. Pulling in of muscles between the ribs with inspiration

Critical Thinking

1. Why is it important to understand the developmental differences of children?

____

____

____

____

2. Why is it important to differentiate between respiratory distress and respiratory failure in the pediatric patient?

____

____

____

____

(continued on next page)

(continued)

3. What is the most common cause of death for infants and children?

4. What is the most common cause of cardiac arrest for infants and children?

The Last Word

The most important focus of prehospital care for infants and children is airway, breathing, and oxygenation. Cardiac events in infants or children are almost always preceded by an obstructed airway or inadequate respirations. A rapid assessment that focuses on appearance, work of breathing, and circulation to the skin begins as soon as you encounter the pediatric patient. Recognizing respiratory distress, respiratory failure, and the signs and symptoms of shock, and then intervening quickly, best improves outcomes for these patients.

Calls involving infants and children are often intimidating to the EMS provider, but using the information provided in this chapter to better understand the differences among age groups as well as to recognize behaviors common to most young children will help you interact more successfully with them and their families. Often, pediatric patients are surrounded by highly emotional or distraught parents or caregivers. Calm, supportive interaction with the family will help you improve interactions with the child.

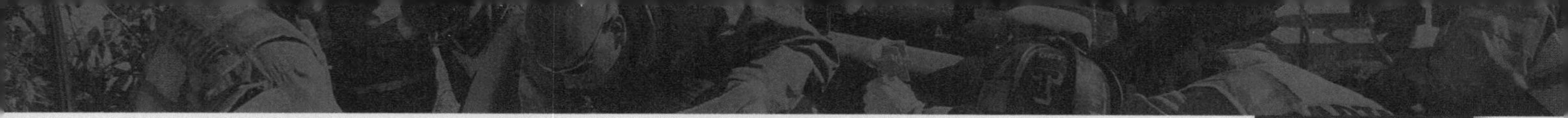

Caring for Geriatric Patients

39

Education Standards

Special Patient Populations: Geriatrics

Competencies

Applies fundamental knowledge of growth, development, aging, and assessment findings to provide basic emergency care and transportation for a patient with special needs.

Objectives

After completion of this lesson, you should be able to:

39-1 Define the key terms introduced in this chapter.

39-2 Describe the general characteristics commonly associated with geriatric patients.

39-3 Describe some of the most common age-related physical changes found in geriatric patients.

39-4 Explain the unique challenges that can arise when assessing and caring for the geriatric patient.

39-5 Describe changes in the approach to care when caring for geriatric patients.

39-6 Describe the common medical problems of geriatric patients.

39-7 Describe common signs and symptoms of abuse and neglect in elder patients.

39-8 Explain the role of the EMT in cases of suspected abuse and/or neglect.

Key Terms

abuse p. 1052
Alzheimer's disease p. 1050
aneurysm p. 1050
beta blocker p. 1041
dementia p. 1050
dysrhythmia p. 1045
geriatric p. 1040
incontinence p. 1043
neglect p. 1052
osteoporosis p. 1046
Parkinson's disease p. 1050

Introduction

This chapter introduces the special considerations necessary in assessing and providing emergency care for elderly patients. There are currently more than 35 million elderly people in the United States, and that number is expected to more than double in the next two decades. Even today, geriatric patients use EMS services more frequently as a population than younger adults. More and more often, you will find yourself providing care for them. Remember that although people are living healthier lifestyles, age-related changes in anatomy and physiology do make the elderly more susceptible to certain illnesses and injuries.

geriatric refers to a person aged 65 or older.

The term **geriatric** refers to people who are elderly, typically over the age of 65. This chapter uses the terms *geriatric* and *elderly* interchangeably to refer to this growing population.

EMERGENCY DISPATCH

"Oh, hey! Watch out!" EMT Brandi Burns grabbed onto the door of the ambulance and steadied her feet. "It's a solid sheet of ice from here over to the steps."

Brandi and her EMT partner, Nancy Purcell, inched their way to the back of the truck, eased the cot out, and continued on to the steps of the single-wide trailer. It was a clear January afternoon, and although the sun stood brightly in the sky, the temperature just wouldn't rise above 30 degrees.

"I'm so glad that you're here!" A man in his mid 50s answered the door after one brief knock. "It's my mom. You need to take her to the hospital."

"Okay." Brandi struggled to get the cot through the narrow doorway. "What's your mom's name and what is she having trouble with today?"

"Her name is Pauline and it's her leg." The man fumbled with his thick glasses, and motioned toward the back of the trailer. "She fell about two weeks ago and it looks infected or something."

The EMTs left the cot in the small living room and carried their bags back to the patient.

"Do you smell that?" Nancy said quietly as they entered the bedroom.

"The nose always knows," Brandi replied, stopping at the bedside of an elderly woman who appeared to be asleep. "Ma'am? Are you awake?"

The woman stirred and her eyes fluttered open. "Darn it, Ralphie!" She pulled the covers up to her neck. "I told you not to call the ambulance people!"

"But Mom," he stammered. "There's something wrong with your leg. Even Doris thought so, remember?"

"I haven't been to a doctor in my entire life," the woman hissed at her son. "And I'm not going to go to one now!"

"Ma'am," Nancy smiled broadly. "Tell you what. Let us just look at your leg and tell you what we think. We can't take you anywhere against your will. You're totally in control, and it won't cost you anything for me to look at it. I just want to see how bad it is. Okay?"

The woman stared at Nancy for a moment, shifted her gaze to the ceiling, and then slowly slid her leg out from under the sheets.

Understanding Geriatric Patients

There is a common misconception that most elderly people are usually ill, hard of hearing, and altered in their mental state to the point of not being able to provide reliable information to caregivers. Understand that this is not true. The vast majority of the elderly lead healthy, active lives and are able to communicate clearly and effectively with those around them (Figure 39-1 ■). Why the misconception, then? Most likely it is because people who are healthy and active rarely require EMS assistance. So when EMS providers are summoned to help an elderly person, the calls frequently come from extended-care facilities where chronically ill and mentally altered geriatric patients are cared for. You should not let frequent calls to those types of facilities distort your view of the geriatric population as a whole.

The majority of the elderly are as healthy and lucid as you are. However, there are some important differences you should keep in mind when dealing with elderly patients. Those differences include anatomical and physiological changes, as well as unique life experiences, the concerns that come with aging, and an awareness of their own mortality.

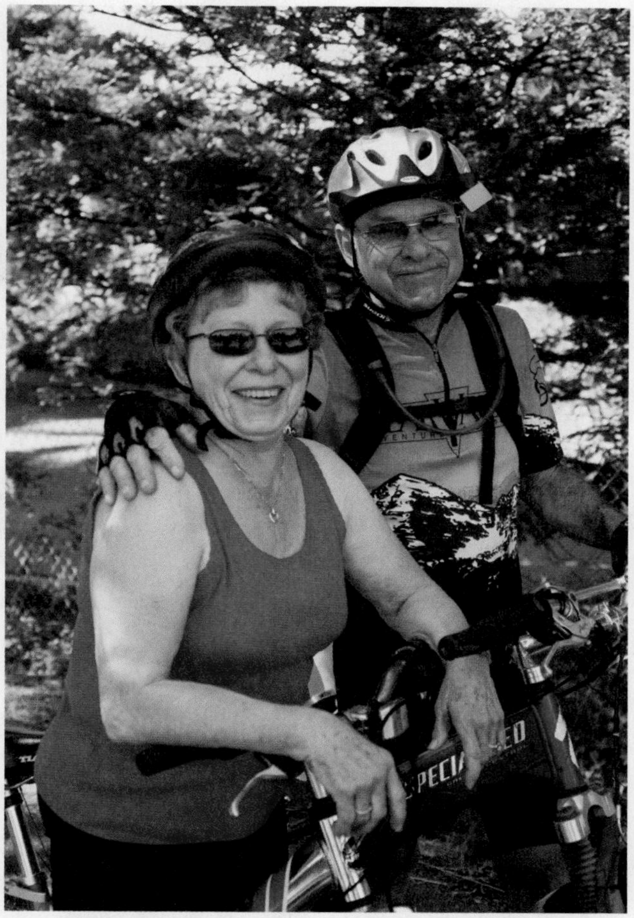

Figure 39-1 The vast majority of senior citizens live active productive lives.

Characteristics of Geriatric Patients

Even though geriatric patients, their bodies, and their specific illnesses change as they age, there are certain generalizations that are fairly consistent across this segment of the population. Being familiar with the following general areas will greatly assist you in understanding your geriatric patients.

Multiple Illnesses

Elderly patients are just as likely to suffer from the same illnesses and disorders as younger adults, but their bodies are less able to defend against them and recover quickly. Elderly people more commonly have multiple medical conditions, illnesses, and diseases at one time. The number tends to increase as the elderly patient ages. Multiple illnesses create a unique challenge for the EMT who is assessing the geriatric patient. The patient may be displaying signs and symptoms from a variety of illnesses, with none of them appearing to be anything specific.

Do not worry. It will not be your job to diagnose all of the patient's medical conditions. It usually takes a physician examining the geriatric patient and ordering a battery of lab tests before a final diagnosis can be made. Your job is to perform a thorough patient assessment and care for the primary complaint as best as you can.

Medications

Directly related to the presence of multiple illnesses, elderly patients tend to take numerous prescription and over-the-counter (OTC) medications each day. Actually, patients age 65 and older take an average of 4.5 medication doses per day (Figure 39-2 ▪). Incorrect medication usage (sometimes caused by forgetfulness or confusion about instructions) can create numerous problems, from overdosing to underdosing. Overdosing will result in toxic medication levels in the patient's system. Underdosing can cause the patient's illness or disease process to get worse. Many elderly patients use a special pillbox to help them remember which medications to take and when (Figure 39-3 ▪).

39-2 Describe the general characteristics commonly associated with geriatric patients.

39-3 Describe some of the most common age-related physical changes found in geriatric patients.

Another common cause of medication misuse is due to the high cost of prescription medications. Elderly patients on fixed incomes may cut their medications in half or take them only every other day in an attempt to get them to last longer than prescribed.

PRACTICAL PATHOPHYSIOLOGY

Due to the effects of aging on the heart and cardiovascular system, many elderly patients take a class of medication called **beta blockers.** Beta blockers inhibit the effect of epinephrine on the sympathetic nervous system. They can inhibit the body's normal compensatory response of increasing the heart rate for such things as blood loss, making the patient more at risk for shock. Thus, do not let the lack of tachycardia (increased heart rate) in a patient on a beta blocker, who otherwise appears to be in shock, confuse you.

beta blocker a class of drugs used primarily to treat heart-related conditions.

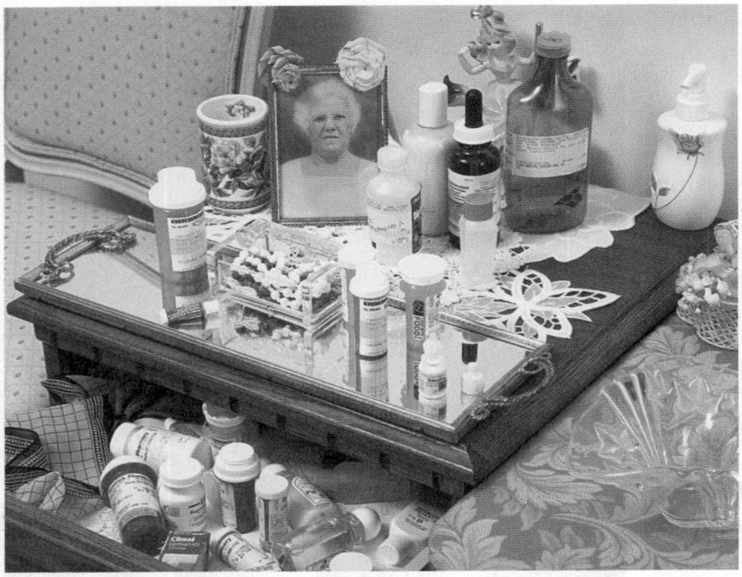

Figure 39-2 Many elderly must take multiple medications, which can be a challenge to keep organized.

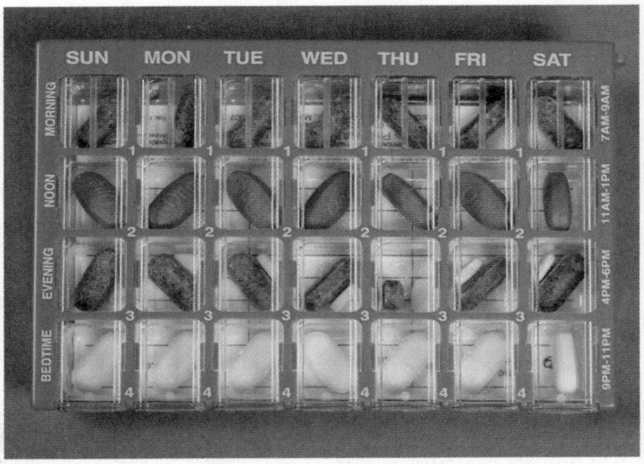

Figure 39-3 One tool to help keep medications organized is a pillbox such as this.

Mobility

Regular exercise is very important. It can help keep aging patients healthy and mobile. However, it is common for some elderly persons to live increasingly sedentary lives. This can be due to illnesses such as arthritis, medications that cause excessive tiredness, or even the fear of injury as their ability to move about becomes more difficult. Having limited mobility can cause many problems for the elderly person, such as:

- Isolation
- Poor nutrition
- Depression
- Difficulty using the bathroom
- Loss of independence
- Higher likelihood for falls or other injuries

In many towns and cities there are special agencies and senior advocacy groups (Meals on Wheels, for example) who look after the elderly and provide needed services such as check-in visits and hot meals (Figure 39-4 ■).

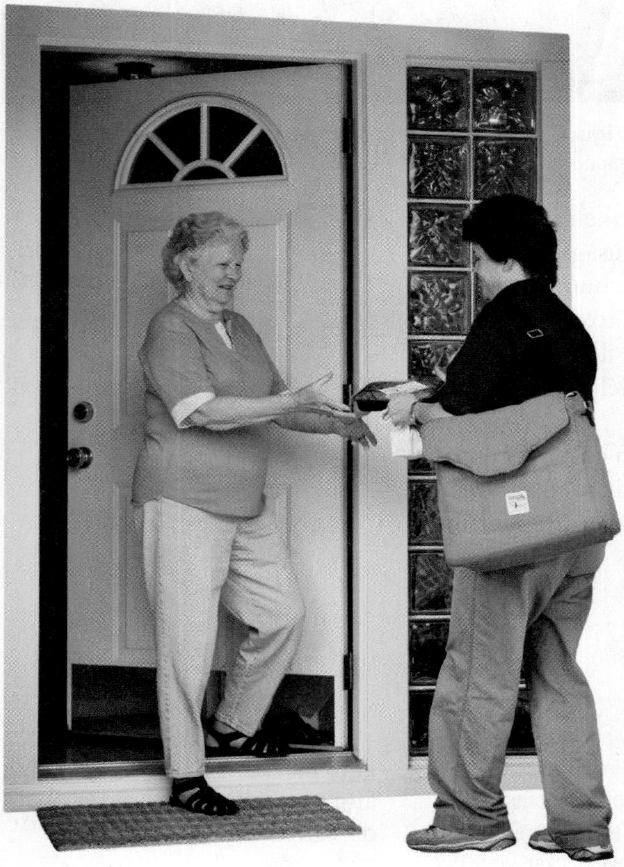

Figure 39-4 Organizations such as Meals on Wheels help bring hot meals to the elderly.

Difficulties with Communication

You will find that many geriatric patients have age-related sensory changes. It is normal for elderly people to experience a lower sensitivity to pain or touch, an altered sense of smell or taste, hearing loss, and impaired vision. Any of those can affect your ability to assess and communicate with the patient. See Table 39-1 for some ideas about how to effectively communicate with an elderly patient.

Incontinence

Not necessarily caused by aging, several factors predispose elderly persons to the inability to retain urine or feces normally.

TABLE 39-1 AGE-RELATED DIFFICULTIES WITH COMMUNICATION

DIFFICULTY	STRATEGY
Poor vision (especially decreased peripheral vision)	Position yourself directly in front of the patient so you can be seen.
	Put your hand on the arm of a blind patient so he knows where you are.
	Locate the patient's glasses, if necessary.
Decreased hearing	Speak clearly. Check hearing aids. Write notes.
	Try letting the patient wear a stethoscope and speak into the head like a microphone.
Inability to speak clearly	Ask the patient to put dentures in (or adjust them), if possible.

Diseases such as diabetes, illnesses that cause diarrhea, and certain medications all can contribute to incontinence. Studies indicate that between 15% and 60% of all elderly people suffer from some form of **incontinence.** Understand that it is important for you *not* make a big deal out of a geriatric patient's chronic incontinence. The need to help maintain the dignity of any patient is important, but for elderly patients, in particular, respect and dignity are extremely vital. However, the sudden development of new onset incontinence can be the sign of an acute illness such as urinary infections or compression of the lower spinal cord by a tumor or other nontrauma-related cause.

incontinence inability to retain urine or feces because of loss of sphincter control.

Confusion or Altered Mental Status

An important thing to remember when you encounter an elderly patient who seems confused or is presenting with an altered mental status is to try to determine if this is normal ("baseline") behavior for the patient or a sudden change. You want to avoid placing too much importance on a patient's confused state if this is the norm for him. On the other hand, new onset confusion or a change in mental status can be a sign of any number of life-threatening emergencies from a heart attack or sepsis to stroke.

When you encounter a geriatric patient with altered mental status, seek out a family member or caregiver who knows the patient's baseline mental status and together determine whether or not the current mental status is a change for the patient.

CLINICAL CLUE

Reading Between the Lines

Patients may be stoic and not admit they are sick. They could feel they are unable to afford care or medications. They may be depressed, or they may be neglected by their families. These are some of the many psychosocial issues the elderly face. Consider such possibilities as you care for your patients. It can make your assessment and care more successful. It also could allow you to identify problems and notify appropriate people in the hospital or community who can help your patients overcome such issues.

Age-Related Physical Changes

Although age-related changes can be determined by genetics and begin at the cellular level, they are greatly affected by lifestyle and environment. As anyone can see, the aging process can differ greatly from person to person. There are, however, some general age-related changes that will be fairly consistent throughout the older population (Figure 39-5 ■). It is important for EMTs to understand the basics of those changes and how they can impact the assessment and care process (Table 39-2).

Respiratory System

As early as the age of 30, without regular exercise, the lungs will begin the aging process with decreased ability to ventilate properly. Aging creates many changes in the respiratory system. For example, the mechanism that helps the body detect low levels of oxygen in the blood becomes increasingly less efficient over time. That means a geriatric patient may become severely hypoxic before the body realizes it and attempts to compensate. Aging also leads to a decrease in the number of cilia in the airway. Cilia are small hairlike structures on the cells lining the airway that help clear

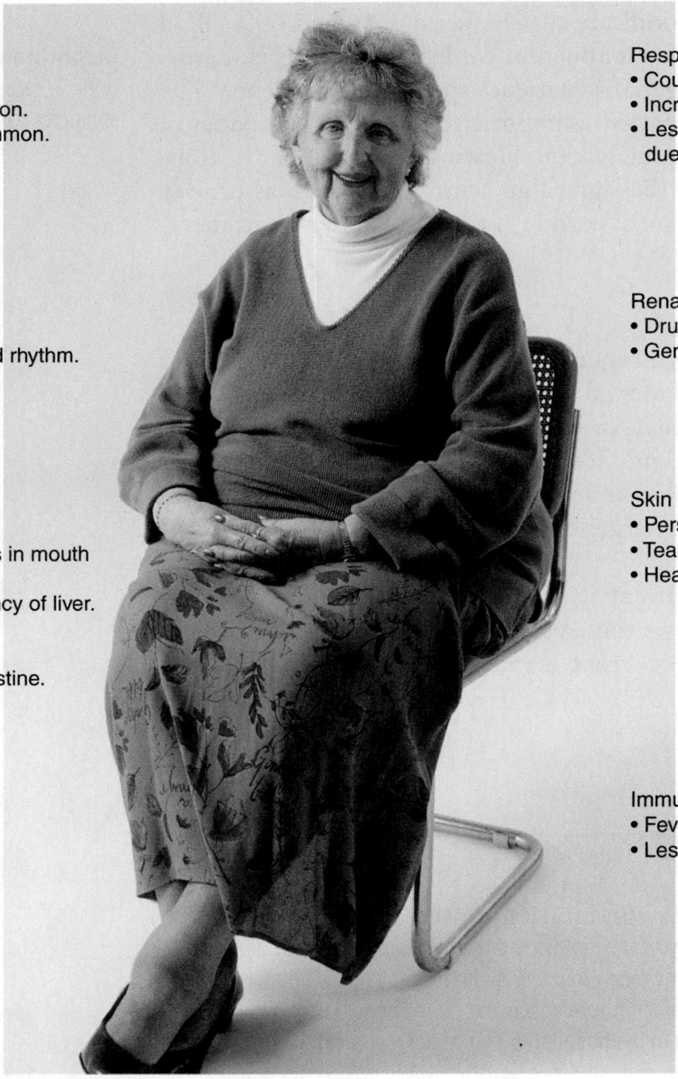
Neurological System
• Brain changes with age.
• Clinical depression common.
• Altered mental status common.
Cardiovascular System
• Hypertension common.
• Changes in heart rate and rhythm.
Gastrointestinal System
• Constipation common.
• Deterioration of structures in mouth common.
• General decline in efficiency of liver.
• Impaired swallowing.
• Malnutrition as result of deterioration of small intestine.
Musculoskeletal System
• Osteoporosis common.
• Osteoarthritis common.
Respiratory System
• Cough power is diminished.
• Increased tendency for infection.
• Less air and less exchange of gases due to general decline.
Renal System
• Drug toxicity problems common.
• General decline in efficiency.
Skin
• Perspires less.
• Tears more easily.
• Heals slowly.
Immune System
• Fever often absent during infections.
• Lessened ability to fight disease.

Figure 39-5 Physiological changes as the body ages.

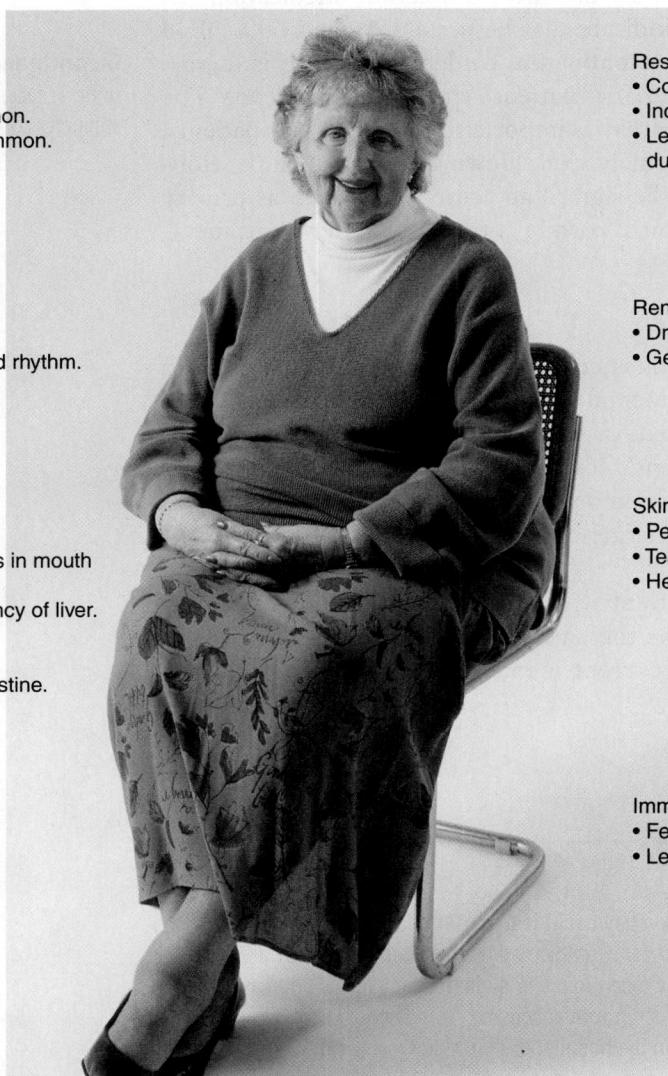

TABLE 39-2 PHYSIOLOGICAL EFFECTS OF AGING AND IMPLICATIONS FOR ASSESSMENT

CHANGE	RESULT	IMPLICATION FOR ASSESSMENT
Depositing of cholesterol on arterial walls that have become thicker	Increased risk of heart attack and stroke, hypertension	Heart attack and stroke more likely
Decreased cardiac output	Diminished activity and tolerance of physical stress	More prone to falls; more complaints of fatigue
Decreased elasticity of lungs and decreased activity of cilia	Decreased ability to clear foreign substances from lungs	Higher risk of pneumonia and other respiratory infections
Fewer taste buds, less saliva; less acid production and slower movement in digestive system	Difficulty chewing and swallowing; less enjoyment of eating; difficulty digesting and absorbing food; constipation; early feeling of fullness when eating	Weight loss; abdominal pain common
Diminished liver and kidney function	Increased toxicity from alcohol and medications; diminished ability of blood to clot	Need for reduced doses of medication; bleeding tendencies
Diminished function of thyroid	Decreased energy and tolerance of heat and cold	Increased risk of hypothermia and hyperthermia
Decreased muscle mass, loss of minerals from bones	Decreased strength	Fall more likely; minor falls more likely to cause fractures
Multiple medical conditions	Many different medications, sometimes prescribed by different physicians	Increased risk of medication error; potentially harmful medication interactions common
Deaths of friends and family	Depression; loss of social support	Increased risk of suicide
Loss of skin elasticity, shrinking of sweat glands	Thin, dry, wrinkled skin	Increased risk of injury (The EMT must handle the patient gently to avoid injuring skin and subcutaneous tissues.)

debris from the airways. Loss of cilia exposes the elderly person to more respiratory illnesses, such as pneumonia. Other respiratory changes due to aging include:

- Reduced strength and endurance of respiratory muscles
- Decreased chest wall flexibility
- Loss of lung elasticity
- Collapse of smaller airway structures

As with any patient, it is important that you continually assess and maintain the geriatric patient's airway and breathing status.

Cardiovascular System

Much of what affects the cardiovascular system seems related to lifestyle. Aging, however, does in itself seem to affect it to a certain degree. Some of the age-related changes in the cardiovascular system include:

- Enlargement of the left ventricle, which can decrease cardiac output
- Stiffening of the aorta, making it more susceptible to tearing
- Degeneration of the heart's electrical system, causing **dysrhythmia**
- Loss of elasticity in the blood vessels, which can result in hypertension and poor circulation

dysrhythmia a disturbance in heart rate or rhythm.

In addition, medications prescribed to elderly patients for heart conditions can prevent effective compensation for blood loss. Geriatric trauma patients who have lost a good amount of blood should be treated for shock even if their signs and symptoms do not indicate it.

PRACTICAL PATHOPHYSIOLOGY

As the heart ages it becomes less responsive to the effects of chemicals called catecholamines, such as epinephrine, which are secreted from the adrenal glands in times of stress. This can limit the ability of the heart to increase heart rate and strength of contractions when an increase in cardiac output is required.

Nervous System

Aging has been shown to affect a person's nervous system in a few key areas. First, the brain loses about 10% of its overall weight between the ages of 20 and 90 years. Although this does *not* mean that elderly patients are less intelligent than younger ones, it does mean that there is more room for destructive bleeding inside the skull following a blow to the head. Also, aging causes a substantial decrease in the overall number of nerve fibers and the speed at which the impulses travel across them. Those deteriorations mean elderly patients may experience some of the following changes over time:

- Decreased reaction times
- Difficulty with recent memory
- Psychomotor slowing

As you examine the geriatric patient, assess for sluggishness, confusion, or any mental status that appears below the level of full coherence. An altered mental status can indicate a wide range of illnesses and injuries, from infection and medication overdose to stroke and head trauma, all of which are very serious conditions. It is important that you summon advanced medical care for any elderly patient who presents with an abnormally altered mental status.

Although it may not be uncommon for an elderly person to seem agitated, confused, or have a decreased level of consciousness, always assume that he is normally coherent and mentally sharp until you can determine otherwise by questioning caregivers, spouse, or family members. If you operate on the assumption that a patient is normally altered, you may fail to properly address an underlying medical or trauma-related problem.

Although not directly related to the physical effects of aging on the nervous system, it is worth mentioning here that depression is a common condition found among elderly patients. In fact, suicides, or suicide attempts, are not unusual in the 65 and older segment of the population, especially among men. Be alert for signs of depression, such as poor hygiene, poor eating habits, and disorderly living environments.

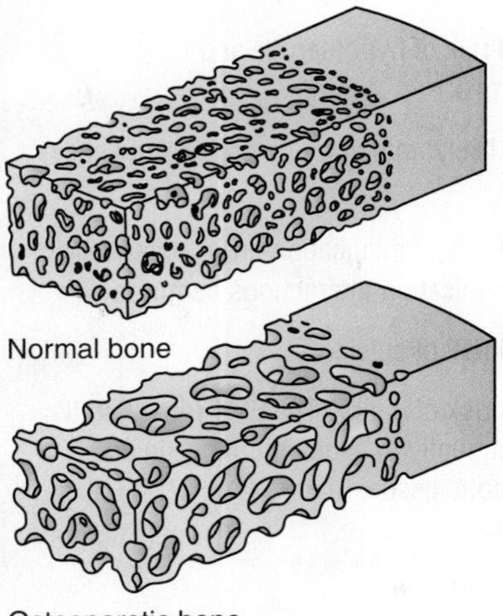

Figure 39-6 Osteoporosis causes a reduction in the bone mineral density, making the bones weak and brittle.

Musculoskeletal System

osteoporosis softening of bone tissue due to the loss of essential minerals, principally calcium.

Age-related changes in the musculoskeletal system can lead to changes in posture, range of motion, and balance. Some elderly people can even lose up to three inches of overall height due to deterioration of the discs between the vertebrae and slow collapse of the vertebrae height due to **osteoporosis** (Figure 39-6 ■). Osteoporosis is the loss of minerals from bones. That loss causes the bones to soften and become weak. If an elderly person falls, he is far more prone to bony injuries such as hip fractures due to more fragile bones. Also keep in mind that age-related changes in the spine can result in curvatures, which can affect your ability to manage a patient's airway or effectively immobilize him following an injury.

PRACTICAL PATHOPHYSIOLOGY

While affecting both men and women, women who have gone through menopause are at a much higher risk for developing osteoporosis. The weakening of the bone structure due to mineral loss makes the bones much more prone to fracture.

Digestive System

With age, the digestive system slows and produces less of the secretions needed to break down food. The sense of taste is diminished, making eating less pleasurable, and the loss of teeth or poorly fitting dentures may make eating difficult. Those factors can lead to poor nutrition, frequent heartburn, excessive gas production, and constipation. Since the stomach empties more slowly, vomiting of stomach contents may occur during illness or injury.

Tooth loss, no teeth, or poorly fitting dentures may make it difficult for an elderly patient to communicate. If the patient is not wearing dentures and you are having difficulty understanding him, ask if he has dentures he can put in.

Ulcers and disorders of the intestinal tract can lead to bleeding. Bleeding from the upper gastrointestinal tract (esophagus and stomach) can result in the patient vomiting blood. Blood that has been exposed to the digestive secretions of the stomach may take on a "coffee grounds" appearance. Bleeding in the lower gastrointestinal tract can lead to blood in the stools. Generally, blood from an upper gastrointestinal source will result in dark (tarry), sticky stools, while blood from lower in the gastrointestinal tract will not undergo those changes and will appear as maroon or bright red in color.

Integumentary System (Skin)

Because of its prominence on the body, age-related changes to the skin are going to be the most obvious to you as an EMT. As people grow older, their skin loses its elasticity and thickness, causing it to be easily torn or injured. You also may notice dark areas of pigment on the skin, usually called "age spots" or "liver spots." The skin of a geriatric patient may be dry and flaky due to a decrease in the production of oils. The ability to perspire tends to decrease as well, making heat-related emergencies more common and the onset of shock more difficult to recognize. As skin grows thinner and weaker, cell reproduction slows down, so that not only are skin injuries worse among the elderly, but healing times also can be greatly extended compared to younger adults.

PERSPECTIVE

Brandi—The EMT

Nancy is always so good with the older patients. Especially the ladies! She's got this big smile and a low voice, you know? And I think she talks to them with a lot of respect and addresses the things that worry them. Like the money. It was good that she built rapport. The patient had a serious case of gangrene. It won't surprise me if she loses part of that leg. Yet she was just stubborn enough that she might have refused to go with us if Nancy hadn't immediately made that connection with her.

STOP, REVIEW, REMEMBER!

Multiple Choice

For each question, place a check next to the correct answer.

1. Which one of the following is an age-related change of the skin?

_____ a. Loss of pigmentation

_____ b. Decreased ability to perspire

_____ c. Increased oil production

_____ d. Increased thickness

2. Which one of the following decreases the elderly patient's ability to compensate for blood loss?

_____ a. Diminished ability to increase the heart rate

_____ b. Increased cardiac output

_____ c. Increased elasticity of the blood vessels

_____ d. Decreased likelihood for dysrhythmia

(continued on next page)

(continued)

3. Age-related changes that affect the musculoskeletal system include all of the following *except:*

_____ a. posture.

_____ b. range of motion.

_____ c. unequal pupils.

_____ d. balance.

4. When confronted with an elderly female patient who has an altered mental status, you should first:

_____ a. determine her baseline mental status.

_____ b. obtain baseline vital signs.

_____ c. evaluate her current medications.

_____ d. obtain a detailed medical history.

5. All of the following are consequences of an increased loss of mobility for the elderly *except:*

_____ a. isolation.

_____ b. poor nutrition.

_____ c. depression.

_____ d. increased desire for food.

Fill in the Blank

For each body system, list at least one age-related change.

Body System	Age-Related Changes
1. Cardiovascular system	____________
2. Respiratory system	____________
3. Musculoskeletal system	____________
4. Digestive system	____________
5. Nervous system	____________

Critical Thinking

1. How do changes in the cardiovascular system affect the signs and symptoms of shock in the elderly patient?

____

____

____

____

2. List at least three barriers to good communication with the elderly and a strategy for overcoming each barrier.

____

____

____

____

Assessment of Geriatric Patients

Your assessment of a geriatric patient will follow the same basic path as any other patient assessment, with a few additional considerations. As always, make sure you begin by taking appropriate BSI precautions.

39-4 Explain the unique challenges that can arise when assessing and caring for the geriatric patient.

39-5 Describe changes in the approach to care when caring for geriatric patients.

Scene Size-up

For geriatric patients as for any other, you must ensure the scene is safe before you enter it. However, for the geriatric patient you also should survey the environment for evidence of the following:

- Inadequate food, shelter, or hygiene
- Lack of a working heating or cooling system
- Potential fall hazards
- Conditions that suggest abuse or neglect

When you approach the patient, always focus on him instead of caregivers or family members who may be present. This will show the patient you respect him as a person and will give him a sense of control over the situation. If the patient is seated or lying on a bed, position yourself at the patient's level and make eye contact before introducing yourself (Figure 39-7 ■).

Another way to show respect to the patient is to use a title and last name, such as "Mrs. Becker." Avoid using generic nicknames such as "dear," "buddy," "sweetie," or "honey." Also avoid using an elderly person's first name (unless you are asked to use it), because doing so could be considered rude or disrespectful.

If appropriate, offer to shake the patient's hand during the introduction. It can help build rapport while also giving you the ability to check the patient's skin signs and mobility in an unobtrusive way.

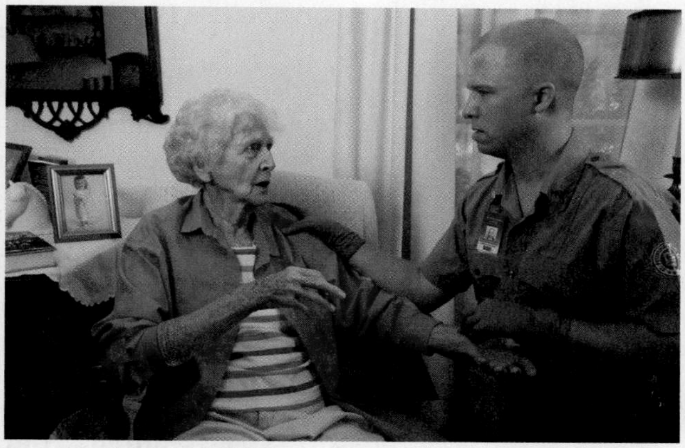

Figure 39-7 Get down at eye level and speak slowly and clearly to maximize the effectiveness of your communication.

> **CLINICAL CLUE**
>
> **Assessment in the Elderly**
>
> Elderly patients can present a series of contradictions when it comes to assessment and determining severity of injury. They can develop infections, but often do not have a fever. They can be injured, but not feel the same degree of pain a younger patient would. And they may have trouble communicating their symptoms and concerns to you. Be patient as you perform your assessment. Obtain a history. Listen to what the patient says and what the patient does not say. Pay attention to body language. And remember the differences between the elderly and younger patients.

Primary Assessment

As with all patients, you will perform a complete primary assessment as the first step in the assessment process. As you approach the patient, make note of his position. Is he sitting up and alert, or is he lying in bed and unresponsive? The patient who is sitting up and aware of his surroundings clearly has a patent airway and is breathing. The patient who presents as unresponsive will require a more aggressive ABC check before you can move on to your secondary assessment.

Confirm that the patient has a clear airway and is breathing with an adequate rate and tidal volume. Confirm that he has an adequate pulse and that there are no immediate threats to life before moving on to your secondary assessment.

Obtaining a History

Unlike the majority of younger patients, gathering a medical history on an elderly person may take quite a bit of time. You will find it helpful to first obtain the patient's medications (prescription and over-the-counter) and then ask why each is taken. Also be aware of the patient's surroundings. Are there medical identification tags or stickers? Oxygen supplies? Is there anything else that would indicate a medical condition? If you are unsure about a patient's answers to your questions, try to verify information with a reliable source, such as a caregiver.

Secondary Assessment

The following considerations are important when examining a geriatric patient:

- Handle elderly patients gently.
- Histories and exams can easily tire elderly patients.
- Always explain what you are going to do before you do it.
- Anticipate numerous layers of clothing (due to problems with temperature regulation).
- Respect the modesty and privacy of elderly patients.

Remember that some geriatric patients may deny or minimize symptoms during the physical exam. Often this is because they fear being hospitalized and losing their independence, if the extent of their condition is "discovered."

PERSPECTIVE

Pauline—The Patient

I just hadn't been feeling right for a while, I guess. Ever since my Raymond passed away, maybe. Raymond was my middle boy. I've lost my husband, a child, and my best friend who I've known since grade school, all in a span of two years. It's hell getting old. I don't know if I'd wish this on my worst enemy. So when I fell and hurt my leg, staying in bed just didn't seem like a bad idea at all. I kind of thought that I might, maybe just, pass on. Or something. But instead I got Ralphie, my youngest, running around like a darn Chicken Little. Calling out those ambulance folks. That boy! I can't be too mad at him, though, my leg really is in bad shape.

39-6 Describe the common medical problems of geriatric patients.

aneurysm the dilation, or ballooning, of a weakened section of the wall of an artery.

dementia the loss of normal cognitive ability.

Alzheimer's disease a form of dementia that is progressive and attacks the brain, resulting in impaired memory, thinking, and behavior. It affects over 5 million adults in the United States.

Parkinson's disease chronic, degenerative nervous disease characterized by tremors, muscular weakness, and rigidity, and a loss of postural reflexes.

Common Medical Problems of Geriatric Patients

As we age and our bodies become less efficient, illnesses become more common. The average geriatric patient may be taking several different medications to help minimize the effects of illnesses related to age.

Illnesses

Common illnesses among the elderly include pneumonia; chronic obstructive pulmonary diseases; cancer; heart failure; **aneurysm**; high blood pressure; stroke; **dementia** (including **Alzheimer's disease**), **Parkinson's disease**; diabetes; bleeding in the stomach, esophagus, or intestines; urinary tract infections; and adverse reactions to medications. Due to the thinning of skin, a decreased ability to perspire and muted physical sensations, heat- and cold-related emergencies are also common among geriatric patients.

Alzheimer's disease affects over 5 million elderly people in the United States and is the most common type of dementia. It is a progressive, degenerative disease that attacks the brain and results in impaired memory, thinking, and behavior. Alzheimer's is a progressive form of dementia that can last from three to 20 years. As the disease progresses, the patient is less able to properly care for himself, often resulting in self neglect. Dementia can cause a person to become more forgetful with regards to taking their prescribed medications. For this reason it is common for these patients to accidently overdose or underdose themselves.

Injuries

Trauma caused by falls is the leading cause of injury death among the elderly. The weakening of bones, deterioration of skin integrity, and loss of blood vessel flexibility all combine to make injuries much more severe for geriatric patients. The risk of death from traumatic injury in older patients is three times higher than in younger adults who suffer the same injury. Add to that the medications taken by many elderly persons, including those that can prevent clotting and make bleeding control extremely difficult. In those cases, a relatively minor injury for a young patient can actually cause a serious injury or even death in an elderly patient.

As an EMT, you should be an advocate for injury prevention among the elderly. Because you will respond to the homes of geriatric patients, remember to look for potential dangers, such as unsecured rugs, loose handrails, unsafely stacked items, and so on, and make a caregiver or family member aware of any safety concerns.

STOP, REVIEW, REMEMBER!

Multiple Choice

For each question, place a check next to the correct answer.

1. You have completed your assessment of an elderly fall victim and are about to roll her onto a long backboard. You should:

_____ a. move her quickly to get it over with.

_____ b. explain exactly what the plan is.

_____ c. obtain another set of vital signs first.

_____ d. ask her to slide herself onto the board.

2. Which one of the following statements regarding trauma in the elderly is *true*?

_____ a. Bones heal more quickly because there is less bone mass.

_____ b. Blood-thinning medications help stop bleeding.

_____ c. The risk of death from a traumatic injury is three times higher than in younger adults.

_____ d. Injury prevention has been proven ineffective for the elderly population.

3. Which one of the following is most accurate regarding Alzheimer's disease?

_____ a. It affects over five million elderly in the United States.

_____ b. It is a sudden and acute illness.

_____ c. It results in blindness and impaired hearing.

_____ d. It typically lasts from three to five years.

4. Changes in the skin make the elderly more susceptible to:

_____ a. bleeding.

_____ b. heart dysrhythmia.

_____ c. heat and cold emergencies.

_____ d. bowel obstructions.

5. An elderly patient may tend to minimize symptoms due to:

_____ a. denial of illness.

_____ b. the low cost of health care.

_____ c. a fear of losing independence.

_____ d. diminished ability to feel pain.

(continued on next page)

(continued)

Fill in the Blank

For each of the following write in "more" or "less" to complete the statement correctly.

1. The elderly patient's skin is ______________________ elastic.
2. The elderly patient is ______________________ able to compensate for shock.
3. Elderly patients have ______________________ medical problems than younger adults.
4. Elderly patients are ______________________ likely to die from trauma than a younger adult.
5. Elderly patients usually take ______________________ medications than younger adults.
6. Elderly patients are ______________________ likely to have a fever with an infection.
7. Elderly patients have ______________________ cilia in their airway.

Critical Thinking

1. You are treating a generally healthy 84-year-old woman who, according to her daughter, seems a bit confused today. What could you do to make communication with this patient effective?

____

____

____

____

2. You are taking the blood pressure of an elderly man. As you pump the cuff up he begins to scream in pain. You look at the gauge and note that it is only at about 120 mmHg. What might be some causes of this discomfort?

____

____

____

____

Elder Abuse and Neglect

39-7 Describe common signs and symptoms of abuse and neglect in elder patients.

Elder **abuse** is the mistreatment of an elderly person. As mentioned earlier, an elderly person is anyone over the age of 65. Elder **neglect** is the abandonment or the deprivation of basic needs such as water, food, housing, clothing, or medical care. There is another form of abuse unique to this population called *self-neglect*. It is characterized by the inability or unwillingness to provide or care for oneself. It can be a deliberate act on the part of the elderly person, who has purposely given up or intentionally stopped caring. It also can be the result of an inability to properly care for oneself due to illness, dementia, or physical limitations.

39-8 Explain the role of the EMT in cases of suspected abuse and/or neglect.

Elder abuse comes in many forms, including:

- *Physical abuse*, such as hitting, pushing, causing unnecessary pain, intentional misuse of medication, causing injury, and unauthorized restraint
- *Sexual abuse*, such as inappropriate exposure, inappropriate sexual advances, inappropriate sexual contact, sexual exploitation, and rape
- *Emotional or verbal abuse*, such as humiliation, threats of harm or abandonment, isolation, non-communication, intimidation
- *Financial abuse*, such as undue influence to change legal documents, misuse of property, and theft or embezzlement

abuse physical or psychological injury by another person.

neglect a person's inability to care for self or a person's caregiver providing inadequate care.

The signs of abuse and neglect are not always obvious and sometimes difficult to identify. In many cases, the injuries or circumstances can be blamed on the normal characteristics of aging, such as dementia, coexisting illnesses, and more frequent falls.

Some clues you might discover during your physical exam that may be indications of abuse or neglect include:

- Sores, bruises, or other wounds
- Unkempt appearance
- Poor hygiene
- Malnutrition
- Dehydration

PERSPECTIVE

Ralph—The Son

Mom's on a fixed income. Isn't that what it's called? Where she only gets social security and Dad's pension each month? Everything's about money with her, you know? "How much is this costin' me?" or "How much is that costin' me?" Get this: She once called me because a pan had caught fire on her stove and she asked me if she'd get charged for calling for a fire truck. I said, "Momma, is the pan still burnin' right now?" and she says, "Oh, yeah, and the drapes by the sink too." Do you believe that? After that, I've visited her a lot more frequently.

Advocating for the Elderly

As an EMT you have a duty to serve as an advocate for your patients, especially those patient populations that may not be able to care or advocate for themselves. When caring for the elderly, be especially diligent when obtaining a history and performing your physical exam. Be sure to evaluate for signs and symptoms that may not necessarily pertain to the chief complaint. Common signs of suspected abuse:

- Unrealistic or vague explanations for injuries
- An obvious delay in seeking care
- Unexplained injuries (past or present)
- Poor interaction between patient and caregiver

Much like any suspected case of abuse or neglect, you have an obligation to carefully and thoroughly document your findings objectively and report all cases of suspected abuse or neglect to the proper authorities. All 50 states have specific guidelines for the reporting of elder abuse and neglect, and your instructor can provide you with the details for your state.

EMERGENCY DISPATCH SUMMARY

Nancy was able to persuade the patient to see a doctor and, due to the ice outside the home, Brandi requested a lift assist from the local fire station. The patient was then transported in a position of comfort to County General where the emergency department physician recommended immediate surgery to remove her lower leg. The patient has since returned home and is receiving in-home physical therapy to assist her in relearning how to walk using a prosthesis.

Chapter Review

To the Point

- The assessment and emergency care of geriatric patients can sometimes be challenging due to normal age-related changes in the human body.
- Many geriatric patients have multiple illnesses, take numerous prescription and over-the-counter medications, have problems with mobility, and may have issues of incontinence.
- The respiratory system can experience a reduction in strength and endurance of the muscles that assist in breathing, a loss of lung elasticity, and collapse of the smaller airway structures, all of which contribute to respiratory challenges.
- The circulatory system can be affected by a thickening of the walls of the heart, a reduction in the effectiveness of the heart's conduction system, and a loss of elasticity of the blood vessels, which can cause everything from reduced cardiac output and dysrhythmia to aneurysms that can burst.
- Age-related deterioration of the nervous system can cause slowing of psychomotor functioning, decreased reaction times, forgetfulness, and loss of sensation and coordination, which is often the cause of falls among the elderly.
- Osteoporosis and degeneration of the musculoskeletal system can cause bone weakness and general instability, which can lead to falls and serious injuries. You also will notice degeneration-related curvature of the spine in some elderly patients, which makes immobilization and airway maintenance a challenge.
- Age changes the skin in several important ways. The skin becomes thinner and weaker, more susceptible to tears and injuries, and yet due to sluggish cellular regeneration, it can be very slow to heal.
- When assessing a geriatric patient, remember to look for things in the patient's environment such as unsafe conditions, nonworking heating and cooling systems, and signs that may indicate abuse or neglect.
- Be respectful when physically examining a geriatric patient, ensuring modesty and privacy.
- Elder abuse can come in many forms, including physical, emotional, sexual, and financial.
- As an EMT you have a legal duty to report suspected cases of abuse and neglect to the appropriate authorities.

Chapter Questions

Multiple Choice

For each question, place a check next to the correct answer.

1. In reference to physiological changes in the respiratory system, all of the following are true *except*:

_____ a. lung tissue becomes more elastic.

_____ b. gag reflexes may be diminished.

_____ c. elderly patients are more prone to pneumonia.

_____ d. strokes and nervous system diseases can cause difficulty swallowing.

2. Medications for high blood pressure and heart conditions may:
   _____ a. prevent the heart rate from increasing to compensate for shock.
   _____ b. cause severe constriction of the vessels.
   _____ c. cause unequal pupils.
   _____ d. cause a buildup of fluid in the sac surrounding the heart.
3. Which one of the following is *true* regarding the senses in the elderly?
   _____ a. All elderly patients have hearing deficits.
   _____ b. A slightly delayed response to a question indicates a hearing problem.
   _____ c. A prior stroke can cause problems with speech.
   _____ d. If the patient cannot see, you should try writing your questions on a piece of paper.
4. Geriatric patients often are less able to defend against illness and may take much longer to recover when they do become ill. This often results in:
   _____ a. multiple simultaneous illnesses.
   _____ b. forgetting doctor appointments.
   _____ c. taking the wrong medications.
   _____ d. hearing loss.
5. The aging process can cause a degeneration of the heart's electrical system, which can lead to:
   _____ a. hearing loss.
   _____ b. vision loss.
   _____ c. dysrhythmias.
   _____ d. stroke (brain attack).
6. Most states have laws that require EMTs to report suspected cases of:
   _____ a. dementia.
   _____ b. abuse and neglect.
   _____ c. Alzheimer's disease.
   _____ d. overdose.
7. You have been called to the home of an elderly person and discover that she is refusing care. She states that she just wants to be left alone. You observe that the patient lives alone, is wearing only undergarments, and has multiple open sores and bruises over her body. These are most likely the signs of:
   _____ a. abuse.
   _____ b. neglect.
   _____ c. self-neglect.
   _____ d. Alzheimer's.
8. While caring for an elderly patient, he shares with you that his caregiver frequently yells at him and refuses to respond to his calls for assistance. This may be a form of what type of abuse?
   _____ a. Physical
   _____ b. Emotional
   _____ c. Financial
   _____ d. Sexual

Critical Thinking

1. You are called to the residence of an elderly patient who has fallen out of bed. She is not injured and refuses transport. You consider this an opportunity to prevent further falls and injury. List three things you can check that might prevent injury in the future.

2. If you were to respond to an elderly patient several times and the complaint always seems minor, what would you look for to determine if the patient is experiencing depression?

Case Study

Your patient is an 89-year-old woman who has an altered mental status. You were called by her daughter who says she checked on her mother the night before and she was fine. You arrive to find the patient sitting quietly in a chair. She tells you she feels "fine, but tired." Her daughter is concerned because of the sudden change in mental status. You perform a history and physical examination for a medical patient. She denies falls or injury, is not diabetic and has eaten, shows no signs of neurological problems, and has no problems completing all components of the Cincinnati Prehospital Stroke Scale. Her vitals are within normal limits. She has a history of high blood pressure and is on a blood thinner because she had a "mini-stroke" several months ago.

1. Based on the information in this chapter and throughout the book, choose two or three possibilities of what could be wrong with this patient.

   ____

   ____

   ____

   ____

2. For each of the possibilities you wrote above, list two ways to examine or explore that problem.

   ____

   ____

   ____

   ____

The Last Word

The number of elderly persons in the United States is growing quickly. Since most EMTs will routinely respond to care for elderly patients, it is important to have an understanding of the unique physical and psychosocial characteristics of the elderly. Although the majority of the elderly lead healthy, active lives, many illnesses become more common with age. Age-related changes make the elderly prone to injuries from falls and motor-vehicle collisions and leave them less able to compensate for illness and injury. Because of this reduced ability to respond and compensate, the patient's illness or injury may be much more serious than it appears. In addition to the physical changes of aging, financial concerns, isolation, substance abuse, and depression all can impact the health of the elderly patient.

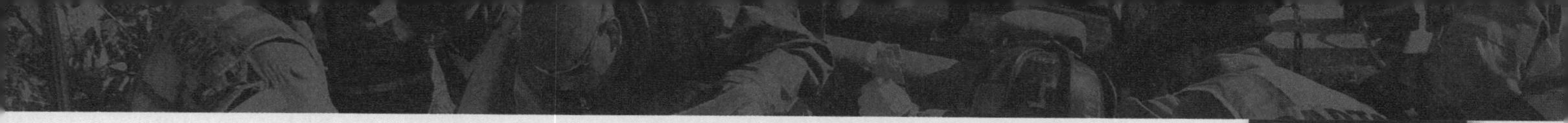

Caring for Patients with Special Challenges

40

Education Standards

Special Patient Populations: Patients with Special Challenges

Competencies

Applies fundamental knowledge of growth, development, and aging and assessment findings to provide basic emergency care and transportation for a patient with special needs.

Objectives

After completion of this lesson, you should be able to:

40-1 Define key terms introduced in this chapter.

40-2 Recognize a variety of special needs patients.

40-3 Describe important principles in the general approach to special needs patients.

40-4 Identify particular health concerns of the obese, homeless, and poor.

40-5 Recognize common medical devices used in the home care of special needs patients.

40-6 Employ effective techniques of communication with special needs patients, their families, and caregivers.

Key Terms

autism spectrum disorders (ASD) p. 1067
automatic implanted cardiac defibrillator (AICD) p. 1077
bariatrics p. 1070
cerebral palsy (CP) p. 1068
colostomy p. 1082
congenital p. 1061
continuous positive airway pressure (CPAP) p. 1074
developmental disability p. 1067
dialysis p. 1080
disability p. 1058
Down syndrome p. 1063
feeding tube p. 1080
left ventricular assist device (LVAD) p. 1078
obesity p. 1070
ostomy bag p. 1082
pacemaker p. 1077
stoma p. 1075
tracheostomy p. 1074
urinary catheter p. 1081
vascular access device p. 1083
ventilator p. 1076

Introduction

The principles of emergency medical care you have learned so far apply to a wide variety of patients. You must adapt those principles to meet the particular health care needs of patients with special challenges. Special challenges include sensory impairments, communication disorders, cognitive impairment, physical limitations, developmental disorders, terminal illness, obesity, homelessness, and poverty. Some patients with special challenges are dependent on medical technology, either in their homes or in health care facilities. Like other vulnerable people, such as the elderly and children, these patients as a group are at higher risk for abuse and neglect.

The health problems associated with special challenges increase the likelihood that these patients will need EMS at one time or another. Patients with chronic illnesses may develop a sudden worsening of the disease that prompts a call to 911. A patient with a chronic disease may develop an acute illness, which can be more difficult to manage than the same disease would be for a patient without a coexisting chronic disease.

Patients with special challenges are sometimes referred to as *special-needs patients*. Patients with many types of challenges require special considerations. One of the few generalizations you can make about caring for such a diverse group is that empathy and respect for the patient, the patient's dignity, and the patient's rights are key.

EMERGENCY DISPATCH

EMTs Joe Davies and Heather Drake were in the process of updating the base protocol binders, when the overhead speakers buzzed loudly several times and were then silent. Both EMTs sat motionless with photocopied pages halfway inserted into plastic sheet protectors in their hands, waiting.

"I guess they didn't need …" Joe began after a long pause, but was interrupted by the dispatcher's amplified voice, booming through the corridors of the quiet fire station.

"EMS Unit four-forty, respond to 1778 Alex Place for a difficulty breathing. Looks like you're going to unit 19B."

"Four-forty copies, 1-7-7-8 Alex Place," Heather responded on the portable, smiling and shrugging her shoulders at Joe as he dropped the protocols in a haphazard stack on the table and grabbed the truck keys.

After a long seven-minute drive through rush hour traffic with the late afternoon sun positioned blindingly at the center of the windshield, they arrived at the Alex Place Apartments. Heather flipped off the siren as they entered the expansive but run-down complex of squat brown buildings, scanning the walls and doorways for anything that would identify unit 19B.

They located the correct building toward the back of the complex, next to what once was a basketball court but now resembled a rusty museum of construction debris left behind when the county refurbished the apartment complex several summers ago.

"Ronnie's in the back bedroom," a woman answered their knock almost immediately, her face flushed and wet with tears. "He fell out of bed and I can't get him up and I don't think he can breathe too good."

Joe and Heather left the gurney in the living room and walked down the dark hallway to the back bedroom where they found a morbidly obese man lying face down on the carpet. He was wedged between the edge of a twin bed and the wall, his large body filling the entire empty space on the floor of the room, and he was breathing in gasps, saying, "Somebody help Ronnie. Somebody help Ronnie."

Patients with Special Challenges

disability a physical, emotional, cognitive, or behavioral condition that interferes with a person's ability to function.

The term **disability** is used to refer to a condition that interferes significantly with a person's ability to engage in activities of daily living, such as working and caring for oneself. Disabilities include vision impairment and loss (Figure 40-1 ■), hearing impairment and loss (Figure 40-2 ■), loss of mobility, and emotional and cognitive impairments. It is preferable to speak of a person having a disability, rather than speaking of a disabled person or using the term *handicapped*.

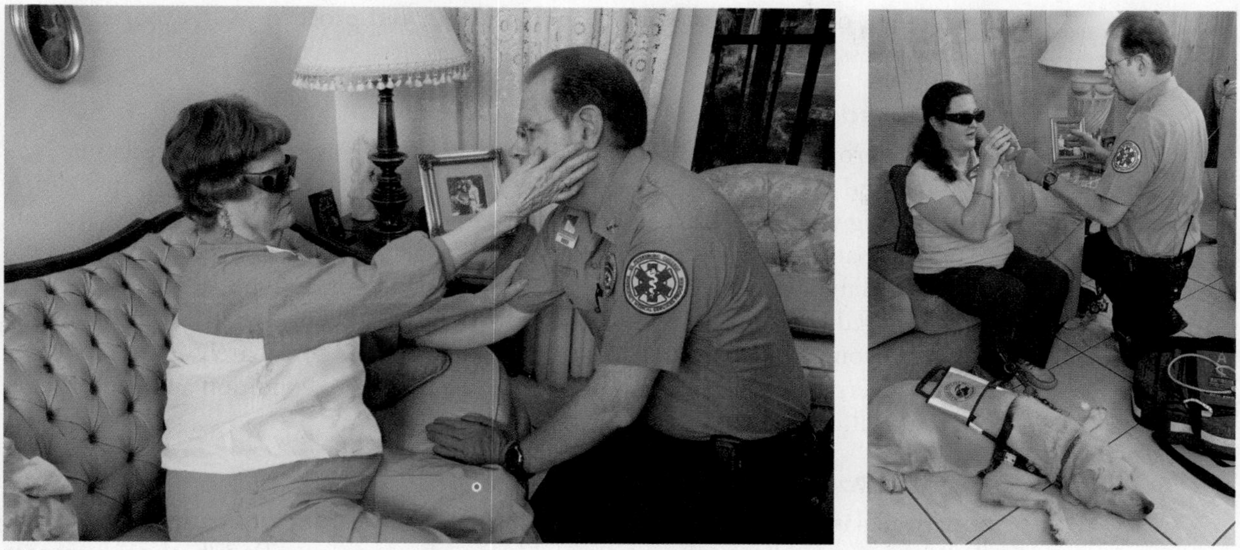

(A) (B)

Figure 40-1 (A) A blind patient may wish to touch the EMT's face. (© Michal Heron) (B) If the blind patient has a guide dog, the EMT must never get between the dog and the patient. (© Michal Heron)

Many patients with disabilities can live independently, often with some type of assistive equipment or accommodations. For example, wheelchair ramps, lowered countertops, handrails, and modified bathrooms help someone who relies on a wheelchair to live alone. Service animals, too, can be of great assistance to people with many different disabilities, increasing their independence.

Some patients with more severe disabilities live at home but require special assistance, such as ventilators, feeding tubes, and home health care services. You may also encounter patients with special needs in a variety of group home and institutional settings.

Assessing and Managing Patients with Special Challenges

40-3 Describe important principles in the general approach to special needs patients.

When a person with a special challenge presents as a patient, do not assume that the reason for requesting EMS is directly related to the disability or special need. However, it is likely that you will have to make some modifications in your approach to accommodate it (Figure 40-3 ■). In other cases, the problem may be directly related to the special challenge. Whichever the situation, perform a scene size-up and primary

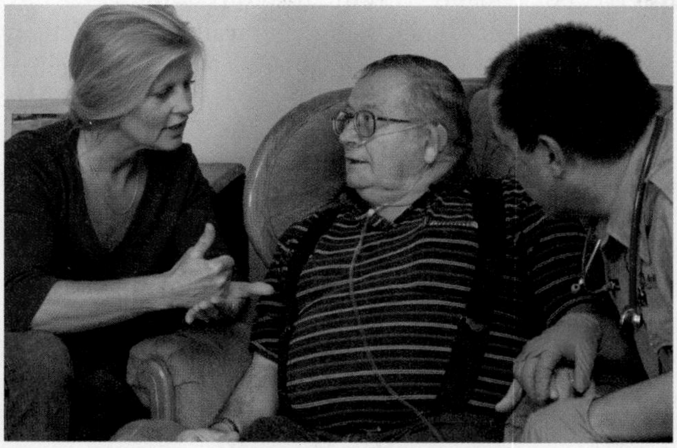

Figure 40-2 Interacting with hearing-impaired patient with a family member who signs.

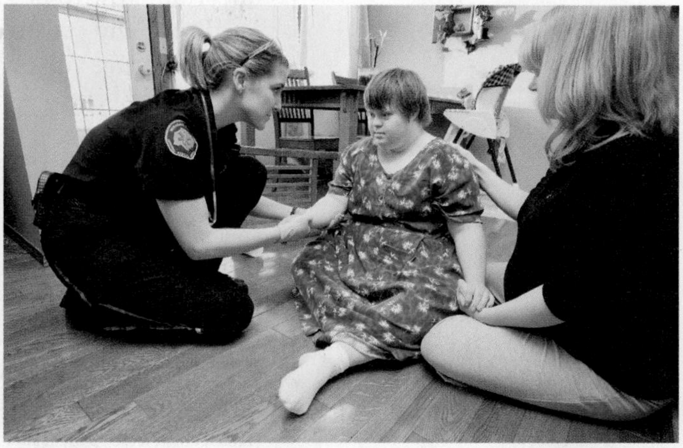

Figure 40-3 Assessing a patient with Down syndrome who has fallen.

assessment, obtain the patient's chief complaint, and proceed with a thorough secondary assessment and history based on the patient's presenting problem.

Be Knowledgeable About Special Challenges

To ensure proper care for a patient with special needs, you must be able to recognize, understand, and evaluate the patient's specific special health care requirements. In addition to increasing your knowledge, you should take steps to be prepared for specific patients or types of patients in your response area. Knowledge is critical, but you also must understand your limitations with regard to the patient's condition and special medical devices.

The medical problems of patients with special challenges can be quite complicated and some types of problems are very uncommon. Fortunately, the patient and his caregivers typically are very knowledgeable about the condition and can provide you with valuable information.

Establish Rapport

As with all patients, an important aspect of successfully caring for a patient with special challenges is establishing rapport with him and his caregiver. Treat both with respect and dignity. Be patient, listen to their concerns, and provide them with information.

Specialized Care Settings and Medical Technology

When you respond to patients with special care needs, you will encounter a variety of medical technology and health care providers, as well as the patients and their families. One example is the presence of a service dog, which helps the patient with various aspects of daily living. By federal law, you must allow the animal to accompany the patient in the ambulance unless the dog poses a threat to others, such as by growling or lunging. However, service animals are well trained and aggressive behavior is unusual. Also remember, as attracted as you may be to a service animal, he is a working animal and it is not appropriate to distract him by petting or playing with him.

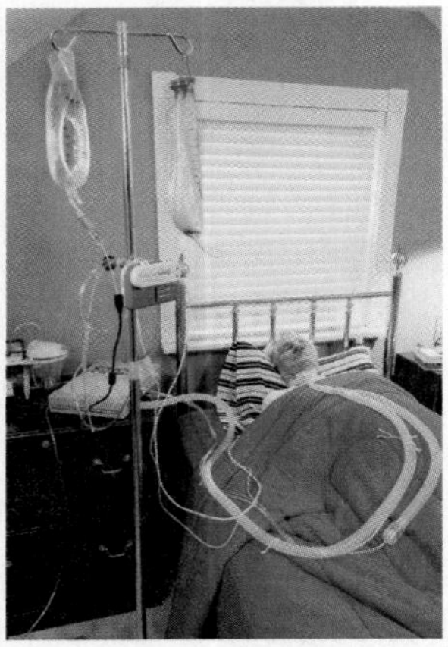

Figure 40-4 Patient on a home ventilator and receiving nutrition by way of a feeding tube.

Patients with special challenges often require the use of medical devices in the home. You will be familiar with some, such as oxygen for home use. However, other devices, such as feeding tubes, mechanical ventilators, and central venous lines, are not used in the EMT scope of practice (Figure 40-4 ■). Consult with medical direction if the treatment or skill required is not something for which you are trained or not specifically addressed by your protocols.

In most cases, the patient or his caregiver is knowledgeable about the patient's medical device. Always ask questions rather than assume you understand an unfamiliar device. If the reason for the 911 call centers around the device and you are uncertain how to proceed, request ALS or consult with medical direction.

Bring any assistive device the patient needs, such as a cane, walker, wheelchair, brace, hearing aid, or glasses along with the patient if transport to a medical facility is necessary.

Settings

EMTs respond to calls at private residences, nursing homes, rehabilitation centers, and specialized care facilities. Take the time to become familiar with all special health care facilities in your community so you can be better prepared for calls of this nature. Your management and medical direction should meet and develop plans with facility representatives to ensure smooth interaction between EMS providers and facility staff during emergency calls. Facility representatives may be able to arrange for you to see various medical devices in operation to familiarize you with them. In some communities, the dispatch center offers a mechanism to identify people who may require additional help with medical devices in case of a disaster or evacuation from a building.

Knowledgeable Patients, Families, and Care Providers

One of the advantages of encounters with patients with special needs is that they often have on site, or are accompanied by, a person who has been trained regarding the patient's devices and conditions. This person may be medically trained, such as a registered nurse, a certified nursing assistant, or a home health aide, but more often it will be a family member or friend. The patient, too, is generally a good source of information about his condition and devices (Figure 40-5 ■).

40-6 Employ effective techniques of communication with special needs patients, their families, and caregivers.

The source of information and your approach to obtaining it depend on the patient's mental status and baseline level of functioning. If the patient has an altered mental status or if medical conditions prevent effective interaction, the family will be the primary source of knowledge. Regardless of the patient's mental status or condition, always explain what you are doing. Even if it appears that the patient is unresponsive, he may be able to hear you. Talking and explaining your actions to the patient may help alleviate any stress the patient may be feeling yet unable to show.

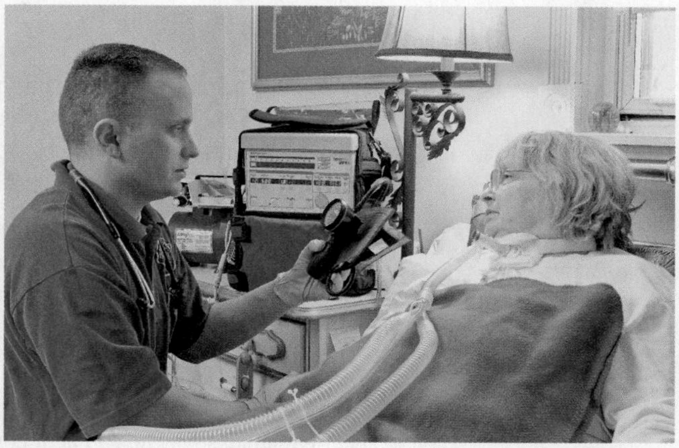

Figure 40-5 The patient is often a good source about her own condition and home medical devices.

Although patients and family members may not have had formal medical education or certification, they are generally very familiar and comfortable with using the devices on which the patient relies. Part of the hospital discharge planning process for patients with special needs is to provide training for the patient and his family or other caregivers. Because they have a vested interest in being competent with the devices, family members usually are very thorough and deliberate with their understanding and use of the devices. A call for EMS generally means that something is occurring beyond their level to address. Seek patient or family input on any problem that may be occurring with devices or the patient's condition. Some general questions should include: Has this problem ever occurred before? If so, what fixed it? Has someone here been taught how to fix this problem? Have you tried to fix the problem? If so, what happened?

Family members do not necessarily expect the arriving members of EMS to know or be familiar with the patient's medical device or condition. They can help guide the EMTs in a device's use and function. So, it is a good idea to assign a member of the EMS team to work with the family member regarding the medical device while others on the team concentrate on assessment, treatment, and moving the patient to the ambulance.

Asking questions (What is the best way to move you? How do you normally move him? Has she ever been transported by ambulance, and what worked well for the transfer?) will allow patients and family members to be part of the solution and retain some sense of control in the situation.

Despite the family's willingness to help you, they will still be apprehensive about the problem that prompted the EMS call. Proceed with deliberate steps and explain all of your actions to the family.

Causes of Disability

A patient may face special challenges because of a variety of diseases or conditions that result in disability. Some conditions include only physical, cognitive, or emotional impairment, while other conditions involve combinations. Table 40-1 describes some impairments associated with particular conditions.

40-2 Recognize a variety of special needs patients.

Diseases or conditions that lead to disability may be **congenital** or acquired. A congenital disease or condition is one that is present at birth. Congenital conditions can arise from a variety of factors, including inherited (genetic) disorders such

congenital existing at birth.

TABLE 40-1 SELECTED CONDITIONS FOR PATIENTS WITH SPECIAL NEEDS

CONDITION	DESCRIPTION	IMPLICATIONS
Autism spectrum disorders	A developmental disorder in which the patient has impaired social functioning and communication. The patient may have repetitive or restricted behaviors.	There is a wide spectrum of autism disorders. Patients with Asperger's syndrome may have social challenges and unusual behaviors, but normal language and intellect. Patients usually have language delays, communication problems, and often intellectual disability.
Cerebral palsy	A permanent impairment in motor control, present within two years of birth. Cerebral palsy is not progressive. Movements are characterized by lack of coordination, exaggerated reflexes, and tightness of muscles.	Although some patients with cerebral palsy may also have cognitive impairment, do not assume this is the case.
Cognitive disabilities	These may result from mental retardation due to a variety of genetic and congenital problems—for example, Down syndrome and fetal alcohol syndrome. It may also result from stroke, dementia, or past traumatic brain injury.	Patients have varying levels of impairment in intellectual functioning, including learning, judgment, problem solving, social skills, and communication with others. Some patients may live independently, whereas others have only limited ability to interact with others.
Hearing impairment	This condition may be congenital, due to trauma, or due to age. Hearing loss may be partial or complete.	Patients may have hearing aids, use TTY devices, or use sign language. Some patients can lip read, so it is important to face the patient and talk to him directly, even if he has complete hearing loss.
Kidney failure	This condition may be a consequence of diabetes, high blood pressure, or other medical problems. Patients can have varying levels of kidney function, and receive dialysis at different frequencies.	Patients are prone to a number of metabolic disturbances, especially if a dialysis appointment is missed. Dialysis access devices (shunts or fistulas) can malfunction and bleed. Do not take a blood pressure in an extremity with dialysis access. Patients with continuous ambulatory peritoneal dialysis will usually know the best way to manage their device.
Neuromuscular disorders	Examples include muscular dystrophy, multiple sclerosis, and Lou Gehrig's disease.	Patients have varying levels of muscular weakness, which can be intermittent or progressive, resulting in paralysis. Complications can include respiratory paralysis, in which the patient depends on a ventilator.
Stroke	Levels of disability vary from mild to incapacitating. Specific problems relate to the area of the brain affected, and may involve emotional, behavioral, communication, intellectual, or physical limitations.	Do not make assumptions about a patient's ability to hear and understand, even though communication skills may be impaired.
Spinal-cord injury	With complete spinal-cord injury, patients experience lack of sensation and function below the level of the injury.	Patients with high spinal-cord injuries may be ventilator dependent. This, combined with an inability to cough, increases the chances of pneumonia. Patients with urinary catheters are also prone to infection. Immobility may result in ischemia of compressed tissues, leading to breakdown of the skin and tissue beneath it (decubitus ulcer, pressure sore, or bedsore).
Vision impairment	This condition may be congenital or acquired, and may be either complete or partial.	Often, visually impaired patients cope well and are able to find their way through familiar surroundings. Ask the patient about the best way to help him navigate. If the patient uses a cane or service animal, be sure to transport them with the patient. Always explain what you are going to do before you do it.

as cystic fibrosis, chromosomal abnormalities such as **Down syndrome**, maternal illness during pregnancy (deafness related to maternal rubella), exposure to toxins during fetal development (fetal alcohol syndrome), or lack of certain nutrients at key points in fetal development (neural tube defects, such as spina bifida). In some cases, such as certain congenital heart defects (malformation of the heart or great vessels that are connected to it), the causes of the condition are incompletely understood and may involve a variety of factors.

Down syndrome a developmental disability that arises from an extra copy of the 21st chromosome and which results in characteristic physical features and medical conditions.

An *acquired disease* or condition is one that occurs after birth and may be the result of exposure to an infectious organism, lifestyle factors, genetic predisposition, or may be the result of another medical condition or trauma. Examples of acquired diseases and conditions include osteoarthritis, coronary heart disease, obesity, COPD, HIV/AIDS, and traumatic spinal-cord injury.

Some patients face special challenges because of psychosocial factors, such as homelessness, poverty, and abuse. Patients with chronic illnesses often face financial stresses that lead to poverty, and patients who are homeless or poor are at higher risk for health problems.

PERSPECTIVES

Joe—The EMT

Wow. That was a new one for me. We get there and not only is the patient morbidly obese, and I mean very, very morbidly obese, but he's also got Down syndrome and was having a really tough time understanding what was going on. He couldn't lift his own weight, was lying on both arms, and the way he was wedged between the bed and the wall was preventing him from breathing adequately. And there was no way for us to get positioned in the little room to move him. That was just a nightmare. Luckily, Heather had the presence of mind to call for a lift assist because I got so focused on trying to find a way to reposition Ronnie that I would have caused a real delay by the time I thought of it.

Sensory Impairment and Communication Disorders

Impairment or loss of one of the special senses or the ability to communicate can create special challenges for people. Hearing impairment, blindness, and speech disorders can complicate the ability for patients to relate their complaints and histories to caregivers, and can complicate the health care provider's ability to provide information to the patient. EMS providers tend to get a lot of information about what people are thinking by interacting with them in ways that involve the senses and ability to communicate.

Keep in mind that an impaired ability to get information through the senses or through speech and language does not mean that a patient's cognitive ability is impaired. It simply means that the patient may not be able to get certain information to inform his thoughts or communicate well with others about his thoughts. However, in some patients, a sensory or communication disorder does coexist with a cognitive disorder. Take the opportunity to assess both the patient's sensory and communication challenges, as well as his cognitive ability without making assumptions about them.

Hearing Impairment

Hearing impairment, or deafness, can be congenital or can develop for a variety of reasons. Because some loss of hearing can occur with aging (presbycusis), hearing loss is more common among the elderly.

Patients have a variety of ways of adapting to deafness. Patients with some types of partial hearing loss can benefit from hearing aids to amplify sound. Hearing aids do not produce normal hearing and in fact can make it difficult to distinguish background noise from conversation and other sounds the patient wishes to hear. For that reason, patients do not always use hearing aids, even when they have them. If a patient uses hearing aids but does not have one in, offer to retrieve the device for the patient to improve communication.

Some patients who are deaf may receive cochlear implants. Such devices replace the function of the ear structures and nerves by converting the mechanical movements of the inner ear structure to electrical impulses, which are transmitted to areas of the brain that interpret the impulses as sound. Although there is a period of learning what all of the conducted sounds (including words) mean, patients with cochlear implants will be able to communicate normally once that learning has occurred.

Patients who are deaf may read lips or communicate using American Sign Language (ASL). Lip reading is prone to misinterpretation, especially when it involves an unfamiliar person and unfamiliar words, such as those that might be used in an emergency. Exaggerating words, slowing speech, or speaking loudly will distort the appearance of words on the lips, which interferes with lip reading. When confronted with someone who has a hearing impairment, face the patient squarely and speak normally to give him the best opportunity to read your lips.

The speech of hearing-impaired patients may or may not be affected. It is often preferable to communicate with hearing-impaired patients, including those whose hearing aids seem not to be functioning, by using writing. Write your questions and statements on a piece of paper, and have the patient do the same.

A family member may be able to serve as an interpreter, but keep in mind that using family members as interpreters in any situation is not the same as getting the information directly from the patient, because information in both directions can be "filtered" by the interpreter. Be sure to document on your prehospital care report that you had to work through an interpreter for the patient history.

Some deaf patients use a TDD/TTY, which stands for Telecommunication Device for the Deaf/TeleTypewriter. The system consists of a keyboard, display screen, and modem connected to an analog telephone line. The user can type in a message and receive a response that is displayed on the screen. Such a device may be how the deaf patient contacted and communicated with the emergency call center when requesting EMS.

Vision Impairment

Vision impairment can be partial or complete (blindness). Blindness can be congenital or acquired. Glaucoma, cataracts, macular degeneration, and diabetes are causes of acquired vision impairment. Blind patients may not use lights in their home or may not notice lights that have burned out. You may need to use your flashlight to provide adequate light to assess, treat, and move the patient.

Speak to a blind patient to let him know you are nearby before touching him, and always explain what you are going to do before you do it. When assisting a blind person in walking, ask how you can best help him navigate. A blind patient usually knows the layout of his home very well and relies on things being in the same place to navigate safely. If you move anything to gain access to or treat the patient, return it to the exact position in which you found it. If the patient has a service dog, follow the guidelines presented earlier in the chapter.

Speech Impairment

Speech impairment falls into four categories: language disorders, articulation disorders, voice production disorders, and fluency disorders. Language disorders involve the inability to understand spoken or written communication. They can result from learning or developmental disorders, stroke, or traumatic brain injury. An articulation order is the inability to speak clearly, despite understanding and being able to use language. It can result from deafness or neurological or neuromuscular disorders. Patients with articulation disorders should be able to write normally. A voice production disorder arises from damage of the larynx or vocal cords. A fluency disorder presents with stuttering speech.

Be patient with persons who have speech impairments. Do not interrupt them when they are speaking. Seek the assistance of family members and, if necessary, have the patient use a pen and paper to communicate with you.

Cognitive Impairment

Cognitive impairment involves a level of difficulty with intellectual functions, such as reasoning, problem-solving, memory, or learning. Cognitive impairment can be mild or profound. Some causes include dementia, mental retardation, stroke, traumatic or hypoxic brain injury, and developmental disorders (for example, Down syndrome and cerebral palsy). The patient's ability to communicate with you is related to the severity of impairment and whether he also has sensory impairment or communication disorders.

Attempt to communicate with the patient first. Adapt your vocabulary and the complexity of speech to achieve understanding. If communication with the patient is severely affected, you must obtain additional information from a caregiver.

Emotional impairment can accompany cognitive impairment and, in some types of cognitive impairment, judgment and inhibition may be affected. Be alert to the potential for violence or other inappropriate behaviors. Understand that the patient may be afraid or anxious and do not separate him from caregivers, if possible.

STOP, REVIEW, REMEMBER!

Multiple Choice

For each question, place a check next to the correct answer.

1. A condition that significantly interferes with a person's ability to engage in the activities of daily living and work is most appropriately referred to as a(n):

_____ a. handicap.

_____ b. disability.

_____ c. disorder.

_____ d. impairment.

2. If you respond to care for a patient who has a service dog, which one of the following best describes how you should manage the dog?

_____ a. Contact your supervisor to determine your employer's policy and insurance coverage regarding having animals in the ambulance.

_____ b. Never allow an animal in a health care setting, including an ambulance.

_____ c. Under federal law, service animals must be transported unless they pose a threat.

_____ d. Call animal control to take possession of the dog while the owner is being transported.

(continued on next page)

(continued)

3. The first source of information about a patient's home medical device that you should consider is:

_____ a. on-line medical direction.

_____ b. the device manufacturer.

_____ c. the patient's physician.

_____ d. the patient.

4. As you approach a patient and begin to ask questions, he makes gestures to indicate that he cannot hear. Neither you nor your partner sign, and the patient cannot seem to read your lips. The best approach to try in this situation is to:

_____ a. try writing your questions on a piece of paper and have the patient respond in writing.

_____ b. speak more slowly.

_____ c. request a sign language interpreter to respond to the scene.

_____ d. pantomime and gesture, even though you do not know American Sign Language.

5. A patient you are trying to communicate with uses words that sound clear, but that do not make sense. Some of the words seem made-up. The most likely explanation is a(n) _____________ disorder.

_____ a. language

_____ b. articulation

_____ c. fluency

_____ d. voice production

Critical Thinking

1. What clues would prompt you to determine whether or not a patient has a cognitive impairment?

____

____

____

____

2. How can blindness interfere with communication?

____

____

____

____

3. What explains the high degree of understanding of medical conditions and devices that the family of a patient with special needs often has, despite not having formal medical education?

____

____

____

____

4. You have responded to care for a patient who has a special implanted pump, which his family refers to as an LVAD. The family is concerned that there is a problem with the device. What are some questions you should ask?

____

____

____

____

5. Describe several ways that can help you communicate well with hearing impaired patients.

____

____

____

____

Developmental Disability

The Centers for Disease Control uses the term **developmental disability** to mean a chronic mental or physical impairment beginning at any age up to 22 years and causing significant impairment in the person's major life activities. The underlying causes of developmental disabilities can be congenital or acquired, and in some cases, the causes are incompletely understood. Developmental disabilities include cerebral palsy, Down syndrome, and autism spectrum disorders (ASD) (Figure 40-6 ■), among others.

developmental disability lifelong physical or mental impairments that begin before the age of 22 years.

Autism

Autism spectrum disorders (ASD) affect approximately 1 in 88 children. Although it is clear that the diagnosis of ASD has increased over recent years, the reasons for that increase are not clear. It may be because of better methods of diagnosis, for example, and not an increase in the number of individuals affected. Because ASD is common and often misunderstood, and because patients with more severe forms of ASD can be difficult to manage, particularly if the initial approach of the health care provider agitates the patient, it is important to learn about it.

autism spectrum disorders (ASD) developmental disorders that affect, among other things, language, social skills, and behavior.

Autism spectrum disorders represent a range of syndromes from patients with Asperger's syndrome (who usually have good language skills, but are socially impaired, being intensely and narrowly focused on a particular interest) to patients with autistic disorder (who have severely impaired language and social skills, exhibit repetitive behaviors, and often have mental retardation and seizures). However, people with ASD are susceptible to the same medical emergencies as the general population, often have coexisting medical conditions such as seizure disorders, and are prone to sustaining certain types of injuries, all of which increase the likelihood of an EMS response.

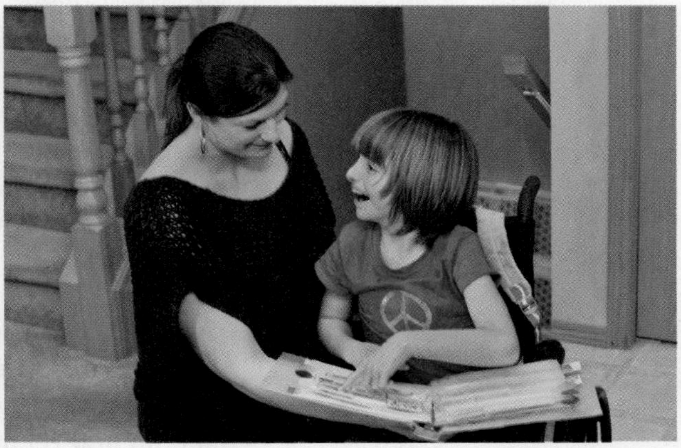

Figure 40-6 A child with developmental delay.

Communicating and building trust with patients who have ASD is likely to be one of the most challenging aspects of care. They often interpret words literally and have difficulty distinguishing patterns of speech such as humor, slang, sarcasm, or idioms. Body language, such as gesturing or facial expressions, also may not be recognized. Understanding the limitations in communication abilities and, as much as possible, accommodating the needs of a patient with ASD provide the best chance of building trust and increasing compliance and cooperation.

Key aspects of dealing with patients with ASD include the following:

- Be aware that patients with ASD can have rigid routines and a strong preference for things to be predictable. Disruption is not well tolerated.
- Keep things basic. Use simple, clear, precise directions. For example, say "Sit down here," pointing at a chair, *not* "Why don't you have a seat?" Use short, closed-ended questions instead of open-ended ones. Allow extra time to answer. Basic also means less "stuff." Radios, pagers, cell phones, flashlights, and other items may overstimulate the senses of people with autism.
- If a person with ASD is behaving aggressively or is escalated, it is rarely from what most of us would refer to as malicious or defiant behavior. The patient with ASD is reacting to extreme stress.
- When dealing with a person who has ASD, particularly if the patient is escalating, remain calm. Assertive body language, loud commands, becoming impatient, or even telling the patient to "calm down" can be ineffective or even counterproductive. Remember that calm creates calm.
- Involving the patient in his own care and accommodating his needs, when possible, will likely build trust and increase compliance and cooperation.

Down Syndrome

Down syndrome (also called *trisomy 21*) is a genetic disorder in which a patient is born with three, instead of the normal two Number 21 chromosomes. Because of their intellectual disabilities, using similar communication and treatment strategies as described for the ASD patient may be helpful when treating patients with Down syndrome.

However, unlike patients with ASD, patients with Down syndrome possess significant anatomical differences that can affect their emergency care. They are physically shorter than the average population. Their tongues are larger in proportion to their mouths and can easily cause upper airway obstruction. Their necks are not only short, which sometimes makes the proper fitting of a cervical collar difficult, but they are also prone to instability and injuries of the upper cervical spine. Patients with Down syndrome have a higher incidence of certain medical conditions that may also trigger an EMS response. They include seizure disorders, heart defects, and the premature development of dementia.

Cerebral Palsy

cerebral palsy (CP) a developmental disorder that affects movement, balance, and posture.

Cerebral palsy (CP) is a group of disorders caused by abnormalities or injuries of the brain that occur as a fetus through two years of age. This results in central nervous system abnormalities that can affect functions such as movement, learning, hearing, seeing, and speech. The effects of CP can range from mild to severe. The most common form is spastic cerebral palsy that manifests in characteristic stiff muscles, stiff or nonmobile joints (called *contractures*) and walking (gait) abnormalities.

Many patients with CP will have speech difficulties that may lead the EMT to presumptively and incorrectly believe the patient is mentally retarded. In fact, mental retardation only occurs in roughly 30% to 50% of patients with CP. When speaking with CP patients, take extra time for them to answer and express themselves. Perhaps the most common reason that patients with CP require EMS services is due to seizures. (They occur in about 50% of patients with CP.) Emergency care for such seizures is the same as for other seizure patients. (See Chapter 19.)

One special consideration in the treatment of CP patients is in the setting of trauma. Falls are common in patients with CP due to their gait disturbances. However, if the mechanism of injury warrants spinal immobilization, be aware that it can be difficult to place a CP patient on a long backboard due to the skeletal contractures. A vacuum immobilization device is ideal in that situation. If a traditional long backboard is used, extensive padding with towels or sheets may be necessary to fill in the gaps of contact and secure the patient to the board.

PERSPECTIVES

Doreen—Ronnie's Mother

Ronnie's my baby and I kept telling those ambulance folks to be careful and talk slow and simple to him because he sometimes gets mean when he gets scared or confused. And, boy, I could tell he was real scared, being stuck like that and with that guy tugging at his shoulder and all. Ronnie's a good boy, as sweet and loving as a mother could ever want, but I don't know how I can keep doing this. I'm getting old and would never be able to help him up anymore. And what if that happened while I was down at the laundromat or at the supermarket? He couldn't breathe. But I don't know what I'd do with my days if I didn't have Ronnie to tend to. He's all I've got.

Physical Disabilities

Physical disabilities may be present at birth (such as a person who is born without one or more limbs) or can arise from amputation of limb or orthopedic trauma. Physical limitations can also result from neuromuscular disorders, such as muscular dystrophy or Parkinson's disease, spinal-cord injury, or various forms of arthritis. Patients who are paralyzed, such as from spinal-cord injury, stroke, or neuromuscular disorders, are susceptible to a number of medical complications, such as pneumonia, urinary tract infections, and pressure sores.

Depending on the extent of paralysis, patients may require varying degrees of assistance in tasks of daily living, and may require the use of devices such as mechanical ventilators and urinary catheters. Patients with mobility limitations may use canes, walkers, wheelchairs, prostheses (artificial limbs), or braces to assist them. Be sure to transport these items with the patient.

CLINICAL CLUE

Paralysis

Patients who are paralyzed are at increased risk of respiratory infection if the paralysis prevents deep breathing and coughing, which normally help clear mucus and debris from the airway. Dependence on a ventilator also increases the risk of respiratory infection. In addition, the use of a catheter increases the risk of urinary tract infection, and the presence of pressure sores can lead to infection as well. Check the patient's skin temperature and, if possible, use a thermometer. An elevated temperature is one of the most common signs of an underlying infection.

Terminally Ill Patients

Terminally ill patients, such as patients with end-stage cancer, heart failure, or kidney failure or those with progressive fatal diseases such as Huntington's disease or Lou Gehrig's disease, may prefer to stay at home under the care of family, possibly with assistance from hospice or home health care providers.

Alternatively, they may spend the final weeks or days of their lives in a specially designated hospice facility. Terminally ill patients may be depending on technology to sustain life or relieve pain. Often, terminally ill patients have advance directives that specify what type of emergency care they are willing to accept. (See Chapter 3 to review the topic of advance directives.) Terminally ill patients and their families also have special emotional needs. (See Chapter 2 to review reactions to death and dying.)

Obese Patients

bariatrics the branch of medicine that deals with preventing and treating obesity.

obesity having too much body fat; a body mass index greater than 30.

Bariatrics is the branch of medicine that deals with the causes, prevention, and treatment of obesity. **Obesity** is defined as a *body mass index (BMI)* of 30 or more. Body mass index is calculated by dividing your weight in pounds by the square of your height in inches, and multiplying by 703. For example, for a woman who weighs 135 pounds and is 5 feet 5 inches tall (65 inches), the calculation is as follows:

$$\text{BMI} = 135/(65 \times 65) \times 703 = 22.46$$

A BMI of up to 24.9 is considered healthy for people over 20 years of age. A BMI of 25 to 29 is considered as overweight, while a BMI of 30 or greater is considered obese. Keep in mind that BMI does not measure body fat directly, and that an extremely muscular person could end up with a BMI of 30 or more without being obese. Recent research using sophisticated diagnostic equipment indicates that BMI may actually underestimate body fat in some patients. For most people, though, BMI is a good indicator of healthy weight.

Obesity is a significant and growing health concern in the United States for both adults and children. Obesity increases the risk of some cancers, type 2 diabetes, hypertension, heart attack, stroke, liver and gallbladder disease, arthritis, sleep apnea, and respiratory problems. Because of the prevalence of obesity and because of the serious health issues related to obesity, you will frequently encounter obese patients (Figure 40-7 ■).

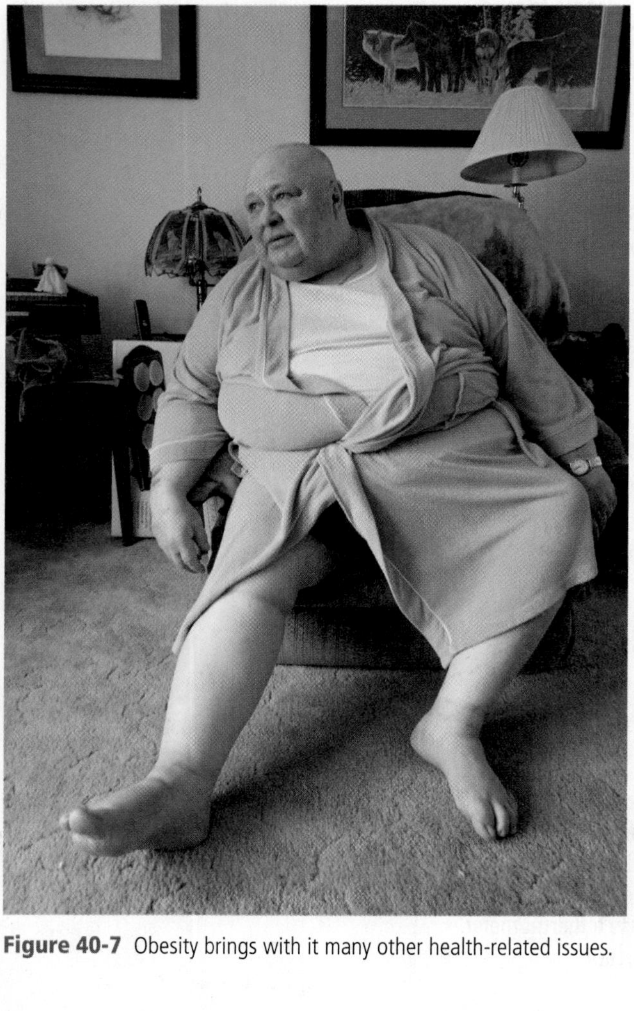

Figure 40-7 Obesity brings with it many other health-related issues.

You must take special measures to care for the obese patient, and you also must take special care in lifting to avoid injury to yourself, your coworkers, and the patient. Very obese patients may have difficulty breathing when they are supine, because of the extra weight that must be moved by the chest wall during inspiration. If possible, allow the patient to assume a comfortable position for breathing. Monitor the patient's oxygen saturation, and provide oxygen and ventilatory assistance as needed. Make sure you have enough assistance when lifting and moving obese patients, and use special equipment if the patient's weight exceeds the maximum load capacity of your stretcher. (See Chapter 8 to review lifting, moving, and positioning patients.)

PERSPECTIVES

Heather—The EMT

Unfortunately, that's becoming more common these days, calls involving really obese people. We've even had some special training days at the department on how to respond to these patients. That poor guy, though, I felt so bad for him. Luckily, we got a lift assist response right away and the fire captain who came out was an amazing problem solver! Since no one could get into the room enough to get any leverage, he says, "Why don't we inch a bed sheet under him and then see if we can pull him out into the living room and lift him there." Worked perfectly! Ronnie was a trooper, though. I love that guy. We had to bring his mom along to the hospital, of course. He made it clear there was no way he was going anywhere without her!

Homelessness and Poverty

40-4 Identify particular health concerns of the obese, homeless, and poor.

Homelessness is a state of not having a regular place to live, often because of an inability to afford or otherwise maintain regular, safe, and adequate housing. The homeless may live in vehicles, parks, on the street, in makeshift dwellings, or in abandoned buildings (Figure 40-8 ■).

In many communities, homeless shelters are available but may not have the capacity to provide for the number of homeless seeking shelter. Many homeless individuals choose not to use shelters even when space is available. The homeless include individual men, women, children, as well as families. Accurate data about the number of homeless is difficult to obtain. However, it has been estimated that between 700,000 and 1.5 million people in the United States may be homeless in any given recent year.

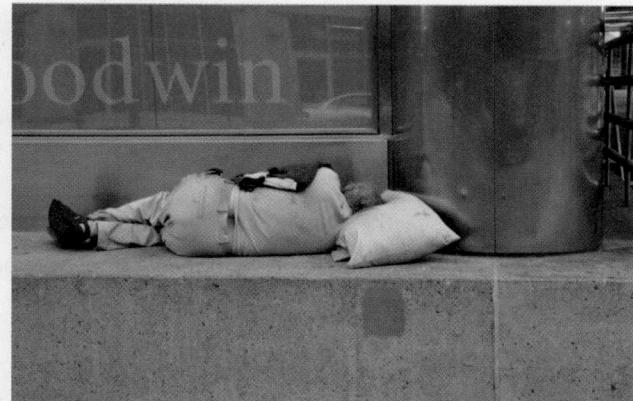

Figure 40-8 A homeless person. (© Edward T. Dickinson, MD)

Several serious health problems are related to homelessness: mental health problems, malnutrition, substance abuse problems, HIV/AIDS, tuberculosis, bronchitis and pneumonia, heat- and cold-related emergencies, wounds, and skin infections. The lack of access to health care also means conditions that begin as minor problems can go untreated until they become emergencies. Underlying chronic health problems and malnutrition can impair the body's ability to respond to injuries and acute illnesses, making them issues of more serious concern than they might otherwise be. In addition, homeless women may be victims of domestic or sexual abuse.

Poverty, which is a contributing factor to homelessness, means that income is not adequate to allow someone a standard of living considered acceptable in society. For 2009, the U.S. Department of Health and Human Services determined the poverty guideline for a single person as an income of $10,830 or less, and $22,050 for a family of four. However, there are also large numbers of individuals and families whose incomes are above this, yet it is not enough to provide all necessities, including health care, health insurance, prescription medications, and adequate nutrition. Therefore, the poor are prone to many of the same health issues as the homeless.

Abuse and Neglect

Patients with special needs can be more vulnerable to physical or sexual abuse, exploitation, and neglect because of their dependence on others and possible difficulty in reporting what has happened. This vulnerable population can include children and adults, especially the elderly. Be alert to this possibility during your scene size-up, history taking, and assessment. Stories that are inconsistent with injuries, multiple injuries in various stages of healing, repeated injuries, and caregiver indifference to the patient should bring to mind the possibility of abuse or neglect.

As with any suspected case of abuse or neglect, do not make accusations. Do your best to get the patient out of the environment and report your suspicions according to the requirements of your jurisdiction. (See Chapter 3 to review reporting situations.)

STOP, REVIEW, REMEMBER!

Multiple Choice

For each question, place a check next to the correct answer.

1. Which characteristic differentiates a developmental disability from other types of disabilities?

_____ a. It is a chronic impairment that begins before the age of 22 years.

_____ b. It always involves cognitive and emotional impairment.

_____ c. The patient"outgrows" it by adulthood.

_____ d. The physical impairments are severe, but cognitive and emotional functions are rarely affected.

2. A four-year-old boy has an autism spectrum disorder that is characterized by good language skills but poor social skills. He has an intense interest in cars. He knows the make and model of nearly every car he sees, and identifies extended family members and family friends by the kind of cars they drive. This description is most characteristic of:

_____ a. Down syndrome.

_____ b. Asperger's syndrome.

_____ c. childhood disintegrative disorder.

_____ d. pervasive developmental disorder that is not otherwise specified.

3. All of the following are characteristics of autism spectrum disorders *except:*

_____ a. repetitive behaviors.

_____ b. high incidence of seizures.

_____ c. inability to appreciate humor and sarcasm.

_____ d. profound muscle weakness.

4. Regardless of the chief complaint and overall presentation, you must take special care to monitor the ___________ when transporting a very obese patient.

_____ a. blood glucose level

_____ b. respiratory status

_____ c. blood pressure

_____ d. pain level

5. Which one of the statements that follows *best* describes homelessness?

_____ a. There are adequate shelters available, but the homeless usually choose not to use them.

_____ b. At any given time, about 5 million individuals are homeless.

_____ c. Illness and injury can be more serious in a homeless person than in a patient who is not homeless.

_____ d. The primary reason for homelessness is refusal to work.

Critical Thinking

1. A 12-year-old boy with an autism spectrum disorder is having a meltdown. What are some possible factors that could be contributing to or worsening the situation?

2. What are some special considerations to keep in mind when responding to a terminally ill patient?

3. What are some of the health complications of obesity?

4. What are some health complications associated with homelessness?

5. What chronic medical conditions can be associated with Down syndrome?

Medical Technology

40-5 Recognize common medical devices used in the home care of special needs patients.

Adaptations and advances in medical technology allow people who otherwise would require hospitalization or residence in a specialized care facility to be in the relative comfort of living and working in a nonhospital environment. When making decisions about how to proceed with regard to a patient's medical device, take into account the answers to these questions: What is the purpose of the device? What does it do for the patient? Is the problem with the device life threatening? Do I have the knowledge to fix this problem? Do I have the supplies needed to fix this problem? Is this within my protocols or within medical direction authorization?

Respiratory Devices

Patients can use a variety of respiratory support devices in the home, ranging from oxygen administered by nasal cannula to mechanical ventilators. While continuing oxygen administration is not a problem for EMTs, making decisions about CPAP, BiPAP, tracheostomy care, and mechanical ventilators can be more challenging.

Continuous Positive Airway Pressure Devices

continuous positive airway pressure (CPAP) a form of noninvasive positive pressure ventilation that consists of a mask that provides air or oxygen under pressure to prevent collapse of the airway or assist with some causes of difficulty breathing.

Continuous positive airway pressure (CPAP) is a form of noninvasive positive-pressure ventilation (NPPV) (Figure 40-9 ▪). It blows oxygen or air under constant low pressure, through a tube and mask, to prevent the patient's airway passages from collapsing at the end of a breath. It is often prescribed to patients who suffer sleep apnea (periods when breathing stops during sleep) to help keep airway passages open as the patient sleeps. CPAP can help such patients prevent exacerbation of other medical conditions and reduce the chronic fatigue and irritability caused by interrupted sleep. CPAP can be used in adults and children.

A related device is the biphasic continuous positive airway pressure (BiPAP) device. Rather than a continuous pressure, BiPAP provides higher pressure during inspiration and lower pressure during expiration.

A patient who uses a CPAP device only at night is unlikely to have a medical emergency directly related to the device and will not need the device during transport. However, hospital personnel should be alerted that the patient uses a CPAP device during sleep.

Tracheostomies and Stomas

tracheostomy a surgical incision into the trachea in order to insert a breathing tube.

A **tracheostomy** is a procedure that creates a surgical opening through the neck into the trachea (Figure 40-10 ▪). A tracheostomy is usually created near the second to

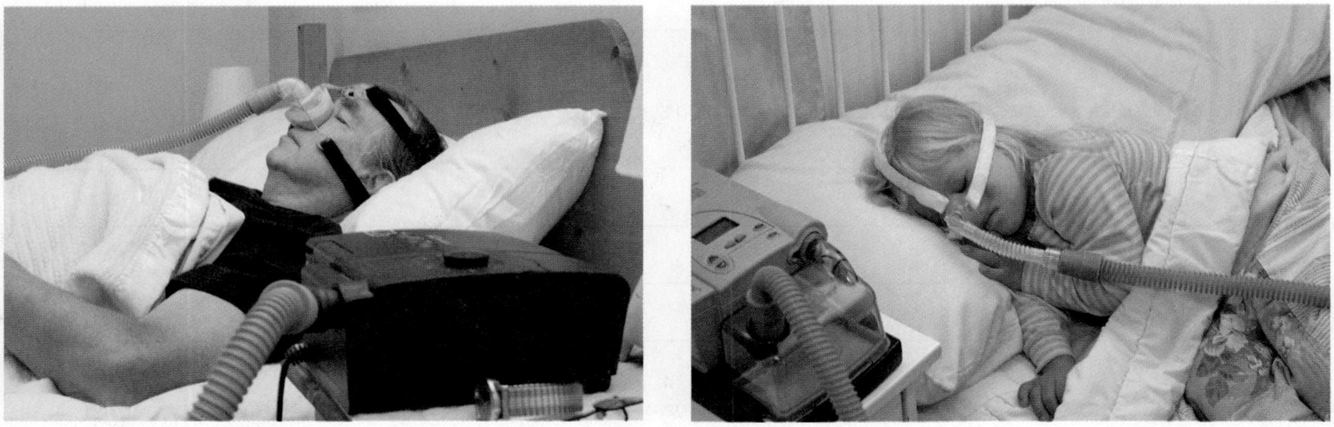

(A) (B)

Figure 40-9 A continuous positive airway pressure (CPAP) device may be prescribed to (A) adults and (B) children.

fourth tracheal ring. It is performed to allow the insertion of a tracheostomy tube in patients who need long-term ventilatory assistance, or as a means of providing an air passage in patients who have undergone a laryngectomy (surgical removal of the larynx). The opening itself is called a **stoma**.

A tracheostomy procedure may be performed in patients who need long-term ventilator assistance, such as those with neuromuscular disorders, spinal-cord injuries, tumors, congenital deformities, coma, and a variety of other conditions that affect the ability to breathe. A patient with a tracheostomy tube may or may not be on a home ventilator. Tracheostomy patients who are on ventilators may be on them all the time or only when sleeping.

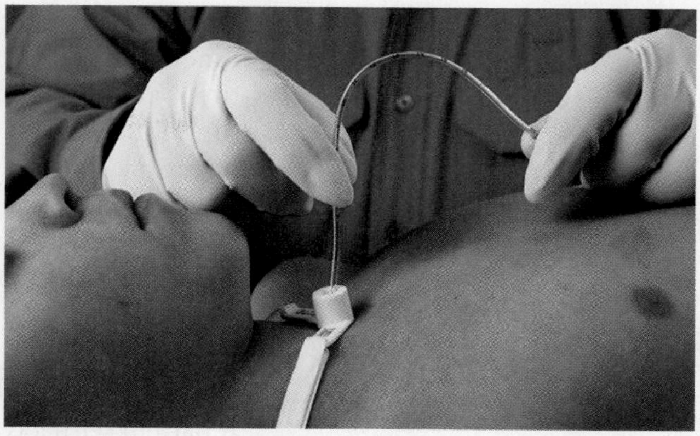

Figure 40-10 Suctioning a tracheostomy tube.

Tracheostomy patients range from newborns to the very elderly. A patient with a tracheostomy may or may not be able to speak, depending on his condition. Some are able to speak by covering the tracheostomy tube briefly and making use of a speaker valve attached to the tube or an electronic box applied to the larynx. Do not assume that a patient with a tracheostomy either can or cannot speak.

stoma a permanent surgical opening in the front of the neck through which the patient breathes.

Tracheostomy Tubes

A tracheostomy tube is a short breathing tube with a collar, called a *flange*, at one end. It is inserted into the airway to allow the patient to breathe through the stoma instead of through the nose and mouth (Figure 40-11 ■). It is often called a trach (pronounced *trayk*) tube.

Tracheostomy tubes used by older children and adults are usually double-cannula devices (a cannula is a hollow tube). A double-cannula tube has an inner cannula (a tube within a tube) that can be locked into place and removed periodically for cleaning. Tracheostomy tubes for young children are usually single-cannula tubes that do not have the removable inner cannula. A bag-mask device can be connected to either type of tracheostomy tube—to the inner cannula of a double-cannula tube or directly to a single-cannula tube.

Tracheostomy tubes usually come with an obturator, which is a long plug that is placed inside the tube to help guide it and prevent mucus from entering and clogging the tube during insertion. The obturator is removed after the tracheostomy tube is in place, but it is usually kept with the patient's supplies. If you need to suction a patient's tracheostomy tube, you will have to measure the depth of suction catheter insertion using the obturator, which is the same length as the tube.

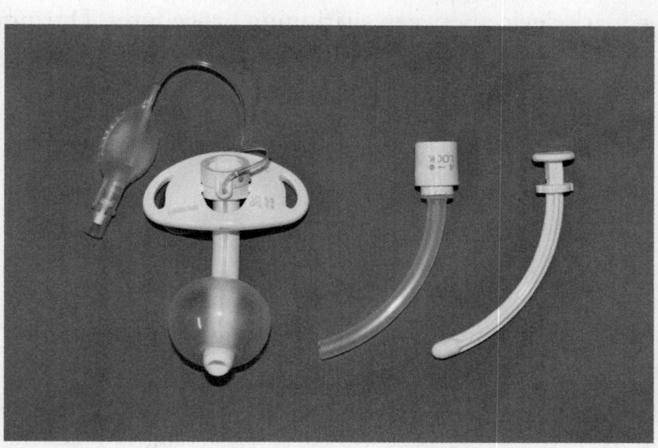

(A)

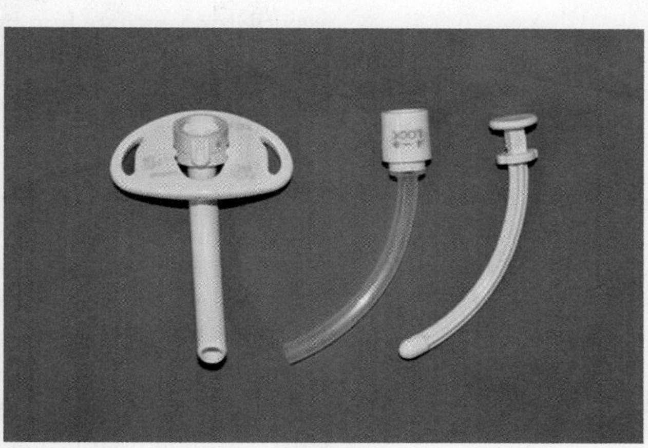

(B)

Figure 40-11 Tracheostomy tubes: (A) cuffed and (B) uncuffed. (© Edward T. Dickinson)

With a tracheostomy, air bypasses the upper airway. Normal upper airway functions, such as filtering and humidifying air and assistance with clearing secretions, are impaired. Consequences include accumulation of mucus in the tracheostomy tube, which may obstruct it and increase the chances of a lower respiratory infection. The tube must be suctioned frequently to remove the mucus. Mucus accumulation is a particular problem during times of distress, the first few weeks after tube insertion, or if the patient has an infection. Other problems with the tube can range from dislodgement to infection around the stoma to general respiratory distress.

Tracheal Suctioning

A patient with a tracheostomy requires meticulous care. Caregivers receive specific training in tracheostomy care, including suctioning and cleaning and changing the tracheostomy tube. Those procedures are not specifically listed in the National EMS Scope of Practice at the EMT level. If your protocols do not specifically address what actions you should take to manage problems, consult with medical direction.

Remember that the stoma or tracheostomy tube serves as the patient's airway. Assess the stoma or tube to ensure the patient has a clear airway. If you see or hear mucus, the patient needs to be suctioned. If the patient requires ventilation or oxygenation, provide several manual ventilations close together to preoxygenate him, if possible, before suctioning.

Soft suction catheters are sterile. Handle them with sterile gloves and avoid contact between the catheter and other surfaces. Use eye and face protection as BSI precautions when suctioning.

To suction obstructions caused by mucus, insert a soft, flexible suction catheter into the stoma or tracheostomy tube. The depth of insertion is determined prior to suctioning by measuring the suction catheter against the length of the obturator (as described earlier). If you cannot locate the obturator for measurement, advance the suction catheter gently until you feel resistance.

Cover the side port of the suction catheter to apply suction as the catheter is being withdrawn, using a twisting motion as it is slowly removed. Limit suction attempts to 10 to 15 seconds. The patient's body may reflexively jerk during this procedure from stimulation of the lower airway. After removing the catheter, resume ventilations and oxygen administration if the patient requires it. Without contaminating the suction catheter, insert the tip into a container of sterile water to remove any mucus left in the catheter, and then repeat suctioning if mucus remains. If the patient is on a ventilator, ventilate him by bag-mask device between suctioning procedures. During transport, the patient should be positioned with his head slightly elevated to allow mucus to drain.

Home Ventilators

ventilator a device that breathes for a patient.

A **ventilator** is a device that breathes for a patient. A home ventilator weighs anywhere from several pounds to over 20 pounds, ranging from the size of a large textbook to the size of a desktop computer. Ventilator settings include ventilator rate, duration of inspiratory and expiratory phases, airway pressures, and the amount of oxygen provided. The ventilator is attached to a corrugated tube called a *ventilator circuit*, which attaches to an endotracheal or tracheostomy tube.

Ventilators are equipped with a number of alarms to alert the patient and caregivers to potential problems. Follow the caregiver's guidance regarding any alarms that sound on the ventilator.

The patient on a home ventilator may require EMS for a variety of reasons. Mucus plugs and secretions in the tracheostomy or endotracheal tube may require suctioning. Respiratory infections are common in ventilator patients, and respiratory distress may develop. Make sure the patient's airway device is clear, suctioning as needed.

Home ventilators require AC electrical power, and power failures may be cause for concern. Ventilators do have backup batteries that generally last an hour or more. In some cases, the patient may require bag-mask assistance during transport to a hospital if his ventilator power source is disrupted. Adjust the rate, volume, and pressure of the bag-mask device to the patient's needs and comfort. Assess the patient's comfort, chest rise, skin color, and oxygen saturation.

Ventilators can be awkward to maintain while moving and transporting patients. If the ventilator is not easily moved with the patient, switch to bag-mask ventilation, at least temporarily. If the ventilator is left attached to the patient, firmly secure it to the stretcher, and once in the ambulance, secure the ventilator to prevent it from moving during transport. During transport, plug the ventilator into the ambulance's inverter, if available, to conserve its battery. If a bag-mask device is used during transport, obtain extra help by asking a firefighter or another rescuer at the scene to ride along in the ambulance so you can continue to provide assessment and care.

> **CLINICAL CLUE**
>
> **Ventilators**
>
> Some patients who are dependent on a ventilator may lead an active life. One of the best examples of this was Christopher Reeve, the actor who once played Superman, who was paralyzed from the neck down in a 1995 horseback riding accident. With the assistance of a ventilator, he was able to lead an active professional and family life until his death in 2004.

Cardiac Devices

The quality and length of life of many patients with severe cardiac disease can be improved with devices that correct electrical abnormalities or assist with the heart's mechanical function of pumping blood. Pacemakers and implanted cardiac defibrillators can treat life-threatening cardiac arrhythmias. A left ventricular assist device can improve cardiac output in patients awaiting a heart transplant. Patients who have one of the devices have had a significant cardiac medical history. They may be on multiple medications and may carry wallet cards or wear bracelets stating that they have one of the devices in use.

Implanted Pacemakers and Cardiac Defibrillators

A cardiac **pacemaker** is a small device that is implanted under the skin. The device generates an electrical impulse that is transmitted to the heart through wires, providing the electrical stimulation the heart muscle needs to contract. Pacemakers are typically used for patients who have a problem with a heart rate that is too slow to meet the body's needs. There are different configurations of pacemakers, depending on a patient's needs.

pacemaker a small device implanted under the skin with wires that are inserted into the heart to ensure a patient maintains a normal heart rate.

The pacemaker delivers a series of low-energy pulses at programmed intervals to stimulate the heart to beat at a faster rate. Neither the patient nor health care providers can feel the pulses. A pacemaker only provides an electrical stimulus to regulate the heart rate. It cannot improve the strength of contraction of the heart if the heart muscle is weakened.

An **automatic implanted cardiac defibrillator (AICD)** also is placed under the skin with wires inserted into the heart. Much like an automatic defibrillator applied to a pulseless patient, an implanted defibrillator detects life-threatening cardiac rhythms, such as ventricular fibrillation and ventricular tachycardia, and delivers a shock. The energy level of the shock is much lower than that delivered by an external defibrillator, because the energy does not have to overcome the impedance to electrical flow provided by the chest wall. The electricity is delivered directly to the heart. Some devices have a pacemaker built in, as well.

automatic implanted cardiac defibrillator (AICD) a small, surgically implanted device that can recognize life-threatening cardiac rhythms and deliver an electrical shock to correct the rhythm.

The AICD delivers a single shock when a life-threatening rhythm is detected. The shock is often very painful to the patient, generally rated as 6 on a pain scale of 10. If the single shock does not correct the rhythm, or if the rhythm returns, other shocks will be delivered, one at a time, until the dysrhythmia is resolved or the machine is turned off. The AICD can be turned off only by a special magnet and generally only in a hospital setting. Depending on the rhythm and the result of the shock, the patient may remain conscious, and the situation can be very traumatizing. Provide emotional support and reassurance to the patient.

Because the amount of energy, though still low, is greater than that delivered by a pacemaker, the electrical stimulus can cause the patient's muscles to twitch. However, you will not receive an electrical shock if you touch the patient.

Patients are usually instructed to call their doctor if they feel fine after a shock. However, if they have any symptoms such as dizziness, chest pain, shortness of breath, not feeling well, or if they are shocked more than twice in any 24-hour period, they should go to the hospital or call EMS for immediate transport to an emergency department.

Pacemakers and AICDs can be affected by certain electromagnetic and radio frequency signals. People with the devices should not stand still in the doorway of a business with an electronic anti-theft device or stand still in a walk-through metal detector, although walking through either without stopping is not harmful. Stereo speakers and cellular telephones should not be held against a pacemaker or AICD device, because the device may turn off without the patient's knowledge. Patients should maintain a distance of at least six inches between the device and appliances or power tools with electric or gas motors when they are running.

Depending on the nature of the call and chief complaint, it may be advisable to request ALS transport for a patient with a pacemaker or AICD. A patient who merely has a pacemaker as part of his medical history may not need ALS, but if the pacemaker is malfunctioning or if an AICD has discharged, the patient is a high-risk cardiac patient and should be treated as such.

Manage the patient according to your protocols for the chief complaint and presentation. The patient may require oxygen and other interventions. Reassess the patient frequently. If cardiac arrest occurs, perform CPR and apply an AED. If an AED is used, keep the pads at least three inches away from the implanted device. Otherwise, use the AED as usual.

left ventricular assist device (LVAD) a battery-powered electrical pump implanted in the body to assist a failing left ventricle in pumping blood to the body.

Left Ventricular Assist Devices

A **left ventricular assist device (LVAD)** improves cardiac output in some patients who have severe left ventricular heart failure while awaiting a heart transplant. The LVAD removes blood from the weakened left ventricle to a special pump inserted in the abdomen by way of a tube inserted into the left ventricle. The pump pressurizes the blood and pumps it into the aorta as the left ventricle usually would do, where it is distributed throughout the body. The connections between the pump and the external power supply are conducted from the pump in the abdomen through special tubing to the outside of the body.

Problems associated with LVADs are infection, air leakage, and battery failure. Keep in mind that the patient requires a properly functioning LVAD to maintain cardiac output. Do not delay in transporting the patient to a hospital.

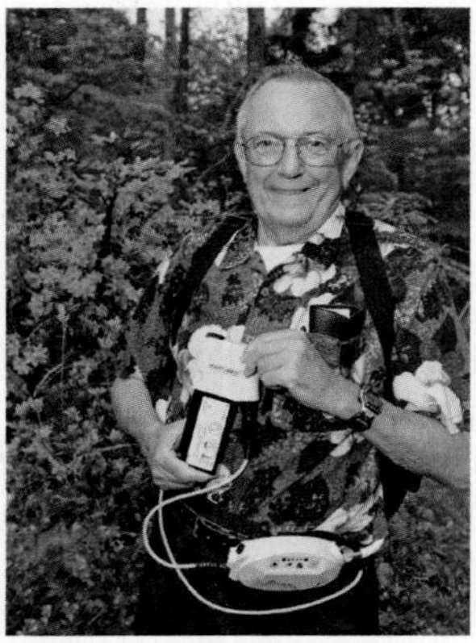

Figure 40-12 Left ventricular assist device (LVAD). (AP Images/George Widman)

LVADs have an external battery pack the size of a small backpack or briefcase (Figure 40-12 ■). Carefully secure it and prevent it from tugging on the attached tubing. If the battery system seems not to be working, plug the unit into an AC source at the scene or the inverter in the ambulance. This will help you determine if the problem is the battery charge or a failure of the unit. If the pump fails, a hand or foot pump is included with the system as a backup. The pump is similar to the bulb on a blood pressure cuff and must be squeezed for each beat of the heart.

If someone in the community has an LVAD, training can often be arranged for EMS providers who may respond for the patient, because the exact operation of the device can vary according to the model.

STOP, REVIEW, REMEMBER!

Multiple Choice

For each question, place a check next to the correct answer.

1. Often used by patients with sleep apnea, a home medical device that provides a single level of pressure to the airway throughout the respiratory cycle by way of a mask sealed over the mouth and nose is called:

_____ a. BiPAP.

_____ b. tracheostomy tube.

_____ c. CPAP.

_____ d. automatic ventilator.

2. An opening in the neck that remains after surgery to provide access to the trachea is called a(n):

_____ a. stoma.

_____ b. trach tube.

_____ c. cannula.

_____ d. obturator.

3. Which one of the principles below applies to tracheal suctioning of a patient with a trach tube?

_____ a. Use a sterile, flexible suction catheter.

_____ b. Remove the trach tube, clean it out, and then replace it.

_____ c. Insert the obturator before suctioning.

_____ d. Suction for 20 to 30 seconds at a time.

4. Which one of the following problems is treated using an LVAD?

_____ a. Slow heart rate

_____ b. Ventricular fibrillation

_____ c. Heart failure

_____ d. Difficulty breathing

5. What precaution should be followed when managing a patient with an AICD?

_____ a. Do not touch the patient if he is wet and the device is delivering shocks.

_____ b. Do not place an automatic external defibrillator on a patient who has an AICD.

_____ c. Do not use a cell phone or radio near the patient.

_____ d. If you apply defibrillator pads, place them at least three inches away from the defibrillator unit.

Matching

Match the term on the left with its applicable use on the right.

1. _____	Pacemaker	A. High spinal-cord injury
2. _____	Ventilator	B. Sleep apnea
3. _____	CPAP	C. Bradycardia

(continued on next page)

(continued)

Critical Thinking

1. Your patient has a pacemaker and a slow heart rate. What could explain this?

2. You have responded to an ice cream shop for an elderly man whose AICD delivered a shock. Employees at the ice cream shop called 911 because the patient reacted to the pain of the shock by dropping onto his knees. The patient says he feels fine and does not want to go to the hospital. Is the patient making an appropriate decision? Explain why or why not.

3. You have responded to a residence for a patient with an LVAD. The family is concerned because their electrical power has been out for over an hour and the battery for the LVAD is low. If the battery fails and you do not have an inverter to plug in the unit during transport, what should you be prepared to do?

Gastrointestinal and Urinary Devices

Patients with difficulty swallowing may need to receive some or all of their nutrition through a feeding tube inserted directly into the stomach or small intestine. Patients who have certain diseases or surgeries of the intestine may require a temporary or permanent ostomy to divert fecal matter from the intestine to a collection pouch outside the body. Patients with urinary continence or retention problems may require constant or intermittent urinary catheterization, while patients with renal failure have special devices for receiving **dialysis.**

dialysis a process of separating blood and a specially formulated fluid by a semipermeable membrane to remove toxins from the blood in patients whose kidneys are not functioning.

feeding tube a device for providing nutrition to the gastrointestinal system in patients who cannot swallow.

Feeding Tubes

A **feeding tube** can be required for short-term situations, such as recovery from surgery, or as part of long-term care for a chronic condition. For short-term use, a nasogastric (NG) tube is used. For longer-term care, a gastric tube (G-tube) or jejunal tube (J-tube) can be used.

A NG tube is inserted through the nose where it passes through the pharynx and esophagus into the stomach. The tube is taped to the patient's nose to prevent it from slipping. Specially prepared liquid nutrient solutions can be poured through the tube into the stomach. Tube feedings can be provided from a bag similar to an IV bag. In this case, the bag must be placed higher than the stomach for the contents to move in the right direction. Between feedings, the tube is clamped to prevent stomach contents from leaking out of the tube. An NG tube is also used to empty the stomach in some cases.

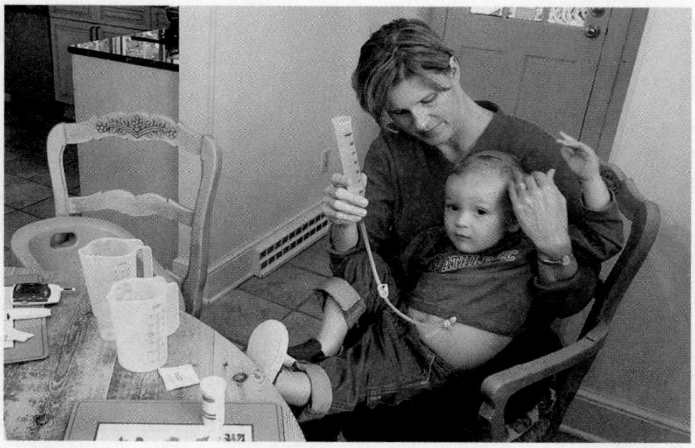

Figure 40-13 Gastric feeding tube in child. (AP Images/David T. Foster III)

A G-tube is surgically implanted through the abdominal wall and into the stomach (Figure 40-13 ■). It is held in place by a balloon inside the stomach. It also can serve to empty the stomach contents in some conditions. A J-tube is placed into the jejunum, the second section of the small intestine, in much the same way as a G-tube is placed.

Common problems with feeding tubes include dislodgement, infection at the site of insertion, or an obstruction that prevents nutrients from being provided to the patient. All of those conditions warrant transport and evaluation in a hospital setting. A particularly serious complication can occur if the end of an NG tube becomes dislodged from the stomach and enters the trachea, or if it was improperly placed to begin with. Any feeding or medications provided through the tube end up in the lungs. Aspiration of a large volume of gastric contents can lead to respiratory distress, hypoxia, severe lung damage, and pneumonia.

urinary catheter a tube used to drain the bladder.

Urinary Catheters

A **urinary catheter** is used for a patient who has lost the ability to urinate or has lost the ability to control when he urinates. An indwelling Foley catheter is a hollow tube with a balloon at its tip that is inserted through the urethra until it enters the bladder. The balloon is filled with sterile water to anchor it in the bladder. Urine is drained through the tube into a collection bag or drain. A bag can be strapped to the patient's leg to allow mobility, while a drain hangs on the side of the bed (Figure 40-14 ■). The collection bag or drain must always be kept lower than the patient's bladder to prevent backflow of contents. If the bag must temporarily be at the patient's level, clamp the tube to prevent backflow. However, you must unclamp the tubing once the device is placed back in position to allow the patient's bladder to empty. If the catheter is not unclamped, the bladder will become distended and painful, and if not promptly corrected, can lead to additional urinary complications.

A condom catheter is an alternative for male patients. The collection tubing connects to a condom-like device that fits over the penis. Other patients do not require constant catheterization, but cannot empty their bladders and need to intermittently catheterize themselves to drain urine from the bladder.

Problems with urinary catheters include urinary tract infection (bacteria can be introduced into the bladder when the catheter is placed), which can lead to sepsis; obstruction (including obstruction from failure to unclamp the tubing), which can prevent urinary outflow and create

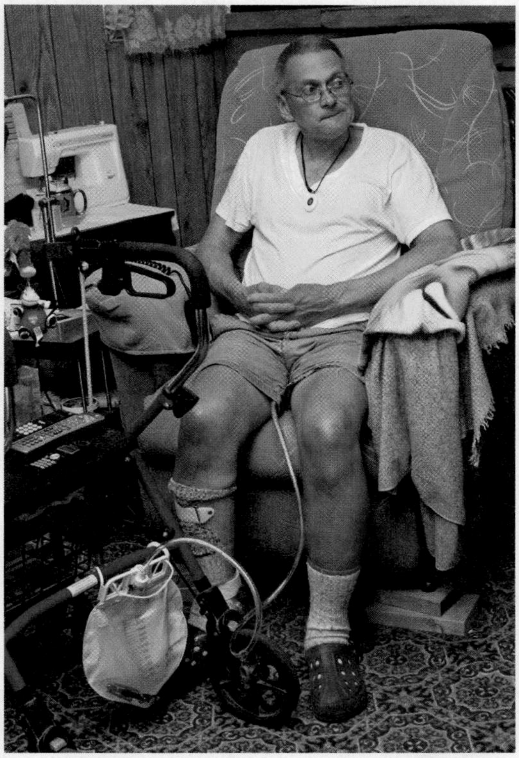

Figure 40-14 Patient with a urinary catheter device.

serious complications if not corrected; and dislodgement of the catheter, which can cause trauma to the bladder or urethra if the catheter is pulled out with the balloon inflated.

Always inspect the urine in a collection device. Cloudy or dark urine can indicate urinary tract infection or other problems. Document the amount of urine and its appearance in your prehospital care report. Collection devices should be emptied when they are one-third to one-half full. If the device is emptied, document the amount that was emptied. Use care that the catheter tubing does not become caught or entangled when you are moving the patient.

Ostomy Bags

ostomy bag a collection device used in conjunction with a colostomy or ileostomy to collect fecal matter.

colostomy a surgical opening that connects a portion of the colon to the external abdominal wall.

An **ostomy bag** is connected to the site of a **colostomy** or an ileostomy. A colostomy or ileostomy is the result of a surgery that brings a section of the intestine through the abdominal wall to divert the flow of stool away from the normal path to the rectum. An ostomy may be necessary because of a medical condition such as Crohn's disease, ulcerative colitis, or colon cancer. An ostomy bag is usually attached to the patient's leg and often will not be visible under clothing. Common problems include infection at the ostomy site, blockage, or, in some cases, dislodgement. Use care when moving a patient if an ostomy bag is present to prevent breakage or dislodgement through rough handling.

Dialysis

Patients who have end-stage renal failure require dialysis. In end-stage renal failure, the kidneys are unable to remove toxic products of metabolism or regulate the amount of water, electrolytes, and other substances in the blood as they usually would. Dialysis is a process of using a semipermeable membrane to filter the blood. However, dialysis cannot be fine-tuned to make the minute-by-minute adjustments to the blood composition that healthy kidneys make. Therefore, dialysis patients never really feel "normal," even when they are compliant with their dialysis regimen.

There are two forms of dialysis: hemodialysis and peritoneal dialysis. *Hemodialysis* is performed by attaching the patient to an external machine called a *dialyzer*. The procedure is usually performed at a dialysis center, although home units do exist. Hemodialysis requires the use of large needles and tubing to remove and return the blood. The needles are inserted into a site where an artery has been surgically connected to a vein. Depending on the configuration, the dialysis access site is called an *arteriovenous (A-V) fistula* or *AV graft* or, in some cases, a *shunt graft*. Common complications encountered with patients on hemodialysis include bleeding from the dialysis access site after dialysis and infection.

The shunt or fistula site is extremely fragile and prone to injury. Never take a blood pressure in an extremity with a dialysis access site. A damaged shunt or fistula cannot be used for dialysis, which the patient relies on. He will need to have a central line placed for dialysis and will require surgery to repair the shunt or fistula, or to create a new one. The repaired or new shunt or fistula cannot be used until it is healed.

If a shunt or fistula ruptures, an external blood loss of 500 mL/min, or even more, can occur. Immediately stop the bleeding with firm direct pressure. The dialysis access site also may bleed beneath the skin, causing substantial swelling. Apply direct pressure to control this bleeding. It is unlikely that bleeding from a dialysis access site will clot, so do not release direct pressure until you have arrived at the hospital and a physician has evaluated the patient. Treat the patient for shock, transport, and reassess frequently.

In *peritoneal dialysis* a catheter is implanted through the abdominal wall and into the peritoneal cavity. Several liters of a specially formulated dialysis solution (dialysate) are infused into the abdominal cavity, where the peritoneal membranes and mesenteries act as a dialysis membrane. After a period of time, the fluid is emptied from the abdominal cavity. The patient can perform this procedure at home, but it must be performed frequently, often several times a day. Common complications include dislodging the catheter and infection in the peritoneal cavity (peritonitis). (See Chapter 25 to review renal emergencies and dialysis.)

Ventriculostomy Shunt

Some patients, mostly children, have a medical condition that results in a buildup of cerebrospinal fluid (CSF) in the brain, called *hydrocephalus*, which causes increased intracranial pressure (ICP). A device called a *ventriculostomy shunt* is surgically placed in one of the ventricles of the brain, allowing excess fluid to be drained through tubing that is tunneled through the tissues into the abdomen, heart, chest, or a blood vessel in the neck. Complications include infection, subdural bleeding, and occlusion. Infection can result in sepsis or encephalitis. Occlusion can cause accumulation of CSF in the brain, and an increase in ICP.

Vascular Access Devices

A patient who receives frequent IV therapy, such as with chemotherapy or total parenteral nutrition (TPN, which is the process of providing all nutrition intravenously), may have one of a variety of **vascular access devices.** Central IV catheters are placed into large central veins (such as the subclavian vein under the clavicle) to prevent a patient who needs frequent or ongoing intravenous access from enduring multiple IV sticks. In addition, some types of medications are too irritating to the smaller peripheral veins, or a patient may have poor peripheral venous access. Critically ill patients in the hospital may have central IV catheters so that large amounts of IV fluids can be delivered rapidly to the central circulation.

vascular access devices a catheter inserted into a central vein or a port implanted under the skin to allow access to the patient's central circulation.

Central IV catheters require a surgical procedure, sometimes assisted by radiographic imaging, for placement. Central venous access devices carry a variety of brand names, such as Groshong, Hickman, or Broviac catheters. These catheters may have one, two, or three external access tubes.

A *peripherally inserted central catheter (PICC)* is inserted into a peripheral vein in the arm and then threaded into the central circulation. An *implanted port* has no external tubing like a central IV line or PICC. The device is a small disc inserted just under the skin of the upper chest to allow access to a central vein. A special needle called a *Huber needle* is used to access the central circulation through the port. Brand names for implanted ports include Port-a-Cath and Mediport.

With all types of central venous access devices, infection is a common and serious problem. In most cases, neither EMS personnel nor a family caregiver will use a central IV catheter to administer medications to the patient or for any other purpose. Use of a central IV catheter is usually restricted to hospital personnel. However, awareness of the presence of a central IV device is important. Exercise caution to avoid any tugging or contamination of the catheter site.

STOP, REVIEW, REMEMBER!

Multiple Choice

For each question, place a check next to the correct answer.

1. Where is the tip of a G-tube when it is properly placed?

_____ a. Colon

_____ b. Jejunum

_____ c. Stomach

_____ d. Esophagus

2. A 79-year-old patient who has a past medical history of a stroke presents with breathing difficulty, which began after a feeding through his NG tube about 30 minutes ago. He is awake, but nonverbal. His eyes are darting about anxiously. He is diaphoretic and has a weak, wet cough. His pulse is 108, respiratory rate is 28, and SpO_2 is 86% on 2 L/min of oxygen by nasal cannula, which was provided by his home health care provider. Of the following, the first thing you should do is:

_____ a. flush the NG tube with a large volume of sterile water.

_____ b. switch the patient to a nonrebreather mask with 15 L/min of oxygen flow.

_____ c. listen to and document the breath sounds.

_____ d. find out what specific feeding formula was introduced through the NG tube and how much.

3. Which one of the following vascular access devices consists of a small disc inserted under the skin of the chest that is accessed by a special needle called a Huber needle?

_____ a. PICC

_____ b. Groshong

_____ c. Implanted port

_____ d. Arterial line

4. You are transporting a patient for a routine medical appointment. He is alert and has no complaints. His Foley catheter collection bag contains 350 mL of cloudy, dark-colored urine. Of the following, you should have the highest suspicion for:

_____ a. urinary tract infection.

_____ b. end-stage renal failure.

_____ c. kidney stone.

_____ d. the catheter being placed incorrectly.

5. You have arrived for a call for "a patient hemorrhaging" to find a 42-year-old man who had hemodialysis earlier in the day. There is spurting blood from his dialysis fistula in his left arm. After taking BSI precautions, you should:

_____ a. apply direct pressure.

_____ b. apply a tourniquet above the site.

_____ c. call for an ALS unit.

_____ d. elevate the patient's arm.

Fill in the Blank

1. In peritoneal dialysis, the patient infuses fluid into his ____________________.

2. Unlike a Foley catheter, a condom catheter does not have to be inserted into the ____________________.

3. The most common complications of peritoneal dialysis are ____________________ and ____________________.

Critical Thinking

1. What are some complications you should anticipate in a patient with chronic renal failure on hemodialysis?

2. What is the difference between a G-tube and a J-tube?

EMERGENCY DISPATCH SUMMARY

The patient was safely removed from the apartment and transported with his mother to Baptist Medical Center in Tower Pines. He was found to have pneumonia and uncontrolled diabetes so he was admitted for care in their bariatric unit. At the urging of social services, Ronnie's mother agreed to allow in-home medical visits for him and, since being released, he has been undergoing treatment for the diabetes, as well as sleep apnea, and has lost nearly 25 pounds. Recently, EMTs Joe Davies and Heather Drake were pleasantly surprised to receive a handmade thank-you card from Ronnie and have scheduled a time to visit him under more favorable circumstances.

Chapter Review

To the Point

- Because patients with special challenges often have underlying health conditions, they have an increased likelihood of requiring emergency medical care.
- Patients with special challenges and their families are usually very knowledgeable about the patient's condition and any special medical devices the patient may use.
- Special challenges include sensory impairment and communication difficulties, cognitive impairment, developmental disabilities, physical disabilities (such as paralysis or limited mobility), terminal illness, obesity, homelessness, poverty, and the need to rely on medical devices.
- Devices you should be familiar with include trach tubes, CPAP, ventilators, pacemakers, AICDs, LVADs, feeding tubes, dialysis devices, urinary catheters, ostomy bags, vascular access devices, and ventriculostomy shunts.

Chapter Questions

Multiple Choice

For each question, place a check next to the correct answer.

1. A 15-year-old boy presents with slurred speech that is difficult for you to understand, although his mother seems to be able to understand what he is saying. This patient most likely has a(n) ____________ disorder.

_____ a. language
_____ b. fluency
_____ c. articulation
_____ d. voice production

2. In order to minimize difficulty breathing, obese patients should be transported in which position?

_____ a. Supine
_____ b. Prone
_____ c. Position of comfort
_____ d. Lateral recumbent

3. Ventriculostomy shunts are placed to:

_____ a. prevent increased intracranial pressure.
_____ b. allow for hemodialysis.
_____ c. assist the pumping mechanism of the heart.
_____ d. drain the bladder.

4. When communicating with a hearing-impaired patient, you should:

_____ a. exaggerate how you articulate your words.
_____ b. shout.
_____ c. speak in a clear, normal voice.
_____ d. speak more slowly than normal.

5. Types of feeding tubes include all of the following *except:*

_____ a. nasogastric tube.
_____ b. G-tube.
_____ c. J-tube.
_____ d. ostomy pouch.

6. A developmental disorder characterized by impaired language skills, poor social skills, repetitive behaviors, and narrow but intense interests is:

_____ a. Down syndrome.
_____ b. autism.
_____ c. cystic fibrosis.
_____ d. cerebral palsy.

Critical Thinking

1. Your patient has Down syndrome. What anatomical challenges can you expect to encounter during your airway management?

____

____

____

____

2. What is the difference between a congenital and an acquired condition? What are some examples of each?

____

____

____

____

3. Why are patients with devices such as tracheostomies and urinary catheters at increased risk of infection?

____

____

____

____

4. Your patient is a 50-year-old woman who receives peritoneal dialysis at home. When you arrive, the patient is allowing fluid to be drained from her abdomen into a collection device. How should you manage the patient and the device?

____

____

____

____

5. Why would a patient with paralysis be more prone to complications such as urinary tract infections, pneumonia, and pressure sores?

____

____

____

____

The Last Word

EMTs encounter patients with special challenges that range from hearing loss to homelessness to dependence on life-sustaining medical technology. To provide the best care, you must understand the patient's needs and how their challenges relate to the reason you were called. Learn as much as you can about particular patient populations in your response area before the need to respond in an emergency arises. The staff of specialty centers can provide you with information about devices such as LVADs.

Patients with communication challenges, cognitive impairment, and developmental disabilities require adaptations to your usual approach to communication and assessment. Be prepared to take additional time to gain the trust and cooperation of patients with autism spectrum disorders.

When called to care for a patient who relies on technology, do not let the presence of the equipment distract you from performing a systematic assessment and appropriately treating the patient. Enlist the assistance of the patient or his caregivers when faced with unfamiliar equipment.

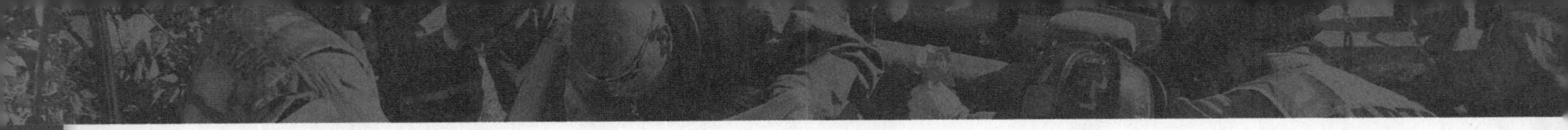

Module 5: Review and Practice Examination for Chapters 38–40

***DIRECTIONS**: Assess what you have learned in this module by placing a check mark in the blank beside the best answer for each multiple-choice question. When you are done, check your answers against the Answer Key at the back of the book.*

1. The fontanels are most obvious in patients who are in which one of the following age groups?
   ____ a. Infants ____ c. Preschoolers
   ____ b. Toddlers ____ d. School age

2. Believing that injury or illness is a punishment for bad behavior is characteristic of which one of the following age groups?
   ____ a. Infants and toddlers
   ____ b. Toddlers and preschoolers
   ____ c. Preschoolers and school-age children
   ____ d. School-age children and adolescents

3. When a pediatric patient suffers cardiac arrest, it is most often due to a(n):
   ____ a. respiratory problem.
   ____ b. birth defect.
   ____ c. poisoning.
   ____ d. electrical shock.

4. The pediatric assessment triangle includes all of the following *except*:
   ____ a. observing the safety of the environment.
   ____ b. general appearance of the patient.
   ____ c. work of breathing.
   ____ d. circulatory status as noted by skin signs.

5. It should take less than ____________ seconds for capillary refill after blanching the back of the hand of the patient.
   ____ a. 10 ____ c. 5
   ____ b. 7 ____ d. 2

6. The absence of tears in the crying pediatric patient should be considered by the EMT to be a(n):
   ____ a. sign of dehydration.
   ____ b. variation of normal.
   ____ c. indication that the illness or injury is not serious.
   ____ d. sign of psychiatric illness.

7. Which one of the following statements concerning respiratory emergencies in pediatric patients is *true*?
   ____ a. Pediatric patients gradually decompensate, providing warning of impending respiratory failure.
   ____ b. The presence of nasal flaring is unlikely to occur in the pediatric patient in respiratory distress.
   ____ c. Grunting with exhalation is a sign of respiratory distress in pediatric patients.
   ____ d. Respiratory distress is always accompanied by cyanosis in the pediatric patient.

8. To maintain an open airway in an unresponsive pediatric patient, the head must be in a ____________ position.
   ____ a. hyperextended
   ____ b. neutral
   ____ c. flexed
   ____ d. sagittal

9. To maintain the airway of an unresponsive pediatric patient, it may be necessary to place a folded towel under the:
   ____ a. head. ____ c. shoulders.
   ____ b. neck. ____ d. back.

10. Which one of the following devices is preferred for *nasal* suctioning of a newborn infant?
    ____ a. Bulb-type suction device
    ____ b. 30-mL medicine syringe
    ____ c. Flexible suction catheter
    ____ d. Rigid suction tip

11. Which one of the following devices is preferred for *oral* suctioning of a newborn infant?
    ____ a. Rigid suction tip
    ____ b. 30-mL medicine syringe
    ____ c. Flexible suction catheter
    ____ d. Bulb-type suction device

12. Inserting a suction tip too far into the mouth of a pediatric patient may result in:
____ a. slowing the heart rate.
____ b. trauma to the lungs.
____ c. the tip entering the stomach.
____ d. airway obstruction.

13. You have responded to a report of a child choking. Your patient is a 20-month-old who is coughing and has stridorous breathing. The patient is alert, his skin color is normal, and his skin is warm and dry. You should:
____ a. inspect the mouth and perform a finger sweep if you can see a foreign object.
____ b. transport, allowing the mother to give him some oxygen by the "blow-by" technique.
____ c. place him across your lap and perform back blows.
____ d. place him on the floor and perform abdominal thrusts.

14. Your patient is a 16-month-old whose grandmother gave her some canned peaches for lunch. The patient started choking while eating and is pale with cyanotic lips. Her respiratory effort is ineffective. You should:
____ a. place her across your lap and perform back blows.
____ b. alternate back slaps and chest thrusts.
____ c. perform abdominal thrusts.
____ d. perform a finger sweep if you cannot see the obstruction.

15. Which one of the following is *true* concerning the use of oropharyngeal airways in pediatric patients?
____ a. They are measured from the corner of the mouth to the earlobe.
____ b. The airway must be rotated as it is inserted.
____ c. Oropharyngeal airways are contraindicated for children under 12 years old.
____ d. Correct head position must be maintained, even with a properly inserted oropharyngeal airway.

16. Which one of the following is *not* a common cause of shock in pediatric patients?
____ a. Blood loss
____ b. Vomiting
____ c. Diarrhea
____ d. Cardiac problems

17. Which one of the following is a late sign of shock in a pediatric patient?
____ a. Pale skin color
____ b. Lack of activity
____ c. Weak peripheral pulses
____ d. Lack of tears when crying

18. Your patient is a nine-month-old with a three-day history of fever and refusing food and fluids. He is pale and limp and does not respond to your presence. His skin is mottled and moist. Which one of the following describes the appropriate sequence of care for this patient?
____ a. Perform a rapid secondary assessment, apply oxygen, take vital signs, perform reassessments
____ b. Perform a secondary assessment, take vital signs, apply oxygen, perform reassessments
____ c. Take vital signs, perform a primary assessment, apply oxygen
____ d. Apply oxygen, vital signs, perform a secondary assessment

19. The leading cause of death in children is:
____ a. sudden infant death syndrome.
____ b. poisoning.
____ c. trauma.
____ d. asthma.

20. The most common cause of blunt trauma in children is:
____ a. falls.
____ b. motor-vehicle crashes.
____ c. child abuse.
____ d. recreational injuries.

21. Which one of the following is *not* a factor in the increased risk of hypothermia in the pediatric population?
____ a. Less body fat
____ b. Greater body surface area
____ c. Few glucose reserves
____ d. Slower metabolism

22. When documenting suspected child abuse, all of the following are appropriate *except:*
____ a. describing the appearance of injuries.
____ b. quoting statements made by caregivers.
____ c. reaching conclusions based on the history and injuries.
____ d. describing the behavior of the child.

23. Which one of the following devices is used to provide nutrition to the pediatric patient who cannot eat or swallow?
____ a. Gastrostomy tube
____ b. Ventral-peritoneal shunt
____ c. Tracheotomy tube
____ d. Central venous line

24. There are currently more than 35 million elderly people in the United States and that number is expected to ____________ in the next 20 years.
____ a. decrease by half
____ b. double
____ c. remain stable
____ d. quadruple

25. Geriatric patients are those aged ____________ years and older.
____ a. 40
____ b. 65
____ c. 70
____ d. 85

26. Which one of the following changes occurs with aging?
____ a. The body is less able to detect changes in oxygen levels.
____ b. The body becomes more sensitive to changes in carbon dioxide levels.
____ c. Lung capacity increases.
____ d. Tissues in the lungs become more elastic.

27. Which one of the following statements regarding the majority of elderly persons in the United States is *true*?
____ a. They live in extended care facilities.
____ b. Their health is generally poor.
____ c. They enjoy active lifestyles.
____ d. They suffer severe problems with memory and thinking.

28. The elderly may be less able to compensate for blood loss due to which one of the following factors?
____ a. Increased elasticity of the blood vessels
____ b. Increased cardiac output
____ c. Taking blood-thinning medications
____ d. Inability to produce red blood cells

29. Which one of the following is *not* a normal age-related change in the nervous system?
____ a. Decreased sensory perception
____ b. Decreased motor reaction time
____ c. Inability to learn new things
____ d. Difficulty with recent memory

30. Which one of the following statements is *true* regarding depression in the elderly?
____ a. The elderly suffer from a high rate of depression.
____ b. Depression may have both biochemical and situational causes.
____ c. There are no warning signs of depression in the elderly.
____ d. It is almost always reversible.

31. Musculoskeletal changes in the elderly include all of the following *except:*
____ a. curvature of the spine.
____ b. changes in posture.
____ c. decreased height.
____ d. increased bone density.

32. Which one of the following does *not* contribute to malnutrition in the elderly?
____ a. Decreased sense of taste and smell
____ b. Poorly fitting dentures
____ c. Depression
____ d. Decreased physical activity

33. Which one of the following is *not* a normal age-related change of the skin?
____ a. Increased elasticity
____ b. Liver spots
____ c. Decreased oil secretion
____ d. Decreased perspiration

34. Which one of the following is *not* a normal age-related change in the senses?
____ a. Altered ability to smell and taste
____ b. Decreased ability to hear
____ c. Loss of peripheral vision
____ d. Increased sensitivity to pain

35. Which one of the following is *not* related to depression among the elderly?
____ a. Living independently
____ b. Needing help with activities of daily living
____ c. Loss of body functions
____ d. Changes in appearance

36. Which one of the following would be a form of neglect among the elderly?
____ a. Exploitation of the elderly person's finances
____ b. Restraint
____ c. Food deprivation
____ d. Degrading comments

37. All of the following may be signs of abuse or neglect in the geriatric patient *except:*
____ a. poor hygiene.
____ b. multiple medications.
____ c. malnutrition.
____ d. unkempt appearance.

38. Which one of the following is *not* a common illness or injury among the elderly population?
____ a. Measles
____ b. Trauma
____ c. Aneurysm
____ d. Diabetes

39. Which one of the following is *not* an injury-prevention measure in the home of an elderly person?
____ a. Installation of smoke detectors
____ b. Reducing the hot water temperature
____ c. Using throw rugs on hard tile or vinyl floors
____ d. Installing railings on steps and stairways

40. Which one of the following should be part of the scene size-up when responding to an elderly patient?
____ a. Quickly obtaining vital signs
____ b. Looking for household hazards
____ c. Collecting medications
____ d. Notifying neighbors of the emergency

41. You have just introduced yourself to a 71-year-old woman. She responds with, "My name is Inez Goldsmith." You should then address her as:
____ a. Inez.
____ b. Mrs. Goldsmith.
____ c. Sweetie.
____ d. Any of the above is acceptable.

42. You have just introduced yourself to an 87-year-old male patient. He responds with, "What's that? I can't hear you." All of the following would be appropriate *except:*
____ a. making sure the patient can see your face when you speak.
____ b. asking if the patient has a hearing aid.
____ c. turning off any background noise, such as a radio or television.
____ d. shouting.

43. Which one of the following is a common reason geriatric patients may tend to hide their symptoms?
____ a. They do not want to bother family members with their care.
____ b. They simply do not understand the severity of their symptoms.
____ c. They are afraid of losing their independence.
____ d. They are concerned about being a burden on the EMS system.

44. When performing a history and physical exam on a geriatric patient, you should:
____ a. focus on gathering information from caregivers only.
____ b. always explain what you are doing before you do it.
____ c. delay the history until you get the patient to the hospital.
____ d. obtain the history only from the medications the patient takes.

45. Changes that occur with the aging of the musculoskeletal system include all of the following *except:*
____ a. decrease in range of motion.
____ b. increase in sensitivity to pain.
____ c. difficulty balancing.
____ d. loss of mobility.

46. Which one of the following is a progressive, degenerative disease that attacks the brain and results in impaired memory, thinking, and behavior?
____ a. Heart failure
____ b. Osteoporosis
____ c. Kyphosis
____ d. Alzheimer's

47. Your patient is a 16-month-old who has experienced a seizure. She takes no medications, has no significant past medical history, and has no signs of trauma. Which one of the following questions is most meaningful in this patient's history?
____ a. Was the patient born full-term?
____ b. Has the patient had a fever or illness recently?
____ c. Does the patient have any allergies?
____ d. Is there a family history of seizures?

48. Your patient is a 12-year-old with a history of asthma. He is awake, noticeably short of breath with audible wheezing, and a respiratory rate of 28. You should:
____ a. initiate oxygen therapy as soon as practical.
____ b. contact the parents before taking any other action.
____ c. insert an oropharyngeal airway and begin bag-mask ventilations.
____ d. transport but do not initiate treatment unless you are able to contact the parents.

49. Your patient is a four-year-old who was run over by a vehicle as she was playing in her driveway. The patient has a capillary refill time of three seconds. The most likely explanation for this finding is:
____ a. she is hypothermic.
____ b. this refill time is normal for a four-year-old.
____ c. she has internal injuries.
____ d. she is frightened.

50. The risk of death from traumatic injury in older patients is ____________ times higher than in younger adults who suffer the same injury.
____ a. two
____ b. three
____ c. five
____ d. eight

51. Which one of the following is characterized by the inability or unwillingness to provide or care for oneself?
____ a. Dementia
____ b. Self abuse
____ c. Self neglect
____ d. Incontinence

52. A congenital disease or condition is one that is present:
____ a. at birth.
____ b. as a result of exposure to an infectious organism.
____ c. within the first few years of life.
____ d. once a person reaches puberty.

53. Coronary heart disease is an example of a(n) ______________ disease.
    ____ a. genetic
    ____ b. immune
    ____ c. acquired
    ____ d. congenital

54. You have been called to the residence of an 84-year-old man. The patient is complaining of abdominal pain that started suddenly about three hours ago. As you begin your assessment, it becomes apparent that the patient suffers from presbycusis. How might you best alter your communication style to ensure that your assessment is complete?
    ____ a. Lean close to the patient's ear and shout.
    ____ b. Write down your questions.
    ____ c. Assume the patient can read your lips.
    ____ d. Use hand gestures.

55. When treating a patient who has an autism spectrum disorder, consider:
    ____ a. overcommunicating.
    ____ b. leaving excess equipment in another room.
    ____ c. asking family to stand back.
    ____ d. explaining exactly how your treatment will help.

56. A person who is obese has a BMI of at least:
    ____ a. 25.
    ____ b. 20.
    ____ c. 10.
    ____ d. 30.

57. A CPAP device works to:
    ____ a. prevent airway passages from collapsing.
    ____ b. increase air volume at inspiration.
    ____ c. continuously breathe for the user.
    ____ d. prevent a complete exhalation.

58. A BiPAP device differs from a CPAP device by:
    ____ a. preventing airway passages from swelling.
    ____ b. increasing air pressure during inspiration.
    ____ c. decreasing air pressure during inspiration.
    ____ d. preventing a complete exhalation.

59. To suction a trach tube, first measure the suction catheter:
    ____ a. from the trach opening to the base of the neck.
    ____ b. the length of the neck.
    ____ c. the depth of the obturator.
    ____ d. from the corner of the mouth to the tip of the earlobe.

60. End-of-life care for terminally ill patients that focuses on comfort and dignity is called:
    ____ a. comfort care.
    ____ b. life support.
    ____ c. advance directive.
    ____ d. hospice.

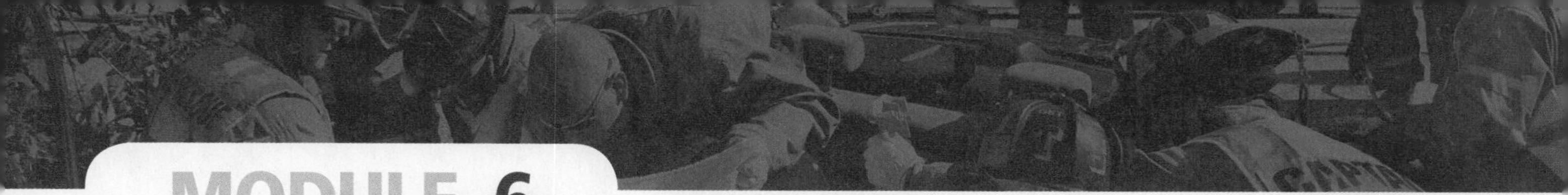

MODULE 6

Ambulance Operations

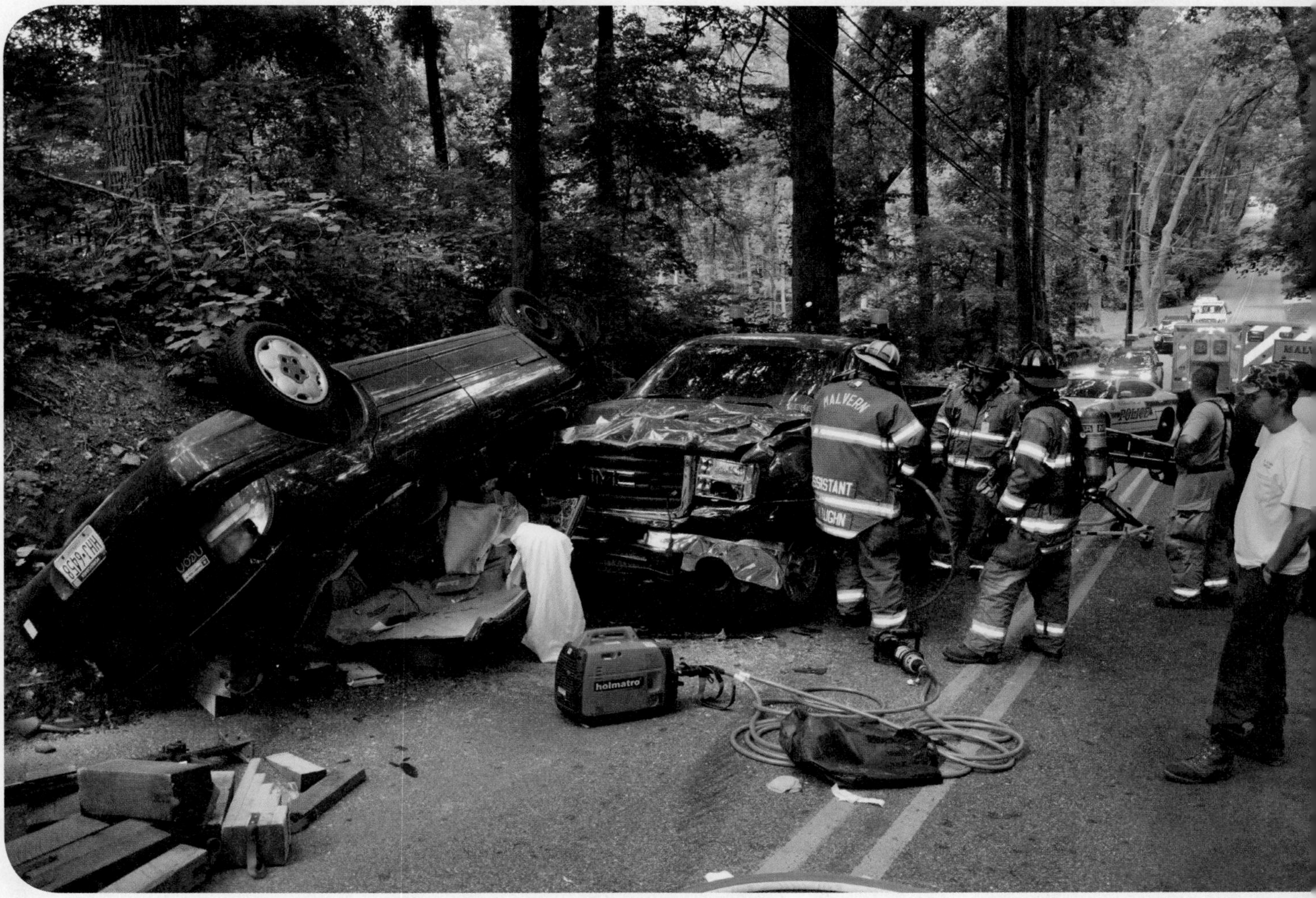

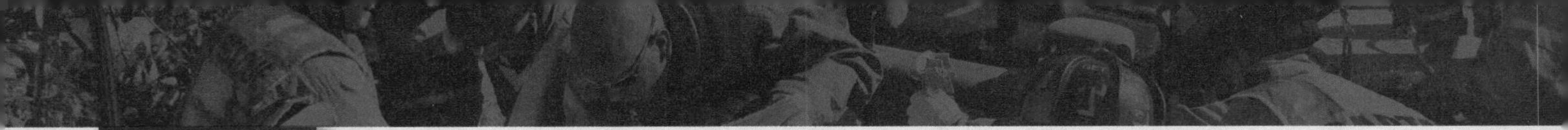

41 Operating and Maintaining Your Ambulance

Education Standards

EMS Operations: Principles of safely operating a ground ambulance

Competencies

Applies knowledge of operational roles and responsibilities to ensure patient, public, and personnel safety.

Objectives

After completion of this lesson, you should be able to:

41-1 Define key terms introduced in this chapter.

41-2 Describe the privileges afforded to EMTs operating emergency vehicles and the precautions that must be observed while using those privileges.

41-3 Give examples of the EMT's responsibilities during each of the major phases of an ambulance call.

41-4 Give examples of habits and behaviors that improve driving safety.

41-5 Discuss factors that can affect your ability to maintain control while driving an ambulance.

41-6 Describe the appropriate use of emergency warning devices, such as lights and sirens.

41-7 Explain precautions that should be taken when driving an ambulance in inclement weather.

41-8 Explain precautions that should be taken when driving an ambulance at night.

41-9 Describe the safety precautions to be taken when working at scenes on and near roadways.

41-10 Describe post-run actions that should be taken to reduce the spread of infection to you, your coworkers, and patients.

41-11 Describe the recommendations of the National Association of Emergency Medical Technicians with respect to EMT security and safety.

41-12 Explain precautions to avoid exposing yourself or others to increased levels of carbon monoxide associated with ambulance operations.

Key Terms

abandonment p. 1119
cleaning p. 1120
disinfecting p. 1120
due regard p. 1109
right of way p. 1108
sirens p. 1108
sterilization p. 1120
warning lights p. 1108

Introduction

When considering safety issues, our thoughts typically go first to knife-wielding criminals bound to do us harm. However, if you look at the statistics, an EMT is far more likely to be injured or killed in a motor-vehicle crash than by any other threat. Your safety and the safety of your crew and patient are directly linked to the safe operation of the ambulance.

41-2 Describe the privileges afforded to EMTs operating emergency vehicles and the precautions that must be observed while using those privileges.

EMTs are afforded a great privilege in the ability to operate an ambulance. In many cases routine traffic laws can be put aside and speed limits ignored. But with this privilege comes great responsibility. Although laws may not apply, judgment and due regard for safety are by far the heavier burden. By sitting behind the wheel, you accept responsibility for the occupants in your ambulance, and their safe delivery is in your hands.

Although afforded many legal protections, the operation of an ambulance is fraught with challenges. Ambulances are driven at all times of the day, in all types of weather, and sometimes under the worst possible conditions. Furthermore, operators of ambulances are frequently taxed physically and emotionally. Fear, excitement, fatigue, and stress can affect the ability to operate a vehicle safely. As an EMT, you must recognize those challenges and take steps to mitigate their effects. Remember, yours is the most precious cargo.

Operating an ambulance safely requires diligent effort at many different phases of day-to-day life. Safety is not limited to the time spent behind the wheel. The professional responsibility you accept as an EMT mandates constant attention to detail and hypervigilance to be prepared, operate safely, and then prepare for the next call. No one element is more important than the other and the combination of all those elements creates a culture grounded in safety.

This chapter discusses safety and how it relates to all the phases of ambulance operation. Particular attention is paid to driver safety, but attention is also given to the larger responsibilities of security and readiness.

EMERGENCY DISPATCH

"Quick, turn up the portable," EMT Rollie Engmeyer said to his partner Marianne Smith. "I think they just called us."

"Oops, sorry," She grinned and adjusted the radio volume before answering the dispatcher.

"Three-three," the dispatcher said. "I need you to respond code three to a rollover MVC on the I-77 service road just south of Vintner."

"Dispatch, 33 copies. We're on our way," Marianne said as they hurried to the ambulance.

"First call of the day, and it's a good one!" Rollie hit the lights and siren and inched out into the heavy morning traffic.

The cars, full of well-dressed, coffee-sipping people on their way to the financial district, pulled this way and that in front of the ambulance but never quite cleared the way. The drivers' heads were shooting from side to side with confused looks on their faces.

"Come on! Move!" Rollie shouted over the siren, hitting the air horn several times. "How difficult is it to just pull to the right?"

"This is weird," Marianne looked at the clotted traffic. "It's almost like … hmm."

"Like what?" Rollie pressed and held the air horn button in an attempt to get the attention of the cars in front of him.

"Like they don't know where we are." Marianne moved her spotlight to look for reflection of the emergency lights in the chrome. Nothing. "We've got no emergency lights."

"What?" Rollie shouted, flipping the console switch off and on. "Look again."

"Still nothing," Marianne said. "Did you check the lights when we got in the truck?"

"Yes, I checked the lights!"

Phases of an Ambulance Call

41-3 Give examples of the EMT's responsibilities during each of the major phases of an ambulance call.

Safety is an ongoing process. It begins long before the call happens and continues not just during the call but after the call as well. Each time you report for duty and respond to an emergency, there is a specific sequence of events that occurs. They can be referred to as the *phases of an ambulance call.* In general, the phases are as follows:

- ***Preparing for the call.*** In this phase the EMTs ensure proper mechanical function and readiness of the ambulance. The supplies and equipment that may be used during the shift also are checked and restocked.
- ***Receiving and responding to the call.*** In this phase, information is relayed to the crew and the response begins. Safety is at its highest priority during this phase because commonly there are many unknowns and specific challenges to safe operation.
- ***Transferring the patient to the ambulance.*** After you assess your patient, make important decisions, and provide emergency care, the patient is transferred to the ambulance. This must be done safely, efficiently, and with regard to the patient's condition.
- ***Transporting the patient to the hospital.*** The patient in the ambulance is transported to the hospital, sometimes with lights and sirens, sometimes not. In any event, operation of the emergency vehicle must be done with regard to safety. The emergency vehicle operator must be aware of the ongoing patient care and how operation of the vehicle can affect that care.
- ***Transferring the patient to hospital staff.*** The patient is brought into the hospital and care is transferred to hospital personnel. This involves transfer of important patient information as well as physically transferring the patient from your stretcher to the hospital gurney.
- ***Terminating the call.*** After transferring the patient, the final stage of the call involves completing documentation, cleaning and disinfecting equipment, and restocking the ambulance.

Preparing for the Call

Preparation for an EMS call includes two very important elements. First, the ambulance itself must be checked. EMTs must ensure proper mechanical operation and inspect exterior warning devices to make sure the vehicle can be operated safely even in the worst of conditions. Secondly, the contents of the ambulance must be checked. Most systems have specific inventory lists to ensure that proper equipment is present. Although there may be formal inventory checks on a regular scheduled basis, each and every shift should start with a review of essential equipment. Think of this review as a readiness operation. In a daily check you are not only accounting for important equipment, but familiarizing yourself with its location and organizing your unit to suit your individual needs.

The following lists are meant to be comprehensive. Your service likely has a regularly scheduled inventory to ensure minimum stocking. Your daily check may or may not include laying eyes on each and every item mentioned. However, at a minimum, you should work to develop a daily check that includes an inventory of the most essential items, with special attention to those items that are perishable, expire, or use batteries.

Your check should also ensure that all equipment is properly secured. In the unfortunate event of a crash, it is vitally important that equipment not be thrown violently throughout the unit. Proper securing will prevent this and should be considered a necessary component of the daily check.

At the end of the day, the responsibility for having the right equipment ready for patient care is yours and yours alone. With this in mind, design your check to make sure that you and your ambulance are ready for whatever call comes next.

Checking the Vehicle

Operating a safe vehicle means the mechanical function of that vehicle must be reliable. Most ambulances, like cars, require routine maintenance and scheduled checkups (Figure 41-1 ■). At a minimum, the following items should be checked daily (Scan 41-1):

- Fuel level
- Oil level
- Engine cooling system
- Battery
- Brakes
- Wheels and tires
- Headlights
- Stoplights
- Turn signals
- Emergency warning lights
- Wipers
- Horn
- Siren
- Doors closing and latching
- Communication systems
- Air conditioning/heating system
- Ventilation systems

In addition to mechanical function, the contents of an ambulance must be checked regularly. The daily check should include a brief inventory of essential supplies and a check to see they are functioning properly. Furthermore, EMTs should familiarize themselves with the placement of these items and make sure that all are properly secured prior to the ambulance moving. The following sections describe items typically carried on an ambulance. Your service, region, and/or state may have more specific lists. Always adhere to local guidelines.

Checking Infection Control and Comfort Supplies

The following list includes supplies needed for infection control and patient comfort:

- Two pillows
- Four pillow cases
- Two spare sheets
- Four blankets
- Six disposable emesis (vomit) bags or basins
- Two boxes of facial tissues
- Disposable bedpan, urinal, and toilet paper
- One package of drinking cups
- One package of wet wipes
- Four liters of sterile water or saline
- Four soft restraining devices (upper and lower extremities) (if local protocol allows)
- Packages of large and small red biohazard bags for waste or severed parts

Ambulance Daily Inventory Check Sheet

For Units Deployed Under Coastal Valleys EMS Agency

Vehicle Number: __________ Unit Identifier: __________ Date: __________

Rig	
Unit Identifier	
Current Registration	
CHP Identification Card	
Insurance Card	
Fuel Card	
Headlights	
Beam Selector/Indicator	
Headlight Flasher (FORD)	
Primary/Secondary Lights	
Turn Signals	
Side Marker Lights	
Stop Lights	
Tail Lights	
Backup Lights	
Inside Cot & Bench Lights	
Defroster/Heater (front and rear)	
Mirrors	
Horn & Siren	
Air Conditioning (front & rear) Area	
Steering & Suspension	
Brake System	
Tires—Including Spare (PSI and wear)	
Jack & Tools	
Fire Extinguisher	
Jumper cables	
Flashlight	
Map Books (Sonoma/Napa, Bay Area, Sac/Solano)	
FasTrak Module	
2 Roadside Safety Vests	
Engine Oil Level	
Transmission Fluid Level (FORD)	
Power Steering Fluid Level	
Break Fluid Level	
Radiator Fluid Level	
Windshield Wiper Fluid	
Hoses & Belts	
Battery Cables Clean	
DOT Handbook	
UHF Radio Check	
Zoll Defib Test@ 30 Joules	
Batteries Rotated	
Memory card erased	
Clipboard with paperwork	

Oxygen	
Medical O_2 (main) __________ psi	
Medical Air (main) __________ psi	
"D" O_2 tank (gumey) __________ psi	
"D" O_2 tank (blue bag) __________ psi	
"D" O_2 tank (spare) (1 for BLS, 2 for ALS)	

Locked / Stocked	Y/N
Cabinet 1	
Cabinet 2	
Cabinet 3	
Cabinet 4	
Cabinet 5	
Cabinet 6	
Cabinet 7	
Cabinet 8	
Cabinet 9	
Cabinet 10	
Cabinet 11	
Cabinet 12	
Cabinet 13	
Cabinet 14	
Cabinet 15 (SPRINTER)	
Area 1	
Area 2	
Area 3	
Area 4 (SPRINTER)	
Area 5 (SPRINTER)	
Behind Passenger Seat (SPRINTER)	
Left Side Door (FORD)	
Bench Seat	
Under Bench Seat	
Gurney	

OD Prep	Y/N
Fuel Above ¾ Full	
Trash Removed	
Front/Back Swept	
Gurney Cleaned	
Surfaces Wiped Down	
Supplies Re-Stocked/Cabs Locked	
O_2 turned off	
Radios Turned Off	
Ending Mileage Entered	
MDT Turned Off	
Rig Mod and Battery Off	
Inverter Light Off	
Ambulance Locked	

Notes (use back of sheet for more space)

Crew ____________________ Emp#: _____ Crew ____________________ Emp#: _____

Figure 41-1 Daily ambulance inventory checklist.

SCAN 41-1 Performing a Daily Ambulance Inspection

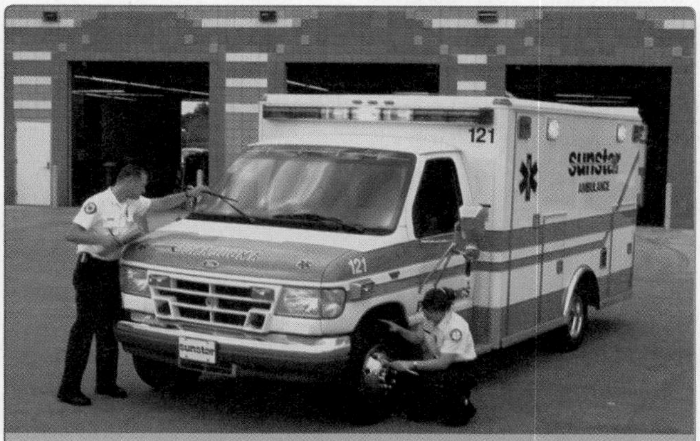

41-1-1 Perform a "walk around" and inspect the exterior of the vehicle including body, lights, wheels, tires, and wipers.

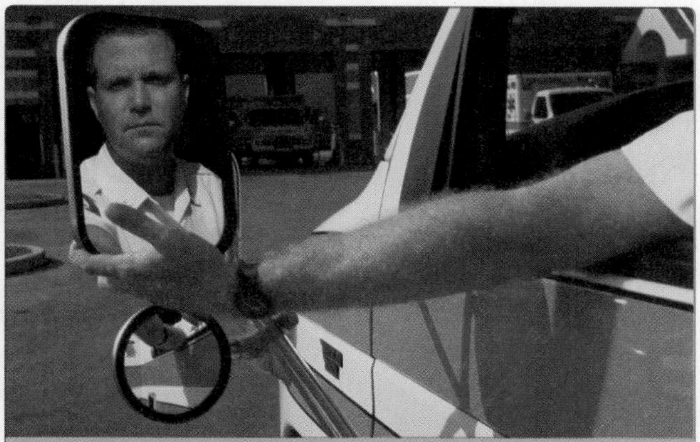

41-1-2 Check windows and doors, and adjust all mirrors.

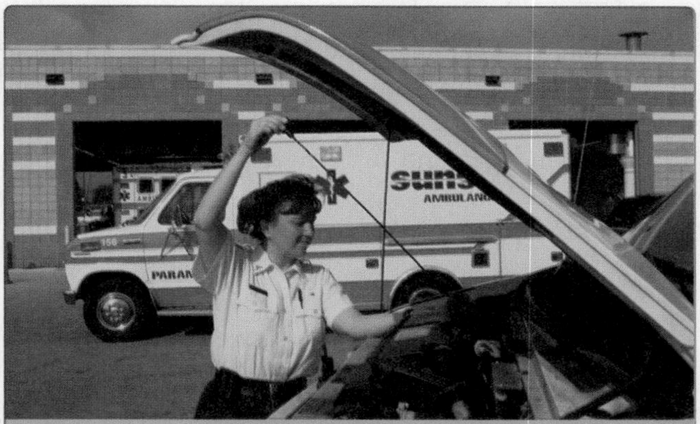

41-1-3 Check all fluid levels.

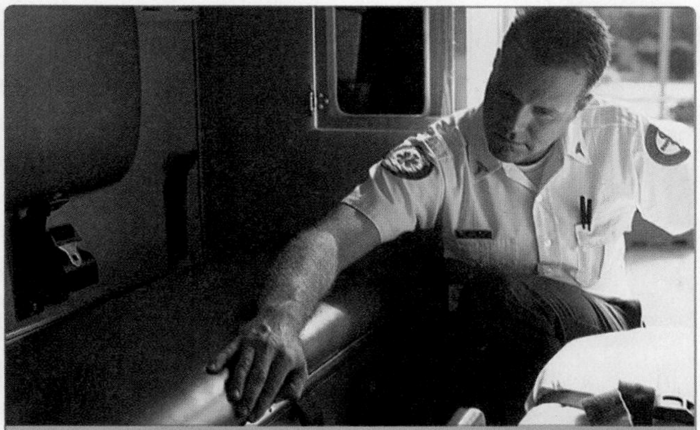

41-1-4 Inspect the interior.

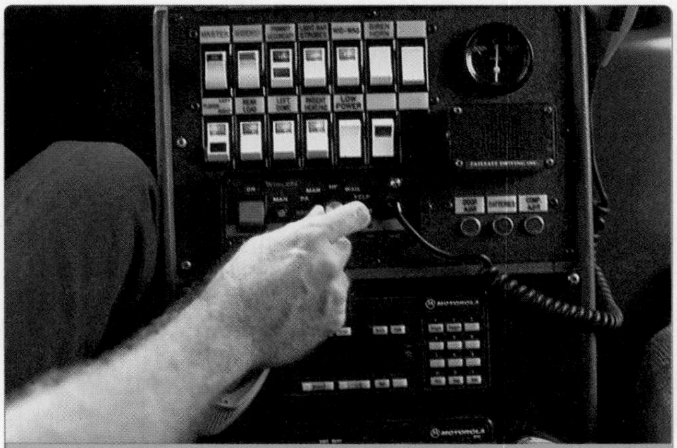

41-1-5 Check the function of all switches, gauges, and communications equipment.

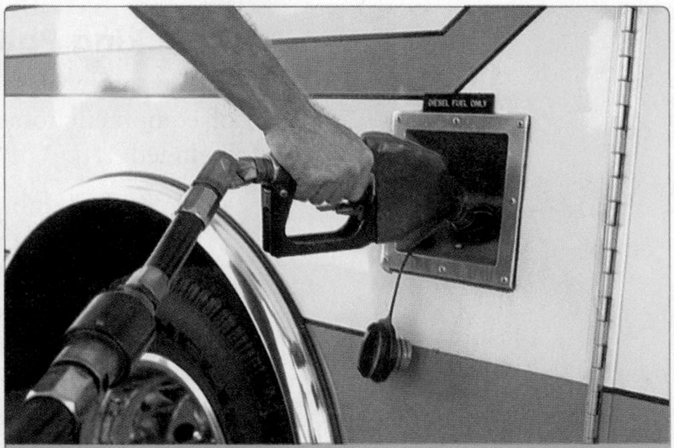

41-1-6 Be sure the fuel tank is topped off at the beginning of each shift.

- One package of large yellow bags for used linens or garbage (or otherwise color-coded or labeled according to your service's exposure control plan)
- EPA-registered, intermediate-level disinfectant (which destroys *mycobacterium tuberculosis*)
- EPA-registered, low-level disinfectant, such as Lysol®
- An empty plastic spray bottle with lines at the 1:100 level, a plastic bottle of water, and a plastic bottle of bleach for cleaning up blood spills. (Measure a fresh mixture of one part bleach to 100 parts water each day as needed.)
- Eye shields or other protective eyewear for each crew member
- Sharps container for the vehicle (BLS or ALS unit) and drug box (ALS unit)
- Disposable latex, vinyl, or other synthetic gloves: a box of each size
- N-95 or HEPA respirator for each crew member

Checking Primary and Secondary Assessment Equipment

Primary and secondary assessment equipment is often portable to allow it to be brought into the patient's home or onto a specific location. It is often organized in a single kit and frequently referred to as a "first-in kit" or "jump bag." The kits come in all shapes and sizes, in hard cases or soft bags. A first-in kit or jump bag should include supplies for the following:

- ***Airway.*** Airway adjuncts, suction, infection control, and personal protective equipment. If permitted for EMT use by local protocols, equipment for adult and pediatric orotracheal intubation or other advanced airways
- ***Breathing.*** Stethoscope, pocket mask with one-way valve and oxygen inlet, bag-mask device, oxygen, and oxygen delivery devices
- ***Circulation.*** Blood pressure cuff, bandages and dressings, occlusive dressings, and automated external defibrillator (AED)
- ***Neck and spine stabilization.*** Set of rigid cervical collars
- ***Exposure.*** Scissors and blankets
- ***Vital signs:***
    - Sphygmomanometer kit with separate cuffs for average-size and obese adults as well as child sizes
    - Adult and pediatric stethoscopes
    - Thermometer and a hypothermia thermometer that goes down to at least 82°F
    - Penlight(s)
    - Pulse oximeter

Checking Patient Transfer Equipment

Safe transfer of the patient is an important concern. Ambulances carry a variety of equipment to assist in this endeavor. The following carrying devices should be included:

- Wheeled ambulance stretcher, designed so that a sick or injured person can be transported in the Fowler's (sitting), supine, or Trendelenburg position. It should be adjustable in height and have detachable supports for intravenous fluid containers. Restraining devices, including straps for the body and for the shoulders, should be provided so that a patient will not fall off the stretcher or slide past the foot end or head end. Also called a *cot* or *gurney*
- Reeves stretcher, used for carrying a patient who must lie supine down stairs when a cot is too heavy or wide
- Folding stair chair, used for moving patients down stairs in a sitting position
- Scoop stretcher, used for picking up patients found in tight spaces with a minimum of movement. Also called an *orthopedic stretcher*

- Stokes or basket stretcher, used for long-distance carries, high-angle, or off-the-road rescues
- Child safety seat, used for transporting infants and small children in the ambulance (optional)

Checking Airway Maintenance, Ventilation, and Resuscitation Equipment

The first-in kit or jump bag typically contains many airway and breathing devices. The ambulance likely contains a number of additional devices used for maintaining an open airway and assisting breathing. Together they include:

- Oropharyngeal airways in sizes suitable for adults, children, and infants
- Soft rubber nasopharyngeal airways in sizes 14 through 30
- Two pocket face masks with one-way valves and filters for times when ventilation is necessary or when you are the only person ventilating a patient who does not have an endotracheal tube inserted
- Three manually operated, self-refilling bag-mask units (infant, child, adult) capable of delivering 100% oxygen to a patient by the addition of a reservoir. Masks of various sizes should be designed to ensure a tight face seal and should have an air cushion. The masks should be clear so you can see vomitus and the clouding caused by exhalations.

Oxygen Therapy and Suction Equipment

An ambulance should have two oxygen supply systems (one fixed, one portable) so oxygen can be supplied to two patients at once:

- Fixed oxygen delivery system supplies oxygen to a patient in the ambulance. A typical installation consists of a minimum 3,000-liter reservoir, regulator, and flow meter. Oxygen delivery tubes, transparent masks, and controls should all be located within easy reach when you are sitting at the patient's head. The system should be capable of delivering at least 15 liters of oxygen per minute and adaptable to the bag-mask units carried on the ambulance.
- Two portable oxygen delivery systems that have a capacity of at least 350 liters. Each system should have a regulator capable of delivering at least 15 liters of oxygen per minute. Many ambulances are equipped with multiple-function regulators that can be used for liter-flow oxygen, suctioning, and positive pressure ventilation. Because this oxygen is used frequently, EMTs must check levels regularly and replace empty tanks or refill depleted systems. Services and regional protocols should describe minimum pressures that indicate replacement.

In addition, an ambulance should have the following:

- Spare D, E, or jumbo D oxygen cylinders with a current hydrostat test date seal imprinted on the tank
- Six adult and four pediatric nonrebreather masks
- Six adult and four pediatric nasal cannulas
- One flow-restricted, oxygen-powered ventilation device
- One automatic transport ventilator (ATV) (optional)
- One noninvasive positive pressure ventilation (NIPPV) device such as CPAP (optional)
- One plastic comic cup for administering blow-by oxygen to a child
- Pulse oximeter

The fixed suction system should be sufficient to provide an air flow of over 30 liters per minute at the end of the delivery tube. A vacuum of at least 300 mmHg should be reached within four seconds after the suction tube is clamped. The suction should be controllable. The installed system should have a large-diameter, nonkinking tube fitted with a rigid tip. There should be a spare nonbreakable, disposable suction bottle and a container of water for rinsing the tubes. There should be an assortment of sterile catheters. The suction system should be usable by a person seated at the head of the patient.

The portable suction unit may be one of the many models powered by battery, hand or foot action, oxygen, or compressed air. The unit should be fitted with a nonkinking connecting tube as well as a large-bore rigid tip catheter.

EMTs should check both on-board and portable suction units daily. Ensure vacuum pressures and change batteries when necessary.

Cardiac Resuscitation Equipment

The following equipment for assisting with cardiopulmonary resuscitation and defibrillation should be carried on the ambulance:

- Short or long backboard to provide rigid support during CPR efforts
- An automated external defibrillator (AED)

Remember that an AED also should have scheduled maintenance. Daily checks should include any routine checks recommended by the manufacturer and a brief check of defibrillation pad expiration.

Immobilization Supplies and Equipment

The ambulance should carry a variety of devices for immobilization of injured extremities and suspected spine injuries:

- Adult and pediatric traction splints (such as the Sager or Hare) for the immobilization of a painful, swollen, or deformed femur
- Padded board splints for the immobilization of upper and lower extremities. Recommended are 2 × 54-inch splints, 2 × 36-inch splints, and 2 × 15-inch splints.
- Variety of splints: air-inflatable splints, vacuum splints, wire ladder splints, cardboard splints, soft rubberized splints with aluminum stays and Velcro fasteners, padded aluminum (SAM) splints, and splints that are inflated with cryogenic (cold) gas
- Tongue depressors to immobilize broken fingers
- Triangular bandages for use with splints and for making slings and swathes
- Several rolls of self-adhering roller bandage for securing the various splints
- Six chemical cold packs for use on injured extremities
- Two long backboards for full-body immobilization, preferably with speed clips or Velcro straps. The long backboard can also be used for patient transfer.
- Rigid cervical collars in a variety of adult and child sizes
- One KED or short backboard for seated patients with possible spine injuries
- Six 9-foot-by-2-inch web straps with aircraft-style buckles or D-rings for securing patients to carrying devices
- Commercial head immobilizer device or a set of rolled blankets or towels for the same purpose

Supplies for Wound Care and Treatment of Shock

A variety of dressings and bandaging materials should be carried on the ambulance:

- Sterile gauze pads (2 × 2 inches and 4 × 4 inches)
- 5 × 9-inch dressings
- Tourniquet and hemostatic dressings

- Sterile universal dressings (multi-trauma dressings) approximately 10 × 36 inches
- Self-adhering roller bandages in 4- and 6-inch width × 5 yards
- Occlusive dressings for sealing open (sucking) chest wounds and eviscerations
- Sterile burn sheets or commercial burn kit
- Adhesive strip bandages for minor wound care (1 × ¾ inch and 1 × ½ inch), individually packaged
- Hypoallergenic adhesive tape (1- and 3-inch rolls)
- Large safety pins for the securing of slings and swathes
- Bandage scissors
- Pneumatic anti-shock garments (PASG) in sizes for adults and children
- Specialized blankets (survival blankets) for maintaining body heat

Supplies for Childbirth

A sterile childbirth kit, either provided by a local medical facility or a commercially available disposable kit, as mandated by your system, should contain the following:

- Several pairs of sterile surgical gloves
- Four umbilical cord clamps
- One pair of sterile surgical scissors
- One rubber bulb syringe (3 ounces)
- Twelve 4 × 4 inch gauze pads
- Five towels
- One baby blanket (receiving blanket)
- Sanitary napkins
- Two large plastic bags
- Two stockinet infant caps

Also carry items that you can wear to minimize contamination of or by the mother and baby during and after childbirth:

- Two surgical gowns
- Two surgical caps
- Two surgical masks
- Two pairs of goggles or eye shields

Special Supplies and Equipment

- Medications as allowed by local protocol, such as oral glucose, aspirin, and EpiPen
- Sterile saline or water for irrigating a patient's eyes or skin
- Elastic bandages for snakebites (if local protocol allows)

Special Equipment for Advanced Providers

Depending on state laws and your medical director, some ambulances are provided with locked kits of supplies and equipment that can be used by advanced EMTs or paramedics, especially in rural areas. This equipment may include supplies for:

- Endotracheal intubation, orotracheal and endotracheal suctioning, and pediatric nasogastric intubation. (In some areas EMTs will be trained to perform these procedures.)
- Chest decompression
- IV medication administration
- Advanced supraglottic airways such as the King Tube™, laryngeal mask airway (LMA), or dual lumen Combitube® airway
- Cricothyrotomy kit
- Cardiac monitoring and defibrillation

Safety and Miscellaneous Equipment

Ambulances should be provided with personal protective equipment: equipment for warning, signaling, and lighting; hazard control devices; and tools for gaining access and disentanglements, including:

- Most current edition of the *Emergency Response Guidebook (ERG)*
- Binoculars
- Clipboard, prehospital care reports (PCRs), and other documentation forms
- Ring cutter
- Multiple-casualty incident management logs
- Triage tags and destination logs
- Reflective vests
- Disposable jumpsuits
- Flares
- Jumper cables
- Set of protective gear (helmet, protective eyewear, gloves) for each crew member
- Large floodlight/spotlight
- Spring-loaded center punch
- Wheel chocks
- Utility rope
- Stuffed animal for child patients

The daily check should also include maps or street books designed to provide the ability to quickly find an address. Some agencies use GPS-based programs that provide on-board directions to calls. Some satellite-based systems also communicate with dispatch centers to identify ambulance locations, ensuring that the closest ambulance is dispatched to a call. All such systems should be checked. You should continue to carry up-to-date maps or street books in case a GPS-based program fails.

Most states require safety equipment such as fire extinguishers, road flares or cones, and tools to assist the crew in the event of a mechanical or other vehicle emergency.

Additional Elements of a Safety Check

41-4 Give examples of habits and behaviors that improve driving safety.

41-5 Discuss factors that can affect your ability to maintain control while driving an ambulance.

All the gadgets and gear are useless without properly trained and prepared men and women. Ambulances should be staffed according to state, regional, or local protocol, but at least one certified EMT should be available to treat the patient in the patient compartment. In many places a minimum of two EMTs are required and that is the preferred staffing level for basic life support (BLS) ambulances. They must be available for emergency calls whether they are stationed at a rescue squad, fire department, or other station. In addition to checking the ambulance, your safety check should include a readiness check of crew members because there are a variety of problems that can impede safe performance on a call. Consider the following issues:

- ***Fatigue.*** Fatigue is a significant threat to the safe operation of an ambulance. Although the rigorous and unpredictable timing of EMS typically promotes being tired, you must carefully assess fatigue's impact on your ability to perform your duty. Safe operation is hampered when providers are sleep deprived and this "sleep debt" can be repaid only by actual uninterrupted sleep. That means providers should not work overloaded schedules and should plan quality sleep between shifts. If an EMT is unable to do so, he should be considered unsafe, particularly if he is behind the wheel of an ambulance. Although this has much to do with scheduling, it must be the responsibility of each EMT to be self-aware and avoid operating in an overly fatigued state.
- ***Stress.*** EMS operations are stressful by nature. As discussed in previous chapters, stress can have both immediate and ongoing effects. Most importantly, stress

can affect judgment and decision making and impair a provider's ability to safely operate an ambulance. Immediate stress can be mitigated by proper training and preparation. However, EMTs should be vigilant and recognize the signs of impairment in both themselves and their crew members.

- ***Illness and injury.*** Illnesses and injuries can impact a provider's ability to carry out a job. EMTs should always avoid situations in which physical maladies could impair their capabilities behind the wheel of an ambulance.
- ***Alcohol, drugs, and other intoxicants.*** It goes without saying that an ambulance should never be operated while the driver is intoxicated. However, many substances can impair driving capabilities. Medications, both prescription and over the counter, can impair driving abilities and should be used with care by EMS providers. Always consult your personal physician to be sure any medication you are taking is compatible with the responsibilities of your job. Remember also that lingering effects of alcohol and other intoxicants can impact performance for prolonged periods. Many services have very specific regulations pertaining to the use of alcohol prior to reporting to duty. Although you may not feel the effects of last night's drinking, your ability to drive and perform tasks as an EMT can be impaired well into your next day's shift.

PERSPECTIVE

Rollie—The EMT

I can't believe that happened. The crew before us said the lights had cut out on them but had come back on. I tested them and they were okay this morning. Wait'll I see them. They should've done more testing before the next shift. Maybe because they didn't want to drive to the shop or miss lunch or something, we couldn't get to the patient. But I get a trip to the repair shop and someone else took our call. Next time when it comes to lights, I'll be checking and rechecking. And we've got to work more like a team across shifts.

STOP, REVIEW, REMEMBER!

Multiple Choice

For each question, place a check next to the correct answer.

1. Which one of the following would be considered a critical element of a *daily* safety check?

_____ a. Inspecting the undercarriage of the ambulance for rust

_____ b. Making sure the exterior of the ambulance is washed and clean

_____ c. Ensuring proper function of all warning devices on the ambulance

_____ d. Inspecting the number of 4 × 4 dressings

2. Which level of training is designed to be the minimum level to staff an ambulance?

_____ a. Emergency medical responder (EMR)

_____ b. Emergency medical technician (EMT)

_____ c. Advanced EMT (AEMT)

_____ d. Paramedic

(continued on next page)

(continued)

3. Vehicle maintenance checks should be performed at least:
   _____ a. daily.
   _____ b. weekly.
   _____ c. biweekly.
   _____ d. monthly.

4. When inspecting your ambulance prior to the beginning of your shift, you notice that the left rear brake light is not working. You should:
   _____ a. immediately notify your supervisor and take the ambulance out of service until the light can be replaced.
   _____ b. complete your check report and begin your shift. After all, you have two brake lights.
   _____ c. Start your shift and fix the light while on post.
   _____ d. Conduct your shift, but double pump the brakes when stopping so drivers will note the good light.

5. You are dispatched to a call upon arriving at the station. As soon as you get into the passenger seat, you notice the odor of alcohol on your partner, the driver. You confront him and he tells you "It's from last night. I'm fine this morning." You should:
   _____ a. continue the call.
   _____ b. stop the call and immediately discuss the situation with a supervisor.
   _____ c. continue the call, but discuss the situation later with a supervisor.
   _____ d. trade places with your partner so that you are driving the ambulance.

Matching

Match the event on the left with a phase of an ambulance call on the right.

1. _____ Moving the patient from your stretcher to the hospital gurney
2. _____ Placing the patient on your stretcher and wheeling it to the ambulance
3. _____ Your morning vehicle checks
4. _____ Completing your documentation
5. _____ Disinfecting the ambulance after an MVC with a patient bleeding
6. _____ Driving to the hospital
7. _____ Stocking the rig after a call
8. _____ The dispatcher radios you with a call
9. _____ Verbally advising the hospital staff about your patient

A. Preparing for the call
B. Receiving and responding to the call
C. Transferring the patient to the ambulance
D. Transport to the hospital
E. Transfer to hospital staff
F. Terminating the call

Critical Thinking

1. You are in a patient's home working a cardiac arrest. You reach for the suction and find that the battery is dead. What do you do? Why did this happen?

____

____

____

____

2. The emergency medical dispatcher gets a few pieces of information initially. They include the patient's location, the complaint, and the call-back number. They are very important. Why?

____

____

____

____

Receiving and Responding to the Call

The wheels of the EMS system begin spinning well before you hear the tones that signal your dispatch for a call. Most EMS responses begin when the patient or patient's family dials 911. Although there are systems that use other emergency numbers, 911 commonly provides the first point of access to the emergency system and puts the calling party in touch with the closest communications center (Figure 41-2 ■).

Many regions use "enhanced 911" systems that allow the dispatcher to not only communicate with the caller, but to also simultaneously gain real time information such as the address of the caller and notes from previous calls to that location.

In some situations, emergency medical dispatch may reach into the community before an emergency occurs. That is, many EMS systems provide education to people in their community on warning signs of serious medical conditions and when and how to contact EMS. In the event of a cardiac arrest, your system's ongoing involvement in the community could ensure that CPR is being performed, a defibrillator is present, and EMS has been activated at the earliest possible moment.

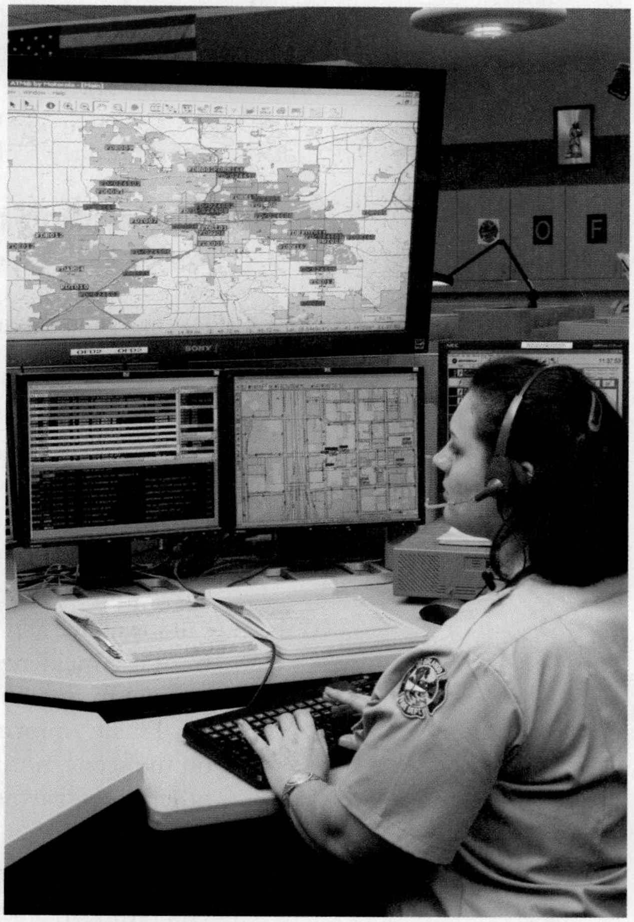

Figure 41-2 A typical EMS dispatch center.

The Initial Dispatch

In most systems, the dispatcher is able to obtain key initial information from the caller including the nature of the request for emergency assistance, the location of the patient, and a call-back number at the location. This information is critical in the event the caller loses consciousness or is disconnected from the dispatcher. Even though enhanced 911 centers display the number the patient is calling from, it is always verified to prevent errors in data entry or technology.

The dispatcher then begins to obtain information on the reason the patient (or family member, coworker, or bystander) called. A few additional focused questions are now asked of the caller. They include:

- What is the current condition of the patient? For example, is he responsive and breathing?
- Are there hazards on the scene, such as pets, traffic, or a crime in progress?

- Will the EMTs be able to get to the patient in the current location? Are car or house doors unlocked? For an EMS call at an apartment complex or large building such as a factory, dispatchers will obtain detailed location information and instruct the caller to send someone to meet the ambulance.

The questions take a relatively short time. In most dispatch centers, a call-taker will obtain the initial information while a second dispatcher simultaneously dispatches the call.

Emergency medical dispatch is rapidly becoming an additional element of most dispatch centers. With this specialized training, dispatchers are able to provide pre-arrival instructions to callers. The instructions may include proper patient positioning, artificial ventilation and CPR, how to stop bleeding, and more. Emergency medical dispatchers providing this information most commonly use a series of cards with prompts determining which questions to ask and the instructions to provide.

The information obtained by dispatchers helps to determine the priority of EMS response, the need for first response (such as a local fire department engine company for serious calls), and whether additional apparatus (for example, fire, heavy-rescue, or hazmat) will be required.

Dispatchers are a vital asset to the EMS system. Their actions provide critical information, which begins the EMS call in the most efficient way possible.

Responding to the Call

Responding to the call is the next phase of the EMS response. This is perhaps the most visible part of what EMTs do and in many cases it is also the most dangerous. During the response, you and your crew should consider who will be responsible for what tasks at the scene. Based on the dispatch information, you may also discuss possible causes of the emergency. For example, if the patient is experiencing chest pain, is that chest pain an acute myocardial infarction or angina or is it being caused by asthma or other breathing problem? Did the patient fall down or get assaulted? Considering different reasons for the call will help you prepare for the questions you may want to ask of the patient on scene.

Additionally during the response, consider whether or not there are any scene hazards or need for police resources. One rule for crew protection states that if you call for police and stage away from the scene, you should do so at least two turns away from the incident so that if the dangerous incident starts to come to you, there will be time for you to get away.

Finally, inform your dispatcher that you are responding to the call. Upon arrival on the scene, notify the dispatcher of both your arrival and any specific information other units may need such as an updated address or obvious hazards.

Operating an Emergency Vehicle

Operating an emergency vehicle is one of the more dangerous tasks performed by an EMT. Although it is a routine element of most day-to-day activities, you must never become complacent about the extreme hazards associated with this task. Motor-vehicle crashes are the leading cause of vocation-related death for EMTs, and as such, extreme care must be demonstrated during all phases of ambulance operation.

EMS commonly responds to calls that are time sensitive. As a result, EMTs rush and look for ways to reach the patient sooner. In most states, **warning lights** and **sirens** on an ambulance are allowed to be operated when responding to a call to communicate urgency to other drivers and request passage of the ambulance through traffic. The warning devices also may be used when responding from the scene to the hospital.

In some cases, lights and sirens legally provide the ambulance driver a **right of way,** or permission to travel through traffic without delay. Some states allow ambulance

warning lights visual warning devices used on an emergency vehicle.

sirens audible warning devices used on an emergency vehicle.

right of way permission to travel through traffic without delay.

drivers going to the scene or leaving for the hospital to use the shoulder, restricted lanes, and other privileges not accorded to nonemergency drivers. However, the lights and sirens of your ambulance never give you a free pass to drive recklessly or at a high rate of speed through traffic. Since each state is different, EMT students should research local and state rules on these matters before attempting to drive an ambulance.

The term **due regard** (or *due caution*) for the safety of others is a term often used to describe the responsibility of the emergency vehicle operator. Although your local statutes may allow the ambulance to be exempt from certain traffic regulations, it is never appropriate to operate that ambulance in a manner that puts other drivers at risk. At all times the ambulance operator must consider the safety of other drivers while conducting a response. Even when laws are put aside, the operator's actions must be reasonable and include a due regard for the safety of those around the ambulance.

due regard functioning in a manner that is precise, cautious, and does not injure anyone else. Also called *due caution.*

Far too often, some EMTs view the legal protections they are afforded as a rationale to drive the ambulance aggressively and sometimes even dangerously. The high risk of driving an ambulance should induce just the opposite type of behavior. Although traffic laws may not apply, driving an ambulance should be completed in a defensive manner and in such a way as to always avoid the risk of collision. Operating an emergency vehicle is a great responsibility and should be given great respect by those granted the privilege.

Ambulances must not be operated recklessly. Ambulance collisions are not only a cause of injury and death to EMS providers, but also a leading cause of lawsuits against EMS systems and the operators themselves. Excess speed, failure to use caution at intersections (especially when proceeding against a red light), and operating in poor weather conditions are significant causes of crashes and the liability that follows.

Training plays an enormous role in creating a culture of safety. Driving an ambulance is different from driving a car, especially in emergency conditions. The skill requires education and practice. Many states now require EMTs who operate ambulances on state roads to have completed a state-approved driver's course that covers topics such as road hazards, defensive driving, and weather-related traffic issues. At a minimum, providers should learn the rigors of ambulance operation before engaging in emergency driving.

Driving an ambulance is an inherently unsafe operation. Although there are many steps a provider can take to make this situation safer, dangers abound. Many factors compound the risk. Fatigue and stress are among them. The time of day and day of the week likely play a role in safety, too. For example, cities experience peak traffic during rush hours Monday through Friday. During the day, there may be an increase in pedestrian traffic in some areas. Weather, including rain, snow, sleet, and ice storms can limit visibility and make the road surface slippery, causing longer stopping distances. Heavy traffic and traffic backups can change the availability of lanes for turns. Drivers may stop in the driving lane because they have nowhere to pull over to let you pass. Construction areas, bridges, and tunnels all have smaller lanes associated with them. They can make driving, turning, and operating your vehicle an increased challenge. In addition, turning an ambulance (which requires a much larger radius than typical vehicles) or simply backing up the ambulance and parking, are all situations where the ambulance has limited visibility for the driver, making accidents more likely (Figure 41-3 ■).

The prepared ambulance operator will know of potential driving problems, such as the times of heavy traffic and construction plans in his area, and will know both main and alternate routes to get to various locations and hospitals.

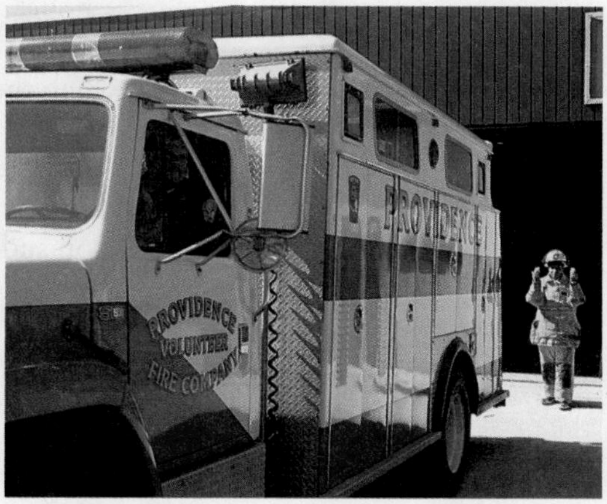

Figure 41-3 It is good practice to always use a spotter when backing the vehicle.

PERSPECTIVE

Marianne—The EMT

I was trying to shrink into my seat when all those people were glaring and shouting at us. We stupidly tried to drive through a big glut of cars that didn't even know where we were. This kind of thing just cannot happen. And it's a safety issue for everyone involved! Any time lost getting to the patient is wrong. Just plain wrong.

Safe Driving

41-6 Describe the appropriate use of emergency warning devices, such as lights and sirens.

Driving an emergency vehicle should always be conducted defensively. At all times the driver should be aware of his surroundings and attempt to maintain the utmost control of the vehicle. In general, drivers should always attempt to anticipate the next, upcoming danger and do their best to predict the moves of others. Always be prepared for the unexpected. Ample room should be left between the ambulance and cars in front of it. This allows adequate time to brake or take evasive action if a dangerous situation arises unexpectedly. Drivers should maintain a safety zone around the ambulance and visualize the road ahead for potential threats. Always leave space in front, behind, and to the sides to maneuver. It is commonly suggested that the ambulance maintain at least two car lengths of following distance at all times. Never tailgate and increase following distances in inclement weather or in situations in which driving conditions are more hazardous.

When operating in emergency mode, take as many steps as possible to warn others. Use all your warning lights and your siren. Your daily safety check should ensure that all lights function and provide a 360-degree zone of visual warning around the ambulance. Many states have specific regulations on warning lights so be sure to review your local regulations. Even in nonemergency situations, make every attempt to let other drivers understand your intentions. Use turn signals and emergency flashers, and avoid operating the ambulance in areas of low visibility of other vehicles.

Although traffic regulations may allow you to exceed the posted speed limit, never travel at speeds that create an unsafe condition. Drive only as fast as conditions allow and reduce speeds in inclement weather and other dangerous circumstances.

Multiple emergency vehicles traveling together create additional risk. Ambulances should not receive escorts to the hospital. This is because the danger of the procedure usually outweighs the benefits. Motorists will see one vehicle moving through an intersection and think that it is safe to proceed, never expecting the second vehicle to come through. It is the vehicle being escorted that usually ends up in a collision. In very few cases, are escorts warranted. Some examples of appropriate escorts might include a situation in which the driver is lost in an unfamiliar district or when the ambulance is transporting a priority patient and loses power to its warning devices, including the sirens and warning lights.

When following an escort vehicle, give the lead vehicle appropriate distance to navigate through traffic without becoming involved in a collision should they have to stop suddenly. Use the warning systems you have available to you (if any), and drive much more cautiously.

Intersections are a hazardous area. When responding to a call with a stop sign or red light at an intersection, ambulance operators should stop and check in both directions prior to entering the intersection. Many times traffic will hear an ambulance but not see it and will race through intersections hoping to beat the ambulance wherever it is going. It does your patient no good if you do not make it to the call or wind up going to the hospital with him.

Another problem with intersections is that separate emergency units may be responding to a call from different directions. In those cases, an emergency vehicle that does not stop for the red light may inadvertently hit another emergency responder. This creates a two-fold problem because two units responding to the incident are now unavailable, their crews possibly injured, and the original call is still in place but understaffed.

If you know that multiple units have been dispatched to a call and will be traveling through the same intersection, use the radio to notify other units that you are approaching the intersection. Use additional caution as you approach the intersection, because your siren will drown out the sirens of other emergency vehicles.

Every ambulance is marked with a visual display of its organization's name. Reckless behavior and collisions involving ambulances are disastrous for those organizations from a public relations and public trust perspective, even when it is not the ambulance operator who was at fault and even when no one is hurt. The public takes note of how you operate your vehicle. It will reflect on both you and your organization.

Specific Driving Hazards

Certain specific circumstances make emergency driving even more dangerous, and driving techniques must be adapted to account for those risks. They include operating in emergency mode, driving at night, inclement weather, highway operations, fatigue, and distracted driving.

41-7 Explain precautions that should be taken when driving an ambulance in inclement weather.

41-8 Explain precautions that should be taken when driving an ambulance at night.

OPERATING IN EMERGENCY MODE

For many EMTs, operating in the emergency mode (using lights and sirens while responding to a call or to the hospital) is a routine practice. Even so, you should never forget the inherent dangers associated with it. According to the National Highway Transportation Safety Administration, operation with lights and sirens increases the risk of collision nearly 600%. Frequently others react dangerously by braking quickly, making abrupt turns, and displaying bad decision-making skills in general. As a result, you must take steps to increase your vigilance while operating in this mode. Defensive driving is an absolute must under these conditions.

The use of lights and sirens is meant to ask other drivers for the right of way but not to demand it. You should anticipate the unsure decisions of other drivers and only take the right of way when it is clearly safe to do so. Furthermore, you should think carefully about when to employ emergency mode. Although there are time-sensitive situations in EMS, they are relatively infrequent. EMTs should reserve emergency transport only to those situations warranting the increased risk. As with many things EMTs do, the use of lights and sirens should come only after a cost–benefit analysis that compares the risks of collision to the benefits of time saving. Consideration should be given to the patient's condition and to the status of interventions being performed. Many systems have specific guidelines for the use of emergency mode. As always, follow local protocol.

DRIVING AT NIGHT

Nighttime operations pose specific risks. Visibility is the largest challenge. Although in many cases visual warning devices may be more visible, dark conditions generally impair visibility. In some cases, headlights and warning lights may actually impair the night vision of other drivers. Other specific hazards include driver fatigue and a higher incidence of impaired driving. Care should be taken to recognize those challenges and take steps to proceed even more cautiously in darkened situations.

INCLEMENT WEATHER

Inclement weather can lead to more difficult driving conditions. For example, snow and ice make roads slippery and can cause the ambulance to lose control during braking and turning. Rain can cause hydroplaning (even at relatively low speeds) and also causes control issues. As a result, drivers must take proactive steps to increase safety when operating in those conditions.

Consider increasing following distances in anticipation of increased braking distances. Slower speeds and longer stopping distances are necessary to maintain control. Beware of hazards that have caused other collisions, because they may affect your vehicle as well. For example, if icy roads have caused multiple vehicles to spin out off the road, care should be taken before driving down the same road. Inclement weather also may require special equipment such as snow tires. Consider proactive steps such as maintaining wiper blades and cleaning headlights regularly.

HIGHWAY OPERATIONS

The high speeds of highways pose significant risks during emergency operation. Audible warnings such as sirens are more difficult to hear and sudden movements pose extreme risk for collision. The most significant areas of danger on the highway are entering and leaving traffic because high speeds provide little margin for error. Remember that entering a highway requires much more space between vehicles. When entering traffic, first await a safe opportunity and then accelerate quickly to the right lane. Use that lane to gain highway speed and allow others to pass you if your speed is not sufficient. Then move to the left lane for emergent travel. When slowing or leaving traffic, beware of oncoming drivers. High speeds leave little reaction time. Leave the high-speed lanes rapidly and allow room for other drivers to pass you if necessary.

FATIGUE

Driving while sleep deprived is a serious safety concern. Not only does this behavior pose the risk of falling asleep at the wheel, but it also causes increased reaction time and poor judgment. Drivers should avoid operating emergency vehicles when these conditions exist.

DISTRACTED DRIVING

Ambulance operators face any number of potential distractions. From unavoidable issues such as patient problems, GPS use, and radio communication to clearly unnecessary distractions such as use of a stereo or cell phone and eating and drinking. All distractions pose a major hazard. Drivers should minimize distractions as best as possible by eliminating unnecessary actions and minimizing the necessary ones.

If a distracting activity is necessary, drivers should always consider the possibility of pulling the vehicle over to accomplish the task and then proceed when they can focus their full attention to the road ahead. In some systems, drivers can find themselves alone in the vehicle. This can be an especially dangerous source of distracted driving. When alone, the driver may have to accomplish all the necessary tasks of operating the vehicle, including navigation and radio communication. Although driving alone may be impossible to avoid, every attempt should be made to minimize its role, and when necessary, steps should be taken to prevent distracting actions.

Arrival and Parking at Emergency Scenes

41-9 Describe the safety precautions to be taken when working at scenes on and near roadways.

Parking at an emergency scene entails many considerations. For example, when you respond to calls at a residence or business, you must park in a place clear of traffic. The position you choose should be convenient to the scene in the event a crew member needs additional equipment and because transfer of the patient between the scene and ambulance should be over the shortest distance safely possible. When responding to motor-vehicle collisions, you must park at least 100 feet away from the collision (Figure 41-4 ■) either in front of or behind the crash site.

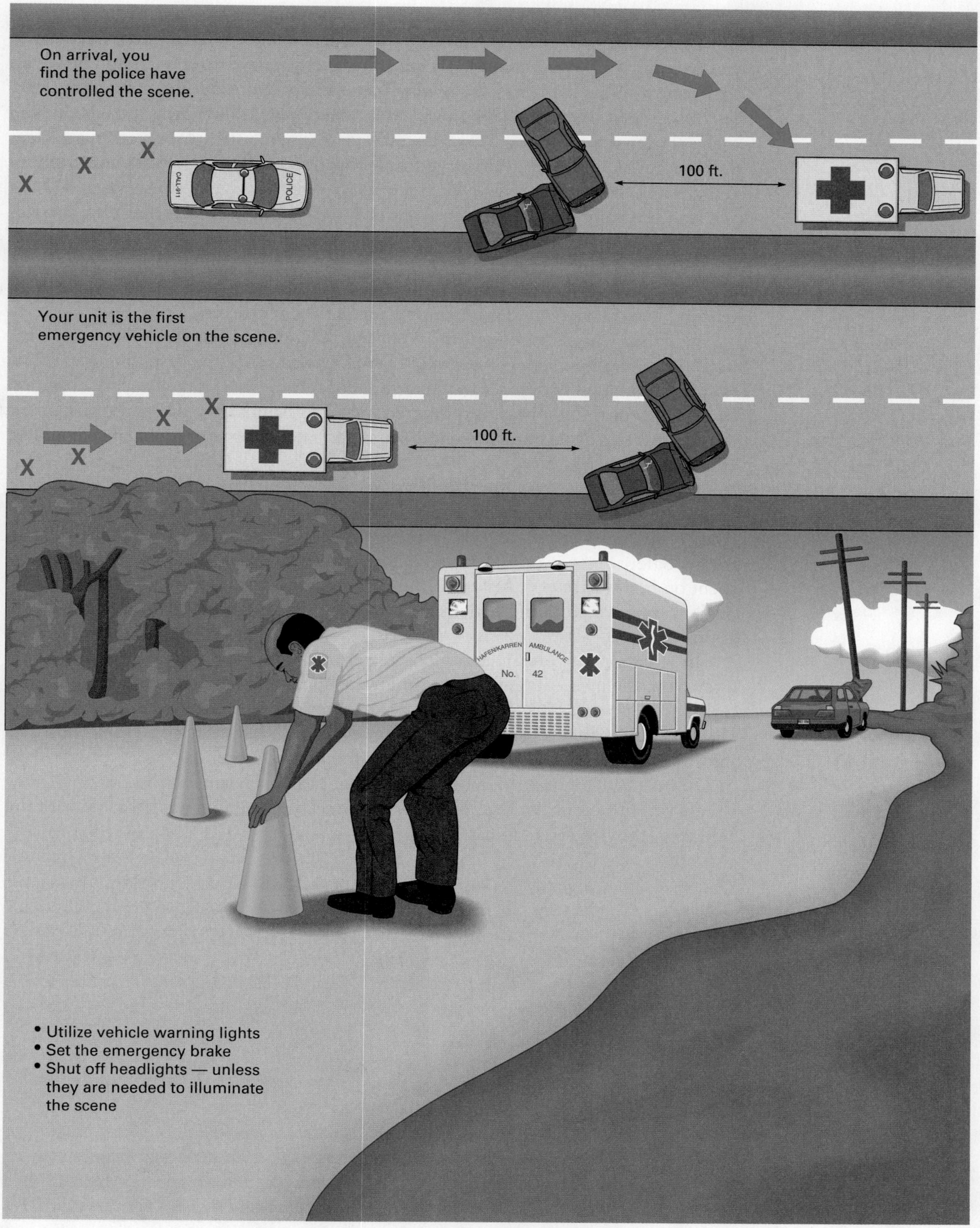

Figure 41-4 Recommendations for positioning your vehicle at the scene of a vehicle collision.

If you elect to park behind the collision (between oncoming traffic and the collision) because you are the first vehicle on scene, additional care must be given to traffic coming up from behind. Traffic cones or reflective devices should be set up to direct traffic away from the collision scene and give direction to oncoming drivers of the need to change lanes away from where you are working. If the collision scene is over the crest of a hill or beyond a curve, you must place warning devices at the other side of the hill or curve to allow proper stopping time for approaching vehicles.

It is generally safer to park in front of the collision because other cars, fire engines, and so on will provide a buffer if another vehicle impacts the scene. Maintain the 100-foot safety distance. Never park so that your headlights distract oncoming drivers. If you must park facing traffic, turn off your headlights and use only those warning devices that will not impair the vision of other drivers.

Whether you park in front of or behind the collision scene, be extremely cautious. Be sure all personnel wear NHTSA-approved reflective vests (Figure 41-5 ■) at roadside scenes. Motorists watching the collision scene are not paying attention to activities in the roadway. Add inattention from cellular phones and other in-car distractions to this mix and it is quite possible that you or your ambulance could be at high risk.

Highway scenes pose even higher risks. The ambulance should be positioned so that loading can take place away from traffic. Crew members should exit the ambulance only after carefully checking oncoming traffic and never turn their backs to traffic. Safety vests are essential here, too. In general, it is safest to minimize time spent on highway scenes. Although this is not always possible, every effort should be made to remove crew and patient from this highly dangerous environment as soon as possible.

In situations involving hazardous materials, park approximately one-half mile away from the incident. Park your ambulance uphill and upwind of a hazardous materials scene to avoid becoming sick from noxious or otherwise dangerous chemicals. Use binoculars to size up the scene from a distance before approaching. (Further information on hazardous materials can be found in Chapter 44.)

At incidents that are not motor-vehicle collisions or hazmat spills, the EMS crew should still fully consider the possibility of the scene becoming unstable and park the vehicle to provide for a rapid exit if needed.

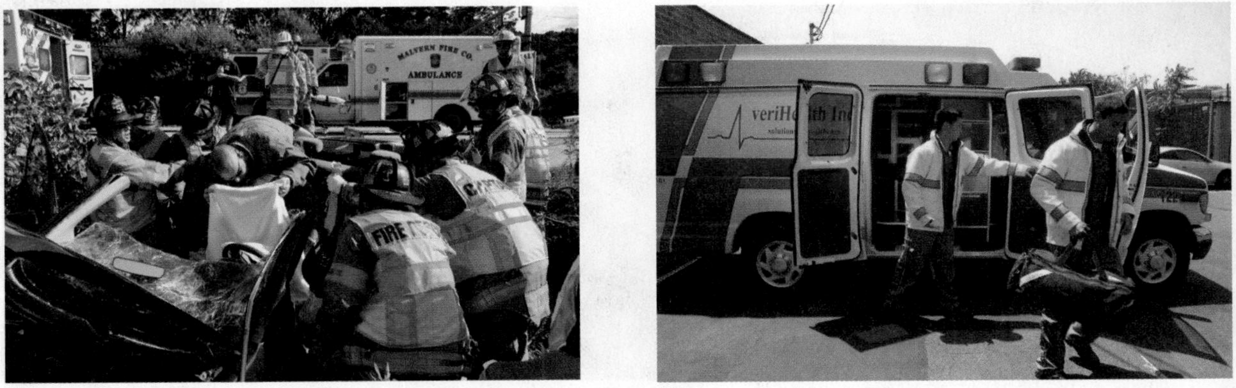

(A) (B)

Figure 41-5 EMS personnel working on an active roadway must wear high-visibility jackets. (A) © Edward T. Dickinson, MD, (B) © Christopher J. Le Baudour.

STOP, REVIEW, REMEMBER!

Multiple Choice

For each question, place a check next to the correct answer.

1. Which one of the following best describes operating an ambulance with due regard?

_____ a. Always obeying all traffic laws and regulations

_____ b. Disregarding traffic laws when necessary but considering the safety of other drivers around you

_____ c. Aggressively driving with no consideration of traffic laws or regulations

_____ d. Disregarding traffic laws based only on patient condition

2. Which one of the following is a specific risk associated with operating an ambulance on a highway?

_____ a. It is difficult for other drivers to hear audible warnings.

_____ b. It is difficult for other drivers to see visual warning devices.

_____ c. Ambulances are not as fast as other vehicles.

_____ d. Radio communication is more difficult in highway areas.

3. You are returning from a call when it begins to snow heavily. To increase safety you should:

_____ a. decrease following distance.

_____ b. disregard the snow because ambulances are designed for all climate use.

_____ c. stop the ambulance because emergency driving is impossible in snow.

_____ d. increase following distance.

4. When parking at an emergency scene, you should place the ambulance at least _____________ feet away from the crash.

_____ a. 25

_____ b. 50

_____ c. 75

_____ d. 100

5. You have been dispatched to a motor-vehicle collision involving two vehicles at the base of a hill. En route the police department notifies you that the hill is very icy and that the cause of the collision was most likely the ice. You should:

_____ a. stop the ambulance at the top of the hill and investigate the scene on foot.

_____ b. start down the hill carefully and stop if conditions are too icy.

_____ c. disregard the police officer's warning.

_____ d. proceed down the hill normally, but allow extra distance for stopping.

Short Answer

1. Describe three general measures you can use to improve safety while driving an ambulance.

____

____

____

____

(continued on next page)

(continued)

2. Discuss how inclement weather might increase the inherent dangers of emergency driving.

3. Describe three common factors that might distract an emergency driver.

Critical Thinking

1. Your state allows you to disregard traffic regulations while operating an emergency vehicle but requires due regard. Please explain what is meant by the term *due regard* and how it applies to emergency operation of a vehicle.

2. You are tasked with responding to a scene alone. Please describe how this situation might have more inherent risk associated with vehicle operation than driving with a partner.

Transferring the Patient to the Ambulance

Multiple ways are available to the EMT and ambulance crew to move patients. The method selected will depend on terrain and the condition of the patient. The stretcher is a mobile bed-like device that can be used to move patients in a supine or semi-sitting position across flat distances. It should be used with caution, because it can easily tip over due to the high center of gravity when wheeled with the patient in the elevated position. One safety consideration is to use stretchers only when you can keep the wheels on the floor or ground. Otherwise, there is likely a better way to move the patient.

The stair chair, as the name suggests, works particularly well over stairs. The stair chair is for patients who will be sitting or semi-sitting during transport but who need to be moved down steps prior to being placed on a stretcher. (See Chapter 8 for more information on the stair chair.)

Unconscious patients or those being transported in a supine position may be moved using any number of devices including long backboards, scoop stretchers, and Reeves stretchers. Each of those devices has its own benefits and drawbacks that must be considered before use. The Reeves stretcher is a flexible, litter-type device that can move unconscious medical patients from upstairs and across areas a wheeled stretcher cannot easily access because of unstable terrain. Long backboards can be useful in those situations, too, but sometimes require additional time to get the patient fully secured to the board.

Once loaded in the ambulance, securing the patient is a significant safety priority. If a crash occurs, injury is best prevented by keeping both occupants and equipment in place. Seat belts and shoulder straps are the best methods of securing the patient in place but work only if they are used on every patient during every transport. All EMTs should embrace a culture of safety that includes not moving the ambulance unless the patient is properly secured. Remember, also, to secure any loose equipment such as oxygen cylinders or pulse oximetry devices.

Make sure that any family member who is riding with the patient is secured with a seat belt in the appropriate position in the ambulance per your local guidelines.

The ambulance operator should drive to the hospital in such a way as to create a sense of comfort for the patient. Remember, in many cases the patient is not in a typical riding position but is either semi-sitting or supine and *backwards*. The driver should keep this in mind while departing for the receiving facility.

As you leave the scene, once again notify dispatch of your change in status. They should know your unit identifier, where you are going, how many patients you are transporting, and your mode of transport (with or without lights and sirens).

Transporting the Patient to the Hospital

Transport to the hospital is performed with the same due regard as discussed earlier in this chapter. The difference is that during response to the hospital, the vehicle will be operated while a patient and crew are in the patient compartment.

The ride in the back of the ambulance is much different than the ride the driver will experience. The center of gravity for those in the patient compartment is high. This causes considerable swaying of the box, which can throw EMTs around. It is safest for EMTs to remain seated and belted during the trip to the hospital. Although this is not always possible, such as when CPR and airway maneuvers must be performed, it should always be the goal. When not belted, the EMT should have "three points" anchored in the ambulance. For example, if you are standing to adjust the oxygen flow rate, you should have both feet on the floor and one hand holding onto the grab rail above the patient.

Important steps to be taken en route to the hospital (Scan 41-2) include checking to see that the patient is belted to the stretcher. The stretcher should be properly secured to the ambulance by the mounting system on the floor. Check this system periodically to ensure that all connecting bolts and latches are secure.

The ride for the patient also has its share of discomforts. Because the patient will be supine on the stretcher (sometimes on a rigid backboard), sitting, or somewhere

SCAN 41-2 Duties While Transporting to the Receiving Hospital

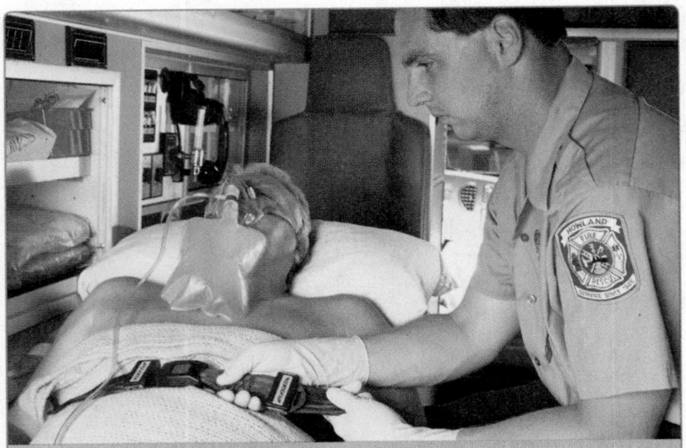

41-2-1 Ensure the patient is properly secured to the stretcher using all available belts and straps.

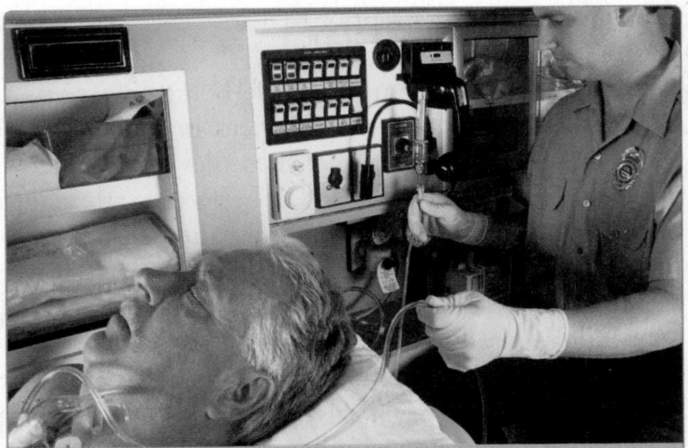

41-2-2 Transfer the patient from the portable oxygen source to the onboard oxygen source when appropriate.

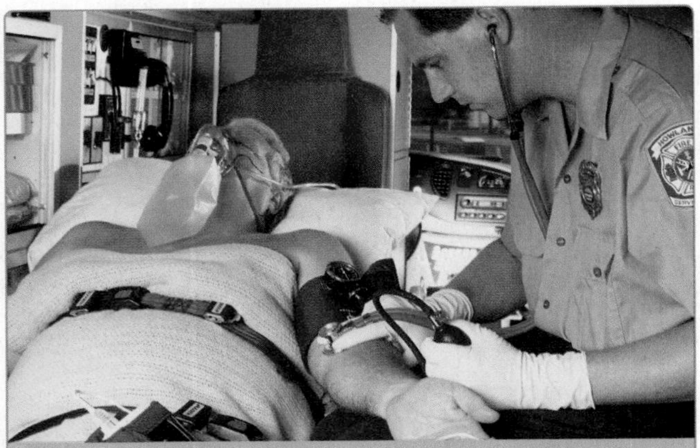

41-2-3 Continue to monitor the patient's condition.

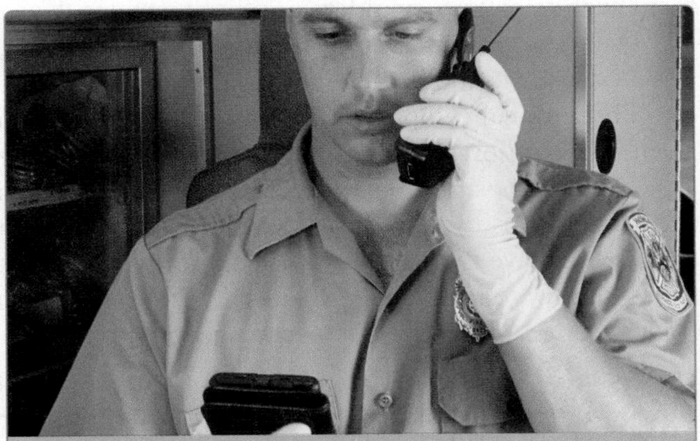

41-2-4 Notify the receiving facility that you are en route with a patient.

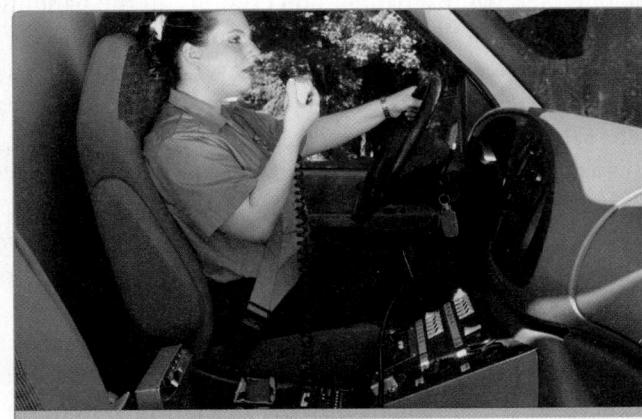

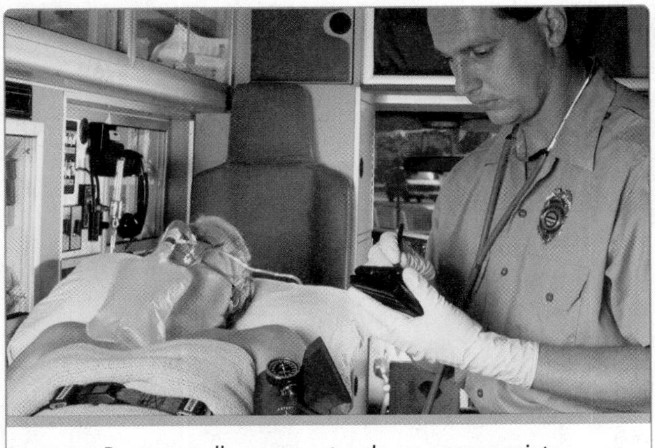

41-2-5 Document all assessment and care as appropriate.

41-2-6 Notify dispatch when you depart the scene and again when you arrive at the hospital.

in between, there is a significant portion of the patient in contact with the ambulance floor (via the stretcher). When EMTs ride in the ambulance, their buttocks touch the seat or bench. A supine patient on a backboard feels bumps in the road over his entire body through a rigid piece of plastic. The patient also acutely feels any swerves or quick turns in an exaggerated fashion. Be sure to avoid last minute turns, lane changes, and abrupt stops unless necessary to avoid a collision.

Perform ongoing assessments en route to the hospital every 5 minutes for the unstable patient and at least every 15 minutes for the stable patient. During the assessment, be sure to check the oxygen, including transfer of the oxygen from the portable cylinder to the onboard oxygen unit.

Also reassure the patient during transport. This will help calm the patient, who is likely anxious from the transport process in addition to the condition that caused his ride to the hospital.

You should provide a radio or cell-phone call-in to the receiving hospital. The exact content of this report is covered in Chapter 10. The report should paint the picture of the patient's condition (generally the patient's signs, symptoms, vital signs, and severity). Should the patient's condition change significantly en route, you should contact the receiving hospital again to advise them of the change.

En route to the hospital communication between the driver and the EMT in the patient compartment is important. The driver may need to notify the EMT in back of traffic delays or construction, poor road conditions, or mechanical problems with the ambulance. The EMT in the back may need to communicate changes in the patient's condition, request to either begin or discontinue use of lights and sirens, or request to pull to the side of the road in cases such as defibrillation, during which the ambulance should be stopped to effectively analyze the heart rhythm.

Not all responses to the hospital require lights and sirens. When determining the need for lights and sirens consider:

- Condition of the patient (stable or unstable)
- Patient's injuries (bumps cause extreme pain in a fractured leg, for instance)
- Effect of lights and sirens on the patient's condition (anxiety worsens chest pain)
- Distance to be traveled
- Traffic along the route
- Type of roadway (highway, urban, rural)

Transferring the Patient to Hospital Staff

On arrival at the receiving location or hospital, the ambulance operator should inform dispatch that the ambulance has reached its destination.

Next is transfer of the patient to the hospital staff. A core concept in transfer of care is the hand off of the patient to a person with equal or higher training than your own. Failure to ensure that patient care has been assumed by hospital staff would be considered **abandonment,** even though you left the patient at the hospital. An example of this situation would be sliding a patient over to a hospital gurney and leaving him without providing a report or ensuring that staff has taken control of the patient. If you were to leave and complete your report while the patient developed an airway problem, you would likely be considered liable for any harm that came to the patient.

abandonment leaving a patient after care has been initiated and before the patient has been transferred to someone with equal or greater medical training.

Generally, a nurse will take your written and verbal report of the situation you found, your assessment, the care you provided, and the patient's responses to your interventions. Make sure you transfer all of the patient's personal belongings that you may have transported, including jewelry, medications, and clothing.

Terminating the Call

41-10 Describe post-run actions that should be taken to reduce the spread of infection to you, your coworkers, and patients.

While this section is called "terminating the call," it could quite reasonably be called "making sure your next call goes well" because the tasks included not only terminate the current call but ensure that your ambulance is ready for the next call. It is by far *not* the most exciting part of EMS, but the few moments it will take to prepare is a large investment in your next call and a sign of integrity and pride in what you do.

At the hospital, after you have transferred care, you should begin to prepare for your next call. That starts with washing your hands. Hand washing is the single best way to avoid disease transmission. It is vital for you to not carry any germs from your first patient to future patients or, just as important, to your crew or family. Then, still at the hospital, the ambulance should be restocked with any equipment that is replaced or exchanged from hospital stock. This varies widely by area. Anything you used on the previous call that will be reused and the ambulance itself should be cleaned and disinfected.

Before leaving the hospital, the EMT should complete the prehospital care report. A copy should be provided to the receiving facility staff. The report should be complete and accurate, describing the patient's condition on your arrival and any changes in the patient's condition en route. You should document all vital signs, the patient's medical history, your assessment findings, the care you provided, and the patient's response to that care. Other fields include run data, mileage, and agency-specific information, which also should be recorded. (Further information on documentation requirements may be found in Chapter 11.)

Then, just as you prepared for the first call of the day by checking the unit over thoroughly, the ambulance must be readied for the next patient. The ambulance should be cleaned as needed to present both a positive image to the public and a clean environment for you and your crew and the next patient.

Many tasks may not be completed at the hospital and are completed while en route to quarters or when you arrive back at quarters (Scan 41-3). When you leave the hospital, notify the dispatcher of your status. You may be ready for the next call or remain out of service because necessary equipment is not available or ready for use. Before completing the call, the ambulance should be fully restocked and refueled as necessary.

Again, you and your partner must wash your hands after finishing with the patient and after cleaning the ambulance. In addition, on the way back from the call, many crews will debrief even minor calls to provide an assessment of the call and consider ways to make the next call go better.

cleaning wiping up blood, body fluids, dirt, or grime that may have come from the patient or the scene.

disinfecting killing some of the microbes that may be on a piece of medical equipment.

sterilization controlled process that, like disinfection, requires its own specific equipment and is usually done under controlled circumstances; all organisms on the piece of equipment are killed.

Regarding cleaning the ambulance, several different terms are sometimes used interchangeably. It is important to note the difference, though, so that proper decontamination can occur. **Cleaning** means to wipe up, such as blood or vomitus that may have come from the patient. **Disinfecting** is killing some of the microbes that may be on a piece of equipment. **Sterilization** is a controlled process that, like disinfection, requires its own specific equipment and is usually done under controlled circumstances.

In sterilization, organisms on the piece of equipment are killed. This is usually done in the hospital by autoclave in which steam is used to sterilize equipment. Occasionally, dry heat or gas systems will be used instead of steam. A few EMS systems use this type of sterilization equipment, but more often they use a chemical to sterilize equipment.

SCAN 41-3 Duties After Each Call

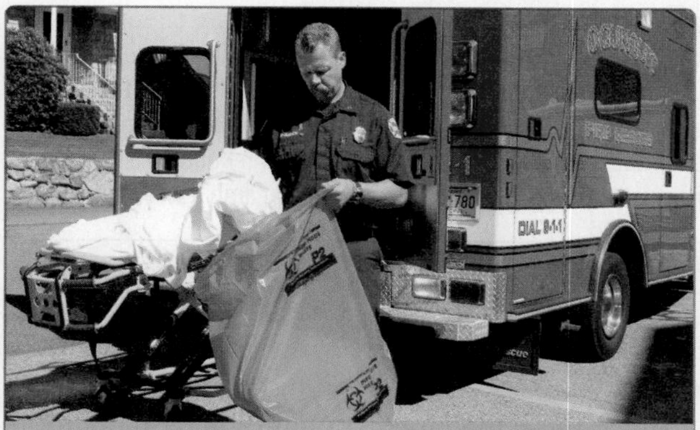

41-3-1 Properly dispose of contaminated and non-contaminated materials.

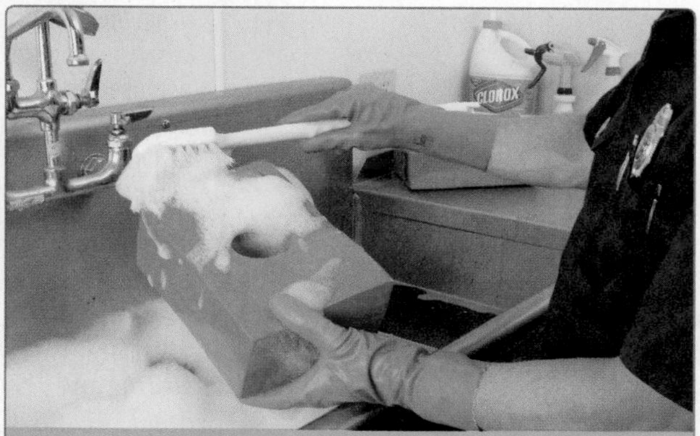

41-3-2 Clean or decontaminate all equipment used on the call.

41-3-3 Clean or decontaminate the inside of the vehicle as appropriate.

41-3-4 Restock all used equipment and supplies.

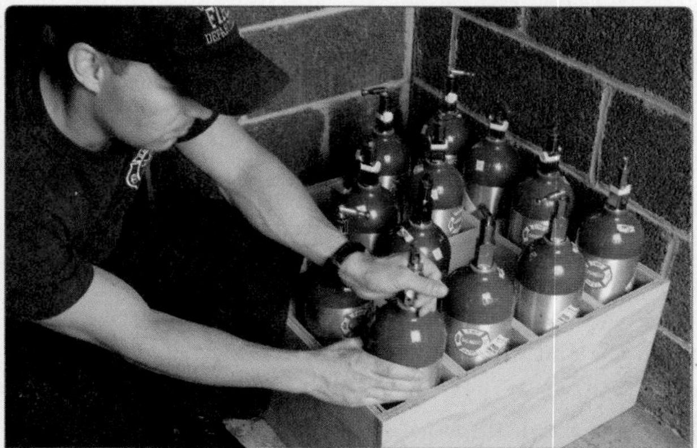

41-3-5 Replace any empty oxygen cylinders.

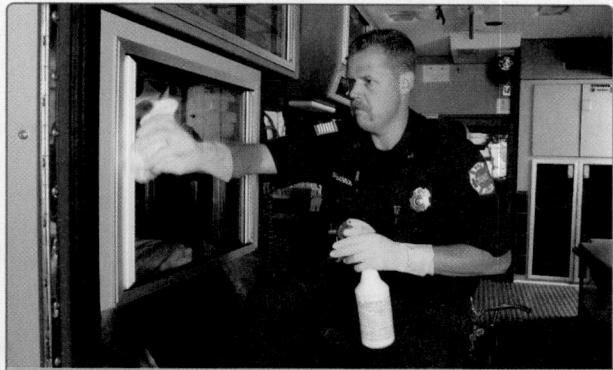

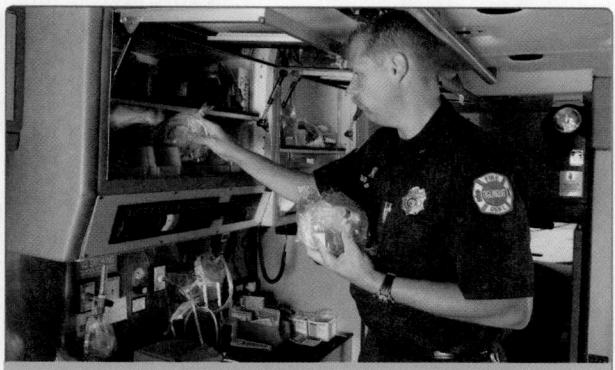

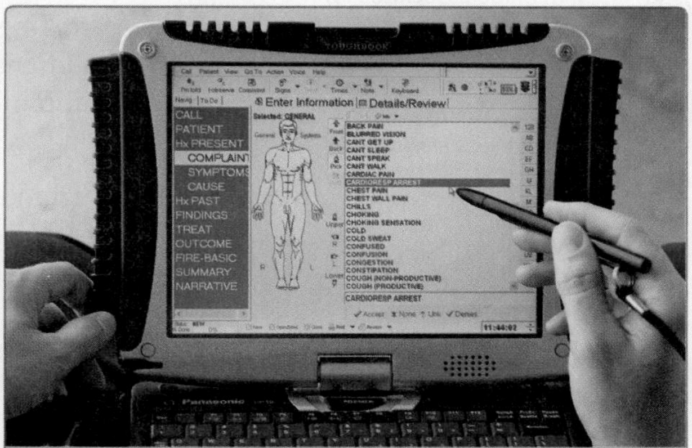

41-3-6 Thoroughly document all assessment and care.

PERSPECTIVE

Russ—The Commuter

What the heck was wrong with those guys? I'm just on my way to work and hear this siren somewhere really close by. I'm looking all over the place and all I can see is a bunch of other people just as confused as I was. The guy I carpool with thought that maybe it was just a car alarm that went crazy or something. So no one on 45th Street knew if we were pulling over or just moving on! So finally, as I'm turning onto Bryant, this ambulance squeezes past me with the siren blaring but no flashing lights or anything. Talk about creating confusion. I wonder what was up with that ambulance.

First and foremost, the crew must protect themselves by using gloves while cleaning and disinfecting. If there is any possibility of splashing fluids, eye and face protection must be used. Additionally, if there is a large amount of body fluid, footwear that is impervious to fluid is important. Footwear should also be equipped with steel toes and nonslip soles.

Basic disinfection can occur with a 1:100 household-bleach-to-water mixture. Clean anything that is visible, and then clean the area again. Towels should be disposable and should be discarded properly once the cleaning is completed.

High-level disinfection is usually applied to equipment involving the airway, such as laryngoscope blades and handles. Generally, they need to be cleaned by special chemicals. In some systems, such as hospital-based services, certain reusable airway items are actually sterilized by placing them in specialized devices such as autoclaves.

Additional Safety Considerations

41-11 Describe the recommendations of the National Association of Emergency Medical Technicians with respect to EMT security and safety.

41-12 Explain precautions to avoid exposing yourself or others to increased levels of carbon monoxide associated with ambulance operations.

Unfortunately, the safety hazards of operating an emergency vehicle are not limited only to driving. There are other situations involving the vehicle that can pose a risk to providers.

Carbon Monoxide

Although not a visible risk, the threat associated with exposure to carbon monoxide is a serious health issue for EMS providers. For many years vehicles were run in and around stations exposing EMTs to relatively high levels of this poisonous gas. Recently, many services have begun to take proactive measures to minimize exposures such as installing ventilation systems and developing guidelines for ambulance storage and maintenance, but risks still are prevalent. As an EMS provider, you should be proactive in minimizing exposure to carbon monoxide whenever possible. Consider the following steps:

- Park a running ambulance only in well-ventilated areas. Avoid running an ambulance in areas such as closed bays or immediately in front of hospital doors. Utilize ventilation systems when possible.
- When parking the ambulance at a scene, consider exposure to exhaust. Parking close to a patient can expose the patient and the crew to dangerous exhaust fumes.
- Check door seals on the ambulance. Leaking door seals can lead to exposure to carbon monoxide–laden engine exhaust. Report and repair any poorly functioning passenger compartment door and pay particular attention to those doors at the rear of the ambulance.
- Keep rear windows closed to avoid accidental inflow of engine exhaust.

Ambulance Security

In recent years the risk of ambulances being used in terrorist activities has increased. This issue has heightened attention on keeping ambulances, and EMS services in general, secure. Although the risk of a terrorist hijacking your unit may be low, employing simple security measures can prevent problems at any number of levels. The National Association of Emergency Medical Technicians has suggested the following security steps:

- EMTs should be briefed and forewarned of any potential security or terror risk. Briefing information should include specific threats and any necessary countermeasures.
- All EMS vehicles, including those placed out of service, should be accounted for and tracked at all times.
- Personal access to emergency vehicles should also be tracked including access during repair.
- Ambulances should be locked and never left open and running.
- Vehicles sold or permanently retired should have markings removed.
- EMS services should protect access to uniform items and take proactive steps to prevent counterfeiting of identification materials.

EMERGENCY DISPATCH SUMMARY

The equipment failure on Rollie and Marianne's truck resulted in their inability to respond safely and quickly. The Post 15 ambulance had to be called in to cover the rollover motor-vehicle collision. Time was lost. Because of this resource move, and concurrent emergency calls around the city, dispatch wasn't able to back-fill Post 15. A subsequent call in the Post 15 area resulted in a 24-minute response time with a patient who should have received care much sooner but did survive.

Chapter Review

To the Point

- Operating an emergency vehicle is a privilege that requires great personal responsibility.
- Operating an emergency vehicle is an inherently unsafe activity. Providers should learn the basic procedures to minimize the dangers and maximize safety.
- Ambulances should be driven defensively with due regard for the safety of others.
- Safe and proper use of an ambulance begins before the call and continues once the patient has been transferred to the hospital.
- Many factors can increase the inherent dangers of emergency vehicle operation. Those factors include fatigue, stress, and distraction.
- External factors, such as night driving, highway conditions, and inclement weather must be accounted for when operating an emergency vehicle.
- The roadside is a particular hazard for EMS providers. Care should be taken to park and exit the ambulance properly, particularly when operating on a highway scene.
- Ambulances must be prepared before the call and then restocked and cleaned after the call. Always leave the ambulance ready for the next call.
- Carbon monoxide is an insidious danger that should be considered when operating an emergency vehicle.
- Proactive steps are necessary to maintain ambulance security.

Chapter Questions

Multiple Choice

For each question, place a check next to the correct answer.

1. Prior to accepting your first call for service at the beginning of your shift, you should:
   _____ a. complete a thorough vehicle inspection.
   _____ b. complete a thorough station inspection.
   _____ c. ensure that you have a good breakfast.
   _____ d. contact dispatch to see what calls are waiting.

2. After transferring the patient to the hospital staff, the most important thing you can do to prevent the spread of disease is to:
   _____ a. wash your hands.
   _____ b. sterilize the ambulance.
   _____ c. continue to wear gloves while at the hospital.
   _____ d. disinfect the ambulance.

3. When operating an emergency vehicle with lights and sirens activated, the operator must exercise ____________ for the safety of other motorists and pedestrians.
   _____ a. some caution
   _____ b. due regard
   _____ c. reasonable caution
   _____ d. determinant prudence

4. When cleaning up blood from the floor of your ambulance, which one of the following is the correct procedure to use?
   _____ a. Wipe the blood up with a towel.
   _____ b. Use a spray cleaner or bleach solution.
   _____ c. Wipe up the visible material and then use a spray cleaner or bleach solution.
   _____ d. Take the ambulance out of service for sterilization at the ambulance garage.

5. Which one of the following should be considered when deciding to use lights and siren to transport a patient to the hospital?
   _____ a. Nature of the patient's condition
   _____ b. Time of day
   _____ c. Amount of traffic
   _____ d. Time until shift change

6. Which one of the following statements is true about transporting patients to the hospital?
   _____ a. Patients do not care how fast you drive as long as they get to the hospital.
   _____ b. The ride on the stretcher is usually the smoothest since the patient is lying down.
   _____ c. The patient can utilize the three-point restraint system to be comfortable in the stretcher.
   _____ d. The patient may suffer anxiety from quick turns or excess bumps.

Critical Thinking

1. What is the difference between disinfection and sterilization?

____

____

____

____

2. Which do you perform when you clean a blood stain on a long backboard, disinfection or sterilization? Explain your answer.

Case Study

You are operating an ambulance with lights and sirens activated en route to a call for a "child choking" at a day care. The following questions are based on that statement.

1. Should the fact that you are responding to a "child choking" change your driving at all compared to other responses? Would it be different if it were a call for a fall or a "sick person"? Explain your answers.

2. What are three considerations you should make in choosing your route to the scene?

3. You are driving to the hospital with lights and sirens while your crew is performing CPR on the child in the back of the ambulance. What driving considerations do you have in regard to the crew working in the back?

The Last Word

EMS is a relatively high-risk profession. Dangers exist at many levels for both your crew and your patients. As many other professionals have done, you must contribute to building a culture of safety in which there are no exceptions when it comes to keeping everyone safe. Although there are many institutional elements involved in building this culture, it really starts with every individual EMT. Every provider is responsible for safety and security. Join in promoting a profession that makes this the first priority.

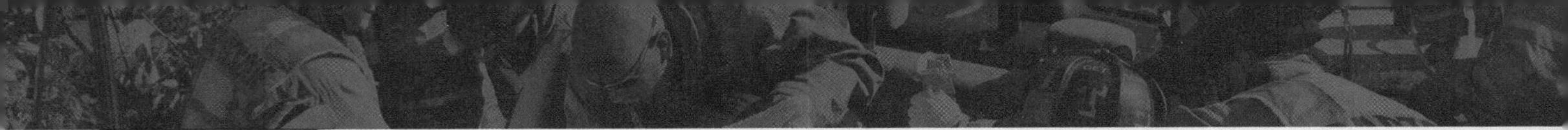

42 Overview of Incident Command and Incident Management Systems

Education Standards

EMS Operations: Multiple-Casualty Incidents

Competencies

Applies knowledge of operational roles and responsibilities to ensure patient, public, and personnel safety.

Objectives

After completion of this lesson, you should be able to:

42-1 Define key terms introduced in this chapter.

42-2 State the purpose of using an organized incident management system.

42-3 List the key elements of a typical incident management system.

42-4 Explain the purposes for establishment of the National Incident Management System (NIMS).

42-5 State the purpose of an incident command system.

42-6 List the key elements of an incident command system.

42-7 Identify responsibilities that may be assigned to EMS (units that might be established) at a multiple-casualty incident.

Key Terms

ambulance strike team p. 1141
base p. 1144
branch p. 1138
camp p. 1144
clear text p. 1135
command staff p. 1131
division p. 1138
EMS task force p. 1141
freelancing p. 1128
general staff p. 1131
group p. 1138
helibase p. 1144
helispots p. 1144
incident action plan (IAP) p. 1135
incident command post (ICP) p. 1133
incident command system (ICS) p. 1128
incident commander (IC) p. 1131
liaison officer p. 1131
multiple-casualty incident (MCI) p. 1127
National Incident Management System (NIMS) p. 1128
public information officer p. 1131
rescue/extrication group p. 1139
safety officer p. 1131
singular command p. 1133
span of control p. 1138
staging area p. 1144
supply unit p. 1139
transportation group p. 1138
treatment group p. 1135
triage group p. 1139
unified command p. 1133
unit p. 1138
unity of command p. 1138

Introduction

Most EMS calls involve relatively simple circumstances and require only basic resources to meet the needs of the emergency. An EMS call typically involves one patient calling 911 and a single ambulance crew responding to the request for help. Occasionally though, an emergency call can be far more complex and require a much larger commitment of resources to meet the needs of the situation. An emergency with more than one patient that exceeds or overwhelms the resources of the EMS system is referred to as a **multiple-casualty incident (MCI)** (Figure 42-1 ■).

multiple-casualty incident (MCI) emergencies involving illness or injuries that exceed or overwhelm EMS and hospital capabilities.

MCIs present very specific challenges to EMS practitioners. First and foremost, there are more patients than the usual resources can handle. Furthermore, the additional resources responding to the scene make management of the overall operation particularly difficult. Problems with leadership, span of control, and accountability are all common. Other unusual situations can cause similar difficulties. Large-scale incidents involving different response agencies or multiple jurisdictions or incidents of an unusual nature, such as hazmat responses, also can create scene management chaos.

Experience with such large-scale incidents has led to the development of the National Incident Management System (NIMS). This management framework helps agencies prepare for, respond to, and recover from otherwise overwhelming incidents. Although it is not a specific response plan, components of NIMS improve and standardize incident management among agencies. NIMS also introduces the incident command system. This standardized structure allows practitioners to organize a response around a known formula and to better coordinate assets. Incident command systems improve span of control, improve management, and make complex situations safer for responders.

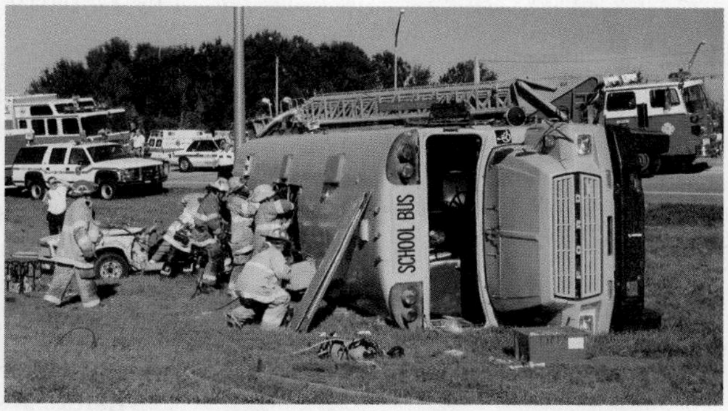

Figure 42-1 An incident involving multiple patients is referred to as a multiple-casualty incident or MCI. (© Craig Jackson/In the Dark Photography)

This chapter offers the principles of an incident management system and describes the role of the EMS professional within that system. Even if you are not in a leadership position, every EMT should be prepared to play a key role within an incident management system. EMS services should understand common terminology and standardized practices so as to improve response

EMERGENCY DISPATCH

"Unit six, come in." There was a hint of uncharacteristic panic in the dispatcher's voice. "Unit six, I need you to cancel off that call and proceed, priority one, to Barker and 12th Avenue. Please advise once on scene."

"Copy that," EMT Jeffrey Clark responded as his partner, Kelli Barnaby, spun the wheel and sped toward the new call.

"That's odd," Kelli said, checking her mirrors and changing lanes. "Didn't they already send Mark's truck there for that motorcycle crash?"

"Yeah, I think you're right," Jeffrey said, pulling two exam gloves from the box between the seats.

As Kelli navigated the final corner onto Barker Street, her jaw fell slack and Jeffrey whistled quietly through his teeth. There were people hurrying around the roadway, swirling through a haze of smoke that just hung in the still air. There was a smashed car over to the left, huge chunks of pavement torn up in front of them, and an ambulance resting on the sidewalk on the right, its front wheels and much of the engine compartment gone. Farther down the road a city bus was sitting diagonally across both lanes with a small green car buried beneath it and about 50 feet past that, in the next intersection, there was a motorcycle down in the street. A figure lay motionless next to it, blood running like a wide, shining ribbon across the intersection and down into a storm drain.

"Hey," Jeffrey's voice broke the silence in the cab. "There's Mark!"

Paramedic Mark Gainer walked shakily toward their truck, carrying his blood-soaked uniform shirt limply in one hand. Jeffrey got out and hurried over to meet him while Kelli grabbed the cot and equipment from the back.

"What happened, man?" Jeffrey asked. Mark looked at him, moved his mouth several times as if to speak, and then just threw his arms around him in a tight hug.

Just then, a firefighter ran over from the direction of the bus, sweat soaking his dark T-shirt. "Hey! We got criticals everywhere! One in that car, two in the green one, about four on the bus, a little girl on the sidewalk just past the ambulance and, uh, I think the motorcycle guy's a black tag. We need more help, quick!"

when multiple resources are involved. Understanding the incident management system prepares practitioners for a role in a large team effort. It also allows EMS to integrate smoothly in a large operation and makes management of a complex situation far simpler.

National Incident Management System

42-2 State the purpose of using an organized incident management system.

42-3 List the key elements of a typical incident management system.

42-4 Explain the purposes for establishment of the National Incident Management System (NIMS).

National Incident Management System (NIMS) system implemented in 2004 by the U.S. Department of Homeland Security that provides a consistent nationwide approach for incident management and requires federal, state, tribal, and local governments to work together before, during, and after incidents.

The **National Incident Management System (NIMS)** was established in 2004 by the U.S. Department of Homeland Security. It is a system that provides a consistent nationwide approach for incident management and requires federal, state, tribal, and local governments to work together before, during, and after incidents. It involves preparing for, preventing, responding to, and recovering from domestic incidents of all sizes and complexities.

The Department of Homeland Security describes NIMS as a core set of concepts, principles, procedures, organizational processes, terminology, and standard requirements that apply to a broad community of users. NIMS helps agencies prepare for major incidents by standardizing their approach. By making responses more systematic in nature, agencies can work together regardless of their background or training level. NIMS promotes smooth interoperability among diverse responders even in the worst circumstances.

The Department of Homeland Security further describes the NIMS as:

- A comprehensive, nationwide, systematic approach to incident management, including the incident command system, multiagency coordination systems, and public information
- A set of preparedness concepts and principles for all hazards
- Essential principles for a common operating picture and interoperability of communications and information management
- Standardized resource management procedures that enable coordination among different jurisdictions or organizations
- Scalable, so it may be used for all incidents (from day-to-day to large-scale)
- A dynamic system that promotes ongoing management and maintenance

incident command system (ICS) the first management system that was developed by an interagency task force working in a cooperative local, state, and federal interagency effort called FIRESCOPE (Firefighting Resources of California Organized for Potential Emergencies). Initial ICS applications were designed for responding to disastrous wildland fires in California.

freelancing situation in which a person on an emergency scene takes action without the knowledge or permission of the incident commander.

Within NIMS, an **incident command system (ICS)** has been developed to assist with the control, direction, and coordination of emergency response resources. EMTs, firefighters, and police officers all utilize ICS to provide an orderly means of communication and information for decision making and accountability of resources. Interactions with other agencies are easier when this system is utilized because of uniform procedures, common terminology, and coordination using business management principles.

Incident command seeks to ensure there is no **freelancing.** Freelancing is when a person on an emergency scene takes action without the knowledge or permission of the incident commander. This behavior is dangerous for those who are inside the incident working without the knowledge of the incident commander. It may also disrupt the normal deployment of resources needed for the incident.

Long before NIMS was established, the first incident command systems were designed for responding to disastrous wildland fires in California. Agencies such as the California Department of Forestry and the U.S. Forestry Service developed them to manage the enormous and widespread resources engaged in battling fires. In 1972, those driving forces formed an interagency task force working in a cooperative local, state, and federal interagency effort called FIRESCOPE (Firefighting Resources of California Organized for Potential Emergencies). FIRESCOPE formalized the incident management system and implemented it statewide in 1980. Early in the development process, four essential requirements became clear:

- The system must be organizationally flexible to meet the needs of incidents of any kind and size.

- Agencies must be able to use the system on a day-to-day basis for routine situations as well as for major emergencies.
- The system must be sufficiently standard to allow personnel from a variety of agencies and diverse geographic locations to rapidly meld into a common management structure.
- The system must be cost effective.

ICS is now widely used throughout the United States by EMS and fire agencies and is increasingly used for law enforcement, other public safety applications, and for emergency and event management. Although many major incidents have occurred in many districts, the major event that led to these changes were the terrorist events of September 11, 2001, and the subsequent 9/11 Commission Report. Increasing the communication of law enforcement and emergency services will lead to a smooth transition when a unified command is established. The buzz word for this is *interoperability*. When NIMS was established in 2004, ICS was incorporated as the backbone of the wider-based federal system (Table 42-1).

TABLE 42-1 HOMELAND SECURITY PRESIDENTIAL DIRECTIVE 5
To prevent, prepare for, respond to, and recover from terrorist attacks, major disasters, and other emergencies, the United States Government shall establish a single comprehensive approach to domestic incident management. The objective of the United States Government is to ensure that all levels of government across the Nation have the capability to work efficiently and effectively together, using a national approach to domestic incident management.

STOP, REVIEW, REMEMBER!

Multiple Choice

For each question, place a check next to the correct answer.

1. Which agency was responsible for developing the national incident management system (NIMS)?

   _____ a. Department of Homeland Security

   _____ b. Office of Domestic Preparedness

   _____ c. Local fire department

   _____ d. An ambulance company

2. Interaction with other agencies is well accomplished when responders use an incident management system because __________ principles guide efficient management of resources and tasks.

   _____ a. uniform

   _____ b. unified

   _____ c. infamous

   _____ d. numerous

3. The abbreviation NIMS stands for:

   _____ a. nationally inventoried business management system.

   _____ b. national incident management sequencing.

   _____ c. national incident management system.

   _____ d. national institute of medicine system.

4. Which one of the following is the term used to describe action taken on an emergency scene without the knowledge or permission of the incident commander?

   _____ a. Incident commanding

   _____ b. Freeloading

   _____ c. Firescoping

   _____ d. Freelancing

(continued on next page)

(continued)

5. Which one of the following best describes the national incident management system (NIMS)?

_____ a. Response plan

_____ b. Communications plan

_____ c. Static system

_____ d. Set of preparedness concepts

Fill in the Blank

Write the terms represented by the abbreviations.

1. NIMS: ______________________________

2. ICS: ______________________________

3. MCI: ______________________________

Critical Thinking

1. When multiple injuries occur at large events, such as a ride collapse at a carnival, use of an incident management system may be necessary. Where in your community does the potential for such events exist?

____

____

____

____

2. Explain why freelancing would be the wrong decision on an MCI.

____

____

____

____

Incident Command System (ICS)

42-5 State the purpose of an incident command system.

The Department of Homeland Security describes ICS as "a fundamental form of management established in a standard format, with the purpose of enabling incident managers to identify the key concerns associated with the incident—often under urgent conditions—without sacrificing attention to any component of the command system." Although this may seem complicated, it is important to remember that every incident or event has certain major management activities or actions that must be performed. Even if the event is small, and only one or two people are involved, the activities still always apply to some degree. Using an incident command system helps manage basic functions and provides essential structure to the leadership elements.

The standardized NIMS incident command system is designed to create a management structure that can be used by any type of agency on every incident no matter the size. By design, it is meant to be used for all incidents. This routine use prepares providers for more complex situations and times when stress levels are increased. To afford this flexibility, ICS is scalable. That is, it can be used on a small incident, but then expanded to increase its size as the scale of the incident widens.

The organization of the ICS is built around five major management functions: command, finance/administration, logistics, operations, and planning (C-FLOP) (Table 42-2). The five ICS functions apply whether you are handling a routine emergency, organizing for a major event, or managing a major response to a disaster. On small incidents, those functions may be managed by one person, the **incident commander (IC).** Large incidents usually require that the incident commander set up separate sections to organize resources and services. A fully expanded ICS system has several **general staff** positions. Each member of the general staff overseas one of the ICS major functional elements and is given the title *section chief.* So in addition to the incident commander, there is the finance/administration section chief, the logistics section chief, the operations section chief, and the planning section chief.

At each level in the ICS organization, individuals with primary responsibility positions have distinctive titles. Those titles are a key component of NIMS, which requires emergency responders to be familiar with common titles and common terminology. Those positions are staffed only when needed and demonstrate the flexibility of the ICS and incident management systems.

TABLE 42-2 MANAGEMENT ACTIVITIES OF THE INCIDENT COMMAND SYSTEM

Command	• Sets objectives and priorities • Has overall responsibility at the incident or event
Finance/ Administration	• Monitors costs related to incident • Provides accounting, procurement, time records, cost analyses
Logistics	• Provides support to meet incident needs • Provides resources and all other services needed to support the incident
Operations	• Conducts tactical operations to carry out the plan • Develops the tactical objectives • Develops the organizational plan • Directs all resources
Planning	• Develops the action plan to accomplish the objectives • Collects and evaluates information/ intelligence (law enforcement) • Maintains resource status

The incident commander also has a **command staff.** The command staff is composed of the liaison officer, the safety officer, and the information officer. The **liaison officer** is responsible for communicating with other agencies. The liaison officer may be the person making the initial contact with an EMS agency. The **safety officer** ensures that incident safety considerations are recognized and has the power to stop activity or remove people immediately from a hazardous situation. The **public information officer** is the only one authorized to release information to the news media after approval by the incident commander (Figure 42-2 ■). Additional positions that may be required for a specific incident may be established by the incident commander.

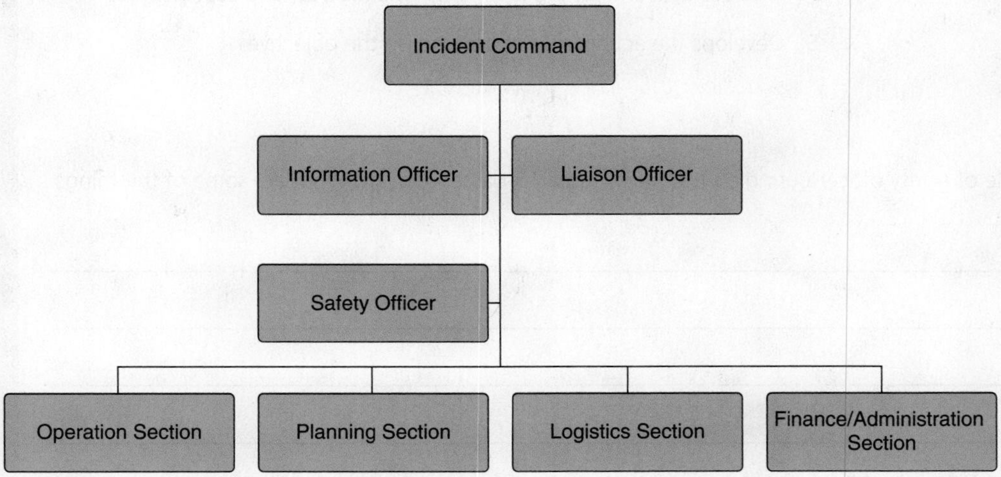

Figure 42-2 The command staff organizational chart.

incident commander (IC) the person in overall charge of an emergency under ICS or incident management system.

general staff the key staff positions that oversee the sections in a fully expanded ICS or incident management system.

command staff the incident commander's staff, which consists of the liaison officer, the safety officer, and the information officer.

liaison officer command staff officer responsible for communicating with other agencies; may be the person making the initial contact with an EMS agency.

safety officer command staff officer who ensures that the incident safety considerations are recognized; has the power to stop activity or remove people immediately from a hazardous situation.

public information officer command staff officer who is the only one authorized to release information to the news media after approval by the incident commander.

STOP, REVIEW, REMEMBER!

Multiple Choice

For each question, place a check next to the correct.

1. In the mnemonic, or memory aid, C-FLOP, "L" refers to:
   _____ a. liaison.
   _____ b. legal.
   _____ c. logistics.
   _____ d. lieutenants.

2. In a fully expanded ICS, the general staff consists of the:
   _____ a. section chiefs.
   _____ b. liaison officers.
   _____ c. operations officers.
   _____ d. planning staff.

3. Which one of the lists that follow include all three major activities of the command staff?
   _____ a. Safety, information, and logistics
   _____ b. Information, safety, and planning
   _____ c. Safety, information, and liaison
   _____ d. Planning, logistics, and safety

4. What is the one ICS position staffed at all incidents?
   _____ a. Division supervisor
   _____ b. Incident commander
   _____ c. Task force leader
   _____ d. Operations section chief

5. Which one of the following would be the most appropriate situation for the use of ICS?
   _____ a. Only on situations with more than one responding agency
   _____ b. On every situation that overlaps jurisdictions
   _____ c. Only on multiple-casualty incidents
   _____ d. Every incident

Matching

Match the term on the left with the applicable definition on the right.

1. _____ Command
2. _____ Operations
3. _____ Planning
4. _____ Logistics
5. _____ Finance/administration

A. Conducts tactical operations to carry out the plan
B. Has overall responsibility at the incident or event
C. Provides resources and all other services needed to support the incident
D. Provides accounting, procurement, time records, and cost analyses
E. Develops the action plan to accomplish the objectives

Critical Thinking

1. You have been assigned the role of safety officer during an MCI involving a 15-passenger van. What are some of the things that you should look for?

____

____

____

____

2. You are approached by members of the media about your role in an MCI. What would you do?

Components of an Incident Command System

All incident command systems have similar components. Some components, such as an incident commander, will be common to all systems, while others will come into play only if the situation warrants them. Ideally, the incident command system allows the management structure to be flexible and to adapt to the specific needs and scope of a particular situation.

42-6 List the key elements of an incident command system.

42-7 Identify responsibilities that may be assigned to EMS (units that might be established) at a multiple-casualty incident.

Incident Command

Any emergency scene, regardless of its size or nature, requires an incident commander (IC). The incident commander is the person in charge. In the words of the NIMS, "He or she is responsible for the overall success and safety of the incident and implements a strategy for handling all current and potential scene issues." In addition to oversight of the incident, the incident commander also is responsible for building the structure of the particular incident command system, adding levels when necessary, and scaling down as the incident concludes.

Typically, the first arriving unit assumes incident command. In fact, this responsibility could fall on a relatively junior member of the response team. That responder, even though inexperienced, would be responsible for completing key initial tasks, which are very simple and quite straightforward. In most cases, command will be transferred quickly as more highly trained personnel arrive. Although a new EMT may not be prepared to assume command over a large-scale incident, it is essential to remember that if you are on the scene alone, you are in command at least until other units arrive. Your initial actions, reports, and requests for additional resources are as important as any other element in the response plan.

Anyone can be an incident commander. Command is immediately established by the first responder on scene. On initial size-up, he reports the need to activate the incident command system, immediately designates himself as the incident commander, and identifies his location. An **incident command post (ICP),** the physical location of the incident commander on or near the incident, is frequently designated so that the incident commander can be found easily.

Two types of command are possible at an emergency incident: singular or unified. Most incidents have a single person in command who carries the authority of the agency or jurisdiction. **Singular command** is for incidents that are small in scope, do not involve outside agencies, and occur within a single jurisdiction. **Unified command** is a team effort that allows all agencies with a jurisdictional responsibility for the incident, either geographical or functional, to play a part in the management of the incident. For example, a school shooting would have a unified command incorporating law enforcement, EMS, and school authorities. However, unified command would still maintain one set of objectives developed for the entire incident. That is accomplished by a cooperative approach to developing the strategies to achieve the incident goals.

incident command post (ICP) a physical location near an incident from which the incident commander oversees all incident operations. Also called the *command post (CP).*

singular command method of command used for incidents that are small in scope, do not involve outside agencies, and occur within a single jurisdiction.

unified command method of command that is a team effort, allowing all agencies with a jurisdictional responsibility for the incident, either geographical or functional, to play a part in the management of the incident.

Initial Responsibilities of Incident Command

The most important responsibility for any incident commander is safety. The incident commander must assess the situation and build a plan that is capable of minimizing risk to responders. The following are two different but related examples of how an incident commander might prioritize safety in an action plan:

Example 1:

You are a new EMT who is the first unit on the scene of a tank truck rollover. As you approach the scene you notice chemicals spilling from the truck and multiple victims. Because you are the first unit on scene, you establish command and request the appropriate resources. By yourself, you are unable to effect any type of rescue, so your initial actions are to direct your partner to cordon off the scene and prevent others from entering. You perform a size-up and relay information of the safest approach back to dispatch. Although you have not initiated a formal response, your immediate actions have been vital to keeping incoming responders safe.

Example 2:

You are an experienced fire chief who is now developing a plan to mitigate the chemical spill described in the previous situation. Incident command was handed off to you from the first arriving EMT and you received a thorough report. You have now designated several additional groups to your incident command structure, including operations and medical. Even with all your other responsibilities, the first and most immediate remains to be safety. To ensure responder well-being, you have designated a safety officer to your command staff and coordinated a plan through your group leaders. You routinely review the progress of your groups and are regularly updated by the safety officer.

Scene Size-up

It is important for the first on-scene unit to conduct a scene size-up on which a brief initial report is based. This is typically the responsibility of the designated incident commander unless the task is delegated by the incident commander. When conducting the scene size-up, the incident commander should systematically look at:

- Scene safety and appropriate personal protective equipment needed
- Exact location or address of the incident
- Nature of the event and severity
- Number of injuries, if known
- Risk factors for EMS responders, such as the presence of hazardous materials or contamination
- Possibility of a crime scene and requirements for scene safety
- Additional resource(s) required
- Possible actions to be taken

After completing a scene size-up, the incident commander should transmit a brief report to the communications center and for other responders. It should be presented as a calm, clear, and concise message that follows the standard format:

- Confirm the address and exact location
- Identify the designation and location of the incident commander and command post
- Describe the event and the situation, including safety issues
- Request additional resources
- State the action you are taking

Communications

Radio communications on an incident should use **clear text**, also known as *plain text* or *common language* (no radio codes). Refer to incident facilities by their incident name (for example, Broadway command post or Second Street staging area). EMTs should refer to personnel by ICS title, not by a numeric code or name of the unit. For example, when calling the treatment area being managed by Medic 4, the title **treatment group** would be used instead of Medic 4.

clear text communications using plain language (not radio codes).

treatment group team that will establish an area where patients can be treated and collected.

Good communication practice at an ICS scene includes repeating information or assignment. For example, if you arrived on scene as Rescue 18 and the incident commander gives you an assignment to report to the treatment group, you would repeat the assignment: "Rescue 18 copies, reporting to treatment group." This practice ensures that the incident commander knows you understood your assignment.

Once the incident appears to require more radio traffic, the incident commander will move the incident onto a tactical frequency or secondary channel, which allows other demands in the EMS system to be met without interrupting the communication at the incident.

Other Responsibilities of Incident Command

Once the scene size-up has been communicated and safety issues have been addressed, the incident commander must focus attention on the incident itself. Of course, every incident will be slightly different, but in general there are common tasks that must be performed. They include:

- Assessing the current situation and establishing incident objectives
- Confirming the request for additional resources
- Determining the need for unified command and forming this command if necessary
- Activating appropriate additional levels of the incident command system

Large-scale events typically have a written or oral **incident action plan (IAP).** It is the incident commander who makes the decision on whether the IAP is written or verbal. For large-scale incidents, the planning section creates and puts together the written action plan with the approval of the incident commander. Essential elements in any written or oral incident action plan are:

incident action plan (IAP) plan for the management of a specific component of incident operations.

- ***Statement of objectives.*** These are appropriate to the overall incident.
- ***Organization.*** It describes what parts of the ICS organization will be in place for each operational period.
- ***Assignments to accomplish the objectives.*** These are normally prepared for each division or group and include the strategy, tactics, and resources to be used.
- ***Supporting material.*** This includes such necessary and helpful information as a map of the incident, the communications plan, the medical plan, traffic plan, and so on.

PERSPECTIVE

Kelli—The EMT

At first there was just complete pandemonium. Everyone was confused, and the firefighter and Mark's partner, Dave, were kind of just jumping around from patient to patient. I knew at that point that Mark should have probably been in charge, since he is the only paramedic on scene and all, but he was in no condition to do it. So, after calling for, like, seven more ambulances and the helicopter, I got on the PA and told all of the people with minor injuries to get over in one place. Oh man, I was so nervous and just on autopilot, you know? There were so many injured people and so much to keep track of, I was so glad when the other ambulances started arriving. Then when that fire captain showed up and put on the incident commander vest and said, "Okay, what do you have for me?" I almost hugged him.

STOP, REVIEW, REMEMBER!

Multiple Choice

For each question, place a check next to the correct answer.

1. An incident action plan will be the responsibility of the:
   _____ a. division leader.
   _____ b. incident commander.
   _____ c. section chief.
   _____ d. branch director.

2. When communicating on the radio in an ICS emergency, the EMT should use:
   _____ a. clear text.
   _____ b. 10 Codes.
   _____ c. 400 Codes.
   _____ d. secret codes.

3. Which one of the following would best describe a unified command situation?
   _____ a. Single incident commander overseeing an emergency scene
   _____ b. Two agencies sharing command functions on an emergency scene
   _____ c. Two separate commanders each working toward a similar objective
   _____ d. Each responding agency retaining an incident commander at the scene

4. The most important responsibility of an incident commander would be:
   _____ a. safety of responders.
   _____ b. developing an action plan.
   _____ c. completing a scene size-up.
   _____ d. delivering an initial report.

5. You are first to arrive on a multiple-casualty motor-vehicle crash. There are several critical patients and a need for technical rescue to extricate victims. After ensuring the scene is safe, you should next:
   _____ a. identify yourself as incident commander and designate your location.
   _____ b. begin triage and report your findings.
   _____ c. request additional resources and begin treatment.
   _____ d. begin rescue efforts using manual tools.

Short Answer

1. According to NIMS, who is qualified to assume the role of incident commander?

____

____

____

____

2. Describe the common components of a scene size-up as conducted by an incident commander.

____

____

____

____

3. Describe the necessary components of an initial report as delivered by an incident commander.

Critical Thinking

1. Think about your community. List the annual events that could be organized with an incident action plan and why.

2. What areas in your community have the capacity to generate a large number of patients or victims?

PERSPECTIVE

Carl Becker—The Dispatcher

Kelli did such a great job on that call. The only thing that I knew about it was that I had dispatched another unit for a truck versus motorcycle collision and then, about five minutes later, I got a cell phone call from them saying that they had been in a collision. I had no idea the extent of it until Kelli got on the radio to call for more units. I've been doing this job for seven years this coming June, and I must say, not until today have I had anyone get on the radio at an MCI and give me such a perfect initial report.

Organizing an Incident

On most large scale incidents, the first responding units will establish command and deliver an initial report, but soon thereafter a more senior command officer will arrive on scene and assume management responsibilities. This process is known as *transfer of command* and it is completed when the first-arriving unit relays the information and current status to a command officer from the fire department, law enforcement, or EMS agency. This places the responsibility of the incident on the new incident commander and makes the first responding resources available to attend to other objectives within the incident.

The size and structure of an incident command system depend on the nature and scale of the emergency. Large-scale incidents will necessitate many resources and may require multiple agencies and overlapping responses. Directing them increases in difficulty as the scale of the incident widens. Generally, incident commanders can manage two to three responders in a small-scale emergency, but have difficulty safely overseeing larger numbers. **Span of control** is a principle of the ICS system that refers to how many organizational elements or people may be directly managed by another person. Specifically, it is designed to limit the number of responders managed by a single commander. Effective span of control may vary from three to seven, although a ratio of one to five reporting elements is commonly recommended. Because appropriate accountability and supervision are very important in high-risk operations, maintaining adequate span of control throughout the ICS organization is essential. The incident command system and its organizational structure are designed to provide a formula for constantly maintaining this span of control.

span of control the number of organizational elements or people that are directly managed by another person; effective span of control may vary from three to seven, although a ratio of one to five reporting elements is commonly recommended.

As the scale and scope of an incident increases and more and more responders enter the scene, the effectiveness of a single incident commander's span of control decreases. To prevent disorganization, the incident commander would add additional leaders to oversee specific sections of the incident and report back directly to him. Rather than overseeing 20 responders himself, the incident commander might create four distinct groups or sections, each with its own leader. Responders would report directly to their section leader, and the section leaders then would report directly to the incident commander. The span of control for the incident commander would then become 1:4 rather than 1:20.

The principle of **unity of command** dictates that each individual in an organization has only one supervisor. This helps to ensure accountability and safety of resources and allows the organization to promote an effective span of control. Sections can be organized around a specific task or around a geographic area, but the key is that one person oversees a manageable span of control while ultimate control of the incident remains in the hands of the incident commander.

unity of command the principle that each individual in an organization has only one supervisor; should not be confused with the term *unified command.*

The structure of the incident command system for a large-scale or complex event is determined by the goals, objectives, and tasks needed to resolve the incident. **Units, groups, divisions,** and **branches** are established as needed to ensure the span of control is maintained:

- Units can function under groups and divisions and are used for a specific task, often involving only one or two people. A unit assignment is staffed by a unit leader or manager. For example, the triage unit is often conducted by one person.
- Groups are designated for functional activities. For example, the treatment group is responsible for treating patients and requesting resources from the **transportation group** for the patients to be transported to the hospital.
- Divisions are geographical in nature. For example, an incident at a concert that has produced casualties on the west side of the location would be called the West Division.
- Branches are either geographical or functional and are used to keep a manageable span of control. For example, a fire in an apartment complex that produces several patients may be divided into a multiple-casualty branch and a fire-suppression branch.

unit team assigned a specific task.

group team assigned to functional activities.

division a team assigned to function in a specific geographical area.

branch management tool for the incident commander that can be either geographical or functional; used to keep a manageable span of control.

transportation group team responsible for obtaining resources to ensure that all patients are transported to the appropriate hospital.

As a responder to a large-scale incident, you will be assigned to a particular role in one of the units, groups, divisions, or branches. Upon arrival, if unassigned, you should report to the incident commander who will give you an assignment. When given an assignment, you would then report directly to a group leader or division supervisor for specific duties. Once assigned a specific task, you should complete it and report back to the officer in charge of that unit, group, division, or branch.

The medical or multiple-casualty branch will have a basic ICS/EMS organizational structure. As an EMT, you can expect to be assigned to one of the following groups or units (Figure 42-3 ■):

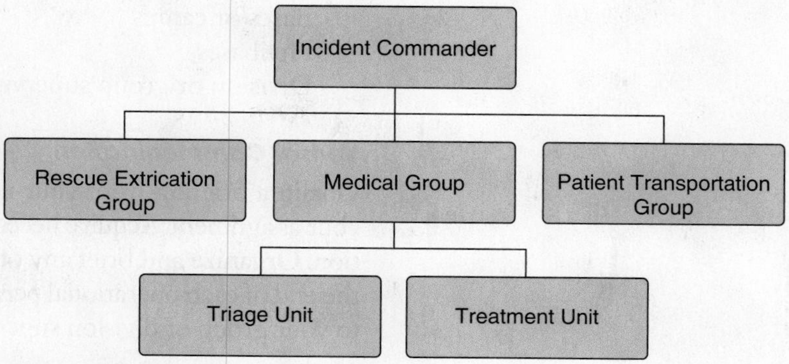

Figure 42-3 The medical branch of ICS.

- ***Command.*** Command directs the overall operation and is responsible for the overall success and safety of the incident.
- ***Medical communications coordinator.*** This responder handles communications with the disaster control facility for the prompt transportation of all patients. He works under the direction of the patient transportation group leader.
- ***Rescue/extrication group.*** The **rescue/extrication group** is responsible for all the operations necessary to remove victims from the hazard zone and place them into the treatment area. Those assigned should have training in vehicle and special rescue techniques.
- ***Triage group.*** The **triage group** is responsible for the sorting and tagging of all patients according to the seriousness and extent of injuries.
- ***Treatment group.*** This group will establish a treatment area in which patients can be collected and treated.
- ***Patient transportation group.*** This group is responsible for obtaining the resources to ensure that all patients are transported to the appropriate hospital.
- ***Staging area manager.*** This responder directs all incoming resources (such as ambulances, rescue equipment, and search and rescue teams) and establishes a traffic plan for ease of outgoing transports.
- ***Supply unit.*** The **supply unit** receives supplies and equipment from staging and issues them to the operational units as requested.
- ***Rehab area.*** The rehab area responders provide rehydration, nutritional support, and medical evaluation and monitoring of members involved in prolonged or strenuous operations.

rescue/extrication group team responsible for all the operations necessary to remove victims from the hazard to the treatment area.

triage group team responsible for the sorting and tagging of all patients according to the seriousness and extent of injuries.

supply unit team that receives supplies and equipment from staging and issues them to the operational units as requested.

Common Responsibilities

If you respond to a large incident or disaster where ICS is in place, there are certain common responsibilities or instructions that all responders should follow. Following them will make your job easier and result in a more effective operation. You will receive your incident assignment from your organization leader. That information should include, at a minimum:

- Reporting location and time
- Likely length of assignment
- Brief description of assignment
- Route information
- Designated communications link, if necessary. (Different agencies may have additional requirements.)

Bring any specialized supplies or equipment required for your job. Be sure you have adequate supplies to last you for the expected stay. Upon arrival, follow the check-in procedure for the incident. Check-in locations may be found at:

- Incident command post
- Staging areas

- Bases or camps
- Helibases
- Division or group supervisors (for direct assignments)

Verbal Communication

Obtain a briefing from your immediate or group supervisor. Be sure you understand your assignment. Acquire necessary work materials and locate and set up your work station. Organize and brief any other EMS personnel assigned to you. Brief your relief at the end of each operational period. Complete required forms and reports and give them to your group or division supervisor before you leave. Demobilize according to plan.

STOP, REVIEW, REMEMBER!

Multiple Choice

For each question, place a check next to the correct answer.

1. An incident commander has established operations in two separate geographic locations. According to NIMS terminology, the operations would be referred to as:

_____ a. units.
_____ b. groups.
_____ c. branches.
_____ d. sectors.

2. Upon responding to a large-scale incident, you are instructed to report to the treatment group. On arrival there you should:

_____ a. find a patient and begin treatment.
_____ b. report to the incident commander.
_____ c. report to the treatment group leader.
_____ d. assess the situation and determine the most appropriate task.

3. The concept of *unity of command* means that:

_____ a. two agencies share command functions.
_____ b. one supervisor has no more than seven subordinates.
_____ c. one person has one supervisor.
_____ d. the incident is divided into functional blocks.

4. The optimal span of control is:

_____ a. one to five.
_____ b. one to 20.
_____ c. one to one.
_____ d. one to 10.

Matching

Match the term on the left with the applicable definition on the right.

1. _____ Command
2. _____ Rescue/extrication group
3. _____ Treatment group
4. _____ Transportation group
5. _____ Triage group

A. Is responsible for all operations necessary to remove victims from the hazard zone and to the treatment area and should have training in vehicle and special rescue techniques
B. Directs the overall operation and is responsible for the overall success and safety of the incident
C. Is responsible for the sorting and tagging of all patients according to the seriousness and extent of injuries
D. Is responsible for obtaining resources to ensure that all patients are transported to the appropriate hospital
E. Will establish a treatment area where patient can be treated and collected

Critical Thinking

1. Why is the incident commander ultimately responsible for the overall operation of the incident?

2. Why might it be advantageous to locate the command post away from the site of the incident?

3. Why is it necessary for the first arriving unit to give an accurate size-up of the incident?

PERSPECTIVE

Jeffrey—The EMT

That whole incident almost doesn't seem real now that I look back on it, you know? It was my first real MCI and one that actually needed an incident commander. I'm really very impressed with how effectively that whole incident command system works. All the pieces that began as a mass of confusion just fell into place. We didn't lose any patients, well, except for the guy on the motorcycle, but he was gone when we arrived on scene.

EMS and ICS

The organization and terminology of ICS are universal and not specific to the fire service or to EMS. However, there are some elements of particular importance to EMS practitioners.

Transportation

The Department of Homeland Security, under the Federal Emergency Management System's support function for medical incidents, has classified EMS resources by two designations: **EMS task force** (Figure 42-4 ■) and **ambulance strike team** (Figure 42-5 ■).

EMS task force any combination of resources within the span of control of three to seven units (such as ambulances, rescues, engines, and squads) assembled for a medical mission, with common communications and a leader (supervisor).

ambulance strike team a group of five ambulances of the same type with common communications and a leader.

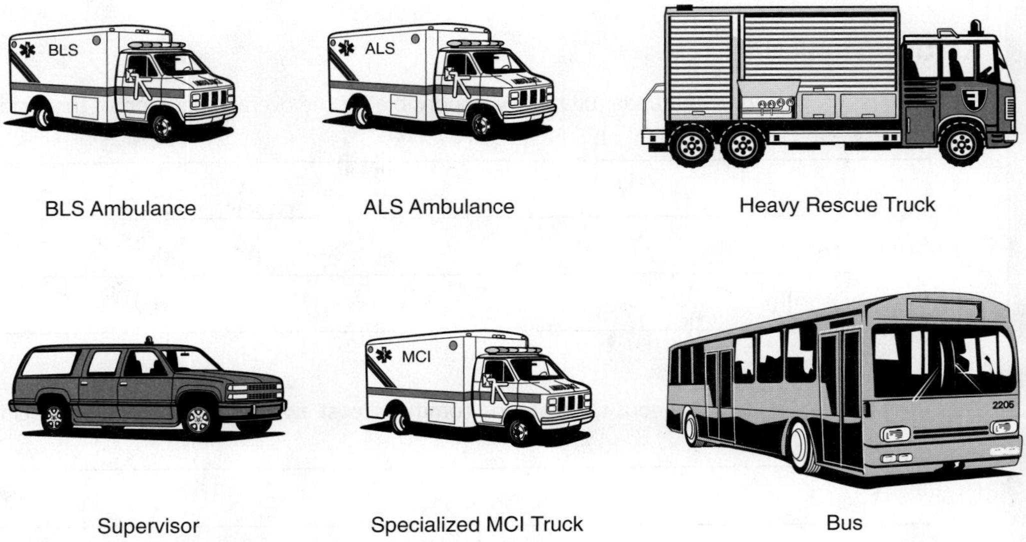

Figure 42-4 Vehicle recourse that makes up a typical EMS task force.

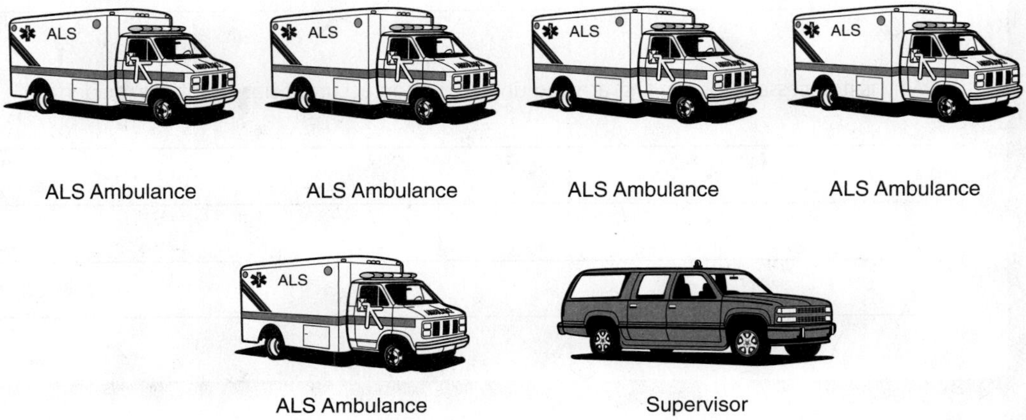

Figure 42-5 Vehicle recourse that makes up a typical ambulance strike team.

A task force is made up of elements of different types of equipment and resources combined to accomplish a specific task. A strike team is made up of several elements of the same type of equipment or resources, usually in a five-piece configuration with a leader.

A task force or strike team should be self-sufficient for 12-hour operational periods, although it may be deployed longer, depending on need. Support elements include fuel, security, resupply of medical supplies, and support for personnel. Table 42-3 provides an overview of the U.S. Department of Homeland Security and Federal Emergency Management Agency's classification of ambulance resources.

An ambulance strike team can work 12-hour shifts. The team will need backup supplies and equipment, depending on the number of patients and the type of incident. Communication equipment may be programmable for interoperability but must be tested and verified in advance. Fuel supply and maintenance support must be available. There should be a plan for augmenting existing communication equipment. Environmental considerations related to temperature control in the patient care compartment and pharmaceutical storage may be necessary for locations with excessive ranges in temperature. Security of vehicle support is needed for periods of standby without crew in attendance. Decontamination supplies and support are required for responses to incidents with potential threat to responding services or transport of infectious patients.

TABLE 42-3 U.S. DEPARTMENT OF HOMELAND SECURITY AND FEDERAL EMERGENCY MANAGEMENT AGENCY CLASSIFICATION OF AMBULANCE RESOURCES

RESOURCE: AMBULANCES (GROUND)

CATEGORY: HEALTH & MEDICAL (EMERGENCY SUPPORT FUNCTION #8)

KIND: TEAM; EQUIPMENT; PERSONNEL; SUPPLIES; VEHICLES

MINIMUM CAPABILITIES	TYPE I*	TYPE II	TYPE III*	TYPE IV	OTHER
EMS team with equipment, supplies, and vehicle for patient transport (Type I–IV) and emergency medical care prehospital	Advanced life support (ALS); Minimum two staff (paramedic and EMT); Transport two-litter patients	Advanced life support (ALS); Minimum two staff (paramedic and EMT); Transport two-litter patients, non-hazmat response	Basic life support (BLS); Minimum two staff (EMT and first responder); Transport two-litter patients	Basic life support (BLS) operations; Minimum two personnel (EMT and first responder); Transport two-litter patients	Nontransporting emergency medical response; Minimum one staff; BLS or ALS equipment supplies

*Type I and Type III: Training and equipment meets or exceeds standards as addressed by EPA, OSHA, and NFPA 471, 472, 473 and 29 CFR 1910, 120 ETA 3–11 to work in HazMat Level B and specific threat conditions; all immunized in accordance with CDC core adult immunizations and specific threat as appropriate.

Rehabilitation

As an EMS resource at the scene of an MCI or large-scale incident, you may be tasked with monitoring the well-being of rescuers. Due to the stressful nature of the events and the physical demand that they require of many rescuers, you may be part of a rehabilitation (rehab) team. As such, you will monitor the well-being of other rescuers by checking vital signs before entry and after exit from an incident. You also will be responsible for providing medical support to any rescuers who require it.

Incident Facilities

ICS facilities will be established, depending on the kind and complexity of the incident or event. It is important to know and understand the names and functions of the principal types of ICS facilities. Not all of those listed here will necessarily be used.

The incident command post (ICP) is the location from which the incident commander oversees all incident operations. There is only one ICP for each incident or event, but every incident or event must have one. On a map it is marked by a square with a diagonal darkened on the lower half.

PERSPECTIVE

Mark—The Paramedic

What an absolute nightmare. I could see the fire truck just up the road at the motorcycle crash. I was putting my gloves on and, you know, going over protocols in my head. Then suddenly there was a car in front of us. I don't know what that driver was thinking! She looked right at us and just turned anyway. When we hit her, all I could see for a few seconds was the blue sky through the cracked windshield, and then we crashed back down and rolled to a stop. I guess there was some sort of chain reaction also. The car we hit crashed into another car, which hit a bus or something. And a little girl got hit on her bike, too. Just a mess. I must've hit my head in there somewhere. I ended up with a pretty good headache and I remember being so confused! At first I did try to treat the lady in the car that we hit. I got my IV start-kit out, but—and this is really weird—I couldn't remember how to start an IV. It's kind of a blur after that.

staging area location or locations at an incident where incoming resources report.

A **staging area** is a location that the incident commander will use to hold resources not immediately needed. Typically, this is an area near the scene where ambulances (for example) would be parked prior to being utilized. The staging area helps prevent unneeded vehicles and personnel from accumulating on scene and promotes accountability and organization. Staging areas are marked on a map by a circle with an "S." Most large incidents have a staging area, and some incidents may have several staging areas.

base location at an incident at which primary service and support activities are performed.

A **base** is a location at the incident at which primary service and support activities are performed. It is marked with a circle with a "B." There is only one base for each incident.

camp location where resources may be kept to support incident operations.

A **camp** is a location where resources may be kept to support incident operations. It is marked with a circle and a "C." A camp differs from a staging area in that essential support operations are done at camps, and resources at camps are not always immediately available for use. Not all incidents will have camps.

helibase locations in or near an incident area at which helicopters may be parked, maintained, fueled, and equipped for incident operations.

helispots temporary locations where helicopters can land, load, and off-load personnel, equipment, and supplies.

If air operations are conducted at the scene of an MCI, activities involved with the takeoff and landing of helicopters are organized under the air operations branch. The air operations branch utilizes a **helibase** and **helispots.** A helibase is a location in or near an incident area at which helicopters may be parked, maintained, fueled, and equipped for incident operations. A helibase is marked as a circle with an "H."

Helispots are temporary locations where helicopters can land and load and off-load personnel, equipment, and supplies. Large incidents may have several helispots. Helispots are marked by a completely darkened circle.

Treatment and triage areas do not have specific symbols. When an ambulance arrives at the scene of a large incident in which maps with symbols are being used, EMTs can expect to be sent to a base, a camp, or an assignment. If the EMS crew remains at the base location, they are often assigned to logistics or the medical unit within the logistics section. The medical unit is staffed at large incidents to provide medical care for the responders. This should not be confused with the medical group supervisor who is within the operations section.

STOP, REVIEW, REMEMBER!

Multiple Choice

For each question, place a check next to the correct answer.

1. Helibases differ from helispots in that:

_____ a. helibases have maintenance supplies for helicopters.

_____ b. helispots have fuel for helicopters.

_____ c. helibases are temporary locations for helicopters to land.

_____ d. helispots are marked on the map with a circled "H."

2. According to the U.S. Department of Homeland Security and Federal Emergency Management Agency Classification of Ambulance Resources, a basic life support ambulance with minimum of two (EMT and emergency medical responder) that is able to transport two-litter patients would be classified as:

_____ a. Type I.

_____ b. Type II.

_____ c. Type III.

_____ d. Type IV.

3. An ambulance strike team is a group of ______ ambulances of the same type with common communications and a leader.

_____ a. two

_____ b. four

_____ c. three

_____ d. five

4. The incident command post is signified on a map with a:

_____ a. square with a diagonal darkened on the lower half.

_____ b. circle with a "B."

_____ c. circle with a "C."

_____ d. circle with an "S."

5. You are the incident commander on a motor-vehicle crash at the end of a narrow one-way street. Your triage report notes a need for three ambulances, but there is only room for one ambulance on the street. You should:

_____ a. designate a staging area and load one at a time.

_____ b. create a camp and hold the ambulances there.

_____ c. carry the patients to the end of the street to the waiting ambulances.

_____ d. designate a helispot and use aeromedical transport.

Critical Thinking

1. Why is it necessary to be able to track patients in an MCI?

____

____

____

____

2. Think about your community. What locations could serve as a helibase or helispot in the event that an earthquake, snowstorm, flood, or tornado temporarily disrupts the transportation network?

____

____

____

____

EMERGENCY DISPATCH SUMMARY

Eight ambulances from several area agencies, along with the University Hospital's Life-Flight helicopter, cooperating under the ICS, treated and transported a total of eight critical and six noncritical patients to local hospitals. All the patients survived, with all but two being discharged within 12 days of the incident. Many are still undergoing physical therapy or reconstructive surgeries. The incident has been hailed as a shining example of the effectiveness of both multiple-agency MCI training and the incident command system. EMTs Kelli Barnaby and Jeffrey Clark have been nominated for a special Mayor's Award for their actions.

Chapter Review

To the Point

- A large-scale or complex incident creates numerous safety, accountability, and resource management difficulties above and beyond the challenges of the typical request for service.
- The difficulties of a large-scale operation can be mitigated by using an incident management system.
- An incident management system is a standardized framework used to organize and manage a response.
- The national incident management system (NIMS) was designed to provide a standardized system of common terminology and resources that could be utilized to improve interoperability and response to large-scale events.
- NIMS highlights the use of the incident command system (ICS) to further improve organization and communication during emergency responses.
- Incident command is the most important element of any incident management system.
- It is the incident commander's responsibility to ensure the safety of responders and direct all action at an emergency scene.
- The ICS is scalable to the needs of an incident. Additional elements can be added as the size or scope of the incident increases.
- A key goal of incident management is a reasonable span of control. The unity of command afforded by an acceptable span of control improves safety and the organization of a response.

Chapter Questions

Multiple Choice

For each question, place a check next to the correct answer.

1. The five major activities around which the ICS is organized are:
   _____ a. command, liaison, operations, communications, and logistics.
   _____ b. command, planning, operations, communications, and logistics.
   _____ c. command, planning, operations, finance/administration, and logistics.
   _____ d. command, liaison, safety, operations, and planning.

2. The general staff consists of operations, planning, and:
   _____ a. information and logistics.
   _____ b. command and logistics.
   _____ c. finance/administration and liaison.
   _____ d. finance/administration and logistics.

3. Safety is a major responsibility of the command staff. What are two other of its major activities?
   _____ a. Public information and logistics
   _____ b. Public information and planning
   _____ c. Public information and liaison
   _____ d. Planning and logistics

4. What is the one ICS position staffed at all incidents?
   _____ a. Division supervisor
   _____ b. Incident commander
   _____ c. Task force leader
   _____ d. Operations section chief

5. Air operations, if activated at an incident, will be at what organizational level?
_____ a. Division
_____ b. Unit
_____ c. Section
_____ d. Branch

6. When would branches be used in the logistics section?
_____ a. In place of units
_____ b. To reduce span of control
_____ c. To maintain unity of command
_____ d. To place personnel with their day-to-day supervisors

7. Each individual reporting to only one supervisor defines:
_____ a. unified command.
_____ b. unity of command.
_____ c. span of control.
_____ d. consolidated command.

8. The ____________ is responsible for tracking incident costs.
_____ a. finance/administration section
_____ b. command section
_____ c. public information section
_____ d. planning section

9. Which one of the following is responsible for providing facilities, services, and materials for the incident?
_____ a. Finance
_____ b. Logistics
_____ c. Liaison
_____ d. Staging

10. An organizational level responsible for operations in a specified geographic area defines:
_____ a. group.
_____ b. division.
_____ c. section.
_____ d. branch.

11. The ICS position that oversees the removal of patients from the wreckage is the:
_____ a. treatment group supervisor.
_____ b. transportation group leader.
_____ c. rescue/extrication group supervisor.
_____ d. medical unit deputy.

12. The information officer is responsible for:
_____ a. bypassing the chain of command when talking with the press.
_____ b. coordinating all incident decisions.
_____ c. establishing the staging area.
_____ d. interfacing with the press and disseminating public information.

13. Effective span of control in ICS may vary from:
_____ a. one to three.
_____ b. two to seven.
_____ c. three to seven.
_____ d. five to seven.

14. The decision to have a written incident action plan is made by the:
_____ a. operations chief.
_____ b. incident commander.
_____ c. planning section chief.
_____ d. safety officer.

15. Operational periods are how long?
_____ a. One hour
_____ b. Six hours
_____ c. 12 hours
_____ d. No fixed length

16. Groups have ____________ responsibility, while divisions have ____________ responsibility.
_____ a. functional; geographic
_____ b. more; less
_____ c. outside; inside
_____ d. geographic; functional

(continued on next page)

(continued)

Critical Thinking

1. Locate your local area disaster plan and identify the role of the EMS provider in the event of a disaster involving large numbers of patients. Who is in charge and what are the capacities of the hospital resources that are listed in that plan?

2. It is 2:00 on a Wednesday afternoon in January, and you and your EMT partner are responding to a reported traffic collision with at least three vehicles involved at a busy downtown intersection. Also dispatched to this incident are the following:

   Rescue 10—A fire department transporting a paramedic unit staffed with two EMT-paramedics
   Engine 2—A fire engine staffed with three EMT-firefighters, including the company officer
   Medic 11—An ambulance with two EMTs from the local private ambulance company

   You arrive on scene first. Your size-up gives you a total of eight patients. Three are critical trauma victims, two have moderate injuries, and three have minor injuries. The two moderate injuries are trapped inside an overturned vehicle. There is a gas leak from one of the vehicles. All the hospitals are within 10 minutes of the scene.

   a. Outline the incident in an organizational chart format that reflects your system. Be specific about the organizational position titles you would fill and who else would fill them.

b. Make a list of potential problems, additional resources needed, and issues and how you would address them.

3. As a group activity locate a piece of plywood and create a small scene using premade plastic buildings that can be purchased in a hobby shop and typically used for model railroading. Configure streets and parking lots. Locate small model cars including a fire truck, ambulance, and any vehicles of interest. As a group, create a model incident and employ the principles described for proper incident management.

Case Study

As the first arriving ambulance, you must take the role of incident commander on the scene of an MCI involving a pickup truck and a 15-passenger van from the local high school carrying band members. Your partner is acting as triage officer. He has performed a size-up of the scene and found 10 passengers in the van and one driver in the pickup who is obviously DOA. Four of the passengers were crawling out of the overturned van on your arrival.

You assign the next ambulance to arrive on scene to treat the wounded. You call the four passengers to a treatment area away from the incident. The remaining passengers are pinned or entrapped in the vehicle. The fire department arrives on the scene and begins extrication of the victims. They estimate it will take 10 to 15 minutes to free the remaining patients.

(continued on next page)

(continued)

You have called for a helicopter to transport two of the most critically injured patients. You have requested two additional transport units to transport the remaining victims. Your supervisor has just arrived on scene and has requested that you turn over command to him. To follow procedure, you must give a summation of your efforts thus far. Write out a verbal report that you would give to your supervisor.

The Last Word

Multiple-casualty incidents (MCIs) are some of the most challenging calls you will experience in your career. Due to the serious nature and legal implications of MCIs, the federal government has mandated that all first responders be managed by the national incident management system (NIMS).

When a structured incident management system is in place, EMTs will have a safer more efficient environment in which to function. EMS and first responders will be able to provide the best patient care when a systematic approach to the sorting and movement of victims is accomplished.

EMTs can be expected to function in part of a large-scale incident. The minimum requirement for first responders is basic understanding of the command and general staff responsibilities under an incident command system. As an EMT, you should look for opportunities to acquire additional ICS or incident management system training. The federal government maintains several resources and training programs on the Internet at NIMS.gov.

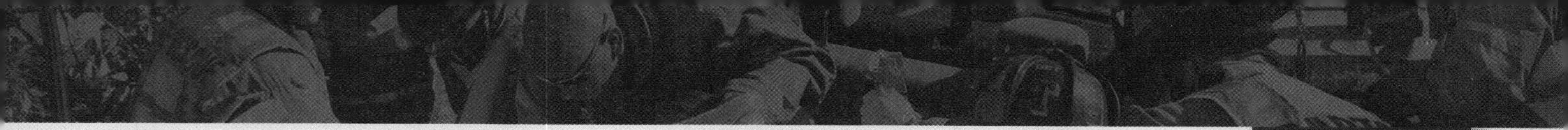

Responses Involving a Multiple-Casualty Incident

43

Education Standards

EMS Operations: Multiple-Casualty Incidents

Competencies

Applies knowledge of operational roles and responsibilities to ensure patient, public, and personnel safety.

Objectives

After completion of this lesson, you should be able to:

43-1 Define key terms introduced in this chapter.

43-2 List situations that might result in a multiple-casualty incident.

43-3 List aspects important to effective management of a multiple-casualty incident.

43-4 List the first actions (the Five S's) that should be taken upon arrival at a multiple-casualty incident.

43-5 Identify responsibilities that may be assigned to EMS at a multiple-casualty incident.

43-6 Describe the principles of a triage system.

43-7 Describe and contrast primary triage with secondary triage.

43-8 Explain the principles and assessment categories used in START triage.

43-9 Explain the principles used in the pediatric JumpSTART triage system.

43-10 Explain the important principles of a patient-tagging system to be used during triage.

43-11 Explain the interrelationship of triage and treatment within the treatment area at a multiple-casualty incident.

43-12 Discuss the logistics of staging and transportation at a multiple-casualty incident.

43-13 Discuss common issues with communications in multiple-casualty incident and disaster situations.

43-14 List measures that can be taken to reduce rescuer stress before, during, and after a multiple-casualty incident.

Key Terms

deceased patients p. 1159
delayed patients p. 1161
immediate-tagged patients p. 1161
mass gathering p. 1152
minor injuries p. 1154
multiple-casualty incident (MCI) p. 1152
preplanning p. 1153
triage p. 1158

Introduction

The facts about multiple-casualty incidents might surprise you. For example, think of an incident with multiple patients. Does a large one involving a plane crash or terrorist strike with hundreds or even thousands of patients come to mind? In fact, you are more likely to respond to a multiple-casualty incident that involves 3 to 10 patients. This chapter introduces the concepts and practices necessary to prepare you to respond to incidents of any size.

EMERGENCY DISPATCH

"Dispatch to ambulance 14, dispatch to ambulance 14. Do you copy?"

"Ambulance 14," EMT Devon Sayers said, trying to keep an ice cream cone from dripping onto his uniform pants.

"Ambulance 14, I need you to respond to a report of a downed private airplane on Horizon Boulevard. Fire and police are both en route."

"Ambulance 14 is responding." Devon put the microphone back into its holder, thought for a moment, and then looked over at DJ Smith. "Did he say a small airplane?"

"No. He said private airplane, but I'm hoping that means small. Now can we get moving?"

Devon tossed her ice cream into a garbage can outside the truck, activated the emergency lights, and headed toward Horizon Boulevard. A single fire truck was already on scene when they arrived and the crew was attempting to extricate the pilot from the small Cessna airplane, which was heavily damaged and sitting awkwardly across several traffic lanes.

"How many patients do we have here?" DJ shouted into the small group of firefighters. He had just climbed from the ambulance and spotted a car and a pickup truck with extensive body damage pulled off to the side of the road.

One of the firefighters looked over at him, shrugged, shook his head as if to say, "I don't know," and went back to stretching a hose line.

"DJ!" Devon called from the opposite side of the chaotic roadway. "There's a van from Sunflower Preschool on its side down in this ditch. I can see movement inside!"

Multiple-Casualty Incidents

43-2 List situations that might result in a multiple-casualty incident.

multiple-casualty incident (MCI) an incident resulting from human or natural causes resulting in illness or injuries that exceed or overwhelm normal EMS and hospital capabilities.

Multiple-casualty incidents (MCIs) are incidents that are caused by humans, or occur naturally and can result in illness or injuries that exceed or overwhelm normal EMS and hospital capabilities. A large multiple-casualty incident is likely to impose a sustained demand for health and medical services rather than the short, intense peak demand typical of less extensive multiple-casualty incidents. Examples of multiple-casualty incidents include:

- Motor-vehicle crashes with multiple victims
- Fires with burn or smoke-inhalation victims
- Environmental disasters
- Public transportation accidents (aircraft, train, bus)
- Mining or construction accidents
- Industrial accidents
- Building collapses
- Hazardous materials incidents
- Chemical, biological, radiological, nuclear, or explosive (CBRNE) incidents
- Planned events, such as celebrations, parades, concerts, or **mass gatherings**

mass gathering any collection of more than 1,000 people at one site or location; applies to all types of events, including concerts and sporting or other large-scale events.

Multiple-casualty incidents are calls that involve multiple patients. While one patient may seem a challenge for the new EMT, a multiple-casualty incident can create an entirely new set of challenges for both the new and the experienced

EMT (Figure 43-1 ■). These calls will stress the resources of a jurisdiction and, in some cases, the resources of a region beyond those normally available for a given call.

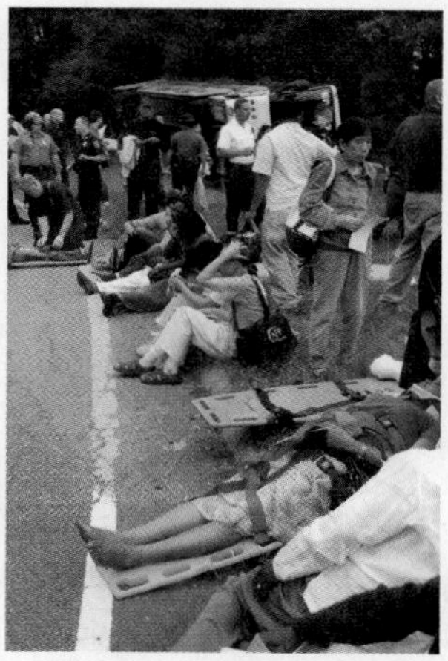

Figure 43-1 An incident involving multiple patients is referred to as a multiple-casualty incident (MCI). (© Mark C. Ide)

In general, multiple-casualty incidents do not have to be as dramatic as airplane crashes or terrorism incidents, but can be a family injured in a house fire or a three-car collision with two patients in each car. How you approach the airplane crash is very similar to how you approach the three-car collision, as you will see.

Multiple-casualty incidents by their very nature are different from everyday calls. Usually, a call involves a single patient. Whether the patient is experiencing chest pain or fell and broke his arm, most of the time it is just one patient you will treat until he is either transported for care or refuses treatment and transport. Multiple-casualty incidents are much more complex and require lots of logistics to manage a variety of resources. Because of this, day-to-day systems will not work, and your procedures must change to facilitate rapid, yet effective, treatment of numerous patients.

Another issue with multiple-casualty incidents is that, more often than not, no one anticipates them. While some multiple-casualty incidents are the result of predictable weather events, such as hurricanes, most are unpredictable, including tornados; earthquakes; fires; vehicle crashes involving trains, planes, and automobiles; and, occasionally, acts of terrorism or other criminal acts. This unpredictability factor makes the EMS job that much harder and necessitates preplanning on the part of EMS organizations for multiple-casualty incidents.

Preplanning can take many forms, but most often it consists of the development of a response plan for future expected or possible incidents that would require a large response of multiple units, personnel, and supervisors. Response plans developed during preplanning are often practiced during multiple-casualty incident drills and then revised based on post-drill debriefing.

preplanning developing a plan for future possible incidents that would require a large response of units, personnel, and supervisors.

As you can see, every call has the possibility of being a multiple-casualty incident, and even what seems like a mundane car crash could be one if it involves more patients than you and your crew can handle.

Goals of Multiple-Casualty Incident Management

43-3 List aspects important to effective management of a multiple-casualty incident.

When, as a new EMT, you arrive on the scene of a multiple-casualty incident, you should keep three overall goals in mind. They are to do the best for the most, to manage very limited resources, and to avoid relocating the disaster. These goals might seem easy enough, but each has a significant challenge associated with it.

Do the Best for the Most

Doing the best for the most means that the goal is to save the greatest possible number of patients. This can mean allowing mortally injured patients to die rather than to exhaust limited resources. Every day EMS responds to medical emergencies with two to eight EMTs for a single patient. In a multiple-casualty incident, the ratio is reversed, and one provider may be treating up to eight patients. How would a single EMT treat four patients, all with significant airway issues? The answer is with great difficulty. Understand that a single paramedic, nurse, or physician would also have difficulty in this situation.

The task may seem impossible, but the first-arriving EMT in fact may have responsibility for all the patients who are having difficulty breathing. In that case, when there are not enough hands to go around, you must concentrate on doing the most you can for those you can help. That means some patients with conditions you might normally treat will not receive extensive resources. Instead, you will tag the patient who is not breathing as "deceased," and triage the patient in extreme pain from two broken legs into a low-priority category.

Manage Very Limited Resources

The second goal of multiple-casualty incident management is to manage scarce or limited resources. Whether it is ambulances, personnel, oxygen masks, or even bandages, all will be in short supply. The only thing that will be in abundance will be patients.

Ultimately, short supplies will include hospital beds and space, which leads to the third goal: During the early stages of the incident, be sure to complete the triage process and focus your attention on the patients most in need of your care. It will be important to have patients with **minor injuries** assist with providing care for the more seriously wounded. Give them simple tasks such as bandaging, moving supplies, and comfort care. Before long, the number of rescuers will increase and you will not have to ration so much.

minor injuries in a triage situation, the term refers to patients with minor injuries who are classified as "minor." Sometimes referred to as *walking wounded.*

Avoid Relocating the Disaster

In a catastrophe, you must not "relocate the disaster" by sending patients to hospitals unable to care for them, or by sending too many patients to the same hospital. Remember that the usual everyday number of people will be using the nearest hospital's resources. The disaster's "walking wounded" will likely be there as well, all asking for medical attention. That hospital may become inundated with patients. Concise communication between on-scene EMTs and hospitals is an essential part of multiple-casualty incident management. Never send all of an incident's patients to a single location unless you know the facility can handle the increased patient load.

You also must resist the temptation to bypass the triage process. Do not put injured patients in ambulances for transport directly from the scene. It is important to maintain triage priorities and follow the order of who gets cared for and transported first.

Initial Actions: The Five S's

43-4 List the first actions (the Five S's) that should be taken upon arrival at a multiple-casualty incident.

Many providers feel overwhelmed when they are riding the first unit to arrive at a multiple-casualty incident. Some describe feeling drowned by a "sea of patients" and unsure about their first steps. The goals of multiple-casualty incident management may be common sense, but how can an EMT attain the most desirable outcome in incidents like these? To help providers limit their normal stress responses and take some charge over the scene, the *Five S's* were developed. They are a set of systematic actions to start handling a multiple-casualty incident. The Five S's are safety, scene size-up, send information, set up incident command, and start triaging.

Safety

The first and most important of the Five S's is *safety.* Whether the call is an auto collision, house fire, or terrorist incident, a multiple-casualty incident by definition has too many patients. Initial EMS responders must be sure to take extra time to consider their own safety as they approach the scene and as they proceed with their assignments. Adding patients to an incident never makes sense. In the case of a multiple-casualty incident in which resources such as EMTs are valuable, it is even more imperative that EMS providers do not themselves become patients.

PERSPECTIVE

DJ—The EMT

That was intense! Oh my gosh! We ended up getting seven patients transported from that scene. And that doesn't include the pilot, because he died there. Surprisingly, we were able to handle it all within our agency. It's weird. Sometimes when something big is going to happen, there is a kind of lull around the rest of the city, you know? Like when the air gets really still and quiet just before a tornado? I couldn't believe it when I gave my initial report to dispatch and he had about five ambulances that he was able to free up and send our way immediately. I think that made a huge difference in the outcome.

Scene Size-up

Scene size-up is the second of the Five S's. It means to consider the incident in its entirety. The initial on-scene report must include a description of the incident so that other crews and personnel will have an idea of how big and how bad the incident might turn out. You must ask yourself questions, such as: Is this a large airliner crash or a small bus crash? How many victims are obvious? What issues are there that incoming responders need to know?

Send Information

Once the scene is sized up, you need to *send information*, the third of the Five S's. Knowing the characteristics of an incident without telling other responders does no good. The initial crew on a multiple-casualty incident must not only assess the scene as they would assess a patient, but they also must inform incoming crews so they will be able to begin work as soon as they arrive.

Inform dispatch of your unit designation, the nature of the incident, and its correct location. Are there any obvious hazards such as fire, entrapment, or lack of structural integrity? Then request additional units that will assist with the scene or have specialized rescue capability. Some EMS systems have specific protocols for larger EMS responses, such as an EMS task force or an EMS strike team that provides specific transport, treatment, and multiple-casualty assistance.

Set up Incident Command

The fourth of the Five S's is *set up incident command* and any necessary structures such as a medical branch, using the incident command system (ICS) as discussed in Chapter 42. It is typically the first responding fire units that establish incident command with dispatch. In rare cases it may be the first responding EMS unit. If an EMS unit establishes incident command, the next fire units on scene will take over command of the incident to allow EMS resources to establish the medical branch.

While setting up a medical branch can seem like a waste of time versus immediately treating patients, the first arriving EMS unit should do it. By starting the incident with this mind-set, there will be organization for the incident, instead of ambulances just showing up, scooping up patients, and going to the closest hospital, which will quickly become overloaded. An organized response leads to a more efficient use of personnel and resources, which will lead to patients being treated more effectively.

PERSPECTIVE

Devon—The EMT

I've never had to triage anybody in real life before. At first I asked myself, "Where do I start?" There was an injured lady in the pickup, a guy next to the car, the pilot, and a whole group of little kids in that van. I really got overwhelmed. I hate to say it, but I actually started to panic a little. I mean, I was afraid that one of the kids would die if I didn't start with the van, but I'd have to walk right past other patients to get to it. I keep remembering the look in that one lady's eyes. It was the one in the pickup. Her eyes showed just terror and confusion, you know? I couldn't just walk past her! But then, all at once I remembered something my instructor said back in my EMT class. She said, "Start where you stand." So I did. It's amazing. Once you get moving, everything just falls into place.

START Triage

Finally, you must know how many patients you have and how badly injured they are right now. This is accomplished with the fifth of the Five S's, the *START triage.* The letters of START stand for Simple Triage and Rapid Transport. Triage enables the transport group supervisor to determine how many patients will need to be transported to how many hospitals and how many personnel will be required to accomplish the task.

STOP, REVIEW, REMEMBER!

Multiple Choice

For each question, place a check next to the correct answer.

1. The first and most important of the Five S's is:

_____ a. scene size-up.

_____ b. safety.

_____ c. send information.

_____ d. START triage.

2. An incident that will overwhelm the initial responding units but *not* the resources of the system is known as a(n) ______________ incident.

_____ a. multiple-casualty

_____ b. controlled

_____ c. minimal-casualty

_____ d. unmanageable

3. After giving dispatch the initial details of a multiple-casualty incident, the first responding unit should immediately:

_____ a. size up the scene.

_____ b. initiate START triage.

_____ c. evaluate safety concerns.

_____ d. set up a medical branch.

4. Developing a plan for future possible incidents that would require a large response of units, personnel, and supervisors is called:

_____ a. forward incident control.

_____ b. resource management.

_____ c. preplanning.

_____ d. preemptive logistics.

5. Which one of the following sets up the medical branch at the scene of a multiple-casualty incident?

_____ a. First ALS unit on scene

_____ b. First supervisor on scene

_____ c. First EMS unit on scene

_____ d. Multiple-casualty strike team

Fill in the Blank

Put the following Five S's in their proper order by writing the order number in the blank space.

1. ______________________ Size-up
2. ______________________ Safety
3. ______________________ START triage
4. ______________________ Send information
5. ______________________ Set up incident command

Critical Thinking

1. What are the three primary goals of EMS during a multiple-casualty incident?

____

____

____

____

2. Explain what the role of the EMT is likely to be in the early stages of a multiple-casualty incident.

____

____

____

____

Command Structure at a Multiple-Casualty Incident

43-5 Identify responsibilities that may be assigned to EMS at a multiple-casualty incident.

Once command has been established at a multiple-casualty incident, it is up to the incident commander (IC) to establish a strategy for handling all patients. Figure 43-2 ■ depicts a commonly used incident command chart and some of the roles and responsibilities that incoming EMS units may be assigned.

All incidents have an IC who is ultimately responsible for the overall incident. Depending on the scale of the incident, the IC may establish an operations section chief who is to oversee all the actual hands-on work during the incident, including staged resources. The staging area manager will keep track of which units are available within the staging area and report directly to the operations section chief. The medical branch director will likely establish a triage group, treatment group, and transport group. Each group's supervisor reports to the medical branch director, who reports to the operations section chief or directly to the incident commander, depending on the scale of the incident.

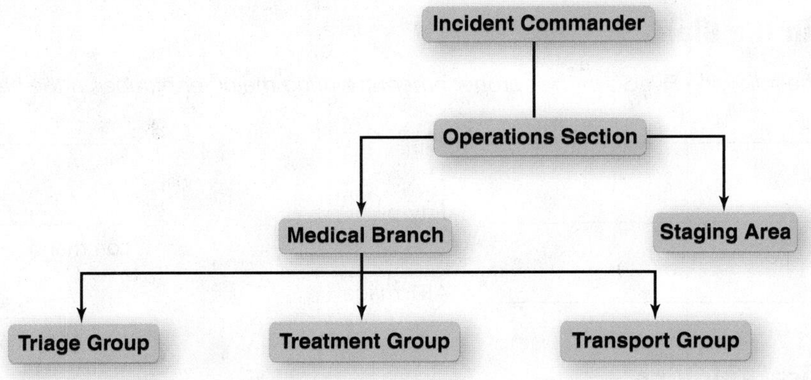

Figure 43-2 Medical components of ICS at a multiple-casualty incident.

As an EMT on an ambulance, you are most likely to be assigned to the triage, treatment, or transport group, and will be required to report to and follow the direct orders of that group's supervisor.

Triage

43-6 Describe the principles of a triage system.

triage the process of sorting patients based on the severity of their injuries and prioritizing them for treatment and transport.

Triage is a French word that means "to sort." As an EMT, you can use any accepted triage system, but one of the most accepted and widely used is the START system, developed in California during the 1980s. The START system uses simple patient assessment to rank the nature of injuries and the need for care, using a color-coded system to identify patient priority categories (Figure 43-3 ■). The colors associated with triage most often are red, yellow, green, and black:

- *Red—Immediate.* These are patients who are salvageable and most in need of care and transport.
- *Yellow—Delayed.* These are patients who are salvageable and do not require immediate care and transport.
- *Green—Minor.* These are patients with minor injuries who will eventually need care but do not require immediate care or transport.
- *Black—Deceased.* These are patients who present with no pulse and/or no breathing. They would require too many resources to attempt to resuscitate, risking the lives of many others.

Triage should start with the first on-scene unit using a public-address or other system to ask patients who can walk under their own power to go to a designated area where another responder from the unit can start to care for them. When those patients move themselves, they do several things for the incident, one of which is to tell you by their actions that they are "walking wounded" and likely have only minor injuries. They can be moved to any easily accessible position or building where a group can receive basic medical care. These patients are immediately classified as *green*.

The walking wounded may be treated and released from the designated area, preventing unnecessary impact on the local hospital. They also may be gathered together and transported by less conventional means (a bus, for example) to a hospital farther away. That tactic supports two multiple-casualty incident goals: not relocating the disaster and doing the most good for the most patients.

When triaging patients, EMTs should remember to work systematically to make sure that everyone is triaged and, depending on local protocol, tied with colored tape and possibly triage tagged. Triage time is kept to a minimum. Each patient encounter

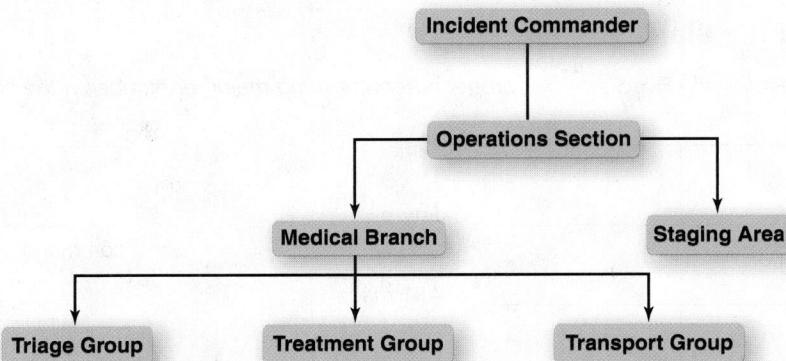

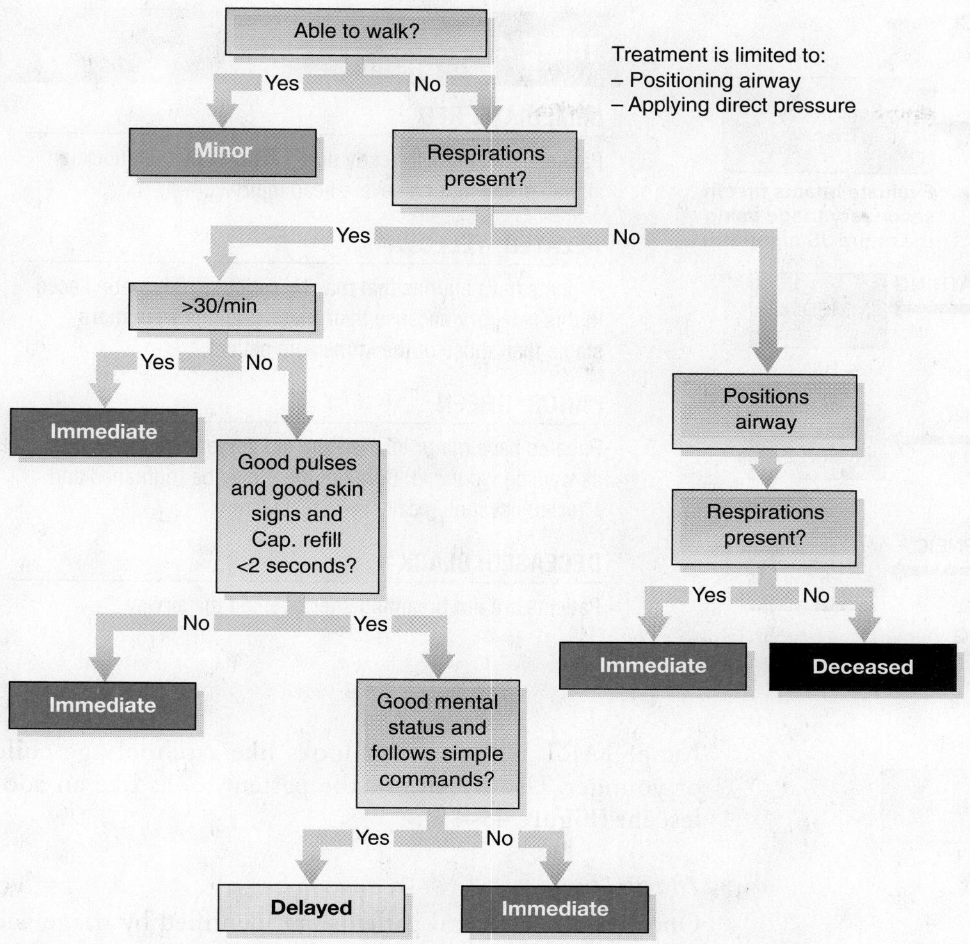

Figure 43-3 The START triage flowchart.

should last only 15 to 30 seconds. Only the most basic care is performed during triage, generally limited to opening airways and controlling severe bleeding. Patients who initially present with no pulse and no breathing are categorized as **deceased patients** and no further care is provided.

deceased patients patients who are not breathing after opening the airway.

A final critical note is to be accurate in your patient count. Many EMS systems will utilize colored surveyor's tape tied to a patient's wrists to indicate the patient's triage status. One way of keeping track of a large number of patients is to then tear off a section and place it in your pocket. At the conclusion of triaging your area, all these small pieces of triage tape will be in your pocket, allowing you to quickly divide them by color and provide the triage group supervisor with an accurate count of patients in each category.

The START triage system itself is simple to use and relies on a condition-based, not an injury-based, system of classification (Table 43-1). For instance, badly burned patients might be tagged black, red, or yellow, depending on how they fit into the criteria. This helps get treatment for the most seriously injured patients and allows resources to be managed more effectively.

43-8 Explain the principles and assessment categories used in START triage.

There are important variations to consider when triaging pediatric patients. One method is the JumpSTART system. Developed by Lou Romig, MD, JumpSTART recognizes that pediatric patients experience cardiovascular compromise differently from adults and prioritizes them accordingly. Use

43-9 Explain the principles used in the pediatric JumpSTART triage system.

JumpSTART Pediatric MCI Triage

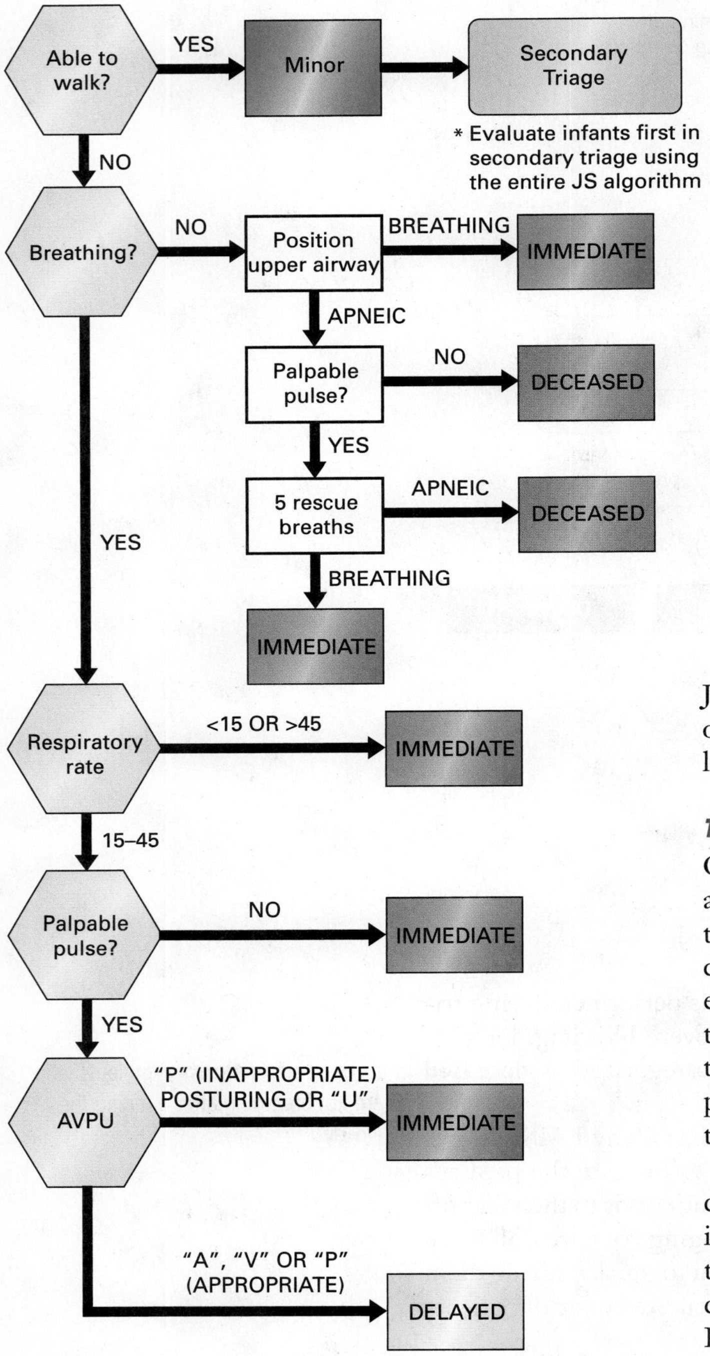

Figure 43-4 The JumpSTART triage flowchart for pediatric patients.
(© Lou Romig, MD, FAAP, FACEP, 2002)

TABLE 43-1 START TRIAGE

IMMEDIATE: RED

Patients are at risk for early death, usually due to shock, an airway problem, or a severe head injury.

DELAYED: YELLOW

Patients have injuries that may be serious. They were placed in this category because their triage findings were more stable than those of the immediate patient.

MINOR: GREEN

Patients have minor injuries and are sometimes referred to as walking wounded. Some of them may be frightened and affected psychologically by the incident.

DECEASED: BLACK

Patients are not breathing after opening the airway.

JumpSTART if the patient looks like a school-age child or younger. Use START if the patient looks like an adolescent (Figure 43-4 ■).

Triage Tags

Once the most critical patients are identified by triage and are moved to the treatment area, be sure each patient has a triage tag, which will document the patient's condition and care provided from that point forward. Triage tags should be easy to read, weatherproof, and contain unique patient identifying numbers or bar codes (Figure 43-5 ■). Many triage tags have portions of the tag that rip off for tracking purposes, or stickers that may be attached to incident logs or to the patient's medical record at the hospital.

Triage tags should be tied directly to the patient using color-coded triage tape in a conspicuous location. In the initial stages of an incident it is not critical to fill in all of the patient's information (such as name, address, and medical history) because it can be gathered later as time allows. However, it is crucial that once a triage tag is tied to a patient that it remains attached to the patient throughout the duration of the incident.

43-10 Explain the important principles of a patient-tagging system to be used during triage.

43-11 Explain the interrelationship of triage and treatment within the treatment area at a multiple-casualty incident.

Treatment Area

Once all patients on scene have been triaged, the immediate- or red-tagged patients should be the first to be moved to the treatment area. The treatment area should be staffed with advanced life support (ALS) providers who can begin providing lifesaving treatment, while the treatment group supervisor and the transport group supervisor coordinate transportation of the most critical patients first. The treatment area is also where secondary triage occurs.

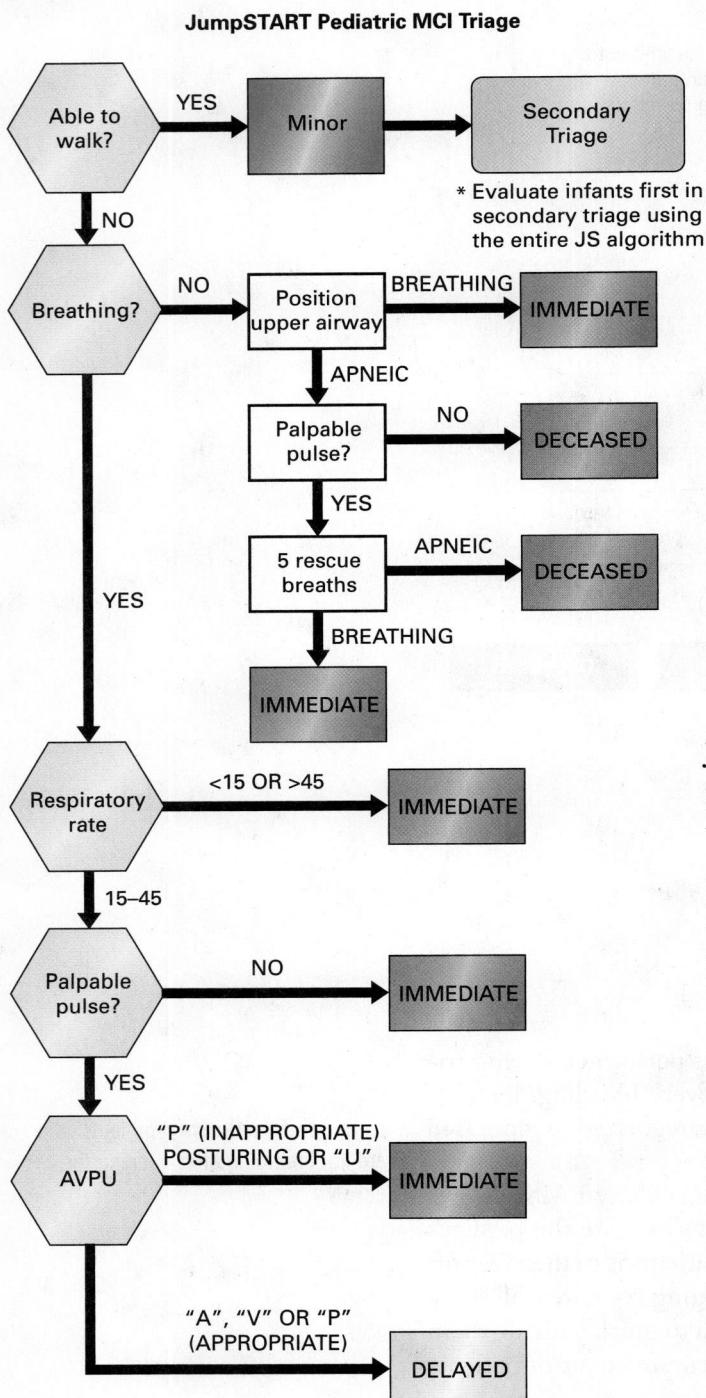

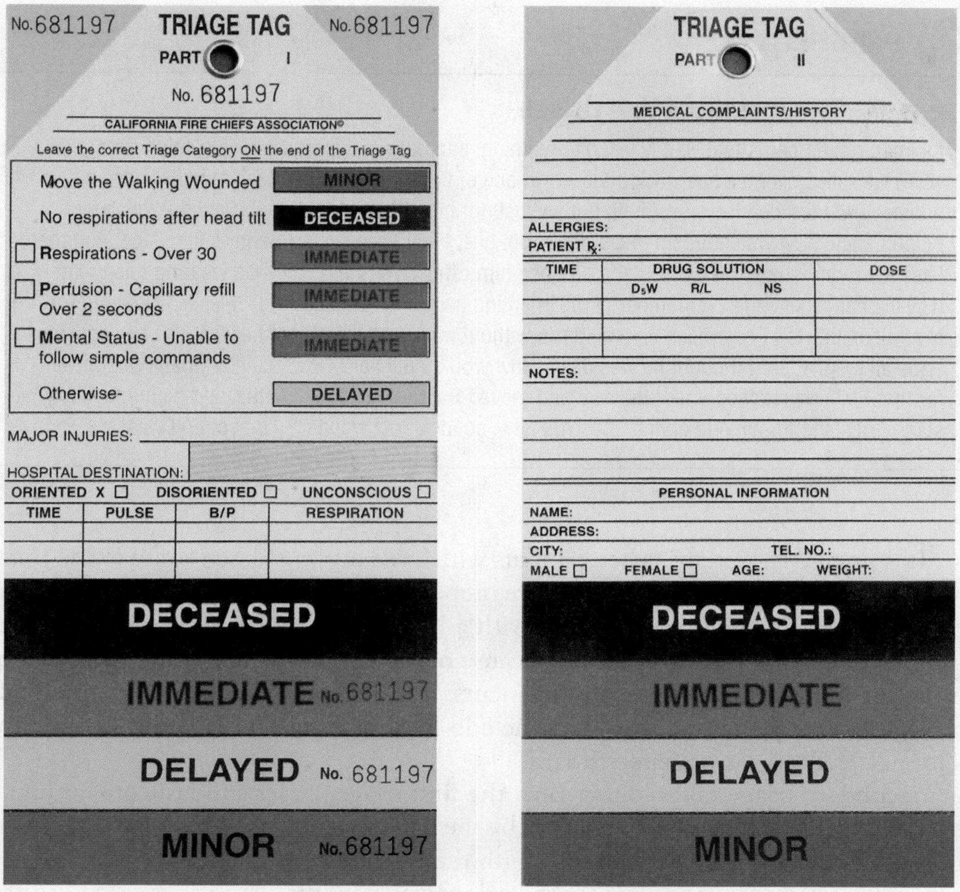

Figure 43-5 A typical triage tag (front/back).

As the immediate-tagged patients are transported out of the treatment area, the triage team can begin sending **delayed patients,** who have yellow tags, to the treatment area. During a multiple-casualty incident, it is helpful to set up a treatment area for each category of patient: immediate, delayed, and minor. The most resources will be dedicated to the **immediate-tagged patients.** However, all patients will be triaged a second time and be monitored for changes in condition.

delayed patients patients who are injured but whose triage findings are more stable than those of the immediate patient.

immediate-tagged patients patients who are at risk for early death, usually due to shock, an airway problem, or a severe head injury.

43-7 Describe and contrast primary triage with secondary triage.

Secondary Triage

During secondary triage, a more thorough assessment of the patient should be conducted for the purpose of locating specific injuries and providing additional lifesaving treatment. Generally, secondary triage will be performed by an ALS provider, such as a paramedic.

As noted earlier, patients who are classified with a red tag are likely to be in shock or may have difficulty maintaining their own airway. Patients with a yellow tag, while significantly injured, probably will have incapacitating injuries that can be treated later in the course of the incident. Patients with a green tag are those whose injuries are minor and who will be able to wait hours before treatment. Patients with a black tag are those with no cardiorespiratory effort.

While initial triage classifies a patient, the patient may need to be reclassified during secondary triage or during emergency care by the treatment group. An example might be a patient with a leg fracture who was classified with a yellow tag initially, and who may be reclassified with a red tag if subsequent evaluation reveals internal injuries and progressing shock.

PERSPECTIVE

Elise—The Preschool Van Driver

All I can remember is that Randy wasn't breathing, and he was this horrible blue color. Somehow when we rolled over, he got stuck underneath one of the seats. I don't understand. He was in a booster and was wearing a seat belt, but we just got hit so hard. I think I blacked out, because I didn't know how we ended up in the ditch. Oh, gee, I just keep seeing Randy's little face. And then I see his mom, you know? When she dropped him off this morning, she was wearing this great new leather jacket, and I remember complimenting her on it. And she said, "Please watch out for my little man. He's never been on a field trip without me." And then there he was with his legs and arms all tangled up. I thought he was dead. How would I tell her? How could I? Thank goodness for that EMT. He reached under the seat and moved Randy's head just a little, and he immediately started gasping for air, and crying, too. You have no idea how wonderful that sound was!

In some EMS systems, when patients with a red tag worsen en route to the treatment area, resuscitation may take place, depending on the size of the incident and the availability of resources. Patients with a black tag on scene during initial triage most likely will not be moved at all. Because of the high probability that there will be investigations of multiple-casualty incidents, it is generally better to leave the body in place for investigators, who may include local and state police, the FBI, or the National Transportation Safety Board.

Secondary triage takes longer than the first triage, but it still lasts only minutes as patients are prioritized for transport by the treatment group. The treatment group supervisor will communicate directly with the transport group supervisor to coordinate transportation to hospitals for the prioritized patients.

Staging and Transportation

43-12 Discuss the logistics of staging and transportation at a multiple-casualty incident.

When the treatment group supervisor communicates the number of priority patients who need transportation to hospitals, the transportation group supervisor will coordinate with the staging area manager. The staging area manager will then direct appropriate transport units into the treatment area to transport the patients according to their triaged priorities. The staging area manager must ensure that the supply of properly equipped and staffed BLS and ALS transport units does not become depleted, and he must communicate his resource needs to the operations section chief. The transportation group supervisor will communicate with area hospitals to determine the number and severity of patients that each facility is equipped to receive.

Communications

43-13 Discuss common issues with communications in multiple-casualty incident and disaster situations.

Multiple-casualty incidents are large chaotic scenes in which radios must be used because face-to-face communication will prove difficult if not impossible. Large numbers of responders, often from multiple different jurisdictions, respond to multiple-casualty incidents. Jurisdictions that normally work together and have mutual aid agreements often have worked out arrangements for interoperability of different radio systems. However, jurisdictions that do not frequently work together may find themselves working side by side and their radios may not be compatible. Disaster management teams at the state, regional, or federal level can be called on to assist with solving communications problems for incidents of long duration.

Beyond the technical problems, it is important that all EMS providers speak the same common language and not use 10-codes or jurisdiction-specific language to communicate at a multiple-casualty incident. The National Incident Management

System (NIMS) emphasizes both the use of common language and that all responders should be trained in the proper use of ICS because it will be implemented at all multiple-casualty incidents.

Rescuer Health and Stress Management

43-14 List measures that can be taken to reduce rescuer stress before, during, and after a multiple-casualty incident.

The best prepared responder for a multiple-casualty incident is one who is physically, emotionally, and spiritually healthy. You must take care of your own needs and the needs of your loved ones on a daily basis before you are appropriately equipped to help others through a stressful tragic incident. While working at the scene of a multiple-casualty incident, ensure that you and your teammates take rehabilitation breaks to rest, eat, and hydrate yourselves. Remember that you will not be able to continue to care for your patients if you become a patient as well.

It is important to realize that even the healthiest and strongest responders can be deeply affected by traumatic incidents. This can manifest itself through physical, emotional, and behavioral symptoms that can be delayed by years. Become familiar with the resources available to you for coping with critical incident stress. You will also be helping your fellow responders, who may be hurting more than you.

STOP, REVIEW, REMEMBER!

Multiple Choice

For each question, place a check next to the correct answer.

1. The JumpSTART triage system was designed for ______________ patients.
   _____ a. unresponsive
   _____ b. critical
   _____ c. "walking wounded"
   _____ d. pediatric

2. The triaging EMT should spend no more than ______________ seconds on each patient.
   _____ a. 10
   _____ b. 30
   _____ c. 60
   _____ d. 45

3. Medical interventions during triage should be limited to opening airways and:
   _____ a. controlling severe bleeding.
   _____ b. performing emergency moves.
   _____ c. spinal immobilization.
   _____ d. performing CPR.

4. START stands for:
   _____ a. Selective Transport after Rapid Triage.
   _____ b. Safe Transport and Radial Triage.
   _____ c. Simple Triage and Rapid Transport.
   _____ d. Split Triage and Responsive Transport.

5. Patients are tagged *black* using START triage when:
   _____ a. their radial pulse is absent.
   _____ b. they are apneic after their airway has been manually opened.
   _____ c. they are unresponsive to painful stimuli.
   _____ d. their carotid pulse is present.

(continued on next page)

(continued)

Fill in the Blank

1. *Triage* is a ____________________ word that means "____________________."

2. During an MCI, more thorough assessments of the patients will be made during the ____________________ triage.

3. Patients whose injuries are ____________________ and who can wait an extended period of time before treatment are tagged ____________________.

Critical Thinking

1. When triaging, what is the difference between START and JumpSTART?

____

____

____

____

2. During an MCI, how would you tag a patient who has a strong pulse but is unable to maintain his airway? Why?

____

____

____

____

EMERGENCY DISPATCH SUMMARY

The FAA investigation of the incident determined that the pilot had suffered a myocardial infarction just after takeoff and had chosen to land on the largest roadway in sight. He suffered an aortic injury during the impact and died during the crash landing. Everyone on the ground survived with moderate injuries, Randy's dislocated femur and mild concussion being the worst. As a result of the uncoordinated initial response to this incident, a system-wide training program was created. The training has greatly improved the ability of law enforcement, fire, and EMS to respond effectively together.

Chapter Review

To the Point

- Multiple-casualty incidents (MCI) vary greatly in scale and nature. The most common are vehicle collisions involving many patients. Often the resources on scene cannot handle the patients, but the resources within a jurisdiction are adequate.
- Multiple-casualty incidents may require resources from multiple jurisdictions to handle large numbers of patients.
- The main goals of multiple-casualty incident management are to do the best for the most patients, manage very limited resources, and avoid relocating the disaster to the closest hospitals.
- The initial unit on a multiple-casualty incident should remember the Five S's to begin managing the situation: safety, scene size-up, send information, set up the medical branch, and START triage.
- Multiple-casualty incidents are most effectively managed by the incident command system (ICS). All incidents will have an incident commander and, depending on the scale of the incident, other likely ICS positions including operations section, medical branch, staging area, triage group, treatment group, and transport group.
- Triage is a method to quickly sort patients by priority. START triage is used on adolescents and adult patients. JumpSTART triage is used on school-age patients and younger. There are four triage categories: immediate or red, delayed or yellow, minor or green (walking wounded), and deceased or black. Patients are labeled with colored tape and triage tags.
- The most critical patients are moved first into the treatment area, where they are triaged for a second time and given life-saving treatment while awaiting transport to a hospital. Large-scale multiple-casualty incidents may have multiple treatment areas for different triage category patients.
- On multiple-casualty incidents, the transport group supervisor must coordinate with area hospitals and the staging area manager to facilitate the transportation of critically injured patients in a timely manner to hospitals that have the capacity to treat them.
- NIMS calls for the use of common language, which can help to ease communication barriers among responders from different jurisdictions. Disaster management teams can be requested to assist with radio incompatibility problems during large-scale, long-term incidents.
- Multiple-casualty incidents can be extremely stressful to EMS responders. It is important that EMTs prepare for duty by maintaining a healthy lifestyle. During an incident, EMTs need to take care of each other by following orders to report to rehabilitation for rest, nourishment, and rehydration. After the incident is over, it is important to access any available resources that may help you begin to cope with a stressful incident.

Chapter Questions

Multiple Choice

For each question, place a check next to the correct answer.

1. Patients with obvious signs and symptoms of shock will most likely be given a ______________ tag during a multiple-casualty incident.

_____ a. black
_____ b. red
_____ c. yellow
_____ d. green

2. A multiple-casualty incident is defined as:

_____ a. an incident with 10 or more patients.
_____ b. an incident that requires heavy or specialty rescue.
_____ c. a terrorist or industrial accident.
_____ d. an incident that exceeds the resources of the initial units on scene.

(continued on next page)

(continued)

3. During initial triage, rescue breaths should be provided only to ____________ patients.
   _____ a. unresponsive
   _____ b. adult
   _____ c. red-tagged
   _____ d. pediatric
4. You ask all patients who are able to walk to move to a particular area. The patients who do are tagged:
   _____ a. green.
   _____ b. yellow.
   _____ c. red.
   _____ d. black.
5. The START triage system relies on ____________-based classification, not ____________-based classification.
   _____ a. injury; condition
   _____ b. patient; incident
   _____ c. condition; injury
   _____ d. system; patient
6. Triage tags:
   _____ a. should be filled out completely upon first patient encounter.
   _____ b. need to be tied in an inconspicuous location due to HIPAA.
   _____ c. are removed from patients as they are transported to the hospital.
   _____ d. are part of the patient's permanent medical record.
7. During multiple-casualty incidents, the transport group supervisor will:
   _____ a. coordinate with area hospitals.
   _____ b. oversee treatment of critically injured patients.
   _____ c. request additional resources from dispatch.
   _____ d. ensure that all patients are triaged appropriately.
8. The treatment area:
   _____ a. is staffed by a basic life support (BLS) provider.
   _____ b. is where secondary triage is performed.
   _____ c. always contains patients tagged as immediate, delayed, and minor.
   _____ d. provides patients with one-on-one patient care.
9. Secondary triage is performed:
   _____ a. en route to the hospital.
   _____ b. by a second provider immediately after the first to verify that the first provider is correct.
   _____ c. because patients' conditions change.
   _____ d. by the transport group to ensure transport of highest priority patients first.
10. How should responders handle the stress of a multiple-casualty incident?
    _____ a. Prepare with healthy habits and participate in debriefings after the incident.
    _____ b. Prepare with healthy habits and resume healthy habits to defuse the stress.
    _____ c. Blow off the stress with fellow providers at the local hangout after the incident.
    _____ d. Nothing, because stress is a natural response to such incidents and will go away with time.

Fill in the Blank

Your ambulance is called to a multiple-car collision on a rainy night along the interstate. You arrive to find five cars all over the road. Traffic is stopped and no hazard from oncoming traffic is present. For each patient, write the correct color code—red, yellow, green, or black—using the START or JumpSTART triage system as appropriate.

1. ______________________ 17-year-old male patient who is sitting in the driver's seat of his car. He has loud, moist gurgling sounds coming from his airway. His pulse is 124 and he responds only to loud verbal stimulus.
2. ______________________ 42-year-old man who says his neck hurts. He is ambulatory and able to follow instructions.

3. ______________ 86-year-old man with a head wound with minor bleeding. He is sitting in his car and appears confused and unable to focus. His pulse is 66, respirations 24.
4. ______________ 79-year-old woman who is the passenger of patient "3." She is unresponsive without respirations or pulse. No obvious injuries. No change when opening her airway.
5. ______________ Six-year-old male patient who is unresponsive with a pulse of 140 and respirations of 50.
6. ______________ 24-year-old, oriented female patient, sitting in her car complaining of neck and abdominal pain. Her pulse is 82 and respirations are 16.
7. ______________ 57-year-old female patient who is oriented and ambulatory, complaining of shoulder pain.
8. ______________ 37-year-old male patient found in the roadway who responds only to painful stimulus. He is breathing irregularly with a slow pulse.
9. ______________ 29-year-old male patient sitting at the roadside who does not believe he is injured at all. His pulse is 120 and respirations are 28. He did not move when ambulatory patients were asked to.
10. ______________ 14-year-old alert male patient who believes he has a broken lower leg. His pulse is 94, respirations 24.

Critical Thinking

1. You are triaging numerous patients following a structure fire, and you find an apneic four-year-old girl. What should you do?

____

____

____

____

2. If a large number of green-tagged patients are on scene and they are beginning to get restless or complain about lack of care, what is the incident commander's best option?

____

____

____

____

3. Do you think it would take longer to triage 15 patients on a rolled-over municipal bus or 15 patients injured after a race car hit a wall and peppered the nearby crowd with flying car parts? Why?

____

____

____

____

Case Study

You are driving home late one evening following a busy day of work for the county ambulance service. You are tired and are looking forward to getting home, relaxing in front of the television for a few minutes, and then going to bed. You are suddenly passed by a semi truck that is going much faster than the posted 55 mph speed limit. As you watch in horror, the semi puts on its right blinker and merges directly over the top of a minivan that is about 100 feet ahead of you. The truck's trailer lurches upward and showers the roadway with sparks as it drags the van sideways, finally crushing it under the wide rear wheels. The semi then veers off onto the shoulder and clumsily rolls over, throwing a huge dust cloud up over the road.

1. If you choose to assist in this situation, what is the very first thing that you should do?

2. Would you still follow all of the Five S's in this situation? Why or why not?

3. When beginning triage, which vehicle should you approach first?

The Last Word

Multiple-casualty incidents require a significantly different response than the typical EMS call. It is the multiple-casualty incident with two to 10 patients that historically catches EMTs unprepared. When a commercial airplane crashes or a passenger train derails, everyone can all agree they need help. But when two cars, each containing three people, collide, or when someone mixes cleaning fluids and eight people get sick, or even when a mother gives birth to premature twins, you have a multiple-casualty incident. Do not be fooled by the small ones.

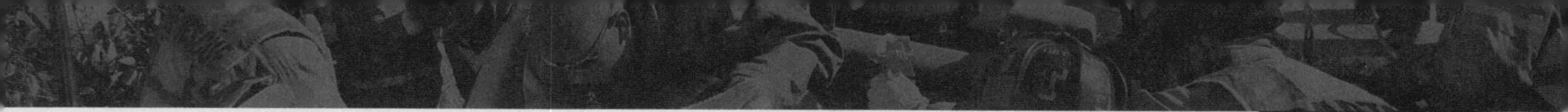

Responses Involving Hazardous Materials

44

Education Standards

EMS Operations: Hazardous Materials.

Competencies

Applies knowledge of operational roles and responsibilities to ensure patient, public, and personnel safety.

Objectives

After completion of this lesson, you should be able to:

44-1 Define key terms introduced in this chapter.

44-2 Explain the U.S. Department of Transportation placard system and the National Fire Protection Association symbols for identifying hazardous materials.

44-3 Explain the purpose of shipping papers and material safety data sheets.

44-4 List sensory indications that a hazardous materials situation may exist.

44-5 Identify resources that can be used in the identification and management of hazardous materials incidents.

44-6 Differentiate between the levels of hazardous materials training identified by the Occupational Safety and Health Administration.

44-7 Describe the safety considerations when responding to hazardous materials incidents.

44-8 Discuss the components of hazardous materials incident management: preincident planning, considerations in implementing the plan, establishing safety zones, and emergency procedures, including decontamination, that should take place in each zone.

44-9 Describe special considerations in responding to and managing patients exposed to or contaminated with radiation.

44-10 Differentiate between radiation sickness, radiation injury, and radiation poisoning.

44-11 List factors that determine the amount of risk to patients and rescuers by a source of radiation.

44-12 Describe the importance of being knowledgeable about terrorist attacks involving weapons of mass destruction.

Key Terms

absorption p. 1188
acute exposure p. 1190
carcinogenic p. 1190
chemical and physical characteristics p. 1189
chronic exposure p. 1190
concentration p. 1189
contained p. 1189
contaminated p. 1187
cross-contamination p. 1187
decontamination p. 1187
dermal exposure p. 1188
direct pathway p. 1189
duration p. 1189
Emergency Response Guidebook (ERG) p. 1178
exposure pathway p. 1189
First Responder Awareness Level p. 1186
form p. 1189
Hazard Class 1, Explosives p. 1180
Hazard Class 2, Gases p. 1180
Hazard Class 3, Flammable liquids, combustible liquids p. 1180

Hazard Class 4, Flammable solids, spontaneously combustible materials, and dangerous when wet materials p. 1180
Hazard Class 5, Oxidizers and organic peroxides p. 1181
Hazard Class 6, Toxic materials and infectious substances p. 1181
Hazard Class 7, Radioactive materials p. 1181
Hazard Class 8, Corrosive materials p. 1181
Hazard Class 9, Miscellaneous dangerous goods p. 1181
hazardous material p. 1171
Hazardous Materials First Responder Operations Level p. 1186
Hazardous Materials Specialist Level p. 1186
Hazardous Materials Technician Level p. 1186
hazardous properties p. 1189
immediate and adverse effects p. 1190
indirect pathway p. 1189
ingestion p. 1188
inhalation p. 1188
injection p. 1188
material safety data sheet (MSDS) p. 1175
mutagenic p. 1190
National Fire Protection Association (NFPA) p. 1172
NFPA 704 p. 1172
occupancy p. 1172
pathways of exposure p. 1189
placard p. 1175
receptor p. 1189
risk p. 1171
routes of entry p. 1188
source p. 1189
teratogenic p. 1190

Introduction

Every day millions of tons of hazardous materials (hazmats) are processed, transported, and used by business and industry. As an EMT you can expect to be involved in patient care or to function in a support role at the scene of a hazmat incident. An accidental release of these materials presents a potential danger to the public and the environment. Most commonly, hazmat incidents require a very specialized response. Teams with specific training and experience are utilized to contain and stop a release. However, all public safety personnel should be minimally trained to recognize and react to a hazmat incident in a first response role. As your training continues you may choose to obtain specialized hazardous materials training, but even at an entry level you should understand your immediate responsibilities. This chapter describes those priorities as well as a general overview of a hazmat response.

EMERGENCY DISPATCH

"Is this thing even working?" EMT Austin Brace tapped on the ambulance's air conditioning control switch.

"Yeah, it works," his partner, Maya, said as she swept a lock of damp hair from her cheek. "But being that it's 110 degrees outside, it's not gonna do much."

"Eight-oh-two," the radio crackled. "Eight-oh-two, I need you to start emergency care for 4908 County Road Fifty-Three for a . . . standby one."

"Oh, please, let it be a call in a nice air-conditioned office building," Austin pulled his seat belt on. "Or a swimming pool. Is that too much to ask?"

"Probably," Maya said. "I think the only thing out that far on C.R. Fifty-Three is the . . ." She was interrupted by the dispatcher.

"Okay, oh-two," the dispatcher added. "It's at the sewage treatment plant at 4908 County Road Fifty-Three for a man down in the parking lot. Was called in by a driver who passed by."

"Hmm, the sewage treatment plant," Maya finished, frowning.

As they turned onto the newly paved county road, a fire truck rolled to a stop at the sewage plant's entrance gate. Four firefighters spilled out and hurried into the parking lot. "How do they do that?" Austin pulled up next to the fire truck. "They are just so fast."

"Uh-oh, Austin," Maya began jabbing her index finger toward the windshield. "Look!"

All four firefighters were now sprawled motionless on the ground next to the treatment plant worker.

"Oh, shoot. Hold on!" Austin slammed the truck into reverse and raced back up the county road as Maya grabbed for the radio.

Hazardous Materials

The U.S. Department of Transportation (DOT) defines a **hazardous material** as any substance or material that poses an unreasonable **risk** to health, safety, and property. Hazardous materials can range from a simple bottle of cleaning supplies stored in the back of a janitor's closet to a railroad tank car filled with chemical waste. Hazardous materials are everywhere and you should always be alert to the potential safety risk they pose. (See Table 44-1 for examples of hazardous materials.)

hazardous material any substance or material in a form that poses an unreasonable risk to health, safety, and property.

risk the chance of injury, damage, or loss.

Although there are many situations in which the hazardous material will be an unknown substance, identification is a very important element of the response. It may not be the most immediate priority and certainly should never take precedence over safety, but identifying the substance provides the best information on how to most appropriately handle the incident. For that purpose, two hazardous materials identification systems have been developed, one for responses to buildings and one for responses to transportation accidents.

TABLE 44-1 EXAMPLES OF HAZARDOUS MATERIALS

MATERIAL	POSSIBLE HAZARD
Benzene (benzol)	Toxic vapors; can be absorbed through the skin; destroys bone marrow
Benzoyl peroxide	Fire and explosion
Carbon tetrachloride	Damages internal organs, long-term cancer risk
Cyclohexane	Explosive; eye and throat irritant
Diethyl ether	Flammable and can be explosive; irritant to eyes and respiratory tract; can cause drowsiness or unconsciousness
Ethyl acetate	Irritates eyes and respiratory tract
Ethylene chloride	Damages eyes
Ethylene dichloride	Strong irritant
Heptane	Respiratory irritant
Hydrochloric acid	Respiratory irritant; exposure to high concentration of vapors can produce pulmonary edema; can damage skin and eyes
Hydrogen cyanide	Highly flammable; toxic through inhalation or absorption
Methyl isobutyl ketone	Irritates eyes and mucous membranes
Nitric acid	Produces a toxic gas (nitrogen dioxide); skin irritant; can cause self-ignition of cellulose products (such as sawdust)
Organochloride (chlordane, DDT, dieldrin, lindane, methoxyclor)	Irritates eyes and skin; fumes and smoke toxic
Perchloroethylene	Toxic if inhaled or swallowed
Silicon tetrachloride	Water-reactive to form toxic hydrogen chloride fumes
Tetrahydrofuran (THF)	Damages eyes and mucous membranes
Toluol (toluene)	Toxic vapors; can cause organ damage
Vinyl chloride	Flammable and explosive; listed as a carcinogen

44-2 Explain the U.S. Department of Transportation placard system and the National Fire Protection Association symbols for identifying hazardous materials.

44-5 Identify resources that can be used in the identification and management of hazardous materials incidents.

National Fire Protection Association (NFPA) the world's leading advocate of fire prevention and an authoritative source on public safety. NFPA 300 codes and standards influence every building, process, service, design, and installation in the United States, as well as many of those used in other countries.

NFPA 704 a standardized system that uses numbers and colors on a sign to indicate the basic hazards of a specific material being stored in large containers or at a manufacturing site.

occupancy the term used to describe a building that may be used to manufacture or process chemicals.

Responses to Buildings

The **National Fire Protection Association (NFPA)** has devised a voluntary marking system to alert emergency responders to the characteristics of hazardous materials stored in stationary tanks and facilities (Figure 44-1 ▪). This system, known as **NFPA 704,** is a standardized system that uses numbers and colors on a sign to indicate the basic hazards of a specific material being stored in large containers or at a manufacturing site.

Occupancy is the term used to describe a building that may be used to manufacture or process chemicals. The occupancy will be marked by a multicolored diamond-shaped sign that indicates characteristics of the stored substance according to the NFPA 704 system. Look for the 704 sign to be mounted on the exterior of the building or fencing around the perimeter of a complex.

The diamond-shaped NFPA 704 label is divided into four parts, or quadrants (Figure 44-2 ▪):

- ***Left quadrant.*** This quadrant is blue, and contains a numerical rating of the substance's health hazard. Ratings are made on a scale of 4 to 0, with a rating of 4 indicating a severe hazard to which a very short exposure could cause serious injury or death. A zero or no code at all in this quadrant means that no unusual health hazard would result from exposure.
- ***Top quadrant.*** The top quadrant of the NFPA symbol is red, and contains the substance's flammability hazard rating. Again, number codes in this quadrant range from 4 to 0, with 4 representing the highest level of potential hazard.
- ***Right quadrant.*** The right quadrant, colored yellow, indicates the substance's instability hazard rating, or its likelihood to explode or react. As with the health

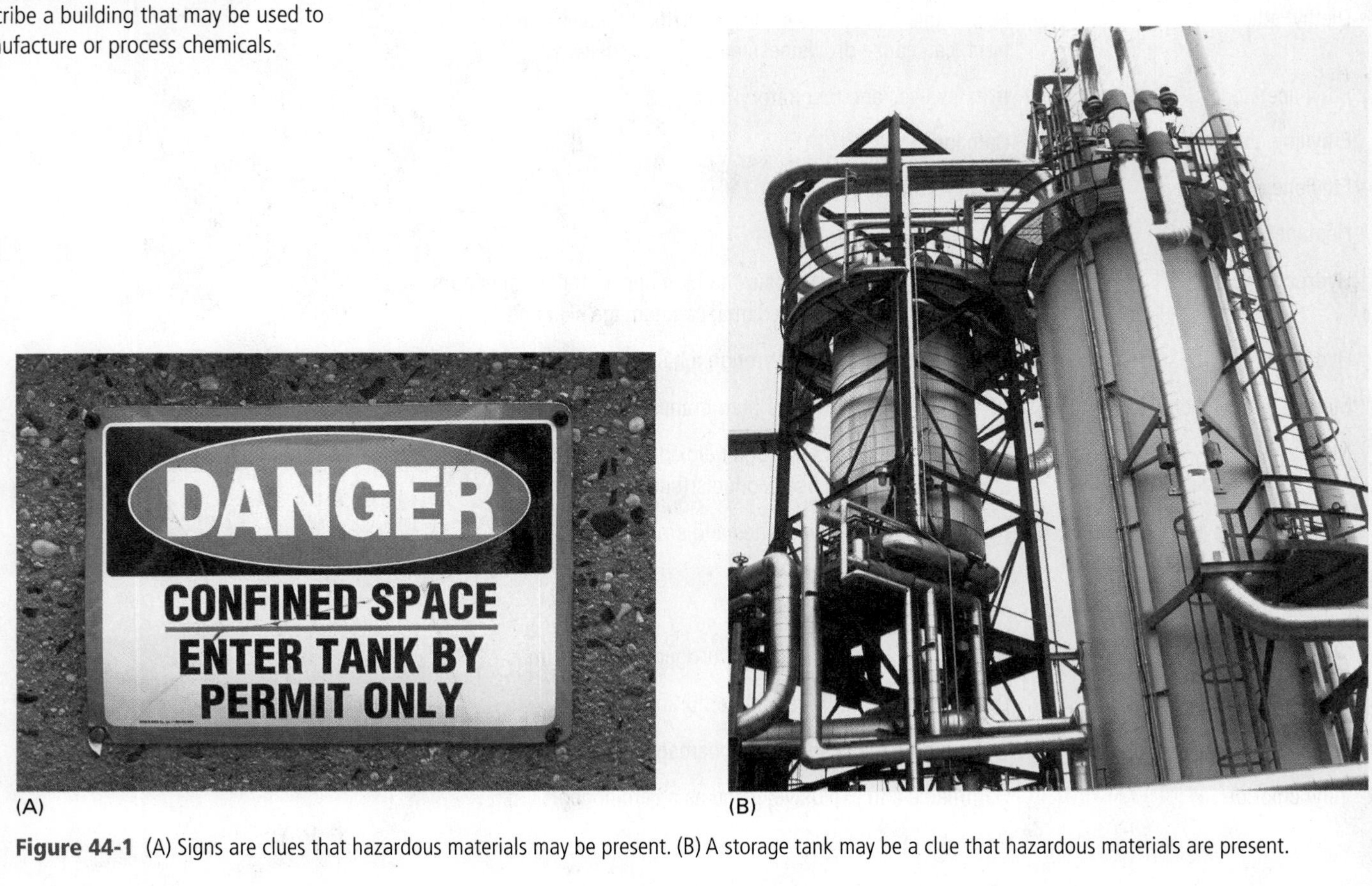

(A) (B)

Figure 44-1 (A) Signs are clues that hazardous materials may be present. (B) A storage tank may be a clue that hazardous materials are present.

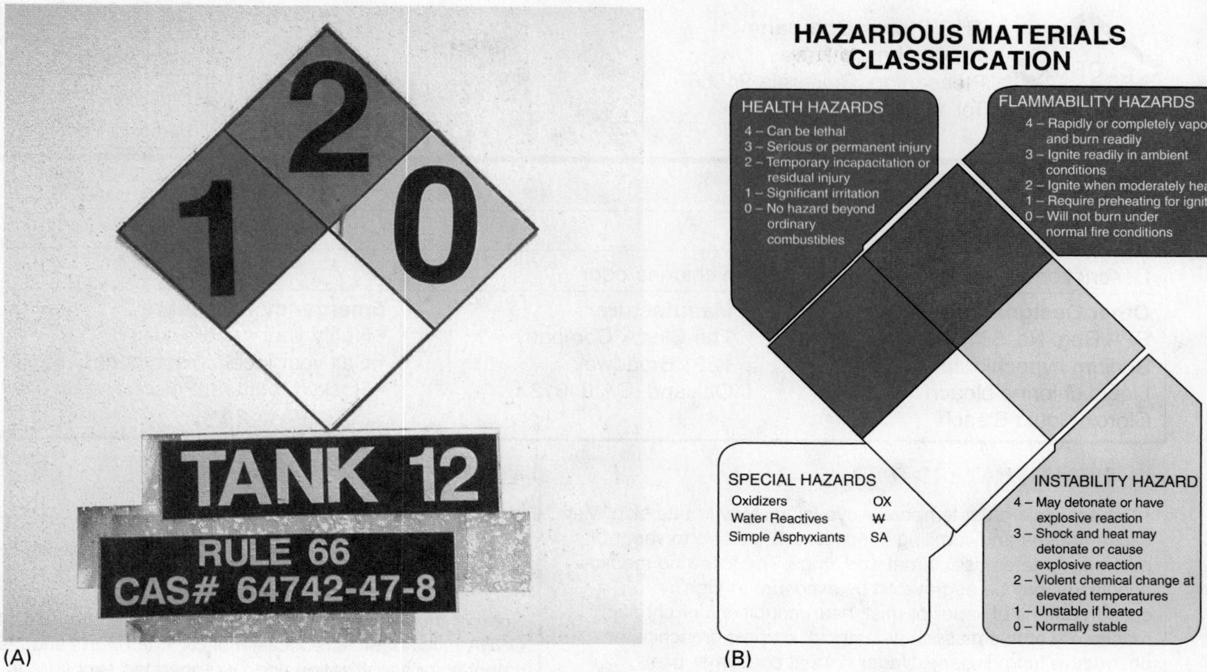

Figure 44-2 (A) A typical NFPA 704 tank placard. (B) The numeric and color classification key for the NFPA 704 hazardous materials identification system.
(Adapted with permission from NFPA 704-2012, System for the Identification of the Hazards of Materials for Emergency Response, Copyright © 2011, National Fire Protection Association. This reprinted material is not the complete and official position of the NFPA on the referenced subject, which is represented solely by the standard in its entirety. The classification of any particular material within this system is the sole responsibility of the user and not the NFPA. The NFPA bears no responsibility for any determinations of any values for any particular material classified or represented using this system.)

hazard and flammability hazard quadrants, ratings from 4 to 0 are used to indicate the degree of hazard. If a 2 appears in this quadrant, the material may readily undergo violent chemical change at elevated temperatures and pressures. A zero in this quadrant indicates that the material is considered to be stable even in the event of a fire.

- ***Bottom quadrant.*** The bottom quadrant is white, and contains information about any special hazards that may apply. There are three possible codes for the bottom quadrant of the NFPA symbol. *OX* means this material is an oxidizer that can easily release oxygen to create or worsen a fire or explosion hazard. The symbol W indicates a material that reacts with water to release a gas that is either flammable or hazardous to health. *SA* indicates the material is a simple asphyxiant.

The EMT needs to pay particular attention to the blue area that denotes the health hazards of the chemicals inside the occupancy. A "4" rating in the blue area of the diamond indicates that the building or container contains chemicals that are deadly.

CLINICAL CLUE

Know the NFPA 704 System

You know the old saying, "If you don't use it, you'll lose it." In the case of hazardous materials this could mean the difference between life and death. Take time once a month to review the NFPA 704 system and practice using it with your partners.

In many cases small quantities of hazardous materials are stored inside buildings. For example, consider the contents of an average broom closet. The shelves typically

THE Clorox Company
7200 Johnson Drive
Pleasanton, California 94566
Tel. (415) 847-6100

Material Safety Data Sheets

Health	2+
Flammability	0
Reactivity	1
Personal Protection	B

I – CHEMICAL IDENTIFICATION

Name	regular Clorox Bleach	CAS No.	N/A
Description	clear, light yellow liquid with chlorine odor	RTECs No.	N/A

Other Designations
EPA Reg. No. 5813-1
Sodium hypochlorite solution
Liquid chlorine bleach
Clorox Liquid Bleach

Manufacturer
The Clorox Company
1221 Broadway
Oakland, CA 94612

Emergency Procedure
- Notify your supervisor
- Call your local poison control center OR
- Rocky Mountain Poison Center (303)573-1014

II – HEALTH HAZARD DATA

- Causes severe but temporary eye injury. May irritate skin. May cause nausea and vomiting if ingested. Exposure to vapor or mist may irritate nose, throat and lungs. The following medical conditions may be aggravated by exposure to high concentrations of vapor or mist: heart conditions or chronic respiratory problems such as asthma, chronic bronchitis or obstructive lung disease. Under normal consumer use conditions the likelihood of any adverse health effects are low. FIRST AID: EYE CONTACT: Immediately flush eyes with plenty of water. If irritation persists, see a doctor. SKIN CONTACT: Remove contaminated clothing. Wash area with water. INGESTION: Drink a glassful of water and call a physician. INHALATION: If breathing problems develop remove to fresh air.

III – HAZARDOUS INGREDIENTS

Ingredients	Concentration	Worker Exposure Limit
Sodium hypochlorite CAS# 7681-52-9	5.25%	not established

None of the ingredients in this product are on the IARC, NTP or OSHA carcinogen list. Occasional clinical reports suggest a low potential for sensitization upon exaggerated exposure to sodium hypochlorite if skin damage (e.g., irritation) occurs during exposure. Routine clinical tests conducted on intact skin with Clorox Liquid Bleach found no sensitization in the test subjects.

IV – SPECIAL PROTECTION INFORMATION

Hygienic Practices: Wear safety glasses. With repeated or prolonged use, wear gloves.

Engineering Controls: Use general ventilation to minimize exposure to vapor or mist.

Work Practices: Avoid eye and skin contact and inhalation of vapor or mist.

V – SPECIAL PRECAUTIONS

Keep out of reach of children. Do not get in eyes or on skin. Wash thoroughly with soap and water after handling. Do not mix with other household chemicals such as toilet bowl cleaners, rust removers, vinegar, acid or ammonia containing products. Store in a cool, dry place. Do not reuse empty container; rinse container and put in trash container.

VI – SPILL OR LEAK PROCEDURES

Small quantities of less than 5 gallons may be flushed down drain. For larger quantities wipe up with an absorbent material or mop and dispose of in accordance with local, state and federal regulations. Dilute with water to minimize oxidizing effect on spilled surface.

VII – REACTIVITY DATA

Stable under normal use and storage conditions. Strong oxidizing agent. Reacts with other household chemicals such as toilet bowl cleaners, rust removers, vinegar, acids or ammonia containing products to produce hazardous gases, such as chlorine and other chlorinated species. Prolonged contact with metal may cause pitting or discoloration.

VIII – FIRE AND EXPLOSION DATA

Not flammable or explosive. In a fire, cool containers to prevent rupture and release of sodium chlorate.

IX – PHYSICAL DATA

Boiling point........212°F/100°C (decomposes)
Specific Gravity (H_2O = 1)........1.085
Solubility in Water........complete
pH........11.4

Figure 44-3 A typical material safety data sheet (MSDS).

house any number of cleaners, solvents, and other potentially dangerous chemicals. Although their presence may not be displayed on the outside of the building, employers are required to maintain a current **material safety data sheet (MSDS)** from the manufacturer for each hazardous chemical in the workplace (Figure 44-3 ■). In a hazmat response, an MSDS can provide vital identification and response information on the substances involved. The Occupational Safety and Health Administration's Hazard Communication Standard (HCS) requires very specific information to be outlined in an MSDS. That information includes:

material safety data sheet (MSDS) document from the manufacturer for each hazardous chemical in the workplace; contains important safety information about each hazardous chemical present.

- Identification and ingredients
- First-aid and firefighting measures
- Handling and storage
- Exposure controls/personal protection

If it can be done safely, obtaining an MSDS can be a useful tool in developing a response plan to a specific hazardous material. Additionally, when a patient is transported from a site where an MSDS is maintained, that sheet should accompany the patient to the hospital so information can be shared with other aspects of the emergency medical team.

Finally, remember that on-site personnel may be the best resource as to the hazardous materials involved in an incident. Workers who handle hazardous materials every day are typically well versed in the dangers and safety precautions associated with them. Always involve workers early in your scene size-up and, when possible, utilize their expertise in developing your response plan.

Responses to Transportation Accidents

Millions of tons of hazardous materials are transported throughout the country in various containers, packages, and specialty vehicles. In fact, over 1,700 different hazardous materials are regulated by the Department of Transportation (DOT) and vehicles carrying them are required to display a warning device in the form of a diamond-shaped sign called a **placard** (Figure 44-4 ■). The law also requires a four-digit code number that identifies the substance to be displayed on vehicles traveling between states. The four-digit ID number, also referred to as the *North American (NA)* or *United Nations (UN) ID number*, may be shown on the diamond-shaped placard or on an adjacent orange panel displayed next to the placard on the ends and sides of a cargo tank, vehicle, or rail car.

44-3 Explain the purpose of shipping papers and material safety data sheets.

placard diamond-shaped sign placed on cargo tanks, vehicles, or rail cars to display one of nine classes of hazardous materials that is being carried.

Information on the hazardous material can be found on the placard, which displays one of nine classes of hazardous materials. For example, a Hazard Class 7 would indicate a radioactive material. In that case the placard would commonly display not only the number 7, but also the word *radioactive* and the symbol for radioactive substances. Additionally, there may be numbers that show a division of the class of hazardous material that is being transported.

Other sources of information on hazardous materials include invoices, shipping papers (barges and trains), and bills of lading (trucks). All of these documents identify the type, quantity, origin, and destination of the hazardous materials. Often they are kept in the wheelhouse of a water-going vessel, the cab of a truck, or with the engineer.

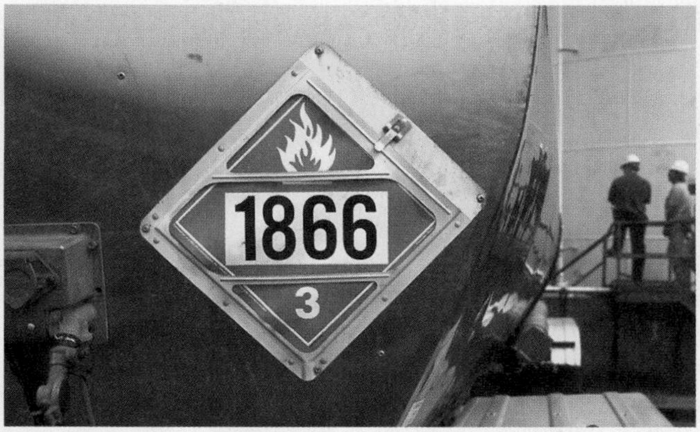

Figure 44-4 Vehicles carrying hazardous materials are required to display placards that identify their contents.

STOP, REVIEW, REMEMBER!

Multiple Choice

For each question, place a check next to the correct answer.

1. The U.S. Department of Transportation (DOT) defines a *hazardous material* as:
   _____ a. a poison or chemical that could harm you.
   _____ b. any substance or material in a form that poses an unreasonable risk to health.
   _____ c. a substance that must be marked with a placard when shipped or stored.
   _____ d. a poison or chemical that is not harmful to you.

2. The National Fire Protection Association Standard 704 system is used to mark ______________ with a multicolored diamond sign.
   _____ a. occupancy
   _____ b. hazardous materials
   _____ c. flammable materials
   _____ d. chemical materials

3. You arrive at a building for a medical call. The red quadrant of the NFPA symbol contains the number 3. This means there is ______________ fire hazard.
   _____ a. no
   _____ b. a minimal
   _____ c. a serious
   _____ d. a moderate

4. When responding to a motor-vehicle collision involving a vehicle that transports hazardous materials, you should look for ______________ during your scene size-up.
   _____ a. material data safety sheets
   _____ b. invoices, shipping papers, and bills of lading
   _____ c. placards
   _____ d. red diamonds

5. A cleaning woman has splashed a cleaning solvent in her eyes. Which one of the following would be the *best* source of information on the product?
   _____ a. Material data safety sheets
   _____ b. Label on the solvent's bottle
   _____ c. Hazardous materials response guidebook
   _____ d. Shipping container containing bottles of solvent

Matching

Match the color on the left with an element of the 704 Placard System on the right.

1. _____ Red		A. Reactivity hazard
2. _____ Blue		B. Health hazard
3. _____ Yellow		C. Fire hazard
4. _____ White		D. Special hazard

Critical Thinking

1. What impact would a hazmat incident have on the local high school? What resources does your jurisdiction have to respond to such an incident?

2. What industries within your community have hazardous chemicals in large quantities?

3. What materials are being shipped through your community by way of all transportation arteries?

General Procedures

44-4 List sensory indications that a hazardous materials situation may exist.

A fundamental principle of scene safety is to enter a scene only after ensuring it is safe to do so. This theory applies strongly to the hazmat response. It is of the utmost importance that you recognize a hazmat situation before exposing yourself to its harmful effects. In some cases this is easy. Dispatch may identify the situation prior to arrival or you may recognize a location as a high-threat area. On the other hand, hazardous materials are present in so many places, it may require conscious thought to actually identify the threat. EMTs should be ever vigilant for the presence of hazardous materials and use a thorough scene size-up before entering any situation. The following is a list of scene clues that might indicate the presence of hazardous materials:

- Known hazardous materials sites (chemical factories, laboratories, and so on)
- Prior incidents at the response site
- Descriptions of vapors, odors, or obvious chemical spills
- Multiple medical patients presenting at the same time (two patients actively seizing or multiple complaints of respiratory distress, for example)

> **CLINICAL CLUE**
>
> **If It Doesn't Smell Right, Get Out**
>
> Be extra alert for unusual odors as you approach the scene. Often your nose will identify the first clue that something is wrong. If you smell unusual odors or begin to experience any kind of irritation to your eyes or nose, retreat immediately and call for the hazmat team.

- Presence of identified or unidentified containers
- Signs, placards, warnings
- Shipping or delivery trucks

In many cases, you will use your senses to identify a hazardous material. Sensory clues, however, are the least dependable and potentially the most dangerous method of recognition and identification. Many materials do not have warning signals such as smell or taste. If you notice that an area has a terrible smell, your eyes water, your skin is irritated, or you begin to cough or feel nauseated, leave immediately and contact your communication center. Police, fire, and local hazmat response teams should be dispatched. If you encounter a suspicious substance, do *not* handle it yourself. Remove the patient to a safe zone, if it is safe to do so, and isolate and deny entry into the area. Visual clues are probably most important because they can be used at the safest distance.

Look for any of the above listed clues but also look at the presentation of the patient. Are there unknown substances such as powders or liquids on or around the patient's body? Does the patient have burns or other injuries consistent with hazardous materials exposure? As stated previously, listening to the reports of both dispatch and of on-site workers can give you an enormous amount of information that will help keep you safe. Other senses are useful as well, but far more dangerous. Be conscious of unusual odors, but be aware that by the time you are able to smell a substance, you are likely already exposed.

Proceed carefully if any of the above listed clues are found. Remember the substance that has harmed the patient can easily harm you and your crew.

> **PRACTICAL PATHOPHYSIOLOGY**
>
> Many toxic vapors, gases, and fumes can cause damage to the lungs upon inhalation. This damage can significantly disrupt normal gas exchange at the alveolar level. Provide supplemental oxygen and support ventilations as necessary during transport. Whenever possible, use a bag-mask device to assist ventilations.

Emergency Response Guidebook (ERG) U.S. DOT's quick-information guide to hazmat responses.

Identification

After recognizing a hazardous materials situation, one of your most important tasks is to identify the substances involved. Your safety is your primary responsibility when responding to a hazmat incident, so this should be attempted only if it is safe to do so. The ambulance should be equipped with basic equipment for a hazmat response and recognition, such as binoculars and the DOT ***Emergency Response Guidebook (ERG)*** (Figure 44-5 ■).

The *Emergency Response Guidebook* was developed jointly by Transport Canada (TC), the U.S. Department of Transportation (DOT), and the Secretariat of Transport and Communications of Mexico (SCT), with the collaboration of CIQUIME (Centro de Información Química para Emergencias) of Argentina for use by firefighters, police, and other emergency services personnel who may be the first to arrive at the scene of a transportation incident involving dangerous goods and hazardous materials. The *Emergency Response Guidebook* provides the names, procedures, physical behavior, medical issues, and evacuation distances for certain chemicals.

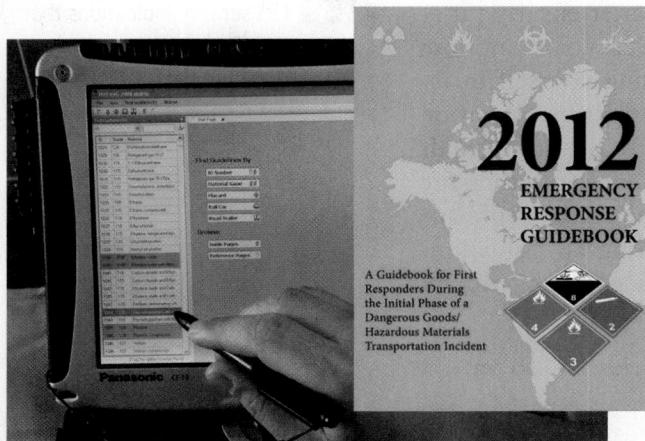

Figure 44-5 The *Emergency Response Guidebook* is updated every four years and contains important information for responders.

The *Emergency Response Guidebook* is divided into four sections:

- The yellow section lists hazardous materials based on a specific identification number.
- The blue section lists hazardous materials by name in alphabetical order.
- The orange section has all the safety recommendations.
- The green section, among other things, provides information on safe distances and is further divided into daytime and nighttime incidences.

The *Emergency Response Guidebook* is the basic resource for all emergency responders. It is designed to help responders get through the first 20 minutes of an incident.

DOT Hazard Classification System

The hazard class of dangerous substances is indicated either by its hazard class (or division) number or name. For a placard corresponding to the primary hazard class of a material, the hazard class or division number must be displayed in the lower corner of the placard (Figure 44-6 ■). No hazard class or division number, however, may be displayed on a placard representing the subsidiary hazard of a material. For other than Hazard Class 7 or the oxygen placard, text indicating a hazard (for example, "corrosive") is not required. Text is shown only in the United States. The hazard class or division number must appear on the shipping document after each shipping name.

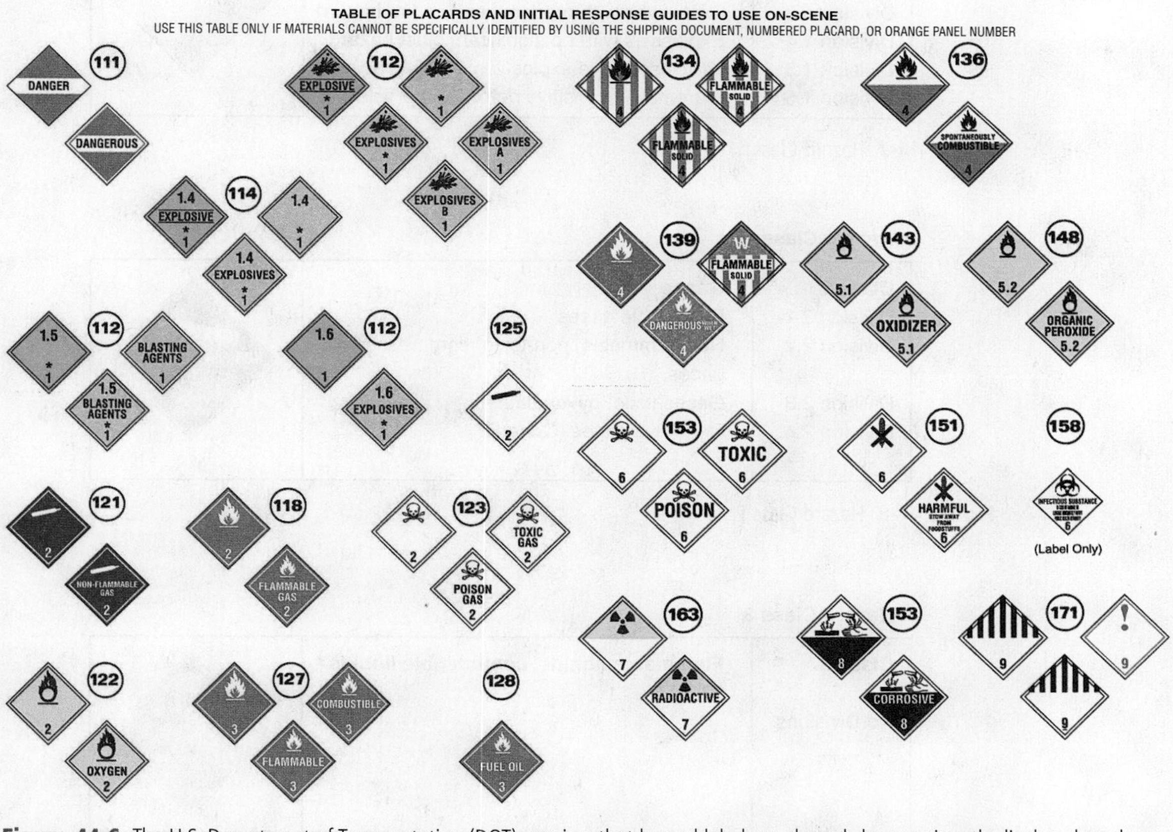

Figure 44-6 The U.S. Department of Transportation (DOT) requires that hazard labels or placards be prominently displayed on the outside of containers, packages, and vehicles during transport.

Hazard Class 1, Explosives one of nine classes of hazardous materials; indicates the hazard can cause injuries by the primary, secondary, and tertiary blasts.

Hazard Class 2, Gases one of nine classes of hazardous materials; indicates the hazard can cause injuries by being toxic or displacing oxygen to cause asphyxiation.

Hazard Class 3, Flammable liquids, combustible liquids one of nine classes of hazardous materials; indicates the hazard can cause injuries by penetrating the skin and attacking internal organs.

Hazard Class 4, Flammable solids, spontaneously combustible materials, and dangerous when wet materials one of nine classes of hazardous materials; indicates the hazard can cause injuries by creating severe and deep burns to tissue. Many of the flammable solids are reactive to water.

The DOT hazard classes and divisions are as follows:

- **Hazard Class 1, Explosives** (Figure 44-7 ■). Explosive injuries produce primary, secondary, and tertiary blast injuries.
- **Hazard Class 2, Gases** (Figure 44-8 ■). Gases cause injury by being toxic or displacing oxygen to cause asphyxiation. Toxic gases can kill by causing irritation of the airway and lungs.
- **Hazard Class 3, Flammable liquids, combustible liquids** (Figure 44-9 ■). Flammable and combustible liquids cause injury by penetrating the skin and attacking internal organs. Vapors or gases can be generated from flammable and combustible liquids that can cause inhalation injury. The ignition of flammable liquids can result in varying degrees of burn injuries.
- **Hazard Class 4, Flammable solids, spontaneously combustible materials, and dangerous when wet materials** (Figure 44-10 ■). Flammable solids cause injuries by creating severe and deep burns to tissue. Many of the flammable solids are reactive to water and create deeper burns when rescuers attempt to flush the material from the skin. Alkaline burns penetrate deep into the tissue and destroy the fat layer under the skin, causing severe tissue destruction. The EMT should contact poison control for treatment procedures and remove powdered or metal materials with a dry brush.

Hazard Class 1

Class 1	**Explosives**	
Division 1.1	Explosives with a mass explosion hazard	
Division 1.2	Explosives with a projection hazard	
Division 1.3	Explosives with predominantly a fire hazard	
Division 1.4	Explosives with no significant blast hazard	
Division 1.5	Very insensitive explosives; blasting agents	
Division 1.6	Extremely insensitive detonating articles	

Figure 44-7 Hazard Class 1.

Hazard Class 2

Class 2	**Gases**	
Division 2.1	Flammable gases	
Division 2.2	Non-flammable, non-toxic* compressed gases	
Division 2.3	Gases toxic* by inhalation	
Division 2.4	Corrosive gases (Canada)	

Figure 44-8 Hazard Class 2.

Hazard Class 3

Class 3	**Flammable liquids, combustible liquids [U.S.]**	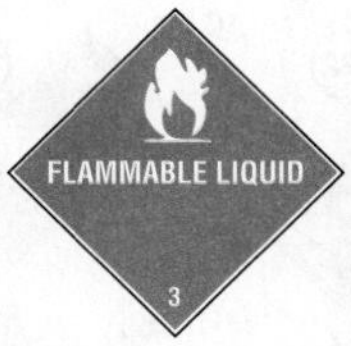
No Divisions		

Figure 44-9 Hazard Class 3.

- **Hazard Class 5, Oxidizers and organic peroxides** (Figure 44-11 ■). Oxidizers can trigger an explosion and can also act as a corrosive, destroying tissue and triggering inflammation in the lungs. Many peroxides can degrade and become explosives, which can result in a blast injury.
- **Hazard Class 6, Toxic materials and infectious substances** (Figure 44-12 ■). Toxic materials involve biological and poisonous substances. Infectious material can include blood products or blood-contaminated materials and plant, virus, bacterial, or other living organisms. Toxic materials can include cellular poisons or other substances that injure or kill.
- **Hazard Class 7, Radioactive materials** (Figure 44-13 ■). Radioactive materials injure or kill by disrupting the nervous system or cellular functions.
- **Hazard Class 8, Corrosive materials** (Figure 44-14 ■). Corrosives injure by destroying and dissolving tissue. They usually involve acids, bases, and some solvents. Alkaline corrosives dissolve fat and connective tissues, creating a waxy appearance. Acids react immediately with the water in the skin and tissue to create acids that may burn or dissolve tissue. Weak acids and bases may only produce signs of irritation or itching.
- **Hazard Class 9, Miscellaneous dangerous goods** (Figure 44-15 ■). Miscellaneous dangerous goods can be a mixed load of materials that do not require specific labels unless they are in the required amount.

Hazard Class 5, Oxidizers and organic peroxides one of nine classes of hazardous materials; indicates the hazard can trigger an explosion and act as a corrosive destroying tissue and triggering inflammation in the lungs.

Hazard Class 6, Toxic materials and infectious substances one of nine classes of hazardous materials; indicates the hazard can involve biological and poisonous substances. Infectious material can include blood products or blood-contaminated materials and plant, virus, bacterial, or other living organisms.

Hazard Class 7, Radioactive materials one of nine classes of hazardous materials; indicates the hazard can injure or kill by disrupting the nervous system or cellular functions.

Hazard Class 8, Corrosive materials one of nine classes of hazardous materials; indicates the hazard can cause injuries by destroying and dissolving tissue. Corrosives usually involve acids, bases, and some solvents.

Hazard Class 9, Miscellaneous dangerous goods one of nine classes of hazardous materials; indicates hazardous materials that do not fit into one of the other hazard classes.

Hazard Class 4

Class 4	**Flammable solids, spontaneously combustible materials, and dangerous when wet materials**	
Division 4.1	Flammable solids	
Division 4.2	Spontaneously combustible materials	
Division 4.3	Dangerous when wet materials	

Figure 44-10 Hazard Class 4.

Hazard Class 5

Class 5	**Oxidizers and organic peroxides**	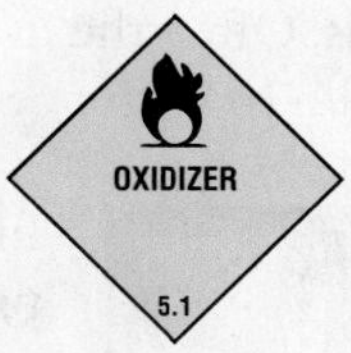
Division 5.1	Oxidizers	
Division 5.2	Organic peroxides	

Figure 44-11 Hazard Class 5.

Hazard Class 6

Class 6	**Toxic* materials and infectious substances**	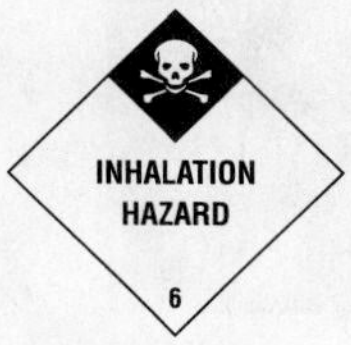
Division 6.1	Toxic* materials	
Division 6.2	Infectious substances	

Figure 44-12 Hazard Class 6.

Hazard Class 7

Class 7 No Divisions	**Radioactive materials**	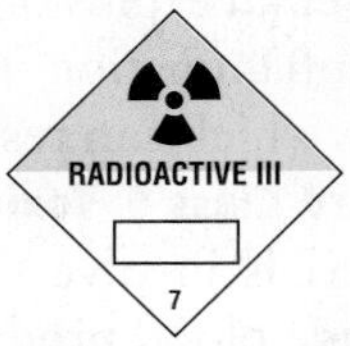

Figure 44-13 Hazard Class 7.

Hazard Class 8

Class 8 No Divisions	**Corrosive materials**	

Figure 44-14 Hazard Class 8.

Hazard Class 9

Class 9 Division 9.1 Division 9.2 Division 9.3	**Miscellaneous dangerous goods** Miscellaneous dangerous goods (Canada) Environmentally hazardous substances (Canada) Dangerous wastes (Canada)	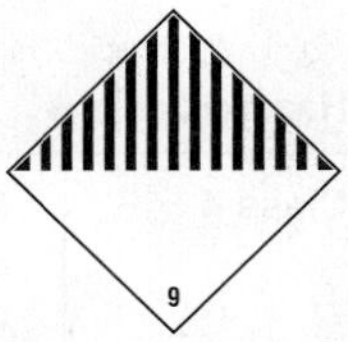

Figure 44-15 Hazard Class 9.

Approaching the Scene

44-7 Describe the safety considerations when responding to hazardous materials incidents.

When responding to a reported hazmat incident, it is good practice to call for a weather report from the local communications center. It is important to park upwind and uphill from the incident at a safe distance. Do not drive through leaking chemicals. Often the first responders assess the scene from a distance with binoculars (Figure 44-16 ■).

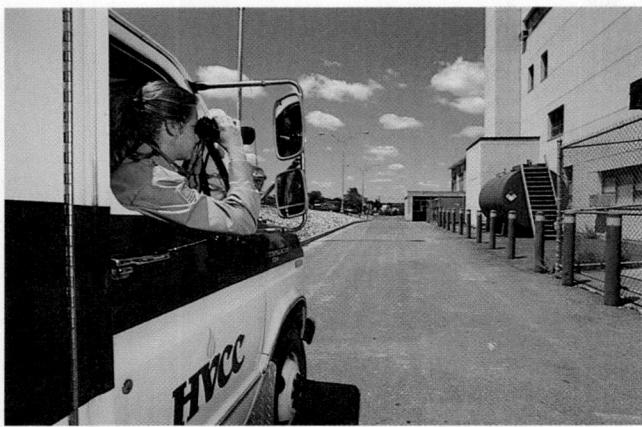

Figure 44-16 If available, use binoculars to try to identify any visible placards.

The first responders to a hazmat scene may include EMS, fire, and police resources. Typically they will not have the protective equipment or specialized expertise to fully react and mitigate a major hazmat situation. As a result, the initial response should involve recognizing the situation and then protecting responding crews and bystanders. The following include key responsibilities of the immediate response:

- Provide bystander safety.
- Identify the materials involved.
- Determine the risk or hazard posed by the spill.
- Call for additional resources, if necessary, to monitor and contain the spill.
- Isolate the scene, restrict or reroute traffic, and conduct evacuation, if necessary.
- Provide first aid, as needed.

- Fight the fire and protect against explosions (if properly trained and equipped).
- Keep the public informed of the hazard that exists, the actions being taken, precautionary measures to take, and evacuation routes and destinations (if necessary).
- Take overall scene safety and management responsibilities.

In many cases, the first responding EMS units will be limited to recognizing the event and then isolating the incident so as to deny entry into the area to all but specially equipped and trained personnel. In some cases you will need to direct patients to a decontamination area. *Do not enter an area contaminated by hazardous materials unless you are trained as a hazardous materials technician and have proper training in SCBA and other protective equipment.*

A 24-hour resource available to emergency responders is CHEMTREC. An emergency responder can call 1-800-424-9300 for immediate support on a hazmat emergency. CHEMTREC services are provided to emergency responders by the Chemical Manufacturers Association. They will provide notification to the shipper and can obtain emergency information from federal and industry resources.

PERSPECTIVE

John—The Firefighter

I can't believe we did that. We've been trained and trained and trained about stuff like that, and yet there we were, just running right in. I was thinking the guy was a full arrest or something, you know? I've been with the department for 22 years and there have never been any problems at that plant. I wasn't thinking hazmat. We just didn't consider all the possibilities. I remember for just a split second I thought I smelled rotten eggs. But then it was gone, just like that. Maybe I imagined it. Well, no, I guess I didn't.

STOP, REVIEW, REMEMBER!

Multiple Choice

For each question, place a check next to the correct answer.

1. You should safely evaluate a motor-vehicle collision with potential hazmat involvement from a distance, using your ______________ to access information on identified placards to set safety and containment zones.

_____ a. BLS

_____ b. MSDS

_____ c. ERG

_____ d. REG

2. A 32-year-old man has been found unconscious in the storeroom of a cleaning supply store. Upon entering the room, you note a strong odor of bleach and find that your eyes are burning. You should:

_____ a. find the patient and then immediately remove him from the building.

_____ b. immediately leave the building and contact the hazmat team.

_____ c. attempt to identify the source of the odor and write down its chemical name.

_____ d. continue treatment but request additional resources in case you are overcome by the fumes.

(continued on next page)

(continued)

3. Which one of the following injures or kills by disrupting the nervous system or cellular functions?
   _____ a. Radioactive materials
   _____ b. Flammable solids
   _____ c. Corrosive materials
   _____ d. Flammable gases

4. Which one of the following can trigger an explosion and also act as a corrosive destroying tissue and triggering inflammation in the lungs?
   _____ a. Flammable gases
   _____ b. Toxic materials and infectious substances
   _____ c. Oxidizers and organic peroxides
   _____ d. Flammable solids

5. Which one of the following would be considered a primary responsibility of first-responding EMS units at an unknown hazardous materials incident?
   _____ a. Controlling the source of the hazmat spill
   _____ b. Restricting access to the scene
   _____ c. Treating contaminated patients within the scene
   _____ d. Entering the scene to identify the specific hazardous material

Matching

Match the term on the left with the applicable definition on the right.

1. _____	Hazard Class 1	A. Miscellaneous
2. _____	Hazard Class 2	B. Corrosive materials
3. _____	Hazard Class 3	C. Radioactive materials
4. _____	Hazard Class 4	D. Toxic
5. _____	Hazard Class 5	E. Oxidizers
6. _____	Hazard Class 6	F. Flammable solids
7. _____	Hazard Class 7	G. Flammable liquids
8. _____	Hazard Class 8	H. Gases
9. _____	Hazard Class 9	I. Explosive

Critical Thinking

1. Why should you evaluate a potentially hazardous scene from a distance using your *Emergency Response Guidebook* and binoculars?

____

____

____

____

2. You have identified an explosive placard in your *Emergency Response Guidebook* that requires a 1,500-foot safety perimeter. Describe the necessary steps to create this perimeter.

____

____

____

____

PERSPECTIVE

Maya—The EMT

That absolutely scared me to death! You should've seen it! Those firefighters were down in a matter of seconds. I really thought they were dead and that Austin and I were next. That hazmat stuff is scary, and it can just sneak up on you, you know? What did I learn? I'll tell you what I learned. To think through all the possibilities of each call before going in. Heck, if those firefighters had stayed conscious for a little longer before they went down, we would have been lying right next to them. I hate to admit it, but I guess I've been in the habit of just following other people into calls. Police, fire, and even my partner. I swear that my size ups are going to be much more thorough from now on!

Operations at a Hazmat Incident

There are many phases to a hazmat response and the complexity of the response plan is directly linked to the level of the threat. Some situations can be handled easily with local resources, while other more dangerous situations will require specialized regional resources. In general, hazmat operations involve the following elements:

44-8 Discuss the components of hazardous materials incident management: preincident planning, considerations in implementing the plan, establishing safety zones, and emergency procedures, including decontamination, that should take place in each zone.

- ***Preincident planning.*** Many response districts contain locations, businesses, and industries that routinely handle hazardous materials. Although the vast majority of them handle them safely, preincident planning can help make a hazmat response far safer and much simpler. Elements of a plan include identification of existing hazards, review of specific handling and safety procedures, response planning, and identification of necessary specialized resources. Most businesses are more than willing to participate in preincident planning sessions because it will likely be their personnel involved if one occurs. Preincident planning should also include high-threat areas such as those considered high risk to terrorist activity.
- ***Considerations in implementing the plan.*** Considerations that must be included in any response plan include safety, securing the scene, and requesting the appropriate type and amount of specialized resources. Any hazmat response plan is significantly enhanced by early identification of the hazardous material. Although this should be done only if safety allows, it should be considered early. Also, remember when enacting a hazmat plan that other affected resources should be notified. Consider early discussion with hospitals, law enforcement, and even environmental protection agencies.

- ***Establishing safety zones.*** One of the most important tactics involved with responding to a hazmat incident is the early establishment of safety zones. As with other dangerous situations, the *hot zone* would include the area where the actual hazardous material is located. Only specially trained and protected personnel will enter it. It is where hazmat technicians will work to contain and stop the hazardous materials leak. The *warm zone* would include areas where contamination is less likely but still possible. Decontamination of patients typically takes place in there. The *cold zone* is the area where no contamination is typically possible and is the safety perimeter established early to prevent further injury. EMS units typically work in the cold zone.

Hazmat incidents require specialized responses. Frequently, a specially trained and equipped hazmat team will handle rescue and any mitigation efforts. Because responses often become a complicated combination of resources, ICS plays a vital role. As stated previously, the first responding units have important responsibilities. Whether they are EMS, fire, or law enforcement, they likely will establish command and restrict access. As more-specialized units respond, command will likely be turned over to better prepared resources.

Within the incident command structure of a hazmat situation EMS can play any number of roles. With specialized training, an EMT might become a member of the hazmat response team. In other situations, an EMS group might be utilized to support, monitor, and provide rehabilitation services to the operations of the entry team. An EMS group also should be utilized to triage and treat patients.

Unless specially trained, EMS generally works in the cold zone. The cold zone is the area free from hazardous materials. If patients have been exposed, the hazmat team will hand them off only after completing the decontamination process.

44-6 Differentiate between the levels of hazardous materials training identified by the Occupational Safety and Health Administration.

First Responder Awareness Level minimum level of hazmat training an EMT should receive; responders are trained to recognize a problem and initiate a response from an agency with operational-level training.

Hazardous Materials First Responder Operations Level level of hazmat training that includes procedures to contain and keep hazardous materials from spreading and to prevent exposures to people, property, and the environment. At this level first responders wear and operate in level B protection.

Hazardous Materials Technician Level level of advanced hazmat training that focuses on controlling a spill and operating in hazardous environments in chemical protective clothing and level A suits.

Hazardous Materials Specialist Level level of hazmat training that includes advanced knowledge of monitoring devices, toxicology, and command and control of large-scale hazmat incidents.

Hazardous Materials Training

The NFPA Standard 473 details the competencies for EMS providers at hazmat incidents and OSHA standard 29 CFR 1910.120 details the four levels of response for emergency responders. Training is required for all responders who may be called to a hazmat incident, with the EMT's employer having the responsibility to decide the level of training for each one.

The four levels of hazardous materials training for emergency responders are:

- The **First Responder Awareness Level,** which is the minimum training EMTs should receive, is designed to protect the first rescuers to respond to the scene. They are trained to recognize a problem and initiate a response from an agency with operational-level training.
- Training for the **Hazardous Materials First Responder Operations Level** includes procedures to contain and keep hazardous materials from spreading and to prevent exposures to people, property, and the environment. Training for the operations level requires first responders to wear and operate in protection and includes understanding how to decontaminate patients who have been exposed to hazardous materials.
- Training for the **Hazardous Materials Technician Level** is advanced training that teaches a first responder to control a spill and operate in hazardous environments in chemical protective clothing and suits.
- The highest level of training is the **Hazardous Materials Specialist Level.** Responders at this level are trained to have advanced knowledge of monitoring devices, toxicology, and command and control of large-scale hazmat incidents.

Decontamination

A person or item that has been exposed to a hazardous material is **contaminated** and can contaminate other people or items, the latter of which is called **cross-contamination.** For example, if you enter your car after being exposed to a toxic substance, you will contaminate your car.

Decontamination is the process of removing or neutralizing contaminants that have accumulated on people and equipment. At hazmat incidents, cold zones (clean areas) must be established and maintained, and materials in contaminated areas must be confined to specific hot zones (Figure 44-17 ▪). Response personnel who have had to enter the middle area—the warm zone (contamination-reduction zone)—must later remove their clothing and equipment, shower in fresh water, be rinsed with neutralizing agents, re-shower, and change into clean clothing (Figure 44-18 ▪). Station yourself in the cold zone, where equipment and other emergency rescuers should be staged adjacent to the warm zone.

The specific procedure for decontamination will vary according to the chemical to which the individual was exposed. Certain items—for example, leather and some plastic and rubber materials—absorb toxic substances so easily that they cannot be completely decontaminated. Those items must be discarded.

contaminated to have some hazardous material on the person or object.

cross-contamination exposure through contact with a contaminated person or object.

decontamination the process of removing or neutralizing contaminants from a person or object.

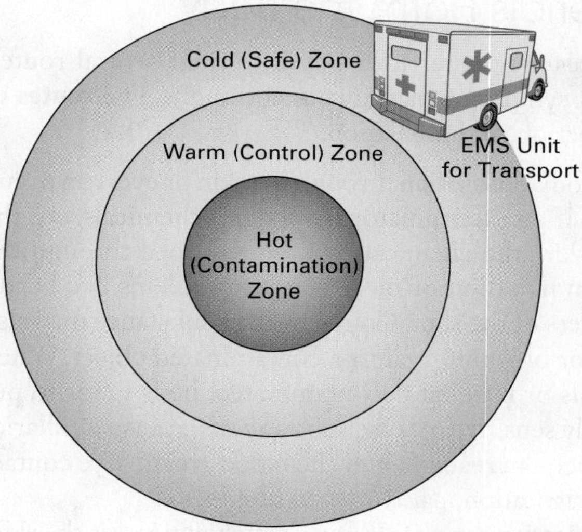

Hot (Contamination) Zone
Contamination is actually present.
Personnel must wear appropriate protective gear.
Number of rescuers limited to those absolutely necessary.
Bystanders never allowed.

Warm (Control) Zone
Area surrounding the contamination zone.
Vital to preventing spread of contamination.
Personnel must wear appropriate protective gear.
Life-saving emergency care is performed.

Cold (Safe) Zone
Normal triage, stabilization, and treatment performed.
Rescuers must shed contaminated gear before entering the cold zone.

Figure 44-17 Safety zones are established around the incident to minimize risk to rescuers.

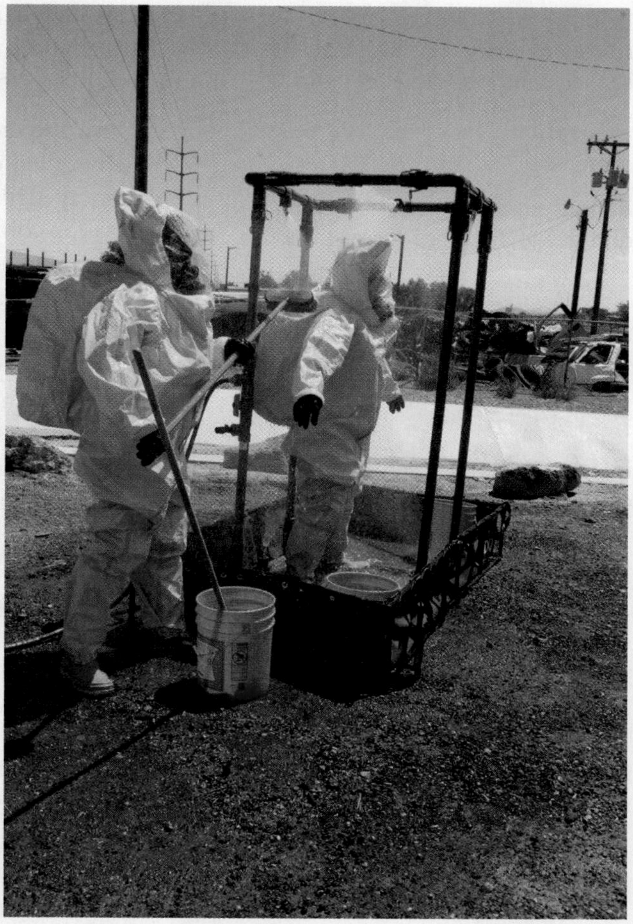

Figure 44-18 Decontamination at the scene of a hazardous materials incident.

Decontamination methods seek to:

- Physically remove contaminants
- Deactivate contaminants by chemical detoxification or disinfection/sterilization
- Remove contaminants through a combination of physical and chemical methods

If you believe the patient may be contaminated and is in need of immediate medical assistance, remove all of the patient's clothing, shower him thoroughly, and place him in a hospital gown. Advise *all* who come in contact with you that you may have been exposed to a toxic substance so they can take proper precautions. To avoid contaminating others, place any exposed clothing in a nonpermeable container without allowing it to contact other materials, and arrange for proper disposal. The steps you must take to decontaminate a patient are:

1. Wash down outer clothing (unless the chemical is water-reactive).
2. Remove clothing, working from the top down.
3. Wash down the entire body (unless the chemical is water-reactive).
4. Wrap up or dress the patient in clean clothing, preferably a hospital gown.
5. Discard contaminated clothing in a well-secured plastic bag.

If you have been or may have been contaminated by contact with the contaminated patient, follow the same steps for yourself.

How Hazardous Materials Harm the Body

Chemicals and hazardous substances may enter the body by any of several routes. The nature and onset of signs and symptoms may vary accordingly. The **routes of entry** are absorption, ingestion, injection, and inhalation.

routes of entry the ways that hazardous materials can enter the body.

absorption entry through the skin or eye.

dermal exposure when a chemical contacts and is absorbed through the skin.

injection entry through a puncture or open skin.

ingestion entry into the digestive system by eating or drinking.

inhalation entry by breathing into the lungs.

- When a chemical contacts the body, **absorption** through the skin or eyes can occur. This is called **dermal exposure.** If an exterminator is spraying chemicals and the overspray strikes unprotected skin, the chemicals will be absorbed through the skin. This could cause mild skin irritation or more serious problems like burns, sores, or ulcers on the outer layers of the skin. Contact with a substance may also occur by spilling it on the skin or brushing against a contaminated object. When a person is exposed to chemicals or is being decontaminated, he is never to put hand to eye. Eyes are particularly sensitive to toxic substances. Because capillaries are near the surface, the substance can readily enter the bloodstream. Eye contact with toxic substances can cause irritation, pain, or even blindness.
- The most familiar example of **injection** is a needle stick, which punctures the skin, allowing the substance to enter the body. Injection also can occur in other ways. For example, if a contaminated can or a piece of glass cuts the skin, the contaminant could be injected into the body. This is a very powerful means of exposure because the contaminant enters the bloodstream immediately.
- **Ingestion** occurs when a patient eats a substance that contains a harmful material and the substance enters the body by means of the digestive system. An example of this is the child who puts a toxic substance in his mouth out of curiosity. People also can ingest residue from chemicals that have been added to food to kill germs or parasites.
- It is also possible to be contaminated by **inhalation** when a patient breathes toxic substances into his lungs. Some chemicals have excellent warning properties. There is the well-known "rotten egg" smell of hydrogen sulfide, for example. But at high concentrations of that gas, the sense of smell is quickly lost. Many toxic substances, such as carbon monoxide, are both colorless and odorless, providing no sensory clues. Inhalation injuries are the most common of hazardous materials exposures and can be the most dangerous.

PERSPECTIVE

Austin—The EMT

Oh, man! Now that was a helpless feeling. I could see those firefighters and that sewer worker, and I knew that they were either dying or maybe already dead. But all I could do was stay with the ambulance and look at them through the binoculars. I sometimes have to remind myself that I'm not invincible, you know? I kept thinking that if I moved quickly enough or drove right up to them, I could get them out of there and still be okay. Of course, I know that's stupid, and safety is critical, but I'm in this job to help people, right? Not to just stand by and watch them die. It's just a really tough position to be in.

Pathway of Exposure

There are a number of ways in which contaminants escaping into the environment from their **source** may reach a living plant or animal, or **receptor.** The specific route a chemical might travel from a source to a receptor is called an **exposure pathway.** The pathway may be either a **direct pathway** or an **indirect pathway.** If an open toxic waste dump were near you, you could inhale the vapors from the toxic material, or your skin could contact toxic contaminants if you walked through the substance. Those are direct means of exposure. The substance also can reach you by an indirect pathway. For example, toxic vapors or particles from a site at which hazardous waste has been illegally discarded could be carried some distance in the air or water and deposited on crops or into the water supply.

Assessing Risk

The amount of risk associated with a particular source depends on the characteristics of the source, the availability of pathways for it to reach a receptor, and the characteristics of the receptors. No single piece of information alone is sufficient, and incomplete information can be highly misleading. Among the key questions that must be asked in determining risk are the following:

- What are the **hazardous properties** of the substance? What effects can it have on living things or the environment?
- What is the **concentration,** or how much of the substance exists at the source? A higher quantity or higher concentration of a toxic substance is more dangerous.
- In what **form** is the substance? Whether the substance is in large blocks or tiny particles, or whether it is a liquid or a vapor, will be important in determining not only how it might travel but also how it could contact and enter the body.
- What are the **chemical and physical characteristics** of the substance? These characteristics determine the environmental pathways in which it is likely to move and how rapidly (for example, whether or not the substance can dissolve easily in water).
- How is the substance **contained?** If a chemical is in old, rusting containers that can leak, the danger is clearly greater than if the container is solid and appropriate to the substance.
- What **pathways of exposure** exist? When scientists study the risk of exposure in any particular situation, they look at all the ways a contaminant could reach the population at risk and make measurements to see how much of it is moving through each identified path. For example, if the source were near a stream, water samples would be taken at several places to see what level of contamination exists at different distances from the source.
- What is the **duration,** or how long did the exposure to the contaminant last? Duration is another key factor in determining risk.

PRACTICAL PATHOPHYSIOLOGY

Chlorine is a chemical found throughout cities and towns. Exposure to chlorine gas causes immediate irritation to the eyes and upper respiratory tract. Eventually, the upper and lower airways begin to swell and the alveoli fill with fluid, disrupting gas exchange.

source initial location of the hazardous material.

receptor living plant or animal that is exposed to a hazardous substance.

exposure pathway specific route by which a chemical might travel from a source to a receptor.

direct pathway exposure resulting from contact with hazardous vapors or substances.

indirect pathway exposure resulting from taking in air, water, or food that has been contaminated by hazardous vapors or substances.

hazardous properties effects the hazardous materials can have on living things or the environment.

concentration how much of the substance exists at the source.

form refers to whether a hazardous material is in large blocks or tiny particles, or whether it is a liquid or a vapor.

chemical and physical characteristics qualities that determine the environmental pathways in which a hazardous material is likely to move and how rapidly.

contained stored.

pathways of exposure all the ways a contaminant could reach the population at risk.

duration how long the exposure to a contaminant lasted.

Toxic Effects

There have been many attempts to categorize or define toxic effects. Generally, the terms *acute* and *chronic* are used to delineate effects on the basis of severity or duration. **Acute exposure** is the exposure to a hazardous substance over a short period of time or at a high dose. A reaction to a chemical can occur at the time of exposure, and might include vomiting, eye irritation, or other symptoms that may be readily linked to a chemical exposure. Those symptoms are known as **immediate and adverse effects.** **Chronic exposure** is the exposure to a hazardous substance over a long period of time. If a carpenter used a stripper regularly and breathed in a little of it eight hours a day for 40 years, that would be a chronic exposure. The term *chronic effect* is often used to cover only three effects: a **carcinogenic** effect, which is an increase in an individual's risk of contracting cancer; a **mutagenic** effect, which is a mutation, or permanent change in the genetic material (DNA), which may be passed along to later generations; and a **teratogenic** effect, which is an increased risk that a developing embryo will have physical defects.

acute exposure exposure to a hazardous substance over a short period of time or at a high dose.

immediate and adverse effects reactions to a chemical that occur at the time of exposure, such as vomiting or eye irritation.

chronic exposure exposure to a hazardous substance over a long period of time.

carcinogenic causing an increased risk of contracting cancer.

mutagenic causing a mutation, which is a permanent change in the genetic material (DNA) that may be passed along to later generations.

teratogenic causing an increased risk that a developing embryo will have physical defects.

44-9 Describe special considerations in responding to and managing patients exposed to or contaminated with radiation.

44-10 Differentiate between radiation sickness, radiation injury, and radiation poisoning.

44-11 List factors that determine the amount of risk to patients and rescuers by a source of radiation.

Special Considerations: Radiation

Unlike many other hazardous materials, radioactive substances pose a risk at many levels. First, the radioactive material itself emits electromagnetic energy that can be powerful enough to kill. People who have come into contact with this type of energy are considered "exposed" to radiation. Secondly, if a radioactive material is transferred onto a patient, the patient himself will carry this radioactivity and emit harmful radiation as long as the substance remains on his body. The transfer of radioactive materials onto a person is considered "contamination." Both situations pose a major health risk and complicate rescue operations significantly.

Radiation is all around us. Each day you are exposed to radiation in the form of sunlight and other nonharmful electromagnetic energy. There are, however, sources of very harmful radiation that pose an immediate risk to well-being. Nuclear power plants, radioactive isotopes used in laboratory settings, and even weaponized radiation are very real concerns. In many cases, local sources of radiation will be identified by preincident planning, but just the same, you should be prepared to respond to situations in the event of an unexpected threat.

There are several dangers associated with exposure to radioactive substances. Because they are inherently unstable, radioactive substances constantly break down and emit energy in the form of radioactive particles and electromagnetic energy. Alpha particles travel only a few centimeters and generally cannot penetrate clothing. Beta particles travel farther and can pose a risk if exposure is long enough. Gamma energy poses the highest risk because these rays are emitted at great speeds and penetrate all but the densest materials. Gamma radiation can destroy and alter cells and is a major health hazard.

Alpha and beta particles can be easily protected against with simple shielding, but pose a great risk if they are inhaled or ingested. Gamma radiation poses its greatest risk simply through exposure to its energy.

The true dangers of radiation are directly linked to its concentration (how much energy is present) and the length of exposure. Some sources, such as X-ray machines emit radiation but pose little risk due to limited exposure.

The U.S. Centers for Disease Control describe the effects of harmful radiation under the umbrella term *acute radiation syndrome (ARS)*. ARS can affect the body in several different ways, over a long period of time and in the short term. Radiation injury results from rapid, high doses of radioactive energy and commonly occurs immediately or in the short-term setting. Typically, radiation injury is considered a local or partial body exposure. This injury most commonly results from direct contact with radioactive materials and causes burn-like injuries including blistering and reddening of the skin. Radiation injuries can be more systemic in nature in the context of massive doses of radiation, such as those caused by radioactive weapons. Radiation sickness and radiation poisoning are closely related and describe the ongoing complications associated with exposure to radiation. In addition to immediate injuries, radiation poisoning can affect any number of other body systems. Delayed effects include nausea, vomiting, hair loss, bleeding, and hypotension. In the long term, radiation sickness can cause higher rates of cancer and other illnesses.

Handling a radioactive situation calls for several special considerations. First, exposure to radiation does not require direct contact with the radioactive substance. Therefore, the safe perimeter may need to be substantially wider than in more common hazmat situations. Secondly, patients contaminated by radioactive materials will emit radiation as long as they remain contaminated. Decontamination is therefore a major concern. Finally, personal protective equipment does little to shield responders from the effects of gamma radiation. Providers must be protected by distance, significant shielding (concrete or lead, for example), or by limiting the time of exposure. These decisions will typically be directed through incident command, but as a first responder you must be aware of the inherent dangers.

44-12 Describe the importance of being knowledgeable about terrorist attacks involving weapons of mass destruction.

Special Considerations: Weapons of Mass Destruction

Unfortunately, not all hazmat situations are caused by accidents. In some cases the release of dangerous materials is done with the purpose of causing harm. Terrorists use hazardous materials to cause widespread injury, illness, and death. Such events also cause panic among populations, which can severely impact an EMS system. (Chapter 46 addresses terrorism incidents in more detail.) With regard to hazardous materials, providers should always consider the possibility of intent. In many ways these situations can be far more difficult to manage because they were specifically designed to cause maximum impact. Safety must be your highest priority.

PERSPECTIVE

Carl—The Hazmat Crew Leader

That's the worst I've seen it. I mean, in my own personal experiences. We got suited up, walked toward the gate, and wham! My H_2S sensor just starts screaming. It showed 500–600 parts per million hydrogen sulfide! And it was right there in the parking lot. That's just nuts! No wonder the fire crew crashed so quickly. They probably didn't even know anything was wrong until they woke up getting bagged. Well, at least they woke up. Obviously not everyone gets so lucky.

STOP, REVIEW, REMEMBER!

Multiple Choice

For each question, place a check next to the correct answer.

1. A patient spilled a toxic substance. He coughed, and his eyes immediately began to water. The patient was experiencing what type of exposure?

_____ a. Acute

_____ b. Chronic

_____ c. Septic

_____ d. Radioactive

2. You have just learned that a chemical to which a patient was exposed is a mutagen. What effect does this chemical have?

_____ a. Increases the risk of cancer

_____ b. Increases the risk of physical defects in a developing embryo

_____ c. Causes a permanent change in genetic material (DNA)

_____ d. Irritates the lining of the throat

(continued on next page)

(continued)

3. Gases can cause injury by displacing oxygen to cause:
   _____ a. CNS (central nervous system) depression.
   _____ b. irritation.
   _____ c. asphyxiation.
   _____ d. corrosion.

4. A farmer was spraying pesticides and not wearing long pants, a long-sleeved shirt, or gloves. The farmer developed nausea, vomiting, and shortness of breath. The poison most likely entered the body primarily by:
   _____ a. absorption.
   _____ b. injection.
   _____ c. ingestion.
   _____ d. inhalation.

5. If you inhale the vapors from toxic material, you have been contaminated by which exposure pathway?
   _____ a. Indirect
   _____ b. Source
   _____ c. Multi-direct
   _____ d. Direct

Matching

Match the term on the left with the applicable definition on the right.

1. _____ Awareness level		A. Includes training in patient decontamination
2. _____ Operational level		B. Teaches a responder to operate in hazardous environments
3. _____ Technician level		C. The minimum training an EMT should receive
4. _____ Specialist level		D. When a chemical is absorbed through the skin
5. _____ Absorption		E. Has advanced knowledge of hazardous materials
6. _____ Ingestion		F. The skin is punctured so that a substance can enter the body
7. _____ Injection		G. Route of entry by inhaling into the lungs
8. _____ Inhalation		H. Enters the body by means of the digestive system

Critical Thinking

1. When transporting a patient from a hazmat scene, it is important to remove all contaminants from the patient prior to transportation. Why?

____

____

____

____

2. What information is needed to assess risk of a hazardous materials exposure?

EMERGENCY DISPATCH SUMMARY

The hazmat crew quickly moved the patients to the green zone where ambulances waited to transport them. They were then able to trace the cause of the leak—an erroneously opened valve—and stop the release of hydrogen sulfide gas. All four firefighters were in respiratory arrest and transported with ventilatory assistance and oxygen. The plant worker, who was in cardiac arrest, was transported by an ALS crew, but never regained a pulse. Fire station 12 recently held a barbecue in honor of the two EMTs, whose quick thinking saved four of their own. And perhaps more.

Chapter Review

To the Point

- Safety is the most important priority in any hazardous materials event.
- Hazardous materials are omnipresent. Emergency responders must have a high index of suspicion and learn to recognize the signs of a hazmat incident.
- Hazardous materials can be recognized through standardized signs and warnings, but also through a thorough scene size-up including the use of all the senses.
- Identification of hazardous materials can greatly improve a response plan. However, this priority should be undertaken only if safety allows.
- Many resources exist to help the EMS provider identify hazardous materials. They include federal labeling requirements and signage, MSDS, and shipping manifests. Responders also should be familiar with the *Emergency Response Guidebook* and other resources at their disposal.
- Entering a hazmat scene requires specialized training and appropriate personal protective equipment.
- Effective strategies for responding to a hazmat situation include preincident planning, recognition, security, identification, response utilizing appropriate resources, and the establishment of safety zones.
- Special circumstances such as radiation and weapons of mass destruction pose increased risk for first responders. EMTs should always consider these possibilities and proceed with the greatest caution.

Chapter Questions

Multiple Choice

For each question, place a check next to the correct answer.

1. When dealing with a radioactive material, contamination generally refers to:
   _____ a. the material being transferred onto the patient.
   _____ b. excessive and prolonged exposure to gamma rays.
   _____ c. short, but powerful exposure to gamma rays.
   _____ d. being near a patient who has been contaminated.

2. You are first on scene at a chemical spill. As you arrive, you observe contaminated workers leaving the building. You should:
   _____ a. tell them to go immediately to the hospital.
   _____ b. gather them in the back of your ambulance.
   _____ c. establish a safety perimeter and have them stay in the warm zone.
   _____ d. tell them to go back into the building until you can identify the hazmat.

3. Responders may work in the warm (control) zone only if:
   _____ a. the patient is not contaminated.
   _____ b. they have entered by way of the cold zone.
   _____ c. they are in the proper protective clothing.
   _____ d. none of the above.

4. According to NFPA standards, which one of the following would be placed on the outside of an occupancy to warn of hazardous materials?
   _____ a. DOT placard
   _____ b. MSDS
   _____ c. Bill of lading
   _____ d. Diamond-shaped sign

5. The U.S. Department of Transportation placard that is approximately half black and half white identifies what hazard class?
   _____ a. Poison/poison gas
   _____ b. Blasting agents
   _____ c. Nonflammable gas
   _____ d. Corrosives

6. Hazards such as toxic gas will cause:
   _____ a. physical discomfort, but usually not permanent injury or death.
   _____ b. death, by causing irritation of the airway and lungs.
   _____ c. health hazards because they are so poisonous.
   _____ d. disease in humans.

7. A 31-year-old male patient has been exposed to a hazardous powder. He complains of burns and skin irritation. He has not yet been decontaminated. Which one of the following describes the correct procedure for decontaminating this patient?
   _____ a. Decontamination should occur only in the cold zone.
   _____ b. Decontamination involves scrubbing down only the outer layers of the patient's clothing.
   _____ c. Treatment of the patient's burns must begin before decontamination.
   _____ d. The patient should be stripped and flushed with water prior to leaving the warm zone.

Critical Thinking

1. What is the difference between a chronic and an acute exposure to a hazardous substance?

____

____

____

____

2. What are the four routes of exposure to a hazardous substance? Briefly describe how exposure through each route occurs.

Case Study

You and your partner have been dispatched to a hazmat incident at a chemical plant to transport victims to the hospital. The scene size-up given over the radio describes a ruptured gas storage tank with about 30 victims.

You arrive at the staging area and your unit is then directed to the decontamination treatment area. Your patient is a 33-year-old man who was exposed to hydrogen sulfide gas that was leaking from a storage tank. Hydrogen sulfide is a gas that smells like rotten eggs, that is slightly heavier than air, and that will stratify at or around the head and shoulders. The primary effect of hydrogen sulfide is that it is a cellular asphyxiant, which means that it stops the cells from correctly processing oxygen. The patient has been decontaminated by the hazmat team. He is dressed in the paper dressing gown from the hazmat team's decontamination area. His hair is wet and he is shivering.

Your patient's vital signs are respirations 30, pulse 118, and blood pressure 138/88. He is coughing and complains of difficulty breathing and nausea. His pupils are equal and reactive to light. His mucous membranes are slightly cyanotic. His neck veins are flat, chest has equal rise and fall, breath sounds reveal some crackles, and abdomen is soft and nontender. The patient obeys all commands and has good pulses to all extremities.

1. What will be the first steps of care you will provide?

2. What is your next step in assessment and action?

The Last Word

Hazmat responses, although rare, do occur in the line of duty. As an EMT you can expect to be involved in patient care or function in a support role in a hazmat incident. Remember that without special training in hazmat operations, your primary responsibility is to protect yourself and the public. Secure the scene safely from a distance. Use your binoculars and *Emergency Response Guidebook* to identify placards. Call in the hazmat response team. Then prepare to treat and transport decontaminated patients.

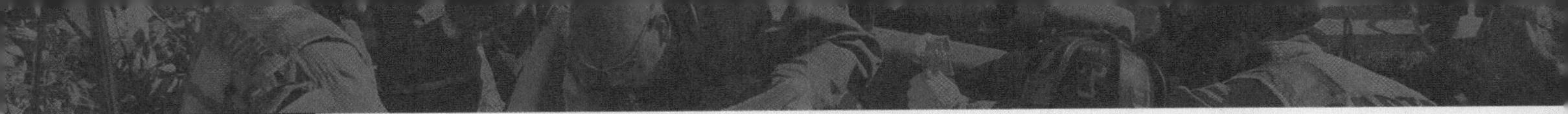

45 Vehicle Extrication and Air Medical Response

Education Standards

EMS Operations: Vehicle Extrication

Competencies

Applies knowledge of operational roles and responsibilities to ensure patient, public, and personnel safety.

Objectives

After completion of this lesson, you should be able to:

45-1 Define key terms introduced in this chapter.

45-2 List the nine classifications of technical rescue incidents identified by the NFPA.

45-3 Describe the elements of a scene size-up that involve a rescue situation.

45-4 Describe the components of a typical rescue response.

45-5 Describe the role of the EMT and basic considerations for caring for a patient entrapped in a vehicle, including the concepts of simple and complex access.

45-6 Describe equipment and methods for stabilizing an upright vehicle, a vehicle on its side, and a vehicle on its roof.

45-7 Describe various methods of accessing, disentangling, and extricating a patient entrapped in a vehicle.

45-8 Describe the common crew configurations within air medical transport.

45-9 Differentiate and discuss the benefits of both fixed-wing and rotor-wing air medical transport.

45-10 Describe the two types of rotor-wing air medical transport missions.

45-11 Explain the common criteria for choosing air medical transport over ground transport.

45-12 Differentiate between visual and instrument flight rules.

45-13 Describe the characteristics of an appropriate helicopter landing zone.

45-14 Explain the safe principles of working around aircraft at the scene of an emergency.

Key Terms

awareness level p. 1197
complex access p. 1203
cribbing p. 1203
crumple zones p. 1203
fixed-wing aircraft p. 1205
helipad p. 1207
instrument flight rules (IFR) p. 1209
interfacility transport (IFT) p. 1206
laminated glass p. 1203
landing zone (LZ) p. 1209
operational level p. 1198
rotor-wing aircraft p. 1205
safety glass p. 1203
scene call p. 1206
simple access p. 1203
step chocks p. 1203
technical rescue incidents p. 1197
technician level p. 1198
visual flight rules (VFR) p. 1208

Introduction

Incidents involving vehicle extrication require unique skills and specialized training and education. As an EMT you may not have the appropriate training to initiate operations but you must know when to call in the appropriate resources. You may be asked to care for a patient during extrication or to assist more highly trained personnel during a specialized operation. This chapter introduces you to the basic concepts related to rescue, extrication, and other common types of special operations.

Air medical resources are a valuable resource when transportation by a ground ambulance may be delayed or extended. This chapter introduces you to the common air medical resources and the guidelines for their use.

EMERGENCY DISPATCH

"Be careful!" a firefighter shouted as the second ambulance on scene rolled to a stop. "There's glass everywhere." EMT Claire Owen stepped from the truck and sized up the scene while pulling on a pair of exam gloves. She stood in the middle of a notorious intersection known as the "Terrible T," a location so well known to local emergency personnel that dispatch would commonly just say, "Accident at the T," when summoning crews.

"It looks like that little car and that glass truck hit head on." Claire's partner, EMT Ray Parker, pointed as they moved the cot toward the busy rescue crew. "But I've never seen anything like that." The glass truck, its racks now empty, sat awkwardly off to one side of the road and the small car was overturned, resting partially up the embankment. The car was surrounded in all directions by large shards of broken glass, embedded upright into the soft soil and pointing skyward. Their clear, sharp blades, glinting brightly in the early morning sunlight, prevented access to the car and its injured driver.

"We've got the guy from the truck," EMT Perry Bose said as he and his partner strapped the bloody man onto a long backboard. "You guys are here for the lady in the car. It's gonna be a few minutes." Claire and Ray stopped at the edge of the road and watched as the fire crew dislodged and removed shard after shard of glass, slowly clearing a path to the overturned vehicle.

"Why isn't anyone helping me?" The woman screamed from the car. "I'm bleeding and my leg is stuck and it really hurts!"

"We're coming, Ma'am," one of the firefighters yelled back, tossing a large piece of glass onto the pile at the edge of the road. "We're going to help you as quickly as we can!"

"Hey Claire," Ray said, peering into the car from different angles. "Can you do me a favor and grab my turnout coat, helmet, and leather gloves? Once they get that thing cribbed, I think I'm going to have to get in through the back window."

Rescue Incidents

According to the National Fire Protection Association (NFPA), the nine classifications of **technical rescue incidents** are:

- Vehicle and machinery rescue
- Wilderness search and rescue
- Water/surf/ice rescue
- Dive rescue
- Trench rescue
- Collapse rescue
- Rope rescue
- Confined space rescue
- Any other rescue operation requiring specialized training

45-2 List the nine classifications of technical rescue incidents identified by the NFPA.

technical rescue incidents rescue situations requiring specialized training and equipment.

Interagency cooperation is essential for the successful completion of many technical rescue incidents. All personnel involved in a complicated rescue operation will most likely be operating under an incident management system (ICS).

Consensus standards from the NFPA identify the need to be trained to the awareness level. Training to the **awareness level** represents the minimum capabilities

awareness level level of training that represents the minimum capabilities of a responder who, in the course of duty, could be called on to respond to or be first on scene of a technical rescue incident.

of a responder who could be called on to respond to or be first on scene of a technical rescue incident. Awareness-level operations may involve search, rescue, and recovery of victims in technical rescue incidents. EMTs trained to this level generally do not act as rescuers but rather as support personnel for the operation.

operational level level of training that is designed for responders who will be responsible for hazard recognition, equipment use, and techniques necessary to conduct a technical rescue.

technician level level of training that is designed for responders who will be capable of hazard recognition, equipment use, techniques necessary to perform, and supervision of a technical rescue incident.

Operational level training is designed for responders who are trained in hazard recognition, equipment use, and techniques necessary to conduct a technical rescue. Rescue operations are usually supervised by a rescuer certified at the **technician level.** Those with technician-level certification are capable of hazard recognition, equipment use, techniques necessary to perform, and supervision of a technical rescue incident.

CLINICAL CLUE

Focus on Patient Care

As an EMT participating in an incident requiring rescue or extrication, your primary role will be one of patient care. In most cases those with specialized training will conduct the rescue and bring the patient to you. In other cases you may be asked to initiate emergency care prior to and during extrication. Be sure to don the appropriate PPE before entering the scene.

Scene Safety

Scene safety at a technical rescue involves the assessment and analysis of victims. A live victim means a rescue with its associated high level of urgency. A deceased victim, however, suggests a far less urgent response. You must follow standard safety procedures when making a rescue. As always, it is critical to ensure your own safety as well as the safety of your team or partner and other responders. Many fatalities of emergency responders have occurred when responders rushed to help victims and entered unsafe environments.

Sizing Up the Scene

45-3 Describe the elements of a scene size-up that involve a rescue situation.

Scene size-up in rescue operations is not much different than what you have already learned. It includes confirming the exact location, the nature of the incident, the number and condition of victims, and the risks versus benefits that will dictate a rescue or a body recovery. The difference is determining the appropriate resources for the type of incident. The sooner you request resources, the sooner they can arrive and help you initiate a safe rescue.

PERSPECTIVE

Perry—The EMT

We were the first ones on scene this morning. Kirk went to check on the guy in the truck, and I was going to check out the overturned car, but all that glass stopped me. I started to kind of kick some of it down but then this one piece cut right through the side of my boot. Oh man, once I saw my sock sticking out, I realized I totally wasn't equipped to do what I was trying to do. So I got on the radio and explained the whole thing to dispatch. They sent out the rescue crew and Claire's ambulance while we started helping the guy in the glass truck. I hope someone got a picture of all that broken glass just standing upright around that car. I've never seen anything like that before.

You need to know the resources for each type of incident and where they are in your local jurisdiction. Call for the appropriate resources as soon as possible. In some EMS systems a predefined response matrix sends a specific set of resources to the scene based on the incident type and information from the reporting party. This may include fire department resources, specialized rescue teams, hazmat teams, and air medical resources. Often public works, utility companies, and law enforcement will be needed at the scene as well.

Vehicle Extrication

Rescuing victims from motor vehicles is the most frequent response for EMS personnel. Each and every incident requires a thorough size up of the scene for immediate and potential hazards.

When approaching a vehicle collision, note the scope and magnitude of the incident. It is a critical function of the EMT to determine if the incident can be handled by the normal responding units or if specialized resources are required. The number, size, and type of vehicles involved are key pieces of information that can help in determining what additional resources are needed. Specialized rescue tools often are required for collisions involving entrapped victims. The integrity of a vehicle and its stability are important pieces of information. A vehicle on its roof is inherently unstable and will almost always have a fluid leak. A vehicle on its side presents the same challenges. The number of victims at the scene dictates the number of ambulances and additional resources to request.

Identify any issues related to accessing patients, such as cars located at the bottom of embankments or vehicles that crashed into a building. Report any hazards to other rescuers and responders, such as downed electrical wires or other exposed utilities, fluid leaks, or traffic (Figure 45-1 ■). Pay special attention to electrical hazards. In older residential developments there are overhead wire systems. In newer developments there are underground systems with pad-mounted electrical transformers set on the ground that, if damaged, can become a significant hazard.

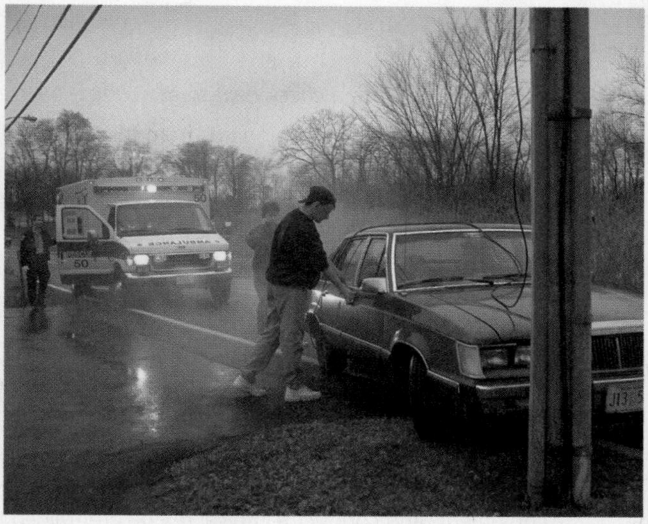

Figure 45-1 Downed power lines are an immediate hazard at the scene of many vehicle collisions. Do not approach the scene until it is safe to do so.

Make sure to note any hazardous traffic conditions. Freeway or highway responses have become one of the most dangerous environments for EMTs and rescue personnel. When placing emergency vehicles at a collision scene, it is important to block approaching traffic with an emergency vehicle parked at a 45-degree angle. In most cases, it is preferred that the blocking vehicle be a fire truck and that the ambulance pull past the blocking vehicle to protect the rescuers who are loading patients (Figure 45-2 ■). The safety zone should be extended when the emergency scene is on the round of a curve, on the opposite side of the crest of a hill, or in poor weather conditions. Vehicles should be uphill and upwind from any fuel leak or hazardous materials release.

Many vehicle and machinery incidents present with unique challenges. For example, hybrid electric vehicles present an electric shock hazard and natural-gas or propane vehicles present explosive hazards.

CLINICAL CLUE

Electrical Hazards

Remember that metal guardrails, other vehicles, and water conduct electricity if they are close to the vehicles that are energized. Do not attempt to move power lines or electrical equipment. Maintain a safe distance and have utility crews cut the power before accessing the crash vehicle.

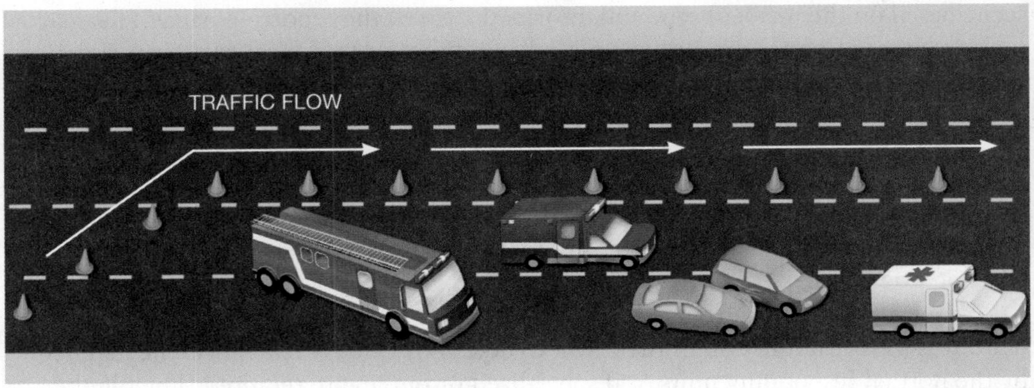

Figure 45-2 Use a larger rescue vehicle to block the scene and place the ambulance ahead for easy patient loading and egress.

STOP, REVIEW, REMEMBER!

Multiple Choice

For each question, place a check next to the correct answer.

1. Based on the consensus standards from the National Fire Protection Association, the minimum training requirement for EMS personnel at a technical rescue incident is the ______________ level.

   _____ a. awareness
   _____ b. operations
   _____ c. technician
   _____ d. specialist

2. Rescuers trained to recognize hazards, utilize specialized equipment, and conduct technical rescue are trained to the ______________ level.

   _____ a. operational
   _____ b. technician
   _____ c. awareness
   _____ d. novice

3. When performing a scene size-up for an extrication or rescue incident, it is especially important to:

   _____ a. respond with lights and sirens.
   _____ b. quickly identify the need for additional resources.
   _____ c. quickly remove patients from the scene.
   _____ d. only enter the scene if law enforcement allows it.

4. All of the following are NFPA-recognized categories of technical rescue incidents *except:*

   _____ a. dive rescue.
   _____ b. search and rescue.
   _____ c. trench rescue.
   _____ d. aircraft rescue.

Fill in the Blank

1. List at least six immediate and potential hazards that may be encountered at a vehicle-collision incident.

____

____

____

____

Critical Thinking

1. You and your partner are the first vehicle to arrive at the scene of a vehicle collision on a blind curve. What should you do?

2. What technical rescue resources are available in your community?

Fundamentals of Patient Extrication

45-4 Describe the components of a typical rescue response.

The role of the EMT is to assist rescuers in the process of removing entrapped patients from vehicles, building collapses, and other scenarios that keep a patient from self-extricating. The following steps make up a typical rescue response:

1. Prepare for the rescue.
2. Size up the situation.
3. Identify and manage hazards.
4. Stabilize the vehicle prior to entering.
5. Gain access to the patient.
6. Perform a primary and secondary assessment.
7. Disentangle the patient.
8. Immobilize and extricate the patient from the vehicle.
9. Provide emergency care and transport.
10. Terminate the rescue.

Preparing for the Extrication

Your role in a vehicle rescue depends on your agency's responsibility and your specific assignment by the on-scene incident commander (IC). As an EMT in a non-rescue role, you are responsible for administering patient care prior to the extrication and for assisting the rescue personnel in determining the most appropriate way to remove the patient. Preventing or minimizing further injury is a primary responsibility of the EMT.

In some cases the EMT is part of the rescue team and, if so, should receive specialized training in vehicle extrication. Vehicle rescue technicians typically receive 40 hours or so of vehicle rescue training. The EMT should cooperate with the activities of the rescuers but not allow those activities to interfere with patient care.

If you are an EMT functioning as part of a rescue team, often you are working under a chain of command and being given direction by fire or rescue squad officers. The chain of command ensures that patient care is coordinated with removing the patient in a way that minimizes further injury.

PERSPECTIVE

Ray—The EMT

I think that extricating patients from overturned vehicles is probably the toughest thing to do in our line of work. I mean, think about it. You've got this injured person with a busted leg—a possible spine injury—and just bleeding everywhere. And, oh, guess what? He's hanging upside down. Think about it for a minute. How do we cut him down and get him out of the car—all while trying to keep that closed fracture closed, maintaining spinal immobilization, and not injuring him more than he already is? Or hurting ourselves. Don't forget that one!

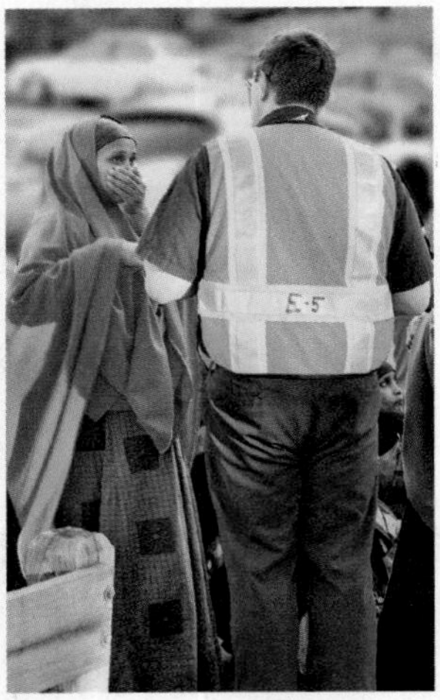

Figure 45-3 High visibility reflective vests are an important safety device when working on active roadways. (© Dan Limmer)

Personal safety is the number-one priority for you and all EMS personnel. Protective clothing that is appropriate for the situation should be used by rescue and EMS personnel (Figure 45-3 ■). If you are involved with extrication, you should wear firefighter turnout or brush clothing, a helmet, and eye protection.

Modern vehicles are made from composite fibers. Glass and composite fibers release particles that are hazardous if inhaled, so EMTs should wear a particle mask when cutting through these materials. When using firefighting gloves for extrication and treating a patient, it is important to wear medical gloves under them to ensure that blood does not soak through and expose the EMT to potential infection. Finally, a federal law that went into effect in 2008 requires all responders to incidents on a roadway to wear an approved high-visibility vest or jacket. Since most vehicle collisions are on the roadway, protect yourself and be alert to the possibility of inattentive or distracted drivers.

Safeguarding the Patient

45-5 Describe the role of the EMT and basic considerations for caring for a patient entrapped in a vehicle, including the concepts of simple and complex access.

Once measures have been taken to ensure responder safety, focus on patient safety. Emergency medical care precedes extrication unless a delay would endanger the life of the patient. If the patient has airway compromise or a life-threatening injury, or if there is a hazard that can cause additional injury or death, you should rapidly remove the patient.

If responsive, the patient should be informed of the extrication process. This helps minimize the fear associated with the noises that accompany a difficult extrication. It also is important that the patient be protected from hazards such as glass and sharp metal during the extrication process.

Precaution should be taken to ensure that air bags, seat belt actuators, and power sources are disabled in vehicles involved in a collision. Firefighters and EMTs have been injured when air bags activated during the rescue process.

If the rescue crews are using hydraulic extrication equipment, the EMT should monitor the action to ensure that metal and glass do not come in contact with the patient. Several techniques or pieces of rescue equipment can be used to protect the patient. Long and short backboards can be positioned as shields. Commercial rescue blankets and lightweight tarps are all acceptable choices to protect the patient during rescue operations.

Stabilizing the Vehicle

Even upright vehicles can be unstable. Make sure the vehicle ignition is turned off as part of securing the scene. A common practice is to deflate the tires and place the car on **step chocks** or **cribbing** (Figures 45-4 ■ and 45-5 ■). Tire deflation is best accomplished by pulling the valve stems to preserve the tire for later investigation. This procedure also prevents any rocking motion created by rescue efforts. Blocks or cribbing should be placed on each side of the vehicle. As an added measure of safety, cribbing can be placed in the front and rear of the vehicle.

Keep in mind that a vehicle on its side is inherently unstable and is a real danger to rescuers but can be stabilized with cribbing and struts (Figure 45-6 ■).

45-6 Describe equipment and methods for stabilizing an upright vehicle, a vehicle on its side, and a vehicle on its roof.

step chocks wooden blocks or other supportive materials placed in a stair-step pattern to assist in stabilizing a vehicle.

cribbing wooden blocks or other supportive materials placed in a box pattern (crib) to assist in stabilizing a vehicle.

Access

There are two types of access to the patient. The first is **simple access,** which does not require equipment. Have the patient unlock doors if possible. Try opening each door yourself, if safe to do so. If the doors do not open, roll down the windows.

Complex access requires the use of tools or special equipment. In complex access, you and the rescuers will follow a step-by-step process to gain access to the patient. The first step is to size up the vehicle design. New vehicle technologies pose new hazards. The front and rear compartments of modern vehicles have been reinforced. They have been designed to deflect the wheels, engine, hood, and trunk away from the passenger compartment. **Crumple zones** that absorb energy are now welded into the frame, minimizing the transmission of crash energy to the passenger compartment. Reinforced dash and side-injury protection bars, designed to encapsulate the passengers, can make access difficult.

If simple access methods do not work, removing glass will be the second action taken to gain access to an entrapped victim. Glass is a significant hazard to the rescuer. There are two types of glass in vehicles: laminated glass and safety glass. **Laminated glass** is present in the front windshield and occasionally in the rear windshield. Laminated glass has a layer of glue, plastic, or mastic sandwiched between two pieces of glass and must be cut. A flat-head axe, saw, or commercial glass cutter can be used to remove laminated glass. **Safety glass** is present in the side windows and often in the rear windows. When struck, safety glass will break into small rounded pieces, not the sharp shards formed by other kinds of glass. When removing either laminated or safety glass, make sure the patient and rescuers are protected.

45-7 Describe various methods of accessing, disentangling, and extricating a patient entrapped in a vehicle.

simple access means of getting into a vehicle that does not require specialized training, tools, or equipment.

complex access means of getting into a vehicle that requires specialized training, tools, or equipment.

crumple zones vehicle parts that are designed to collapse, allowing for the crash energy to be absorbed rather than being transmitted to the passenger compartment.

laminated glass type of glass that has a layer of glue, plastic, or mastic sandwiched between two pieces of glass.

safety glass type of glass that, when struck, will break into small pieces. Also called *tempered glass.*

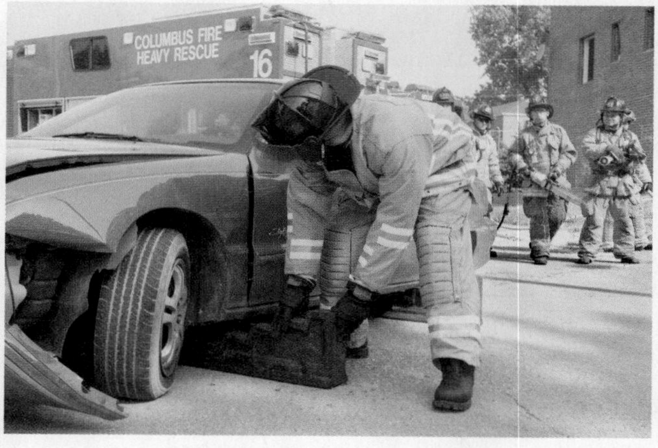

Figure 45-4 Step blocks are an efficient means for stabilizing a vehicle.

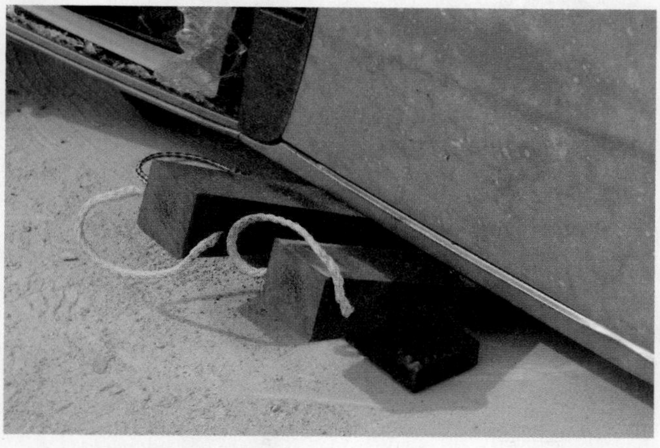

Figure 45-5 Cribbing can be used to stabilize a vehicle prior to extrication.

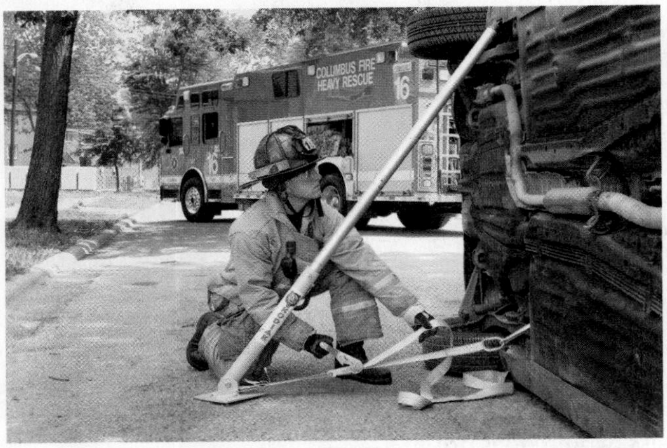

Figure 45-6 Specialized struts are used to stabilize a vehicle on its side prior to extricating the patients.

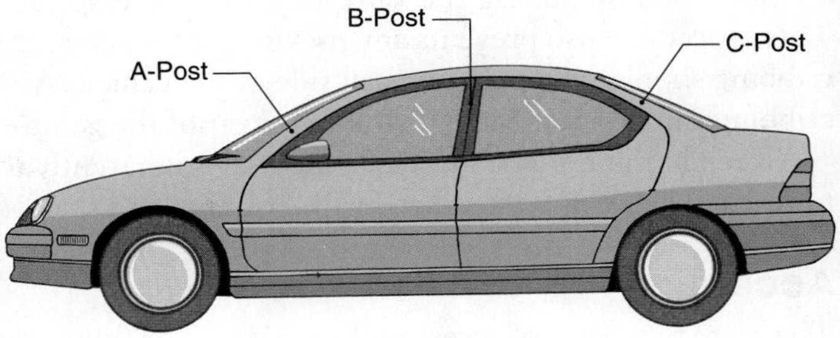

Figure 45-7 Vehicle doorpost designations.

If access cannot be achieved by breaking glass, rescuers can pry open a door. An assortment of tools are made for this procedure. In most cases a pry bar, saw, or hydraulic spreader can force the latching mechanism. However, the side-injury protection bars in some vehicles make it difficult to pry the door open.

If forcing the door becomes too time consuming, you and the rescuers may opt to remove the roof and lift the patient out. The A and B posts in modern vehicles are very strong, being designed to support the weight of the vehicle if it turns upside down (Figure 45-7 ■). So, removing the roof requires a hydraulic cutter or reciprocating saw to cut through the A and B posts, with a relief cut to the roof behind the B post to fold the roof back. When cutting the B post, rescuers should be cautious not to cut the seat belt tensioner. The seat belt tensioner is a pressurized cylinder that can explode if it is cut. Also, the roof should be secured with rope to prevent the wind from flapping it back onto the rescue team. Glass should be removed to prevent injury.

A final procedure that may be necessary for severely trapped patients is a dash roll-up. In some collisions, the dash pins the patient's lower extremities and pelvis. The rescue team will make a relief cut to weaken the metal on both sides close to the bottom of the front hinge after the door has been removed. A hydraulic ram is then placed in the door panel and the dash is pushed off the patient. Often this creates an obstruction, and the patient may need to be lifted vertically to a long backboard. You must constantly check in with your patient to ensure you are not causing undo discomfort.

STOP, REVIEW, REMEMBER!

Multiple Choice

For each question, place a check next to the correct answer.

1. Which one of the following is an example of a simple access technique?

_____ a. Cutting door posts

_____ b. Prying a door open

_____ c. Unlocking and opening a door

_____ d. Asking the patient to self-extricate

2. A window in a vehicle that has a layer of plastic, glue, or mastic between two sheets of glass is called _____________ glass.

_____ a. laminated

_____ b. safety

_____ c. lexan

_____ d. impact-resistant

3. During a complicated extrication, the patient should be protected from glass and metal with:

_____ a. a sheet.

_____ b. some plastic.

_____ c. a rescue blanket.

_____ d. nothing, because a cover will frighten the patient.

Labeling

Identify the doorpost designations used for vehicle extrication.

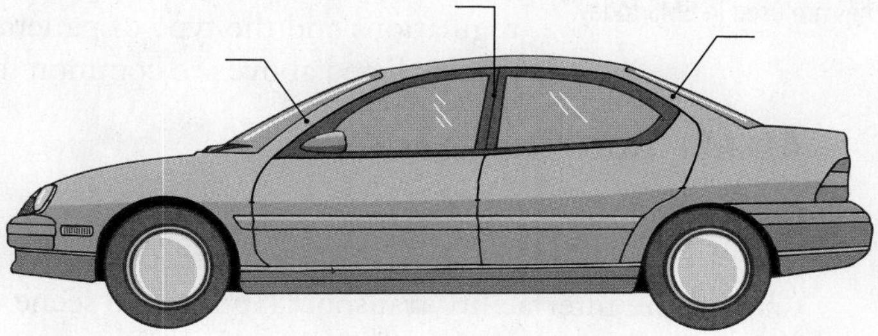

Critical Thinking

1. What are the potential dangers to rescuers that can occur during a vehicle rescue operation?

___

___

___

___

2. What is the sequence for gaining access to a vehicle?

___

___

___

___

Air Medical Operations

Many EMS systems across the United States use air medical resources such as **rotor-wing aircraft** (helicopters) and **fixed-wing aircraft** (airplanes) to transport critically ill and injured patients (Figure 45-8 ■). It is estimated that there are approximately 500,000 patients transported by helicopter and another 150,000 transported by airplane each year. Although it is uncommon for an EMT to be hired to work on an EMS aircraft, your current training can be the first step in becoming qualified to eventually gain employment with an air medical organization. However, as an EMT, you may be in a position to request a helicopter or at the very least assist in the landing of a helicopter at the scene of an emergency.

rotor-wing aircraft a helicopter.

fixed-wing aircraft an airplane.

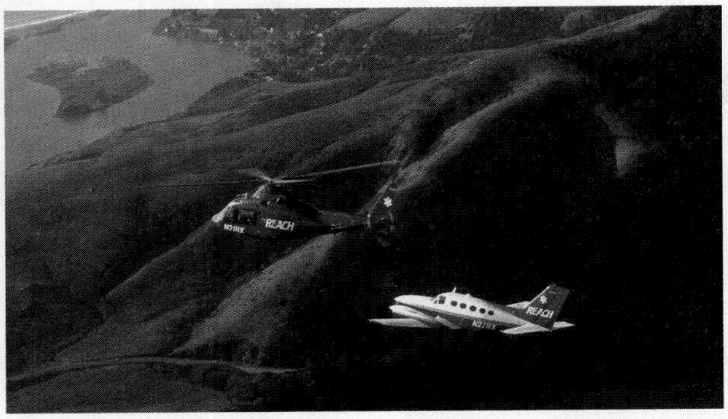

Figure 45-8 Both helicopters and airplanes are used in EMS today. (© REACH Air Medical Services, LLC/Tony Irvin)

Crew Configurations

The majority of EMS aircraft being flown in the United States are staffed with a nurse and a paramedic. The following is a list of other common medical crew configurations:

- Nurse and paramedic
- Nurse and nurse
- Doctor and nurse
- Nurse and respiratory therapist
- Paramedic and paramedic.

The specific crew configuration is often determined by local regulations and the type of patient being cared for. The configurations listed above are common for both helicopters and planes.

45-8 Describe the common crew configurations within air medical transport.

45-9 Differentiate and discuss the benefits of both fixed-wing and rotor-wing air medical transport.

45-10 Describe the two types of rotor-wing air medical transport missions.

scene call an emergency scene that occurs outside of a hospital.

Air Medical Resources

Rotor-Wing Resources

Most rotor-wing resources in EMS (helicopters) fly two types of missions: the **scene call** and the interfacility transport (IFT). The scene call is made when a helicopter is requested to respond to the scene of an emergency, such as a vehicle collision or a drowning incident at a lake or the beach. In those cases, the helicopter is requested to respond to the scene just as a ground ambulance might. If all goes well, the helicopter will land near the patient, allowing the medical crew to exit the aircraft, begin caring for the patient, and prepare him for transport (Figure 45-9 ■).

> **CLINICAL CLUE**
>
> **Safe Operations**
>
> Helicopter scene call operations are very risky. It is important to use an experienced person to help choose an appropriate landing zone and assist with landing the helicopter. Position yourself so that you are always within eyesight of the pilot.

interfacility transport (IFT) the transportation of a patient from one hospital to another, typically for a higher level of care.

The **interfacility transport (IFT)** occurs when a patient is already at a hospital but needs to be transported to another hospital. In most cases, the patient is in need of a higher level of care than the sending hospital is capable of providing. For example, a patient with significant trauma transported by ground ambulance to a hospital five minutes away may need to be transported to the regional trauma center 60 miles away. An interfacility transport by aircraft would be required.

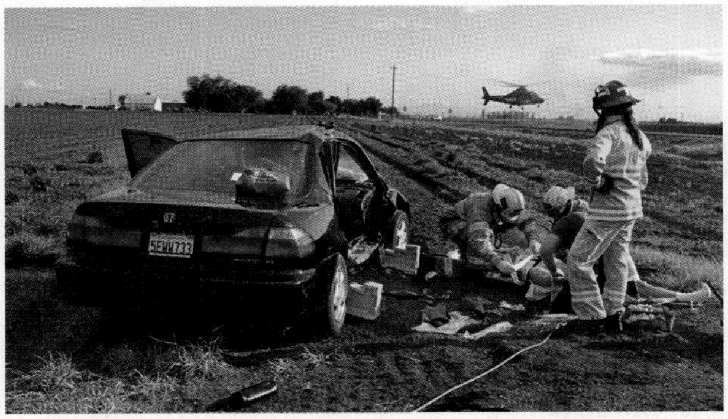

Figure 45-9 In many cases, a helicopter can land right at the emergency scene. (© REACH Air Medical Services, LLC/Rick Roach)

There are many different types of EMS helicopters in use today. They differ in many ways, including size, shape, number of engines, and how high or fast they can fly (Figure 45-10 ■). Regardless of size or performance capabilities, EMS helicopters all share one very important characteristic: they are designed to carry critically ill or injured patients. The vast majority of helicopters are configured to carry just one patient lying on a stretcher. Although some can carry two patients, the ability to provide care while in flight is greatly minimized due to the limited space. Because a helicopter can fly from hospital pad to hospital pad, it is ideal for short transports (under 200 miles).

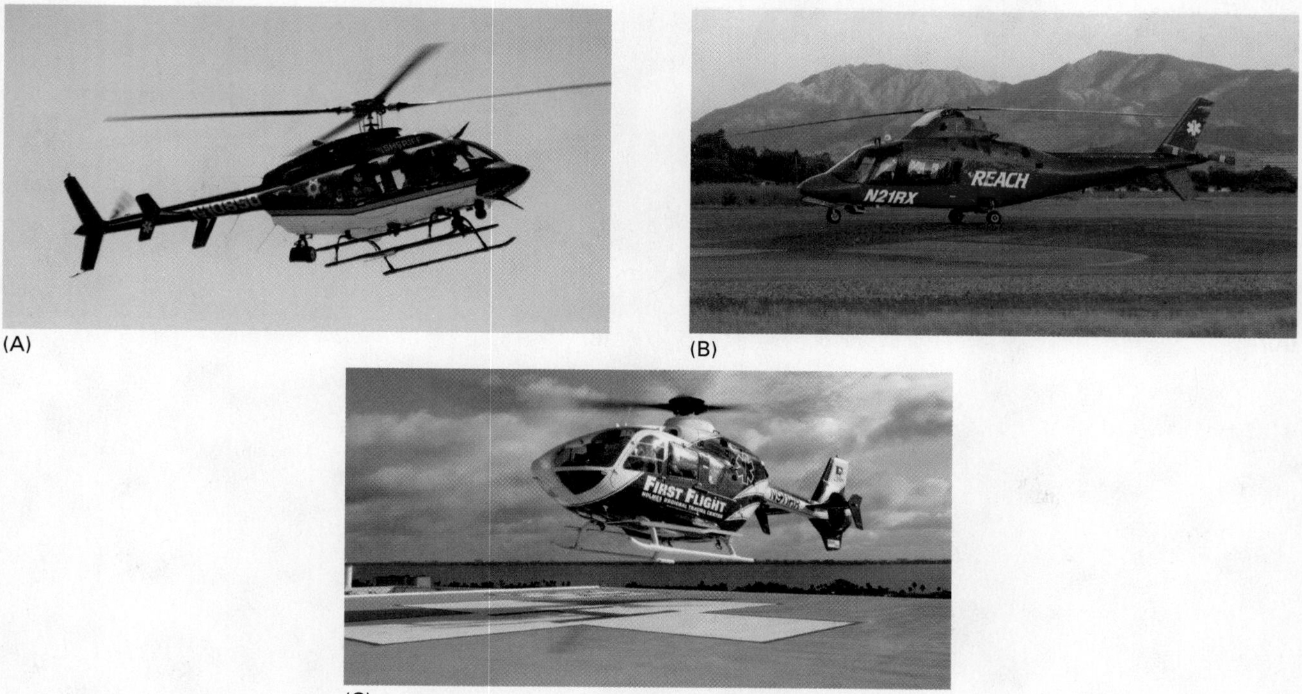

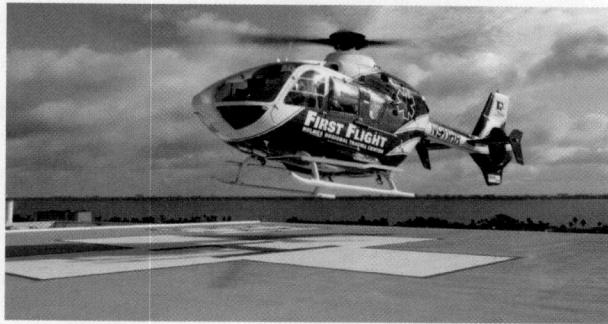

(A) (B) (C)

Figure 45-10 EMS helicopters come in many shapes and sizes. (A) Bell 407. (© REACH Air Medical Services, LLC) (B) Agusta 109. (© REACH Air Medical Services, LLC) (C) Eurocopter EC 135. (© REACH Air Medical Services, LLC)

Fixed-Wing Resources

Like helicopters, fixed-wing resources (airplanes) vary in size and performance capabilities and include jets, turboprops, and piston-driven aircraft (Figure 45-11 ■). The reason to choose an airplane over a helicopter is most often distance. Airplanes can fly much faster and farther than the typical helicopter, due largely to their ability to carry much more fuel. The airplane is ideal when there is no **helipad** at either the sending or receiving hospital and the two hospitals are more than 200 miles apart. Unlike the helicopter, the airplane is only capable of performing interfacility transports. This is due to the fact that it is not feasible for an airplane to land at the scene of an emergency. It can, however, land at an airport and meet a waiting ambulance.

helipad a designated location for a helicopter landing.

Note that all fixed-wing transports require a ground ambulance at each end of the transport. One ambulance will be necessary to bring the patient from the sending hospital to the airport, and another to take the patient from the receiving airport to the receiving hospital.

PERSPECTIVE

The Patient

That was the worst thing that I've ever gone through. I'm just so thankful that I had already dropped my daughter off at day care. I was just driving to work like I had done a million times before, you know? And I got this weird feeling in my stomach as I came up to that intersection, but I was running late and had spilled my coffee. The next thing I see is headlights and then I was just spinning through the air. It's like it was in slow motion, like a movie or something. The air bag might have been the worst part. I can still smell it. It probably saved my life, though. I don't know. It seemed like it took forever before they got to me in my car. My leg was caught between the steering wheel and the dash and blood just kept dripping from somewhere. I'm still not sure where it all came from! And I heard sirens and men talking and stuff, but no one was helping me. Yet I know they were trying. Did I say that I was so glad that my daughter was already at day care?

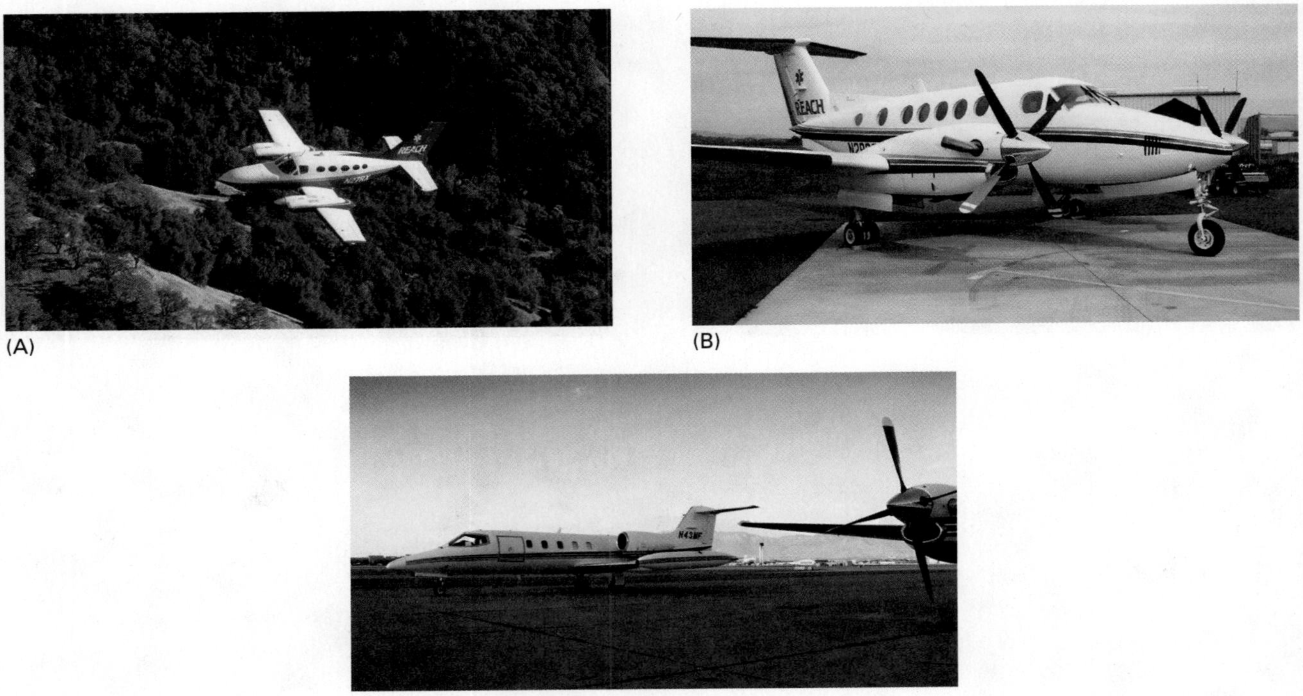

(A) (B) (C)

Figure 45-11 Fixed-wing aircraft (airplanes) are used for longer transports: (A) Cessna 421. (© REACH Air Medical Services, LLC) (B) KingAir B200. (© REACH Air Medical Services, LLC) (C) Lear Jet.(© Med Flight Air Ambulance)

Requesting Air Medical Resources

45-11 Explain the common criteria for choosing air medical transport over ground transport.

In most cases, it is the first responding units that determine the need for a helicopter response. That is why it is important for you as an EMT to become familiar with the air medical resources in your region and understand their capabilities and limitations. In most cases, a helicopter is appropriate whenever expedient transport is necessary or advanced providers are required. Most helicopter medical personnel receive specialized training over and above their counterparts on an ambulance or in a hospital. The training gives them an advanced scope of practice and allows them to deliver medications and perform procedures beyond the typical nurse or paramedic.

Most EMS systems with air medical resources will have specific protocols or guidelines for deciding when it is appropriate to activate an air resource. They often define specific patient types, such as severe trauma and critical medical. They also may define areas of the region that are remote and thus may take hours for a typical ground ambulance transport. It is important that you familiarize yourself with your local protocols for the use of air medical resources.

Just because you request a helicopter does not mean that one will respond. EMS helicopters are a limited resource, and many things can prevent them from responding to your request. They could be committed to another emergency and therefore may be unable to respond, or there could be weather in the area of the scene or at the receiving hospital that would prevent the pilot from completing the transport safely and legally.

Visual Flight Rules

45-12 Differentiate between visual and instrument flight rules.

visual flight rules (VFR) rules defined by the Federal Aviation Administration regarding the operation of an aircraft when weather is not a factor.

All pilots must operate aircraft based on specific and clearly defined rules established by the Federal Aviation Administration (FAA). The ability to fly any particular mission will depend on at least two factors: the training and capabilities of the pilot, and the design and configuration of the aircraft. It is safe to say that most EMS aircraft operate under what are known as **visual flight rules (VFR).** That means conditions along the intended route must be clear and free of weather, such as fog or clouds.

A VFR mission can be flown day or night so long as there is no significant weather anywhere along the intended route of flight.

Instrument Flight Rules

Many EMS air medical programs have specially trained pilots and specially configured aircraft so they can accept a request for transport even when the weather is bad. The rules that must be followed are called **instrument flight rules (IFR).** Being IFR capable allows the pilot to fly into and through known weather along the route of flight. There are limitations to the type and extent of weather in which an IFR pilot can fly. For instance, there must be at least some visibility on the ground for the pilot to take off and land safely. In conditions in which fog is so thick that visibility is no more than a few hundred yards, the pilot may decline the request due to extreme weather conditions.

instrument flight rules (IFR) rules defined by the Federal Aviation Administration regarding the operation of an aircraft in inclement weather.

Note that there are many more requirements that must be met for a team to safely complete a patient transport under IFR rules. The planning and preparation for an IFR flight may include extra weather checks and additional fuel, which can add to the time it takes to launch and get to the scene or hospital.

What Happens After a Request Is Made?

EMS flight programs use specially trained dispatchers called the *flight communication specialist* (Figure 45-12 ▪). It is the communication specialist who receives the request for transport, provides an estimated time of arrival (ETA) to the caller, and relays the request to the flight crew in the form of a dispatch. Once the flight crew receives a dispatch, several events must take place prior to the launch of the aircraft. The pilot will perform a weather check and confirm that weather conditions along the intended route of flight are within acceptable minimums. The medical crew will gather any needed equipment and head to the aircraft. In many programs, a specific risk assessment is performed prior to each flight to ensure the highest level of safety.

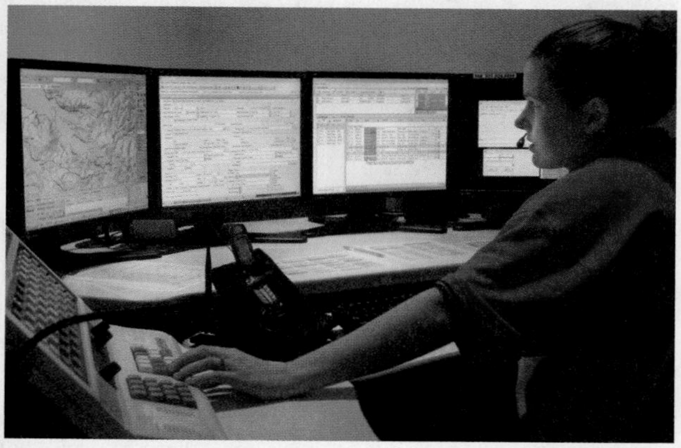

Figure 45-12 Flight communication specialists are responsible for dispatching and tracking EMS aircraft on each mission. (© Chris Le Baudour)

If the weather is acceptable and the medical crew has everything they need, all crew members approach the aircraft and perform a series of specific preflight safety checks prior to engine start and launch. If all goes well, they will be in the air and headed to their destination within minutes.

Occasionally, there will be factors that require the team to decline a request. Some of the most common reasons a crew might decline a request are poor weather conditions, mechanical failure, or patient size and weight.

Selecting an Appropriate Landing Zone

One of the characteristics that make helicopters so versatile is their ability to land nearly anywhere. However, they do require a clear, flat space to set down. An appropriate space for a helicopter to land is referred to as a **landing zone (LZ)**. The following landing zone characteristics are general guidelines and may differ slightly from program to program. It is best to learn the specific requirements of the programs operating in your area (Figure 45-13 ▪).

45-13 Describe the characteristics of an appropriate helicopter landing zone.

landing zone (LZ) a temporary location for the landing of a helicopter, typically at the scene of an emergency.

Characteristics of a good landing zone include:

- As close to the incident as possible
- 100 feet × 100 feet for daytime use, or 125 feet × 125 feet for nighttime use
- Little or no slope
- Free of dry sand or dirt and loose debris

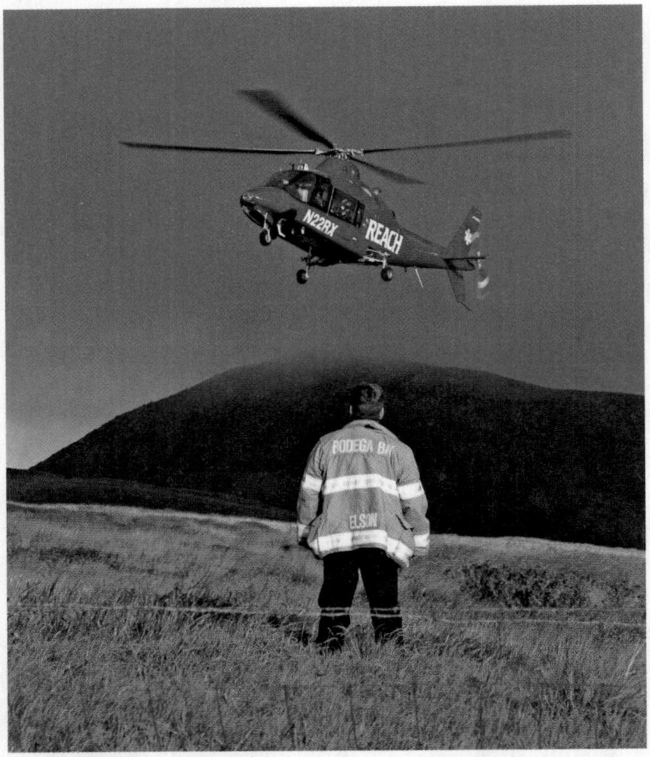

Figure 45-13 To ensure a safe landing, an EMT should assist in the landing process. (© REACH Air Medical Services, LLC)

- Free of utility wires near or around the site
- Free of tall trees or poles around the site
- Free of roaming animals

One of the most important things you can do as an EMT at the scene where a helicopter has been requested is to provide the dispatch center with accurate GPS coordinates (latitude and longitude). If the flight crew can find the scene from the air based on your coordinates, they may be able to see other areas near the scene that could serve as ideal landing zones.

Once an LZ has been selected, it is important to perform a quick checklist and report the findings to the flight crew. The acronym HOTSAW is a common tool used to remember this LZ checklist:

H—Hazards. Be sure the area is free of obvious hazards such as loose debris and traffic.

O—Obstacles. Confirm that there are no obstacles such as tall trees, poles, or wires.

T—Terrain. Ensure that the area selected is firm and even.

S—Slope. Ensure that the area is as flat as possible.

A—Animals. Check to see that there are no roaming animals in the area.

W—Wind. Estimate wind speed and direction and relay that information to the flight crew.

If the area chosen for the LZ is a dirt surface, try to wet the area down prior to landing to avoid a dust storm caused by the downwash from the rotor blades. An excessive amount of dirt or snow can cause the pilot to lose site of the ground, which can be very dangerous.

In most instances, a single person will be designated as the landing officer for the aircraft. This person should maintain radio contact with the flight crew during the entire landing phase whenever possible. He should stand at one side of the LZ and wave his arms to signal to the flight crew that he is the landing officer. It is important for the landing officer and others to wear proper eye and ear protection whenever working around a helicopter.

If the helicopter is to land at night, *never* shine any kind of light, such as a flashlight, at the aircraft. This could temporarily blind the pilot, which could have catastrophic consequences. In most cases, the lights of your emergency vehicle will be all the pilot needs to locate the scene.

Once the aircraft is safely on the ground, maintain direct eye contact with the pilot or other flight crew members. Do not approach the aircraft until someone from the flight crew has specifically directed you to do so.

Safety Around the Aircraft

45-14 Explain the safe principles of working around aircraft at the scene of an emergency.

Depending on several factors, the pilot will decide to shut down at the scene or remain "hot" with the rotors spinning. Regardless of the circumstances, follow these important guidelines when working around an aircraft at an LZ:

- Never approach an aircraft unless specifically directed to do so by the flight crew.
- Never shine any light at the aircraft.
- Never walk behind an aircraft, regardless of whether or not it is shut down.
- If on a slight slope, never approach the aircraft from the uphill side.
- Always remove your hat before approaching the aircraft.

STOP, REVIEW, REMEMBER!

Multiple Choice

For each question, place a check next to the correct answer.

1. The most common crew configuration for air medical operations in the United States is:
   _____ a. nurse/nurse.
   _____ b. nurse/paramedic.
   _____ c. paramedic/paramedic.
   _____ d. paramedic/EMT.

2. The two most common types of missions conducted by EMS air medical operations are scene calls and:
   _____ a. interfacility transports.
   _____ b. rescue missions.
   _____ c. search missions.
   _____ d. training missions.

3. Helicopter resources are best for flights up to _____________ miles.
   _____ a. 50
   _____ b. 100
   _____ c. 200
   _____ d. 500

4. Air medical missions conducted in clear weather often operate under:
   _____ a. visual flight rules.
   _____ b. instrument flight rules.
   _____ c. restricted flight rules.
   _____ d. the direction of a control tower.

5. Air medical resources are most often requested by:
   _____ a. law enforcement.
   _____ b. bystanders.
   _____ c. air traffic control.
   _____ d. the first responding EMS units.

Matching

Match the term on the left with the applicable definition on the right.

1. _____ Fixed-wing aircraft
2. _____ Helipad
3. _____ Instrument flight rules (IFR)
4. _____ Landing zone (LZ)
5. _____ Rotor-wing aircraft
6. _____ Visual flight rules (VFR)

A. Rules defined by the Federal Aviation Administration (FAA) for flight into inclement weather
B. Helicopter
C. Designated location for a helicopter landing
D. Rules defined by the FAA for flight in good weather
E. Temporary location for a helicopter landing, typically at the emergency scene
F. Airplane

(continued on next page)

(continued)

Critical Thinking

1. List two circumstances for which an air medical resource might be appropriate.

____

____

____

____

2. List the characteristics of an ideal landing zone for a helicopter at the scene of an emergency.

____

____

____

____

EMERGENCY DISPATCH SUMMARY

After the glass was cleared, the patient—suffering from an obviously broken right leg and numerous lacerations—was quickly extricated from the vehicle. She was secured to a long backboard, placed on supplemental oxygen, and transported to the Dobbs County Memorial Hospital. Once in the emergency department, she was found to have a pelvic fracture, a ruptured spleen, and a concussion. A precautionary CT scan of her head later showed an acute subdural hematoma. The patient underwent several surgeries—one to remove her spleen, one to drain the subdural hematoma, and two to reconstruct her leg—and has since been discharged. She is still undergoing daily physical therapy. The police issued a citation to the driver of the glass truck for failing to stop at the stop sign and for traveling at excessive speed.

Chapter Review

To the Point

- The NFPA has identified nine categories of technical rescue operations. They are vehicle/machinery, wilderness, water/surf/ice, dive, trench, collapse, rope, confined space, and other rescue operations.
- In addition to general safety, rescue operations involve a more detailed scene size-up that requires understanding the unique needs of the incident and requesting the appropriate resources as soon as possible.
- The components of a typical rescue response are: preparation, size up, hazard mitigation, vehicle stabilization, access, patient assessment, disentanglement, immobilization and extrication, emergency care and transport, and termination.
- Before ever attempting to access a patient, you must ensure that the scene is safe and that you are properly equipped to safely access the patient. It is often appropriate to access the patient and begin care before and during the actual extrication process.
- Access to patients may be divided into two categories: simple access and complex access. Simple access requires no special tools and can be accomplished by the EMT. Complex access takes more time and planning and requires special expertise and equipment to accomplish.
- It is important to stabilize a vehicle prior to access. Simple methods for stabilizing a vehicle include flattening the tires, using step blocks, cribbing, and struts.
- EMS air medical operations include both helicopters and airplanes. Helicopters are best used for short flights and emergency scenes much like ambulances. Airplanes are used to transport critically ill patients long distances between hospitals.
- EMS helicopters typically fly two types of missions: scene calls and interfacility transports. Airplanes only fly interfacility transports.
- Air medical resources are typically utilized when the patient requires the skills of a critical care team and must travel a distance not easily covered by a ground ambulance. Aircraft are a great resource when the patient's condition is time sensitive.
- All EMS aircraft are capable of flying in good weather under visual flight rules. Some aircraft and pilots are capable of flying on instruments and this is known as instrument flight rules.
- In order to safely land an EMS helicopter at the scene of an emergency it must have access to a site close to the scene that is flat and clear of any tall obstructions, loose dirt or gravel, and wires. It also must be at least 100 × 100 feet for daytime operations.
- Aircraft are inherently dangerous. You must exercise great caution when working around them. Always remain in eye contact with the pilot and never approach an aircraft unless the pilot or other crew member has requested that you do so. Never approach a helicopter from the rear because most have a spinning rail rotor that is not easily seen when in motion.

Chapter Questions

Multiple Choice

For each question, place a check next to the correct answer.

1. You are performing a scene size-up at a motor-vehicle collision. You note that there are two vehicles involved in a T-bone collision. There are two victims, both entrapped. Fluids are leaking from one of the vehicles. Which one of the following statements is the best scene size-up to be given over the radio to dispatch?

_____ a. Unit 14 to dispatch, on the scene with a two-vehicle MVC with two victims.

_____ b. Unit 14 to dispatch, on the scene of an MVC, T-bone type, with fluids leaking.

_____ c. Unit 14 to dispatch, on the scene of a two-vehicle MVC, two victims, both entrapped, fluids leaking from one vehicle. Dispatch heavy rescue and fire department to this location.

_____ d. Unit 14 to dispatch, on the scene of an MVC involving two vehicles, one van and one passenger car. There is one male victim and one female victim, both victims entrapped, fluids leaking from the van. There are no power lines down. Please dispatch heavy rescue to this location.

(continued on next page)

(continued)

2. You are inside a vehicle assessing a patient who was involved in an MVC. The fire department is preparing to extricate her, and the fire captain tells you that they are going to have to pop the windows to gain access. After you inform the patient of what is about to happen, what precautions should you take to protect her?
   _____ a. Cover the patient with a rescue blanket.
   _____ b. Cover the patient with a sheet.
   _____ c. Cover the patient with a plastic bag.
   _____ d. Exit the vehicle and let the fire department pop the glass.
3. You are on the scene of a motor-vehicle collision. The driver is sitting inside the car with all windows up. When you attempt to open the doors, you find that they are locked. Given this situation, which one of the following statements made to the patient is most appropriate?
   _____ a. Remain still. I am calling for the rescue truck to remove the door of your car.
   _____ b. Very carefully roll down the window.
   _____ c. Shield your eyes. I am going to break the window so we can open the door.
   _____ d. Without moving your head or neck, try to unlock the door.
4. You have been given an order to assist with cutting through the C posts of a car with a trapped passenger. As an EMT with knowledge of vehicle extrication, you cut the posts located at which areas of the roof?
   _____ a. Front
   _____ b. Middle
   _____ c. Rear
   _____ d. Top
5. Which one of the following is *not* one of the nine categories of technical rescue as defined by the NFPA?
   _____ a. Open space
   _____ b. Confined space
   _____ c. Trench
   _____ d. Rope
6. It is recommended that rescue operations be supervised by someone trained at the _______________ level.
   _____ a. awareness
   _____ b. operations
   _____ c. technician
   _____ d. command
7. Which one of the following actions is appropriate when using a helicopter on the scene of an emergency?
   _____ a. Point a spotlight at the helicopter to indicate the location of the landing zone.
   _____ b. Always approach the helicopter from the front and never from behind.
   _____ c. Keep all rescue personnel at least 10 feet from the helicopter as it lands.
   _____ d. Always approach the helicopter from behind and never from the front.
8. You are assisting with the setup of the daytime landing zone for the arriving helicopter. You must ensure that the spot you have selected is level and at least _______________ feet.
   _____ a. 100 × 100
   _____ b. 125 × 125
   _____ c. 150 × 150
   _____ d. 175 × 175
9. An unresponsive patient is in a car with the doors locked and the windows up. Which one of the following actions is most appropriate when attempting to gain access to the patient?
   _____ a. Use a crowbar to break the lock on the door.
   _____ b. Break the window opposite the patient.
   _____ c. Break the patient's window by striking it with a crowbar.
   _____ d. Call for a rescue truck to forcibly remove a door.
10. On the scene of a motor-vehicle collision, which one of the following is an example of complex extrication of the patient?
   _____ a. Asking the patient to exit the vehicle
   _____ b. Prying the door open
   _____ c. Entering through an open window
   _____ d. Pulling open an unlocked door

Labeling

Label the following parts in the diagram: A post, B post, C post, and side-injury protection bar.

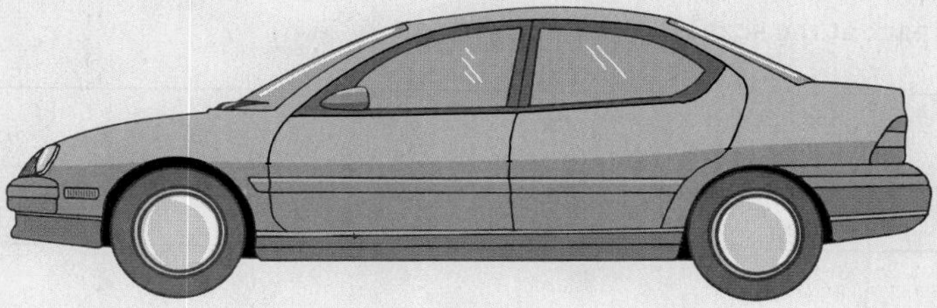

Critical Thinking

1. You have been dispatched to a motor-vehicle collision. On scene you find that a minivan has completely sheared a wooden utility pole. The electrical wires are draped over the hood of the minivan. The driver is screaming that she is hurt and wants to get out of the vehicle. Further observation of the wires reveals that they are not moving, arcing, or making any noise. What will you say to the woman in the car?

____

____

____

____

2. You have just arrived on the scene of a motor-vehicle collision in which a car rolled several times at a high rate of speed. The car is on its wheels and the restrained driver appears to be unresponsive in his seat. What will you do to ensure your safety? What will you do first for the patient?

____

____

____

____

Case Study

Your ambulance has been called to a collision scene on a four-lane interstate highway. You note that two lanes are blocked by the crash. Traffic is backed up but moving past the scene in the two open lanes.

1. Where should the ambulance park at the scene?

____

____

____

____

2. How should personnel at the scene be protected?

____

____

____

____

The Last Word

It is important to understand that training over and above the EMT's initial training is required to safely operate in rescue situations. You should strive to achieve awareness-level training in all of the areas of special rescue operations, which will give you the fundamental education you need to operate safely at a rescue. As you know by now, safety is the paramount concern for all responders in any response.

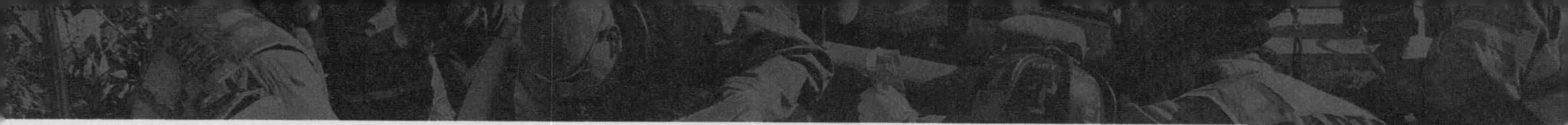

Responses Involving Terrorism

46

Education Standards

EMS Operations: Terrorism and Disaster

Competencies

Applies knowledge of operational roles and responsibilities to ensure patient, public, and personnel safety.

Objectives

After completion of this lesson, you should be able to:

46-1 Define key terms introduced in this chapter.

46-2 Explain the mnemonics CBRNE and B-NICE and describe the characteristics of the various types of weapons of mass destruction.

46-3 Explain the importance of preplanning a response to terrorism involving weapons of mass destruction.

46-4 Discuss the components that should be included in a plan for responding to terrorism involving weapons of mass destruction.

46-5 Recognize indications that a response may involve terrorism with weapons of mass destruction.

46-6 Describe the EMT's role when responding to terrorism involving weapons of mass destruction.

46-7 Describe types of injuries that may occur from conventional explosives and incendiary devices.

46-8 Discuss the effects of exposure to and explain the appropriate medical care for each of the following types of chemical agents: cyanide, nerve agents, pulmonary agents, riot-control agents, toxic industrial chemicals, and vesicants.

46-9 Differentiate between primary exposure and fallout associated with a nuclear explosion.

46-10 Explain blast injuries and thermal burns as mechanisms of injury from nuclear explosions.

46-11 Differentiate between a nuclear weapon and a radiological dispersal device (RDD, or "dirty bomb").

46-12 Discuss assessment and care of patients affected by nuclear detonation and radiation injuries.

46-13 Explain issues of personal protection and patient decontamination in connection with chemical, biological, and radiological/nuclear weapons exposure.

Key Terms

B-NICE p. 1224
bacteria p. 1224
biological weapons (BW) p. 1224
CBRNE p. 1224
chemical weapons (CW) p. 1227
dermal contact p. 1225
improvised nuclear device (IND) p. 1225
incubation period p. 1225
index of suspicion p. 1220
ingestion p. 1225
inhalation p. 1225
lacrimation p. 1229
lethality p. 1224
nuclear weapon (NW) p. 1225
persistence p. 1224
radiological dispersal device (RDD) p. 1226
secondary devices p. 1221
simple radiological device p. 1226
SLUDGEM p. 1229
terrorism p. 1219
toxins p. 1224
transmissibility p. 1224
vapor pressure p. 1228
vector p. 1225
virulence p. 1224
viruses p. 1224
weapons of mass destruction (WMDs) p. 1224

Introduction

The unfortunate reality for today's EMS practitioner is that terrorism is now an everyday danger. The first attack on the World Trade Center in 1993, the Murrah Federal Building in Oklahoma City in April, 1995, the devastating attacks of September 11, 2001, and the October, 2005, anthrax attacks on U.S. government facilities have all proven that public safety professionals are at risk and must be ready to respond to a diverse array of potential threats (Figures 46-1 ■ and 46-2 ■). Explosives, incendiaries, chemicals, biological agents, and even radioactive materials are all realities EMTs must be prepared to face. Prehospital practitioners must integrate an alertness to the risks of terrorism into their routine situational awareness and learn to recognize the signs of a potential terrorist incident. Furthermore, today's EMT must be prepared to respond to threats that are not just dangerous, but designed to cause maximum harm and injury.

Weapons of mass destruction (WMD) are no longer just a potential danger, but rather a very realistic threat to the health and well-being of all public safety responders. Incidents of this level require a combination of specialized resources, but they also can quickly overwhelm the capabilities of even the most advanced EMS systems. Although it is not possible to prepare for every contingency, broad-based training in an all-hazards approach can improve response and make it safer.

The hazards posed by terrorism are vast and ever changing and although this chapter provides a basic overview of recognition, preplanning, and response, it is essential that EMTs continue the lessons through ongoing education.

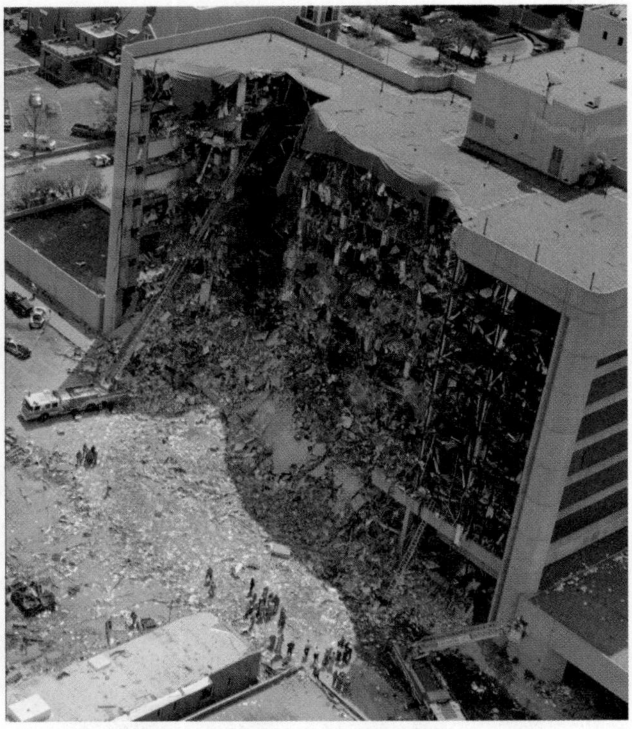

Figure 46-1 The scene of the 1995 bombing of the Alfred P. Murrah Federal Building in Oklahoma City. (AP Images)

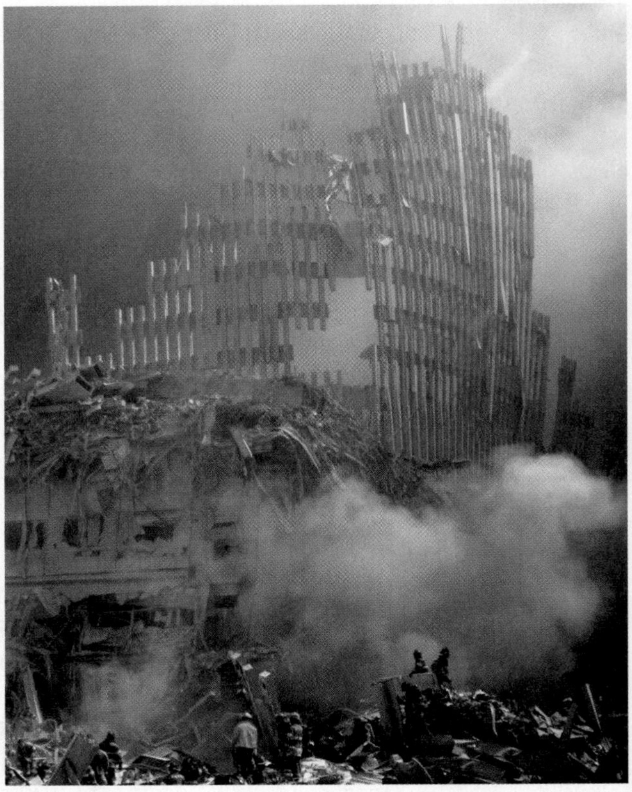

Figure 46-2 Ground zero following the destruction of the World Trade Center on September 11, 2001. (AP Photo/Shawn Baldwin)

EMERGENCY DISPATCH

"Station three, rescue . . . Station three, medical," the dispatcher's voice echoed through the fire station from the polished concrete floors to the well-stocked kitchen. "Proceed, priority one to West Avendell for a semi-truck versus the Cinema 16 building."

The search-and-rescue crew scrambled through the hallways, donning turnouts while piling into the truck, and then disappeared in a cloud of diesel exhaust and screaming sirens.

"Come on, Terry!" EMT Joelle Havens pounded on the bathroom door. "We've got a call!"

"I know! I know!" came the muffled reply. "Get the truck started and I'll be there in two seconds!"

Joelle started the ambulance and inched out of the building, nervously tapping on the steering wheel. A minute later Joelle's paramedic partner, Terry Edwards, jumped into the passenger seat, still trying to buckle his belt.

"There's no better way to jinx a nice, quiet afternoon!" he said. "So, what do we have?"

"A big rig into the Cinema 16 building," Joelle said, carefully clearing a busy intersection before proceeding.

"Really?" Terry said, suddenly serious. "That's odd. Big trucks aren't even allowed on those downtown streets. How bad is it?"

"I don't know." Joelle sounded the air horn at a taxi that seemed oblivious to them. "But once Rescue Three got there, they called for a lot of fire support."

"Well, once we get there, go slow." Terry could just make out the roof of the Cinema 16 building across town and thick, dark smoke was beginning to boil up into the sky above it.

As they turned onto West Avendell, Terry leaned forward and covered his mouth with his hand. "Oh, brother, there is no way that's an accident." The box trailer of a semi-truck was jutting from the destroyed lobby entrance of the newly remodeled movie theater and black smoke poured from the gaping opening. The Rescue Three truck was parked near the rear of the trailer and about seven police cars were situated haphazardly along the road around it. Crowds of screaming moviegoers, blackened from the smoke, streamed from the emergency exits and disappeared in all directions as police officers tried in vain to direct them.

Joelle stopped about a hundred feet from the theater entrance and Terry picked up the radio microphone. Several more fire trucks rounded the corner at the other end of the street. "Something's not right, Jo! I'm serious. Back up, quick!" Terry then keyed the mic. "Headquarters, medical three. We need to set up a perimeter. Don't send anyone else downtown. I repeat . . ."

The radio transmission ended abruptly as the semi's trailer buckled and then disappeared in a huge explosion that rattled windows as far as 25 miles away.

What Is Terrorism?

Terrorism is an illegal act that is dangerous to human life and performed with intent to intimidate or coerce a government or civilian population in the furtherance of a political or social agenda. Terrorists frequently use violence to further their goals, but also use threats of violence to cause enough fear to initiate some kind of change. Terrorists are considered to hold extreme ideas and philosophies and are intolerant of the viewpoints of others. There are different types of terrorism, both international and domestic, representing a wide array of both political and religious motivations. Targets of terrorism can be people, places, or infrastructure.

Perhaps the most dangerous element of terrorism is the desire to have maximum impact in striking widespread fear and disrupting the confidence of the population. Often such a desire leads to the use of WMDs and the targeting of public safety responders. Incidents involving WMDs are associated with massive destruction and harm that rapidly overwhelm resources and are difficult to respond to safely. These threats require specialized training and preparation.

46-3 Explain the importance of preplanning a response to terrorism involving weapons of mass destruction.

terrorism an illegal act that is dangerous to human life, with intent to intimidate or coerce a government or civilian population in the furtherance of a political or social agenda.

Preoperational Considerations

When considering a response to a terrorist attack, the actions taken prior to the event are extremely important. By definition, terrorist attacks disrupt, confuse, and overwhelm resources. Such a scene presents an enormous safety and management challenge. Best practices and historical lessons have clearly demonstrated that the most effective responses have resulted from well-practiced plans. Having practiced tactics, including taking the time to recognize an incident before fully committing to a response, affords the best chances of safety, security, and success.

Preplanning

46-4 Discuss the components that should be included in a plan for responding to terrorism involving weapons of mass destruction.

Preparation for responding to a terrorist attack of WMDs must encompass the entire community. It should begin with a review of high-risk locations such as political offices, religious organizations, controversial businesses, and specific high-profile events and mass gatherings. A review of specific response tactics, incident command structures, communication plans, and details of each particular location should be included. In addition to that research, preplanning highlights considerations for dealing with the massive destruction and harm WMDs can cause.

The benefit of preplanning is that it allows multiple agencies (law enforcement, fire, and EMS) to work together to create a plan for identifying why, when, and how to respond to a WMD situation should one occur. Often preplanning is addressed in the community's disaster response plan as required by the national incident management system (NIMS).

NIMS defines preparedness as a continuous cycle of planning, organizing, training, equipping, exercising, evaluating, and taking corrective action in an effort to ensure effective coordination during incident response. All preplanning should include those elements. More specifically, NIMS requires local planners to conduct the following assessments as they begin to build their response plans:

- Identify facilities and transportation routes of extremely hazardous substances.
- Describe emergency response procedures, on and off site.
- Designate a community coordinator and facility coordinators to implement the plan.
- Outline emergency notification procedures.
- Describe how to determine the probable affected area and population.
- Describe local emergency equipment and facilities and the persons responsible for them.
- Outline evacuation plans.
- Provide a training program for emergency responders (including schedules).
- Provide methods and schedules for exercising emergency response plans.

Scene Size-up

46-5 Recognize indications that a response may involve terrorism with weapons of mass destruction.

46-6 Describe the EMT's role when responding to terrorism involving weapons of mass destruction.

As an EMT, you play a variety of roles at the scene of a terrorist event. As a first responder, you may be tasked with taking command and assessing the situation. As described in Chapter 42, your immediate actions are critically important to the success of the incident command system. You may be the first to recognize the event and initiate changes to the response to keep providers safe. A WMD event will likely involve multiple casualties, so as an EMT, you may be further tasked with triage and treatment responsibilities.

Perhaps the most important consideration when responding to a potential terrorist act is scene size-up. A proper scene size-up can identify a terrorist act and help keep responders safe in a very dangerous and dynamic situation. As a public safety responder, you must develop a high **index of suspicion** for potential terrorist-related situations. In many cases this suspicion is a natural extension of the preplan, but in other cases it will be related to scene assessment and situational awareness.

index of suspicion a mental trigger that will help an EMT recognize an emergency call as a potential terrorist event.

Often location plays a critical role. Incidents involving a location with symbolic or historic significance, such as places of public assembly (arenas or stadiums), controversial facilities (some political headquarters), locations involving critical infrastructure (for example, the New York Stock Exchange), and government installations are considered common targets for terrorists (Figure 46-3 ■) and should immediately raise your level of concern during a response. Specific dates also can help identify terrorist incidents. For example, the Murrah Federal building in Oklahoma City was bombed on the anniversary of the deadly conclusion to the siege in Waco, Texas. Specific birthdays, anniversaries, and holidays may be important indicators of terrorist activity.

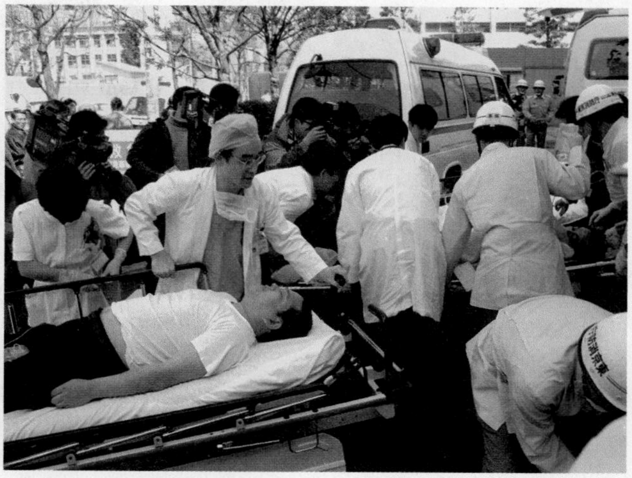

Figure 46-3 The scene of the Tokyo subway following the poison gas attack by terrorists. (AP Images/Chikumo Chiaki)

Ideally, emergency personnel will be advised if there has been a threat. However, this may not always be the case. Upon arrival or when receiving the dispatch report, look for physical indicators of a potential terrorist incident, such as:

- A report of mass casualties with minimal trauma or without a known traumatic cause
- Explosions that disrupt the transportation and communication systems, including the emergency services or critical infrastructure
- A debris field or severe structural damage to a building
- First-responder casualties, dead animals, or dead vegetation
- Unusual smells, color of smoke, and vapor clouds indicating the need for immediate respiratory protection and evacuation from the scene
- Incidents that involve large crowds of people, such as concerts or sports events, that have multiple patients injured or showing illness from an unknown cause

CLINICAL CLUE

Signs of Terrorism

Certain types of injuries and complaints point to terrorism. For example, multiple patients seizing at the same time is so unusual that it should always be considered a result of a poison or toxin and an indicator of terrorism. Consider also multiple simultaneous respiratory complaints as a "red flag situation."

Approaching the Scene

As you approach any emergency scene, consider the possibility of a terrorist event if there is more than one indicator present. Assess scene safety. If, on approach to the scene, you notice that other first responders (law enforcement, firefighters, and EMS) have become incapacitated, consider that someone has purposely targeted the emergency responders. First responders have sometimes been intentionally targeted, as in the Atlanta Abortion Clinic bombing where **secondary devices** were placed specifically to target the emergency personnel responding to the incident. The best way to minimize the risk of a secondary device is not to do what the terrorists expect of you in a response to a terrorist event. Instead of rushing into the scene, stop and consider the best approach.

secondary devices devices used to intentionally disrupt rescue and to injure emergency responders after an initial attack has taken place.

When indicators are present, assume command of the scene if no one has done so. Conduct a scene size-up and request resources. Do not park your ambulance in a location closest to the event. Look for suspicious packages, such as backpacks, packages, or things that look out of place or appear to be recently left in a location. Secondary devices may be hidden in trash cans, bushes, shrubbery, or planted vehicles. If you identify a secondary device, immediately move to a safe distance, and notify dispatch or the incident commander to have the bomb squad neutralize the device.

Requesting Additional Resources

Terrorist events require a specialized response with very specific resources. As described later in this chapter, WMDs often involve chemicals, radiation, or other hazardous materials. It is important for first-responding practitioners to identify those hazardous substances early to prevent the exposure of other incoming responders. Multiple indicators of hazardous materials can demonstrate the presence of terrorism and at a minimum should identify the need for personal protective equipment and

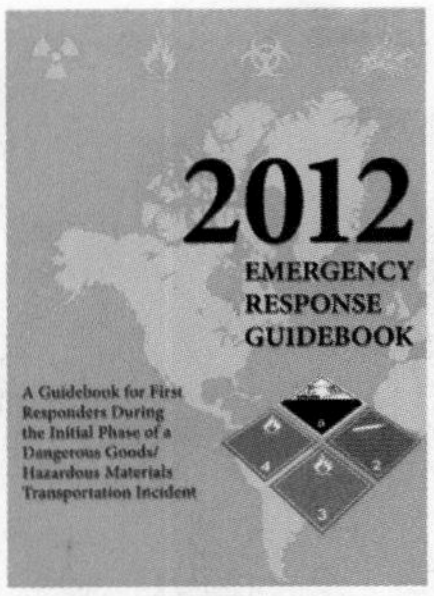

Figure 46-4 The DOT's *Emergency Response Guidebook* can help responders identify safety precautions when faced with known hazardous chemicals.

possibly respiratory protection. (For more information on hazardous materials and specific protective measures, it may be helpful to review Chapter 44.)

If you suspect a terrorist incident, make immediate contact with law enforcement for coordination. Approach the scene uphill and upwind and ask your dispatch center for a weather report. Make sure you have a quick, unimpeded exit route and are working with a partner. Avoid situations in which the response is being funneled into an area that will bottleneck or congest vehicles, making it difficult to withdraw to a safe position if a secondary device or attack on rescue personnel is launched.

Identify a rally point to meet and regroup in the event a secondary device detonates or another attack is conducted on emergency responders. Identify safe staging areas for other EMS, fire, and police units. Isolate and deny entry to nonemergency personnel, referring to DOT's *Emergency Response Guidebook (ERG)* (Figure 46-4 ■) for a safe minimum distance if an identified hazardous material is present. Consider the need for additional resources and that the site is a potential crime scene. Notify the hospital of the situation and the number of patients to expect from the incident.

STOP, REVIEW, REMEMBER!

Multiple Choice

For each question, place a check next to the correct answer.

1. Terrorism can be best defined as:
   _____ a. an illegal act that is dangerous to human life.
   _____ b. violence or the threat of violence, because it is fear that initiates a change in a population.
   _____ c. the use of a bomb or chemical weapon to kill or injure a population.
   _____ d. an illegal act of violence to kill or injure a population.

2. Which one of the following reports would prompt the highest index of suspicion of a terrorist attack?
   _____ a. Report of a single-vehicle motor-vehicle collision involving a tanker truck
   _____ b. Report of multiple victims unresponsive in a train station
   _____ c. Report of an explosion in a grain-storage bin in an isolated rural area
   _____ d. Report of an explosion of a factory

3. A secondary device is an explosive device designed to:
   _____ a. kill bystanders when they come to look at the damage caused by the initial event.
   _____ b. injure hospital personnel when victims are transported to their facility.
   _____ c. kill first responders when they respond to the initial event.
   _____ d. kill those who did not die initially.

4. You are called to a local church where, during a service, multiple people have begun to complain of shortness of breath and difficulty breathing. On arrival the crowd in front of the building waves and directs you to help the people inside. You should:
   _____ a. enter the church carefully and assess for any clouds or odors.
   _____ b. enter the church only long enough to remove the patients who cannot walk.
   _____ c. direct members of the crowd to go back into the church and bring the patients out.
   _____ d. stage outside and await a hazmat team.

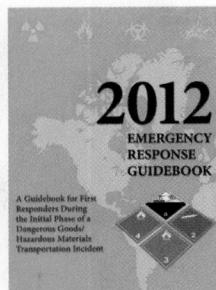

5. An explosion has occurred at an office building. You are the first arriving unit. After arriving, you should next:

_____ a. establish a security perimeter and command.

_____ b. enter the building and begin triage.

_____ c. leave the scene and await law enforcement.

_____ d. initiate a treatment area for those victims who have already escaped.

Ordering

Indicate the correct sequence—1 to 7—of the following recommended steps of a response to a potential terrorist attack.

1. _____
2. _____
3. _____
4. _____
5. _____
6. _____
7. _____

A. Ask your dispatch center for a weather report.

B. Look for situations in which the response is being funneled into an area that will bottleneck.

C. Make immediate contact with law enforcement for coordination.

D. Identify a rally point to meet and regroup in the event of a secondary device.

E. Identify safe staging areas for other EMS, fire, and police units.

F. Approach the scene uphill and upwind.

G. Make sure you have a quick, unimpeded exit route.

Critical Thinking

1. List potential terrorist targets in your community.

____

____

____

____

2. When responding to a potential terrorist event, the EMT must be aware of secondary devices. What can you do to minimize the threat to you from secondary devices?

____

____

____

____

46-2 Explain the mnemonics CBRNE and B-NICE and describe the characteristics of the various types of weapons of mass destruction.

46-7 Describe types of injuries that may occur from conventional explosives and incendiary devices.

weapons of mass destruction (WMDs) variety of explosive, chemical, biological, nuclear, and other devices used by terrorists to strike at government and high-profile or high-population targets; designed to create a maximum number of casualties.

B-NICE mnemonic used to categorize weapons of mass destruction; the letters stand for biological, nuclear, incendiary, chemical, and explosive.

CBRNE mnemonic used to categorize weapons of mass destruction; the letters stand for chemical, biological, radiological, nuclear, and enhanced explosives.

biological weapons (BW) devices designed to release either living organisms or toxins produced by living organisms that are deliberately distributed to cause disease and death.

bacteria single-celled organisms without a true nucleus or cell organelles.

viruses pathogenic organisms made of nucleic acid inside a protein shell, which must utilize a host cell for growth and reproduction.

toxins poisonous substances produced by animals or plants.

persistence length of time an agent stays in the environment.

virulence the power of infection once started.

transmissibility the ease with which an agent or disease can spread from person to person.

lethality the ability of an agent or disease to cause death; the percentage of those who die from an agent or disease.

PERSPECTIVE

Terry—The Paramedic

I can't believe what happened. I just can't believe it! Right there at the movie theater that I've taken my kids to a hundred times. There were probably kids in there today. Why do this? Why here? Has anyone heard from Rescue Three, yet? I know they couldn't have made it, but I still hope. And why did everyone just rush in? I couldn't have been the only one with that uneasy feeling, could I? It was just all wrong. A semi couldn't accidentally crash into the lobby of that movie theater. There was just no way. Did I know that it would explode? Hell no! I was afraid of some chemical agent in the smoke, actually. I never in a million years thought that it'd blow up.

Weapons of Mass Destruction

Weapons of mass destruction (WMDs) can be found in many different forms and designs. However, they are commonly created to inflict either great harm or great emotional impact. For many years, some of the most common WMDs have been simple explosives and incendiary devices. Improvised explosives can be created easily and inexpensively and inflict significant blast damage. WMDs also can utilize other nontraditional methods such as chemicals or radioactive materials. The mnemonic **B-NICE** outlines the categories of WMDs into the following areas: biological, nuclear, incendiary, chemical, and explosive. Another common mnemonic is **CBRNE** or chemical, biological, radiological, nuclear, and enhanced explosives. Each type of weapon has a specific delivery method and accompanying signs and symptoms of the attack. As an EMT, you must understand the physical principles of these weapons and recognize when they have been deployed.

Biological Weapons

Biological weapons (BW) are accessible to terrorists and are relatively easy to produce. Their effects usually go undetected for days until large numbers of the population begin to present with a similar pattern of symptoms. There are three types of biological agents: **bacteria** (such as anthrax), **viruses** (such as smallpox), and **toxins** (such as botulism or ricin).

Biological agents are dispersed as either wet or dry agents. Dry agents can be dispersed into heating, ventilation, and air conditioning (HVAC) systems or appear in packages with no visible evidence of their contents. The EMT should be on the lookout for visible foggers, sprayers, or aerosolizing devices. Naturally occurring biological outbreaks start with a few cases and slowly progress to a peak weeks or perhaps a month or more later. In contrast, a biological terrorism event will have a sudden peak in patients in a very short period of time, because most people will have been exposed at the same time and will become sick within a similar time frame.

How long an agent stays in the environment is known as **persistence.** Persistency depends on exposure to sunlight, temperature, and humidity. **Virulence** is the power of infection once started. The more rapid the onset and the greater the severity of the disease, the more virulent the agent is said to be. **Transmissibility** is the ease with which an agent or disease can spread from person to person. Finally, the EMT must understand the **lethality** of an agent, which is usually expressed as a percentage of those who die from the agent or disease.

Despite the inherent differences among various types of biological agents, some common characteristics are shared among bacteria, viruses, and toxins. Since biological agents are nonvolatile (do not evaporate), they must be dispersed in aerosols as 1- to 5-micron-size particles (1/30,000 the diameter of a hair follicle), which may remain suspended in the air for hours, depending on weather conditions. The primary route of infection would be **inhalation.** When inhaled, the particles deposit themselves deep into the alveoli of the lungs, causing disease.

inhalation entrance of a substance into the respiratory system.

A biological agent is a naturally occurring microorganism. The difference is that it has been deliberately altered to be used as a weapon. Biological agents commonly enter the body through one of four routes of entry as follows:

- Inhalation into the respiratory system, which is an easy target because of the vast surface area of the lungs and the warm, wet environment of the lungs that allows the organism to grow.
- **Ingestion** into the gastrointestinal tract is not as effective as inhalation. Only about 1% of municipal water is consumed, and filtration with chlorine or ultraviolet light reduces the threat. More probable is the contamination of food products.
- **Dermal contact** (contact with the skin) is another route by which a weapon can be disseminated. While most biological agents are stopped by the skin, the mucus membranes and breaks in the skin can permit absorption and contamination.
- A **vector** is an animal, insect, or person that carries a disease. Exposure to a vector-borne disease can occur from a bite, a sneeze, or person-to-person contact. When transmission is human to human, called *cross-contamination*, it becomes a contagious disease.

ingestion entrance of a substance into the digestive system.

dermal contact entrance of a substance through the skin or mucous membranes.

vector a carrier, such as animals, insects, or people who have a disease.

Signs and Symptoms of Biological Agent Exposure

Immediately after exposure to a biological agent, there is a period of time before signs and symptoms occur. It is called the **incubation period.** During this period, the agent multiplies and overwhelms the host. At the end of the period, the victim presents with signs and symptoms of the illness. For a bacteria or virus, the incubation period is measured in days. For a toxin, the time frame is much shorter. When compared to chemical weapons, whose effects tend to be immediate, the ill effects from biological weapons are delayed. Therefore, it is more difficult to detect a biological weapon.

incubation period the period of time from exposure until signs and symptoms occur.

The EMT who suspects a biological agent should take immediate precautions and obtain the following information from the patient:

- Travel history: Where has the patient been?
- Infectious contacts: Has the patient been around any sick people?
- Employment history: Where does the patient work?
- Activities over the preceding three days: What has the patient been doing?

46-11 Differentiate between a nuclear weapon and a radiological dispersal device (RDD, or "dirty bomb").

Protection from Biological Threats

Compliance with the Occupational Safety and Health Administration's (OSHA's) Bloodborne Pathogen Standard (29 CFR 1910.1030) and your organization's exposure control plan generally provides adequate protection. Standard precautions include surgical gloves, a high-efficiency particulate air (HEPA) mask of the type used against TB, splash goggles, and an appropriate dermal ensemble. They should be worn when contacting victims of a suspected biological attack.

46-12 Discuss assessment and care of patients affected by nuclear detonation and radiation injuries.

Nuclear and Radiological Agents

Nuclear and radiological agents have three basic forms of delivery that the EMT should know about. The first form of delivery is a **nuclear weapon (NW)** or **improvised nuclear device (IND).** It is a device that can produce a nuclear explosion, such as those that occurred in Hiroshima and Nagasaki during World War Two. The reaction from fission and fusion of radioactive materials produces a powerful explosion that is far more devastating than traditional explosives. In addition to explosive force, nuclear weapons emit gamma, beta, and alpha radiation (Figure 46-5 ■). The detonation of a

nuclear weapon (NW) device designed to release the energy generated during splitting (fission) or combining (fusion) of heavy nuclei to form new elements that are deliberately distributed to cause harm or death; a weapon that can produce an actual nuclear explosion.

improvised nuclear device (IND) device that can produce a nuclear explosion.

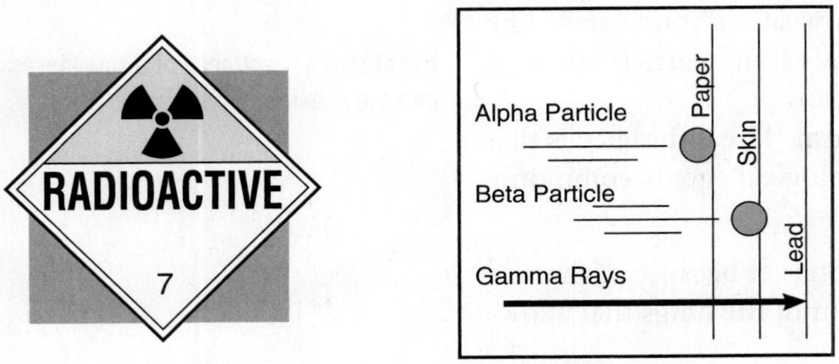

Figure 46-5 The effects of radiation depend on the type and the ability to penetrate through protective barriers.

nuclear device would identify itself by the classic mushroom cloud along with radiation that would accompany the event.

The second form of delivery is a **radiological dispersal device (RDD),** or "dirty bomb." It is a conventional (not nuclear) bomb laced with radioactive material. Although far less powerful than an actual nuclear explosion, the RDD is designed primarily to disperse the radioactive material into the atmosphere, not for its destructive force. An RDD would appear to be a conventional explosion, but signs of radiation sickness would appear among the victims who were exposed.

The third form of delivery is a **simple radiological device,** which disperses radioactive particles without any explosion at all. Such a device affects a population group that would begin to exhibit signs and symptoms of radiation sickness.

radiological dispersal device (RDD) a conventional bomb laced with radioactive material. Also called a *dirty bomb.*

simple radiological device device that disperses radioactive particles without explosion.

46-9 Differentiate between primary exposure and fallout associated with a nuclear explosion.

46-10 Explain blast injuries and thermal burns as mechanisms of injury from nuclear explosions.

Signs and Symptoms of Radiation Exposure and Sickness

The powerful explosion of a nuclear device causes a blast wave and thermal pulse that can cause burns, traumatic injuries, and death immediately. In many ways, the blast injuries are similar to the traditional effects of explosives and incendiary devices. An RDD also can cause blast-related injuries, although its explosive capability is not nearly as powerful as a nuclear device. A nuclear blast (or theoretically the dispersal of an RDD) also causes *primary exposure* to radioactive particles and rays that are emitted from the explosion.

In addition to this primary exposure, a nuclear blast or RDD also distributes radioactive particles into the atmosphere and onto the surrounding area. Those radioactive particles are referred to as *fallout*. Either of these two types of radiation dispersal can cause significant harm to exposed persons. The severity of radiation sickness depends on the total amount of radiation absorbed. Signs and symptoms of radiation exposure can vary from loss of appetite, nausea, vomiting, fatigue, and diarrhea with a low-dose exposure to fever, respiratory distress, and increased excitability with a higher dose. This is the stage at which most victims seek medical care. (For more on radiation sickness, please review Chapter 44.)

PRACTICAL PATHOPHYSIOLOGY

In addition to severe burns, acute exposure to high doses of radiation can cause rapidly developing illness. Symptoms of acute radiation sickness also include nausea and vomiting, headache, and diarrhea. At very high doses, rapid changes in mental status and blurred vision are common.

Protection from Nuclear Threats

The best way for the EMT to guard against radiation exposure is to follow the rules of time, distance, shielding, and quantity as follows:

46-13 Explain issues of personal protection and patient decontamination in connection with chemical, biological, and radiological/nuclear weapons exposure.

- ***Time.*** The shorter the time in a radiation field, the less the radiation exposure. Work quickly and efficiently. A rotating-team approach can keep individual radiation exposures to a minimum.
- ***Distance.*** The farther a person is from a source of radiation, the lower the radiation dose. Do not touch radioactive materials. Use shovels, brooms, and the like to move materials without physical contact.
- ***Shielding.*** Although not always practical in emergency situations, shielding offered by barriers can reduce radiation exposure. At a minimum, personal protective equipment should prevent radioactive particles from touching the skin or entering the respiratory or GI system. Remember, however, that gamma radiation rapidly penetrates protective clothing and can cause injury unless you are shielded by much denser barriers.
- ***Quantity.*** Limit the amount of radioactive material in the working area to decrease exposure.

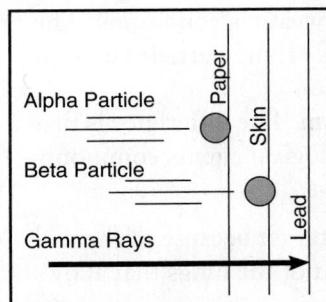

Incendiary Weapons

Incendiary weapons have been used as WMDs for literally thousands of years because they cause fire and burns to the people who come in contact with them. Modern terrorists often combine explosives with flammable substances to cause large fires and maximum damage. Incendiary weapons are most commonly recognized by the fire they produce, but also can be identified by the flammable substance they employ. Substances such as petroleum products (gasoline and kerosene, for example) are frequently associated with these types of weapons.

Burns are the most common types of injuries resulting from incendiary devices. Remember, however, that these types of weapons are frequently paired with explosives, so blast injuries are also common. (For more information on the treatment of burns, refer to Chapter 32.)

> **CLINICAL CLUE**
>
> **Too Hot to Handle**
>
> Some incendiary weapons burn at far hotter temperatures and are much more difficult to extinguish than others. That is because substances such as white phosphorus and certain fuel products (jet fuel and alcohols, for example) may be very difficult to stop with water. If a substance cannot be extinguished by using traditional means, immediately suspect an incendiary weapon and terrorism.

Responders can protect themselves from incendiary agents by avoiding the fire and heat source. Commonly, fire protective equipment such as bunker gear is sufficient to protect a responder from dangerous effects. However, it should be remembered that many incendiary devices utilize substances that emit heat in far greater quantity than typical fires. Although it may be very difficult to determine this in a scene size-up, clues include strange colors of smoke and flames, excessive heat, and unusual odors. When encountering such situations, traditional fire protective gear may be ineffective and avoidance may be the only sufficient protection.

Chemical Weapons

46-8 Discuss the effects of exposure to and explain the appropriate medical care for each of the following types of chemical agents: cyanide, nerve agents, pulmonary agents, riot-control agents, toxic industrial chemicals, and vesicants.

Chemical weapons injure by the dispersal of harmful substances onto the skin or into the internal systems of the body itself. **Chemical weapons (CW)** differ from biological weapons (BW) in that the chemical agent is a nonliving compound. Chemical agents can cause immediate signs and symptoms, unlike biological agents, which require an incubation period. Chemical agents can be aerosolized and cause local or systematic effects. Onset may be rapid from inhalation or ingestion or delayed from agents absorbed through the skin. Victims of a chemical weapons attack can experience a variety of signs and symptoms, depending on the agent used in the attack.

chemical weapons (CW) devices designed to release a range of simple to sophisticated chemicals that are deliberately distributed to cause harm or death.

One of the most effective ways to dispense a chemical agent is to disseminate it into the respiratory system. The respiratory system is an easy target because of the vast surface area of the lungs. The smaller the size of the particles, the easier it is to aerosolize the agent. Dispersal can occur with explosives, spraying equipment, or natural currents created by the movement of equipment. The heating of agents often creates vapors and that can increase the penetration to the lung tissue. Greater velocity of air movement can move a greater amount of an agent into the lungs as well, making it more effective.

vapor pressure the pressure exerted by a chemical against the atmosphere.

Vapor pressure, a factor with chemical agents, is the pressure exerted by a chemical against the atmosphere. The higher the vapor pressure, the greater the tendency to evaporate (give off a vapor). The higher the vapor pressure, the less persistent the agent is in the environment.

Terrorists have ample access to chemicals used in the community. For example, chlorine can be found in large quantities in most communities and could be used as a weapon. Chemical agents are commonly classified into the following categories:

- ***Nerve agents.*** Nerve agents disrupt the function of the nervous system. They kill by stopping basic autonomic functions such as breathing and cardiac output. Nerve agents are closely related to some fertilizers (specifically organophosphates) and can be found in many common pesticides. Weaponized nerve agents are far more powerful variations. Nerve agents are frequently absorbed through the skin, but also can be inhaled or ingested.
- ***Vesicants.*** Also known as blister agents, vesicants harm by causing irritation and burns to the skin and mucous membranes. Severe topical injury is common and simple contact is enough to cause harm.
- ***Blood agents.*** Blood agents harm the patient by way of the bloodstream. Cyanide is the most well-known blood agent and causes harm by disrupting oxygen exchange at the level of the hemoglobin. Cyanide is produced naturally as a by-product of combustion and can be found in many house fires. However, as a weapon, it is very effective. Blood agents can be absorbed through the skin and also inhaled or ingested.
- ***Pulmonary agents.*** Pulmonary agents target the respiratory system. They disrupt the patient's ability to breathe. Also known as *choking agents*, they cause irritation and destruction in the airway. Most commonly, they are aerosolized and inhaled.
- ***Riot-control agents.*** Riot-control agents are similar to pulmonary agents. However, they are not typically intended to cause long-term harm. Capsicum (pepper spray) and chemical mace are used to temporarily incapacitate by irritating the airway and mucous membranes. Exposure causes difficulty breathing and irritation to the eyes and nose, but is typically limited in its effect. Although painful, these effects are not life threatening.
- ***Toxic industrial chemicals.*** Chemical weapons can be derived from any potentially harmful chemical. Commonly used industrial products can be used in a weapon form if they are able to cause harm. Unfortunately, this list is literally endless and the effects are specific to the chemical itself.

As part of the medical response to a terrorist event, an EMT may be assigned to help with mass decontamination of victims. Decontamination procedures are broken down into three levels: gross, primary, and secondary decontamination. Gross decontamination is done on scene and is aimed at getting most of the material off the victim. Primary decontamination is done in a shower area, possibly with special chemical agents. Secondary decontamination is conducted at the hospital and includes cleaning wounds and a thorough scrubbing of the skin. Special chemical antidotes may be applied by hospital emergency department staff. The steps for on-scene decontamination include locating the decontamination area or corridor upwind and uphill from the site.

Signs and Symptoms of Chemical Weapons Attack

Several signs and symptoms indicate a terrorist chemical attack. The EMT should be suspicious of unresponsive victims with minimal or no trauma. Blistered, red, discolored, or irritated skin can indicate exposure to vesicants or other toxic chemicals. **SLUDGEM** is the mnemonic used to describe the common signs and symptoms of exposure to nerve agents based on organophosphate pesticides, which are as follows:

S—Salivation (saliva production)
L—**Lacrimation** (tear production)
U—Urination
D—Defecation
G—Gastrointestinal motility (overactive digestion)
E—Emesis (vomiting)
M—Miosis (constricted pupils)

SLUDGEM mnemonic for the common signs and symptoms of exposure to nerve agents based on organophosphate pesticides; the letters stand for salivation, lacrimation, urination, defecation, gastrointestinal motility, emesis, and miosis.

lacrimation abnormal or excessive secretion of tears.

PRACTICAL PATHOPHYSIOLOGY

Nerve agents disrupt the breakdown of the neurotransmitter acetylcholine. As a result, their effects continue without regulation. Areas most profoundly affected include skeletal muscle, the smooth muscle of the GI tract, and the airway. Unregulated acetylcholine causes prolonged contraction and uncontrolled muscle activity. This dysfunction is the underlying cause of the widespread excretion of body fluids. A patient affected by a nerve agent will literally be excreting fluids from every possible source. In addition, the uncontrolled acetylcholine also causes jerking movements in the skeletal muscle and status seizures if left uncorrected.

Protection from Chemical Agents

First responders wearing chemical protective gear or firefighting turnout gear with self-contained breathing apparatus (SCBA) may approach victims to rescue or guide them through the decontamination corridor. EMTs should avoid direct contact with any liquids, victims' clothing, or other potentially contaminated surfaces. Victims should be separated into symptomatic and nonsymptomatic or walking and nonwalking. A small number of patients can be decontaminated with a single hoseline from a fire truck, while a large number of patients will require a decontamination corridor to be established. This can be accomplished by placing two engines side by side.

Explosives

Explosives are simple, affordable, and effective means of creating a WMD, and they are the most common type. Explosives cause harm by creating a rapid chemical reaction that forms heat and displaces air. Injuries are caused by a shock wave of pressure (*primary blast injury*); fragments, otherwise known as *shrapnel* ejected from the explosion (*secondary blast injury*); and by the patient being violently thrown by the explosion (*tertiary blast injuries*). In some cases, the explosive will be used to disperse a chemical, biological, or radiological agent. The heat and combustion generated by an explosive will also potentially cause injury. These additional effects are sometimes referred to as the *quaternary blast effects*.

Explosives can be found in a variety of forms from high-grade military substances to homemade agents derived from common household products. The explosive force is often related to both the quantity and quality of the explosive. Improvised explosive devices are common explosives made by enhancing existing explosive devices to maximize their lethality. This can include increasing their explosive quantity or by altering their intended purpose to increase their deadly impact.

PERSPECTIVE

Joelle—The EMT

Terry saved my life. I don't know how we made it. That building collapsed right next to us and it totaled the truck. But we walked away from it. I'm numb right now. Just completely numb. I know that many of my friends are still buried out there, and I'll never, never see them again. But it hasn't sunk in yet, you know? It never crossed my mind that that truck was a weapon—even after 9-11, not even a suspicion, nothing. I mean, this is still America. And to think that whoever built that thing actually meant for us to get there before it went off. That terrifies me. I don't know what I'm supposed to do with this whole thing. This event. I can't talk anymore right now. Is that okay?

STOP, REVIEW, REMEMBER!

Multiple Choice

For each question, place a check next to the correct answer.

1. Anthrax is a:
   _____ a. chemical agent.
   _____ b. biological agent.
   _____ c. toxin.
   _____ d. radiological agent.

2. Biological weapons need to:
   _____ a. be dispersed in an aerosol.
   _____ b. enter through dermal or oral routes.
   _____ c. be relatively easy to disseminate.
   _____ d. Any one of the above.

3. Biological agents that can be used as a terrorist weapon are _____________ and toxins.
   _____ a. viruses and bacteria
   _____ b. chemicals and bacteria
   _____ c. proteins and bacteria
   _____ d. viruses and proteins

4. The disruption of the breakdown of acetylcholine is a common characteristic of:
   _____ a. vesicants.
   _____ b. nerve agents.
   _____ c. blood agents.
   _____ d. pulmonary agents.

5. Which one of the following would be an example of a blood agent?
   _____ a. Sarin gas
   _____ b. Ricin
   _____ c. Cyanide
   _____ d. Capsicum spray

Fill in the Blank

1. What does each letter in the mnemonic SLUDGEM stand for?

____

____

____

____

2. List at least three things to do when responding to a terrorist attack.

Critical Thinking

1. You have responded to a potential radiological weapons attack. What is the best way to protect yourself?

2. You are transporting a patient who possibly has been exposed to a chemical weapon during a terrorist attack. He currently has no symptoms. What are the signs and symptoms that you should be alert for that would tend to confirm exposure to a chemical agent?

PERSPECTIVE

Michael—Local Resident and Survivor

I was walking my dog to the park over on Bundle Street when I heard all the sirens. I got kind of curious, and it wasn't really out of my way, you know? So I crossed over to Avendell, about a mile from the theater. I could see the flashing lights and the smoke, but I couldn't really tell what was going on. It definitely was crazy though. People were running everywhere down there. And then there was this big bright flash. I couldn't see anything else for a second. And then it felt like when you fall on your back and the wind gets knocked out of you, you know? I just couldn't breathe. And then I got thrown to the ground really, really hard. Next came the sound. It was so loud that I can't even describe it, but it just seemed to go on forever. I think that was the strangest part for me. I can still hear it, over and over again. It came so long after the blast. Am I making any sense? I think my dog ran away, too. I don't know where he is.

Emergency Care for WMD Victims

One of the first responsibilities of the EMT when responding to a possible WMD attack is not to become a victim. Once you have ensured your personal safety and the safety of the scene, you may proceed to provide patient care. No matter the cause of a WMD attack, there are some basic tenets of patient care that do not change. The primary responsibility of the EMT is to manage the patient's ABCs.

Blast-Injury Victims

In a terrorist attack of explosives, the victims will have many of the injuries that have been discussed in the trauma care module of this text (Figure 46-6 ■). Emergency care is the same as if they had been injured in a motor-vehicle crash. In a patient with a traumatic mechanism of injury, cervical-spine precautions must be considered. Blast injuries also frequently are associated with penetrating trauma from shrapnel, blunt trauma from the pressure wave, and barotrauma such as pneumothorax and perforated eardrums. Treatment is not specific to the terrorist incident and should be accomplished by adhering to the basic principles of trauma care.

In a terrorist attack, the EMT must be aware that most likely there will be multiple victims, and the scene will be classified as a multiple-casualty incident (MCI). The EMT must follow the local disaster plan and implement the triage and treatment

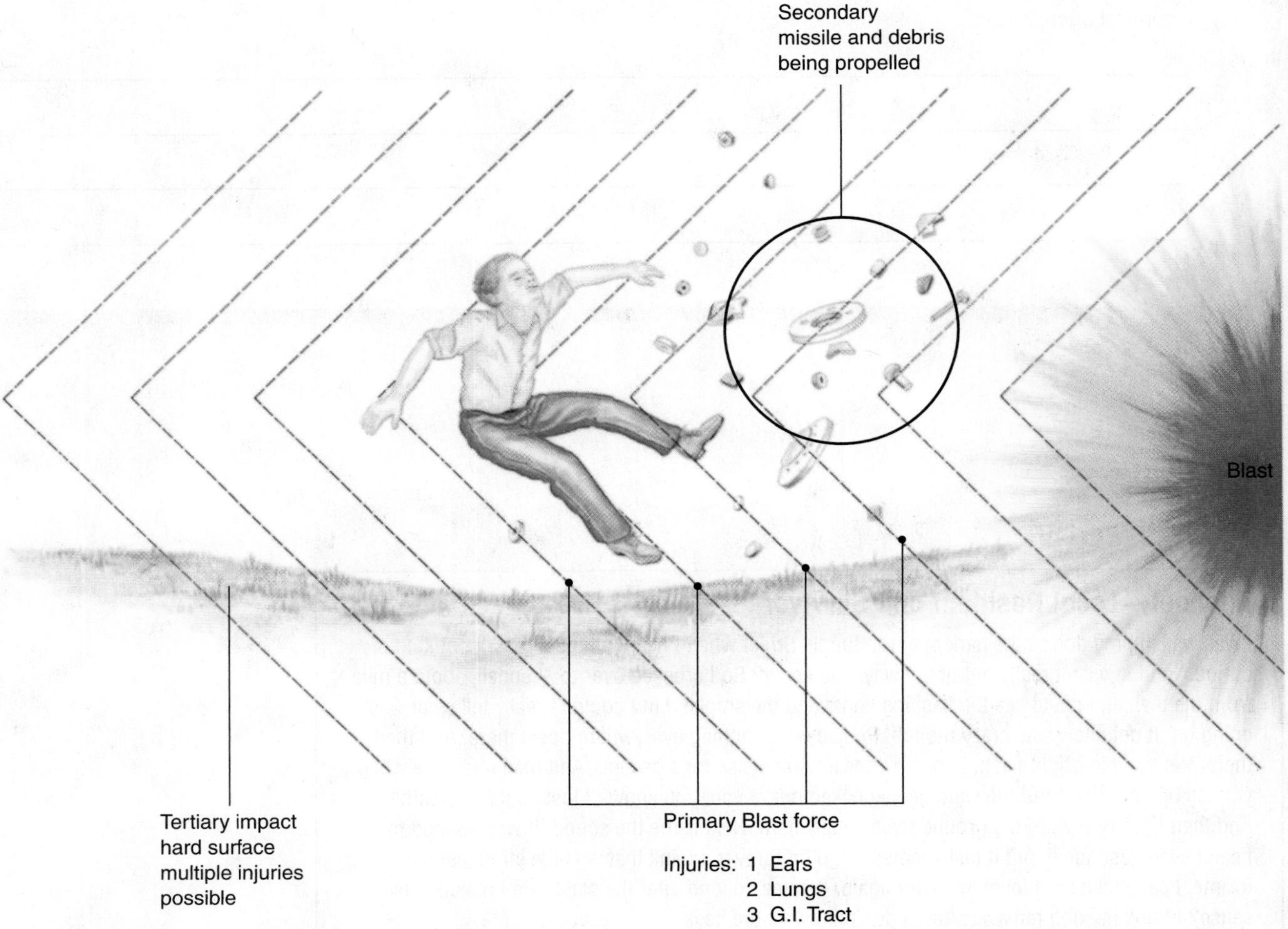

Figure 46-6 Blast injuries can cause injury from the initial blast wave, which involves being hit by debris and from being thrown by the blast.

outlined in it. Remember that during an MCI, resources are limited and must be used to benefit the maximum number of patients.

Chemical Weapons Victims

During a chemical weapons attack, the scene is unsafe and there will be multiple victims suffering from a variety of symptoms. Once the victims have been decontaminated, you may safely begin to treat them. Remember, chemical weapons often target the respiratory system. Therefore, many victims of a chemical attack will require aggressive airway management. Chemical weapons also can induce seizures and cause burns to the skin.

Chemical weapons require specific treatments, depending on the offending agent. For example, nerve agents/organophosphate-pesticide-based chemical exposures can be treated using a Mark I antidote kit (Figure 46-7 ■). This kit utilizes an auto-injector similar to an Epi-Pen to inject atropine and pralidoxime chloride. Both medications are used to reverse the effects on the nervous system. It is important to remember that as an EMT, you may be able to use this medication as a self-protective measure in the event of a nerve agent exposure. As always, follow local protocol and utilize manufacturer's instructions on actual administration.

Other chemical agents may have specific antidotes. Cyanide-based chemical exposures can be treated with a cyanide antidote kit, which is usually administered by advanced life support (ALS) personnel. Many urban centers that have been listed as potential terrorist targets have the antidote kits stockpiled for distribution in the event of an attack. If you are required to assist in the administration of an antidote kit, you will receive training for that responsibility.

PRACTICAL PATHOPHYSIOLOGY

Blast injuries can cause a wide range of trauma. The pressure wave created by the blast can be particularly harmful to gas-filled organs such as the lungs. Assess carefully for signs of rupture after exposure to a massive pressure change. Look for signs of pneumothorax and other damage associated with high pressure. Consider also the potential for penetrating trauma as a result of flying shrapnel.

CLINICAL CLUE

Signs of the Cause

The physical effects of a chemical often help identify the substance that has caused the harm. Particular chemicals demonstrate specific effects. SLUDGEM signs are associated with nerve toxins. Skin irritation and burns are associated with vesicants and blood agents, which will cause a rapid and otherwise unexplained drop in oxygenation and perfusion in the patient. Although findings may not be absolutely specific, recognizing the cardinal presentations of various chemical exposures can be helpful in tracking down the agent.

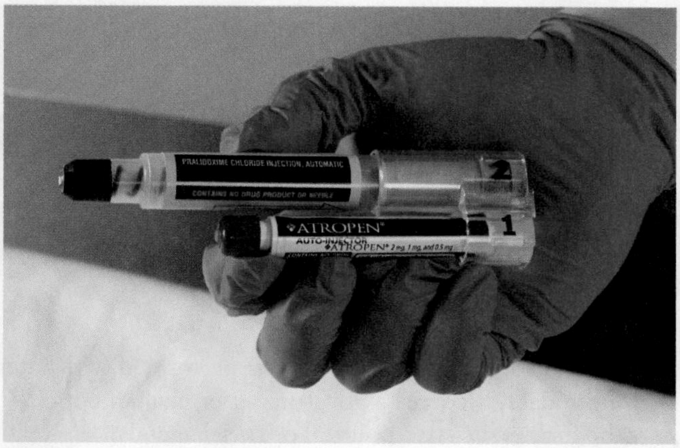

Figure 46-7 A typical nerve agent antidote kit provided to EMS personnel.

Biological Weapons Victims

Of all the types of WMDs, biological agents are the most difficult to detect. Many of the common signs and symptoms are similar to those for the flu. As discussed earlier, the most significant sign of a biological agent is the sudden spike in the number and acuity of patients suffering flu-like symptoms with a common location of exposure.

Remember that when you are treating potential victims of a biological agent, you should don an approved N-95 respirator and take all appropriate BSI precautions. The EMT's care should focus on the ABCs and supportive measures. As with chemical weapons, the specific treatment depends on the agent used. For example, a bacterium like anthrax requires an antibiotic. Remember that some types of biological agents have no treatment, and the only way to manage the patient is with supportive care at the scene and in the hospital.

Radiological Weapons Victims

Radiological weapons can cause a wide range of injuries. In many cases, the most immediate injury may be related to the explosives used to disperse the radiation. As Chapter 44 described, radiation sickness can present in many different forms often over a large time frame. High doses of radiation can cause burns, but exposure can lead to more chronic illnesses developed over time. It is essential to remember that a contaminated patient must be decontaminated before being handled. Furthermore, a patient exposed to radioactive particles may himself remain radioactive (and thus very dangerous) until those particles are removed.

EMERGENCY DISPATCH SUMMARY

A total of 112 people died that day, including 19 emergency personnel. Although several foreign and domestic terrorist organizations claimed responsibility for the incident, the FBI has yet to conclude the investigation. Joelle Havens has become a vocal advocate for terrorism preparedness, speaking at EMS conventions and consulting with educators nationwide. Terry Edwards remains a paramedic with the city fire department and is happy to see that crews have begun to rebuild the downtown area.

Chapter Review

To the Point

- Terrorism is an illegal act that is performed with intent to intimidate or coerce a government or civilian population in the furtherance of a political or social agenda.
- Terrorists use WMDs to inflict maximum harm and to cause an emotional reaction in the populace.
- Terrorist events overwhelm resources and cause mass chaos. The best responses are those that are planned.
- Preplanning for a WMD response should include recognition, command, communications, and resource management.
- EMTs must develop a high index of suspicion for terrorist incidents and use scene clues to identify otherwise unknown situations.
- Scene size-up should be used to identify a terrorist incident and to provide safety and security to future responding units.
- CBRNE and B-NICE are mnemonics that describe the different categories of WMDs.
- EMTs should be familiar with the basic characteristics of each of the CBRNE and B-NICE categories.
- Explosive and incendiary weapons cause common traumatic injuries. Specific patterns can be used to identify their cause.
- Chemical weapon effects are directly related to the type of chemical used in the attack. EMTs should learn the cardinal presentations to help them better identify the root cause.
- Radiological events can be either nuclear or simply radiological in nature.
- Biological weapons are difficult to identify because their effects are not immediate. These weapons are typically identified by the emerging patterns of illness that develop.
- Personal protection and safety are primary concerns when responding to a WMD incident.

Chapter Questions

Multiple Choice

For each question, place a check next to the correct answer.

1. The treatment an EMT would provide for a chemical or biological weapon exposure is:
   _____ a. supportive, including the ABCs.
   _____ b. not indicated. Pronounce victims dead, because they are very contagious.
   _____ c. decontamination.
   _____ d. to call the nearest level I trauma center and have the burn center prepared.

2. Ten patients have been recently diagnosed with an unusual illness. Their symptoms are similar and all have developed within a similar time frame. These findings most likely indicate a:
   _____ a. chemical weapon.
   _____ b. blood agent.
   _____ c. pulmonary agent.
   _____ d. biological weapon.

3. Single-celled microorganisms are known as:
   _____ a. viruses.
   _____ b. chemicals.
   _____ c. toxins.
   _____ d. bacteria.

4. Bacteria, viruses, and toxins are examples of:
   _____ a. drugs found in a doctor's office.
   _____ b. WMDs that have no treatment options.
   _____ c. things a terrorist might be afraid of.
   _____ d. biologicals that a terrorist might use in a WMD.

5. Inhalation, absorption, ingestion, and injection are all:
   _____ a. ways a level C suit can be permeated.
   _____ b. types of anaphylaxis.
   _____ c. routes of exposure.
   _____ d. problems you will likely encounter while in a level A suit.

6. Identification, isolation, and notification are the duties of a(n):
   _____ a. informant.
   _____ b. task force manager.
   _____ c. hazmat technician.
   _____ d. hazmat awareness responder.

7. Terrorism is best described as:
   _____ a. hijackers on an aircraft with unlawful weapons posing as airline pilots.
   _____ b. an intimidation of an entire group of people or government for monetary gain and recognition.
   _____ c. the unlawful use of force or violence against persons or property to intimidate or coerce a government or civilian population in furtherance of political or social objectives.
   _____ d. a third-world country with disgruntled citizens trying to take control of their government.

8. Miosis, copious secretions, muscle twitching, convulsions, and GI effects are symptoms of:
   _____ a. food poisoning.
   _____ b. tetanus and diphtheria.
   _____ c. nerve agents.
   _____ d. hoof and mouth disease.

9. The letters in the mnemonic SLUDGEM stand for:
   _____ a. slobbering, lacrimation, urination, decreased respirations, gas, ecchymosis, meningitis.
   _____ b. shaking, loss of bladder control, urination, defecation, gas, embolism, miosis.
   _____ c. salivation, lacrimation, urination, defecation, gastrointestinal motility, emesis, miosis.
   _____ d. slurred speech, lacrimation, uncontrollable bowels, decreased respiration, gangrene, emesis, miosis.

Matching

Match the term on the left with the applicable definition on the right.

1. ____ Index of suspicion
2. ____ Secondary devices
3. ____ Weapons of mass destruction (WMDs)
4. ____ Nuclear weapon (NW)
5. ____ Biological weapon (BW)
6. ____ Chemical weapon (CW)
7. ____ Vapor pressure
8. ____ Improvised nuclear device (IND)
9. ____ Radiological dispersal device (RDD)
10. ____ Simple radiological device

A. Variety of chemical, biological, nuclear, or other devices used by terrorists to strike at government or high-profile targets; designed to create a maximum number of casualties

B. Mental trigger that, when called to an event, will help an EMT recognize it as a potential terrorist event

C. Device used to intentionally disrupt rescue and to injure emergency responders

D. Device designed to release either living organisms or toxins produced by living organisms that are deliberately distributed to cause disease and death

E. Device designed to release the energy generated during splitting (fission) or combining (fusion) of heavy nuclei to form new elements that are deliberately distributed to cause harm or death

F. Device that can produce an actual nuclear explosion

G. Device designed to release a range of simple to sophisticated chemicals that are deliberately distributed to cause harm or death

H. Pressure exerted by a chemical against the atmosphere

I. Device that disperses radioactive particles without explosion

J. Bomb laced with radioactive material; also called a *dirty bomb*

Critical Thinking

1. Describe the two most probable terrorism scenarios that could take place in your community and explain why you think they are the most probable.

____

____

____

____

2. Name the three types of biological agents and give an example of how each can be used as an agent of terrorism.

____

____

____

____

3. Do the signs and symptoms of biological weapon exposure make it easier or more difficult to identify compared to other types of WMDs? Explain your answer.

____

____

____

____

Case Study

It is 8:30 on a Thursday morning in July. It is partly cloudy, humid, and the temperature is 90°F. There have been various militia groups arriving in the city to demonstrate over the weekend and for the Fourth of July parade. An EMS unit, a fire engine, and fire investigator have been dispatched to the south end of the city on an "assist the police" call. The information over the mobile data terminal or by way of a secured transmission indicates this call is for a "suspicious device."

At 8:45 your EMS unit is dispatched to the center of the city to the local government offices for difficulty breathing. Upon arrival, you see approximately 15 people outside the main door to the government building coughing, tearing, and in respiratory distress.

1. What are the elements of your scene size-up that you would want to relay to dispatch?

2. How will you proceed with caring for the victims?

The Last Word

In the United States, terrorism is now perceived as an everyday threat to which EMTs are on the front line. It is important to understand that terrorists use acts of violence toward a political or social end, with the intent to intimidate or coerce a government or civilian population in the furtherance of their agenda. Your job as an EMT is to help make the response effective and safe.

Remember that WMDs come in many nuclear, biological, and chemical forms. One of your primary responsibilities is to guard against becoming a victim yourself. Each weapon has a specific delivery method and accompanying signs and symptoms. After you have donned appropriate personal protective equipment, you can safely begin treating patients. Your duty is to provide care to the victims of a WMD attack, focusing on the ABCs and providing supportive care.

During your initial EMT training, you may not have the opportunity to train to respond to a WMD attack. However, as an EMT you may have the opportunity to participate in your local community's disaster drill. Take advantage of the training to prepare yourself for a possible terrorist attack. Additional training is offered free of charge by the Federal Emergency Management Agency (FEMA). This training is available online at *www.fema.gov*.

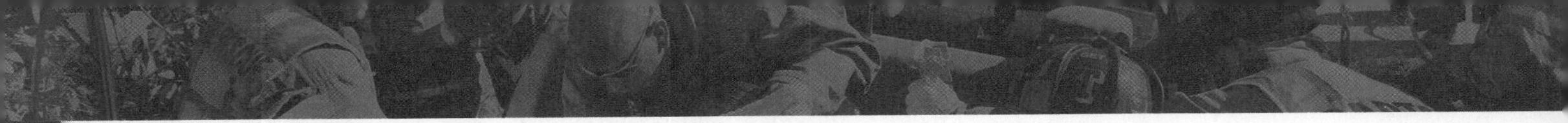

Module 6: Review and Practice Examination for Chapters 41–46

DIRECTIONS: *Assess what you have learned in this module by placing a check mark in the blank beside the best answer for each multiple-choice question. When you are done, check your answers against the Answer Key at the back of the book.*

1. The phase of an ambulance call in which you complete documentation of your call is called:
   ____ a. preparing for the call.
   ____ b. transfer to hospital staff.
   ____ c. terminating the call.
   ____ d. receiving and responding to the call.

2. Which one of the following items is included when checking the mechanical condition of an ambulance?
   ____ a. AED ____ c. Bandaging supplies
   ____ b. Maps ____ d. Brakes

3. When responding to a call, which one of the following is *least* important for an EMT to know?
   ____ a. Patient's ethnic group
   ____ b. Nature of the request for assistance
   ____ c. Current condition of the patient
   ____ d. Hazards at the scene

4. Which one of the following principles should be followed by EMTs when driving an ambulance?
   ____ a. Have due regard for the safety of all others.
   ____ b. Always pass other vehicles on the right.
   ____ c. Ambulances have the right of way in all circumstances.
   ____ d. EMTs are held harmless from liability due to ambulance collisions.

5. Which one of the following is the correct order of the phases of an EMS call?
   1. Caring for the patient
   2. Dispatch
   3. Responding
   4. Preparation for the call

   ____ a. 2, 4, 3, 1
   ____ b. 2, 3, 4, 1
   ____ c. 4, 3, 1, 2
   ____ d. 4, 2, 3, 1

6. For which one of the following patients is the use of a stair chair most appropriate?
   ____ a. 75-year-old man who fell out of bed is complaining of back and neck pain
   ____ b. 68-year-old man complaining of shortness of breath
   ____ c. 60-year-old woman in cardiac arrest
   ____ d. 25-year-old woman in hemorrhagic shock

7. You are preparing to return to service following a call. The patient you transported had a laceration to his leg, and there is a moderate amount of blood on your stretcher. Which one of the following is appropriate?
   ____ a. Cleaning and disinfection
   ____ b. Disinfection only
   ____ c. Cleaning and sterilization
   ____ d. Cleaning only

8. You have just arrived at the scene of a roll-over motor-vehicle collision. A sedan is on its side in the intersection. You can hear a child crying inside the vehicle. Rescue has a two-minute ETA. Your obligations as an EMT are best met by which of the following actions?
   1. Stay about 12 feet back from the vehicle and make a better determination of what the situation in the vehicle is.
   2. Check the scene for additional vehicles, patients, and hazards.
   3. Determine the best way to immediately remove the child from the vehicle.

   ____ a. 1, 2 ____ c. 2
   ____ b. 1 ____ d. 2, 3

9. NIMS is best described as:
   ____ a. a consistent nationwide approach in responding to events requiring coordinated public safety response.
   ____ b. a multiple-casualty incident.
   ____ c. EMS personnel "freelancing" at the scene of an emergency.
   ____ d. a designated disaster medical response team.

10. NIMS is overseen by the:
____ a. Department of Health and Human Services.
____ b. Department of Defense.
____ c. Department of Homeland Security.
____ d. Justice Department.

11. In an incident command system, the area responsible for developing tactical objectives is:
____ a. command.
____ b. operations.
____ c. planning.
____ d. logistics.

12. In an incident command system, the area responsible for providing support and resources is:
____ a. operations.
____ b. planning.
____ c. logistics.
____ d. finance/administration.

13. In a smaller incident, the person in charge of all major activities is the:
____ a. general staff.
____ b. safety officer.
____ c. information officer.
____ d. incident commander.

14. The number of people or elements that can be effectively managed by a single individual in an ICS is referred to as:
____ a. unity of command.
____ b. incident action plan.
____ c. span of control.
____ d. staging.

15. The incident management element that is geographical in nature is a(n):
____ a. division. ____ c. cluster.
____ b. unit. ____ d. group.

16. In ICS, the individual responsible for management of the entire scene is the:
____ a. public information officer.
____ b. safety officer.
____ c. triage sector leader.
____ d. incident commander.

17. By definition, an event that exceeds the capabilities of an EMS system is called a(n):
____ a. disaster. ____ c. ICS.
____ b. MCI. ____ d. CBRNE.

18. A mass gathering is an assembly of ____________ or more people in a single location.
____ a. 100 ____ c. 10,000
____ b. 1,000 ____ d. 100,000

19. An incident that involves more than one patient and cannot be managed by the normal responding units but can be handled by the resources of a single system is a ____________ casualty incident.
____ a. mass- ____ c. multiple-
____ b. major- ____ d. minor-

20. Which one of the following is a management goal for MCIs?
____ a. Relocate the disaster to a controlled environment.
____ b. Do the greatest good for the largest number of patients.
____ c. Send all patients to the same hospital.
____ d. Assign two to three patients to each provider.

21. Which one of the following is the first of the "Five S's" for initial actions at the scene of an MCI?
____ a. Scene size-up
____ b. Send information
____ c. Start triage
____ d. Safety

22. The act of sorting patients into categories for treatment and transport based on the severity of condition is known as:
____ a. triage.
____ b. assessment.
____ c. classification.
____ d. deployment.

23. At the scene of an MCI you encounter a patient who is not breathing. You should first:
____ a. open the airway.
____ b. tag the patient black.
____ c. tag the patient red.
____ d. begin rescue breathing.

24. At the scene of an MCI you encounter a patient who is responsive to verbal stimuli, is breathing 28 times per minute, and has a carotid pulse but no radial pulse. This patient should be tagged:
____ a. green. ____ c. red.
____ b. yellow. ____ d. black.

25. At the scene of an MCI you encounter a five-year-old patient who has a pulse but is not breathing. You have opened the airway and the patient is still not breathing. Which one of the following should you do next?
____ a. Give five rescue breaths.
____ b. Tag the patient black.
____ c. Tag the patient red.
____ d. Move on to the next patient.

26. In MCIs, the first patients to be transported are those tagged:
____ a. black. ____ c. white.
____ b. red. ____ d. green.

27. Extrication, triage, treatment, and transportation sectors in an MCI are part of the ____________ section.
____ a. planning ____ c. rescue
____ b. operations ____ d. finance

28. The individual at an MCI who ensures that ambulances are directed to the appropriate receiving hospital is the ____________ officer.
____ a. staging
____ b. sector
____ c. communications
____ d. commanding

29. When rescuers responding to an MCI operate outside the incident command system, it is known as:
____ a. mutiny. ____ c. freelancing.
____ b. rebellion. ____ d. free contracting.

30. Of the following, the greatest benefit of NIMS is:
____ a. it is a commonly understood way of structuring response to large-scale incidents.
____ b. it allows control of all major incidents by the federal government.
____ c. it encourages response by lay rescuers without creating delays caused by unnecessary rules.
____ d. it makes it unnecessary for local agencies to create a disaster response plan.

31. In an MCI, triage is based on the principle of:
____ a. providing the same care as when treating a single patient.
____ b. treating the youngest patients first.
____ c. transporting to the closest hospital.
____ d. providing the best care for the greatest number of patients.

32. Any substance or material that poses an unreasonable risk to health, safety, and property is a(n):
____ a. chemical substance.
____ b. hazardous material.
____ c. inert matter.
____ d. vapor compound.

33. Substances stored in stationary tanks and facilities, such as at swimming pools, are marked using a voluntary marking system known as:
____ a. DOT placards.
____ b. Emergency response guides.
____ c. NFPA 704.
____ d. U.S. Radiologic Survey.

34. You have noted a diamond-shaped sign on a storage tank behind a hospital. The top quadrant of the diamond contains the numeral "4." This means the substance stored inside the tank poses a(n):
____ a. extreme risk of fire.
____ b. low risk of fire.
____ c. extreme risk of explosion.
____ d. low risk of explosion.

35. You have noted a diamond-shaped sign on a storage tank at a farm supply company. The bottom quadrant of the diamond contains a letter "W" with a line through it. This means:
____ a. the tank contains an inert substance.
____ b. the tank contains a dry substance rather than a liquid or wet substance.
____ c. the tank contains an oxidizer.
____ d. mixing water with this substance creates a hazard.

36. The diamond-shaped symbol on a transportation container, such as a tanker truck, is called a:
____ a. bill of lading.
____ b. placard.
____ c. hazard notice.
____ d. material safety data sheet.

37. Employers must keep paperwork on all potentially hazardous substances in the workplace. Those papers are called:
____ a. material safety data sheets.
____ b. placards.
____ c. manifests.
____ d. ORM-Ds.

38. The blue quadrant of an NFPA diamond contains information about a substance's:
____ a. special considerations.
____ b. health risks.
____ c. fire hazard.
____ d. explosive potential.

39. You have been dispatched to a railroad yard for a "sick person." On your arrival you note that there are three individuals on the ground next to a tank car. Using binoculars to inspect the tank, you should compare the information you gather to that found in the:
____ a. *Emergency Response Guidebook.*
____ b. *Hazmat Manual.*
____ c. bill of lading.
____ d. material safety data sheet.

40. Under what circumstances is it permissible for an EMT to approach a hazardous materials scene?
____ a. The EMT is a firefighter and is wearing turnout gear.
____ b. The EMT is trained as a hazardous materials technician and is wearing SCBA.
____ c. The EMT is trained at the hazardous materials awareness level and is wearing a HEPA mask.
____ d. The EMT has immediate access to a decontamination shower upon leaving the area.

41. A flammable solid is considered a DOT hazard class:
____ a. 1.
____ b. 2.
____ c. 3.
____ d. 4.

42. DOT hazard class 9 indicates:
____ a. flammable liquids.
____ b. explosives.
____ c. miscellaneous dangerous goods.
____ d. corrosives.

43. When a chemical substance makes contact with the skin or mucous membranes, it can enter the body by way of:
____ a. injection.
____ b. ingestion.
____ c. absorption.
____ d. amalgamation.

44. You have responded to a small furniture factory. Three employees are experiencing coughing and watery eyes after one of them spilled a can of paint solvent. To find out more about the material spilled, you should locate the:
____ a. NFPA 704 placard.
____ b. U.S. DOT placard.
____ c. material data safety sheet.
____ d. manifest.

45. The first phase of a rescue operation is:
____ a. gaining access to the patient.
____ b. preparing for the rescue.
____ c. sizing up the situation.
____ d. providing initial patient assessment.

46. Devices placed on either side of the tires of a vehicle to stabilize it are called:
____ a. chocks.
____ b. props.
____ c. jacks.
____ d. buttresses.

47. You are able to access a patient entrapped in a motor vehicle following a collision without the use of equipment. This is known as ____________ access.
____ a. complex
____ b. intricate
____ c. easy
____ d. simple

48. Generally, a fixed-wing resource will be used to transport a patient when the receiving facility is ____________ than ____________ miles away.
____ a. more/200
____ b. less/150
____ c. more/150
____ d. less/300

49. The FAA allows pilots to use ____________ to fly day and night as long as no significant weather exists along its intended route.
____ a. IFR
____ b. IBR
____ c. VFR
____ d. GTR

50. A daytime helicopter landing zone should be at least ____________ feet.
____ a. 115 × 115
____ b. 100 × 100
____ c. 125 × 125
____ d. 75 × 75

51. Terrorism is different from other types of threatened or actual violence in which one of the following ways?
____ a. It always involves more victims than other acts of violence.
____ b. It is carried out to further a political or social agenda through intimidation or coercion.
____ c. It relies solely on the use of explosive devices.
____ d. By definition, it is not committed by U.S. citizens.

52. Which one of the following is *most* suspicious for an act of terrorism being committed?
____ a. Explosion at a place of worship
____ b. Explosion in a residence
____ c. Motor-vehicle collision between a car and a tanker truck
____ d. Dozen people becoming ill at a wedding reception

53. In regard to a biological agent being released, its *persistence* refers to how:
____ a. long people becoming infected remain ill.
____ b. effective the agent is in producing death.
____ c. easily one person can spread the disease to another.
____ d. long the agent stays in the environment.

54. A conventional explosive spiked with radioactive material is known as a(n):
____ a. improvised nuclear device.
____ b. radiological dispersal device.
____ c. simple radiological device.
____ d. smart bomb.

55. Aerosolized anthrax is an example of a ____________ weapon.

____ a. biological ____ c. nuclear
____ b. chemical ____ d. radioactive

56. You and your partner are responding to a report of an explosion at a doctor's office. Which of the following are appropriate actions?

1. Park well away from the building.
2. Consider the possibility of a second explosion inside the building.
3. Enter and search the building for victims.
4. Consider the possibility of a second explosion outside the building.

____ a. 1, 2, 3, 4 ____ c. 1, 2, 4
____ b. 1, 2 ____ d. 2, 4

57. A simple, homemade explosive device containing radioactive material is sometimes referred to as a(n):

____ a. improvised nuclear weapon.
____ b. dirty bomb.
____ c. simple radiological device.
____ d. weapon of mass destruction.

APPENDIX 1
Final Practice Review

***DIRECTIONS:** Assess what you have learned by placing a check mark in the blank beside the best answer for each multiple-choice question. When you are done, check your answers against the Answer Key at the back of the book.*

1. Which one of the following levels of EMS responder is nationally recognized by the U.S. DOT?
   ____ a. Emergency medical responder
   ____ b. Cardiac technician
   ____ c. Advanced paramedic
   ____ d. Paramedic specialist
2. EMS personnel staffing the ambulance must be trained to at least the level of:
   ____ a. CPR certification.
   ____ b. paramedic.
   ____ c. cardiac technician.
   ____ d. EMT.
3. Which one of the following components of an EMS system is demonstrated by EMS providers giving training classes in their communities?
   ____ a. Health education and screening
   ____ b. Citizen education resources
   ____ c. Public information and education
   ____ d. Medical direction
4. The survivor of a disaster experiences an emotional reaction a year after the event. This is an example of a(n) ____________ stress response.
   ____ a. delayed
   ____ b. atypical
   ____ c. cumulative
   ____ d. tardy
5. In which one of the following situations should an EMT wear a HEPA mask?
   ____ a. Responding to a hazardous materials incident
   ____ b. Caring for a patient with suspected tuberculosis
   ____ c. Reporting for duty with a cold, flu, or other respiratory infection
   ____ d. Caring for a patient who is spitting at the EMS providers
6. Which one of the following patients can be treated under implied consent?
   ____ a. 22-year-old woman who is unresponsive after hitting her head on the ground during a football game
   ____ b. 45-year-old man with chest pain who states he smoked some marijuana an hour ago
   ____ c. 18-year-old high school student who was injured in a motor-vehicle collision
   ____ d. 75-year-old man who knows his name and where he is but is not sure of the day of the week and is complaining of abdominal pain
7. You have just arrived on the scene of a 16-year-old female patient who reportedly took an overdose of over-the-counter medications. Her eyes are closed and she is not responding to verbal stimuli. Your partner believes the patient is just trying to get attention and is not truly unresponsive. He says to you, "Watch this. This will teach her a lesson." He then pinches the patient's arm hard enough to leave a bruise. This may be considered:
   ____ a. battery. ____ c. damages.
   ____ b. assault. ____ d. abandonment.
8. Your patient has a laceration to the outside of his right leg. What side of the leg is that?
   ____ a. Medial ____ c. Distal
   ____ b. Lateral ____ d. Proximal
9. The primary function of platelets is to:
   ____ a. help blood clot.
   ____ b. carry oxygen.
   ____ c. carry carbon dioxide.
   ____ d. detoxify waste products.
10. Which one of the following is a characteristic of a child's airway anatomy when compared to that of an adult?
    ____ a. The tongue is proportionally smaller.
    ____ b. The trachea is rigid and inflexible.
    ____ c. Children primarily use their intercostal muscles to breathe.
    ____ d. The cricoid cartilage is less well-developed.

11. The valve that separates the left atrium from the left ventricle is the ______________ valve.

____ a. mitral ____ c. pulmonic
____ b. tricuspid ____ d. bilateral

12. Some blood vessels have sensors that regulate the level of internal pressure by sending messages to the nervous system to adjust their size. What are these sensors called?

____ a. Size receptors
____ b. Size sensors
____ c. Stretch receptors
____ d. Barrel receptors

13. The age of a neonate spans from birth to:

____ a. 28 days. ____ c. 18 months.
____ b. one year. ____ d. six months.

14. You are on the scene of a one-car motor-vehicle collision. The vehicle is wedged against a tree at the driver's door. The driver is unresponsive with inadequate respirations. The front seat passenger is alert and oriented with minor complaints, but you cannot get to the driver without first moving the passenger. Which one of the following is appropriate to move the passenger?

____ a. Emergent move
____ b. Non-emergent move
____ c. Non-urgent move
____ d. Elective move

15. You have responded to the home of a 60-year-old man who is complaining of nausea and diarrhea and says he gets light-headed when he stands up. The patient weighs about 350 pounds. The last time you called for assistance in lifting a patient, the responding crew got very upset with you and your partner. Which one of the following is the best course of action?

____ a. Tell the patient you will help him walk to the ambulance and that if he gets light-headed, to let you know so he can sit down and rest.
____ b. Call for help and deal with the other crew's reaction later if they are upset about it.
____ c. Make the patient comfortable on the cot, then, using good communication and body mechanics, lift the cot with your partner's assistance.
____ d. See if you can find a neighbor or family member to help lift the patient.

16. Which one of the following is a patient symptom?

____ a. Nausea
____ b. Deformed extremity
____ c. Low blood pressure
____ d. Laceration

17. Which one of the following is a patient sign?

____ a. Dizziness ____ c. Pale skin
____ b. Nausea ____ d. Itching

18. Trending is best described as:

____ a. keeping up on the latest knowledge and skills in EMS.
____ b. following a fad in patient treatment without consulting medical direction.
____ c. a cluster of signs and symptoms related to a specific type of medical problem.
____ d. comparing each set of patient vital signs to the sets before it.

19. A patient who breathes six times in a 30-second period has a respiratory rate of:

____ a. 6. ____ c. 18.
____ b. 12. ____ d. 24.

20. The amount of air that moves in and out of the lungs with each respiration is referred to as the ______________ volume.

____ a. tidal ____ c. resting
____ b. minute ____ d. lung

21. When assessing the pulse of an unresponsive adult, the preferred site is the ______________ artery, located in the ______________.

____ a. brachial; neck
____ b. radial; wrist
____ c. femoral; groin
____ d. carotid; neck

22. Blood pressure should be assessed in all patients ______________ old or older.

____ a. six months
____ b. one year
____ c. three years
____ d. five years

23. Which one of the following best describes systolic blood pressure?

____ a. The reading on the blood pressure gauge when the first sound is heard through the stethoscope as the blood pressure cuff is deflated
____ b. The difference between the top number of the blood pressure reading and the bottom number of the blood pressure reading
____ c. The reading on the blood pressure gauge when sounds are no longer heard though the stethoscope as the blood pressure cuff is deflated
____ d. The lower pressure exerted against arterial walls when the heart is relaxed between contractions

24. Jaundice is best described as:
____ a. redness or flushing of the skin.
____ b. bluish discoloration of the skin due to poor oxygenation.
____ c. yellowish discoloration of the skin.
____ d. black, blue, or purple discoloration of the skin due to bruising.

25. When the pupils are described as "dilated," this means they:
____ a. are larger than normal.
____ b. do not react to light.
____ c. are unequal in size.
____ d. are smaller than normal.

26. A pulse oximetry reading of less than ____________ is considered abnormal and may be indicative of early hypoxia.
____ a. 100% ____ c. 96%
____ b. 98% ____ d. 94%

27. Which one of the following best describes a portable radio?
____ a. It is carried by the EMT.
____ b. It is mounted in the ambulance.
____ c. It is located on a tower to receive and amplify radio signals.
____ d. It is used only by ALS personnel to send ECG signals to the physician at the hospital.

28. A prehospital care report in which events and observations are recorded in the order they occurred best describes the ____________ method of documentation.
____ a. SOAP
____ b. chronological
____ c. CHART
____ d. physiological

29. The best way to protect yourself and your crew from hazards at a scene is:
____ a. performing a scene size-up.
____ b. always responding with a crew of at least three EMS providers.
____ c. wearing body armor.
____ d. refusing to respond without a law enforcement escort.

30. It is usually best to call for additional resources at a scene when you:
____ a. are absolutely certain you need them.
____ b. arrive at the scene and begin your scene size-up.
____ c. perform a complete assessment of all patients.
____ d. consult with medical direction.

31. Which one of the following is a disadvantage of mouth-to-mask ventilation with no supplemental oxygen?
____ a. Inadequate volume of ventilation
____ b. Low delivered-oxygen concentration
____ c. Requires extensive training
____ d. Difficult to maintain an adequate seal by one rescuer

32. Your patient is an elderly man who is ill. You find him unresponsive with snoring respirations. You should:
____ a. place a pillow under his head to flex the neck.
____ b. insert an oropharyngeal airway.
____ c. suction the mouth and pharynx.
____ d. use a head-tilt/chin-lift maneuver.

33. Your patient is suspected of taking an overdose of sleeping pills. He is snoring. Which one of the following is most likely responsible for this noise?
____ a. There is fluid in his lungs.
____ b. He has vomited and has fluid in his pharynx.
____ c. His tongue is obstructing his airway.
____ d. His dentures are obstructing his airway.

34. Aspiration is best described as:
____ a. drawing air into the lungs during normal breathing.
____ b. inhaling foreign material, such as liquids, into the lungs.
____ c. air leaving the lungs during breathing.
____ d. using a suction device to clear fluids from the mouth.

35. When suctioning an adult patient's mouth, suction should be applied for no more than ____________ seconds.
____ a. 5 ____ c. 15
____ b. 10 ____ d. 20

36. When suctioning the mouth of an infant, suction should be applied for no more than ____________ seconds.
____ a. 5 ____ c. 15
____ b. 10 ____ d. 20

37. Which of the following is the correct sequence for suctioning a patient's mouth?
1. Activate suction on the suction unit.
2. Place the tip of the catheter in the mouth.
3. Take BSI precautions.
4. Remove the suction tip from the mouth.
5. Connect the suction catheter to the suction tubing.
____ a. 3, 5, 1, 2, 4
____ b. 5, 1, 3, 2, 4
____ c. 3, 5, 2, 1, 4
____ d. 1, 5, 3, 2, 4

38. Which of the following steps are required for nasal suctioning of an adult patient but *not* for oral suctioning?
   1. Take BSI precautions.
   2. Measure the catheter from the tip of the nose to the earlobe.
   3. Use a water-based lubricant on the suction catheter.
   4. Suction for no more than 15 seconds.

   ____ a. 1, 3 ____ c. 1, 3, 4
   ____ b. 2, 3 ____ d. 1, 4

39. A bulb-type device is the best choice for:
   ____ a. oropharyngeal suctioning of an adult patient.
   ____ b. clearing food, teeth, or other solid objects from the airway.
   ____ c. suctioning the mouth and nose of newborns and infants.
   ____ d. inflating the large balloon of a Combitube.

40. Which one of the following statements regarding oropharyngeal airways is true?
   ____ a. They must not be used in patients with facial or head trauma.
   ____ b. They eliminate the need for manually opening the airway.
   ____ c. They must never be used in patients with a gag reflex.
   ____ d. They must not be used in patients under 12 years old.

41. The proper way to measure an oropharyngeal airway is from the ____________ to the earlobe.
   ____ a. tip of the nose
   ____ b. nostril
   ____ c. corner of the mouth
   ____ d. center of the mouth

42. You are attempting to deliver ventilations to your patient with a bag-mask device, but there is significant resistance to airflow. You should:
   ____ a. suction the patient's airway.
   ____ b. remove the oropharyngeal airway you have inserted and replace it with a different size.
   ____ c. initiate rescue breaths using a pocket mask.
   ____ d. perform abdominal thrusts.

43. Compared to insertion of basic airway adjuncts into the oral cavity, insertion of basic adjuncts into the nares carries a *decreased* risk of:
   ____ a. bleeding.
   ____ b. infection.
   ____ c. inducing a gag reflex.
   ____ d. failed ventilation.

44. The preferred technique of ventilating a patient when a single rescuer is present is:
   ____ a. one-rescuer bag-mask.
   ____ b. two-rescuer bag-mask.
   ____ c. demand-valve device.
   ____ d. mouth-to-mask.

45. The best device for ventilating through a stoma is a:
   ____ a. nonrebreather mask and supplemental oxygen.
   ____ b. Combitube and bag-mask device.
   ____ c. bag-mask device using an infant mask.
   ____ d. demand valve.

46. When caring for a patient with significant trauma, the scene time should be kept to a maximum of ____________ minutes.
   ____ a. 5 ____ c. 15
   ____ b. 10 ____ d. 30

47. Which of the following is *not* performed during the rapid assessment of a trauma patient?
   ____ a. Taking vital signs
   ____ b. Checking the chest for deformities
   ____ c. Checking the patient's back for significant injuries
   ____ d. Assessing for potentially life-threatening injuries

48. Your patient is a 48-year-old woman with pain in the right lower quadrant of her abdomen. Which one of the following is the best approach to the assessment and history of this patient?
   ____ a. Perform a rapid physical examination followed by a medical history.
   ____ b. Perform a thorough head-to-toe examination, and then obtain a SAMPLE history.
   ____ c. Obtain a medical history, and then perform a focused secondary assessment.
   ____ d. Perform a primary assessment and obtain a history, but defer further assessment to the physician at the emergency department.

49. The name of a drug that describes its composition is its ____________ name.
   ____ a. chemical ____ c. trade
   ____ b. official ____ d. generic

50. Which one of the following best describes the trade name of a drug?
   ____ a. Describes the elemental makeup of the drug
   ____ b. Used in the *United States Pharmacopeia* to reference the drug
   ____ c. Used by all companies that market the drug
   ____ d. Given by the company that first markets the drug

51. Which one of the following medications would have its effect most quickly?
____ a. Subcutaneous injection of epinephrine
____ b. Oral glucose gel
____ c. Tylenol tablet
____ d. Puff of albuterol

52. Which one of the following best describes contraindications of a drug?
____ a. Unwanted effects of the drug
____ b. Reasons why the drug should be given
____ c. Desired effects of the drug
____ d. Reasons why someone should *not* be given a drug

53. Nitroglycerin is a drug that can come in multiple forms. Both common forms—spray and tablet—are administered:
____ a. as a subcutaneous injection.
____ b. intramuscularly.
____ c. by injection.
____ d. sublingually.

54. Your patient is a 22-year-old man. You should consider his respiratory rate normal if it is ____________ per minute.
____ a. 60 ____ c. 12
____ b. 48 ____ d. 28

55. Cheyne-Stokes respirations are characterized by:
____ a. regular, deep, rapid respirations.
____ b. alternating cycles of very deep respirations followed by shallow respirations and a period of apnea.
____ c. an irregular, chaotic pattern.
____ d. shallow, gasping respirations.

56. Respiratory failure is best defined as:
____ a. use of accessory muscles during breathing.
____ b. sensation of shortness of breath.
____ c. inability of the body to compensate for illness or injury, resulting in an inadequate supply of oxygen to the body.
____ d. constriction of the bronchioles, resulting in wheezing and coughing.

57. Fine, crackling sounds in the lungs indicate the presence of which one of the following?
____ a. Thick mucus in the bronchi
____ b. Swelling in the upper airway
____ c. Fluid in the alveoli
____ d. Narrowing of the bronchioles

58. Asthma is characterized by:
____ a. air trapped in the lungs due to breakdown of the walls of the alveoli.
____ b. constriction of the small airways leading to the alveoli.
____ c. chronic increased mucus production and cough due to smoking.
____ d. pockets of pus in the lungs due to bacterial infection.

59. Which one of the following devices delivers tiny droplets of medication over an extended period of time through a mask or mouthpiece?
____ a. Nebulizer ____ c. Aspirator
____ b. Inhaler ____ d. Vaporizer

60. The function of the epiglottis is to:
____ a. allow food to pass from the pharynx to the stomach.
____ b. keep air flowing into the trachea during swallowing.
____ c. make the trachea more rigid.
____ d. prevent food and liquids from entering the trachea.

61. You have just assisted a patient with the use of an albuterol inhaler. Upon reassessing vital signs, you note the pulse rate has increased from 92 to 112. The patient's hands are shaking, but she is alert and her respiratory rate has decreased from 44 to 30. Which one of the following is most likely?
____ a. The patient received an adequate dose of the medication.
____ b. The patient is becoming hypoxic.
____ c. You are making the patient nervous.
____ d. She is having an allergic reaction to the medication.

62. A dangerous side effect of nitroglycerin is that it can cause:
____ a. constriction of the coronary arteries.
____ b. a drop in blood pressure.
____ c. psychotic behavior.
____ d. blood clots.

63. The aorta is best described as:
____ a. a large vein in the neck.
____ b. an artery in the chest and abdomen.
____ c. the largest vein in the body.
____ d. a large artery in the groin.

64. The circulation of well-oxygenated blood to the cells of the body is known as:
____ a. perfusion. ____ c. distribution.
____ b. metabolism. ____ d. exchange.

65. A myocardial infarction is a:
____ a. cardiac arrest.
____ b. heart failure.
____ c. heart attack.
____ d. stroke.

66. Which one of the following is a contraindication for the administration of nitroglycerin to a patient with chest pain?
____ a. The patient took Cialis earlier in the day.
____ b. The blood pressure is 130/90.
____ c. The patient took a nitroglycerin tablet before you arrived.
____ d. The patient's pulse is otherwise "normal."

67. Defibrillation is designed to work in which one of the following situations?
____ a. There is no electrical activity in the heart.
____ b. There is chaotic electrical activity in the heart.
____ c. The patient is having chest pain.
____ d. The patient has an irregular pulse.

68. Most automatic defibrillators are programmed to deliver ____________ shock(s) during the first cycle.
____ a. one
____ b. two
____ c. three
____ d. four

69. A seizure that affects both sides of the brain can be referred to as a ____________ seizure.
____ a. complex
____ b. simple partial
____ c. generalized
____ d. postictal

70. A blood clot in or rupture of a blood vessel in the brain leading to signs and symptoms such as headache, paralysis, and slurred speech best describes:
____ a. seizure.
____ b. myocardial infarction.
____ c. epilepsy.
____ d. stroke.

71. For which one of the following situations would you most likely receive an order to administer activated charcoal?
____ a. Patient has a known allergy to bees and has just been stung by a bee.
____ b. Diabetic has taken his insulin but did not eat lunch.
____ c. Patient took an overdose of seizure medications within the last 30 minutes.
____ d. Patient complaining of chest pain has a prescription for the drug.

72. You are called to a marina where you are directed to a 46-year-old woman who slipped on a portable staircase while boarding her boat. When she fell, her abdomen struck the boat's railing. Her vitals are pulse 136, respiration 24, and blood pressure 80/60. After completing the primary assessment, you should next:
____ a. initiate transport.
____ b. utilize OPQRST to further examine chief complaint.
____ c. obtain SAMPLE history.
____ d. conduct secondary assessment.

73. Prior to being diagnosed, a patient with diabetes will most likely have which one of the following conditions?
____ a. Hyperglycemia
____ b. Hypoglycemia
____ c. Diabetic coma
____ d. Insulin effect

74. Your patient is a 40-year-old woman who is allergic to shellfish. Immediately after eating some stew at a friend's house, she experienced swelling of her face, severe difficulty breathing, light-headedness, and low blood pressure. This is most likely:
____ a. a mild allergic reaction.
____ b. hives.
____ c. anaphylaxis.
____ d. food poisoning.

75. Another word for epinephrine is:
____ a. insulin.
____ b. glucose.
____ c. adrenalin.
____ d. bile.

76. While obtaining a SAMPLE history on a 68-year-old man who has been involved in a significant fall while shopping, you learn that he is taking Coumadin (warfarin). Based on this information where would you transport him?
____ a. Nearest emergency department
____ b. Cardiac center
____ c. Trauma center
____ d. Stroke center

77. Your patient is a 22-year-old woman who is breathing rapidly, clutching her chest, and begging you not to let her die. Her roommate tells you that the patient has a history of panic attacks. Which one of the following is an appropriate approach to the patient?

____ a. Look the patient directly in the eye and say, "You need to get a hold of yourself. There's no reason for you to be panicked."

____ b. Stand back from the patient and ask whether or not she wants to go to the hospital.

____ c. Get on the patient's level and say, "I'm an EMT with the ambulance service. Let's see what we can do to help you."

____ d. Place your hand on the patient's shoulder and let her know that EMTs are not trained to handle psychiatric problems and that she should contact her psychiatrist.

78. You have just assisted with the delivery of a full-term infant. You have suctioned his mouth and nose and have clamped and cut the cord, but the infant is not breathing. Which one of the following should you do next?

____ a. Insert an oropharyngeal airway and ventilate the patient with a bag-mask device.

____ b. Utilize tactile stimulation to get him to breathe.

____ c. Perform mouth-to-mask ventilations.

____ d. Administer supplemental oxygen.

79. Shock is best described as:

____ a. hypoperfusion.

____ b. low blood pressure.

____ c. bleeding.

____ d. internal hemorrhage.

80. Which one of the following statements about shock is true?

____ a. Once a patient is in shock, death is inevitable.

____ b. Shock is progressive without intervention.

____ c. Definitive treatment for the patient in shock is supplemental oxygen.

____ d. All blood loss leads to shock.

81. Your patient is a 32-year-old male motorcycle rider who struck a parked vehicle and was thrown over the handlebars of the motorcycle. He has contusions on both thighs from contact with the handlebars as he was ejected. Which one of the following best explains why you should be concerned with this finding?

____ a. The patient is likely experiencing a crush injury.

____ b. It indicates the patient is at risk for shock.

____ c. Contusions are extremely painful.

____ d. The wounds may become contaminated if not properly dressed and bandaged.

82. Your patient has cut her hand with a knife and has bright red bleeding that seems to be pumping out under pressure. This is most likely ____________ bleeding.

____ a. venous

____ b. capillary

____ c. arterial

____ d. mixed venous and capillary

83. Your patient is a 12-year-old who cut his anterior elbow when he ran through a glass door with his arms outstretched. The patient is bleeding severely. You have tried direct pressure without success. You should:

____ a. apply a tourniquet.

____ b. elevate the limb and put pressure on the brachial artery.

____ c. apply a pressure point.

____ d. place pressure on the brachial artery, and then elevate.

84. The purpose of a dressing is to:

____ a. cover a wound to control bleeding and prevent contamination.

____ b. prevent motion of an injured extremity.

____ c. relieve pain and reduce swelling.

____ d. hold gauze pads in place over a wound.

85. Crush-force trauma would most likely occur in which one of the following situations?

____ a. A hunter is accidentally shot in the back with an arrow.

____ b. A soldier steps on a land mine.

____ c. A man falls from a fifth floor balcony onto a parked car below.

____ d. A construction worker is pinned by a forklift that rolled over on his legs.

86. Partial-thickness burns are characterized by:

____ a. redness and with no blisters.

____ b. redness with blisters.

____ c. charring.

____ d. white, leathery appearance.

87. Your patient is a 15-month-old who pulled a deep-fryer full of hot oil off a countertop. She has burns to her entire head, face, neck, and anterior torso. The percentage of body surface area involved is:

____ a. 9%. ____ c. 24%.

____ b. 18%. ____ d. 27%.

88. Burns are considered more serious if they affect which one of the following body parts?

____ a. Chest ____ c. Hand

____ b. Arm ____ d. Leg

89. Your patient is a 25-year-old male who was soldering two pieces of metal together when the soldering gun slipped and created a full-thickness burn about the size of a penny on his forearm. This burn would be considered:

____ a. severe. ____ c. moderate.
____ b. intense. ____ d. mild.

90. Your patient is a factory-worker whose face was splashed with an acid. You should:

____ a. transport him to the hospital for proper decontamination.
____ b. flush with large amounts of water.
____ c. wipe the chemical away with a damp cloth.
____ d. find an antidote to the chemical and apply it to the affected areas.

91. Which one of the following statements concerning electrical burns is true?

____ a. The greatest risk with electrical burns is thermal burns to a large percentage of body surface area.
____ b. Electrical burns can be associated with cardiac and respiratory problems.
____ c. Exposure to electrical current does not cause a burn on entry, but causes massive burns where it exits the body.
____ d. Electricity generally travels across the skin rather than internally through the body.

92. Your patient is a 15-year-old who received partial-thickness burns to 50% of his body and full-thickness burns to 20% of his body. Which of the following should be your greatest concern in the immediate care of this patient?

____ a. Hypothermia
____ b. Blood loss
____ c. Infection
____ d. Heart failure

93. The pleural layers and the fluid between them are important in providing:

____ a. suction between the chest wall and lungs.
____ b. friction between the chest wall and lungs.
____ c. trapped air in the thorax.
____ d. protection from blunt trauma.

94. An adult male patient was stabbed in the left anterior chest at the nipple-level just next to his sternum. The knife has a three-inch blade. It would be *least* likely to have injury to the patient's:

____ a. kidney. ____ c. liver.
____ b. heart ____ d. bronchus.

95. A flail chest is characterized by:

____ a. two or more consecutive ribs, each fractured in two or more places.
____ b. a collapsed lung.
____ c. air entering the pleural cavity through an open wound in the chest wall.
____ d. an accumulation of blood in the pleural cavity.

96. The primary concerns with damage to hollow organs of the abdomen are:

____ a. irritation of the peritoneum and infection.
____ b. bleeding and hemorrhagic shock.
____ c. swelling and pain.
____ d. vomiting and diarrhea.

97. Which one of the following is the best example of injury caused by indirect force?

____ a. The driver of a small truck strikes his knees on the dash in a frontal collision and suffers a fractured femur.
____ b. An elderly man has bone cancer. He coughs and sustains a fracture of a thoracic vertebra.
____ c. A football player has his foot planted when he is struck by another player, causing him to rotate around the planted foot, resulting in a fracture to his tibia and fibula.
____ d. A police officer is shot in the thigh with a large caliber projectile that fractures his femur.

98. Overstretching a muscle results in a:

____ a. fracture. ____ c. sprain.
____ b. strain. ____ d. dislocation.

99. Your patient is a 30-year-old woman who slipped on a wet floor and fell, injuring her wrist. The most appropriate approach to this patient is a:

____ a. rapid secondary assessment.
____ b. focused medical history.
____ c. focused secondary assessment.
____ d. detailed history and focused assessment.

100. For which one of the following patients would a rapid secondary assessment be appropriate?

____ a. 40-year-old who stepped off a curb, twisted her ankle, and fell to her knees.
____ b. Nine-year-old who fell 15 feet from a tree house and has a deformed right arm.
____ c. 75-year-old who stood up from her chair, felt a "snap" in her hip, and fell back into the chair.
____ d. Seven-year-old who has a deformed forearm after performing a cartwheel in gymnastics class.

101. Which one of the following does *not* adequately explain the purpose of splinting a swollen, painful, deformed extremity?
____ a. Splinting reduces pain associated with movement.
____ b. It makes the patient feel as if you are doing something for him but it serves little medical purpose.
____ c. Bleeding can be reduced by splinting.
____ d. Stabilizing bone ends reduces the possibility of further tissue damage.

102. Your patient has a swollen, deformed, painful wrist. A properly applied splint should start at the patient's ____________ and extend to ____________.
____ a. hand; just below the elbow
____ b. fingers; just above the elbow
____ c. hand; the shoulder
____ d. wrist; the shoulder

103. A traction splint is designed to be used for which one of the following injuries?
____ a. Open fractures of the tibia
____ b. Deformed mid-shaft humerus fractures
____ c. Injuries to the knee
____ d. Suspected femur fractures

104. A swathe is a useful adjunct to a sling in splinting which one of the following injuries?
____ a. Injured shoulder
____ b. Fractured pelvis
____ c. Suspected femur fracture
____ d. Swollen, deformed, painful finger

105. Your patient is a 12-year-old boy who fell 20 feet from a tree house to the ground. He is sitting up with his back against the tree, crying. He has a badly deformed humerus. Your priority in caring for this patient is:
____ a. checking the distal circulation, sensation, and motor function.
____ b. immobilizing the injured part.
____ c. minimizing the patient's pain.
____ d. assessing for and managing life-threatening conditions.

106. The floor of the cranial vault is described as the ____________ skull.
____ a. frontal ____ c. occipital
____ b. basilar ____ d. parietal

107. The weakest area of the skull is (are) the ____________ bone(s).
____ a. maxillary ____ c. parietal
____ b. temporal ____ d. occipital

108. Of the following, the highest priority in the care of the trauma patient is:
____ a. controlling bleeding.
____ b. determining the mechanism of injury.
____ c. providing manual stabilization of the cervical spine.
____ d. ensuring an open airway.

109. The skull is made up of the:
____ a. cranium and scalp.
____ b. cranium and face.
____ c. carpals and metacarpals.
____ d. carpals and ilium.

110. The cervical vertebrae are located:
____ a. in the back at the level of the ribs.
____ b. in the neck.
____ c. at the very base of the spine.
____ d. at the level of the pelvis.

111. The first step in proper spinal immobilization is:
____ a. manual stabilization of the head and neck.
____ b. placing a properly sized cervical collar.
____ c. using a short spinal immobilization device.
____ d. log rolling the patient onto a long backboard.

112. Your patient is a 21-year-old driver who was involved in a significant lateral-impact collision. She denies neck pain and is stable, but she is crying, she says she is cold, and it is taking you too long to get her into the ambulance. You should:
____ a. use rapid extrication to get her out of the vehicle.
____ b. use a short spinal immobilization device, and then remove her from the vehicle onto a long backboard.
____ c. contact medical direction for permission to skip spinal immobilization.
____ d. place the long backboard on the stretcher and have the patient place herself on it.

113. When responding to a victim of a deep-water diving emergency, you should keep in mind the location of the nearest:
____ a. hyperresonance compartment.
____ b. hypothermic resuscitation unit.
____ c. hyperbaric chamber.
____ d. hydrotherapy response team.

114. It is a cold morning, but it is clear and there is no wind. Your patient is a 48-year-old found lying on the frozen ground without a coat. He is losing heat mostly due to:

____ a. conduction and radiation.
____ b. evaporation and conduction.
____ c. convection and evaporation.
____ d. convection and radiation.

115. Your patient was hiking in the desert and was bitten on the ankle by a rattlesnake. You should:

____ a. keep the foot lower than the level of the patient's heart.
____ b. elevate the foot on pillows.
____ c. apply a tourniquet above the bite.
____ d. apply ice to the area of the bite.

116. When a pediatric patient suffers cardiac arrest, it is most often due to:

____ a. a respiratory problem.
____ b. a birth defect.
____ c. poisoning.
____ d. electrical shock.

117. Which one of the following is included in the pediatric assessment triangle?

____ a. Observing the safety of the environment
____ b. General appearance of the patient
____ c. Parent reaction to the child's condition
____ d. Pupillary reaction

118. Which one of the following statements concerning respiratory emergencies in pediatric patients is true?

____ a. Pediatric patients gradually decompensate, providing warning of impending respiratory failure.
____ b. The presence of nasal flaring is unlikely to occur in the pediatric patient in respiratory distress.
____ c. Grunting with exhalation is a sign of respiratory distress in pediatric patients.
____ d. Respiratory distress is always accompanied by cyanosis in the pediatric patient.

119. Which one of the following devices is preferred for nasal suctioning of an infant?

____ a. Bulb syringe
____ b. 30-mL medicine syringe
____ c. Flexible suction catheter
____ d. Rigid suction tip

120. You are called to a home day care center where an eight-month-old placed the wheel of a toy car in his mouth. The frantic day care provider hands you a baby who appears blue around the lips and is minimally moving air. Which one of the following is appropriate for this patient?

____ a. Perform back blows (slaps) and chest thrusts.
____ b. Perform abdominal thrusts.
____ c. Observe the patient in case he coughs up the wheel.
____ d. Perform a finger sweep.

121. The most common cause of trauma in children is:

____ a. falls.
____ b. motor-vehicle crashes.
____ c. child abuse.
____ d. recreational injuries.

122. Which one of the following is *not* a factor in the increased risk of hypothermia in the pediatric population?

____ a. Less body fat
____ b. Greater body surface area
____ c. Few glucose reserves
____ d. Slower metabolism

123. A gastrostomy tube is used to:

____ a. drain excessive cerebrospinal fluid from the skull into the abdomen.
____ b. provide a means of mechanical ventilation through an opening in the neck.
____ c. provide nutrition to a patient who cannot eat or swallow.
____ d. provide access to the central circulation for the administration of medications.

124. Medically, patients over the age of 65 are referred to as:

____ a. old.
____ b. geriatric.
____ c. seniors.
____ d. mature.

125. Which one of the following is a normal age-related change in the nervous system?

____ a. Increased sensitivity of the skin
____ b. Decreased motor reaction time
____ c. Inability to learn new things
____ d. Weight gain

126. Your 85-year-old female patient is obviously short of breath but is refusing to be transported to the hospital. You should:

____ a. find out if a family member has power of attorney to consent to the patient's transport.
____ b. contact medical direction for advice.
____ c. find out why the patient does not want to go the hospital.
____ d. have the patient sign a refusal of treatment and transport form.

127. You are taking a report from a nurse who describes the patient as obese. You recognize this means that the patient has a BMI of at least:

____ a. 30 ____ c. 35
____ b. 25 ____ d. 40

128. When responding to a call with light and siren, it is most important to ____________ at red lights.

____ a. slow to 10 mph
____ b. stop
____ c. look each direction
____ d. use the horn

129. NIMS is best described as:

____ a. a consistent nationwide approach in responding to events requiring coordinated public safety response.
____ b. a multiple-casualty incident.
____ c. EMS personnel "freelancing" at the scene of an emergency.
____ d. a designated disaster medical response team.

130. As you begin to classify patients at an MCI, what is the first group or color tag you should address?

____ a. Red ____ c. Black
____ b. Yellow ____ d. Green

131. Patients are tagged red using START triage when:

____ a. capillary refill time is over two seconds.
____ b. their radial pulse is above 60.
____ c. they are unresponsive to verbal stimuli.
____ d. they can walk away from the incident.

132. Any substance or material that poses an unreasonable risk to health, safety, and property is a(an):

____ a. chemical substance.
____ b. hazardous material.
____ c. inert matter.
____ d. vapor compound.

133. Substances stored in stationary tanks and facilities, such as at swimming pools, are marked using a system known as:

____ a. DOT placards.
____ b. Emergency Response Guides.
____ c. NFPA 704.
____ d. U.S. Radiologic Survey.

134. You have noted a diamond-shaped sign on a storage tank behind a hospital. The top quadrant of the diamond contains the numeral "1." This means the substance stored inside the tank poses a(an):

____ a. extreme risk of fire.
____ b. low risk of fire.
____ c. extreme risk of explosion.
____ d. low risk of explosion.

135. You have noted a diamond-shaped sign on a storage tank at a farm supply company. The bottom quadrant of the diamond contains a letter "W" with a line through it. This means:

____ a. the tank contains an inert substance.
____ b. the tank contains a dry substance rather than a liquid or wet substance.
____ c. the tank contains an oxidizer.
____ d. mixing water with this substance creates a hazard.

136. The diamond-shaped symbol on a transportation container, such as a tanker truck, is called a:

____ a. bill of lading.
____ b. placard.
____ c. hazard notice.
____ d. material safety data sheet.

137. Employers must keep paperwork on all potentially hazardous substances in the workplace called:

____ a. material safety data sheets.
____ b. placards.
____ c. manifests.
____ d. ORM-Ds.

138. The blue quadrant of an NFPA diamond contains information about a substance's:

____ a. special considerations.
____ b. health risks.
____ c. fire hazard.
____ d. explosive potential.

139. You have been dispatched to a railroad yard for a "sick person." On your arrival, you note that there are three individuals on the ground next to a tank car. Using binoculars to inspect the tank, you should compare the information you find to that found in the:

____ a. *Emergency Response Guidebook.*
____ b. hazmat manual.
____ c. bill of lading.
____ d. material safety data sheet.

140. Under what circumstances is it permissible for an EMT to approach a hazardous materials scene?

____ a. The EMT is a firefighter and is wearing turnout gear.
____ b. The EMT is trained as a hazardous materials technician and is wearing SCBA.
____ c. The EMT is trained at the hazardous materials awareness level and is wearing a HEPA mask.
____ d. The EMT has immediate access to a decontamination shower upon leaving the area.

141. A flammable solid is considered a DOT hazard class:

____ a. 1. ____ c. 3.
____ b. 2. ____ d. 4.

142. DOT hazard class 9 indicates:
____ a. flammable liquids.
____ b. explosives.
____ c. miscellaneous dangerous goods.
____ d. corrosives.

143. Situations calling for wilderness search and rescue, water rescue, rope rescue, and other types of events requiring special training and equipment are called __________ rescue situations.
____ a. USAR ____ c. tactical
____ b. operational ____ d. technical

144. The first phase of a rescue operation is:
____ a. gaining access to the patient.
____ b. preparing for the rescue.
____ c. sizing up the situation.
____ d. providing initial patient assessment.

145. Devices placed on either side of the tires of a vehicle to stabilize it are called:
____ a. chocks. ____ c. jacks.
____ b. props. ____ d. buttresses.

146. You are not able to access a patient entrapped in a motor vehicle following a collision without the use of equipment. This is known as ____________ access.
____ a. complex ____ c. easy
____ b. intricate ____ d. simple

147. According to the NFPA, all technical rescue incidents involve:
____ a. SCBA equipment.
____ b. trenches or other confined spaces.
____ c. special ropes and ladders.
____ d. specialized training.

148. The period of time it takes for a biological agent to start manifesting itself is called the:
____ a. dormant life.
____ b. gestation period.
____ c. transmission state.
____ d. incubation period.

149. In which one of the following settings might you suspect terrorism?
____ a. Hospital where multiple patients are suffering from the same illness
____ b. Large sporting event where large numbers of people are showing signs of illness
____ c. Patrons of an auto race that were struck by debris
____ d. Industrial site dealing with an MCI after an equipment explosion

150. What weapon does *not* fall into a B-NICE category for weapons of mass destruction?
____ a. Nuclear ____ c. Improvised
____ b. Biological ____ d. Chemical

APPENDIX 2

ALS Assist Skills

Objectives

After completion of this lesson, you should be able to:

A2-1 Define key terms introduced in this appendix.

A2-2 List the various skills the EMT is able to assist an ALS provider with performing.

A2-3 Discuss the role of the EMT when assisting the ALS provider with medication administration.

A2-4 Differentiate the purpose of a three- or four-lead ECG and a 12-lead ECG.

A2-5 Describe the proper electrode placement for three- and four-lead ECG analysis.

A2-6 Describe the proper electrode placement for a 12-lead ECG analysis.

A2-7 Differentiate between an endotracheal tube and the various types of supraglottic airways used in EMS.

A2-8 List the tools necessary for endotracheal intubation.

A2-9 Differentiate between the Mac and Miller style of laryngoscope blades.

A2-10 Describe the various ways to confirm placement of an advanced airway.

A2-11 Describe the proper technique for securing an advanced airway in place.

A2-12 List the common IV fluids used in EMS.

A2-13 Differentiate between macro and micro drip sets.

A2-14 Describe how to set up an intravenous line for infusion of fluids.

A2-15 Describe the purpose of a saline lock.

Key Terms

capnography p. 1259
ECG p. 1255
endotracheal tube (ETT) p. 1259
end-tidal CO_2 p. 1259
vallecula p. 1259

Introduction

It is often said that while both EMTs and ALS providers save lives, EMTs also save ALS providers. In any given emergency there are many different challenges that the EMS team must face. The ability to work together as a smooth and efficient team is critical to excellent patient care. The EMT is a valuable team member. The ALS provider must learn to depend on EMT assistance in order to provide prompt and efficient care.

Assisting with ALS Care

A2-2 List the various skills the EMT is able to assist an ALS provider with performing.

While many EMTs work together with other EMTs and emergency medical responders, there also are systems that utilize an ALS/BLS transport team such as an ALS provider and EMT. In this configuration, the EMT must learn additional skills that will maximize the effectiveness of the ALS provider and the care provided. Those skills include:

- Patient assessment
- **ECG** lead placement
- Advanced airway management
- Intravenous access and fluid therapy

ECG electrocardiogram. Also called *EKG*.

BLS Before ALS

All patients must receive appropriate BLS care if there is any hope that ALS care will be beneficial. In other words, BLS before ALS. This is an important mantra for all EMS teams to remember and practice. Many of the advanced skills that an ALS provider is able to perform will not make a difference if the most basic BLS skills have been neglected. For instance, an advanced airway and medications will not be of benefit if the patient has not had proper BLS airway management and proper ventilations.

The EMT can be instrumental in assisting with many of the elements of the patient assessment. Both the primary and secondary assessments are skills that can be accomplished as a team, making the process much faster. This in turn means that necessary interventions can be initiated sooner. Other BLS skills such as spinal immobilization and bleeding control are essential and do not differ from EMT to ALS provider.

Assisting with Medication Administration

A2-3 Discuss the role of the EMT when assisting the ALS provider with medication administration.

In many EMS systems EMTs may assist the patient with the administration of certain medications such as nitroglycerin (NTG), aspirin, metered-dose inhalers, and some nebulized medications. When every second counts, the patient experiencing a cardiac or respiratory emergency greatly depends on both the EMT and ALS provider to deliver life-saving care. Cardiac patients require a combination of treatments, such as rapid medical assessment and administration of medications. While it may be outside the EMT's scope of practice to administrator the NTG and aspirin, the EMT can assist the patient with the medication. Afterward, it is important for the EMT to assist the ALS provider with obtaining follow-up vital signs and observing for signs and symptoms of any reactions to the medication or changes in the patient's condition.

There are numerous considerations to make when administering medications. Prehospital care is almost always in a high-stress environment. Therefore, it is appropriate to think that medication errors and mistakes can and will be made. As an EMT you can assist the ALS provider and decrease the likelihood of a potential medication administration error. Simply managing the patient's other medical needs while the ALS provider gives consideration to the proper drug, dosage, and route is one way to help. Another is to gather up the equipment such as the proper syringe, needle, fluid, tubing, and perhaps reminding the ALS provider to review the five "rights" of medication administration before administering the medication.

Many prehospital medication dosages are calculated based on the patient's body weight. For the purpose of medication dosing, body weight is calculated in kilograms. As an EMT you can help serve your ALS partner by becoming proficient in converting pounds to kilograms. As a quick refresher, there are 2.2 kg per pound. For instance, a typical 180 lb adult man would weigh 81.6 kg.

Cardiac Monitoring

A2-4 Differentiate the purpose of a three- or four-lead ECG and a 12-lead ECG.

An important tool in the assessment of the suspected cardiac patient is the cardiac monitor. Depending on the type and model, the cardiac monitor may be capable of obtaining several different "views" of the electrical activity of the heart. A view is simply a look at the electrical activity of the heart from a specific angle. This advanced skill has proven time and time again to be one of the determining factors of whether or not the patient is experiencing a myocardial infarction.

Many times as the ALS provider is obtaining important medical history from the patient or family members, the EMT can begin applying the ECG leads on the patient. Depending on the capabilities of the cardiac monitor and the number of leads applied to the patient, the ALS provider will have anywhere from a single view (three leads) to 12 views (10 leads) of the electrical activity of the heart. The 12-lead ECG provides one

SCAN A2-1 Placement of a Three-Lead ECG

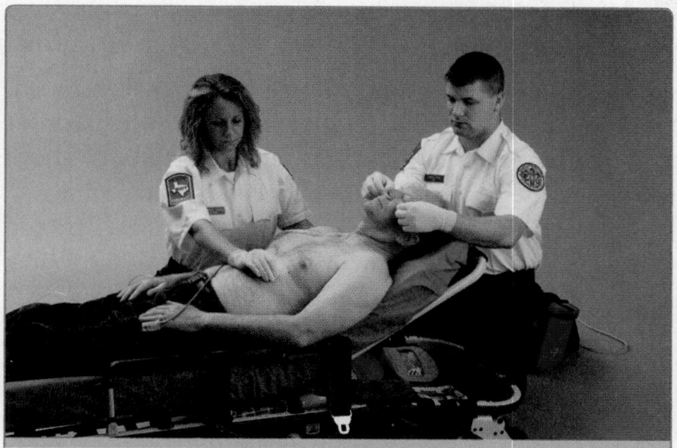

A2-1-1 Expose the patient's chest and ensure that it is dry and clean.

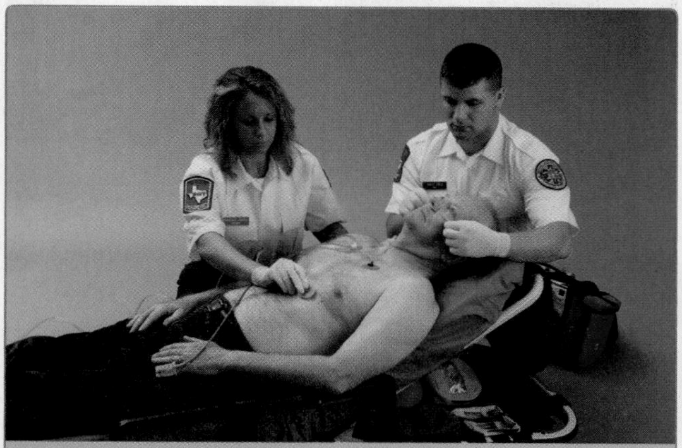

A2-1-2 Apply the three limb leads according to the manufacturer's recommendation.

of the most comprehensive views of the heart and often can reveal the presence of a variety of cardiac abnormalities including a myocardial infarction.

Three- and Four-Lead Electrode Placement

A2-5 Describe the proper electrode placement for three- and four-lead ECG analysis.

Depending on the particular monitor you are using, you may have either three or four leads that must be attached to the patient in order to obtain a view of the electrical activity of the heart. These leads are often referred to as *limb leads* because they are placed on or very near three or four of the patient's limbs.

The first step to ensure a proper view of the heart is proper electrode placement. An old saying used to remind the EMT of the proper three-lead placement is "white to the right and smoke over fire." This represents the correct placement of the three electrodes and leads, which are white, black, and red. It is important to remember that the white lead is labeled, *RA* (right arm). The black lead is labeled *LA* (left arm), and the red lead is labeled *LL* (left leg). These leads are actually placed on the patient's chest near the respective limb. The white lead is placed on the right side near or at the patient's clavicle or first intercostal space. The black lead is placed directly across from the white lead in the same location but on the left side. The red lead is placed below the black lead at or near the seventh intercostal space (Scan A2-1).

A five-lead ECG is becoming more and more common in EMS and utilizes a fifth lead that can be placed in different locations on the chest to reveal different views.

12-Lead Electrode Placement

A2-6 Describe the proper electrode placement for a 12-lead ECG analysis.

The 12-lead ECG is becoming quite common in the prehospital setting and is by far the most comprehensive tool for examining the electrical activity of the heart. It has been in use in hospitals for many years but only in the past 10 years has it become more common in EMS. Not all cardiac monitors are capable of performing a 12-lead ECG (Figure A2-1 ■).

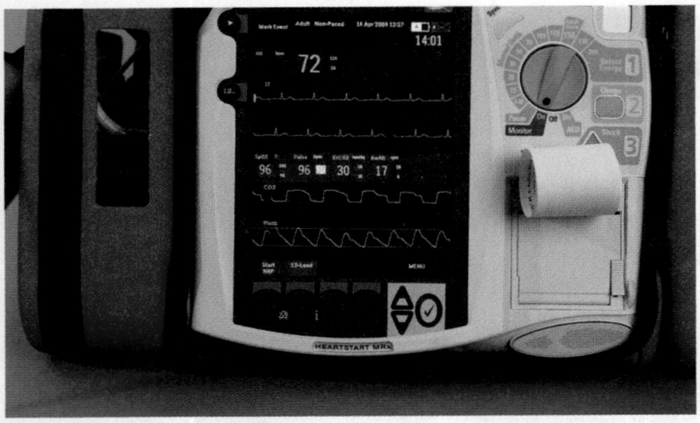

Figure A2-1 A typical cardiac monitor capable of obtaining a 12-lead ECG.

Having the ability to put all the pieces of the puzzle together at once certainly allows you to understand the complete picture. Obtaining a 12-lead ECG allows you to do just that. The application requires six chest leads and four limb leads. The six chest leads are labeled V1, V2, V3, V4, V5, V6 and the four limb leads are labeled LL, LA, RL, RA.

The limb leads are applied according to their labels. The LL (left leg) is placed just above the left foot and the LA (left arm) is placed on the left wrist. The RL (right leg) is placed just above the right foot, and the RA (right arm) is placed on the right wrist.

The V leads are placed on the patient's chest wall. V1 should be placed just lateral to the sternum on the right side at the fourth intercostal space. Moving across the sternum to the left side, V2 should also be placed at the fourth intercostal space. V3 is skipped and V4 is placed over the fifth intercostal space directly on the midclavicular line. Then V3 is placed midway between V2 and V4. V5 should be placed at the fifth intercostal space on the anterior axillary line. V6 should be placed at the fifth intercostal space on the mid-axillary line (Figure A2-2 ■).

Assisting with Advanced Airway Management

A2-7 Differentiate between an endotracheal tube and the various types of supraglottic airways used in EMS.

Proper management of a patient's ABCs is essential for survival. The EMT can deliver care to the patient who needs an airway only up to a certain point. Patients that present with a difficult airway or patients needing a more reliable airway require skills that only the ALS provider can perform in the field. Skills such as endotracheal intubation, rapid sequence induction, and the use of a ventilator are all procedures the EMT might be able to lend a useful hand.

The EMT can assist with maintaining an open airway and basic maneuvers such as ventilating with a bag-mask device, while the ALS provider prepares the patient for the insertion of an advanced airway. In many situations in which the patient is in need of an advanced airway, the EMT can direct other rescuers at the scene about BLS airway management and ventilation. That can free up the EMT to begin gathering the necessary equipment for the ALS provider. Selecting a device of the proper size, assembling the device, assembling the laryngoscope with the requested blade, and gathering the necessary tools for verifying placement are all ways the EMT can assist the ALS

Lead V_1 The electrode is at the fourth intercostal space just to the right of the sternum.
Lead V_2 The electrode is at the fourth intercostal space just to the left of the sternum.
Lead V_3 The electrode is at the line midway between leads V_2 and V_4.
Lead V_4 The electrode is at the midclavicular line in the fifth interspace.
Lead V_5 The electrode is at the anterior axillary line at the same level as lead V_4.
Lead V_6 The electrode is at the midaxillary line at the same level as lead V_4.

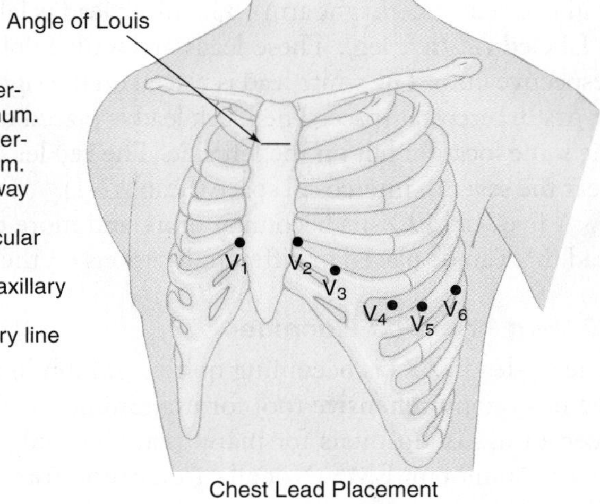

Figure A2-2 Proper placement of the chest leads for a 12-lead ECG.

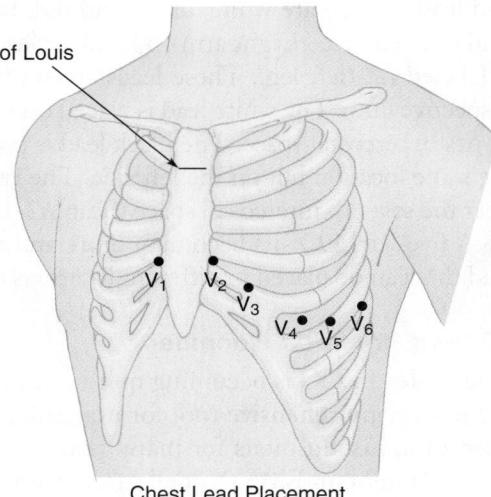

provider with placement of an advanced airway. (Refer to Appendix 3 for more information regarding advanced airway placement.)

The **endotracheal tube** is most commonly referred to as an ETT or ET tube. The ETT is a common advanced airway used by many ALS providers, respiratory therapists, and physicians. The ETT has long been the gold standard of advanced airways and is often compared to other devices used in EMS such as supraglottic airway devices.

endotracheal tube (ETT) an advanced airway that is placed directly into the trachea.

The ETT requires specialized training and technique because it must be placed directly into the trachea to ventilate the lungs. If this is not done correctly, the patient will become more and more hypoxic and die.

Supraglottic airways can range from triple-lumen tubes to a single device. They are commonly used by BLS providers as well as advanced providers. Though specialized training is needed to utilize a supraglottic airway, seating it in the trachea is not as important as it is for the ETT. Supraglottic airways can be blindly placed into the oral cavity and seated in or near either the esophagus or trachea. The provider simply ventilates to obtain chest rise and fall.

A2-8 List the tools necessary for endotracheal intubation.

Properly preparing the patient for an endotracheal intubation is an essential and vital step toward a successful outcome. Many mistakes can be made by simply not taking the time to thoroughly assess the patient and spending ample time assessing the patient's airway. In addition, many times providers find themselves in a bad situation because they either forgot what equipment they needed or did not take the time to gather all the proper equipment in advance.

Depending on the patient's condition and your local protocol, there may be a slight difference in procedure or equipment to gather. Common equipment needed is as follows:

- ETT appropriate for the patient's age and size
- Laryngoscope with either a Miller or Macintosh blade
- Stylet for guiding the ETT
- 10-cc syringe
- Securing device
- Colorimetric or **capnography** device

capnography the monitoring of the concentration or partial pressure of carbon dioxide (CO_2) in respiratory gases.

The Laryngoscope

The laryngoscope is a device that is used to facilitate endotracheal intubation and is composed of a handle, blade, and a light. Laryngoscope blades are long, smooth, dull devices that come in two different types—the Miller and Macintosh. The Miller blade is straight and the Macintosh blade is curved. For most providers it is simply personal preference as to which blade they prefer. The Macintosh (curved) blade is placed at the **vallecula** and anterior to the epiglottis. This allows for the lifting and visualization of the glottic opening. The Miller blade is positioned posterior to the epiglottis, allowing exposure to the glottis and vocal cords.

A2-9 Differentiate between the Mac and Miller style of laryngoscope blades.

vallecula a depression between the root of the tongue and the epiglottis.

Once the ETT is secured, it is important to confirm it is in the correct place. That can be done by auscultation of the lung fields, placing a colorimetric CO_2 detection device on the end of the ETT or by way of capnography. During auscultation you should hear air movement over the right and left and upper and lower lung fields. If breath sounds cannot be heard in any lung field, it is likely that the tube is not placed properly and will have to be removed.

A2-10 Describe the various ways to confirm placement of an advanced airway.

The colorimetric CO_2 detection device has three colors—yellow, tan, and purple. It is placed on the end of the ETT. Normal **end-tidal CO_2** is $>2\%$. Purple implies $ETCO_2$ of $<0.5\%$. Tan implies $ETCO_2$ of 0.5% to 2%. Yellow implies $ETCO_2$ of $>2\%$. In simple terms purple people die, yellow means yes, and tan means trouble.

end-tidal CO_2 the concentration of carbon dioxide (CO_2) contained in the respiratory gases at the end of each exhaled breath.

Capnography is a great tool in conjunction with intubation or other airway adjunct devices that allow $ETCO_2$ measurement. The process of $ETCO_2$ begins at the cellular level. Food is turned into energy; both O_2 and CO_2 are transported from the cells to the pulmonary capillaries and into the alveoli. Once in the alveoli, ventilation and gas exchanges take place. Patients with lung diseases may have prior damage to the alveoli, causing a decrease in gas exchanges. This could play a significant role in the severity of respiratory failure.

Most transport monitors are equipped with $ETCO_2$ capabilities. This is a great resource for monitoring the patient in respiratory failure during transport. Simply connect the CO_2 detection device to the ETT or airway device. The advanced provider can then monitor the waveforms and parameters. Normal $ETCO_2$ parameters should fall within 35 to 37 mmHg.

A2-11 Describe the proper technique for securing an advanced airway in place.

Properly securing an advanced airway is one of the many important aspects to maintaining a patent airway. Without it, the risk of the ETT tube dislodging greatly increases. There are several different devices or methods available to secure an advanced airway. Some advanced airways may come prepackaged with a securing device. This is the approved method by the manufacturer and should always be considered as the preferred way to secure the device.

Other devices can be placed in the patient's mouth and tightly secured to the patient's head and neck. The tube is then secured in the center of the holder. This type of securing device also serves as a bite block that prevents the patient from inadvertently chewing on the tube and causing a compromise.

Some advanced airways are designed so that once they are seated in the correct position, they are secured. As with any advanced airway, the manufacturer's methods and recommendations should always be followed first.

A careful and thorough assessment should always be done before, during, and after the advanced airway is secured. Documentation should include the fact that the lung fields were assessed and equal breath sounds were heard, or that some form of $ETCO_2$ monitoring was used to confirm proper placement. Ensuring proper placement should be a part of reassessment. Some systems require the use of multiple methods to confirm tube placement.

Assisting with Intravenous Therapy

A2-12 List the common IV fluids used in EMS.

One of the most common skills an EMT can assist with is setting up an intravenous (IV) line. Once requested by the ALS provider, the EMT can select the proper solution, proper bag, and proper tubing. The two most common reasons an IV is established are medication administration and fluid replacement.

There are three commonly used IV fluids in EMS. They are normal saline (0.9% sodium chloride solution), lactated Ringer's solution, and D5W (5% dextrose in water).

Normal saline is the most commonly used among the three. For the most part, that is because it does not cause significant fluid or electrolyte shifts within the cells. Normal saline is used for the temporary expansion of the vascular volume by replacing water and electrolytes. Lactated Ringer's solution is commonly used in burn and hypovolemia patients.

D5W is a common solution used for many medical patients. D5W is most commonly used for IV access or to dilute medications to be given intravenously over a period of time.

Intravenous Tubing

A2-13 Differentiate between macro and micro drip sets.

In order to establish an IV you must have a way to get the solution from the solution bag to the patient. This is accomplished by way of IV tubing or an "administration set." Administration sets come in two common types—macro drip and micro drip. They are differentiated based on the number of drops it takes to deliver a single milliliter of fluid (gtt/mL). A micro or "mini" set requires 60 gtt/mL. A macro set comes in several sizes including 10-, 15-, and 20-drip variations. The ability to control the drip rate allows the ALS provider to control the amount of fluid being delivered to the patient. A macro set is capable of delivering more fluid faster, while the micro set allows for very controlled and precise delivery of fluid. There are several components common to most administration sets. They are as follows:

- Piercing spike
- Drip chamber
- Flow regulation clamp
- Drug administration port
- Connector end

The piercing spike is at the top of the drip chamber and is used to pierce the solution bag to begin the flow of fluid into the drip chamber. Down the line from the drip chamber are one or more administration ports that can be used to infuse medications or add additional fluids in a "piggy back" fashion. The end of the tube has a hard plastic port (connector end) that connects to the IV catheter inserted into the patient's vein. About halfway down the tubing is a small device called the *flow regulation clamp*. It is a small ribbed wheel locked inside a tapered housing. When the wheel is moved from one end of the housing to another, it can control flow by clamping or unclamping the tube.

A2-14 Describe how to set up an intravenous line for infusion of fluids.

When the ALS provider has instructed you to set up a specific solution, you must repeat back the order and confirm the type of drip tubing requested (micro or macro). Then perform the following steps to set up the solution and administration set (Scan A2-2):

1. Confirm the correct fluid and expiration date.
2. Open the proper administration kit and unwrap the tubing.
3. Close the flow regulation clamp on the tubing.
4. Remove the protective caps from both the IV bag and the piercing spike on the drip chamber.
5. Force the spike into the exposed port on the solution bag and give the soft drip chamber a couple of squeezes to draw the solution into the chamber. Be sure not to allow too much fluid into the chamber. There should be at least half an inch between the water line and the drip port inside the drip chamber.
6. Open the flow regulation clamp all the way to allow the solution to fill the tubing and push out all the air. If necessary, you may have to remove the protective cap from the end of the tubing to allow the free flow of fluid. Once all the air is out of the tubing, close the flow clamp and place the protective cap back on the end.

A2-15 Describe the purpose of a saline lock.

Another task that the EMT is commonly called on to perform is the securing of the IV catheter once it has been inserted. This typically involves the strategic placement of small strips of tape to ensure that the catheter does not become easily dislodged from the vein. There are several strategies for securing an IV catheter and most ALS providers have their preferred method. Be sure to ask your ALS partners what their preferences are before the need arises.

The Saline Lock

There are times when a patient is not in immediate need of fluids or medications but the clinical team would like to have convenient access to a vein should the need arise. A common tool for those patients is called a *saline lock*. A saline lock is a small access port that is connected to the end of the standard IV catheter with a special cap over the access port (Figure A2-3 ▪). The device is taped

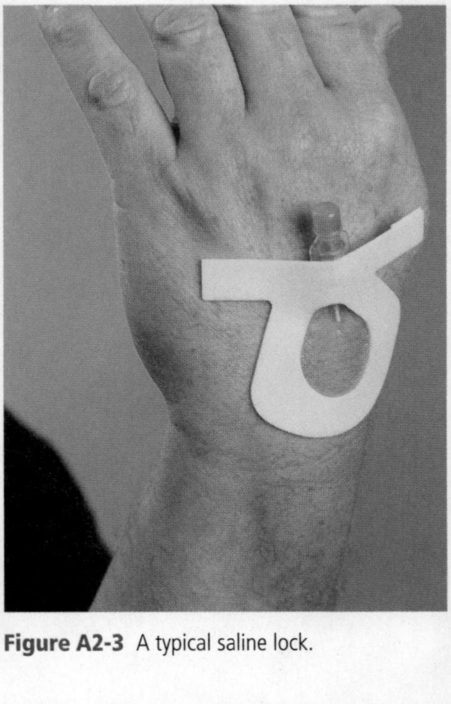

Figure A2-3 A typical saline lock.

SCAN A2-2 Preparing an IV Solution with Administration Set

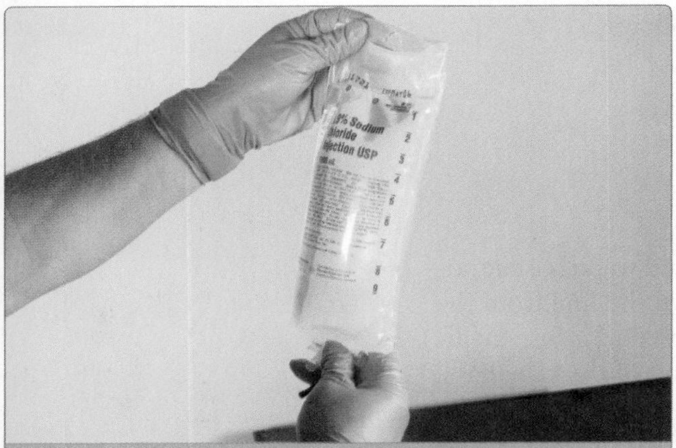

A2-2-1 Confirm the correct solution and expiration date.

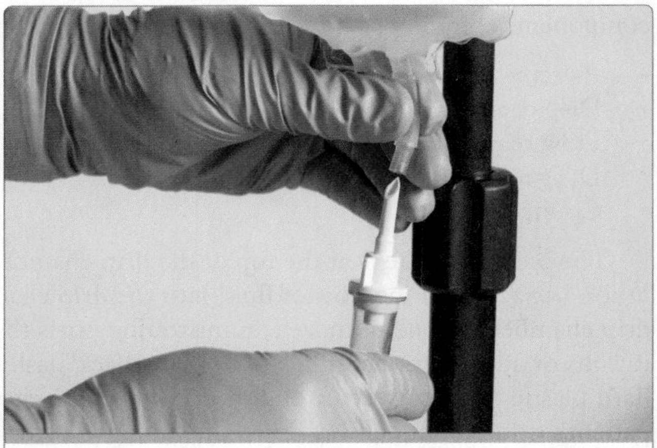

A2-2-2 Remove the protective cap on both the solution bag and the drip chamber, and then insert into the bag.

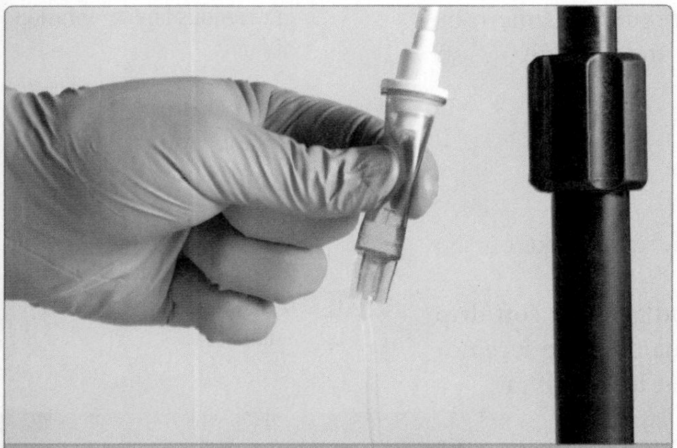

A2-2-3 Squeeze the drip chamber a couple of times to fill with fluid. Do not overfill.

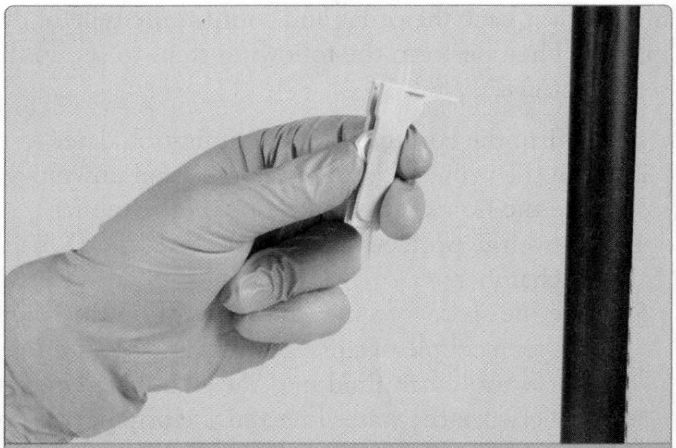

A2-2-4 Open the flow clamp to allow the solution to completely fill the tubing and push out the air. Close the clamp when tubing is full.

in place and provides quick and easy venous access should the patient require immediate medications or fluid replacement.

As the EMT you will most likely be responsible for the securing of the saline lock once the ALS provider inserts it. You will secure it to the site with tape and monitor it during transport to make sure it does not get pulled out accidentally.

The Last Word

This appendix covers some of the more common tasks an EMT performs to assist ALS partners. It is very important that you never forget your primary role on the team as the "BLS expert" and the one your ALS partner can count on to monitor the patient's ABCs and provide BLS care when appropriate. There are many other smaller tasks you will learn and integrate into the team dynamic, depending on the experience and willingness of your ALS partner. Many of those tasks will be afforded you based on the trust and confidence that can come only with time and running many calls together.

APPENDIX 3
Advanced Airway Management

Objectives

After completion of this lesson, you should be able to:

A3-1 Define key terms introduced in this appendix.
A3-2 Identify and describe the anatomy of the airway.
A3-3 Describe the indications for advanced airway management.
A3-4 Differentiate between endotracheal tubes and supraglottic airways.
A3-5 List the equipment required for orotracheal intubation.
A3-6 Differentiate the intended use of a curved and straight blade.
A3-7 Describe the methods for selecting the appropriately sized endotracheal tube.
A3-8 Discuss the purpose of the stylet in orotracheal intubation.
A3-9 List common complications associated with advanced airway management.
A3-10 Describe the steps of orotracheal intubation.
A3-11 Describe various methods for confirming tube placement.
A3-12 Describe the method for securing the endotracheal tube.

Key Terms

alveoli p. 1266
bronchi p. 1266
bronchioles p. 1266
Broselow tape p. 1271
capnographer p. 1276
capnography p. 1276
capnometer p. 1276
conchae p. 1265
cricoid cartilage p. 1266
endotracheal intubation p. 1268
endotracheal tube (ETT) p. 1268
end-tidal carbon dioxide ($ETCO_2$) detector p. 1276
epiglottis p. 1265
esophageal detector device (EDD) p. 1276
esophageal tracheal combitube (ETC) p. 1274
esophagus p. 1271
glottis p. 1266
laryngeal mask airway (LMA) p. 1275
laryngopharynx p. 1266
laryngoscope p. 1268
larynx p. 1266
Macintosh p. 1268
Miller p. 1268
nares p. 1265
nasal vestibule p. 1265
nasopharynx p. 1265
oropharynx p. 1265
orotracheal intubation p. 1268
pulse oximeter p. 1277
pulse oximetry p. 1276
Sellick's maneuver p. 1273
soft palate p. 1265
stylet p. 1271
trachea p. 1266
vallecula p. 1268
vocal cords p. 1266

Introduction

You can only be successful with advanced airway management skills after you have mastered the basic skills described in Chapters 13 and 17. Because ensuring a patent airway is the your highest priority in managing any patient, learning about when and how to use advanced airway skills will be a benefit to your patients—and a tremendous responsibility for you.

As an EMT, your protocols may allow you to use one or more of the airway devices and procedures described in this appendix. Use of these skills requires initial training, continuous practice, and frequent use in the field to maintain proficiency. As you learn and begin to practice advanced airway skills, *never, never, never* forget the importance of basic airway skills.

Airway Anatomy Review

In Chapter 5 you were introduced to general airway anatomy and physiology. To successfully use advanced airway devices, you must understand even more (Figure A3-1 ■).

The upper airway extends from the mouth and nose to the **epiglottis.** The beginning of the nasal upper airway is formed by the **nares,** also known as *nostrils*. They are the opening to the nasal cavity. As air enters the nasal cavity, it first passes through the **nasal vestibule,** which is made of flexible tissue in the anteriormost portion of the nasal cavity. Within the nasal cavity there are coarse hairs intended to filter foreign particles and stop them from entering the airway. The nasal cavity also contains **conchae** or what are commonly referred to as *turbinates*.

The conchae are positioned one on top of another and are designed to create a swirling air path across and through each level on inspiration. This swirling of air helps to warm and humidify the air before it enters the lower airways. The conchae are highly vascular and contain multiple nerve endings. Because of this, any procedure involving the nares must be done with an awareness for potential bleeding and pain.

Be cautious of the conchae when using a nasopharyngeal airway or nasogastric tube. Many EMTs insert a nasal airway using an upward and posterior technique. The advised insertion technique is to insert the airway adjunct straight back, because upward insertion will irritate the conchae, causing pain and bleeding.

Air passes from the **nasopharynx,** which is the posteriormost portion of the nasal cavity, over the **soft palate.** (When a person swallows, the soft palate lifts up, closing off the **oropharynx** from the nasopharynx.) From the soft palate, air moves to the oropharynx, which is the portion of the pharynx that lies directly behind the oral cavity—specifically, behind the base of the tongue.

A3-2 Identify and describe the anatomy of the airway.

epiglottis leaf-shaped structure that covers the glottis to prevent food and foreign matter from entering the trachea.

nares the opening to the nasal cavity. Also called *nostrils*.

nasal vestibule the anteriormost portion of the nasal cavity.

conchae tissue within the nasal cavity that causes a swirling air path. Also called *turbinates*.

nasopharynx the section of the pharynx directly posterior to the nose.

soft palate tissue designed to lift up when a person swallows, closing off the oropharynx from the nasopharynx.

oropharynx the section of the pharynx directly posterior to the mouth.

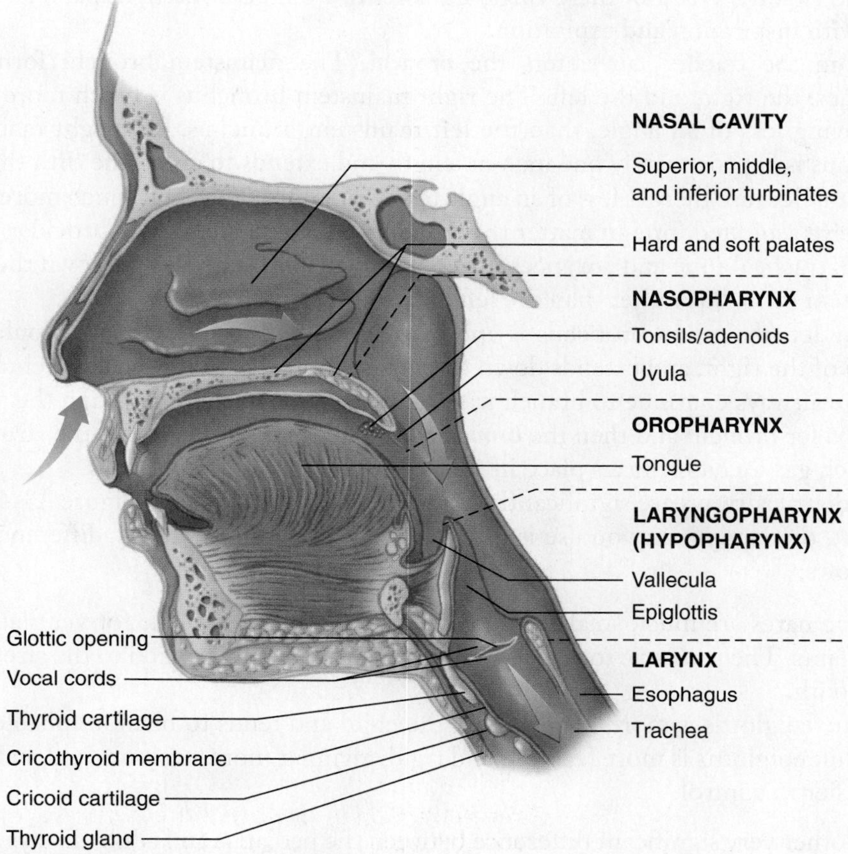

Figure A3-1 Anatomy of the upper airway.

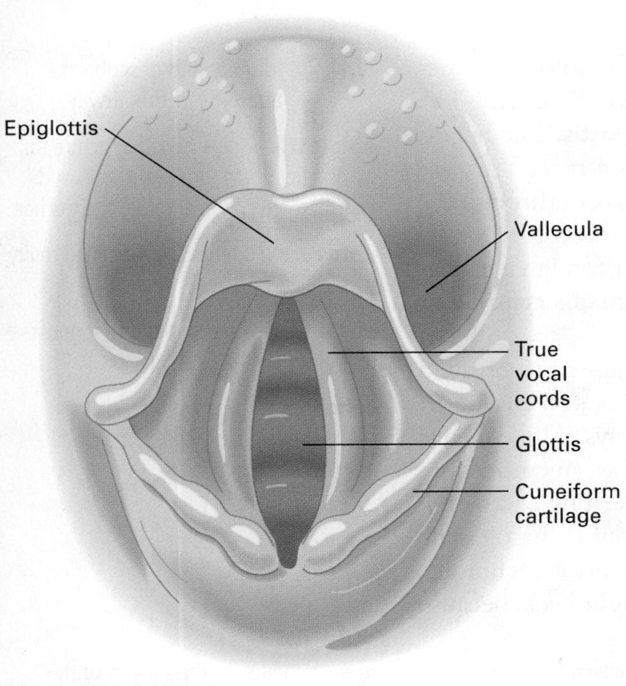

Figure A3-2 Epiglottis and vocal cords.

laryngopharynx the portion of the pharynx that connects the oropharynx to the larynx. Also called the *hypopharynx*.

alveoli the microscopic sacs of the lungs where gas exchange with the bloodstream takes place.

larynx structure located between the laryngopharynx and the trachea; houses the glottis and the vocal cords. Also called the *voice box*.

glottis opening between the vocal cords that separates the upper airway from the lower airway. Also called the *glottic opening*.

trachea the structure that connects the pharynx to the lungs. Also called the *windpipe*.

vocal cords tissue found within the larynx that opens and closes the glottis to produce sound vibrations.

cricoid cartilage the ring-shaped structure that circles the trachea at the lower edge of the larynx.

bronchi the two large sets of branches that come off the trachea and enter the lungs. There are right and left bronchi. Singular, *bronchus*.

bronchioles the smallest bronchi.

Air enters through the mouth as well and into the oropharynx. It then passes through the **laryngopharynx** (also called the *hypopharynx)*. From the laryngopharynx, air advances to the lower airways.

The lower airway begins with the epiglottis and terminates at the **alveoli.** The primary function of the epiglottis is to protect the airway by covering the glottic opening during swallowing (Figure A3-2 ■). When a person swallows, the muscles of the neck contract, and the **larynx** is elevated. When the larynx moves up, the epiglottis folds back over the **glottis,** and the **trachea** is covered.

The glottis is the opening from the upper airway that leads into the lower airway. It is at the level of the **vocal cords** and is at the very top of the trachea. As air passes through the glottis, it is channeled through the larynx, or voice box. To speak, air passes through the larynx and causes vibration of the vocal cords, producing sound.

On the inferior aspect of the larynx is the **cricoid cartilage.** It serves as a protective mechanism for the glottis and trachea and gives support to the larynx. After air moves through the larynx, it advances to the trachea. The cricoid cartilage is sometimes thought of as the first—and only complete—tracheal cartilage.

The trachea (Figure A3-3 ■), otherwise known as the *windpipe*, is a tough but flexible tube with a diameter of about 2.5 centimeters (one inch) and a length of about 11 centimeters (four and a quarter inches). It is flexible because it is made up of about 20 incomplete rings of cartilage that provide structure and support of the trachea with no rigidity. Without these rings, the trachea would constantly expand and contract with inspiration and expiration.

From the trachea, air enters the **bronchi.** The mainstem bronchi form two branches, the right and the left. The right mainstem bronchus is much more vertical, having less of an angle, than the left mainstem bronchus. The right mainstem bronchus is approximately one inch in length and extends to about the fifth thoracic vertebra. Because there is less of an angle to the right bronchus, it is much more likely to receive aspirated foreign matter than the left. Likewise, if an EMS provider places an endotracheal tube and advances it too far, it will almost always go down the right mainstem bronchus rather than the left.

The left mainstem bronchus is approximately two inches in length, double the length of the right, and extends down to the level of the sixth thoracic vertebra.

The airways continue to branch from the mainstem bronchi, through the gradually smaller bronchi and then the **bronchioles.** They end at the alveoli, the structures in which gas exchange takes place in the lungs.

Pediatric airways are significantly different from adult airways (Figure A3-4 ■). As a result, the equipment you use is different as well. Pediatric airway differences are as follows:

- The nares are much smaller and constitute the primary route for ventilation in infants. The pediatric tongue is proportionally larger in relation to the size of the mouth.
- The epiglottis is more U-shaped in the child and tends to be more pliable. The adult epiglottis is more leaf-like and rigid, giving it more structure and making it easier to control.

Another very significant difference between the pediatric and adult airways is that the narrowest portion of the adult airway is at the glottic opening and the narrowest portion of the pediatric airway is more inferior at the level of the cricoid cartilage.

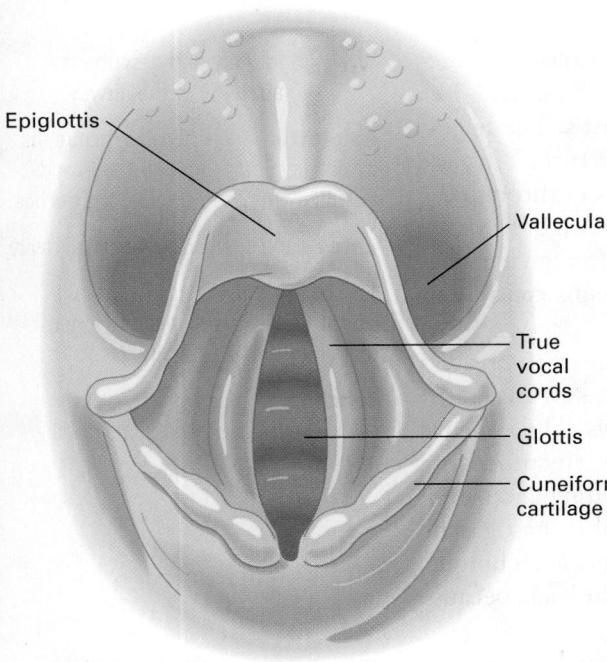

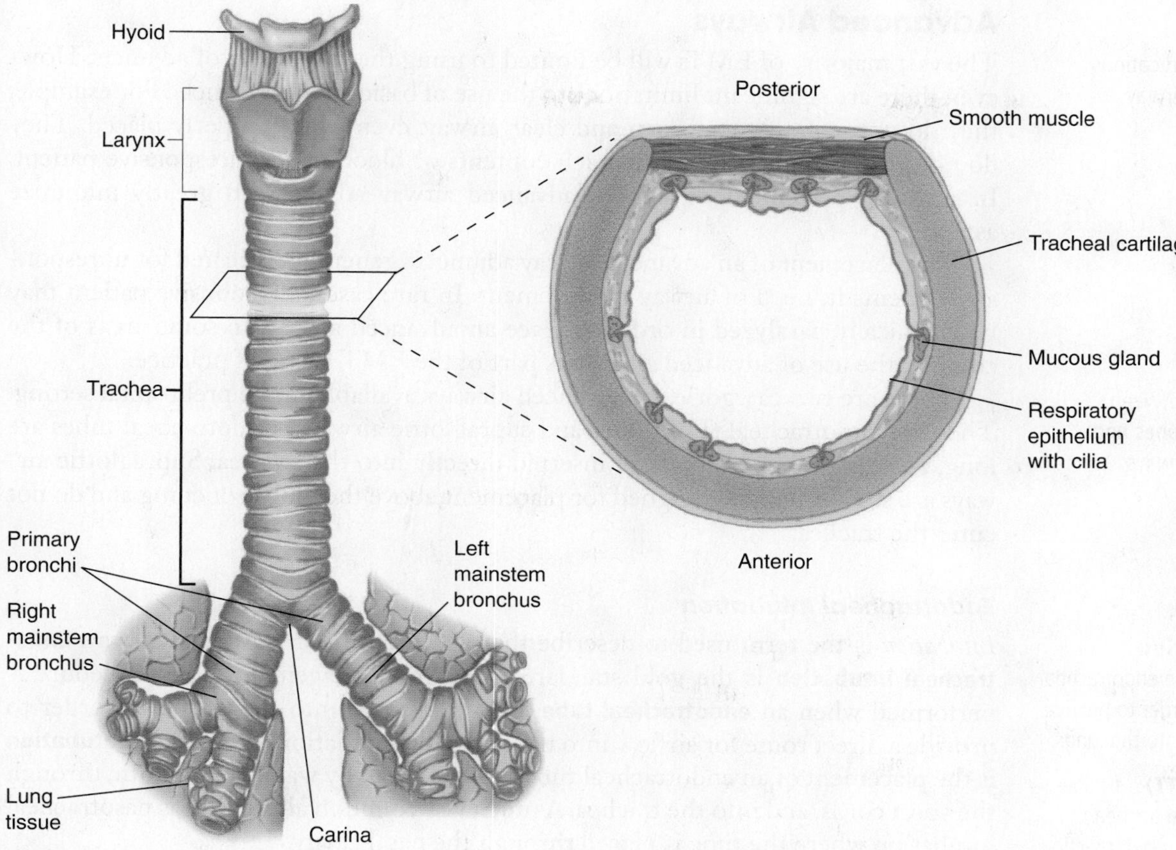

Figure A3-3 Anatomy of the trachea.

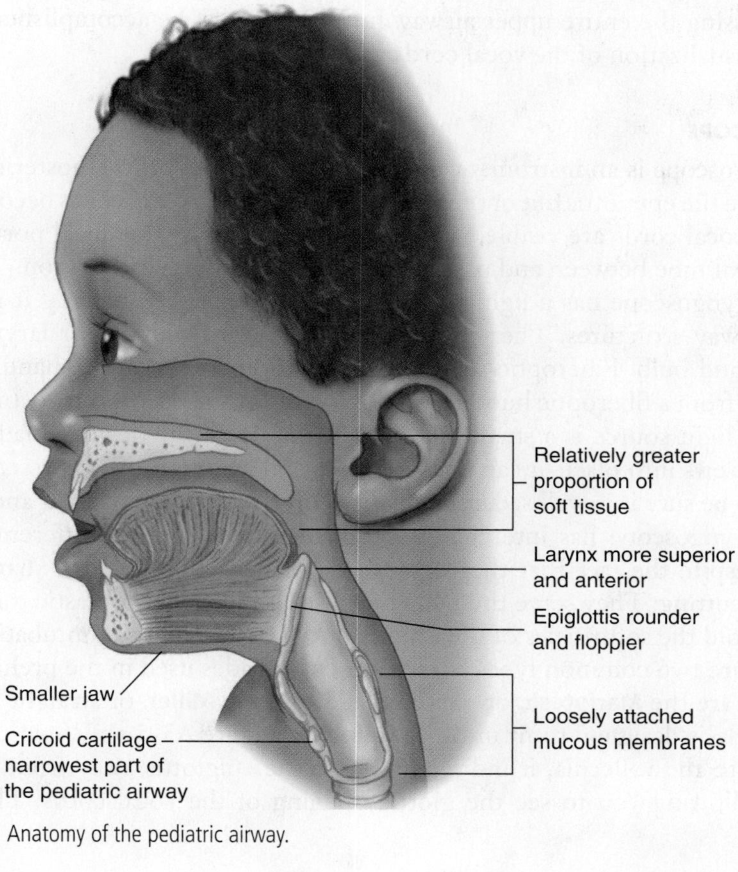

Figure A3-4 Anatomy of the pediatric airway.

Advanced Airways

A3-3 Describe the indications for advanced airway management.

The vast majority of EMTs will be limited to using the most basic of adjuncts. However, there are significant limitations to the use of basic airway adjuncts. For example, they do not guarantee an open and clear airway, even when properly placed. They do not prevent aspiration of stomach contents or blood in an unresponsive patient. In contrast, placement of a more advanced airway adjunct can greatly minimize aspiration.

The placement of an advanced airway adjunct is generally indicated for unresponsive patients in need of airway management. In rare cases, a responsive patient may be chemically paralyzed in order to place an advanced airway. In some areas of the country, the use of advanced airways is part of the EMT scope of practice.

A3-4 Differentiate between endotracheal tubes and supraglottic airways.

There are two categories of advanced airways available in the prehospital setting. They are endotracheal (ET) tubes and supraglottic airways. Endotracheal tubes are long, thin, hollow tubes that are inserted directly into the trachea. Supraglottic airways are similar but are designed for placement above the glottic opening and do not enter the trachea.

Endotracheal Intubation

endotracheal intubation technique used to place an endotracheal tube into the trachea in order to provide a direct route for airflow into the lungs.

endotracheal tube (ETT) flexible tube that is placed into the trachea to provide ventilation and airway protection.

orotracheal intubation the placement of an endotracheal tube orally, by way of the mouth, then through the vocal cords and into the trachea.

laryngoscope instrument used to lift the tongue off the posterior pharynx and move the epiglottis out of the visual field so that the vocal cords are visible.

Intubation is the term used to describe the placement of an advanced airway. **Endotracheal intubation** is the gold standard in airway management. The procedure is performed when an **endotracheal tube (ETT)** is inserted into the trachea in order to provide a direct route for airflow into the lungs for ventilation. **Orotracheal intubation** is the placement of an endotracheal tube orally; that is, by way of the mouth, through the vocal cords, and into the trachea. A much less common alternative is nasotracheal intubation where the tube is placed through the nasal cavity.

The greatest benefit to intubation is that the procedure provides definitive airway protection, meaning it allows direct ventilation of the lungs through the endotracheal tube, bypassing the entire upper airway. Intubation must be accomplished with and by direct visualization of the vocal cords with a **laryngoscope.**

LARYNGOSCOPE

A3-5 List the equipment required for orotracheal intubation.

The laryngoscope is an instrument used to lift the tongue off the posterior pharynx and to move the epiglottis out of the visual field so that the vocal cords become visible. Once the vocal cords are visible, it will be possible to pass the distal portion of the endotracheal tube between and past the cords under direct visualization.

The laryngoscope has a light that illuminates the airway, making it possible to see the airway structures. There are two types of light sources for laryngoscopes: fiberoptic and bulb. Fiberoptic scopes have the light source in the handle, and the light emits from a fiberoptic bundle at the tip of the laryngoscope blade. In bulb-type scopes the light source is a small lightbulb at the tip of the device's blade. Because the bulb screws into place, it can become loose and lessen its brightness. Always test the bulb to be sure it is well secured and gives off a bright light ("tight and bright").

A3-6 Differentiate the intended use of a curved and straight blade.

Macintosh a type of laryngoscope blade. Also called a *curved blade*.

Miller a type of laryngoscope blade. Also called a *straight blade*.

vallecula space between the tongue and epiglottis.

The laryngoscope has interchangeable blades that come in different sizes and shapes. Despite the fact that they are called "blades," they are not sharp and not meant for cutting. They serve the same purpose as a wooden or plastic tongue blade and help hold the soft tissues of the tongue out of the way during intubation.

There are two common types of laryngoscope blades used in the prehospital setting. They are the **Macintosh,** or curved blade, and the **Miller,** or straight blade. The curved blade is designed to fit into the **vallecula** (Figure A3-5 ■). When the blade is inserted into the vallecula, it indirectly moves the epiglottis away from the glottic opening, allowing you to see the glottic opening of the vocal cords. The straight

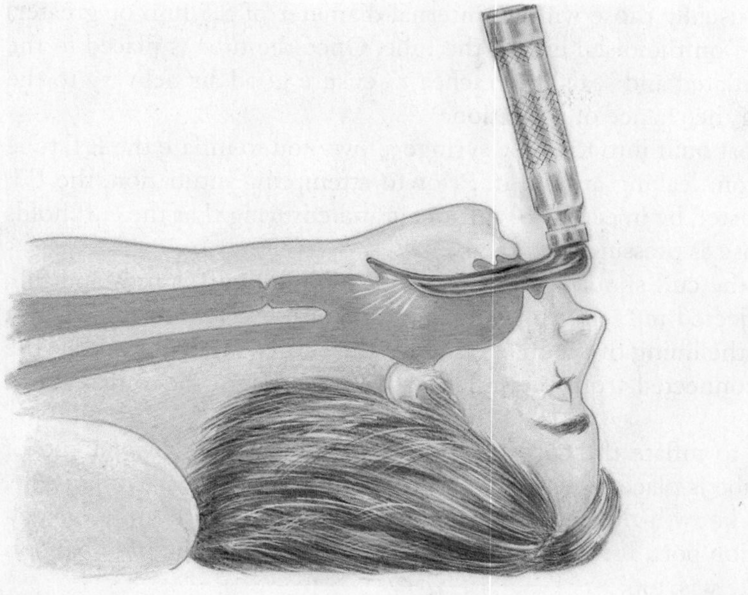

Figure A3-5 The tip of the Macintosh (curved) blade is placed into the vallecula during intubation.

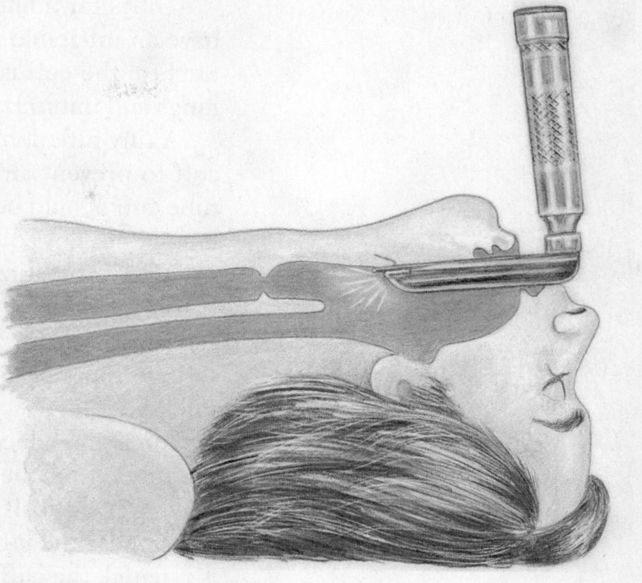

Figure A3-6 The tip of the Miller (straight) blade is placed under the epiglottis during intubation.

blade is designed to slide under the epiglottis and directly lift the epiglottis away from the glottic opening (Figure A3-6 ■). Because the straight blade directly manipulates the epiglottis, it is the ideal choice when managing a pediatric airway in which the epiglottis is soft and difficult to move indirectly.

ENDOTRACHEAL TUBE

The endotracheal (ET) tube (Figure A3-7 ■) is a flexible tube that is placed into the trachea to provide ventilation and airway protection. The ET tube is available with internal diameters ranging from 2.5 to 9 mm. These diameters represent the tube size.

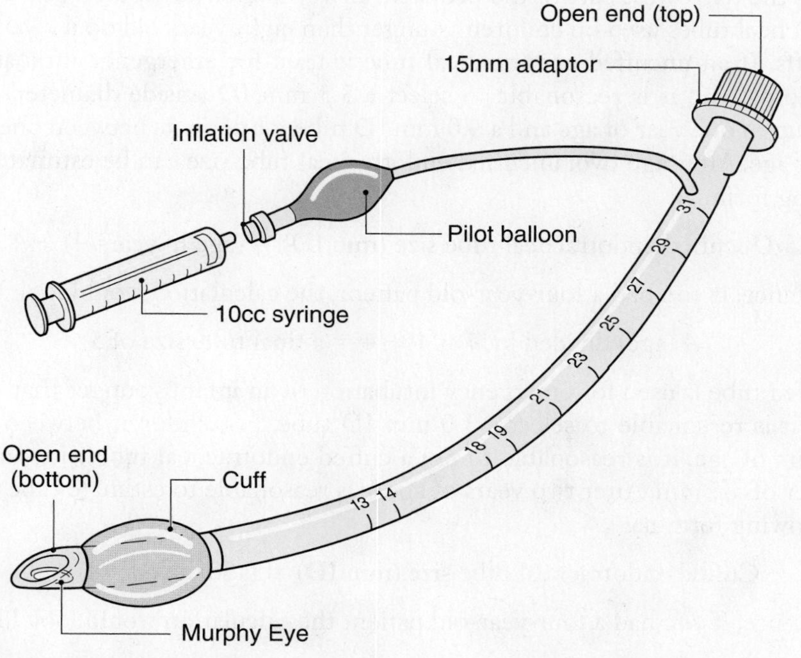

Figure A3-7 A typical endotracheal tube.

Tubes for adults (usually those with an internal diameter of 5.5 mm or greater) have an inflatable cuff on the distal end of the tube. Once the tube is placed in the trachea, the cuff is inflated and seals the trachea to ensure good air delivery to the lungs and minimizing the chance of aspiration.

A tiny inflation port built into the tube syringe allows you to inflate the ET tube cuff to prevent air from leaking around it. Prior to attempting intubation, the ET tube cuff should be tested by injecting 10 mL of air and ensuring that the cuff holds it and does not collapse as pressure is exerted.

After intubation, the cuff should be inflated until the pilot cuff is firm and full. If too much air is injected into the cuff, however, pressure exerted on the trachea can cause damage to the lining of the trachea. Once the cuff is inflated properly, the syringe must be disconnected from the inflation valve to ensure the cuff remains inflated.

Air is introduced to inflate the cuff by way of a port near the proximal end of the tube. After the tube is placed, the distal end of the tube and cuff are not visible, making it difficult to know if the cuff remains inflated. The pilot balloon is a small pouch near the inflation port. It represents the status of the cuff. If the pilot balloon is inflated, the cuff likely is, too.

ENDOTRACHEAL TUBE SIZING

A3-7 Describe the methods for selecting the appropriately sized endotracheal tube.

As a general rule, most adult male patients will accommodate between an 8.0 mm and a 9.0 mm ET tube, and most adult female patients can receive between a 7.0 mm and 8.0 mm ET tube. There are, however, variations to these recommendations. Studies in children have shown the most effective way to estimate the endotracheal tube size is by mathematical formula. All people are created differently. Therefore, it is also wise to have an additional criterion that can be used to select tube size. The diameter measured is the distance from one side of the internal wall of the tube to the other, and is called the *internal diameter (ID)*.

PEDIATRIC CONSIDERATIONS

Because the narrowest part of the pediatric airway is inferior to the vocal cords, the endotracheal tubes used on children younger than eight years old do not have inflatable cuffs. If an uncuffed endotracheal tube is used for emergency intubation of a pediatric patient, it is reasonable to select a 3.5 mm ID (inside diameter) tube for infants up to one year of age and a 4.0 mm ID tube for patients between one and two years of age. After age two, uncuffed endotracheal tube size can be estimated by the following formula:

$$\text{Uncuffed endotracheal tube size (mm ID)} = (\text{age in years}/4) + 4$$

For instance, if you had a four-year-old patient, the calculation would look like this:

$$4\ (\text{age}) \text{ divided by } 4 = 1 + 4 = \text{a final tube size of } 5$$

If a cuffed tube is used for emergency intubation of an infant younger than one year of age, it is reasonable to select a 3.0 mm ID tube. For children between one and two years of age, it is reasonable to use a cuffed endotracheal tube with an internal diameter of 3.5 mm. After two years of age it is reasonable to estimate tube size with the following formula:

$$\text{Cuffed endotracheal tube size (mm ID)} = (\text{age in years}/4) + 3$$

For instance, if you had a four-year-old patient the calculation would look like this:

$$4\ (\text{age}) \text{ divided by } 4 = 1 + 3 = \text{a final tube size of } 4$$

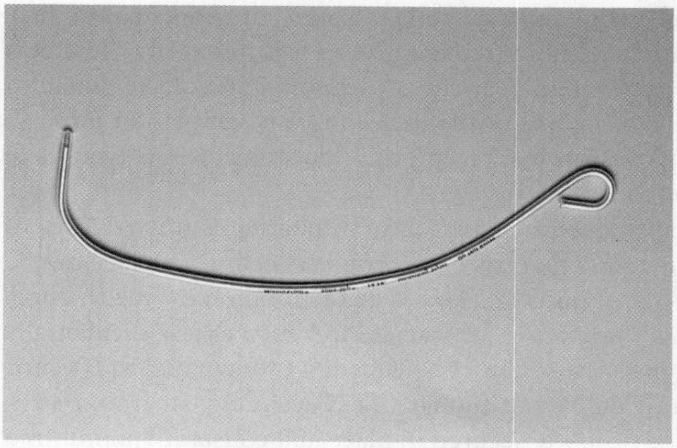

Figure A3-8 A typical stylet used for intubation.

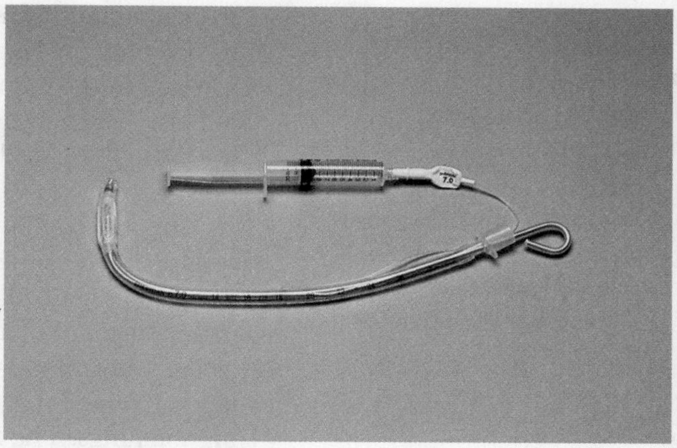

Figure A3-9 An ET tube with stylet in place.

This formula will allow the EMT to identify the most likely ET tube to be used in a specific age group. Because the pediatric airway does not accommodate a cuffed ET tube well, the EMT must also have a larger and smaller tube readily available to be sure of achieving the best fit during intubation.

STYLET

The **stylet** (Figure A3-8 ■) is a moldable wire that can be inserted into the ET tube to stiffen and shape it to facilitate tube placement when the airway is narrow or difficult to access. The most common method for stylet manipulation is molding the tube into a hockey-stick shape (Figure A3-9 ■). Be careful about placing the stylet. If it is advanced beyond the distal end of the ET tube, it could cause trauma to the tissue of the airways. Stylets are often not used in pediatric intubations, especially in newborns and infants.

A3-8 Discuss the purpose of the stylet in orotracheal intubation.

stylet moldable wire that can be inserted into an endotracheal tube to facilitate tube placement.

CLINICAL CLUE

Pediatric Intubation Sizing

In some EMS systems, a standard pediatric measuring device, such as the **Broselow tape,** should be used in determining the appropriate ET tube size for a child.

Broselow tape a measurement tape that provides approximate height and weight ratios in infants and children; used to estimate ET tube sizes and drug dosages for pediatric patients.

As an EMT you may be permitted by your medical director to perform endotracheal intubation. Endotracheal intubation requires great skill and, if your system allows you to perform it, you will need hours of additional training beyond your regular EMT course before you will become proficient in the procedure.

POSSIBLE COMPLICATIONS

Intubation can be a life-saving intervention, but an endotracheal tube that is mistakenly placed in the **esophagus** will result in your patient's death unless you immediately recognize the error. Due to the complex nature of this skill and the fact that it is often attempted during a stressful emergency, proper placement can sometimes be difficult. The most common complication associated with endotracheal intubation is improper placement of the tube.

A3-9 List common complications associated with advanced airway management.

esophagus tube connecting the laryngopharynx to the stomach.

There are only two places the tube can go during insertion— the trachea or the esophagus. Because visualization of the airway can be difficult, it is quite easy

> **CLINICAL CLUE**
>
> **Proper Placement**
>
> Whenever you are anything less than 100% sure that the endotracheal tube has been properly placed, immediately remove the tube and ventilate the patient with 100% oxygen by way of bag-mask device.

to inadvertently insert the tube into the esophagus. This is an immediately life-threatening mistake for the patient. Failure to recognize an endotracheal tube that is inserted in the esophagus will result in the patient's death. Insertion of the tube into the esophagus means that the patient will not be receiving any ventilation into the lungs at all. Instead, the air and oxygen will be entering the stomach and eventually cause significant gastric distention.

Another complication associated with endotracheal intubation is the inadvertent displacement of the tube. Even a tube that has been properly secured in place can be accidentally pulled or pushed out of position. This is most common during the normal movement of a patient when preparing for transport. A tube that is accidentally pushed down too far may slip into one of the two mainstem bronchi and thus ventilate only one lung. A tube that is pulled out too far will prevent any air from reaching the lungs. The tube must be properly secured in place and constantly monitored during transport to ensure proper placement at all times. The proper placement of the endotracheal tube should be verified after each patient move.

OROTRACHEAL INTUBATION PROCEDURE

A3-10 Describe the steps of orotracheal intubation.

Follow these steps to perform an orotracheal intubation:

1. Take proper BSI precautions.
2. Gather all necessary equipment. Choose the appropriately sized endotracheal tube. Make certain the cuff (for patients older than eight years) holds air and does not leak. Then test the laryngoscope to ensure the lightbulb is "tight and bright."
3. Preoxygenate the patient with several closely spaced ventilations.
4. Place the patient's head in a sniffing position, if there is no trauma. The sniffing position is accomplished by first flexing the neck forward and then extending the head backward. If there is a suspicion of trauma, the procedure must be performed using an in-line position with manual stabilization of the neck.
5. Perform laryngoscopy.
   - *Macintosh (curved) blade technique:* Open the patient's mouth with the right hand and remove any dentures. Grasp the laryngoscope in the left hand, spread the patient's lips, and insert the blade between the teeth, being careful not to break them. Insert the blade along the tongue to the right, and rest the tip of the blade at the base of the tongue. (This technique should be accomplished with a simultaneous leftward sweeping action. The leftward sweep moves the tongue away from the visual field.) Lift the laryngoscope upward and forward, without changing the angle of the blade, to expose the vocal cords.
   - *Miller (straight) blade technique:* Open the patient's mouth with the right hand and remove any dentures. Grasp the laryngoscope in the left hand, spread the patient's lips, and insert the blade between the teeth, being careful not to break them. Insert the blade directly into the laryngopharynx and lift the laryngoscope upward and forward, without changing the angle of the blade, to expose the vocal cords.
6. After visualizing the glottis and vocal cords, gently advance the tube through the vocal cords and into the trachea. Stop advancing the tube when all of the balloon is just past the cords.
7. Either you or your assistant should carefully hold the ET tube and prevent movement, which could dislodge the tube or force it deeper into the trachea.
8. Connect an end-tidal CO_2 detector to the tube to verify tube placement. (Some EMS systems will use an esophageal detector device [EDD] to verify tube placement.)

9. If either device indicates proper tracheal placement of the endotracheal tube, use the syringe to inflate the cuff with 10 mL of air. Then detach the syringe from the inflation valve.
10. Attempt ventilation of the patient using 100% oxygen and a bag-mask device.
11. Confirm tube placement by auscultating first over the epigastrium and then over the lung fields. If sounds are heard over the epigastrium, immediately stop ventilating the patient and remove the tube.
12. If the initial endotracheal tube placement is unsuccessful, immediately remove the tube, ventilate, and reoxygenate the patient with a bag-mask device. Reattempt intubation and again verify tube placement with an end-tidal CO_2 detector or EDD. Then listen for breath sounds and make sure there are no sounds over the stomach.
13. Once the tube is properly placed, note the centimeter mark at the lips. This ensures that the EMT can easily identify a change in tube depth.
14. Secure the tube with tape or a commercial tube-securing device.

CLINCAL CLUE

Orotracheal Intubation

Do not waste too much time attempting to intubate. You should only make two attempts at intubation. If both attempts fail, insert an oral airway, continue to ventilate the patient with oxygen by way of bag-mask, and suction the airway as necessary.

SELLICK'S MANEUVER

Sellick's maneuver is a technique that can be used to assist with improving visualization of the vocal cords during intubation (Figure A3-10 ■). It is most often performed by a second rescuer at the scene who applies downward pressure on the cricoid cartilage. This promotes more effective visualization of the cords during endotracheal intubation. Sellick's maneuver is no longer recommended as a technique for minimizing gastric inflation during ventilations.

Sellick's maneuver technique of applying downward pressure on the cricoid cartilage; used to help visualize the vocal cords.

Supraglottic Airways

Supraglottic or rescue airways do not require the use of the laryngoscope and can be inserted "blindly." They may be used in place of ET tubes or when attempts at endotracheal intubation fail. The following are examples of supraglottic airways: King airway, Combitube, laryngeal mask airway (LMA), pharyngeo-tracheal lumen airway (PTL), and the Cobra perilaryngeal airway (PLA).

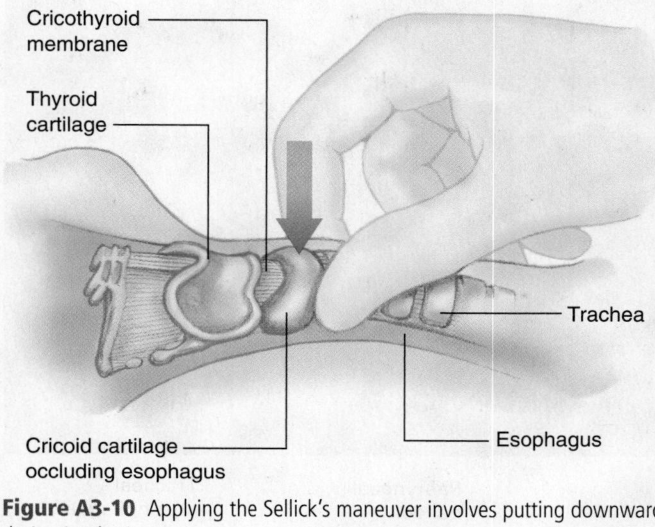

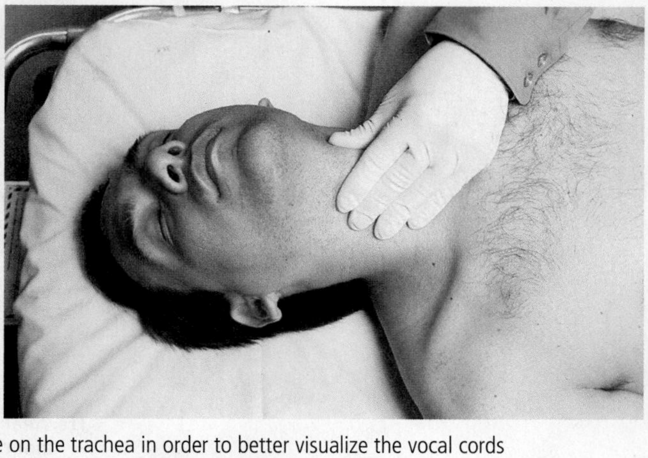

Figure A3-10 Applying the Sellick's maneuver involves putting downward pressure on the trachea in order to better visualize the vocal cords during intubation.

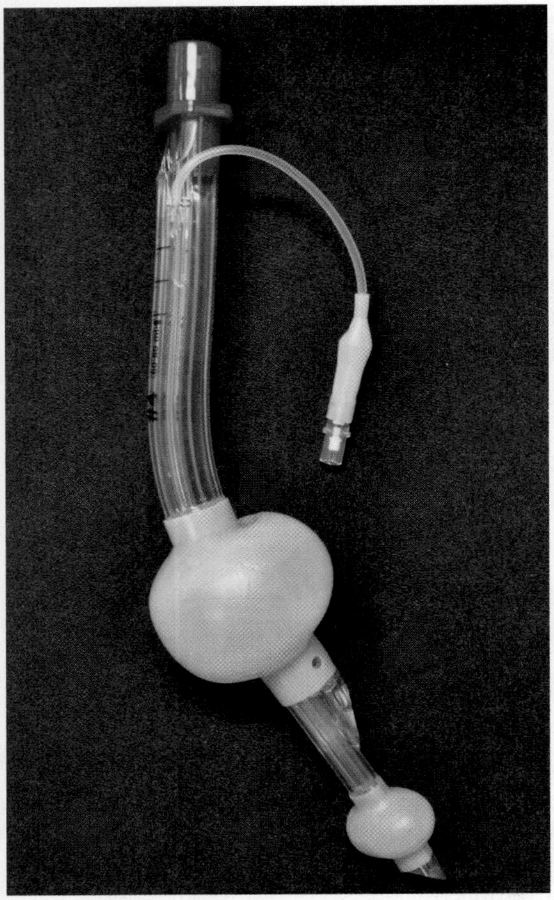

Figure A3-11 The King LT-D disposable airway.
(© Edward T. Dickinson, MD)

esophageal tracheal combitube (ETC) type of dual-lumen airway used to provide ventilations and help protect the airway.

KING AIRWAY

Manufactured by King Systems, the King LT-D supraglottic airway is one of the newest entries to the rescue airway market (Figure A3-11 ■). The King airway is designed with a large proximal pharyngeal cuff and a smaller distal cuff that occludes the esophagus. Between the two cuffs is the ventilation port where air exits the tube and enters the glottic opening and into the lungs.

King airways come in five sizes. The LTS-D model is designed with an additional lumen that allows for gastric suctioning.

COMBITUBE AIRWAY

The Combitube, also known as an **esophageal tracheal combitube (ETC),** is a dual-lumen airway (side-by-side tubes) with a ventilation port for each lumen (Figure A3-12 ■). One tube is closed-ended but has multiple holes that can be ventilated through. The other tube is open like an ET tube.

When inserted, the device will enter the esophagus 90% of the time or the trachea 10% of the time. Regardless of whether the tube enters either the esophagus or trachea, the patient can be ventilated.

There is a large high-volume inflatable cuff near the center of the device. This cuff is designed to be positioned in the oropharynx to prevent air from escaping through the mouth and nose when the device is being used. Near the distal tip of the device is another smaller volume inflatable cuff. When the ETC is placed in the esophagus, this smaller cuff occludes the esophagus, preventing both the passage of air into the esophagus and the regurgitation of the stomach contents up into the airway. When the ETC is placed in the trachea, this distal cuff acts

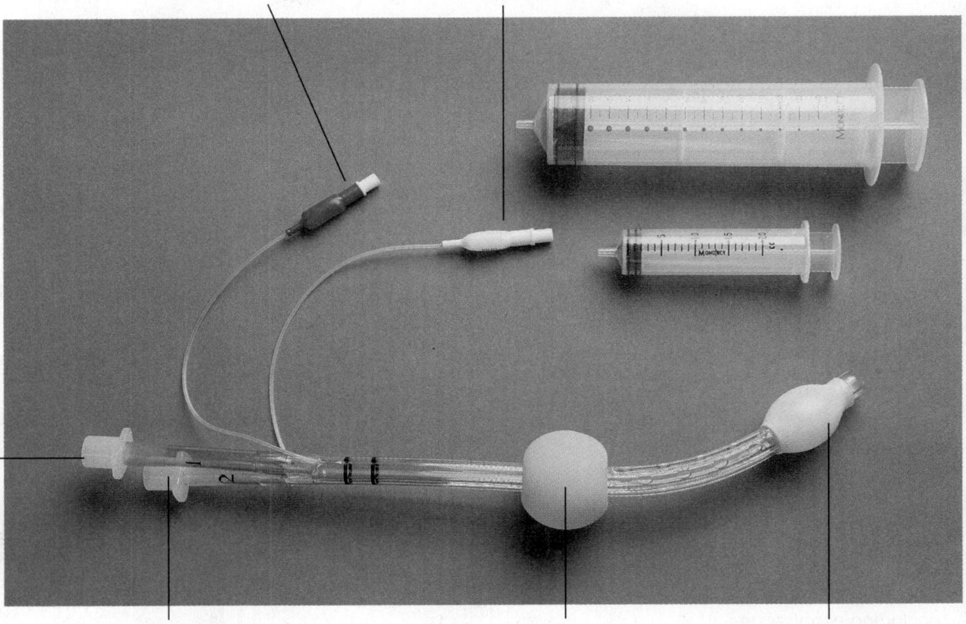

Figure A3-12 The Combitube airway.

like a normal endotracheal tube cuff and fits snugly up against the walls of the trachea.

Combitubes come in two sizes, 37 French (Combitube SA) for patients from four to six feet tall, and 41 French for patients from six to seven feet tall.

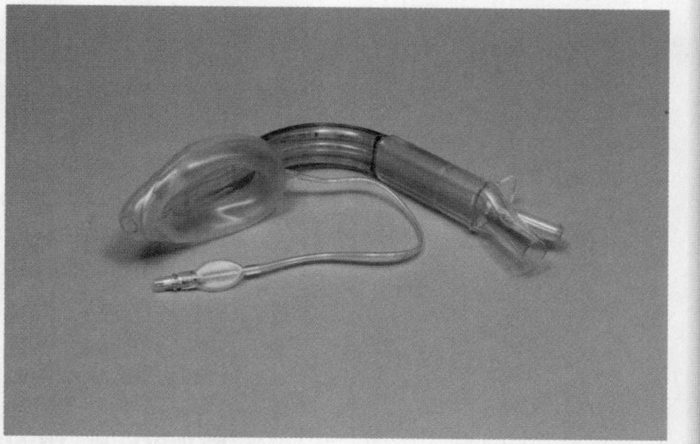

Figure A3-13 The laryngeal mask airway (LMA).

LARYNGEAL MASK AIRWAY (LMA)

The **laryngeal mask airway (LMA)** was initially designed for use in a controlled environment such as the operating room (Figure A3-13 ■). A large oblong cuff is placed in the laryngopharynx and pointed directly over the glottic opening. The biggest difference between the LMA and an ET tube or Combitube is that it does *not* effectively provide airway protection. LMA masks come in various sizes in both reusable and disposable models.

laryngeal mask airway (LMA) type of airway used to provide ventilations and help protect the airway.

INSERTING A SUPRAGLOTTIC AIRWAY

1. Have a partner ventilate the patient while you prepare the equipment.
2. Lubricate the tube with water-soluble lubricant.
3. Direct your partner to stop ventilations.
4. Grasp the patient's lower jaw with your left hand and insert the tube along the natural curve of the mouth and throat. Stop when the teeth are between the two black rings. Do not force the tube into place.
5. Inflate the appropriate cuff or cuffs.
6. Ventilate through the appropriate port and look and listen for lung sounds.
7. If you do not hear lung sounds when performing step #6, attach your bag-mask device to the alternate port, if applicable, and attempt to ventilate. Listen for lung sounds.
8. If ventilation of neither tube results in breath sounds, deflate both balloons, remove the device, and ventilate the patient with a bag-mask device.

CONFIRMATION OF TUBE PLACEMENT

A3-11 Describe various methods for confirming tube placement.

Confirming placement of an advanced airway device, whether it is an endotracheal tube or a supraglottic airway, must be performed consistently and accurately. If improper placement of a device goes unidentified, the patient will certainly die. The following methods may be used to confirm tube placement during and following insertion:

- Direct visualization (only with endotracheal tube)
- Auscultation of the epigastrium
- Visualization of chest rise
- Auscultation of breath sounds
- Monitoring of end-tidal CO_2
- Use of an esophageal intubation detection device (only with an endotracheal tube)
- Use of pulse oximetry

The first method of confirming proper ET tube placement is positive visualization of the tube passing through the vocal cords. After visualizing the tube passing through the cords, the EMT should watch for chest rise and fall. It is also imperative that epigastric and lung sounds be auscultated immediately following placement of an advanced airway device. When properly placed, the endotracheal tube will result in equal breath sounds over both sides of the chest and no sounds over the epigastrium. If you listen to the epigastrium first, you may identify an esophageal intubation and be able to stop ventilating the stomach before the patient vomits. Lung sounds that are present on the right side but absent or diminished on the left may indicate that the airway device has been advanced too deeply and has entered the right mainstem bronchus. An end-tidal CO_2 detector or another device approved by your medical director must be used in addition to auscultation to confirm tube placement.

Although rare, absent or decreased lung sounds could indicate a bronchial obstruction or a pneumothorax. Absent lung sounds throughout the chest indicate an esophageal intubation until proven otherwise. Finally, if the patient regains consciousness following placement of a tube into the trachea through the vocal cords, the EMT should understand that the patient will not be able to communicate because the cords cannot move enough to create sound.

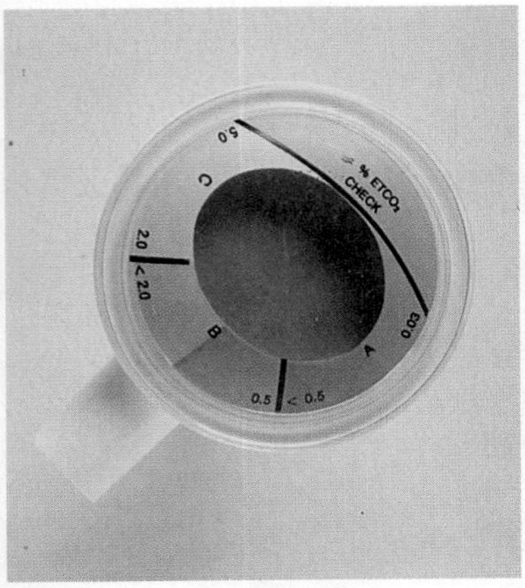

Figure A3-14 A colorimetric $ETCO_2$ detector.

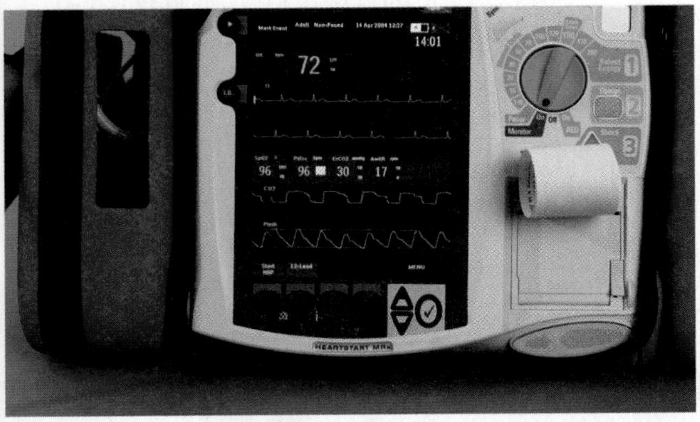

Figure A3-15 A waveform $ETCO_2$ detector built into a cardiac monitor.

MONITORING END-TIDAL CO_2

End-tidal carbon dioxide ($ETCO_2$) detector devices come in the form of simple presence (colorimetric) detectors (Figure A3-14 ■), as well as quantifying detectors (Figure A3-15 ■). **Capnography** has been designed to distinguish between esophageal and tracheal intubation. Exhaled carbon dioxide can be present only if the tube has entered the trachea, which leads to the lungs. Exhaled carbon dioxide will not be present if the tube has entered the esophagus, which leads to the stomach.

A colorimetric device contains filter paper saturated with a colorless liquid base and a pH-sensitive medium. The color in the device changes when the paper comes into contact with carbon dioxide and returns to normal when the carbon dioxide is gone. Thus a colorimetric device is able to show the presence of CO_2 but not the amount. A **capnometer** is an electronic device that quantifies the amount of carbon dioxide through a probe attached at the end of an endotracheal tube. A **capnographer** will quantify the amount of carbon dioxide being exhaled, but displays a continuous waveform to indicate levels of carbon dioxide over time.

End-tidal CO_2 detectors are not always reliable in the cardiac-arrest environment. In the cardiac-arrest patient, there is no perfusion to the lungs, so carbon dioxide is not produced. Therefore, the detector will not show the presence of carbon dioxide even if the tube is correctly placed in the trachea.

In most situations, end-tidal CO_2 detectors are of great benefit. It is, however, important to remember that capnography, just like **pulse oximetry,** should be used as just one differential diagnosis tool in conjunction with the patient's clinical presentation.

An **esophageal detector device (EDD)** (Figure A3-16 ■) is used in some regions as a way to verify the placement of an endotracheal tube in the prehospital setting. Unlike end-tidal CO_2 detectors, the EDD cannot be used on supraglottic airway devices. The esophageal detector device works because of anatomical variations in the trachea and esophagus. The trachea remains rigid and patent because of the cartilaginous rings that run the entire length of it. The esophagus, however, has no supporting rings and is therefore collapsible. The principle of the EDD is that the esophagus will collapse when a negative pressure is applied to its lumen, whereas the trachea will not. There are two common types of EDDs—a syringe type and a bulb type.

The syringe-type EDD works by using an adapter to attach a 60 mL syringe to the endotracheal tube. Once the syringe is attached, the EMT should pull back on the plunger to attempt to withdraw air. If resistance is met, then the tube is in the esophagus and the esophagus collapsed as air was removed.

end-tidal carbon dioxide ($ETCO_2$) detector device used to detect the presence or the amount of carbon dioxide in exhaled air.

capnography recording or display indicating the presence or quantity of exhaled carbon dioxide concentrations.

capnometer electronic device that uses infrared light to quantify carbon dioxide in exhaled air.

capnographer device that uses infrared light to evaluate exhaled carbon dioxide and displays a continuous waveform to indicate levels of carbon dioxide over time.

pulse oximetry noninvasive and continuous means of determining arterial oxygen saturation.

esophageal detector device (EDD) mechanical device that uses negative pressure to differentiate tracheal from esophageal placement of an endotracheal tube.

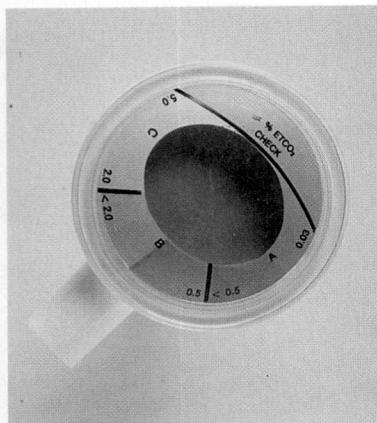

The bulb-type EDD is attached to the endotracheal tube while the bulb is fully compressed. If the bulb reinflates when it is released, then the tube is in the trachea. If it does not reinflate, then the tube is in the esophagus and the vacuum created by release of the bulb has collapsed the soft walls of the esophagus.

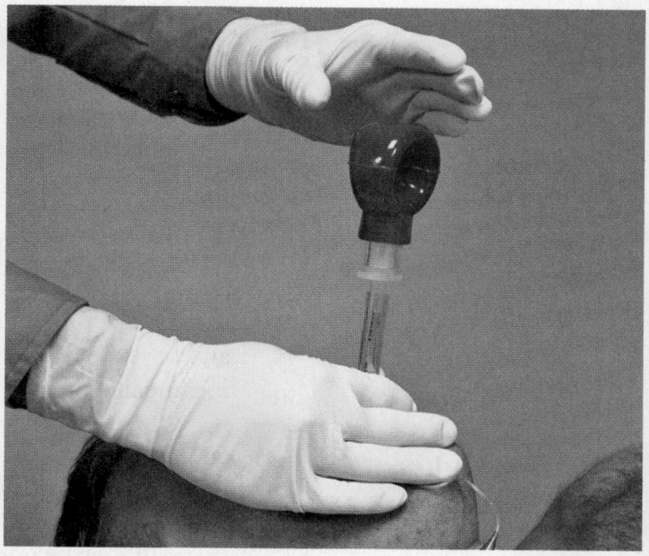

Figure A3-16 An esophageal detector device being used to confirm placement of an inserted ET tube.

PULSE OXIMETRY

Pulse oximetry is a noninvasive and continuous means of determining arterial oxygen saturation. The **pulse oximeter** uses infrared light to determine the oxygen saturation of hemoglobin. The oximeter probe is attached to the patient's finger. The infrared light is emitted through the probe, and a sensor placed at the backside of the probe determines how much of the light was able to pass through the capillary beds. Hemoglobin without oxygen bound to it or with low concentrations of oxygen allows more light through the capillaries than oxygen-saturated hemoglobin.

Standard pulse oximeters generally overestimate true arterial hemoglobin oxygen saturation in the setting of carbon monoxide toxicity. By understanding how pulse oximetry works, it is easy to understand how carbon monoxide can produce a false positive reading. Carbon monoxide has a greater affinity to hemoglobin than oxygen does and allows easy passage of infrared light just as oxygen would. The newer co-oximeters can detect both oxygen saturation and hemoglobin bound to carbon monoxide.

Patients with advanced airway devices in place should have their oxygen saturation continuously monitored.

pulse oximeter device that uses infrared light to determine arterial oxygen saturation.

CLINICAL CLUE

Pulse Oximetry

It should be understood that pulse oximetry is not the definitive answer to diagnostic tools of respiration. Pulse oximetry should be used as only one differential diagnosis tool in conjunction with the patient's clinical presentation.

A3-12 Describe the method for securing the endotracheal tube.

SECURING THE DEVICE

After placement, the next most important step in the use of an advanced airway is ensuring that it remains in place. You must take very specific care to make certain that it does not move or get pulled out during movement and transport of the patient.

One of the most effective tools for securing the tube in place is a commercial device such as the one shown in Figure A3-17 ■. This device is placed around the tube and secured with a clamp. It also has Velcro straps that wrap around the head to secure the device in place.

There are several variations of the commercial securing devices available on the market today. In the absence of a commercial device, tape can be used to effectively secure the tube in place.

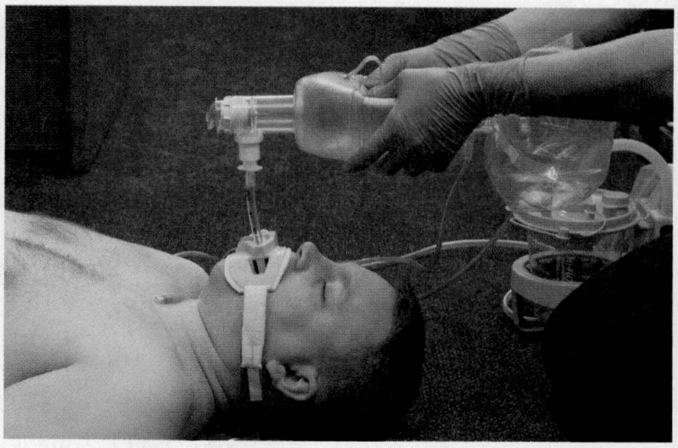

Figure A3-17 A typical commercial ET tube-securing device in place on a patient.

APPENDIX 4

Your Successful Career in EMS

Introduction

If you are reading this, you are probably just completing your EMT training and about to take your certification exams. You are probably also interested in some of the things that EMS has to offer you. Of course, you may be anywhere in your training and have a curiosity about what happens after your class. So read on. If you are reading ahead, you are not alone. Many in your class are likely doing the same.

Obtaining certification or licensure as an EMT is merely the beginning of what could potentially be a lifelong journey. You have learned much in your class. There is more to learn in the field. The purpose of this appendix is to provide information to help you begin and succeed in EMS and to explore some of the career possibilities that will now be open to you. EMS is practiced in a number of ways and in a variety of places. Your EMT certification is the beginning of many opportunities.

Training Complete, What Happens Next?

Very soon you will be completing your EMT training program and taking the state certification exam. In most states, this is the National Registry exam. In other states it is most likely an exam that has been developed by the state, and all EMTs within that state must pass before becoming certified. Regardless of which exam you may be required to take, it is very important to sign up to take the exam. You will never be as prepared to successfully pass the exam as you are immediately after your EMT training. That means you should schedule to take the exam as soon as possible. A study conducted by the UCLA Center for Prehospital Care suggested that the highest pass rates were achieved when students take the exam within 15 days following the completion of the program. Do not let fear stop you from jumping right in and taking the exam.

In most states, simply passing the state or national certifying exam is just one step in a multiple-step process to becoming a state-certified EMT. It is important to ask your instructor or contact your local EMS agency for all the details regarding becoming certified. Many states require fingerprinting and a thorough background check. At the very least, you will be required to complete an official application in the state, region, or system where you will be working.

Ambulance Driver's Certificate

Depending on the state you will be working in and the employer, you may be required to obtain an ambulance driver's license or certificate. This in itself can require several additional steps that all cost money. For instance, in some states the Department of Motor Vehicles requires a written exam, medical examination, and fingerprinting prior to issuance of an ambulance driver's certificate. Your instructor or local DMV office should be able to provide the specific details regarding this requirement in your state.

Many employers require that you have all the necessary certifications and documentation before applying for a job. Not having everything in place could get your application rejected. Be ready for work before you submit your application.

Success in EMS

Your EMT course taught you much of importance. You listened to lectures, participated in discussions, responded to simulated patients, practiced skills, and perhaps did some hospital or ambulance ride time as part of your training. You have likely wondered, "How will I be able to do this on an ambulance?" or "What happens if I get out there and have a horrible accident on my first call?" Or even, "What if I see something overwhelming and get sick on the job?" You are not alone. These are questions every new EMT asks. A few tips that have helped many new EMS providers begin a successful EMS career follow. But before proceeding, note that there is a strong volunteer component to EMS in the United States. Some EMTs volunteer, some are paid, and many do both. The term "career" is used to represent your experience in EMS, whether volunteer or paid. Both are done with significant pride and professionalism. Both treat patients using the same skills.

The following tips are designed to help you enjoy EMS for the long haul:

- ***Identify and connect with a mentor.*** Beginning any job is stressful enough. But being an EMT is not just any job. Many people who succeed in EMS have someone who showed them "the ropes." You will have new questions, issues, and feelings. A mentor will help you find answers and provide advice to you at important times (Figure A4-1 ■). Your mentor also can help guide you through all your options and save you hours of wasted time and energy in your quest for the perfect EMS career path.

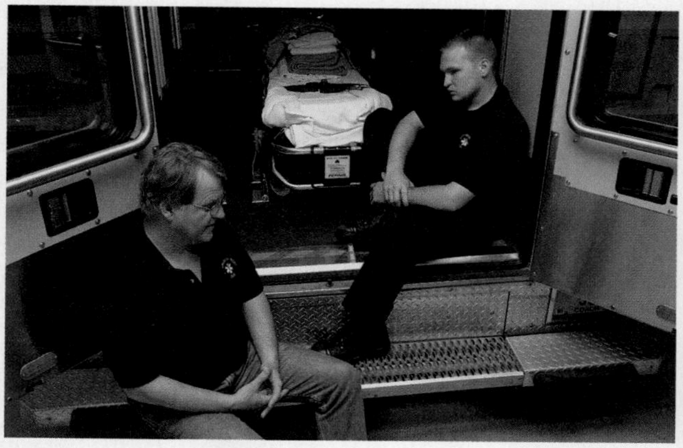

Figure A4-1 Identifying and connecting with a mentor can greatly help you start your EMS career. (© Dan Limmer)

- ***Jump right in.*** Begin your search even before you complete your training and let as many people as possible know what you want to do. Look for any opportunity to gain experience as an EMT, even if it means volunteering. Do not hold out for the 911 ambulance job when a BLS transport opportunity is immediately available. There is still much to learn about being an excellent EMT and waiting for the ideal job while allowing less appealing jobs pass you by is never a good idea.
- ***Strive for confidence.*** Many people feel that they cannot ride as the EMT in charge of a call until they know everything. You will never know everything. Confidence was once defined as knowing how to handle almost everything that comes your way and knowing when and where to look for help on the calls that stump you. You will not simply have confidence because you decide to have it. Confidence comes through experience and experience takes time.
- ***Get along with everyone.*** There is a name for people who are overconfident. That name is "cocky." When you are a new EMT, demonstrate respect for people who have experience. Pay attention. Ask good questions. The person who is training you will look at thoughtful questions as a sign you are interested. There are many EMTs with great skills and potential who got out or were pushed out of EMS because they could not get along with others. It is not difficult, but it does take effort.
- ***Cultivate a beginner's mind.*** This is not as easy as it may sound. As a new EMT who gets a job right away, it only takes a few months before you think you have this EMT thing in the bag. Other more experienced EMTs will see you as overconfident or arrogant and may not want to work with you. Everyone has more to learn, and everyone loves to work with someone interested in learning more. A wise old EMT once said, "Cultivate a beginner's mind, because there is no room for improvement in an expert's mind." There is much to learn from everyone you encounter, even from those who are not the most respected. You must be deliberate in your desire to learn from everyone and every situation.

- ***Engage in the profession.*** Your journey to becoming the best EMS professional that you can be begins when you start to respond to real calls and interact with real patients, and it never ends. One of the best ways to become engaged in the profession is to subscribe to the two primary EMS trade journals, *EMS World* (www.emsworld.com) and the *Journal for Emergency Medical Services (JEMS)* (www.jems.com). Both journals offer free six-month subscriptions to new EMTs. Ask your instructor or contact the journals directly for more information. They will keep you connected to the latest research and information related to the profession and ensure you are always up to date on the latest happenings in the profession around the country.
- ***There is honor in all labor.*** EMS is not all about 911 emergencies and lights and sirens. As a matter of fact, most ambulances around the country serve as nonemergency (BLS) transport units. When you do work on a 911 ambulance, there will be long stretches of "routine" calls (routine to us but important to our patients). Television portrays EMS as constant heart-pounding, lights-and-siren excitement. It is not! Finding satisfaction in doing all calls well will keep you in EMS longer than if you live for the thrill. Many of the most routine calls are significant events in the lives of patients. Do your best to treat every interaction as though the patient was one of your own family members. Be proud of the role you play in EMS.
- ***You are more than a technician.*** You have most likely been introduced to the term "critical thinking." It refers to the process of assembling all available facts in a given situation, interpreting them, and making a correct decision. It is one of the most important skills that will help you make the leap from simply a "technician" to a true clinician. Clinicians are always anticipating what may happen next, and how the patient is going to respond to any given injury, illness, or treatment. They plan ahead and manage problems before they are out of control, all while providing the best customer service to their patients.
- ***EMS is about relationships.*** This profession is about you, the people you work with and, of course, your patients. Regardless of a patient's attitude, odor, socioeconomic class, or medical condition (or apparent lack of same), treating patients well is perhaps one of the most important things you will do. Treat your partners and crews with that same respect.
- ***Be nice.*** Patients may not remember whether you gave them oxygen or checked their distal pulses. But they will remember how they were treated. The act of calming and reassuring a patient is one of the core skills of an EMT. And there are medical benefits to calming your patient. Treating a patient as you would want yourself or a family member treated is a gold standard of EMS (Figure A4-2 ▪).

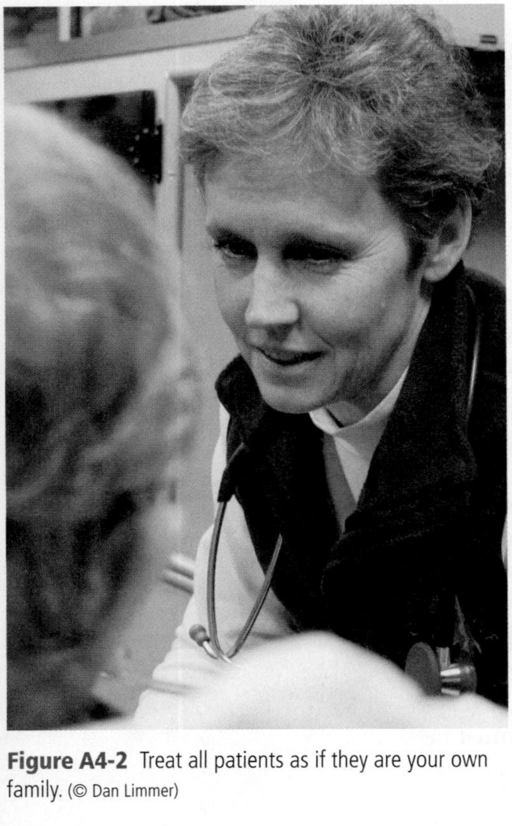

Figure A4-2 Treat all patients as if they are your own family. (© Dan Limmer)

Next Steps

When you read Chapter 1 of this textbook, you probably were not thinking about moving up to the next level of EMS certification as described there. Most students focus on passing the EMT class first. However, you may have the opportunity to become an advanced provider such as an advanced EMT (AEMT) or a paramedic (Tables A4-1 and A4-2).

The AEMT is an intermediate step between the EMT and the paramedic. The AEMT level of certification varies widely from state to state, but generally involves advanced airway techniques, intravenous fluids, and some medications. The amount of training for the AEMT level is significantly less than that for a paramedic. The AEMT level is often found in rural areas where recruiting and training personnel is challenging and in cities where transport times to the hospital are very short.

TABLE A4-1	ADVANCED EMT SKILLS
	• In-depth patient assessment and critical thinking skills • Advanced airway insertion • IV insertion and administration • Medication administration *Note:* Skills and medications vary by state and region.

TABLE A4-2	PARAMEDIC SKILLS
	• Advanced knowledge in anatomy, physiology, pathophysiology, and pharmacology • Advanced assessment and decision-making skills • Advanced airway skills (ETT, Combitube, LMA, and in some systems cricothyrotomy and medication-facilitated intubation) • IV medication administration • Subcutaneous and intramuscular injections • Cardiac monitoring • Wide range of medications including drugs used to relieve pain, treat heart failure, reverse dangerous cardiac rhythms, and treat cardiac arrest

The paramedic is the highest level prehospital provider. Training involves over 1,000 hours and sometimes substantially more. Paramedics can do all the skills of the intermediate level but also can provide a much larger range of medications and more invasive skills.

It should be noted that the responsibilities of advanced providers are not advanced skills alone. Advanced providers also perform all the basic skills you perform as an EMT, including airway management, patient assessment, and the very important reassurance and kindness each patient should receive.

But I'm Just an EMT!

EMTs are the foundation of the emergency medical services (EMS) system. Although there are levels of training above the EMT, it is the EMT who provides the core life-saving skills such as airway management, ventilation, suction, oxygen administration, automated defibrillation, spinal immobilization, bleeding control, and more (Figure A4-3 ■). Without them, advanced skills would not stand a chance of success. A paramedic uses more EMT skills than paramedic skills every day. So, when you hear someone say, "I'm *only* an EMT," consider responding with this: "Paramedics save patients. EMTs save paramedics." It refers to the fact that advanced skills would not make a difference without a solid foundation of basic skills.

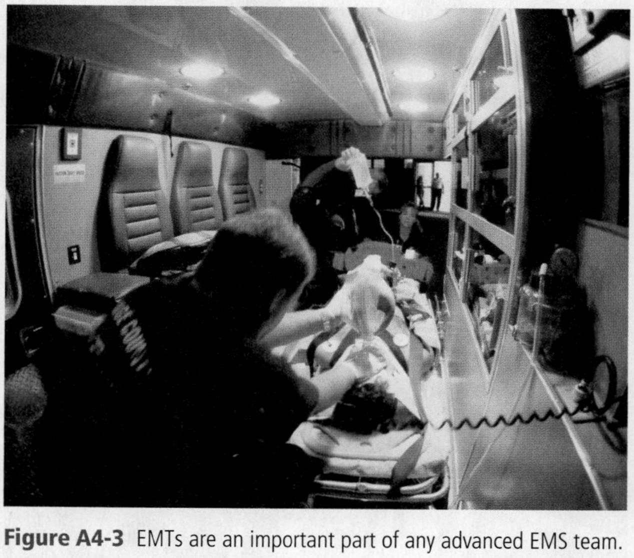

Figure A4-3 EMTs are an important part of any advanced EMS team. (© Craig Jackson/In the Dark Photography)

Where Do EMTs Work or Volunteer?

Where do EMTs work or volunteer? You may think that the answer is simple—on an ambulance, of course. But that is only part of the answer. EMTs work and volunteer in a number of other settings including fire departments, rescue squads, industrial response teams, summer camps, and hospitals.

The EMT training you have taken is one of the few courses that instantly qualifies you for a job upon obtaining your certification. You may choose to begin full-time work, part-time work while a student or at another job, or volunteering. Here are some of the opportunities others who have completed an EMT course have found:

- ***Ambulances.*** Most people think of EMTs working on ambulances (Figure A4-4 ■). As a matter of fact, when the EMT certification was originally developed it was

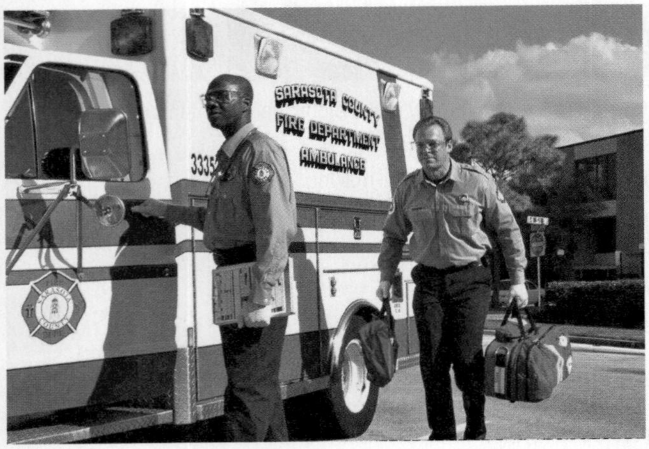

Figure A4-4 Being an EMT is the minimum qualification for working on most ambulances.

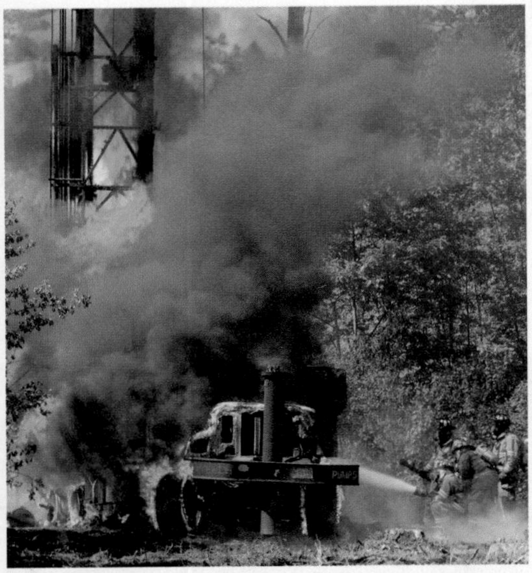

Figure A4-5 Many fire departments require their firefighters to be EMTs. (© Dan Limmer)

called "EMT-A" for EMT-Ambulance. In most areas, the EMT is the minimum level of certification required for an ambulance to respond to a call. There are many types of ambulance services including municipal (third service), private, volunteer, and fire-based.

- ***Fire departments*** (Figure A4-5 ▪). Many fire departments provide EMS. Many government officials believe that this is an ideal setup, since there are strategically placed fire stations throughout any area. Personnel are cross-trained as both firefighters and EMTs. In many areas fire service jobs are desirable because of the pay and retirement plans offered. Many, if not most, fire departments require all personnel to be EMTs. Some require certification even to take the entrance examination.
- ***Communications*** (Figure A4-6 ▪). You may find that you are interested in becoming a communications specialist/ dispatcher for an EMS or public service agency. Your EMT training will be well regarded in this arena.

- ***Industrial emergency response*** (Figure A4-7 ▪). Many employers value EMT certification in their employees. The ability to have someone available to respond in the event of an emergency until the ambulance arrives is beneficial to the employer and the patient. In many professions, there are events for which a planned emergency response team is created and staffed by EMTs. Examples include industrial plants with heavy equipment, dangerous machinery, or hazardous chemicals.
- ***Disaster response and search and rescue*** (Figure A4-8 ▪). Over the past several years there have been terrorist incidents, natural disasters, and large-scale accidents to which emergency personnel have been called from around the country. Many EMTs have taken on additional roles in those situations, including heavy rescue, trench rescue, building collapse, search and rescue, and positions on Federal Disaster Medical Assistance Teams (DMATs).

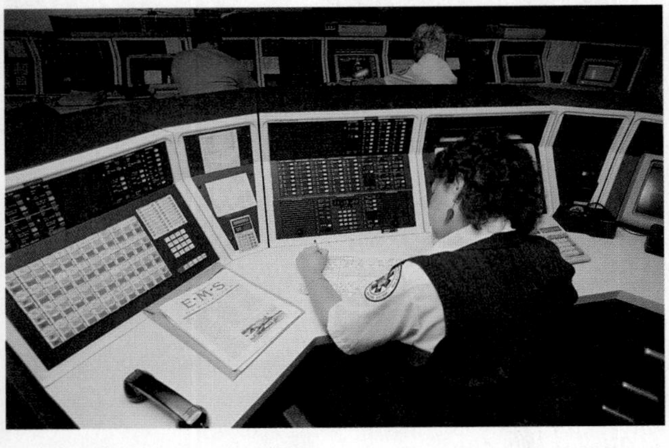

Figure A4-6 Many communication centers recommend or require dispatchers to be EMTs.

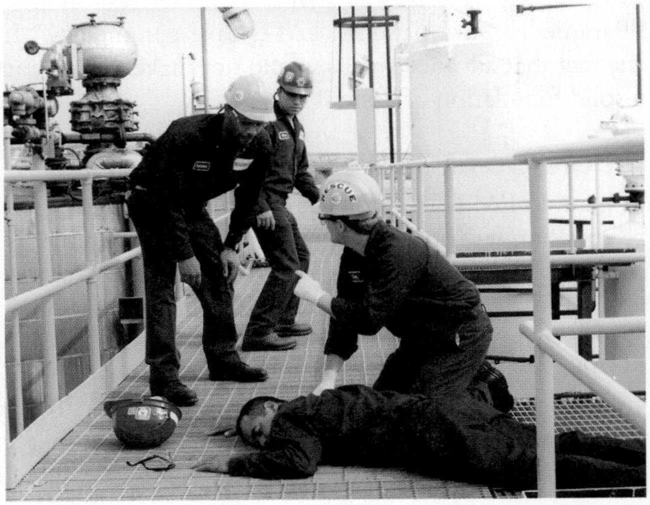

Figure A4-7 Many large industrial sites employ EMTs for the safety of their workers.

- ***Hospital jobs.*** Some of the skills you have learned in EMT class—such as taking vital signs, interviewing patients, and providing comfort—can translate to the hospital setting. Many hospitals hire EMS personnel as emergency department technicians. People holding this position were previously called "orderlies," because they moved patients around and generally kept order. Skills have been added to this position, including taking vital signs, processing paperwork, and others. Some hospitals provide training in additional skills such as drawing blood or obtaining ECGs.
- ***A step toward additional health care training.*** Many take an EMT course to "test the health care waters" to see if a career in health care is a good fit. Other times it is the EMT course that causes students to realize that they may be interested in another career in health care. There are many programs available that offer advanced standing or additional credit for paramedics toward a nursing degree. Experience in a patient care setting such as EMS is generally considered favorably by admissions committees when applying to nursing or medical schools.
- ***Training new EMTs.*** After you have some experience under your belt, you may choose to help in EMT and EMR training. Your class had a lead instructor and probably had some guest lecturers and lab assistants. Those opportunities may be open to you in the future if you choose.

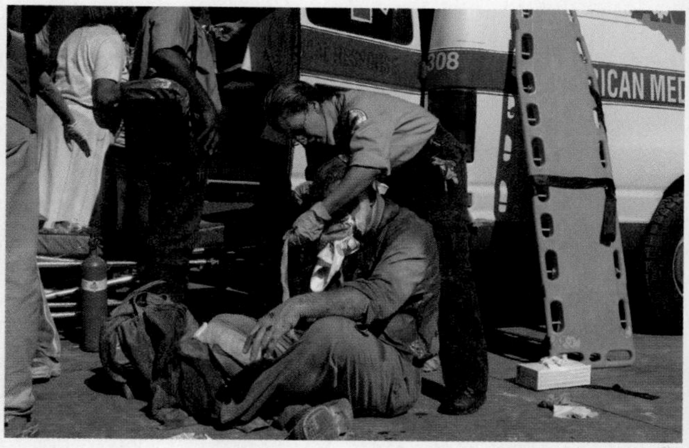

Figure A4-8 Many states and government agencies utilize EMTs as part of their disaster response teams. (AP Images/Amy Sancetta)

Not every opportunity listed is for you. Each one has a set of pros and cons that you will have to evaluate. For example, if you only want to provide EMS and not fight fires, the fire service may not be for you.

Hitting the Streets

There are a few realities in EMS you should be aware of. One of them is the salary offered to EMTs in some areas. It is not unusual for students to obtain their certification and find they cannot make enough money as a full-time EMT, so they choose to volunteer or work part-time instead. In some cases EMTs work full time and supplement their income with overtime. It is an unfortunate reality, but it is improving.

You can help the salary situation in both local and global perspectives. If you want the status and pay of a professional, you must act like a professional. In the big picture, get involved in national organizations and support legislation and causes that benefit the profession as a whole. *This is EMS.*

You also will find that EMS is a 24-7 business, holidays included. And while your training program may have cancelled class because of inclement weather, ambulances are often busier in bad weather. You should plan to work or volunteer on some nights, weekends, and holidays. It's inevitable. You will work in very hot and very cold weather, in the rain and in the snow. You will lift patients, be vomited on, and called names. Patients will die. *This is EMS.*

Even with all that being true, never forget the good you can do for your patients and fellow EMTs, the fun you can have, and the lives you will save. Remember? No job is perfect. EMS is no different. What EMS offers that many jobs do not is a chance to use what you have learned for the good of others. EMS offers the opportunity to hold the hand of a scared child or an elderly patient, to feel the highs of saving a life and the sadness when one is lost, to regularly be in the homes of strangers, rich or poor, and see almost every walk of life in the best and worst lights. You may be there when something big happens. See yourself on the news at 11 p.m., delivering a baby on one call, or listening to a lonely senior citizen with nothing wrong on the next.

EMS is a profession that can get hold of you and your dreams. Hang on, especially if you recognize and embrace the contradictions you will find. Not the best pay but big responsibility. Very sick people and those who abuse the system. Vivid excitement followed by days of monotony. Sincere gratitude from some patients, abuse from others. *This is EMS.*

Be proud of what you have accomplished in your course and look forward to using your skills in the field. We wish you the best. Good luck.

Additional Resources

The Internet is a source of volumes of information—and some of it is reliable. Your best sources are EMS-related professional organizations. Do consider subscribing to an EMS journal, as well, so you can stay up to date on current news, clinical updates, and new ideas each month. Some journals provide continuing education (CE) opportunities. Also attend local, regional, state, and national EMS conferences. Your agency or a regional or state EMS agency will have additional information on them. Here are some Web sites you should explore:

- The National Registry of Emergency Medical Technicians at *www.nremt.org*
- The National Association of Emergency Medical Technicians at *www.naemt.org*
- Journal of Emergency Medical Services (JEMS) at *www.jems.com*
- EMS World Magazine at *www.emsworld.com*

GLOSSARY

A

abandonment a legal term referring to leaving a patient after care has been initiated and before the patient has been transferred to someone with equal or greater medical training.

abdominal aortic aneurysm (AAA) the abnormal bulging of an artery wall.

abrasions injuries to the skin that involve the wearing down or removal of the superficial layers of the skin.

abruptio placentae a condition in which the placenta prematurely separates from the uterine wall and causes pain and bleeding.

absence seizure a seizure common in children, characterized by a blank stare and unresponsiveness. Also called *petit mal seizure.*

absorbed poisons poisons taken into the body through the skin.

absorption entry through the skin or mucous membranes.

abuse physical or psychological injury by another person.

accessory muscles muscles in the neck, chest, back, and abdomen used to assist ventilations during respiratory distress.

acronym a word created from the first letters of each word in a series of words.

actions the desired responses in the body a medication may cause. Also called the *desired effect*.

activated charcoal a medication used to treat certain cases of poisoning or overdose; it binds with the ingested substance inside the gastrointestinal tract and reduces the amount the body can absorb.

active external rewarming application of an external heat source to rewarm the body of a hypothermic patient.

acute sudden-onset. Opposite of *chronic*.

acute exposure exposure to a hazardous substance over a short period of time or at a high dose.

acute medical condition the sudden onset of a new illness or worsening of an existing (chronic) medical condition.

acute stress response stress reactions that are most commonly linked to sudden, unexpected catastrophic events.

adenosine triphosphate (ATP) a byproduct of cellular respiration and responsible for the transport of chemical energy for metabolism.

adhesions internal scar tissue that connects tissues that are not normally connected.

adolescent a child between 12 and 18 years of age.

adsorb the binding of molecules to a substance such as activated charcoal; the attachment of a substance to the surface of another material.

advance directive a legal statement of a patient's wishes regarding his own health care.

advanced EMT (AEMT) the next level of EMS training beyond the EMT level, which provides for the addition of a minimum level of advanced life support (ALS), such as the initiation of intravenous (IV) lines, advanced airway techniques, and administration of some medications.

aerobic metabolism the cellular process by which oxygen is used to metabolize glucose, and energy is produced in an efficient manner with minimal waste products.

agitated delirium a dangerous condition of extreme anxiety and agitation usually associated with drug abuse and withdrawal.

air embolism a bubble of air that enters the circulatory system.

albuterol a medication used to dilate bronchioles in patients who have respiratory disorders.

alcohol intoxication alteration of normal mental status as a result of ingestion of ethanol.

alcohol withdrawal syndrome a spectrum of physical reactions (that can include anxiousness, tremors, seizures, and even hallucinations) caused when chronic alcoholics suddenly stop their normal consumption of ethanol.

allergens a substance that when introduced into the body causes an allergic reaction.

allergic reaction the body's exaggerated response when exposed to specific substances to which it has been sensitized.

altered mental status (AMS) a condition in which a patient appears to be abnormally sleepy, confused, violent, or even completely unresponsive; change in alertness and awareness.

alveoli the microscopic sacs of the lungs in which gas exchange with the bloodstream takes place.

Alzheimer's disease a form of dementia that is progressive and attacks the brain, resulting in impaired memory, thinking, and behavior.

ambulance strike team a group of five ambulances of the same type with common communications and a leader.

amniotic sac fluid-filled sac surrounding the developing fetus. Also called the *bag of waters.*

amputation injury resulting in the loss of a limb or part of a limb.

anaerobic metabolism the cellular process by which glucose is metabolized without oxygen, and energy is produced in an inefficient manner with many waste products.

anaphylactic shock progression of a severe allergic reaction that can result in death.

anaphylaxis sudden, severe allergic reaction.

anatomical position the standard reference position for the body in the study of anatomy; a position in which the body is standing erect, facing the observer, with arms down at the sides and palms of the hands forward.

anatomy of injury the term used in the National Trauma Triage Protocol to identify life-threatening injuries, which require the highest level of transport priority and emergency care.

anatomy the study of the basic structures of the body.

anemia lack of a normal number of red blood cells in the circulation.

aneurysm the dilation, or ballooning, of a weakened section of the wall of an artery.

angina literally a pain in the chest; occurs when one or more of the coronary arteries are unable to provide an adequate supply of oxygenated blood to the heart muscle. Also called *angina pectoris.*

angioedema swelling that occurs in the dermis and subcutaneous layers of the skin and the mucus membranes following an allergic response.

anterior fontanels soft spots lying between the cranial bones.

anterior the front of the body or body part. Opposite of *posterior*.

antibodies protein molecules used by the immune system to identify and neutralize foreign bodies such as viruses and bacteria.

antidote a substance that will neutralize a poison of its effects.

antigen a substance that when introduced into the body stimulates the production of antibodies.

anxiety a state characterized by excess worry or fears.

aorta the largest artery in the body, which transports blood from the left ventricle to begin systemic circulation.

aortic valve a structure between the left ventricle and aorta that opens and closes to permit the flow of a fluid in only one direction.

APGAR score system for evaluating a newborn's physical condition; letters stand for *appearance*, *pulse*, *grimace*, *activity*, and *respirations*.

aphasia a condition in which the patient loses the ability to express speech.

apnea absence of any breathing or respiratory effort.

apparent life-threatening event (ALTE) episode in which an infant or child younger than two years of age has an episode of apnea, skin color change (cyanotic, pale, or redness), loss of muscle tone, or choking or gagging not associated with feeding or a foreign body aspiration.

appendicitis inflammation of the appendix.

arachnoid membrane web-like layer of tissue located between the dura mater and the pia mater.

arrhythmia any variation from the normal rate or rhythm of the heart. Also called *dysrhythmia*.

arteries blood vessels that carry blood away from the heart.

arterioles the smallest arteries.

aspiration the drawing of a foreign substance into the lungs during inhalation.

aspirin a medication used for a variety of conditions, including pain relief and to minimize the effects of a heart attack.

assault a legal term referring to the threat to use force on another.

asthma a disease that causes bronchoconstriction and mucus production with significant difficulty breathing.

asystole the state of no electrical activity within the heart; not an AED shockable rhythm. Also known as *flat line*.

ataxic (Biot's) respirations pattern of respirations characterized by deep, gasping breaths separated by periods of apnea.

atria the two upper chambers of the heart. Singular *atrium*.

attempted suicide an attempt or threat to take one's own life.

aura a particular symptom experienced just prior to the onset of a migraine or seizure; often manifested as a strange light, unpleasant smell or taste, or strange thoughts.

auscultation assessment technique of listening, usually with a stethoscope.

autism spectrum disorders (ASD) developmental disorders that affect, among other things, language, social skills, and behavior.

automated external defibrillator (AED) an electrical device that analyzes the heart rhythm and, if appropriate, provides a measured dose of electricity through the heart in an attempt to defibrillate or convert the heart into a normal rhythm.

automatic implanted cardiac defibrillator (AICD) a small, surgically implanted device that can recognize life-threatening cardiac rhythms and deliver an electrical shock to correct the rhythm.

automaticity the ability of the heart muscle to generate and conduct electrical impulses on its own.

autonomic nervous system a division of the peripheral nervous system; controls functions that are involuntary.

AVPU scale a method for classifying a patient's level of responsiveness, or mental status; letters stand for *alert*, *verbal*, *painful*, and *unresponsive*.

avulsions injuries in which the skin and/or underlying tissue is forcibly torn away.

awareness level level of training that represents the minimum capabilities of a responder who, in the course of duty, could be called on to or be first on scene of a technical rescue or hazardous materials incident.

B

bacteria single-celled organisms without a true nucleus or cell organelles.

bag-mask device a handheld device with a face mask and self-refilling bag that can be squeezed to provide artificial ventilations to a patient; delivers air from the atmosphere or oxygen from a supplemental oxygen supply.

ball-and-socket joint a type of joint in which the ball-shaped head of one bone fits into a rounded receptacle or socket formed by another bone; type of joint with the greatest range of motion.

bariatrics the branch of medicine that deals with preventing and treating obesity.

baroreceptors stretch-sensitive sensors in the aorta and carotid arteries that monitor blood pressure.

base station radios two-way radios at fixed sites such as a hospital or dispatch center.

baseline vital signs the very first set of vital signs obtained on a patient.

basilar artery an artery arising from the vertebral arteries of the spine at the base of the skull.

basilar skull portion of the skull that forms the floor of the skull.

basket stretcher a metal or plastic basket designed to move patients over uneven terrain. Also called a *Stokes basket*.

battery a legal term referring to the carrying out of a threat to use force on another.

Battle's sign bruising behind the ears (over the mastoid process) indicative of a basilar skull fracture.

behavioral emergency a situation in which a patient's behavior becomes intolerable, dangerous, or bizarre enough to cause the concern of family, bystanders, or the patient; a situation in which emotional issues interrupt normal life activities.

beta blocker a class of drugs used primarily to treat heart-related conditions.

beta$_2$ agonist a class of medications that cause smooth muscle relaxation resulting in dilation of the bronchioles and vessels.

bilateral on both sides.

bile chemical that assists in the digestion of fat.

biological weapon (BW) device designed to release either living organisms or toxins produced by living organisms that are deliberately distributed to cause disease and death.

bipolar disorder a behavioral condition characterized by extreme increases in mood and activity contrasted by periods of depression.

birth canal passageway that extends from the cervix to the vaginal opening through which the baby is born. Also called the *vagina*.

bladder anatomical structure that stores urine until excretion.

bleeding out refers to the loss of blood and is not specific to internal or external blood loss.

blood clot a clumping together of blood cells.

blood pressure the pressure exerted by blood against the walls of blood vessels.

bloody show the initial discharge of blood and mucus at the beginning of labor.

blow-by technique providing supplemental oxygen by holding the mask or tubing near an infant or child's face.

B-NICE mnemonic used to categorize weapons of mass destruction; letters stand for *biological*, *nuclear*, *incendiary*, *chemical*, and *explosive*.

body mechanics the proper use of one's body to facilitate lifting and moving in such a way as to minimize risk of injury.

body substance isolation (BSI) precautions the practice of using appropriate barriers to infection at the emergency scene, such as gloves, masks, gowns, and protective eyewear.

body surface area (BSA) the amount of body surface area affected by burns.

BP-DOC an assessment mnemonic used primarily for the trauma patient; letters stand for *bleeding*, *pain*, *deformity*, *open wounds*, and *crepitus*.

brachial artery the major artery of the upper arm.

brachial pulse pulse point felt in two locations: on the inside of the upper arm and over the medial aspect of the anterior elbow.

bradycardia a pulse rate below 60 beats per minute.

brain tumor an abnormal growth of cells within the brain.

brainstem portion of the brain located at the base, responsible for vital activities such as respiration, cardiac function, and blood pressure.

branches management tool for the incident commander that can be either geographical or functional; used to keep a manageable span of control.

breech presentation refers to the buttocks or both lower extremities as the presenting part at the vaginal opening. Also called a *breech birth*.

bronchi the two large sets of branches that come off the trachea and enter the lungs. Singular *bronchus*.

bronchioles smallest branches of bronchi.

bronchoconstriction constriction or narrowing of the bronchioles in the lungs, caused by allergies, respiratory infections, exercise, or emotion.

Broselow tape a measurement tape that provides approximate height and weight ratios in infants and children; used to estimate ET tube sizes and drug dosages for pediatric patients..

C

capacity the ability of a patient to fully comprehend the medical situation and the potential consequences of refusal of care or transport.

capillaries tiny vessels that connect arterioles and venules; thin-walled, microscopic blood vessels in which oxygen, carbon dioxide, nutrients, and waste are exchanged with the body's cells.

capillary refill test a test used to assess perfusion status in the extremities.

capillary refill time how long it takes for the blood to return after blanching tissue and releasing it; normally, this takes no more than two seconds.

capnographer device that uses infrared light to evaluate exhaled carbon dioxide and displays a continuous waveform to indicate.

capnography the monitoring of the concentration or partial pressure of carbon dioxide (CO_2) in respiratory gases; recording or display indicating the presence or quantity of exhaled carbon dioxide concentrations.

capnometer electronic device that uses infrared light to quantify carbon dioxide in exhaled air.

carbohydrate source of fuel for the body.

carbon dioxide a byproduct of cellular metabolism found in the blood and exchanged with oxygen in the lungs.

carcinogenic causing an increased risk of contracting cancer.

cardiac arrest the stopping of the heart, resulting in a loss of effective circulation.

cardiac contusion bruising of the heart tissue typically as the result of blunt trauma.

cardiac muscle specialized involuntary muscle found only in the heart.

cardiac output (CO) the amount of blood ejected from the heart in one minute (heart rate × stroke volume).

cardiogenic shock type of shock caused when the heart can no longer pump blood adequately, resulting in a decrease in cardiac output and thus a decrease in perfusion.

cardiovascular system the system made up of the heart (*cardio*), the blood vessels (*vascular*), and the blood. Also called the *circulatory system*.

carotid artery a large neck artery that carries blood from the heart to the head; one on each side of the neck.

carotid pulse the pulse point located on either side of the anterior neck lateral to the trachea.

carpals the wrist bones.

cartilage tough elastic connective tissue found in various parts of the body such as the joints, ears, nose, and larynx.

CBRNE mnemonic used to categorize weapons of mass destruction; letters stand for *chemical*, *biological*, *radiological*, *nuclear*, and *enhanced explosives*.

cell membrane outer covering of the cell that protects and selectively allows water and other substances into and out of the cell.

central nervous system (CNS) part of the nervous system that is composed of the brain and spinal cord.

central neurogenic hyperventilation pattern of respirations characterized by deep, rapid respirations; condition caused by damage or injury to the brainstem.

central perfusion the supply of oxygen to and removal of wastes from central circulation.

central venous line intravenous catheter placed close to the heart for long-term fluid or medication administration.

cephalic refers to the head.

cerebellum portion of the brain that lies behind and under the cerebrum; responsible for coordination, posture, and equilibrium.

cerebral palsy a developmental disorder that affects movement, balance, and posture.

cerebrospinal fluid (CSF) liquid found around the brain and spinal cord that helps cushion them.

cerebrum largest portion of the brain, responsible for conscious activities, personality, and sensory input.

cervical vertebrae the seven vertebrae that begin at the head and meet the thoracic vertebrae.

cervix the neck (opening) of the uterus.

cesarean section procedure that surgically removes the baby from the uterus. Also called a *C-section*.

CHART a method of documentation in which each letter stands for a specific portion of the narrative: *chief complaint*, *history*, *assessment*, *Rx (or treatment)*, and *transport*.

chemical and physical characteristics qualities that determine the environmental pathways in which a hazardous material is likely to move and how rapidly.

chemical asphyxiants chemicals, such as carbon monoxide, that asphyxiate patients at the cellular level by massively deranging normal cellular utilization of oxygen.

chemical burn a type of burn caused when the skin is exposed to substances such as acids, bases, and caustics.

chemical name the name that reflects the chemical structure of the medication.

chemical weapon (CW) device designed to release a range of simple to sophisticated chemicals that are deliberately distributed to cause harm or death.

chemoreceptors chemical sensors in the brain and blood vessels that identify changing levels of oxygen and carbon dioxide.

Cheyne-Stokes respirations pattern of respirations characterized by gradually increasing and then decreasing tidal volumes with a period of apnea.

chief complaint the patient's perception of the problem or emergency in his own words.

cholecystitis inflammation of the gall bladder.

chronic slow-onset or long-term. Opposite of *acute*.

chronic bronchitis condition in which the lining of the bronchiole is inflamed, and excess mucus is formed in the airway, with accumulation becoming severe.

chronic exposure exposure to a hazardous substance over a long period of time.

chronic medical condition an existing, recurrent medical condition.

circulatory system the system made up of the heart, the blood vessels, and the blood. Also called the *cardiovascular system* (*cardio* referring to the heart; *vascular* referring to the blood vessels).

circumferential burns burns that completely surround a body part such as a finger, arm, leg, or chest.

clavicles the collarbones.

clear text communications using plain language (not radio codes).

clonic the contraction and relaxation of muscles during a seizure.

closed head injury a head injury that involves damage to the skull or brain by a traumatic force that does not cause an open injury of the skin or cranium.

closed skeletal injury skeletal injury not associated with any break in the overlying skin.

clotting factors proteins produced in the liver that aid in the formation of clots.

cluster headache intense pain typically "clustered" or confined to one area of the head or face that may be accompanied by nausea, vomiting, and facial tenderness.

coagulopathy a lack of normal clotting.

coccygeal vertebrae fused vertebrae making up the coccyx or tailbone.

colostomy a surgical opening that connects a portion of the colon to the external abdominal wall.

coma a deep state of unconsciousness lasting more than six hours.

combining form a root word used to create a compound word.

command staff the incident commander's staff, which consists of the liaison officer, the safety officer, and the information officer.

commotio cordis cardiac arrest caused by bunt force trauma to the chest.

communication the exchange of common symbols that are written, spoken, or otherwise exchanged.

compartment syndrome a condition caused by the compression of nerves, vessels, and other soft tissue within a closed space within the body.

compensate the body's ability to temporarily counteract s problem such as a decrease in perfusion due to blood loss.

compensated shock a condition that occurs when the patient is developing shock but the body is still able to maintain perfusion.

competent a legal term that describes the ability of an adult to make informed and rational decisions about his own well-being.

complex access means of getting into a vehicle that requires specialized training, tools, or equipment.

complex partial seizure a seizure that involves just one hemisphere of the brain; typically lasts a few seconds to two minutes and the patient is unaware that it is occurring. Also called *psychomotor seizure* or *temporal lobe seizure*.

compression mechanism of injury caused by direct force from the top or the bottom, causing vertebrae to jam together.

concentration how much of a substance exists at the source.

conchae tissue within the nasal cavity that causes a swirling air path. Also called *turbinates*.

concussion type of injury causing a jarring to the brain and temporary signs and symptoms including confusion and loss of memory about the incident.

conduction pathway the path of electrical impulses through the heart, which causes the heart to beat.

conduction system specialized tissue that provides the electrical stimulus that makes the heart beat.

conductive tissue a system of specialized muscle tissues that conduct the electrical impulses that stimulate the heart to beat.

confined space a small, closed-in area with poor access and egress.

congenital existing at birth.

congestive heart failure (CHF) an overload of fluid in the body's tissues that results when the heart is unable to pump an adequate volume of blood. Also called *heart failure*.

consent permission from the patient for care or other action by the EMT. See also *expressed consent; implied consent*.

constricted pupils pupils that are smaller than normal.

contact dermatitis localized rash or irritation of the skin.

contained stored.

contaminated to have some hazardous material on the person or object.

continuous positive airway pressure (CPAP) a form of noninvasive positive pressure ventilation consisting of a mask that provides air or oxygen under pressure to prevent collapse of the lower airway or assist with some causes of difficulty breathing.

contractions repeated tightening of the uterus to expel the baby during childbirth.

contraindication situation in which a medication should not be administered because it could do more harm than good.

contributory negligence any behavior on the part of the patient that may have led to the injuries being described in a negligence lawsuit.

contusions injuries resulting when the tissues below the epidermis are damaged and cause bleeding into the surrounding tissues following a blunt trauma or crushing force. Also called *bruises*.

convulsion full body muscle contractions.

coronary arteries arteries that branch off the aorta and provide blood supply directly to the heart.

crackles lung sounds caused by fluid in the lungs; usually heard on inspiration as fine crackling or bubbling sounds.

cranial vault portion of the skull containing the brain and composed of the temporal, frontal, parietal, and occipital bones. Also called the *cranial skull*.

crepitus the grating, crackling, or popping sounds and sensations that can be heard and felt beneath the skin.

cribbing wooden blocks or other supportive materials placed in a box pattern (crib) to assist in stabilizing a vehicle.

cricoid cartilage the ring-shaped structure that circles the trachea at the lower edge of the larynx.

critical incident stress debriefing (CISD) held one to 10 days after a highly stressful incident, a process in which teams of professional and peer counselors provide emotional and psychological support to EMS personnel who are or were involved.

critical incident stress management (CISM) a comprehensive, integrated, multicomponent crisis intervention system.

cross-contamination exposure through contact with a contaminated person or object.

croup viral illness characterized by inspiratory and expiratory stridor and a seal-barklike cough.

crowning refers to the baby's head becoming visible at the vaginal opening.

crumple zones vehicle parts that are designed to collapse, allowing for crash energy to be absorbed rather than transmitted to the passenger compartment.

crush injuries injuries typically caused when a patient or a part of the patient's body becomes trapped between two surfaces and the pressure from both sides causes damage to the soft tissues and/or internal organs.

cumulative stress response a type of stress reaction that results from the accumulation of recurring low-level stressors over many years.

Cushing's triad three signs—increased blood pressure, decreased pulse, and abnormal respirations—when combined, indicate increased intracranial pressure.

cyanosis a blue or gray color resulting from lack of oxygen in the body.

D

dead air space air that occupies the space between the mouth and alveoli, but does not actually reach the area of gas exchange. Also called *dead space*.

deceased patients a category of triage for patients who are not breathing after opening the airway.

decerebrate patient posture characterized by stiff extended arms at the elbows and pronated forearms; often occurs following severe head injury.

decompensate become unable to compensate for low blood volume or lack of perfusion.

decompensated shock a condition that occurs when the body can no longer compensate for low blood volume or lack of perfusion.

decompression sickness a condition that arises when dissolved gases come out of solution inside the body during depressurization. Also called *dysbarism* or *the bends*.

decontamination the process of chemically removing or neutralizing contaminants from a person or object.

decorticate patient posture characterized by stiff flexed arms at the elbows, clenched fists, and extended legs; often occurs following severe head injury.

defusing small-group discussion held within hours of a critical incident, designed to address acute symptoms of stress.

dehydration an abnormally low amount of water in the body.

delayed patients a category of triage for patients who are injured but whose triage findings are more stable than those of the "immediate" patient.

delayed stress response stress reactions that may not appear for days, months, or even years following an event.

delirium tremens (DTs) the most severe type of alcohol withdrawal during which the patient experiences visual hallucinations.

delusions false beliefs.

demand-valve device a device that uses oxygen under pressure to deliver artificial ventilations to adult patients. Also called a *flow-restricted, oxygen-powered ventilation device (FROPVD)*.

dementia a condition involving gradual development of memory impairment and cognitive disturbance; the loss of normal cognitive ability.

dependent lividity pooling of blood in the lower parts of the body after death.

depression profound sadness or feeling of melancholy; may affect major portions of the patient's life including work, relationships, weight changes, sleeping difficulties, feeling of worthlessness and guilt, and occasionally the desire to die.

dermal contact entrance of a substance through the skin or mucous membranes.

dermal exposure when a chemical contacts and is absorbed through the skin.

dermis the inner (second) layer of the skin found beneath the epidermis.

developmental disability lifelong physical or mental impairments that begin before the age of 22 years.

diabetes mellitus (DM) a group of metabolic disorders that cause patients with the disease to have an abnormally high blood-glucose level.

diabetic ketoacidosis (DKA) a potentially life-threatening condition in which the body begins to burn fat for energy rather than glucose, causing high acid levels in the blood.

dialysis the process by which toxins and excess fluid are removed from the body by a medical system independent of the kidneys.

diaphoretic perspiring, sweaty, moist; a characterization of skin condition.

diaphragm the large flat muscle responsible for breathing; forms the upper border of the abdominal vault.

diastolic the pressure remaining in the arteries when the left ventricle of the heart is relaxed and refilling.

dilated pupils pupils that are larger than normal.

direct force the force caused by a direct blow to an area of the body.

direct pathway exposure resulting from contact with hazardous vapors or substances. See also *indirect pathway*.

direct pressure pressure applied using the fingers, palm, or entire surface of one hand to help control bleeding.

disability a physical, emotional, cognitive, or behavioral condition that interferes with a person's ability to function.

disinfecting the use of a chemical or process to kill the microbes that may be on a piece of medical equipment.

dislocation displacement of the bones that make up a joint, such as the elbow, shoulder, knee, or hip.

displaced fracture a fracture of the spinal column that results in displacement of the broken bones.

distal farther away from the torso. Opposite of *proximal*.

distention the state of being stretched beyond normal dimensions.

distraction mechanism of injury caused by pulling forces such as in a hanging.

division a team assigned to function in a specific geographical area.

do not resuscitate (DNR) order a legal document, usually signed by the patient and his physician, which states that the patient has a terminal illness and does not wish to prolong life through resuscitative efforts.

dorsal refers to the back of the body or the back of the hand or foot. Synonym for *posterior*.

dorsalis pedis artery artery supplying the foot, lateral to the large tendon of the big toe.

dorsalis pedis (pedal) pulse pulse point located over the anterior foot.

dose the amount of medication that is to be administered.

Down syndrome a developmental disability that arises from an extra copy of the 21st chromosome, resulting in characteristic physical features and medical conditions.

dressings sterile or nonsterile material placed directly over an open wound.

drowning the process of experiencing respiratory impairment after submersion or immersion in a liquid.

due regard functioning in a manner that is precise, cautious, and does not injure anyone else. Also called *due caution*.

dura mater fibrous layer of tissue lining the inside of the cranial vault.

duration how long the exposure to a contaminant lasted.

duty to act a legal obligation to provide care to a patient.

dysmenorrhea pain during menstruation.

dysphasia a condition in which a patient is not able to generate clear and understandable speech.

dyspnea shortness of breath.

dysrhythmia any variation from the normal rate or rhythm of the heart. Also called *arrhythmia*.

E

ECG electrocardiogram. Also called ***EKG***.

eclampsia a complication related to pregnancy characterized by severe hypertension (high blood pressure), convulsions, and coma.

ectopic pregnancy a pregnancy in which the fetus implants in an area other than the uterus.

edema swelling associated with the movement of water into the interstitial space.

electrical burns burns caused when the body becomes exposed to an electrical current.

electrolyte a substance that, in water, separates into electrically charged particles.

elevation refers to the location of an injury site above the level of the patient's heart to reduce the amount of pressure at the site and make it easier for bleeding to be controlled.

emancipated minor a child under the age of 18 years of age who has become legally independent from his parents or legal guardians.

embolism a clot, particle, or air bubble that travels from its original site to another location in the body.

embryo the stage of fetal development between the zygote and the fetus.

emergency medical dispatcher (EMD) specially trained dispatchers who provide prearrival medical instructions for emergency care, including instructions for CPR, artificial ventilation, and bleeding control.

emergency medical responder (EMR) a level of EMS training designed for the person who often is first at the scene of an emergency; training emphasizes activating the EMS system and providing immediate care for life-threatening injuries or illnesses, controlling the scene, and preparing for the arrival of the ambulance.

emergency medical services (EMS) system a highly specialized chain of resources designed to minimize the impact of sudden injury and illness on society.

emergency medical technician (EMT) a level of EMS training with emphasis on assessment, care, and transport of the ill or injured patient and in most areas is considered the minimum level of certification for ambulance personnel.

Emergency Medical Treatment and Active Labor Act (EMTALA) passed in 1986, this act requires hospitals to provide care to anyone needing emergency health care treatment regardkess of citizenship, legal status, or ability to pay.

Emergency Response Guidebook (ERG) U.S. Department of Transportation's quick-information guide to hazardous materials responses.

emergent move a category of patient moves performed when there is an immediate risk of death or serious injury to the patient or when access to another patient in need of life-saving care is blocked.

emphysema condition in which the walls of the alveoli break down and lose surface area.

EMS task force any combination of resources within the span of control of three to seven units (such as ambulances, rescues, engines, and squads) assembled for a medical mission, with common communications and a leader (supervisor).

endometriosis development of uterine-lining cells outside the uterus; typically on the external surface of the uterus and the ovaries.

endometritis an infection of the lining of the uterus.

endoplasmic reticulum structure within the cell that synthesizes protein.

endotracheal intubation technique used to place an endotracheal tube into the trachea in order to provide a direct route for airflow into the lungs.

endotracheal tube (ETT) an advanced airway that is placed directly into the trachea.

end-stage renal disease (ESRD) irreversible renal failure to the extent that the kidneys can no longer provide adequate filtration and fluid balance to sustain life; survival with ESRD usually requires dialysis.

end-tidal carbon dioxide ($ETCO_2$) detector device used to detect the presence or the amount of carbon dioxide in exhaled air.

end-tidal CO_2 the concentration of carbon dioxide (CO_2) contained in the respiratory gases at the end of each exhaled breath.

enteral administered through the GI system.

epidermis the outer layer of the skin.

epidural hematoma collection of blood between the dura mater and the skull.

epiglottis a leaf-shaped structure that covers and prevents food and foreign matter from entering the larynx and trachea.

epiglottitis abnormal swelling of the epiglottis.

epilepsy a neurological disorder characterized by sudden recurring attacks of motor, sensory, or mental malfunction with or without loss of consciousness or convulsive seizures.

epinephrine a hormone produced by the body; a medication that constricts blood vessels and dilates respiratory passages and is used to relieve severe allergic reactions. Also known as *adrenaline*.

epistaxis a simple nosebleed.

error of commission action that should not have been taken, especially an action that causes harm to a patient.

error of omission something that was not done that should have been, resulting in harm to the patient.

erythema redness of the skin.

esophageal detector device (EDD) mechanical device that uses negative pressure to differentiate tracheal from esophageal placement of an endotracheal tube.

esophageal tracheal combitube (ETC) type of dual-lumen airway used to provide ventilations and help protect the airway.

esophageal varices an increase in pressure and exposure of the blood vessels of the esophagus.

esophagus the tube that connects the mouth to the stomach.

ethics the study of principles that define behavior as right, good, and proper.

evisceration an injury to the abdomen resulting in the protrusion of the intestinal organs through the abdominal wall.

excretion elimination of waste products from the large intestine.

exhalation a passive process in which the intercostal (rib) muscles and the diaphragm relax, causing the chest cavity to decrease in size and air to flow out of the lungs. Also called *expiration*.

exposure pathway specific route by which a chemical might travel from a source to a receptor.

expressed consent consent given by adults who are of legal age and have the mental capacity to make a rational decision in regard to their medical well-being. See also *consent; implied consent*.

extension the movement of a joint that results in increased angle between two bones or body surfaces at a joint.

F

facial bones bones that combined make up the structures of the face.

fallopian tube anatomical structure that extends from the ovary to the uterus. Female counterpart to the vas deferens.

falsification documentation of false information in a prehospital care report.

febrile seizure a seizure common in young children, caused by a sudden spike in fever.

feeding tube a device for providing nutrition to the gastrointestinal system in patients who cannot swallow.

femoral artery the major arteries supplying the lower extremities.

femoral pulse pulse point located deep in the groin between the hip and the inside of the upper thigh.

femur the large bone of the thigh.

fertilization the combining of a sperm and an egg; usually occurs in the fallopian tube.

fetus the clinical term for an unborn baby.

fibrinolytic therapy the use of specialized drugs to dissolve blood clots in patients with suspected myocardial infarctions and certain types of strokes.

fibrinolytics specialized drugs used to dissolve blood clots. Also known as *thrombolytics*.

fibula the lateral and smaller bone of the lower leg.

fimbriae fingerlike projections that propel ova into the fallopian tubes.

FiO_2 fraction of inspired oxygen; the concentration of oxygen in the air we breathe.

First Responder Awareness Level minimum level of hazardous materials training an EMT should receive; responders are trained to recognize a problem and initiate a response from an agency with operational-level training.

first stage of labor refers to the time of the beginning of uterine contractions until full dilation of the cervix.

five rights memory aid for all things an EMT must check when administering a medication to the patient; they include right medication, right dose, right route, right patient, and right time.

fixed-wing aircraft an airplane.

flail chest two or more ribs broken in two or more places.

flexible stretcher a lightweight device used for carrying supine patients down stairs or through tight spaces. Also known as a *flat stretcher* or *Reeves stretcher*.

flexion decrease in the angle between the bones forming a joint; tilting the head forward.

floating ribs the two lowest ribs that are connected to vertebrae but not to the sternum.

flushed a reddish skin color commonly seen when someone is embarrassed or is suffering a heat-related emergency.

focused secondary assessment a variation of the secondary assessment during which the EMT focuses on the specific body part or region affected; the part of the secondary assessment that is performed on stable medical and trauma patients.

form refers to whether a hazardous material is in large blocks or tiny particles, or whether it is a liquid or a vapor.

Fowler's position a position in which the patient is sitting fully upright.

fracture broken bone; can be as minor as a hairline crack all the way to a badly shattered bone that appears deformed.

freelancing situation in which a person at a multiple-casualty incident takes action without the knowledge or permission of the incident commander.

frostbite local cold injury; damage to local tissues from exposure to cold temperatures.

frostnip early or superficial frostbite.

full-thickness burns burns that extend beyond all layers of the skin, causing damage to underlying muscle, bone, nerves, and vital organs. See also *superficial burns* and *partial-thickness burns.*

G

gall bladder an organ in the form of a sac on the underside of the liver that stores bile produced by the liver.

gastric refers to the stomach.

gastroenteritis an inflammation and breakdown of the lining of the stomach and intestines, resulting in diarrhea.

gastrointestinal (GI) refers to the digestive system, including the stomach and intestines.

gastrostomy tube (G-tube) a tube placed directly into the stomach or upper small intestine through the abdominal wall to provide nutrition to a patient who cannot eat or swallow.

gel jelly-like form of medication.

general impression an element of the patient assessment that includes gender, approximate age, and level of distress.

general staff the key staff positions that oversee the sections in a fully expanded incident management system.

generalized seizure a seizure that involves both hemispheres of the brain and is characterized by a loss of consciousness and convulsions. Also called *grand mal seizure.*

generic name the medication name found in the *United States Pharmacopoeia.*

genitalia male or female reproductive organs.

geriatric refers to a person aged 65 or older.

geriatrics refers to older adults, or more specifically, the branch of medicine dealing with care of the elderly.

gestation length of time from conception to birth.

gestational diabetes a temporary condition that results in abnormally high glucose levels during pregnancy.

Glasgow Coma Scale (GCS) a widely used objective assessment tool or objective scale for rating a patient's level of responsiveness.

gliding joints a type of joint in which one bone end slides on another, such as the wrist or ankle.

glottic opening the opening of the trachea in the hypopharynx. Also known as the *glottis.*

glottis opening between the vocal cords that separates the upper airway from the lower airway. Also called the glottic opening.

glucagon a hormone produced by the pancreas.

glucose a simple form of sugar that is required by all cells as fuel for metabolic processes.

Good Samaritan laws laws, varying in each state, designed to provide limited legal protection for citizens and some health care personnel when they are administering emergency care.

guarding the act of contracting the abdominal muscles in response to pain.

gurgling intermittent low-pitched sounds indicative of fluids in the upper airway.

H

hallucinations sensory perceptions without an external stimulus.

Hazard Class 1, Explosives one of nine classes of hazardous materials; indicates the hazard can cause injuries by the primary, secondary, and tertiary blasts.

Hazard Class 2, Gases one of nine classes of hazardous materials; indicates the hazard can cause injuries by being toxic or displacing oxygen to cause asphyxiation.

Hazard Class 3, Flammable liquids, combustible liquids one of nine classes of hazardous materials; indicates the hazard can cause injuries by penetrating the skin and attacking internal organs.

Hazard Class 4, Flammable solids, spontaneously combustible materials, and dangerous when wet materials one of nine classes of hazardous materials; indicates the hazard can cause injuries by creating severe and deep burns to tissue. Many of the flammable solids are reactive to water.

Hazard Class 5, Oxidizers and organic peroxides one of nine classes of hazardous materials; indicates the hazard can trigger an explosion and act as a corrosive destroying tissue and triggering inflammation in the lungs.

Hazard Class 6, Toxic materials and infectious substances one of nine classes of hazardous materials; indicates the hazard can involve biological and poisonous substances. Infectious material can include blood products or blood-contaminated materials and plant, virus, bacterial, or other living organisms.

Hazard Class 7, Radioactive materials one of nine classes of hazardous materials; indicates the hazard can injure or kill by disrupting the nervous system or cellular functions.

Hazard Class 8, Corrosive materials one of nine classes of hazardous materials; indicates the hazard can cause injuries by destroying and dissolving tissue. Corrosives usually involve acids, bases, and some solvents.

Hazard Class 9, Miscellaneous dangerous goods one of nine classes of hazardous materials; indicates hazardous materials that do not fit into one of the other hazard classes.

hazardous material any substance or material in a form that poses an unreasonable risk to health, safety, and property.

Hazardous Materials First Responder Operations Level level of hazmat training that includes procedures to contain and keep hazardous materials from spreading and to prevent exposures to people, property, and the environment. At this level first responders wear and operate in level B protection.

Hazardous Materials Specialist Level level of hazmat training that includes advanced knowledge of monitoring devices, toxicology, and command and control of large-scale hazmat incidents.

Hazardous Materials Technician Level level of advanced hazmat training that focuses on controlling a spill and operating in hazardous environments in chemical protective clothing and level A suits.

hazardous properties effects the hazardous materials can have on living things or the environment.

head-tilt/chin-lift maneuver a means of opening the airway by tilting the head back and lifting the chin; used when no trauma, or injury, is suspected.

Health Insurance Portability and Accountability Act (HIPAA) federal legislation enacted in 1996 that protects the privacy of patient health care information.

heat cramps a progressive heat injury caused by dehydration and electrolyte depletion; characterized by pain in large muscle groups.

heat exhaustion a progressive heat injury characterized by cool skin, syncope, and fatigue.

heat stroke a progressive heat injury characterized by altered mental status, hot skin, and shock.

helibase locations in or near an incident area at which helicopters may be parked, maintained, fueled, and equipped for incident operations.

helipad a designated location for a helicopter landing.

helispots temporary locations where helicopters can land, load, and off-load personnel, equipment, and supplies.

hematemesis the vomiting of blood.

hematochezia the passing of blood through the feces.

hematomas areas of localized swelling caused by the accumulation of blood and other fluids beneath the skin.

hemiparesis weakness on one side of the body.

hemiplegia paralysis of one side of the body.

hemodialysis the clearing of blood toxins and waste products in patients with renal failure by placing the patient on a machine that filters the blood externally and then returns the filtered blood to the body.

hemoglobin molecule within the red blood cell that carries oxygen to the cells and carbon dioxide away from the cells.

hemorrhagic shock type of shock caused by loss of blood.

hemorrhagic stroke stroke caused by a ruptured blood vessel.

hemostatic dressing a specialized gauze dressing treated with a chemical agent that promotes clotting.

hemothorax a condition in which blood accumulates within the pleural space.

hernia a protrusion of abdominal organs through a membranous wall such as the diaphragm.

herniation tissue protrusion outside the area in which it is normally contained.

high-angle rescue a vertical or above-ground rescue situation requiring specialized training and equipment.

hinge joints a type of joint that moves in only one direction, such as a finger or toe.

histamine a chemical mediator that triggers an inflammatory response by the immune system.

history of present illness the medical history related to the patient's chief complaint.

hives red, itchy, possibly raised blotches on the skin; can be from insect bites or food allergy.

home ventilator a mechanical device that moves air in and out of the lungs.

hormones chemicals involved in regulation of body functions.

humerus the bone of the upper arm, between the shoulder and the elbow.

hydrostatic pressure the push of water out of the bloodstream as a result of the pressure within the vessel.

hypercarbia excessive carbon dioxide in the blood.

hyperextension extreme or abnormal extension or increase in the angle between bones of a joint.

hyperglycemia abnormally high levels of blood glucose.

hypersensitivity an exaggerated response by the immune system to a particular substance.

hyperthermia abnormally elevated core body temperature.

hyperventilation breathing that is abnormally rapid and deep.

hyperventilation syndrome an abnormal respiratory condition characterized by rapid deep respirations; often associated with anxiety that can be psychologically or physiologically based.

hypocarbia abnormally low carbon dioxide levels in the blood that leads to constriction of the cerebral blood vessels

hypoglycemia abnormally low levels of blood glucose.

hypoperfusion inadequate distribution of blood to an organ or organs of the body. Also called *shock*.

hypopharynx the back of the throat superior to the opening of the trachea.

hypothermia abnormally low core body temperature.

hypovolemic shock type of shock caused by a sudden decrease in body fluids (blood or other body fluids).

hypoxia an insufficiency of oxygen in the body's tissues.

hypoxic drive when the stimulus to breathe is the amount of oxygen in the blood, rather than the normal drive to breathe, which is related to the amount of carbon dioxide in the blood.

I

ilium the superior and widest portion of the pelvis.

immediate and adverse effects reactions to a chemical that occur at the time of exposure, such as vomiting or eye irritation.

immediate-tagged patients triaged patients who are at risk for early death, usually due to shock, an airway problem, or a severe head injury.

immunoglobulin E (IgE) a class of antibody that is responsible for causing the most severe allergic reactions.

impaled object penetrating trauma in which the object remains in the body.

implantation the attachment of a fertilized egg to the uterine lining.

implied consent the consent it is presumed a patient or patient's parent or guardian would give if he could, such as for an unconscious patient or by a parent who cannot be contacted when care is needed. See also *consent; expressed consent.*

improvised nuclear device (IND) device that can produce a nuclear explosion.

incident action plan (IAP) plan for the management of a specific component of incident operations.

incident command post (ICP) a physical location near an incident from which the incident commander oversees all incident operations. Also called the *command post (CP)*.

incident command system (ICS) a tool used for the systematic command, control, and coordination of a large scale event or incident.

incident commander (IC) the person in overall charge of an emergency under an incident management system.

incontinence inability to retain urine or feces because of loss of sphincter control.

incubation period the period of time from exposure to a pathogen until signs and symptoms occur.

index of suspicion an awareness or suspicion that there may be injuries based on the evaluation of the mechanism of injury; also refers to recognizing a potential terrorist event.

indication reason a medication is administered.

indirect force the force that occurs when energy is transferred along a bone, usually proximal to the site of impact.

indirect pathway exposure resulting from taking in air, water, or food that has been contaminated by hazardous vapors or substances. See also *direct pathway*.

infant a child from birth to one year of age.

inferior away from the head; usually compared with another structure that is closer to the head (for example, the lips are inferior to the nose). Opposite of *superior*.

inflammatory headache a symptom of an associated neurological problem such as hemorrhagic stroke, meningitis, or tumor.

ingested poisons poisons that are swallowed.

ingestion entry into the digestive system by eating or drinking.

inhalation an active process in which the intercostal (rib) muscles and the diaphragm contract, expanding the size of the chest cavity and causing air to flow into the lungs. Also called *inspiration*.

inhaled bronchodilators medication used to open up bronchioles that are constricted due to a respiratory disease such as asthma.

inhaled poisons poisons that are breathed in.

inhaler a spray device with a mouthpiece that contains an aerosol form of a medication a patient can spray into his airway.

injected poisons poisons that are inserted through the skin.

injection entry through a puncture or open skin.

instrument flight rules (IFR) rules defined by the Federal Aviation Administration regarding the operation of an aircraft in inclement weather.

insulin a hormone produced by the pancreas or taken as a medication by many diabetics that helps the body use glucose as fuel.

interfacility transfer (IFT) the transportation of a patient from one hospital to another, typically for a higher level of care.

interventions anything that the EMT does to comfort or provide care for the patient.

intracerebral hemorrhage bleeding within the brain matter.

intracranial pressure increasing pressure within the cranial vault due to bleeding or swelling.

intramuscular within a muscle.

intraperitoneal within the peritoneal cavity.

involuntary muscle muscle that responds automatically to brain signals but cannot be consciously controlled. Also called *smooth muscle*.

ischemia an inadequate blood supply to an organ or part of the body, especially the heart muscles.

ischemic stroke the most common kind of stroke; caused by an interruption in the flow of blood to the brain by a blocked vessel.

ischium the lower, posterior portions of the pelvis.

islets of Langerhans the region of the pancreas responsible for monitoring blood glucose and producing hormones such as glucagon and insulin.

J

jaundice the yellowing of the skin and mucous membranes caused by a buildup of bilirubin; a condition that is commonly associated with liver failure.

jaw-thrust maneuver a means of correcting blockage of the airway by moving the jaw forward without tilting the head or neck; used when trauma, or injury, is suspected.

jugular vein distention (JVD) an abnormal bulging of the neck veins commonly caused by a compromise of the circulatory system.

K

kidney stones small rock-like structures formed in the kidneys of certain patients; cause symptoms of flank pain when they become lodged in the ureter.

kidneys a pair of organs that filters the blood to remove excess water and waste.

Kussmaul's respirations rapid, deep ventilations usually caused by very acidic blood such as in some diabetic conditions and aspirin overdose.

L

labia soft tissues that protect the exterior entrance to the vagina.

labor the physiological process characterized by increasingly intense contractions of the uterus, whereby the fetus is expelled from the uterus of a pregnant woman.

lacerations open wounds that can have either jagged or straight edges.

lacrimation the secretion of tears.

laminated glass type of glass that has a layer of glue, plastic, or mastic sandwiched between two pieces of glass.

landing zone (LZ) a temporary location for the landing of a helicopter, typically at the scene of an emergency.

large intestine organ that is a muscular tube that removes water from waste products received from the small intestine and removes anything not absorbed by the body toward excretion from the body. Also called the *colon*.

laryngeal mask airway (LMA) type of airway used to provide ventilations and help protect the airway.

laryngopharynx the area in the back of the throat just inferior to the epiglottis. Also called *hypopharynx*.

laryngoscope instrument used to lift the tongue off the posterior pharynx and move the epiglottis out of the visual field so that the vocal cords are visible.

larynx the structure that contains the vocal cords and is connected to the superior portion of the trachea.

lateral to the side, away from the midline of the body.

lateral recumbent position lying on one side. Also called the *recovery position*.

left ventricular assist device (LVAD) a battery-powered electrical pump implanted in the body to assist a failing left ventricle in pumping blood to the body.

left refers to the patient's left.

lethality the ability of an agent or disease to cause death; the percentage of those who die from an agent or disease.

liaison officer command staff officer responsible for communicating with other agencies during a multiple-casualty incident; may be the person making the initial contact with an EMS agency.

life expectancy the average number of additional years a person is expected to live, based on current age.

lift-in stretcher a type of wheeled stretcher that must be lifted by at least two rescuers to be placed into the ambulance.

ligaments tissues that connect bone to bone.

light burns burns caused by high-intensity light sources including the sun and lasers.

limb presentation refers to a single limb presenting at the vaginal opening during the birth process.

liver organ that produces bile to assist in breakdown of fats and in the metabolism of various substances in the body.

lobes sections of the lung; the left lung has two lobes and the right lung has three lobes.

long backboard a rigid device, usually made of plastic or a composite material, that is used to stabilize a patient with a suspected spine injury. Also called a *long spine board.*

low-angle rescue a rescue situation involving shallow heights and requiring specialized training and equipment.

lumbar vertebrae the five vertebrae that form the lower back.

lungs the primary organs of respiration.

M

Macintosh a type of laryngoscope blade. Also called a *curved blade.*

mandible the lower jaw bone.

manual stabilization method of stabilization in which the EMT firmly grasps the patient's head with both hands and attempts to keep it from moving.

mass gathering any collection of more than 1,000 people at one site or location; applies to all types of events, including concerts and sporting or other large-scale events.

material safety data sheet (MSDS) document from the manufacturer for each hazardous chemical in the workplace; contains important safety information about each hazardous chemical present.

maxilla the upper jaw bone, which is formed by two bones fused together.

mechanism of action the specific biochemical interaction that is caused by a medication to produce a pharmacological effect.

mechanism of injury (MOI) a force or forces that may have caused injury.

meconium fecal matter excreted by a baby while still in the uterus.

medial toward the midline of the body.

medical assessment the examination of someone with an illness.

medical direction oversight of the patient-care aspects of an EMS system by a licensed physician who is referred to as the *medical director*.

medical director a physician who assumes ultimate responsibility for the patient care aspects of an EMS system.

medical patient a patient whose chief complaint is related to an acute illness or disease process.

medulla oblongata portion of the brain that directly connects to the spinal cord. Also called the *medulla.*

melena black tarry feces associated with blood in the stool.

meninges three membranes that surround and protect the brain and spinal cord: the dura mater, the pia mater, and the arachnoid membrane.

menstrual cycle monthly recurrent changes in the female reproductive system.

mentation the mental activity of a patient.

metabolic acidosis the accumulation of excess lactic acid in the bloodstream as a result of hypoperfusion of the body's cells.

metabolism the conversion of glucose into energy in the form of adenosine triphosphate (ATP).

metacarpals the hand bones.

metatarsals the foot bones.

metered-dose inhaler a device that patients use to breathe in medication.

midaxillary line an imaginary line drawn vertically from the middle of the armpit to the hip.

midclavicular line the imaginary line drawn vertically through the center of each clavicle.

midline an imaginary line drawn down the center of the body, dividing it into right and left halves.

migraine severe, throbbing headache often characterized initially by an aura and accompanied by sensitivity to light, sweating, nausea, and vomiting. Also called *vascular headache*.

Miller a type of laryngoscope blade. Also called a *straight blade.*

minor injuries in a triage situation, refers to patients with minor injuries who are classified as "minor." Sometimes referred to as *walking wounded*.

minute volume the volume of air moved in one minute by the lungs (tidal volume × respiratory rate).

mitochondria structure within the cell that produces energy.

mitral valve a structure between the left atrium and left ventricle that opens and closes to permit the flow of a fluid in only one direction.

mnemonic a memory aid.

mobile data terminals (MDTs) computers that are mounted in a vehicle and connected to the base station by radio modem.

mobile radios two-way radios that are used or are affixed in a vehicle.

motor nerves portion of the nervous system that carries information from the brain through the spinal cord and to the body.

mottling uneven coloration or spotting of the skin; commonly caused by poor perfusion to the skin.

multiple birth delivery of more than one baby. Also called *multiple gestations.*

multiple-casualty incident (MCI) an emergency involving illness or injuries that exceed or overwhelm EMS and hospital capabilities.

multisystem trauma injury to multiple organ systems within the body.

mutagenic causing a mutation, which is a permanent change in the genetic material (DNA) that may be passed along to later generations.

myocardial infarction (MI) occlusion or blockage of one or more of the coronary arteries, resulting in damage to the heart muscle. Also called a *heart attack*.

N

nares external openings in the nasal cavity; nostrils.

nasal bones the bones that form the upper third, or bridge, of the nose.

nasal cannula a device that delivers low concentrations of oxygen through two prongs that rest in the patient's nostrils.

nasal flaring the extended opening or flaring of nostrils.

nasal vestibule the anteriormost portion of the nasal cavity.

nasopharyngeal airway (NPA) a soft flexible tube inserted into the patient's nose and into the pharynx to help maintain an open airway.

nasopharynx the area directly posterior to the nose.

National EMS Education Standards standards developed by NHTSA that define what each level of EMS training must include.

National Fire Protection Association (NFPA) the world's leading advocate of fire prevention and an authoritative source on public safety.

National Highway Traffic Safety Administration (NHTSA) a division of the U.S. Department of Transportation (DOT), which develops the National Standard Curricula for various levels of EMS providers.

national incident management system (NIMS) system implemented in 2004 by the U.S. Department of Homeland Security that provides a consistent nationwide approach for incident management and requires federal, state, tribal, and local governments to work together before, during, and after incidents.

National Standard Curriculum (NSC) the curriculum developed by the U.S. Department of Transportation as the foundation for the scope of practice for all EMS personnel.

National Trauma Triage Protocol a systematic approach for assessing and categorizing trauma patients developed by the CDC; used to determine whether or not a patient should be transported directly to a trauma center.

nature of illness (NOI) what is medically wrong with a patient.

nebulized process of mixing air and medication to produce a mist, which is inhaled.

nebulizer a device used to administer medications in the form of a fine mist.

neglect a person's inability to care for self, or a person's caregiver providing inadequate care.

negligence a legal finding of failure to act properly in a situation in which there was a duty to act, needed care as would reasonably be expected of the EMT was not provided, and harm was caused to the patient as a result.

neonate a child from the moment of birth up until one month of age (28 days). Also called a *newborn*.

nerve agents chemicals (often used as weapons) that incapacitate and kill by deranging normal function of the central nervous system.

neurogenic hypotension decreased blood pressure secondary to a disruption of sympathetic nervous system messaging; usually resulting from a spinal-cord injury.

neurogenic shock type of shock caused when the vessels dilate abnormally in response to injury to the spinal cord.

NFPA 704 a standardized system that uses numbers and colors on a sign to indicate the basic hazards of a specific material being stored in large containers or at a manufacturing site.

nitroglycerin a medication used to treat chest pain.

nondisplaced fracture a fracture that results in no displacement of the broken bones.

nonemergent move a category of patient moves performed when there is no need to expedite due to the patient's condition or hazards at the scene.

nonrebreather mask a face mask and reservoir bag device that delivers high concentrations of oxygen.

nonsignificant mechanism of injury a mechanism of injury that does not result in a high likelihood of life-threatening injury.

normothermic normal body temperature.

nuclear weapon (NW) device designed to release the energy generated during splitting (fission) or combining (fusion) of heavy nuclei to form new elements that are deliberately distributed to cause harm or death; a weapon that can produce an actual nuclear explosion.

nucleus structure within the cell that contains DNA.

O

obesity having too much body fat; a body mass index greater than 30.

objective information information that you have personally observed and can measure or attest to.

obstructive shock a form of shock that blocks the forward movement of blood within the circulatory system.

occipital posterior (back) region of the skull.

occlusive dressing a dressing that does not allow air to move through it; an airtight dressing. Also called a *nonporous dressing*.

occult refers to something that is hidden, such as bleeding within the skull.

off-line medical direction instructions consisting of protocols and standing orders, which allow EMTs to give certain medications or perform certain procedures without speaking directly to the medical director or another physician.

on-line medical direction instructions consisting of orders from the on-duty physician or designee given directly to an EMT in the field by radio or telephone.

on-scene time the time spent on scene assessing, caring for, and preparing the patient for transport.

open head injury head injury in which there is a break in the skin and cranium.

open pneumothorax air within the pleural space that is accumulating due to a penetration of the chest wall.

open skeletal injury skeletal injury in which the skin is damaged causing an open soft-tissue wound in connection with the injury.

operational level (hazardous materials) level of training that is designed for responders who will be responsible for hazard recognition, equipment use, and techniques necessary to conduct a technical rescue.

OPQRST a mnemonic for the questions asked to get a description of the present illness; letters stand for *onset*, *provocation*, *quality*, *region and radiate*, *severity*, and *time*.

oral glucose a medication used to treat patients with suspected low blood sugar.

orbits the bony structures around the eyes; the eye sockets.

organic caused by medical or traumatic etiology, as opposed to a psychiatric origin.

organic headache a symptom of an associated neurological problem such as hemorrhagic stroke, meningitis, or tumor.

oropharyngeal airway (OPA) a curved device inserted into the patient's mouth and the pharynx to help maintain an open airway.

oropharynx the area directly posterior to the mouth.

orotracheal intubation the placement of an endotracheal tube orally, by way of the mouth, then through the vocal cords and into the trachea.

orthostatic vital signs a test in which vital signs are measured before and after a patient moves from a supine to a sitting or a sitting to a standing position.

osteoporosis softening of bone tissue due to the loss of essential minerals, principally calcium.

ostomy bag a collection device used in conjunction with a colostomy or ileostomy to collect fecal matter.

ova female sex cell; female counterpart to the sperm. Singular *ovum.*

ovarian cyst the development of a fluid-filled sac on the outside of the ovaries.

ovaries internal glands producing ova (eggs); female counterpart to the testicles.

ovulation the release of an ovum (egg) from the ovary.

ovum an unfertilized egg. Plural, *ova*.

oxygen a gas necessary to life that makes up 21% of the air we breathe; a medication administered to increase the amount of circulating oxygen in the bloodstream.

P

pacemaker site within the heart that originates an electrical impulse; a small device implanted under the skin with wires that are inserted into the heart to ensure a patient maintains a normal heart rate.

pale a whitish skin color indicative of poor perfusion.

palmar refers to the palm of the hand.

palpation the act of examining by feeling with the hands; a technique used for obtaining a blood pressure reading.

pancreas a gland located behind the stomach that produces insulin and juices that assist in digestion of food in the duodenum of the small intestine.

pancreatitis inflammation of the pancreas.

panic attack sudden onset of a fear or discomfort including symptoms such as sweating, trembling, palpitations, feelings of shortness of breath or chest tightness, nausea and vomiting, and fears of dying or loss of control.

paradoxical movement a sign found on the chest wall where a flail segment of the chest moves in a direction opposite from the rest of the chest during inspiration and expiration.

paralysis suffering temporary or permanent loss of muscular power or sensation.

paramedic a level of EMS training that requires significantly more training than an EMT, specifically in advanced life support procedures including insertion of endotracheal tubes, initiation of IV lines, administration of a variety of medications, interpretation of electrocardiograms, and cardiac defibrillation.

paranoia a delusion in which the patient believes he is being followed, persecuted, or harmed.

parenteral administered outside of the GI system.

paresthesia a sensation of tingling, burning, pricking, or numbness in an extremity.

parietal peritoneum the outermost layer of the peritoneum attached to the wall of the abdomen.

parietal pleura a membrane that is attached to the chest wall.

Parkinson's disease chronic, degenerative nervous disease characterized by tremors, muscular weakness, rigidity, and a loss of postural reflexes.

partial-thickness burns burns that extend down beyond the epidermis and into the dermis. See also *superficial burns* and *full-thickness burns*.

passive rewarming covering a hypothermic patient and taking other steps to prevent further heat loss and to help the body rewarm itself.

past medical history the medical history related to prior illness or events.

patella the kneecap.

patent open and clear; free from obstruction.

patent airway open and clear, without interference to the passage of air into and out of the body.

pathogens organisms that cause disease, such as viruses and bacteria.

pathophysiology the study of how disease processes affect the function of the body.

pathways of exposure all the ways a contaminant could reach the population at risk.

patient assessment overall evaluation of a patient for life-threatening and non-life-threatening conditions.

patient data all the information about the patient (name, address, date of birth), insurance, and details of the patient's complaint, assessment, care, and vital signs.

patient tagging affixing to a patient a triage tag that identifies his triage category.

pediatrics refers to children up to the age of 18, or more specifically, the branch of medicine dealing with the development and care of children.

pelvic inflammatory disease (PID) refers to processes (typically sexually transmitted diseases) that cause inflammation of the uterus, ovaries, and the fallopian tubes.

pelvis the basin-shaped bony structure that supports the spine and is the point of proximal attachment for the lower extremities.

penetration injuries injuries caused by an object that passes through the skin or other body tissues.

penis external male genitalia that contains the urethra.

percutaneous transluminal coronary angiography (PTCA) a procedure in which a wire catheter is inserted through the femoral or brachial artery directly into the coronary arteries in order to visualize the status and condition of the vessels.

perfusion the supply of oxygen to and removal of wastes from the cells and tissues of the body as a result of the flow of blood through the capillaries.

pericardial tamponade a form of cardiac compromise caused by a collection of blood in the sac surrounding the heart.

perineum the skin between the vagina and the anus.

peripheral nervous system (PNS) the nerves that enter and leave the spinal cord and those that extend from brain to organs without passing through the spinal cord.

peripheral pulses pulses in the distal circulation such as the radial pulse and the pedal pulse.

peritoneal dialysis the clearing of blood toxins and waste products in patients with renal failure by placing specialized dialysis fluid into the peritoneal cavity and then draining the fluid out in an exchange.

peritoneum the membrane of connective tissue that lines and separates the abdominal cavity.

peritonitis bacterial infection within the peritoneal cavity.

PERRL a mnemonic used to evaluate a patient's pupils; letters stand for *pupils equal and round, reactive to light*.

persistence length of time an agent stays in the environment.

personal protective equipment (PPE) equipment that protects the EMS worker from infection and exposure to the dangers of rescue operations.

phalanges bones of the fingers and toes.

pharmacodynamics the study of the biochemical and physiological effects of medications on the body.

pharmacology the study of drugs—their sources, characteristics, and effects.

pharynx passageway that extends from nose and mouth to trachea.

phobia an unfounded or intense fear of an object or situation.

physiology the study of body function.

pia mater layer of tissue directly covering the brain.

placard diamond-shaped sign placed on cargo tanks, vehicles, or rail cars to display one of nine classes of hazardous materials that is being carried.

placenta anatomical structure that provides nutrition to the fetus and eliminates fetal waste.

placenta previa a condition in which the placenta is attached to the uterine wall over the opening of the cervix, but in the wrong position.

plane a flat surface formed when slicing through a solid object.

plantar refers to the sole of the foot.

plasma the fluid portion of the blood.

plasma oncotic pressure the pull exerted on water in and around the body cells into the bloodstream by large proteins in the plasma portion of blood.

platelets components of the blood; membrane-enclosed fragments of specialized cells involved in clotting. Also called *thrombocytes*.

pleura two tissue layers that line the chest wall and cover the lungs.

pleural space potential space between the two tissue layers that line the chest wall and cover the lungs.

pneumonia a respiratory condition caused by inflammation of a lung secondary to infection.

pneumothorax an abnormal collection of air in the pleural space that separates the lung from the chest wall.

poisons substances that can harm the body by altering cell function or structure.

polydipsia excessive thirst.

polyuria excessive urination.

popliteal pulse pulse point located over the posterior aspect of the knee.

portable radios handheld two-way radios.

portable stretcher a lightweight device made of canvas or plastic with two poles extended from each side for easy carrying.

position of function position of the hands and feet when they are at rest.

positional asphyxia death of a patient who has been inappropriately restrained; a condition often associated with extreme exertion (long foot chases or struggling against restraints), drug or alcohol use, and hog-tie or hobble restraints.

posterior the back of the body or body part. Opposite of *anterior.*

posterior tibial artery artery supplying the foot, behind the medial ankle.

posterior tibial pulse pulse point located over the medial ankle just posterior to the ankle bone.

postictal the state after a seizure during which the patient may exhibit decreased respirations and altered mental status.

postictal phase the state that occurs when a seizure has stopped and the brain is attempting to recover, characterized by unconsciousness.

postpartum refers to the mother and the period of time beginning immediately following the birth of the child.

power grip gripping with as much hand surface as possible in contact with the object being lifted; palms are up, all fingers are bent at the same angle, and hands are at least 10 inches apart.

power lift a lift from a squatting position with weight to be lifted close to the body. Also called the *squat-lift position*.

preeclampsia a complication of pregnancy characterized by hypertension (high blood pressure) and edema.

prefix a word or part of a word added to the beginning of another word to add description.

prehospital care report (PCR) written documentation of the call and patient encounter. Also called a *patient care report* or a *run report*.

premature birth birth before the baby has fully developed, which occurs prior to a 38-week gestation.

prenatal refers to a time before birth.

preplanning developing a plan for future possible incidents that would require a large response of units, personnel, and supervisors.

preschooler a child between three and six years of age.

presenting part the part of the baby that first becomes visible at the vaginal opening during the process of birth.

pressure dressing a dressing that applies pressure to control bleeding from a wound to an extremity that is still actively bleeding. Also called a *pressure bandage*.

priapism persistent erection of the penis that may result from spine injury and some medical problems.

primary assessment a component of the overall patient assessment; the main objective is to identify and treat any immediate life threats to the patient.

primary seizures seizures that are thought to be caused by a genetic disorder or an unidentified cause.

prolapsed cord refers to the umbilical cord entering the birth canal before the baby's head.

prone a position in which the patient is lying face down on the stomach. Opposite of *supine*.

proteins source of amino acids, the building blocks of the body.

protocols written guidelines for patient care approved by the medical director of an EMS system.

proximal closer to the torso. Opposite of *distal.*

pruritus itching of the skin.

psychogenic shock type of shock caused by a sudden and temporary dilation of the blood vessels from psychological causes.

psychosis unusual or bizarre behavior indicating a lack of touch with reality.

puberty the process of physical changes by which a child's body matures and becomes capable of reproduction.

pubis the medial anterior portion of the pelvis.

public information officer command staff officer who is the only one at the scene of a multiple-casualty incident who is authorized by the incident commander to release information to the news media.

public safety answering point (PSAP) the agency responsible for answering 911 calls.

pulmonary arteries vessels that carry oxygen-poor blood from the right ventricle to the lungs.

pulmonary contusion bruising of the lung tissue typically as the result of blunt trauma.

pulmonary edema a condition of fluid in the lungs.

pulmonary embolism a blockage of the main artery of the lung.

pulmonary veins vessels that carry oxygen-rich blood from the lungs to the left atrium.

pulmonic valve a structure between the right ventricle and pulmonary arteries that opens and closes to permit the flow of a fluid in only one direction.

pulse the pumping of the heart as a pressure wave felt over an artery.

pulse oximeter device that uses infrared light to determine arterial oxygen saturation.

pulse oximetry use of an electronic device, a pulse oximeter, to determine the amount of oxygen carried by the hemoglobin in the blood, known as the oxygen saturation or SpO_2.

pyelonephritis an infection of the kidney.

Q

quality improvement (QI) a process of continuous self-review with the purpose of identifying and correcting aspects of the system that require improvement.

R

raccoon eyes bruising around the eyes indicative of a basilar skull fracture.

radial artery artery of the lower arm.

radial pulse the pulse point located over the lateral aspect of the anterior wrist.

radiation burn a type of burn from sources of radiation such as nuclear fallout or radioactive materials used in medicine.

radiological dispersal device (RDD) a conventional bomb laced with radioactive material. Also called a *dirty bomb*.

radius the lateral bone of the forearm.

rapid extrication the rapid removal of a patient from a vehicle when the patient's condition or the situation does not permit use of a short backboard or vest-type extrication device.

rapid secondary assessment a variation of the secondary assessment that is performed on unstable patients and on patients who have sustained a significant mechanism of injury.

reassessment the component of the patient assessment that is repeated at regular intervals and designed to monitor the status of the ABCs, vital signs, mental status, and effectiveness of interventions.

receptor living plant or animal that is exposed to a hazardous substance.

recovery position a position in which the patient is lying on one side. Also called a *lateral recumbent position*.

red blood cells specialized blood cells containing hemoglobin.

referred pain pain that is perceived at a site other than that of the painful stimulus.

renal failure loss of the kidneys' ability to filter the blood and remove toxins and excess fluid from the body.

repeaters devices that allow long-distance transmissions by picking up signals from lower-power radio units, such as mobile and portable radios, and retransmitting them at a higher power.

rescue/extrication group team responsible for all the operations necessary to remove victims from the hazard to the treatment area at a multiple-casualty incident.

respiration inhalation and exhalation. Also called *ventilation*.

respiration (cellular) the movement of oxygen and waste products at the cellular level.

respiratory arrest the absence of breathing.

respiratory distress the body's attempts to compensate for an inadequate gas exchange (perfusion).

respiratory failure the condition that occurs when the body is no longer able to adequately compensate for inadequate oxygenation; the reduction of breathing to the point at which oxygen intake is not sufficient to support life.

respiratory/metabolic shock a form of shock caused by a disruption in the ability of cells to utilize oxygen effectively.

retraction muscles pulling in between the ribs and above th clavicles and below the ribs upon inspiration.

retroperitoneal space referring to the area behind or outside the abdominal cavity; the kidneys are located here.

rhinitis nasal irritation or inflammation.

rhonchi low-pitched snoring or rattling sounds caused by secretions in the larger airways; may be seen in chronic lung diseases and possibly pneumonia.

rib fracture any break in a rib.

ribs the 12 pairs of bones that help form the thoracic cavity.

right refers to the patient's right. See also *left*.

right of way permission to travel through traffic without delay.

rigor mortis body stiffness or rigidity that occurs after a person has been dead for a period of time.

risk the chance of injury, damage, or loss.

roll-in stretcher a type of wheeled stretcher that can be rolled into the ambulance without lifting.

root word the main part of a word with all prefixes and suffixes removed.

rotor-wing aircraft a helicopter.

route how a medication is administered.

routes of entry the ways that hazardous materials can enter the body.

rule of nines a method of estimating the body surface area (BSA) burned based on dividing the body into areas of approximately 9% each.

rule of palm a method of estimating the body surface area (BSA) burned based on the principle that a patient's palm is equal to approximately 1% of BSA.

run data information about the call itself, such as the name of the unit and crew members responding, the date and time of the call, and the name of the ambulance service.

run report written documentation of the call and patient encounter. Also called a *prehospital care report* or a *patient care report*.

S

sacral spine vertebrae that form the posterior pelvis.

sacral vertebrae fused vertebrae that help to form the pelvis.

sacrum fused vertebrae that help to form the pelvis. Also called *sacral vertebrae*.

safety glass type of glass that, when struck, will break into small pieces. Also called *tempered glass*.

safety officer command staff officer who ensures that the incident safety considerations are recognized at the scene of a multiple-casualty incident.

SAMPLE an acronym used to help remember the components of a patient history; letters stand for *signs and symptoms, allergies, medications, past pertinent medical history, last oral intake*, and *events leading to the injury or illness*.

saturated filled, as hemoglobin with oxygen.

scapulae the shoulder blades. Singular *scapula*.

scene call an emergency scene that occurs outside of a hospital.

scene safety an awareness that you must continually ensure your own safety and the safety of your crew and patient.

scene size-up the component of the patient assessment during which the following factors are assessed: safety, number of patients, need for resources, nature of illness or mechanism of injury, and need for spinal precautions.

schizophrenia a condition that involves unusual or bizarre thoughts, behaviors, speech, and auditory hallucinations.

school-age child a child between six and 12 years of age.

scoop stretcher a device that separates in two and can be used to "scoop" the patient off the ground. Also called an *orthopedic stretcher.*

scope of practice a detailed description of the specific care and actions EMTs are allowed to perform.

second stage of labor refers to the time of full dilation of the cervix until delivery of the baby.

secondary assessment the component of the patient assessment during which the medical history and physical exam are performed.

secondary devices devices used to intentionally disrupt rescue and to injure emergency responders after an initial attack has taken place.

secondary seizure a seizure that is directly caused by a known source such as a medical condition or injury.

secreting releasing of substances.

seizure a temporary electrical disturbance in the brain that is sometimes characterized by a loss of consciousness and convulsions.

Sellick's maneuver technique of applying downward pressure on the cricoid cartilage; used to help visualize the vocal cords.

semi-Fowler's position a semi-sitting position.

sensitization the production of antibodies to a specific allergen.

sensory nerves portion of the nervous system that carries information from the body back to the central nervous system.

septic shock type of shock caused by severe infections that abnormally dilate the blood vessels.

shock inadequate perfusion of blood to an organ or organs. Also called *hypoperfusion*.

shock position refers to the patient lying supine with feet elevated 12 to 18 inches.

sickle cell anemia (SCA) an inherited disease in which a genetic defect in the hemoglobin results in abnormal structure of the red blood cells.

side effects any action of a drug other than the desired action.

sign something that the EMT can see or observe or has a value that can be recorded.

significant mechanism of injury a type of mechanism of injury that has a strong likelihood for multiple organ system injury.

simple access means of getting into a vehicle that does not require specialized training, tools, or equipment.

simple asphyxiants chemicals, such as carbon monoxide, that cause injury by their presence in an environment, rather than the presence of normal levels of atmospheric oxygen.

simple partial seizure a seizure that involves just one side of the brain and often produces a jerky spasm of a specific part of the body. Also called *focal motor seizure*.

simple radiological device device that disperses radioactive particles without explosion.

singular command method of command used for multiple-casualty incidents that are small in scope, do not involve outside agencies, and occur within a single jurisdiction.

sinoatrial node beginning of the cardiac conduction pathway, located at the top of the heart near the right atrium.

sirens audible warning devices used on an emergency vehicle.

skeletal muscle See *voluntary muscle*.

SLUDGEM mnemonic for the common signs and symptoms of exposure to nerve agents based on organophosphate pesticides; letters stand for *salivation, lacrimation, urination, defecation, gastrointestinal motility, emesis*, and *miosis*.

small intestine organ that digests solid foods and absorbs nutrients through the intestinal wall; composed of the duodenum, jejunum, and ileum.

small-volume nebulizer (SVN) a device that continuously administers a vaporized medication, as opposed to the inhaler that provides a one-time dose.

smooth muscle See *involuntary muscle*.

smooth-muscle relaxant a medication that relaxes smooth muscles, for example, as nitroglycerin relaxes the muscle in blood vessels and permits an increased blood flow.

snoring intermittent low-pitched sounds heard during inhalation, and often indicative of partial upper airway obstruction caused by the tongue and associated soft tissue.

SOAP a method of documentation in which each letter stands for a specific portion of the narrative: *subjective, objective, assessment*, and *plan*.

sodium potassium pump a cellular process that is responsible for regulating the concentration of sodium and potassium ions within the cell and uses ATP to power the active transport of those ions.

soft palate tissue designed to lift up when a person swallows, closing off the oropharynx from the nasopharynx.

source initial location of a hazardous material.

sovereign immunity a legal term used to describe the exemption provided to a governmental entity from being sued in its own courts without permission.

span of control the number of organizational elements or people that are directly managed by another person during a multiple-casualty incident; effective span of control may vary from three to seven, although a ratio of one to five reporting elements is commonly recommended.

sperm male sex cell; male counterpart to the ovum.

spinal column the 33 stacked bones that extend from the base of the skull to the pelvis and contain the spinal cord.

spinal cord the central nervous system (CNS) pathway responsible for transmitting sensory input from the body to the brain and for conducting motor impulses from the brain to the body muscles and organs.

spinal shock a temporary, concussion-like injury to the spinal cord.

spontaneous abortion the expulsion of the developing fetus prior to full gestation. Also called *miscarriage*.

spontaneous pneumothorax an abnormal collection of air in the pleural space that occurs with no apparent cause.

sprain injury caused by the stretching or tearing of the ligaments and tendons that support the joint.

stable refers to a patient who is not likely to get worse in the immediate future.

staging area location at an incident where incoming resources report.

stair chair a chair-style device used to move patients in a sitting position up and down stairs.

stale air air that has become trapped in the alveoli and contains no oxygen.

standard of care a modified scope of practice specifically designed to meet the needs of a specific area or region.

standard precautions Centers for Disease Control and Prevention (CDC) guidelines and practices based on the awareness that all patients are potentially infectious regardless of diagnosis or presumed infection. Also called *universal precautions*.

standing orders a type of protocol that allows the EMT to provide specific types of treatment or medications for specific patients.

status asthmaticus prolonged, life-threatening asthma attack, often one that does not respond to the patient's own medications.

status epilepticus a condition characterized by seizures lasting more than five minutes or recurrent seizures with no period of consciousness.

statute of limitations the maximum time after an event that legal proceedings based on that event may be initiated.

step chocks wooden blocks or other supportive materials placed in a stair-step pattern to assist in stabilizing a vehicle.

sterilization controlled process that, like disinfection, requires its own specific equipment and is usually done under controlled circumstances; all organisms on the piece of equipment are killed.

sternum the breastbone.

Stokes basket a metal or plastic basket designed to move patients over uneven terrain. Also called a *basket stretcher*.

stoma a permanent surgical opening in the anterior (front) of the neck through which the patient breathes.

stomach organ that receives food from the esophagus.

strain injury caused when a muscle is pulled or torn, causing severe pain.

stress any event or situation that places extraordinary demands on a person's mental or emotional resources.

stretch receptors specialized sensors in certain blood vessels that sense pressure within the vessel.

stridor a harsh high-pitched sound that can occur during inhalation or exhalation, indicative of partial upper airway obstruction.

stroke a condition that occurs when the blood supply to an area of the brain is interrupted. Also called *cerebral vascular accident* or *brain attack*.

stroke volume (SV) the volume of blood ejected from the heart in one contraction.

stroke volume amount of blood ejected into the aorta with each heartbeat.

stylet moldable wire that can be inserted into an endotracheal tube to facilitate tube placement.

subarachnoid hemorrhage bleeding into the cerebrospinal fluid surrounding the brain.

subcutaneous emphysema air that has become trapped beneath the skin; characterized by crepitus.

subcutaneous layer the deepest layer of the skin.

subdural hematoma collection of blood between the dura mater and the arachnoid membrane.

subjective information information that is not firsthand or that is subject to interpretation.

sublingual beneath the tongue.

sudden infant death syndrome (SIDS) the sudden death of healthy infants in the first year of life.

suffix a word or part of a word added to the end of another word to add description.

superficial burns burns that affect the outermost layer of skin, the epidermis. See also *partial-thickness burns* and *full-thickness burns*.

superior toward the head (for example, the chest is superior to the abdomen). Opposite of *inferior*.

supine a position in which a patient is lying face up on the back. Opposite of *prone*.

supine hypotensive syndrome a condition that occurs when the pregnant patient lies flat and the fetus compresses the inferior vena cava, which reduces blood flow back to the heart and causes significant hypotension.

supply unit team that receives supplies and equipment from staging at a multiple-casualty incident and issues them to the operational units as requested.

supportive care interventions in cases of poisonings or toxic exposures, such as keeping the airway clear by suctioning, providing supplemental oxygen or ventilation, and treatment for shock.

suspension solid medication mixed in a fluid; must be shaken before giving.

sympathetic nervous system part of the nervous system that activates the fight-or-flight response.

symptom something that is experienced and described by the patient as it pertains to his chief complaint. See also *sign*.

syncope a sudden and temporary loss of consciousness; fainting.

systemic vascular resistance the pressure in the peripheral blood vessels that the heart most overcome to pump blood.

systolic the pressure created when the left ventricle contracts and forces blood out into the arteries.

T

tablet small disk-like compressed form of medication.

tachycardia a pulse rate greater than 100 beats per minute.

tarsals the ankle bones.

technical rescue incidents rescue situations requiring specialized training and equipment.

technician level level of training that is designed for responders who will be capable of hazard recognition, equipment use, techniques necessary to perform, and supervision of a technical rescue incident.

temperature regulation the body's ability to maintain a stable core temperature.

temporal bones bones that form part of the side of the skull.

temporomandibular joint the movable joint formed between the mandible and the temporal bone. Also called the *TM joint*.

tendons tissues that connect muscle to bone.

tension headaches pain that has a gradual onset caused by muscle tension that leads to a "squeezing" sensation in various regions of the head, often radiating to the neck and shoulders.

tension pneumothorax an abnormal collection of air in the pleural space that results in a build up of pressure significant enough to impair breathing or circulation.

teratogenic causing an increased risk that a developing embryo will have physical defects.

terrorism an illegal act that is dangerous to human life, with intent to intimidate or coerce a government or civilian population in the furtherance of a political or social agenda.

testicles external male gland that produces the sperm.

therapeutic communication the face-to-face communication process that focuses on advancing the physical and emotional well-being of the patient.

therapeutic hypothermia the intentional and controlled cooling of the body in order to slow metabolism and the demand for oxygen.

thermal burn a type of burn most commonly caused by exposure to fire, steam, hot objects, and hot liquids. Also called a *heat burn*.

third stage of labor refers to the time from the birth of the baby until delivery of the placenta.

thoracic cavity the area that lies inferior to the clavicles and superior to the diaphragm.

thoracic vertebrae the 12 vertebrae that help form the thoracic cage.

thrill a vibration felt on gentle palpation, such as that which typically occurs within an arterial-venous fistula.

thrombus a blood clot that forms in a vessel and remains there.

thyroid cartilage prominence in the anterior neck. Also called the *Adam's apple*.

tibia the medial and larger bone of the lower leg.

tidal volume the amount of air moved in and out with each breath.

time on scene the time spent on scene assessing, caring for, and preparing the patient for transport.

timeline narration method of telling the story of the call as it happened in a step-by-step, chronological narrative. Also called *sequential narration*.

toddler a child between one and three years of age.

tonic prolonged muscle contractions as seen with generalized seizures.

tonic-clonic seizure a seizure that is characterized by intermittent muscle contractions and relaxation.

tourniquet method designed to stop all blood flow past the point at which it is applied.

toxicology the medical study of toxins and how they affect living organisms.

toxin a noxious or poisonous substance produced by animals or plants.

trachea the structure that connects the pharynx to the lungs. Also called the *windpipe*.

tracheostomy a surgical incision into the trachea in order to insert a breathing tube.

tracheostomy tube tube placed through a surgical opening in the neck to provide an airway.

traction headache a symptom of an associated neurological problem such as hemorrhagic stroke, meningitis, or tumor.

trade name the medication name a pharmaceutical company gives to a drug. Also called *brand name*.

transdermal through or by way of the skin.

transection a complete severing of the spinal cord.

transient ischemic attack (TIA) a condition for which signs and symptoms similar to a stroke go away, usually within 24 hours.

transmissibility the ease with which an agent or disease can spread from person to person.

transportation group team responsible for obtaining resources at a multiple-casualty incident to ensure that all patients are transported to the appropriate hospital.

trauma assessment a variation of the secondary assessment that is performed on a patient who has an injury.

trauma centers specially designated trauma receiving hospitals that are staffed and equipped to manage victims of trauma.

trauma patient a patient whose chief complaint is related to a sudden injury.

traumatic asphyxia a condition in which a severe blunt force or weight is placed on the chest, forcing blood from the right atrium up into the circulation of the head and neck.

treatment group team that will establish an area where patients can be treated and collected at a multiple-casualty incident.

Trendelenburg position a position in which the patient's feet and legs are higher than the head.

trending the comparing of multiple sets of vital signs over a period of time in order to reveal a trend in the patient's condition.

triage the process of sorting patients based on the severity of their injuries and prioritizing them for treatment and transport.

triage group team responsible for the sorting and tagging of all patients according to the seriousness and extent of injuries.

tricuspid valve a structure between the right atrium and right ventricle that opens and closes to permit the flow of a fluid in only one direction.

triggers allergies, respiratory infections, exercise, or emotion that may cause bronchoconstriction.

trimester division of the pregnancy period, usually 13 weeks, or about one-third of the pregnancy.

tripod position a position that may be assumed during respiratory distress to facilitate breathing; the patient usually sits or may stand or crouch, leaning forward with hands placed on the bed, chair, table, or knees.

twisting force the force that occurs when one end of a limb is stationary and the other end moves in a circle.

type 1 diabetes mellitus a type of diabetes mellitus that results from an insufficiency of insulin production and requires a daily administration of insulin.

type 2 diabetes mellitus a type of noninsulin dependent diabetes mellitus.

U

ulcers points within the stomach where the inner lining has been worn thin or destroyed.

ulna the medial bone of the forearm.

ultrasound an examination technique that uses sound to produce a visual image.

umbilical cord an anatomical structure that connects the fetus to the placenta.

unified command method of command that is a team effort, allowing all agencies with a jurisdictional responsibility for a multiple-casualty incident, either geographical or functional, to play a part in the management of the incident.

unit team assigned a specific task.

United States Pharmacopoeia (USP) government listing of all medications.

unity of command the principle that each individual in an organization has only one supervisor; should not be confused with the term *unified command*.

unstable refers to a patient who has a high likelihood of getting worse in the immediate future.

ureters an anatomical structure that transports urine from the kidneys to the bladder.

urethra an anatomical structure that transports urine from the bladder to be excreted outside the body.

urinary catheter a device usually placed in the urethra of patients who have lost the ability to drain their bladder either due to obstruction or loss of necessary neurological control of the bladder.

urticaria hives.

uterine rupture a tearing of the muscular wall of the uterus.

uterus the muscular abdominal organ in which the fetus develops. Also called the *womb*.

V

vagina the birth canal; the tubular structure leading from the uterus to the outer body.

vallecula a depression or space between the root of the tongue and the epiglottis.

vapor pressure the pressure exerted by a chemical against the atmosphere.

vas deferens carries the sperm from the testicles to the urethra.

vascular access device a catheter inserted into a central vein or a port implanted under the skin to allow access to the patient's central circulation.

vasovagal response an exaggerated response by the parasympathetic nervous system, causing syncope.

vector a carrier, such as animals, insects, or people who have a disease.

veins blood vessels that return blood to the heart.

vena cava either of two major veins that carry oxygen-poor blood from the body to the right atrium. Plural *venae cavae*.

ventilation the movement of oxygen and carbon dioxide at the alveolar level.

ventilation/perfusion match (V/Q match) the coupling of appropriate amounts of air in the alveoli with a sufficient blood supply so as to promote gas exchange.

ventilator a device that breathes for a patient.

ventral referring to the front of the body. Synonym for *anterior*.

ventricles the two lower chambers of the heart.

ventricular fibrillation (VF) one of the most common electrical rhythms associated with sudden cardiac arrest in which the ventricles of the heart contract spontaneously and in an uncoordinated manner, thus preventing the heart from circulating any meaningful amount of blood. Also called *V-fib*.

ventricular tachycardia (VT) a rapid and uncoordinated life-threatening electrical rhythm that originates in the ventricles. Also called *V-tach*.

ventriculoperitoneal (VP) shunt a device that drains excess cerebrospinal fluid from the brain to the abdomen.

venules the smallest veins.

vertebrae the 33 bones of the spinal column. Singular *vertebra*.

virulence the power of infection once started.

viruses pathogenic organisms made of nucleic acid inside a protein shell, which must utilize a host cell for growth and reproduction.

visceral peritoneum innermost lining of the peritoneum adhered to the abdominal organs.

visceral pleura a membrane that is attached to the lung surface.

visual flight rules (VFR) rules defined by the Federal Aviation Administration regarding the operation of an aircraft when weather is not a factor.

vocal cords tissue found within the larynx that opens and closes the glottis to produce sound vibrations.

voluntary muscle muscle that can be consciously controlled. Also called *skeletal muscle*.

W

weapons of mass destruction (WMDs) variety of explosive, chemical, biological, nuclear, and other devices used by terrorists to strike at government and high-profile or high-population targets; designed to create a maximum number of casualties.

wheeled stretcher the most commonly used device for moving patients. Also called *cot* or *gurney*.

wheezing high-pitched, musical lung sounds created by air moving through constricted air passages.

white blood cells specialized blood cells that produce substances that help the body fight infection.

withdrawal the severe physical reaction that results when a person who chronically uses drugs, such as alcohol or narcotics, is deprived of those drugs.

work of breathing effort needed for adequate ventilation.

Z

zygomatic bone the facial bone that forms the cheek.

ANSWER KEY

Chapter 1

STOP, REVIEW, REMEMBER! *(p. 10)*

Multiple Choice

1. b (p. 6)
2. c (p. 8)
3. d (p. 9)

Fill in the Blank

1. emergency medical responder (EMR) (p. 9)
2. U.S. Department of Transportation (DOT) (p. 9)
3. emergency medical services (EMS) system (p. 6)
4. emergency medical technician (EMT) (p. 9)
5. National Highway Traffic Safety Administration (NHTSA) (p. 6)

Critical Thinking

1. Student answers will vary, depending on their location. (pp. 6–8)
2. The emergency medical responder (EMR) is the most basic level of nationally recognized care, requiring 40 hours of training. EMRs often are the first responders at the scene of an emergency and are therefore trained to identify potential hazards, identify and treat immediate life threats, and assist other EMS personnel at the scene. They also are trained to function with a minimum of equipment. (p. 9)
3. Student answers will vary, depending on location. (p. 9)

STOP, REVIEW, REMEMBER! *(p. 15)*

Multiple Choice

1. d (p. 11)
2. a (p. 11)
3. d (pp. 11–12)
4. b (p. 12)
5. c (p. 14)

Matching

1. B (p. 11)
2. C (pp. 11–12)
3. A (p. 11)
4. F (pp. 11–12)
5. E (p. 12)
6. D (p. 12)

Critical Thinking

1. Student answers will vary, depending on location. (p. 11)
2. Student answers will vary. (pp. 13–14)
3. Student answers will vary, depending on location. (p. 14)

CHAPTER REVIEW *(p. 18)*

Multiple Choice

1. d (pp. 6–8)
2. a (p. 6)
3. c (p. 9)
4. b (p. 13)
5. c (p. 14)
6. d (pp. 6–8)
7. a (p. 9)
8. b (pp. 13–14)
9. c (p. 11)
10. d (pp. 11–12)

Matching

1. B (p. 12)
2. C (pp. 11–12)
3. E (p. 14)
4. A (p. 9)
5. D (p. 11)

Critical Thinking

1. Changes in medicine and the science behind medicine change frequently. This is especially true in the area of resuscitation. 2010 saw major changes in the emergency care of patients in cardiac arrest. EMTs must seek out current research in order to understand and implement those important changes. (p. 14)
2. Student answers will vary. (p. 8)
3. The EMT is allowed to do everything an EMR can do, plus in nearly all areas of the United States receives the minimum level of training for providing care on an ambulance. Unlike the advanced EMT and paramedic, the EMT can assist only with certain prescribed medications and cannot perform advanced procedures except where allowed by local protocol. (p. 8)
4. Specialty hospitals include trauma centers, pediatric centers, burn centers, reattachment centers, hyperbaric centers, and neurosurgery centers. (p. 11)
5. Medical direction can be off-line or on-line direction. Off-line direction includes written protocols and standing orders. On-line direction includes orders given to the EMT in person, over the phone, or by radio. (p. 11)
6. Unlike traditional dispatchers, the emergency medical dispatcher (EMD) is trained to provide pre-arrival medical care instructions until the EMS units arrive. (p. 12)

CASE STUDIES

Case Study 1

1. You must respectfully inform the patient that local protocol does not allow you to puncture her blisters. You may offer her a place to rest and perhaps offer her some adhesive bandages or gauze to help relieve discomfort. (p. 11)
2. When in doubt, contact medical direction or your immediate field supervisor for instructions. (p. 12)
3. It is always important to document patient care. Good care along with good documentation helps to ensure patients receive the most appropriate care during their path to recovery. (p. 13)

Case Study 2

1. Safety is your first priority at every emergency scene. (p. 13)
2. The immediate hazard is traffic, because you are on a blind curve of a well-traveled highway. You must keep your warning lights on and place flares or reflectors a good distance from the scene in both directions. You also must be alert for spilled fuel and the potential for fire. (p. 13)
3. Your personal safety comes before that of anyone else at the scene. It is your duty to remain safe and to do what you can to minimize threats to anyone else who may enter the scene, even if the result is delayed care to the patient. (p. 13)

Chapter 2

STOP, REVIEW, REMEMBER! *(p. 27)*

Multiple Choice

1. b (p. 24)
2. d (pp. 25–26)
3. a (p. 26)
4. c (p. 26)
5. a (p. 26)

Matching

1. b (p. 25)
2. d (p. 26)
3. a (p. 26)
4. c (p. 26)

Critical Thinking

1. Student answers will vary. (pp. 24–25)
2. Student answers will vary. (pp. 24–25)
3. Student answers will vary. (p. 25)

STOP, REVIEW, REMEMBER! *(p. 32)*

Multiple Choice

1. b (p. 30)
2. c (p. 30)
3. d (p. 31)
4. a (pp. 31–32)
5. c (p. 31)

Matching

1. b (p. 30)
2. c (p. 30)
3. a (p. 30)
4. e (p. 31)
5. d (p. 31)

Critical Thinking

1. Student answers will vary. (pp. 29–30)
2. Being proactive about the management of stress in your life means that you are doing things in advance to better prepare yourself to handle stress when it appears. That may include eating a balanced diet, exercising regularly, and being open and honest about your feelings when your job becomes stressful. (pp. 28–30)
3. Resiliency refers to the ability to recover quickly from the stress caused by illness, change, or misfortune. Being resilient requires that you learn to

manage stress before it happens and develop habits that will help you cope when stress becomes acute. (p. 31)

STOP, REVIEW, REMEMBER! *(p. 41)*

Multiple Choice

1. c (p. 34)
2. a (p. 37)
3. b (p. 35)
4. a (p. 34)
5. c (p. 37)

Critical Thinking

1. In most cases that involve patient care, taking proper BSI precautions means using the appropriate PPE for the situation. PPE such as gloves, masks, and eye protection are all a part of BSI precautions. (pp. 34–37)
2. You would want to wear specialized suits and self-contained breathing apparatus (SCBA) in some cases prior to entry. (pp. 39–40)
3. When entering a potential crime scene, you must begin with being careful where you walk and step. Be careful not to disturb potential crime evidence. (pp. 40–41)
4. (pp. 34–37)

Situation	Gloves	Glasses	Mask	Gown
Minor bleed to the left hand	X	X		
Suctioning a vomiting patient	X	X	X	
Assisting with a birth	X	X	X	X
Cleaning a bloody backboard	X	X		
Taking a blood pressure on a medical patient	X			
Major bleed of the lower leg with spurting blood	X	X	X	
Cleaning the back of the ambulance after a call	X			

CHAPTER REVIEW *(p. 43)*

Multiple Choice

1. c (pp. 29–30)
2. c (p. 32)
3. b (p. 26)
4. d (pp. 40–41)
5. a (p. 32)
6. b (p. 34)

Critical Thinking

1. Student answers will vary. (pp. 28–30)
2. Student answers will vary. (pp. 28–30)
3. Student answers will vary. (pp. 30–31)

CASE STUDIES

Case Study 1

1. It is not a bad idea to engage Will in a conversation about the call so long as he does not reveal any information that might identify the patient. Be sensitive to the fact that talking about it is healthy but Will may not feel comfortable at this time. When appropriate, encourage Will to talk about the event with a supervisor or peer counselor. (pp. 24–32)
2. Many people who have experienced a stressful event will become quiet and somewhat distant in their behavior. They may not have a normal appetite and may want to be alone. They also may get angry easily and lash out for little or no reason. (pp. 24–32)
3. The most important thing you can do is be a good listener when he is willing to talk. Do not judge him or criticize him for anything relating to the incident. (pp. 24–32)

Case Study 2

1. You might be having trouble sleeping and are probably not eating well. You also may not be exercising. You may become angered easily and this leads to others seeing you as having a negative attitude. (pp. 24–31)
2. At some point you will not be able to cope and may end up experiencing an emotional and/or physical breakdown. (pp. 24–31)
3. This begins with working a reasonable number of hours. You cannot work every shift, at least not for long. Be sure to eat as healthily as you can, get plenty of sleep, and exercise regularly, even if it is only a nice long walk. (pp. 24–31)

Chapter 3

STOP, REVIEW, REMEMBER! *(p. 52)*

Multiple Choice

1. a (p. 49)
2. b (p. 49)
3. c (p. 51)
4. c (p. 49)
5. a (p. 52)

Matching

1. F (p. 49)
2. G (p. 49)
3. E (p. 49)
4. B (p. 49)
5. C (p. 49)
6. D (p. 51)
7. A (p. 52)

Critical Thinking

1. The answer is most likely "yes." The standard of care is defined by local protocols, which may allow you to do more or less than the training you will receive in this class. (p. 49)
2. A legal duty to provide care is determined by law and applies to most EMTs who work for a provider agency regardless if it is volunteer or paid. An ethical duty may apply to the EMT who is off duty and comes upon someone who is injured. The EMT also has an ethical duty to always do what is best for the patient and not let personal desires interfere with that care. (pp. 49–51)
3. Good Samaritan laws exist in some form in all 50 states and are designed to encourage the passerby to stop and render care. These laws minimize the exposure to liability for acts and omissions while providing care at the scene of an emergency so long as the caregiver is not being compensated. (p. 52)

STOP, REVIEW, REMEMBER! *(p. 60)*

Multiple Choice

1. d (p. 54)
2. a (pp. 56–58)
3. c (pp. 55–56)
4. b (pp. 56–57)
5. a (pp. 58–59)
6. c (p. 51)

Matching

1. F (p. 54)
2. G (p. 54)
3. A (pp. 55–56)
4. B (p. 54)
5. D (p. 51)
6. C (pp. 58–60)
7. E (pp. 59–60)

Critical Thinking

1. A responsive adult with capacity may provide consent in verbal form by simply saying "yes" to your request to provide care. Consent also can be nonverbal if you have asked for permission and the patient's behavior indicates he wants you to help, even though he has not stated so verbally. (p. 54)
2. In situations where a patient's mental status is altered either by injury, illness, or substance, it may be difficult to determine if he has the capacity to understand the situation and therefore refuse care. (pp. 54–55)
3. It is best to contact medical direction as soon as possible and, when practical, initiate care until the DNR can be confirmed. (pp. 58–60)

STOP, REVIEW, REMEMBER! *(p. 67)*

Multiple Choice

1. b (p. 63)
2. c (pp. 62–63)
3. c (p. 62)
4. d (pp. 64–65)
5. a (p. 62)

Matching

1. G (p. 63)
2. F (p. 63)
3. B (p. 62)
4. E (p. 62)
5. C (p. 62)
6. D (p. 62)
7. A (p. 62)

Critical Thinking

1. The term *assault* refers to the threat to use force against another person. The term *battery* refers to the actual carrying out of that threat. (p. 63)

2. There are many examples of how an EMT may be accused of negligence. Examples include performing skills that are clearly outside the scope of care for an EMT or abandoning a patient before someone of equal or higher training takes over. (p. 62)
3. After providing the appropriate care for the patient, you should advise the medical personnel at the hospital of your findings. You should immediately document all of your findings including the care that you provided. You must then contact your supervisor or law enforcement officer to report your findings. The specific steps may vary in your system. Follow local laws and protocols. (p. 65)

CHAPTER REVIEW *(p. 69)*

Multiple Choice

1. b (p. 49)
2. a (p. 60)
3. c (p. 54)
4. a (pp. 62–63)
5. a (p. 65)
6. c (pp. 55–56)
7. c (p. 66)
8. c (pp. 65–66)
9. d (p. 49)
10. b (p. 63)

Critical Thinking

1. It may become necessary to use force to restrain a patient if he poses a risk to himself or anyone else attempting to care for him. While it is not your duty to forcibly restrain patients, it may become unavoidable if the patient suddenly becomes violent. If you are able, it is appropriate to retreat and call for law enforcement. (p. 63)
2. The answer to this question will vary depending on the laws in your state. (p. 51)
3. Your care should not change simply because of the fact that the patient is a potential organ donor. However, you will want to advise the receiving hospital of the fact in case the patient dies and the family wishes to donate the organs. (p. 66)

CASE STUDIES

Case Study 1

1. Your legal obligation to stop and render care will depend on the state where you reside. Ask your instructor how the laws in your state pertain to this scenario. (p. 51)
2. The legal ramifications of not stopping to render care will depend on the state where you reside. Research the information or ask your instructor how the laws in your state pertain to this scenario. (p. 51)
3. In most states, the fact that you began care established a legal duty to stay at the scene and continue to provide care to the best of your ability. You could be accused of abandonment if you leave the patient before someone of equal or higher training takes over. Ask your instructor how the laws of your state pertain to this situation. (p. 51)

Case Study 2

1. If in doubt, you should contact medical direction for advice. (pp. 58–60)
2. A DNR order can appear in many forms including a formal signed document and written orders on a patient's chart. Most states recognize medical identification jewelry as an acceptable form of a legal DNR order. Check with your instructor regarding your state. (pp. 58–60)
3. In the presence of a valid DNR it is appropriate to stop care. You must then provide comfort and compassionate care for the family members. (pp. 58–60)

Chapter 4

STOP, REVIEW, REMEMBER! *(p. 77)*

Multiple Choice

1. a (pp. 75–76)
2. b (p. 76)
3. c (pp. 75–76)
4. d (pp. 75–76)
5. a (p. 76)
6. d (p. 76)
7. d (p. 76)

Matching

1. B (p. 76)
2. E (p. 76)
3. G (p. 76)
4. A (p. 76)
5. F (p. 76)
6. C (p. 76)
7. D (p. 76)

Fill in the Blank

1. neo (neonate) (p. 76)
2. leuko (leukocyte) (p. 76)
3. -itis (cholecystitis) (p. 76)
4. eryth (erythema) (p. 76)
5. hyper (hyperthermia) (p. 76)

Critical Thinking

1. Water/fluid on the brain (excessive CSF) (pp. 75–76)
2. Narrowing of the aorta (pp. 75–76)
3. Excessive urination. Students should use a dictionary to help them identify "uria," which refers to urination. (p. 76)
4. Blood in vomit (pp. 75–76)
5. Double vision. Students should use a dictionary to help them identify "oplia," which refers to vision. (pp. 75–76)

STOP, REVIEW, REMEMBER! *(p. 87)*

Multiple Choice

1. b (p. 80)
2. c (p. 80)
3. d (p. 81)
4. b (p. 80)
5. c (p. 81)
6. a (p. 79)

Labeling

(pp. 80–83)

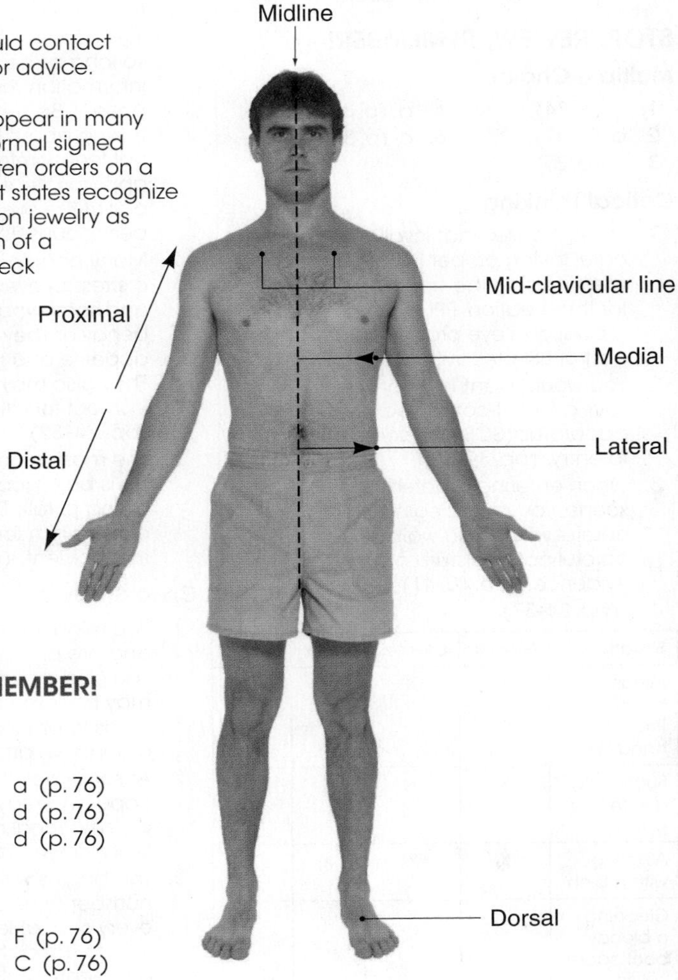

Fill in the Blank

1. proximal, distal (p. 83)
2. midline (p. 80)
3. midclavicular line (p. 81)
4. midaxillary line (p. 81)
5. bilateral (p. 80)

Critical Thinking

1. Posterior forearm, proximal to the wrist (pp. 81–83)
2. Posterior lower leg, distal to the knee (pp. 81–83)
3. Right lower quadrant, periumbilical (pp. 81–82)
4. Forehead, superior to the right eye (p. 83)
5. Plantar surface (p. 81)

CHAPTER REVIEW *(p. 90)*

Multiple Choice

1. c (p. 74)
2. b (p. 83)
3. d (p. 83)
4. b (pp. 74–75)
5. a (pp. 75–76)
6. b (p. 80)
7. b (p. 80)
8. d (p. 81)
9. a (p. 86)
10. a (pp. 83–84)

Matching

1. E (p. 76)
2. A (pp. 75–76)
3. K (pp. 75–76)
4. C (p. 75)
5. G (pp. 75–76)
6. J (p. 75)
7. H (p. 75)
8. F (pp. 75–76)
9. D (pp. 75–76)
10. B (p. 75)
11. I (p. 75)
12. O (p. 75)
13. L (p. 76)
14. M (p. 76)
15. N (p. 76)

Critical Thinking

1. Pain in the right upper quadrant just inferior to the ribs (p. 80)
2. Deformity to the distal forearm, proximal to the wrist (p. 83)
3. Posterior hand, proximal to the knuckles (pp. 81–83)

CASE STUDY

1. Patient is complaining of pain to the right lateral chest and there is no obvious bruising or deformity. (p. 80)
2. Your son was struck on his right side and has pain over the right side of his chest. He may have injured some of the ribs on his right side. (p. 85)
3. Using technical terms with people unfamiliar with them can further confuse or frighten them. (p. 85)

Labeling

(p. 109)

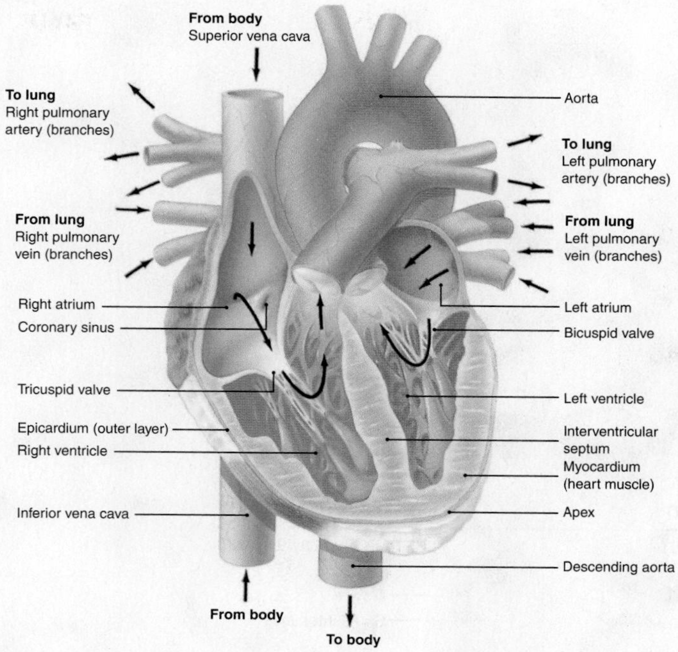

Chapter 5

STOP, REVIEW, REMEMBER! *(p. 103)*

Multiple Choice

1. b (pp. 96–98)
2. d (p. 101)
3. a (pp. 96–98)
4. c (pp. 97–98)
5. d (pp. 98, 100–101)
6. d (pp. 100–101)
7. a (pp. 97–98)

Fill in the Blank

1. radius, ulna (pp. 96–98)
2. floating (p. 97)
3. hinged (pp. 97–98)
4. coccyx (pp. 98, 100)
5. smooth, involuntary (pp. 100–101)

Critical Thinking

1. Protection, structure, movement. (p. 97)
2. Temperature regulation, protection, and impact absorption. (p. 102)

STOP, REVIEW, REMEMBER! *(p. 114)*

Multiple Choice

1. c (p. 105)
2. d (p. 109)
3. c (p. 105)
4. b (p. 113)
5. b (p. 105)

Fill in the Blank

1. alveoli (p. 105)
2. nasopharynx (p. 105)
3. Arteries (p. 110)
4. Capillaries (p. 110)
5. atria, ventricles (p. 108)
6. radial (p. 108)

Critical Thinking

1. Air, blood, adequate blood pressure, adequate supply of oxygen (pp. 104–105)
2. Good perfusion occurs when there is an adequate supply of oxygen and nutrients coupled with the appropriate removal of waste products. Poor perfusion, also known as hypoperfusion, occurs when there is a disruption in normal perfusion such as in the case of shock. (pp. 104, 113)
3. Any three of the following: smaller airways; proportionately larger tongue; a trachea that is narrower, softer, more flexible; less developed cricoid cartilage; softer chest wall; increased oxygen consumption (pp. 107–108)

STOP, REVIEW, REMEMBER! *(p. 123)*

Multiple Choice

1. c (p. 119)
2. c (p. 119)
3. d (p. 116)
4. a (p. 119)
5. b (p. 116)
6. c (p. 116)
7. d (p. 119)

Fill in the Blank

1. autonomic (p. 116)
2. Sensory (p. 116)
3. Motor (p. 116)
4. insulin (p. 116)
5. esophagus (p. 119)
6. brain, spinal cord (p. 116)

Critical Thinking

1. It is the counterbalance to the sympathetic nervous system and is responsible for relaxation, dilation of blood vessels, decrease in heart rate (p. 116)
2. Fluid regulation, filtration, pH regulation (p. 119)

CHAPTER REVIEW *(p. 125)*

Multiple Choice

1. c (p. 112)
2. a (p. 97)
3. a (p. 97)
4. c (p. 105)
5. a (p. 109)
6. b (p. 109)
7. a (p. 116)
8. d (p. 116)
9. c (p. 119)
10. a (p. 100)

Matching

1. K (pp. 97–98)
2. A (pp. 97–98)
3. E (pp. 97–98)
4. O (pp. 97–98)
5. B (p. 97)
6. C (pp. 97–98)
7. M (pp. 97–98)
8. H (pp. 97–98)
9. N. (p. 97)
10. I (pp. 97–98)
11. L (pp. 97–98)
12. J (pp. 97–98)
13. G (pp. 97–98)
14. D (pp. 97–98)
15. F (pp. 97–98, 100)

Labeling

(Chapter 4, p. 81)

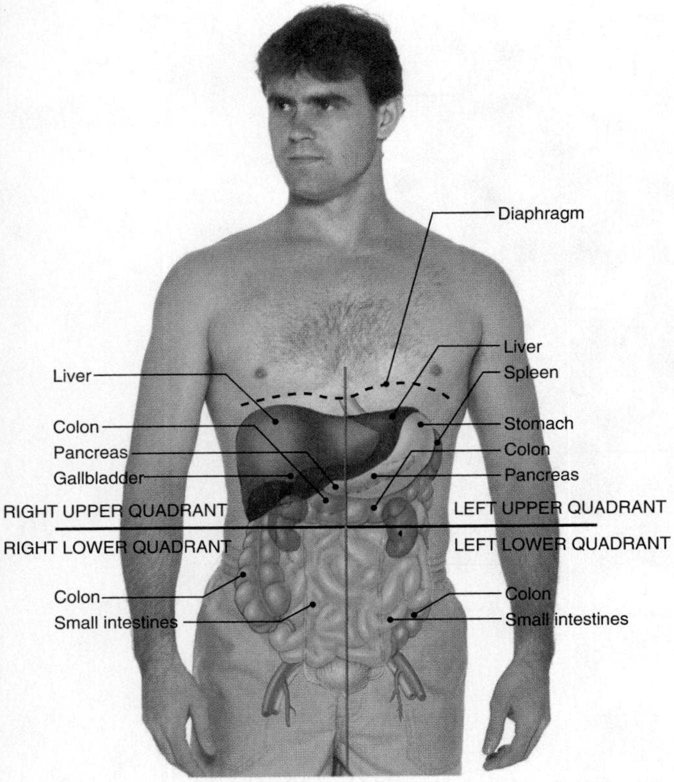

Ordering

1. 9, 6, 8, 10, 5, 7, 2, 12, 1, 3, 4, 11

Critical Thinking

1. Blood pressure is created by the pumping action of the heart. Pressure waves can be felt each time the heart contracts. These waves can be felt in the form of a pulsation (pulse) at certain locations on the body, such as the radial pulse. (p. 108)
2. Air is moved during inhalation by the creation of negative pressure. Diaphragm contracts, the chest wall expands, and air is pulled in. (pp. 105–106)
3. Perfusion is created by a constant supply of oxygen and nutrients and the removal of waste products. Necessary components include enough blood, pressure in the system, an intact pump, and air getting in and out of the alveoli. (pp. 104–105)

CASE STUDY

1. Lungs, heart, great vessels (pp. 105–112)
2. Lungs, liver, gall bladder, pancreas, colon (pp. 105–106, 119–120)
3. Injuries to internal organs will cause blood loss, which will lead to a drop in blood pressure and poor perfusion. Injury to the chest wall or lungs will lead to inadequate breathing, which will lead to poor oxygenation of the blood and then poor perfusion. (pp. 104–105, 108, 113)

Chapter 6

STOP, REVIEW, REMEMBER! *(p. 135)*

Multiple Choice

1. d (p. 132)
2. c (p. 131)
3. a (p. 132)
4. a (p. 133)
5. a (p. 134)
6. b (p. 134)

Fill in the Blank

1. endoplasmic reticulum (p. 132)
2. Electrolytes (p. 133)
3. Edema (p. 135)
4. interstitial (p. 134)
5. cell membrane (p. 132)

Critical Thinking

1. Aerobic metabolism uses sufficient quantities of oxygen in the conversion of glucose to ATP. Anaerobic does not. (p. 133)
2. Water, oxygen, glucose (p. 133)
3. The brain and kidneys regulate thirst and elimination of excess fluid, the large proteins in our blood plasma pull fluid into the bloodstream, and the permeability of both cell membranes and the walls of capillaries help determine how much water can be held in and pushed out of cells and blood vessels. (p. 134)

STOP, REVIEW, REMEMBER! *(p. 147)*

Multiple Choice

1. a (p. 134)
2. c (p. 137)
3. a (p. 137)
4. d (pp. 139–140)
5. d (p. 140)
6. b (p. 134)
7. c (p. 142)

Fill in the Blank

1. stretch receptors (p. 142)
2. systemic vascular resistance (p. 143)
3. preload (p. 143)
4. Contractility (p. 143)
5. perfusion (p. 144)

Critical Thinking

1. Increased respiratory rate, increased tidal volume. During assessment, you might see increased respiratory rate. (p. 146)
2. Increased heart rate, increased contractility, vasoconstriction, increased respiratory rate. During assessment, you might see increased pulse, pale skin, delayed capillary refill time, increased respiratory rate. (pp. 145–146)
3. Pediatric patients use rate more than contractility and vasoconstrict well. During assessment, you might see fast heart rates, pale skin, and delayed capillary refill time. (p. 146)

STOP, REVIEW, REMEMBER! *(p. 151)*

Multiple Choice

1. a (p. 150)
2. c (p. 149)
3. b (p. 150)
4. d (p. 150)
5. b (p. 150)

Fill in the Blank

1. vomiting and diarrhea (p. 150)
2. white blood cells, antibodies (p. 150)
3. hypersensitivity reaction (p. 150)
4. stroke (p. 149)
5. endocrine system (p. 150)

Critical Thinking

1. Medical problems and trauma (p. 149)
2. Overproduction of hormones and underproduction of hormones (p. 150)
3. Dehydration and malnutrition (p. 150)

CHAPTER REVIEW *(p. 153)*

Multiple Choice

1. a (p. 132)
2. d (p. 133)
3. a (p. 133)
4. c (p. 133)
5. b (p. 133)
6. c (p. 134)
7. d (pp. 134–135)
8. a (p. 140)
9. b (p. 146)
10. d (p. 146)

Matching

1. E (p. 137)
2. C (p. 142)
3. B (p. 149)
4. G (p. 150)
5. A (p. 150)
6. F (p. 150)
7. D (p. 151)

Critical Thinking

1. Elimination, large proteins in the blood, permeability of the vessels. (p. 134)
2. The systems must work in concert to match a sufficient supply of air at the alveoli with a sufficient supply of blood in the capillaries surrounding the alveoli. (pp. 144–146)
3. Increased heart rate, increased contractility, vasoconstriction, increased respiratory rate. (pp. 145–147)

CASE STUDY

1. Hypoperfusion caused by not enough oxygen reaching the system would lead to acidosis secondary to anaerobic metabolism. (pp. 133, 145)
2. You would expect to see an increased pulse and respiratory rate and efforts to increase tidal volume. (pp. 140, 146)

Chapter 7

STOP, REVIEW, REMEMBER! *(p. 161)*

Multiple Choice

1. c (p. 159)
2. d (p. 158)
3. b (p. 160)
4. a (p. 159)
5. b (p. 160)

Critical Thinking

1. A typical six-month old infant sits upright; supports upper body with arms; tries to imitate sounds; makes one-syllable sounds; grasps objects; sees and recognizes familiar objects at a distance. (p. 161)
2. Undeveloped accessory muscles can lead to fatigue and rapid progression to respiratory failure; airway is proportionally narrower and less rigid than an adult's so can more easily become obstructed. Tongue is proportionally larger therefore less swelling can block airway. (p. 160)
3. See Table 7-1. (p. 159)

CHAPTER REVIEW *(p. 169)*

Multiple Choice

1. a (p. 168)
2. d (p. 159)
3. c (p. 163)
4. b (p. 159)
5. c (p. 167)

Matching

1. D (p. 158)
2. B (p. 158)
3. F (p. 158)
4. C (p. 158)
5. E (p. 158)
6. A (p. 158)

Critical Thinking

1. For a three-year-old, first engage the parents or caregivers so the child sees you are trusted by them, allow the parent to hold the child, begin examination at the extremities and slowly work upward, provide lots of reassurance and very simple explanations, allow the child to touch or hold equipment before you use it on them. For a 12-year-old, follow the child's wishes about having parents present or not during your assessment, be considerate of the patient's modesty and privacy, speak using language the child will understand. (pp. 163, 166)
2. Student answers will vary. (pp. 158, 168)
3. Consider interviewing the patient away from her parents. Make sure you are using medical terminology she understands, that you are not threatening, and that she understands you are there to help her. (pp. 165, 166)
4. Decreased perception of pain; decline in the ability to hear and see; overlapping illnesses and medications; unknown baseline mental status; presence of caregivers; fear of losing independence; fear of medical bills. (pp. 167, 168)

CASE STUDIES

Case Study 1

1. Chronic dementia (this is the patient's baseline mental status), hypothermia from lying on the tile floor, head injury from the fall, shock (inadequate perfusion from injury or cardiac disturbance), medication overdose. (pp. 167, 168)
2. Ask the patient's daughter if he is behaving normally, or if the confusion is new for him. (pp. 167, 168)
3. Some blood pressure medications cause a low heart rate, so it may be normal to find a slow or even bradycardic pulse. Since you know the patient has a history of high blood pressure, you might expect to find an elevated blood pressure, or if his hypertension is controlled with medications, you might find a normal blood pressure, or if his medication levels are too high, you might even find hypotension. (pp. 167, 168)
4. Trip and fall due to decreased balance and coordination; dizziness or syncope due to low blood pressure or low cardiac output; hip fracture due to osteoporosis; medication error. (pp. 167, 168)

Case Study 2

1. Nine-month-old: heart rate 100–160, respiratory rate 20–40; four-year-old: heart rate 80–120, respiratory rate 20–30; adult: heart rate 60–100, respiratory rate 12–20; elder: same as adult without knowing any medical history. (p. 159)
2. Nine-month-old: 70; four-year-old: 80; adult: 120 (note, while a systolic blood pressure of 120 is considered normal for most adults, EMTs usually do not consider someone hypotensive until their systolic blood pressure falls below 90–100); elder: same as adult without knowing any medical history. (p. 159)

Chapter 8

STOP, REVIEW, REMEMBER! *(p. 185)*

Multiple Choice

1. a (p. 180)
2. b (p. 175)
3. b (p. 178)
4. a (p. 177)
5. c (pp. 182–183)
6. c (pp. 182–183)
7. d (p. 185)
8. b (p. 178)
9. b (pp. 180, 183)
10. c (p. 175)

Fill in the Blank

1. right, left (p. 185)
2. emergent (p. 178)
3. supine (pp. 182–183)
4. comfort (p. 185)
5. armpit-forearm (pp. 177, 179)

Critical Thinking

1. An emergent move is used when there is an immediate threat to life (such as with a car on fire or hazardous materials). A nonemergent move is indicated in every other situation. A stable patient in a safe environment would be an example of a nonemergent move. (pp. 178–180)
2. The five factors that you must consider before deciding how to move your patient are urgency, size and weight, number of available rescuers, distance, and terrain. (pp. 175–176)

STOP, REVIEW, REMEMBER! *(p. 192)*

Multiple Choice

1. d (pp. 174–175)
2. a (pp. 191–192)
3. d (pp. 187–189)
4. c (pp. 189–190)
5. b (p. 190)
6. b (p. 187)

Matching

1. b (pp. 191–192)
2. a (p. 191)
3. d (pp. 189–190)
4. c (pp. 187–189)
5. e (p. 191)

Critical Thinking

1. A. The power grip involves ensuring as much as possible of your palm and fingers are in contact with the object being lifted, and that your hands are placed about 10 inches apart. (p. 177)
   B. The power lift involves placing your feet a comfortable width apart, distributing the weight evenly on both feet, and keeping your back in a straight and locked position. (pp. 176–177)
2. It is important to have at least three rescuers when moving a patient with a stair chair. One rescuer should be behind the chair facing down the stairs, one rescuer should be in front of the chair facing the patient, and the third rescuer should act as a spotter for the downhill rescuer. (pp. 189–190)
3. The greatest risk for performing a move too quickly or with the wrong device is injury to the rescuer or the

patient should either fall. In addition, using the wrong device may make the patient's condition worse. (pp. 174–178, 187–192)

CHAPTER REVIEW *(p. 195)*

Multiple Choice

1. c (pp. 176, 191–192)
2. d (p. 175)
3. b (pp. 187–189)
4. a (p. 176)
5. b (p. 191)
6. c (pp. 174–175)
7. b (p. 178)
8. c (pp. 190–191)
9. d (p. 181)
10. c (pp. 191–192)

Matching

1. E (p. 185)
2. D (p. 185)
3. C (p. 185)
4. B (p. 185)
5. A (p. 185)

Labeling

1a. supine (p. 183)
1b. prone (p. 183)
1c. recovery position (p. 183)
2a. portable stretcher (flat stretcher) (p. 192)
2b. stair chair (p. 190)
2c. flexible stretcher (p. 190)
2d. scoop stretcher (p. 191)

CASE STUDIES

Case Study 1

1. d (p. 178)
2. b (p. 178)

Case Study 2

1. Due to the fact that CPR is in progress, you must move this patient quickly. Before doing so, you will want to position the patient and backboard on the wheeled stretcher so that CPR can continue. Have at least two rescuers control the stretcher as it is moved. Also make sure the path out to the ambulance is clear before you begin the move. (pp. 176, 180, 187, 190–191)
2. It will be necessary to use additional rescuers to help guide and control the stretcher as it is rolled across the grass. It must remain in contact with the ground so that CPR can continue without interruption. (pp. 175–176, 187–190)
3. Answers may vary. Generally, the EMTs would carry some equipment on the stretcher (strapped in or in specially designed carriers). One rescuer could carry the bag not strapped to the stretcher as he assists the crew carrying the stretcher. If necessary, one rescuer could reenter the residence quickly after the patient has been loaded in the ambulance. If the police or other rescuers show up, they can assist in this as well.

Case Study 3

1. Your first call should be to your dispatch center to request a "lift assist." This is a common request when additional help is needed to lift or move a patient. Your dispatch center may call out the local fire department to assist. (pp. 175–176, 189)
2. Depending on the weight limit of your stretcher, you may need a special (bariatric) stretcher designed to hold this weight. This may cause additional issues such as moving the patient through small doorways, and so on. If the patient must be transported down stairs, you may need special Reeves stretchers or stair chairs. (p. 189)

Chapter 9

STOP, REVIEW, REMEMBER! *(p. 209)*

Multiple Choice

1. a (p. 203)
2. c (p. 206)
3. d (pp. 204–209)
4. b (p. 208)
5. b (p. 207)

Fill in the Blank

1. sign (p. 203)
2. symptom (p. 203)
3. pupils (p. 204)
4. baseline (p. 204)
5. Respirations (p. 207)

Critical Thinking

1. It is important for trending purposes so that EMTs can determine if a patient's condition is changing over time and how quickly it is changing. (p. 204)
2. A sign is something that you, as the EMT, can see, such as a bruise or pale skin. A symptom is something the patient describes, such as pain or nausea. (p. 203)
3. Baseline is the name given to the very first set of vital signs taken on a patient. It is the basis for which all subsequent vital signs will be compared in order to spot a trend in the patient's condition. (p. 203)

STOP, REVIEW, REMEMBER! *(p. 220)*

Multiple Choice

1. b (p. 212)
2. d (p. 212)
3. c (p. 218)
4. b (p. 218)
5. a (p. 204)

Matching

1. F (p. 214)
2. D (p. 211)
3. G (p. 213)
4. B (p. 215)
5. H (p. 214)
6. A (p. 211)
7. E (p. 215)
8. C (p. 213)

Critical Thinking

1. When a patient's blood pressure drops as in the case of shock, the pulses farthest from the heart will become difficult if not impossible to feel. Therefore, it is important to confirm the absence or presence of a pulse at one of the central pulse points (carotid or femoral) before beginning CPR. (p. 211)
2. Asking a patient what his blood pressure is normally before you take it could provide you with some idea about what can be expected. (p. 218)
3. The systolic pressure is the pressure in the arteries as the heart beats. The diastolic pressure is the pressure that remains in the arteries between beats as the heart rests momentarily. (p. 215)

STOP, REVIEW, REMEMBER! *(p. 228)*

Multiple Choice

1. b (p. 221)
2. b (p. 222)
3. a (p. 226)
4. d (p. 226)
5. a (p. 226)

Fill in the Blank

1. temperature (p. 221)
2. oral mucosa (p. 221)
3. on the inside of the eyelid (p. 221)
4. jaundiced (p. 222)
5. diaphoretic (p. 222)

Matching

1. C (p. 222)
2. D (p. 222)
3. E (p. 222)
4. A (p. 222)
5. B (p. 222)

Critical Thinking

1. The skin of the face, fingers, and toes for capillary refill, conjunctiva around eyes, mucus membranes of mouth. (p. 222)
2. Pale—shock. Cyanotic—hypoxia from respiratory distress or shock. Flushed—heat exhaustion. Jaundiced—poor liver function. (p. 222)
3. The recommended method for assessing a patient's skin signs for temperature and moisture is to pull the glove off the back of one hand and lay the exposed skin of your hand against the patient's forehead or face. This will allow you to feel the temperature and moisture status of the patient's skin. The normal characteristic for temperature and moisture is warm and dry. (p. 222)

STOP, REVIEW, REMEMBER! *(p. 233)*

Multiple Choice

1. a (p. 230)
2. b (p. 230)
3. c (p. 230)
4. d (p. 231)
5. a (p. 231)

Matching

1. H (p. 222)
2. D (p. 222)
3. E, F, G (pp. 222–223)
4. B, C (p. 223)
5. I (p. 223)
6. A (p. 223)

Critical Thinking

1. One good technique for investigating the existence of a prior medical condition is to ask about medications. A patient may deny the existence of a medical problem but tell you they take insulin and a pill for high blood pressure. They do not always see existing medical conditions as "problems" since they have lived with them so long. (pp. 231–232)
2. Is your pain sharp or dull? Is your pain steady or does it come and go? Have you ever felt this pain before? What did it feel like the first time you experienced it? (pp. 222–223)

CHAPTER REVIEW *(p. 236)*

Multiple Choice

1. b (p. 204)
2. c (p. 204)
3. d (pp. 206–207)
4. a (p. 206)
5. d (p. 211)
6. b (p. 211)
7. a (p. 212)
8. c (p. 222)
9. d (p. 222)
10. b (p. 224)
11. a (p. 222)
12. c (p. 219)
13. d (p. 205)
14. c (p. 215)
15. c (p. 203)

Labeling *(p. 212)*

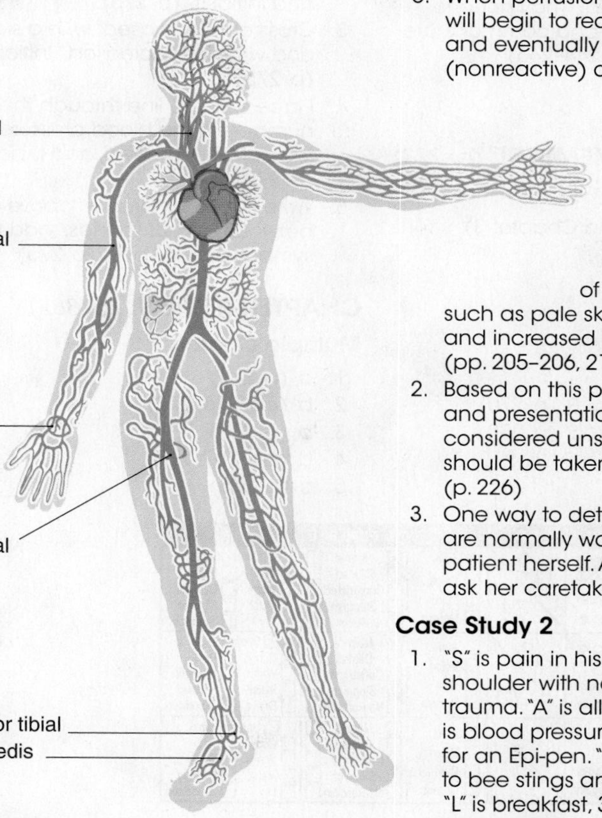

Critical Thinking

1. Time is essential when differentiating multiple sets of vital signs from the same patient. Recording time allows you to compare one set of vitals to another and spot trends in the condition of the patient based on changes. (p. 204)
2. As the time of the sample you are taking decreases, so does the accuracy of the minute rate. The most accurate way to measure heart rate and breathing would be to count for a full minute. Short samples are especially inaccurate when the rhythm is irregular; therefore, you must use a longer sample in these cases. (p. 207)
3. An auscultated blood pressure is taken by listening with a stethoscope. A palpated pressure is taken by feeling the pulse in the wrist. The palpated method is used when the environment is too noisy to allow for the use of a stethoscope or when time is critical and you have several patients. (p. 215)
4. To properly assess skin color in dark-skinned patients you will have to observe alternative areas such as the conjunctiva, nail beds, and the inside of the mouth (mucus membranes). Those areas should be pink and moist or show adequate capillary refill. (p. 221)
5. When perfusion is poor, the pupils will begin to react more sluggishly and eventually will become fixed (nonreactive) and dilated. (p. 225)

CASE STUDIES

Case Study 1

1. Based on the woman's baseline vital signs alone, she has several of the signs of shock, such as pale skin, rapid heart rate, and increased respiratory rate. (pp. 205–206, 213, 222)
2. Based on this patient's history and presentation, she should be considered unstable; therefore, vitals should be taken every five minutes. (p. 226)
3. One way to determine what her vitals are normally would be to ask the patient herself. Another would be to ask her caretaker. (pp. 202, 218)

Case Study 2

1. "S" is pain in his right elbow and shoulder with no obvious signs of trauma. "A" is allergy to bee stings. "M" is blood pressure pill and prescription for an Epi-pen. "P" is history of reaction to bee stings and high blood pressure. "L" is breakfast, 30 minutes ago. "E" is heading out to mow the lawn. (pp. 231–232)
2. Due to his altered mental status and potential for a reaction to a bee sting, this man should be treated as an unstable patient. (pp. 231–232)

Chapter 10

STOP, REVIEW, REMEMBER! *(p. 249)*

Multiple Choice

1. a (p. 246)
2. d (p. 246)
3. b (p. 248)
4. c (p. 248)

Critical Thinking

1. Depending on the resources available and the methods routinely used by the patient, you may try writing questions on paper, enlisting a friend or relative to use sign language and translate, or the patient may read lips. (p. 245)
2. One method will be to work through the mother to get answers from the child. Another method would be to distract the child with a toy or tool, such as a stethoscope. Attempt to gain the trust of the child, who might then begin to allow you to assess and care for him. (p. 247)

STOP, REVIEW, REMEMBER! *(p. 253)*

Multiple Choice

1. b (pp. 250–251)
2. b (p. 250)
3. d (p. 250)
4. c (p. 250)
5. b (p. 252)

Matching

1. B (p. 250)
2. D (p. 252)
3. A (p. 250)
4. C (p. 250)

Critical Thinking

1. A portable radio is small and designed to be carried on one's person. A mobile radio is mounted in a vehicle such as the ambulance. Base station radios are in a building such as the dispatch center or hospital. (p. 250)

STOP, REVIEW, REMEMBER! *(p. 258)*

Multiple Choice

1. c (pp. 254–255)
2. c (pp. 254–255)
3. b (p. 255)
4. d (pp. 256–257)
5. d (pp. 257–258)

Critical Thinking

1. Identify your unit (ambulance identifier) and your level of certification—in this case, EMT; your estimated time of arrival (ETA); the patient's age and sex; the patient's chief complaint; a brief, pertinent history of the present illness or injury; relevant past medical history; vital signs, including mental status; pertinent findings of your examination; the care you have provided; the patient's response to your care. (pp. 254–255)
2. The hand-off can focus on changes in the patient's condition that have occurred since the radio report, if the receiver is familiar with the information. The hand-off report is done in person,

and the call-in is done via radio. (pp. 257–258)

3. A hurried and incomplete radio report can suggest hurried and incomplete patient care. This reflects on you and your agency. Disorganization in the report can cause hospital personnel to feel they have to check the care you provided, even if the care was excellent. (pp. 254–256)

CHAPTER REVIEW *(p. 260)*

Multiple Choice

1. b (p. 251)
2. c (p. 245)
3. d (p. 256)
4. c (p. 250)
5. d (p. 245)

Critical Thinking

1. Get down at the patient's level. Speak to the patient clearly and make sure that there are no barriers to her understanding what you say (hearing, language, and so on). Listen to her to determine why she will not go. You then will be able to address some of her fears. (pp. 245–246)
2. The dispatcher records these events either on paper or in a computer system. The information is used for documentation, research, quality improvement, and in the event of a lawsuit. (p. 252)
3. Not listening or looking at the patient implied disrespect, carelessness, or indifference (or all of these). You would likely feel as if the provider did not care. This is not only rude and inconsiderate, it also raises the potential for liability. (p. 246)
4. You would confirm the order by repeating it back to the physician and then waiting for acknowledgment back from the physician. You would say: "Confirming you would like me to assist the patient with one spray of nitroglycerin sublingually and to have the patient chew four low-dose aspirin, which is 324 mg. Over." (pp. 256–257)
5. You would ask for an order for a medication. You would tell the physician whether or not the patient had used the medication already. You would verify that the patient was not allergic to the medication. You would explain the signs and symptoms (indications) for the medication. You would realize that vital signs have additional relevance in this situation. (pp. 256–257)
6. Information transmitted over the radio may be heard on scanners and violate the patient's privacy. Radio information should be limited to what is pertinent to allow others to use the radio frequency. (p. 251)
7. Most would expect quality clinical care with time spent to reassure and comfort the patient. (p. 246)

RECONSTRUCT THE RADIO REPORT

Radio Report 1 *(pp. 254–255)*

8, 2, 5, 6, 3, 1, 4, 9, 7

Radio Report 2 *(pp. 254–255)*

6, 4, 9, 7, 2, 8, 1, 3, 10, 5

CASE STUDY

1. Yes, as long as the son is calm and reliable. If not, you may wish to find another person who will be calmer (for example, a trusted neighbor). (pp. 244–246)
2. You can ensure accuracy by taking your time. Determine if the answers you receive match other factors such as injuries, level of distress of the patient, and mechanism of injury. (pp. 244–246)
3. Your assessment will likely be slower because of the time it will take to have everything said and interpreted twice. This time is worthwhile when it leads to accurate assessment and care. In serious trauma you may need to expedite transport and communicate on the move. (pp. 244–246)

Chapter 11

STOP, REVIEW, REMEMBER! *(p. 273)*

Multiple Choice

1. d (pp. 265, 267, and Chapter 3)
2. b (pp. 268–269)
3. b (p. 268)
4. a (p. 269)
5. d (pp. 269, 272)

Labeling

1. S (p. 270)
2. O (p. 270)
3. O (p. 270)
4. S (p. 270)
5. S (p. 270)
6. O (p. 270)

Fill in the Blank

VITAL SIGNS: TIME	RESP	PULSE	B.P.	LEVEL OF CONSCIOUSNESS	R PUPILS L	SKIN
1117	Rate: 22 [ ] Regular [ ] Shallow [X] Labored	Rate: 94 [X] Regular [ ] Irregular	112/74	[ ] Alert [ ] Voice [ ] Pain [ ] Unresp.	[X] Normal [ ] [ ] Dilated [ ] [ ] Constricted [ ] [ ] Sluggish [ ] [ ] No-Reaction [ ]	[ ] Unremarkable [X] Cool [ ] Pale [ ] Warm [ ] Cyanotic [X] Moist [ ] Flushed [ ] Dry [ ] Jaundiced
1122	Rate: 20 [ ] Regular [ ] Shallow [X] Labored	Rate: 88 [X] Regular [ ] Irregular	108/70	[ ] Alert [ ] Voice [ ] Pain [ ] Unresp.	[X] Normal [ ] [ ] Dilated [ ] [ ] Constricted [ ] [ ] Sluggish [ ] [ ] No-Reaction [ ]	[ ] Unremarkable [X] Cool [ ] Pale [ ] Warm [ ] Cyanotic [ ] Moist [ ] Flushed [X] Dry [ ] Jaundiced
	Rate: [ ] Regular [ ] Shallow [ ] Labored	Rate: [ ] Regular [ ] Irregular	/	[ ] Alert [ ] Voice [ ] Pain [ ] Unresp.	[ ] Normal [ ] [ ] Dilated [ ] [ ] Constricted [ ] [ ] Sluggish [ ] [ ] No-Reaction [ ]	[ ] Unremarkable [ ] Cool [ ] Pale [ ] Warm [ ] Cyanotic [ ] Moist [ ] Flushed [ ] Dry [ ] Jaundiced

Critical Thinking

1. Documentation can help minimize liability but only if it is done in conjunction with high quality, patient-centered prehospital care. (p. 267)

STOP, REVIEW, REMEMBER! *(p. 279)*

Multiple Choice

1. c (p. 274)
2. a (pp. 265, 267)
3. c (p. 275)
4. b (pp. 276–277)
5. b (p. 275)
6. c (p. 269)
7. b (pp. 276–277)
8. a (pp. 276–277)
9. c (pp. 278–279)

Critical Thinking

1. Since the form has already been left at the hospital and likely sent to other agencies, simply crossing out and correcting the error is not enough. Follow your local rules for sending amended copies to agencies that have received copies of the original. (p. 275)

Make It Right

1. Cross out the "1" with a single line and initial it. (p. 275)
2. Place a single line through the sentence, note the patient's allergies, and initial it. (p. 275)
3. Cross out "increased" with a single line and write in "decreased." Initial it. (p. 275)
4. Place a single line through the numbers in the blood pressure, write in the correct numbers, and initial it. (p. 275)
5. Write the word "breath" above and between "equal sounds," add the ^ symbol, and initial it. (p. 275)

CHAPTER REVIEW *(p. 382)*

Multiple Choice

1. a (p. 274)
2. b (pp. 276–277)
3. b (p. 275)
4. d (pp. 269–270)
5. c (p. 275)

Critical Thinking

1. The report could be used for reference in the emergency department, referenced in other units in the hospital where the patient stays, for prehospital research, in quality improvement. (pp. 265, 267)
2. Document that the patient vomited en route and that you could not obtain a second set of vitals because of a short transport time and the fact that you were providing airway care to the patient. Never make false statements on any report for any reason. (p. 275)
3. Because there are many patients and often not enough EMTs, there will be minimal time for documentation. Because of this, it is acceptable to make brief but important notes on triage tags instead of filling out a full report for each patient. Full documentation may be required after the call is completed. (pp. 278–279)

Name That Error

1. O (p. 275)
2. O (p. 275)
3. C (p. 275)
4. O (p. 275)
5. C (p. 275)

CASE STUDY

1. Answers may vary. Your feelings may range from hurt and insult to anger. You may have done nothing, spoken to the EMTs about it, or made a complaint to their agency's leadership. (p. 274)
2. This breach of patient confidentiality is serious and unprofessional. There are obviously many factors ranging from where the complaint is filed to the allegations themselves. Suffice it to say that a violation of HIPAA statutes could result in a federal complaint with substantial fines. Personnel issues such as retraining, suspension, or dismissal also could occur. (p. 274)

Module 1

REVIEW AND PRACTICE EXAMINATION

1. d (p. 6) Objective 1-3
2. b (p. 8) Objective 1-3
3. d (p. 10) Objective 1-4
4. c (p. 10) Objective 1-4
5. a (p. 6) Objective 1-3
6. a (p. 12) Objective 1-5
7. b (p. 13) Objective 1-7
8. c (p. 14) Objective 1-9
9. b (p. 26) Objective 2-5
10. c (p. 26) Objective 2-4
11. a (p. 28) Objective 2-6
12. b (p. 31) Objective 2-9
13. d (p. 31) Objective 2-8
14. d (p. 34) Objective 2-10
15. b (p. 34) Objective 2-10
16. c (p. 34) Objective 2-11
17. b (p. 37) Objective 2-10
18. c (p. 38) Objective 2-12
19. b (p. 40) Objective 2-14
20. a (p. 41) Objective 2-14
21. b (p. 49) Objective 3-2
22. d (p. 49) Objective 3-2
23. c (p. 50) Objective 3-4
24. a (p. 51) Objective 3-6
25. a (p. 52) Objective 3-7
26. c (p. 55) Objective 3-8
27. b (p. 55) Objective 3-9
28. b (p. 56) Objective 3-10
29. d (p. 56) Objective 3-10
30. c (p. 58) Objective 3-11
31. a (pp. 58–60) Objective 3-12
32. d (p. 63) Objective 3-17
33. c (pp. 64–65) Objective 3-18
34. d (p. 76) Objective 4-5
35. d (p. 75) Objective 4-5
36. c (p. 75) Objective 4-5
37. b (p. 81) Objective 4-3
38. c (pp. 75–76) Objective 4-5
39. a (p. 75) Objective 4-5
40. c (p. 80) Objective 4-3
41. a (p. 83) Objective 4-3
42. d (p. 81) Objective 4-3
43. c (p. 105) Objective 5-10
44. b (p. 105) Objective 5-10
45. a (p. 108) Objective 5-11
46. d (pp. 108–113) Objective 5-12
47. b (p. 112) Objective 5-14
48. d (p. 112) Objective 5-13
49. c (p. 113) Objective 5-14
50. b (p. 112) Objective 5-13
51. b (p. 97) Objective 5-4
52. a (p. 98) Objective 5-6
53. d (p. 100) Objective 5-6
54. b (p. 100) Objective 5-7
55. c (p. 100) Objective 5-7
56. b (p. 116) Objective 5-16
57. a (p. 102) Objective 5-8
58. a (p. 101) Objective 5-8
59. d (p. 119) Objective 5-20
60. c (p. 119) Objective 5-21
61. b (p. 145) Objective 6-12
62. b (p. 104) Objective 5-9
63. c (p. 140) Objective 6-11
64. d (p. 136) Objective 6-6
65. c (p. 143) Objective 6-20
66. a (p. 133) Objective 6-3
67. c (p. 158) Objective 7-2
68. b (p. 163) Objective 7-4
69. a (p. 160) Objective 7-3
70. b (p. 166) Objective 7-4
71. a (pp. 142–143) Objective 6-18
72. a (p. 144) Objective 6-5
73. c (p. 137) Objective 6-9
74. a (pp. 189–190) Objective 8-11
75. a (p. 191) Objective 8-11
76. c (p. 178) Objective 8-8
77. d (p. 182) Objective 8-10
78. b (p. 203) Objective 9-2
79. a (p. 203) Objective 9-2
80. c (p. 204) Objective 9-3
81. a (p. 207) Objective 9-6
82. c (p. 208) Objective 9-6
83. d (p. 208) Objective 9-6
84. a (p. 211) Objective 9-8
85. c (p. 212) Objective 9-10
86. b (p. 214) Objective 9-12
87. c (p. 222) Objective 9-13
88. c (p. 222) Objective 9-12
89. a (p. 225) Objective 9-16
90. b (p. 232) Objective 9-21
91. a (p. 204) Objective 9-3
92. d (p. 244) Objective 10-3
93. c (p. 250) Objective 10-13
94. b (p. 269) Objective 11-6
95. c (p. 274) Objective 11-8
96. d (p. 275) Objective 11-8
97. d (p. 137) Objective 6-7
98. c (p. 208) Objective 9-7
99. a (p. 222) Objective 9-13
100. c (p. 226) Objective 9-17

Chapter 12

STOP, REVIEW, REMEMBER! *(p. 303)*

Multiple Choice

1. d (pp. 295–296)
2. b (p. 301)
3. c (p. 302)
4. a (pp. 296–298)
5. a (p. 299)

Short Answer

1. Hazardous chemicals can burn, explode, be toxic for inhalation, and pose many other dangers. Call for assistance from the fire department and/or hazmat team. (pp. 298–299, 302)
2. Intoxicated people can exhibit unpredictable behavior. In this case yelling is a possible sign of agitation or aggression. Call for law enforcement. (pp. 298–299, 302)
3. The vehicle on its side is unstable and must be stabilized to keep it from falling on others or further injuring the people inside. Call for a rescue team and additional ambulances, depending on the number of patients. (pp. 298–299, 302)
4. Dangers include falling and injuries to the rescuers. A high-angle rescue team may be necessary. You also may need a Stokes basket for transport and additional personnel for lifting and moving over distances. (pp. 298–299, 302)

Critical Thinking

1. Make sure you and your partner stay together. If at any time you feel that your safety or the safety of anyone at the scene is at risk, retreat to your vehicle and request law enforcement. (p. 299)
2. It is possible to become distracted by patient care once you enter the scene. The sooner you request resources, the sooner they will arrive and manage any hazards. You also may need additional patient

care resources, such as extrication resources, that must arrive quickly to ensure patient care in a timely manner. (p. 302)

STOP, REVIEW, REMEMBER! *(p. 310)*

Multiple Choice

1. b (p. 307)
2. c (p. 309)
3. b (p. 308)
4. b (p. 309)
5. c (p. 309)

Fill in the Blank

1. scene size-up (p. 307)
2. immediate life threats (p. 305)
3. general impression (p. 307)
4. general impression (p. 307)
5. event (p. 308)
6. verbal (p. 308)

Critical Thinking

1. The purpose of the primary assessment is to identify and care for any immediate life threats to the patient. You should not feel compelled to perform a thorough physical examination of the patient if an immediate life threat exists. Your time and effort must be spent dealing with the life threat and not performing less important tasks. (p. 307)
2. An unresponsive patient will need a more aggressive primary assessment, looking for a patent airway, adequate breathing, and adequate circulation. (pp. 309–310)
3. A patient who has problems with the airway, breathing, or circulation will need all your attention placed on correcting those problems. The secondary assessment will be conducted only when the ABCs are corrected. (p. 306)

STOP, REVIEW, REMEMBER! *(p. 316)*

Multiple Choice

1. c (p. 312)
2. a (p. 312)
3. a (p. 313)
4. b (p. 314)
5. c (p. 313)

Matching

1. B (p. 311)
2. A (p. 314)
3. E (p. 312)
4. C (p. 314)
5. D (p. 314)

Critical Thinking

1. The assessment of the airway of a responsive patient is as simple as asking him a question or two and observing his ability to speak. If he is responsive and able to speak, it can be concluded that his airway is patent. For the unresponsive patient, you must watch the chest for rise and fall. If you see, hear, and feel evidence of breathing, the airway is clear. If you do not see evidence of breathing, you must provide assisted ventilations and see the chest rise and fall with each breath. (p. 312)
2. The adequacy of breathing is determined by two factors: the depth of breathing (tidal volume) and the rate. A patient who is breathing adequately will be breathing at least 10 to 12 times each minute and you will see obvious chest rise and fall with each breath. (p. 312)
3. It is safe to say that most patients who are experiencing a medical or trauma emergency will benefit from supplemental oxygen. You must assess their level of distress, mental status, and vital signs to determine just how much you should give. Ultimately, the decision to provide oxygen is up to the EMT, guided by local protocol. (p. 313)

CHAPTER REVIEW *(p. 318)*

Multiple Choice

1. b (p. 301)
2. d (pp. 313–314)
3. a (pp. 305–306)
4. d (pp. 305–306)
5. a (p. 308)
6. b (p. 308)

Listing

1. Scene safety (pp. 295–296)
2. Body substance isolation (BSI) precautions (pp. 295–296)
3. Additional resources (pp. 295–296)
4. Number of patients (pp. 295–296)
5. Mechanism of injury/nature of illness (pp. 295–296)
6. Consider the need for spinal immobilization (pp. 295–296)

Critical Thinking

1. (1) Obstructed airway: Without a clear airway, a patient will be unable to breathe and could die within minutes. (2) No breathing: A patient may have a patent airway but still not be breathing. Without an adequate supply of oxygen, death will soon follow. (3) No pulse: It is safe to assume that if the patient has no pulse, breathing also has stopped. With adequate circulation, a patient will experience brain death within minutes. (4) Severe bleeding: The body must have an adequate supply of blood volume in order to maintain a blood pressure and adequate perfusion. Without it, the patient will go into shock and death will soon follow. (p. 306)
2. Student answers will vary. Discuss answers with your instructor. (p. 306)
3. One of the main reasons for forming a general impression with each patient is to establish as early as possible the need for immediate care and transport. You are trying to quickly categorize the patient as either "big sick" or "little sick" so that you can act accordingly. (p. 307)
4. One of your goals is to be a fact finder and remain as objective as possible during your assessment of the patient. By using the patient's own words and descriptions, you remain true to this concept. (p. 311)

CASE STUDIES

Case Study 1

1. You can call out to the patient and attempt to get him to respond verbally. If he responds, then you know he at least has an open airway, is breathing, and has a pulse. You also may attempt to observe the patient from outside the vehicle to see if he is breathing or not. (pp. 307, 308)
2. If the patient is responsive, then about the only element you will not be able to easily assess is severe bleeding. If he is unresponsive, then assessing both pulse and bleeding become very difficult by observation only. (pp. 313–314)

Case Study 2

1. You should begin by kneeling beside the patient and observing for adequate chest rise and fall to confirm the patient has an airway and is breathing. You can do this initially without moving the patient. You can simply observe the patient for obvious bleeding. (pp. 312–314)
2. If you are unable to confirm an open airway and breathing, you will have to carefully roll the patient onto her back and open the airway. (p. 312)
3. You must assess the pulse at the carotid artery in the neck before assuming she is in cardiac arrest. As blood pressure falls, the pulses farthest from the heart become weak and difficult to feel. (p. 314)

Chapter 13

STOP, REVIEW, REMEMBER! *(p. 335)*

Multiple Choice

1. d (pp. 326–329)
2. a (p. 327)
3. b (p. 331)
4. a (p. 334)
5. c (p. 333)

Critical Thinking

1. Several things to look for in both responsive and unresponsive patients include adequate chest rise and fall (tidal volume), adequate rate, ability to speak in full sentences, and good skin signs. (p. 326)
2. When a patient is in respiratory distress, the body is still attempting to compensate by increasing the rate and volume of breathing. When failure sets in, these compensatory mechanisms begin to fail and

breathing rate and volume decrease and the mental status decreases as well. (pp. 327–329)

3. You must do your best to manage the airway of a trauma patient by minimizing movement of the neck. If possible, keep the head and neck in a neutral position and place an appropriate airway adjunct. Suction fluids as necessary. If these measures do not result in an open airway, attempt the jaw thrust maneuver. If the jaw thrust does not result in an open airway, reposition the head with slight extension until an open airway is achieved. In this case an open airway takes priority over the possibility of aggravating an existing neck injury. (pp. 339–344)

COMPLETE THE TABLE *(pp. 327–328)*

Sign	Distress	Failure
Increased respiratory rate	X	
Decreased respiratory rate		X
Altered mental status	X	X
Use of accessory muscles	X	X
Nasal flaring	X	
Cyanosis		X
Agonal respirations		X

STOP, REVIEW, REMEMBER! *(p. 345)*

Multiple Choice

1. c (p. 337)
2. a (p. 337)
3. b (p. 340)
4. d (p. 345)
5. c (p. 339)

Matching

1. e (p. 337)
2. d (p. 338)
3. b (p. 339)
4. a (p. 340)
5. c (p. 344)

Critical Thinking

1. Whenever you are manually ventilating a patient, regardless of how good of an airway you may have, there is a strong likelihood that some air will enter the patient's stomach. This increases the chances that the patient may vomit. Have suction ready to help minimize the chances of aspiration. (p. 337)
2. These airway adjuncts are designed to "assist" the EMT in maintaining a patent airway and do not guarantee an open airway when inserted. You must constantly reassess the airway and maintain manual support of the airway (head-tilt/chin-lift or jaw-thrust) when appropriate. (pp. 339–340)
3. NPAs are contraindicated in patients with significant facial trauma because such injuries could be an indication of a skull fracture. There is a possibility that an NPA inserted into a patient with a skull fracture could result in the device entering the skull and causing damage and infection. (p. 345)

STOP, REVIEW, REMEMBER! *(p. 356)*

Multiple Choice

1. b (p. 326)
2. c (p. 349)
3. d (p. 356)
4. a (p. 352)
5. d (p. 350)

Critical Thinking

1. This patient's respirations are inadequate for two reasons. They are below the acceptable rate and tidal volume. You must provide assisted ventilations with an appropriate device such as a bag-mask with supplemental oxygen. You can squeeze the bag whenever the patient attempts to breathe, enhancing his breath. You also must add additional breaths to bring his rate up to the minimum 12 per minute necessary. (p. 347)
2. The ideal device will be a pediatric-size bag-mask. The correct size will minimize the chances that you will overinflate the patient, causing a buildup of air in the stomach. (pp. 350–352)
3. You must ensure that you have the proper size mask to ensure a good seal. The head needs only to be extended slightly to ensure an open airway. (pp. 354–355)

COMPLETE THE TABLE *(pp. 349–353)*

Situation	Mouth-to-Mask	Two-Rescuer Bag-Mask	Demand Valve	One-Rescuer Bag-Mask
You are alone and off duty with an unresponsive nonbreathing infant.	X			
You, your partner, and a firefighter are ventilating a patient as you carry him down a flight of stairs on a portable stretcher.		X	X	X
You and a firefighter are ventilating an adult male in the back of an ambulance.		X	X	X
You are alone in the back of an ambulance and ventilating an eight-year-old drowning victim.				X
You are ventilating a 20-year-old male who is the third patient from an accidental carbon monoxide poisoning.			X	X

STOP, REVIEW, REMEMBER! *(p. 368)*

Multiple Choice

1. b (p. 358)
2. c (p. 358)
3. d (p. 360)
4. a (p. 366)
5. c (p. 363)
6. b (p. 365)
7. c (p. 368)
8. d (p. 363)
9. a (pp. 330, 350)
10. d (p. 366)

Matching

1. e (p. 355)
2. c (p. 340)
3. d (p. 363)
4. a (p. 366)
5. b (p. 350)

Critical Thinking

1. Medical oxygen is 100% oxygen, while the air we breathe is approximately 21% oxygen. (p. 358)
2. For a patient who is not getting enough oxygen due to inadequate rate or volume, increasing the concentration of oxygen will compensate. (p. 364)
3. The nonrebreather mask does not create an airtight seal around the face; therefore, it allows room air to enter the mask and mix with the oxygen. When the air mixes with the oxygen, it lowers the overall concentration. (p. 364)

CHAPTER REVIEW *(p. 371)*

Multiple Choice

1. c (p. 327)
2. b (p. 324)
3. a (p. 325)
4. a (p. 334)
5. a (p. 339)
6. b (p. 338)

7. c (p. 350)
8. b (p. 354 and Chapter 12, p. 306)
9. d (p. 337)
10. c (p. 363)

Critical Thinking

1. The best way to determine if the flow rate on a nonrebreather mask is appropriate is when the reservoir bag is able to refill completely between breaths. (p. 364)
2. Passive oxygen delivery devices, such as a nonrebreather mask or cannula, require that the patient be breathing adequately in order to be effective. They simply increase the concentration of available oxygen that must be breathed in by the patient to provide benefit. In contrast a demand valve or bag-mask are used to breathe for a patient who is either not breathing or breathing inadequately. (p. 362)
3. Due to the fact that a nonrebreather mask is not airtight, it will always allow some ambient air in around the seal. For this reason, a nonrebreather mask is not capable of providing a breathable oxygen concentration of 100%. In a best case, a properly fitted nonrebreather mask may deliver a breathable concentration of approximately 90% oxygen. (p. 364)

CASE STUDIES

Case Study 1

1. Your first priority will be to clear this man's airway and begin providing assisted ventilations with supplemental oxygen. Due to the mechanism of injury, you must do so while taking the appropriate spinal precautions. (pp. 331–335)
2. The best way to address his airway and breathing problems is to have someone manually stabilize his head and neck while suctioning his airway, and then insert an airway adjunct. You then should assist his breathing with manual ventilations. (pp. 337–345)
3. The most appropriate device is most likely a bag-mask; however, a pocket mask with supplemental O_2 or a demand valve could also be used. (pp. 349–352)

Case Study 2

1. If you can rule out the possibility of trauma, you can use the head-tilt/chin-lift maneuver to open her airway. (pp. 333–334)
2. Yes, assisted ventilations are most likely needed since her tidal volume is so poor. A bag-mask is the most appropriate device for this patient; however, a pocket mask with supplemental oxygen or a demand valve could also be used. (pp. 349–352)

Chapter 14

STOP, REVIEW, REMEMBER! *(p. 379)*

Multiple Choice

1. b (p. 375)
2. a (p. 375)
3. b (p. 376)
4. b (p. 376)
5. d (p. 378)

Matching *(p. 378)*

Sign or Symptom	Category
1. Alert and oriented	S
2. No major complaint of chest or abdominal pain	S
3. Significant MOI	U
4. Uncontrolled bleeding	U
5. Difficulty breathing	U
6. Absence of recent trauma	S
7. Vital signs that are within normal limits	S
8. Abnormal vital signs	U
9. Altered mental status	U
10. Normal breathing characteristics	S

Critical Thinking

1. You must do your best to determine if your patient is unstable early in the process because this will likely change the urgency with which you decide to transport your patient. (p. 378)
2. You must always be monitoring the status of your patient, looking for signs that he is getting worse (unstable). If a patient suddenly becomes unstable, you must address immediate life threats and expedite transport to the hospital. (p. 378)

STOP, REVIEW, REMEMBER! *(p. 389)*

Multiple Choice

1. a (p. 382)
2. b (p. 382)
3. a (p. 380)
4. c (p. 387)
5. b (p. 383)

Matching

1. C (p. 385)
2. A (p. 385)
3. E (p. 389)
4. D (p. 385)
5. F (p. 385)
6. B (p. 388)

Critical Thinking

1. The criterion for performing a rapid secondary assessment on a medical patient is that he is unstable. An unstable medical patient may have one of more of the following signs or symptoms: difficulty breathing, cardiac chest pain, altered mental status, signs of a stroke. (pp. 382–387)
2. When assessing the neck of a medical patient, you should be looking for pain, jugular vein distention, a stoma, accessory muscle use, medical identification jewelry, pulse. (p. 385)
3. When assessing the abdomen of a medical patient, you should be looking for pain, distention, rigidity, guarding, referred pain, pulsating mass, scars, and rashes. (p. 385)

STOP, REVIEW, REMEMBER! *(p. 403)*

Multiple Choice

1. b (p. 393)
2. b (p. 398)
3. d (p. 391)
4. d (p. 391)
5. a (p. 391)

Critical Thinking

1. Answers will vary. Example responses are as follows. Medical: a patient who is having difficulty breathing; a patient with an altered mental status. Trauma: a patient who fell and injured a hip; a patient who was caught under a collapsed structure. (p. 376)
2. How old is the patient? How far did he fall? What caused the fall? What type of surface did he land on? How did he land? Did he lose consciousness? (pp. 392–393)
3. a. significant; b. nonsignificant; c. significant; d. significant; e. nonsignificant (pp. 393–394)

CHAPTER REVIEW *(p. 405)*

Multiple Choice

1. a (p. 391)
2. c (p. 376)
3. b (p. 385)
4. b (pp. 391–393)
5. d (p. 391)
6. c (p. 403)
7. d (p. 403)
8. a (p. 387)
9. b (p. 391)
10. c (p. 387)
11. b (pp. 388–389)
12. d (p. 386)
13. a (p. 376)
14. a (p. 402)
15. b (p. 383)

Matching

1. E (p. 397)
2. C (p. 396)
3. D (p. 385)
4. A (p. 394)
5. B (p. 397)

Critical Thinking

1. Answers will vary. Example responses are as follows: Trauma: a patient involved in a vehicle collision, a patient who fell from the roof of a house, and a patient who suffered an injury to the leg playing soccer. Medical: a patient who was having chest pain, a patient who was having an asthma attack, and a patient with a sudden onset of abdominal pain. (p. 376)
2. The medical patient is assessed based on his chief complaint, with care focusing on the signs and symptoms he is presenting with at the time. A thorough history of both the present illness and past medical problems is important. In contrast, the trauma patient is assessed and cared for primarily based on the MOI. (p. 376)

3. The objective of the reassessment is to reevaluate the ABCs to ensure that no life-threatening conditions develop. It also includes an assessment of vital signs and interventions. (pp. 401–402)
4. a. Cardiac and respiratory systems; b. digestive and renal systems; c. cardiac system; d. respiratory, skin, and immune systems; e. nervous system (p. 381)

CASE STUDIES

Case Study 1

1. Noisy respirations are a strong indication of a partially obstructed airway. In this case the gurgling may be an indication of fluid buildup in the oropharynx. (p. 378)
2. Changes in the patient's airway status require that you abandon the less important secondary assessment and manage the airway immediately. This patient may need suctioning. (p. 378)

Case Study 2

1. Since this man is responsive and able to answer questions, the most appropriate assessment path is the focused secondary assessment. (p. 387)
2. O: What were you doing when the pain began? Has this ever happened before? P: Does anything you do make the pain worse? Does anything you do make the pain better? Q: Can you describe your pain for me? Is the pain sharp or dull? Is it steady or does it come and go? R: Can you point with one finger to where the pain is the most? Does the pain radiate anywhere else? S: On a scale of 1 to 10, how would you rate your pain right now? On a scale of 1 to 10, what was your pain when it first began? T: When did the pain first begin? Has it gotten better or worse since it first began? (p. 389)

Case Study 3

1. You will examine the outside of the vehicle to assess the amount of damage and intrusion into the passenger compartment. If possible, you also will want to determine if the patient was wearing a seat belt of any kind and if the car had air bags that had deployed. (p. 391)
2. Due to the significant MOI, the most appropriate assessment path is the rapid secondary assessment. (p. 391)
3. Based on the fact that the patient is unresponsive, you must determine that she has an open airway and that she is breathing adequately. This must be accomplished while maintaining spinal precautions. You must immediately control any external bleeding and maintain a high index of suspicion for internal bleeding. (pp. 391, 393)

Case Study 4

1. You will want to confirm that the cause of the fall was "mechanical" in nature. In other words, she tripped and did not fall as a result of some underlying medical problem such as a seizure. You also will want to determine if she hit her head or lost consciousness. Ask her to describe exactly how she fell and what hit the ground first. (p. 391)
2. It appears that this patient did not sustain a significant MOI; therefore, the most appropriate assessment path would be a focused secondary assessment. (pp. 393–394)

Module 2

REVIEW AND PRACTICE EXAMINATION

1. a (p. 296) Objective 12-2
2. c (p. 295) Objective 12-3
3. d (pp. 295–296) Objective 12-3
4. b (p. 299) Objective 12-4
5. b (p. 299) Objective 12-5
6. c (pp. 300–301) Objective 12-6
7. c (p. 305) Objective 12-9
8. c (p. 301) Objective 12-7
9. d (p. 326) Objective 13-5
10. b (p. 326) Objective 13-4
11. c (p. 326) Objective 13-4
12. b (p. 326) Objective 13-6
13. d (p. 329) Objective 13-6
14. a (p. 329) Objective 13-5
15. b (p. 333) Objective 13-10
16. c (p. 334) Objective 13-10
17. d (p. 337) Objective 13-11
18. b (p. 332) Objective 13-8
19. c (p. 339) Objective 13-11
20. a (p. 339) Objective 13-11
21. a (p. 338) Objective 13-13
22. d (p. 340) Objective 13-15
23. c (p. 343) Objective 13-15
24. a (p. 350) Objective 13-18
25. a (p. 349) Objective 13-18
26. d (p. 349) Objective 13-18
27. d (p. 349) Objective 13-18
28. c (p. 350) Objective 13-18
29. c (p. 350) Objective 13-18
30. c (p. 352) Objective 13-20
31. a (p. 355) Objective 13-22
32. b (pp. 355–356) Objective 13-23
33. c (p. 360) Objective 13-25
34. a (p. 360) Objective 13-26
35. b (p. 361) Objective 13-27
36. c (p. 363) Objective 13-29
37. b (p. 363) Objective 13-29
38. a (p. 364) Objective 13-29
39. d (p. 363) Objective 13-29
40. c (p. 363) Objective 13-16
41. b (p. 367) Objective 13-29
42. c (p. 366) Objective 13-29
43. a (p. 366) Objective 13-29
44. b (p. 366) Objective 13-29
45. a (p. 337) Objective 13-12
46. b (p. 351) Objective 13-18
47. c (p. 328) Objective 13-4
48. d (pp. 350–352) Objective 13-18
49. d (p. 358) Objective 13-24
50. c (p. 358) Objective 13-3
51. a (p. 326) Objective 13-3
52. a (p. 328) Objective 14-2
53. a (p. 326) Objective 13-3
54. b (p.203) Objective 9-2
55. a (p. 203) Objective 9-2
56. a (p. 327) Objective 13-3
57. c (p. 328 and Chapter 9, p. 208) Objective 13-4
58. d (p. 332) Objective 13-8
59. c (p. 313) Objective 12-11
60. d (p. 314) Objective 12-11
61. c (p. 376) Objective 14-1
62. b (p. 389) Objective 14-11
63. c (p. 308) Objective 12-11
64. a (p. 375) Objective 14-3
65. b (p. 393) Objective 14-12
66. c (p. 382) Objective 14-8
67. b (p. 385) Objective 14-14
68. c (p. 387) Objective 14-11
69. d (p. 382) Objective 14-9
70. d (p. 388) Objective 14-11
71. b (p. 389) Objective 14-11
72. d (p. 327) Objective 13-3
73. c (p. 308) Objective 14-6
74. c (p. 382) Objective 14-14
75. c (p. 385) Objective 14-10

Chapter 16

STOP, REVIEW, REMEMBER! *(p. 428)*

Multiple Choice

1. c (p. 426)
2. d (p. 426)
3. c (p. 426)
4. a (p. 426)
5. a (p. 426)

Matching

1. B (p. 426)
2. A (p. 426)
3. E (p. 426)
4. D (p. 426)
5. C (p. 426)

Critical Thinking

1. A metered-dose inhaler is a device used to deliver a powder aerosolized to be inhaled in a single dose. A nebulized medication is typically a liquid mixed with air to create a vapor that is inhaled over a period of time. (p. 426)
2. Nitroglycerin is a generic name for the medication. Nitrostat is a brand name of nitroglycerin that may come in either a tablet or spray form. (p. 426)
3. Medication meant for sublingual administration will enter the bloodstream much faster if it is allowed to dissolve under the tongue. If it is chewed and swallowed, it may take longer to enter the bloodstream. (p. 426)
4. a. trade, b. chemical, c. generic, d. generic, e. trade, f. generic, g. trade, h. generic (p. 426)

STOP, REVIEW, REMEMBER! *(p. 439)*

Multiple Choice

1. c (p. 434)
2. a (p. 431)
3. d (p. 442)
4. b (p. 434)
5. a (p. 435)

Matching

1. C (p. 432)
2. D (p. 434)
3. B (p. 432)
4. E (p. 434)
5. G (p. 436)
6. B (p. 432)
7. A (p. 430)
8. F (p. 427)

Critical Thinking

1. Student answers will vary.
2. Inhalers are typically powders that are aerosolized so they can be inhaled and absorbed in the lungs. (p. 437)

STOP, REVIEW, REMEMBER! *(p. 444)*

Multiple Choice

1. b (p. 441)
2. c (p. 427)
3. d (p. 442)
4. a (p. 432)
5. b (p. 438)

Short Answer

1. Right medication refers to the appropriate indication to administer the medication. Is the medication I am about to administer the medication I believe it is? Have I checked and rechecked the label to verify this? Is the medication current (not expired)? (p. 441)
2. Right patient refers to the necessity to confirm the medication belongs to the patient who will receive it. This is also another opportunity to be sure your indications are correct. (p. 441)
3. Right dose refers to how much of the medication you will administer. (p. 441)
4. Right route refers to how the medication will be administered and how the medication will enter the body. (p. 441)
5. Right time refers to ensuring that you have an appropriate indication to give the drug before giving it. Will the medication treat the patient's condition? (p. 441)

Critical Thinking

1. Student answers will vary. The typical manner in which an EMT in the field might contact medical direction is by way of radio or telephone. (p. 442)
2. Because IV drug administration is not typically in the EMT scope of practice, you should clarify the order and make sure the physician knows you are an EMT. You might question the route of administration and discuss alternatives that are within your scope of practice. (p. 443)
3. You should document the specific medication (including correct spelling). You should also document the dose, route, and time of administration. Finally, you should document any changes in the patient after administration including assessment findings and vital signs. (p. 442)

CHAPTER REVIEW *(p. 447)*

Multiple Choice

1. b (p. 443)
2. a (p. 427)
3. c (p. 431)
4. d (p. 443)
5. d (p. 441)

Matching

1. B (p. 427)
2. F (p. 426)
3. E (p. 441)
4. A (p. 442)
5. D (p. 442)
6. C (p. 427)

Critical Thinking

1. A side effect is an action that may be negative to the patient. A contraindication is a situation in which a medication should not be administered. (pp. 427, 442)
2. You should reassess the patient's condition. Look for any changes (especially those you would anticipate). Reassessment should also include repeating vital signs and comparing them to previous readings. (p. 433)
3. You may not use another person's inhaler. It could have been prescribed for very different reasons than the situation at hand. (p. 441)
4. Right medication: Is this the right medication for the patient's condition? Right dose: Am I giving the correct amount of medication? Right route: Am I giving the medication through the correct route? Right patient: Does this medication belong to the patient I am about to give it to? Right time: Is it the right time to give the medication? In other words should I wait a little longer before repeating a dose? (p. 441)

CASE STUDY

1. General Hospital, this is unit B533. We are on scene with a 67-year-old man with a chief complaint of chest pain that started approximately 10 minutes prior to our arrival while he was mowing his lawn. Patient states he has a history of angina, and he states his pain started as an 8 and is now a 5. Vitals are as follows: RR 20, GTV and slightly labored, HR 96 S/R, BP 124/86; skin is pale, cool, and moist. Request permission to administer a single dose of nitroglycerin for the chest pain. (pp. 442–443)
2. Common side effects from nitroglycerin include headache, drop in blood pressure, light headedness, dizziness, and increased heart rate. (p. 433)

Chapter 17

STOP, REVIEW, REMEMBER! *(p. 454)*

Multiple Choice

1. d (p. 452)
2. b (p. 452)
3. c (p. 452)
4. d (p. 452)
5. b (p. 452)
6. a (p. 452)

Fill in the Blank

1. oropharynx (p. 452)
2. alveoli (p. 452)
3. epiglottis (p. 452)
4. parietal, visceral (p. 452)
5. dead space (p. 452)
6. nose, mouth (p. 452)
7. trachea (p. 452)
8. carina (p. 452)

Critical Thinking

1. Air passes through the mouth and nose through the oropharynx and nasopharynx into the larynx. Air passes the epiglottis and enters the trachea through the vocal cords. Air travels from the trachea through the mainstem bronchi and into the bronchioles until air reaches the alveoli where gas exchange takes place. (p. 452)
2. The respiratory system obtains air from the environment, filters and warms it through the nose and mouth, and delivers it to the alveoli for exchange of gases. Oxygen is transferred to the cells while carbon dioxide is removed. (p. 452)
3. The medulla and pons are both responsible for inspiration and expiration as well as rate and depth of respirations. The medulla controls inspiration and expiration. Without this function we would constantly have to tell ourselves to breathe. The pons is responsible for coordinating the transition between inhalation and exhalation and defines the respiratory rate or prolonged inhalations. (p. 454)

STOP, REVIEW, REMEMBER! *(p. 469)*

Multiple Choice

1. b (p. 458)
2. d (p. 458)
3. d (p. 457 and Chapter 9, p. 222)
4. c (p. 461)
5. a (p. 464)
6. b (p. 464)
7. c (p. 465)
8. a (p. 468)
9. a (p. 468)
10. b (p. 464)

Fill in the Blank

1. onset, provocation, quality, radiation, severity, time (p. 459)
2. tell me what you were doing when the distress began (p. 459)

3. tripod (p. 457)
4. rate, depth (p. 457)
5. nonrebreather mask (pp. 457–458)

Critical Thinking

1. This can provide a significant amount of information for the current problem. For example, if a patient is complaining of respiratory distress and he has a history of emphysema and has prescribed medications, this is very pertinent. (p. 458)
2. The history generally provides the most information about a medical patient's condition. The onset of the symptoms, the description of the pain or distress, and the past history generally provide the most valuable information. (p. 458)
3. Epiglottitis is among one of the least common but most deadly respiratory conditions. It is a bacterial infection that causes excessive edema, which can obstruct the airway. Patients with epiglottitis, usually children, must be handled so as not to agitate them or force them into an uncomfortable position. Careful consideration should be taken before separating pediatric patients from their caregivers, which could upset them, thus increasing the chances of swelling and further obstructing the airway. The delivery of oxygen may also be challenging; administering by blow-by may be the best option. (pp. 457–458)

STOP, REVIEW, REMEMBER! *(p. 478)*

Multiple Choice

1. b (p. 474)
2. a (p. 474)
3. b (p. 458)
4. c (p. 474)
5. d (p. 475)

Fill in the Blank

1. small-volume nebulizer (p. 473)
2. medical direction (p. 475)
3. spacer (spacer device or aerochamber) (p. 475)
4. sitting (p. 471)
5. prescribed (p. 474)

Critical Thinking

1. Right patient, dose, medication, route, time. (p. 474)
2. You should administer oxygen to every patient with respiratory distress. A true hypoxic drive is rare. It is even rarer to "knock out" the patient's respiratory drive, especially in the relatively short time the patient is in the care of EMS. Give oxygen to patients who need it. (p. 461)

CHAPTER REVIEW *(p. 480)*

Multiple Choice

1. d (p. 463)
2. a (pp. 457–458)
3. c (p. 474 and Chapter 16, p. 437)
4. a (p. 452)
5. c (p. 471)
6. b (p. 474)
7. c (p. 466)
8. c (pp. 457–458)
9. d (p. 475)
10. c (p. 452)

Matching 1

1. B (p. 458)
2. C (p. 463)
3. D (p. 463)
4. A (p. 463)

Matching 2

1. A (pp. 457–458)
2. A (pp. 457–458)
3. B (p. 458)
4. B (p. 458)
5. B (p. 458)
6. A (pp. 457–458)
7. A (pp. 457–458)
8. A (pp. 457–458)
9. A (pp. 457–458)
10. A (pp. 457–458)

Critical Thinking

1. Remember that breathing requires adequate rate and depth. If breathing is very slow or very fast and shallow, the patient is moving so little air that it is not enough to support life (inadequate breathing). Ventilation with a bag-mask or pocket mask is necessary. (pp. 457–458)
2. A patient in severe respiratory distress will have some or all of the following signs that can be observed as you approach: increased work of breathing, tripod position, use of accessory muscles, pale skin, inability to speak in complete sentences. (p. 457)
3. Increasing the heart rate is one of the body's ways to compensate for hypoxia. (Note that infants and children often exhibit a slowed heart rate.) Because the body is short of oxygen, it tries to move more blood to increase oxygen distribution. The sweaty skin (often pale and cool) is a sign that the body is in significant distress and the nervous system is taking drastic actions to survive. (pp. 457–459)

CASE STUDIES

Case Study 1

1. Marie is breathing adequately based on her mental status, ability to speak long, full sentences and skin color. Obtaining an actual respiratory rate will also help confirm this decision. (pp. 458–460)
2. Marie would likely be a candidate for a nasal cannula. Her distress is not severe and this level of supplemental oxygen may be sufficient. If your protocols require it, a higher level of oxygen could be administered. (pp. 457–458)
3. If the husband falls, he could become a patient. You must prevent that. Your responsibility is not only to treat the patient, but you must also remain aware of the scene and control it. He is probably concerned about his wife and wants to help. Reassure him and tell him that you are helping Marie. Try to get him to sit down while you care for his wife. Speak to him throughout the call. Call for the nursing staff if necessary to help him around. (p. 457)
4. Marie has distress. It may be minimal, but it is distress. Complete a thorough assessment and begin transport. After giving the report to the hospital, you can ask medical direction if they believe it would benefit the patient to use the inhaler. If you have the ability to ease even minor distress, you should consider doing so. (p. 473)

Case Study 2

1. b (p. 457)
2. b (p. 473)

Case Study 3

1. c (p. 471)
2. b (p. 460)
3. a (Chapter 14, p. 402)

Chapter 18

STOP, REVIEW, REMEMBER! *(p. 495)*

Multiple Choice

1. c (p. 489)
2. b (p. 487)
3. b (p. 486)
4. a (pp. 493–494)
5. d (p. 495)

Fill in the Blank

1. Perfusion (p. 487)
2. atria (p. 487)
3. Automaticity (p. 487)
4. arteries, veins (pp. 488–489)
5. CPR, advanced care (p. 491)
6. angina, congestive heart failure (CHF) (p. 493)

Critical Thinking

1. You can evaluate a patient's perfusion status by assessing his mental status, vital signs, capillary refill, and skin signs. (p. 487)
2. When the heart becomes damaged from an MI, its ability to pump blood is compromised. This decrease in the heart's ability to pump blood is what affects perfusion and leads to the signs and symptoms of cardiac compromise. (pp. 493–493)
3. When a patient experiences an MI, a portion of the heart muscle (myocardium) is damaged. Angina results when blood flow to a portion of the heart is diminished but not cut off completely. (pp. 493–493)

STOP, REVIEW, REMEMBER! *(p. 504)*

Multiple Choice

1. b (p. 502)
2. b (p. 500)
3. c (p. 497)
4. a (p. 501)
5. d (p. 503)

Signs and Symptoms *(pp. 493–495)*

Condition	Signs	Symptoms	Treatment
Congestive heart failure	Pedal edema Sacral edema Jugular vein distention when sitting	Shortness of breath that may increase when lying down May have chest pain or discomfort	Take appropriate BSI precautions. Perform an appropriate primary assessment. Administer supplemental oxygen. Obtain a thorough SAMPLE history, using the OPQRST assessment mnemonic. Obtain a baseline set of vital signs. Perform a secondary assessment. Assist with the administration of the patient's prescribed nitroglycerin. (Follow local protocol.) Perform regular reassessments and adjust your care as appropriate. Transport as soon as practical and consider the need for an ALS backup or intercept.
Myocardial infarction	Fainting Vomiting	Chest, back, arm, or jaw pain not relieved by rest With angina, often relieved by rest Shortness of breath Nausea Dizziness Weakness Abdominal pain Fatigue Indigestion	Take appropriate BSI precautions. Perform an appropriate primary assessment. Administer supplemental oxygen. Obtain a thorough SAMPLE history, utilizing the OPQRST assessment mnemonic. Obtain a baseline set of vital signs. Perform an appropriate secondary assessment. Assist with the administration of the patient's prescribed nitroglycerin. (Follow local protocol.) Perform regular reassessments and adjust your care as appropriate. Transport as soon as practical and consider the need for an ALS backup or intercept.
Angina	Fainting Vomiting	Chest, back, arm, or jaw pain not relieved by rest With angina, often relieved by rest Shortness of breath Nausea Dizziness Weakness Abdominal pain Fatigue Indigestion	Take appropriate BSI precautions. Perform an appropriate primary assessment. Administer supplemental oxygen. Obtain a thorough SAMPLE history, utilizing the OPQRST assessment mnemonic. Obtain a baseline set of vital signs. Perform an appropriate secondary assessment. Assist with the administration of the patient's prescribed nitroglycerin. (Follow local protocol.) Perform regular reassessments and adjust your care as appropriate. Transport as soon as practical and consider the need for an ALS backup or intercept.

Critical Thinking

1. Edema is caused by an accumulation of fluids within the tissues. The fluid is backing up into the tissues as a result of a decrease in efficiency of the heart. Edema develops in the ankles in patients who are sitting for a long period of time because gravity pulls the fluid to the lowest part of the body. It accumulates in the sacral area of patients who are bedridden. (p. 497)
2. Cardiac arrest occurs when the heart stops pumping blood effectively. Myocardial infarction is when a portion of the heart dies due to lack of sufficient blood and oxygen. Most patients suffering an MI remain responsive and if they receive proper care in time will go on to survive the event. (pp. 493–494)
3. S–Can you describe the feeling that you are having? A–Do you have any allergies to medications that you know of? M–Are you currently taking any medications? P–Do you have any past medical history such as lung or heart problems, seizures, or diabetes? L–When and what did you last eat? E–What were the events that led up to you calling for an ambulance? (pp. 501–502)

STOP, REVIEW, REMEMBER! *(p. 509)*

Multiple Choice

1. c (p. 358)
2. c (p. 491)
3. d (p. 509 and Chapter 16, p. 433)
4. b (p. 509)
5. a (p. 509)

Fill in the Blank

1. prescription (p. 508)
2. expired (p. 508)
3. 24 to 72 (p. 509 and Chapter 16, p. 434)
4. systolic, 100 (p. 509)

Critical Thinking

1. Nitroglycerin is a smooth muscle relaxant, and causes the blood vessels to dilate thereby increasing the blood supply to the heart muscle and reducing the workload of the heart. (p. 506)
2. Because nitroglycerin is a potent vasodilator, the patient must have a blood pressure above 100 mmHg systolic prior to administration. This will minimize the chances that the patient may have an unacceptable drop in blood pressure. Another contraindication is if the patient has taken Viagra or other erectile dysfunction medication. Such medications cause the blood vessels to dilate and when taken in conjunction with nitroglycerin may cause a severe drop in blood pressure. (p. 509)

3. Providing supplemental oxygen to a patient presenting with cardiac compromise will increase the percentage of oxygen available to him and therefore compensate somewhat for the decrease caused by the compromise of the circulatory system. (p. 358)

STOP, REVIEW, REMEMBER! *(p. 514)*

Multiple Choice

1. d (p. 512)
2. c (p. 491)
3. a (p. 512)
4. a (p. 513)

Fill in the Blank

1. minimize or reduce (p. 509)
2. second (p. 491)
3. ventricular fibrillation (p. 512)
4. trauma (p. 514)

Critical Thinking

1. They are easy to operate because the software takes out all the guesswork. There is no need to have to interpret a heart rhythm; the device does it all. (p. 513)
2. Research has shown that the longer a patient who is in VF goes without a shock, the less their chances of survival. It is estimated that for every minute following collapse without a shock, there is a 10% less chance of survival. (p. 492)
3. AEDs use adhesive electrode pads that are clearly labeled as to the proper location and once placed they are used to analyze the rhythm and deliver the shocks. AEDs also interpret the patient's rhythm automatically with little or no input or training on behalf of the rescuer. (p. 513)

CHAPTER REVIEW *(p. 521)*

Multiple Choice

1. c (p. 489)
2. a (p. 508)
3. d (p. 509)
4. b (p. 497 and Chapter 16, p. 433)
5. b (p. 493)
6. c (p. 520)
7. c (p. 518)
8. a (p. 519)
9. a (p. 516)
10. d (p. 518)

Critical Thinking

1. A heart attack (myocardial infarction) occurs when a portion of the heart muscle dies due to an insufficient supply of well-oxygenated blood. In the majority of cases the heart-attack patient remains responsive and complains of chest pain or discomfort. In the case of cardiac arrest, the heart has stopped pumping blood effectively and the patient becomes unresponsive with no pulses and no breathing. Death will soon follow. (pp. 493–494)
2. As an EMT you will play an important part in the first three links in the chain. You may be the one calling 911 and you will be expected to perform CPR and attach an AED, if one is available. (p. 491)
3. Once the AED is turned on and the pads are properly placed, the fully automatic AED will analyze and deliver shocks as necessary without any further input from the operator. At a minimum, the semi-automatic AED requires the operator to press a button to initiate a shock and some require that a button be pressed to initiate the analyze phase as well. (p. 515)
4. The software that runs the AED will recognize ventricular fibrillation and rapid ventricular tachycardia as shockable rhythms. (pp. 512–513)
5. In most states, medical direction is required for the implementation of an AED program. The medical director must approve the policies, procedures, protocols, and training that are a part of every AED program. In addition, the medical director must review all cases where an AED has been used. (p. 520)

CASE STUDIES

Case Study 1

1. You must continue to ventilate this man at a rate of at least 10–12 breaths per minute. You should use a bag-mask device with supplemental oxygen and constantly monitor his pulse. (p. 501)
2. You must immediately begin CPR and attach the AED as soon as possible. Once the AED is attached, you must stop compressions and initiate the analyze phase of the AED. (pp. 513–514)
3. The AED will pause for two minutes while you resume CPR. Now is the time to get the patient on the stretcher and prepare for transport. (p. 518)

Case Study 2

1. The first thing is to place this man on supplemental oxygen by nonrebreather mask and call for ALS backup, if available. You need to complete a thorough SAMPLE history, including OPQRST. (p. 506)
2. Based on his presentation and history, this man appears to be a candidate for nitroglycerin. You have already confirmed that his systolic pressure is adequate. Confirm that the medication is his, that it has not expired, and that he has not taken any erectile dysfunction medications within the last 24 to 72 hours. (pp. 506–509)

Chapter 19

STOP, REVIEW, REMEMBER! *(p. 532)*

Multiple Choice

1. b (p. 526)
2. c (pp. 526–527)
3. a (p. 527)
4. d (p. 528)
5. c (p. 529)

Matching

1. B (p. 529)
2. C (p. 528)
3. A (p. 529)
4. E (p. 529)
5. D (pp. 528–529)

Critical Thinking

1. There is little the EMT can do for a patient who is actively seizing other than protect him from further harm. Restraining the patient may cause tissue or skeletal injuries. Move objects away from the patient and place something soft under his head to protect against injury. (p. 530)
2. Primary seizures are thought to be caused by genetic disorders or other unidentified causes. Secondary seizures are directly caused by a known source such as fevers, withdrawal, and head injury. (p. 529)

STOP, REVIEW, REMEMBER! *(p. 535)*

Multiple Choice

1. b (p. 533)
2. c (p. 535)
3. b (p. 534)
4. a (p. 534)

Short Answer

1. If you are with the patient during the event, help him to lie down. This will increase perfusion to the brain. After the event, encourage him to remain lying down to allow for circulation to return to normal. (p. 535)
2. Two common serious causes of syncope in older adults are a reaction from multiple medications and cardiac dysrhythmia. (p. 534)

Critical Thinking

1. The parasympathetic nervous system is responsible for a rapid dilation of blood vessels that results in a sudden drop in blood pressure and reduced perfusion to the brain. (pp. 533–534)

CHAPTER REVIEW *(p. 537)*

Multiple Choice

1. a (p. 529)
2. b (p. 529)
3. d (p. 534)
4. a (p. 530)
5. c (p. 527)
6. a (p. 526)

Short Answer

1. A febrile seizure is most common in small children and is caused by a rapid spike in fever. (p. 529)

2. Any four: dizziness, loss of vision, nausea, weakness, sweating (p. 533)

Critical Thinking

1. Care for the postictal patient includes assessing the airway (suction, if necessary), rolling the patient onto his side to allow for drainage of any secretions, administration of oxygen, performing a secondary assessment, and obtaining a medical history. (p. 530)
2. A patient may fall and strike his head or torso on any number of items, including the ground. Extra care should be taken to ensure proper spinal precautions when palpating the abdomen, chest, head, neck, and back. (p. 528)

CASE STUDY

1. I will carefully and gently control the patient's head and ask one of the friends for his jacket to place beneath the patient's head. I will direct one of the other friends to call 911 from his cell phone. I will instruct two of the others to go to the curb and flag down the responding units. (pp. 530–532)
2. Yes. Trying to restrain or inserting objects into the patient's mouth can cause unnecessary injury. It is best to remove any surrounding objects that the seizing person could injure himself on and place a soft item under his head. (pp. 530–532)
3. The first thing to check is the patient's airway. Make sure it is open and the patient is breathing. After that, address any other injuries. (pp. 530–532)

Chapter 20

STOP, REVIEW, REMEMBER! *(p. 545)*

Multiple Choice

1. b (pp. 542–544 and Chapter 12, p. 305)
2. d (p. 544)
3. a (p. 544)
4. c (p. 402)
5. d (p. 545)

Fill in the GCS Score

1. 4, 4, 5 (13) (p. 544)
2. 2, 2, 4 (8) (p. 544)
3. 1, 1, 1 (3) (p. 544)

Critical Thinking

1. Possible answers include, but are not limited to, the following: hypoglycemia, hyperglycemia, seizure, stroke, poisoning, trauma or significant blood loss, infection, kidney failure, psychosis, brain tumor, dementia, alcohol and drug abuse. (p. 542)
2. Patient history may confirm that mental status is "at baseline" in dementia patients, for example, but until proven otherwise a new onset of altered mental status should be treated as a medical emergency and considered a high priority for transport. (p. 541)
3. Patients should be positioned to maintain a patent airway. Placing the patient in the recovery position is often most effective. (pp. 544–545)

STOP, REVIEW, REMEMBER! *(p. 550)*

Multiple Choice

1. c (pp. 548–550)
2. b (p. 547)
3. a (p. 548)
4. d (p. 550)
5. d (p. 550)

Critical Thinking

1. An ischemic stroke occurs when blood flow to the brain is interrupted by a blocked artery. A hemorrhagic stroke occurs when the blood flow to the brain is interrupted by a ruptured artery. (pp. 548–550)
2. The range of stroke signs and symptoms include altered mental status, hemiparesis, hemiplegia, facial droop, difficulty swallowing, dysphasia, unequal or sluggish pupils, blurred or double vision, dizziness, loss of bowel or bladder control, and seizures. A transient ischemic attack (TIA) closely resembles those signs and symptoms but it usually resolves within 24 hours. Because TIA and stroke are indistinguishable in the early stages, all patients with stroke-like symptoms should be considered a high priority. (pp. 547–550)

CHAPTER REVIEW *(p. 556)*

Multiple Choice

1. b (pp. 548–549)
2. c (p. 552)
3. b (p. 553)
4. a (p. 553)
5. a (p. 555)
6. c (p. 553)
7. d (p. 550)
8. b (p. 545)
9. a (p. 545)
10. a (p. 215)

Critical Thinking

1. Quickly obtain a thorough history and assessment, record time of stroke symptom onset, obtain a blood glucose level, and support airway and ventilation as necessary. Proceed to nearest hospital designated as a stroke center, and provide early notification of possible stroke. (pp. 551–555)
2. The patient with a severe migraine requires a history and assessment, which includes a thorough pain assessment. Monitor the patient's airway and provide supplemental oxygen and seizure pads as necessary. Remove stimuli that may further aggravate migraine pain (such as noise and light). Provide supportive care and comfort and monitor for changes in mental status en route. (pp. 555–556)

CASE STUDIES

Case Study 1

1. Gather a SAMPLE history, specifically asking about hypertension. Also perform an OPQRST pain assessment and question if the patient experienced an aura prior to the headache. (p. 553)
2. Migraine (p. 555)
3. Reassessment with serial vital signs, and protect the patient from noise and light. Transport, continuing to monitor for changes in mental status. (pp. 555–556)

Case Study 2

1. Facial droop, arm drift, and abnormal speech (p. 552)
2. Symptoms are on the right side of her body; therefore, the stroke is likely located on the left side of her brain. (p. 553)
3. SAMPLE history, physical assessment with the Cincinnati Prehospital Stroke Scale, blood glucose check, serial vital signs, and continued monitoring for changes in neurological presentation and airway assessment during transport. Support airway and ventilation as appropriate and transfer to a stroke center, providing early notification of possible stroke. (pp. 551–555)

Chapter 21

STOP, REVIEW, REMEMBER! *(p. 564)*

Multiple Choice

1. c (p. 565)
2. d (p. 562)
3. d (p. 561)
4. c (p. 564)

Matching

1. C (p. 562)
2. A (p. 562)
3. D (p. 562)
4. B (p. 562)

STOP, REVIEW, REMEMBER! *(p. 576)*

Multiple Choice

1. b (p. 562)
2. c (pp. 574–576)
3. b (p. 567)
4. c (p. 564)
5. d (p. 570)
6. a (pp. 563–564)

Short Answer

1. Toxicology is defined as the study of the harmful interaction between humans and toxic substances. (p. 564)
2. The four portals of entry for toxins into the body are ingestion, absorption, injection, and inhalation. (p. 562)
3. The four general mechanisms by which inhaled poisons exert their toxic effects on the body are simple asphyxiants, chemical asphyxiants, physical particulates, and chemical irritants. (p. 569)

Critical Thinking

1. It is immediately evident that there is a large-scale chemical emergency that has the magnitude to render multiple victims in an unresponsive state. Despite the urge to help the patients, it would be appropriate to not enter the scene until it is rendered safe by a hazmat team. It is of critical importance that you radio a concise report of your

scene size-up to your dispatch and ensure that appropriate resources are responding to the scene. You should make certain that your unit is then staged upwind and at a safe distance away because it is reasonable to assume that the toxic agent involved may be airborne. (pp. 561, 563)

2. Fortunately, in this case the store manager is immediately able to identify the substance involved as dry lime. The patient will still need to be decontaminated prior to transport. Unlike many contaminants, dry lime should be brushed off, not washed off the contaminated patient. It is important to ensure that personnel do not expose themselves to the inhalation of dry lime while decontaminating the patient. (p. 574)

STOP, REVIEW, REMEMBER! *(p. 583)*

Multiple Choice

1. d (p. 582)
2. d (p. 581)
3. a (p. 581)
4. b (p. 579)
5. c (p. 574)

Short Answer

1. Salivation, lacrimation, urination, diarrhea, GI symptoms, emesis (p. 582)
2. Chest pain and loss of consciousness (p. 581)

Critical Thinking

1. The Mark 1 auto-injector should be used for the patient who is in severe respiratory distress because he is more likely to survive than the patient who has already suffered a cardiac arrest from the organophosphate poisoning. (p. 582)
2. Oxygen is the drug of choice for patients with carbon monoxide poisoning. It should be administered in the highest possible concentration by way of a nonrebreather mask at 10 to 15 L/minute. (p. 581)

CHAPTER REVIEW *(p. 585)*

Multiple Choice

1. c (p. 582)
2. b (p. 581)
3. b (p. 582)
4. d (p. 581)
5. a (p. 581)
6. d (p. 561)
7. b (p. 567)
8. a (pp. 567, 569)
9. d (p. 562)
10. b (p. 562)

Short Answer

1. Contaminated needles, weapons, potentially violent patients, intoxicated patients (p. 573)
2. Narcotics, organophosphates, nerve agents, cyanide, carbon monoxide (p. 582)
3. Inhalation, ingestion, absorption, injection (p. 562)
4. Visual hallucinations and profound disorientation (p. 579)
5. Initial signs and symptoms are restlessness, tremulous hands, elevated pulse, and elevated blood pressure as early as six to eight hours after cessation of chronic drinking. Over 24 to 48 hours the patient may develop seizures. After three to five days delirium tremens (DTs) may develop. (pp. 578–579)

Critical Thinking

1. Carbon monoxide (CO) asphyxiates the patient at the level of the cell by disrupting normal cell metabolism (a chemical asphyxiant). Carbon dioxide (CO_2) asphyxiates the patient by displacing oxygen in the atmosphere, not allowing the patient enough inhaled oxygen to survive (a simple asphyxiant). (pp. 570, 581)
2. Both patients with asthma and COPD have reactive airways that can go into bronchospasm when irritated by inhaled physical particulates, causing increased shortness of breath and wheezing (p. 569)

CASE STUDIES

Case Study 1

1. The patient cannot legally refuse treatment because his intoxication has resulted in the loss of his capacity to fully understand his situation and the risks of refusal. An EMT would never leave an intoxicated patient in the care of other intoxicated individuals. (Chapter 3, pp. 54–56)
2. The patient's active vomiting and evident facial trauma make securing a clear and open airway the highest and most evident priority during assessment. Suction should be immediately available to clear blood from his airway and be ready if he vomits again. (p. 564)
3. Intoxication may alter his ability to sense pain. In this case the patient has sustained an obvious significant facial impact and could potentially have a cervical-spine injury and deny any neck pain. So, in addition to careful monitoring of his airway and having suction equipment ready, patients who are intoxicated and have a significant mechanism of injury should be placed in a cervical collar and be fully immobilized on a long backboard, even if he reports no neck pain and has no neck tenderness on physical examination. (p. 578)

Case Study 2

1. Your inexperienced partner should never have pulled up directly in front of the call location. Knowing the call history of the location, it is appropriate to stage a safe distance from it until law enforcement arrives on scene and ensures safe entry. It is the responsibility of more experienced EMTs to educate and protect the well-being of less experienced providers. (pp. 563, 580)
2. Specific hazards you might expect to encounter on the scene include weapons, contaminated hypodermic needles, and irrational patients or bystanders secondary to drug intoxication. In addition, the building itself may not be structurally sound due to neglect. Thus, stairs and floor may be rotten and unsafe. (p. 572)
3. Knowing that supportive care is the basis of most toxicology-related emergencies, suctioning equipment, oxygen, bag-mask, and so on should always be brought to the potential overdose patient. In this specific case you also should be prepared to manage an injury, including a stab wound or gunshot wound. Finally, because of the second-floor location and the need to minimize time spent in the structure due to the multiple hazards on scene, you should bring in a stair chair or Reeves-type carrier to facilitate the extrication of the patient from the second floor. (p. 563)

Chapter 22

STOP, REVIEW, REMEMBER! *(p. 596)*

Multiple Choice

1. b (p. 593)
2. c (p. 593)
3. a (p. 595)
4. c (p. 594)
5. a (p. 592)

Matching

1. B (p. 593)
2. A (p. 593)
3. C (p. 593)
4. E (p. 593)
5. D (p. 593)

Critical Thinking

1. Hollow-organ pain usually results from peristaltic movement against an obstruction or from spasm of a hollow vessel. (p. 594)
2. Organs of the abdomen are rich in blood supply and generally vulnerable to trauma and to pathophysiologies that make bleeding likely. (p. 595)
3. Referred pain is felt in an area different from where the affected organ is located. (p. 594)

STOP, REVIEW, REMEMBER! *(p. 602)*

Multiple Choice

1. a (p. 598)
2. a (p. 598)
3. c (p. 598)
4. c (p. 599)
5. d (p. 600)

Critical Thinking

1. Scene assessment can provide valuable clues such as smells, medications, last meal, and alcohol. (p. 598)

2. Fast heart rate, tachypnea, absent pulses, pale skin, delayed capillary refill time. (p. 598)
3. Many abdominal-complaint patients will be sicker than they appear to be. Because their disorders present subtly, their status may not initially be identified. Furthermore, because of dynamic problems such as internal bleeding, patient status can rapidly worsen. (p. 598)
4. You would not complete a secondary assessment for a patient with an immediate life threat such as an esophageal bleed that compromises the airway. (p. 599)
5. A SAMPLE history can help identify patterns that point to specific abdominal disorders. (p. 601)

STOP, REVIEW, REMEMBER! *(p. 610)*

Multiple Choice

1. c (p. 594)
2. a (p. 594)
3. b (p. 608)
4. d (p. 607)
5. a (p. 609)

Critical Thinking

1. The first life threat of esophageal varices is profound blood loss. The second is bleeding into the airway. (p. 598)
2. Lower GI bleeds tend to show digested blood in the form of melena (unless bleeding is severe). Upper GI bleeds tend to show blood in vomit. (p. 606)
3. The pain is increased as the peristaltic motion of the intestine puts pressure on the obstructed area. (p. 608)
4. Unilateral, sharp pain in the lower abdominal quadrant, referred pain in the shoulder, and possibly shock and vaginal bleeding. (p. 595)
5. Gastroenteritis breaks down the inner lining of the stomach and intestine, which is responsible for absorption of water. (pp. 608–609)

CHAPTER REVIEW *(p. 612)*

Multiple Choice

1. a (p. 593)
2. b (p. 605)
3. a (pp. 608–609)
4. c (p. 605)
5. a (p. 609)
6. c (p. 607)
7. b (p. 595)

Fill in the Blank

1. parietal (p. 593)
2. spleen (p. 593)
3. endometritis (p. 609)

Critical Thinking

1. Liver, gall bladder, intestine (p. 593)
2. Acute myocardial infarction, pancreatitis (pp. 607, 609)
3. Abdominal aortic aneurysm (p. 606)
4. (a) Liver, intestine, gall bladder, kidney (retroperitoneal); (b) stomach, spleen, intestine, pancreas, kidney (retroperitoneal); (c) appendix, intestine, ovaries, fallopian tubes, uterus, bladder; (d) intestine, ovaries, fallopian tubes, uterus, bladder (p. 593)

CASE STUDY

1. Important immediate information would include history of the present illness and any past medical history, especially as it pertains to the vomiting of blood. How long has he felt this way? How much blood has he lost? (p. 601)
2. The most immediate assessment concern for this patient should be the primary assessment. Is his airway threatened, are there any concerns with breathing, and most importantly are there any signs of shock? (p. 598)
3. Tachypnea and tachycardia most likely indicate shock. (p. 605)
4. The most important treatment concern should be to initiate rapid transport because this patient likely has internal bleeding and is in shock. Other considerations should be a supine position if tolerated and oxygen if indicated. (p. 599)
5. Other assessment elements include the secondary assessment and reassessment. This patient seems to be very sick and can change rapidly. The secondary assessment, including both a comprehensive physical examination and a more thorough patient history, can help identify more subtle life threats. A vigilant reassessment would identify patient decompensation. (pp. 599, 604)

Chapter 23

STOP, REVIEW, REMEMBER! *(p. 624)*

Multiple Choice

1. a (p. 622)
2. d (p. 623)
3. c (p. 623)
4. b (p. 617)
5. a (p. 618)

Matching

1. D (p. 617)
2. E (p. 619)
3. B (p. 623)
4. A (p. 622)
5. C (p. 620)

Critical Thinking

1. Without an adequate supply of insulin, glucose will remain in the bloodstream and continue to increase in concentration causing hyperglycemia. Insulin acts as the "bridge" that allows glucose to cross over from the blood to the tissues and cells where it can be used for energy. (p. 619)
2. Hypoglycemia has a faster onset and begins with an altered mental status, and then signs similar to shock. Hyperglycemia has a much slower onset and presents with altered mental status, abdominal pain, ketone smell on the breath, and rapid deep respirations. (pp. 622–623)
3. Insulin is produced by the pancreas in response to high blood-glucose levels and glucagon is produced in response to low blood glucose levels. (p. 619)

STOP, REVIEW, REMEMBER! *(p. 628)*

Multiple Choice

1. b (p. 619)
2. d (p. 620)
3. a (p. 622)
4. b (p. 627)
5. c (p. 627)

Fill in the Blank

1. 80 to 120 (p. 620)
2. polyuria, polydipsia, polyphagia (p. 619)
3. Hyperglycemia, hypoglycemia (pp. 622–623)

Critical Thinking

1. When glucose levels get too high, the sympathetic nervous system response is to release epinephrine. This release causes shock-like signs such as increased pulse, pale skin, and sweating. (p. 622)
2. Hyperglycemia is an abnormally elevated blood glucose level, which can be easily treated by hospital personnel. If hyperglycemia is left untreated, it can lead to diabetic ketoacidosis during which the body begins to burn fat instead of glucose. (p. 623)
3. The care should begin with a primary assessment to ensure a patent airway and adequate breathing. Then you will perform a secondary assessment and history. Provide supportive care, place in the recovery position, and provide oxygen. If the patient is responsive, you may administer oral glucose. Follow local protocols. (p. 626)

CHAPTER REVIEW *(p. 630)*

Multiple Choice

1. c (p. 623)
2. a (p. 622)
3. d (p. 626)
4. c (p. 627)
5. d (p. 620)
6. c (p. 627)
7. a (p. 625)
8. b (p. 620)
9. c (p. 626)
10. b (p. 620)

Critical Thinking

1. The diabetic patient who is hyperglycemic will become dehydrated due to fluid loss that accompanies the elimination of glucose in the urine. The body rids itself of the excess glucose by dumping it into the urine. The glucose carries with it large amounts of water making the patient dehydrated. Thus the patient urinates a lot and tries to replace the fluid by drinking more. (p. 618)
2. The primary concern with any patient who has an altered mental status is ensuring a patent airway. This is why it is contraindicated to give a diabetic patient with an altered mental status oral glucose. (p. 626)

CASE STUDIES

Case Study 1

1. Since you already know that the man is diabetic, you will want to try to determine if the man has taken his insulin today and if so, when. You will also want to know if he has had anything at all to eat and if so, what and when. (p. 626)
2. Based on the fact that he is a diabetic, that he has taken his insulin, and that he has had nothing to eat, he is very likely suffering an episode of hypoglycemia. (p. 622)
3. Begin by establishing a baseline set of vitals. Then you can provide him with oral glucose. Provide glucose or a similar substance only if he is able to swallow and is capable of managing his own airway. Provide supplemental oxygen and transport. (p. 626)

Case Study 2

1. You must manage this patient's airway and breathing before moving on to a secondary assessment. Suction the airway, attempt to insert an airway adjunct, and initiate supplemental oxygen. (p. 626)
2. Because this patient is a type 1 diabetic, she most likely takes daily injections of insulin. You will want to know if she took her medication today and what she has had to eat in the past 12 hours or so. You will also want to know if the family obtained a blood glucose level before your arrival. (p. 626)
3. Based on the fact that she is unresponsive with rapid deep respirations, she is most likely suffering from a severe case of hyperglycemia. You should smell her breath for the presence of a sweet (acetone) smell indicating diabetic ketoacidosis. (p. 623)

Chapter 24

STOP, REVIEW, REMEMBER! *(p. 639)*

Multiple Choice

1. b (p. 635)
2. c (p. 636)
3. a (p. 638)
4. d (p. 639)
5. a (pp. 636–637)

Fill in the Blank

1. Allergic reactions (p. 635)
2. allergens (p. 635)
3. Mild reactions (pp. 636–637)
4. anaphylaxis (p. 638)
5. anaphylactic shock (p. 638)

Critical Thinking

1. Allergens are substances foreign to the body that can cause an exaggerated response by the body's immune system, resulting in a reaction that can range from mild and localized to a severe reaction affecting the entire body. (p. 635)
2. A mild reaction usually involves some localized swelling at the site of injury but does not involve a systemic reaction. A severe reaction (anaphylaxis) is characterized by swelling to the face, neck, throat, tongue, hands, and/or feet as well as tightness in the chest and difficulty breathing. If not treated promptly, anaphylaxis can be life threatening. (pp. 636–638)
3. There are two primary mechanisms at work during an anaphylactic reaction. The exaggerated immune response is causing the blood vessels to dilate while causing the airway passages to constrict. As the blood vessels dilate, blood pressure drops, which decreases the perfusion to the brain and other vital organs. At the same time, the body is struggling to bring in an adequate supply of oxygen because the air passages are progressively getting smaller. (pp. 638–639)

CHAPTER REVIEW *(p. 649)*

Multiple Choice

1. d (pp. 643–644)
2. b (p. 642)
3. c (p. 643)
4. d (p. 644)
5. b (pp. 638–639)
6. b (pp. 638–639)
7. b (pp. 638–639)
8. b (p. 647)
9. a (p. 638)
10. b (pp. 638–639)

Critical Thinking

1. The care for a patient with a mild reaction must include a thorough secondary assessment and history to ensure that the patient has not experienced a severe reaction in the past. Often a cool gauze or ice pack will help with the pain, swelling, and itching. The patient must be observed for and informed of the signs of a severe reaction before being allowed to go about his way, if he does not want to be transported. A patient with signs of a severe reaction must receive supplemental oxygen and rapid transport. The use of an Epi-Pen may be indicated, if allowed by local protocols. (pp. 643–644)
2. Epinephrine acts on the blood vessels by causing them to constrict, thus helping to maintain an adequate blood pressure. It acts on the airways, causing them to dilate, making it easier for the patient to breathe. (p. 644)
3. Immediately following the administration of epinephrine the patient should be closely observed for indications of improvement in his condition. If the patient responds well to the medication, he will become more responsive and breathing will be easier. It should be noted that epinephrine is rather short acting (10 to 20 minutes) and transport should not be delayed even if the patient is showing signs of improvement. (pp. 644–647)

CASE STUDIES

Case Study 1

1. Your first concern for this woman given her history and presentation will be to ensure that she has a clear airway and adequate breathing. (p. 643)
2. Given that her rate is only 10 per minute and shallow, this woman will need supplemental oxygen via nonrebreather mask at a minimum. You must watch her respiratory status carefully and if her rate drops anywhere below 10 per minute, you will have to assist her with manual ventilations using a bag-mask device. (p. 643)
3. Questions such as: Does she have any known history of allergic reactions in the past? If so, to what? Does she have an Epi-Pen prescribed to her and if so, where is it? Did anyone see what may have caused the bite/sting? Does she have any past pertinent medical history? (p. 642)

Case Study 2

1. You will want to assess his respiratory status for adequate rate and tidal volume as well as his mental status and any signs of shock. (pp. 641–642)
2. Based on his presentation and the fact that it has been nearly 30 minutes since he was stung, it appears that this patient is only experiencing a mild allergic reaction. He has no signs of respiratory distress, shock, or altered mental status. (p. 636)
3. There is no reason why you should not transport this patient, since the parents are insisting. You must follow local protocol in this instance. To be on the safe side it would be appropriate to transport him with one parent in the ambulance and ask the other parent to follow behind in his or her own car. You can provide supplemental oxygen to the patient, if he will tolerate it. Closely monitor for signs of shock or respiratory distress during transport. (p. 642)

Chapter 25

STOP, REVIEW, REMEMBER! *(p. 659)*

Multiple Choice

1. d (p. 658)
2. b (p. 658)
3. c (p. 656)
4. d (p. 657)
5. b (p. 659)

Short Answer

1. Any three: stroke, loss of spleen, chest syndrome, sickle cell pain crisis, priapism, jaundice (p. 658)

2. Any two: advanced liver disease, hemophilia, von Willebrand's disease (p. 655)
3. Any two: chronic gastrointestinal bleeding, chronic heavy menstrual periods, diseases of the bone marrow (p. 657)

Critical Thinking

1. Patients with SCA suffer from destruction of their spleen over time. Since the spleen is crucial in immune system function, these patients are more prone to certain types of infection. (p. 658)
2. The body's clotting factors are made in the liver. Patients with advanced liver disease cannot manufacture normal amounts of clotting factors so they often suffer from coagulopathies. (p. 656)

STOP, REVIEW AND REMEMBER! *(p. 667)*

Multiple Choice

1. b (p. 663)
2. c (p. 661)
3. c (p. 660)
4. a (p. 665)
5. c (p. 663)

Matching

1. C (p. 663)
2. D (p. 661)
3. E (p. 666)
4. B (p. 663)
5. A (p. 665)

Fill in the Blank

1. Pyelonephritis (p. 661)
2. bacterial infection (p. 661)

Short Answer

1. Turbid, like chicken broth (p. 666)
2. The vibration felt over a dialysis access site on the extremity (p. 663)

Critical Thinking

1. UTIs are more common in female patients because the relatively short length of their urethra puts them at greater risk for bacterial invasion of the bladder. (p. 661)
2. Acute renal failure can be reversed if caught in time and the underlying insult to the kidneys is controlled. Chronic renal failure is not reversible and results in the patient needing dialysis in order to survive. (pp. 661, 663)
3. Complications of missed dialysis include fluid overload and the buildup of excessive potassium in the bloodstream. Signs and symptoms include edema of the body, shortness of breath due to fluid accumulation in the lungs, and palpitations or even sudden death due to the effect of high potassium on the heart. (p. 665)

CHAPTER REVIEW *(p. 670)*

Multiple Choice

1. b (p. 654)
2. a (p. 655)
3. c (pp. 663, 665)
4. c (p. 655)
5. a (p. 658)
6. b (p. 655)
7. c (p. 655)
8. a (p. 668)
9. d (p. 663)
10. c (pp. 661, 663)

Short Answer

1. SCA is a genetic disorder that affects the structure of red blood cells, giving them a characteristic "C" or sickle shape. (p. 658)
2. Sludging in patients with SCA is due to the inability of sickle-shaped red blood cells to pass easily in small blood vessels, causing them to pile up and sludge. (p. 668)
3. Anemia is an abnormally low number of red blood cells in the circulation. (p. 657)
4. A kidney stone is a small rock-like mass that develops in the kidney. (p. 661)
5. Patients of African descent are most likely to have the sickle cell gene. (p. 657)

Critical Thinking

1. Signs and symptoms of fluid overload seen in both renal failure patients and patients with congestive heart failure include edema and swelling of the ankles, shortness of breath, coarse breath sounds at the bases of the lungs on auscultation, jugular vein distention, and inability to lie flat without increased shortness or breath. (p. 665)
2. Yes, because Plavix is a medication that inhibits normal clotting, this patient with a head injury is at high risk for intracranial bleeding. She should be transported to a trauma center. (p. 656)
3. Patients with sickle cell disease are more prone to strokes than other patients due to the potential for sludging of red cells in the brain's blood supply, blocking adequate blood flow. (p. 658)
4. Because SCA destroys the patient's spleen, they are at increased risk for serious infections because the protective immune function of the spleen is gone. (p. 658)

CASE STUDIES

Case Study 1

1. I disagree with my partner. Patients with SCA do frequently have narcotic addiction problems, but this is because of their frequent and extremely painful sickle cell crises. All sickle cell patients with pain are presumed to be having a sickle cell crisis and should be treated accordingly. (p. 658)
2. The patient should be placed on supplemental oxygen and transported to the hospital. You should discuss your concerns with your partner after the call is completed to educate him about sickle cell anemia. (p. 658)

Case Study 2

1. Perform a primary assessment to look for immediate life threats. (p. 666)
2. Patients on hemodialysis are prone to both complications of their dialysis (such as infections in their bloodstream) as well as complications of their underlying diseases such as diabetes (prone to high and low blood sugars and stroke) and hypertension (prone to stroke). (p. 666)
3. Obtain full vitals signs and perform a secondary assessment. (p. 666)
4. Place the patient on supplemental oxygen and monitor for development of inadequate breathing, which may require ventilations. (p. 666)
5. Your assessment as an EMT is that this patient is having an acute, potentially life-threatening medical emergency. You should inform the staff of your assessment and plan for emergency transport to an emergency department, not to dialysis. If there is further conflict with the facility staff, contact medical direction for assistance. (p. 666)

Chapter 26

STOP, REVIEW, REMEMBER! *(p. 682)*

Multiple Choice

1. c (p. 678)
2. b (p. 679)
3. b (pp. 677–678)
4. d (p. 677)
5. a (p. 681)

Short Answer

1. A situation in which a patient's behavior becomes intolerable, dangerous, or bizarre enough to cause the concern of family, bystanders, or the patient (p. 677)
2. Hypoxia, hypoglycemia, stroke, infection, brain injury (p. 677)
3. Single, widowed, or divorced; depression; substance abuse; suicide plan; experienced prior suicide; previous attempts (p. 680)

Critical Thinking

1. (a) A medical history of diabetes or seizures may be uncovered. (b) The patient may be on medications that can cause the problem if stopped or taken in excess. (c) The patient may have a history of psychiatric problems. (d) Vital signs may show signs of medical or traumatic conditions. (pp. 677–678)
2. The exact words will be up to you. Everyone may say something a little different. Respect that the patient is in distress and do not downplay the situation. An example may be: "I can help take care of you and will treat you well. I can see you have a lot going on and I want to help." (p. 681)

STOP, REVIEW, REMEMBER! *(p. 690)*

Multiple Choice

1. a (p. 685)
2. b (p. 684)
3. c (p. 688)
4. a (p. 684)
5. b (p. 685)

Short Answer

1. Person over 18 who is alert and oriented and capable of understanding consequences (p. 687)
2. Unusual or bizarre behavior indicating a lack of touch with reality (p. 679)
3. Restraints made of soft materials unlikely to cause harm in the process of restraining the patient (p. 688)

Critical Thinking

1. (a) Place an oxygen mask or surgical mask on his face. (b) Don eye and face protection for yourself. (pp. 676–677)
2. When a patient realizes what may happen, he may reconsider and comply. Secondly, the patient must know what you are doing. By explaining, the patient may be less anxious and combative and if he chooses to cooperate, he can. (p. 688)
3. Positional asphyxia as it applies to EMS is the death of a patient while restrained. It can be prevented by restraining a patient face up, and through constant monitoring of the patient's respirations and mental status. (pp. 688–689)

CHAPTER REVIEW *(p. 693)*

Multiple Choice

1. a (p. 688)
2. b (p. 678)
3. d (p. 689)
4. c (p. 679)
5. d (p. 689)

Matching

1. F (p. 678)
2. A (p. 679)
3. E (p. 679)
4. D (p. 679)
5. B (p. 679)
6. C (p. 679)

Critical Thinking

1. While some patients may end up requiring restraint, there is a wide variety of interpersonal techniques that can calm patients and help prevent the need for restraint. This is always the goal (along with safety). You should disagree with the statement. (p. 688)
2. The history and physical exam will be the key. Determine if the patient is up to date on medications and has eaten, and use a blood glucose monitor if you are allowed to do so. Observe the patient for signs of hypoglycemia such as diaphoresis. (p. 677)
3. No. Let the police enter first. Explain to the parent why you are waiting. Take the time to be sure you are in a safe position and to obtain a history of the events today. (p. 684)

CASE STUDY

1. Conduct a mental status examination. Attempt to identify the patient's medical history. Identify any medications that the patient may be taking. (pp. 677–678)
2. Delusions are false beliefs such as being a famous or religious figure. (p. 679)
3. Warning signs of escalation include a change in voice or speech, pacing, violent hand movements, or other increased patient activity. (p. 687)
4. A firm but respectful attitude is often successful in this situation. Patients in crisis often respond positively to structure. (p. 686)

Chapter 27

STOP, REVIEW, REMEMBER! *(p. 709)*

Multiple Choice

1. a (p. 702)
2. b (p. 699)
3. b (p. 703)
4. a (p. 707)
5. d (p. 705)

Short Answer

1. Treat for shock. Apply absorbent pads, do not insert anything into the vagina, consider possible causes. (p. 703)
2. Increase in size of uterus, changing hormone levels, breast size increase, cessation of menstrual cycle (pp. 699–700)
3. Death of the fetus, often accompanied by bleeding, infection, and expulsion of the fetus (pp. 705–706)

Critical Thinking

1. If at all possible, you do not want a woman who has been the victim of a possible sexual assault to use the toilet or clean herself. This will eliminate or destroy possible evidence. You must use your best bedside manner and compassionately explain the reason for not allowing her to use the toilet or shower. (p. 704)
2. The general care for soft-tissue injuries is the same, no matter where on the body it occurs. However, when these injuries involve the genitalia, you must remain very aware of the patient's modesty and maintain a high degree of privacy for the patient while properly managing the injury. (p. 704)

STOP, REVIEW, REMEMBER! *(p. 718)*

Multiple Choice

1. b (p. 712)
2. d (p. 700)
3. c (p. 711)
4. c (p. 711)
5. c (p. 712)

Sorting

1. 1 (p. 711)
2. 3 (p. 711)
3. 2 (p. 711)
4. 2 (p. 711)
5. 1 (p. 711)
6. 1 (p. 711)

Critical Thinking

1. When is your due date? Did your waters break? Do you feel the urge to push? Are you aware of any complications with this pregnancy? How far apart are your contractions? (p. 712)
2. Take control of the scene and ask all nonessential bystanders to leave. Remove the mother's pants and underwear. Position her appropriately, open the OB kit, and place clean drapes over the mother and under her buttocks. (p. 714)

STOP, REVIEW, REMEMBER! *(p. 727)*

Multiple Choice

1. a (p. 727)
2. d (p. 724)
3. c (p. 724)
4. a (p. 707)
5. d (p. 725)

Short Answer

1. You must prepare for the delivery and care of two infants. It is best to have one rescuer available to care for each infant delivered just in case resuscitation is necessary. (p. 713)
2. At 32 weeks the infant is still considered premature. Premature infants are at high risk for complications, so you must prepare to resuscitate the infant immediately following delivery. (p. 726)
3. It is not possible to deliver a breech baby in the field. You must transport immediately to the nearest hospital. (p. 725)
4. Prenatal care is an important part of identifying potential problems with the infant or the delivery ahead of time. A mother who has not had prenatal care has no idea about the condition or position of the infant. It is best to transport this patient to the nearest hospital rather than attempt a field delivery. (p. 713)

Critical Thinking

1. Appearance—the color of the baby; pulse—obtain a pulse rate; grimace—response to irritation; activity—is the baby moving; respirations—what is the respiratory rate? (p. 720)
2. (p. 721)

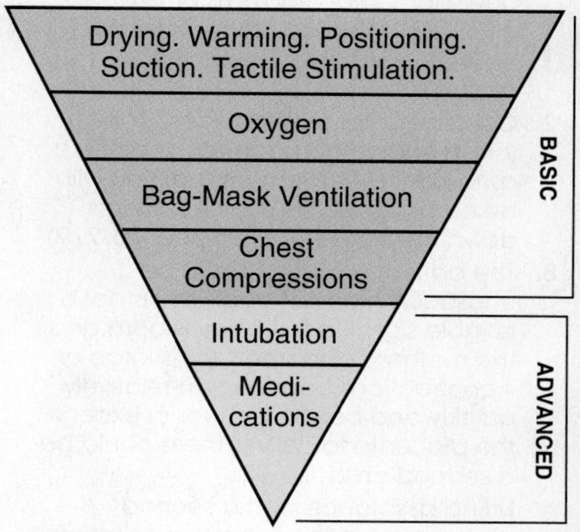

CHAPTER REVIEW *(p. 730)*

Multiple Choice

1. a (p. 714)
2. b (p. 702)
3. c (p. 722)
4. a (p. 717)
5. c (p. 722)

Matching

1. D (p. 727)
2. E (p. 725)
3. I (p. 707)
4. C (p. 726)
5. B (p. 726)
6. A (p. 723)
7. F (p. 725)
8. H (p. 707)

Critical Thinking

1. Many mothers have prenatal care. Prenatal care includes regular visits to an obstetrician and ultrasounds to determine the number of infants and in some cases birth defects. Prenatal care will usually mean that the mother will be aware of her estimated due date. Obtaining this information in the history is crucial to determine whether additional resources will be needed, if the baby will be premature or will possibly require resuscitation. (p. 726)
2. Newborns have a greater surface area than adults, do not have the fat layers for insulation, have minimal temperature regulation abilities, and they are born wet, which can cause evaporation and significant cooling. (p. 717)
3. Gloves, face protection, gown; drapes to cover the mother; clamps or ties for the umbilical cord; scissors to cut the umbilical cord; towels to dry the newborn, and also may include bag for the placenta, absorbent pads to place under the mother, and bulb syringes for suction of the newborn. (p. 714)

CASE STUDY

1. Maria could be expecting twins or triplets, or experiencing premature labor. The baby may also have developmental problems or positioning that could complicate delivery and subsequent care. (p. 713)
2. Call for additional resources. Call for an engine company or another ambulance. Remember that you will be carrying two (or more) patients down the stairs—not just one. (p. 719)
3. The patient may appear to be unusually large although this is not a reliable sign. If a first baby is born and the mother's abdomen still is large or if contractions begin again relatively quickly and before you would expect the placenta to deliver, there could be a second child. (p. 726)
4. Lifting assistance and a second ambulance in the event resuscitation of the newborn is needed. Multiple births would increase the personnel needed because you will now have three (or more) patients. (p. 726)

Module 3

REVIEW AND PRACTICE EXAMINATION

1. d (p. 426) Objective 16-3
2. a (p. 426) Objective 16-3
3. c (p. 426) Objective 16-5
4. b (p. 427) Objective 16-7
5. c (p. 427) Objective 16-10
6. a (p. 443) Objective 16-8
7. a (p. 432) Objective 16-7
8. c (p. 474) Objective 17-14
9. d (p. 460) Objective 17-5
10. d (p. 461) Objective 17-6
11. c (p. 464) Objective 17-10
12. d (p. 458) Objective 17-11
13. a (p. 475) Objective 17-13
14. d (p. 463) Objective 17-9
15. a (p. 457) Objective 17-3
16. c (p. 487) Objective 18-3
17. b (p. 509) Objective 18-6
18. a (p. 493) Objective 18-8
19. c (p. 493) Objective 18-8
20. b (p. 493) Objective 18-8
21. a (p. 497) Objective 18-8
22. d (pp. 508–509) Objective 18-13
23. b (p. 622) Objective 23-6
24. b (p. 622) Objective 23-5
25. c (p. 526) Objective 19-2
26. c (p. 528) Objective 19-8
27. d (p. 548) Objective 20-8
28. d (p. 553) Objective 19-12
29. c (p. 543) Objective 20-7
30. c (p. 569) Objective 21-2
31. b (p. 562) Objective 21-3
32. a (p. 563) Objective 21-4
33. b (p. 564) Objective 21-5
34. c (p. 563) Objective 21-8
35. a (p. 574) Objective 21-11
36. d (p. 573) Objective 21-13
37. c (p. 571) Objective 21-14
38. c (p. 593) Objective 22-2
39. b (p. 595) Objective 22-4
40. b (p. 592) Objective 22-3
41. a (p. 598) Objective 22-6
42. d (p. 605) Objective 22-6
43. a (p. 609) Objective 22-8
44. c (p. 606) Objective 22-5
45. a (pp. 638–639) Objective 24-6
46. c (p. 645) Objective 24-10
47. b (p. 655) Objective 25-2
48. a (p. 654) Objective 25-2
49. a (p. 655) Objective 25-4
50. c (p. 657) Objective 25-5
51. c (p. 656) Objective 25-6
52. b (p. 657) Objective 25-7
53. a (p. 658) Objective 25-8
54. a (p. 660) Objective 25-10
55. d (pp. 660–661) Objective 25-11
56. b (p. 661) Objective 25-12
57. b (p. 663) Objective 25-13
58. c (p. 666) Objective 25-16
59. a (p. 665) Objective 25-15
60. b (p. 679) Objective 26-5
61. d (p. 681) Objective 26-8
62. c (p. 687) Objective 26-5
63. d (p. 711) Objective 27-8
64. c (p. 714) Objective 27-8
65. b (p. 721) Objective 27-14
66. d (p. 707) Objective 27-11
67. c (p. 512) Objective 18-17
68. b (pp. 513–514) Objective 18-16
69. a (p. 516) Objective 18-16
70. a (p. 699) Objective 27-1
71. c (p. 702) Objective 27-2
72. d (p. 702) Objective 27-3
73. b (p. 702) Objective 27-3
74. b (p. 703) Objective 27-5
75. a (p. 711) Objective 27-6
76. c (p. 711) Objective 27-6
77. a (p. 725) Objective 27-7
78. b (p. 722) Objective 27-9)
79. a (p. 724) Objective 27-11
80. d (p. 725) Objective 27-11
81. a (p. 717) Objective 27-13
82. c (p. 721) Objective 27-15
83. a (p. 721) Objective 27-15
84. d (p. 722) Objective 27-15
85. b (p. 721) Objective 27-15

Chapter 29

STOP, REVIEW, REMEMBER! *(p. 756)*

Multiple Choice

1. b (p. 751)
2. a (p. 750)
3. b (p. 754)
4. c (p. 753)
5. d (p. 753)

Fill in the Blank

1. Trauma (p. 750)
2. well-oxygenated (p. 751)
3. mental status (p. 751)
4. hypoperfusion (p. 751)
5. chest (p. 754)

Critical Thinking

1. The mechanism of injury is one of the first indicators for possible internal injury and bleeding. When the mechanism of injury is significant enough and involves areas such as the chest, abdomen, and pelvis, you must maintain a high index of suspicion for internal bleeding. (p. 755)
2. Internal bleeding occurs deep within the body and is concealed from view by the skin. For this reason patients can lose a significant amount of blood without realizing it and thus may die before they can receive the necessary care. (p. 754)
3. Anxiety, anxiousness, confusion, altered mental status, increasing pulse rate, increased respiratory rate, decreasing blood pressure, skin that is pale, cool, and clammy, and history of significant MOI. (p. 755)

CHAPTER REVIEW *(p. 765)*

Multiple Choice

1. c (p. 751)
2. a (p. 762)
3. b (p. 760)
4. c (p. 762)
5. a (pp. 762, 764)
6. d (p. 754)
7. b (p. 755)
8. d (p. 753)
9. a (p. 757)
10. d (p. 757)

Matching

1. F (p. 760)
2. C (p. 753)
3. A (p. 753)
4. D (p. 753)
5. E (p. 753)
6. B (p. 760)

Critical Thinking

1. When a patient loses enough blood, the blood pressure drops and can no longer perfuse the tissues with an adequate supply of well-oxygenated blood. In addition, the waste products from the cells cannot be adequately removed. This causes a decrease in cell function, which in turn causes the affected organ systems to fail resulting in the death of the patient. (p. 760)
2. The body is capable of compensating well for the loss of blood up to a point. During the compensatory phase, the increase in pulse rate and redistribution of fluids into the core can maintain a normal blood pressure for some time. Late in the process when so much blood is lost that the body can no longer compensate, a major drop in blood pressure occurs. (pp. 751, 760)
3. The signs and symptoms of internal bleeding and those of shock are essentially the same. With internal bleeding you may have additional signs such as blood in the vomit or in the stool. (p. 755)

CASE STUDIES

Case Study 1

1. The fact that this man suffered blunt trauma to the chest and now is showing signs and symptoms of shock is a strong indication that he may be bleeding internally. (p. 755)
2. You should get this man into a supine position, place him on supplemental oxygen, and get a baseline set of vital signs. You also should maintain a comfortable body temperature and transport him immediately. (p. 762)
3. Based on his deteriorating condition, this man should be considered unstable and therefore should receive reassessments every five minutes. (p. 762)

Case Study 2

1. This boy has a clear history of trauma as well as obvious signs of injury (abrasions) to his left abdomen. His pulse is rapid and weak and his breathing rate is elevated. He is nauseous and vomiting. (p. 755)
2. The fact that this boy has what is likely a normal blood pressure for his age and that his skin still appears normal are signs that his body is still in the compensatory state of shock. (p. 760)
3. In the upper left abdomen is part of the liver, the spleen, the pancreas, and the stomach. The lower left quadrant contains mostly the small intestine. (p. 592)

Chapter 30

STOP, REVIEW, REMEMBER! *(p. 775)*

Multiple Choice

1. b (p. 771)
2. a (p. 773)
3. c (p. 771)
4. d (p. 775)
5. c (p. 775)

Fill in the Blank

1. Perfusion (p. 751)
2. vital signs (p. 751)
3. moist (p. 789)
4. left ventricle (p. 771)
5. internal (p. 773)

Critical Thinking

1. Perfusion is directly related to blood pressure. Assuming all other factors (breathing and heart rate) are functioning properly, a person with a good blood pressure will be perfusing well. (pp. 770–771)
2. A patient who is not perfusing well will have signs and symptoms of shock that include an altered mental status, increased pulse rate, increased breathing rate, and eventually a dropping blood pressure. (p. 770)
3. Being able to assess external blood loss is similar to evaluating the mechanism of injury for a trauma patient. It will provide valuable information as to the amount of blood loss and therefore allow you to make a better determination of the severity of the patient's condition. (p. 775)

STOP, REVIEW, REMEMBER! *(p. 785)*

Multiple Choice

1. a (p. 777)
2. c (p. 777)
3. b (p. 778)
4. d (p. 778)
5. c (p. 787)

Fill in the Blank

1. Arteries (p. 777)
2. capillaries (p. 778)
3. dark (p. 777)
4. elevating (p. 778)
5. proximal (p. 780)

Critical Thinking

1. Bleeding from arteries is often more difficult to control because the pressure in arteries is much greater than that of veins or capillaries. This pressure makes it difficult for an adequate clot to form at the injury site. The control of arterial bleeding often requires the combination of direct pressure, elevation (if possible), and a tourniquet (only for life-threatening bleeding). (p. 777)
2. A pressure dressing is used to help control bleeding that is not easily managed by direct pressure and elevation alone. By placing a pressure dressing over the wound it will free up your hands should you need to apply a tourniquet later. (pp. 779–780)
3. Anytime you are placing a bandage completely around a limb (circumferentially), there is the possibility of creating a tourniquet effect and cutting off all blood flow past the bandage. This is especially true when applying pressure dressings. Be sure to assess circulation, sensation, and motor function before and after application of a pressure dressing. Consider loosening the bandage if circulation is lost following application. (p. 780)

CHAPTER REVIEW *(p. 790)*

Multiple Choice

1. d (p. 777)
2. a (p. 778)
3. c (p. 780)
4. d (p. 788)
5. d (p. 774)
6. a (p. 775)
7. c (p. 775)
8. a (p. 777)
9. b (p. 778)
10. c (p. 780)

Matching

1. F (p. 773)
2. C (p. 773)
3. E (p. 773)
4. A (p. 773)
5. G (p. 773)
6. B (p. 778)
7. D (p. 778)

Critical Thinking

1. Large wounds have the potential to cause arterial, venous, and capillary bleeding. In most cases treat for the worst and assume there is arterial bleeding even if the blood appears dark or is not spurting. Providing direct pressure, elevation (if possible), and a pressure dressing should easily control most external bleeding. (pp. 777–778)
2. Arteries are under higher pressure than veins or capillaries. Because the pressure inside the arteries results in a greater flow of blood at the opening, arterial bleeding can be difficult to control. (p. 777)
3. Pale, moist skin, which is caused when the circulation to the skin is redirected to the vital organs in the core of the body. Increased pulse rate, which results as the heart tries to maintain an adequate blood pressure by increasing the rate. Decreasing blood pressure is the result when blood loss exceeds the body's ability to compensate. Increased respiratory rate is the body's attempt to compensate for poor perfusion. Altered mental status occurs as a result of poor perfusion. (p. 774)

CASE STUDIES

Case Study 1

1. Your priority of care for Monique is to control the bleeding as soon as possible. You must expose the wound and attempt to control the bleeding as appropriate. (p. 778)
2. Based on the presentation of her hand, it appears that she has arterial, venous, and capillary bleeding. The best way to manage this injury is to place medium-size trauma dressings on both sides of the hand and put fingertip pressure on the spurting wound on her palm. Keep the hand elevated as best you can and apply a pressure dressing as appropriate. (p. 778)
3. You must keep her lying flat, provide her with supplemental oxygen, and transport as soon as possible, monitoring her body temperature along the way. (p. 783)

Case Study 2

1. As you attempt to stop the bleeding from this man's wound, you must consider the possibility of a skull fracture and use only the amount of pressure necessary to control the bleeding. Also consider the need for spinal precautions. (p. 787)
2. Use sterile dressings and direct pressure for this wound. If possible use roller gauze or cravats to secure the dressings to the wound. (p. 787)
3. Keep the patient lying down with his head slightly elevated to minimize the pressure at the site of injury. Place him on supplemental oxygen and monitor for signs of shock during transport. (p. 783)

Chapter 31

STOP, REVIEW, REMEMBER! *(p. 801)*

Multiple Choice

1. a (p. 795)
2. d (p. 795)
3. c (p. 797)
4. a (p. 797)
5. c (p. 799)

Matching

1. b (p. 795)
2. c (p. 795)
3. a (p. 795)
4. g (p. 799)
5. e (p. 797)
6. d (p. 797)
7. f (p. 797)
8. h (p. 797)

Critical Thinking

1. The skin serves as protection from injury for the underlying structures as well as protection from infection. It helps regulate temperature and houses the sensory nerves that allow us to feel hot, cold, and pain. It also serves as an important fluid barrier that keeps moisture in. (p. 795)
2. The primary reason closed injuries have a greater potential for being life threatening is because they are likely to hide dangerous bleeding that is not easily managed. (p. 797)
3. A contusion, also known as a bruise, is often seen as a reddish blue discoloration of the skin most often caused by blunt trauma. A hematoma is a swelling beneath the skin seen as a raised area or bump caused by an accumulation of fluid beneath the skin. Hematomas are also most often caused by blunt trauma. (p. 797)

STOP, REVIEW, REMEMBER! *(p. 804)*

Multiple Choice

1. c (p. 799)
2. b (p. 799)
3. a (p. 796)
4. c (p. 803)
5. d (p. 803)

Sorting

1. B (p. 803)
2. F (pp. 798, 803, and Chapter 28)
3. G (p. 803)
4. D (p. 803)
5. A (p. 803)
6. I (p. 803)
7. E (p. 803)
8. H (p. 803)
9. C (p. 803)

STOP, REVIEW, REMEMBER! *(p. 809)*

Multiple Choice

1. d (p. 805)
2. a (p. 808)
3. c (p. 805)
4. b (p. 808)
5. d (p. 805)

Matching

1. B (p. 805)
2. C (p. 805)
3. A (p. 797)

Critical Thinking

1. An impaled object creates a challenge because in most instances it must be left in place for transport. It also has caused damage and bleeding to internal soft tissue and organs that cannot be treated by the EMT. Impaled objects that interfere with the patient's airway or with attempts to resuscitate the patient should be removed in order to allow for proper care. (p. 805)
2. Damage to major blood vessels in the neck can result in significant blood loss. An open wound to the neck can result in an air embolism entering one of the large vessels of the neck, resulting in possible death. It also can affect the airway and make it difficult for the patient to breathe adequately. (p. 808)
3. An amputation of the hand should be managed by first controlling any active bleeding at the injury site with direct pressure, elevation (if possible), pressure dressing, and tourniquet (for life-threatening bleeding). You must then place the amputated part in a plastic bag, and then placing cool packs side by side with the bagged part. (pp. 806–807)

CHAPTER REVIEW *(p. 816)*

Multiple Choice

1. b (p. 811)
2. b (p. 811)
3. c (p. 814)
4. a (p. 812)
5. d (pp. 813, 814)
6. a (p. 795)
7. c (p. 795)
8. d (p. 797)
9. b (p. 799)
10. a (p. 799)

Fill in the Blank

1. bleeding, infection (pp. 810–811)
2. dressing (p. 811)
3. Adhesive (p. 811)
4. Occlusive (p. 811)
5. bandage (p. 812)
6. position of function (p. 814)

Critical Thinking

1. A dressing, which is typically sterile, is designed to be placed directly on a wound and cover it on all sides. A dressing absorbs blood and helps in the formation of a clot. A bandage is designed to secure a dressing in place and can be tied in such a way as to hold pressure against the wound over the dressing. (pp. 810–811)
2. The proper application of dressings and bandages is an important skill that all EMTs must learn. It aids in minimizing external blood loss and infection of the wound. (pp. 810–811)
3. A pressure dressing is different from other types of dressings in that its main purpose is to maintain pressure over a bleeding wound in an attempt to control bleeding. Other dressings and bandages are applied to wounds where bleeding has already been controlled and the main purpose is to minimize infection. (p. 814)

CASE STUDIES

Case Study 1

1. Given that the mechanism of injury was a fall from a 12-foot height, and the fact that this man is conscious and breathing, your top priority should be maintaining spinal precautions. He should be quickly secured to a long board, given supplemental oxygen, and monitored for signs of shock or any change in breathing during transport. (p. 798)
2. This man has clearly sustained blunt trauma as a result of the fall from 12 feet up. He has high potential for spine injuries as well as internal injuries to the abdomen due to the fall onto the bucket. (p. 797)

Case Study 2

1. Your number-one priority will be to minimize the loss of blood while maintaining spinal precautions. Even

though he has no obvious injury to the head, neck, or torso, the MOI suggests possible spine injury. (p. 803)

2. Given the severity of the injury, you must control the bleeding as quickly as possible. If direct pressure, elevation, and pressure dressings fail, you must apply a tourniquet just above the wound to stop the bleeding. (p. 803)
3. Cover the open end with a moist sterile dressing and then carefully place the amputated leg into a plastic bag. Common red biohazard bags work well for this type of transport. Transport the limb with the patient, and if possible, place cool packs around the limb during transport. (pp. 805–808)

Chapter 32

STOP, REVIEW, REMEMBER! *(p. 826)*

Multiple Choice

1. c (p. 824)
2. a (p. 822)
3. b (p. 825)
4. d (p. 821)
5. a (pp. 825-825)

Fill in the Blank

1. source, depth, body surface area (pp. 821, 828)
2. thermal (p. 821)
3. Chemical (p. 821)
4. superficial (p. 824)
5. dermis (p. 824)
6. full-thickness (p. 824)

Critical Thinking

1. Student answers will vary, depending on the environment in which the student works.
2. Student answers will vary, depending on the environment in which the student works.
3. Patients who have experienced a full-thickness burn will have surrounding tissue that has sustained either partial-thickness or superficial burns. For this reason, the areas surrounding the full-thickness burns will likely be very painful. (p. 825)

STOP, REVIEW, REMEMBER! *(p. 836)*

Multiple Choice

1. d (p. 828)
2. c (p. 829)
3. d (p. 831)
4. a (p. 831)
5. c (p. 828)

Matching

1. C (p. 824)
2. D (p. 828)
3. B (p. 829)
4. E (p. 831)
5. A (p. 831)

Critical Thinking

1. Airway patency and adequacy of breathing, depth of injury, percentage of body surface area (BSA) affected, location of the injury, patient's age, preexisting medical conditions (p. 828)
2. Airway patency and adequacy of breathing: As with any patient, airway and breathing are first and foremost in your assessment. Without an open airway and adequate breathing, the patient will quickly die. Depth of injury: The greater the depth of injury, the more severe the injury will be from a standpoint of tissue damage and infection. Percentage of body surface area (BSA) affected: The greater the BSA, the more severe the burn. Location of the injury: Minor burns can be complicated by location, especially if they affect the face, airways, hands, feet, and genitalia. Patient's age: The very old and very young have a much more difficult time recovering from burns. Preexisting medical conditions: A great many medical conditions and medications can complicate the recovery from burns. (pp. 828-830)
3. The source of the burn is still a hazard: You must mitigate the source yourself if appropriate or call for the appropriate resources to do so. Objects on or around the patient may be hot: Avoid touching these or wear protective garments when doing so. (p. 831)

CHAPTER REVIEW *(p. 838)*

Multiple Choice

1. c (p. 824)
2. a (p. 824)
3. d (p. 824)
4. b (p. 824)
5. c (p. 825)
6. c (p. 824)
7. a (pp. 825-826)
8. a (p. 834)
9. d (p. 834)
10. b (p. 829)

Matching

1. b (p. 821)
2. a (p. 821)
3. e (p. 822)
4. c (p. 822)
5. d (p. 822)

Critical Thinking

1. Once you have confirmed that the burning has stopped and that the ABCs are okay, you must cover both arms with dry sterile dressings. You may want to place sterile gauze between the fingers of each hand before wrapping the entire hand with sterile gauze. (pp. 832, 825)
2. Circumferential burns are burns that encircle the entire body area or body part. When this happens, the swelling of the tissues either restricts movement as in the case of a circumferential burn to the chest, or it can severely restrict circulation, as in the case of an arm, hand, or finger. (p. 835)

CASE STUDIES

Case Study 1

1. This boy has burned approximately half of each arm (4.5% × 2 = 9%) and his face (6%) for a total of approximately 15%. (p. 828)
2. You should place sterile dressings between each of his fingers, and then wrap both hands and forearms with roller bandages. (pp. 832, 825)
3. The burns to his face indicate he might have inhaled superheated air or smoke and therefore could experience swelling of his air passages. This will make it difficult for him to breathe and could result in total blockage of his airway. He must be transported immediately in the event his airway begins to swell. (pp. 831, 832)

Case Study 2

1. Front of one leg = 9% × both legs = 18%. One-half of the anterior torso = 9%. Total = 27% (p. 828)
2. Entire head = 18%. Entire right arm = 9%. Total = 27% (p. 828)
3. Entire back = 18%. Back of one arm (4.5%) × both arms = 9%. Total = 27% (p. 828)

Chapter 33

STOP, REVIEW, REMEMBER! *(p. 855)*

Multiple Choice

1. a (p. 844)
2. d (p. 849)
3. c (p. 851)
4. d (p. 853)
5. a (pp. 848-849)

Matching

1. d (p. 849)
2. a (p. 848)
3. c (pp. 848-849)
4. e (p. 852)
5. b (p. 847)

Critical Thinking

1. Both are potentially serious and will require supplemental oxygen and care for shock. However, the open chest wound also will require the application of an occlusive dressing. (pp. 846-854)
2. Sealing the dressing on three sides (or sealed on four sides with one corner left untaped) creates a "flutter valve," which allows air to escape during exhalation or when pressure increases while preventing air from entering during inhalation. (p. 853)

STOP, REVIEW, REMEMBER! *(p. 864)*

Multiple Choice

1. d (p. 860)
2. c (p. 860)
3. c (p. 844)
4. c (p. 856)
5. a (p. 859)

Matching

1. h (Chapter 5, p. 119)
2. a (Chapter 5, p. 119)
3. e (Chapter 5, p. 119)
4. g (Chapter 5, p. 119)
5. f (p. 593)
6. b (Chapter 5, p. 119)
7. d (Chapter 5, p. 119)

Critical Thinking

1. Unlike closed wounds, open abdominal wounds have the potential to expose abdominal organs,

which can result in damage to the organs, infection, and evisceration. Note that closed wounds also have the potential for further injury, including internal bleeding. Care for both conditions involves care for shock. (pp. 858, 860)

2. Student answers will vary. Refer to Table 33-1 for answers. (p. 857)

CHAPTER REVIEW *(p. 866)*

Multiple Choice

1. b (p. 854)
2. a (p. 852)
3. c (pp. 853–854)
4. c (p. 860)
5. b (p. 850)

Fill in the Blank

1. tamponade (p. 852)
2. saline (p. 860)
3. retroperitoneal (p. 856)

Critical Thinking

1. The major organ of concern is the liver. This is a solid organ that can cause profuse internal bleeding. The gall bladder and portions of the stomach and duodenum (small intestine) may also be injured. (p. 857)
2. The patient may experience sudden onset of one-sided sharp chest pain and increasing shortness of breath. Auscultation of the chest may reveal unequal breath sounds (diminished on the side of the pneumothorax). (p. 849)
3. The pulse pressure is the difference between the systolic and diastolic pressures. It will narrow (become smaller) in tension pneumothorax as well as in other conditions that cause shock. (pp. 848–849)

CASE STUDY

1. After the airway opening and suctioning the patient should receive an oral airway (if he did not have a gag reflex). The patient would require assisted ventilations with a bag-mask device or pocket mask with supplemental oxygen. The airway should be constantly monitored. (p. 850)
2. Observe and palpate the chest. Remember that the muscles of the chest will create a splint and reduce the "classic" paradoxical motion. If two or more ribs are broken in two or more places, it is a flail segment. (p. 847)
3. The patient could experience a pneumothorax, tension pneumothorax, hemothorax, and lacerations or damage to great vessels and the heart. (pp. 847–849)

Chapter 34

STOP, REVIEW, REMEMBER! *(p. 873)*

Multiple Choice

1. c (p. 870)
2. b (p. 870)
3. a (p. 871)
4. d (p. 873)
5. a (p. 873)

Labeling

(p. 871)

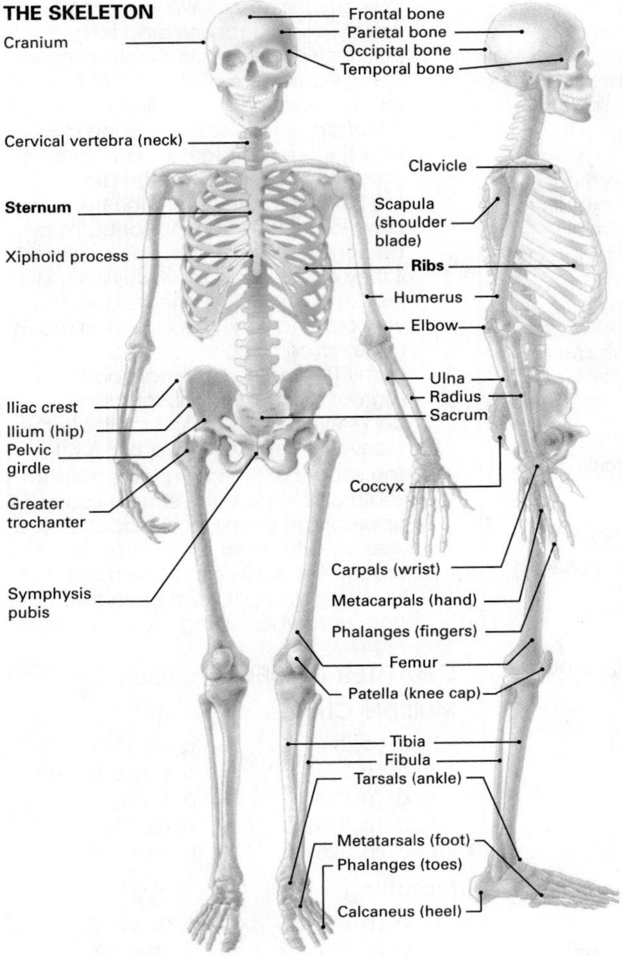

Critical Thinking

1. A strain is an injury involving a muscle, typically caused when the muscle is stretched beyond normal limitations. A sprain occurs at a joint and results when the joint and the associated supportive tissue (ligaments and tendons) are stretched beyond their normal limitations. (p. 873)

STOP, REVIEW, REMEMBER! *(p. 879)*

Multiple Choice

1. b (p. 875)
2. c (p. 875)
3. a (p. 876)
4. d (pp. 877–878)
5. a (p. 873)

Fill in the Blank

1. pain (p. 875)
2. joints (p. 875)
3. closed (p. 875)
4. skin (p. 875)
5. mechanism of injury (p. 876)

Critical Thinking

1. In most cases an injury to a joint will result in the patient being unable to move the joint. This requires immobilization of the injured extremity in the position in which it is found. (p. 877)
2. Assuming that the ABCs are okay, the emergency care priorities for an open skeletal injury include controlling bleeding, keeping the open wound clean, and immobilizing the extremity. (p. 875)
3. An injured extremity with abnormal distal CSM findings could indicate damage to the blood vessels or nerves that feed the extremity. Abnormal findings might include the absence of a pulse, the presence of numbness and tingling, and weakness or the inability to move the distal extremity appropriately. (p. 878)

STOP, REVIEW, REMEMBER! *(p. 896)*

Multiple Choice

1. d (p. 881)
2. a (pp. 881–882)
3. c (pp. 881–882)
4. b (pp. 888, 890–892)
5. d (p. 883)

Fill in the Blank

1. fracture (p. 873)
2. elevated (p. 881)
3. movement (p. 881)
4. manual stabilization (p. 881)
5. position of function (p. 883)

Critical Thinking

1. The most common signs and symptoms of a closed skeletal injury include pain, tenderness, deformity, swelling, discoloration, crepitation, and the inability to move the joint. (p. 877)
2. The objective is to immobilize the knee in the position in which it is found. This can be accomplished by placing adequate support beneath the knee and either securing a rigid splint on either side to form a triangle or securing the ankle of the injured extremity to the uninjured extremity. In any case it is best to place the patient on a carrying device such

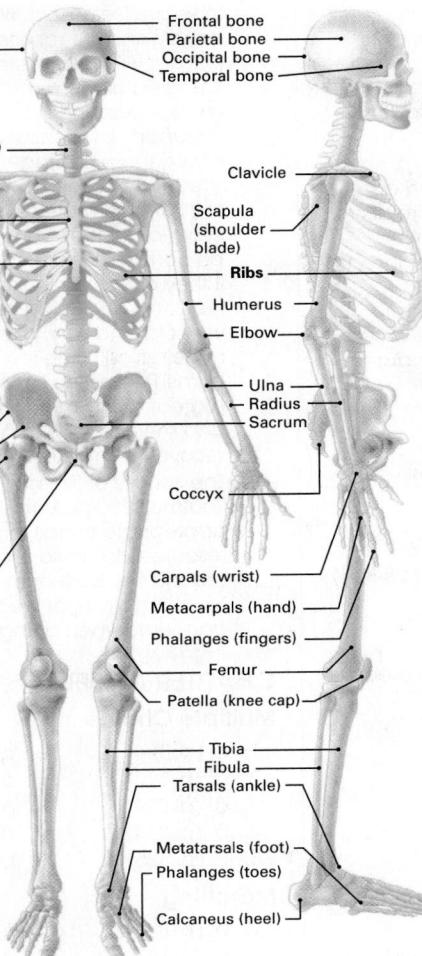

as a long backboard for easy transport. (p. 883)

3. Immobilizing the joints adjacent to the suspected fracture site helps ensure that the bones at the injury site remain immobile, thereby minimizing pain and additional soft-tissue damage and swelling. (pp. 881–882)

CHAPTER REVIEW *(p. 898)*

Multiple Choice

1. c (pp. 883–884)
2. a (p. 884)
3. b (p. 884)
4. b (p. 885)
5. d (p. 887)
6. c (p. 887)
7. d (p. 871)
8. a (p. 877)
9. c (p. 895)
10. a (p. 894)

Matching

1. e (pp. 887–888, 892)
2. a (pp. 887–888, 892)
3. d (p. 885)
4. c (p. 885)
5. b (p. 884)
6. f (p. 884)

Critical Thinking

1. The most common signs and symptoms of an open skeletal injury include pain, tenderness, open wound, external bleeding, deformity, swelling, and crepitation. (pp. 875–877)
2. A shoulder injury can be easily immobilized by using a sling and swathe. If properly placed, the sling can immobilize the elbow and the swathe immobilizes the shoulder joint. (p. 887)
3. In most cases you will discover a difference in push/pull strength or grip strength from side to side as you assess motor function. This is typically attributed to pain in the injured extremity. (pp. 878–879)

CASE STUDIES

Case Study 1

1. With the ABCs addressed, your next priority will be to maintain manual stabilization of the head while you package this patient in full spinal precautions on a long backboard. Also provide supplemental oxygen as you package him. (p. 876)
2. Due to the significant MOI, you will most likely immobilize the extremities as a package when you secure the patient to the long backboard. Given his mental status and the MOI, he is a high priority for rapid transport. (pp. 886–887)
3. While this patient may be a candidate for a traction splint, it will not be your top priority. He needs to be packaged on a long backboard and transported immediately. If you have enough resources at the scene or in transport, you might apply a traction splint to his left leg. (p. 886)

Case Study 2

1. Because her ABCs are okay and there is no need for spinal precautions, your attention should be focused on properly immobilizing the injured arm. As always, pay attention to any changes in her condition that would indicate the need for spinal precautions. (p. 876)
2. You can carefully attempt to align the arm and place it in a splint. Be sure to monitor the status of circulation, sensation, and motor function throughout the process. Whether circulation returns or not, you should transport this patient as soon as is practical. (p. 887)
3. One way to immobilize this injury will be to place it in a three-sided cardboard splint that extends from the wrist to just past the elbow. Secure the splint in place with lots of padding, and then place the arm in a sling and swathe. (p. 887)

Chapter 35

STOP, REVIEW, REMEMBER! *(p. 906)*

Multiple Choice

1. d (p. 904)
2. a (p. 905)
3. d (p. 904)
4. c (pp. 905, 916)
5. c (p. 905)

Matching

1. e (p. 905)
2. d (p. 905)
3. a (p. 905)
4. a (p. 905)
5. f (p. 905)
6. c (p. 905)
7. b (p. 905)
8. e (p. 905)

Critical Thinking

1. A vault is technically defined as a container. The brain is contained within the skull or cranial vault. (p. 904)
2. The brain is covered with three membranes or layers. The dura mater is a fibrous layer that lines the inside of the cranial vault. The pia mater lies directly over the brain tissue. Between these two layers is a very thin, weblike layer called the arachnoid membrane. These three layers are called the meninges and also cover the spine. (p. 905)

STOP, REVIEW, REMEMBER! *(p. 914)*

Multiple Choice

1. c (p. 912)
2. d (p. 910)
3. a (p. 912)
4. c (p. 904)
5. b (p. 913)

Labeling

(p. 904)

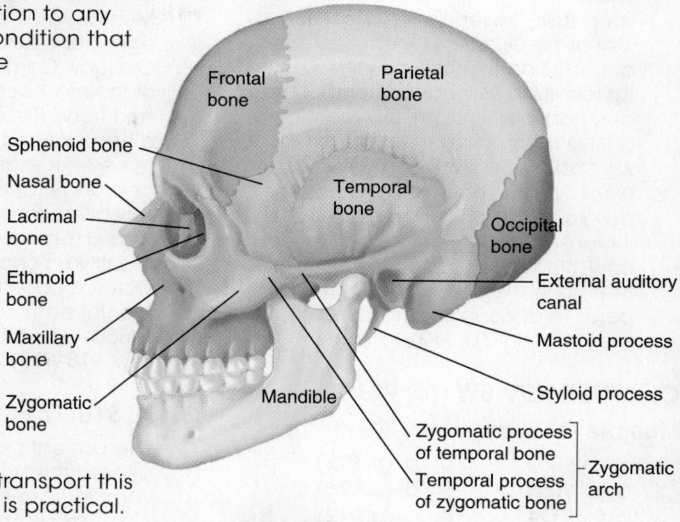

Critical Thinking

1. Patients taking anticoagulants (such as Coumadin) and antiplatelet agents are more likely to develop life-threatening bleeding after trauma than are other patients. In the case of head injury this is even more critical because even a small amount of bleeding within the cranium can be life threatening. These patients can be expected to have exaggerated heavy bleeding from scalp and facial wounds as well. (p. 912)
2. No, these are signs and symptoms of hypovolemic shock and are almost certainly being caused by hemorrhage from some other injury. Remember that you cannot lose enough blood into the head to cause shock. Based on the mechanism of injury, injury to the chest, abdomen, or pelvis is a more likely cause of the patient's current condition. The head injury may still be serious, but it likely is not causing the vitals you see. (p. 912)

STOP, REVIEW, REMEMBER! *(p. 920)*

Multiple Choice

1. d (p. 918)
2. d (pp. 916, 918)
3. c (p. 916)
4. b (p. 919)
5. c (p. 918)

Fill in the Blank

1. 13 (p. 918)
2. 6 (p. 918)
3. 15 (p. 918)
4. 3 (p. 918)
5. 8 (p. 918)

Critical Thinking

1. Your protocols will require you to take the distance to each hospital into

consideration. The ability to control the patient's airway, whether or not you need to ventilate the patient, and your ability to ventilate adequately as well as his Glasgow Coma Scale score are additional considerations. External factors such as weather conditions and transport times (early morning or during commuting times, for example) will also play a part. (pp. 918–920)

2. Probably not. The vital signs indicate developing shock (increased pulse, increased respirations, agitation, and cool, clammy skin). Look for possible trauma to the chest, abdomen, and pelvis to account for this patient's presentation. (p. 912)

CHAPTER REVIEW *(p. 923)*

Multiple Choice

1. a (p. 905)
2. d (p. 905)
3. b (p. 912)
4. a (p. 910)
5. d (p. 918)
6. b (p. 912)
7. d (p. 918)
8. c (p. 912)
9. b (p. 920)
10. b (p. 918)

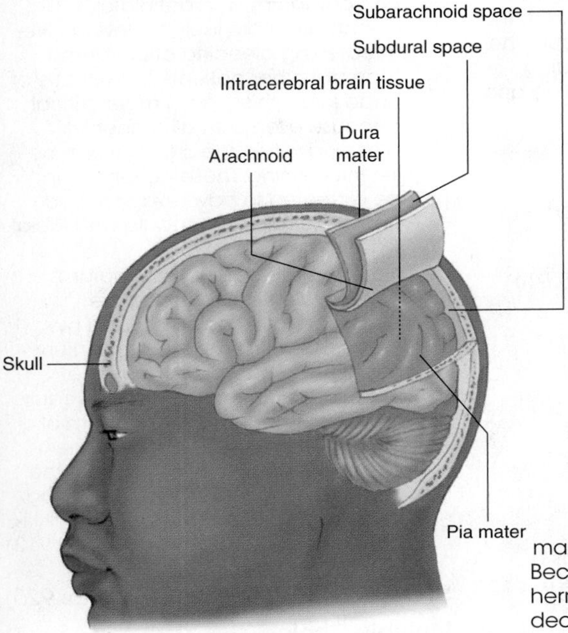

Labeling

(p. 905)

Critical Thinking

1. A concussion is an injury that causes jarring to the brain, resulting in temporary signs and symptoms. A contusion is a bruising of brain tissue. The bleeding in this injury is limited but significant enough to cause altered mental status and other signs and symptoms lasting longer than those of a concussion. In the field it will not be possible to distinguish one condition from another. Most importantly, remember that all patients with signs of head trauma of any type should receive hospital examination and care. (p. 909)
2. Mental status is thought of as the most significant indicator of head injury. The Glasgow Coma Scale score is one of the most common ways to assess and trend the mental status of a head-injured patient. Always remember that the brain works best under certain conditions. Any alteration in oxygen levels, pressure, glucose, or pH quickly results in a change in mental status. A patient with an altered mental status is considered serious—period. (pp. 918–919)

CASE STUDY

1. The patient's clammy skin, altered mental status, and vomiting are all indications of problems. Together they are a giant red flag waving at you that you are dealing with a high-priority, unstable patient who requires your help. (pp. 910, 919)
2. The patient is having some sort of intracranial bleeding, either from old trauma he does not recall or possibly spontaneous rupture of a vessel or vessels around or within the brain. (pp. 909–910)
3. Promptly transport to a facility capable of handling this emergency (a trauma center), if available. Call for ALS assistance if necessary. The patient will require airway maintenance due to the vomiting. Because the patient has signs of herniation including posturing, decreasing GCS, unresponsiveness, and fixed pupils, you should ventilate the patient at 20/minute. (pp. 915, 919)

Chapter 36

STOP, REVIEW, REMEMBER! *(p. 935)*

Multiple Choice

1. a (p. 934)
2. d (p. 929)
3. a (p. 929)
4. b (p. 929)
5. d (p. 930)

Critical Thinking

1. Evaluation of the mechanism of injury plays an important role in determining the most appropriate care for the patient with a suspected spine injury.

Labeling

(Chapter 5, p. 101)

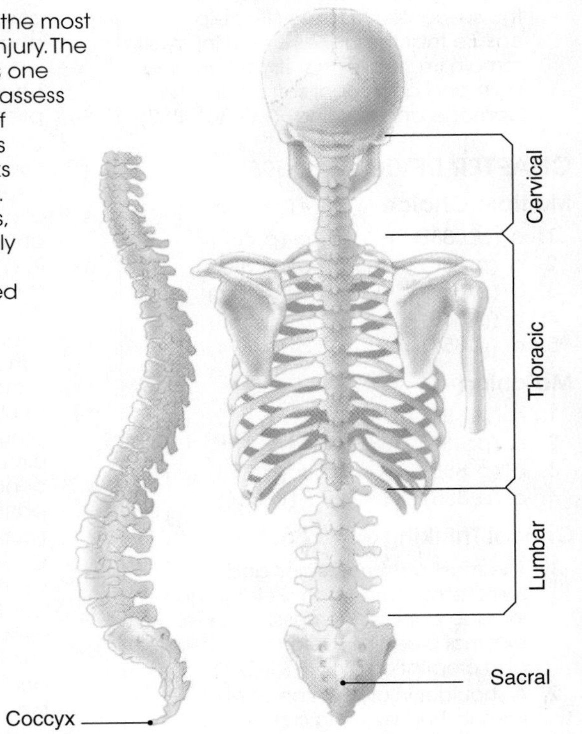

Unlike suspected fractures, in which pain is the primary indicator for injury, the presence or absence of pain alone is unreliable in predicting injury to the spine. If the MOI is consistent with a potential spine injury, then you must provide the appropriate care, despite the absence of pain or neurological deficit. (p. 932)

2. The central nervous system consists of the brain and spinal cord and is responsible for the control of all basic body functions. The peripheral nervous system consists of an elaborate network of motor and sensory fibers that connect the central nervous system to the rest of the body. (p. 928)
3. While it may be impossible to assess and care for a patient with a suspected spine injury without moving him at all, it is essential to keep movement to a minimum. Inappropriate movement of such a patient could make the injury worse, increasing the potential for permanent damage to the spinal cord and paralysis. (pp. 930–931)

STOP, REVIEW, REMEMBER! *(p. 950)*

Multiple Choice

1. b (p. 937)
2. c (p. 937)
3. b (p. 939)
4. a (p. 942)
5. d (p. 948)

Labeling

(p. 933)

DISTRACTION INJURY

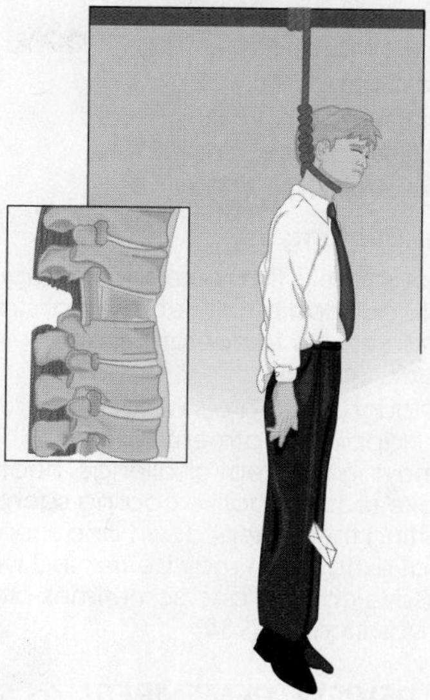

FLEXION INJURY

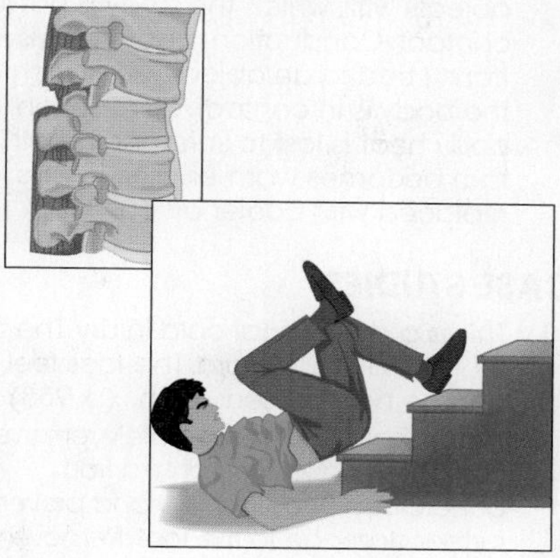

COMPRESSION INJURY

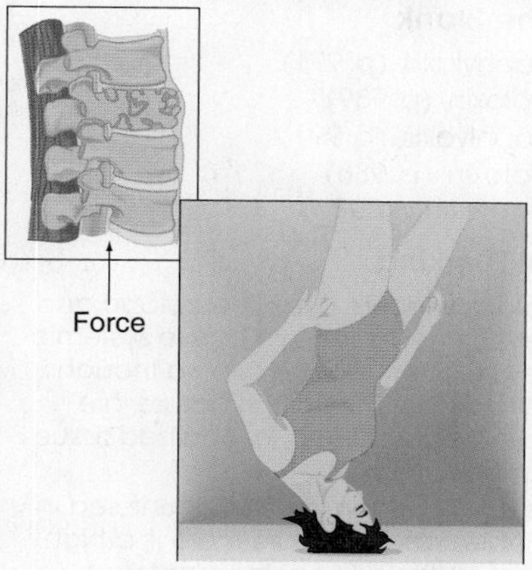

EXTENSION INJURY

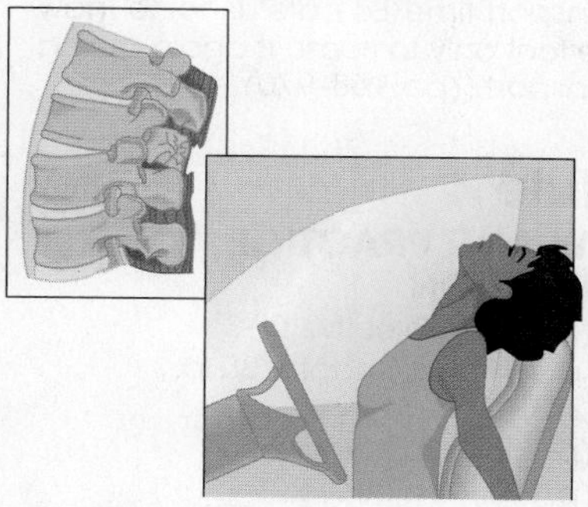

Critical Thinking

1. Your first clue that a patient may have suffered a spine injury is the mechanism of injury. After assessing the MOI, you can then assess for pain along the spine or numbness and tingling in any of the extremities. (pp. 932, 935)
2. All factors relating to the MOI can help you determine the likelihood of a spine injury such as the force involved, the surface the patient struck, loss of consciousness, and obvious external trauma. When the MOI is unknown, you must assume the worst and treat for suspected spine injury. (pp. 930, 932)
3. It is important to minimize movement of the head and neck of a patient with a suspected spine injury. For this reason you must make every attempt to use the jaw-thrust maneuver when opening and maintaining the airway of these patients. (p. 937)

CHAPTER REVIEW *(p. 958)*

Multiple Choice

1. c (p. 928)
2. d (p. 928)
3. a (p. 955)
4. c (pp. 932, 934)
5. c (p. 932)
6. a (p. 955)
7. c (p. 930)
8. b (p. 938)
9. d (p. 948)
10. b (p. 942)
11. a (p. 954)
12. a (p. 946)
13. b (p. 948)
14. d (p. 937)

Fill in the Blank

1. spinal cord (p. 928)
2. peripheral (p. 928)
3. cervical spine (p. 929)
4. 12 (p. 928)
5. lumbar (p. 928)
6. below (p. 930)
7. compression (p. 932)
8. third (p. 930)

Critical Thinking

1. Rapid extrication is necessary when the patient has life-threatening problems related to the ABCs that cannot be managed easily while he remains in the vehicle. It also is indicated when hazards at the scene threaten either the patient or the rescuers. (p. 954)
2. During rapid extrication the priorities of proper spinal immobilization and the need for movement must be balanced. An emphasis is placed on manual stabilization of the head, neck, and spine to accommodate rapid movement of the patient. (p. 954)
3. First and foremost your priority is to ensure that the ABCs are all okay. You must do this while maintaining manual stabilization of the head. In most cases it is better to leave the helmet and shoulder pads in place in order to keep the head properly aligned. If you remove the helmet and not the pads, the head will fall into a hyperextended position. If you remove the helmet, you must remove the shoulder pads as well in order to keep the spine in neutral alignment. (p. 955)

CASE STUDIES

Case Study 1

1. Due to the obvious mechanism of injury and wound to the head, this man is definitely a candidate for spinal immobilization. The absence of pain is not justification for assuming he does not have a neck or spine injury. (p. 932)
2. It will be important to know this man's mental status by asking if he lost consciousness and determining if he is A&O × 4. Also determine if he was wearing a seat belt and if the vehicle had an air bag that deployed. (pp. 916, 938)
3. Given that the man is standing when you find him, the best approach will be to get him onto a backboard from the standing position. Once he is secured to the board, you can control bleeding from open wounds and complete a more detailed physical exam. You also will want to start him on supplemental oxygen. (pp. 939–940)
4. Given that this man is found in the standing position, the long backboard would be most appropriate for taking full spinal precautions. You must begin by placing an appropriate-size cervical collar. (pp. 944–948)

Case Study 2

1. Your first priority for this patient will be to establish an open airway and begin artificial ventilation. (p. 938)
2. Yes, you must roll this patient onto his back in order to manage his airway and begin to stabilize his spine. One of you must hold manual stabilization of the head, while the other gently rolls the patient onto his back. (pp. 939–940)
3. Yes, you must remove the helmet in order to gain proper access to the airway and to ventilate this patient. Both rescuers should hold the head stable. The rescuer at the top of the patient holds the helmet, while the other rescuer places her hands beneath the helmet at the base of the skull. Then the first rescuer pulls the straps and slips the helmet off, while the second rescuer slides her hands up to maintain control of the head. Once the helmet is removed, the first rescuer takes over control of the head. (pp. 955–957)
4. This patient should have a cervical collar placed and be properly secured to a long backboard. (pp. 941–948)

Chapter 37

STOP, REVIEW, REMEMBER! *(p. 978)*

Multiple Choice

1. b (p. 966)
2. a (p. 966)
3. d (p. 970)
4. c (p. 965)
5. a (p. 966)

Matching

1. B (p. 966)
2. B (p. 966)
3. E (p. 966)
4. A (p. 966)
5. D (p. 966)
6. E (p. 966)

Critical Thinking

1. Hyperthermia occurs when the body retains more heat than it gives off. Hypothermia occurs when the body gives off more heat than it retains. Hyperthermia is an emergency involving abnormally high body temperature. Hypothermia is an abnormally low body temperature. (p. 966)
2. The patient could be moved to the shade and his clothing removed. The patient may be sprayed with water and/or fanned. All help to reduce body temperature. (p. 966, 984)

STOP, REVIEW, REMEMBER! *(p. 985)*

Multiple Choice

1. c (p. 983)
2. b (p. 984)
3. c (pp. 980–981)
4. a (p. 966)
5. c (p. 983)

Fill in the Blank

1. Heat stroke (p. 983)
2. Heat stroke (p. 983)
3. Heat exhaustion (p. 982)
4. Heat cramps (p. 982)
5. Heat stroke (p. 983)
6. Heat exhaustion (p. 982)
7. Heat stroke (p. 983)

Critical Thinking

1. Heat stroke is the more severe stage distinguished by altered mental status, extreme core temperature, and severe shock. (p. 983)
2. Although there are several overlapping treatments such as removing the heat challenge, heat stroke requires active cooling such as wetting the patient down and fanning. Heat exhaustion may be treated with passive cooling and sometimes oral rehydration. (p. 984)

STOP, REVIEW, REMEMBER! *(p. 995)*

Multiple Choice

1. c (p. 988)
2. d (p. 991)
3. c (p. 989)
4. a (p. 989)
5. a (p. 990)

Fill in the Blank

1. anaphylaxis (p. 991)
2. cytotoxin (p. 989)
3. anaphlyaxis (p. 991)
4. cytotoxin (p. 988)
5. neurotoxin (p. 987)

Critical Thinking

1. A black widow's bite is neurotoxic and therefore more likely to cause systemic effects. Brown recluse bites, although they can be systemic in nature, are more likely confined to localized tissue damage. (pp. 987–988)
2. Fire ants are generally encountered in colonies and therefore there is a high risk of multiple (if not hundreds) of bites. (p. 991)
3. The poison of the nematocysts must be neutralized immediately. Rinsing in vinegar or a baking soda slurry can neutralize the toxin. Nematocysts can then be scraped away. Monitor closely for anaphylaxis and transport. (p. 992)

CHAPTER REVIEW *(p. 997)*

Multiple Choice

1. a (p. 982)
2. a (p. 974)
3. a (p. 988)
4. a (p. 965)
5. a (p. 993)
6. b (p. 989)

Critical Thinking

1. In a setting where there will be a delay in getting a patient to medical care (for example, storms or wilderness) you may actively rewarm a local cold injury. This would be done by warm (not hot) water. (p. 968)
2. Geriatric age, pediatric age, medications, certain medical conditions (heart disease, diabetes, fever, fatigue, obesity, dehydration) (p. 980)
3. Radiation: body heat is lost to nearby objects with which the body is not in contact. Conduction: body heat is transferred to an object with which the body is in contact. Convection: body heat is lost to surrounding air that becomes warmer, rises, and is replaced with cooler air (p. 966)

CASE STUDIES

1. This is a deep local cold injury. The foot is white and hard. The toes feel stiff and he has lost sensation. (p. 968)
2. Thom should be immediately removed from the cold to protect him from generalized hypothermia and prevent further damage to the foot. Remove wet clothes and cover the foot with warm materials. Splint the extremity. Do not rub the foot or break blisters. (p. 968)
3. Thom's foot could be actively rewarmed because of the extended transport time. Be careful not to thaw the foot only to freeze it again during transport. (pp. 968–970)

Module 4

REVIEW AND PRACTICE EXAMINATION

1. a (p. 751) Objective 29-3
2. c (p. 754 and Chapter 35, p. 912) Objective 29-4
3. b (p. 755) Objective 29-5
4. b (p. 751) Objective 29-7
5. d (p. 771) Objective 30-2
6. b (p. 771) Objective 30-2
7. a (p. 773) Objective 30-2
8. b (pp. 773–775) Objective 30-4
9. a (p. 775) Objective 30-5
10. c (p. 777) Objective 30-6
11. d (p. 778) Objective 30-7
12. d (p. 778) Objective 30-7
13. a (p. 780) Objective 30-7
14. c (p. 781) Objective 30-8
15. b (p. 788) Objective 30-11
16. a (p. 795) Objective 31-2
17. c (p. 795) Objective 31-2
18. b (p. 797) Objective 31-6
19. d (p. 797) Objective 31-6
20. c (pp. 797–798) Objective 31-6
21. b (p. 799) Objective 31-7
22. a (p. 805) Objective 31-9
23. d (pp. 805–807) Objective 31-9
24. b (p. 811) Objective 31-10

25. c (p. 803) Objective 31-8
26. b (p. 821) Objective 32-2
27. b (p. 824) Objective 32-5
28. d (p. 825) Objective 32-5
29. c (pp. 831–832) Objective 32-7
30. c (pp. 828–829) Objective 32-6
31. b (pp. 828–829) Objective 32-6
32. d (pp. 828–829) Objective 32-6
33. c (p. 829) Objective 32-7
34. c (p. 831) Objective 32-7
35. b (p. 834) Objective 32-10
36. a (pp. 834–835) Objective 32-13
37. d (pp. 823, 826, 832, 836) Objective 32-8
38. a (p. 845) Objective 33-2
39. b (p. 851) Objective 33-6
40. b (p. 844) Objective 33-2
41. d (p. 847) Objective 33-5
42. c (p. 849) Objective 33-5
43. d (p. 853) Objective 33-7
44. a (p. 856) Objective 33-8
45. b (p. 858) Objective 33-9
46. c (p. 860) Objective 33-11
47. c (p. 870) Objective 34-2
48. d (p. 872) Objective 34-3
49. d (p. 873) Objective 34-4
50. d (p. 876) Objective 34-5
51. b (p. 876) Objective 34-6
52. a (pp. 878, 882) Objective 34-8
53. b (pp. 882, 884) Objective 34-8
54. c (p. 892) Objective 34-8
55. d (p. 886) Objective 34-10
56. a (p. 895) Objective 34-10
57. a (p. 878) Objective 34-5
58. c (p. 904) Objective 35-2
59. b (p. 904) Objective 35-2
60. a (p. 905) Objective 35-4
61. c (p. 905) Objective 35-4
62. d (p. 908) Objective 35-5
63. b (p. 909) Objective 35-5
64. c (p. 910) Objective 35-5
65. b (p. 910) Objective 35-5
66. b (p. 916) Objective 35-7
67. c (p. 920) Objective 35-7
68. d (p. 910) Objective 35-7
69. d (p. 928) Objective 36-2
70. a (p. 929) Objective 36-2
71. d (p. 932) Objective 36-3
72. d (p. 932) Objective 36-3
73. a (p. 932) Objective 36-9
74. c (p. 953) Objective 36-9
75. b (p. 954) Objective 36-11
76. a (p. 955) Objective 36-12
77. c (p. 991 and Chapter 24, pp. 639, 645) Objective 37-24
78. b (p. 965) Objective 37-7
79. c (p. 966) Objective 37-4
80. c (p. 967) Objective 37-6
81. d (p. 973) Objective 37-12
82. b (p. 973) Objective 37-12
83. a (p. 968) Objective 37-10
84. c (p. 983) Objective 37-21
85. d (p. 982) Objective 37-20
86. a (p. 970) Objective 37-24

Chapter 38

STOP, REVIEW, REMEMBER! *(p. 1016)*

Multiple Choice

1. a (p. 1012)
2. a (p. 1013)
3. c (p. 1014)
4. c (p. 1011)
5. b (p. 1013)

Fill in the Blank

1. airway, breathing (p. 1013)
2. central pulses (p. 1016)
3. decompensates (p. 1016)

Critical Thinking

1. School-age children are able to recall and retell what they have seen or experienced but may not understand what it means. Also, speaking to the adolescent respectfully and nonjudgmentally will improve your ability to obtain an accurate history. (pp. 1012–1013)
2. In both cases, look for how the patient interacts with the environment and family members. Does he make eye contact or respond to a parent's voice? Observe the child's work of breathing and listen for audible respiratory noises such as wheezing or grunting. Observe for retractions, nasal flaring, and respiratory rate. (pp. 1012–1013, 1015)
3. The head and tongue are proportionally larger than an adult's. The trachea is thin and flexible. The nose does not have much supporting cartilage, so nasal flaring is an early sign of respiratory distress. See also Table 38-2 for a more comprehensive listing. (pp. 1013, 1015)

STOP, REVIEW, REMEMBER! *(p. 1025)*

Multiple Choice

1. a (pp. 1018, 1019)
2. d (p. 1013)
3. c (p. 1014)
4. c (p. 1018)

Critical Thinking

1. In most cases the easiest way to evaluate rate of a crying child is to count the number of times he inhales or takes a breath. The breathing pattern will most likely be irregular due to the crying. (p. 1014; Chapter 9, pp. 206–207; Ch 13, pp. 326–327)
2. Allow a family member to hold the child. Allow the child to examine your stethoscope. Allow the child to hold a favorite toy. (p. 1011)
3. Deciding on which oxygen delivery device to use for the pediatric patient is a process identified by local protocol. However, in general, the patients described would benefit from the following choices: (a) blow-by technique; (b) nonrebreather mask; (c) assisted artificial ventilation; (d) nonrebreather mask. (p. 1020)

STOP, REVIEW, REMEMBER! *(p. 1034)*

Multiple Choice

1. a (p. 1030)
2. b (p. 1025)
3. b (p. 1032)
4. c (p. 1033)

Fill in the Blank

1. shock (p. 1024)
2. tongue (pp. 1013, 1014, 1027)
3. airway, immobilization (p. 1028)
4. febrile (p. 1029)

Critical Thinking

1. Children have smaller stores of glucose in their bodies, and less fat to insulate them. The lack of fat predisposes them to becoming hypothermic, thus increasing glucose consumption. Keeping the child warm will help minimize both hypothermia and hypoglycemia. (p. 1028)
2. Remember to report objectively, identifying specific things you saw or heard, not what you think might have happened. Do not delay transport to accuse or confront a suspected negligent or abusive caregiver. (p. 1032)
3. Student answers will vary. However, exposure to the care of children in all settings, getting as much practice as possible with assessing the infant and child, and becoming familiar with the equipment used in their care, will improve provider confidence. (p. 1033)

CHAPTER REVIEW *(p. 1036)*

Multiple Choice

1. b (p. 1028)
2. a (pp. 1015, 1018)
3. c (p. 1020)
4. a (p. 1019)
5. c (p. 1024)

Matching

1. f (p. 1014)
2. b (p. 1014)
3. c (p. 1015)
4. e (p. 1018)
5. a (p. 1031)
6. d (p. 1024)

Critical Thinking

1. Children of different ages will respond differently to their environment, caregivers, and strangers. Understanding those differences can give you important clues that will aid with your assessment and interventions. (p. 1011)
2. Recognizing respiratory distress and intervening appropriately and quickly can help prevent respiratory failure. (p. 1018)
3. Blunt trauma most commonly caused by motor-vehicle crashes (p. 1026)
4. An obstructed airway or inadequate respirations are the most common causes of cardiac arrest. Opening the airway and providing supplemental oxygen by the appropriate means is the best way to avoid cardiac arrest in these patients. (pp. 1014, 1017)

Chapter 39

STOP, REVIEW, REMEMBER! *(p. 1047)*

Multiple Choice

1. b (p. 1047)
2. a (p. 1046)
3. c (p. 1046)
4. a (p. 1043)
5. d (p. 1042)

Fill in the Blank

1. Decreased cardiac output, heart failure, changes in the blood vessels including atherosclerosis and aneurysm, high blood pressure, syncope (p. 1045)
2. Lung tissue becomes less elastic, hypoxia can develop unchecked for some time, less able to fight respiratory infection (p. 1044)
3. Osteoporosis, shrinking of discs in the spine, changes in posture and balance, falls (p. 1046)
4. Slowed digestion, decreased taste sensation, dentures make eating difficult (pp. 1046–1047)
5. Decreased sensory perception, decreased reaction time, changes in balance and coordination (p. 1046)

Critical Thinking

1. Elderly patients are not able to compensate for shock as efficiently because they cannot constrict blood vessels or elevate the heart rate in the same manner a younger patient can. (p. 1046)
2. Hearing loss: Get down at eye level with the patient and speak slowly and clearly; speak closer to the good ear if possible. Poor vision: Position yourself so the patient can see you straight on; maintain a gentle touch so the patient is aware of your presence. Inability to speak clearly: Be patient; if the patient wears dentures, make sure they are in place in the mouth; use another caregiver for information if available. (p. 1043)

STOP, REVIEW, REMEMBER! *(p. 1051)*

Multiple Choice

1. b (p. 1050)
2. c (p. 1051)
3. a (p. 1050)
4. c (p. 1047)
5. c (p. 1050)

Fill in the Blank

1. less (p. 1045)
2. less (p. 1041)
3. more (p. 1040)
4. more (p. 1051)
5. more (p. 1041)
6. less (p. 1044)
7. less (p. 1044)

Critical Thinking

1. Get down to the patient's level, speak slowly and clearly, ask one question at a time, and allow the patient time to formulate a response and answer. Of course the amount of time you can realistically take depends on the patient's condition. Serious patients should be promptly moved to the ambulance for transport. Obtain additional information en route. (p. 1043)
2. Elderly patients may have alterations in pain sensation. The pressure of the cuff may in fact be painful to this patient. In other cases dementia may cause the patient to yell out because he does not understand what is happening. (pp. 1042, 1047, 1051)

CHAPTER REVIEW *(p. 1054)*

Multiple Choice

1. a (pp. 1044, 1045)
2. a (p. 1041)
3. c (p. 1043 and Chapter 20, pp. 547–548)
4. a (p. 1041)
5. c (p. 1045)
6. b (p. 1053)
7. c (p. 1053)
8. b (p. 1053)

Critical Thinking

1. The risk of burns and falls can be reduced by taking safety measures in the home, such as reducing the temperature of the hot water heater, using nonskid rugs, wearing shoes with nonslip soles, and installing handholds in the shower. (p. 1051)
2. The fact that the patient seems to call for nonemergent reasons may be from loneliness. This is one indicator. Talk of all her friends dying, a depressed effect, isolation, recent changes in independence or dependence on medical equipment, incontinence, or other quality-of-life issues may be triggers for the depression. (p. 1043)

CASE STUDY

1. A complaint of fatigue should cause you to consider the possibility of a cardiac problem. Remember that women and elderly patients may not present with chest pain. Also check her medications to rule out overdose, either accidental or intentional. Finally, because of her history of stroke, you should consider stroke a possibility. (pp. 1041, 1043, 1045)
2. The cardiac problem can be assessed by asking about fatigue, chest discomfort, or heaviness, if the patient is having any trouble breathing (including sleeping on more pillows at night or having trouble breathing on exertion). Examine her ankles for fluid accumulation. For her medications check the bottles or other containers to see if the remaining dose matches what should be left. Further evaluation for stroke will be difficult. The patient should be transported anyway because altered mental status is a serious finding. Take note that the resolution of this scenario is as follows: It was determined that the patient's daughter set out medications in a plastic container with four compartments for each day. Instead of taking the medications from the compartments vertically, the patient took three doses horizontally (morning meds for three days), resulting in tripling her anti-anxiety medication dose for the day. She was transported, treated, and released. Her daughter is keeping a closer eye on the medications. You need to remember to always ask about a patient's medication regimens. (pp. 1041, 1043, 1045, 1049)

Chapter 40

STOP, REVIEW, REMEMBER! *(p. 1065)*

Multiple Choice

1. d (p. 1058)
2. c (p. 1060)
3. d (p. 1061)
4. a (p. 1064)
5. a (p. 1063)

Critical Thinking

1. A patient who is confused, disoriented, exhibiting problems with memory, having difficulty understanding or answering questions despite absence of hearing or speech disorders may have a cognitive impairment. Of course, you should make sure through your history and assessment that the problems are not being caused by an acute medical problem or injury. Pay attention to the content of the patient's speech, which will give you clues to whether his fund of knowledge is appropriate to his age. (p. 1065)
2. A person who cannot see misses much of the nonverbal communication that assists in understanding messages from others. For example, usually, when you touch another person, he can see that you are going to touch him and anticipates it. With a blind person, unannounced touching can be startling and can undermine trust. (p. 1063)
3. The well-being of a loved one depends on the use of the device, making the family (or patient) highly motivated to be knowledgeable about it. Note that part of discharge planning for patients who have special medical devices includes teaching the patient and family what the device does, how it works, and how to use and troubleshoot it. (p. 1061)

4. Has this problem occurred before? If so, how was the problem solved? What do you think the problem is with the device? Have you tried to fix the problem? What happened? What instructions have you received about the device? (p. 1061)
5. Communicating well with hearing impaired patients might include the utilization of sign language, the use of Telecommunication Device for the Deaf/TeleTypewriter, and writing your questions and allowing the patient to respond in writing as well. (pp. 1063–1064)

STOP, REVIEW, REMEMBER! *(p. 1072)*

Multiple Choice

1. a (p. 1067)
2. b (p. 1067)
3. d (pp. 1067–1068)
4. b (p. 1070)
5. c (p. 1071)

Critical Thinking

1. Anything that is unusual, out of routine, or overstimulates the senses can lead to a meltdown. Keep the patient in familiar surroundings, disperse unnecessary personnel and bystanders, minimize sensory stimulation, and be calm. (p. 1068)
2. The patient may have special medical devices, including ventilators, devices to administer high doses of pain medications, feeding tubes, catheters, vascular access devices, and other equipment. The patient and family may be under incredible stress and require emotional support. There are medical/legal considerations concerning advance directives. (p. 1070)
3. Obesity is associated with an increased risk of some cancers, diabetes, hypertension, heart attack, stroke, liver and gallbladder disease, arthritis, sleep apnea, and respiratory problems. (p. 1070)
4. The homeless are at increased risk of mental health problems, malnutrition, substance abuse, certain infectious diseases, heat- and cold-related emergencies, wounds, and complications of untreated chronic illnesses. (p. 1071)
5. Down syndrome patients may suffer from associated chronic medical conditions that include seizure disorders, heart defects, and the premature development of dementia. (p. 1068)

STOP, REVIEW, REMEMBER! *(p. 1079)*

Multiple Choice

1. c (p. 1074)
2. a (p. 1075)
3. a (p. 1076)
4. c (p. 1078)
5. d (p. 1078)

Matching

1. C (p. 1077)
2. A (p. 1076)
3. B (p. 1074)

Critical Thinking

1. Although uncommon, a pacemaker or AICD can malfunction or inadvertently be turned off. If the patient is symptomatic (altered mental status, chest pain, hypotension), call for ALS, if available. (p. 1078)
2. When an AICD delivers a shock, it is doing what it is designed to do. Usually, when only a single shock is delivered, the patient has been advised to call his physician. However, if more than one shock was delivered, if repeated shocks occur within a 24-hour period, or if the patient does not feel well, he should be transported for evaluation. (p. 1078)
3. LVADs have a backup manual pump that can be operated by hand or foot pressure in an emergency. If you are not familiar with how to use it, have the family show you before you leave the scene. (pp. 1078–1079)

STOP, REVIEW, REMEMBER! *(p. 1084)*

Multiple Choice

1. c (p. 1081)
2. b (pp. 1081–1082 and Ch 17, p. 460)
3. c (p. 1083)
4. a (pp. 1081–1082)
5. a (p. 1082)

Fill in the blank

1. peritoneal cavity (p. 1083)
2. urethra (p. 1081)
3. dislodged catheter, peritonitis (p. 1083)

Critical Thinking

1. Bleeding from the graft or fistula site, infection, fluid overload, and electrolyte-related emergencies in those who have missed their scheduled dialysis treatments. (pp. 1082–1083 and Chapter 25, pp. 665–666)
2. A G-tube is a feeding tube that is inserted through the abdominal wall into the stomach, while a J-tube is inserted through the abdominal wall into the second section of the small intestine, the jejunum. (p. 1081)

CHAPTER REVIEW *(p. 1086)*

Multiple Choice

1. c (pp. 1064–1065)
2. c (p. 1070)
3. a (p. 1083)
4. c (p. 1064)
5. d (p. 1081)
6. b (pp. 1067–1068)

Critical Thinking

1. Patients with Down syndrome have proportionally larger tongues and shorter necks than other patients. (p. 1068)
2. A congenital condition is one a person is born with, while an acquired condition develops at some point during the life span. Some conditions can occur congenitally and be acquired. For example, deafness can be congenital due to genetic reasons or exposure to infection during fetal development, or can occur from occupational exposure to noise, traumatic brain injury, or aging. HIV/AIDS can be present at birth in babies born to infected mothers, but is usually acquired. (pp. 1061, 1063)
3. A tracheostomy is a surgical procedure that produces a wound that can become infected. Even after the opening has healed, the protective functions of the upper airway are bypassed. Bacteria can be introduced into the urinary bladder as a catheter is passed through the urethra. (pp. 1076, 1081)
4. Ask the patient about the procedure and how long it will take to empty the fluid from the abdomen. Ask about the feasibility of moving the patient at this point in the procedure, and what can be done if the patient must be moved before the procedure is complete. (p. 1083)
5. Patients who are paralyzed must spend long hours sitting or lying down because of their immobility, which can create enough pressure in the tissues to result in ischemia. The tissue damage results in pressure sores. In addition to immobility, paralysis is often accompanied by lack of sensation, preventing the patient from detecting the discomfort of increased tissue pressure and tissue damage. Paralysis can also prevent the deep breathing and coughing needed to clear the lungs of mucus and debris, which can result in pneumonia. Use of a ventilator can increase the risk. An inability to efficiently empty the bladder, or to know when the bladder is full, can increase the risk of urinary tract infection; use of a catheter increases the risk as well. (p. 1069)

Module 5

REVIEW AND PRACTICE EXAMINATION

1. a (p. 1011) Objective 38-3
2. b (p. 1011) Objective 38-6
3. a (p. 1013) Objective 38-5
4. a (p. 1014) Objective 38-5
5. d (p. 1015) Objective 38-5
6. a (p. 1011) Objective 38-5
7. c (p. 1018) Objective 38-5
8. b (p. 1019) Objective 38-8
9. c (p. 1019) Objective 38-8
10. a (p. 1019) Objective 38-8
11. d (p. 1019) Objective 38-8
12. a (p. 1019) Objective 38-8
13. a (p. 1020) Objective 38-8
14. c (p. 1020) Objective 38-8

15. a (p. 1021) Objective 38-8
16. d (p. 1024) Objective 38-9
17. c (p. 1024) Objective 38-9
18. a (p. 1024) Objective 38-11
19. c (p. 1026) Objective 38-11
20. b (p. 1026) Objective 38-14
21. d (p. 1028) Objective 38-11
22. c (p. 1032) Objective 38-13
23. a (p. 1033) Objective 38-11
24. b (p. 1040) Objective 39-2
25. b (p. 1040) Objective 39-2
26. a (p. 1044) Objective 39-3
27. c (p. 1041) Objective 39-2
28. c (p. 1046) Objective 39-4
29. c (pp. 1042, 1046) Objective 39-3
30. a (p. 1046) Objective 39-6
31. d (p. 1046) Objective 39-3
32. d (pp. 1042, 1046) Objective 39-3
33. a (p. 1047) Objective 39-3
34. d (p. 1042) Objective 39-3
35. a (pp. 1043–1044) Objective 39-2
36. c (pp. 1042, 1052) Objective 39-7
37. b (p. 1052) Objective 39-7
38. a (pp. 1050–1051) Objective 39-6
39. c (p. 1051) Objective 39-6
40. b (p. 1051) Objective 39-8
41. b (p. 1049) Objective 39-5
42. d (p. 1049) Objective 39-5
43. c (p. 1050) Objective 39-5
44. b (p. 1050) Objective 39-4
45. b (pp. 1042, 1046) Objective 39-5
46. d (p. 1050) Objective 39-5
47. b (p. 1029) Objective 38-11
48. a (p. 1024) Objective 38-9
49. c (p. 1024) Objective 38-10
50. b (p. 1051) Objective 39-5
51. c (p. 1052) Objective 39-5
52. a (p. 1061) Objective 40-3
53. c (p. 1063) Objective 40-3
54. b (p. 1064) Objective 40-4
55. b (p. 1068) Objective 40-5
56. d (p. 1070) Objective 40-7
57. a (p. 1074) Objective 40-10
58. b (p. 1074) Objective 40-10
59. c (p. 1076) Objective 40-10
60. d (p. 1070) Objective 40-11

Chapter 41

STOP, REVIEW, REMEMBER! *(p. 1105)*

Multiple Choice

1. c (p. 1097)
2. b (p. 1104 and Chapter 1, p. 9)
3. a (p. 1097)
4. a (pp. 1096, 1097)
5. b (p. 1105)

Matching

1. E (p. 1096)
2. C (p. 1096)
3. A (p. 1096)
4. F (p. 1096)
5. F (p. 1096)
6. D (p. 1096)
7. F (p. 1096)
8. B (p. 1096)
9. E (p. 1096)

Critical Thinking

1. You would find other means to deal with the airway problem. This may include finger sweeps initially followed by manual suction devices or getting a portable unit from another ambulance. Not having suction can cause the patient to aspirate and worsen his condition. Most likely this occurred because the unit was not checked or was not checked thoroughly at the beginning of the shift. (p. 1097, plus Chapter 12, p. 312 and Chapter 13, p. 337)
2. These pieces of information allow the dispatcher to get the call out to the ambulance quickly and give the ability to get the caller back on the line in the event he is disconnected. (pp. 1107–1108 and Chapter 1, p. 12)

STOP, REVIEW, REMEMBER! *(p. 1115)*

Multiple Choice

1. b (p. 1109)
2. a (p. 1112)
3. d (p. 1112)
4. d (p. 1112)
5. a (p. 1112)

Short Answer

1. Drive defensively. Anticipate the actions of other drivers. Leave room to react. (pp. 1111–1112)
2. Slippery conditions from snow, ice, or hydroplaning cause loss of control of the vehicle. Poor visibility. (pp. 1111–1112)
3. Radio/computer/GPS use; fatigue, stress; stereo/phone use. (p. 1112)

Critical Thinking

1. Due regard means considering the safety of others regardless of the traffic regulations. It means a provider can never operate a vehicle in a manner that is reckless or unsafe. (p. 1109)
2. Driving alone requires the driver to conduct all the tasks associated with responding to a scene including navigation, driving, communication, and so on. Any of these essential components could be considered a distraction to safe operation. (p. 1112)

CHAPTER REVIEW *(p. 1124)*

Multiple Choice

1. a (p. 1096)
2. a (p. 1120)
3. b (p. 1109)
4. c (p. 1120)
5. a (p. 1119)
6. d (p. 1119)

Critical Thinking

1. Disinfection kills most organisms on a surface. Sterilization is designed to kill all microorganisms including those spore-forming organisms that are very difficult to kill. (p. 1120)
2. You disinfect the surface of the backboard. Sterilization is not necessary on a backboard and would be very difficult in a prehospital environment. (pp. 1120–1122)

CASE STUDY

1. Every experienced EMT will acknowledge that a serious call involving a child gets his pulse going. If that pulse affects important decisions such as driving safely, you and your crew may never make it to the patient. Drive safely *every time* you activate the lights and sirens regardless of the type of call. (p. 1110)
2. Choosing your route to the scene is important to ensure a safe and minimal response time. Considerations include choosing a direct route, time of day and traffic, construction, or other delays. (p. 1109)
3. In short, you will need to balance prompt transportation to the hospital with providing a safe and practical working environment in the back of the moving ambulance. You should avoid sudden stops, sharp turns, swerving, and other actions that could both throw the crew around as well as prevent care of the patient. Careful attention to traffic conditions, road surfaces, and vehicle motion will help to accomplish this goal. (pp. 1117, 1119)

Chapter 42

STOP, REVIEW, REMEMBER! *(p. 1129)*

Multiple Choice

1. a (p. 1128)
2. a (p. 1128)
3. c (p. 1128)
4. d (p. 1128)
5. d (p. 1128)

Fill in the Blank

1. national incident management system (p. 1128)
2. incident command system (p. 1128)
3. multiple-casualty incident (p. 1127)

Critical Thinking

1. This list should include, but not be limited to, manufacturing facilities, major traffic intersections, and chemical/petrochemical storage facilities. A discussion on this topic should raise the awareness of the potential for the need of a working local incident management system. (pp. 1127–1129)
2. Freelancing puts the rescuer at risk because the incident commander is not aware of his presence at the scene. Also his presence may interfere with the normal deployment of resources at the scene. (p. 1128)

STOP, REVIEW, REMEMBER! *(p. 1132)*

Multiple Choice

1. c (p. 1131)
2. a (p. 1131)
3. c (p. 1131)
4. b (p. 1131)
5. d (p. 1130)

Matching

1. B (p. 1131)
2. A (p. 1131)
3. E (p. 1131)
4. C (p. 1131)
5. D (p. 1131)

Critical Thinking

1. You should make sure that all responders have donned PPE and that the safety of the crew and of the victims is being taken into account during the operation. (p. 1131)
2. Refer the media to the public information officer or incident commander. (p. 1131)

STOP, REVIEW, REMEMBER! *(p. 1136)*

Multiple Choice

1. b (p. 1135)
2. a (p. 1135)
3. b (p. 1133)
4. a (p. 1134)
5. a (p. 1133)

Short Answer

1. Any provider is qualified, although less-qualified individuals will likely quickly transfer command when more-qualified individuals arrive. (p. 1133)
2. Scene safety and appropriate personal protective equipment needed; exact location or address of the incident; nature of the event and severity; number of injuries if known; risk factors for EMS responders, such as hazardous material or contamination; possibility of a crime scene and requirements for scene safety; additional resources required; actions you are taking. (p. 1134)
3. Confirm the address and exact location; designation and location of the incident commander and command post; describe the event and the situation, including safety issues; request additional resources; state the action you are taking. (p. 1134)

Critical Thinking

1. This list would be specific to the student's region. (p. 1135)
2. This list would be specific to the student's region. (pp. 1133–1135)

STOP, REVIEW, REMEMBER! *(p. 1140)*

Multiple Choice

1. c (p. 1138)
2. c (p. 1139)
3. c (p. 1138)
4. a (p. 1138)

Matching

1. B (p. 1139)
2. A (p. 1139)
3. E (p. 1139)
4. D (p. 1139)
5. C (p. 1139)

Critical Thinking

1. In order to prevent chaos, the incident must be resolved with a single vision. (p. 1138)
2. Keeping the command post apart from the incident allows for uninterrupted command in the event of a collapse or secondary explosion. Also, the command post often serves as a site for the media and bystanders to gather. (pp. 1138–1140)
3. To determine scene safety, exact location, additional resources (for example, fire department, power company, law enforcement), the number of patients, and mechanism of injury/nature of illness. (p. 1134)

STOP, REVIEW, REMEMBER! *(p. 1144)*

Multiple Choice

1. a (p. 1144)
2. c (p. 1143)
3. d (p. 1142)
4. c (p. 1144)
5. a (p. 1144)

Critical Thinking

1. It is vitally important to know which hospital receives each patient so that no one facility becomes overwhelmed. It is also important so that family members can be properly notified. (pp. 1127, 1138–1139)
2. Answers will vary. (p. 1144)

CHAPTER REVIEW *(p. 1146)*

Multiple Choice

1. c (p. 1131)
2. d (p. 1131)
3. c (p. 1131)
4. b (p. 1133)
5. d (p. 1144)
6. b (p. 1138)
7. b (p. 1138)
8. a (p. 1131)
9. b (p. 1131)
10. d (p. 1138)
11. c (p. 1139)
12. d (p. 1131)
13. c (p. 1138)
14. b (p. 1135)
15. c (p. 1142)
16. a (p. 1138)

Critical Thinking

1. Answers will vary. (p. 1139)
2. Answers will vary. (p. 1131)
3. Answers will vary. (p. 1134)

CASE STUDY

Answers will vary and are meant to encourage discussion.

Chapter 43

STOP, REVIEW, REMEMBER! *(p. 1156)*

Multiple Choice

1. b (p. 1154)
2. a (p. 1152)
3. a (p. 1155)
4. c (p. 1153)
5. c (p. 1155)

Fill in the Blank

1. 2 (p. 1155)
2. 1 (p. 1154)
3. 4 (p. 1156)
4. 5 (p. 1155)
5. 3 (p. 1155)

Critical Thinking

1. Do the best for the most, effectively manage the limited resources, and avoid relocating the disaster. (p. 1153)
2. Early on in the process of dealing with a multiple-casualty incident, the EMT must focus on scene safety and ensure that both bystanders and other responding units understand what they are responding to. They must size up the scene as best as they can and provide a detailed report of the scene to dispatch. (pp. 1154–1155)

STOP, REVIEW, REMEMBER! *(p. 1163)*

Multiple Choice

1. d (p. 1159)
2. b (p. 1159)
3. a (p. 1159)
4. c (p. 1156)
5. b (p. 1160)

Fill in the Blank

1. French, to sort (p. 1158)
2. secondary (p. 1161)
3. minor, green (p. 1160)

Critical Thinking

1. The START triage system is designed for adult MCI patients, whereas JumpSTART is specific to children and infants. JumpSTART also focuses more on the respiratory status of the patient than the START system does. (p. 1159)
2. A patient who is unable to maintain an airway following the assistance of the triaging EMT should be tagged black. A patient who cannot maintain an airway will unfortunately require more time and effort than can be afforded during the initial triage period. (p. 1159)

CHAPTER REVIEW *(p. 1165)*

Multiple Choice

1. b (p. 1160)
2. d (p. 1152)
3. d (p. 1160)
4. a (p. 1160)
5. c (p. 1159)
6. d (p. 1160)
7. a (p. 1160)
8. b (p. 1160)
9. c (p. 1162)
10. a (p. 1163)

Fill in the Blank

1. red (p. 1160)
2. green (p. 1160)
3. red (p. 1160)
4. black (p. 1160)
5. red (p. 1160)
6. yellow (p. 1160)
7. green (p. 1160)
8. red (p. 1160)
9. yellow (p. 1160)
10. yellow (p. 1160)

Critical Thinking

1. Open the child's airway and check for spontaneous breathing. If there is none, give five rescue breaths and reevaluate for spontaneous breathing. If the child starts to breathe on her

own, she would receive a red tag and if she does not, she should receive a black tag. You would then move on to the next patient. (p. 1160)

2. In a situation in which the numerous "walking wounded" start to disrupt a scene (or simply leave) due to boredom or perceived lack of care, a good solution is to call in buses from local transit companies or schools. The noncritical patients can then be loaded onto the buses and not only be removed from the scene, but also delivered to the most appropriate receiving facilities. (p. 1158)
3. It will most likely take longer to triage the patients on the bus because, due to crowded conditions, some patients will have to be moved following evaluation before other patients can be reached. (p. 1155)

Case Study

1. Determine scene safety. There are many hazards in this type of situation: two damaged vehicles, a dust-obscured roadway, darkness of night, potential for hazardous cargo on the truck, and so on. (p. 1154)
2. You would follow four of the five. You would obviously determine scene safety, size-up the scene, and send the incident information to dispatch by calling 911. As an off-duty EMT in your personal vehicle, you would forego setting up the medical branch. Following the phone call to dispatch, you would begin triage. (pp. 1154–1156)
3. The vehicle nearest to you that appears safe to approach. Be mindful of fires, dripping fluids, and unstable positioning. (p. 1154)

Chapter 44

STOP, REVIEW, REMEMBER! *(p. 1176)*

Multiple Choice

1. b (p. 1171)
2. a (p. 1172)
3. d (p. 1172)
4. c (p. 1175)
5. a (p. 1175)

Matching

1. c (p. 1172)
2. b (p. 1172)
3. a (p. 1172)
4. d (p. 1173)

Critical Thinking

1. Schools are typically areas with a high concentration of people depending on the day of the week and time of day. Exposure to a large number of students and faculty could quickly overwhelm the local resources. This will vary from community to community. For example, take into consideration gas and chemical plants. (p. 1152)
2. This answer will vary from community to community.
3. This answer will vary from community to community.

STOP, REVIEW, REMEMBER! *(p. 1183)*

Multiple Choice

1. c (p. 1178)
2. b (p. 1178)
3. a (p. 1181)
4. c (p. 1181)
5. b (p. 1182)

Matching

1. I (p. 1180)
2. H (p. 1180)
3. G (p. 1180)
4. F (p. 1180)
5. E (p. 1181)
6. D (p. 1181)
7. C (p. 1181)
8. B (p. 1181)
9. A (p. 1181)

Critical Thinking

1. It is essential to approach any potential hazardous incident with great caution. Binoculars allow one to see into the scene from a safe distance and in some instances attempt to identify the substance in question. When a hazardous materials placard is visible, the *ERG* can be used to identify the material and the recommended precautions. (p. 1178)
2. Isolate the scene, restrict or reroute traffic, and conduct evacuation, if necessary. (p. 1182)

STOP, REVIEW, REMEMBER! *(p. 1191)*

Multiple Choice

1. a (p. 1190)
2. c (p. 1190)
3. c (pp. 1181, 1188)
4. a (p. 1188)
5. d (p. 1189)

Matching

1. C (p. 1187)
2. A (p. 1187)
3. B (p. 1187)
4. E (p. 1187)
5. D (p. 1188)
6. H (p. 1188)
7. F (p. 1188)
8. G (p. 1188)

Critical Thinking

1. To prevent cross-contamination (p. 1187)
2. What are the hazardous properties of the substance, what is the concentration, in what form is the substance, what are the chemical and physical characteristics of the substance, how is the substance contained, what pathways of exposure exist, and what was the duration of exposure? (p. 1189)

CHAPTER REVIEW *(p. 1194)*

Multiple Choice

1. a (p. 1190)
2. c (p. 1186)
3. c (p. 1187)
4. d (p. 1187)
5. d (p. 1182)
6. b (p. 1180)
7. d (p. 1186)

Critical Thinking

1. An *acute exposure* is the exposure to a hazardous substance over a short period of time or at a high dose. A *chronic exposure* is the exposure to a hazardous substance over a long period of time. (p. 1190)
2. Absorption (through the skin or eye): When a chemical contacts the skin (dermal exposure), it can be absorbed into the body. Injection: The most familiar example of injection is that of needlestick. Ingestion: The substance enters the body by means of the digestive system (eating or drinking). Inhalation: A patient breathes the substance into his lungs. (p. 1188)

Case Study

1. Despite the fact that you know the patient has been properly decontaminated, you must still don the proper PPE prior to caring for this patient. Then focus your care on his chief complaint of difficulty breathing. Oxygen by nonrebreather mask and keeping him in a position of comfort will be your top priorities. (pp. 457–458 and Chapter 2, p. 34)
2. Once you have ensured that your patient has a clear airway, is breathing adequately, and has a good pulse, you can perform a secondary assessment during transport to the hospital. You will look for additional signs of exposure such as redness to the skin and possible injuries. Closely monitor his airway and breathing throughout transport. (pp. 377, 400)

Chapter 45

STOP, REVIEW, REMEMBER! *(p. 1200)*

Multiple Choice

1. a (pp. 1197–1198)
2. a (p. 1198)
3. b (p. 1198)
4. d (p. 1197)

Fill in the Blank

1. Traffic, spilled fuel/chemicals, downed power lines, broken glass, undeployed air bags, and fire (pp. 1199, 1202)

Critical Thinking

1. Call for additional resources. Park the emergency vehicle so that the emergency lights can be seen easily by oncoming traffic. Ensure the scene is safe before approaching to care for patients. (pp. 1198–1199)
2. This answer should include a list of rescue squads and fire departments and their rescue capabilities.

STOP, REVIEW, REMEMBER! *(p. 1204)*

Multiple Choice

1. c (p. 1203)
2. a (p. 1203)
3. c (p. 1202)

Labeling

(p. 1204)

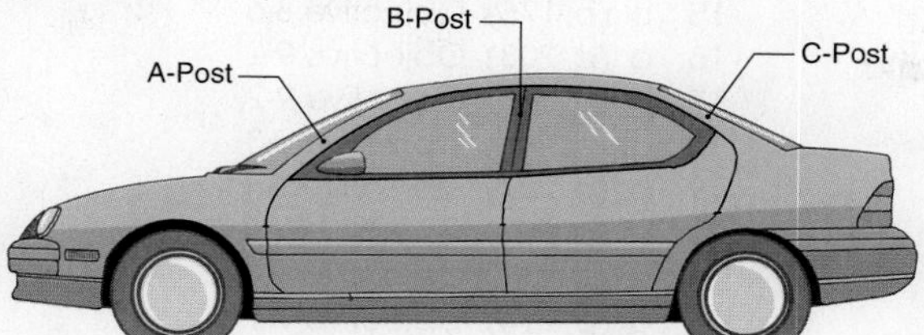

Critical Thinking

1. There are hazards from the vehicle such as sharp metal, glass, fuel and fluids from the vehicle, fire, traffic moving around the vehicle, rescue equipment being used on the vehicle, and utility hazards (power and gas lines). (pp. 1199, 1202)
2. Prepare for the rescue, size up the situation, identify and manage hazards, stabilize the vehicle prior to entering, gain access to the patient, perform a primary and secondary assessment, disentangle the patient, immobilize and extricate the patient from the vehicle, provide emergency care and transport, terminate the rescue. (pp. 1201–1204)

STOP, REVIEW, REMEMBER! *(p. 1211)*

Multiple Choice

1. b (p. 1206)
2. a (p. 1206)
3. c (p. 1206)
4. a (p. 1208)
5. d (p. 1208)

Matching

1. F (p. 1207)
2. C (p. 1207)
3. A (p. 1209)
4. E (p. 1209)
5. B (p. 1206)
6. D (p. 1208)

Critical Thinking

1. An air medical resource would be appropriate if the patient was critical and ground transport was too far away or the patient required the advanced skills of the air medical team. (p. 1208)
2. The characteristics of an ideal landing zone include a flat, paved surface at least 100 × 100 feet for daytime or 125 × 125 feet for nighttime; close to the incident; clear of utility poles, wires, and tall trees; and free of roaming people or animals. (pp. 1209–1210)

CHAPTER REVIEW *(p. 1213)*

Multiple Choice

1. c (pp. 1198-1199)
2. a (p. 1202)
3. d (p. 1203)
4. c (p. 1204)
5. a (p. 1197)
6. c (p. 1198)
7. b (p. 1210)
8. a (p. 1209)
9. b (p. 1213)
10. b (p. 1204)

Labeling

(p. 1204)

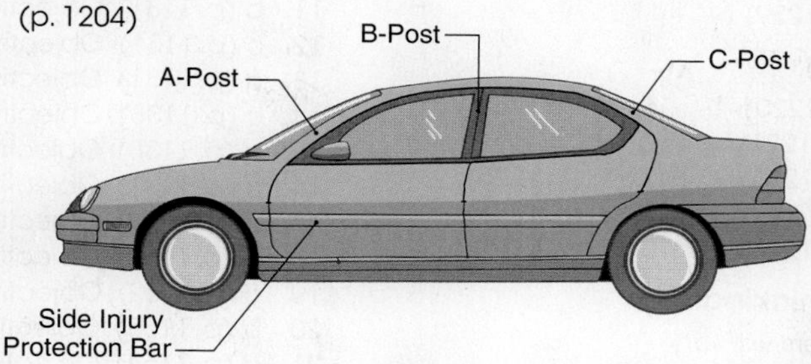

Critical Thinking

1. You must instruct the woman to remain in the car because there is extreme danger if she should try to exit her vehicle. Advise her that additional help is on the way and that you will remain at the scene with her. Instruct her to not touch any surface inside the car. (pp. 1198–1199, 1202)
2. You must ensure that traffic is not a hazard, the car is on stable ground, and that there are no fuel leaks. When it is safe, you must access the vehicle to perform a primary assessment of the patient. You will be able to provide minimal care until the patient is safely extricated. (pp. 1198–1199)

CASE STUDY

1. The ambulance should park past the scene, if possible, to allow access to the rear doors for patient loading without risk of being struck. The ambulance should also park uphill and upwind from any potentially hazardous materials. (p. 1199)
2. The scene is ideally protected by a large piece of fire apparatus physically blocking rescue efforts from approaching traffic. Alternatively, in work areas or when available, highway crews may provide signage, barricade vehicles, and other warning devices. (p. 1199)

Chapter 46

STOP, REVIEW, REMEMBER! *(p. 1222)*

Multiple Choice

1. a (p. 1219)
2. b (p. 1220)
3. c (p. 1221)
4. d (pp. 1221–1222)
5. a (p. 1221)

Ordering

1. C (p. 1222)
2. F (p. 1222)
3. A (p. 1222)
4. G (p. 1222)
5. B (p. 1222)
6. D (p. 1222)
7. E (p. 1222)

Critical Thinking

1. Because this is a community-specific list, student answers will differ.
2. When sizing up the scene, do not park in a location closest to the event. Take the time to size up the scene; look for suspicious packages (for example, backpacks, packages, or things that look out of place). These are often hidden in trash cans, bushes, or shrubbery or in planted vehicles. If you identify a secondary device, immediately move to a safe distance and notify dispatch or the incident commander to have the bomb squad neutralize it. (p. 1221)

STOP, REVIEW, REMEMBER! *(p. 1230)*

Multiple Choice

1. b (p. 1224)
2. d (p. 1224)
3. a (p. 1224)
4. b (p. 1228)
5. c (p. 1228)

Fill in the Blank

1. The letters in the mnemonic SLUDGEM stand for salivation, lacrimation, urination, defecation, GI motility, emesis, and miosis. (p. 1222)
2. For three things to do when responding to a terrorist attack, your answers may include: Ask your dispatch center for a weather report. Look for situations in which the response is being funneled into an area that will bottleneck. Immediately contact law enforcement for coordination. Identify a rally point to meet and regroup in the event of a secondary device. Identify safe staging areas to which other EMS, fire, and police units can respond. Approach the scene uphill and upwind. Make sure you have a quick unimpeded exit route. (p. 1229)

Critical Thinking

1. The best way for the EMT to guard against radiation exposure is to follow the rules of time, distance, shielding, and quantity. (p. 1226)
2. Blistering, red, discolored, or irritated skin or any signs or symptoms of SLUDGEM. (pp. 1228–1229)

CHAPTER REVIEW *(p. 1235)*

Multiple Choice

1. a (p. 1233)
2. d (p. 1224)
3. d (p. 1224)
4. d (p. 1224)
5. c (p. 1225)
6. d (p. 1182)

7. c (p. 1219)
8. c (p. 1229)
9. c (p. 1229)

Matching

1. B (p. 1220)
2. C (p. 1221)
3. A (p. 1218)
4. E (p. 1225)
5. D (p. 1224)
6. G (p. 1227)
7. H (p. 1228)
8. F (p. 1225)
9. J (p. 1226)
10. I (p. 1226)

Critical Thinking

1. Answers will vary.
2. Bacteria, viruses, and toxins. Biological agents enter the body through one of four common routes of entry: inhalation, ingestion, dermal, or vector borne. They can be introduced in the air, community water sources, on broken skin wounds, and through animals and insects. (pp. 1224–1225)
3. There are no signs during the incubation period, immediately after exposure to a biological agent. The agent multiplies and overwhelms the host. At the end of this period the victim will present with signs and symptoms of the illness. For bacteria or viruses that produce infection, this period is measured in days. For a toxin, the timeframe is much shorter. When compared to chemical weapons, the ill effects from biological weapons would be delayed. Therefore, it is more difficult to detect a biological agent. (p. 1225)

CASE STUDY

1. You must advise dispatch of the approximate number of patients and presenting signs that may be consistent with a toxic exposure. Look for and report any signs of an explosion such as smoke or burns on the victims. Call for additional resources including a hazmat team. (pp. 1220–1222)
2. You must find a safe location that is upwind from the scene and verbally direct the victims toward your ambulance. Don appropriate PPE such as gloves, mask, and a gown. Observe the victims for signs of toxic exposure and avoid direct contact with the victims. (pp. 1222, 1223)

Module 6

REVIEW AND PRACTICE EXAMINATION

1. c (p. 1096) Objective 41-3
2. d (p. 1097) Objective 41-4
3. a (p. 1107) Objective 41-4
4. a (p. 1109) Objective 41-4
5. d (p. 1096) Objective 41-3
6. b (p. 1117) Objective 41-3
7. a (p. 1220) Objective 41-10
8. a (p. 1134) Objective 41-9
9. a (p. 1128) Objective 42-4
10. c (p. 1128) Objective 42-4
11. b (p. 1131) Objective 42-4
12. c (p. 1131) Objective 42-4
13. d (p. 1131) Objective 42-6
14. c (p. 1138) Objective 42-7
15. a (p. 1138) Objective 42-6
16. d (p. 1131) Objective 42-6
17. b (p. 1152) Objective 43-2
18. b (p. 1152) Objective 43-2
19. c (p. 1152) Objective 43-2
20. b (p. 1153) Objective 43-3
21. d (p. 1154) Objective 43-4
22. a (p. 1158) Objective 43-6
23. a (p. 1159) Objective 43-8
24. c (p. 1160) Objective 43-8
25. a (p. 1160) Objective 43-10
26. b (p. 1158) Objective 43-6
27. b (p. 1158) Objective 43-5
28. a (p. 1162) Objective 43-13
29. c (p. 1128) Objective 43-14
30. a (p. 1128) Objective 42-4
31. d (p. 1153) Objective 43-6
32. b (p. 1171) Objective 44-6
33. c (p. 1172) Objective 44-1
34. a (p. 1172) Objective 44-5
35. d (p. 1173) Objective 44-5
36. b (p. 1175) Objective 44-1
37. a (p. 1175) Objective 44-2
38. b (p. 1172) Objective 44-5
39. a (p. 1178) Objective 44-4
40. b (p. 1186) Objective 44-6
41. d (p. 1180) Objective 44-5
42. c (p. 1181) Objective 44-5
43. c (p. 1188) Objective 44-8
44. c (p. 1175) Objective 44-2
45. c (p. 1198) Objective 45-3
46. a (p. 1203) Objective 45-6
47. d (p. 1203) Objective 45-7
48. a (p. 1207) Objective 45-9
49. c (p. 1208) Objective 45-12
50. b (p. 1209) Objective 45-13
51. b (p. 1219) Objective 46-4
52. a (p. 1219) Objective 46-4
53. d (p. 1224) Objective 46-1
54. b (p. 1226) Objective 46-1
55. a (p. 1224) Objective 46-1
56. c (p. 1221) Objective 46-5
57. b (p. 1226) Objective 46-1

Appendix 1

FINAL PRACTICE REVIEW

1. a (p. 9) Objective 1-4
2. d (p. 9) Objective 1-4
3. c (p. 8) Objective 1-4
4. a (p. 26) Objective 2-5
5. b (p. 34) Objective 2-11
6. a (p. 55) Objective 3-8
7. a (p. 63) Objective 3-17
8. b (p. 80) Objective 4-3
9. a (p. 112) Objective 5-14
10. d (p. 108) Objective 5-12
11. a (p. 109) Objective 5-13
12. c (p. 142) Objective 6-20
13. a (p. 158) Objective 7-2
14. a (p. 178) Objective 8-8
15. b (p. 175) Objective 8-6
16. a (p. 203) Objective 9-2
17. c (p. 203) Objective 9-2
18. d (p. 204) Objective 9-3
19. b (p. 207) Objective 9-4
20. a (p. 207) Objective 9-6
21. d (p. 211) Objective 9-8
22. c (p. 214) Objective 9-11
23. a (p. 215) Objective 9-11
24. c (p. 222) Objective 9-13
25. a (p. 224) Objective 9-16
26. d (p. 882) Objective 9-19
27. a (p. 250) Objective 10-13
28. b (p. 270) Objective 11-7
29. a (p. 295) Objective 12-2
30. b (p. 296) Objective 12-2
31. b (p. 349) Objective 13-8
32. d (pp. 332, 333) Objective 13-8
33. c (p. 332) Objective 13-8
34. b (pp. 333, 348) Objective 13-9
35. c (p. 339) Objective 13-14
36. a (p. 339) Objective 13-23
37. c (p. 339) Objective 13-14
38. b (p. 339) Objective 13-14
39. c (p. 339) Objective 13-14
40. c (p. 340) Objective 13-15
41. c (p. 342) Objective 13-15
42. c (pp. 349, 352) Objective 13-15
43. c (pp. 343–344) Objective 13-15
44. d (p. 349) Objective 13-18
45. c (pp. 355–356) Objective 13-23
46. b (p. 391) Objective 14-3
47. a (p. 391) Objective 14-9
48. c (p. 387) Objective 14-10
49. a (pp. 425–426) Objective 16-3
50. d (p. 426) Objective 16-3
51. d (p. 426) Objective 16-6
52. d (p. 427) Objective 16-7
53. d (p. 431) Objective 16-6
54. c (p. 457) Objective 17-5
55. b (p. 460) Objective 17-6
56. c (p. 461) Objective 17-8
57. c (p. 463) Objective 17-6
58. b (p. 463) Objective 17-10
59. a (p. 475) Objective 17-13
60. d (p. 452) Objective 17-10
61. a (pp. 468, 474) Objective 17-15
62. b (p. 509) Objective 18-13
63. b (p. 489) Objective 18-3
64. a (p. 490) Objective 18-15
65. c (p. 493) Objective 18-8
66. a (p. 509) Objective 18-13
67. b (p. 512) Objective 18-16
68. a (p. 516) Objective 18-16
69. c (p. 528) Objective 19-5
70. d (p. 547) Objective 20-9
71. c (p. 567) Objective 21-8
72. a (p. 603) Objective 22-6
73. a (p. 617) Objective 23-2
74. c (p. 638) Objective 24-4
75. c (p. 643) Objective 24-10
76. c (p. 656) Objective 25-5

77. c (pp. 679, 685) Objective 26-5
78. b (p. 721) Objective 27-8
79. a (p. 751) Objective 29-4
80. b (p. 757) Objective 29-8
81. b (p. 753) Objective 29-5
82. c (p. 777) Objective 30-6
83. a (p. 780) Objective 30-7
84. a (p. 811) Objective 30-7
85. d (p. 797) Objective 31-6
86. b (p. 825) Objective 32-5
87. d (p. 828) Objective 32-6
88. c (p. 829) Objective 32-7
89. d (p. 824) Objective 32-5
90. b (p. 834) Objective 32-13
91. b (p. 835) Objective 32-13
92. a (p. 836) Objective 32-4
93. a (p. 845) Objective 33-2
94. a (p. 857) Objective 33-11
95. a (p. 847) Objective 33-5
96. a (p. 858) Objective 33-9
97. a (p. 872) Objective 33-12
98. b (p. 873) Objective 34-4
99. c (p. 876) Objective 34-5
100. b (p. 876) Objective 34-6
101. b (p. 882) Objective 34-8
102. b (p. 888) Objective 34-9
103. d (p. 886) Objective 34-10
104. a (p. 885) Objective 34-10
105. d (p. 876) Objective 34-6
106. b (p. 904) Objective 35-2
107. b (p. 904) Objective 35-2
108. d (p. 916) Objective 35-7
109. b (p. 904) Objective 35-2
110. b (p. 929) Objective 36-2
111. a (p. 937) Objective 36-10
112. b (p. 948) Objective 36-10
113. c (p. 994) Objective 37-30
114. a (p. 966) Objective 37-4
115. a (pp. 989–990) Objective 37-24
116. a (p. 1017) Objective 38-10
117. b (p. 1014) Objective 38-5
118. c (p. 1014) Objective 38-7
119. a (p. 1019) Objective 38-8
120. a (p. 1020) Objective 38-12
121. b (p. 1027) Objective 38-3
122. d (p. 1028) Objective 38-11
123. c (p. 1015) Objective 38-13
124. b (p. 1040) Objective 39-2
125. b (p. 1046) Objective 39-3
126. c (p. 1050) Objective 39-7
127. a (p. 1070) Objective 40-7
128. b (p. 1110) Objective 41-4
129. a (p. 1128) Objective 42-4
130. d (p. 1158) Objective 43-9
131. a (p. 1160) Objective 43-8
132. b (p. 1171) Objective 44-2
133. c (p. 1172) Objective 44-1
134. b (p. 1171) Objective 44-1
135. d (p. 1173) Objective 44-1
136. b (p. 1175) Objective 44-1
137. a (p. 1175) Objective 44-2
138. b (p. 1172) Objective 44-1
139. a (p. 1178) Objective 44-4
140. b (p. 1186) Objective 44-5
141. d (p. 1180) Objective 44-1
142. c (p. 1181) Objective 44-1
143. d (p. 1197) Objective 44-5
144. c (p. 1198) Objective 45-4
145. a (p. 1203) Objective 45-6
146. a (p. 1203) Objective 45-7
147. b (p. 1197) Objective 45-2
148. d (p. 1225) Objective 46-1
149. b (p. 1221) Objective 46-4
150. c (p. 1225) Objective 46-1

INDEX

Page numbers followed by *f* indicate figures; those followed by *t* indicate tables.